The American Journal of Medicine

VOLUME 61

JULY—DECEMBER 1976

DUN • DONNELLEY PUBLISHING CORPORATION
666 Fifth Avenue, New York, New York 10019

Printed in the United States of America

JULY 1976

The American Journal of Medicine

VOLUME 61

NUMBER 1

CONTENTS

EDITORIALS

Cytodestructive Mechanisms Provoked by Lymphocytes. *Wojciech Konstanty Podleski* 1

Ketogenesis and Its Regulation. *J. Denis McGarry, Daniel W. Foster* 9

CLINICAL STUDIES

Splenectomy for Palliation of Chronic Myelocytic Leukemia. *German A. Gomez, Joseph E. Sokal, Arnold Mittelman, C. William Aungst* 14

Torulopsis glabrata Infections in Patients with Cancer. Increasing Incidence and Relationship to Colonization. *Joseph Aisner, Stephen C. Schimpff, John C. Sutherland, Viola M. Young, Peter H. Wiernik* 23

Felty's Syndrome. Effect of Lithium on Granulopoiesis. *Ramesh C. Gupta, William A. Robinson, John E. Kurnick* 29

The Gamut of Paracoccidioidomycosis. *Angela Restrepo, Mario Robledo, Roberto Giraldo, Humberto Hernández, Fernando Sierra, Fernando Gutiérrez, Fernando Londoño, Roberto López, Gonzalo Calle* 33

Bartter's Syndrome: A Disorder Characterized by High Urinary Prostaglandins and a Dependence of Hyperreninemia on Prostaglandin Synthesis. *John R. Gill, Jurgen C. Frölich, Robert E. Bowden, Addison A. Taylor, Harry R. Keiser, Hannsjorg W. Seyberth, John A. Oates, Frederic C. Bartter* . . 43

Low Dose Radioiodide Thyroid Ablation in Postsurgical Patients with Thyroid Cancer. *K. David McCowen, Robert A. Adler, Nasser Ghaed, Thomas Verdon, Fred D. Hofeldt* 52

Body Composition and Skeletal Metabolism Following Pituitary Irradiation in Acromegaly. *John F. Aloia, Zrinko Petrak, Kenneth Ellis, Stanton H. Cohn* 59

The Investigation and Treatment of Renal Bone Disease. *G. R. D. Catto, M. MacLeod* 64

Effects of an Inhaled Bronchodilator on Gas Distribution and Over-All Ventilatory Efficiency in Patients with Chronic Obstructive Pulmonary Disease. *Antonio Cutillo, Rodolfo Perondi, Maurizio Turiel, Stefano Monti* 74

REVIEW

Diagnosis of Obstruction of the Upper and Central Airways. *Meir Kryger, Frederick Bode, Ral Antic, Nicholas Anthonisen* 85

CLINICOPATHOLOGIC CONFERENCE

Mixed Cryoimmunoglobulinemia (Washington University School of Medicine) 95

FEATURED REPORT

The Coroner Describes the Manner of Dying in New York City, 1784–1816. *Abraham Blinderman* . 103

CASE REPORTS

Bartter's Syndrome. Study of a 52 Year Old Man with Evidence for a Defect in Proximal Tubular Sodium Readsorption and Comments on Therapy. *David J. Tomko, Betty P. Y. Yeh, William F. Falls, Jr.* 111

Hypercalcemia of Acute Renal Failure. Clinical Significance and Pathogenesis. *Antoine de Torrente, Thomas Berl, Peter D. Cohn, Ernest Kawamoto, Phillip Hertz, Robert W. Schrier* 119

Primary Empty Sella Syndrome with Visual Field Defects. *Maire T. Buckman, Muhammed Husain, Thomas J. Carlow, Glenn T. Peake* 124

The Syndrome of Multiple Endocrine Gland Insufficiency. *Gerald B. Appel, Donald A. Holub* . . . 129

Ectopic Hyperparathyroidism (Pseudohyperparathyroidism) in Esophageal Malignancy. Report of a Case and a Review of the Literature. *Martin Grajower, Uriel S. Barzel* 134

Primary Hyperparathyroidism and Breast Cancer. *Apichati Vichayanrat, Avraam Avramides, Bernard Gardner, Stanley Wallach, Anne C. Carter* 136

Fever with Dissecting Aneurysm of the Aorta. *Henry W. Murray, John J. Mann, Abraham Genecin, Victor A. McKusick* 140

Thrombocytopenia, Macrothrombocytopathia, Nephritis and Deafness. *J. Bernheim, M. Dechavanne, P. A. Bryon, M. Lagarde, S. Colon, N. Pozet, J. Traeger* 145

Instructions for Authors 94

Abstracts of papers in this issue A41,A44,A46,A47,A63

AUGUST 1976

The American Journal of Medicine

VOLUME 61

NUMBER 2

CONTENTS

EDITORIALS

Flexible Fiberoptic Bronchoscopy. *M. Anees Khan, Michael E. Whitcomb, Gordon L. Snider* . . . 151

Primary Medical Care and Training Programs in General Internal Medicine. *Robert H. Crede* . . . 156

CLINICAL STUDIES

Malaria—The Mime. Recent Lessons From a Group of Civilian Travellers. *B. H. Kean, Philip C. Reilly, Jr.* . . . 159

The Mechanism of Increase in Total Lung Capacity During Acute Asthma. *Leonard Peress, Gerhart Sybrecht, Peter T. Macklem* . . . 165

Neurologic Involvement in Seven Patients with Behçet's Disease. *J. Desmond O'Duffy, Norman P. Goldstein* . . . 170

Hereditary Antithrombin III Deficiency. Effect of Antithrombin III Deficiency on Platelet Function. *Angelina Carvalho, Leonard Ellman* . . . 179

Renal Responses to PTH in Patients with Hormone-Resistant (Pseudo) Hypoparathyroidism. *Arnold M. Moses, Neil Breslau, Richard Coulson* . . . 184

Etiology and Prognosis in Acute Post-Transplant Renal Failure. *Carl M. Kjellstrand, Robert E. Casali, Richard L. Simmons, Jeffrey R. Shideman, Theodore J. Buselmeier, John S. Najarian* . . . 190

Recurrent Nephrolithiasis: Natural History and Effect of Phosphate Therapy. A Double-Blind Controlled Study. *Bruce Ettinger* . . . 200

Irreversible Acute Renal Failure in Idiopathic Nephrotic Syndrome. *Leopoldo Raij, William F. Keane, Arthur Leonard, Fred L. Shapiro* . . . 207

Comparative Effects of Lidocaine and Procainamide on Acutely Impaired Hemodynamics. *Jeffrey R. Burton, M. Thomas Mathew, Paul W. Armstrong* . . . 215

REVIEW

Idiopathic Late-Onset Immunoglobulin Deficiency. Clinical Observations in 50 Patients. *Paul E. Hermans, Jose A. Diaz-Buxo, John D. Stobo* . . . 221

CLINICOPATHOLOGIC CONFERENCE

Hodgkin's Disease with Nervous System Manifestations (Washington University School of Medicine) . . . 239

COMBINED CLINICAL AND BASIC SCIENCE SEMINAR

Male Pseudohermaphroditism: The Complexities of Male Phenotypic Development (New York Hospital-Cornell Medical Center) Lecturers: *Julianne Imperato-McGinley, Ralph E. Peterson* . . . 251

CASE REPORTS

Echocardiographic Detection of Fungal Vegetations in Candida Parasilopsis Endocarditis. *Joseph A. C. Gomes, Jaime Calderon, Fouad LaJam, Hideki Sakurai, Howard S. Friedman, with the technical assistance of Joseph S. Tatz* . . . 273

Tuberculous Arthritis. A Report on Two Cases with Review of Biopsy and Synovial Fluid Findings. *Richard Wallace, Alan S. Cohen* . . . 277

Therapy for Disseminated Coccidioidomycosis with Transfer Factor from a Related Donor. *Russell W. Steele, Barry E. Sieger, Theodore R. McNitt, Layne O. Gentry, William L. Moore, Jr.* . . . 283

Allopurinol Hypersensitivity. Granular Deposition of IgM at the Dermal-Epidermal Junction. *Peter D. Utsinger, William J. Yount* . . . 287

A Case of Bilateral Escherichia coli Endogenous Endophthalmitis. *W. Lee Fanning, James Stubbert, E. S. Irwin, Mark D. Aronson* . . . 295

Malignant External Otitis: A Severe Form of Otitis in Diabetic Patients. *Dawlat A. Zaky, David W. Bentley, Karl Lowy, Robert F. Betts, R. Gordon Douglas, Jr.* . . . 298

Information for Authors . . . 238

Abstracts of papers in this issue . . . A62, A64, A69, A73

SEPTEMBER 1976

The American Journal of Medicine

VOLUME 61

CONTENTS

NUMBER 3

EDITORIALS

Cellular Origins of Autoantibody—A Perplexing Question. *A. D. Bankhurst, R. C. Williams, Jr.* 303

Acute Renal Success. The Unexpected Logic of Oliguria in Acute Renal Failure. *Klaus Thurau, John W. Boylan* 308

CLINICAL STUDIES

IgM Pyroglobulinemia with Erythrocytosis Presenting as Hyperviscosity Syndrome. I. Clinical Features and Viscometric Studies. *Shaun R. McCann, Horace H. Zinneman, Martin M. Oken, Michael C. Leary, William R. Swaim, Mark Moore* 316

IgM Pyroglobulinemia with Erythrocytosis Presenting as Hyperviscosity Syndrome. II. Biochemical Properties and Mechanisms of Pyrogel Formation. *Shaun R. McCann, Horace H. Zinneman, Martin M. Oken, Akhouri A. Sinha* 321

Diagnosis of Cytomegalovirus Pneumonia in Compromised Hosts. *Paul S. Abdallah, James B. D. Mark, Thomas C. Merigan* 326

Clinical and Laboratory Evaluation of Elderly Patients with Heterophil-Antibody Positive Infectious Mononucleosis. Report of Seven Patients, Ages 40 to 78. *Charles A. Horwitz, Werner Henle, Gertrude Henle, Marvin Segal, Thomas Arnold, F. Bruce Lewis, David Zanick, Patrick C. J. Ward* 333

Clinical, Epidemiologic and Bacteriologic Observations of an Outbreak of Methicillin-Resistant Staphylococcus aureus at a Large Community Hospital. *Joseph J. Klimek, Frederick J. Marsik, Raymond C. Bartlett, Barbara Weir, Patricia Shea, Richard Quintiliani* 340

Sepsis Associated with Decubitus Ulcers. *Jeffrey E. Galpin, Anthony W. Chow, Arnold S. Bayer, Lucien B. Guze* 346

Metastatic Infection Secondary to Genitourinary Tract Sepsis. *Mike B. Siroky, Robert A. Moylan, George Austen, Jr., Carl A. Olsson* 351

The Cardiac Conduction System in Progressive Systemic Sclerosis. Clinical and Pathologic Features of 35 Patients. *Ren L. Ridolfi, Bernadine H. Bulkley, Grover M. Hutchins* 361

REVIEW

Jaundice in Pregnancy—1976. *R. Thomas Holzbach* 367

CLINICOPATHOLOGIC CONFERENCE

American Burkitt's Lymphoma (Washington University School of Medicine) 377

COMBINED CLINICAL AND BASIC SCIENCE SEMINAR

Vasculitis Syndromes: Clinical and Experimental Models (New York Hospital-Cornell Medical Center) *Lecturers: Charles L. Christian, John S. Sergent* 385

CASE REPORTS

Immunodeficiency, Xanthomas and Obstructive Liver Disease. *J. Nevin Isenberg, Russell F. Hanson, Gail C. Williams, James Zavoral, Arthur R. Page, Harvey L. Sharp* 393

Goodpasture's Syndrome in a Patient with the Nail-Patella Syndrome. *John J. Curtis, Dinyar Bhathena, Richard P. Leach, John H. Galla, Bruce A. Lucas, Robert G. Luke* 401

The Appearance of Nonlinear Deposits of Immunoglobulins in Goodpasture's Syndrome. *Lawrence C. Y. Agodoa, Gary E. Striker, C. R. P. George, Richard Glassock, Leonard J. Quadracci* 407

Splenosis: Autotransplantation of Splenic Tissue. *C. Richard Fleming, E. Rolland Dickson, Edgar G. Harrison, Jr.* 414

Regression of Atherosclerotic Stenosing Lesions of the Renal Arteries and Spontaneous Cure of Systemic Hypertension Through Control of Hyperlipidemia. *Lotfy L. Basta, Chad Williams, J. Michael Kioschos, Arthur A. Spector* 420

Arthritis with an Inflammatory Dermatosis Resembling Sweet's Syndrome. Report of a Unique Case and Review of the Literature on Arthritis Associated with Inflammatory Dermatoses. *David E. Trentham, Alfonse T. Masi, George F. Bale* 424

Absence of Immune Deficiencies in a Case of Progressive Multifocal Leukoencephalopathy. *David Rockwell, Frederick L. Ruben, Alan Winkelstein, Harvey Mendelow* 433

Sickle Cell-β^0 Thalassemia Variant with High Hemoglobin F and Mild Clinical Course. *Joseph R. Shaeffer, Joel L. Moake* WITH THE TECHNICAL ASSISTANCE *of Lois Kleve* 437

Thrombotic Thrombocytopenic Purpura—Remission Following Splenectomy. Report of a Case and Review of the Literature. *Patricia M. Reynolds, John M. Jackson, John A. S. Brine, A. Brian Vivian* 439

Information for Authors 448

Abstracts of papers in this issue A51, A55, A61, A70, A72, A88

OCTOBER 1976

The American Journal of Medicine

VOLUME 61

NUMBER 4

CONTENTS

EDITORIAL

Ventricular Rhythm Disorders and Sudden Cardiac Death. *B. Levitt, N. A. Cagin, J. C. Somberg, J. J. Kleid* . . . 449

CLINICAL STUDIES

The Short- and Long-Term Prognosis of Patients with Transmural and Nontransmural Myocardial Infarction. *David S. Cannom, William Levy, Lawrence S. Cohen* . . . 452

Idiopathic Portal Hypertension. *J. P. Villeneuve, P.-M. Huet, J.-G. Joly, D. Marleau, J. Côté, A. Légaré, M. Lafortune, P. Lavoie, A. Viallet* . . . 459

Ascites in Patients Undergoing Maintenance Hemodialysis. Report of Six Cases and Physiopathologic Approach. *Lazaro Gotloib, Ciro Servadio* . . . 465

Nephrotic Syndrome in Hodgkin's Disease. Evidence for Pathogenesis Alternative to Immune Complex Deposition. *A. Vishnu Moorthy, Stephen W. Zimmerman, Peter M. Burkholder* . . . 471

Effects of Alternating Phosphorus and Calcium Infusions on Osteoporosis. *Mordecai M. Popovtzer, Melvyn Stjernholm, William E. Huffer* . . . 478

Steroid Myopathy in Connective Tissue Disease. *Ali Askari, Paul J. Vignos, Jr., Roland W. Moskowitz* 485

Simultaneous Antibiotic Levels in "Breakthrough" Gram-Negative Rod Bacteremia. *Elizabeth T. Anderson, Lowell S. Young, William L. Hewitt* . . . 493

Serious Infections in Adults Due to Group B Streptococci. Clinical and Serotypic Characterization. *Arnold S. Bayer, Anthony W. Chow, Bascom F. Anthony, Lucien B. Guze* . . . 498

The Course of Pregnancy in Patients with Artificial Heart Valves. *Carlos Ibarra-Perez, Noel Arevalo-Toledo, Octavio Alvarez-De La Cadena, Luis Noriega-Guerra* . . . 504

REVIEW

Splenic Abscess. Report of 10 Cases and Review of the Literature. *Jeffrey D. Chulay, Mohammad R. Lankerani* . . . 513

CLINICOPATHOLOGIC CONFERENCE

Metastatic Catecholamine-Secreting Paraganglioma (Extra-Adrenal Pheochromocytoma) (Washington University School of Medicine) . . . 523

CASE REPORTS

Acute Unilateral Adrenal Hemorrhage Following ACTH Administration in a Patient with Cushing's Syndrome. *John F. Redman, Fred H. Faas* . . . 533

Unusual Electrocardiographic Finding—Bifascicular Block Due to Hyperkalemia. *James P. O'Neil, Edward K. Chung* . . . 537

Bilateral Scalp Necrosis in Temporal Arteritis. A Rare Complication of Horton's Disease. *Carl W. Soderstrom, James R. Seehafer* . . . 541

Chronic Intravascular Coagulation Associated with Chronic Myelocytic Leukemia. Use of Heparin in Connection with a Surgical Procedure. *Harold J. German, Jeanne A. Smith, John Lindenbaum* . 547

Immunoblastic Lymphadenopathy. Evolution into a Malignant Lymphoma with Plasmacytoid Features. *Richard I. Fisher, Elaine S. Jaffe, Raul C. Braylan, Judith C. Andersen, Henry K. Tan* . . . 553

C1q Deficiency Associated with Urticarial-Like Lesions and Cutaneous Vasculitis. *R. J. Marder, Rosemarie Rent, E. Y. C. Choi, H. Gewurz* . . . 560

Purpura Fulminans. *Thomas E. Spicer, Jerold M. Rau* . . . 566

A Complement Independent Erythropoietic Inhibitor Acting on the Progenitor Cell in Refractory Anemia. *G. P. Browman, M. H. Freedman, M. A. Blajchman, J. A. McBride* . . . 572

Hypertension, Hyperreninemia and a Solitary Renal Cyst in an Adolescent. *H. Josephine Rose, Albert W. Pruitt* . . . 579

Letters to the Editor . . . 583, 584

Information for Authors . . . A70

Abstracts of papers in this issue . . . A79, A82a, A83, A87, A89

NOVEMBER 1976

The American Journal of Medicine

VOLUME 61

NUMBER 5

CONTENTS

EDITORIAL

Intravascular Coagulation Associated with the Adult Respiratory Distress Syndrome. *Roger C. Bone, P. Bailey Francis, Alan K. Pierce* 585

CLINICAL STUDIES

Diagnosis and Evaluation of Patients with an Enlarged Sella Turcica. *Leon A. Weisberg, Earl A. Zimmerman, Andrew G. Frantz* 590

The Effect of Anti-Inflammatory Agents and Inflammation on Granulocyte Adherence. Evidence for Regulation by Plasma Factors. *Rob Roy MacGregor* 597

Effect of Sodium Depletion on Plasma Renin Concentration Before and During Adrenergic β-Receptor Blockade with Propranolol in Normotensive Man. *Per Omvik, Erik Enger, Ivar Eide* 608

A Nationwide Outbreak of Reye's Syndrome. Its Epidemiologic Relationship to Influenza B. *Lawrence Corey, Robert J. Rubin, Michael A. W. Hattwick, Gary R. Noble, Edward Cassidy* 615

Pulmonary Aspergilloma. A Rational Approach to Treatment. *Basil Varkey, Harold D. Rose* 626

Visceral Fungal Infections Due to Petriellidium boydii (Allescheria boydii). In Vitro Drug Sensitivity Studies. *Larry I. Lutwick, John N. Galgiani, Rudolph H. Johnson, David A. Stevens* 632

Atrial Pacing in Patients with Sinus Node Dysfunction. *Melvin M. Scheinman, Frederick W. Kunkel, Robert W. Peters, David S. Hirschfeld, Philippe L. Schoenfeld, Joseph A. Abbott, Gunnard Modin* 641

Local Characteristics of the Normal and Asynergic Left Ventricle in Man. *Monty M. Bodenheimer, Vidya S. Banka, Robert G. Trout, George A. Hermann, Homayoon Pasdar, Richard H. Helfant* 650

Pulmonary Hypertension and Foreign Body Granulomas in Intravenous Drug Abusers. Documentation by Cardiac Catheterization and Lung Biopsy. *Charles H. Robertson, Jr., Rolland C. Reynolds, James E. Wilson, III* 657

REVIEW

The Cardiovascular Effects of Lithium in Man. A Review of the Literature. *Ara G. Tilkian, John S. Schroeder, John Jue Kao, Herbert N. Hultgren* 665

CLINICOPATHOLOGIC CONFERENCE

Systemic Mastocytosis (Washington University School of Medicine) 671

COMBINED CLINICAL AND BASIC SCIENCE SEMINAR

Prostaglandins and Blood Pressure Control (New York Hospital-Cornell Medical Center). *Moderator: Henry O. Heinemann; Lecturer: James B. Lee* 681

CASE REPORTS

Influenza A Viral Infection Associated with Acute Renal Failure. *Adel Shenouda, Fred E. Hatch* 697

Herpesvirus Hominis Type 2 Meningoencephalitis Following Renal Transplantation. *Calvin C. Linnemann, Jr., M. Roy First, Mariano M. Alvira, J. Wesley Alexander, Gilbert M. Schiff* 703

Diurnal Pattern of Water and Electrolyte Excretion and Body Weight in Idiopathic Orthostatic Hypotension. The Effect of Three Treatments. *C. Davidson, D. Smith, D. B. Morgan* 709

Post-Transplant Malignant Lymphoma. Distinctive Morphologic Features Related to Its Pathogenesis. *Arthur J. Matas, Bruce F. Hertel, Juan Rosai, Richard L. Simmons, John S. Najarian* 716

SYMPOSIUM ON HYPERTENSION

Introduction to Part II of the Hypertension Symposium. Prorenin, Renal Hypertension; Diuretics and Hyperlipidemia; Angiotensin Receptors and Blocking Drugs; A New Treatment System. *John H. Laragh* 721

Methodologic Problems in Plasma Renin Activity Measurements. *Anne Delorme, Phan Tam Guyene, Pierre Corvol, Joel Menard* 725

Plasma Prorenin: Cryoactivation and Relationship to Renin Substrate in Normal Subjects. *Jean E. Sealey, Carol Moon, John H. Laragh, Michael Alderman* 731

Hypertension Associated with Early Stage Kidney Disease. Complementary Roles of Circulating Renin, the Body Sodium/Volume State and Duration of Hypertension. *Carlo Beretta-Piccoli, Peter Weidmann, Rudolf De Chátel, François Reubi* 739

Elevation of Serum Lipid Levels During Diuretic Therapy of Hypertension. *Richard P. Ames, Peter Hill* 748

Angiotensin Receptors in Vascular Tissue. *Marie-A. Devynck, Philippe Meyer* 758

Vascular Angiotensin Receptors and Their Role in Blood Pressure Control. *H. Thurston* 768

Beta-Adrenergic Receptor Blocking Drugs in Spontaneous Hypertension. *Joseph V. Levy* 779

Estimating Renin Participation in Hypertension: Superiority of Converting Enzyme Inhibitor Over Saralasin. *David B. Case, John M. Wallace, Hans J. Keim, Michael A. Weber, Jan I. M. Drayer, Robert P. White, Jean E. Sealey, John H. Laragh* 790

Modern System for Treating High Blood Pressure Based on Renin Profiling and Vasoconstriction-Volume Analysis. A Primary Role for Beta Blocking Drugs Such as Propranolol. *John H. Laragh* 797

Information for Authors 696

DECEMBER 1976
The American Journal of Medicine
VOLUME 61

CONTENTS

NUMBER 6

EDITORIAL

Labile Hypertension. Precursor of Sustained Essential Hypertension? *Robert M. Carey, Carlos R. Ayers* . . . 811

CLINICAL STUDIES

Body Fat: Its Relationship to Coronary Heart Disease, Blood Pressure, Lipids and Other Risk Factors Measured in a Large Male Population. *Roland L. Weinsier, Robert J. Fuchs, Thomas D. Kay, John H. Triebwasser, Malcolm C. Lancaster* . . . 815

Plasma Arginine Vasopressin in the Syndrome of Antidiuretic Hormone Excess Associated with Bronchogenic Carcinoma. *Paul L. Padfield, James J. Morton, Jehoiada J. Brown, Anthony F. Lever, J. Ian S. Robertson, Martin Wood, Ruth Fox* . . . 825

Candida Peritonitis. Report of 22 Cases and Review of the English Literature. *Arnold S. Bayer, Michael J. Blumenkrantz, John Z. Montgomerie, Jeffrey E. Galpin, Jack W. Coburn, Lucien B. Guze* . . . 832

Clinical Manifestations of Mannosidosis—A Longitudinal Study. *Jorge J. Yunis, Raymond C. Lewandowski, Jr., Sylvester J. Sanfillippo, Michael Y. Tsai, Iancu Foni, Heinz H. Bruhl* . . . 841

Chronic Neutropenia in Childhood. Analysis of 16 Cases and a Review of the Literature. *Stephanie H. Pincus, Laurence A. Boxer, Thomas P. Stossel* . . . 849

Skin Capillary Abnormalities As Indicators of Organ Involvement in Scleroderma (Systemic Sclerosis), Raynaud's Syndrome and Dermatomyositis. *Hildegard R. Maricq, George Spencer-Green, E. Carwile LeRoy* . . . 862

Benign Hepatic Tumors and Oral Contraceptive Pills. *Tejinder M. S. Kalra, Jagdish C. Mangla, Elise W. DePapp* . . . 871

The Myeloproliferative Disorders. Correlation Between Clinical Evolution and Alterations of Granulopoiesis. *Peter Greenberg, Beth Mara, Ine Bax, Remy Brossel, Stanley Schrier* . . . 878

Mediastinal Irradiation for Chronic Lymphocytic Leukemia. *Arthur Sawitsky, Kanti R. Rai, Isamettin Aral, Richard T. Silver, Arvin S. Glicksman, Robert W. Carey, Salvatore Scialla, C. J. Cornell, Jr., Barbara Seligman, Lorne Shapiro* . . . 892

REVIEW

Are Agents Affecting Platelet Functions Clinically Useful? *M. Verstraete* . . . 897

CLINICOSOCIOLOGIC CONFERENCE

Decisions Regarding the Provision or Withholding of Therapy (Washington University School of Medicine) . . . 915

FEATURED REPORTS

Factors Involved in Immunization Program for Swine Influenza. *Goronwy O. Broun, Sr., Dennis O'Connor, Rose Rita Schmidt, Barbara Puder* . . . 925

Recommendations for Screening Programs for Congenital Hypothyroidism. Report of a Committee of the American Thyroid Association. *D. A. Fisher, G. N. Burrow, J. H. Dussault, D. R. Hollingsworth, P. R. Larsen, E. B. Man, P. G. Walfish* . . . 932

CASE REPORTS

Propionibacterium acnes: Pathogen in Central Nervous System Shunt Infection. Report of Three Cases Including Immune Complex Glomerulonephritis. *B. A. Beeler, J. G. Crowder, J. W. Smith, A. White* . . . 935

Extrinsic Allergic Alveolitis After Aspergillus fumigatus Inhalation. Evidence of a Type IV Immunologic Pathogenesis. *Michael W. Yocum, Alan R. Saltzman, Douglas M. Strong, John C. Donaldson, George W. Ward, Francis M. Walsh, Orr M. Cobb, Jr., Robert C. Elliott* . . . 939

Tuberculous Pseudotumors of the Liver. *Robert D. Zipser, James E. Rau, Richard R. Ricketts, Lynn C. Bevans* . . . 946

Multiple Endocrine Adenomas in a Patient with the Maffucci Syndrome. *Adrian M. Schnall, Saul M. Genuth* . . . 952

Monoclonal IgE with Renal Failure. *Adrian O. Vladutiu, Romesh K. Kohli, Anthony P. Prezyna* . . . 957

Information for Authors . . . 924

Author Index . . . 963

Subject Index . . . 966

JULY 1976

The American Journal of Medicine

VOLUME 61

NUMBER 1

EDITORIALS

Cytodestructive Mechanisms Provoked by Lymphocytes

WOJCIECH KONSTANTY PODLESKI, M.D., Ph.D.
Denver, Colorado

Of all man's miseries the bitterest is this, to know so much and to have control over nothing. (The words which Herodotus put into the mouth of the Persian who talked with Thersander at Thebes.)

A number of experimental observations are consistent with the concept that lymphocytes express a direct and specific killer property [1–3]. Although the interaction between lymphocytes or their product and target cells is an intricate phenomenon, it appears possible to reduce the apparent complexity to three different mechanisms, each of which culminate in the cytolysis of the target cells involved. These models are diagrammatically summarized in Figure 1. Basically, we can divide lymphocyte-mediated cytotoxicity as (A) specific cytolysis of antigen-bearing target cells by either one of two alternative mechanisms (type I and type II), and (B) nonspecific cytolysis of antigenically-unrelated target cells (type III). Specific cytolysis, at the level of cell surface antigen recognition, may be further subdivided into effector function achieved by direct lymphocytotoxicity (type I) or by antibody-dependent cell-mediated cytotoxicity (type II). This classification of type I, II and III is unrelated to that proposed by P. G. H. Gell and R. R. A. Coombs.

Type I mechanisms occur when sensitized T cells act directly on target cells bearing the membrane antigens [4]. This reaction is specific and requires intimate contact between reacting cells. Although there is no concrete evidence [5] that during this membrane-membrane interaction some diffusible factor is released causing destruction of target cells, the existence of an early lymphotoxin locally delivered is possible in human subjects [6,7]. When histocompatibility antigens are involved, it happens that two distinct subsets of T cells are cooperating in elaborating the cytotoxic function [8–11].

From the Department of Medicine, Section of Allergy and Clinical Immunology, National Jewish Hospital and Research Center, 3800 East Colfax Avenue, Denver, Colorado 80206; and the Department of Medicine, Division of Clinical Immunology, University of Colorado Medical Center, 4200 East Ninth Avenue, Denver, Colorado 80220. Requests for reprints should be addressed to Dr. W. K. Podleski, Department of Medicine, Section of Allergy and Clinical Immunology, National Jewish Hospital and Research Center, 3800 E. Colfax Avenue, Denver, Colorado 80206. Manuscript accepted October 9, 1975.

One of these precursors of killer T cells recognizes the antigen by having a recognition unit of similar specificity toward the antigen and differentiates into effector killer T cells. A second subpopulation of T cells acts by amplifying those "pre-killer" cells which are responsible for the cytotoxic allograft reaction in vitro. There is also evidence that in tumor immunity, transfer factor may amplify killer T cells in human subjects [12]. Very recently, the demonstration of functional inactivation of killer T cells by other cytotoxic T cells specifically directed against them confirms the concept of a separate entity related to lytic mechanisms among T cells [13]. There is also evidence that under certain conditions, human circulating lymphocytes are capable of transforming into killer cells in vitro and of effectuating lysis of xenogenic target cells [14].

The existence of more than one pathway leading to the production of sensitized effector lymphoid cells capable of lymphocyte-mediated cytolysis has been postulated [15]. In addition, experimental evidence indicates that acquisition of histamine type II receptor units on the surface of cytolytically active T cells is related to certain immunosuppressive functions, perhaps linked with the control of killer T cell proliferation [16].

Type II mechanisms occur via a reaction termed antibody-dependent cell-mediated cytotoxicity (ADCC). This system requires recognition of target cells by antibody and the subsequent recognition of the reacting antibody by unsensitized "normal inactive" effector cells. Several cell types have been involved in this type of cytolysis, but they all share a common property, namely, receptors for the Fc fragment of the mediating IgG antibodies. Among the most important effector cells in this type of cytolysis are "null" cells, monocytes, macrophages and polymorphonuclear leukocytes [17–29]. Recently, a subclass of lymphocytes termed killer or K cells, but unrelated to the direct killer T cells mentioned (in type I reaction), perhaps a variant of an immature form of B cells, has also been shown to destroy the target cells under these circumstances [30,31]. Antibodies as products of the immune cells in this assay or from exogenous sources, interact specifically with the target cell's antigens [32]. Lysis is induced following bridging between the effector cell and its surface receptors for Fc fragment and antibody-coated target cells. Several cascade reactions are required until such cells can function as cytotoxic effector cells. Some data indicate that ADCC is an extensively dynamic process in the cell membranes of interacting cells [33]. Unfortunately, the phenomenon has been studied under variable conditions and utilizing different effector cells, target cells and antibodies, and uniform interpretation of the mechanism involved in this type of cytotoxic reaction is difficult [34,35]. However, certain hard facts concerning this process include direct binding between effector cells and antibody-coated target cells, the noninvolvement of complement, and active energy requirements of the effector cell [36,37].

The type III mechanism involves a set of conditions in which the cytotoxicity can be expressed nonspecifically by products of lymphocytes. By this nonspecific mechanism, lymphocytes which are activated under certain in vitro conditions release substances which have been termed "mediators of cellular immunity," lymphocyte effector molecules or lymphocyte's associated products [38]. Lymphokines can be released in response to various stimuli. The first is an exposure of specifically sensitive lymphocytes to antigen—a process of specific activation. The second is a stimulation of nonsensitive lymphocytes with a number of nonspecific agents like mitogens, antilymphocytic serum, antigen-antibody complexes and bacterial antigens. A recent finding suggests that both B and T cells are able to produce these mediators [39–41]. One of the lymphocyte effector molecules, a lymphotoxin, exerts a particular function related to the lysis of antigenically-unrelated target cells [42]. However, a wide range of target cell susceptibility to lymphotoxin has been observed [43,44]. Such a process of cell destruction is nonspecific, and contact between activated lymphoid cells and target cells may [45] or may not be required [46]. There is no satisfactory explanation, at present, as to how cytolysis occurs. The process of cytoplasmic fragmentation and membrane destabilization during the action of lymphotoxin molecules on target cells has nevertheless been observed [47].

It has been demonstrated that activated lymphocytes release mitogenic factors which recruit other lymphocytes to transformation. Therefore, nonspecific cytotoxicity, at the induction level, expressed by lymphotoxin release represents an early event in the continuous process of lymphocyte transformation. A combination of these two secretory events might reflect a recruitment phenomenon by which a cell-mediated cytotoxic effect may be amplified nonspecifically [48].

An intriguing issue has been raised by recent experiments which have utilized antibodies against human lymphotoxin [49,50]. Although it appeared that all lymphocytes kill through the same lymphotoxin molecule [49], the recent observation strongly suggests [6,7] that lymphotoxin might express activity by early and late lymphotoxin—antigenically and functionally different lymphotoxins. The early lymphotoxin is detected within 9 hours after adding phytohemagglutinin (PHA) [6]; it may be a good candidate as the molecular mediator of direct T lymphocyte cytotoxicity (type I reaction) in human subjects. The late lymphotoxin (alfa-toxin) appears after 24 to 36 hours in culture and may possess suppressive function for lymphocytes through the expression of toxicity against a selected subpopulation of T cells [7]. In other words, T suppressor function may be mediated through lymphotoxin. This preliminary assumption seems to be in accordance with some experimental data suggesting that thymic suppressor activity is mediated by a diffusible mediator of lymphotoxin-like properties [51].

Details of lymphokine interaction are as yet lacking. We can, however, reasonably assume that such a process of control and immunoregulation among them effectively exists and is operative. Increasing evidence indicates that lymphocyte chalones are the most suitable candidates in limiting the misleading spurious "anarchy" of lymphokines release [52,53].

Some of these experimental approaches have been translated into clinical application, in particular the use of several of the in vitro assay systems mentioned. As a result it has been shown that mechanisms similar to those previously described operate in the cases of autoimmune diseases, transplantation, tumor immunity and certain infectious and/or parasitic diseases. However, there it is important to view the interpretation and clinical significance of the observed results in the light of the natural evolution of disease and its therapeutic modification. Experimental models rarely may be compared with the true clinical picture in this field. These factors are of special importance regarding duration and intensity of antigenic stimulation in vivo during different phases of immune response. Finally, it should be remembered that in vitro models which, despite some convincing parallelism with the in vivo reaction, may in many ways be misleading.

During the last years, one of the classic examples of autoimmune disease, namely, Hashimoto's thyroiditis, has been the object of particular attention. The demonstration of specific cytotoxic lymphocytes in this illness [54,55] appeared to provide a human prototype of the experimental model of direct cytolysis mediated by killer T cells (type I). However, as yet there is only indirect in vitro demonstration that such a subpopulation of human T cells operate in this illness. Increasing evidence suggests that antibody-dependent cell-mediated cytotoxicity (type II) in Hashimoto's thyroiditis may be a more appropriate model in vitro to define a new important cytophilic antibody toward human thyroglobulin [56,57]. Clear distinction of its real significance is difficult in the light of participation of nonspecific mechanisms mediated by lymphotoxin (type III). Thus, when lymphocytes from patients with chronic thyroiditis are activated with thyroid antigens in vitro, they release soluble effector molecules which destroy xenogenic cells [46]. Such spontaneous nonspecific cytolysis by lymphocytes has already been reported in patients with Graves' disease [58]. Additional observations (Podleski et al., unpublished results) indicate that those nonspecific reactions, probably mediated by lymphotoxin, correlate well with the high level of serum circulating long-acting thyroid stimulator (LATS). It has also been demonstrated that PHA-stimulated lymphocytes from patients with Graves' disease are able to release LATS in vitro [59]. Further careful studies on the lymphotoxin-like activity of the LATS immunoglobulin G (IgG) molecule are required. However, human lymphotoxin purification and characterization suggests its immunologic cross-reactivity with IgG globulin [60]. There is also evidence that the inhibition of lymphocytic cytotoxicity in Hashimoto's thyroiditis by dibutyryl cyclic AMP in vitro [61] may resemble in many instances, the control of secretory processes by the already well documented cyclic AMP action in experimental models [62]. In such situations, immune-sensitized lymphocytes react as quasi endocrine cells. In conclusion, the observations mentioned suggest a combination of all three basic mechanisms of lymphocytotoxicity in thyroid autoimmunity, but their exact sequences and significance in the development of disease remain to be established.

There are also several observations proving the presence of cytotoxic lymphocytes in systemic lupus erythematosus (SLE) [63] as well as in muscle diseases [64–67] and in rheumatoid arthritis [68] suggesting that those findings might directly reflect the observed tissue destruction in vivo. Reduced antibody-dependent lymphocyte cytotoxicity (type II reaction) demonstrated in active SLE [69] could result from masking of a receptor for Fc fragment, by steric hindrance phenomenon, of well documented antibody against lymphocyte membranes in SLE [70]. An extensive search for its specific antigen is in progress and perhaps smooth muscle contractile protein in the lymphocytes microvilli should be considered [71].

Immunologic studies in patients with chronic active hepatitis showed [72,73] that circulating lymphocytes express specific cytotoxicity against liver cells. This supports the concept of autoimmune origin of this disease. Interestingly, in active chronic ulcerative colitis and in patients with Crohn's disease, lack of tissue specificity expressed by lymphotoxin elaboration has been observed [74].

There is a special interest in defining the circum-

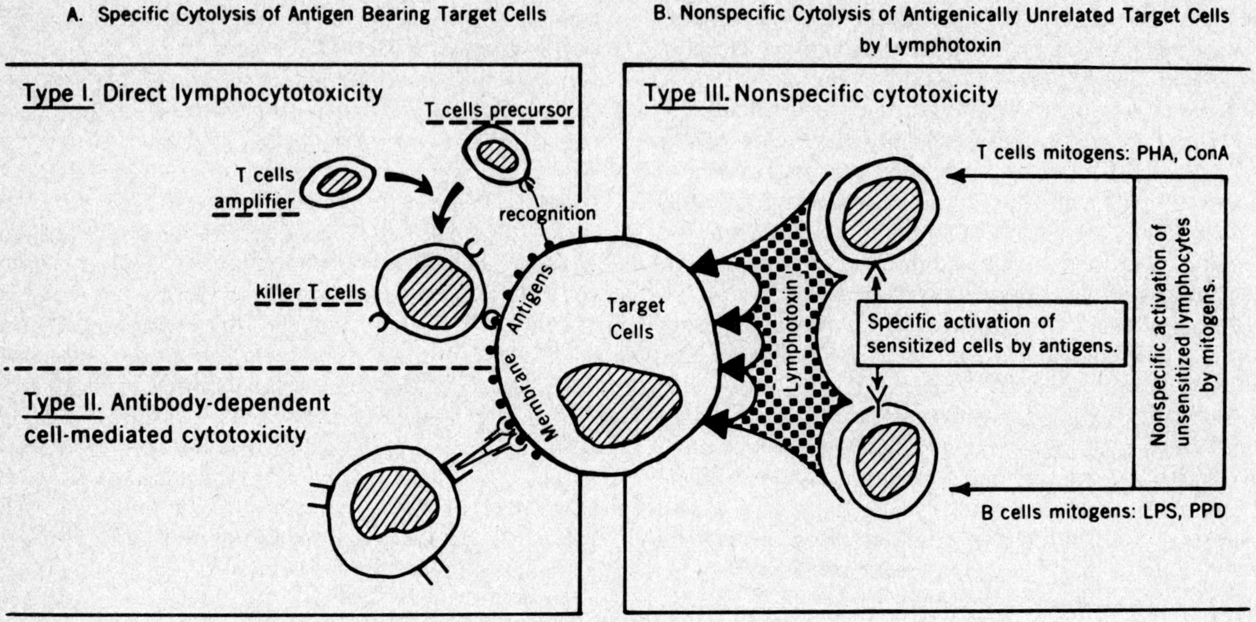

Figure 1. *Basic cytodestructive mechanisms provoked by lymphocytes.*

stances by which lymphocytes in autoimmune diseases acquire such killer properties. An attractive concept of the lack of an independent intracellular control normally provided by homeostatic mechanisms of cyclic AMP is most probably the case. However, we cannot exclude some participation of defective suppressor function probably mediated by separate subsets of T cells and/or their soluble products. Further experiments and clinical observations are necessary to document whether autoimmunity occurs when a selective deficiency of certain suppressors of T cells are present [75–77].

Pregnancy is the natural model of an allogeneic confrontation. Several studies have been undertaken to understand why maternal lymphocytes do not reject their fetus. It is of particular interest that lymphotoxin production by cord blood lymphocytes is markedly diminished [78]. This phenomenon, which appears to be a stage in the maturation of lymphotoxin producing lymphocytes, may be comparable with the recent observation that there is a high percentage of suppressor cells (of T origin?) in umbilical cords of human newborns [79]. A possible role for immunoglobulin D (IgD) in the regulation of the immune response remains to be determined at this point. However, from the evolutionary standpoint of Homo sapiens it is hard to believe that the most important protective function related to preserve cell-mediated-immunity is impaired in the mother at the expense of pregnancy. The biologic activity of the female provides her all necessary and possible mechanisms to protect the progenity of our species. It seems rather that the observed temporary depression of cell-mediated immunity in pregnancy [80] is the consequence of immunosuppressive abilities transferred to the mother from the fetus.

Various cytotoxic assays have been satisfactorily used to detect the presensitization in a group of prospective renal transplant recipients to a group of potential donors. There is impressive evidence that a variety of mixed cytodestructive processes are of high clinical significance [81–85]. With respect to the appropriate selection of donors, it appears that those assays satisfy better the histocompatibility criteria than comparison with complement-dependent cross-match tests.

Antagonism and synergism between serum factors and cytotoxic lymphocytes in the field of tumor immunology appear, at present, to be the most challenging subject. There is no doubt about the expression of cytotoxicity by patients' lymphocytes in several neoplastic manifestations [86–88]. However, the effectiveness of cytolytic potency of circulating lymphocytes toward tumor cells is variably blocked by a serum factor [89–91] of an as yet undefined nature. In those circumstances, effector cells are unable to recognize foreign neoantigens on the surface of neoplastic cells. No intracellular defect of lymphotoxin release has been documented. An original therapeutic approach has recently been shown by injection of an in vitro elaborated lymphokine into in vivo breast cancer tissue [92]. Expected tumor regression was achieved. The purification and preliminary characterization of human lymphotoxin makes such an approach very plausible [6,7,60].

The demonstration of circulating cytotoxic lymphocytes in patients with tuberculosis [93] emphasizes the possible induction and/or amplification of killer lymphocytic property by Bacille Calmette-Guérin vaccination. There is also evidence that in schistosomiasis [25], listeriosis [94] and toxoplasmosis [95], many types of cytotoxic reactions may occur. However, as yet we have no convincing data of how those infestations or viral infections [96–102] can either impair or be beneficial to the host immunoregulatory function (protective immunity).

A few clinical examples of the numerous observations in this field provide clear evidence that for practical and didactical purposes, an illustrated schematical simplification (Figure 1) may clarify and offer some help in the distinction and interpretation of certain clinical pictures.

The vast majority of in vitro assay systems for monitoring lymphocytes mediating cytotoxicity are relatively easy and could be adapted in routine diagnostic tests. Although the complexity of the discussed reactions may not be immediately and satisfactorily elucidated on the basis of clinical material, some valuable principles should be of increasing help for the establishment of critical points in diagnosis and therapy.

The basic questions which emerge from these and other studies are: Can the cytotoxic potential of lymphocytes be evidenced in vitro? Is the destructive process specific (type I versus type II) or nonspecific (type III)? What is the relevance of in vitro observation facing the mystery of Natura artis magistra?

In such a complex field, the direction of future research and its critical clinical confrontation are matters of paramount concern and should concentrate on a few standardized technics rather than to proliferate, difficult to unify, observations. This clearly far reaching implication should increase our ability to evaluate the full significance of our findings.

ACKNOWLEDGMENT

I am deeply indebted to Dr. David S. Rowe for his encouragement and kind support during attempts to indoctrinate some of the issues presented into the field of clinical immunology. The helpful review of this manuscript by Drs. Richard S. Farr and Jacques Chiller is gratefully acknowledged.

ADDENDUM

Since this paper was submitted for publication, an observation, termed spontaneous lymphocyte-mediated cytotoxicity expressed by normal human lymphocytes, has been considered. (Podleski WK: Spontaneous lymphocyte-mediated cytotoxicity (Letter to the Editor). Lancet 2: 1315, 1975).

REFERENCES

1. Cerottini JC, Brunner KT: Cell-mediated cytotoxicity, allograft rejection, and tumor immunity. Adv Immunol 18: 67, 1974.
2. Henney CS: Killer T cells. N Engl J Med 291: 1357, 1974.
3. Cerottini JC, MacDonald HR, Engers HD, Brunner KT: Differentiation pathway of cytolytic T lymphocytes: in vivo and in vitro studies, chap 2. Progress in Immunology, 2nd ed, vol 3 (Brent L, Holborow J, eds), Amsterdam-Oxford, North-Holland Pub. Co., 1974, p 153.
4. Brunner KT, Simpson E: T cell cytotoxicity in vitro. (Workshop reports.) Progress in Immunology, 2nd ed, vol 3 (Brent L, Holborow J, eds), North-Holland Pub. Co., 1974, p 343.
5. Henney CS, Gaffney J, Bloom BR: On the relation of products of activated lymphocytes to cell-mediated cytolysis. J Exp Med 140: 837, 1974.
6. Reed WP, Lucas ZJ: Cytotoxic activity of lymphocytes. V. Role of soluble toxin in macrophage-inhibited cultures of tumor cells. J Immunol 115: 395, 1975.
7. Walker SM, Lee S-C, Lucas ZJ: Cytotoxic activity of lymphocytes. VI. Heterogeneity of cytotoxins in supernatants of mitogen-activated lymphocytes. J Immunol 116: 807, 1976.
8. Wagner H, Rollinghoff M, Shortmann K: Evidence for T-T cell synergism during in vitro cytotoxic allograft responses, chap 2. Progress in Immunology, 2nd ed, vol 3 (Brent L, Holborow J, eds), Amsterdam-Oxford, North-Holland Pub. Co., 1974, p 111.
9. Stobo JD, Paul WE, Henney CS: Functional heterogeneity of murine lymphoid cells. IV. Allogeneic mixed lymphocyte reactivity and cytolytic activity as functions of distinct T cell subsets. J Immunol 110: 652, 1973.
10. Cantor H, Simpson E: Regulation of the immune response by subclasses of T lymphocytes. I. Interactions between pre-killer T cells and regulatory T cells obtained from peripheral lymphoid tissues of mice. Eur J Immunol 5: 330, 1975.
11. Sabbadini E: Regulation of cell-mediated cytotoxicity. II. Synergism of two types of thymus dependent cells in vivo. Cell Immunol 18: 76, 1975.
12. Levin AS, Byers VS, Fudenberg HH, Wybran J, Hackett AJ, Johnston JO, Spitler LE: Osteogenic sarcoma—immunologic parameters before and during immunotherapy with tumor-specific transfer factor. J Clin Invest 55: 487, 1975.
13. Golstein P: Sensitivity of cytotoxic T cells to T-cell mediated cytotoxicity. Nature (Lond) 252: 81, 1974.
14. Behelak Y, Richter M: Immunocompetent cells in man. III. The killer cell activity of normal circulating lymphocytes. Clin Immunol Immunopathol 4: 286, 1975.
15. Berke G, Amos DB: Mechanism of lymphocyte-mediated cytolysis. The LMC cycle and its role in transplantation immunity. Transplant Rev 17: 71, 1973.
16. Plaut M, Lichtenstein LM, Henney CS: Properties of a subpopulation of T cells bearing histamine receptors. J Clin Invest 55: 856, 1975.
17. Perlmann P, Maclennan ICM: Non-T cytotoxicity in vitro. (Workshop reports.) Progress in Immunology, 2nd ed, vol 3 (Brent L, Holborow J, eds), Amsterdam-Oxford, North-Holland Pub. Co., 1974, p 347.
18. Papamichail M, Temple A: Characterization of the human effector cell causing antibody-mediated cytotoxicity. Clin Exp Immunol 20: 459, 1975.
19. Schirrmacher V, Rubin B, Pross H, Wigzell H: Cytotoxic

immune cells with specificity for defined soluble antigens. IV. Antibody as mediator of specific cytotoxicity. J Exp Med 139: 93, 1974.
20. Gale RP, Zighelboim J: Modulation of polymorphonuclear leukocyte-mediated antibody-dependent cellular cytotoxicity. J Immunol 113: 1793, 1974.
21. Michaelsen TE, Wisløff F, Natvig JB: Structural requirements in the Fc region of rabbit IgG antibodies necessary to induce cytotoxicity by human lymphocytes. Scand J Immunol 4: 71, 1975.
22. Trinchieri G, Bauman P, DeMarchi M, Tokes Z: Antibody-dependent cell-mediated cytotoxicity in humans. I. Characterization of the effector cell. J Immunol 115: 249, 1975.
23. Scornik JC, Cosenza H: Antibody-dependent cell-mediated cytotoxicity. III. Two functionally different effector cells. J Immunol 113: 1527, 1974.
24. Gale RP, Zighelboim J, Ossorio RC, Fahey JL: A comparison of human lymphoid cells in antibody-dependent cellular cytotoxicity (ADCC). Clin Immunol Immunopathol 3: 377, 1975.
25. Butterworth AE, Sturrock RF, Houba V, Rees PH: Antibody-dependent cell-mediated damage to schistosomula in vitro. Nature (Lond) 252: 503, 1974.
26. Wisløff F, Frøland SS, Michaelsen TE: Antibody-dependent cytotoxicity mediated by human Fc-receptor-bearing cells lacking markers for B-and T-lymphocytes. Int Arch Allergy 47: 139, 1974.
27. Yust I, Smith RW, Dickler HB, Wunderlich J, Mann DL: Human lymphocyte dependent antibody mediated cytotoxicity: adherence of lymphocytes to antibody treated target cells. Cell Immunol 18: 176, 1975.
28. Pross HF, Tracey DE, Wigzell H, Schirrmacher V: Antibody-dependent cell-mediated cytotoxicity in the mouse. I. Surface characteristics of an effector cell. Scand J Immunol 3: 769, 1974.
29. Sanderson CJ, Clark IA, Taylor GA: Different effector cell types in antibody-dependent cell-mediated cytotoxicity. Nature (Lond) 253: 376, 1975.
30. Calder EA, Irvine WJ, Ghaffer A: K-cell cytotoxic activity in the spleen and lymph nodes of tumour-bearing mice. Clin Exp Immunol 19: 393, 1975.
31. Peter HH, Pavie-Fischer J, Fridman WH, Aubert C, Cesarini JP, Roubin R, Kourilsky FM: Cell-mediated cytotoxicity in vitro of human lymphocytes against a tissue culture melanoma cell line (IGR3). J Immunol 115: 539, 1975.
32. Blair PB, Lane MA: Non-T cell killing of mammary tumor cells by spleen cells. Secretion of antibody and recruitment of cells. J Immunol 115: 184, 1975.
33. Schirrmacher V, Halloran P, Ross E, Festenstein H: A new sensitive assay for antibody against cell surface antigens based on inhibition of cell-dependent antibody-mediated cytotoxicity. II. Mechanism. Cell Immunol 16: 362, 1975.
34. Kovithavongs T, Rice G, Thong KL, Dossetor JB: Effector cell activity in antibody mediated cell dependent immune lysis. II. Evidence for different populations of effector cells for different targets. Cell Immunol 18: 167, 1975.
35. Zighelboim J, Gale RP: Interspecies variability in antibody-dependent cellular cytotoxicity (ADCC). J Immunol 113: 1145, 1974.
36. Van Boxel JA, Paul WE, Green I, Frank MM: Antibody-dependent lymphoid cell-mediated cytotoxicity: role of complement. J Immunol 112: 398, 1974.
37. Trinchieri G, DeMarchi M: Antibody-dependent cell-mediated cytotoxicity in humans. II. Energy requirement. J Immunol 115: 256, 1975.
38. Lymphokines. Lancet 1: 1490, 1973.
39. Yoshida T, Sonozaki H, Cohen S: The production of migration inhibition factor by B- and T-cells of the guinea pig. J Exp Med 138: 784, 1973.
40. Shacks SJ, Chiller J, Granger GA: Studies on in vitro models of cellular immunity. The role of T and B cells in the secretion of lymphotoxin. Cell Immunol 7: 313, 1973.
41. Stejskal V, Härfast B, Holm G, Perlmann P: Cytotoxicity of human lymphocytes induced by pokeweed mitogen or in mixed lymphocyte culture. Specificity and nature of effector cells. Eur J Immunol 4: 126, 1974.
42. Daynes RA, Granger GA: The regulation of lymphotoxin release from stimulated human lymphocyte cultures. The requirement for continual mitogen stimulation. Cell Immunol 12: 252, 1974.
43. Kramer SL, Granger GA: The role of lymphotoxin in target cell destruction by mitogen-activated human lymphocytes. I. The correlation of target cell sensitivity to lymphotoxin and the intact lymphocyte. Cell Immunol 15: 57, 1975.
44. Eifel PJ, Walker SM, Lucas ZJ: Standardization of a sensitive and rapid assay for lymphotoxin. Cell Immunol 15: 208, 1975.
45. Asherson GL, Ferluga J, Janossy G: Non-specific cytotoxicity by T cells activated with plant mitogens in vitro and the requirement for plant agents during the killing reaction. Clin Exp Immunol 15: 573, 1973.
46. Amino N, DeGroot LJ: Concentration of cultured medium to detect small amounts of lymphotoxin induced by PHA, PPD, and thyroid antigens. Cell Immunol 11: 188, 1974.
47. Rosenau W, Goldberg ML, Burke GC: Early biochemical alterations induced by lymphotoxin in target cells. J Immunol 111: 1128, 1973.
48. Butterworth AE: Nonspecific cytotoxic effects of antigen-transformed lymphocytes. Kinetics, cell-requirements and the role of recruitment. Cell Immunol 7: 357, 1973.
49. Walker SM, Lucas ZJ: Inhibition of T and B lymphocyte mediated cytotoxicity by heterologous antiserum to human lymphotoxin. Proceedings of the Eighth Leucocyte Culture Conference Lymphocyte Recognition and Effector Mechanisms, Academic Press, 1974, p 389.
50. Walker SM, Lucas ZJ: Cytotoxic activity of lymphocytes. IV. Preparation of heterologous antibody to human lymphotoxin. J Immunol 113: 813, 1974.
51. Ha TY, Waksman BH, Treffers HP: The thymic suppressor cell. II. Metabolic requirements of suppressor activity. Immunol Commun 3: 351, 1974.
52. Lozzio BB: Regulators of cell division. A review. I. Endogenous mitotic inhibitors of hematopoietic cells. Exp Hematol 1: 309, 1973.
53. Houck JC, Attallah AM, Lilly JR: Immunosuppressive properties of the lymphocyte chalone. Nature (Lond) 245: 148, 1973.
54. Podleski WK: Cytotoxic lymphocytes in Hashimoto's thyroiditis. Clin Exp Immunol 11: 543, 1972.
55. Calder EA, Penhale WJ, Barnes EW, Irvine WJ: Cytotoxic lymphocytes in Hashimoto thyroiditis. An in vitro assay system using ^{51}Cr-labelled chicken red blood cells coated with thyroglobulin. Clin Exp Immunol 14: 19, 1973.
56. Podleski WK, Podleski UG: Antibody-dependent peritoneal-cell-mediated cytotoxicity in man. (Letter to the Editor.) Lancet 1: 1389, 1973.
57. Wasserman J, VonStedingk LV, Perlmann P, Jonsson J: Antibody-induced in vitro lymphocyte cytotoxicity in Hashimoto thyroiditis. Intern Arch Allergy 47: 473, 1974.
58. Podleski WK, Brunner KT, Lemarchand-Beraud T, Scazziga BR, Rowe D, Vannotti A: Cytotoxic lymphocytes in Graves' and Hashimoto's diseases (abstract). Isr J Med

Sci 8: 1881, 1972.
59. Wall JR, Good BF, Forbes IJ, Hetzel BS: Demonstration of the production of the long acting thyroid stimulator (LATS) by peripheral lymphocytes cultured in vitro. Clin Exp Immunol 14: 555, 1973.
60. Amino N, Linn ES, Pysher TJ, Mier R, Moore GE, DeGroot LJ: Human lymphotoxin obtained from established lymphoid lines. Purification characteristics and inhibition by anti-immunoglobulin. J Immunol 113: 1334, 1974.
61. Podleski WK, Podleski UG: Dibutyrul cyclic AMP and cytotoxic lymphocytes in Hashimoto's thyroiditis. J Lab Clin Med 84: 459, 1974.
62. Bourne HR, Lichtenstein LM, Melmon KL, Henney CS, Weinstein Y, Shearer GM: Modulation of inflammation and immunity by cyclic AMP. Receptors for vaso-active hormones and mediators of inflammation regulate many leukocyte functions. Science 184: 19, 1974.
63. Podleski WK, Podleski UG: Circulating sensitized lymphocytes in systemic lupus erythematosus. Nature (Lond) 241: 278, 1973.
64. Dawkins RL, Mastaglia FL: Cell-mediated cytotoxicity to muscle in polymyositis. Effect of immunosuppression. N Engl J Med 288: 434, 1973.
65. Kott E, Genkins G, Rule AH: Leukocyte response to muscle antigens in myasthenla gravis. Relationship to clinical severity and presence of circulating antibodies. Neurology 23: 374, 1973.
66. Haas DC, Arnason BGW: Cell-mediated immunity in polymyositis. Arch Neurol 31: 192, 1974.
67. Mori R, Kawanami S: Destruction of cultured thymus cells by autologous lymphocytes from a patient with myasthenia gravis. (Letter to the Editor.) Lancet 1: 210, 1973.
68. Person DA, Sharp JT, Lidsky MD: Cytotoxicity of rheumatoid mononuclear cells for synovial cells (abstract). Clin Res 23: 24, 1975.
69. Schneider J, Chin W, Friou GJ, Cooper SM, Harding B, Hill RL, Quismorio FP: Reduced antibody-dependent cell-mediated cytotoxicity in systemic lupus erythematosus. Clin Exp Immunol 20: 187, 1975.
70. Lies RB, Messner RP, Williams RC Jr: Relative T-cell specificity of lymphocytotoxins from patients with systemic lupus erythematosus. Arthritis Rheum 16: 369, 1973.
71. Fagraeus A, Lidman K, Biberfeld G: Reaction of human smooth muscle antibodies with human blood lymphocytes and lymphoid cell lines. Nature (Lond) 252: 246, 1974.
72. Paronetto F, Vernace S: Immunological studies in patients with chronic active hepatitis. Cytotoxic activity of lymphocytes to autochthonous liver cells grown in tissue culture. Clin Exp Immunol 19: 99, 1975.
73. Wands JR, Isselbacher KJ: Lymphocyte cytotoxicity to autologous liver cells in chronic active hepatitis. Proc Natl Acad Sci USA 72: 1301, 1975.
74. Shorter RG, Huizenga KA, Spencer RJ, Weedon D: Lymphotoxin in nonspecific inflammatory bowel disease lymphocytes. Digest Dis 18: 79, 1973.
75. Fudenberg HH: Autoimmune disease and malignancy due to selective T-cell deficiency. Critical Factors in Cancer Immunology, vol 10 (Schultz J, Leif RC, eds), Proceedings of Miami Symposia, Jan 13–17, 1975, New York, Academic Press, 1975, p 179.
76. Goldman AS, Lord RA, Dupree E, Goldblum RM, Smith CW, Dahl EV: Lack of suppression of certain immunoglobulin-producing lymphocytes in T-lymphocyte deficiency. Clin Immunol Immunopathol 3: 69, 1974.
77. Jacobson EN, Zembala M: Inhibitory T-cells. (Workshop reports.) Progress in Immunology, 2nd ed, vol 3 (Brent L, Holborow J, eds), Amsterdam-Oxford, North-Holland Pub. Co., 1974, p 351.
78. Eife RF, Eife G, August CS, Kuhre WL, Staehr-Johansen K: Lymphotoxin production and blast cell transformation by cord blood lymphocytes: dissociated lymphocyte function in newborn infants. Cell Immunol 14: 435, 1974.
79. Olding LB, Benirschke K, Oldstone MBA: Inhibition of mitosis of lymphocytes from human adults by lymphocytes from human newborns. Clin Immunol Immunopathol 3: 79, 1974.
80. Immunological changes in women. Lancet 1: 909, 1974.
81. Ting A, Terasaki PI: Lymphocyte-dependent antibody cross-matching for transplant patients. Lancet 1: 304, 1975.
82. Strom TB, Tilney NL, Carpenter CB, Busch GJ: Identity and cytotoxic capacity of cells infiltrating renal allografts. N Engl J Med 292: 1257, 1975.
83. Balfour IC, Evans CA, Middleton VL, Pegrum GD: Observations on the cytotoxicity of lymphocytes to a target cell system. Clin Exp Immunol 10: 67, 1972.
84. Hersey P, Culen P, MacLennan ICM: Lymphocyte-dependent cytotoxic antibody activity against human transplantation antigens. Transplantation (Baltimore) 16: 9, 1973.
85. Lightbody JJ, Rosenberg JC: Antibody-dependent cell-mediated cytotoxicity in prospective kidney transplant recipients. J Immunol 112: 890, 1974.
86. Wybran J, Hellström I, Hellström KE, Fudenberg HH: Cytotoxicity of human rosette-forming blood lymphocytes on cultivated human tumor cells. Int J Cancer 13: 515, 1974.
87. O'Toole C, Stejskal V, Perlman P, Karlsson M: Lymphoid cells mediating tumor-specific cytotoxicity to carcinoma of the urinary bladder. Separation of the effector population using a surface marker. J Exp Med 139: 457, 1974.
88. Moore GE: Cell lines from humans with hematopoietic malignancies, chap 11. Human Tumor Cells In Vitro (Fogh J, ed), New York, Plenum Pub. Co., 1975, p 322.
89. Hellström KE, Hellström I: Lymphocyte-mediated cytotoxicity and blocking serum activity to tumor antigens. Advances in Immunology, vol 18 (Dixon FJ, Kunkel HG, eds), New York, Academic Press, 1974, p 209.
90. Nelson K, Pollack SB, Hellström KE: Specific anti-tumor responses by cultured immune spleen cells. I. In vitro culture method and initial characterization of factors which block immune cell-mediated cytotoxicity in vitro. Int J Cancer 15: 806, 1975.
91. Saksela E, Penttinen K, Pyrhönen S: "Nonspecific" blocking of human ovarian carcinoma-associated cellular cytotoxicity in vitro. Scand J Immunol 3: 781, 1974.
92. Papermaster BW, Holtermann OA, Rosner D, Klein E, Dao T, Djerassi J: Regressions produced in breast cancer lesions by a lymphokine fraction from a human lymphoid cell line. Res Commun Chem Pathol Pharmacol 8: 413, 1974.
93. Podleski WK, Podleski UG: Circulating cytotoxic lymphocytes in human tuberculosis. Am Rev Respir Dis 108: 791, 1973.
94. Campbell PA, Martens BL, Cooper HR, McClatchy JK: Requirement for bone marrow-derived cells in resistance to Listeria. J Immunol 112: 1407, 1974.
95. Rose NR, Zeschke RH, Podleski WK: Specific and nonspecific mechanisms of immunity in Toxoplasmosis. The Immune System and Infectious Diseases: 4th International Convocation on Immunology, Buffalo, New York, June 1974 (Neter E, et al., eds), Basel, S. Karger, 1975, p 524.
96. Lamon EW, Skurzak HM, Klein E, Wigzell H: In vitro cytotoxicity by a non-thymus-processed lymphocyte popu-

lation with specificity for a virally determined tumor cell surface antigen. J Exp Med 136: 1072, 1972.

97. Rola-Pleszczynski M, Hurtado RC, Woody JN, Sell KW, Vincent MM, Hensen SA, Bellanti JA: Identification of the cell population involved in viral-specific cell-mediated cytotoxicity in man. Evidence for T cell specificity. J Immunol 115: 239, 1975.

98. Härfast B, Andersson T, Perlmann P: Human lymphocyte cytotoxicity against mumps virus-infected target cells. Requirement for non-T cells. J Immunol 114: 1820, 1975.

99. Greenberg SB, Criswell BS, Couch RB: Lymphocyte-mediated cytotoxicity against influenza virus-infected cells. An in vitro method. J Immunol 115: 601, 1975.

100. Vesikari T, Kanra GY, Buimovici-Klein E, Cooper LZ: Cell-mediated immunity in rubella assayed by cytotoxicity of supernatants from rubella virus-stimulated human lymphocyte cultures. Clin Exp Immunol 19: 33, 1975.

101. Svedmyr E, Jondal M: Cytotoxic effector cells specific for B cell lines transformed by Epstein-Barr virus are present in patients with infectious mononucleosis. Proc Natl Acad Sci USA 72: 1622, 1975.

102. Hutt LM, Huang YT, Dascomb HE, Pagano JS: Enhanced destruction of lymphoid cell lines by peripheral blood leukocytes taken from patients with acute infectious mononucleosis. J Immunol 115: 243, 1975.

Ketogenesis and Its Regulation

J. DENIS McGARRY, Ph.D.
DANIEL W. FOSTER, M.D.
Dallas, Texas

The ketotic state has been of major interest to biochemists, physiologists and clinicians for many years. It is our purpose here to review recent advances that provide new insights into the mechanisms by which ketogenesis is regulated. To this end, we shall briefly discuss current understanding of the biochemical physiology of ketogenesis, the hormonal induction of ketosis and clinical implications.

THE BIOCHEMICAL PHYSIOLOGY OF KETOGENESIS

It is now clear that enhanced production of ketone bodies in the intact organism requires changes in the metabolic patterns of both adipose tissue and liver. The substrate for acetoacetate and β-hydroxybutyrate synthesis by the liver is long chain fatty acids. The latter are readily provided from triglycerides stored in adipose tissue through the operation of a hormone-sensitive lipase [1] which is activated in conditions such as starvation, exercise and uncontrolled diabetes. The released free fatty acids (and glycerol) are transported via plasma to the liver and other tissues. In the liver the incoming fatty acids have essentially two fates. They may be esterified to form triglycerides (for storage or release in very low density lipoprotein particles) or they may be oxidized [2–4]. Partitioning between the two pathways determines the rate of ketogenesis. If the rate of fatty acid oxidation is high, overproduction of ketones results. The important point is that rapid rates of fatty acid oxidation (and ketogenesis) do not passively follow the increased delivery of free fatty acids to the liver; direct activation of the oxidative sequence is also required. Evidence for this conclusion has been discussed elsewhere [5].

The nature of the change that "turns on" the ketogenic machinery can now be described in some detail. It was early noted that the hepatic metabolism of long and medium chain fatty acids was distinctly different in normal and ketotic states. Octanoate, a medium chain fatty acid, was shown to be oxidized at equal rates in livers taken from fed, fasted and diabetic animals whereas oleate, representative of physiologic long chain fatty acids, was oxidized at low rates in livers from fed animals and at high rates in livers from starved or diabetic rats [3,6]; the converse situation obtained with regard to the quantity of oleic acid entering the triglyceride pathway. Both types of fatty acid are oxidized intramitochondrially by enzymes of the β-oxidation sequence, but their transport into the mitochondrion occurs by different mechanisms. As shown in Figure 1, octanoate traverses the mitochondrial membrane directly whereas oleate requires activation to oleyl coenzyme A (CoA) in the cytosol and transesterification to carnitine at the outer aspect of the inner mitochondrial membrane for transfer across the restrictive barrier. Re-esterification to CoA occurs on the inner side [7–9]. On the basis of these findings it seemed likely that the control site for ketogenesis from long chain fatty acids was localized to the single step unique to their oxidation, namely, the coupled carnitine acyltransferase system.

From the Departments of Internal Medicine and Biochemistry, The University of Texas Health Science Center at Dallas, Dallas, Texas 75235. Requests for reprints should be addressed to Dr. J. Denis McGarry. Manuscript accepted December 10, 1975.

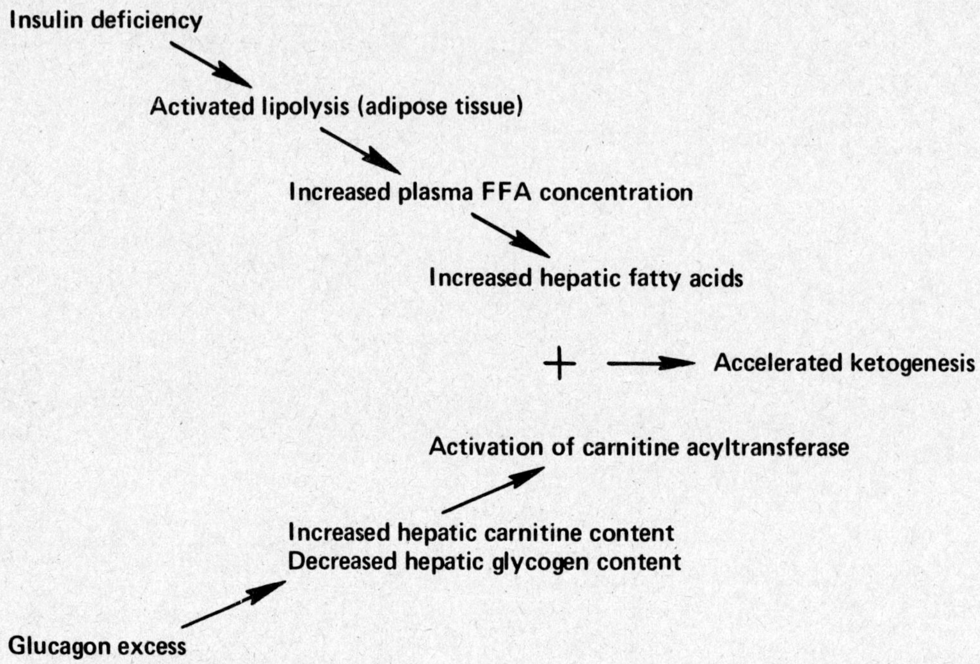

Figure 1. *Reactions involved in hepatic oxidation of oleic acid, octanoylcarnitine and octanoic acid. Steps 1 and 2 represent carnitine acyltransferase I and II, respectively. Steps 3 and 4 refer to the sequences of β-oxidation and the HMG-CoA cycle for ketogenesis, respectively [5]. The carnitine acyltransferases are bound to the inner membrane in vivo but for clarity the reactions are drawn away from the membrane.*

Direct evidence supporting this hypothesis has now been obtained [10]. As noted herein, the nonphysiologic substrate, octanoic acid, does not require esterification to carnitine to enter the mitochondrion and therefore bypasses the carnitine acyltransferase step. However, if octanoate is esterified to carnitine it cannot be oxidized unless it is transesterified to CoA by carnitine acyltransferase II. We have found that ketone body production from (−)-octanoylcarnitine, in contrast to free octanoic acid, is low in perfused livers from fed animals and enhanced in all circumstances in which ketogenesis from oleate is elevated; i.e., in all animals exhibiting ketosis in vivo. Thus, octanoate can be made to act as a long chain fatty acid by imposing a requirement for carnitine acyltransferase action prior to oxidation, a finding strongly supporting a central role for the transferase reaction in the control of ketogenesis.

A reasonable interpretation of the data is as follows: the capacity for oxidation of CoA derivatives of fatty acids inside the mitochondrion is fixed, large and nonrate limiting for the generation of acetyl CoA. Since utilization pathways of acetyl CoA apart from ketogenesis (tricarboxylic acid cycle, fatty acid synthesis) are relatively low capacity systems [6], high rates of acetyl CoA generation yield high rates of ketone synthesis. The rate of acetyl CoA generation is primarily determined by the rate of fatty acid oxidation; this, in turn, is controlled by the activity of the carnitine acyltransferase system*. Once the latter is activated, the restriction to entry of fatty acids into the mitochondrion is removed and the rate of ketogenesis is determined in first order fashion by the rate of delivery of free fatty acids to the liver. In short, the liver is potentially ketogenic when carnitine acyltransferase is activated and actually ketogenic to the degree that substrate is supplied.

HORMONAL CONTROL OF KETOSIS

Historically, the ketotic state has been considered to be the result of a single hormone disturbance, namely, insulin deficiency. It is now clear that such an interpretation is oversimplified and that the ketotic state requires for its development not only a deficiency of insulin but also an inappropriate increase in the blood concentration of glucagon. The evidence supporting this conclusion can be summarized as follows. If fed (nonketotic) rats are given intravenous infusions of anti-insulin serum, a diabetic state develops with hyperglycemia and ketosis, whereas an infusion of glucagon under similar circumstances produces only a transient hyperglycemia without ketosis [12]. Anti-

* Detailed examination of mitochondria taken from livers from nonketotic and ketotic rats showed no significant change in the total quantity of carnitine acyltransferase [11]. It thus seems likely that in the intact liver the activity rather than the amount of this enzyme is subject to metabolic control.

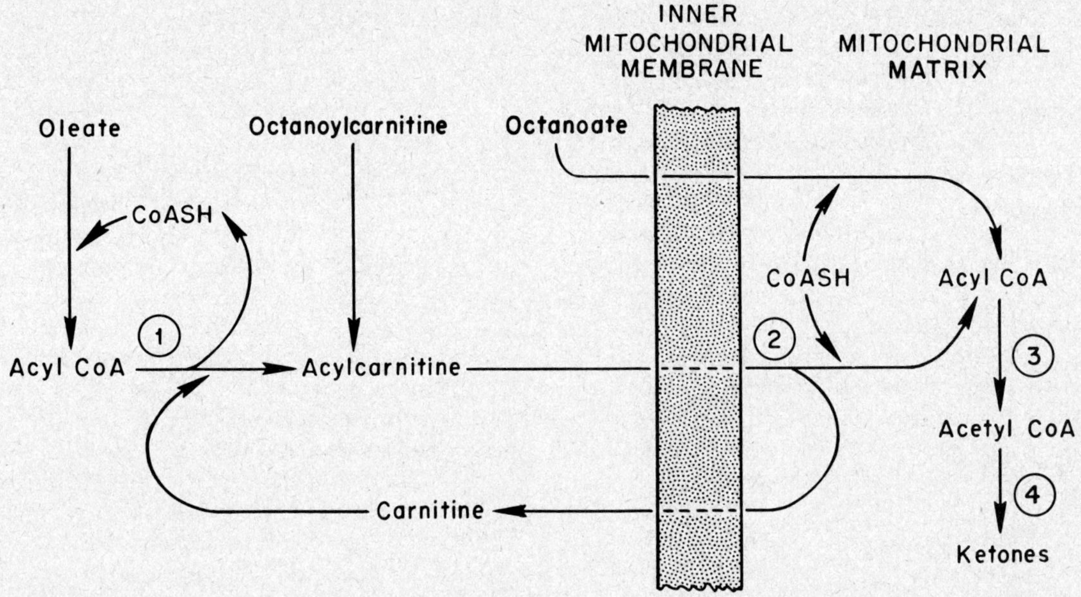

Figure 2. *Presumed roles of insulin deficiency and glucagon excess in the regulation of ketogenesis.*

insulin serum diminishes plasma insulin and increases plasma glucagon whereas a glucagon infusion increases plasma levels of both hormones. Despite the fact that anti-insulin serum treatment produced ketosis and glucagon treatment did not, when the livers were subsequently isolated and perfused with fatty acids, *both* types showed activated fatty acid oxidation and accelerated acetoacetate and β-hydroxybutyrate synthesis. In other words, we had produced a "ketogenic" liver in a nonketotic animal by a 1 hour infusion of glucagon alone. The absence of ketosis in these rats was shown to be due to the fact that plasma free fatty acid concentrations were very low, presumably as a result of insulin secretion secondary to hyperglycemia produced by the glycogenolytic action of glucagon on the liver. When free fatty acid levels were artificially elevated in vivo, ketonemia promptly developed in the glucagon-treated animals but not in the control group [12].

On the basis of these findings it appears likely that activation of the ketogenic process in the liver is mediated primarily by glucagon excess, since it can be produced in the face of "normal" insulin concentrations by infusion of glucagon. In contrast, the primary site for manifestation of insulin deficiency is considered to be adipose tissue in which accelerated lipolysis would assure sufficient fatty acid substrate to supply the activated hepatic ketogenic machinery*.

* Although the ketogenic change can be induced without lowering peripheral plasma insulin concentrations, we wish to make clear that it cannot be definitely stated that insulin plays no direct role in the control of hepatic ketogenic mechanisms. It remains an open possibility that the glucagon:insulin ratio is the operational hormonal unit for regulation of liver metabolism [13].

Strong support for the key role of glucagon in regulating ketogenic potential has come from studies with somatostatin in insulin-dependent diabetic patients. This hormone, which is a potent inhibitor of glucagon release from the pancreas, has the capacity to retard the appearance of ketosis when administered to such subjects after withdrawal of insulin [14]. It has also been shown that glucagon enhances the ketogenic response to a fatty acid load in diabetic man [15].

How does glucagon excess increase the ketogenic potential of the liver? In accord with the cited studies in starvation and diabetes, 1 hour of treatment of fed animals with glucagon was found to increase the ability of the liver to oxidize oleic acid and (−)-octanoylcarnitine to the same degree, indicating activation of the carnitine acyltransferase system [12]. The mechanism by which this is accomplished is not completely understood. Our initial hypothesis was that hepatic ketogenic capacity was related in some way to the glycogen content of the liver since, as had been found in many earlier studies in the literature [16,17], an inverse relationship was always found between the two parameters [12,18]. It was considered that the activity of carnitine acyltransferase might be suppressed by some component of carbohydrate metabolism in the liver that fluctuates in parallel with the glycogen level. However, since glucagon failed to activate ketogenesis when added directly to the medium perfusing livers from fed rats, despite its prompt induction of glycogenolysis [12], it was apparent that glycogen depletion of the tissue could not be the sole mechanism through which anti-insulin serum and glucagon enhanced hepatic ketogenic potential in the intact animal. This suggested that some additional factor mediated the effects of such hormonal manipulations in vivo. Of particular interest in this regard is our recent observation that all ketogenic states are accompanied by an increase in hepatic carnitine content [19]. This increase can be produced rapidly by glucagon or anti-insulin serum and is likewise seen in starvation and experimental diabetes. More important, it was demonstrated that carnitine has the capacity to activate ketogenesis in the isolated perfused liver from fed animals. No other substance has been found to have a similar capability. We do not yet know whether the increased carnitine content represents de novo synthesis in the liver or whether it (or a precursor) is transported from peripheral tissues to the liver in the same way that amino acids and fatty acids are mobilized for gluconeogenesis and ketone production*.

Figure 2 represents an overview of the system and indicates the bihormonal nature of its control. The lipolytic component produced by insulin deficiency seems straightforward, but the connecting link between glucagon excess and activation of carnitine acyltransferase must be considered tentative. It seems probable that both increased hepatic carnitine and decreased levels of hepatic glycogen (or a related component of carbohydrate metabolism) are required for full activation of the ketogenic machinery.

CLINICAL IMPLICATIONS

Based on the formulations given, it is clear that clinical ketotic states can best be understood by considering the interaction between the lipolytic rate in adipose tissue, which determines substrate supply, and the capacity for fatty acid oxidation in the liver, which determines ketone body production from the fatty acid substrate. By way of illustration, a normal man fasted for several days has only modest ketosis (2 to 6 mmol/liter total ketones) because, despite activation of the hepatic ketogenic sequence, fatty acid delivery to the liver is only moderately increased. On the other hand, certain alcoholic patients, with identical starvation-induced changes in the liver, have ketoacidosis equivalent to that seen in uncontrolled diabetes because of greatly increased plasma fatty acid concentrations [20]. The latter may well result from a genetically determined propensity for an abnormally brisk lipolytic response to alcohol in a small percentage of the alcoholic population at risk. Patterns of reversal in ketotic states can also be explained by the model. Rapid reversal of starvation ketosis by infusion of glucose (with consequent endogenous insulin release) or small amounts of exogenous insulin would be due to diminished lipolysis at the level of the adipocyte. On the other hand, the antilipolytic action of insulin in diabetic ketoacidosis would generally have little immediate effect on hepatic ketone production because hepatic triglycerides are markedly increased under these circumstances and can function as substrate for fatty acid oxidation for a several hour period even when plasma fatty acid levels are returned to normal [21]. In this situation response doubtless requires depletion of hepatic triglycerides or deactivation of the carnitine acyltransferase system, accounting for the protracted recovery period that characterizes diabetic ketoacidosis [5]. We presume that deactivation operates via lowering of glucagon levels (and/or increasing the insulin:glucagon ratio) with consequent reduction of hepatic carnitine content and replenishment of tissue glycogen stores.

To summarize, the development of the ketotic state involves two organ systems, adipose tissue and liver, and is controlled primarily by the interactions of two hormones, insulin and glucagon. For maximal ketogenesis to occur alterations are required in both hormones and both organs; unilateral changes will not suffice. Since Unger and associates [22–24] and others [14] have found that the hyperglycemia of uncontrolled diabetes is related to glucagon excess, the work described here invites the generalization that essentially all the metabolic abnormalities of diabetic ketoacidosis reflect changes in the relative concentrations of glucagon and insulin.

* Examination of Figure 1 indicates that an increase in carnitine content would be expected to stimulate the carnitine acyltransferase I reaction. On the other hand, the oxidation of (−)-octanoylcarnitine should be independent of the carnitine concentration. Since the oxidation of both long chain fatty acids and (−)-octanoylcarnitine is enhanced in the ketotic liver it is likely that the two transferases are under coordinate control.

REFERENCES

1. Khoo JC, Steinberg D, Thompson B, Mayer SE: Hormonal regulation of adipocyte enzymes. The effects of epinephrine and insulin on the control of lipase, phosphorylase kinase, phosphorylase and glycogen synthase. J Biol Chem 248: 3823, 1973.
2. Mayes PA, Felts JM: Regulation of fat metabolism in the liver. Nature (Lond) 215: 716, 1967.
3. McGarry JD, Foster DW: The regulation of ketogenesis from oleic acid and the influence of antiketogenic agents. J Biol Chem 246: 6247, 1971.
4. Ontko JA: Metabolism of free fatty acids in isolated liver cells. Factors affecting the partition between esterification and oxidation. J Biol Chem 247: 1788, 1972.
5. McGarry JD, Foster DW: Regulation of ketogenesis and clinical aspects of the ketotic state. Metabolism 21: 471, 1972.
6. McGarry JD, Foster DW: The regulation of ketogenesis from octanoic acid. The role of the tricarboxylic acid cycle and fatty acid synthesis. J Biol Chem 246: 1149, 1971.
7. Fritz IB: Factors influencing the rates of long chain fatty acid oxidation and synthesis in mammalian systems. Physiol Rev

41: 52, 1961.
8. Kopec B, Fritz IB: Comparison of properties of carnitine palmitoyl-transferase I with those of carnitine palmitoyltransferase II, and preparation of antibodies to carnitine palmitoyltransferases. J Biol Chem 248: 4069, 1973.
9. Brosnan JT, Kopec B, Fritz IB: The localization of carnitine palmitoyltransferase in the inner membrane of bovine liver mitochondrion. J Biol Chem 248: 4075, 1973.
10. McGarry JD, Foster DW: The metabolism of (−)-octanoylcarnitine in perfused livers from fed and fasted rats. Evidence for a possible regulatory role of carnitine acyltransferase in the control of ketogenesis. J Biol Chem 249: 7984, 1974.
11. DiMarco JP, Hoppel C: Hepatic mitochondrial function in ketogenic states. Diabetes, starvation and after growth hormone administration. J Clin Invest 55: 1237, 1975.
12. McGarry JD, Wright PH, Foster DW: Hormonal control of ketogenesis. Rapid activation of hepatic ketogenic capacity in fed rats by anti-insulin serum and glucagon. J Clin Invest 55: 1202, 1975.
13. Parilla R, Goodman MN, Toews CJ: Effect of glucagon: insulin ratios on hepatic metabolism. Diabetes 23: 725, 1974.
14. Gerich JE, Lorenzi M, Bier DM, Schneider V, Tsalikian E, Karam JH, Forsham PH: Prevention of human diabetic ketoacidosis by somatostatin. Evidence for an essential role of glucagon. N Engl J Med 292: 985, 1975.
15. Schade DS, Eaton RP: Glucagon regulation of plasma ketone body concentration in human diabetes. J Clin Invest 56: 1340, 1975.
16. Blixenkrone-Møller N: Respiratorischer stoffwechsel und Ketonbildung der Leber. Z Physiol Chem 252: 117, 1938.
17. Mirsky IA: The etiology of diabetic acidosis. JAMA 118: 690, 1942.
18. McGarry JD, Meier JM, Foster DW: Effects of starvation and refeeding on carbohydrate and lipid metabolism in vivo and in the perfused rat liver. J Biol Chem 248: 270, 1973.
19. McGarry JD, Robles-Valdes C, Foster DW: The role of carnitine in hepatic ketogenesis. Proc Natl Acad Sci 72: 4385, 1975.
20. Levy LJ, Duga J, Girgis M, Gordon EE: Ketoacidosis associated with alcoholism in nondiabetic subjects. Ann Intern Med 78: 213, 1973.
21. Van Harken DR, Dixon CW, Heimberg M: Hepatic lipid metabolism in experimental diabetes. V. The effect of concentration of oleate on metabolism of triglycerides and on ketogenesis. J Biol Chem 244: 2278, 1969.
22. Unger RH: Alpha- and beta-cell interrelationships in health and disease. Metabolism 23: 581, 1974.
23. Unger RH, Orci L: The essential role of glucagon in the pathogenesis of diabetes mellitus. Lancet 1: 14, 1975.
24. Sakurai H, Dobbs R, Unger RH: Somatostatin-induced changes in insulin and glucagon secretion in normal and diabetic dogs. J Clin Invest 59: 1395, 1974.

Splenectomy for Palliation of Chronic Myelocytic Leukemia

GERMAN A. GOMEZ, M.D.
JOSEPH E. SOKAL, M.D.
ARNOLD MITTELMAN, M.D.
C. WILLIAM AUNGST, M.D.
Buffalo, New York

Sixty patients with chronic myelocytic leukemia (CML) (most, in the "terminal phase" of the disease) were subjected to splenectomy because of symptomatic splenomegaly, thrombocytopenia or anemia for which they required frequent transfusions. Surgical morbidity and mortality were high when the procedure was performed on a "casual" basis, but both were reduced sharply after care of these patients was restricted to a single medical-surgical-nursing team and improved technics of surgery and perioperative management were developed. Significant hematologic and clinical benefit was achieved in half of the patients and temporary arrest of the disease was often observed, but in most patients, the basic evolution of CML was not greatly altered. In eight patients, however, long-lasting improvement (one to nine years) was recorded. Measurement of the doubling time of circulating leukemic cells and other observations were consistent with the hypothesis that, in some patients, the spleen contains a more rapidly proliferating and "more malignant" population of leukemic cells than the marrow. We conclude that splenectomy is often a useful palliative procedure in advanced stages of CML, and that it may be strikingly beneficial in 10 to 15 per cent of such cases.

The role of splenectomy in the management of chronic myelocytic leukemia (CML) is controversial. Attitudes recorded in the literature range from cautious palliative application of the procedure [1] to routine use of early splenectomy as an important feature of a program attempting to eradicate the disease [2].

Splenectomy was tested as a therapeutic measure in leukemia more than 100 years ago [3]. However, the discouraging morbidity and mortality recorded in the early experience at several centers [4] resulted in abandonment of the procedure. More recently, improved surgical technics and effective antimicrobial and supportive therapy have resulted in a marked decrease in operative mortality, and splenectomy is now often considered for certain complications of CML. These include splenic infarction, manifestations of "hypersplenism" (i.e., anemia, thrombocytopenia) and mechanical symptoms from massive splenomegaly [5,6]. Splenectomy has been recommended for treatment of patients with busulfan toxicity [7]. Splenectomy early in the disease is being recommended by some clinicians as prophylaxis against complications associated with the progressive enlargement of the spleen which characterizes its later stages. One group has suggested that early splenectomy may delay the onset of myeloblastic transformation [8]. Relatively little information has been recorded regarding the effects of splenectomy in the terminal stages of CML, and most authorities appear to believe that the procedure would be too dangerous in such cases [7,9].

This report presents our experience with splenectomy among 60 patients with CML, principally in the "accelerated" or "blastic" stage of the disease.

From the Department of Medicine B and the General Clinical Research Center, Department of Surgery, Roswell Park Memorial Institute, New York State Department of Health, Buffalo, New York 14263. This study was supported in part by Grant RR-262 from the General Clinical Research Centers Program of the Division of Research Resources, National Institutes of Health. Requests for reprints should be addressed to Dr. German A. Gomez, Medicine B, Roswell Park Memorial Institute, 666 Elm Street, Buffalo, New York 14263. Manuscript accepted November 24, 1975.

CLINICAL MATERIAL AND METHODS

A total of 60 patients with CML underwent splenectomy at this Institute between January 1, 1950, and December 1, 1974. Most of these patients had "typical" CML at the time of diagnosis, but some had unusual manifestations, such as leukemic tumor masses, marked eosinophilia or basophilia, and the like. One patient was classified as having chronic eosinophilic leukemia. In addition to standard hematologic and clinical studies, chromosomal analysis of bone marrow and/or peripheral blood specimens was undertaken in 52 patients. The Ph′ chromosome was found in 49 of these; the remaining three patients were Ph′-negative. In 57 patients, bone marrow aspiration was performed both during the three weeks before splenectomy and after the procedure. Splenic aspiration or imprints from the spleen were obtained in 18 patients before or at the time of splenectomy. Chromosomal analysis was performed on splenic specimens from 15 patients.

There were 35 men and 25 women in this series; at the time of splenectomy, they ranged in age from 16 to 82 years, with a median of 46 years. The time from diagnosis of CML to splenectomy ranged from one month to 10 years, with a median of 30 months. These patients had received considerably varied treatment for their CML before splenectomy, including radiation therapy and chemotherapy with conventional or investigational agents. Thirty-one patients received immunotherapy [10] as part of their management before and/or after splenectomy. All patients had clinical and hematologic abnormalities at the time of splenectomy, but their over-all status varied considerably. A few patients appeared to have responsive disease, with one or more troublesome complications. Most were in the "resistant" or "accelerated" stage of CML, and some were in frank myeloblastic transformation. In a few patients, spleens were impalpable or barely palpable; in most, they were moderately to greatly enlarged.

The major reasons for performing splenectomy were splenic infarction or persistent abdominal discomfort associated with marked splenomegaly; thrombocytopenia, requiring platelet transfusions or limiting the administration of antileukemic chemotherapy; symptomatic anemia, requiring relatively frequent transfusions; and progressively increasing splenomegaly, resistant to antileukemic chemotherapy. In most patients, two or more of these indications were present.

Surgical Technic. The operative technics used prior to 1964 varied. Since then, a standardized surgical procedure [6] has been used and splenectomies have been performed by the same surgical team. Patients are instructed preoperatively in the breathing and coughing exercises they will be asked to perform after surgery. A central venous pressure catheter, a nasogastric tube and a Foley catheter are inserted before the operation. The splenectomy is carried out through a long midline incision. The spleen is palpated; adhesions are lysed by sharp and blunt dissection. The organ is then delivered out of the abdomen. The pedicle is serially clamped and divided, starting at its lower pole and using a double clamp technic. After splenic removal and securing of the main pedicle, careful search for an accessory spleen is made and all bleeding points are controlled. When indicated, a liver biopsy is performed. The incision is then closed. Drains are not used unless the pancreas or stomach has been injured.

In 1968, routine use of epsilonaminocaproic acid (EACA), to prevent fibrinolytic hemorrhage, was adopted. EACA is given by slow intravenous infusion, 5 g during the 12 hours before surgery and 5 g during the first 12 hours thereafter. There is suggestive evidence that this reduces the incidence and severity of bleeding during surgery and the immediate postoperative period [11]. Fresh whole blood or plasma, as well as routine platelet and erythrocyte infusions, were often used during and immediately after surgery among high-risk patients.

Leukemic Cell Doubling Times. In some patients the doubling time of circulating leukemic cells [12] was estimated before and after splenectomy. This was possible when patients had had sufficiently long periods of observation without chemotherapy. The absolute number of cells capable of reproduction (myeloblasts, promyelocytes and myelocytes) was calculated from serial blood counts. These numbers were plotted on semilogarithmic graph paper, and the doubling time was determined from a straight line drawn to fit these points as closely as possible, by visual estimation.

RESULTS

Surgical Complications and Mortality. Ten splenectomies were performed prior to 1964 by different surgical teams. These were associated with a high rate of complications and four deaths. One patient died two days after surgery, with myocardial infarction and pulmonary edema; he also had intra-abdominal bleeding. Two patients died of subphrenic abscess and portal vein thrombosis, 60 and 75 days after splenectomy. One patient died of intestinal obstruction, presumably secondary to postoperative adhesions, eight months after splenectomy.

During 1964–1974 (50 splenectomies), when patients were managed by a single medical-surgical-nursing team and an improved operative procedure was used, surgical morbidity was substantially less. There were two deaths attributable to operative complications (4 per cent). One patient died two days after surgery, with bleeding from multiple sites, and the second patient died at 32 days with multiple thromboses, including thrombosis of the portal system. Patients in frank blastic crisis tolerated surgery as well as those with less advanced disease.

Prior to the routine use of EACA, mean blood loss during surgery was 1,166 ml; after that, it was 585 ml. Although this difference is due in part to the improved surgical technic used during the latter period, it is our impression from this and another series of splenectomies in hematologic neoplasms [11] that administration of an inhibitor of fibrinolysis contributed significantly. This conclusion is supported by one experience (Case 32) in which EACA infusion was erroneously omitted from the preoperative routine; it was started during surgery. The patient bled in the recovery room and required additional transfusions. Bleeding ceased within a few hours, however, at about the time when a thera-

TABLE I Patients with "Controllable" Leukemia

Case No.	Age (yr), Sex	Before Splenectomy: Duration of CML	Before Splenectomy: Other Features	Spleen, Below Costal Margin	Hb or Hct: Before Splenectomy	Hb or Hct: After Splenectomy	Platelets (thousand/mm³): Before Splenectomy	Platelets (thousand/mm³): After Splenectomy	Survival After Splenectomy	Remarks
1	44,F	25 mo	Ph'-pos	Tip	45%	45%	20*	500	35+ mo	Alive, in excellent remission; k
2	60,M	42 mo	Ph'-pos	Tip	40%	40%	30	200	13 mo	No chemotherapy, 3 mo; good control 9 mo
3	34,M	13 mo	Ph'-pos	10 cm	41%	45%	85	400	9+ mo	Alive, blastic; k
4	44,M	15 mo	Ph'-pos	Tip	26%*	42%	20*	150	7+ mo	Alive, in good remission; k
5	50,M	20 mo	Splenic pain	17 cm	9.4 g	10.6 g	118	120	6 mo	Died of another cause
6	34,M	31 mo		24 cm	8.4 g	6.4 g* (sepsis)	160	200	2½ mo	No antileukemic therapy; died of postoperative sepsis

NOTE: CML = chronic myelocytic leukemia; Hb = hemoglobin; Hct = hematocrit; k = immunotherapy.
* Transfusions required.

peutic effect of EACA would have been expected. Subsequent studies demonstrated fibrinolytic activity in the patient's blood.

Patients With "Controllable" Leukemia. Six patients were believed to be in a responsive stage of CML at the time of splenectomy, without significant numbers of blast forms or promyelocytes in peripheral blood (Table I). Two had greatly enlarged spleens and anemia; one of them also had mild thrombocytopenia. One had a moderately enlarged spleen and thrombocytopenia. Two had barely palpable spleens, with thrombocytopenia as the only overt hematologic abnormality. The sixth patient (Case 4, spleen tip palpable) had anemia and thrombocytopenia probably due, at least in part, to busulfan toxicity. Thrombocytopenia was corrected in all four patients with this abnormality, one of whom remains in excellent clinical and hematologic remission 35 months later. Anemia was corrected in one of the two patients who could be evaluated for such an effect.

Patients With "Accelerated" Disease. Thirty-one patients (Table II) were not overtly "blastic," but exhibited one or more poor prognostic signs [13,14] prior to splenectomy. All but four were anemic, and 17 had platelet counts below 100,000/mm³.

Significant diminution in anemia and/or thrombocytopenia was recorded in 17 patients. This was of transient duration (two months or less) in four, but sufficiently prolonged to constitute a meaningful contribution to the subsequent management of the other 13 patients. A decrease in the dosage of antileukemic agents required to control leukocytosis was recorded in nine patients; two of these (Cases 7 and 11) received no chemotherapy for six months after splenectomy. In eight patients, unequivocal clinical and hematologic improvement lasted six months or more after splenectomy. One of these patients (Case 7) died of another cause, with leukemia still in excellent control, nine years after splenectomy.

TABLE II Patients with "Accelerated" Disease

Case No.	Age (yr), Sex	Before Splenectomy: Duration of CML	Before Splenectomy: Other Features	Spleen, Below Costal Margin	Hb or Hct: Before Splenectomy	Hb or Hct: After Splenectomy	Platelets (thousand/mm³): Before Splenectomy	Platelets (thousand/mm³): After Splenectomy	Survival After Splenectomy	Remarks
7	55,F	13 mo	Ph'-pos, a	14 cm	7.7 g*	14.0 g	25	300	107 mo	Good control of leukemia; less chemotherapy; died of another cause
8	22,M	15 mo	Ph'pos, b,k	7 cm	45%	52%	30	500	21 mo	Better control, 18 mo; less chemotherapy; k
9	68,M	30 mo	c	12 cm	6.6 g*	14.0 g	27	1,000	20 mo	Good control, 19 mo; less chemotherapy
10	40,F	41½ mo	Ph'-pos, b,d,k	15 cm	33%	33%	150	500	16 mo	Better control, 6 mo; k

(continued)

TABLE II (cont'd) Patients with "Accelerated" Disease

Case No.	Age (yr), Sex	Before Splenectomy		Spleen, Below Costal Margin	Hb or Hct		Platelets (thousand/mm^3)		Survival After Splenectomy	Remarks
		Duration of CML	Other Features		Before Splenectomy	After Splenectomy	Before Splenectomy	After Splenectomy		
11	55,M	24 mo	Ph'-pos, a,b,k	9 cm	26%*	29%	30	100	11½ mo	No antileukemic therapy, 6 mo; good control, 9 mo; k
12	24,F	32½ mo	Ph'-pos	13 cm	7.6 g*	10.0 g	200	800	10½ mo	Better control, 10½ mo; died of interstitial pneumonia
13	47,F	18 mo	Ph'-neg, b,c,d,k	6 cm	23%	25%*	120	>500	10 mo	Better control, 8 mo
14	53,F	29½ mo	Ph'-pos, a,k	6 cm	45%	37%	130	500	9 mo	Better control, 2 mo
15	47,F	30½ mo	Ph'-pos, a,b,c,e	10 cm	5.9 g*	10.0 g	300	500	8 mo	Less chemotherapy, 5 mo
16	82,F	22 mo	Ph'-pos, b,c	23 cm	5.4 g*	10.0 g	70	300	8 mo	Good control, 8 mo; less chemotherapy; died of intestinal obstruction
17	44,F	32 mo	Ph'-pos, b,c	23 cm	7.6 g*	10.0 g	300	500	8 mo	Better control, 3 mo
18	39,F	36 mo	f	10 cm	7.1 g	10.0 g	250	500	7 mo	Better control, 5 mo
19	39,M	38 mo	Ph'-pos, f,g,k	6 cm	41%	36%	1,000	1,000	7 mo	k
20	64,F	27 mo	g,c	8 cm	7.9 g	7.5 g*	46	52	7 mo	. . .
21	62,F	60½ mo	Ph'-pos, c,k	15 cm	24%*	30%	90	300	6½ mo	Better control, 5 mo; less transfusion; k
22	44,M	3½ mo	Eosinophilic Ph'-neg,d	10 cm	6.9 g*	7.0 g*	27	30	5½ mo	Rapid hematologic deterioration
23	28,M	43 mo	Ph'-pos, c,g,k	12 cm	7.5 g	10.0 g	45	200	5 mo	k
24	19,M	24 mo	Ph'-pos, a,k	10 cm	24%*	23%*	35	30	4½ mo	k
25	41,M	47 mo	Ph'-pos, a,b,c,k	19 cm	19%*	27%	400	1,000	4½ mo	No transfusions for 3 mo; k
26	46,M	2 mo	Ph'-pos,f	6 cm	9.0 g	9.0 g	30	50	3½ mo	Hypercalcemia; f; k
27	67,F	83 mo	Ph'-pos, c,f	0	4.9 g*	10.0 g	50	500	3 mo	Good control; died of GI bleeding
28	25,M	32 mo	Ph'-pos, c,d,g,h,k	13 cm	6.1 g*	9.0 g	15*	10*	2½ mo	. . .
29	54,F	72 mo	Ph'-pos,a	18 cm	15%*	40%	60	200	2 mo	Good control; died of neurologic disorder
30	55,M	21½ mo	c,f	18 cm	4.8 g*	6.7 g*	25	38	2 mo	. . .
31	64,M	102 mo	c	20 cm	6.2 g*	8.0 g*	300	700	2 mo	Subphrenic abscess, thrombosis of portal vein
32	42,M	29 mo	Ph'-pos, d,k	13 cm	45%	33%	45	30	2 mo	Rapid progression; e
33	27,M	18 mo	Ph'-pos,b	8 cm	4.9 g*	7.6 g*	7*	12	1½ mo	Rapid progression
34	64,F	30 mo	Ph'-pos, b,c,g	15 cm	25%	25%*	165	400	1 mo	Differential improved; died of interstitial pneumonia
35	40,F	53 mo	Ph'-pos, a,c	10 cm	6.6 g*	5.4 g*	217	650	1 mo	Rapid deterioration
36	53,M	39 mo	Ph'-pos, a,b,c	15 cm	26%	21%*	700	1,000	1 mo	Massive postoperative clotting and GI bleeding
37	62,M	64 mo	g	11 cm	9.7 g*	. . .	200	. . .	0	Postoperative death

NOTE: a = fever; b = myelofibrosis; c = blast forms, 6–24%; d = aneuploidy; e = bone pain; f = extramedullary leukemic tumor; g = basophilia over 20%; h = double Ph'; k = immunotherapy.

* Transfusions required.

Three of these 32 patients (Cases 32, 33 and 35) exhibited rapid clinical and hematologic deterioration after splenectomy and died in blastic crisis one to two months later. One patient (Case 22, eosinophilic leukemia) also had prompt progression to the blastic state but lived five and a half months after splenectomy.

Patients With "Blastic" Disease. Criteria for the diagnosis of "myeloblastic transformation" vary at different centers. We classified 23 patients in this category; 20 had 30 to 50 per cent blast forms plus promyelocytes in blood and/or marrow and three had more advanced disease. Data for these patients are presented in Table III. Diminution in anemia and/or thrombocytopenia was recorded in 12 patients. Remission was not induced in any of the three patients in advanced myeloblastic transformation, and they died three to six months after surgery. Two of them required significantly fewer platelet or erythrocyte transfusions after splenectomy, however.

Among the 19 patients with less advanced myelo-

TABLE III Patients with "Blastic" Disease

Case No.	Age (yr), Sex	Before Splenectomy: Duration of CML (mo)	Before Splenectomy: Other Features	Spleen, Below Costal Margin (cm)	Hb or Hct: Before Splenectomy	Hb or Hct: After Splenectomy	Platelets (thousand/mm³): Before Splenectomy	Platelets (thousand/mm³): After Splenectomy	Survival After Splenectomy (mo)	Remarks
					Blast Forms + Promyelocytes >50%					
38	53,F	12	Ph′-pos	9	6.9 g*	7.0 g*	5*	50	6	Fewer platelet transfusions; k
39	65,F	67	Ph′-pos	3	6.1 g*	9.0 g	25*	400	3½	No further transfusions
40	70,M	15	Ph′-pos	11	9.0 g	8.5 g*	15	50	3	k
					Blast Forms + Promyelocytes, 30–50%					
41	25,M	4	Ph′-pos	24	5.5 g*	14.0 g	70	1,000	47	Myeloblasts predominated in spleen; excellent control, 44 mo; k
42	32,M	30	Ph′-pos	21	9.0 g	14.0 g	95	200	39	Marker chromosome in spleen; excellent control, 36 mo; k
43	64,M	1	Ph′-neg	Tip	43%	43%	3*	100	23	Excellent control, 6 mo; good clinical status, 15 mo; k
44	43,M	14	Ph′-pos, d,e	12	6.7 g*	6.7 g*	100	100	12	. . .
45	16,F	48	Ph′-pos	9	15%*	25%*	16*	200	11	Less transfusion; good control, 8 mo; k
46	43,M	28½	Ph′-pos, k	6	18%*	25%*	100	350	10½	Less transfusion; good control, 7 mo; k
47	30,F	28	Ph′-pos, k	3	16%*	21%*	35	200	8½	Less transfusion; good control, 7 mo; k
48	60,M	19	Ph′-pos, a,b	21	16%*	29%	35	80	8+	No chemotherapy for 6 mo; less transfusion; alive
49	52,F	15	Ph′-pos, b,d	12	11.0 g	10.0 g	10*	150	7	Better control, 6 mo
50	45,F	30½	Ph′-pos, b,d,k	4	19%*	27%	27	50	6½	Less transfusion, 3 mo
51	54,M	51	Ph′-pos, d,g,k	10	6.5 g*	7.0 g*	4*	10*	4	. . .
52	51,M	119	Ph′-pos, d,h,k	3	13.0 g	10.5 g	15*	5*	4	. . .
53	42,M	81	Ph′-pos	4	18%*	22%*	35	80	4	k
54	26,M	40	Ph′-pos,k	14	13.0 g	10.0 g	200	100	4	k
55	63,F	51	Ph′-pos	13	12.0 g	12.0 g	150	150	3	. . .
56	32,M	12	Ph′-pos,b	7	10.0 g	8.9 g	30	40	3	f; k
57	20,M	64	Ph′-pos, d,h	24	5.0 g*	7.0 g*	20	10*	2	. . .
58	43,F	26	Ph′-pos,k	3	28%	30%	300	300	2	k; died of cytomegalovirus infection
59	56,F	77	Ph′-pos	15	5.9 g*	8.0 g*	25	30*	2	Rapid progression
60	68,M	89½	Ph′-pos,k	4	22%*	. . .	10	. . .	0	Postoperative death

NOTE: b = myelofibrosis; d = aneuploidy; e = bone pain; f = extramedullary leukemic tumor; h = double Ph′; j = erythroleukemia; k = immunotherapy.

* Transfusions required.

blastic transformation, reversion to an easily controlled chronic stage of the disease occurred in two (Cases 41 and 42) who were maintained in excellent remission for three years after splenectomy. In one of these (Case 42), karyotypic analysis demonstrated an abnormal clone of leukemic cells in the spleen, not present in the marrow; this was permanently eradicated by splenectomy [15]. Karyotypic studies of spleen cells were not performed in the other patient but it is noteworthy that myeloblasts constituted the predominant cell type in the spleen, but accounted for only 24 per cent of the marrow cells. A third patient (Case 43, Ph'-negative) also appeared to show reversion to a chronic stage, but for a shorter period of time. Ten patients survived more than six months after splenectomy. Of interest is that one patient (Case 48), who was given a very brief course of chemotherapy after splenectomy, required no further treatment for six months.

Leukemic Cell Doubling Times. Calculation of the doubling time of circulating leukemic cells, before and after splenectomy, was possible in 14 patients (Table IV). A significant increase in doubling time was observed in nine of these, no change was recorded in four and the doubling time was shortened in one. Although survival could not be predicted accurately from these determinations, there was a significant correlation between postoperative doubling time and survival ($p < 0.01$), and between increase in doubling time after splenectomy and survival ($p < 0.001$).

Of particular interest are the patients whose preoperative doubling times were less than five days, values associated with a grave near-term prognosis [12]. There were nine such patients. Four who showed no improvement postoperatively died in three to six months, whereas five who exhibited significant prolongation, survived from eight to 47 months ($p < 0.02$).

Marrow and Spleen Aspirations. In the 18 examinations of paired marrow and spleen specimens, major differences were documented in two instances (Cases 41 and 42, already described). Chromosomal examination of splenic material was not performed in the former; thus, the latter (Case 42) is the only one in which a karyotypic discordance between marrow and spleen was identified. In several other patients with karyotypic abnormalities, different proportions of abnormal clones were found in the two sites, but they were clearly present in both spleen and marrow.

The splenic aspirates all showed leukemic infiltration and nucleated red blood cells. Megakaryocytes were seen in several specimens, confirming the presence of myeloid metaplasia (not an uncommon finding in advanced CML).

The effect of splenectomy on marrow cytology could not be evaluated, since most patients received chemotherapy during the interval between pre- and post-splenectomy marrow aspirations.

TABLE IV **Doubling Time of Circulating Immature Cells and Survival**

Case No.	Doubling Time (days): Before Splenectomy	Doubling Time (days): After Splenectomy	Survival After Splenectomy (mo)
No Increase After Splenectomy			
40	1.5	1.5	3
38	1.5	1.5	6
51	1.5	2.0	4
54	4.0	1.5	4
30	6.0	7.0	2
Significant Increase After Splenectomy			
41	1.5	11	47
9	2.5	22	20
8	3.0	6	21
15	3.5	9	8
42	3.5	14	39
20	5.0	9	7
16	5.0	24	8*
7	8	31	107*
5	25	39	6*

* Death not a direct consequence of leukemia.

Survival After Splenectomy. None of the six patients classified as having "controllable" disease (Table I) showed hematologic deterioration during the first six months after splenectomy. Of the four patients followed more than six months, two progressed to the blastic state subsequently, whereas two are alive and doing well (at seven and 35 months).

The other 54 patients had exhibited one or more poor-risk signs prior to splenectomy. Forty-five of them had met the criteria of Karanas and Silver [14] for the "terminal phase" of CML. Figure 1 presents a life-table plot of the survival of these 45 patients after splenectomy, compared with the survival of the 67 patients of Karanas and Silver from onset of the terminal phase. Also shown are the median survivals (from treatment) of two groups of patients meeting the same criteria and treated more recently than the latter series by members of Acute Leukemia Group B (ALGB) [16]. The latter report does not state what proportion of the patients treated were blastic, and this may have been higher than that among our 45 patients (51 per cent). Nonetheless, it is noteworthy that the longest survivor among the ALGB patients died at six months—the median for our patients. The superior survival of our patients cannot be attributed solely to splenectomy; there were other major differences among these three series. In particular, our chemotherapeutic routines were quite different from those used in the ALGB study. However, the temporary improvement in disease control recorded in many of these patients postoperatively (Tables II and III) suggests that splenectomy contributed significantly to the better survival of this group of "terminal" patients.

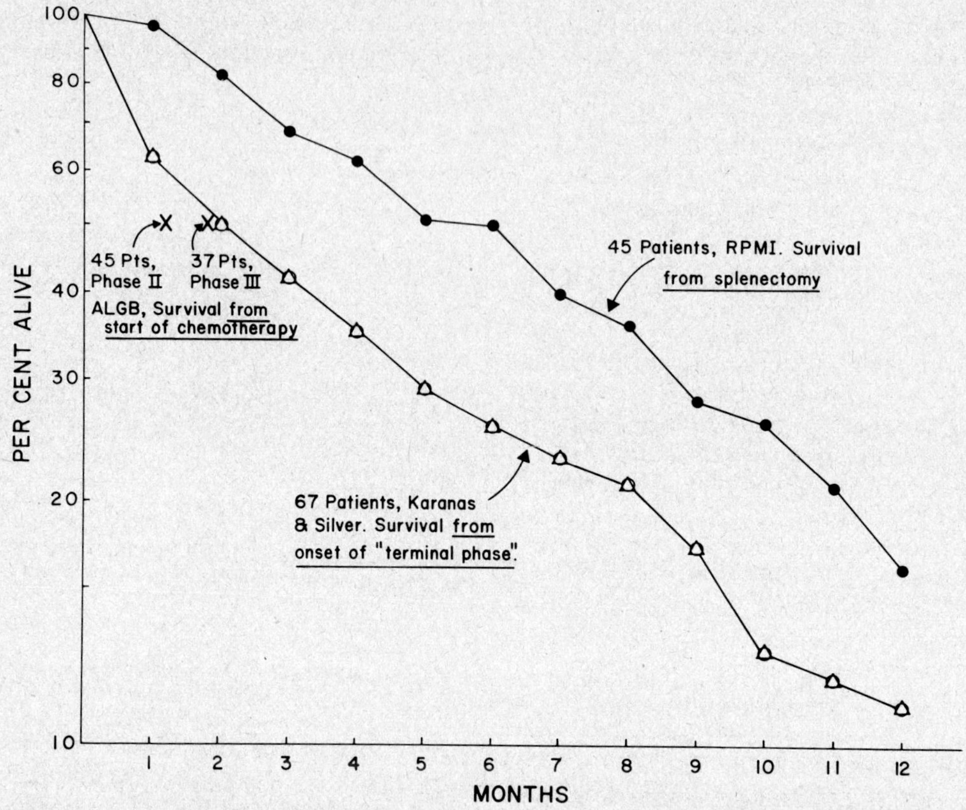

Figure 1. *Survival from splenectomy of 45 patients who had met the criteria of Karanas and Silver [14] for the "terminal phase" of leukemia prior to splenectomy. This is compared with the survival from onset of the terminal phase of patients of Karanas and Silver, and with median survival from start of chemotherapy of patients meeting these criteria and treated by the Acute Leukemia Group B [16].*

The survival pattern of the other nine patients classified as having "accelerated" disease was not significantly different from that shown in Figure 1. This testifies to the validity of poor-risk criteria [13] identified since the study of Karanas and Silver.

Approximately half of our patients received immunotherapy before and/or after splenectomy. To determine whether this had a significant effect on their terminal course, we compared the survival of poor-risk patients who had, or had not, received immunotherapy. For these comparisons, patients who died of postoperative complications and patients whose terminal course was not managed by us were excluded. This provided relatively homogeneous populations of patients, treated in a generally similar way. Survival was compared from (1) onset of the terminal phase and (2) splenectomy. Neither comparison showed a significant difference between the patients who had received immunotherapy and those who had not. Thus, it appears that the immunotherapy schedules used among these patients, which may have delayed progression to the terminal phase of leukemia in some [10], did not affect the course of end-stage disease.

Correlations With Preoperative Findings. Table V summarizes correlations between pre- and post-splenectomy findings in the 55 patients in whom the effects of splenectomy could be evaluated; five patients who died soon after splenectomy of surgical complications or infection are excluded. A significant diminution in anemia was achieved in 44 per cent of patients with this abnormality. Thrombocytopenia was ameliorated in 74 per cent. Control of leukemia was significantly better in 53 per cent.

Anemia was present in 80 per cent of patients whose spleens extended more than 10 cm below the costal margin, and splenectomy was associated with significant improvement in this parameter in 12 patients (60 per cent). Anemia was somewhat less frequent among patients with smaller spleens (63 per cent), and diminished in only 26 per cent after splenectomy. There was no correlation between the severity of anemia and the response to splenectomy. However, the correlation between spleen size and diminution in anemia was significant ($p < 0.05$). This constituted the only statistically significant correlation found among the pre- and postoperative parameters.

Patients with major karyotypic abnormalities (especially, double Ph′ and hyperdiploidy) appeared to benefit

TABLE V Correlation of Pre- and Postsplenectomy Findings in 55 Patients

		Anemia		Thrombocytopenia		Control of Leukemia and Survival			
Parameter	Patients (no.)	Patients (no.)	Diminished	Patients (no.)	Improved (platelets >100,000)	Patients (no.)	Better Control (for 1 yr)	Lived 6 mo. (lived 1 yr)	Median Survival (mo.)
Postoperative course evaluable	55	39	44%	38	74% (53%)	55	53% (15%)	56% (18%)	6½
Duration of CML less than 30 mo	28	18	28%	22	77% (50%)	28	54% (18%)	68% (21%)	7½
Duration of CML 30 mo or more	27	21	57%	16	69% (56%)	27	52% (11%)	44% (14%)	4½
Spleen palpable 0–10 cm	30	19	26%	22	68% (50%)	30	50% (13%)	59% (13%)	7
>10 cm	25	20	60%	16	81% (56%)	25	56% (16%)	52% (24%)	6
Anemia									
Not transfused	8	8	50%	4	75% (50%)	8	63% (13%)	63% (13%)	6½
Transfused	31	31	42%	24	71% (50%)	31	55% (10%)	55% (13%)	6½
Thrombocytopenia									
Not transfused	27	21	43%	27	78% (52%)	27	59% (19%)	54% (22%)	6
Transfused	11	7	43%	11	64% (55%)	11	46% (18%)	54% (18%)	6
Circulating blast forms, >5%	36	29	38%	25	72% (48%)	36	48% (11%)	47% (11%)	5½
Myelofibrosis	13	10	30%	7	71% (43%)	13	69% (8%)	68% (15%)	8
Aneuploidy	11	6	33%	7	43% (14%)	11	36% (0)	45% (18%)	5½

NOTE: Improvement is listed only if sustained for three months (or till death, if earlier); for previously transfused patients, no transfusion must have been given for at least three months postoperatively.

least from splenectomy, but two of the patients with aneuploidy lived more than a year after the procedure.

COMMENTS

Few of the patients in this series would have been classified as good surgical risks, and splenectomy might have been deemed "contraindicated" in many. Such evaluation appeared to be valid, for the patients operated upon prior to 1964; surgical morbidity was substantial and four of 10 patients died of early or delayed operative complications. However, the subsequent improvements in surgical technic and pre- and postoperative management have made splenectomy a feasible procedure for virtually any patient with CML at our Institute. The operative mortality of 4 per cent, since 1964, is quite acceptable in view of the poor status of these patients and their gloomy outlook with conventional therapy.

Significant hematologic and clinical benefit was seen in slightly over half of these patients. Abdominal discomfort was relieved, transfusion requirements were significantly reduced, and functional status improved. The lasting improvement in hemoglobin and platelet counts observed in several patients indicates that "hypersplenism" may occasionally be responsible for manifestations which are usually considered to indicate progression to the terminal stage of leukemia [14]. Management of such patients with splenectomy, rather than aggressive combination chemotherapy, would obviously be desirable. Unfortunately, our data do not indicate how they can be identified preoperatively.

Except for the positive correlation between spleen size and diminution in anemia, we found no criteria which were useful in predicting response to splenectomy (Table V). Unlike our experience in lymphoproliferative disease [11], there was no correlation between the severity of anemia and the response to splenectomy. As in the former study, improvement in the platelet count was frequent—but unpredictable. Thus, selection for splenectomy on the basis of spleen size would result in significant palliation of anemia and thrombocytopenia in the majority of cases, and would relieve the abdominal discomfort and gastrointestinal symptoms which often accompany major splenomegaly. However, such selection would deny splenectomy to some patients who could obtain long-lasting benefit from the procedure (e.g., Cases 1, 2, 8 and 43). Of three patients with double Ph′ chromosomes, only one derived any hematologic benefit (Case 28, diminution in anemia) and none survived more than four months, suggesting that this karyotypic abnormality might constitute a contraindication to splenectomy. However, we hesitate to make a recommendation on the basis of such limited experience.

Of particular interest are the patients in this series in whom the spleen appeared to contain a "more malignant" population of leukemic cells than the marrow. Morphologic [17], cytogenetic [18] and functional [19] differences between marrow and spleen cells have been described in CML. Brandt [20–22] presented evidence that granulocytes from the spleen may have greater proliferative activity than marrow cells. Our experience is consistent with these observations, and suggests that in some cases, removal of the splenic compartment of leukemic cells may result in a substantial change in the near-term course of the disease. We observed a significant increase in the doubling time of circulating immature cells in nine of the 14 patients in whom such comparisons were possible (Table IV); these are obviously not representative of the entire series, however. There was significant reduction in the chemotherapy requirement of a number of patients; and in some there was an unequivocal decrease in circulating immature cells and a marked reduction in the rate of leukemic cell proliferation, attributable to splenectomy alone; four patients required no chemotherapy for two to six months after surgery. In one patient, we obtained cytogenetic evidence that splenectomy eliminated an abnormal clone of leukemic cells.

Although striking and long-lasting beneficial effects were obtained in some patients, we must emphasize that in most patients, splenectomy did not exert a major effect on the course of leukemia. Improvement in platelet counts facilitated additional trials of chemotherapy, and a reduction in transfusion requirements was advantageous, but most patients went on to die with blastic disease during the first postoperative year.

The median survival of these 60 patients after splenectomy was six months. This was longer than might have been expected for such a poor-risk group, but it does not represent a very large gain. The question might therefore be asked, is it worth the effort? The answer to this, obviously, depends on one's viewpoint. An appropriate analogy might be current practice in the management of carcinoma of the lung. At our Institute, all patients with pulmonary lesions not proved to be unresectable are subjected to thoracotomy and, if possible, excision of tumor. This surgical procedure is a more formidable undertaking than splenectomy, and carries an operative mortality of 10 to 15 per cent. Median survival of those patients is less than a year, not greatly different from that in this splenectomy series. The percentage of long-term survivors, of course, is significantly higher among the patients with lung cancer, since some of them are cured. Balancing off the greater immediate morbidity and mortality of one procedure with the poorer long-term results of the other, the two would appear roughly comparable in cost-to-benefit ratio.

We conclude that splenectomy is hazardous in late-stage CML, when performed on a "casual" basis (as at our Institute, prior to 1964). However, the procedure is feasible even in advanced blastic crisis, when sophisticated support facilities are available and patients are managed by an experienced medical-surgical-nursing team. In half of the patients, short-term hematologic and clinical improvement is obtained, hospitalization for supportive treatment is reduced and additional trials of chemotherapy may become feasible on an outpatient basis. In a small but measurable minority, substantial and prolonged benefit is achieved. Therefore, at institutions in which the procedure can be performed safely, it would appear worth undertaking as part of an effort to palliate "late-stage" disease.

REFERENCES

1. Whitby LEH, Britton CJC: The leukemias (leucoses). Disorders of the Blood (Britton CJC, ed), New York, Grune & Stratton, Inc., 1969, p 535.
2. Dowling MD, Hopfan S, Knapper WH, Vaartaja T, Gee T, Hagbin M, Clarkson BD: Attempt to induce true remission in chronic myelogenous leukemia (CML) (abstract 822). Proc Am Soc Clin Oncol 15: 189, 1974.
3. Bryant T: Case of excision of the spleen for an enlargement of the organ, attended with leucocythaemia. Guy's Hosp Reports 12: 444, 1866.
4. Johnston GB: Splenectomy; report of six cases, together with a statistical summary of all the reported operations up to the year 1908. Ann Surg 48: 50, 1908.
5. Strumia MM, Strumia PV, Bassert D: Splenectomy in leukemia. Hematological and clinical effects on 34 patients and review of 299 published cases. Cancer Res 26: 519, 1966.
6. Mittelman A, Elias EG, Wieckowska W, Jones R Jr, Stutzman L, Grace JT Jr: Splenectomy in patients with malignant lymphoma or chronic leukemia. Cancer Bull 22: 10, 1970.
7. Canellos GP, Nordland J, Carbone PP: Splenectomy for thrombocytopenia in chronic granulocytic leukemia. Cancer 29: 660, 1972.
8. Spiers ASK, Baikie AG, Galton DAG, Richards HGH, Wiltshaw E, Goldman JM, Catovsky D, Spencer J, Peto R: Chronic granulocytic leukemia. Effect of elective splenectomy on the course of disease. Br Med J 1: 175, 1975.
9. Rundles WR: Chronic granulocytic leukemia. Hematology (Williams WJ, ed), New York, McGraw-Hill Book Co., 1974, p 689.
10. Sokal JE, Aungst CW, Grace JT Jr: Immunotherapy in well-controlled chronic myelocytic leukemia. NY State J Med 73: 1180, 1973.
11. Adler S, Stutzman L, Mittelman A, Sokal JE: Splenectomy for hematologic depression in lymphocytic lymphoma and leukemia. Cancer 35: 521, 1975.
12. Stryckmans PA, Manaster J, Peltzer T, Socquet M, Vamecq G: Cell proliferation in chronic myeloid leukemia under discontinuous treatment from diagnosis to blastic crisis. Recent Results Cancer Res 30: 156, 1970.
13. Theologides A: Unfavorable signs in patients with chronic myelocytic leukemia. Ann Intern Med 76: 95, 1972.
14. Karanas A, Silver RT: Characteristics of terminal phase of chronic granulocytic leukemia. Blood 32: 445, 1968.
15. Gomez G, Hossfeld DK, Sokal JE: Removal of an abnormal clone of leukemic cells by splenectomy. Br Med J 2: 421, 1975.
16. Hayes DM, Ellison RR, Glidewell O, Holland JF, Silver RT: Chemotherapy for the terminal phase of chronic myelocytic leukemia. Cancer Chemother Rep 58: 233, 1974.
17. Moeschlin S, Klinisch E: Diagnostiche und hematologische engebnisse der milz punktion. Helvet Med Acta 12: 459, 1945.
18. Mittelman F, Brandt L, Nilsson PG: Cytogenetic evidence for splenic origin of blastic transformation in chronic myeloid leukemia. Scand J Haematol 13: 87, 1974.
19. Brandt L: Studies in the phagocytic activity of neutrophilic leukocytes with special reference to chronic myeloproliferative conditions and megaloblastic anemia. Scand J Haematol Suppl 2: 1, 1967.
20. Brandt L: Differences in the proliferative activity of myelocytes from bone marrow, spleen and peripheral blood in chronic myeloid leukemia. Scand J Haematol 6: 105, 1969.
21. Brandt L, Schnell CR: Granulopoiesis in bone marrow and spleen in chronic myeloid leukemia. Scand J Haematol 6: 65, 1969.
22. Brandt L: Difference in uptake of tritiated thymidine by myelocytes from bone marrow and spleen in chronic myeloid leukemia. Scand J Haematol 11: 23, 1973.

Torulopsis glabrata Infections in Patients with Cancer

Increasing Incidence and Relationship to Colonization

JOSEPH AISNER, M.D.
STEPHEN C. SCHIMPFF, M.D.
JOHN C. SUTHERLAND, M.D.
VIOLA M. YOUNG, PhD.
PETER H. WIERNIK, M.D.
Baltimore, Maryland

Torulopsis glabrata, an opportunistic pathogen, was found to be the etiologic agent of infections in patients with cancer. This observation prompted a retrospective review to determine the incidence and underlying factors of infection with this organism. This study showed that T. glabrata had been cultured frequently and that the incidence of infection has been progressively increasing. During a 48-month period (9/70–8/74), T. glabrata was cultured from routine surveillance and diagnostic cultures in 167 patients, 27 of whom had either presumed or documented infection. Review of clinical and necropsy records implicated T. glabrata infections as a contributory factor in the death of 14 of the 27 patients. Etiologic diagnosis of infection was established antemortem in only three patients. Pulmonary isolation in pure growth occurred in 24 of the 27 patients. Seventeen of 19 infected patients who had prior routine surveillance cultures were colonized prior to infection. Infection occurred in the setting of far advanced malignancy or leukopenia and followed the use of systemic, broad spectrum antibiotics. T. glabrata is a frequently overlooked opportunistic pathogen which, in the proper setting, appears to be producing increasing numbers of infections.

Torulopsis glabrata is a yeast-like organism of low virulence which is a commensal in the vagina of some normal women [1]. Attempts to establish infection in animal models have generally been unsuccessful [2]. This organism is an opportunistic pathogen in man, and clinical infections are uncommon. T. glabrata has been reported to cause esophagitis [3], endometritis [1], cystitis [4–6], pyelonephritis [5,6], wound infection [5] and fungemia [1,4–14]. This yeast had also been implicated as the cause of a fatal pneumonia [3], and we have recently reported three cases of pneumonitis caused by this organism, one of which was fatal [15]. T. glabrata has previously been recovered at the Baltimore Cancer Research Center from surveillance cultures, diagnostic cultures and necropsy specimens, but it had not been clinically appreciated. A retrospective analysis was thus undertaken to define the occurrence of T. glabrata infection among patients with various forms of advanced cancer and to determine the relationship of predisposing factors to infection.

From the Section of Medical Oncology, Research Microbiology, and Pathology, National Cancer Institute, Baltimore Cancer Research Center at the University of Maryland Hospital, Baltimore, Maryland. This study was presented in part at the 32nd, annual National Meeting, American Federation for Clinical Research, Atlantic City, N.J. May 4, 1975. Requests for reprints should be addressed to Dr. Joseph Aisner, Section of Medical Oncology, Baltimore Cancer Research Center, 22 South Greene Street, Baltimore, Maryland 21201. Manuscript accepted October 31, 1975.

TABLE I Culture of T. glabrata (TG) by Patient Distribution

Disease Category	No.	No. with TG on Surveillance	No. with Infection
Solid tumors	227	40	12
Brain tumors	115	17	2
Lymphomas	398	48	6
Myeloma	17	4	0
Acute leukemia	158	52	7
Chromic leukemia	42	6	0
Total	957	167	27

MATERIALS AND METHODS

Computerized microbiology records, necropsy data and clinical records were reviewed for a 48-month period (September 1970 to August 1974). All results of surveillance cultures, diagnostic cultures and necropsy cultures of specimens from all sites were indexed for those patients in whom T. glabrata was isolated from any site. Clinical records and necropsy specimens were reviewed to determine which patients had infection with this organism. Histologic sections were examined using hematoxylin and eosin, silver methenamine and periodic acid-Schiff stains.

Specimens from the rectum, gingiva, axilla, nose and urine were regularly obtained for surveillance cultures on admission and twice weekly for patients with leukemia, leukopenia or those hospitalized in the intensive care unit [16]. The sampled population was thus somewhat biased towards the more ill patients. All surveillance cultures were routinely streaked onto multiple plating media and tubes, some of which were neither selective for nor inhibitory to T. glabrata growth. Specimens for diagnostic cultures were obtained as clinically indicated. Specimens for postmortem cultures were obtained at necropsy by seering the lung surface prior to evisceration, then obtaining an aspiration biopsy specimen from each lobe. Other organs were similarly cultured. It is the policy of our laboratory to subculture and speciate all morphologically distinct isolates of bacteria and fungi. No changes in laboratory protocol for culture of the organism were made during the 48-months under consideration, and there were no changes in either the basic patient population or in treatment philosophy, or in the necropsy rate.

Infection with T. glabrata was defined as (1) a pure culture positive for T. glabrata obtained from clinical material such as blood, pleural fluid, transtracheal aspirate, bronchial brushing or tissue scrapings associated with clinical evidence of infection, or (2) a culture positive for T. glabrata in pure growth obtained from postmortem lung aspirates taken from areas of pneumonia with histologic demonstration of the organism or concomitant isolation from other organs.

Presumed infection was defined as a pure culture of T. glabrata obtained by postmortem aspiration from areas of subsequently proved pneumonia, but in which the organism could not be demonstrated histologically.

T. glabrata isolated from surveillance cultures, diagnostic cultures with mixed flora, necropsy cultures with mixed flora or necropsy cultures in the absence of histologic evidence of inflammation was considered as colonization only and not evidence of infection.

RESULTS

During the 48-month period, 9/1/70–8/31/74, 957 patients with cancer were admitted one or more times to the Baltimore Cancer Research Center (Table I). T. glabrata was cultured from one or more sites in 167 patients (17 per cent); 17 (2 per cent) were found to have been infected and 10 (1 per cent) were presumed to be infected on the basis of the definitions given herein. Infection with T. glabrata was thought to be a contributory cause of death in 14 of these 27 patients.

The means of microbiologic diagnosis are shown in Table II. One patient with perineal cellulitis had lesions suggestive of candidal infection, and scrapings showed small budding yeasts. Review of cultures later disclosed pure growth of T. glabrata. Blood cultures were positive for T. glabrata in four patients; one had T. glabrata in pleural fluid and two had pure growth from subsequent postmortem lung aspirates. Although the fungemia was recognized antemortem in these four patients, identification of the organism was not complete until after their death.

Transtracheal aspirate cultures revealed a pure growth of T. glabrata in four other patients, each of whom had clinical evidence of pneumonia. In one patient, previously described [15], the organism was identified antemortem from the transtracheal aspi-

TABLE II Cultural Diagnosis of T. glabrata Infection

Site Cultured	Patients		
Cellulitis	1		
Blood	4		
Alone		1	
Plus pleural fluid		1	Pure growth pulmonary isolation 24
Plus postmortem lung aspirates		2	
Transtracheal aspiration	4		
Alone		1	
Plus blood, urine* and postmortem lung aspirates		1†	
Plus postmortem lung aspirates‡		2	
Bronchial brushing	2†		
Postmortem lung aspiration	16		
Alone‡		10¶	
Plus histologic evidence of organism		4	
Plus other organ bxs		2	
Total	27		

* Pure growth of $>10^5$ organism/ml.
† Organism identified antemortem.
‡ Two patients in each group had mixed funguria-bacteriuria (see text) with $>10^5$ organism/ml of each.
¶ Presumed infections (see text).

rate and subsequently from blood, urine and postmortem lung aspirate. In the other three patients, two of whom also had subsequent positive cultures, the association of T. glabrata and pulmonary infection was not recognized until after death.

In two patients, previously reported to have T. glabrata pneumonia [15], the diagnosis was made by bronchial brushing performed via the cricothyroid membrane [17]. Both patients, believed clinically to have pneumonias, had pure culture isolation of T. glabrata from multiple brushes, and both had resolution of their infection following improvement in their white blood cell count.

In 16 patients T. glabrata was isolated in pure culture from areas of gross and histologically documented pneumonia. In four of these 16 patients, the organism was also identified by special stains; in two of these 16, cultures of other organs were also positive. In 10 patients, pure cultures of T. glabrata were obtained postmortem in lung aspirates from areas of subsequently documented pneumonia, however, the organism could not be demonstrated histologically, and the infection thus was not fully documented. Twenty-four of the 27 patients thus had pure cultures of T. glabrata from the respiratory tract or lungs.

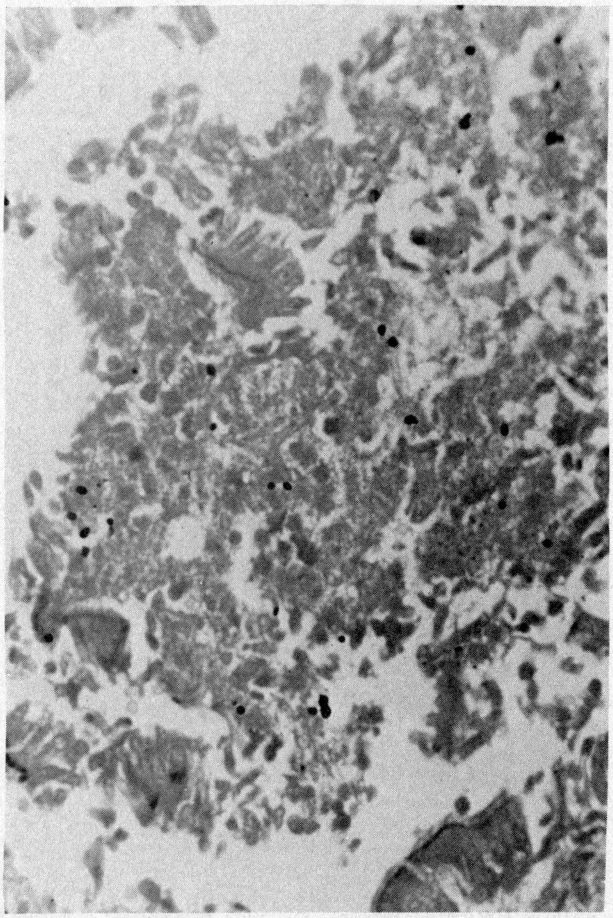

Figure 1. *Small yeast compatible with T. glabrata seen in area of pneumonia. Silver methenamine stain; original magnification X 450, reduced by 50 per cent.*

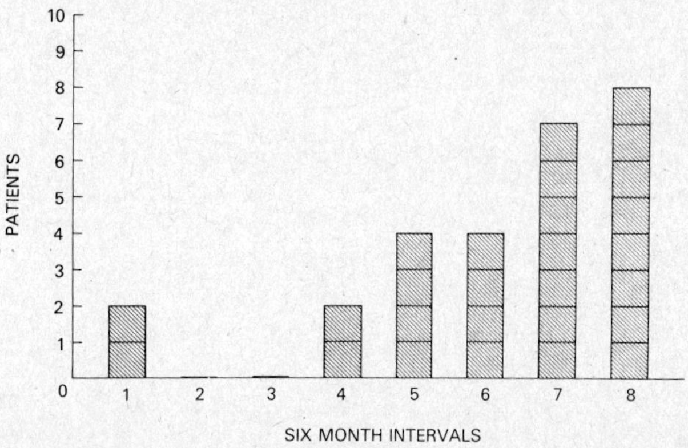

Figure 2. *Occurrence of T. glabrata infection per six month interval.*

The organisms were difficult to identify on histologic sections. Small budding ovoid yeast forms 2 to 3 by 3 to 4 μ were seen on some sections (Figure 1). These yeasts were smaller than Candida spp. forms and no pseudohyphae were found. Thus, these small yeast forms were compatible with Torulopsis sp. as previously described [1].

Infections (both documented and presumed) with T. glabrata appear to be increasing in frequency in our patients (Figure 2). During the 48 months under consideration, 24 (89 per cent) of the infections occurred in the last 24 months, and 17 (63 per cent) in the last 12 months. These infections tended to occur late in a patient's course as a terminal or near terminal event or else after a period of marked leukopenia (i.e., white blood cell count $<1,500/mm^3$). All infected patients had previously been receiving myelosuppressive therapy, and 18 were leukopenic. Twenty-five of the 27 patients had been receiving systemic broad-spectrum antibiotics prior to the development of T. glabrata infection. Only five patients had been receiving corticosteroids and only one was diabetic.

On the basis of the definitions given, nine additional patients in whom T. glabrata was isolated from postmortem lung biopsy specimens were not considered to be infected. The lung biopsy specimens from four of these patients had concomitant growth of other organisms, and five histologic sections failed to reveal evidence of pneumonia. Similarly, wound cultures from two patients grew T. glabrata as well as other organisms and were thus not considered to be infected.

T. glabrata was recovered in concentrations of $>10^5$ organisms/ml urine in five patients, but only one had T. glabrata as a single organism (Table II).

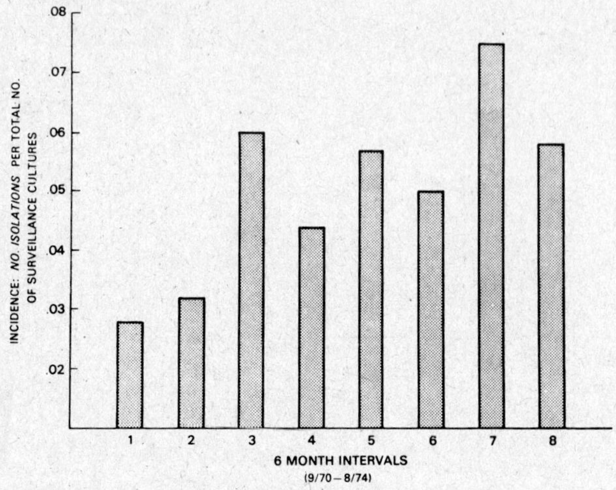

Figure 3. *Incidence of isolation of T. glabrata from all sites per six month intervals.*

The other four patients had concomitant heavy growth of other organisms. All five of these patients had other evidence of infection with T. glabrata, one had a positive blood culture and subsequently a positive lung aspirate, two had positive transtracheal aspirates, and two patients with mixed bacteriuria and funguria later had positive cultures from postmortem lung aspirates (Table II).

Surveillance cultures during these 48 months were positive for T. glabrata from one or more sites in 167 patients, and the frequency of isolation of the organism may have risen slightly (Figure 3). Although the vagina was not routinely cultured, sequential surveillance cultures in both sexes suggested that most patients tended to acquire this organism during their hospital stay. The organism was grown most frequently in samples from the urinary tract and orotracheal area (Table III). Patients who carried this yeast in the sputum, throat and rectum had the highest percentage of subsequent infection. Patients who had a high concentration ($>10^5$/ml) of the organisms in the urine were also found to have a high percentage of subsequent infection. Surveillance cultures were available prior to the day of infection in 19 of the 27 infected patients. Only three of these 19 presented with T. glabrata initially on surveillance cultures, whereas 17 eventually carried the yeast (Table IV). In those patients who subsequently became infected, most carried the organism in multiple sites, and 10 of these patients had positive cultures in three to 10 sites (five patients had ≥five sites). On the other hand, 140 patients who were colonized but not infected tended to carry the organism at few sites. Only 24 of these 140 patients had positive cultures at three to five sites and in none were more than five sites positive. The association of multiple positive sites and infection is statistically significant ($p < 0.0005$).

COMMENTS

Torulopsis glabrata is a frequently overlooked opportunistic pathogen which has been seen frequently on surveillance cultures and has caused increasing numbers of infections among patients with advanced cancer at our center. Infections, both presumed and documented, were rigidly defined resulting in the exclusion of nine patients with positive cultures of postmortem lung aspirates and four patients with funguria. Since co-infection with other organisms is possible and has been described [1,6], and since

TABLE III **Distribution of Colonization with T. glabrata**

Site	Patients with Positive Culture at Site	Patients with Positive Site Who Had Subsequent Infection*
Surveillance		
Axilla	12	2
Rectum	39	8
Urine	60	6
Nose	16	4
Mouth and gums	54	5
Vagina†	13	2
Diagnostic		
Stool	13	2
Throat	30	8
Sputum	54	11
Urine ($>10^5$)	5	4
All others	16	2

* Documented or presumed.
† Not routinely cultured.

TABLE IV **Effect of Colonization with T. glabrata on Infection**

	Sites Colonized			
	≤2	>2	Total	
Colonized* patients infected	7	10	17	
Patients colonized not infected	116	24	140	$\chi^2 = 12.53$ $p < 0.0005$
Infected/ colonized	7/123 (6%)	10/34 (29%)	17/157 (11%)	

* 19 patients in whom prior surveillance cultures were obtained. Two of 19 infected were not found to have previous colonization.

myelosuppressed patients may have a diminished inflammatory response [18], the actual number of infections during this 48-month period may be underestimated.

Infection with T. glabrata tended to occur in the setting of far advanced disease or myelosuppression following the use of broad-spectrum antibiotics. This setting is similar to the predisposing factors seen in other opportunistic fungal infections such as candidiasis, aspergillosis and phycomycosis in patients with cancer [19]. Diabetes and corticosteroid usage, however, could not be associated with infection in this study. Colonization with T. glabrata appears to be an important factor in subsequent infections. As has previously been demonstrated with other organisms, susceptible patients tend to become infected with the organisms which they harbor or acquire [18,20]. Those patients who became infected with this yeast tended to carry the organism in multiple sites. Thus, isolation of T. glabrata from multiple sites should raise the index of suspicion for possible infection.

Indwelling urinary and intravenous catheters are routinely avoided and scalp vein needles are changed frequently at our center. Therefore, with one possible exception, these are not likely a source of infection in this series. T. glabrata was frequently isolated from urines in low concentrations in asymptomatic patients which probably represents colonization. Five patients had isolation of $>10^5$ organisms/ml, all of whom had infections evidenced in other sites. Temporal analysis of cultures indicated that the urinary tract did not seem to be the major portal of entry in this study. Funguria with large numbers of organisms, however, was associated with systemic infection.

In 24 of the 27 patients, pure growth of T. glabrata was recovered from the respiratory tract. Although transient fungemia from other sites with pulmonary or other organ seeding is a distinct possibility, a pulmonary portal of entry is strongly suggested in such patients with advanced cancer. Ten of these 24 were found to have pure growth of T. glabrata in postmortem lung aspirates. Although no organism was documented histologically, material for culture had been taken from areas of pneumonia. Postmortem contamination would most likely yield multiple organisms, and postmortem overgrowth of an organism colonizing the tracheobronchial tree could not explain the histologic findings of pneumonia. Therefore, these findings were considered to be significant, and although not representing a documented infection by the stringent definitions employed, they were classified as presumed infection.

Despite the increasing rate of T. glabrata infection, only three pneumonias were recognized antemortem as having been caused by T. glabrata. Bodey et al. [21] and Sickles et al. [22] noted that the organism responsible for pneumonia was diagnosed during life in 20 to 25 per cent of patients with acute leukemia. More aggressive diagnostic technics, such as transtracheal aspiration [23] and bronchial brushing [17] if applied early in the course of infection, may lead to earlier diagnosis and clinical trials of appropriate therapeutic agents such as amphotericin B [24] or 5-fluorocytosine [5,7,24].

ACKNOWLEDGMENT

We gratefully acknowledge Mr. John Gerster and Mr. Larry Robinson for their assistance with the computer records, and Mr. Norman Friedman for obtaining surveillance cultures.

REFERENCES

1. Grimley PM, Wright LD Jr, Jennings AE: Torulopsis glabrata infection in man. *Am J Clin Pathol* 43: 216, 1965.
2. Wickerman LJ: Apparent increase in frequency of infections involving Torulopsis glabrata. *JAMA* 165: 47, 1957.
3. Bodey GP: Fungal infections complicating acute leukemia. *J Chronic Dis* 19: 667, 1966.
4. Marks MI, Langston C, Eickhoff TC: Torulopsis glabrata. An opportunistic pathogen in man. *N Engl J Med* 283: 1131, 1970.
5. Steer PL, Marks MI, Klite PD, Eickhoff TC: 5-Flourocytosine: an oral anti-fungal compound. *Ann Intern Med* 76: 15, 1972.
6. Kauffman CA, Tan JS: Torluopsis glabrata renal infection. *Am J Med* 57: 217, 1974.
7. Vandevelde AG, Mauceri AA, Johnson JE: 5-Fluorocytosine in the treatment of mycotic infections. *Ann Intern Med* 77: 43, 1972.
8. Rodrigues RJ, Shinya H, Wolf WI, Puttlitz D: Torulopsis glabrata fungemia during prolonged intravenous alimentation therapy. *N Engl J Med* 284: 540, 1971.
9. Lees AW, Rao SS, Garrett JA, Boot PA: Endocarditis due to Torulopsis glabrata. *Lancet* 1: 943, 1971.
10. Hahn H, Condie F, Bulger RF: Diagnosis of Torulopsis glabrata infection. *JAMA* 203: 835, 1968.
11. Louria DB, Blevins A, Armstrong D, Burdick R, Lieberman P: Fungemia caused by "non pathogenic" yeasts. *Arch Intern Med* 119: 247, 1967.
12. Katz D, Pickard RE: Systemic Torulopsis glabrata infection causing shock, fever and coma. *Am J Med* 43: 151, 1967.
13. Edebo L, Johnson LE, Hallen A, Lindbom G: A fatal case of Torulopsis glabrata fungemia. *Acta Chir Scand* 131: 473, 1966.
14. Minkowitz S, Koffler D, Zak FG: Torulopsis glabrata septicemia. *Am J Med* 34: 252, 1963.
15. Aisner J, Sickles EA, Schimpff SC, Young VM, Green WH, Wiernik PH: Torulopsis glabrata pneumonitis in patients with cancer. Report of three cases. *JAMA* 230: 584, 1974.
16. Schimpff SC, Young VM, Greene WH, Vermeulen GD, Moody MR, Wiernik PH: Origin of infection in acute non-

lymphocytic leukemia. *Ann Intern Med* 77: 707, 1972.
17. Aisner J, Kvols L, Sickles EA, Schimpff SC, Wiernik PH: Transtracheal selective bronchial brushing for pneumonitis in patients with cancer. *Chest* 69: 367, 1976.
18. Levine AS, Schimpff SC, Graw RG Jr, Young RC: Hematologic malingancies and other marrow failure states. Progress in the management of complicating infections. *Semin Hematol* 11: 141, 1974.
19. Hart PD, Russell E Jr, Remington JS: The compromised host and infection II. Deep fungal infection. *J Infect Dis* 120: 169, 1969.
20. Schimpff SC, Moody MR, Young VM: Relationship of colonization with Pseudomonas aeruginosa to development of Pseudomonas bacteremia in cancer patients. *Antimicrob Agents Chemother* 9: 240, 1970.
21. Bodey GP, Powell RD, Hersch EM: Pulmonary complications of acute leukemia. *Cancer* 19: 781, 1966.
22. Sickles EA, Young VM, Greene WH, Wiernik PH: Pneumonia in acute leukemia. *Ann Intern Med* 79: 528, 1973.
23. Kalinske RW, Parker RH, Brandt D: Diagnostic usefulness and safety of transtracheal aspiration. *N Engl J Med* 276: 604, 1967.
24. Bennett JE: Chemotherapy of systemic mycosis. *N Engl J Med* 290: 30, 320, 1974.

Felty's Syndrome

Effect of Lithium on Granulopoiesis

RAMESH C. GUPTA, M.D.
WILLIAM A. ROBINSON, M.D., Ph.D.
JOHN E. KURNICK, M.D.
Denver, Colorado

The effect of lithium carbonate upon granulopoiesis was studied in eight patients with Felty's syndrome. Absolute granulocyte counts increased in all patients receiving 900 mg lithium carbonate daily for six weeks. Increased urinary and serum granulocyte colony-stimulating activity was observed in all patients during lithium therapy. A causal relationship between increases in colony-stimulating activity and increased granulocytes is postulated.

Lithium salts are now in common use for the treatment of certain psychiatric disorders [1]. Several reports have documented the occurrence of reversible leukocytosis in patients treated with lithium [2–4]. The leukocytosis is predominantly due to an increase in granulocytes and is observed within a week of initiating therapy. The increase in the white cell count does not persist when the administration of lithium is discontinued [2–4]. Lithium carbonate given to patients with rheumatoid arthritis and granulocytopenia (Felty's syndrome) results in increases in the absolute granulocyte count which, likewise, are not persistent when administration of the drug is discontinued [5].

The mechanism by which lithium increases the granulocyte counts in hematopoietically normal psychiatric patients or in patients with Felty's syndrome is undetermined. Tisman and associates [6] studied serum levels of vitamin B_{12} binding protein in psychiatric patients receiving lithium carbonate as well as the effect of lithium on granulocyte colony growth in vitro. They concluded that the granulocytosis was due to a genuine increase in the total body granulocyte pool and not merely to a demargination of circulating granulocytes. It has recently been shown that granulopoietic activity as measured by the ability of urine to stimulate granulocyte colony formation in vitro is decreased in Felty's syndrome [7].

The present study of serum and urine colony-stimulating activity in patients with Felty's syndrome receiving lithium carbonate shows that an increased granulopoietic activity accompanies the lithium-induced improvement in granulocyte levels.

From the Divisions of Rheumatology and Hematology, Department of Medicine, University of Colorado Medical Center and the Denver Veterans Administration Hospital, Denver, Colorado 80220. This study was supported by grants from the National Institutes of Health, National Cancer Institute (1R01CA11305-6 and CA-05058-10), the American Cancer Society (DT-15E), Veterans Administration Research (5074-1) and General Clinical Research Centers Program of the Division of Research Resources of the National Institutes of Health (RR-51). Requests for reprints should be addressed to Dr. John E. Kurnick, University of Colorado Medical Center, 4200 East Ninth Avenue, Denver, Colorado 80220. Manuscript accepted November 18, 1975.

MATERIALS AND METHODS

The eight patients described here were seen at the University of Colorado Medical Center. The diagnosis of Felty's syndrome in each was based on a history of classic rheumatoid arthritis, clinical splenomegaly and spontaneous sustained neutropenia. After informed consent was obtained, all patients were given lithium carbonate orally in a dose of 300 mg three

TABLE I Hematologic Findings in Patients with Felty's Syndrome Before and During the Administration of 900 mg Daily of Lithium Carbonate

Subject No.	Age (yr) and Sex	Duration of Felty's Syndrome (yr)	Bone Marrow*	Mean Granulocyte Count Before Lithium† (per mm³)	Mean Granulocyte Count During Lithium‡ (per mm³)	% Increase in Granulocytes on Lithium	Range of Serum Lithium Concentration (meq/liter)
1	55, M	1	Maturation arrest	746	1,034	38	0.25–0.40
2	57, M	2	Hyperplasia, maturation arrest	959	1,477	135	0.5–0.85
3	47, F	5	–	2,403	4,491	86	0.43–0.58
4	54, F	1	Hyperplasia, maturation arrest	440	2,718	517	0.35–0.78
5	47, M	6	–	569	940	45	0.53–0.87
6	57, F	2	Hyperplasia, maturation arrest	2,692	4,402	63	0.88–1.00
7	58, F	1/2	Hyperplasia, maturation arrest	1,380	2,403	74	0.51–0.80
8	30, F	4	Normal to hyperplasia	1,652	2,350	49	0.25–0.93

*Description related to granulocyte series.
† Mean of three weekly determinations.
‡ Mean of six weekly determinations.

times daily for six weeks. A weekly hemogram with a differential white cell count and a morning serum lithium level by atomic absorption spectrophotometry were obtained in each patient. A blood sample and 24-hour urine were also collected for the determination of colony-stimulating activity.

The methods for determining serum and urine colony-stimulating activity have been published in detail elsewhere [8,9]. In brief, 0.1 ml of untreated serum or 0.15 ml of dialyzed, sedimented, filter sterilized urine is placed in triplicate 35 mm plastic Falcon petri dishes to which is added a mixture of 0.3 per cent agar in McCoy's 5A medium containing 75,000 nucleated bone marrow cells from the femurs of C57/bl mice. The total volume in each petri dish is 1 ml. After mixing the serum and/or urine with culture medium, the plates are allowed to gel at room temperature and then incubated at 37°C in a fully humidified atmosphere containing 7.5 per cent carbon dioxide. Colony counts are performed after seven days as an index of the level of granulopoietic material present in the specimen. Only colonies containing 50 or more cells are counted. Previous data have shown a linear relationship between the number of such colonies and the amount of granulopoietic activity present, allowing quantitation of the colony-stimulating activity present in the serum or urine sample [9].

RESULTS

The clinical and hematologic details of eight patients with Felty's syndrome are presented in Table I. As shown in this table, the majority of patients had hyperplasia with maturation arrest in the granulocyte series in the bone marrow biopsy studies. Absolute granulocyte counts increased in all patients during lithium carbonate administration, with the percentage increase varying between 38 and 517 per cent. The morning serum lithium concentration varied between 0.25 and 1.0 meq/liter.

Figure 1A shows the mean levels of urine colony-stimulating activity of all patients before and during lithium therapy. The mean urine colony-stimulating activity in the pre-lithium period was 5.2; during lithium therapy it increased to 22.6. This increase is highly significant ($P < 0.01$). The mean value for normal urinary colony-stimulating activity in our laboratory is 13 with a standard deviation of 7.

Figure 1B shows the mean levels of serum colony-stimulating activity of all patients before and during lithium therapy. The mean serum colony-stimulating activity during the pre-lithium period was 6.1 and during lithium therapy 36.5, again showing a highly significant ($P < 0.01$) increase in colony-stimulating activity. The mean value for normal serum colony-stimulating activity in our laboratory is 5 with a standard deviation of 3.

COMMENTS

It has been assumed that the granulocytopenia in Felty's syndrome is the result of a hypersplenic state; on this basis, splenectomy has frequently been performed as a mode of treatment in this group of patients. However, certain features point to a de-

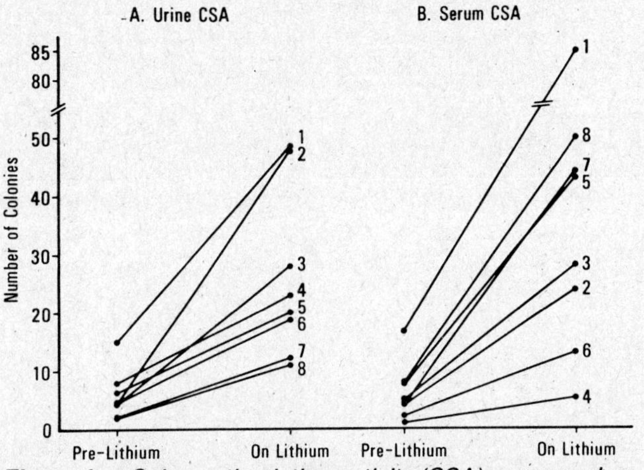

Figure 1. *Colony-stimulating activity (CSA) expressed as granulocyte colonies per 75,000 nucleated C57/bl mouse bone marrow cells in patients with Felty's syndrome before and during administration of 900 mg lithium carbonate daily. Each line represents an individual patient, and each point is the mean value of at least three weekly determinations before the administration of lithium and at least six weekly determinations during lithium therapy.* ***A****, urinary colony-stimulating activity. Normal mean with standard deviation 13 ± 7.* ***B****, serum colony-stimulating activity. Normal mean with standard deviation 5 ± 3.*

creased granulocyte turnover in many patients with Felty's syndrome. Splenectomy fails to remedy the leukopenia in about one third of the cases [10], and in some series there is an additional 30 per cent relapse after initially beneficial results [11,12]. The results of the present study, as well as the observations of Greenberg and Schrier [13] showing decreased granulocytic proliferative capacity in Felty's syndrome, thus combine with the clinical data to suggest strongly that hypersplenism is not the sole factor in the production of neutropenia in the majority of patients with Felty's syndrome.

Increased serum cortisol levels have been reported in psychiatric patients receiving lithium, and this has been offered as an explanation of the leukocytosis in these patients [2–4]. However, Halmi and colleagues [14] showed that although lithium blunts the diurnal variation in serum cortisol secretion, it does not result in consistently increased levels. Moreover, in Felty's syndrome, treatment with corticosteroids has produced only transient and variable effects upon granulocyte counts [11,12]. Therefore, it would be most unlikely that lithium would exert its effect on granulopoietic activity in Felty's syndrome via cortisol. Simple release of mature granulocytes from marrow reserves is also an unlikely mechanism for the action of lithium in Felty's syndrome, since markedly diminished granulocyte reserves have been documented in this condition [15].

Lithium carbonate therapy in our patients increased granulocyte counts along with increases in urine and serum colony-stimulating activity in all cases. Although the per cent increase in colony-stimulating activity levels from those existing before the administration of lithium were not proportionate to the per cent increase in absolute granulocyte count, in a majority of the patients colony-stimulating activity values rose to normal or above during lithium therapy. The mechanism whereby lithium exerts its effect upon colony-stimulating activity has yet to be clarified. Harker and associates [16] have shown that lithium chloride appears to stimulate colony-stimulating activity production by living cells, but that it does not enhance colony formation in the absence of colony-stimulating activity-producing cells. Our results support these conclusions and those reached by Tisman et al. [6], using similar technics in hematopoietically normal psychiatric patients, that lithium induces granulocyte proliferation via enhanced colony-stimulating activity production. This effect serves to correct a defect which we believe plays an important role in the pathogenesis of the neutropenia observed in Felty's syndrome. The clinical potential of the observed findings remains to be determined. The present studies have been of insufficient duration to determine whether long-term administration of lithium salts to patients with Felty's syndrome will decrease the incidence of infections.

REFERENCES

1. Schou M: Lithium in psychiatric therapy and prophylaxis. J Psychiat Res 6: 67, 1968.
2. O'Connell RA: Leukocytosis during lithium carbonate treatment. Int Pharmacopsychiat 4: 30, 1970.
3. Shopsin B, Friedmann R, Gershon S: Lithium and leukocytosis. Clin Pharmacol Ther 12: 923, 1971.
4. Murphy DL, Goodwin FG, Bunney WE Jr: Leukocytosis during lithium treatment. Am J Psychiatry 127: 1559, 1971.
5. Gupta RC, Robinson WA, Smyth CJ: Efficacy of lithium in rheumatoid arthritis with granulocytopenia (Felty's syndrome). Arthritis Rheum 18: 179, 1975.
6. Tisman G, Herbert V, Rosenblatt S: Evidence that lithium induces human granulocyte proliferation: elevated serum vitamin B_{12} binding capacity in vivo and granulocyte colony proliferation in vitro. Br J Hematol 24: 767, 1973.
7. Gupta RC, Robinson WA, Albrecht D: Granulopoietic activity in Felty's syndrome. Ann Rheum Dis 34: 156, 1975.
8. Robinson WA, Pike BL: Leukopoietic activity in human urine. The granulocytic leukemias. N Engl J Med 282: 1291, 1970.
9. Stanley ER, Metcalf D: Partial purification and some properties of the factor in normal and leukaemic human urine stimulating mouse bone marrow colony growth in vitro. Aust J Exp Biol Med Sci 47: 467, 1969.

10. Moore RA, Brunner CM, Sandusky WR, Leavell BD: Felty's syndrome. Ann Intern Med 75: 381, 1971.
11. Ruderman M, Miller LM, Pinals RS: Clinical and serologic observation on 27 patients with Felty's syndrome. Arthritis Rheum 11: 377, 1968.
12. Barnes CG, Turnbull AL, Vernon-Roberts B: Felty's syndrome: a clinical and pathological survey of 21 patients and their response to treatment. Ann Rheum Dis 30: 359, 1971.
13. Greenberg PL, Schrier SL: Granulopoiesis in neutropenic disorders. Blood 41: 753, 1973.
14. Halmi KA, Noyes R Jr, Millard SA: Effect of lithium on plasma cortisol and adrenal response to adrenocorticotropin in man. Clin Pharmacol Ther 13: 699, 1972.
15. Kimball HR, Wolff SM, Talal N, Plotz PH, Decker JL: Marrow granulocyte reserves in the rheumatic diseases. Arthritis Rheum 16: 345, 1973.
16. Harker GW, Rothstein G, Clarkson DW, Athens JW: Stimulation of neutrophil production by lithium (abstract). Clin Res 23: 103A, 1975.

The Gamut of Paracoccidioidomycosis

ANGELA RESTREPO, Ph.D.
MARIO ROBLEDO, M.D.
ROBERTO GIRALDO, M.D.
HUMBERTO HERNÁNDEZ, M.D.
FERNANDO SIERRA, M.D.
FERNANDO GUTIÉRREZ, M.D.
FERNANDO LONDOÑO, M.D.
ROBERTO LÓPEZ, M.D.
GONZALO CALLE, M.D.
Medellín, Colombia

Paracoccidioidomycosis is a systemic mycosis of importance in Latin America. Because of its polymorphic manifestations, it is not always suspected and patients are sometimes misdiagnosed. Case histories of patients with paracoccidioidomycosis are presented in order to illustrate its various manifestations, with emphasis on the primary pulmonary localization.

When originally described, paracoccidioidomycosis was considered to be a disease characterized by a special tropism for the skin and the mucous membranes [1]. Since that time, however, experience has shown that this malady can be quite variable in its clinical manifestations [2–5]. Because of this, a certain number of cases will be misdiagnosed unless the physician is fully alert and has the proper laboratory assistance. Selected cases are used in the present report to illustrate the gamut of paracoccidioidomycosis. In each case the disease is classified according to the form described in another publication [6].

MATERIAL AND METHODS

The pertinent records for 13 patients with paracoccidioidomycosis were selected and reviewed for presentation. Ten of these were chosen from among the 46 patients diagnosed as having this disease between 1970 and 1974, as described before [6]. The remaining three patients were selected from among 115 patients whose records were in the files of the University Hospital and who had been followed at the Mycology Laboratory. The diagnosis was established by direct examination and culture of exudates, sputum samples and other pathologic specimens. The study of biopsy specimens stained by Grocott's silver methenamine method was often used for this purpose. Also, serologic procedures (complement fixation and agar gel immunodiffusion) were systematically used as aids in establishing the diagnosis [7–9]. Other diagnostic procedures included chest roentgenograms and, in some cases, direct and cultural studies for Mycobacterium tuberculosis [10].*

The patients, all males and of Colombian nationality, had sought medical care at either the University Hospital, the Regional Center for Respiratory Diseases or the Chest Hospital during the period indicated.

CASE REPORTS

PARACOCCIDIOIDOMYCOSIS INFECTION

Latent (or Residual) Form

Case A-1. (Paracoccidioidoma): A 42 year old clerk and farm owner sought medical attention in 1961 because of cough and malaise. The chest roentgenogram revealed a nodule in the lower left lung, which was promptly removed by a surgeon, placed in 10 per cent formalin and sent for histologic

* Studies conducted in the Bacteriology Section, School of Medicine, University of Antioquia, Medellín, Colombia.

From the Departments of Microbiology, Pathology and Internal Medicine, School of Medicine and the University Hospital, University of Antioquia; the Regional Health Center for Respiratory Diseases, the Chest Hospital; and the Colombian Institute of Social Security, Medellín, Colombia. Requests for reprints should be addressed to Dr. Angela Restrepo, Department of Microbiology, School of Medicine, Apartado aéreo 883, Medellín, Colombia. Manuscript accepted December 31, 1975.

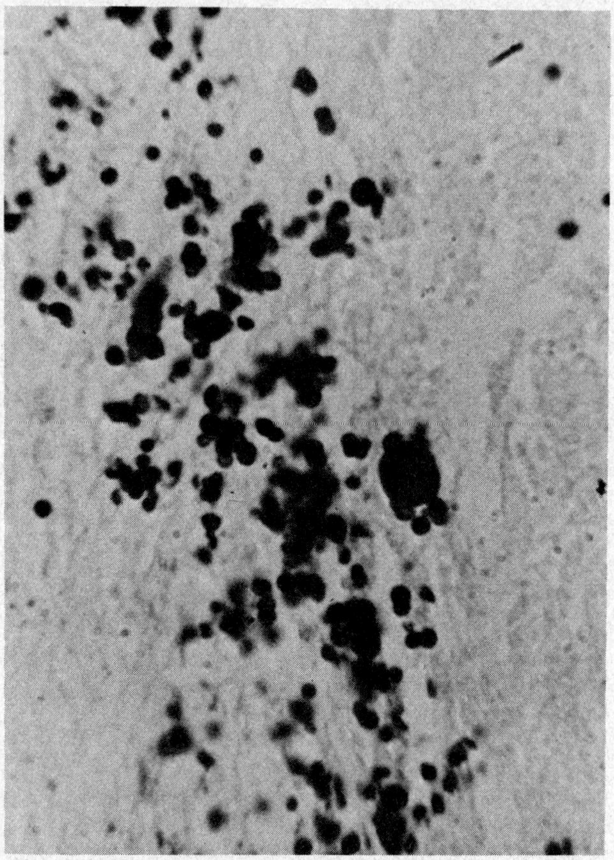

Figure 1. *Case A-1. Nodular lung lesion (paracoccidioidoma). Note the presence of P. brasiliensis multiple budding cells. Grocotts' stain, magnification X 400.*

study. The nodule was surrounded by a fibrotic capsule and presented a necrotic center. The initial diagnosis was residual histoplasmosis. The patient was not treated and has remained asymptomatic since then. In 1970 the surgically removed specimen was restudied, and it became clear that the fungus observed in the lesions was not Histoplasma capsulatum but rather Paracoccidioides brasiliensis. The fungal cells were very abundant but relatively small for this fungus (10 to 15 μ in diameter) and close observation was required before the multiple budding process was demonstrated (Figure 1). The patient was contacted and serologic and intradermal tests gave the following results: complement fixation, negative; immunodiffusion, one weak precipitin band with paracoccidioidin; paracoccidioidin skin test: 46 mm induration.*

PARACOCCIDIOIDOMYCOSIS DISEASE

Acute (or Subacute) Progressive Forms

Case B-1a. (Pulmonary lymphonodular): A 10 year old rural student, the youngest patient in this series, was admitted to the hospital in July 1974. For the previous three months he had experienced generalized malaise, weight loss, vesperal fever and enlarged cervical lymph nodes. The clinical examination revealed involvement of the cervical, preauricular, axillary, inguinal and mesenteric lymph nodes. The spleen and the liver were clinically normal. Initial diagnosis included tuberculosis and lymphoma. Histopathologic studies showed that the process was paracoccidioidomycosis. There was little tissue reaction but numerous P. brasiliensis cells (Figure 2). The fungus was isolated in culture from two bronchial secretion samples, although no lung involvement was observed clinically or roentgenologically. Serologic tests revealed a complement fixation titer of 1:2048 and two precipitin bands with paracoccidioidin. The patient received amphotericin B therapy (1,500 mg) and showed substantial improvement. At the time of this report he is taking sulfa drugs (1.0 g sulfa methoxypyridazine/day) and appears to be in good condition.

Case B-1b. (Pulmonary lymphonodular hepatosplenic): A 17 year old agricultural worker sought medical care at the hospital in August 1972 for enlarged bilateral cervical lymph nodes. This enlargement had first been noticed two months before and it had been accompanied by general malaise, fatigue and vesperal fever. Clinical examination disclosed involvement of other lymph nodes (axillary, inguinal, mesenteric); upon palpation, the spleen and the liver felt enlarged.

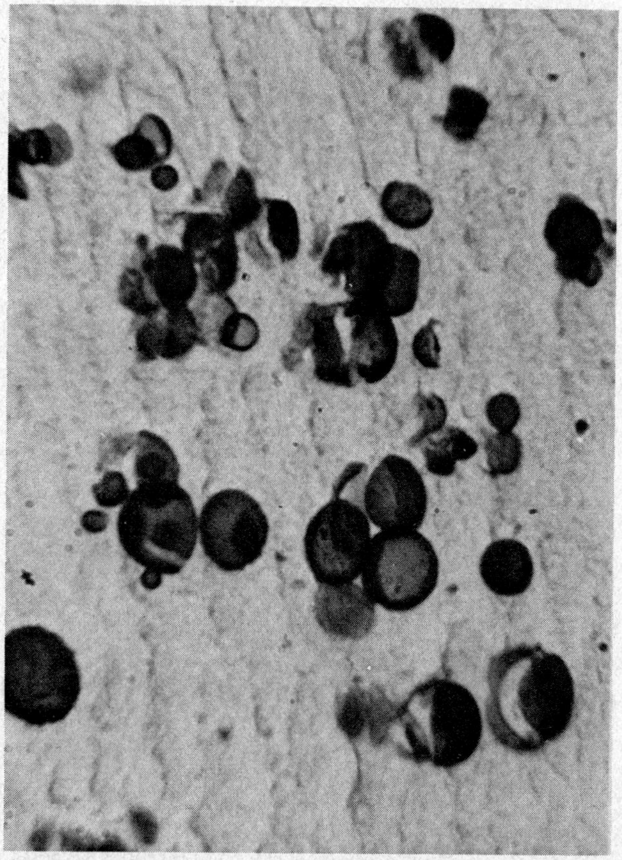

Figure 2. *Case B-1a. P. brasiliensis yeast cells in cervical lymph node. Grocotts' stain, magnification X 650.*

* A paracoccidioidin reaction is considered positive when the induration measures 5 mm or more.

No skin or mucosal lesions were recorded. Differential diagnoses took into account tuberculosis, Hodgkin's disease and mycoses. The chest roentgenogram was reported to be within normal limits. A lymph node biopsy specimen established the diagnosis of paracoccidioidomycosis. There were granulomas containing yeast cells (Figure 3) which, with the fungal stains, revealed multiple budding. The etiologic agent was subsequently observed and isolated from lymph node tissue and from two sputum samples. Serologic tests were positive for paracoccidioidomycosis, although at low titers. As in the previous case, combined amphotericin-sulfa treatment was employed. The patient is back at work and is being maintained on sulfa drugs.

Case B-1c. (Pulmonary fungemic): A 15 year old rural student was brought to the emergency unit in June 1971. For the previous four months he had experienced increasing fatigue, weight loss, fever, sweating, generalized pains and epistaxis. The patient looked emaciated. Multiple enlarged lymph nodes were found in the cervical, axillary and inguinal areas; the spleen and the liver felt enlarged upon palpation, and there were numerous acneiform lesions on the face (Figure 4). The patient was hospitalized with the diagnoses of leukemia, lymphoma or sarcoidosis. A chest roentgenogram revealed disseminated miliary foci suggestive of tuberculosis (Figure 5). Osteolytic lesions were also discovered in the hip area (Figure 6). No mucosal lesions were detected. A lymph node biopsy specimen established the diagnosis of paracoccidioidomycosis. P. brasiliensis was then seen and/or isolated from sputum samples, facial lesions, blood and bone marrow. All serologic tests, on the contrary, were negative. The patient died a few days later from overwhelming disseminated disease. Relatives denied permission to perform an autopsy.

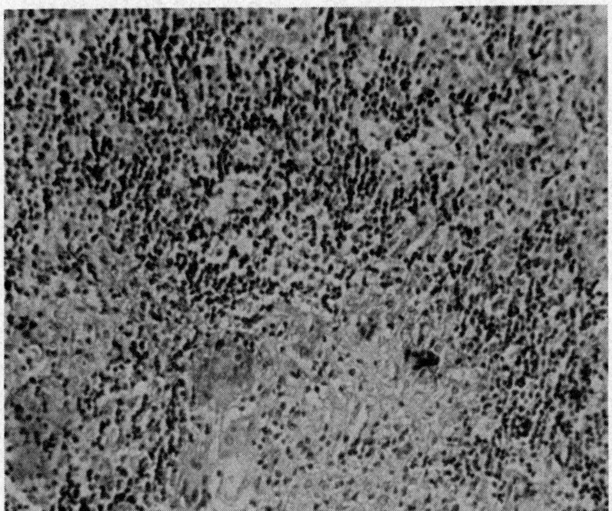

Figure 3. *Case B-1b. Lymph node biopsy specimen. Observe tissue reaction and presence of yeast cells. Hematoxylin and eosin stain, magnification X 100.*

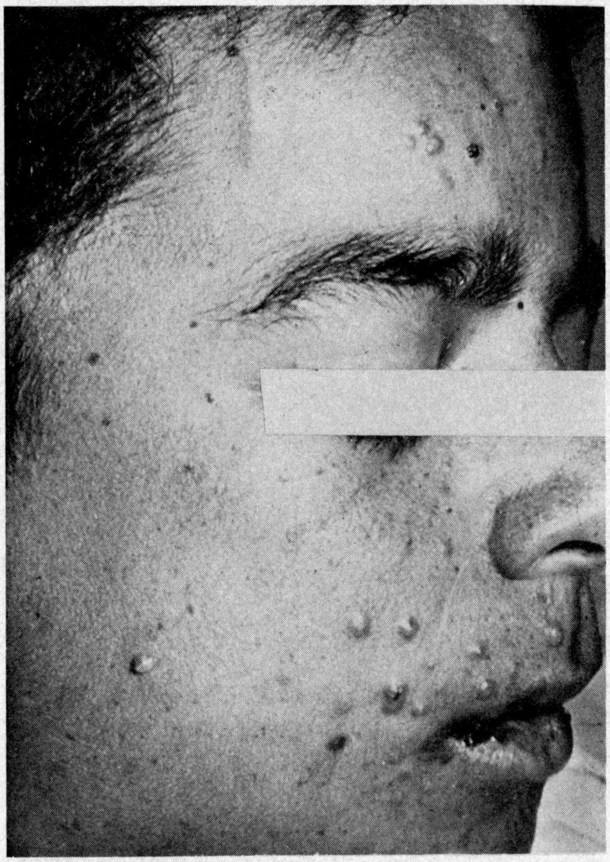

Figure 4. *Case B-1c. Disseminated skin lesions of acneiform appearance.*

Chronic Progressive Forms

Case B-2a. (Pulmonary localized): A rural butcher, 37 years old, was seen in May 1972 after a year's treatment for tuberculosis prescribed on the basis of an abnormal chest roentgenogram. Anamnesis revealed that for the previous 16 months the patient had experienced cough accompanied by mucoid expectoration, dyspnea, vesperal fever and malaise. Review of the original clinical history disclosed that in the six sputum samples examined no acid-fast bacilli had been seen or isolated on culture. In other words, there had never been any substantation of the tuberculosis diagnosis. Clinically, the only abnormal findings were in the lungs, which exhibited signs of diminished ventilation and rales. P. brasiliensis was observed and isolated from sputum samples. The

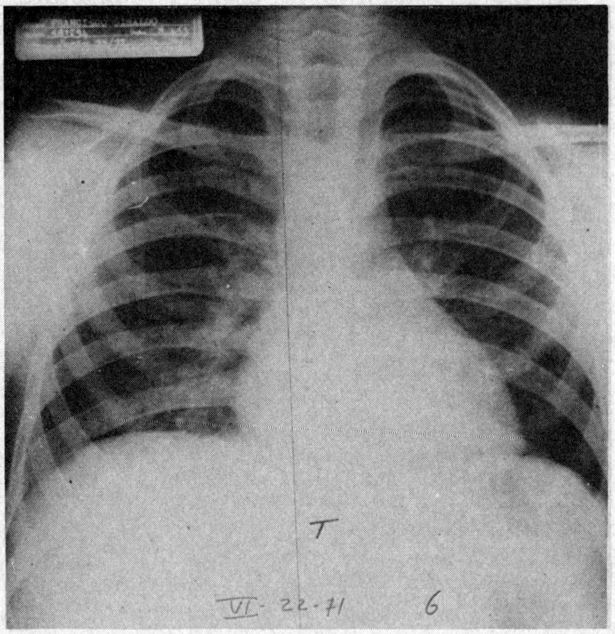

Figure 5. *Case B-1c. Chest film showing disseminated miliary focci.*

original film, taken in 1971, showed bilateral infiltrations with a tendency to coalesce, a few nodular lesions and fibrosis (Figure 7). The film obtained in 1972 showed fewer infiltrative lesions, but fibrotic processes were now more apparent. The patient was treated with sulfamethoxypyridazine alone (2.0 g/day for six months) with success. He is under supervision and maintained on sulfa therapy (1.0 g/day), but in good general condition.

Case B-2b. (Pulmonary localized): A 40 year old urban tailor was seen in March 1972 because of persistent cough, fever, malaise, weight loss, chest pain and moderate dyspnea. The symptoms had been present for over a year, but their severity had increased in the last four months.

Early in 1971 he attended a neighboring health center; a chest roentgenogram was taken and various sputum samples were examined but no diagnosis was made or treatment recommended. Shortly thereafter the patient consulted a different health center. A new chest film was ordered and the findings were considered to be evidence of a tuberculous process. The corresponding treatment was begun, but as no improvement was observed three months later, the patient was referred to us for mycologic studies. The only clinically demonstrable alterations were in the lungs. The chest film showed some infiltration, abundant fibrotic lesions in both fields, early bullae and some pleural involvement (Figure 8). No fungi were seen in direct preparations from sputum samples, but serologic tests gave positive results (two precipitin bands and a complement fixation titer of 1:2048). Three weeks later the culture showed colonies of P. brasiliensis. This patient was also treated with sulfa drugs alone. His condition improved and he is back at work although the residual fibrosis incapacitates him somewhat.

Case B-2c. (Pulmonary with dissemination clinically restricted to mucous membranes): This 44 year old agricultural worker consulted the outpatient clinic of a rural hospital in 1973 for oral ulcerations, which had first appeared a year earlier. In view of the clinical impression of a malignant process, a biopsy specimen was taken and sent for study. The diagnosis was mycosis, there being granulomas and pseudoepitheliomatous hyperplasia; with special stains, yeast cells with the characteristics of P. brasiliensis were observed. The patient was then referred to the University Hospital for treatment. Examination there revealed multiple ulcerations in the oral cavity (sublingual, tonsils, gums), altered breath sounds and dyspnea. There were no skin lesions or enlarged lymph nodes. Adynamia, cough and purulent sputum had been noticed by the patient for eight months prior to the original consultation. The chest film showed bilateral micronodular infiltration, some fibrosis and a cavity in the upper right lung (Figure 9). P. brasiliensis was observed and isolated from the mucosal lesions and serial sputum samples. The serologic tests were also positive (three precipitin bands and a 1:1024 complement-fixation titer). M. tuberculosis was not recovered from culture although several sputum samples were processed. Sulfamethoxypyridazine was selected as the treatment of choice. The patient is still under treatment at the time of this report but his condition has markedly improved, both clinically and roentgenologically.

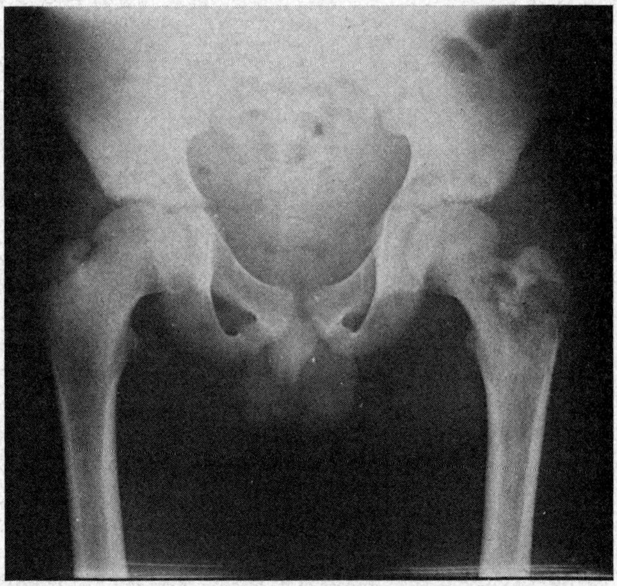

Figure 6. *Case B-1c. Osteolytic lesions in the hip area.*

Case B-2d. (Pulmonary with clinical dissemination to the skin and larynx): A 56 year old male rural laborer, sought medical attention in June 1972 because of ulceration in the scrotum and progressive dysphonia, which had been present for over a year. Anamnesis revealed that in 1967 during an antituberculosus campaign a chest film had been considered "positive." He was then treated for tuberculosis for one year. Five years later, at the time of this consultation, sputum examination for acid-fast bacilli gave negative results. This fact, together with the roentgenologic picture, prompted a search for P. brasiliensis. The roentgenogram showed extensive fibrosis in both fields and basal bullae. The spacing between the ribs in the right side was diminished and some pleural reaction was also noticeable. These indicated a long-term established process (Figure 10). The earliest clue was furnished by the paracoccidioidin serologic tests which showed two precipitin bands and a complement-fixation titer of 1:1024. The fungus was later isolated from two sputum samples and observed in biopsy specimens from scrotal and laryngeal lesions. Treatment consisted of amphotericin B (2,000 mg total dose) followed by sulfa drugs. The patient is back to work although his voice has remained altered and his physical capacity is now restricted.

Case B-2e. (Pulmonary with dissemination clinically restricted to lymph nodes): This 37 year old rural policeman sought medical advice in April 1968 because of persistent cough, dyspnea, fever, weight loss and malaise of eight months' duration. Clinical examination indicated an affection

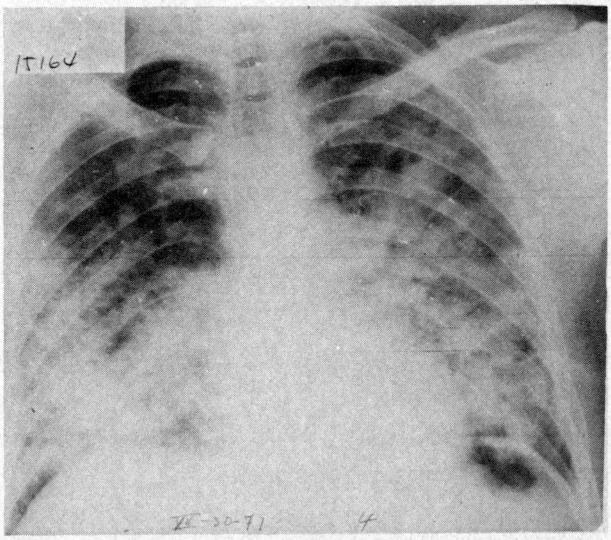

Figure 7. *Case B-2a. Chest film showing coalescent bilateral infiltrations, nodular lesions and fibrosis.*

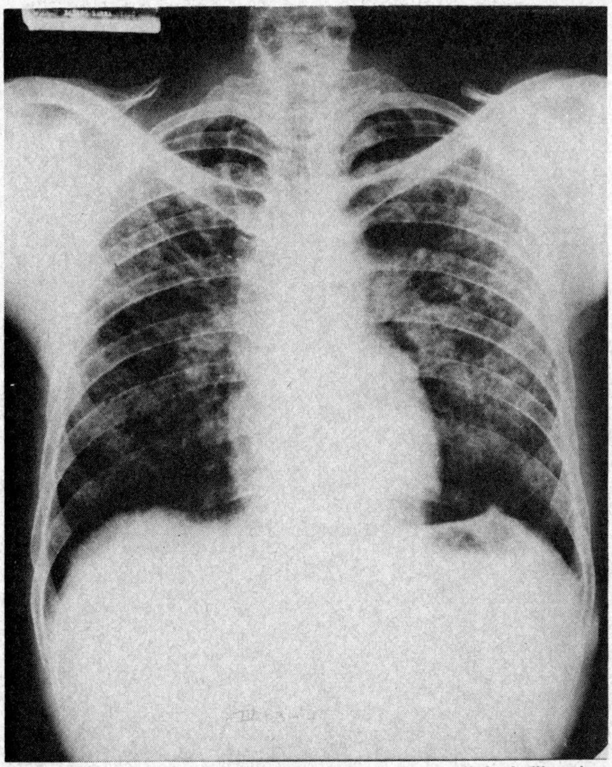

Figure 8. *Case B-2b. The chest film reveals light infiltration, nodular lesions and fibrosis.*

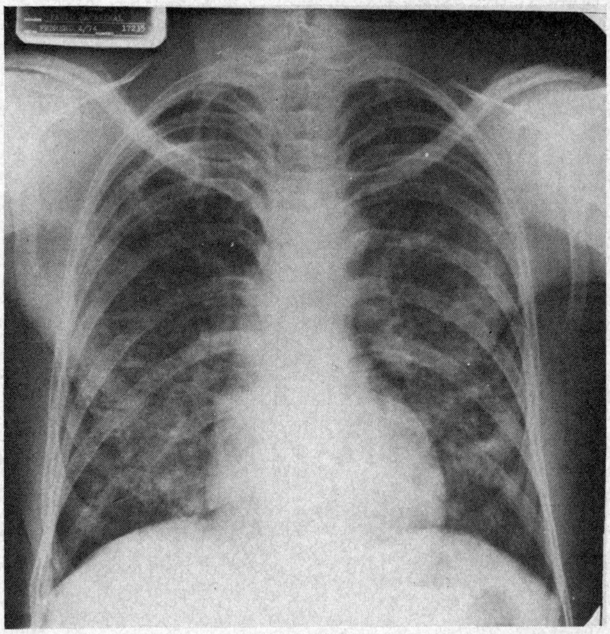

Figure 9. *Case B-2c. Chest film. Note bilateral micronodular infiltrations, fibrosis and a cavity in the upper right lung.*

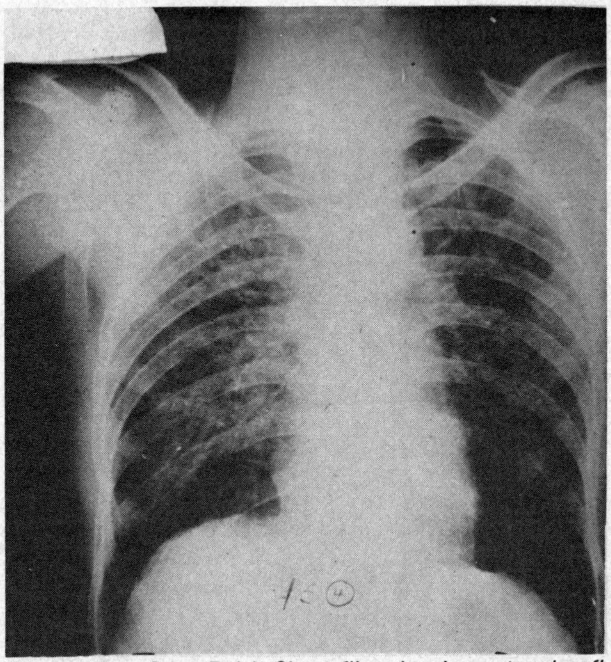

Figure 10. *Case B-2d. Chest film showing extensive fibrosis, basal bullae and pleural reaction.*

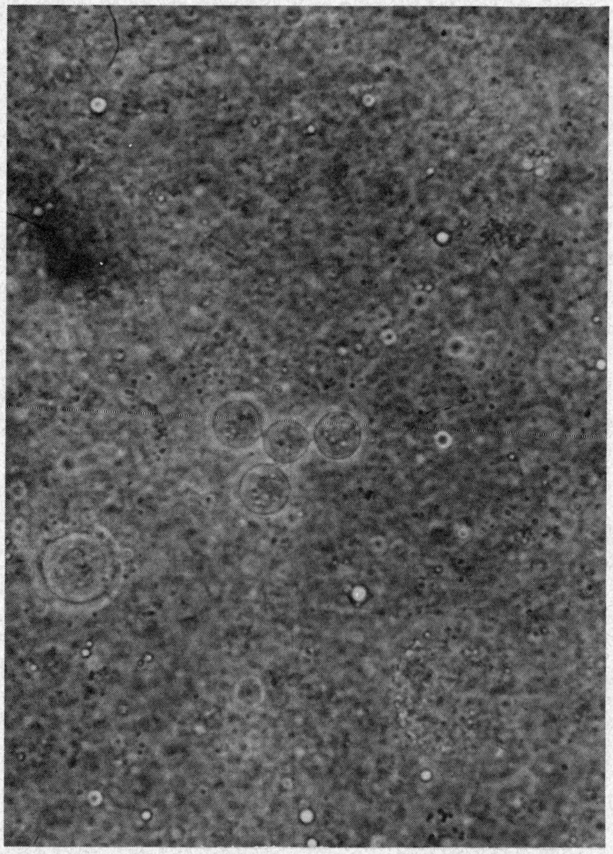

Figure 11. Case B-2e. Direct (KOH) examination of sputum sample. Note the multiple budding P. brasiliensis cell. Magnification X 400.

restricted to the lungs. The chest roentgenogram revealed extensive micronodular infiltration in both fields with the exception of the apical regions. Acid-fast bacilli were not found in serial sputum samples, but P. brasiliensis yeast cells were seen (Figure 11) and later the fungus was recovered from culture. The patient began the prescribed therapy (sulfa drugs alone) and was instructed to continue with this program for two years. However, because of marked improvement, he took the initiative to discontinue treatment one year after diagnosis. In January 1970 the appearance of an enlarged cervical adenopathy prompted a new consultation. Abundant P. brasiliensis cells were seen on examination, and the culture proved to be positive. Re-initiation of the specific therapy was followed by clinical improvement. The patient completed five years of sulfa drug therapy and is being periodically examined. Presently he is in good physical condition.

Case B-2f. (Pulmonary with clinical dissemination to skin, mucous membranes and reticuloendothelial system): A 35 year old agricultural worker sought medical attention in September 1966 because of ulcerations in the oral mucosa (Figure 12) accompanied by increasing dysphagia and dysphonia of seven months' duration. The patient also complained of cough, blood-tinged sputum, fever and general malaise. Medical examination confirmed these symptoms and revealed cutaneous granulomatous lesions in the chest, multiple cervical and inguinal microadenopathies and hepatomegaly. Chest film showed bilateral micronodular infiltration. Histologically, the skin lesions showed pseudoepitheliomatous hyperplasia; P. brasiliensis was observed in biopsy specimens and isolated from sputum, mucosal ulcers, skin lesions and lymph nodes. Serologic tests with paracoccidioidin were nonreactive in the complement fixation test but revealed a band of precipitate in the agar-gel procedure. Amphotericin B treatment was initiated but not completed as the patient left the hospital against medical advice. Six years later (1972) he was brought back in much worse condition. A new amphotericin treatment program was instituted with better results. He is presently receiving sulfa drugs and his condition seems to be improved.

Case B-2g. (Pulmonary with clinical dissemination to the mucous membranes and probably the lymph nodes): A 33 year old truck driver sought medical consultation in March 1973 for painful mouth ulcerations which were noticed eight months previously. Anamnesis revealed that six months previously a cervical nodule had been excised but not examined [1]. Cough and expectoration had been present for the last two years. The patient had lost 10 kg and had asthenia, dysphagia, dysphonia and vesperal fever of approximately four months' duration. Physical examination disclosed a somewhat dyspneic patient with multiple lesions in the oral cavity including the tonsils. Laryngoscopic examination revealed lesions in the vocal cords as well. At the time of consultation there was no clinical evidence of involvement of the reticuloendothelial system. The skin showed no lesions either. Diagnosis was established by biopsy of the oral lesions and isolation of P. brasiliensis. Concomitantly, M. tuberculosis was recovered from sputum cultures. Chest roentgenograms showed confluent micronodular infiltrations in the central and lower fields and some fibrotic lesions; the

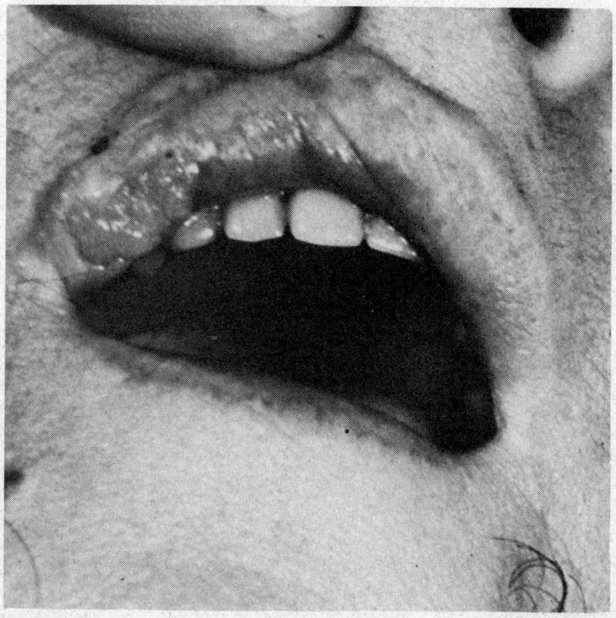

Figure 12. Case B-2f. Mucosal lesions with granulomatous appearance.

right apex revealed a dense shadow and pleural thickness (Figure 13). Dual treatment for both diseases was initiated and completed successfully.

Case B-2h. (Pulmonary with dissemination to the adrenal glands): This patient, a 46 year old agricultural worker who had been hospitalized for the previous two months with adrenal insufficiency, was seen in January 1974. His problems had begun in May 1973, after a severe "cold" when he became very weak, lost weight, noticed increased tegumentary pigmentation and hair loss. Shortly thereafter he experienced serious gastrointestinal disturbances followed by dizziness. A diagnosis of Addison's syndrome was made on the basis of clinical and laboratory evidence; the suspected tuberculous etiology remained unconfirmed despite repeated studies. Treatment for adrenal insufficiency was undertaken with adequate response. The patient had a normal chest film. In a search for other causes of the ailment, serologic tests for fungi were ordered and the results indicated P. brasiliensis as the etiologic agent (two precipitin bands with paracoccidioidin and a complement-fixation titer of 1:128). From bronchial washings, microscopic observation did not reveal presence of the fungus, but P. brasiliensis was recovered twice from cultures made with different bronchial washings. The patient received amphotericin B treatment (2,000 mg) and is presently taking sulfa drugs. When last seen (May 1975) he was in good physical condition.

Case B-2i. (Pulmonary with clinical dissemination to the vascular system): A 54 year old rural carpenter came to the Emergency Unit of the University Hospital in January 1970 with acute abdominal distress. Initial examination led to a diagnosis of a renal calculus, and because signs of an abdominal syndrome requiring surgery were apparent, the patient was taken to surgery. The operation revealed massive mesenteric thrombosis but no ureteral stone. A large portion of the intestine was removed and sent for histopathologic examination. The report indicated severe arteritis due to P. brasiliensis (Figure 14). Fungal spores were abundant in the thrombi and arterial walls. A chest film taken just before surgery showed bilateral micronodular infiltration in the central and lower fields. P. brasiliensis was observed and recovered from sputum samples, although there were no records in the clinical history of previous respiratory complaints. The patient died a few weeks after the diagnosis was established.

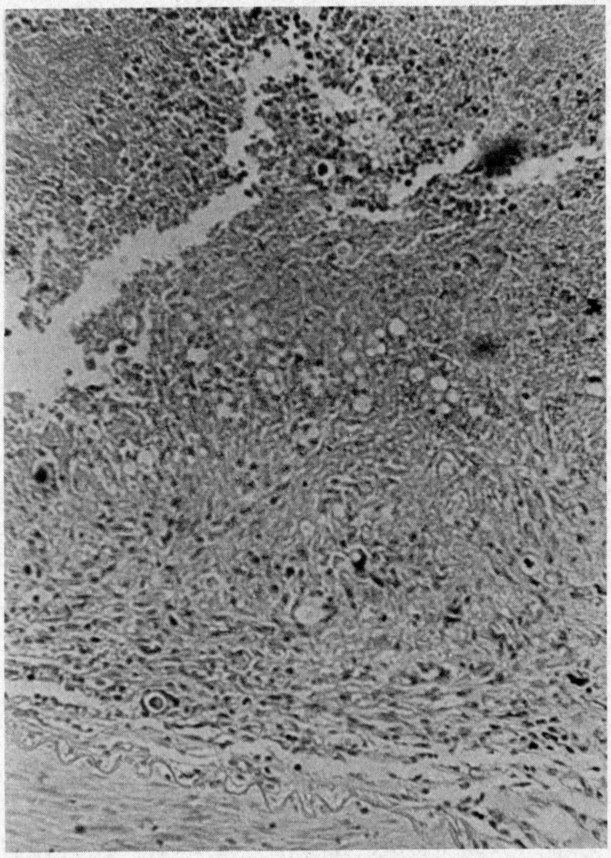

Figure 14. *Case B-2h. Histologic aspect of an involved artery. Note thrombus occluding the lumen and fungal cells. Hematoxylin and eosin stain, magnification X 100.*

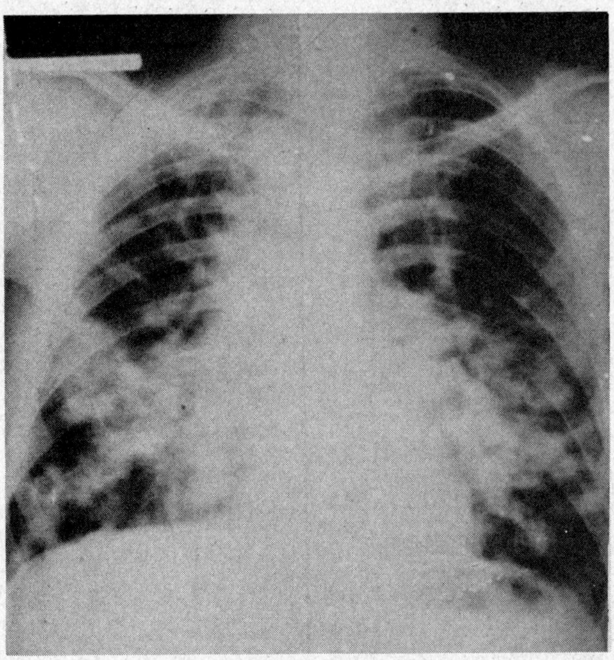

Figure 13. *Case B-2g. Chest film. Confluent micronodular infiltrations, fibrosis and pleural thickness. This patient was found to have both paracoccidioidomycosis and tuberculosis.*

COMMENTS

The examples just given illustrate most of the forms we have proposed for paracoccidioidomycosis [6] and, at the same time, show that this disorder is quite polymorphic. The "juvenile type" of disease, as exemplified by Cases B-1a, B-1b and B-1c, varies in severity depending on the degree of fungal invasion which, in turn, is conditioned by host and environmental factors. The fact that P. brasiliensis was isolated from blood and bone marrow in Case B-1a clearly indicates that the fungus is able to produce an acute, hematogenous dissemination. It is interesting to observe the difference between the skin lesions in this 15 year old patient and those in the older patients, for example, Case B-2a. The multiple lesions in the younger patient had an acneiform appearance, were all at the same stage of development, and had developed relatively soon after the process began. The other more typical lesions in the older patient were slow in developing, had a granulomatous appearance, and were of different sizes and forms. Cases B-1b and B-1c are less severe examples of the acute-subacute progressive form, with varying yet predominant involvement of the reticuloendothelial system. Although clinically and roentgenologically the lungs appeared to be unaffected, in two of the three patients, P. brasiliensis was recovered from their bronchial secretions. Since the patients had no lesions of the oral mucosa, these isolations are clear proof of pulmonary colonization. It is understandable why in such critically ill patients, with manifestations greatly outweighing the importance of those in the lungs, an effort is seldom made to look for the fungus at this site. The finding of the causative agent in the respiratory tract in the absence of demonstrable lesions gives support to the suggestions of Negroni [4], Londero [11] and others [12,13] that the pulmonary lesions might not be readily visible on chest roentgenograms. It is also noteworthy that the younger patients exhibit the most serious acute forms of paracoccidioidomycosis [4,14,15]. It appears imperative to find out what makes these young persons such easy prey. Could it be that they have some serious impairment in the immune responses [16,17] in some way connected with the hormonal balance at the time of puberty?

In the adult patients the clinical pattern was extremely variable, ranging from solitary skin lesions to extensive clinically disseminated disease, with involvement of more than one system. Equally variable, was the number and localization of the tegumentary lesions, as reported by Sampaio [5], and the frequency and multiplicity of lymph node involvement [14]. The type of alterations observed in the chest films, although polymorphic, followed a pattern similar to the one described by others [15,18,19]. However, the lesions may be so minor as to escape detection on the roentgenogram. Case B-2h, in addition to those already mentioned, illustrates this point. The patient did not have respiratory symptoms nor did the chest film reveal any abnormalities. Nevertheless, P. brasiliensis was found to be colonizing the respiratory tissue. The existence of this asymptomatic, or mildly symptomatic, invasion would explain why the initial site of infection was so elusive [20,21].

The similarity in pathogenesis as well as in the clinical and roentgenologic manifestations between this fungal process and tuberculosis, explains why some of our patients (Cases B-2a, B-2d) were treated with tuberculostatics despite negative laboratory findings. In countries like ours, where tuberculosis is still rampant, this is the first logical diagnosis. Nevertheless, physicians must keep paracoccidioidomycosis in mind. Another difficulty is the joint presence of mycobacterial and fungal diseases in the same patient as demonstrated by Case B-2g. As was observed in this series, such association occurs in from 10 to 20 per cent of the cases previously reported [2,4,11].

Serology is frequently decisive in establishing the diagnosis of paracoccidioidomycosis. Our patient with the Addison's syndrome is a case in point. He did not have lesions readily amenable to biopsy or direct examination. Without serologic tests, the suspected mycotic disorder would probably have remained untraceable and no efforts would have been made to demonstrate the fungus in the respiratory tract. It would appear desirable, at least in our areas, to search for P. brasiliensis in patients with adrenal insufficiency in view of the fact that this gland has been shown to be frequently involved [2,11,22]. It may be pertinent to recall that in paracoccidioidomycosis serologic tests have proved to be extremely specific and sensitive tools. Using P. brasiliensis yeast filtrate antigen, one finds a positive immunodiffusion test practically only in patients with paracoccidoidomycosis [8,23]. The complement fixation test is equally sensitive but less specific than the former procedure, as cross reactions occur in cases of histoplasmosis; these are, however, of low order [8,23]. Asymptomatic persons residing in the endemic areas do not normally show circulating antibodies to P. brasiliensis as was revealed by the study of over 3,000 serum specimens collected at random [8]. Consequently, the presence of the characteristic precipitin bands [24], accompanied or not by a reactive complement fixation test, indicates paracoccidioidomycosis. Although high complement fixation titers and/or multiple precipitin bands are not required to make such a diagnosis, the reliability of the tests is increased if they are strongly positive [8,23].

The latent infection demonstrated so well by Angulo-Ortega [25], although not very commonly seen, proves that paracoccidioidomycosis is not always a progressive disease. Case A-1 corroborates this point; it shows that the patient's defenses were powerful enough to restrict the fungal growth. The nodule's histologic aspect indicates that the primary infection had taken place at some time in the past.

It is interesting to compare blastomycosis (North American) with paracoccidioidomycosis as they have features in common. For quite a long time, the former was also considered to be acquired by trauma as mucocutaneous lesions were one of the most frequent manifestations of the disease process. It was not until

1951 that Schwarz and Baum [26] showed that the disease was acquired via the respiratory route. Later on, with the description of cases of primary cutaneous inoculations—proved beyond doubt—by Wilson, Cawley, Weidman and Gilmer [27], it became clear that inoculation by trauma produced a chancriform syndrome, differing greatly from the granulomatous skin lesions exhibited by most patients with blastomycosis. As in paracoccidioidomycosis [2,11], pulmonary involvement is an almost constant necropsy finding in blastomycosis [28,29]; only 60 per cent of the patients with the latter disorder demonstrate roentgenographic abnormalities during life [29], a finding that was also observed in some of the patients described in the present report. Blastomycosis and paracoccidioidomycosis share some other problems, such as the elusive natural habitats of the respective agents, Blastomyces dermatitidis and P. brasiliensis [2,29]. As stated by Chick [30] all this is reminiscent of histoplasmosis 30 years ago, when knowledge concerning pathogenesis, epidemiology and ecology of this disorder was scanty.

On the whole, the results of the present study bear out the paramount importance of the respiratory tract in paracoccidioidomycosis. Although it cannot be denied that some patients can acquire the disease by routes other than inhalation (trauma, for instance), such cases appear to be rare and evidence in support of the extrapulmonary route of infection should be iron-clad. Clearly more precise knowledge about the external habitat of P. brasiliensis is needed in order to conclusively demonstrate that the lungs are indeed the portal of entry. It is hoped, however, that the present report will help to clarify issues concerning the primary site of infection so that previous misconceptions will be no longer perpetuated in the medical literature.

ACKNOWLEDGMENT

Appreciation is expressed to Drs. A. Zapata, L. García and G. González for their kindness in referring patients to our diagnostic unit. The cooperation offered by Dr. F. Díaz in examination for M. tuberculosis is acknowledged. Mr. I. Gómez kindly reviewed some of the clinical histories for us. The excellent technical assistance offered by Luz H. Moncada, Herta Vélez and Lucía Uribe is greatly appreciated. Muriel Vasconcellos kindly revised the manuscript.

REFERENCES

1. Ajello L: Paracoccidioidomycosis: a historial review. Proceedings of the First Pan American Symposium on Paracoccidioidomycosis, Pan American Health Organization Scientific Publication No. 256, 1972, p 3.
2. Angulo-Ortega A, Pollak L: Paracoccidioidomycosis. Chapt 10. The Pathological Anatomy of the Mycoses, Human Infections with Fungi, Actinomycetes and Algae (Baker RD, ed), Berlin, Springer-Verlag, 1971.
3. Lacaz CS: Paracoccidioidomycose, micosis profundas. Chapt 6. Micologia Medica, Sao Paulo, Saravier, 1973.
4. Negroni P: Micosis profundas. vol 3, Las Blastomicosis y Coccidioidomicosis, Comisión Investigación Cientifica, Provincia de Buenos Aires, La Plata, 1966.
5. Sampaio SAP: Clinical manifestations of paracoccidioidomycosis. Proceedings of the First Pan American Symposium on Paracoccidioidomycosis. Pan American Health Organization Scientific Publication No. 254, 1972, p 101.
6. Giraldo R, Restrepo A, Robledo M, Londoño F, Gutiérrez F, Hernández H, Sierra F, Calle G: Pathogenesis of paracoccidioidomycosis: a model proposed on the study of 46 cases. Submitted for publication.
7. Restrepo A, Robledo M, Gutiérrez F, Sanclemente M, Castañeda E, Calle G: Paracoccidioidomycosis (South American blastomycosis). A study of 39 cases observed in Medellín, Colombia. Am J Trop Med Hyg 19: 68, 1970.
8. Restrepo A, Moncada LH: Serologic procedures in the diagnosis of paracoccidioidomycosis. Proceedings, International Symposium on Mycoses. Pan American Health Organization Scientific Publication No. 205, 1970, p 101.
9. Robledo M: Paracoccidioidomycosis: some clinical, pathological and therapeutic considerations. Proceedings of the International Symposium on Mycoses. Pan American Health Organization Scientific Publication No. 205, 1970.
10. Kubica GP, Dye WE: Laboratory methods for clinical and public health mycobacteriology. U.S. Department of Health, Education & Welfare, Public Health Service Publication No. 1547, 1967.
11. Salfelder K, Doehnert C, Doehnert HR: Paracoccidioidomycosis: anatomic studies with complete autopsies. Virchows Arch (Path Anat) 348: 51, 1969.
12. Londero AT, Ramos CD: Paracoccidioidomycosis: a clinical and mycologic study of 41 cases observed in Santa María, RS, Brazil, Am J Med 52: 771, 1972.
13. Fialho A: Patogenia da blastomicose pulmonar. Rev Brasil Tuberc 24: 1531, 1956.
14. Padilha-Goncalvez A: Adenopatia de micose de Lutz, Thesis for professorship in Dermatology, Rio de Janeiro, School of Medicine and Surgery, Copicentro, Rio de Janeiro, 1971.
15. Negroni P, Negroni R: Nuestra experiencia de la Blastomicosis Sudamericana en la Argentina. Mycopathologia 26: 264, 1965.
16. Mendes E, Raphael A: Impaired delayed hypersensitivity in patients with South American blastomycosis. J Allergy 41: 17, 1971.
17. Muchmore HG, Mckwon BA, Mohr JA: Effect of steroid hormones on the growth of P. brasiliensis. Proceedings of the First Pan American Symposium on Paracoccidioidomycosis. Pan American Health Organization Scientific Publication No. 254, 1972, p 300.
18. Machado Filho J, Miranda JL: Consideracoes relativas á Blastomicose Sudamericana. Da participacao pulmonar em 338 casos consecutivos. Hospital (Rio) 58: 431, 1960.
19. Gutiérrez F: Clinical and radiological follow-up in five cases of paracoccidioidomycosis. Proceedings of the First Pan American Symposium on Paracoccidioidomycosis. Pan American Health Organization Scientific Publication No. 254, 1972, p 182.
20. González-Ochoa A: Theories regarding the portal of entry of P. brasiliensis. A brief review. Proceedings of the First Pan American Symposium on Paracoccidioidomycosis. Pan American Health Organization Scientific Publication No.

254, 1972, p. 278.
21. Furtado T: Infection vs. disease in paracoccidioidomycosis. Proceedings of the First Pan American Symposium on Paracoccidioidomycosis. Pan American Health Organization Scientific Publication No. 254, 1972, p 271.
22. Marsiglia F, Pinto J: Adrenal cortical insufficiency associated with paracoccidioidomycosis (South American blastomycosis). J Clin Endocrinol Metab 26: 1109, 1966.
23. Kaufmann L: Evaluation of serological tests of paracoccidioidomycosis: preliminary report. Proceedings of the First Pan American Symposium on Paracoccidioidomycosis. Pan American Health Organization Scientific Publication No. 254, 1972, p 221.
24. Restrepo A, Moncada LH: Characterization of the precipitin bands detected in the immunodiffusion test for paracoccidioidomycosis. Appl Microbiol 28: 138, 1974.
25. Angulo-Ortega A: Calcifications in paracoccidioidomycosis. Are they the morphological manifestions of sub-clinical infection? Proceedings of the First Pan American Symposium on Paracoccidioidomycosis. Pan American Health Organization Scientific Publication No. 254, 1972, p 129.
26. Schwarz J, Baum GL: Blastomycosis. Am J Clin Pathol 21: 999, 1951.
27. Wilson JW, Cawley EP, Weidman FD, Gilmer WJ: Primary cutaneous North American Blastomycosis. Arch Dermatol 71: 39, 1955.
28. Schwarz J, Baum GL: North American blastomycosis. Sem Roentgenol 5: 40, 1970.
29. Amstrong JD: Common fungal diseases of the lungs. Radiol Clin North Am 11: 169, 1973.
30. Chick EW: Blastomycosis. Chest 60: 2, 1971.

Bartter's Syndrome: A Disorder Characterized by High Urinary Prostaglandins and a Dependence of Hyperreninemia on Prostaglandin Synthesis

JOHN R. GILL, Jr. M.D.
Bethesda, Maryland

JURGEN C. FRÖLICH, M.D.
Nashville, Tennesee

ROBERT E. BOWDEN, M.D.
ADDISON A. TAYLOR, M.D.
HARRY R. KEISER, M.D.
Bethesda, Maryland

HANNSJORG W. SEYBERTH, M.D.
JOHN A. OATES, M.D.
Nashville, Tennessee

FREDERIC C. BARTTER, M.D.
Bethesda, Maryland

Urinary prostaglandins E_2 and $F_{2\alpha}$ were measured by gas chromatography-mass spectrometry in three adult women and an adolescent girl with Bartter's syndrome. On a constant metabolic diet prostaglandin E_2 ranged from 293 to 1,221 ng/day (mean, 640 ng/day) and exceeded the normal range for adults of 76 to 281 ng/day in all patients. Prostaglandins $F_{2\alpha}$ ranged from 291 to 1,061 ng/day (mean, 747 ng/day) in the adult women. Only in a young girl did prostaglandins $F_{2\alpha}$ (1,677 ng/day) clearly exceed the normal range for adults of 422 to 871 ng/day. Treatment with indomethacin, which decreased urinary prostaglandin E-like material by 69 per cent or more, did not affect blood pressure. Plasma renin activity, which ranged from 5.2 to 22.2 ng/ml/hour (patients supine) and from 23.3 to 30.4 ng/ml/hour (patients upright), and urinary aldosterone, which ranged from 14.0 to 45.6 ng/day, decreased by 79, 65 and 52 per cent, respectively. The clearance of creatinine was lower for the eight or nine days of treatment, the balances of sodium and potassium were positive, and serum potassium was higher than in control. Ibuprofen, an inhibitor of prostaglandin synthetase which differs in structure from indomethacin, produced metabolic effects which were qualitatively similar to those of indomethacin. The results indicate that the renal synthesis of prostaglandins is increased in Bartter's syndrome and that prostaglandins mediate the hyperreninemia and hyperaldosteronism which characterize the disorder. The overproduction of prostaglandins by the kidney could be a proximal cause of the syndrome, or secondary to intrarenal changes of an unknown nature. This study provides additional evidence for an important role for prostaglandins in the release of renin.

From the Hypertension-Endocrine Branch, National Heart and Lung Institute, Bethesda, Maryland; and the Department of Medicine and Pharmacology, Vanderbilt University, Nashville, Tennessee. Requests for reprints should be addressed to Dr. Frederic C. Bartter, Hypertension-Endocrine Branch, National Heart and Lung Institute, Bethesda, Maryland 20014. Manuscript accepted March 24, 1976.

Bartter's syndrome is characterized by renal juxtaglomerular hyperplasia, hyperreninemia, hyperaldosteronism and normal blood pressure [1]. In addition to these characteristics, patients with the syndrome exhibit two other important features. First, the blood pressure response to angiotensin II or norepinephrine, given intravenously, is subnormal [1,2]. Second, there is an abnormality in the renal tubular reabsorption of sodium, such that a greater than normal fraction of filtered sodium is delivered to sites in the distal nephron where potassium is secreted

[1] and a greater than normal fraction of sodium delivered to the distal nephron is excreted in the urine [3]. The explanation for these two abnormalities and the nature of their relationship to other aspects of the syndrome are unknown.

Results of studies from a number of laboratories indicate that prostaglandins may stimulate the release of renin from the kidneys [4–8] and inhibit the tubular reabsorption of sodium [9–11]. In addition to their effect on the kidney, prostaglandins may also stimulate biogenesis of aldosterone directly [12] and exert vasodepressor effects [4,13]. These properties of the prostaglandins suggested that they could be involved in either a primary or intermediary role in the pathogenesis of Bartter's syndrome. Indeed, the clinical features of Bartter's syndrome have been observed in a patient with hyperplasia of renomedullary interstitial cells and, presumably, with overproduction of prostaglandins [14]. As urinary prostaglandins reflect prostaglandin synthesis by the kidney [15], we have measured prostaglandins in the urine of patients with Bartter's syndrome and have determined, in the same patients, the metabolic effects of inhibiting prostaglandin synthetase with indomethacin and, in one case, with ibuprofen in order to explore further the role of prostaglandins in the syndrome.

MATERIALS AND METHODS

The subjects of the study were two women aged 39 and 46 years (Cases 1 and 3) and a girl aged 14 years (Case 2) who exhibited resistance to angiotensin II (83.5, 20 and 17.6 ng/kg/min of angiotensin II, administered intravenously, were required to increase blood pressure 20 mm Hg in Cases 1, 2 and 3, respectively) and the histologic findings of hyperplasia of the juxtaglomerular apparatus in addition to the clinical features of Bartter's syndrome as presented in subsequent figures and tables. The patients were given constant metabolic diets which contained 9 to 15 meq/day of sodium and 36 to 61 meq/day of potassium. In addition, they were given 100 meq/day of sodium as sodium chloride and 202 meq/day of potassium as potassium chloride. Fluid intake was constant throughout. After four days of control observations indomethacin, 100 to 200 mg/day in divided doses, was administered for eight to nine days followed by postcontrol observations for four to eight days. In a fourth patient, a 40 year old woman with Bartter's syndrome, ibuprofen, 1,600 mg/day, was given for four days. Urine was collected daily in Teflon® containers and stools were collected in four-day aliquots. Aliquots of serum were analyzed for sodium, potassium, chloride, carbon dioxide content and creatinine, and aliquots of urine were analyzed for creatinine by methods previously described [16]. Urinary, fecal and dietary sodium and potassium were determined by internal standard flame photometry. Venous blood for the estimation of plasma renin activity (PRA) by radioimmunoassay [17,18] was taken at 8:00 A.M. when the patients had been supine for at least an hour and at 11:00 A.M. when they had been walking or standing for 3 hours. Urinary aldosterone (aldo) was determined by radioimmunoassay [19].

Analysis of Urinary Prostaglandins. Urinary prostaglandins E_2 (PGE_2) and $F_{2\alpha}$ ($PGF_{2\alpha}$) were determined for one or two days for each of the study periods by gas chromatography-mass spectrometry (GC-MS) as follows: Immediately after completion of the urine collection, 1.76 μg of 3,3,4,4, tetradeutero PGE_2 and 1.53 μg of 3,3,4,4 tetradeutero $PGF_{2\alpha}$ were added to a 75 ml aliquot to serve as internal standards. The sample was stored frozen. Prior to analysis, tritiated PGE_2 and tritiated $PGF_{2\alpha}$ (Amersham-Searle Corp., Arlington Heights, Ill.; specific activity 60 and 15 Ci/mmol, respectively) were added to serve as tracers during extraction and purification. Extraction and separation were carried out essentially as described previously [15,20] by "high-performance" liquid chromatography on a microparticle silicic acid column [20]. Derivatization of the PGE fraction to the PGE-methylester-methyloxime-*bis*-acetate and of the PGF fraction to the PGF-methylester-*tris*-trimethylsilylether, and gas chromatography were performed as described previously [15]. Analysis was accomplished on a Hewlett-Packard dodecapole mass spectrometer (Model 5930A) employed in the selected-ion monitoring mode.

To follow changes in urinary prostaglandins throughout the study, urinary prostaglandin E-like material (iPGE) was also determined by radioimmunoassay on a daily basis as follows [21]:

Approximately 2,000 dpm of prostaglandin (H^3) E_1 (3 to 4 pg) was added to separate 10 ml aliquots of urine and extracted in triplicate at neutral pH with 15 ml of hexane to remove neutral lipids. The hexane layer was discarded, and the urine was adjusted to pH 3.5 and extracted with chloroform; the urine was discarded. The chloroform layer was dried under nitrogen.

Column chromatography was adapted from previously described methods [22,23]. Sephadex LH_{20} (Pharmacia, N.J.) was swelled with a 1:1 mixture of chloroform and methanol, defined and dried overnight at 40°C. The Sephadex was then reconstituted in an excess of a 100:100:2:30 solution of heptane, chloroform, acetic acid and ethanol. The Sephadex was poured into 13 by 1.75 cm columns and the solution drained off. The columns were washed with 15 ml of a 100:100:2:10 solution of heptane, chloroform, acetic acid and ethanol. The samples were reconstituted in 0.2 ml of this latter solution and added to the columns. An additional 0.2 ml was used to wash the tubes, and this was added to the columns. After adsorption of the samples to the columns, 15 ml of the 100:100:2:10 heptane, chloroform, acetic acid and ethanol solution were added and discarded. Then, 12.5 ml of a 100:100:2:20 solution of heptane, chloroform, acetic acid and ethanol were added and also discarded. The PGE peak was collected by the addition of 10 ml of 100:100:2:25 solution of heptane, chloroform, acetic acid and ethanol, and dried under nitrogen.

The prostaglandins of the E series were converted to the B series with a 0.1 N methanolic potassium hydroxide solution, purified in a 0.5 g silicic acid column, then dried under nitrogen and radioimmunoassayed with a prostaglandin B antibody, as previously described [21,24].

Analysis of PGE Metabolite. The chief PGE metabolite, 7 α-hydroxy-5,11-diketotetranorprostane-1, 16-dioic acid

TABLE I Excretion Rates of Prostaglandins E_2 (PGE_2) and $F_{2\alpha}$ ($PGF_{2\alpha}$) and of a Major Metabolite of Prostaglandins of E Series (PGE-M) in Patients with Bartter's Syndrome Before, During and After Treatment with Indomethacin or Ibuprofen

	Control			Drug Therapy			Post-Control		
Case No.	PGE_2 (ng/day)	$PGF_{2\alpha}$ (ng/day)	PGE-M (μg/day)	PGE_2 (ng/day)	$PGF_{2\alpha}$ (ng/day)	PGE-M (μg/day)	PGE_2 (ng/day)	$PGF_{2\alpha}$ (ng/day)	PGE-M (μg/day)
				Indomethacin					
1	601	291	8.84	47	96	1.28	624	264	9.32
	537	...	9.25						
2	293	1,526	3.74	114	1,250	0.77	293	1,800	3.44
	431	1,828	4.25	58	901	0.40	222		3.92
3	1,221	778	32.03	51	390	7.08	1,171	810	32.82
	1,104	835	29.92						
				Ibuprofen					
4	483	769	8.36	153	672	3.3	863	1,068	4.9
	452	1,061	7.68						
Mean ± SD	640 ± 314*	1,012 ± 515	13.01 ± 10.56	85 ± 43	662 ± 399	2.57 ± 2.47	635 ± 354	968 ± 553	10.9 ± 11.2
Normal women 40–60 years old									
Mean ± SD	185 ± 81	560 ± 141	7.3 ± 3.2						
Normal range	76 – 281	422 – 871	3.2 – 14.2						

* $P < 0.05$.

(PGE-M) was also determined in urine by the method of Hamberg [25]. This method is based on the use of the *bis*-(D_3-methyloxime) *bis*-methylester, trimethylsilyl derivative as internal standard, and on the determination of the ratio between unlabeled and deuterium-labeled molecule by selected-ion monitoring with a gas chromatograph-mass spectrometer-computer system (GC-MS). The deuterium-labeled internal standard was prepared by biosynthesis from infusion of 11 α-hydroxy-9,15-diketoprostanoic acid into a rabbit. After purification and isolation from urine, PGE-M was methylated and converted to the *bis*-(D_3-methyloxime). Before this internal standard was added to a sample, electrolytes and protein were removed from the urine by XAD-2 chromatography. The ethanol eluate was evaporated and the residue was treated with diazomethane and then with methoxyamine hydrochloride. After ether extraction, the internal standard was added and the derivatized PGE-M was purified and isolated by reversed-phase partition chromatography and thin-layer chromatography. Finally, the *bis*-methyloxime, *bis*-methylester of PGE-M was converted to the trimethylsilyl derivative and analyzed on an LKB 9000 GC-MS instrument operated in the selected-ion monitoring mode with data acquisition and handling by a PDP-12 computer [26]. Quantitative analysis was performed by obtaining the ratio of the areas under the ion profile of mass to charge ratio (m/e) 365 and 368. The recovery of PGE-M from urine was 93 ± 3 per cent (mean ± SEM) [27].

RESULTS

Urinary Prostaglandins. The values for urinary PGE_2 were high in all four patients with Bartter's syndrome, and the mean value of 640 ± 119 (SD) ng/day for the patients was significantly ($p < 0.05$) greater than the mean value of 185 ± 81 ng/day for normal women 40 to 60 years of age (Table I). As values for PGE_2 in young women aged 20 years do not differ from those in the control group of older women, the values for PGE_2 in one patient (Case 2), aged 14 years, probably are in fact supranormal. The values for urinary PGE-M, however,

TABLE II A Comparison of the Analysis of Urine for Prostaglandins E_2 (PGE_2) by Mass Spectrometry and for Prostaglandin E-like Material (iPGE) by Radioimmunoassay Before, During and After Treatment with Indomethacin or Ibuprofen

Case No.	Mode of Analysis	Control (ng/day)	Treatment (ng/day)	% Decrease	Post-Control (ng/day)
1	PGE_2	569 ± 32	47	92	624
	iPGE	3,336 ± 216	696	79	2,616
2	PGE_2	362 ± 69	86 ± 28	76	258 ± 36
	iPGE	700 ± 0	218 ± 48	69	310 ± 99
3	PGE_2	1,221	51	96	1,171
	iPGE	3,600	1,392	61	4,824
4	PGE_2	452	153	66	863
	iPGE	3,096	1,430	54	2,314

NOTE: All figures are the mean ± SEM.

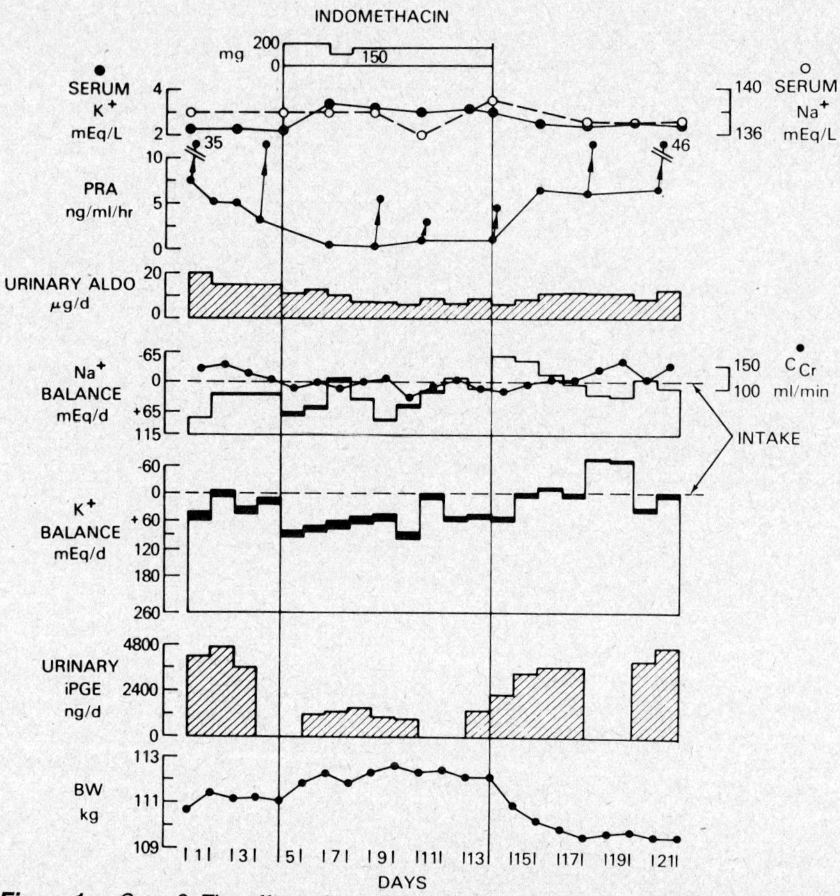

Figure 1. *Case 3. The effect of treatment with indomethacin on serum potassium (K^+) and sodium (Na^+), plasma renin activity (PRA), urinary aldosterone (aldo), creatinine clearance (Ccr), sodium and potassium balances, urinary immunoreactive prostaglandin E-like material (iPGE) and body weight (BW). Note that indomethacin produced an immediate decrease in creatinine clearance and in sodium and potassium excretion, but a gradual decrease in urinary aldosterone. The arrows on the graph of PRA indicate the values obtained after upright posture.*

were high only in Case 3, in which the values for PGE_2 were highest (six times the mean normal value). The values for $PGF_{2\alpha}$ were at the upper limit of, or slightly above, the normal range in only one of the three adult women, but they were three times the mean normal value for women aged 40 to 60 years in the young girl (Case 2). As data on urinary $PGF_{2\alpha}$ are not available for normal girls aged 12 to 18 years, it is not certain that the apparently high values in Case 2 are abnormal. Measurement of urinary PGE-like material by radioimmunoassay (iPGE) was also performed, and a comparison of the values obtained with the values for PGE_2 measured by mass spectrometry in the same urine collection are presented in Table II. The values for iPGE are two (Case 2) to six (Case 4) times the values for PGE_2 obtained by mass spectrometry, and this suggests that the radioimmunoassay procedure employed is a less specific method for quantification of PGE_2. Within a given patient the values for iPGE are reasonably consistent, however, and the percentage decrease in iPGE with indomethacin is only 7 to 13 per cent less than the percentage decrease in PGE_2 (Table II, Figure 1). The results indicate that whereas iPGE may not give a specific measure of total urinary PGE_2, it may be of use in determining the effect of a prostaglandin synthetase inhibitor in relation to time during the course of the study (Figure 1).

Metabolic Effects of Indomethacin. The plan of the study and the results in Case 3 are presented in Figure 1. Treatment with indomethacin, 100 to 200 mg/day for nine days, was associated with a 69 per cent decrease in urinary iPGE by the second day of indomethacin therapy, and this degree of suppression was sustained until administration of the drug was stopped.

PRA, which ranged from 3.2 to 7.5 ng/ml/hour (patient supine) and from 11.5 to 35.1 ng/ml/hour (patient upright) in the control period decreased to 0.33 to 0.80 ng/ml/hour (supine) and to 3.2 to 5.4 ng/ml/hour (up-

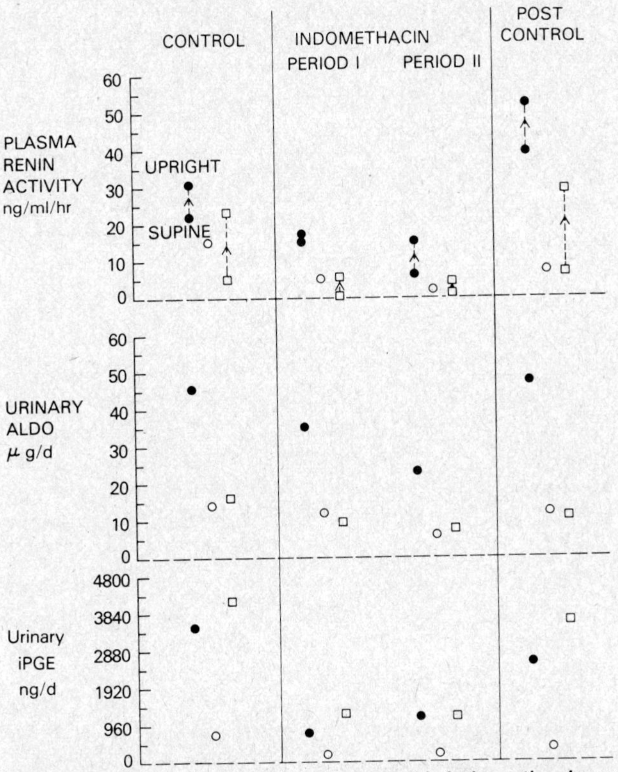

Figure 2. *The effects of treatment with indomethacin on PRA, urinary aldosterone (aldo) and urinary immunoreactive prostaglandin E-like material (iPGE). Values for PRA after 3 hours of standing were not obtained in Case 2. Note that the decrease in PRA, urinary aldosterone and urinary iPGE were sustained throughout the period of treatment. ● = Case 1, ○ = Case 2, □ = Case 3.*

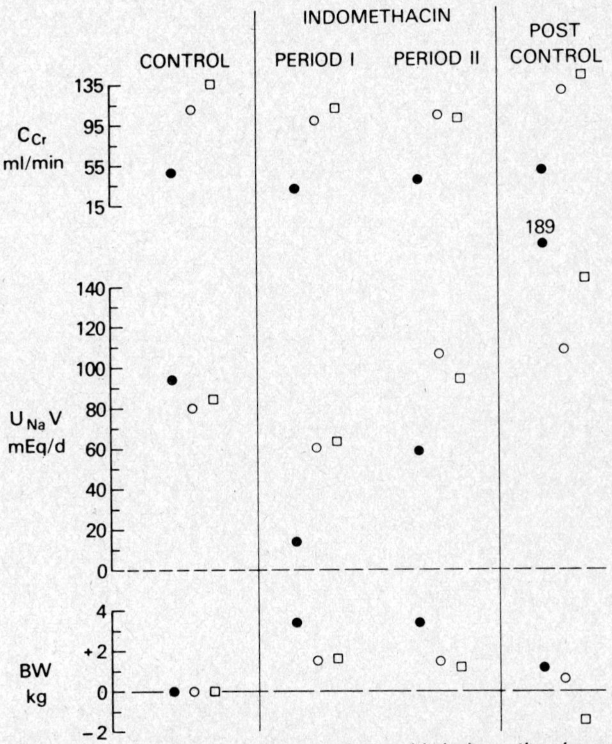

Figure 3. *The effects of treatment with indomethacin on creatinine clearance (Ccr), sodium excretion ($U_{Na}V$) and body weight (BW). ● = Case 1, ○ = Case 2, □ = Case 3.*

right). Urinary aldosterone, which ranged from 14.6 to 20.2 μg/day in the control period, decreased to 6.2 to 11.3 μg/day. The lowest values were observed during the last four days of treatment. Sodium excretion decreased on the first day of indomethacin therapy and, except for the third day when the dosage of indomethacin was decreased to 100 mg, remained less than intake until the eighth day. The positive sodium balance was associated with a gain in body weight of 1.6 kg and a decrease in creatinine clearance (Ccr) by 22 per cent. Potassium balance tended to parallel sodium balance: it became positive with indomethacin and remained so (except for the eighth day) throughout the course of indomethacin therapy. Serum potassium increased promptly with indomethacin therapy to 3.4 meq/liter, then decreased slightly during the remainder of the treatment period.

When indomethacin therapy was stopped, PRA and, to a lesser extent, urinary aldosterone increased toward control values. Sodium and potassium balance became negative, with a loss of body weight and a further decrease in serum potassium. Ccr returned to control values.

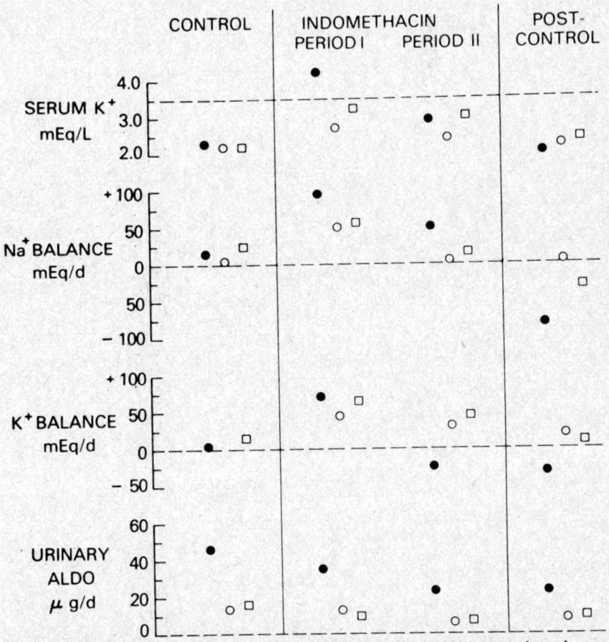

Figure 4. *The effects of treatment with indomethacin on serum potassium (K^+), sodium (Na^+) balance, potassium (K^+) balance and urinary aldosterone. Note that during period II of indomethacin therapy, sodium and potassium balances are less positive and serum potassium is lower than during period I. ● = Case 1, ○ = Case 2, □ = Case 3.*

TABLE III Effect of Indomethacin on Supine Blood Pressure in Patients with Bartter's Syndrome

Case No.	Control (mm Hg)	Indomethacin Period I (mm Hg)	Indomethacin Period II (mm Hg)	Post-Control (mm Hg)
1	91/64 ± 4/1	92/55 ± 6/2.5	85/56 ± 2.5/2.0	92/58 ± 2.8/1.5
2	107/69 ± 2/1.5	110/68 ± 2/2.5	105/69 ± 1.5/3.0	111/70 ± 3.5/2.0
3	144/81 ± 3/1.5	140/82 ± 4/2.5	141/80 ± 4.5/1	136/77 ± 3/1

NOTE: All values are mean ± SEM.

The effects of treatment with indomethacin for all three patients are presented in Figures 2, 3 and 4 as the means for period 1 (days 1 through 4 or 5 of indomethacin) and period 2 (days 5 or 6 through 8 or 9 of indomethacin). Mean control values for PRA ranged from 5.2 to 22.2 ng/ml/hour (supine) and from 23.3 to 30.4 ng/ml/hour (upright) in Cases 3 and 1, respectively (Figure 2). PRA was not determined in Case 2 while the patient was upright. Urinary aldosterone ranged from 14 (Case 2) to 45.6 (Case 1) μg/day. Treatment with indomethacin, 100 to 200 mg/day, decreased urinary iPGE by 69 per cent in Case 1, by 73 per cent in Case 2 and by 74 per cent in Case 3 during period 1, and this degree of inhibition was maintained during period 2. PRA (supine and upright) tended to decrease throughout treatment, and the lowest values were observed during period 2 (6 ng/ml/hour supine, 15 ng/ml/hour, upright in Case 1; 2 ng/ml/hour supine in Case 2; 0.8 ng/ml/hour supine, 3.8 ng/ml/hour upright in Case 3). Urinary aldosterone also decreased throughout treatment and the lowest values were observed during period 2 (23 μg/day in Case 1; 6 μg/day in Case 2; 7.5 μg/day in Case 3). Indomethacin therapy produced an immediate decrease in Ccr (by 33 per cent in Case 1, 10 per cent in Case 2 and 22 per cent in Case 3) and in sodium excretion (Figure 3). Whereas the changes in creatinine clearance persisted throughout treatment, sodium excretion approached or exceeded that of control values during period 2. Body weight reflected the changes in sodium and potassium excretion, with gains of 3.4 kg in Case 1, 1.5 kg in Case 2 and 1.6 kg in Case 3 during period 1, but with no further change during period 2. Potassium balance, like sodium balance, was positive during period 1, but was less positive during period 2 (Figure 4). Serum potassium was highest at the end of period 1 and lower at the end of period 2. When the administration of indomethacin was stopped, values for the several variables tended to return towards those of the control period (Figures 2, 3 and 4).

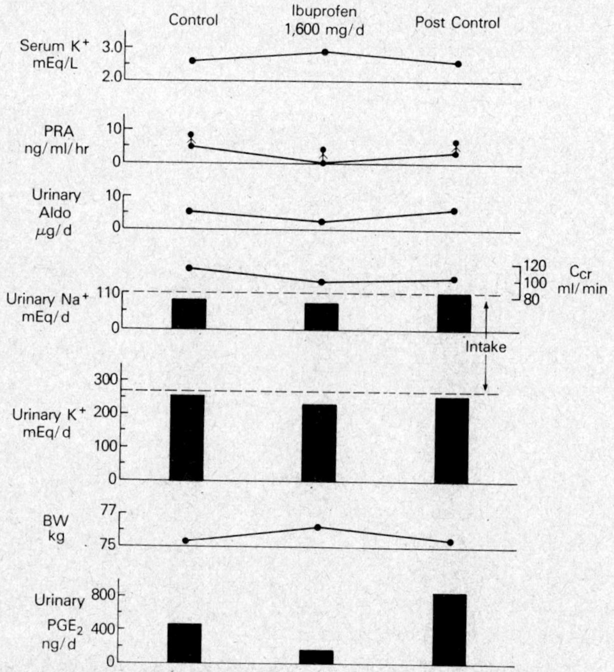

Figure 5. Case 4. The effects of treatment with ibuprofen on serum potassium (K^+), plasma renin activity (PRA), urinary aldosterone (aldo), urinary sodium (Na^+), creatinine clearance (Ccr), urinary potassium (K^+), body weight (BW) and urinary prostaglandin E_2 (PGE_2). Note that the changes are qualitatively similar to those produced by indomethacin.

Effects of Indomethacin on Blood Pressure. Mean control blood pressure was 91/64 ± 4/1 (SEM) mm Hg in Case 1, 107/69 ± 2/1.5 mm Hg in Case 2 and 144/81 ± 3/1.5 mm Hg in Case 3. Blood pressure decreased slightly with treatment only in Case 1, in which it fell to 92/55 ± 6/2.5 mm Hg in period 1 and to 88/56 ± 2.5/2.0 mm Hg in period 2 (Table III).

Metabolic Effects of Ibuprofen. Treatment with ibuprofen, 1,600 mg/day, for four days, was associated with a 67 per cent decrease in urinary PGE_2 (Figure 5). Control PRA, which was 4.0 ng/ml/hour (patient supine) and 7.7 ng/ml/hour (patient upright) decreased to 0.27 and 4.3 ng/ml/hour, respectively; control urinary aldosterone, 5.3 μg/day, decreased to 2.8 μg/day. A decrease in urinary sodium excretion with ibuprofen was associated with a gain in body weight of 0.8 kg and a decrease in Ccr by 14 per cent. Urinary potassium excretion also decreased with ibuprofen therapy and was associated with a rise in serum potassium to 2.9 meq/liter. When the administration of ibuprofen was stopped, the variables reverted to control values.

COMMENTS

Treatment of three patients with Bartter's syndrome with indomethacin at a dosage sufficient to decrease urinary iPGE by 69 per cent or more, for eight or nine days, partially or completely corrected their hyperreninemia and hyperaldosteronism (Figures 1 and 2). Urinary sodium decreased abruptly on the first day of treatment and remained less than intake for four to seven days (Figures 1 and 3). Ccr also decreased on the first day of treatment and did not return to normal values until the administration of indomethacin was stopped; thus a decrease in the filtered load of sodium was one factor in the decreased excretion of sodium (Figures 1 and 3). As blood pressure showed essentially no change with indomethacin therapy (Table III), renal vasoconstriction, which has been suggested as an explanation for the indomethacin-induced decrease in renal blood flow in the anesthetized dog [28], probably explains the decrease in Ccr. Renal vasoconstriction, if it increased filtration fraction, and, in turn, the concentration of plasma proteins in the peritubular capillaries, may have led to an increase in the tubular reabsorption of sodium by a mechanism which remains to be clarified and thereby accounts for the decrease in sodium excretion [29–31].

As regards a direct effect of prostaglandins on the tubular transport of sodium in man, very little is known. PGE, or arachidonic acid, the precursor of prostaglandins, infused into a renal artery of the dog produces renal sodium loss [9–11], and this is associated with a decrease in proximal tubular reabsorption of sodium. As noted, this effect could stem from changes in Starling forces in peritubular vessels [29–31]. If, however, it results from a direct action of PGE on the proximal tubules (and if such an action plays a role in man), the retention of sodium with indomethacin could represent the abolition of such an action. In the dog, prostaglandins of renal origin appear to stimulate sodium reabsorption in the distal nephron [32,33]. If this relationship holds for man, then any indomethacin-induced decrease in the distal tubular reabsorption of sodium may have failed to increase sodium excretion because an increase in proximal tubular sodium reabsorption was the predominant effect on over-all tubular sodium reabsorption.

Potassium balance, which tended to parallel sodium balance, showed retention during period I of indomethacin treatment (Figure 4). During period II of indomethacin treatment, when aldosterone excretion was at its lowest, potassium balance was less positive and in Case 1, actually negative, and serum potassium at the end of period II was lower than at the end of period I (Figure 4). Thus, indomethacin appears to mediate changes in potassium balance largely as a consequence of changes in tubular reabsorption of sodium. A similar interrelationship between sodium and potassium balance in Bartter's syndrome was previously observed in response to the intravenous infusion of human serum albumin, which presumably led to an increase in the tubular reabsorption of sodium as a consequence of an increase in concentration of albumin in peritubular capillaries, as urinary aldosterone did not change [1,29]. In the previous studies with albumin and in the present studies with indomethacin, the decrease in urinary potassium and increase in serum potassium could be explained if the increase in the tubular reabsorption of sodium and water limited the delivery of tubular fluid to the sites in the nephron where potassium is secreted [34].

Aldosterone excretion decreased throughout treatment with indomethacin, and paralleled the decrease in PRA. Whereas a direct effect of prostaglandins on the biogenesis of aldosterone (which could be blocked by indomethacin) remains a possibility [12], the major factor in the decline of urinary aldosterone was most likely the decrease in PRA, which was seen in all patients, both at bedrest and during standing. The retained sodium, chloride and water with expansion of the volume of extracellular fluid, normally a stimulus which suppresses PRA, probably was not an important factor in the changes in PRA. In early studies, expansion of the volume of extracellular fluid by the intravenous infusion of albumin had little effect on the excretion of aldosterone [1] and, more recently, such infusions given to patients with the syndrome did not suppress PRA [34].

The more likely explanation, that indomethacin caused the decrease in PRA by inhibiting prostaglandin synthetase, is supported by a body of evidence which indicates that prostaglandins are in some way involved in the release of renin. Infusion of PGE_1 into the aorta of dogs [5] and infusion of arachidonic acid, the natural precursor of PGE_2 and $PGF_{2\alpha}$, into the aorta of rabbits [6], reportedly increases PRA activity. The studies with arachidonic acid provide evidence that intrarenally generated prostaglandins share with exogenous prostaglandins the capacity to stimulate renin secretion or release. In in vitro studies, PGE_2 was also found to release renin from a suspension of rabbit renal cortex cells [35], and arachidonic acid to release renin from rabbit cortical slices [36]. Such observations suggest that the effects of prostaglandins, either exogenous or generated intrarenally, on renin release are probably direct, and not secondary to sodium loss or renal hemodynamic changes.

Indomethacin, an inhibitor of prostaglandin synthesis, has been observed to decrease PRA in the rabbit [6] and to attenuate the release of renin which occurs in response to a decrease in renal arterial pressure [36]. In normal man, the administration of indomethacin also appears to decrease PRA [7] and to attenuate the response of PRA to standing [37] and to treatment with orally [37] or intravenously administered furosemide [7]. Thus, the relationship of prostaglandins to renin release observed in normal animals and in man appears to extend to patients with Bartter's syndrome. In support of this notion is the observation that ibuprofen, a drug which is structurally different from indomethacin but which also inhibits prostaglandin synthetase, inhibited the release of renin and produced other metabolic changes qualitatively similar to those of indomethacin in a fourth patient with Bartter's syndrome (Figure 5). How prostaglandins effect the release of renin remains to be elucidated, but if the observations that prostaglandins release renin in vitro [35,36] are indicative of what happens in the intact organism, then the explanation is more complex than renal hemodynamic changes.

Considerable evidence indicates that the urinary prostaglandins measured in our patients are of renal origin. When prostaglandins are infused intravenously, the excretion of primary prostaglandins changes very little; this finding excludes glomerular filtration as a major determinant of primary prostaglandins in the urine [38,39]. Infusion of arachidonic acid, a precursor of prostaglandins, into a renal artery of a dog increases the excretion of prostaglandins by the infused kidney but not by the contralateral kidney [15]. Infusion of angiotensin II into a renal artery also produced an ipsilateral but not a contralateral increase in prostaglandin excretion [15]. Thus, the high values for urinary prostaglandins in Bartter's syndrome indicate an increased rate of synthesis of prostaglandins by the kidneys of these patients. Whereas control excretion of PGE_2 was high in all four patients with the syndrome, PGE-M was high only in the patient with the highest value for urinary PGE_2 (Table I). These findings suggest that an increase in the synthesis of PGE_2 by the kidneys occurs before or without an equivalent increase in the synthesis of PGE by the whole body, as reflected by the urinary excretion of a major metabolite of the E series. Thus, the results of studies of urinary prostaglandins in these four patients provide further evidence of a role for prostaglandins in Bartter's syndrome.

The recent description of a patient with the clinical features of Bartter's syndrome and with hyperplasia of renomedullary cells in addition to hyperplasia of the juxtaglomerular apparatus suggests that an overproduction of prostaglandins could be a proximal cause of the syndrome [14]. Measurements of urinary prostaglandins were not reported, but correction of the hyperreninemia, hyperaldosteronism and hypokalemia, and of the resistance to the pressor effects of angiotensin II by treatment with indomethacin is consistent with this hypothesis. In the present studies, the administration of indomethacin or ibuprofen did not produce a sustained correction of hypokalemia. Whereas serum potassium may increase to normal with prolonged correction of hyperaldosteronism, a failure to do so may also indicate that the defect in tubular sodium reabsorption which favors potassium excretion [1,3] may not be corrected by inhibiting prostaglandin synthesis and may be a proximal cause of the syndrome. In this case the excessive synthesis of prostaglandins by the kidney may be stimulated by intrarenal changes of an unknown nature.

The initial hypothesis of impairment of vascular responsiveness to vasopressor agents as the proximal event also remains as a possibility. If there were a defect in resistance arterioles, such that angiotensin II or norepinephrine evoked an excessive release of prostaglandins and thereby produced less than normal arteriolar constriction [40–44], then release of renin might be expected to increase to compensate for the decreased effectiveness of angiotensin II and norepinephrine. Somewhat against this sequence of events is the finding of normal values for PGE-M, an index of whole body synthesis of prostaglandins E, in three of the four patients.

Whether Bartter's syndrome is a heterogeneous disorder characterized by several sequences of events, such as those outlined herein, or a homogeneous disorder, cannot be answered at present, but must await the results of further studies. It does seem clear, from the published data cited herein and the results of the present studies, that prostaglandins are intimately related to the release of renin.

ACKNOWLEDGMENT

We are grateful to Brian J. Sweetman, Ph.D. for his help and to Ms. Susan L. Fulcher, Ms. Annetta Cooper and Mr. James Lee Morgan for their skillful assistance. We are also grateful to Prof. R. Verberckmoes of Louvain, Belgium for an opportunity to review a preprint of his manuscript.

We thank Udo Axen and John Pike, Upjohn Co., Kalamazoo, Michigan, for providing us with a supply of deuterated standards. This work was supported in part by NIH Grants HL 14192, HL 16489 and GM 15431.

REFERENCES

1. Bartter FC, Pronove P, Gill JR Jr, MacCardle RC: Hyperplasia of the juxtaglomerular complex with hyperaldosteronism and hypokalemic alkalosis. Am J Med 33: 811, 1962.
2. Gill JR Jr, Bartter FC: Hyperplasia of the juxtaglomerular complex with hyperaldosteronism and hypokalemic alkalosis. Water and Electrolyte Metabolism (III) (deGraeff J, Leijnse B, eds), Amsterdam, Elsevier Publishing, 1964.
3. Bartter FC, Delea CS, Kawasaki T, Gill JR Jr: The adrenal

cortex and the kidney. Kidney Int 6: 272, 1974.
4. Carlson LA, Eklund LG, Oro L: Circulatory and respiratory effects of different doses of prostaglandin E_1 in man. Acta Physiol Scand 75: 161, 1969.
5. Werning C, Vetter W, Weidmann P, Schweikert HV, et al.: Effect of prostaglandin E_1 on renin in the dog. Am J Physiol 220: 852, 1971.
6. Larsson C, Weber P, Änggård E: Arachidonic acid increases and indomethacin decreases plasma renin activity in the rabbit. Europ J Pharmacol 28: 391, 1974.
7. Frölich JC, Hollifield JW, Wilkinson GR, Oates JA: Effect of indomethacin on furosemide stimulated renin and sodium excretion. Circ Res 52 (suppl II): 99, 1975.
8. Frölich JC, Hollifield JW, Oates JA: Effect of indomethacin on isoproterenol induced renin release. Clin Res 24: 9A, 1976.
9. Martinez-Maldonado M, Saparas N, Ekkoyan G, Suki WN: Renal actions of prostaglandins: comparison with acetylcholine and volume expansion. Am J Physiol 222: 1147, 1972.
10. Gross JB, Bartter FC: Effects of prostaglandins E_1, A_1 and $F_{2\alpha}$ on renal handling of salt and water. Am J Physiol 225: 218, 1973.
11. Tannenbaum J, Splawinski JA, Oates JA, Nies AS: Enhanced renal prostaglandin production in the dog. 1. Effects on renal function. Circ Res 36: 197, 1975.
12. Saruta T, Kaplan NM: Adrenocortical steroidogenesis: the effects of prostaglandins. J Clin Invest 51: 2246, 1972.
13. Larsson C, Anggard E: Arachidonic acid lowers and indomethacin increases the blood pressure of the rabbit. J Pharm Pharmacol 25: 653, 1973.
14. Verberckmoes R, Clement J, Michielsen P, Van Damme B: Bartter's syndrome with hyperplasia of renomedullary interstitial cells. Successful treatment with indomethacin. Kidney Int 9: 302, 1976.
15. Frölich JC, Wilson TW, Sweetman BJ, et al.: Urinary prostaglandins. Identification and origin. J Clin Invest 55: 763, 1975.
16. Williams GC, Young DS, Stein MR, Cotlove E: Biological and analytic components of variation in long-term studies of serum constituents in normal subjects. Clin Chem 16: 1016, 1970.
17. Menard J, Catt KJ: Measurement of renin activity, concentration and substrate in rat plasma by radioimmunoassay of angiotensin I. Endocrinology 90: 422, 1972.
18. Mroczek WJ, Finnerty FA, Catt KJ: Lack of association between plasma renin and history of heart attack or stroke in patients with essential hypertension. Lancet 2: 464, 1973.
19. Sealey JE, Buhler FR, Laragh JH, et al.: Aldosterone excretion. Physiological variations in man measured by radioimmunoassay or double isotope dilution. Circ Res 31: 367, 1972.
20. Carr K, Sweetman BJ, Frölich JC: High performance liquid chromatography of prostaglandins. Biological applications. Prostaglandins 11: 3, 1976.
21. Halushka PV, Alexander RW, Loeffler LJ, et al.: A method for extraction and radioimmunoassay of urinary prostaglandins E and F. Submitted for publication.
22. Änggård E, Bergkvist H: Group separation of prostaglandins on Sephadex-LH_{20}. J Chromatogr 48: 542, 1970.
23. Jouvenaz GH, Nugteren DH, Van Dorp DA: Gas chromatographic determination of nanogram amounts of prostaglandins E and F. Prostaglandins 3: 175, 1973.
24. Alexander RW, Kent KM, Pisano JJ, et al.: Regulation of post-occlusive hyperemia by endogenously synthesized prostaglandins in the dog heart. J Clin Invest 55: 1174, 1975.
25. Hamberg M: Inhibition of prostaglandin synthesis in man. Biochem Biophys Res Commun 49: 720, 1972.
26. Watson JT, Pelster DR, Sweetman BJ, et al.: Display-oriented data system for multiple ion detection with gas chromatography-mass spectrometry in quantifying biomedically important compounds. Anal Chem 45: 2071, 1973.
27. Seyberth HW, Sweetman BJ, Frölich JC, Oates JA: Quantification of the major urinary metabolite of the prostaglandins by mass spectrometry. Evaluation of the method's application to clinical studies. Prostaglandins 11: 381, 1976.
28. Aiken JW, Vane JR: Intrarenal prostaglandin release attenuates the renal vasoconstrictor activity of angiotensin. J Pharmacol Exp Therap 184: 678, 1973.
29. Martino JA, Earley LE: Demonstration of a role of physical factors as determinants of the natriuretic response to volume expansion. J Clin Invest 46: 1963, 1967.
30. Brenner BM, Troy JL: Postglomerular vascular protein concentration: evidence for a causal role in governing fluid reabsorption and glomerulotubular balance by the renal proximal tubule. J Clin Invest 50: 336, 1971.
31. Falcuk K, Brenner BM, Tadokoro M, Berliner RW: Oncotic and hydrostatic pressures in peritubular capillaries and fluid reabsorption by proximal tubule. Am J Physiol 220: 1427, 1971.
32. Gill JR Jr, Alexander RW, Halushka PV, et al.: Indomethacin inhibits distal nephron sodium reabsorption in the dog. Clin Res 23: 431A, 1975.
33. Kirschenbaum MA, Stein JH: The effect of inhibition of prostaglandin synthesis on urinary sodium excretion in the conscious dog. J Clin Invest 57: 517, 1976.
34. Khwii RN, et al.: Effects of flow rate and potassium intake in distal tubular potassium transfer. Am J Physiol 228: 1249, 1975.
35. Dew ME, Michelakis AM: Effect of prostaglandins on renin release in vitro. The Pharmacologist 16: 198, 1974.
36. Änggård E, Larsson C, Weber P: Interactions between the renal prostaglandins and the renin-angiotensin system. International Conference on Prostaglandins, Florence, 1975.
37. Rumpf KW, Frenzel S, Lowitz HD, Scheler F: The effect of indomethacin on plasma renin activity in man under normal conditions and after stimulation of the renin angiotensin system. International Conference on Prostaglandins, Florence, 1975.
38. Granström E: On the metabolism of prostaglandin E_1 in man. Prostaglandins and related factors. Prog Biochem Pharmacol 3: 89, 1967.
39. Granström E, Samuelsson B: The structure of a urinary metabolite of prostaglandin $F_{2\alpha}$ in man. J Am Chem Soc 91: 3398, 1969.
40. Aiken JW: Effects of prostaglandin synthesis inhibitors on angiotensin tachyphylaxis in the isolated coeliac and mesenteric arteries of the rabbit. J Pharmacol Pharm 26: 217, 1974.
41. Terragno DA, Crowshaw K, Terragno NA, McGiff JC: Prostaglandin synthesis by bovine mesenteric arteries and veins. Circ Res 36 and 37 (suppl), 1, 1975.
42. Vane JR: Inhibition of prostaglandin synthesis as a mechanism for aspirin-like drugs. Nature [New Biol] 231: 232, 1972.
43. Ferreira SH, Moncada S, Vane JR: Indomethacin and aspirin abolish prostaglandin release from the spleen. Nature [New Biol] 231: 237, 1971.
44. Hedqvist P: Effect of prostaglandins and prostaglandin synthesis inhibitors on norepinephrine release from vascular tissue. Prostaglandin Synthetase Inhibitors (Robinson H, Vane JR, eds), New York, Raven Press, 1974, p 303.

Low Dose Radioiodide Thyroid Ablation in Postsurgical Patients with Thyroid Cancer

K. DAVID McCOWEN, M.D.*
ROBERT A. ADLER, M.D.
NASSER GHAED, M.D.
THOMAS VERDON, M.D.
FRED D. HOFELDT, M.D.†
Denver, Colorado

Sixty-four patients with well-differentiated carcinoma of the thyroid were treated with initial high (80 to 100 mCi) or low (less than 30 mCi) doses of I^{131} after bilateral subtotal thyroidectomy. A total of 36 patients in the various histologic categories were initially treated with the low dose of I^{131} (group 1), and a total of 28 patients were treated with the higher dose (group 2). Disease-free criteria were no visible tissue in the neck or body, a protein-bound radioactive iodine (PBI^{131}) of less than 0.005 per cent per liter at seven days and/or whole body retention of less than 3 per cent at seven days. Of the patients receiving less than 30 mCi (group 1), 56 per cent with papillary carcinoma, 67 per cent with follicular carcinoma and 56 per cent with mixed carcinoma of the thyroid were rendered disease-free after this initial dose. Of the patients receiving the higher dose of I^{131} (group 2), 67 per cent with papillary carcinoma, 50 per cent with follicular carcinoma and 67 per cent with mixed carcinoma of the thyroid were rendered disease-free after this initial dose. Disease-free mean follow-up time was 5.17 years (group 1) and 5.82 years (group 2). There was no statistical difference in these mean follow-up times, nor was there a statistical difference in the net (total minus initial) dose of I^{131} needed to render the patient disease-free. These data demonstrate that low dose I^{131} therapy is as effective as the larger more routine doses of I^{131} given in this disease.

The approach to well-differentiated thyroid carcinoma is multidisciplinary. Initial therapy is generally considered to be surgical. Many investigators believe that a bilateral subtotal thyroidectomy combined with a more conservative modified neck dissection or "node picking" operation is appropriate [1–6]. Postsurgical medical management of these patients has been extremely variable and controversial as to the role of postsurgical radioactive iodine (I^{131}) therapy versus prolonged medical management with thyroid hormone alone. I^{131} may be used to complete the thyroidectomy only after a bilateral thyroidectomy has been performed without using very large doses of radioiodine [7]. In some cases, occult metastases have become evident with radioimaging only after ablation of the postsurgical thyroid bed tissue [8,9]. I^{131} ablation in patients with well-differentiated thyroid carcinoma has been shown to increase survival in patients over 40 years of age [10] and in patients with metastatic and/or extrathyroidal cervical disease [11–13]. Although there is controversy as to the appropriate postsurgical ablative dose of I^{131}, there are attentive dose-related radiation

From the Endocrine Service, Department of Medicine and Nuclear Medicine Service, Department of Radiology, Fitzsimons Army Medical Center, Denver, Colorado 80240. The opinions contained herein are the private views of the author(s) and are not to be construed as official or as reflecting the views of the Department of Army or Department of Defense. Requests for reprints should be addressed to Dr. K. David McCowen. Manuscript accepted October 31, 1975.

* Present address: Clinical Research Service, Box 99, Madigan Army Medical Center, Tacoma, Washington 98431.

† Present address: Division of Endocrinology and Metabolism, Department of Medicine, University of North Dakota School of Medicine, Grand Forks, North Dakota 58201.

risks [13], including leukemia [15]. There is also the requirement that (under current AEC license and NCRP guidelines*) doses of 30 mCi and greater must be administered to inpatients under isolation precautions. This study examines the efficacy of initial low dose I^{131} therapy (less than 30 mCi) to complete thyroid ablation in postsurgical patients who have undergone bilateral thyroidectomy.

MATERIALS AND METHOD

Between 1960 and 1974, 76 patients with histologically proved carcinoma of the thyroid were referred to the Endocrinology Service after bilateral subtotal thyroidectomy. Sixty-four of these patients underwent postsurgical I^{131} thyroid ablation and were variously assigned to initial high dose (group 1) or initial low dose (group 2) treatment regimens regardless of histologic type. Nine patients had surgery alone and were treated with thyroid hormone suppression for various reasons, usually because of the patients' desire to complete childbearing. Three patients had medullary carcinoma of the thyroid and were not included in this study. There were no cases of anaplastic carcinoma of the thyroid. After surgery, the patients were treated with tri-iodothyronine (T3), 25 μg three times a day for six weeks. At the end of this period, T3 therapy was stopped for 14 days, and the patient underwent base line studies which included whole body scanning, neck scanning, PBI^{131} conversion rates and/or whole body retention studies. Diagnostic I^{131} doses were 1 to 2 mCi. Neck scanning was performed with a rectilinear scanning device. Whole body scanning and whole body retention rates were performed using the Anger camera as a whole body counter [16]. PBI^{131} conversion rates were determined by an anion exchange method [17]. Following base line studies, the patients were treated with initial low doses (25 to 29.7 mCi) or initial high doses (greater than 30 mCi—generally between 80 and 150 mCi) of I^{131} regardless of whether neck nodes noted at surgery were either positive or negative. The patients were then given high dose thyroid suppression therapy consisting of 0.2 to 0.3 mg of L-thyroxine daily which was stopped six weeks prior to repeat diagnostic studies. When L-thyroxine therapy was discontinued, the patient was treated with L-tri-iodothyronine (Cytomel®). Administration of this drug was discontinued two weeks prior to repeat diagnostic studies. Repeat diagnostic studies were conducted at three month intervals by the methods and I^{131} doses used to obtain the base line parameters. Criteria for total thyroid ablation were (1) negative whole body and neck scan, (2) PBI^{131} conversion rate of less than 0.005 per cent per liter in seven days and/or (3) whole body retention of less than 3 per cent in seven days. After the first post-therapeutic evaluation, if the patient did not meet the criteria described for total thyroid ablation, further therapy was then given, usually in dose ranges of an additional 100 mCi. Repeat diagnostic studies were performed at three-month intervals and additional I^{131} was given if required. After satisfying ablative criteria, the patients were evaluated at six-month intervals. When the present data were extracted, all patients entered in the study had satisfied the criteria for total ablation and were considered disease-free. All patients survived and are continuing under medical surveillance.

* U.S. Atomic Energy Commission Byproduct Material License No. 05-00046-13, Amend. 34, Condition No. 7, and National Council on Radiation Protection and Measurement, Report No. 37, Chapter 4, "Release from the hospital of patients containing radioactive material," 1970.

RESULTS

Clinical summaries of the patients are presented in Table I. The average age of the patients was 33.35 years (the average age in group 1 patients was 35.0 years and the average age in group 2 patients was 31.25 years). Of the patients studied, 41 per cent were men and 59 per cent women. Histologic categories were as follows: papillary carcinoma 42 per cent, follicular carcinoma 26 per cent and mixed papillary-follicular carcinoma 28 per cent. The number of years the patients were disease-free was 5.17 $\pm$ 0.552 years (mean $\pm$ SEM) in group 1 and 5.82 $\pm$ 0.759 years in group 2. The number of years the patients were disease-free was not statistically significant between the two groups. For comparison purposes, the patients were divided into the three histologic types previously noted. Patients in group 1 are presented in Table II. Of 13 patients with papillary carcinoma, seven (56 per cent) had thyroid ablation after a single dose less than 30 mCi. Of 12 patients with follicular carcinoma, eight (67 per cent) had thyroid ablation after the single low dose; of 11 patients with mixed carcinoma, six (56 per cent) had thyroid ablation after a single low dose. The patients in group 2 are presented in Table III. Of 15 patients with papillary carcinoma, 10 (67 per cent) required only one dose; of four patients with follicular carcinoma, two (50 per cent) required one dose, and of nine patients with mixed carcinoma of the thyroid, six (67 per cent) required one dose of I^{131} for ablation of residual tissue.

In order to assess the value of utilizing whole body retention studies and PBI^{131} conversion rates for assessment of ablation effectiveness, these values were compared with the presence or absence of scannable tissue in the neck or body. The PBI^{131} conversion rate with scannable tissue revealed a mean of 0.04 per cent $\pm$ 0.012 per cent per liter; the PBI^{131} conversion rate in patients without scannable tissue was 0.0052 per cent $\pm$ 0.0014 per cent per liter. There was a statistically significant difference in the PBI^{131} conversion in patients with a positive scan and in patients with a negative scan ($P < 0.003$). Whole body retention, using the Anger camera, was also compared with the presence or absence of visible tissue in patients. Whole body re-

TABLE I Clinical Summaries of Study Group (patients in group 1)

Case No.	Age (yr) at Diagnosis and Sex	Histologic Type*	First Dose (mCi)	Second Dose (mCi)	Total Dose† (mCi)
1	35, F	F	29.7	...	35
2	14, M	F	25	105	182
3	53, M	P	29.3	...	35
4	23, M	F	29.5	...	34
5	35, F	F	25	...	26
6	51, F	P	29	...	35
7	26, F	P	29	101.5	237
8	36, M	M	25	...	32
9	42, M	P	27.5	...	32
10	23, M	F	25	100	127
11	40, F	P	29.5	...	31
12	14, F	M	29	100	133
13	38, F	P	29.7	100	134
14	48, M	P	29.5	100	133
15	48, F	F	25	...	29
16	49, F	F	23	100	129
17	21, M	M	28	100	135
18	28, F	P	29.7	100	136
19	19, F	P	29	100	135
20	38, M	P	29	100	133
21	45, F	M	29	...	34
22	63, M	F	25	...	31
23	46, M	P	29	...	34
24	35, M	M	29	100	235
25	23, F	M	29	100	133
26	27, M	F	29	...	39
27	50, M	M	29.5	100	232
28	28, M	P	29	...	35
29	29, F	M	29.4	...	34
30	60, F	P	29.5	...	33
31	26, F	F	29	...	32
32	36, F	F	29	...	32
33	38, F	M	25	100	130
34	22, F	P	29	...	34
35	15, F	M	29	...	33
36	36, M	M	25	...	31
37	21, F	P	50	150	398
38	22, M	P	89	...	92
39	39, F	M	115	100	222
40	38, M	P	100	22	133
41	23, M	P	100	...	103
42	32, F	P	100	100	205
43	39, F	M	70	...	74
44	37, F	M	100	...	114
45	35, F	P	60	...	64
46	21, M	M	100	100	229
47	29, M	M	111	...	114
48	27, F	P	100	...	104
49	38, M	M	100	...	105
50	22, M	F	88	100	191
51	21, F	P	60	...	64
52	25, F	M	100	...	106
53	21, M	P	100	75	720
54	30, F	P	150	...	158
55	43, M	P	100	...	103
56	32, F	P	50	...	55
57	38, F	P	75	100	178
58	38, F	M	100	...	105
59	54, F	F	115	...	118
60	30, F	P	100	...	103
61	21, F	M	100	100	205
62	28, F	P	100	...	153
63	27, F	P	100	...	103
64	44, F	F	100	100	205

*F = follicular, M = mixed, P = papillary.

† Total dose includes therapeutic and diagnostic I^{131} over follow-up period.

TABLE II Summary of Results of Initial Low Dose I^{131} Therapy (patients in group 1)

Histologic Type	Extent of Disease	Total No. Patients	Required Ablative Dose and Follow-Up Time: <30 mCi No.	<30 mCi Years Disease-Free Mean	<30 mCi Years Disease-Free Range	<30 mCi plus Additional I^{131} No.	<30 mCi plus Additional I^{131} Years Disease-Free Mean	<30 mCi plus Additional I^{131} Years Disease-Free Range
Papillary	(−) nodes	8	4	3.25	2–4	4	3.15	1–5
	(+) nodes	5	3	3	4–12	2	6	3, 9
	Total	13	7	...	...	6	...	...
Follicular	(−) nodes	8	6	6.83	3–14	2	3.5	3, 4
	(+) nodes	4	2	7.5	7, 8	2*	4	2, 6
	Total	12	8	...	...		...	...
Mixed	(−) nodes	6	4	5.75	2–15	2	3.5	3, 4
	(+) nodes	5	2	5	5, 5	3	3.6	3–4
	Total	11	6	...	...	5	...	...
Total		36	21			15		

*Both patients had lung metastases at time of diagnosis.

TABLE III Summary of Results of Initial High Dose I^{131} Therapy (patients in group 2)

Histologic Type	Extent of Disease	Total No. Patients	Required Ablative Dose and Follow-Up Time: High Dose Once No.	High Dose Once Years Disease-Free Mean	High Dose Once Years Disease-Free Range	High Dose plus Additional ^{131} No.	High Dose plus Additional ^{131} Years Disease-Free Mean	High Dose plus Additional ^{131} Years Disease-Free Range
Papillary	(−) nodes	10	8	9.5	2–14	2	7	4, 10
	(+) nodes	5	2	5.5	2, 9	3*	5	2–7
	Total	15	10	...	...	5	...	...
Follicular	(−) nodes	4	2*	7	1, 13	2	6.5	6, 7
	(+) nodes	0	0	...	...	0	...	...
	Total	4	2	...	...	2	...	...
Mixed	(−) nodes	8	6	5	4–9	2	6	4, 8
	(+) nodes	1	0	...	...	1*	5	...
	Total	9	6	...	...	3	...	...
Total		28	18	...	...	10	...	...

*Patients with lung metastasis at time of diagnosis.

TABLE IV Comparison of Total and Net (Total Minus Initial) Dose of I^{131} (mCi) Required for Thyroid Ablation

Histologic Type	Dose Group	N	Mean Initial Dose (mCi)	Mean Total Dose ± SEM (mCi)	P Value	Mean Net Dose ± SEM (mCi)	P Value
Papillary	1	13	29.08	82.61 ± 18.23	<0.04	44 ± 17.68	N.S.
	2	15	88.93	172.2 ± 44.79		75.93 ± 42.56	
Follicular	1	12	26.74	80.82 ± 17.73	<0.004	38.75 ± 15.37	N.S.
	2	4	113.25	166.75 ± 19.61		53.25 ± 29.3	
Mixed	1	11	27.86	96.54 ± 24.45	N.S.	67.36 ± 24.42	N.S.
	2	9	99.55	141.55 ± 19.77		41.44 ± 18.07	
All types	1	36	27.99	85.05 ± 11.80	<0.004	52.02 ± 10.93	N.S.
	2	28	96.17	159.99 ± 24.05		61.89 ± 25.14	

NOTE: Group 1 = patients who received an initial low dose, group 2 = patients who received an initial high dose.

tention studies in patients with scannable tissue revealed a mean of 5.059 per cent ± 0.01 per cent, and whole body retention studies in patients with no scannable tissue revealed a mean of 1.03 per cent ± 0.2 per cent. There was a statistically significant difference in the whole body retention of patients with a positive scan and in patients with a negative scan ($P < 0.001$). There was, however, no significant correlation between PBI^{131} conversion and whole body retention when these were compared in the same patients (positive scan, $R = 0.34$; negative scan, $R = 0.06$). There was no significant difference in the PBI^{131} values after treatment with the first low dose (0.0145 per cent ± 0.0038 per cent per liter) or the first high dose (0.0125 per cent ± 0.0061 per cent per liter). Likewise, there was no significant difference in the whole body retention of patients treated with an initial low dose (1.771 per cent ± 0.564 per cent) compared to those treated with an initial high dose (6.116 per cent ± 3.02 per cent).

The differences in total and net (total minus initial) amounts of I^{131} required for thyroid tissue ablation in the various categories are presented in Table IV. Significant differences in the total amount of I^{131} required for thyroid ablation of the patients in both groups are noted in the papillary and follicular types, but not in the mixed category. When all histologic types are compared, however, the difference between the total I^{131} required in group 2 (159.9 mCi ± 24.05 mCi) and group 1 (85.05 ± 11.8 mCi) is significant ($P < 0.004$). In all three histologic categories, there was no statistical significance in the net dose required. Likewise, when all patients in both groups were compared, there was again no statistical significance in the amount of I^{131} required to ablate the thyroid bed after the initial dose.

COMMENTS

Although Berierwaltes et al. [10] demonstrated a significant increase in survival in patients with carcinoma of the thyroid receiving I^{131} therapy, there have been widely variable approaches to the operative and postoperative management of these patients. The controversy of the appropriate management of these patients is further contributed to by the lack of true controls in most reported studies of the medical management of this disease. Likewise, in the surgical literature, disagreement exists as to whether or not bilateral thyroidectomy is necessary [14,18–21], particularly in patients with papillary carcinoma of the thyroid. It is our belief that complete ablation of residual thyroid tissue is desirable because of: (1) the reported multicentric origin of these carcinomas [22–26], (2) the ease of follow-up after ablation has been accomplished, (3) the reports of occult metastases discovered with whole body scanning only after the residual neck tissue has been ablated [8,9] and (4) the reports of anaplastic carcinoma associated with well-differentiated carcinoma [26–28]. One of the major objections to bilateral thyroidectomy, when the carcinoma appears confined to one lobe, is the increased risk of surgical hypoparathyroidism [20]. With the availability of I^{131} for postsurgical ablation of residual tissue, the surgeon can leave a thin rim of posterior thyroid bed intact and preserve the parathyroid glands. By complete ablation therapy, it is easier to avoid the dilemma presented by the patient who is status postpartial thyroidectomy* for his thyroid cancer and presents with new masses or visible tissue in the neck: Does this new tissue represent extension of the carcinoma? When complete ablation of thyroid tissue has been accomplished, there is reliable thyroid-free base line data with which to compare the newly discovered tissue by the original diagnostic procedures. Once the decision for ablation has been made, it is desirable to treat with the lowest dose I^{131} necessary to achieve this goal. Doses of <30 mCi can be given to outpatients according to current AEC and NCRP guidelines and would theoretically lessen the risk of aplastic and hypoplastic anemia, leukemia, pulmonary fibrosis and genetically-induced radiation effects. This approach also has the obvious advantage that should more I^{131} be required, initial low dose therapy in no way precludes the patient from receiving larger subsequent doses. The difference in the net dose of I^{131} required for ablation after the initial treatment with high or low doses is not significant between the two groups (Table IV). When these data are viewed in light of the significant difference in the total I^{131} dose required for ablation in these two groups, it would appear that the only difference lies in the initial therapeutic dose received. The difference between the percentage of patients treated with an initial low dose of I^{131} requiring retreatment (41.6 per cent) and the percentage of patients treated with an initial high dose of I^{131} requiring retreatment (35.7 per cent) is small, as can be noted in Tables II and III.

Imaging remains the most reliable criterion for determining the presence or absence of thyroid tissue, be it normal or well-differentiated carcinoma. Fifty to 80 per cent of well-differentiated thyroid carcinomas have been said to take up I^{131} after neck tissue is ablated [8]. PBI^{131} conversion rates and whole body retention may be used as adjunctive parameters to

* Patient's status after a partial thyroidectomy has been performed. That is, after an operation in which the majority (but not all) of the thyroid gland has been removed.

verify the presence or absence of residual tissue. Studies [29] assessing ablation status by urinary I^{131} excretion have shown this method to be unreliable, and it should not be used as criteria for further ablative therapy despite the recommendation of some [5,13,30]. The modification of the Anger camera for whole body counting provides reproducible accurate retention data. This procedure can be performed easily and inexpensively in most Nuclear Medicine facilities, and can serve as a check on scanning procedures [31]. As presented, the difference between whole body retention values in the presence and absence of scannable tissue is quite significant. The difference in PBI^{131} conversion rates between patients with a positive scan and patients with a negative scan is also significant and correlates well with data published by Pochin [8]. We believe both technics utilizing the physiologic and biochemical properties of thyroid to concentrate I^{131} are valuable in the postoperative assessment of these patients.

A possible weakness in this study is the use of only 1 to 2 mCi for diagnostic purposes. The "initial low dose I^{131} approach" has an additional advantage in that high-density neck and whole body scanning may be accomplished when the patient receives the therapy. This has been carried out in the last few patients who have not been included because of the short follow-up time (<1 year) and will continue to be a part of this ongoing protocol.

In summary, the results obtained with the initial low dose (<30 mCi) I^{131} ablation technics are at least comparable to those achieved with much higher doses in patients thus far followed. The advantages to the patient, both medical and economic, are obvious and such an approach does not deny the patient further therapy if needed. We believe that low dose therapy should be restricted to ablative therapy of the thyroid residual bed after a bilateral subtotal thyroidectomy and not utilized in the treatment of extracervical metastases, such as lung, brain, etc. Although the natural history of well-differentiated thyroid carcinoma is benign compared to other cancers, for reasons previously noted, we do believe surgical, followed by I^{131}, thyroid ablation has a definite role. Our data establish a role for initial low dose I^{131} therapy in selected patients with well-differentiated thyroid carcinoma. A continuing evaluation of the long-term results of this new approach on these slow growing thyroid carcinomas is being conducted.

ACKNOWLEDGMENT

We wish to acknowledge the technical assistance of Anne Dolbow and John Pesut; the Department of Clinical Investigation, Fitzsimons Army Medical Center; and the many physicians who have assisted in the management and study of these patients, particularly Drs. Charles R. Hartman, George J. Ellis, J. W. Anderson, Eugene Morita and Edward Lufkin.

REFERENCES

1. Hardin WJ, Hardy JD: Carcinoma of the thyroid gland. Surg Gynecol Obstet 132: 450, 1971.
2. Selenkow JA, Karp PJ: An approach to diagnosis and therapy of thyroid tumors. Semin Nucl Med 1: 461, 1971.
3. Pittman JA, Pittman CS: Thyroid nodules and cancer. Semin Nucl Med 1: 534, 1971.
4. Payne JE, Hendrick DJ: Thyroid cancer, a review of 46 cases. Med J Aust 1: 5, 1972.
5. Sedgwick CE: Considerations in the management of thyroid malignancy. Surg Clin North Am 53: 125, 1973.
6. Wright HK, Gerard GN, Spaulding S, Sheahan DG: Current therapy of thyroid nodules. Surg Clin North Am 54: 277 1974.
7. Fawell WN, Catz B: Attempt at thyroid ablation with radioactive iodine for the treatment of ophthalmopathy in Grave's disease. Am J Med Sci 265: 467, 1973.
8. Pochin EE: Radioiodine therapy of thyroid carcinoma. Semin Nucl Med 1: 503, 1971.
9. Henk JM, Kirkman S, Owen GM: Whole body scanning and I-131 therapy and management of thyroid carcinoma. Br J Radiol 45: 369, 1972.
10. Varma VM, Berierwaltes WH, Nofal MM, Nishiyama RH, Kopp JE: Treatment of thyroid cancer. Death rates after surgery and after surgery followed by sodium I-131. JAMA 214: 1437, 1970.
11. Jackson GL, Blosser NM: Surgical and radioiodide therapy in thyroid carcinoma. Pa Med 74: 77, 1971.
12. Leeper RD: The effect of I-131 on survival of patients with metastatic, papillary or follicular thyroid carcinoma. J Clin Endocrinol Metab 36: 1143, 1973.
13. Bricout P, Kilber RS: Experience in the management of thyroid carcinoma by I-131. J Can Assoc Radiol 24: 323, 1973.
14. Strong EW: Management of cancer of thyroid: a summary. Proc Natl Cancer Conf 7: 179, 1973.
15. Brincker H, Hansen HS, Andersen AP: Induction of leukemia by I-131 treatment of thyroid carcinoma. Br J Cancer 28: 232, 1973.
16. Verdon TA, McCowen KD, Hofeldt FD: Use of the Anger-type scintillation camera. A method for determining I^{131} uptakes. J Nucl Med (in press).
17. Fields T, Kinnory DS, Kaplan E, Oester YT, Bowser EN: The determination of protein bound iodine (I-131) with anion exchange column. J Lab Clin Med 47: 333, 1956.
18. Esselstyn CB, Crile G: Indications for surgical therapy in thyroid disease. Semin Nucl Med 1: 474, 1971.
19. Buckwalter JA, Thomas CG: Selection of surgical treatment for well-differentiated thyroid carcinoma. Ann Surg 176: 565, 1972.
20. Tollefson HR, Shah JP, Huvos AG: Papillary carcinoma of the thyroid. Recurrence in thyroid gland after initial surgical treatment. Am J Surg 124: 468, 1972.
21. Tollefson HR, Shah JP, Huvos AG: Follicular carcinoma of the thyroid. Am J Surg 126: 523, 1973.
22. McDonald I, Kotin P: Surgical management of papillary carcinoma of the thyroid gland. The care for total thyroidectomy. Ann Surg 137: 156, 1953.
23. Rundle FF, Basier AG: Stump recurrence in total thyroidectomy and papillary thyroid cancer. Cancer 9: 692, 1956.
24. Frazell EL, Foot FW: Papillary thyroid carcinoma: a review

of 25 years of experience. Cancer 11: 895, 1958.
25. Clark RL, Ibanez ML, White EC: What constitutes an adequate operation for carcinoma of the thyroid? Arch Surg 92: 23, 1966.
26. Ibanez ML, Russel WO, Albores-Saavedra J, Lampertico P, White EC, Clark RL: Thyroid carcinoma. Biological behavior and mortality. Cancer 19: 1039, 1966.
27. Tollefson HR, DeCosse JJ, Hunter RVP: Papillary carcinoma of the thyroid: a clinical and pathological study of 70 fatal cases. Cancer 17: 1035, 1964.
28. Braverman LE, Vickery AL: Rapidly enlarging cervical mass 12 years after thyroidectomy for carcinoma. N Engl J Med 293: 186, 1975.
29. Verdon TA, Hofeldt FD, Hartman CR, Lufkin EG: I-131 urinary excretion studies: invalidity in thyroid cancer. Rocky Mt Med J 70: 47, 1973.
30. Powell MR: Thyroid testing in vivo with radioisotopes. Laboratory Tests in Diagnosis of Investigation of Endocrine Functions, 2nd ed (Escamilla RF, ed), Philadelphia, F. A. Davis, 1971, p 82.
31. Verdon TA, McRae JR, Anger HO, Yano Y: Whole body distribution of commonly used radionuclides in man. Display presented at Society of Nuclear Medicine Meeting, Boston, Mass., July 1972.

Body Composition and Skeletal Metabolism Following Pituitary Irradiation in Acromegaly

JOHN F. ALOIA, M.D.
ZRINKO PETRAK, M.D.*
East Meadow, New York

KENNETH ELLIS, Ph.D.
STANTON H. COHN, Ph.D.
Upton, New York

The change in body composition in acromegaly that resulted from pituitary irradiation was examined using the technic of total body neutron activation analysis. Before treatment, increased ratios of total body P:Ca, P:K and Na:K were noted. After pituitary irradiation, the total body levels of P, Na and K were reduced in a proportion that indicated restoration of body composition towards normal. Skeletal mass (total body calcium) decreased into the range observed in osteoporosis in several patients. Trabecular bone mass, as reflected by the Singh Index, was consistently reduced, and two patients had vertebral compression fractures. Local bone mass as determined by photon absorptiometry was reduced when the values were normalized for age, sex and body size.

It is postulated that in untreated acromegaly there is differential bone remodelling with an increase in cortical bone accompanied by a reduced trabecular bone mass. When reduction of hGH levels is accomplished with treatment, cortical apposition may decrease. Since the increased cortical bone mass probably aids in preventing vertebral compression fractures, the treated acromegalic patient may incur an increased risk of fractures. This risk may be increased further by the hypogonadism which may arise secondary to pituitary irradiation or surgery. It would be prudent to ensure that the hypogonadal acromegalic patient receives an adequate calcium intake and sex hormone replacement therapy.

Acromegaly is associated with alterations in body composition that are consistent with the anabolic effects of growth hormone (hGH) administration [1,2]. An increase in fat-free protoplasm is noted with increases in total body levels of potassium (TB-K), chloride (TB-Cl), phosphorus (TB-P) and sodium (TB-Na) [1]. TB-Na is increased to a greater extent than TB-K (which reflects lean body mass), and is associated with an increase in total body water [1,3].

Skeletal metabolism is of particular interest in this disorder. Patients with acromegaly have an increased total exchangeable calcium pool with an accelerated calcium turnover, increased periosteal apposition and increased resorption of trabecular bone [1,4–10].

The current study was undertaken to further elucidate the nature of acromegalic bone disease and to determine if the alterations in body composition are reversed when growth hormone levels are reduced by pituitary irradiation.

From the Department of Medicine, Nassau County Medical Center, East Meadow, and the Medical Research Center of the Brookhaven National Laboratory, Upton, New York. This research was supported by the U.S. Energy Research and Development Administration and the Meadowbrook Medical Education and Research Foundation. Request for reprints should be addressed to Dr. John F. Aloia, Department of Medicine, Nassau County Medical Center, 2201 Hempstead Turnpike, East Meadow, New York 11554. Manuscript accepted October 31, 1975.

* Present address: Lederle Laboratories, Medical Advisory Department, Pearl River, New York 10965.

TABLE I Initial Clinical Characteristics

Case	Sex and Age (yr)	Height (cm)	Weight (kg)	Duration Disease (yr)	hGH (ng/ml)
1	M, 60	177	81.3	12	22
2	M, 44	188	93.1	18	18
3	F, 50	173	76.6	25	36
4	M, 52	179	69.0	19	36
5	M, 50	162	76.3	4	3
6	M, 39	179	115.0	34	120
7	M, 41	184	91.8	12	115
8	M, 23	191	101.3	10	5
9	F, 50	157	63.6	29	50
Mean	45	176	85.3	18	45
±SD	±9.9	±10	±15.4	±9	±41

MATERIALS AND METHODS

Routine Studies. Clinical characteristics of the nine patients are indicated in Table I. Anterior pituitary function was assessed by measurement of serum levels of thyroxine (competitive protein binding), triiodine (T_3) resin uptake, and by urinary assays of 17-ketogenic and 17-ketosteroids and pituitary gonadotropins. Serum testosterone (competitive protein binding) was determined in the male patients.

The nine patients were studied at varied intervals after treatment. Serum was obtained at varied intervals and at the final evaluation; it was frozen for analysis for hGH, immunoreactive parathyroid hormone (iPTH) and 25-hydroxycholecalciferol (25-OHD_3) [11–13]. All samples were analyzed at the same time. On the final examination, roentgenograms of the hip were obtained in seven patients for grading according to the Singh Index, a roentgenographic system which evaluates trabecular bone [14].

Total Body Neutron Activation Analysis (TBNAA) and Whole Body Counting. The details of the technic of in vivo TBNAA and the characteristics of the Brookhaven 54-detector whole body counter have been described [15]. With this technic, it is possible to simultaneously determine total body calcium (TB-Ca), phosphorus (TB-P), sodium (TB-Na) and chloride (TB-Cl). Calibration with an anthropormorphic phantom indicated an accuracy and precision of the present technic of ±1.1, 1.8, 2.1 and 3.9 per cent (SD) for the measurement of calcium, sodium, chloride and phosphorus, respectively [16]. Thus, in repeated measurements on the same patients, a difference of twice the values is significant at the 95 per cent level. Total body potassium (TB-K) was also measured in the whole body counter via its naturally occurring isotope, ^{40}K.

TB-Ca was normalized by comparing the observed value to a predicted value. The predicted total body calcium (TB-Ca_p) was calculated from empirically derived equations based on observations in normal human subjects. TB-Ca can be predicted with an accuracy of ±10 per cent at the 95 per cent confidence level. Predicted values for total body postassium (TB-K_p) were calculated from equations derived from over 3,000 determinations in normal subjects [18].

Photon Absorptiometry. The bone mineral content (BMC) and bone width (BW) of the radius were measured in seven patients with a Norland-Cameron Absorptiometer at varying intervals after the initial evaluation [19,20]. The 8 cm site was used in these patients. Five patients also had determinations at the 3 cm radius site. The BMC was normalized for age, sex and body size by comparing the observed value to that predicted from empirically derived formulae (BMC_p) [21].

RESULTS

Laboratory Values. The endocrine evaluations of these patients and their response to pituitary irradiation have, in part, been described previously [22]. Hypogonadotropic hypogonadism was present in two patients (Cases 6 and 8) before they received radiation therapy and developed after pituitary irradiation in four others (Cases 1, 2, 4 and 7). (Each of these patients had a normal response to metyrapone administration.) Three patients (Cases 6, 7 and 8) were treated with parenteral testosterone during the course of this study.

Roentgenograms of the hip (Singh Index) were assessed as II in four patients (Cases 2, 4, 5 and 7) and as III in three others (Cases 1, 3 and 6). In addition to the typical acromegalic changes, roentgenograms of the spine revealed compression of the first lumbar vertebra and decreased density of the spine in one patient (Case 7), and anterior wedge compression of the sixth, seventh and eighth dorsal vertebrae in another (Case 2). Decreased density of the dorsal and lumbosacral spine was also present in two (Cases 4 and 5).

The serum calcium decreased slightly after pituitary irradiation in each patient except one (Case 4), the patient who had an elevated serum iPTH level. Mean serum iPTh levels were 296 ± 122 pg/ml on the first analysis and 328 ± 181 pg/ml (SD) on the final analysis (normal iPTH values are 365 ± 200 pg/ml). The change in serum iPTH was not statistically significant. Mean serum hGH levels in the same samples were 24.4 ± 12.5 ng/ml and 12.6 ± 7.4 ng/ml (SD), respectively. There was no significant change in 25-OHD_3 levels. Initial levels of 25-OHD_3 were 19 ± 6.2 and the final concentration was 21.5 ± 13 ng/ml (SD). Normal values for 25-OHD_3 are 29.9 ± 10 ng/ml (11).

Body Composition. The initial values for total body composition along with the percentage changes after radiation therapy are given in Table II. On the initial evaluation, mean TB-Ca was only 6 per cent greater than predicted. The initial Na:K, P:Ca and P:K ratios were increased when compared with a normal contrast group [17]. The Ca:K ratio was increased in two patients (Cases 6 and 8). The mean Ca:K ratio of 8.81 ± 1.20 compares favorably with an expected

TABLE II Initial Body Composition (and Percentage Change)*

		Grams					Ratios						
Case	Mo†	TB-Ca (%Δ)	TB-K (%Δ)	TB-Na (%Δ)	TB-P (%Δ)	TB-Cl (%Δ)	Ca_{Index}‡	K_{Index}	Ca:K	Na:K	Na:Cl	P:Ca	P:K
1	31	1,359 (−6.2)	146.4 (−3.7)	125.1 (−15.8)	721 (−12.6)	118.0 (−11.4)	1.162	1.102	9.28	0.85	1.06	0.53	4.92
2	9	1,249 (0)	165.7 (−1.9)	100.8 (+1.6)	551 (+5.9)	103.6 (+3.1)	0.970	1.038	7.54	0.61	0.97	0.44	3.32
3	43	1,057 (−10.7)	105.0 (−2.6)	107.5 (−2.8)	611 (13.4)	90.9 (+6.2)	1.055	1.006	10.07	1.02	1.18	0.58	5.82
4	34	1,020 (−14.5)	122.5 (−16.7)	109.3 (−17.2)	585 (−28.2)	105.2 (−7.2)	0.943	0.957	8.33	0.89	1.04	0.57	4.78
5	41	967 (+2.2)	129.7 (−8.4)	96.5 (−26.3)	561 (−37.9)	83.6 (−0.4)	0.961	1.170	7.46	0.74	1.15	0.58	4.31
6	16	1,654 (−13.1)	160.8 (−0.9)	145.1 (−9.9)	867 (+5.9)	130.4 (−6.5)	1.336	0.939	10.29	0.90	1.11	0.52	5.39
7	29	1,166 (−10.7)	159.7 (−7.6)	122.7 (−10.3)	662 (−22.2)	116.0 (+5.6)	0.921	0.996	7.30	0.77	1.06	0.57	4.15
8	31	1,591 (−2.9)	174.8 (−1.4)	150.4 (−21.2)	800 (−20.3)	134.7 (+1.8)	1.154	0.931	9.10	0.86	1.12	0.50	4.58
9	12	900 (−16.7)	90.0 (+0.6)	98.2 (+1.4)	485 (−17.1)	103.4 (−4.9)	1.069	1.083	10.00	1.09	0.95	0.54	5.39
Mean	27	(−8.1)	(−4.7)	(−6.4)	(−15.5)	(−1.6)	1.063	1.024	8.81	0.85	1.07	0.54	4.74

NOTE: TB-Ca = total body calcium, TB-K = total body potassium, TB-Na = total body sodium TB-P = total body phosphorous, TB-Cl = total body chloride.
*The values in parentheses indicate the per cent change in the representative elements from the value observed initially to the final value.
†Mo indicate the number of months between the initial and final evaluation.
‡Ca_{Index} = TB-Ca/Ca_p, K_{Index} = TB-K/K_p.

TABLE III Photon Absorptiometry in Acromegaly (8 cm site)

Case	BMC* (g/cm)	BMC:BW* (g/cm²)	BMC:BMC_p*	DM:MM†
1	1.104	0.749	0.839	
2	1.288	0.866	0.884	1.782
3	0.998	0.651	0.886	
4	0.950	0.624	0.783	1.068
5	1.235	0.801	1.099	1.546
7	0.880	0.568	0.615	1.479
8	1.665	0.951	1.064	1.474
Mean	1.160	0.744	0.881	1.470
±SD	±0.260	±0.138	±0.164	±0.257

*BMC represents bone mineral content, BW represents bone width and BMC_p represents predicted BMC.
†DM:MM represents the ratio of BMC:BW at the diaphyseal (DM) and metaphyseal (MM) sites.

normal value (corrected for age and sex) of 8.41 ± 0.90 [17].

After pituitary irradiation there was a much greater decrease in TB-Ca in seven patients (Cases 1, 3, 4, 6, 7, 8 and 9) than would have been expected from involutional osteopenia [17]. The reduction in TB-K was less remarkable than the decrease in TB-Ca. There was a greater decrease in mean TB-P than in TB-Ca, and TB-Na decreased to a greater extent than TB-Cl. The change in hGH levels were significantly correlated with the changes in TB-P ($P < 0.005$) and TB-Na ($P < 0.001$).

Photon Absorptiometry. The BMC at the 8 cm site (see Table III) was less than that predicted from the normative data of Mazess and Sorenson [23] except in two patients (Cases 3 and 8). The mean BMC of 1.160 ± 0.158 was slightly less than the mean of 1.23 ± 0.158 predicted on the basis of age and sex [23]. When the BMC was normalized for body size ($BMC:BMC_p$), local bone mass was found to be decreased in five of seven patients. The ratio of diaphyseal to metaphyseal bone mineral (DM:MM) was slightly increased in one patient (Case 2) and slightly decreased in another (Case 4), but the mean value was within the normal predicted range (1.449 ± 0.175) [24].

COMMENTS

The anabolic effects of the administration of hGH to normal adults have been demonstrated using the classic balance technic [25]. Both phosphorus and potassium are retained in relation to nitrogen in a proportion predicted by an increment in fat-free muscle protoplasm. In addition to its anabolic effects, hGH promotes the renal retention of sodium and phosphorus [2]. Sodium and body water are disproportionately increased in relation to potassium [2]. We have previously reported an increase in the TB-

TABLE IV A Comparison of Osteoporotic and Acromegalic Bone Disease*

Technics	Parameters	Acromegaly	Osteoporosis
Quantitative microradiography	Trabecular width	H	N
	Bone formation		
	Trabecular	N	N
	Cortical	H	N
	Bone resorption		
	Trabecular	H	H
	Cortical	H	H
Photon absorptiometry†	Cortical bone mass	H, N	L
Singh Index	Trabecular bone mass	L	L
Tracer kinetics / Hydroxyproline	Total bone turnover	H	N
TBNNA‡	Skeletal mass	N, H, L	L

*N = normal, H = high and L = low.
†When cortical bone mass is corrected for body size it may be reduced in acromegaly.
‡TBNAA = total body neutron activation analysis.

Na:K ratio in acromegaly; in the current study we further note an increase in TB-P in relation to both skeletal mass (TB-P:Ca) and lean body mass (TB-P:K) [1]. Pituitary irradiation resulted in a reversal of these changes, i.e., a disproportionately greater loss of sodium than potassium accompanied by a decrease in phosphorus was observed. Thus, treatment of acromegaly is successful in restoring body composition towards normal.

It has generally been held that acromegaly is associated with osteoporosis. Several recent roentgenographic and densitometric studies, however, have failed to disclose evidence of osteoporosis [6,10,26,27]. There are, indeed a number of differences between acromegalic bone disease and osteoporosis (see Table IV). Riggs and others [1,4] have observed the following in acromegaly: (1) bone mineral content, as measured by photon absorptiometry, is normal or increased at the mid-radius site, (2) formation surfaces predominate in cortical bone and resorption surfaces predominate in trabecular bone, and (3) the Singh Index (femoral trabecular pattern) is reduced.

Acromegaly and idiopathic osteoporosis are similar in that resorption surfaces (quantitative microradiography) predominate in trabecular bone and that the Singh Index (tabecular bone) is reduced. There appears to be differential skeletal remodelling in acromegaly with an increase in periosteal apposition accompanied by an increase in trabecular bone resorption [4,28]. This is believed to represent reactivation of skeletal remodelling characteristic of the growth phase with the constraint that apposition of bone must occur radially [4].

Although our studies confirm the decreased value for the Singh Index in acromegaly, we did not find a disproportion between diaphyseal and metaphyseal bone mineral content as might have been expected if differential changes in cortical and trabecular bone mass were present [24]. However, although the distal radius site has relatively more trabecular bone than the 8 cm site, it still consists predominately of cortical bone [29]. It may be that only the marked reduction in trabecular bone mass produced by hyperparathyroidism results in an alteration of the DM:MM ratio. Patients with idiopathic osteoporosis also have a normal DM:MM ratio, despite evidence of a greater reduction in trabecular than cortical bone in osteoporosis [24].

Our finding of a reduced $BMC:BMC_p$ also appears to be in conflict with the various reports that cortical bone mass is normal or increased in acromegaly [10,27]. However, the $BMC:BMC_p$ ratio normalizes local bone mass not only for age and sex, but also for body size. Therefore, despite the differences between acromegalic and osteoporotic bone disease, some people with acromegaly may have a reduced bone mass in relation to their increased body size. These patients may be susceptible to fractures.

It has been suggested that the acromegalic vertebra is probably less susceptible to fracture than the osteoporotic vertebra because the increased cortical apposition results in a larger value and greater strength than if both cortical and trabecular bone were reduced. The increase in trabecular width in acromegaly may also protect against vertebral fracture [1,4]. Nonetheless, in three of our patients (Cases 4, 7 and 9), skeletal mass decreased to a level observed in osteoporotic patients (when normalized for body size), and two patients had vertebral compression fractures. Riggs and his colleagues [4] observed increased vertebral radiolucency in 11 of 28 of their patients, and anterior wedge compression fractures in two patients.

Further reduction of hGH levels after treatment of acromegaly could eventually lead to reduced bone strength and compression fractures of the spine as a result of a reduction in cortical apposition. In addition, hypogonadism is a complication of the treatment of acromegaly, and may, as suggested by Albright [30], further accelerate the loss of trabecular bone. It would appear prudent to ensure treated patients with acromegaly an adequate calcium intake and sex steroid replacement therapy.

Finally, the relationship between acromegaly, PTH

secretion and vitamin D metabolism should be considered. Hypercalcemic hyperparathyroidism occurs in the syndrome of multiple endocrine adenomatosis [31]. One of the patients in the present study had an elevated serum calcium level accompanied by high serum iPTH levels. Normocalcemic hyperparathyroidism was not present in any of the patients. This is consistent with our previous findings that normocalcemic hyperparathyroidism is not present in acromegaly [32]. It is difficult to interpret the inter-relationship between PTH, vitamin D and hGH from the limited data available in the present study. Investigations of the effects of hGH on serum protein binding of calcium, and of hGH-induced tubular phosphate reabsorption on vitamin D metabolism would be of great interest. The lack of correlation between serum hGH levels and serum iPTH levels (or TB-Ca) in the present study may reflect the poor correlation of a single serum hGH level with either hGH secretory rate or somatomedin production.

REFERENCES

1. Aloia JF, Roginsky MS, Jowsey J, et al.: Skeletal metabolism and body composition in acromegaly. J Clin Endocrinol Metab 35: 543, 1972.
2. Raben MS: Physiology of growth hormone. JAMWA 23: 689, 1968.
3. Ikkos D, Ljunggren H, Luft R: The relation between extracellular water in acromegaly. Acta Endocrinol 21: 211, 1956.
4. Riggs BL, Randall RV, Wahner HW, Jowsey J, Kelly PJ, Singh M: The nature of the metabolic bone disorder in acromegaly. J Clin Endocrinol Metab 34: 911, 1972.
5. Eisenberg E, Gordan GS: Skeletal dynamics in man measured by nonradioactive strontium. J Clin Invest 40: 1809, 1961.
6. Nadarajah A, Hartog M, Redfern B, Thalassinos N, Wright AD, Joplin GF, Fraser TR: Calcium metabolism in acromegaly. Br Med J 4: 797, 1968.
7. Bell NH, Bartter FC: Studies of ^{47}Ca metabolism in acromegaly. J Clin Endocrinol Metab 27: 178, 1967.
8. Haymovitz A, Horwith M: The miscible calcium pool in metabolic bone disease—in particular acromegaly. J Clin Endocrinol 24: 4, 1964.
9. Haddad JG, Couranz S, Avioli LV: Nondialyzable urinary hydroxyproline as an index of bone collagen formation. J Clin Endocrinol Metab 30: 282, 1970.
10. Ikkos DG, Ntalles K, Velentzas C, Katsightis P: Cortical bone mass in acromegaly. Acta Radiol 15: 134, 1974.
11. Rosen, JF, Roginsky MS, Natheson G, Finberg L: 25-Hydroxyvitamin D: Plasma levels in mothers and their premature infants with neonatal hypocalcemia. Am J Dis Child 127: 220, 1974.
12. Kleerekoper M, Ingham JP, McCarthy SW, Posen S: Parathyroid hormone assay in primary hyperparathryoidism: experience with radioimmunoassay based on commercially available reagents. Clin Chem 20: 369, 1974.
13. Catt K, Tregear GW: Solid-phase radioimmunoassay in antibody-coated tubes. Science 158: 1570, 1967.
14. Singh MD, Nagrath AR, Maini PS: Changes in trabecular pattern of the upper end of the femur as an index of osteoporosis. J Bone Joint Surg 52: 457, 1970.
15. Cohn SH, Dombrowski CS, Pate HR, Robertson JS: A whole body counter with an invariant response to radionuclide distributor and body size. Phys Med Biol 14: 645, 1969.
16. Cohn SG, Dombrowski CS: Measurement of total body calcium, sodium, chloride, nitrogen and phosphorus in man by in-vivo neutron activation analysis. J Nucl Med 12: 499, 1971.
17. Cohn SH, Vaswani A, Aloia JF, Roginsky MS, Zanzi I, Ellis KJ: Changes in body chemical composition with age measured by total-body neutron activation. BNL No. 20061, 1975.
18. Ellis KJ, Shulka KK, Cohn SH: A predictor for total-body potassium in man based on height, weight, sex and age: Application in metabolic disorders. J Lab Clin Med 83: 716, 1974.
19. Cameron JR, Sorenson J: Measurement of bone mineral in-vivo: an improved method. Science 142: 230, 1963.
20. Johnston CC, Smith DM, Yu PL: In-vivo measurement of bone mass in the radius. Metabolism 17: 1140, 1968.
21. Cohn SH, Ellis KJ, Wallach S, Zanzi I, Atkins HL, Aloia JF: Absolute and relative deficit in total skeletal calcium and radial bone mineral content in osteoporosis. J Nucl Med 15: 428, 1974.
22. Aloia JF, Roginsky MS, Archambeau JO: Pituitary irradiation in acromegaly. Am J Med Sci 267: 81, 1974.
23. Mazess RB, Cameron JR: International Conference on Bone Mineral Measurement, DHEW Publication No. (NIH) 75-683, p 228.
24. Hahn TJ, Boisseau VC, Avioli LV: Effect of chronic corticosteroid administration on diaphyseal and metaphyseal bone mass. J Clin Endocrinol Metab 39: 274, 1974.
25. Rudman D, Chyatte SB, Patterson JH, Gerron GG, O'Beirne I, Barlow J, Ahman P, Jordan A, Mosteller RC: Observations on the responsiveness of human subjects to human growth hormone. J Clin Invest 50: 1941, 1971.
26. Juliani G, Agat G, Molinatti GM: Symposium Ossium, London, E & S Livingstone, 1970, p 173.
27. Doyle FH: Nonparathyroid Endocrine Bone Disease. Proc R Soc Med 60: 1131, 1967.
28. Erdeheim J: Zur normalen und pathologischen histolagie der glandula threidea, parathyroidea und hypophysis. Beitr Pathol 33: 158, 1903.
29. Manzke EM, Chestnut CH, Wergedal JE, Baylink DJ, Nelp WB: Relationship between local and total bone mass in osteoporosis. Metabolism 24: 605, 1975.
30. Albright F, Reifenstein EC: The Parathyroid Glands and Metabolic Bone Disease. Baltimore, Williams & Wilkins Co, 1948.
31. Summers VK, Hunter WR, Hipkin LJ, Davis JC: Hyperparathyroidism in acromegaly. Case reports. Lancet 2: 601, 1966.
32. Aloia JF, Powell D, Mendizibal E, Roginsky MS: Parathyroid function in acromegaly. Horm Res (in press).

The Investigation and Treatment of Renal Bone Disease

G. R. D. CATTO, M.D., M.R.C.P.*
M. MacLEOD, M.D., F.R.C.P.E.
Aberdeen, Scotland

Neutron activation analysis of a hand has been used to monitor changes in skeletal calcium content of patients undergoing maintenance hemodialysis. Assessed by this technic supplementary magnesium therapy was of value in reducing the progressive losses of skeletal calcium in a proportion of the patients receiving maintenance hemodialysis. Oral calcium supplements produced a decrease in the skeletal calcium losses of all the patients studied. 1-alpha-hydroxycholecalciferol, a potent vitamin D analogue, caused a significant increase in the calcium content of bone in three patients receiving maintenance hemodialysis; it may prove to be a safe and effective form of therapy for azotemic osteodystrophy.

For more than a century it has been known that in patients with chronic renal failure a form of metabolic bone disease may develop. Virchow [1] not only described five patients with severe nephritis, destructive skeletal disease and metastatic calcification, but also emphasized the importance of the renal lesions in the pathogenesis of the condition. Thereafter, many similar cases were described [2–5]; the patients became known as "renal dwarfs" [6] and the condition as "renal rickets" [7]. Although similarities to nutritional rickets were noted by many observers [8–11], treatment with vitamin D in physiologic doses was found to be ineffective [12]. Large doses of vitamin D or dihydrotachysterol may produce a diminution in the osteodystrophy of patients with chronic renal failure, but the dangers of vitamin D toxicity are known to be considerable [13–16].

In 1970, Fraser and Kodicek [17] discovered that a potent metabolite of vitamin D is produced in the kidney. This substance, 1,25-dihydroxycholecalciferol, was shown to stimulate calcium absorption in nephrectomized animals [18] and to induce a diminution in clinical renal osteodystrophy [19]. 1-alpha-hydroxycholecalciferol, a vitamin D analogue which is more readily synthesized than 1,25-dihydroxycholecalciferol, was also shown to be of value in the treatment of renal bone disease [20] and "is likely to be the drug of choice in the treatment of patients who may lack sufficient 1-hydroxylating activity in their kidneys" [21].

The vitamin D derivatives were discovered only recently and are not yet readily available, however, the value of calcium supplements in the treatment of patients with azotemic osteodystrophy was investigated by several groups of workers [22–24]. De Wardener and his colleagues [22–24] established that, although patients with renal failure absorb only small quantities of calcium when partaking a typical diet, the oral administration of large amounts of calcium increased calcium absorption [23,24].

From the Department of Medicine, University of Aberdeen, Foresterhill, Aberdeen, AB9 2ZD. Requests for reprints should be addressed to Dr. G. R. D. Catto, Department of Medicine, University of Aberdeen, Foresterhill, Aberdeen AB9 2ZD.
Manuscript accepted November 17, 1975.

* Present address: Renal Division, Peter Bent Brigham Hospital, 721 Huntington Avenue, Boston, Massachusetts 02115.

TABLE I Clinical Details of Patients Studied

Case No.	Age (yr)	Time on Dialysis (mo)	Bone Pain	Plasma Alkaline Phosphatase (IU/liter)	Roentgenologic Findings: Osteomalacia	Hyperparathyroidism	Decreased Bone Density	Vascular Calcification	No. of Fractured Ribs
1	41	81	2+	182	—	4+	—	2+	0
2	32	75	—	287	—	1+	—	1+	0
3	43	74	—	92	—	—	—	—	2
4	41	67	—	114	—	2+	2+	2+	0
5	50	65	—	230	—	—	1+	2+	0
6	45	52	—	156	—	—	2+	1+	0
7	54	50	2+	92	—	—	3+	2+	0
8	42	48	1+	84	—	—	—	—	2
9	34	47	—	72	—	—	—	1+	0
10	43	44	—	114	—	1+	—	—	0
11	22	40	+	420	—	3+	—	1+	0
12	32	36	—	156	—	—	—	—	1
13	29	35	1+	140	—	1+	—	1+	1
14	49	28	3+	230	—	3+	—	2+	2
15	41	28	—	240	—	2+	—	—	0
16	32	25	—	78	—	—	—	—	0
17	39	22	—	64	—	1+	1+	—	0
18	31	20	—	44	—	—	—	—	0
19	23	18	—	96	—	—	—	—	0
20	43	10	—	77	—	—	1+	1+	0
21	26	10	—	28	—	—	—	—	0
22	27	9	—	66	—	1+	—	1+	0
23	21	8	—	62	—	—	—	—	0

Alimentary calcium balance studies on patients receiving maintenance hemodialysis have provided results similar to studies on conservatively treated patients; a small net calcium loss has usually been noted [25]. Supplementary calcium may be administered with beneficial effects to patients with metabolic bone disease by increasing the calcium content of the dialysate to a minimum of 1.5 mmol/liter [25, 26]. Clinical osteodystrophy has not been encountered [27] in one large renal unit in which the concentration of calcium in the dialysis fluid is maintained at 1.5 mmol/liter and, in addition, large oral doses of calcium are given to the patients [28].

Supplementary magnesium therapy was also advocated in the treatment of renal bone disease. It was shown in man that increasing the plasma magnesium concentration above the normal range suppresses parathyroid activity [29]; Heierli and Hill [30] suggested that a high magnesium concentration in the dialysate might, by reducing the plasma concentration of parathyroid hormone, retard the progress of the metabolic bone disease. Raisz [31], however, showed in vitro that the action of parathyroid hormone on bone is inhibited by a low concentration of magnesium in the culture medium.

Studies on dialysis patients treated with a dialysis fluid containing a low concentration of magnesium ($\leq$0.05 mmol/liter) revealed no significant evidence of magnesium depletion in plasma, erythrocyte or bone biopsy samples, although the plasma magnesium concentration was reduced temporarily after hemodialysis treatment [32]. Nevertheless, an increase in the concentration of plasma magnesium was shown to cause a reduction in the plasma concentration of parathyroid hormone; it remained possible that the temporary decrease in plasma magnesium concentration induced by hemodialysis might be important in provoking an increased response from the parathyroid glands thus exacerbating any tendency to metabolic bone disease.

This study was undertaken to assess the prevalence of azotemic osteodystrophy in the Aberdeen Renal Unit and to evaluate the effect of therapy with (1) supplementary calcium; (2) supplementary magnesium and (3) 1-alpha-hydroxycholecalciferol on the progressive osteodystrophy of patients with chronic renal failure receiving maintenance hemodialysis.

Patients and Methods

Clinical details of the patients studied are given in Table I; the mean age was 36.5 years and the mean length of time they received maintenance hemodialysis was 38.8 months. For the most part, the patients were dialyzed on multipoint dialyzers with a surface area of 1 m^2 for a total of 22 hours/week. Oral aluminum hydroxide was prescribed as required to maintain plasma phosphate concentrations within normal limits. All the patients gave informed consent to the investigations.

Investigations. Blood samples, obtained from a forearm vein without the use of a tourniquet, were collected into plastic

TABLE II Mean Results of Dietary Survey and Recommended Allowances

	Calcium (mg/day)	Magnesium (mg/day)	Phosphate (mg/day)	Vitamin D (IU/day)
Mean values obtained	347.0	127.7	682.7	113.7
Range	237–608	70–242	977–430	19–248
SE	24.9	9.0	33.7	10.3
Recommended allowances*	800	350	800	400

* From Davidson, Passmore and Brock [43].

tubes containing lithium heparin, and the plasma was separated by centrifugation at 2,000 "g" for 15 minutes.

Plasma calcium was measured by an automated cresol saline method, plasma magnesium by atomic absorption spectrophotometry [33] using an E.E.L. Atomic Absorption Spectrophotometer, and plasma phosphate by the vanadate method [34]. Plasma alkaline phosphatase was determined by an automated modification of the method of Kind and King [35]. The magnesium concentration of erythrocytes was calculated by the method of Bruyn, Mink and Calje [36] after 1 ml of whole blood had been digested by concentrated nitric and perchloric acids [37], and the magnesium concentration of the solution was measured by atomic absorption spectrophotometry.

At intervals of six months, each patient underwent a roentgenologic examination of hands, forearms, lateral skull, chest, dorsal and lumbosacral spine, pelvis and feet. To ensure that similar exposures were obtained on each occasion, the same radiologist was used.

Bone biopsy specimens were obtained by a modification of the technic of Williams and Nicholson [38] before treatment and at intervals of six months thereafter. Cylinders of bone were taken from the left iliac crest by a Gardner needle and were prepared for histologic examination by the method of Tripp and MacKay [39].

The calcium content of a hand of each patient was measured by a neutron activation technic [40]. The neutrons, provided by a 25 Ci source of ^{241}americium and ^{9}beryllium, produced the radioisotope ^{49}Ca, from the ^{48}Ca naturally present in the bones of the hand; by detecting and quantitating the gamma radiation from the induced ^{49}Ca, an assessment of the calcium content of the hands was made.

Nineteen patients receiving maintenance hemodialysis were asked to weigh and record accurately all the food they consumed during a period of seven days. The total quantities of calcium, magnesium, phosphorus and vitamin D ingested by each patient during the week were calculated from published tables [41]. The results (Table II) are expressed as the quantity of each substance consumed daily.

The Prevalence of Azotemic Osteodystrophy. To assess the prevalence of osteodystrophy in patients receiving maintenance hemodialysis, each of 19 dialysis patients were subjected to a clinical examination, a biochemical investigation, a roentgenographic skeletal survey and a bone biopsy. Clinical details of the patients (Cases 1 through 19) are shown in Table I; the mean age was 38 years and the mean length of time on hemodialysis was 45 months. The concentration of calcium in the dialysis fluid was 1.35 mmol/liter.

THE EFFECT OF CALCIUM SUPPLEMENTS

This study was undertaken over a period of 10 months to evaluate the effect of supplementary calcium therapy on the progressive osteodystrophy of patients with chronic renal failure receiving maintenance hemodialysis.

Patients and Methods

Clinical details of the 14 patients studied (Cases 1, 3, 4, 7, 10, 11, 12, 13, 14, 15, 16, 17, 18 and 19) are given in Table I.

Prior to the start of the study the dialysis fluid, which was prepared by diluting a concentrate with mains tap water, contained calcium in a concentration of 1.35 mmol/liter. During the first 12 weeks of this study the calcium concentration of the dialysate was increased to 1.9 mmol/liter; from the 13th week the concentration was reduced to 1.5 mmol/liter recommended by Wing [25].

Oral calcium, administered as a flavored, aqueous suspension of calcium carbonate (1 g elemental calcium = 5 ml of suspension) was prescribed for each patient in a daily dose of 2 g.

After four months the dosage was increased to 3 g calcium daily, and after eight months it was increased again to 4 g, daily. For those patients unwilling to consume calcium carbonate solution, calcium carbonate powder was incorporated into specially prepared biscuits (1 g elemental calcium = 1 biscuit).

During the period of this study the diets contained 50 to 70 g protein, and none of the patients received magnesium-containing drugs or vitamin D supplements. Eight activation analyses were performed on each patient during the period of 18 months before treatment with calcium was instituted; a further four studies were made in the 10 months after the start of therapy. Student's t-test was used to assess the significance of the alteration in the rate of calcium loss detected by neutron activation analysis following therapy with calcium (Table III).

THE EFFECT OF MAGNESIUM SUPPLEMENTS

This study was undertaken over a period of 10 months to evaluate the effect of supplementary magnesium therapy on the progressive osteodystrophy of six patients with chronic renal failure receiving maintenance hemodialysis.

Patients and Methods

Clinical details of the six patients studied (Cases 5, 9, 20, 21,22 and 23) are given in Table I.

For 60 months before the start of this study no magnesium was included in the concentrate which was diluted with mains tap water to form the dialysis fluid. Thus, the final concentration of magnesium in the dialysate was the same as the concentration of magnesium in the local tap water (≤0.05 mmol/liter). During the period of this study, the concentration of magnesium in the dialysate was increased to 0.8 mmol/

liter while the concentration of calcium remained unaltered at 1.35 mmol/liter. None of the patients were given either oral calcium or vitamin D supplements; the diets contained 50 to 70 g protein daily.

Eight activation studies were performed on two patients (Cases 5 and 9) during a period of 18 months before treatment with magnesium began; four patients (Cases 20, 21, 22 and 23) were studied on five occasions during a 10 month period before treatment. A total of four further studies were made on each patient in the 10 months after the start of treatment.

Nerve conduction studies were performed on all six patients before and 10 months after treatment with magnesium supplements was initiated. The conduction studies, which were made before a dialysis treatment, were made on the radial, median and peroneal nerves in order to maintain representative results from sensory, mixed and motor nerves.

Plasma and erythrocyte magnesium concentrations were determined in all the patients at the beginning and at the end of the study. Plasma calcium, phosphate and alkaline phosphatase concentrations in each patient were determined from the routine blood samples obtained monthly before a hemodialysis treatment. Student's t-test was used to assess the significance of both the increase in plasma magnesium concentration and the alteration in the rate of calcium loss detected by neutron activation analysis after therapy with magnesium.

THE EFFECT OF 1-ALPHA-HYDROXYCHOLECALCIFEROL

This study was undertaken to evaluate the effect of 1-alpha-hydroxycholecalciferol (obtained from Dr. E. Kodicek, Strangeways Laboratories, Cambridge) on the progressive osteodystrophy of three patients with chronic renal failure undergoing maintenance hemodialysis.

Patients and Methods

Clinical details of the patients studied (Cases 2, 6 and 8) are presented in Table I. The dialysis fluid, prepared by diluting a concentrate with mains tap water, contained calcium in a concentration of 1.5 mmol/liter. Magnesium, to a final concentration of 0.8 mmol/liter was added to the dialysate for one patient (Case 2) only. All three patients were given a daily dietary supplement of 2 g calcium as calcium carbonate; none was given aluminum hydroxide.

Nine activation analyses were performed on each patient during the period of 18 months before treatment with 1-alpha-hydroxycholecalciferol was instituted; a further five studies were made at varying intervals after the start of therapy.

1-alpha-hydroxycholecalciferol, dissolved in arachis oil, was administered orally to each patient in a dose of 2 μg/day. After three weeks, the treatment for one patient (Case 8) was discontinued for two weeks and then restarted in a daily dose of 1 μg. The dosage of 1-alpha-hydroxycholecalciferol administered to another patient (Case 2) was increased to 4 μg daily after 12 weeks. Student's t test was used to assess the significance of the alteration in the rate of calcium loss after therapy with 1-alpha-hydroxycholecalciferol (Table III).

TABLE III Rate of Change in Skeletal Calcium Measured by Neutron Activation Analysis in Patients Receiving Maintenance Hemodialysis Before and After Therapy (per cent/week + SE)

Case No.	Before Therapy	After Therapy	p Value
		Calcium	
1	−0.44 ± 0.04	Deceased	–
3	−0.24 ± 0.11	+0.05 ± 0.19	0.20 < p < 0.30
4	−0.58 ± 0.05	+0.44 ± 0.11	< 0.001
7	−0.42 ± 0.06	Deceased	–
10	−0.37 ± 0.10	+0.32 ± 0.22	0.005 < p < 0.01
11	−0.36 ± 0.12	+0.17 ± 0.45	0.2 < p < 0.3
12	−0.31 ± 0.05	−0.07 ± 0.08	0.01 < p < 0.05
13	−0.20 ± 0.06	−0.08 ± 0.19	0.1 < p < 0.2
14	−0.33 ± 0.05	+0.08 ±0.08	0.001 < p < 0.005
15	−0.47 ± 0.09	+0.61 ± 0.16	p < 0.001
16	−0.33 ± 0.04	−0.07 ± 0.13	0.05 < p < 0.1
17	−0.36 ± 0.03	−0.01 ± 0.13	0.01 < p < 0.05
18	−0.39 ± 0.04	+0.00 ± 0.28	p < 0.001
19	−0.44 ± 0.09	+0.25 ± 0.07	p < 0.001
		Magnesium	
5	−0.31 ± 0.10	−0.20 ± 0.12	0.4 < p < 0.5
9	−0.31 ± 0.08	−0.35 ± 0.27	0.8 < p < 0.9
20	−0.70 ± 0.16	−0.13 ± 0.18	0.01 < p < 0.05
21	−0.92 ± 0.16	+0.25 ± 0.16	p < 0.001
22	−1.44 ± 0.35	+0.18 ± 0.24	0.005 < p < 0.01
23	−0.47 ± 0.18	+0.16 ± 0.31	0.05 < p < 0.10
		1-alpha-hydroxycholecalciferol	
2	−0.42 ± 0.04	+0.44 ± 0.13	< 0.001
6	−0.48 ± 0.04	+0.77 ± 0.23	< 0.001
8	−0.37 ± 0.04	+0.80 ± 0.23	< 0.001

RESULTS

Prevalence of Azotemic Osteodystrophy. On direct questioning, six of the 19 patients studied (32 per cent) admitted to episodes of bone pain. Although none of the patients had an abnormally increased plasma calcium concentration before dialysis, 13 (68 per cent) demonstrated an increase in plasma calcium after dialysis; this finding was reported previously in patients receiving maintenance hemodialysis [42]. Plasma phosphate concentrations decreased significantly after dialysis, as expected. In this study, nine patients (47 per cent) had abnormally increased plasma alkaline phosphatase concentrations.

The roentgenographic skeletal surveys were assessed for features of osteomalacia, hyperparathyroidism, diminution in bone density and ectopic or vascular calcification [48]. Only three patients (16 per cent) showed no abnormality on skeletal survey. Subperiosteal erosions, which were the most commonly found abnormality, were detected in 47 per cent of the patients. None of the patients had definitive roentgenologic evidence of osteomalacia, and only 26 per cent had decreased bone density.

The bone biopsy samples were assessed histologi-

TABLE IV Plasma and Erythrocyte Magnesium Concentrations in Six Patients Receiving Maintenance Hemodialysis Before and After Magnesium Therapy (mmol/liter)*

	Before Treatment				After Treatment			
	Plasma Magnesium		Erythrocyte Magnesium		Plasma Magnesium		Erythrocyte Magnesium	
Case No.	Before Dialysis	After Dialysis	Before Dialysis	After Dialysis	Before Dialysis	After Dialysis	Before Dialysis	After Dialysis
5	1.8	1.1	7.9	6.8	2.7	2.6	6.6	5.8
9	1.8	0.8	9.3	9.0	2.3	2.5	6.5	7.4
20	1.7	0.7	10.2	9.4	2.6	2.8	9.8	10.0
21	2.0	1.1	7.4	7.6	2.9	3.0	8.1	7.7
22	1.9	1.0	7.6	7.4	3.1	2.8	8.3	8.0
23	2.1	1.3	8.3	8.0	3.0	2.7	8.9	9.1

*Results obtained before and after dialysis are recorded.

cally for evidence of osteomalacia, osteitis fibrosa, osteosclerosis and osteoporosis. All the patients studied had evidence of osteomalacia as shown by increased quantities of uncalcified osteoid; even in the 17 patients (89 per cent) with evidence of osteitis fibrosa, osteomalacia remained the predominant abnormality.

Roentgenologically, abnormalities were detected in 84 per cent of the patients. All the patients studied had histologic evidence of azotemic osteodystrophy; histologically, osteomalacia was the predominant pathologic lesion even in the patients with marked roentgenographic features of secondary hyperparathyroidism. Thus, although symptomatic bone disease was present in only 32 per cent of the patients, histologic features of renal osteodystrophy were detected in all 19 patients receiving maintenance hemodialysis studied in the Aberdeen Renal Unit.

Results of Dietary Survey

The mean results of the dietary survey on the 19 patients, and the recommended daily allowances for each substance [43], are shown in Table II. The diets of almost all the patients studied were deficient in all the substances estimated; in particular, the quantities of calcium, less than half the recommended values, were inadequate for patients experiencing the unpredictable calcium losses caused by hemodialysis.

Results of Treatment with Calcium Supplements

During the course of this study two patients died. One patient (Case 1) had metastatic tumor from an anaplastic carcinoma of the breast; the other patient (Case 7), who was known to have hyperlipoproteinemia (type IV), died from a myocardial infarction five months after the study started.

No significant differences were detected in the plasma concentrations of calcium and phosphate measured before and during the study; both remained essentially within normal limits. In none of the patients consuming 4 g calcium daily did hypercalcemia develop at any time. Five of the 12 surviving patients (42 per cent) had an abnormally increased plasma alkaline phosphatase concentration prior to the start; this compares with an increased plasma alkaline phosphatase concentration in 33 per cent of the surviving patients at the end of the investigation.

The results from the activation analyses, expressed as the percentage changes from the original ^{49}Ca counts obtained from the hands, showed an increase in the calcium content of a hand in eight of the 12 surviving patients after treatment with calcium. This therapy caused a significant alteration in the rate of change in the calcium content of the hands in six of the surviving patients (50 per cent) and a highly significant alteration in the calcium content of the hands in four patients (33 per cent). These results are presented in Table III.

When these results are assessed collectively, the mean rate of decrease in skeletal calcium measured by neutron activation analysis before calcium therapy started was −0.37 per cent per week. The mean rate of increase after calcium therapy, +0.14 per cent per week, is significantly different ($p < 0.001$).

Roentgenographically only one patient had a detectable change after the start of therapy; in this patient (Case 3) a slight increase in vascular calcification was noted. The results of the histologic assessments of the bone biopsy samples indicated that an improvement was noted in the specimens of four patients (33 per cent), no change in specimens of six patients (50 per cent) and a further deterioration in the specimens of two patients (17 per cent).

Results of Treatment with Magnesium Supplement

Plasma and erythrocyte magnesium concentrations, which were measured before and after a hemodialysis treatment in all the patients prior to the start and at the end of the study, are shown in Table IV. There was a significant increase in the plasma magnesium concentrations after treatment ($p < 0.001$); the decrease in plasma magnesium concentration, which was detectable before the addition of the magnesium supplement, was abolished. However, there was no significant change in the erythrocyte magnesium concentrations ($p > 0.1$).

No significant differences were detected in the plasma concentrations of calcium and phosphate measured before and during the study. In none of the patients did hypercalcemia develop; only one patient had an abnormally increased alkaline phosphatase concentration, and this was present both before and after the magnesium supplement was added to the dialysate.

One month after treatment with magnesium supplements began, clinical evidence of a peripheral, predominantly motor neuropathy, developed in one patient (Case 23). Conduction in the median and peroneal nerves slowed from approximately 50 meters/sec to less than 10 meters/sec. No change was detected in the results obtained in any of the remaining five patients.

The results of the activation analyses, expressed as the per cent change from the original ^{49}Ca counts of the hands, show a continuing decrease in the calcium content of the hands in three patients (50 per cent) after treatment with magnesium was started (Table III). Magnesium therapy caused a significant change in the rate of calcium loss in the hands of three patients (50 per cent).

When the results are assessed collectively, the mean rate of change of skeletal calcium measured by neutron activation analysis before the start of magnesium therapy was −0.69 per cent per week. The mean rate of change after the start of magnesium therapy, − 0.15 per cent per week, is significantly different ($0.01 < p < 0.05$).

Roentgenologically, the only changes noted in these patients during the period of this study were slight increases in the subperiosteal erosions in one (Case 5) and capsular calcification in the fingers of another (Case 21). Histologically, no change was noted in the bone biopsy specimens of any of the patients during the 10 month period of magnesium therapy.

Results of Treatment with 1-alpha-hydroxycholecalciferol

Serial measurements of the plasma concentrations of both calcium and phosphorus from two patients (Cases 2 and 6) did not change after treatment with 1-alpha-hydroxycholecalciferol. However, the results in another patient (Case 8) indicated that the hypercalcemia which developed shortly after therapy started did not persist when administration of the drug was withdrawn and did not recur when the vitamin D analogue was recommenced at a daily dose of 1 μg. The results from the activation analyses expressed as the percentage changes from the original ^{49}Ca counts show an increase in the calcium contents of the hands in all three patients after treatment was started with 1-alpha-hydroxycholecalciferol (Figure 1). This therapy caused a significant alteration in the rate of change in the calcium content of each hand (Table III). The results, marked with a circle, (Figure 1) are inaccurate; the fault was due to a leak in the standard used to calibrate the equipment, but the recorded values were used in the calculations for Table III.

Roentgenologically there was no evidence of progressive demineralization in any of these patients. The increased quantities of uncalcified osteoid tissue noted histologically in the bone biopsy samples of two patients (Cases 6 and 8) before treatment, decreased considerably after therapy with 1-alpha-hydroxycholecalciferol for a period of three months. A diminution was also observed in the biopsy specimen from another patient (Case 2), but quantities of uncalcified osteoid remained.

The increased plasma alkaline phosphatase values obtained in Case 6 returned to normal after treatment with 1-alpha-hydroxycholecalciferol; the plasma alkaline phosphatase concentrations in Case 8 were never above normal. The plasma alkaline phosphatase levels in Case 2, however, have remained abnormally elevated despite therapy.

The dose of 1-alpha-hydroxycholecalciferol administered to the patient in Case 2 was doubled after 12 weeks from 2 μg to 4 μg daily. Although the skeletal calcium content measured by neutron activation analysis increased significantly (Figure 1), the concentration of plasma alkaline phosphatase remained abnormally increased after treatment for a further 12 weeks. Alkaline phosphatase isoenzyme studies suggest that this may be more related to hepatic than bone disease, and results of liver function tests on the blood of one patient (Case 2) have been abnormal for the last five years.

COMMENTS

The technic of partial body neutron activation analysis used in this study was shown to be a more sensitive indicator of the rate of progression of or diminution in renal bone disease than either skeletal roentgenography or photon absorption by a radius [44]. The coefficient of variation was assessed by repeated measurements of anatomic specimens and for clinical studies is between 4 per cent and 5 per cent [40]. Since the activation technic does not distinguish between calcium in bone and soft tissue, it is possible that the results obtained in this study were influenced by changes in ectopic or vascular calcification. Although investigations of total body calcium by neutron activation analysis were complicated in this way, it was suggested that the contribution of ^{49}Ca counts from ectopic calcium may

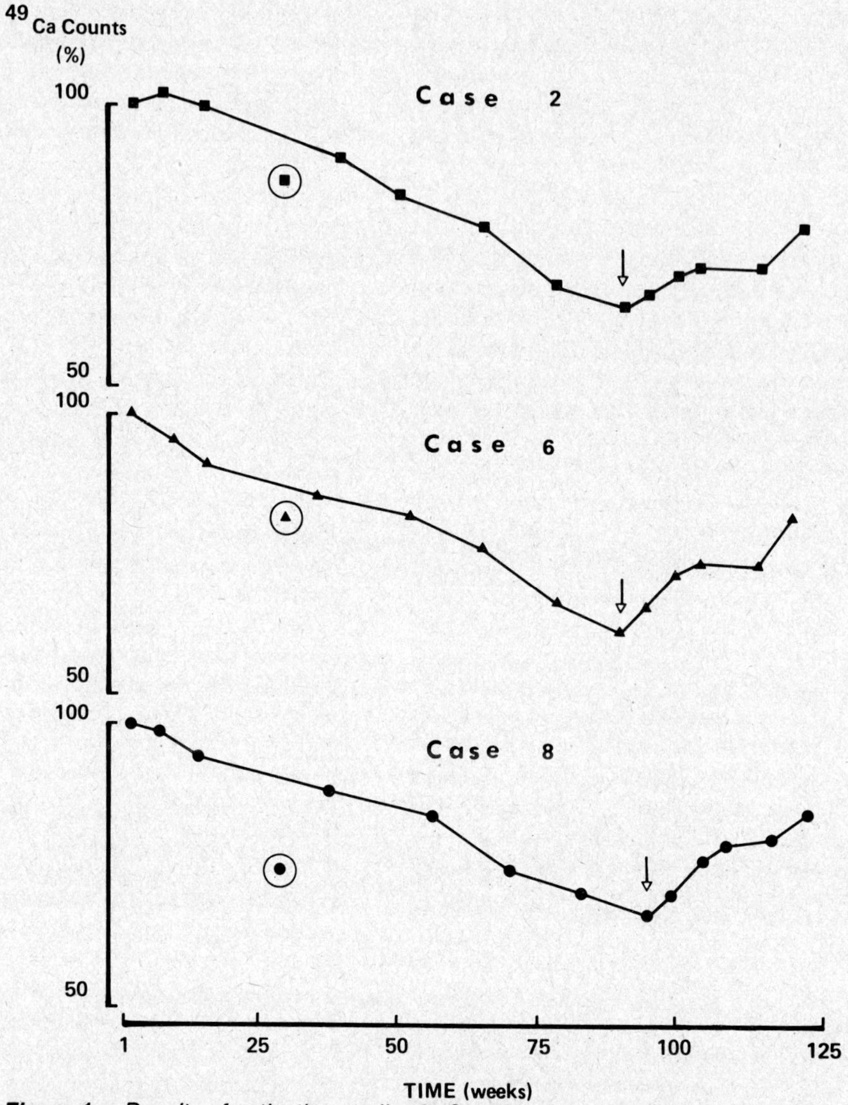

Figure 1. *Results of activation studies in Cases 2, 6 and 8. The arrows indicate the start of therapy with 1-alpha-hydroxycholecalciferol.*

be less in activation analyses of a hand as the ratio of soft tissue to bone is less in the hand than in the body as a whole [40].

As the roentgenologic features of azotemic osteodystrophy have frequently been observed first in the fingers, it was thought that a sensitive method of detecting small changes in the calcium content of a hand might prove of value in assessing the efficacy of different forms of treatment for progressive renal bone disease. Although the activation method employed was not used to measure absolute quantities of calcium, accurate measurements of the relative changes in calcium content, occurring over a period of time in an individual patient, were thought to be of more value when monitoring calcium metabolism in an organ of such variable size as a hand [40]. When the rate at which patients receiving maintenance hemodialysis were losing skeletal calcium was ascertained (Table III), therapy was started in an attempt to limit or reverse the demineralizing process.

The results of the dietary survey in the dialysis patients showed that they all consumed a diet which contained an inadequate quantity of calcium. This confirmed previous findings [45,46]; the deficient diet was attributed to a combination of anorexia and the imposition of a low protein, salt-restricted diet which limited the quantities of dairy produce ingested by the patients. Since Clarkson and her colleagues [45] demonstrated that patients with renal failure could adsorb an important amount of calcium when ingested in large quantities, oral supplements of calcium carbonate were supplied to 14 patients. Caution was exercised in supplying oral calcium therapy because of the severe symptomatic hypercalcemia reported to occur in some patients taking oral calcium carbonate in doses of 3 g to 6 g daily [47]. In the present study hypercalcemia was not detected when the daily dose of calcium was maintained at 4 g or less.

In an attempt to suppress parathyroid overactivity in the 14 patients undergoing maintenance hemodialysis, the concentration of calcium in the dialysate was increased from 1.35 mmol/liter to 1.9 mmol/liter for three months. After that time the concentration of calcium in the dialysate was reduced to the 1.5 mmol/liter recommended by Wing [25]; this was done to prevent the possible formation of ectopic calcification from the continued infusion of large quantities of calcium at each dialysis treatment [48]. Unfortunately, measurements of plasma parathyroid hormone concentration were not available.

None of the surviving patients had significant changes in the plasma concentrations of calcium or phosphorus when therapy with calcium commenced; in one patient an increased plasma alkaline phosphatase concentration decreased to normal levels. The only roentgenologic change noted in the patients during the study was an increase in vascular calcification detected in one (Case 3). As progressive demineralization was detected by radiology in only a minority of the patients prior to therapy [44], it is suggested that the apparent lack of improvement during treatment confirms the relative insensitivity of the roentgenographic technic in monitoring changes in skeletal calcium. Histologic improvement was detected in bone biopsy specimens from 33 per cent of the patients, and no further deterioration was noted in 50 per cent. These results provide a fair measure of agreement with the activation technic; prior to the introduction of therapy, serial bone biopsy specimens revealed only histologic features of progressive osteodystrophy.

The results of the neutron activation studies indicate that the combined supplementary calcium therapy was effective in reducing the skeletal calcium losses in all the patients and promoted an increase in skeletal calcium in 67 per cent of them. Thus, it is concluded that the calcium therapy used was effective in the treatment of azotemic osteodystrophy and that oral calcium supplements, as calcium carbonate, should be supplied to all patients undergoing maintenance hemodialysis. A daily dose of 4 g elemental calcium appears to be both safe and effective; it is also suggested that the concentration of calcium in the dialysate should not be less than 1.5 mmol/liter.

When the results of supplementary magnesium therapy are considered, the neutron activation studies indicate (Table III) that treatment was effective in limiting the progressive loss of skeletal calcium in three patients (Cases 20, 21 and 22) (50 per cent) but of little value in two (Cases 5 and 9). Unfortunately, this conclusion is complicated by clinical differences in the patients selected for the study; it was considered that it would not be justifiable to withhold supplementary calcium from patients with severe osteodystrophy. Thus only two patients (Cases 5 and 9) who failed to demonstrate a significant response to the magnesium therapy had been adequately established on maintenance hemodialysis prior to the start of the study; four others (Cases 20, 21, 22 and 23) had been on the dialysis program for only 8 to 10 months. It is, therefore, possible that the decreases in the rate of skeletal calcium loss monitored in this latter group of patients were associated not with the introduction of magnesium therapy but with the start of maintenance hemodialysis. Alternatively, it may be that parathyroid overactivity was more readily suppressed in patients who had not been established on maintenance hemodialysis for a long period of time. Whatever the correction explanation, it would appear from this study on a very small number of patients that supplementary magnesium therapy may decrease the rate of skeletal calcium loss in a proportion of patients undergoing maintenance hemodialysis. No adverse effects of treatment were noted; no roentgenologic or histologic deterioration was noted in any of the patients nor was any increase in ectopic or vascular calcification detected.

Fleming, Lenman and Stewart [49] concluded that nerve conduction improved when the plasma magnesium concentrations of patients with chronic renal failure undergoing maintenance hemodialysis were reduced by treatment with a dialysate containing a low concentration of magnesium. In the present study a peripheral neuropathy developed in one patient but the nerve conduction in the remaining patients did not alter at a time when plasma magnesium concentrations increased significantly. Thus this study on a small number of patients failed to confirm that magnesium is a major factor in the pathogenesis of uremic neuropathy, although the possibility remains that it may be of importance to a particular subject.

The three patients treated with 1-alpha-hydroxycholecalciferol were selected for this therapy because of the histologic features of osteomalacia observed in the bone biopsy samples and the rapid rate of skeletal demineralization quantitated by the activation technic during the 18 months before treatment was started (Figure 1). Therapy with 1-alpha-hydroxycholecalciferol was evaluated for five months. The reversal of the demineralizing process in all three patients studied is a significant result (Table III). The rate at which the calcium content of the hands increased in patients previously refractory to therapy with calcium supplements alone, suggests that the vitamin D derivative was effective in reversing the demineralizing process.

In this study it was shown that 1-alpha-hydroxycholecalciferol in doses of 1 μg to 4 μg/day is effective in promoting the deposition of calcium in bone. Symptomatic hypercalcemia developed in one patient (Case 3). The rapid reduction in plasma calcium concentration to normal levels when therapy was temporarily stopped is of clinical importance as it may indicate that the toxic effects of inadvertent overdosage are of short duration. If confirmed, this would represent a substantial advantage over conventional vitamin D therapy.

ACKNOWLEDGMENT

We wish to thank Dr. E. Kodicek, Strangeways Laboratories, Cambridge, Dr. B. Pelc, M.R.C. Mineral Metabolism Unit, Leeds, for supplies of 1-alpha-hydroxycholecalciferol; Professor J. Mallard, Mr. J. A. R. McIntoch, Dr. K. Ettinger and Dr. P. Sharp, Department of Medical Physics, University of Aberdeen for encouragement and facilities; Dr. A. MacDonald, Department of Radiology, Dr. T. Anderson and Dr. A. Fraser, Department of Pathology for assistance, Dr. A. W. Downie, Department of Medicine for performing nerve conduction studies and Miss K. Deans for technical help.

REFERENCES

1. Virchow R: Kalk-metastasen. Arch Pathol Anat Physiol 8: 103, 1855.
2. Fletcher HM: Case of infantilism with polyuria and chronic renal disease. Proc R Soc Med 4: 95, 1911.
3. Parsons L: Infantilism associated with chronic interstitial nephritis. Br Med J 2: 481, 1911.
4. Miller, R: Chronic interstitial nephritis with infantilism. Proc R Soc Med 5: 38, 1911.
5. Naish AE: Chronic interstitial nephritis with infantilism—Discussion. Proc R Soc Med 5: 38, 1911.
6. Barber H: The bone deformities of renal dwarfism. Lancet 1: 18, 1920.
7. Shipley PG, Park EA, McCollum EV, Simmonds N: Is there more than one kind of rickets? Am J Dis Child 23: 91, 1922.
8. Barber H: Renal dwarfism. Q J Med 14: 205, 1921.
9. Barber H: Two cases of adolescent rickets. Guy's Hosp Rep 72: 62, 1922.
10. Green CH: Bilateral hypoplastic cystic kidney. Am J Dis Child 24: 1, 1922.
11. Hunt FC: Renal infantilism. Am J Dis Child 34: 234, 1927.
12. Parsons LG: The bone changes occurring in renal and coeliac infantilism and their relationship to rickets. Arch Dis Child 2: 1, 1927.
13. Ogg CS: Parathyroidectomy in the treatment of secondary renal hyperparathyroidism. Kidney Int 4: 168, 1973.
14. Stanbury SW: Azotaemic renal osteodystrophy. Br Med Bull 13: 57, 1957.
15. Dent CE, Harper CM, Philpot GR: Treatment of renal-glomerular osteodystrophy. Q J Med 30: 1, 1961.
16. Fletcher RF, Jones JH, Morgan DF: Bone disease in chronic renal failure. Q J Med 32: 321, 1963.
17. Fraser DR, Kodicek E: Unique biosynthesis by kidney of a biologically active vitamin D metabolite. Nature (Lond) 228: 764, 1970.
18. Boyle IT, Gray RW, Omdahl JL, DeLuca HF: Calcium control of the in vivo biosynthesis of 1,25-dihydroxy-vitamin D_3: Nicholaysen's endogenous factor. Proceedings of the Third International Symposium on Endocrinology, London, Heinemann Medical Books Ltd., 1971.
19. Henderson RG, Russel RGG, Ledingham JGG, Smith R, Oliver DO, Walton RJ, Small DG, Preston C, Warner GT, Norman AW: Effects of 1,25-dihydroxycholecalciferol on calcium absorption, muscle weakness and bone disease in chronic renal failure. Lancet 1: 379, 1974.
20. Catto GRD, MacLeod M, Pelc B, Kodicek E: 1-alpha-hydroxycholecalciferol: a treatment for renal bone disease. Br Med J 1: 12, 1975.
21. DeLuca HF: The kidney as an endocrine organ involved in calcium homeostasis. Kidney Int 4: 80, 1973.
22. Liu SH, Chu HI: Studies of calcium and phosphorus metabolism with special reference of pathogenesis and effects of dihydrotachysterol (A.T.10) and iron. Medicine (Baltimore) 22: 103, 1943.
23. McDonald SJ, Clarkson EM, de Wardener HE: The effect of a large intake of calcium citrate in normal subjects and patients with chronic renal failure. Clin Sci 26: 27, 1964.
24. Clarkson EM, McDonald SJ, de Wardener HE: The effect of a high intake of calcium carbonate in normal subjects and patients with chronic renal failure. Clin Sci 30: 425, 1966.
25. Wing AJ: Optimum calcium concentration of dialysis fluid for maintenance haemodialysis. Br Med J 4: 145, 1968.
26. Goldsmith RS, Furszyfer J, Johnson WJ, Fournier AE, Arnaud CD: Control of secondary hyperparathyroidism during long term haemodialysis. Am J Med 50: 692, 1971.
27. Eastwood JB, Curtis JR, Gower PE, Roberts AP, de Wardener HE: Maintenance Haemodialysis. Lancet 1: 365, 1974.
28. Curtis JR, de Wardener HF, Gower PE, Eastwood JB: The use of calcium carbonate and calcium phosphate without vitamin D in the management of renal osteodystrophy. Proc Eur Dial Transplant Assoc 7: 141, 1970.
29. Pletka P, Bernstein DS, Hampers CL, Merrill JP, Sherwood LM: Effects of magnesium on parathyroid hormone excretion during chronic haemodialysis. Lancet 2: 462, 1971.
30. Heierli C, Hill AVL: The relationship between the magnesium concentration in the dialysis fluid used and in the plasma and erythrocytes of patients with chronic renal failure being treated by regular haemodialysis. Clin Sci 43: 779, 1972.
31. Raisz LG: Parathyroid gland metabolism. Arch Intern Med 124: 389, 1969.
32. Catto GRD, Reid I, MacLeod M: The effect of low magnesium dialysate on plasma, ultrafiltrable, erythrocyte and bone magnesium concentrations from patients on maintenance haemodialysis. Nephron 5: 372, 1974.
33. Willis JB: The determination of metals in blood serum by atomic absorption spectroscopy. Spectrochim Acta 16: 299, 1960.
34. Davies JL, Andrews GS, Miller R, Owen HG: Comparison of the stannous chloride and variadate methods for estimation of serum inorganic phosphorus by use of the "SMA 12/60." Clin Chem. 19: 411, 1973.
35. Kind PRN, King EJ: Estimation of plasma phosphatase by determination of hydrolysed phenol with aminoantipyrine. J Clin Pathol 7: 322, 1954.
36. Bruyn GW, Mink CJK, Calje JF: Biochemical studies in Huntington's chorea: erythrocyte magnesium. Neurology (Minneap.) 15: 455, 1965.
37. Pybus J: Determination of calcium and magnesium in serum and urine by atomic absorption spectrophotometry. Clin

Chim Acta 23: 309, 1969.
38. Williams JA, Nicholson GI: An improved biopsy drill for outpatient use. Lancet 1: 1408, 1963.
39. Tripp EJ, MacKay EH: Silver staining of bone prior to decalcification for quantitative determination of osteoid in sections. Stain Technol 47: 129, 1972.
40. Catto GRD, MacIntosh JAR, MacLeod M: Partial body neutron activation analysis in vivo: a new approach to the investigation of metabolic bone disease. Phys Med Biol 18: 508, 1973.
41. McCance RA, Widdowson EM: The composition of food. Special Report Series (H.M.S.O.) No. 297, 1960.
42. Danesh BJNZ, Walker CHM, Mathers P: The relationship of post dialysis plasma calcium and magnesium to the dialysate levels and to changes in blood pH. N Engl J Med 282: 771, 1970.
43. Davidson S, Passmore R, Brock JF: Human Nutrition and Dietetics, 5th ed, Edinburgh and London, U.K., Churchill Livingstone, 1972.
44. Catto GRD, McIntosh JAR, MacDonald AF, MacLeod M: Haemodialysis therapy and changes in skeletal calcium. Lancet 1: 1150, 1973.
45. Clarkson EM, Eastwood JB, Koutasaimainis KG, de Wardener HF: Net intestinal absorption of calcium in patients with chronic renal failure. Kidney Int 3: 258, 1973.
46. Coburn JW, Koppel MH, Brickman AS, Massry SG: Study of intestinal absorption of calcium in patients with renal failure. Kidney Int 3: 264, 1973.
47. Ginsburg DS, Kaplan EL, Katz AI: Hypercalcaemia after oral calcium carbonate therapy in patients on chronic haemodialysis. Lancet 1: 1271, 1973.
48. Stanbury SW: Azotaemic renal osteodystrophy. Clin Endocrinol Metab 1: 267, 1971.
49. Fleming LW, Lenman JAR, Stewart WK: Effect of magnesium on nerve conduction velocity during regular dialysis treatment. J Neurol Neurosurg Psychiat 35: 342, 1972.

Effects of an Inhaled Bronchodilator on Gas Distribution and Over-All Ventilatory Efficiency in Patients with Chronic Obstructive Pulmonary Disease

ANTONIO CUTILLO, M.D.
RODOLFO PERONDI, M.D.
MAURIZIO TURIEL, M.D.
STEFANO MONTI, M.D.
Milan, Italy

The effects of an inhaled bronchodilator on the distribution of inspired gas and over-all efficiency of ventilation were studied by the nitrogen washout technic in 16 patients with chronic obstructive pulmonary disease; three normal subjects and two patients with asymptomatic asthma (and normal spirometric values) were also studied. In normal and asthmatic subjects and in patients with chronic obstructive pulmonary disease and mild to moderate functional impairment, the nitrogen clearance did not vary significantly or showed changes suggesting less uniform gas distribution and reduced ventilatory efficiency. In most patients with advanced chronic obstructive pulmonary disease, the bronchodilator caused changes suggesting more uniform distribution of inspired gas and increased efficiency of ventilation. Multiple regression analysis showed that the behavior of the nitrogen clearance after treatment was also related to the response of the anatomic dead space. The effects of the bronchodilator varied with time. The results are consistent with the assumption that the changes in nitrogen clearance after bronchodilator therapy reflect the concourse of multiple factors, which may be expected to have favorable or unfavorable effects on the distribution of inspired gas and the efficiency of ventilation.

Although the pulmonary function response to bronchodilators has been studied extensively in patients with chronic obstructive pulmonary disease, there are relatively few reports regarding the effects of these drugs on intrapulmonary distribution of ventilation. The available data mainly concern the response of regional ventilation, measured with radioactive gas methods [1,2] or estimated from the behavior of the alveolar nitrogen plateau [3,4]. Little is known about the over-all effect of the regional changes on ventilatory efficiency following bronchodilator therapy. On the other hand, theoretical considerations and experimental results suggest that contrasting factors (such as the decrease in airway resistance and the increase in anatomic dead space) may concur to determine the effect of bronchodilators on distribution and efficiency of ventilation [5]. Although an added dead space has been shown to affect pulmonary nitrogen clearance [6], the relative importance of an increased anatomic dead space in response to bronchodilator therapy has not been estimated.

This study was thus designed to investigate the effects of an inhaled bronchodilator on the regional distribution of inspired gas and over-all

From the Istituto di Clinica Medica II and Istituto di Ricerche Cardiovascolari, University of Milan; and Centro di Ricerche Cardiovascolari, Consiglio Nazionale delle Ricerche, Milan, Italy. Requests for reprints should be addressed to Dr. Antonio Cutillo, Istituto di Clinica Medica II and Istituto di Ricerche Cardiovascolari, Via Francesco Sforza, 35, 20122 Milano (Italy). Manuscript accepted November 24, 1975.

efficiency of ventilation in patients with chronic obstructive pulmonary disease. The response of the anatomic dead space to the bronchodilator was also studied, with particular reference to its relationship to the changes in gas distribution and ventilatory efficiency. Other factors to which these changes may be related (degree of respiratory impairment, time course of response and time of testing, inhalation technic, etc.) were considered. These factors may also be of practical importance in the clinical assessment of bronchodilator therapy.

METHODS

The main group of subjects consisted of 16 patients with mild to advanced chronic obstructive pulmonary disease; three normal subjects and two patients with bronchial asthma were also studied. At the time of study, the asthmatic patients were asymptomatic; their spirometric values fell within the normal range. The spirometric data obtained in our subjects are given in Table I; the functional residual capacity (FRC) was measured by the closed circuit helium method. Other measurements of FRC were made during the studies of response to the bronchodilator, using the nitrogen dilution method. Predicted values were calculated from the equations of Goldman and Becklake [7] for the static lung volumes, and Berglund et al. [8] for the forced expiratory volume in one second (FEV_1). The subjects were studied in the seated position.

The distribution of inspired gas and the efficiency of ventilation were studied by the open-circuit nitrogen washout technic. The subject inspired from a bag containing from 150 to 200 liters of oxygen. The expired gas was collected in a recording Tissot spirometer. The nitrogen concentration of respired gas sampled at the mouthpiece was continuously measured with a nitrogen meter (Nitralyzer, Model 300 AR), calibrated with standard gas mixtures. To allow continuous control of the breathing pattern, inspiratory flow was measured by a flowmeter connected to a differential pressure transducer (Statham, PM 5), and a volume tracing was obtained by electrical integration of the flow signal; the volume tracing was automatically zeroed by a relay at the end of each inspiration. The nitrogen concentration and volume tracings were displayed on the multitrace oscilloscope screen of a polygraph (Electronics for Medicine, Model DR-8) and photographically recorded. The volume tracing was also reproduced on an oscilloscope (DuMont, Type 322-A) placed in front of the subject. The breathing of oxygen was started at the end of a normal expiration and was continued until the end-tidal nitrogen concentration reached a minimum value (less than 1 per cent) and remained relatively constant. At the end of the washout, the subject delivered a maximal expiration to give a sample of alveolar gas.

The washout data were corrected for inspired nitrogen concentration and tissue nitrogen elimination. The lung clearance index [9] was calculated as the total ventilation of oxygen, per unit FRC, required to reduce the end-tidal nitrogen concentration to 1.5 per cent [10]. The value of FRC was obtained from the total volume and the nitrogen concentration of gas collected in the Tissot spirometer, with a correction for the "alveolar" nitrogen concentration at the end of the washout. The nitrogen washout curves (semilogarithmic plots of end-tidal nitrogen concentration versus breaths number) were analyzed by the methods of Fowler et al. [11] and Briscoe and Cournand [12], and the pulmonary clearance delay [11] was estimated.

TABLE I Physical Characteristics and Spirometric Data

Case No.	Sex and Age (yr)	VC (% predicted)	RV (% predicted)	TLC (% predicted)	FEV_1 (% predicted)
Patients with Chronic Obstructive Pulmonary Disease					
1	M, 67	77	201	128	57
2	M, 68		140		
3	M, 69	83	121	102	56
4	M, 61	90	100	100	50
5	M, 62	88	219	137	26
6	M, 42	97	119	111	54
7	M, 60	38	163	83	17
8	F, 57	100	147	118	73
9	F, 25	31	176	75	13
10	F, 42	72	190	113	
11	M, 64	71	100	89	69
12	M, 72	48	105	80	26
13	M, 49	102	93	100	73
14	F, 28	86	193	117	41
15	M, 55	89	237	144	58
16	M, 64	88	165	118	42
Patients with Asymptomatic Asthma					
17	M, 26	114	105	109	88
18	F, 62	92	101	98	85
Normal Subjects					
19	M, 51	90	91	91	75
20	M, 54	80	119	95	81
21	F, 65	75	119	93	73

NOTE: VC = vital capacity; RV = residual volume; TLC = total lung capacity; FEV_1 = forced expiratory volume in 1 second.

The volume of the anatomic dead space was determined in 14 subjects (two normal subjects and 12 patients with chronic obstructive pulmonary disease). The tidal volume was measured using a spirometer equipped with a potentiometer or by integration of the flow signal. The carbon dioxide concentration of respired gas was continuously measured with an infrared analyzer. Tidal volume and carbon dioxide concentration were simultaneously recorded by the DR-8 poligraph. After correction for the response time of the carbon dioxide analyzer, the tracings were analyzed according to the graphic method of Fowler [13]. Each value of anatomic dead space was calculated as the average of five or more determinations.

In seven subjects (one normal subject and six patients with chronic obstructive pulmonary disease) pulmonary resistance was also measured by a method of electrical subtraction [14], using an esophageal balloon to estimate pleural pressure [15]. Each value of pulmonary resistance was obtained from the analysis of at least five pressure-flow tracings, photographically recorded by the DR-8 poligraph.

The subjects were required not to take bronchodilators for at least 8 hours before the study. They were preliminarily familiarized with the apparatus and instructed to breathe regularly with the aid of the inspiratory volume tracing. Control determinations were carried out in the following order: (1) pulmonary resistance and/or (2) anatomic dead space; (3) nitrogen washout. The determinations were repeated in the

TABLE II Pulmonary Resistance, Anatomic Dead Space and Nitrogen Washout Data Before and After Orciprenaline Inhalation

Case No.	Study Period*	R_L (cm H_2O/liter/sec)	V_D:V_T (%)	V_T (liters)	Frequency (breaths/min)	FRC (liters)	LCI	PCD (%)
				Patients with Chronic Obstructive Pulmonary Disease				
1	C	7.8		0.517	20	6.175	17.9	369
	B	8.2		0.550	20	6.626	14.6	206
2	C		29	0.536	24	4.004	17.1	186
	B		26	0.460	24	4.110	13.9	176
3	C	5.9	29	0.657	21	5.670	14.9	162
	B	3.3†	30	0.721	22	5.354	13.8	202
4	C		19	0.951	11	2.966	11.0	58
	B		17	0.882	13	2.593	12.4	87
5	C		19	0.527	23	3.966	20.6	388
	B (15′)			0.522	27	3.929	23.7	436
	(50′)		23	0.484	29	3.966	19.0	294
6	C		33	0.645	26	3.395	13.1	91
	B		34	0.723	31	4.483	14.0	167
7	C		32	0.666	14	4.508	19.4	331
	B		38‡	0.641	13	4.126	20.1	410
8	C	9.5		0.449	17	2.683	13.3	405
	B	5.9†		0.448	18	2.730	13.1	133
9	C		40	0.374	29	3.260	53.1	1,108
	B		42	0.391	30	3.280	45.1	838
10	C		19	0.500	16	2.547	12.2	165
	B		19	0.494	18	2.491	12.1	174
11	C	3.1	29	0.506	20	2.597	17.3	174
	B (14′)			0.563	20	3.128	17.5	227
	(72′)	3.0	33‡	0.549	21	3.605	15.9	186
	(157′)			0.518	20	3.288	13.7	173
12	C		34	0.457	20	2.751	26.4	586
	B		42†	0.489	22	2.876	26.2	747
13	C			0.876	9	3.074	8.0	148
	B			0.903	9	2.914	9.5	224
14	C			0.777	15	3.110	20.4	167
	B			0.917	15	2.802	19.2	55
15	C	5.5	27	1.213	11	4.159	11.3	47
	B	4.4‡	31	1.272	10	4.495	11.3	52
16	C	2.9	31	0.831	17	3.921	13.5	168
	B (27′)	2.5	38†	0.766	19	4.055	15.3	149
	(64′)	2.4†	37†	0.859	18	4.251	14.6	164
	(89′)	2.0†	36†	0.855	18	3.961	12.4	99
	(145′)		34‡	0.942	18	4.087	13.3	115
				Patients with Asymptomatic Asthma				
17	C			0.440	24	3.287	11.9	100
	B			0.497	24	3.659	14.8	103
18	C			0.569	18	2.227	8.8	26
	B			0.547	19	2.119	9.5	41
				Normal Subjects				
19	C	3.8		1.459	14	1.675	9.3	56
	B	3.7		1.219	13	1.503	10.7	166
20	C		23	0.725	13	3.217	7.6	34
	B		22	0.648	15	2.780	8.4	18
21	C		22	0.550	19	2.490	8.6	
	B		22	0.554	19	2.171	8.9	

NOTE: R_L = pulmonary resistance; V_D:V_T = dead space:tidal volume ratio; V_T = tidal volume; FRC = functional residual capacity; LCI = lung clearance index; PCD = pulmonary clearance delay.

*C = control; B = after bronchodilator. For the subjects studied with multiple nitrogen washout determinations, the respective testing times are also reported (data in parentheses); the associated values of R_L and V_D:V_T were obtained 10 to 20 minutes before the times indicated. Values of V_T, frequency and FRC are those measured during the nitrogen washout determinations. Significance of differences between mean values of R_L or V_D:V_T (analysis of variance); bronchodilator versus control.

†P <0.01.

‡P <0.05.

same order after inhalation of 1 ml of 2 per cent orciprenaline (metaproterenol sulfate, Alupent®). The bronchodilator was administered using a nebulizer (Bird Micronebulizer) driven by compressed air. Generally, pulmonary resistance and/or anatomic dead space were measured from 10 to 15 minutes after the administration of the aerosol. The nitrogen washout was started 40 to 50 minutes after inhalation. In three patients repeated measurements of the lung clearance index and pulmonary clearance delay were performed at various intervals from inhalation, to study the time course of the response to the bronchodilator. In five experiments performed in four patients anatomic dead space, lung clearance index and pulmonary clearance delay were also determined before and after inhalation of 1 ml of distilled water or saline solution by the same technic used for the bronchodilator studies.

The experimental data were analyzed by current statistical methods [16].

RESULTS

The nitrogen washout data obtained before and after inhalation of orciprenaline are given in Table II. Generally, the bronchodilator caused no important changes in tidal volume, respiratory frequency and FRC. The

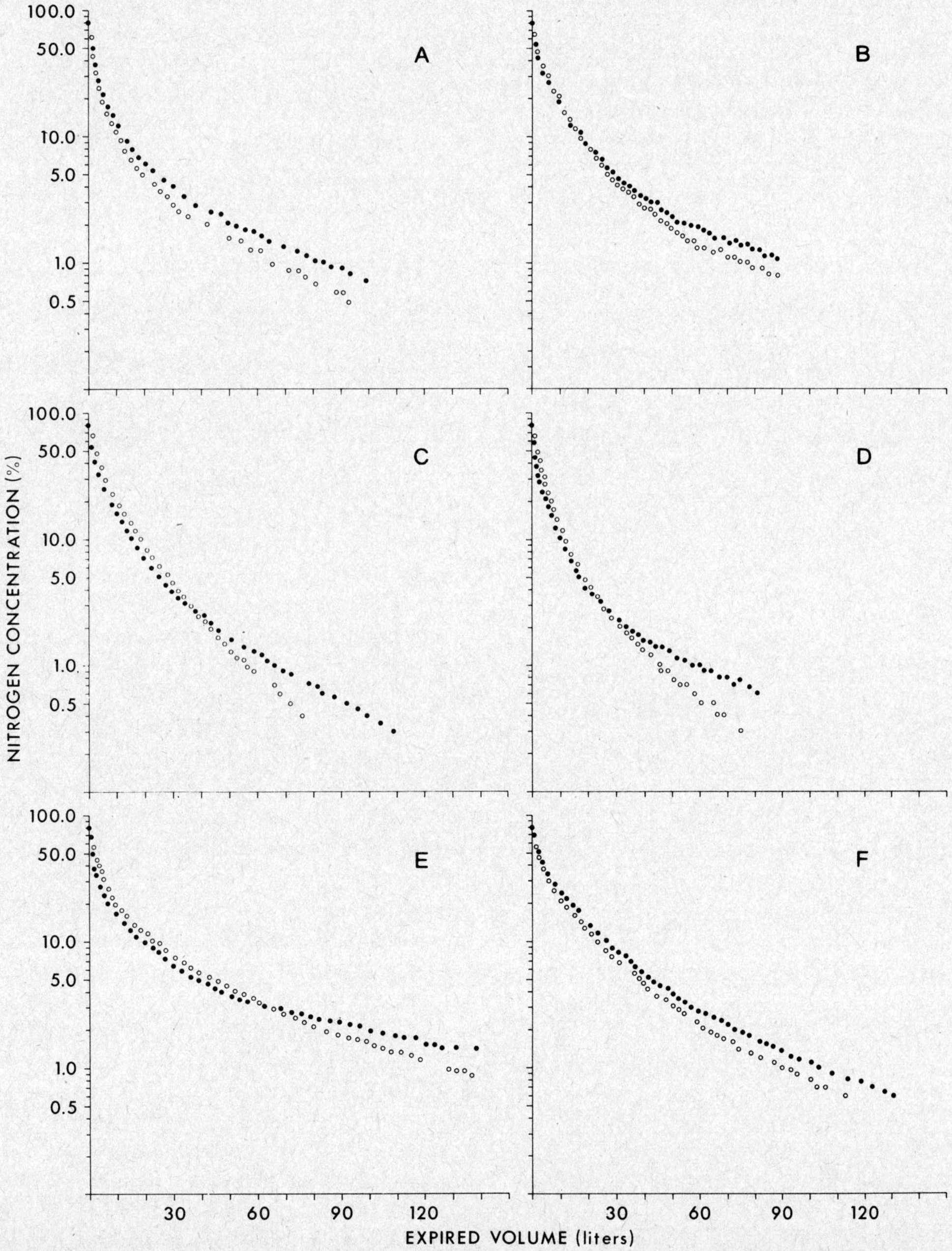

Figure 1. *Nitrogen washout curves before and after orciprenaline inhalation in six patients with chronic obstructive pulmonary disease.* ● *control;* ○ *after bronchodilator. A, Case 14. B, Case 2. C, Case 16. D, Case 8. E, Case 1. F, Case 3.*

response of lung clearance index and pulmonary clearance delay was found to be related to the degree of functional impairment (as expressed by spirometric and lung mechanics data, control values of lung clearance index, pulmonary clearance delay and other pulmonary function data). In the subjects with normal pulmonary function tests (including the two asthmatic subjects) and in those with chronic obstructive pulmonary disease and mild to moderate functional impairment, the lung clearance index and pulmonary clearance delay showed no significant changes or a moderate increase (indicating less uniform distribution of inspired gas and reduced efficiency of ventilation). In most patients with advanced chronic obstructive pulmonary disease a decrease in the lung clearance index and/or pulmonary clearance delay was found (more uniform gas distribution and increased efficiency of ventilation). The washout curves obtained in six of these patients are shown in Figure 1. The absolute change in the lung clearance index was correlated with the pretreatment values of the lung clearance index (correlation coefficient, r = −0.844, P <0.01) and pulmonary clearance delay (r = −0.765, P <0.01), and with the values of vital capacity (VC), expressed as per cent predicted (r = 0.612, P <0.01) and FEV_1, per cent predicted (r = 0.508, P <0.05). The change in pulmonary clearance delay was correlated with the control values of the lung clearance index (r = −0.490, P <0.05) and pulmonary clearance delay (r = −0.530, P <0.05). In most experiments the lung clearance index and pulmonary clearance delay showed a concordant behavior after the administration of bronchodilator. In some subjects, the pulmonary clearance delay increased or decreased whereas the lung clearance index did not change appreciably; in other experiments the lung clearance index only was found to vary after bronchodilator treatment. However, no important discrepancies between the two indexes (for instance, a marked decrease in pulmonary clearance delay associated with a marked increase in the lung clearance index) were observed in the present investigation.

TABLE III Volume and Alveolar Ventilation of the Slow Space Before and After Orciprenaline Inhalation in Patients with Chronic Obstructive Pulmonary Disease

Case No.	Study Period*	Volume (% total lung volume)	Alveolar Ventilation per Unit Lung Volume (times/min)
1	C	60	0.14
	B	49	0.17
2	C	44	0.29
	B	31	0.26
3	C	47	0.31
	B	41	0.38
4	C	49	0.81
	B	46	0.72
5	C	53	0.21
	B (15′)	49	0.17
	(50′)	41	0.22
6	C	45	1.03
	B	54	0.85
7	C	35	0.17
	B	37	0.27
8	C	53	0.19
	B	57	0.19
9	C	71	0.06
	B	64	0.09
10	C	37	0.36
	B	24	0.28
11	C	42	0.39
	B (14′)	46	0.35
	(72′)	49	0.35
	(157′)	42	0.37
12	C	45	0.12
	B	46	0.10
13	C	23	0.26
	B	30	0.20
14	C	40	0.29
	B	21	1.13
15	C	55	0.76
	B	50	0.64
16	C	47	0.42
	B (27′)	51	0.54
	(64′)	57	0.61
	(89′)	53	0.77
	(145′)	51	0.71

*C = control; B = after bronchodilator. For the subjects studied with multiple determinations, the testing times are reported in parentheses.

In accordance with the data presented, the analysis of the washout curve on the basis of the multicompartment model described by Fowler et al. [11] and by Briscoe and Cournand [12] did not show a uniform pattern of response to the bronchodilator. The slope of the slow component of the curve increased in some subjects (suggesting increased ventilation of poorly ventilated lung spaces) and decreased or remained unchanged in others. The data concerning the behavior of the poorly ventilated lung compartment (slow space) in the patients with chronic obstructive pulmonary disease are presented in Table III. The fast and intermediate components (mainly reflecting the nitrogen clearance of more ventilated lung spaces) also showed a variable response to the bronchodilator.

After orciprenaline inhalation, the value of the ratio of dead space to tidal volume (V_D:V_T, expressing V_D as per cent of V_T) increased in some subjects and remained unchanged in others (Table II). No simple correlation was found between the changes in distribution and efficiency of ventilation and the response of dead space. However, the multiple regression analysis showed that the change in the lung clearance index after bronchodilator treatment was related to the control value of the lung clearance index or pulmonary clearance delay (P <0.01), as already indicated by the simple correlation coefficient, and to the change in V_D:V_T ratio (P <0.05). The regression equations were Y = 2.208

$- 0.202 X_1 + 0.218 X_2$ (Y = absolute change in lung clearance index, X_1 = control value of lung clearance index and X_2 = absolute change in $V_D:V_T$ ratio) and $Y = 0.475 - 0.008 X_1 + 0.313 X_2$ (Y and X_2 as above, X_1 = control value of pulmonary clearance delay).

The data concerning the time course of the response of the lung clearance index and pulmonary clearance delay to orciprenaline in three patients with chronic obstructive pulmonary disease are reported in Table II and illustrated in Figure 2. In these patients, the lung clearance index and pulmonary clearance delay increased initially (within 15 to 30 minutes from inhalation) and then decreased, the whole duration of the effect being at least 1 to 2 hours. The response of pulmonary clearance delay was substantially similar to that of the lung clearance index. In Figure 3, the changes in lung clearance index and pulmonary clearance delay observed in one patient at various times from orciprenaline inhalation are compared with the response of anatomic dead space, pulmonary resistance and heart rate.

The inhalation of distilled water or saline solution caused no significant changes in V_T, respiratory frequency and FRC. After inhalation, one patient showed an appreciable increase in pulmonary clearance delay (130 per cent) and lung clearance index (15 per cent), and one patient showed an increase in pulmonary clearance delay (61 per cent). A significant decrease in the $V_D:V_T$ ratio (from 33 per cent to 28 per cent) was found in another experiment. The pulmonary clearance delay, lung clearance index and the $V_D:V_T$ ratio did not change appreciably in the remaining subjects.

COMMENTS

In the present investigation, the response of the lung clearance index and the pulmonary clearance delay could not be tested statistically in individual subjects

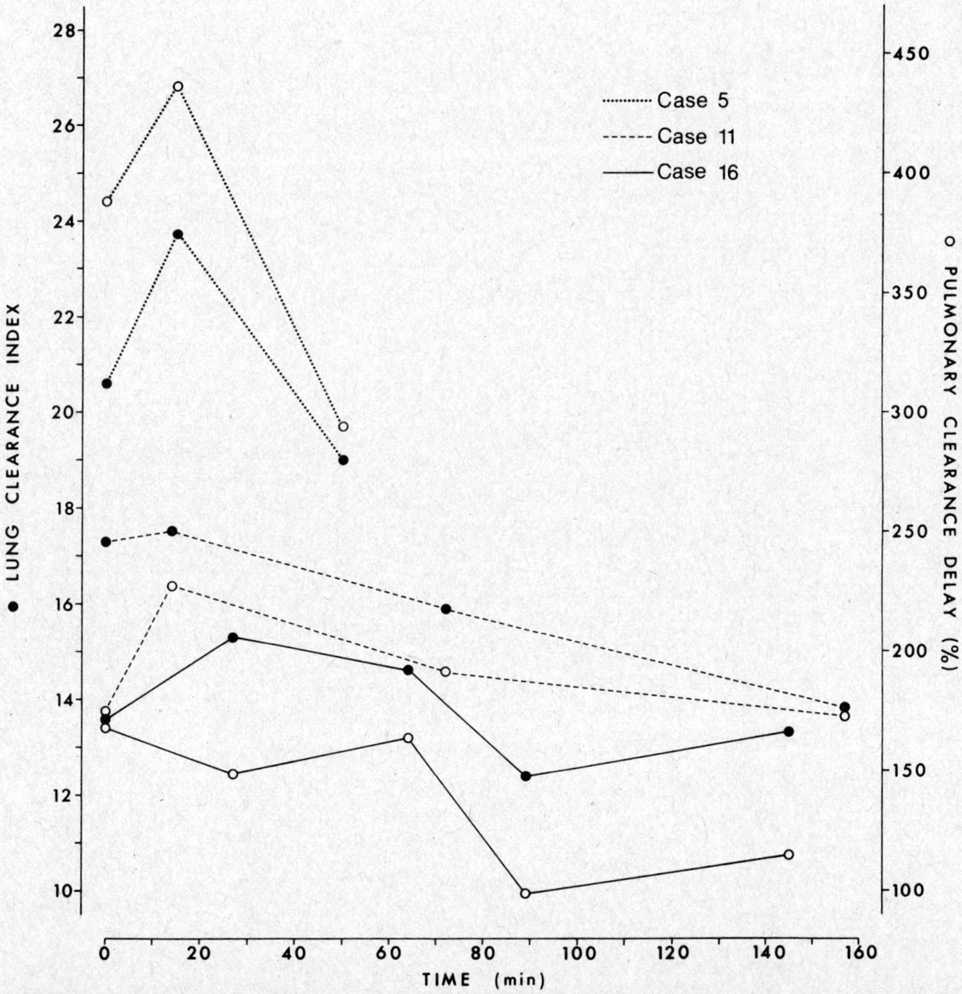

Figure 2. Time course of the changes in lung clearance index and pulmonary clearance delay observed after orciprenaline inhalation in three patients with chronic obstructive pulmonary disease. ● *lung clearance index;* ○ *pulmonary clearance delay.*

because the duration of the nitrogen washout precluded a procedure based on multiple determinations. However, separate studies performed to estimate the reproducibility of the nitrogen washout data showed that the per cent difference between repeated measurements was, on the average, 7.6 ± 4.9 per cent for lung clearance index and 23.4 ± 12.7 per cent for pulmonary clearance delay. On the basis of these data, it appeared reasonable to assume that a change in lung clearance index ≥ 15 per cent and a change in pulmonary clearance delay ≥ 40 per cent (with the exception of the values of pulmonary clearance delay close to zero) were probably significant. According to these criteria, one would conclude that the lung clearance index and/or pulmonary clearance delay decreased, after bronchodilator therapy, in seven patients with chronic obstructive pulmonary disease and increased or remained unchanged in the other subjects.

Watanabe et al. [2] found that the ventilation of individual lung regions may increase, decrease or remain unchanged after inhalation of isoproterenol. These investigators concluded that the over-all response to the bronchodilator, estimated on the basis of changes simultaneously occurring in six lung regions, was "unfavorable" in all but one of their patients with asthma or chronic obstructive pulmonary disease. Our data suggest that in chronic obstructive pulmonary disease an increase in over-all efficiency of ventilation after inhalation of a bronchodilator is more common than indirectly estimated on the basis of regional function studies. This conclusion is supported by the results of the analysis of the washout curve according to the multicompartment model, suggesting that the favorable effects of orciprenaline on over-all ventilatory efficiency may reflect changes in the relative volume as well as in the ventilation of the various lung compartments;

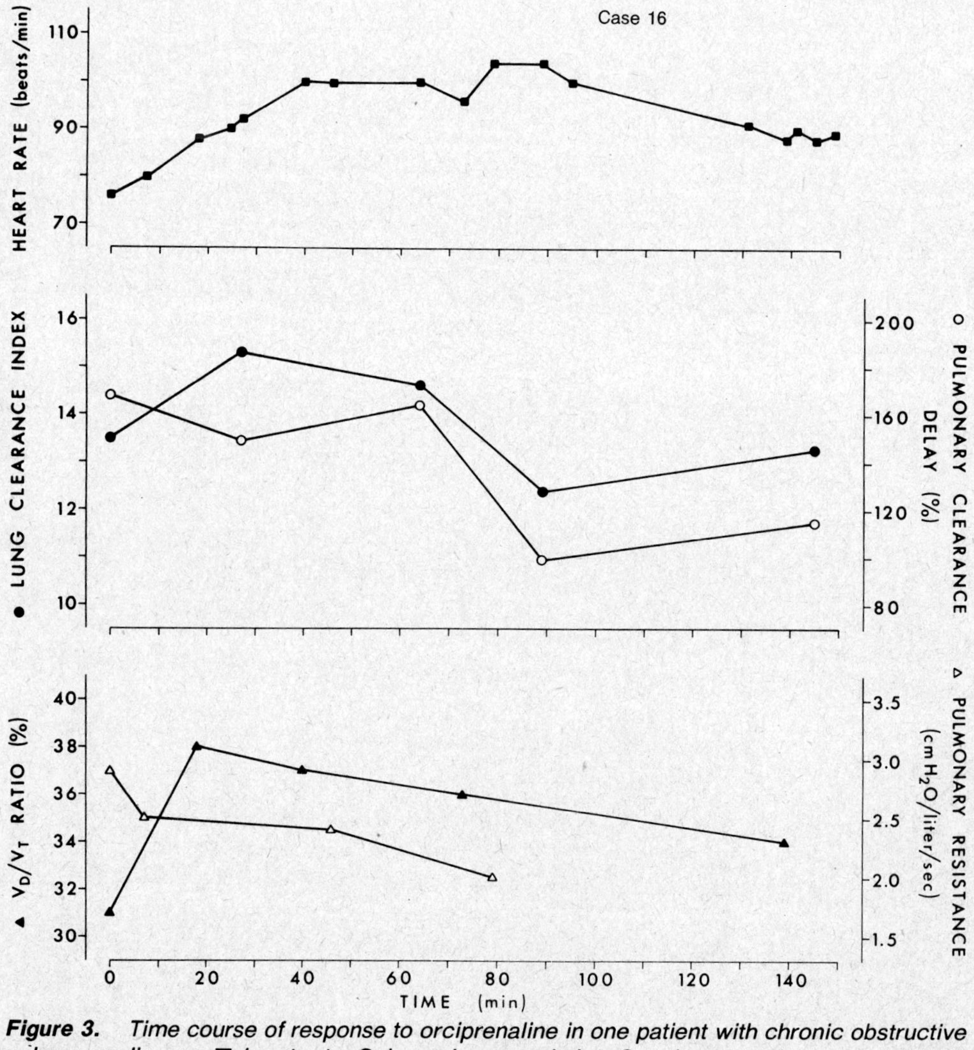

Figure 3. *Time course of response to orciprenaline in one patient with chronic obstructive pulmonary disease.* ■ *heart rate;* ● *lung clearance index;* ○ *pulmonary clearance delay;* ▲ V_D:V_T *ratio;* △ *pulmonary resistance.*

similar data have been obtained by McFadden and Lyons [17] in asthmatic subjects. However, the discrepancy between our results and those of Watanabe et al. [2] may partly be due to differences concerning the bronchodilator used, the dose administered and the patients studied (in the present investigation the effect of the bronchodilator therapy on the distribution of inspired gas and efficiency of ventilation was found to be related to the severity of pulmonary impairment).

The variable response to inhaled bronchodilators may be explained by assuming that the effect of these drugs on regional distribution of inspired gas and efficiency of ventilation results from the interaction of several contrasting factors. In an unevenly ventilated lung the bronchodilator treatment may be expected to have favorable effects on the distribution and efficiency of ventilation to the extent that it causes a decrease in the resistance of poorly ventilated units and, consequently, an increase in the ventilation of these units [2]. In accordance with this view, our data indicate that the beneficial effects of orciprenaline on over-all ventilatory efficiency mainly reflect an increased ventilation and/or a decreased volume of the poorly ventilated compartment. On the other hand, it is likely that in patients with obstructive pulmonary disease inhaled bronchodilators preferentially follow low-resistance pathways and are mainly delivered to well ventilated lung units [18]. Such regional distribution of the aerosol may result in an increased unevenness and reduced efficiency of ventilation.

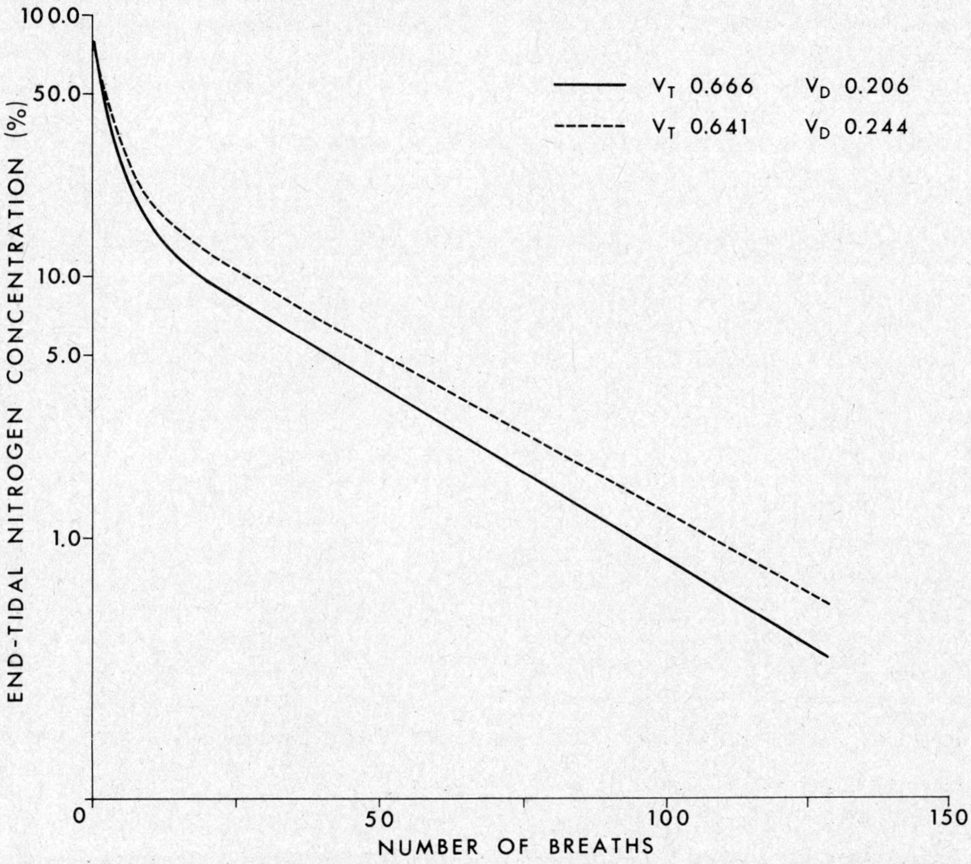

Figure 4. *Effect of anatomic dead space on nitrogen clearance in an unevenly ventilated lung model consisting of two parallel units with a common dead space. The nitrogen washout curves illustrated in the figure were obtained from equation 2 of Nye [25], for the values of tidal volume and dead space:tidal volume ratio observed in one patient before and after orciprenaline inhalation. The distribution of inspired gas between the two units was assumed to be markedly uneven, with the poorly ventilated compartment (75 per cent of the total volume of the lung model) receiving only 15 per cent of the total tidal volume. This pattern of gas distribution was common to both nitrogen washout curves. Thus, the differences between the two curves could be almost entirely attributed to the value of anatomic dead space. Other assumptions concerning the lung model were made according to Nye [25]. As calculated from the theoretic nitrogen washout curves, the increase in dead space was associated with an increase in lung clearance index (from 12.7 to 14.1) and a decrease in pulmonary clearance delay (from 157 per cent to 133 per cent).*

As shown by the multiple regression analysis, the effect of orciprenaline on the lung clearance index was also related to the behavior of the $V_D:V_T$ ratio. This finding, which suggests that a post-treatment increase in the $V_D:V_T$ ratio tends to increase the value of the lung clearance index (that is, to decrease the efficiency of ventilation), is consistent with theoretic and experimental data concerning the influence of anatomic dead space on the nitrogen clearance in a parallel ventilated lung model [6,19–21] (Figure 4). No relationship could be demonstrated between the effect of the bronchodilator on pulmonary clearance delay and the response of the $V_D:V_T$ ratio. An increase in the $V_D:V_T$ ratio might be expected to decrease the value of pulmonary clearance delay [6,20] (Figure 4); presumably, this possible effect of dead space was concealed by the influence of other factors.

The data obtained in normal subjects and in patients with asymptomatic asthma or mild chronic obstructive pulmonary disease (no significant changes or slight increase in the lung clearance index and pulmonary clearance delay after bronchodilator) may reflect the influence of an increase in the anatomic dead space and a preferential distribution of the aerosol to better ventilated lung spaces. Presumably, these unfavorable consequences of bronchodilator treatment tend to counterbalance the effects of mechanical changes promoting a better distribution of ventilation. On the contrary, the influence of factors favorably affecting gas distribution may prevail in patients with advanced chronic obstructive pulmonary disease.

The results concerning the time course of the changes in the lung clearance index and pulmonary clearance delay after orciprenaline inhalation suggest that the relative importance of the factors involved in the response to bronchodilators may vary with time. Enlargement of the anatomic dead space and preferential aerosol distribution may be responsible for the early increase in lung clearance index and pulmonary clearance delay. In conformity with this hypothesis, the analysis of the nitrogen washout curves according to the multicompartment model suggested an increased ventilation of the fast spaces with little changes in the behavior of the slow space. Conversely, the relatively late decrease in the lung clearance index and pulmonary clearance delay appears to reflect an increase in the ventilation of poorly ventilated lung units, as suggested by the analysis of the washout curve, which showed an increased ventilation or reduced volume of the slow compartment. This favorable effect of orciprenaline might be partly due to that fraction of the inhaled dose which is absorbed by the patient. The observation that the maximum decrease in the lung clearance index and pulmonary clearance delay was coincident with the maximum effect of the bronchodilator on heart rate (Figure 3) appears to be consistent with this contention. The absorbed bronchodilator may be expected not to act preferentially on the well ventilated lung spaces, so that an appreciable increase in the ventilation of the poorly ventilated units seems conceivable at this stage.

As shown in Table II, the response of the lung clearance index and pulmonary clearance delay to the bronchodilator was not necessarily associated with significant changes in pulmonary resistance and/or $V_D:V_T$ ratio; on the other hand, in some subjects pulmonary resistance decreased and/or $V_D:V_T$ increased whereas the lung clearance index and pulmonary clearance delay did not change significantly. Similar data concerning the response of several pulmonary function tests to bronchodilators or other bronchoactive agents have been reported [22–25]. The discrepancy observed in the present study may be partly due to errors of measurement and to differences in sensitivity of the various indexes. Furthermore, it seems likely that this finding to some extent reflects the discussed influence of bronchodilator-induced changes in lung mechanics and dead space volume on over-all ventilatory efficiency. However, on the basis of published data [17,26—30], the discrepancy may also be explained by assuming that the changes in the lung clearance index, pulmonary clearance delay, pulmonary resistance and anatomic dead space reflect responses occurring at different levels of the bronchial tree. The decrease in the lung clearance index and pulmonary clearance delay observed in some subjects may, to a large extent, be due to the effect of orciprenaline on peripheral airways, whereas the increase in anatomic dead space and the decrease in pulmonary resistance are likely to reflect the response of the large airways.

The clinical and therapeutic implications of the present results deserve some comments. From a practical point of view, it is of interest that the inhalation of orciprenaline may exert beneficial effects on the distribution of inspired gas and efficiency of ventilation in patients with advanced chronic obstructive pulmonary disease. Our findings support the conclusion reached by some investigators [31,32] on the basis of spirometric and lung mechanics measurements, that the administration of bronchodilators should be recommended in the management of chronic obstructive pulmonary disease. As regards bronchial asthma, the present results and those of McFadden and Lyons [17] suggest that the bronchodilators favorably affect the distribution and efficiency of ventilation when inhaled during acute attacks of bronchospasm whereas, in this respect, they are apparently of no benefit in asymptomatic patients with normal spirometric values. The increase in lung clearance index and pulmonary clearance delay observed in some subjects after orciprenaline inhalation appears to be of little clinical significance, compared with the favorable mechanical effects of the bronchodilator treatment. No immediate adverse reactions to orciprenaline, excepting a generally moderate increase in heart rate, were noted in the present experiments. However, the systematic use of bronchodilators might be limited by adverse effects, especially those resulting from stimulation of cardiovascular receptors.

Mushin [33] found that the effect of nebulized orciprenaline on FEV_1 was maximum at 30 to 60 minutes after inhalation. The data of other investigators are substantially similar [34–37]. As pointed out by Mushin [33], the bronchial response to long-acting bronchodilators, such as orciprenaline, should be tested 60 minutes after administration. Our results suggest that the time-factor is even more critical when testing the effect of orciprenaline inhalation on distribution and efficiency of ventilation.

The discrepancy observed between the behavior of the lung clearance index and pulmonary clearance delay after orciprenaline inhalation and the response of pulmonary resistance and anatomic dead space indicate that the effects of bronchodilators on distribution and efficiency of ventilation are not predictable from determinations of the anatomic dead space or airflow resistance and, possibly, from other pulmonary function measurements. However, a large increase in anatomic dead space may be expected to oppose the favorable effects of bronchodilation on ventilatory efficiency.

In accordance with other published data [38–41], our results suggest that nebulized water or saline solution delivered by ordinary aerosol generators may affect the bronchial tone causing bronchoconstriction with regional inequality of gas distribution. It is of interest that the most marked response was observed in a case of chronic obstructive pulmonary disease characterized by frequent attacks of bronchospasm. The possible adverse effects of nebulized water or saline solution should be taken into account when therapeutic measures involving inhalation of nebulized mists are instituted in patients with chronic obstructive pulmonary disease, especially when bronchial hyperreactivity is present.

SUMMARY

The effects of an inhaled bronchodilator on the distribution of inspired gas and over-all efficiency of ventilation were studied by the nitrogen washout technic in 16 patients with chronic obstructive pulmonary disease; three normal subjects and two patients with asymptomatic asthma (and normal spirometric values) were also studied. The response of anatomic dead space and/or pulmonary resistance to the bronchodilator was measured in 17 subjects and compared with the behavior of gas distribution and ventilatory efficiency. The effects of orciprenaline on nitrogen clearance were related to the degree of functional impairment. In normal and asthmatic subjects and in patients with chronic obstructive pulmonary disease and mild to moderate functional impairment, the nitrogen clearance did not vary significantly or showed changes suggesting less uniform gas distribution and reduced ventilatory efficiency. In most patients with severe chronic obstructive pulmonary disease the bronchodilator caused changes suggesting more uniform distribution of inspired gas and increased efficiency of ventilation. Multiple regression analysis showed that the behavior of the nitrogen clearance following bronchodilator treatment was also related to the response of the anatomic dead space. No relationship was found between the changes in nitrogen clearance and those in pulmonary resistance. The effect of orciprenaline on gas distribution and efficiency of ventilation was found to vary with time, the whole duration of the response being at least 1 to 2 hours. In two subjects, the inhalation of distilled water or saline solution caused changes in the nitrogen clearance suggesting more uneven gas distribution. The present results are consistent with the assumption that the changes in nitrogen clearance following bronchodilator treatment reflect the concourse of multiple factors, which may be expected to have favorable or unfavorable effects on the distribution of inspired gas and the efficiency of ventilation.

REFERENCES

1. Matthys H, Rühle KH, Schlehe H, Konietzko N, Adam WE: Ventilation-perfusion relationship studied with ^{133}xenon before and after bronchodilating drugs in patients with obstructive lung disease. Bull Physiopathol Respir (Nancy) 8: 599, 1972.
2. Watanabe S, Renzetti AD Jr, Bigler A: Bronchodilator and corticosteroid effects on regional and total airway resistance in patients with asthma, chronic bronchitis, and chronic pulmonary emphysema. Am Rev Respir Dis 106: 392, 1972.
3. Simonsson BG: Clinical and physiological studies on chronic bronchitis. IV. Effect of isoprenaline aerosol on the "alveolar nitrogen plateau." Acta Allergol 20: 349, 1965.
4. Quanjer Ph H, Tammeling GJ: Lung volumes and mixing indices before and after bronchodilation. Bull Physiopathol Respir (Nancy) 8: 591, 1972.
5. Widdicombe JG, Nadel JA: Airway volume, airway resistance, and work and force of breathing: theory. J Appl Physiol 18: 863, 1963.
6. Bouhuys A, Jönsson R, Lundin G: Influence of added dead space on pulmonary ventilation. Acta Physiol Scand 39: 105, 1957.
7. Goldman HI, Becklake MR: Respiratory function tests: normal values at median altitudes and the prediction of normal results. Am Rev Tuberc 79: 457, 1959.
8. Berglund E, Birath G, Bjure J, Grimby G, Kjellmer I, Sandqvist L, Söderholm B: Spirometric studies in normal subjects. I. Forced expirograms in subjects between 7 and 70 years

of age. Acta Med Scand 173: 185, 1963.

9. Becklake MR: A new index of the intrapulmonary mixture of inspired air. Thorax 7: 111, 1952.
10. Cutillo A, Omboni E, Delgrossi S: Effects of respiratory frequency on distribution of inspired gas in normal subjects and in patients with chronic obstructive lung disease. Am Rev Respir Dis 105: 756, 1972.
11. Fowler WS, Cornish ER Jr, Kety SS: Lung function studies: VIII. Analysis of alveolar ventilation by pulmonary N_2 clearance curves. J Clin Invest 31: 40, 1952.
12. Briscoe WA, Cournand A: Uneven ventilation of normal and diseased lungs studied by an open-circuit method, J Appl Physiol 14: 284, 1959.
13. Fowler WS: Lung function studies: II. The respiratory dead space. Am J Physiol 154: 405, 1948.
14. Mead J, Whittenberger JL: Physical properties of human lungs measured during spontaneous respiration. J Appl Physiol 5: 779, 1953.
15. Milic-Emili J, Mead J, Turner JM, Glauser EM: Improved technique for estimating pleural pressure from esophageal balloons. J Appl Physiol 19: 207, 1964.
16. Snedecor GW, Cochran WG: Statistical Methods, 6th ed, Ames, Iowa, The Iowa State University Press, 1967.
17. McFadden ER Jr, Lyons HA: Airway resistance and uneven ventilation in bronchial asthma. J Appl Physiol 25: 365, 1968.
18. Knudson RJ, Constantine HP: An effect of isoproterenol on ventilation-perfusion in asthmatic versus normal subjects. J Appl Physiol 22: 402, 1967.
19. Weber J, Bouhuys A: Theoretical considerations on lung clearance. Acta Physiol Pharmacol Neerlandica 8: 121, 1959.
20. Nye RE Jr: Theoretical limits to measurement of uneven ventilation. J Appl Physiol 16: 1115, 1961.
21. Safonoff I, Emmanuel GE: The effect of pendelluft and dead space on nitrogen clearance: mathematical and experimental models and their application to the study of the distribution of ventilation. J Clin Invest 46: 1683, 1967.
22. Nadel JA, Colebatch HJH, Olsen CR: Location and mechanism of airway constriction after barium sulfate microembolism. J Appl Physiol 19: 387, 1964.
23. Colebatch HJH, Olsen CR, Nadel JA: Effect of histamine, serotonin, and acethylcholine on the peripheral airways. J Appl Physiol 21: 217, 1966.
24. McFadden ER Jr, Newton-Howes J, Pride NB: Acute effects of inhaled isoproterenol on the mechanical characteristics of the lungs in normal man. J Clin Invest 49: 779, 1970.
25. Bouhuys A, van de Woestijne KP: Respiratory mechanics and dust exposure in byssinosis. J Clin Invest 49: 106, 1970.
26. Macklem PT, Mead J: Resistance of central and peripheral airways measured by a retrograde catheter. J Appl Physiol 22: 395, 1967.
27. Brown R, Woolcock AJ, Vincent NJ, Macklem PT: Physiological effects of experimental airway obstruction with beads. J Appl Physiol 27: 328, 1969.
28. Severinghaus JW, Stupfel M: Respiratory dead space increase following atropine in man, and atropine, vagal or ganglionic blockade and hypothermia in dogs. J Appl Physiol 8: 81, 1955.
29. Woolcock AJ, Vincent NJ, Macklem PT: Frequency dependence of compliance as a test for obstruction in the small airways. J Clin Invest 48: 1097, 1969.
30. Hughes JMB, Greene RE, Iliff LD, Milic-Emili J: Distribution of inspired gas in early bronchitis. Thorax 26: 491, 1971.
31. Payne CB Jr, Chester EH, Hsi BP: Airway responsiveness in chronic obstructive pulmonary disease. Am J Med 42: 554, 1967.
32. Ayres SM, Griesbach SJ, Reimold F, Evans RG: Bronchial component in chronic obstructive lung disease. Am J Med 57: 183, 1974.
33. Mushin GJ: Time factor in measurement of response to bronchodilators. Thorax 22: 538, 1967.
34. Holmes TH, Morgan B: A comparative clinical trial of metaproterenol and isoproterenol as bronchodilator aerosols. Clin Pharmacol Ther 9: 615, 1968.
35. Ishikawa S, Cherniack RM: The effect of nebulized bronchodilators on air flow resistance in chronic airways obstruction. Am Rev Respir Dis 99: 703, 1969.
36. Freedman BJ, Hill GB: Comparative study of duration of action and cardiovascular effects of bronchodilator aerosols. Thorax 26: 46, 1971.
37. Hurst A: Metaproterenol, a potent and safe bronchodilator. Ann Allergy 31: 460, 1973.
38. Abernethy JD: Effects of inhalation of an artificial fog. Thorax 23: 421, 1968.
39. Cheney FW Jr, Butler J: The effects of ultrasonically-produced aerosols on airway resistance in man. Anesthesiology 29: 1099, 1968.
40. Pflug AE, Cheney FW Jr, Butler J: The effects of an ultrasonic aerosol on pulmonary mechanics and arterial blood gases in patients with chronic bronchitis. Am Rev Respir Dis 101: 710, 1970.
41. Waltemath CL, Bergman NA: Increased respiratory resistance provoked by endotracheal administration of aerosols. Am Rev Respir Dis 108: 520, 1973.

Diagnosis of Obstruction of the Upper and Central Airways

MEIR KRYGER, M.D.*
FREDERICK BODE, M.D., USAF MC†
RAL ANTIC, M.D.‡
NICHOLAS ANTHONISEN, M.D.§
Denver, Colorado

Patients with obstruction of the upper airways are often treated for long periods of time for other disorders. Correct diagnosis is important since treatment is quite specific. Such patients may present with a characteristic history and findings on physical examination. Certain physiologic tests such as flow-volume loops with and without helium help to prove the diagnosis. Patients with upper airway obstruction may also have sleep apneas and the sleep deprivation syndrome. Methods of diagnosis of upper airway obstruction are presented and three instructive cases are reviewed.

Upper airway obstruction is frequently unrecognized. Patients with this condition are often treated for years for asthma, chronic bronchitis, emphysema or recurrent pulmonary infections. In patients with upper airway obstruction, correct diagnosis is critical since definitive therapy often requires surgery. Once diagnosed and properly treated, gratifying results with relief of most of the symptoms are the rule.

CLINICAL FEATURES

Symptoms of upper airway obstruction in the adult are usually nonspecific. Often the patient will complain of wheezing and dyspnea, particularly during exercise. These symptoms may be related to posture, and the patient may notice that breathing appears to be blocked in certain body positions. With some tumors, the patient will be able to localize the lesion because of pain in the chest wall. Dyspnea in the course of a viral respiratory tract infection may be related to upper airway edema. A trial of inhaled or oral vasoconstrictors may help in the diagnosis and treatment. Occasionally the sole complaint may be that sleep is difficult in certain positions and that several times during the night the patient may awaken with dyspnea. Because of poor-quality nocturnal sleep, daytime somnolence may be a prominent feature. The patient may complain of peripheral edema related to cor pulmonale.

An important physical finding with extrathoracic obstruction is inspiratory stridor. Maneuvers to increase flow (hyperventilation, forced inspiration) will accentuate stridor. The voice may be hoarse, and the cough may sound unusual. Unusual wheezes may be heard by putting the bell of the stethoscope over the patient's trachea.

From the Division of Pulmonary Medicine, University of Colorado, Denver, Colorado, and the Royal Victoria Hospital, Montreal, Quebec. Requests for reprints should be addressed to Dr. Meir Kryger. Manuscript accepted October 31, 1975.

* American Lung Association Fellow.

† Present address: 802 Firefly, San Antonio, Texas.

‡ Present address: 40 Meakins-Christie Laboratories, McGill University Montreal, Quebec, Canada

§ Present address: Division of Pulmonary Medicine, University of Manitoba, Department of Medicine, Winnipeg, Manitoba, Canada.

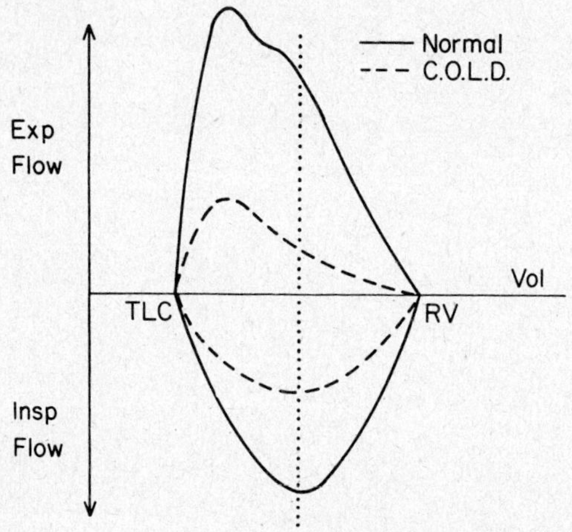

***Figure 1.** Maximal inspiratory and expiratory flow-volume curves in normal subjects (**solid line**), and in those with chronic obstructive peripheral lung disease (**dashed line**). The stippled line represents 50 per cent of vital capacity. In normal subjects the ratio of expired to inspired flow at this lung volume is about 1. In those with chronic obstructive lung disease this ratio is about 0.3.*

When evaluating patients with diseases of the upper airway one must bear in mind that once symptoms or physiologic derangements are present, the obstruction is quite advanced. Early upper airway obstruction produces few symptoms and is difficult to diagnose. A peripheral lung disease may also develop because of an abnormal cough mechanism or aspiration of necrotic tumor fragments.

LABORATORY INVESTIGATIONS

During a forced expiration from total lung capacity the maximal flow achieved in expelling the first 25 per cent of the vital capacity is dependent on effort. An increase in driving pressure due to an increase in effort will increase flow at this lung volume. In the remaining 75 per cent of vital capacity, flow is limited in such a way that an increase in effort with an increased pleural pressure will also compress airways. Thus, maximal flow at the lower 75 per cent of vital capacity is limited by this dynamic compression of airways, is determined by the mechanical properties of the lung and is thus not dependent on effort. With an upper airway obstruction, flow at higher lung volumes may be limited by the obstruction. At lower lung volumes, even in the presence of upper airway obstruction, flow may be limited not by the obstruction but by the dynamic compression of airways as described. Generally, flow measurements made at low lung volumes reflect the function of peripheral airways only, whereas those made at high lung volumes reflect both upper and lower airway function. It thus follows that some tests that measure parameters that occur below 75 per cent of vital capacity may not be sensitive to upper airway obstruction. Thus the forced expiratory volume in 1 second (FEV_1) is a rather insensitive test in upper airway obstruction, since a large part of the vital capacity range it examines reflects dynamic compression of peripheral airways. Experimentally, in subjects breathing through orifices of decreasing size, FEV_1 remained above 90 per cent of control until a 6 mm orifice was used [1]. The peak expiratory flow rate (PEFR) and maximal voluntary ventilation (MVV or MBC) were found to be more sensitive in detecting obstruction than FEV_1.

The finding of a reduction in PEFR, MVV and FEV_1, with none of the other abnormalities one expects in chronic obstructive lung disease (involving the peripheral airways), may be the first clue to upper airway obstruction. With peripheral airway disease one can often demonstrate abnormal lung volumes, diffusing capacity and distribution of ventilation as measured by a single- ("closing volume") or multiple-breath nitrogen washout. These should be normal in pure upper airway obstruction [2]. If the patient has paroxysmal airway obstruction without having an improvement in flow studies after use of a bronchodilator during an "attack," again one should be alerted to the possibility of upper airway obstruction, since most patients with asthma will respond to a bronchodilator. Hypoxemia at rest is unusual, but it may be present during exercise [3]. Carbon dioxide retention is unusual. Even though awake studies may be normal, serious hypoventilation may occur during sleep. The only clue in these patients may be erythrocytosis as a response to the nocturnal hypoxemia.

Ventilatory response to inhaled carbon dioxide may be abnormal with severe upper airway obstruction, and this may become normal following surgical relief [4–6]. In upper airway obstruction an ill-understood loss of lung elasticity may develop with an increase in functional residual capacity (FRC) [7]. Compliance (the relation of volume and the pressure distending the lungs) should drop with increasing respiratory frequency with lower but not upper airway obstruction.

Flow-volume loops (Figure 1) which represent flow at various lung volumes are very useful in the diagnosis of upper airway obstruction, and they have been studied extensively by Miller and Hyatt at the Mayo Clinic [1,8]. The subject inhales to total lung capacity (TLC) then does a forced expiratory vital capacity maneuver. He then inhales as quickly as possible back to TLC. The portion of the expiratory curve near TLC is effort-dependent and that near residual volume (RV) is independent of effort, with flow being limited by dynamic compression of airways. At 50 per cent of vital capacity the ratio of expired to

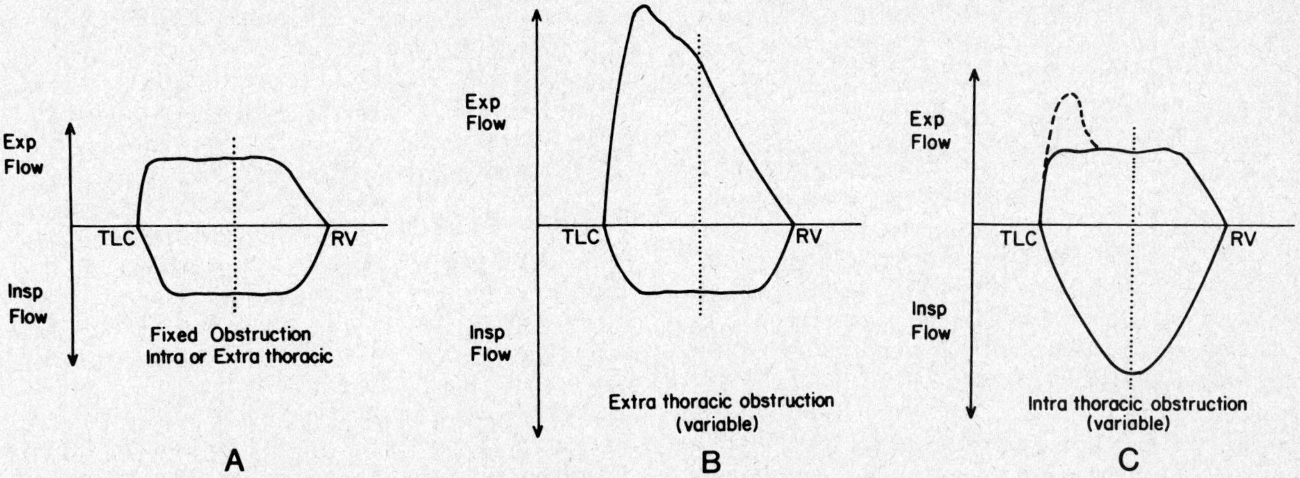

Figure 2. *Maximal inspiratory and expiratory flow-volume curves in fixed obstruction (**A**), extrathoracic variable obstruction (**B**) and intrathoracic variable obstruction (**C**). The dashed line represents a flow transient that occasionally is observed just before the plateau in intrathoracic obstruction. See text for full description.*

inspired flow (the mid-VC ratio) in normal subjects is about 0.9 [8]. This ratio is useful in diagnosis.

Using flow-volume loops, upper airway obstruction can be subdivided into three functional groups: (1) fixed obstruction, (2) variable extrathoracic obstruction, and (3) variable intrathoracic obstruction.

The most common cause of a **fixed obstruction** is a benign stricture resulting from previous endotracheal intubation. A goiter may also result in this functional disorder. With a fixed obstruction (Figure 2A), the airway diameter at the site of the lesion does not change with inspiration or expiration. Constant flow represented by a plateau will be seen on the expiratory curve in the effort-dependent portion near TLC with very little change in the effort-independent portion near RV. The inspiratory part of the curve also shows a plateau indicating constant flow, around 50 per cent of vital capacity. Since the functional disturbance affects both inspiration and expiration, the mid-VC ratio is about 1, within normal limits, and the forced expiratory volume in 1 second (FEV_1) will be about the same as the forced inspiratory volume in 1 second (FIV_1). A straight line in the

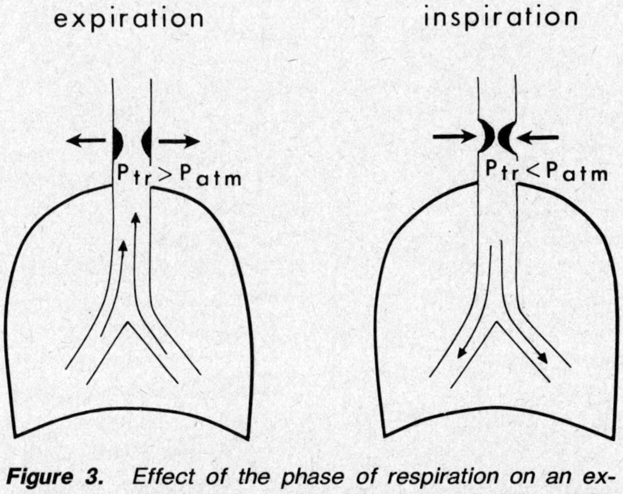

Figure 3. *Effect of the phase of respiration on an extrathoracic variable obstruction. Direction of airflow is indicated by the long thin arrows. During forced expiration the intratracheal pressure (P_{tr}) is greater than the pressure around the airway (P_{atm} = atmospheric pressure), resulting in a decrease of the obstruction. During forced inspiration when the pressure around the airway exceeds the intratracheal pressure the obstruction is increased.*

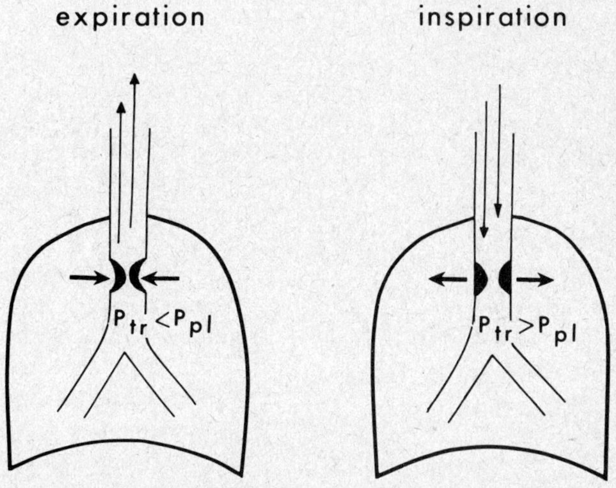

Figure 4. *Effect of the phase of respiration on an intrathoracic variable obstruction. Direction of airflow is indicated by the long thin arrows. During forced expiration the pressure acting around the airway (P_{pl} = pleural pressure) may be greater than the intratracheal pressure (P_{tr}), resulting in an increase in the obstruction. During forced inspiration the intratracheal pressure is greater than the pleural pressure thus decreasing the obstruction.*

timed spirogram gives similar information as the plateau in the flow-volume curve. However, flow must be inferred from the slope of the spirogram, and this seems more difficult than examining a flow-volume curve.

When obstruction caused by a lesion changes with the respiratory cycle, it is called a **variable obstruction.** The physiologic findings will depend on whether the lesion is intrathoracic or extrathoracic. Vocal cord paralysis makes up the majority of cases of **extrathoracic variable obstruction;** but scars, cancers, enlarged lymph nodes and fat deposits may also cause extrathoracic obstruction [8–10]. With the extrathoracic obstruction, during forced inspiration (Figures 2B and 3), the pressure within the airway is markedly negative compared to the atmospheric pressure around the airway. The resultant transmural pressure will tend to decrease the diameter of the airway so that the net effect of forced inspiration is to increase the obstruction so that constant flow ensues, manifested as a plateau on the inspiratory part of the curve. During forced expiration, the marked positive pressure within the airway will tend to decrease the obstruction, so that the expiratory curve may be normal. Thus FEV_1 will be greater than FIV_1, and the mid-VC ratio will be greater than 2.

Tumors make up the majority of **variable intrathoracic obstructions.** Structural abnormalities such as "floppy airways" may occasionally be seen. The pressure acting around an intrathoracic obstruction is pleural pressure. During forced expiration the pleural pressure is markedly positive and greater than the intratracheal pressure. This will tend to decrease the diameter of the airway, and thus increase the obstruction; a plateau indicating constant flow will be seen in the expiratory flow-volume loop (Figures 2C and 4). This plateau probably indicates that the lumen of the trachea at the area of the lesion has assumed its minimal size. This plateau may occur at certain lung volumes, and a peak (indicating that the obstruction may not affect flow until a certain volume is reached) may precede the plateau. During forced inspiration, the pressure acting around the obstruction is markedly negative, so that the effect will be to decrease the obstruction, and the inspiratory flow-volume loop may be normal. This decrease in expiratory relative to inspiratory flow causes the ratio of the two, the mid-VC ratio, to be very low (about 0.3). The FEV_1 is much less than the FIV_1. The mid-VC ratio and FIV_1 to FEV_1 relationship in intrathoracic obstruction is similar to that seen in chronic obstructive lung disease (COLD). However, the shape of the forced expiratory flow curve is entirely different, with the curve in the latter being most abnormal in the effort-independent part of the curve near RV (indicating dynamic compression of abnormal airways) and having a characteristic curvilinear shape (compare Figure 2C to the curve with COLD, Figure 1).

Resistance in any tube can be measured by dividing the pressure drop along the tube by the flow [11]. In man, resistance across the upper airway is about 1 cm water/liter/sec [12], whereas most patients with symptomatic upper airway obstruction are found to have a resistance between 4 and 15 cm water/liter/sec while breathing quietly. Inference from experimental data suggests that the upper airway in such patients is similar functionally to a 5 to 6 mm orifice [1]. The resistance of the upper airway is not constant and with increasing flow (such as during exercise) there is a disproportionate rise in the resistance, probably explaining the dyspnea on exertion of these patients [3].

It appears that flow in the upper airways is turbulent whereas in the peripheral airways it is laminar. In laminar flow, resistance is independent of the density of the gas breathed whereas in turbulent flow resistance is dependent on gas density. Thus in chronic obstructive lung disease, when the obstruction is peripheral and when flow is laminar, there should be little or no change in dynamic lung function with a change in gas density [13], and indeed this has been found in patients breathing 80 per cent helium and 20 per cent oxygen mixtures [14]. However some investigators have reported a small decrease in resistance with helium-oxygen mixtures in similar patients [15].

In contrast, flow in the central and upper airways is turbulent and hence density-dependent. Thus resistance should be reduced in the presence of upper airway obstruction when breathing a less dense gas mixture such as a helium-oxygen mixture. In an excellent study in animals, Barnett [16] showed that with an upper airway obstruction the pulmonary resistance decreased on breathing a helium-oxygen mixture. He also showed that when the obstruction was peripheral (histamine-induced) bronchoconstriction, the resistance was not density-dependent. By examining the effect of helium on the maximum expiratory flow-volume curve Despas et al. [14] showed that the obstruction in asthma may be peripheral in some patients, and in the larger airways in others. It follows that measurement of flow-volume curves breathing gases of different densities should be useful in identifying patients with upper airway obstruction; however, we are unaware of a series of such patients in which the effect of gas density on dynamic lung function has been studied systematically.

Visualization by roentgenologic means including

TABLE I Pulmonary Functions (Case 1)

	Air	Helium	Post Bronchodilator	Predicted
Vital capacity (liters)	3.15			2.6 ± 0.52 (SEE)*
Functional residual capacity (liters)	3.55			2.28 ± 0.39 (CV)†
Total lung capacity (liters)	5.45			4.0 ± 0.44 (CV)
Residual volume (liters)	2.3			1.4 ± 0.34 (CV)
Resistance (cm water/liter/sec)	4.0		4.1	1–2
FEV_1 (liters)	1.25	1.50	1.35	1.98 ± 0.47 (SEE)
FIV_1 (liters)	2.35	2.45	2.65	2.23‡
FEV_1:FIV_1	0.53	0.61	0.51	0.89 ± 0.09§ (SD)¶
Mid-maximal expiratory flow rate (liters/sec)	0.42	0.87	0.70	2.53 ± 0.8 (SEE)

NOTE: FEV_1 = forced expiratory volume in 1 sec; FIV_1 = forced inspiratory volume in 1 sec.
*SEE = standard error of the estimate.
† CV = coefficient of variation.
‡ Standard deviation not available; derived from [28].
§ From [28].
¶ SD = standard deviation.

tomography and contrast studies or direct visualization by endoscopy are most important in the management of this group of patients. Both the radiologist and the endoscopist can appreciate the dynamic nature of the lesion with the respiratory cycle and during forced expiration and inspiration.

Some patients with upper airway obstruction are found to completely occlude the upper airway during sleep. This can be documented by performing polygraphic studies during sleep, monitoring electroencephalograph, airflow at the nose and mouth, activity of the respiratory muscles, and electrocardiogram. These patients may be found to obstruct the upper airway in a periodic manner—cessation of airflow will occur with continuation of respiratory muscle movements. Resumption of airflow will occur with a snort and an arousal pattern on the electroencephalogram, sometimes with a preceding bradyarrhythmia. The recurrent central nervous system arousals are believed to result in a sleep deprivation syndrome and somnolence. Unaccountably, such patients may report that sleep is normal. The nocturnal hypoventilation may be sufficient to cause cor pulmonale. Periodic upper airway obstruction may be an important factor in the pathophysiology of the Pickwickian syndrome [17,18]. Recurrent nocturnal airway obstruction causing a sleep disorder and sometimes cor pulmonale has been described with obesity [9,10,17,18], micrognathia [5,19], and enlarged adenoids and tonsils [20–24].

A diagnosis of upper airway obstruction can easily be made in the modern pulmonary function laboratory. One must keep in mind that symptoms and, thus, diagnosis often occur once the obstruction is severe. If definitive therapy is used the results are usually excellent.

We present three illustrative cases that we have recently studied to show the clinical application of some of the principles outlined.

CASE REPORTS

Case 1. A 53 year old white woman was admitted to the hospital with complaints of episodic wheezing and dyspnea of three years' duration. She was thought to have asthma and bronchitis related to cigarette smoking and was treated with bronchodilators. She did not respond to therapy. Previously, several pulmonary infections were treated successfully with antibiotics. The dyspnea was intermittent, was related to posture and was quite bothersome when she was supine. The patient complained of "a blockage in the upper chest," and of a sensation of choking and "closing of the windpipe" when she coughed or expired with force. One episode of coughing up bright red blood two weeks prior to admission was reported.

The physical examination revealed inspiratory and expiratory sonorous rhonchi best heard directly over the sternum. No sibilant rhonchi were present in the rest of the lung zones. The remainder of the physical examination was within normal limits.

Mechanics and flow studies are presented in Table I. They reveal hyperinflation, air trapping and increased total pulmonary resistance. Loss of elastic recoil measured by a pressure-volume curve was also found.

Flow studies during expiration were abnormal, with minimal response to bronchodilator. The expiratory flow-volume curve (Figure 5) showed an initial peak followed by a segment in which flow rates were variable. At certain lung volumes a constant flow was maintained. On other flow-volume tracings the flow fell to zero at certain lung volumes. A marked response to helium at the effort-dependent segment of the flow-volume curve was demonstrated. Airway closure occurred at 20 per cent of vital capacity. The slope of the alveolar plateau (phase III) was steep.

Chest roentgenograms and tomograms revealed a broad-based intratracheal mass projecting into the lumen. Cinetracheogram showed complete apposition of the tra-

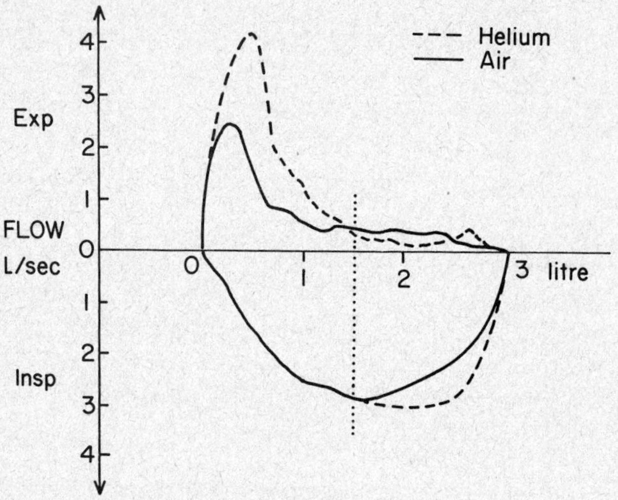

Figure 5. *Case 1. Maximal flow-volume curve. Note the flow transient just below TLC (volume equal to 0). The variation in flow with decreasing lung volume is irregular, with plateaus in contrast to the smooth exponential curve of COLD (Figure 1), in which a similar mid-VC ratio is seen.*

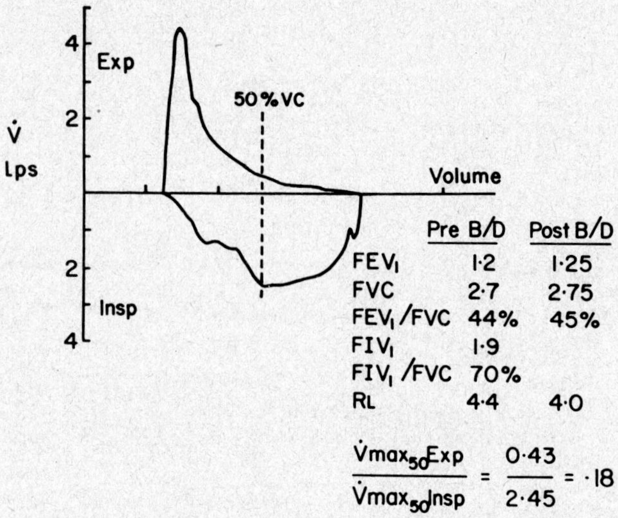

Figure 7. *Case 2. Maximum flow-volume curves. The "ragged" and irregular appearance of the forced curves is different from the smooth curve seen with pure peripheral airway obstruction. TLC is at the left and RV at the right side of the curves. The data represent flow studies before and after bronchodilator ($\dot{V}$ = flow, FVC = forced vital capacity, R_L = total pulmonary resistance, $\dot{V}_{max_{50}}$ = flow at 50 per cent of vital capacity).*

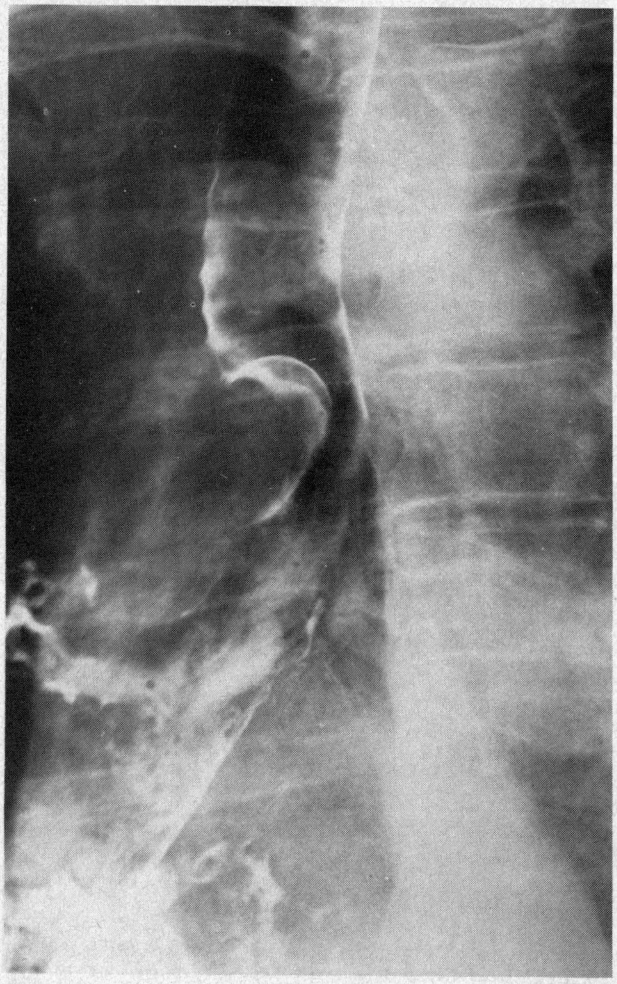

Figure 6. *Case 1. Contrast tracheogram demonstrates the obstructing tumor.*

cheal wall with the neoplasm during forced expiration and coughing. Thoracotomy was performed with excision of the tumor and five rings of the trachea (Figure 6). The pathologic diagnosis was adenocystic basal cell carcinoma of the trachea.

Comment: The history and physical findings were suggestive of upper airway obstruction. The physiologic studies suggested both upper and lower airway obstruction. The flow-volume curves showed that at different lung volumes the tracheal lumen at the site of the lesion assumed its minimal diameter. With chronic obstructive lung disease, the contour of the curve is different from what we obtained. Eighteen months after operation, a flow-volume curve of completely normal contour was obtained.

This case illustrates that examination of the entire flow-volume curve is more helpful than depending upon a specific value for the mid-VC ratio as the sole criterion for diagnosis. On serial flow-volume curves, flow fell to zero at different lung volumes, clearly indicating the variable nature of the obstruction.

Case 2. A 60 year old man was admitted to the hospital because a routine roentgenogram had shown collapse of the lower lobe of the left lung. For more than 20 years he was noticed to have a bizarre, prolonged rasping cough. He was a smoker and had been told that he had chronic bronchitis. For the past 10 years he had noticed slowly progressing shortness of breath. He had not experienced frequent bouts of pulmonary infection.

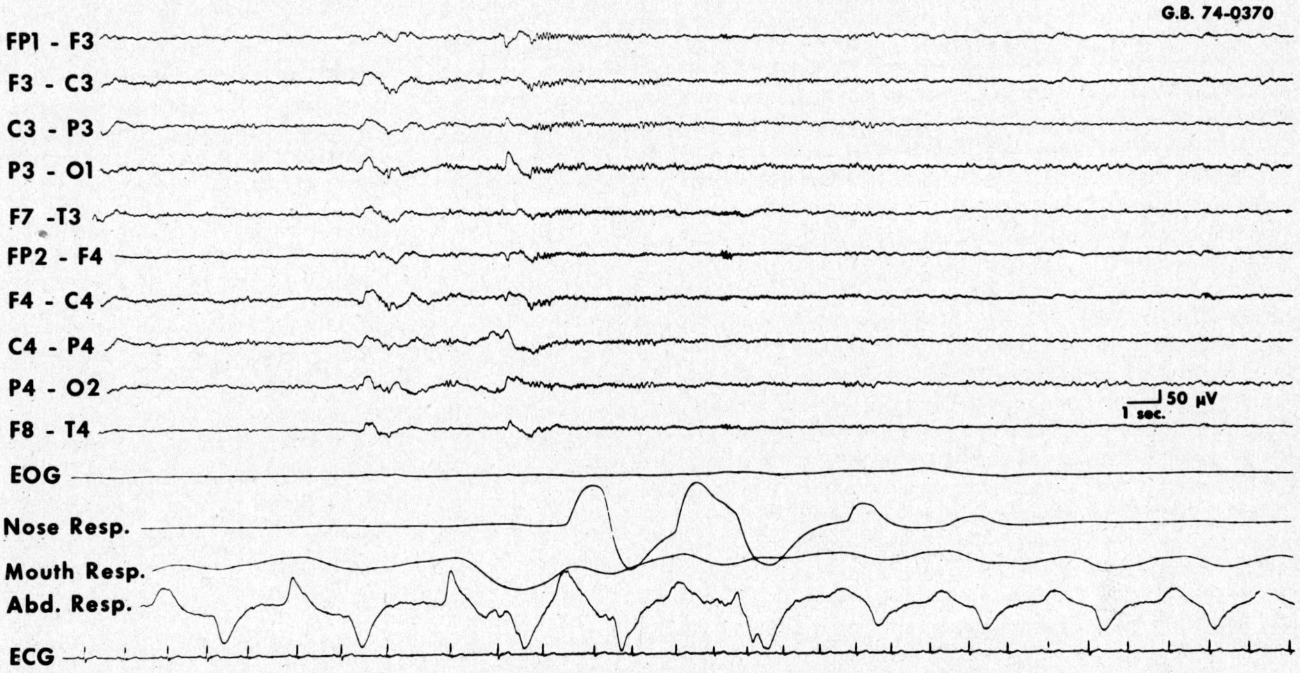

Figure 8. *Case 3. Polygraphic sleep recording. Monitored were electroencephalograph (Channels 1–10), electroculogram (EOG), air flow through nose ("nose resp."), airflow through mouth ("mouth resp."), respiratory muscle activity ("abd. resp.") and electrocardiogram (ECG). Complete obstruction of the upper airway is seen when airflow is absent in the presence of respiratory muscle activity. Onset of unobstructed ventilation occurs together with a nervous system arousal seen on the electroencephalogram.*

Physical examination revealed an elderly man in no acute distress, with normal color and a respiratory rate of 16/min. A slight increase in the anteroposterior diameter of the chest, decreased breath sounds throughout both lung fields and inspiratory rales at the base of the left lung were found. No localized wheeze was heard.

The chest roentgenogram obtained on admission revealed the diameter of the tracheal air column to be markedly increased. Cinebronchogram showed marked collapse of the trachea and bronchi during forced expiration and cough.

Tests of pulmonary mechanics were carried out; they showed hyperinflation and marked loss of recoil on the static volume-pressure curve. These findings were consistent with marked generalized emphysema. The flow-volume curve is shown in Figure 7. The ratio of expiratory to inspiratory flow at 50 per cent of vital capacity was 0.18 and consistent with both emphysema and variable intrathoracic obstruction. The curves on inspiration and expiration were ragged and suggested that central airways obstruction was also present.

At bronchoscopy it was noted that the obstruction of the lower lobe of the left lung was due to severe redundancy of the bronchial mucosa and collapse of the walls. The widely dilated trachea and major bronchi contained copious amounts of purulent secretions. Following this procedure the patient was treated with physiotherapy and positive-pressure breathing. Contrast material and secretions were slowly eliminated from the left side of the chest, but the lower lobe of the left lung did not re-expand.

Comment: The characteristic clinical features of tracheobronchiomegaly, the "Mounier-Kuhn syndrome" [25–27], are well demonstrated in this case. They include a loud, rasping, prolonged, remarkably ineffective cough, abnormally wide trachea and major bronchi, and association with chronic infection of the respiratory tract. The natural history of the syndrome is admittedly unknown, but the pooling of secretions seen on bronchoscopy and bronchography, and the ineffectiveness of the cough, may lead to chronic infection superimposed on the congenitally defective airways. Exaggerated collapse of the trachea and bronchi during forced expiration was easily appreciated during bronchoscopy and resulted in the predictable abnormalities seen during the pulmonary mechanics studies. The combination of the endoscopic findings, the abnormal flow-volume curves and the remarkably abnormal static volume-pressure curve were proof of the central and lower airway obstruction, respectively.

Case 3. A 51 year old man weighing 143 kg (approximately 200 per cent of his ideal weight) was admitted for evaluation of somnolence. This had been present for three months prior to admission, the patient claiming he had fallen asleep while conducting interviews and while driving. Members of his family and friends had told the patient that he snored very loudly and that he appeared to stop breathing at times during sleep. A nonsmoker, the patient denied breathlessness, paroxysmal nocturnal dyspnea, peripheral edema or wheezing. Except for the massive obesity, the physical examination was within normal limits. During sleep, observers noted periods of apnea.

Blood gases revealed mild hypoxemia and a normal carbon dioxide tension. The carbon dioxide response curve was normal. Total pulmonary resistance was 5 cm water/liter/sec in the sitting position and 6 to 7 cm in the supine position. The slope of the single-breath nitrogen washout was normal with airways closure demonstrated at 15 per cent of vital capacity. Polygraphic studies were performed while the patient was sleeping (Figure 8). Monitored were electroculograph, airflow through the nose and mouth using thermisters, and respiratory muscle activity using strain sensors around the thoracoabdominal region. It was found that the patient had episodes of periodic apnea. Some of these apneas were accompanied by respiratory muscle activity indicating airway obstruction; others were true central apneas with neither airflow nor respiratory muscle activity recorded. Prior to the onset of airflow (at the end of an apneic period) an arousal pattern was seen on the electroencephalogram and sometimes a slight bradycardia was noted. Deep stages of sleep were markedly decreased. In two nights of monitoring, only 15 seconds of rapid eye movement were recorded.

After discharge, the patient was placed on a diet. After losing 8 to 10 kg, the somnolence disappeared. He continues to lose weight and has no complaints.

Comment: The increased airway resistance with no history or findings of pulmonary disease and a one-breath nitrogen washout that was normal suggest that the increased resistance was in the upper airway. Polygraphic data showed periodic obstructive and true apneas, and an abnormal sleep electroencephalogram. It is believed that in patients with some forms of upper airway obstruction (in this case presumably fat deposition) obstructive apneas will develop as well as a sleep disorder related to this. Relief of the obstruction will cure the syndrome.

Fortunately this patient had a characteristic history and normal carbon dioxide response curve, and he was successful at losing weight with rapid improvement in his symptoms. Our previous experience with polygraphic tracings led to early diagnosis of the etiology of his symptoms. Since these patients share in common many of the features of the Pickwickian syndrome, the diagnosis is often missed. If weight reduction is not successful, other therapeutic measures such as tracheostomy may become necessary [9,10,18].

ACKNOWLEDGMENT

We are indebted to Dr. P. Gloor and Dr. L. F. Quesney, who performed the polygraphic study at the Montreal Neurological Hospital, and to Dr. T. Petty, Dr. J. V. Weil and Dr. C. Zwillich for their critical review of the manuscript.

REFERENCES

1. Miller RD, Hyatt RE: Obstructing lesions of the larynx and trachea. Clinical and physiological characteristics. Mayo Clin Proc 44: 145, 1969.
2. Sackner MA: Physiological features of upper airway obstruction. Chest 62: 414, 1972.
3. Al-Bazzaz F, Grillo H, Kazemi H: Response to exercise in upper airway obstruction. Am Rev Respir Dis 111: 631, 1975.
4. Milic-Emili J, Tyler JM: Relation between work output of the respiratory muscles and end-tidal CO_2 tension. J Appl Physiol 18: 497, 1963.
5. Valero A, Alroy G: Hypoventilation in acquired micrognathia. Arch Intern Med 115: 307, 1965.
6. Ingram RH, Bishop JB: Ventilatory response to carbon dioxide after removal of chronic upper airway obstruction. Am Rev Respir Dis 102: 645, 1970.
7. Buhain WJ, Brody JS, Fisher AB: Effect of artificial airway obstruction on elastic properties of the lung. J Appl Physiol 33: 589, 1972.
8. Miller RD, Hyatt RE: Evaluation of obstructing lesions of the trachea and larynx by flow-volume loops. Am Rev Respir Dis 108: 475, 1973.
9. Kryger M, Quesney LF, Holder D, Gloor P, McLeod P: The sleep deprivation syndrome of the obese patient. Am J Med 56: 530, 1974.
10. Walsh RE, Michaelson ED, Harkleroad LE, Zighelboim A, Sackner MA: Upper airway obstruction in obese patients with sleep disturbance and somnolence. Ann Intern Med 76: 185, 1972.
11. Dubois AB: Resistance to breathing, Handbook of Physiology, section 3: Respiration, vol. I (Fenn WO, Rahn H, eds), Washington, American Physiological Society, 1964, p 451.
12. Ferris BG Jr, Opie L, Mead J: Partioning of respiratory resistance in man (abstract). Fed Proc 19: 377, 1960.
13. Gold M, Marks A, Bocles JS: Effects of reduction in air density on dynamic function in obstructive airway disease (abstract). Am Rev Respir Dis 90: 316, 1964.
14. Despas PJ, Leroux M, Macklem PT: Site of airway obstruction in asthma as determined by measuring maximal expiratory flow breathing air and a helium-oxygen mixture. J Clin Invest 31: 3235, 1972.
15. Grapé B, Channin E, Tyler JM: The effect of helium and oxygen mixtures on pulmonary resistances in emphysema. Am Rev Respir Dis 81: 823, 1960.
16. Barnett TB: Effects of helium and oxygen mixtures on pulmonary mechanics during airway constriction. J Appl Physiol 22: 707, 1967.
17. Gastaut H, Tassinari CA, Duron B: Etude polygraphique des manifestations épisodiques (hypnique et respiratoire) diurnes et nocturnes, du syndrome de Pickwick. Rev Neurol (Paris) 112: 568, 1965.
18. Kuhlo W, Doll E: Pulmonary hypertension and the effect of tracheotomy in a case of Pickwickian syndrome. Bull Physiopathol Respir (Nancy) 8: 1205, 1972.
19. Tammeling GJ, Blokzijl EJ, Boonstra S, Sluiter HJ: Micrognathia, hypersomnia and periodic breathing. Bull Physiopathol Respir (Nancy) 8: 1229, 1972.
20. Massumi RA, Sarin RK, Pooya M, Reichelderfer TR, Fraga JR, Rios JC, Ayersterian E: Tonsillar hypertrophy, airway obstruction, alveolar hypoventilation, and cor pulmonale in twin brothers. Dis Chest 55: 110, 1969.

21. Luke MJ, Mehrizi A, Folger GM, Rowe RD: Chronic nasopharyngeal obstruction as a cause of cardiomegaly, cor pulmonale, and pulmonary edema. Pediatrics 37: 762, 1966.
22. Levy AM, Tabakin BS, Hanson JS, Narkewicz RM: Hypertrophied adenoids causing pulmonary hypertension and severe congestive heart failure. N Engl J Med 277: 506, 1967.
23. Ainger LE: Large tonsils and adenoids in small children with cor pulmonale. Br Heart J 30: 356, 1968.
24. Bland JW Jr, Edwards FK, Brinsfield D: Pulmonary hypertension and congestive heart failure in children with chronic upper airway obstruction. Am J Cardiol 23: 830, 1969.
25. Mounier-Kuhn P: Dilatation de la trachée. Lyon Med 150: 106, 1932.
26. Katz I, Levine M, Herman P: Tracheobronchiomegaly. The Mounier-Kuhn syndrome. Am J Roentgenol 88: 1084, 1962.
27. Johnston RF, Green RA: Tracheobronchiomegaly. Am Rev Respir Dis 91: 35, 1965.
28. Jordanoglou J, Pride NB: A comparison of maximum inspiratory and expiratory flow in health and lung disease. Thorax 23: 38, 1968.

INFORMATION FOR AUTHORS

PREPARATION OF MANUSCRIPTS

Manuscripts should be typed on one side of the sheet, doublespaced, on white bond paper, 8½ by 11 inches, with margins of 1 inch. Two copies of the manuscript and illustrations should be sent to the Editor at 666 Fifth Avenue, New York, New York 10019. Title page should include full name, degrees and affiliation of all authors, the source from which the article emanates, and the name and address of the person to whom requests for reprints should be addressed.

All manuscript pages including tables and legends should be numbered consecutively in the upper right hand corner.

The number of manuscript pages, the number of illustrations and the number of tables should be indicated at the bottom of the covering letter.

Every article must be preceded by an abstract (not to exceed 350 words). This obviates the need for a summary. In addition, for the convenience of our readers, we require a brief abstract (not exceeding 100 to 125 words) and key words for indexing purposes. These brief abstracts appear in the back of the *Journal* in the same issue in which the paper appears.

Since all manuscripts submitted for publication in the *Journal* are sent out for review before a final decision is made, there is generally a lapse of three to six weeks before contributors are notified. If you have received an acknowledgment of receipt, there is no need to call the *Journal* office; your manuscript has not gone astray. The decision will be forthcoming shortly.

PREPARATION OF ILLUSTRATIONS AND TABLES

Illustrations must be black and white glossy prints or professional drawings in india ink; they should be unmounted. The name of the lead author and the title of the article should be typed on a label and affixed to the back of each illustration; the top should be indicated.

Reference to all illustrations should be inserted in the text in consecutive order. Legends for the illustrations should be typed, double spaced, on a separate sheet with numbers corresponding to those on the photographs or drawings. They should not be attached to the pictures.

Tables should be typed on separate sheets and should be set up in accordance with the style of the Journal. Units of measure should be confined to column headings. Abbreviations should be kept to a minimum and should conform with those used by the *Journal* or listed as acceptable in the Council of Biology Editors Style Manual. Any variations should be explained. All vertical rules should be omitted.

The publisher allows a fixed amount towards the reproduction of illustrations and tables. Charges in excess of this amount must be assumed by the authors. The Editor reserves the right to limit the number of illustrations and/or tables.

PREPARATION OF BIBLIOGRAPHY

Bibliographic references should be listed chronologically on a separate sheet (not in footnotes) as referred to in the text and should be typed (double-spaced) in accordance with the style and abbreviations (open punctuation) used by Index Medicus; only the first page of the journal citation is necessary. Examples follow:

For periodical references:

22. Theologides A, Kennedy BJ: Toxoplasmic myocarditis and pericarditis. Am J Med 47: 169, 1969.

For book references (with chapter):

18. Schiebler GL, Van Mieron LHS, Krovetz LJ: Diseases of the tricuspid valve, chap 2. Heart Disease in Infants, Children and Adolescents (Moss AJ, Adams F, eds), Baltimore, Williams & Wilkins, 1968.

For book references (without chapter):

13. Berne E: Principles of Group Treatment, New York, Oxford University Press, 1966, p 26.

Authors are responsible for the accuracy of all references.

REPRINTS

Price schedules and order cards for reprints are mailed to the person so listed in the footnote on the title page.

The American Journal of Medicine, **666 Fifth Avenue, New York, New York 10019**

Mixed Cryoimmunoglobulinemia

Stenographic reports, edited by Philip E. Cryer, M.D. and John Kissane, M.D., of weekly clinicopathologic conferences held in Barnes and Wohl Hospitals, are published in each issue of the Journal. These conferences are participated in jointly by members of the Departments of Internal Medicine and Pathology of Washington University School of Medicine.

A 50 year old woman was admitted to Barnes Hospital for the last time on July 7, 1975, because of fever, chills and pleuritic chest pain. She died two weeks later.

Joint pain, morning stiffness and occasional fever led to a diagnosis of rheumatoid arthritis in 1965. Glucocorticoid therapy was administered then and intermittently thereafter. No diagnosis was made on a left cervical lymph node excised in 1967; another lymph node was removed from the same region in 1969 and interpreted as demonstrating mixed histiocytic lymphoma. There was, however, some reservation about that diagnosis. A lymphangiogram was abnormal, and irradiation therapy to the neck, right iliac and periaortic areas was administered. After radiation therapy the patient complained of a dry mouth and dry eyes, and hypothyroidism developed and was treated. Raynaud's phenomenon first occurred in 1973. Later that year a violaceous maculopapular rash appeared over the lower part of the abdomen, buttocks and legs, and later over the arms. A biopsy specimen of the skin demonstrated vasculitis.

Persistence of the skin rash and the finding of serum cryoglobulins prompted hospitalization in April 1974. The hematocrit value and white blood cell count were within normal limits, but the erythrocyte sedimentation rate was 66 mm/hour. A filling defect in the spleen was noted on scans. Pulmonary function tests demonstrated mild airway obstruction; the pulmonary diffusing capacity was normal. Evidence of sinusitis, with an air-fluid level in the left maxillary sinus, was noted roentgenographically. Studies of her serum cryoglobulin demonstrated a homogeneous immunoglobulin M (IgM) paraprotein (kappa light chains) and a heterogeneous immunoglobulin G (IgG) paraprotein (kappa and lambda chains). A rheumatoid factor titer of 1:40 (when the cryoglobulins were removed, the titer increased to 1:640), a low titer of antithyroid antibodies and a weakly positive Coombs' test were also detected. A repeat lymphangiogram showed enlarged nodes in the iliac, periaortic and paracaval chains. The earlier lymph node biopsy sections were reviewed and thought not to represent lymphoma. The possibility of Waldenström's macroglobulinemia was raised by the pathologist, but bone marrow sections were not characteristic of that disorder. Chlorambucil and prednisone were administered and the patient was discharged.

Microscopic hematuria with red blood cell casts, scattered white blood cells and granular casts in the urine sediment, and 3+ proteinuria were detected over the next several months. Penicillamine was added to the therapeutic regimen. Generalized seizures prompted the patient's hospitalization in July 1974. The hematocrit value was 25 per cent and the bone marrow was hypoplastic. The creatinine clearance was 60 ml/min. Intermittent fever was noted, and because of congestive heart failure the patient was treated with digoxin and furosemide. The patient was hospitalized three times, twice with pulmonary edema and once with digitalis intoxication, over the next year.

Fever, chills and right pleuritic chest pain led to her final admission on July 7, 1975. The blood pressure was 178/78 mm Hg, the pulse rate 92/min and the initial temperature 37.7°C. Subsequently, the temperature ranged up to 40°C. In addition to a Cushingoid appearance, petechiae over the legs and a flame-shaped hemorrhage in one fundus were noted. There was dullness at the base of the right lung. Bilateral basilar rales were more prominent on the right; tubular breath sounds were heard over the right lung posteriorly. There was a grade 2/6 systolic murmur along the left sternal border. The hemoglobin level was 6.9 g/100 ml, the hematocrit value 19 per cent and the white blood cell count 5,900/mm^3. There were more than 50 red blood cells and 10 white blood cells/hpf in the urine sediment. The urine contained 4.1 g of protein/24 hours and the creatinine clearance was 31 ml/min. The serum albumin was 2.9 g/100 ml; the serum bilirubin, alkaline phosphatase, glutamic-pyruvic transaminase and lactic dehydrogenase were within normal limits.

Gentamicin and blood transfusions were administered. Fever persisted. Bronchoscopy and transbronchial lung biopsy were performed on July 12. The specimen demonstrated only acute and chronic inflammation. Cephazolin therapy was added. An open lung biopsy specimen, obtained on July 16, demonstrated a nonspecific alveolar injury pattern. On July 18 the hematocrit value was 19 per cent with burr cells on the peripheral smear. The platelet count was 9,000/mm^3, the prothrombin time was 22 seconds, the fibrin degradation product level was 64 μg/ml (normal less than 8 μg/ml), and a protamine sulfate precipitation test was weakly positive. The fibrinogen level was 380 mg/100 ml. Because of increasing dyspnea with bibasilar rales, the patient was treated with morphine and furosemide on July 20. Recurrent hemoptysis began. A Swan-Ganz catheter was inserted; the wedge pressure was 0 to 3 mm Hg. Progressive hypotension was followed by cardiopulmonary arrest.

CLINICAL DISCUSSION

Dr. Eduardo Slatopolsky: In summary, we have a 50 year old woman who had a long history of rheumatoid arthritis. An enlarged lymph node in her cervical area was histologically consistent with, but not diagnostic of, lymphoma. She was admitted in 1973 because of vasculitis, Raynaud's phenomenon and cryoglobulinemia. She was treated with chlorambucil and prednisone, with some improvement. From July 1974 to July 1975, she had several admissions to the hospital because of complications, mainly vasculitis, renal insufficiency, seizures and congestive heart failure. In July 1975, she was admitted to Barnes Hospital because of chest pain, fever and chills. She had an infiltrate in her lungs; respiratory insufficiency developed and she died two weeks later. Dr. Forrest, would you please review the roentgenograms for us?

Dr. John Forrest: A chest film in August 1974 showed a moderate degree of cardiomegaly with prominence and blurring of the pulmonary vasculature. Two weeks later, there was considerable resolution. These findings are those of resolving congestive heart failure. In May 1975, she had florid pulmonary edema roentgenographically. A few days later, there was almost complete resolution. A film obtained on her final admission showed consolidation of the lower lobe of the right lung which was not present before. A week later, there was the onset of diffuse lung disease, similar to the pulmonary edema pattern seen before. Three days later, the diffuse lung disease was considerably worse. In summary we have recurrent congestive heart failure with episodes of pulmonary edema, consolidation in the lower lobe of the right lung during her final admission, which would be most compatible with acute pneumonia, and finally the development of extensive diffuse lung disease a few days before death. This diffuse lung disease could be pulmonary edema from congestive heart failure, disseminated infection, or the hemorrhage and edema seen in disseminated intravascular coagulation.

The lymphangiogram obtained in April 1974 showed abnormal lymph nodes in the pelvis. This lymphadenopathy could be malignant or nonmalignant.

Also in April 1974, a spleen scan revealed a large central filling defect. A repeat examination four months later showed that the spleen had decreased in size as had the filling defect. This was at the time of the patient's chlorambucil chemotherapy.

Dr. Slatopolsky: Basically, we have to deal with three main problems. The first problem is related to the interpretation of her lymph node biopsy specimens and bone marrow aspirates. Lymphoma and Waldenström's macroglobulinemia were the main diagnoses considered. The second problem is related to the nature of her cryoglobulinemia and the third one, the type of respiratory insufficiency and the cause of her death.

Dr. Kornfeld, why do you think the pathologists changed their mind? First, they interpreted the lymph node biopsy specimen as a mixed histiocytic lymphoma; then they changed the diagnosis to Waldenström's macroglobulinemia. However, the bone marrow was not consistent with Waldenström's macroglobulinemia. Do you think that she had either one of these two conditions or, perhaps for unknown reasons, that there was an antigenic challenge to her immunologic system and that an immunoproliferative disorder developed which was neither lymphoma nor Waldenström's macroglobulinemia?

Dr. Stuart Kornfeld: Let me mention Waldenström's macroglobulinemia first. This disease is characterized by the proliferation of a clone of B lymphocytes which produce large amounts of IgM paraprotein. Depending upon the physical-chemical characteristics of the paraprotein, various clinical manifestations may occur, such as the hyperviscosity syndrome, coagulation defects and Raynaud's phenomenon. These patients usually have lymphadenopathy and hepatosplenomegaly, and always have bone marrow infiltration with lymphocytes that classically are plasmacytoid in appearance but that may look like mature lymphocytes or mature plasma cells. The diagnosis, then, depends on the bone marrow picture and the presence of circulating IgM paraprotein. The lymph nodes may show abnormalities but I do not think that one can make the diagnosis without the characteristic bone marrow findings. I have reviewed the slides of her bone marrow aspirates and they are nondiagnostic. Thus, we can exclude the diagnosis of Waldenström's macroglobulinemia.

The question of a malignant lymphoma is much more difficult to resolve. Clinically, she very well could have had a lymphoma. About 5 per cent of patients with lymphoma have a circulating IgM paraprotein; some of these paraproteins result in cryoglobulin formation and symptoms similar to those of this patient. In this situation, the diagnosis must be made on the basis of the histology of the lymph node. This can be very difficult in certain instances. I reviewed the lymph node biopsy slides with Dr. Tillack of our Surgical Pathology Department and he is of the opinion that the biopsy specimens do not represent a malignant lymphoma. Therefore, I would agree with the diagnosis of some form of immunologic disorder resulting in the production of an IgM paraprotein and the symptoms that she experienced.

Dr. Slatopolsky: In 1966, Meltzer and Franklin [1] studied 29 patients with cryoglobulinemia. Several of the patients, who had only IgG cryoglobulins, had multiple myeloma. Most of the patients who had IgM cryoglobulins had a form of lymphoma. However, they found 11 patients (10 of them female) with mixed IgG-IgM cryoglobulins with a rheumatoid factor. Most of the patients had purpura, vasculitis and renal insufficiency. I am wondering if we are not dealing here with a situation similar to that described by Meltzer and Franklin.

Dr. Little, would you address yourself to the possible nature of the cryoglobulinemia in this patient? Could it be of help in the diagnosis and what symptoms would you expect to see in patients with cryoglobulinemia?

Dr. J. Russell Little: Almost all clinically significant cryoglobulinemias contain some immunoglobulin in the cryoprecipitate which determines the property of insolubility in the cold. Some investigators have therefore suggested that these complexes be referred to as cryoimmunoglobulins [2]. Very rarely, serum cryoprecipitates may contain only cryofibrinogen, C-reactive protein or other nonimmunoglobulin proteins. The cryoimmunoglobulins can occur in three different forms: (1) About 25 per cent of the patients exhibit the so-called "monoclonal type" in which a cryoprecipitate includes a single homogeneous immunoglobulin. It may be either IgM, IgG, IgA or even a Bence Jones protein, and that is the order of the frequency of their occurrence. The most common one is IgM occurring in patients with Waldenström's macroglobulinemia. IgG, IgA or Bence Jones cryoglobulins occur in multiple myeloma, and each of these monoclonal type cryoprecipitates usually results in a large amount of cryoprecipitate. (2) The second type is the "mixed type" of cryoglobulin in which two or more immunoglobulins are found in the cold precipitate, one of which is a homogeneous immunoglobulin and the other heterogeneous. The most common pattern within the mixed type is one in which the cryoprecipitate contains IgM and IgG. This is the case in our patient in whom the IgM was the homogeneous component. In other words, these are cold-insoluble rheumatoid factors that bind IgG through determinants on the Fc portion of the IgG component of the cryoprecipitate. The antigen portion of this antigen-antibody complex is the heterogeneous IgG component and the antibody is the cold-insoluble IgM. (3) The third group of cryoimmunoglobulinemias is a "polyclonal type" in which the cold-precipitable complex contains one or more classes of immunoglobulins, none of which is homogeneous. Therefore, the light chains of both kappa *and* lambda types would be detected in the cryoglobulin in this third and biggest category of cryoglobulinemias. Unfortunately, although it comprises the largest group of patients, it is probably the one about which the least is known. In general, however, it is associated with very small amounts of cold-precipitable immunoglobulins in the serum. In the "mixed type" cryoimmunoglobulinemia, there may be relatively large amounts of cryoprecipitate or there may be amounts in the general range of 3 to 5 mg/ml, which our patient displayed.

In order to be included within this classification, there must be more than 80 μg/ml of cryoglobulin in the serum. Amounts of less than 80 μg/ml are found with remarkable frequency even in the serum of totally asymptomatic persons. Probably half of the people in this room would have detectable cryoglobulins in their serum, but presumably they would all be present at a very low concentration. Therefore, what we see in polyclonal cryoglobulinemia may be an exaggeration of some physiologic process.

I think that our patient clearly fits into the "mixed type" cryoglobulinemia category, and I believe we must next consider the characteristics and subclassification of this group. At the top of the list of diseases in which "mixed type" cryoglobulins occur is the syndrome that Dr. Slatopolsky just mentioned, essential mixed cryoglobulinemia, or the Meltzer-Franklin syndrome. This is a generalized autoimmunity syndrome in which one characteristically finds an IgM-kappa cryoglobulin which is homogeneous, has rheumatoid factor activity and binds a heterogeneous population of IgG molecules included in the cryoprecipitate. Second, but extremely uncommonly, there have been reported examples of Waldenström's macroglobulinemia in which the Waldenström protein had rheumatoid factor activity and coprecipitated with IgG. That is a theoretic possibility in our case, but one would expect larger amounts of the pathologic protein to be included in the cold precipitate. Mixed cryoglobulins also occur in a group of other generalized autoimmunity syndromes including systemic lupus erythematosus and rheumatoid arthritis, which some might regard as indistinguishable from the first category (essential mixed cryoglobulinemia). Fourth, and I think irrelevant to our patient, is the occurrence of mixed type cryoimmunoglobulinemia secondary to certain kinds of infection, particularly viral infections.

Dr. Slatopolsky: Do you think she had a Sjögren's syndrome?

Dr. Little: The essential mixed cryoglobulin syndrome has been reported very often in patients who exhibit some of the symptoms or signs of Sjögren's syndrome; I think it is a semantic problem whether one considers it Sjögren's syndrome with atypical features or a separable entity of essential mixed cryoglobulinemia with features of Sjögren's syndrome. I do not think we have enough information to make the diagnosis of Sjögren's syndrome in this case.

Dr. Slatopolsky: Dr. Hoffsten, mild renal insufficiency developed in this patient. She had 4 g of protein and red blood cell casts in the urine. Knowing that she had a mixed cryoglobulinemia with a rheumatoid factor, do you think an immune-complex glomerulonephritis developed? Can we rule out a second disease, such as polyarteritis nodosa or amyloidosis?

Dr. Phillip Hoffsten: The characteristic glomerular lesion seen in patients with essential cryoglobulinemia is proliferative glomerulonephritis which is immune complex positive when examined by immunofluorescence microscopy. This patient's course is entirely similar to that in the cases of essential cryoglobulinemia described by Meltzer and Franklin. Amyloidosis is not a feature of essential cryoglobulinemia and, thus, the presence of amyloid in her glomeruli would not be expected. In addition, renal amyloidosis is usually associated with the nephrotic syndrome and more proteinuria than she had. The vasculitis seen in her skin biopsy specimen is compatible with essential cryoglobulinemia, and the diagnosis of polyarteritis nodosa need not be invoked to explain the vasculitis. The presence of red blood cell casts in the urine strongly favors a glomerulopathy; thus, an arteritis alone does explain her entire syndrome. Although we cannot rule out polyarteritis nodosa, I think the renal lesion will be proliferative immune-complex glomerulonephritis.

Dr. Slatopolsky: In July 1975, the patient was admitted to the hospital because of chills, fever, pain, anemia and a low platelet count. She received at least 20 platelet transfusions; however, on the 11th hospital day, she had a platelet count of only 9,000/mm^3. She had a prolonged prothrombin time, the partial thromboplastin time and fibrinogen level were within normal limits, fibrinogen degradation products were increased (64 μg/ml) and a protamine sulphate precipitation test was weakly positive. I think this patient had disseminated intravascular coagulation. Dr. Kornfeld, do you agree with this diagnosis and, if that is the case, do you think that disseminated intravascular coagulation developed because of infection, that it was secondary to her immunoproliferative disorder or that we are missing a malignancy?

Dr. Kornfeld: I agree that these laboratory values are essentially diagnostic of disseminated intravascular coagulation. Another finding consistent with that diagnosis was the presence of fragmented burr cells in her blood film, indicating the development of a microangiopathic hemolytic anemia. The most likely cause of the disseminated intravascular coagulation in this patient would be sepsis. Other possibilities include an accelerated phase of her vasculitis or the presence of an occult malignancy. In addition to the thrombocytopenia and the microangiopathic changes seen in the red cells, it should be noted that the reticulocyte count was low and that the white blood cell count fell to low levels during her hospital stay. This indicates a poor bone marrow response to the peripheral destruction of the various blood cell elements, most probably reflecting bone marrow suppression caused by the long-term chemotherapy.

Dr. Slatopolsky: It seems that the major difficulty the patient had was related to her respiratory failure. An infiltrate developed in the right lung and then in the left one. The chest film was consistent with the diagnosis of pulmonary edema; however, when a Swan-Ganz catheter was placed, the pressures obtained were not consistent with congestive heart failure. Dr. Bruce, do you think that the picture in her lungs was consistent with bleeding secondary to disseminated intravascular coagulation or infection? If infection was responsible,

Pneumocystis carinii should be ruled out. I believe we should also consider other possible explanations, such as vasculitis, paraprotein infiltration or a fungal infection. Which of these possibilities is the most likely one?

Dr. Robert Bruce: On admission, opportunistic infection had to be and was strongly considered. This woman had severely compromised host defenses both from her disease and the treatment that she had received. She was febrile and had collapse of the lower lobe of the right lung. However, atelectasis cleared dramatically with bronchoscopy. No pathologic organisms were recovered either from spontaneously expectorated sputum or from the bronchial washings. Adequate material was sent to the laboratory. Negative cultures exclude the possibility of the more usual forms of bacterial infection. The fever, of course, could be explained by the presence of vasculitis or infection elsewhere in the body that might not be reflected in examination of the lung secretions. Transbronchial biopsy has been helpful in establishing the diagnoses of Pneumocystis carinii as well as fungal infections in the lung. I gather that this procedure was nondiagnostic and I think the correct step, an open lung biopsy, was taken. This was accomplished under extremely difficult circumstances. She was receiving blood transfusions and platelet packs at the time. A small biopsy specimen from the right lung was obtained. If it was representative of the rest of the lung, one can safely say she did not have Pneumocystis carinii. There was no evidence of granuloma formation or of fungal infection. The subsequent cultures did not reveal a pathogen.

The lung biopsy specimen showed acute alveolar injury manifested by proliferation of the type II or granular pneumocytes along with increased thickening of the alveolar walls. The pathology report described what was initially thought to be fibrosis, but there was homogeneous eosinophilic material not only in the interstitial spaces but also in the alveolar spaces. That, along with the rapid roentgenographic appearance of the infiltrates and the fact that her lung compliance remained fairly good, argue against the presence of fibrosis. What was this material in the interstitial and in the alveolar spaces? There are several possibilities. Amyloid has been mentioned several times, but this distribution in the lung is very unusual for amyloid. Could this be deposition of the cryoglobulin, the circulating immune complex? This has not been reported previously, and would be an unlikely although very exciting possibility which could be investigated with immunofluorescence on the tissue. Since the biopsy specimen was obtained during an ongoing disseminated intravascular coagulation, it is very likely that this material represented fibrin in the lung. I think that this is the most likely explanation for this material.

The lung biopsy also helps us to understand the problems that the physicians were having at the bedside. Pulmonary edema, to many clinicians, elicits a reflex equaling it with left ventricular failure. Pulmonary edema means increased lung water. Lung water can be increased by causes other than elevated left atrial pressures. The Swan-Ganz catheterization made it quite clear that the patient was not in left heart failure. Leaking capillaries could be the explanation, and probably were the major reason that the lung water was increased clinically and roentgenographically. Capillary leaking is part of diffuse alveolar injury. There are many causes of diffuse alveolar injury. Rheumatoid arthritis can do it. Chlorambucil can do it. Oxygen can do it. She had all three of these. Disseminated intravascular coagulation can do it and would be my first bet.

The patient died essentially of pump failure. It was clear from the Swan-Ganz catheterization that she was hypovolemic despite the fact that she was in pulmonary edema. She died of low cardiac output despite attempts at volume expansion and use of pressor agents. I wonder what shape the myocardium was in at the time of death. Did she have a myocardial infarction, did she have the myocardiopathy that is associated with essential macroglobulinemia, was there myocarditis?

Dr. Slatopolsky: Do you think she had subacute bacterial endocarditis?

Dr. Bruce: She may have had a marantic endocarditis. We had no evidence in terms of blood cultures to support the diagnosis of bacterial endocarditis.

Dr. Slatopolsky: I would like now to give you my impression of her clinical course. I think that this patient, for some unknown reason, had an antigenic challenge—perhaps viral in nature—which was responsible for the development of an immunoproliferative disorder with an increased plasmacytoid lymphocytic response. However, I do not believe that this patient had lymphoma or Waldenström's macroglobulinemia. I believe she had essential mixed IgG-IgM cryoglobulinemia. Secondary to this abnormality, she had an immune-complex glomerulonephritis. Light microscopy may show diffuse glomerulonephritis with a basement membrane-like material within the glomeruli. Electron microscopy may show annular or cylindrical bodies within the capillary wall and, if immunofluorescence studies were performed, perhaps we will find irregular staining for IgM and IgG. Obviously, the impairment in renal function was not severe enough to produce her death. I believe that she had disseminated intravascular coagulation, most likely secondary to a gram-negative infection; however, an immunoproliferative disorder or malignancy may have played a role. The pathologic process in her lungs was extremely complicated and probably was secondary to disseminated intravascular coagulation with bleeding into her lungs. Vasculitis and infection also may have contributed to her respiratory insufficiency. If infection played a role Pneumocystic carinii, Klebsiella and Candida should be considered.

In summary, I believe the diagnosis in this patient is essential mixed IgG-IgM cryoglobulinemia.

PATHOLOGIC DISCUSSION

Dr. Thomas Tillack: The first biopsy performed on this patient was in 1969; a biopsy specimen of an enlarged parotid salivary gland was obtained that showed changes typical of Mikulicz's disease, with myoepithelial islands and profound lymphocytic infiltrates in the gland. Later in 1969, an enlarged cervical node was biopsied, and on reviewing the sections of that node, I was unable to unequivocally establish a diagnosis of lymphoma. The node was certainly atypical and had some features which were similar to a femoral node obtained at biopsy in 1974. In 1973, a skin biopsy specimen showed allergic vasculitis. In 1974, an enlarged femoral node was biopsied. The over-all architecture was somewhat altered in that germinal centers could not be identified in the node. The capsule was intact, however, and the capsular sinuses were open. The node was almost entirely made up of plasma cells at various stages of maturity (Figure 1). The cytoplasm of the cells was pyroninophilic and many contained periodic acid-Schiff–positive material. Some paraamyloid deposits were present in the node. We interpreted the appearance of this node as being consistent with an immunoproliferative disorder, perhaps Waldenström's macroglobulinemia, although a subsequent bone marrow biopsy specimen failed to show the lymphocytic and plasmacytoid infiltrates characteristic of that disease.

Since this case, we have seen lymph node biopsy specimens from two other patients with essential mixed cryoglobulinemia; these lymph nodes had a histologic appearance identical to that in the present case. In reading about the clinical findings in patients with essential mixed cryoglobulinemia, it is often mentioned that the patients have lymphadenopathy; however, the histologic characteristics of these nodes have not been adequately described. In summary, the best designation for the histologic changes seen in this patient's lymph node biopsy specimens would be that of an immunoproliferative disorder, and we should not classify this as lymphoma.

Dr. Kissane will discuss the autopsy findings.

Dr. John Kissane: At autopsy lymph nodes throughout the body were moderately enlarged. A representative node shows, at low magnificant (Figure 2), preservation of general architecture. Germinal centers are evident and the corticomedullary and sinusoidal structures are intact. At higher magnification, the nodal architecture was altered by the infiltration of sheets of well-differentiated plasma cells in varying stages of maturity. In these plasma cells both cytoplasmic and nuclear periodic acid-Schiff–positive granules can be identified, and

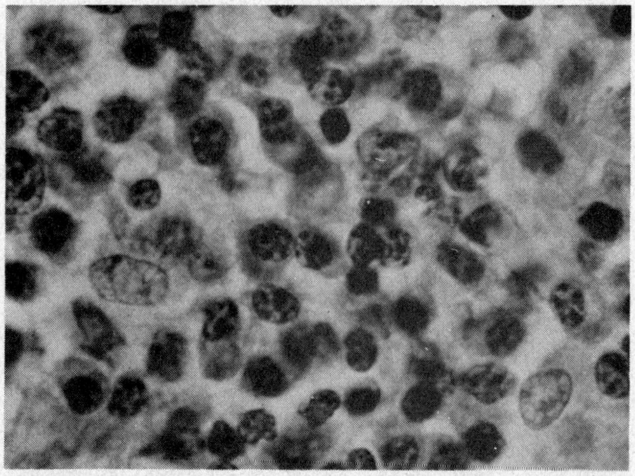

Figure 1. *Micrograph showing a plasmacytic infiltrate that was present throughout the entire lymph node.*

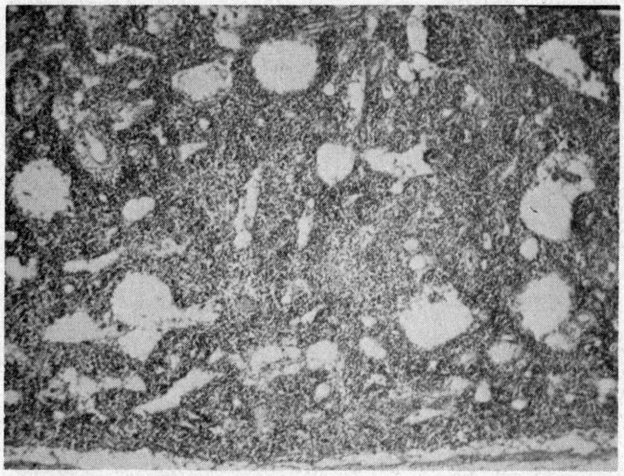

Figure 2. *Photomicrograph of lymph node showing general preservation of architecture. Hematoxylin and eosin stain; magnification × 150, reduced by 15 per cent.*

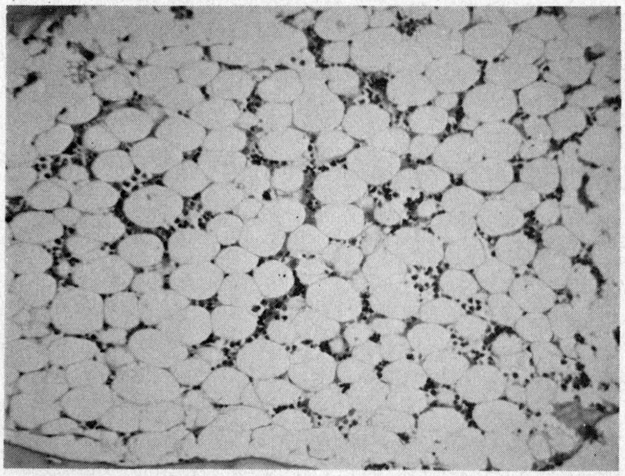

Figure 3. *Photomicrograph of vertebral marrow showing panhypocellularity. Hematoxylin and eosin stain; magnification × 150, reduced by 15 per cent.*

the cells stain positively with methyl-green-pyronine, reflecting active secretion of immunoglobulins. This appearance has been described in peripheral lymph nodes of patients with macroglobulinemia but, failing demonstration at that time of involvement of bone marrow, remains nonspecific. Bone marrow available at autopsy was extremely hypocellular (Figure 3).

The spleen at autopsy was not markedly enlarged (260 g). Microscopically, red and white pulp were poorly demarcated. We attribute the central lucency on the spleen scan to a primary splenic cyst into which there had been hemorrhage (Figure 4) irrelevant to the underlying disease. Littoral cells of the spleen contained hemosiderin reflecting either hemolysis of transfusions or both. Elsewhere in the spleen were peritrabecular infiltration of mononuclear cells, a useful microscopic clue to immune-complex mediated disease. We cannot render a diagnosis of malignant lymphoma on the spleen or lymph nodes in this case.

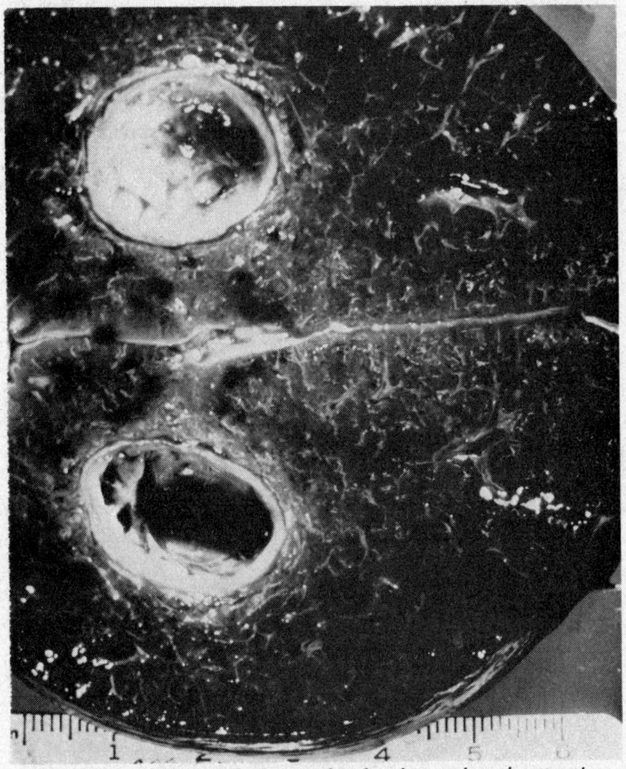

Figure 4. *Gross photograph of spleen showing cyst.*

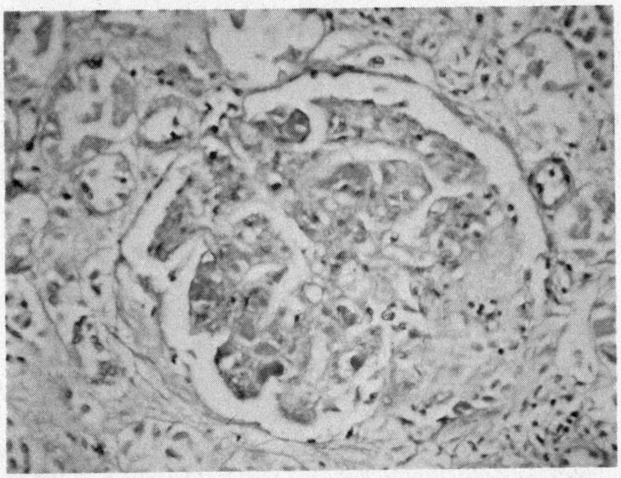

Figure 5. *Photomicrograph of kidney showing hypercellularity and a partially sclerotic crescent. Periodic acid-Schiff stain; magnification × 300, reduced by 15 per cent.*

The thyroid gland was contracted and fibrotic consistent with inclusion of the gland within portals of radiation therapy.

The skin showed microscopic patches of hemosiderosis about dermal vessels consistent with a remote dermal vasculitis.

The bulky (2,990 g) lungs were grossly hemorrhagic. Microscopically, there was extensive intra-alveolar hemorrhage. Bacterial colonization was widespread suggesting Pseudomonas sepsis. Pseudomonas aeruginosa, and Serratia marcesans were in fact, cultured from lung. Postmortem immunofluorescent study of pulmonary tissue, demonstrated perivascular localization of IgM and IgG, but not complement.

The kidneys were enlarged (190 and 240 g) and mottled by cortical petechiae. Microscopically, interstitial hemorrhages were present. Glomeruli were diffusely hypercellular, and occasionally epithelial crescents were identified (Figure 5). These changes resemble those in the three patients described by Meltzer and Franklin with mixed cryoglobulinemia who died in acute failure.

Other findings at autopsy included minimal resolving vasculitis in gut, liver, kidney, thyroid and lung. Extensive necrotizing tracheobronchitis was attributed to demonstration of gram-negative rods, gram-positive cocci, candidial yeast and hyphal elements.

In summary we believe the morphologic features of the sequential biopsies and the autopsy in this case suggest the syndrome of mixed cryoglobulinemia [1]. There was no morphologic evidence that her cyroglobulinemia was secondary to a morphologically identifiable disease process such as Waldenström's macroglobulinemia or to infectious diseases that have been mentioned.

Final pathologic diagnoses were extensive pulmonary consolidation and intra-alveolar hemorrhage with unaltered blood in the tracheobronchial tree (history of IgM-IgG mixed cryoglobulinemia, long-term Chlorambucil therapy and secondary leukopenia, thrombocytopenia and anemia); deposition of IgM and IgG around small pulmonary arteries by immunofluorescence (no staining for complement); bronchopneumonia (extensive), multiple colonies of gram-negative rods and gram-positive cocci identified in sections of lung, gastrointestinal tract, and small vessels of the brain and heart (postmortem blood culture growth of Pseudomonas aeruginosa and Serratia marcesans); resolving vasculitis involving scattered small arteries of the lung, kidney, small bowel, liver and thyroid (history of vasculitis on skin biopsy in 1973); proliferative glomerulonephritis (history of nephritis with creatinine clearance = 20 cc/min); generalized massive infiltration of lymph nodes by plasma cells and plasmacytoid lymphocytes; hypocellular bone marrow; dermal hemorrhage and hemosiderin deposition (history of purpura and Raynaud's phenomenon); necrotizing tracheobronchitis (extensive)—colonization with gram-negative rods, gram-positive cocci and yeast and hyphal element of Candida; necrotizing esophagitis; ulceration of the posterior tongue; resolving hematoma and siderosis of the spleen (history of multiple transfusions and weakly positive direct Coombs' test); submucosal hemorrhage of the urinary bladder, right renal pelvis and stomach; hyperemia of the rectal mucosa; pneumatosis of the gastric mucosa; small subpleural hematoma—right middle lobe of the lung (chest tube, in place, right posterior chest wall); fibrin thrombus adherent to right atrium, right ventricle and Swan-Ganz catheter (Swan-Ganz catheter, in place, in main pulmonary artery); status: Foley catheter, in place; 5 cm right forearm cutdown site—recent; 15 cm right posterior thoracic incision—recent.

REFERENCES

1. Meltzer M, Franklin EC: Cryoglobulinemia. A study of 29 patients. I. IgG and IgM cryoglobulins and factors affecting cryoprecipitability. Am J Med 40: 828, 1966.
2. Grey H, Kohler P: Cryoimmunoglobulins. Semin Hematol 10: 87, 1973.
3. Cordonnier D, Huguette M, Groslambert P. Micouin C, Chenais, F, Stoebner P: Mixed IgG-IgM cryoglobulinemia with glomerulonephritis. Immunochemical, fluorescent and ultrastructural study of the kidney and in vitro cryoprecipitate. Am J Med 59: 867, 1975.

The Coroner Describes the Manner of Dying in New York City, 1784–1816

ABRAHAM BLINDERMAN, Ph.D.
Levittown, New York

Our country is celebrating its 200th anniversary. It is proud of its progress and its accomplishments. How much progress has been made in medicine, science and humanity? We may not appreciate how much. This article will enlighten us; it will remind us of how much progress has indeed been made, and it will, hopefully, stimulate us so that we may stimulate the future generation to continue the work, to make the methods more precise and the writing more succinct, lest that in 2176 our writings will induce smiles and smirks, and remarks about how much progress has been made.

Inquest, May 1, 1795, on an Unknown Corpse. A woman without either head or legges and entire naked—was this morning found drifting up near the air furnace at the North River. How or by what means she came to her Death or her Body separated from the Head and Leggs is to them /the jurors\ unknown, but they are induced to believe she died a natural death and separated by some Surgeon or Surgeons and this Part thereof committed to the River.

The laboratories of modern medical examiners are manned by teams of scientists and technicians who employ sophisticated instrumentation to help them establish the causes of the accidental or violent deaths of their silent clients. Doctors and lawyers specializing in forensic medicine scrutinize autopsy findings carefully for conclusions that might have bearings on their specific legal, scientific or criminalogic interests. Perhaps the greatest debate on a postmortem inquest in modern history still rages as skeptics of the validity of the Warren Commission Report insist in books and on television forums that the complete autopsy reports of President Kennedy's assassination be made public.

Throughout history, religion, superstition and cosmetic vanity have inhibited men from supporting the physician's scientific insistence for the right to practice dissection of human bodies. The unsavory practice of body-snatching arose from the need of medical men to study terminal pathologic states of the bodily organs and from their need to teach anatomy precisely to their students. Ghoulish literature has benefited from the historic proscription of dissection. Charles Dickens in "A Tale of Two Cities" and Mary Shelley in "Frankenstein," in illustration, have effectively depicted the illegal indulgence of physicians in the body-snatching trade.

Physicians have advocated dissection of human bodies since 1000 B.C. Susruta, an eminent Indian surgeon urged his colleagues

From the original coronors' reports in manuscript at the Historical Collections Department, Queens College, Kissena Blvd., Queens, New York. Requests for reprints should be addressed to Dr. A. Blinderman, 47 Tanager Lane, Levittown, New York 11756. Manuscript accepted December 9, 1975.

to study the corpse for clues to the origins of disease, a practice advocated by the eminent Roman physician Celsus about a thousand years later [1]. It was Celsus who said of the Alexandrian physicians, Herophilus and Erasistratus, who first publicly dissected the human body, that "they procured criminals out of prison by royal permission, and dissecting them alive, contemplated, while they were yet breathing, the parts which nature had before concealed" [2]. A heinous indictment but not without probability in light of the abominable experiments performed by Nazi physicians upon living beings in the heyday of Hitler's hegemony over much of Europe.

Paradoxically, it was a law school and not a medical school that first sanctioned autopsies in the Middle Ages. Perhaps forensic medicine originated at the University of Bologna where the Bolognese jurists directed physicians to perform postmortems in cases of suspicious deaths [3]. But not until Leonardo da Vinci scientifically dissected corpses to advance anatomic knowledge and wrote that "those who study only old authors and not the works of Nature are stepsons, not sons of Nature," did medicine step out of medievaldom [4]. The Renaissance anatomists, Vesalius, Fallopius, Servetus, Francisco Diaz, Fabricius Hildanus and Ambrose Paré, daringly demonstrated that medical science could not advance without knowledge of the human body's pathology.

Legal medicine was a prominent discipline in 17th century Italy. Treatises on poisoning were popular, possibly because of the frequent employment of fatal drugs as instruments of political action by hostile factions. Paolo Zaccha's "Queastions-Medico-Legales" was a landmark book in forensic medicine [5].

Another watershed book in anatomy was Joseph Lieutand's "Historia Anatomicomedica." This 18th century anatomist described 3,500 autopsies and taught fervently that the examination of corpses was vital to the advancement of medicine [6]. But after 1800, Anglo-Saxon peoples opposed autopsies. The poor, especially, objected to the use of corpses for teaching purposes, and in many instances their hatred for dissectors impeded medical progress [7].

Generally, little legal attention was given throughout the ages to the specific causes of accidental or violent deaths. Since almost all of the world's population, even in Anglo-Saxon nations, lived marginally, officials were not overly concerned to establish the scientific causes of the unexplained deaths of the masses. The coroner's office had its origins in political and financial concerns of the English monarch. As early as 1000 A.D. the coroner was an important official who added to the king's wealth by executing the confiscation of lands of certain criminals, especially the estates of murderers [8]. By 1300, during the reign of Edward I, the coroner's duties included determining whether a murder was committed by felony or misdemeanor. Given the right to interview witnesses, acquire weapons, hold inquests and appoint jurors, the coroner was now a powerful official of the realm. To qualify for this sinecure, the appointee had to have high social status, a known reputation for loyalty to the crown and a willingness to serve without remuneration [9]. Under George II, the coroner was paid 20 shillings per inquest and allowed 9 pence per mile for travel expenses. His chief function now was to hold inquests over bodies of persons who died unnaturally or violently. To make his office workable, the king granted the coroner the right to issue subpoenas and to make arrests [10]. Unfortunately, the coroner had the power to hold or dismiss the accused, a privilege probably abused by incompetent and corrupt coroners [11]. By 1800, the coroner's power was taken from him; he ranked no higher than a dog-catcher and became an unenvied minor official [12]. Dismayed by the degradation of what he believed should be an office of dignity, Thomas Wakely, editor of the famed *Lancet,* wrote vigorously to reform the corrupt and ignorant coroner's office. But his campaign to have only physicians appointed as coroners was premature. Unhappily, the Coroners Act of 1877 did not require coroners to be physicians; in addition, the act gave the coroner the powers of judge, jury and constable, privileges hardly consonant with the objectivity that the office required [13].

Postmortems in colonial America were unusual events. Gradually, the public began to accept postmortems but not anatomic dissections performed by medical students. In 1765, there was a riot against Dr. Shippen's school of anatomy, but the resourceful surgeon quieted the mob by assuring them that he dissected only bodies of murderers, suicides and paupers who had died from diseases deserving special study [14].

In 1766, Dr. Thomas Bond of Philadelphia advocated autopsy as the scientific way to check speculative theories on the nature of disease. But the public was still not impressed with scientific logic. As late as 1788, a mob objected to the alleged display of a human limb hanging out of a window of the Doctor's Hospital in New York. The people did not object to the dissection of the corpses of blacks or strangers, but they resented the mutilation of the corpses of respectable persons. The mob smashed the interior of the hospital; the doctors fled to the local jail for protection; and finally the militia was called out to repel the mob. This they did, only after killing three rioters and wounding many others [15].

A year before Parliament legalized dissection in 1832, Massachusetts passed a similar law. But most American states did not legislate dissection laws until after the Civil War [16].

THE CORONER'S REPORTS OF NEW YORK CITY, 1784–1816

Through the kindness of Professor Leo Hershkowitz, curator of the Historical Documents Department of Queens College, I was privileged to examine hundreds of coroners' reports of post-Revolutionary New York City. In quaint language, often redundant, the coroners describe how Americans died 200 years ago. There are accounts of murders, suicides, accidental deaths, infanticides, unexplained deaths and deaths by visitation of God. Usually, the inquest was held in the home of a respectable citizen. The coroner, an appointee, was paid per inquest. The jurors were chosen from respectable, middle class citizens. Physicians were called infrequently to dignify an inquest that posed problems. As the samplings from the archives reveal, the reports are hardly illustrative of objective, scientific investigations into the causes of the subject's death. To illustrate the form and style of the typical report of this period, I shall reproduce in its entirety the coroner's report of 26 March, 1805, of the murder of Margaret Bancks:

"Upon the view of the body of Margaret Bancks, then and their lying dead upon the oaths of /six jurors\ they do say upon their oaths that a certain person unknown, not having God before his eyes but being moved and seduced by the instigation of the Devil, on the twenty-fifth day of March and year above written at about the fifth hour of the afternoon of the same day, with force of arms at the house of the said Margaret Bancks in the seventh ward of the City and County aforesaid, in and upon the aforesaid Margaret Bancks, then and there being in the peace of God and of the said People, feloniously, voluntarily, and of his malice aforethought, made an assault—and the said person unknown, then and there with some blunt-edged instrument which he, the said person unknown, then and there held in his right hand, the aforesaid Margaret Bancks in and upon the top of the head somewhat to the left side thereof, then and there violently, feloniously, with malice forethought struck and pierced and gave the said Margaret Bancks one mortal wound of the breadth of an eighth of an inch, and of the depth of three inches, with part of the skull drove in the brain, and the said jurors further say that the aforesaid person unknown, in and upon the aforesaid Mrs. Bancks, another assault did make then and there with a certain rasor of steel of the value of three cents, which the said person unknown, then and there held in his right hand, the aforesaid person, in an upon the throat of the aforesaid Mrs. Bancks, then and there feloniously, voluntarily . . . struck, Cutt, and pierced and gave to the said Margaret Bancks, one mortal wound, beginning from a little below the left ear and so deep, as to cut asunder both the windpipe and the right main artery and to the neck bone of her the said Mrs. Bancks of which two mortal wounds the aforesaid M. Bancks instantly died [17]."

Inquests on Murder. Many inquests on victims of alleged murder failed to name the assailant. For example, "David Colden Cooper came to his death at a place and time to the person aforesaid unknown but the jurors believe from the testimony offered before them that the said David Colden Cooper came to his death at some place west of the Hudson River by a wound occasioned by a Ball and that from the examination of the said wound the said David Colden Cooper must have died without languishing at any time."

A boxing match, of motive unknown, led to the watery death of one James Duffield on December 21, 1816:

"James Duffield, on the evening of the day above written, in the City and County aforesaid, on the brig Rebecca of Liverpool, Thomas Manlove Master, lying at Beekman Slip . . . the ward aforesaid, was then and there boxing with a certain Edward Leighton, cook of the said Brig—that the said Edward Leighton, him the said James, one blow or push did give, by which blow, or push the said James was knocked or pushed into the River called the East River, immediately drowned, and the aforesaid Edward Leighton, in manner, by the means aforesaid, him the said James, did Slaughter and Kill, and afterwards did flee away and conceal himself against the People of this State and their Dignity."

Modern medical examiners probably would have been more circumspect in their inquest over the body of Mary Storm than the jurors, physician and coroner were who investigated the cause of her death on March 2, 1810. Although the depositions of the three witnesses suggest the culpability of Daniel Storm, the deceased's husband, the investigators attributed Mrs. Storm's death to a Visitation of God. The verbatim report of the coroner would not satisfy the curiosity of a modern district attorney or medical examiner:

Evidence taken at the Holding and Inquest over the body of Mary Storm in the Seventh Ward, March 2, 1810.

"Ann Bentley deposeth and saith that she lives in the house with Daniel Storm, the husband of the deceased, that she has frequently heard Daniel Storm disputing or wrangling with the Deceased that last evening after 7 o'clock Mr. Storm came into her Room, said that his wife was dead or was dying, she went in saw the deceased breathe twice and there expire, he immediately sent for a doctor, Mr. Bailry came and tryed to bleed the deceased but could not get any blood, Storm seemed very anctious the Doctor might do something that might help the deceased.

Naome Beck wittness deposeth and Saith that she lives in the same floor with Daniel Storm that last evening first instant she heard Mr. Storm say I will Nock you down but cannot say who was in the Room with him as I was in my own apartment I heard somebody fall and soon heard a heavy groaning and went into the Room found Mrs. Storm was dead. He seemed to be anctious for the Doctor to do something for his wife.

Phebe Doughty deposeth and saith that on the March 1 instant Mary Storm called in at her house and informed this deponent that Storm had made the deceased an offer if she would consent to part with him, that the oldest child might be put to board with the deponent and he would pay the board and find the child clothes and give the deceased all the furniture including the bead. She said she thought she would agree to his proposal."

Jurors' Report. We the subscribers, Physician summoned to examine the body of Mrs. Mary Storm, cannot discover those evident marks which would guide us in our opinion that the defunct came to her death otherwise than by Providence of God.

Sam Nesbitt
Samuel Akerly
William Bäilley

Coroner's Report. Mary Storm was seized with violent spasms or fits of which spasms or fits she died by the Visitation of God.

Strange are the ways of manslaughterers! John L. Dewbois, "with a certain Windsor chair of the value of ten cents . . . in and upon the top of her hand and on the left temple then and there violently feloniously voluntarily and of his malice aforethought struck and pierced and gave to the said Catherine Dewbois . . . two mortal wounds of which wounds the aforesaid Catherine Dewbois died."

Arsenic was subtly used by one Diana Sollick to remove Hatty Johnson from their precints. Hapless Diana Sollick, "not having God before her eyes but seduced by the instigation of the Devil, a certain quantity of arsenic mixed in gin, in a certain bowl of the value of six cents which she then and there had in her hand, and which arsenic she knew to be a deadly poison, feloniously willfully, and of her malice aforethought did mix with the said gin and sweetening it with sugar—and the said Diana Sollick, the poison mixed as aforesaid . . . did offer and give to her the said Hatty Johnson to take and swallow down by means whereof the said Hatty Johnson having taken down and swallowed the said poison, did then and there become sick and distempered in her body, of which sickness and distemper she did languish until the day of taking of this inquisition and then died. January 8, 1815."

Inquests on Infanticide and Childbirth Neglect. The saddest inquests in any age are those held over the bodies of unwanted babies. A large number of post-Revolutionary coroners' reports deal with the cruelties perpetrated by adults upon their offspring. The coroners' words are devoid of sentiment but the pathos of each case cited is implicit in the narration of each crime:

(November 26, 1808) A certain person or persons . . . did make an assault upon the said female infant unknown . . . and did take and carry to the door of No. 83 Chatham Street and her did lay on the cold stone steps of the Door of which cold it languished and died.

(May 3, 1805) Upon the view of the body of a certain female infant of one Elizabeth Stephens now or late of the seventeenth ward of the City and County aforesaid, then and there lying dead upon the oaths of —— who say upon their Oaths that the said Elizabeth Stephens being alone in the perilous time of Child Birth without help—it so happened that accidentally, casually, and by misfortune that she the aforesaid infant, strangled suffocated and died.

(October 12, 1805) . . . A certain person or persons unknown not having God before his eyes, did make an assault upon the said male infant unknown . . . him did take and carry to the arched bridge on the Sandy Hill Road in the said eighth ward, and him did lay under the said bridge of which cold and Wett it languished and died.

(October 14, 1814) A new born male infant unknown was found floating in the water of the Coffee House Slip—that a certain person or persons unknown with force and arms did make an assault upon the said new born unknown and did take him and carry to a privy and afterwards was thrown into the river. . .

Unhappy laboring women frequently cast their new born infants into privies, cut the umbilical cord without tying it to prevent the infant's bleeding to death, or merely neglected to feed or warm the helpless infants. The medical report of Dr. William McIntosh on the death of an unknown infant is almost naive in its formulation: "Being called upon by the coroner to an inquest, held on the body of an infant child, to examine into the cause of its death if any—it was examined by me, and no marks of violence except the umbilical cord which appeared to have been tore in too rather than cut, neither did it appear to have had any precausions taken to prevent the loss of blood which is absolute to the preservation of life."

The inquisition held to determine the death of Jane Curry's bastard child includes a quaint denial by the mother that the deposition of Catherine Rogers, "duly sworn on the Holy Evangelist of Almighty God," was accurate. Jane Curry insisted that Catherine Rogers had mistaken her seasonal obesity for pregnancy, that she had not given birth, but the testimony of Dr. Isaac Ledyard negated her contrived excuse. She had given birth to a mature child that was alive at the commencement of her labor. The coroner's jury concluded that she was delivered of her child unassisted in a garret room, that she had thrown the live bastard child out of the window, and that she was guilty of feloniously killing and murdering her child.

Inquests on Suicide. It seemed to be the consensus of the coroners of this period that all suicides were either insane, melancholy or deranged. Then as now, suicides employed poisons, guns, knives and ropes to rid themselves of life; others jumped out of buildings or drowned themselves, but Daniel Leffingwell insured his death by drinking laudanum and shooting himself through his right ear. Although the coroner's report is long, it is a fine example of the quaint official rhetoric of his office and is reproduced here with minor deletions:

An inquisition . . . taken for the People of the State of New York, at the first Ward of the City of New York the ninth day of October in the year of Our Lord one thousand eight hundred and four before me John Burger Coroner, for the City and County aforesaid, on view of the body of Daniel Leffingwell then and there lying dead upon the oaths of —— —— good and lawful men of the said City and County who having been sworn and charged the inquiry for the said People, When, Where, How, and after what Manner the said Daniel Leffingwell came to his death do say upon their oaths, that the said Daniel Leffingwell on the eighth day of December and year above written having the fear of God before his eyes being moved and seduced by the instigation of the Devil at the first Ward in the City and County aforesaid, the said Daniel Leffingwell being then and there . . . with a certain Vessel of poison commonly called laudanum of the value of six cents, which he then and there held in his hand and to his mouth did put, and voluntarily and feloniously and of his malice forethought did drinck, and that he then and there still being alone with two certain Pistols of the Value of two dollars, charged and loaded with gun powder and balls, which he the said Daniel Leffingwell held the One in his left and the other in his right-hand, which said pistol in his right hand, to, at, and against or in his own ear on the right side of his head, did put, and voluntarily, feloniously, and of his malice forethought—did then and there shoot off and discharge, by means where of he the said Daniel Leffingwell voluntarily, feloniously, and of his malice aforethought did then and there give himself one mortal wound of which he instantly died, and so the Jurors aforesaid do say that the said Daniel Leffingwell in manner and form and by the means aforesaid as a felon of himself, feloniously, voluntarily and of his malice aforethought himself killed poisoned shot and murdered against the peace of the People of the State of New York and their dignity.

Catherine Shakell, committed to a hospital as insane, hanged herself by her garter; Thomasin Woods who was "of a melancholy and insane mind . . . cast herself into a cistern of water and drowned herself;" Andrew Morrison, "at the time of his death and long before was a lunatic and person of insane mind, and being a lunatic did then and there with a razor cut his own throat;" Mary Hopper, being a person of an insane mind . . . being alone in the third story of the House of . . . John Hopper, did then by her own effort throw herself out of a door of the said third story facing the street, struck on the stone pavement of said street which throwing and striking on the said pavement she instantly died;" and Sally Lockwood . . . with a certain portion of poison commonly called opium of the value of six cents which the said Sally then and there held in her hand and into her mouth did put and the said opium did eate of which eating the said Sally suffocated and died."

Not all attempts at suicide immediately release the sufferer from his anguish. Christopher Manly . . . "feloniously voluntarily and of his malice forethought made an assault, and that the said Christopher Manly then and there with a certain knife of the vallue of one penney which he then and there had and held in his hand, and as a fellen to himself, in and upon his belly, then and there feloniously, and of his malice aforethought did strike and gave to himself upon his belly two mortal wounds of the length of an half inch and depth of two inches of which mortal wounds he the said Christopher Manly languished and languishing lived from the said eighth day of May until the eleventh day of May instant, and then and there of the mortal wounds aforesaid died."

Inquests on Accidental Deaths. Then as now unfortunate people died by drowning, falls, vehicular accidents, imbibing of fatal medicines, accidental gunshots, and choking on food. Since much of the commuting in the environs of Manhattan island was by waterways, the incidence of death by drowning was high. The waters near Hellgate were treacherous and many small boats were capsized by the strong currents in the vicinity. For example, on June 23, 1789, "Sarah Baker and Lucretia Sherman were passengers on board Josiah Lecounts boat, then on their passage from New Rochelle to New York that the aforesaid Sarah Baker and Lucretia Sherman were in the cabbins of said boat, that when the said boat was in helgate, she was upset by a violent gale of wind, when the aforesaid Sarah Baker and the aforesaid Lucretia Sherman were drownded in the waters then in the cabbin of the aforesaid boat." Another unfortunate, John Stevenson, "on the 16th day of June (1814), while sailing in the Narrows, it so happens that accidentally, casually, and by misfortune the said John Stevenson was knocked overboard by the boom in the act of jibing in the said river, there suffocated and drowning, he the said John Stevenson then and there instantly died."

Occasionally, a coroner's report inadvertently reflects the social conditions of his age. The plight of the very poor of New York City is strikingly depicted in the report of Coroner John Bloodgood, June 9, 1813: "Rachel Still died of a Typhus Fever, occasioned by a fall and wounds received on the hand and Bruises on the arm and the loathesome confined celleur living in, Being eight or ten together, as doeth appear by the Testimony of Doctor Schenck and not otherwise."

Although self-propelled vehicles were not yet decimating its population, deaths resulting from injuries sustained in horse-drawn vehicles were common. In illustration, Jacob Snydecker, cartman, "on the First Day of August (1814) at the tenth ward in Sherriff Street, being negligently Driving a cart, and then and there accidentally, casually, and by misfortune, fell from the said cart and received a violent contution on his head and body of which said contution he then and there instantly died." A curious grammatical construction describes the unhappy death of Barney Mullen "who came to his death by falling off a horse hanging by one foot in the stirrup and the horse kicking him between the hours of 2 and 3 o'clock."

Tebelon Congdon came to a painful end while eating his supper. He "did then and there choak, strangle and suffocated, of which said choaking, strangling, and suffocation the said Tebelon Congdon there instantly died." William Stimson, not mindful of the condition of his window, "was caught with his head in a window between the sill and sash thereof, in which situation before any aid was afforded him, he did choak and suffocate, of which choaking and suffocation he did die."

An unlabeled bottle was the undoing of James McBride, cabinet maker, on June 28, 1815: "At the house known by the name of Mechanic Hall, in the third ward, occupied as a boarding house by Anthony V. Marcellin about the hour of seven in the afternoon, /James McBride\ being in the employ of Kelly Cabinet Makers engaged in fixing a bottom to a bedstead—a certain vessel containing poison being corrosive sublimate, dissolved in spirits, and contained in a bottle being in the room where the said James was at work, he the said James, not knowing the same to be poison, the said bottle to his mouth did put and of said poison did drink, of which drinking he immediately sickened and languished, languishing for twenty hours he died."

An accidental shooting of a militiaman on parade brought grief to John Adams, a friend of the deceased. Ephraim Brasher, Coroner, reported this tragedy at length:

> On the 28th day of September, 1787, a body of the Militia of the City aforesaid /New York City\ under the command of Lieut. Colonel Sebastian Beauman were paraded for the purpose of Review and sham fighting, that after the said Body of Militia had been reviewed in the field commonly called the Raceground . . . by Brigadier General William Malcolm, the aforesaid body of militia were divided in two parties, to wit, the Corps of Artilery and Horse were marched in the Fort in the rear of Colonel Morgan Lewis's house, and there stationed under the command of Major Reed, that the other party of the Militia under the command of the aforesaid Colonel Beauman as the besieged parteys were then firing with blank cartridges, the aforesaid John Loudon then on horseback with the besiegers close under aforesaid fort was then and there by accident shot thro the body and killed by a ramrod ball, or some other instrument of matter and by some person unknown.

The death of John Loudon grieved John Adams who wrote emotionally to his friend, James Greenleaf, of Loudon's strange passing: "The melancholy fate of our friend John Loudon, killed in a sham fight of militia, of which he was adjutant, is a subject on which I cannot dwell."

Inquests on Deaths by Visitation of God. For want of more accurate findings, coroners and jurors conveniently ascribed deaths to Visitations by God, a euphemism for natural deaths or unexplained deaths. For example, "Betsey, an infant was seized with violent spasms or fits, by the Visitation of God, it died in a natural way." Apparently, the coroner did not think it necessary to have an autopsy performed on Betsey's corpse to determine the cause of her spasms or fits. Similarly, Jane Kelly was "seized with Violent Apoplectick fits of which fits she died;" again, the coroner did not deem it advantageous legally or medically to establish the reasons for her apoplexy. In the case of Captain Robt. W. Osborn, a medical reason was given for his death by the Visitation of God "in a natural way." An abscess of the liver "bursted and discharged the contents in the chest of the stomach;" this finding was either a physician's report of emergency treatment or a postmortem analysis—or both. Other cases of death by Visitation of God were ascribed to the "bursting of the left ventricle of the heart," to "a Natural disease called pneumonia," to a "quinsey sore throat," to a "spasm or cramp in the stomach by drinking cold water," and to debility caused by lack of medical assistance in jail.

Inquests on Deaths Occasioned by Intemperance. Overdrinking was a problem in post-Revolutionary America as it is today. The coroners' reports include inquests on deaths ascribed to alcoholism and to accidental deaths resulting from drunkenness. So, Marianne Gillespie "came to her death from a life of dissipation which brought on debility," Elizabeth Goodell "came to her death through intemperance and debility," Thomas Taylor died on February 24, 1784, "by taking too much strong liquor," and John Richards "from the want of bedding, cloathing, and the common necessaries of life and the two frequent use of spiritous, liquors, he languished and died." Another imbiber "while in liquor, fell and broke his neck," Hannah Hall who "was in liquor . . . by accident fell into the fire by which accident the aforesaid Hannah was burned in the right side of the breast, and side, . . . and lingering lived until the eleventh day of May," and Philas Johnson, "after the exertion of dancing, and immoderately drinking of strong liquor was taken ill and suddenly died."

Inquests on Medical Malpractice and Dissections. Coroners' inquests do not concern themselves with instances of medical malpractice. Few such cases are cited in the archives, probably because governmental and professional supervision of medical practice was minimal. For example, it is doubtful that Dr. William Nobes received a reprimand for his negligence in his treatment of Hannah McCalvey: "One William Nobes, Physician, in giving medicine to the said Hannah it so happened the said William Nobes gave Hannah some corrosive sublimate (instead of bilious powders) of which said medicine so taken she the said Hannah was casually, accidentally and by misfortune killed."

That doctors performed anatomical operations upon the corpses of unknowns is evident in the following excerpts from bizarre reports: The "unknown died a natural death that after his death some person or persons who are also unknown, cut off the legs, one of the arms, opened the bowels, and performed other operations. And that afterwards the said body and limbs were put into a bag and thrown into the river." How the coroner determined that the deceased had died a natural death is incomprehensible in view of his anonymity and the mutilation of his body. Another macabre case of supposed medical tampering with unknown corpses was reported in 1799 by Coroner Charles Dickinson. The unidentified corpse with "Scull sawed off, arms and legs cutt off, and the body opened," influenced the jury to entertain the opinion that "the body was a dead Corps, opperated on by some Doctor or Doctors to try experiments and afterwards thrown in to the river." On May 1, 1810, a coroner's jury attested that an unknown colored girl who had died in the State prison on the tenth day of April "was delivered to some Doctor or Doctors, after they had her in their possession some time put her in a box and threw her into the North River and so the jurors do say that the aforesaid coloured girl came to her death." In none of these reports is there a hint of suspicion that the deceased might have come to their deaths by foul play.

Inquests on Unexplained Deaths of Blacks. In four instances at least, it seems that coroners' juries were reluctant to give more than cursory attention to the deaths of blacks. An unknown black woman, "then and there being in a common river called Hudson, herself voluntarily and feloniously drowned." But on what evidence? Another unidentified black woman "was found on the night of the fifth instant (September 5, 1792) by Jonathan Dunn who where then fishing with a Net in Hudson River, commonly called and known by the name of North River, nearly opposite to W. George Campbell's Tavern, and appeared to have lain in the water some months, but how she came to her death, they /the jurors\ could not find out." Another black woman, a "Negro wench Betty came to her Death today upon the oaths of —— that the aforesaid Betty, the property of Ebenezer Wilson—was yesterday morning found lying naked in the Water, in the Old Slip, near the house where the said Wilson lived." How could the jurors be certain that an "unknown black man . . . with a bag of stone fastened about his neck, himself did throw in the east river, of which he Voluntarily and feloniously drowned?" Perhaps it was easier to write off a case as suicide than to expend time and money in detective work in behalf of justice for common folk.

CONCLUSION

Lacking today's sophisticated scientific apparatus and technics, the post-Revolutionary coroners could not investigate unexplained deaths with the precision of modern medical examiners. The coroner's office was a sinecure granted for political favors or allegiances. Although the new nation had repudiated monarchy, many of its eminent leaders were still aristocratic in temper. Why, then, should local governments expend their budgets and energies in seeking causes for the violent and accidental deaths of its ordinary citizens? The coroners' juries were carefully chosen from the middle or upper classes; probably, they were justified in their frequent superficial documentation of the causes of death in those cases they considered in view of the limited investigatory means at their disposal.

The coroners' reports of the period 1788–1816 are valuable records of the ways of death in early republican America, of the social mores then extant, and of the quaint rhetoric of minor officials in law and medicine. Unfortunately, men today still are "moved and seduced by the instigation of the Devil" to do harm and to affront "the dignity of the People of the state" by their felonies committed upon themselves and upon their victims.

REFERENCES

1. Castiglioni A: A History of Medicine, New York, Alfred A. Knopf, 1958, p 95.
2. Robinson V: The Story of Medicine, New York, Tudor Publishing Co., 1935, p 67.
3. Ibid, p 220.
4. Ibid, p 249.
5. Castiglioni A: A History of Medicine, New York, Alfred A. Knopf, 1958, p 557.
6. King LS: The Medical World of the Eighteenth Century, Chicago, The University of Chicago Press, 1958, p 265.
7. Shryock RH: The Development of Modern Medicine, Philadelphia, University of Pennsylvania Press, 1936, p 38.
8. Martin ME: The Doctor Looks at Murder, Garden City, Doubleday & Co., 1937, p 10.
9. Ibid, p 13.
10. Ibid, p 15.
11. Ibid, p 16.
12. Ibid, p 14.
13. Ibid, p 19.
14. Shafer HB: The American Medical Profession, New York, The AMS Press, 1966, p 57.
15. Ibid, p 57.
16. Shryock RH: The Development of Modern Medicine, Philadelphia, University of Pennsylvania Press, 1936, p 39.
17. All of the coroners' reports cited in this paper are verbatim copies of the original archives in the Historical Documents Collection of Queens College of New York City.

Bartter's Syndrome

Study of a 52 Year Old Man with Evidence for a Defect in Proximal Tubular Sodium Reabsorption and Comments on Therapy

DAVID J. TOMKO, M.D.
BETTY P. Y. YEH, M.D.
WILLIAM F. FALLS, Jr., M.D.
Richmond, Virginia

A patient with Bartter's syndrome in whom the disease was recognized at 52 years of age is described. Studies of his renal function suggest that the basic pathophysiologic defect was an abnormality in proximal tubular sodium reabsorption which led to extracellular fluid volume depletion and consequent stimulation of the renin-angiotensin-aldosterone axis. After comparing the physiologic studies in this patient with those in other reported cases, we postulate that Bartter's syndrome may represent the end result of different pathophysiologic processes which share in common juxtaglomerular hyperplasia, increased renin release and secondary hyperaldosteronism. Therapy with B-adrenergic blocking agents produced adverse effects, but the patient responded well to more conventional measures.

In 1962 Bartter et al. [1] described a five year old retarded boy and a 25 year old immature man, both of whom had hypokalemia, metabolic alkalosis, normotension, increased plasma angiotensin concentration, increased urinary aldosterone excretion and a renal biopsy specimen showing hyperplasia of the juxtaglomerular apparatus. The appellation of "Bartter's syndrome" has been given to this constellation of findings, and a number of reports of similar patients have appeared [2–23]. Most of the cases [2–15] have been noted in the pediatric age group, but an occasional young adult [16–23] with the disorder has also been described. The syndrome has seldom been recognized in middle or late life, the occurrence of severe hypokalemia in this age group usually being traced to surreptitious use of diuretics or laxatives by mentally disturbed persons [24,25].

Despite numerous studies, the pathogenesis of Bartter's syndrome is not clearly understood; and there is, indeed, question as to the homogeneity of the disease process among the reported cases. The basic defect proposed by Bartter et al. [1] was a vascular insensitivity to the pressor action of angiotensin leading to a tendency to vasodilatation with resultant renal hypoperfusion and a tonic stimulation of the renin-angiotensin-aldosterone system. According to this hypothesis the hypokalemia and alkalosis were a direct result of excessive aldosterone release. Recently, Bartter's

From the Medical Service, Veterans Administration Hospital and Department of Medicine, Medical College of Virginia, Health Sciences Division, Virginia Commonwealth University, Richmond, Virginia. Requests for reprints should be addressed to Dr. W. F. Falls, Jr., Medical Service, Veterans Administration Hospital, Richmond, Virginia 23249. Manuscript accepted November 20, 1975.

thesis has been questioned, and evidence has been presented suggesting renal tubular sodium wasting as the basic defect in some patients [3-5,10,11,13-16,19]. Both the proximal tubule [3-5,13-15] and the thick ascending limb of Henle's loop [10,16,21] have been implicated as the site of defective sodium reabsorption.

Several therapeutic modalities including the administration of potassium supplements [1-6,8,13,16,19,21], spironolactone [1-6,8,16,19-21]; and, more recently, the use of propranolol [18] have been tried with varying success in patients with Bartter's syndrome.

The case report which follows is of interest because of its implications regarding the age at which a diagnosis of the syndrome must be considered, the origin of the abnormalities in urinary acidification and sodium wasting observed, the hazards of propranolol therapy and the possible heterogeneity of pathogenetic processes which may comprise Bartter's syndrome.

CASE REPORT

A 52 year old white man was admitted to the McGuire VA Hospital for the first time on January 7, 1974, with a four-day history of severe generalized weakness and muscle pain. The first such episode had occurred at age 13 and had cleared spontaneously following bedrest. Subsequently, the patient functioned normally, serving in the military service and working as a merchant seaman until he sustained a head injury in 1952. Thereafter he became unable to hold a steady job because of frequent episodes of nervousness, weakness and nausea, which were usually associated with physical effort. Lifelong polyuria, nocturia and occasional enuresis were also annoying symptoms and led to a transurethral resection of the prostate in 1958 without improvement. Because of these symptoms and the inability to cope with his life situation, he was admitted to the VA Domiciliary, Kecoughtan, Virginia, in the early 1960's. During the next few years he was admitted to the Neuropsychiatric Section of the hospital on several occasions because of "nervousness and weakness"; a diagnosis of chronic anxiety was made, and therapy with large doses of chlorpromazine was initiated. Hypokalemia was first recognized on December 23, 1971, when he was admitted to the Medical Service of the hospital complaining of severe weakness. No replacement therapy was given, and the symptoms gradually subsided with bedrest. On three occasions during 1973 and 1974 he was again admitted because of generalized weakness, leg pains, and slight swelling and tenderness of the muscles of both legs. Serum potassium levels varied from 1.7 to 2.8 meq/liter; no specific therapy was given to correct the hypokalemia, and the weakness gradually subsided on each occasion with therapy consisting of bedrest, a hospital diet and chlorpromazine, 100 mg four times a day. Throughout this period the patient specifically denied frequent or sustained vomiting; diarrhea; or ingestion of laxatives, diuretics or licorice. A brother, sister and three children were in good health, and, like other family members, had never experienced muscle weakness.

Physical examination revealed a well-developed and nourished white man who was profoundly weak. He could neither lift his head nor walk, and he was dysarthric. The pulse rate was 100/min and regular, the blood pressure 95/65 mm Hg, the respiration rate 12/min, the height 5′6″ and the weight 142 pounds. Examination of the heart, chest and abdomen revealed no abnormalities. Abnormal physical findings were limited to the neurologic examination which showed generalized weakness and hyporeflexia, more marked in the lower extremities.

Pertinent studies of the blood and serum revealed a normal hemoglobin level, hematocrit value, white blood cell count, and total protein, albumin, calcium, phosphorus, uric acid, creatinine, bilirubin and alkaline phosphatase levels. Twenty-four hour urinary 17-hydroxycorticosteroid and 17-ketosteroid levels were normal. The serum glutamic oxaloacetic transaminase (SGOT) was 17 units (normal, less than 50 units) and lactic dehydrogenase (LDH) 250 units (normal, less than 225 units). The blood urea nitrogen was 10 mg/100 ml and the serum glucose 115 mg/100 ml. On admission the serum electrolytes included sodium 134 meq/liter, potassium 1.6 meq/liter, chloride 95 meq/liter and bicarbonate 29 meq/liter. The serum magnesium was 1.5 meq/liter. The urinalysis was negative for protein and sugar with only an occasional white blood cell in the sediment. Toxicologic screening for diuretic agents was negative.

Following admission the patient was treated with large doses of potassium chloride (greater than 200 meq/day) with a slow return of the serum potassium concentration to 2.5 meq/liter. In association with this improvement in the serum potassium concentration, the patient's muscle strength rapidly returned, and he was able to be up and about. Polyuria persisted with urine volumes in the range of 5 to 7 liters/24 hours despite improvement in the serum chemical values. An intravenous urogram showed bilateral dilatation of the collecting systems and some blunting of the calyces without evidence of obstruction. A number of special studies were performed and the results are recorded in Table I. Investigation of various aspects of renal function was carried out over the next several weeks; the results are described herein.

On March 14, 1974, an open renal biopsy was performed without difficulty. The biopsy specimen revealed moderate separation of tubules suggesting interstitial edema, normal appearing vessels and numerous glomeruli which showed slight diffuse mesangial cell proliferation. Juxtaglomerular hyperplasia of varying degrees was noted among the glomeruli; in some instances it was quite marked (Figure 1).

The constellation of hypokalemia, relative hypotension, increased renin activity (Table I), increased aldosterone excretion (Table I) and juxtaglomerular hyperplasia substantiated the diagnosis of Bartter's syndrome. After failure of a therapeutic trial with propranolol (vide infra) the patient was ultimately discharged on March 27, 1974, on a regimen of spironolactone, 50 mg four times a day, potassium chloride, 60 meq four times a day and chlorproma-

TABLE I Special Studies

U_{max}*	
Before elevation of serum potassium	374 m0sm/kg H_2O
After elevation of serum potassium	527 m0sm/kg H_2O
Plasma renin activity	29 ng/ml/hour (N = 0.0–3.3)†
Urine aldosterone excretion	27–40 μg/24 hours (N = 2–26)‡
Clearance of sodium iothalamate	116 ml/min
Clearance of PAH	675 ml/min
$^{35}SO_4$ space	8,953 liters 10 meq sodium diet 10,251 liters 300 meq sodium diet
24 hour urine α amino nitrogen	220 mg/24 hours (N = 50–200)

* U_{max}: Maximum urine concentration after 10 hours fluid restriction and 0.5 cc vasopressin in oil.
† Range for normal persons excreting 300 meq sodium daily as was the patient at the time of measurement.
‡ Represents values in normal persons on an unrestricted intake of sodium.

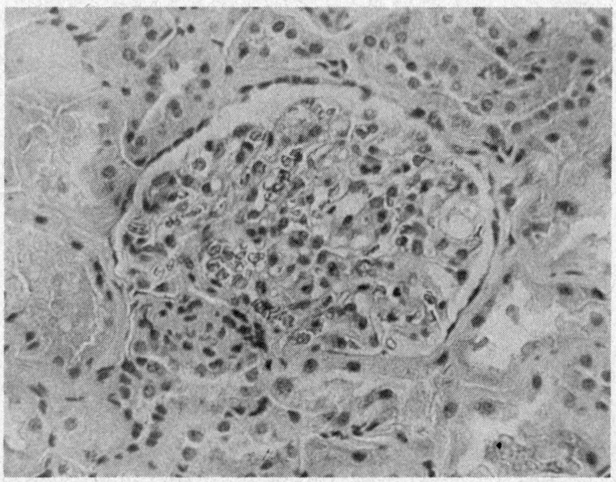

Figure 1. Representative glomerulus showing mild mesangial hypercellularity and marked hyperplasia of the juxtaglomerular apparatus.

zine, 100 mg four times a day. On this regimen the serum potassium concentration returned to normal and the patient did well for seven months. At the end of this period he voluntarily discontinued all medications. There was an abrupt recurrence of weakness necessitating his rehospitalization in December 1974. The serum potassium concentration was 2.2 meq/liter. Further renal function studies were performed, and the patient was discharged improved on his previously successful therapeutic regimen.

In March 1975 the patient was electively readmitted for further studies of his ability to handle an acid load. Serum electrolytes at the time of admission and after completion of the studies were essentially within normal limits except for slightly reduced levels of serum sodium and potassium.

METHODS

Serum and urine determinations of electrolytes, creatinine, urea nitrogen and osmolality were performed by methods routine to this laboratory [26]. Plasma renin activity was measured by a modification of the method of Cohen et al. (Squibb Angiotensin I Immunotope Kit) [27]. Urinary aldosterone and α amino nitrogen were measured by Bio-Science Laboratory, Philadelphia, Pennsylvania. An angiotensin infusion test was performed by the method of Kaplan and Silah [28]. Sulfate space was measured by a modification of the method of Walser et al. [29]. Solute free water clearance (C_{H_2O}) and sodium clearance (C_{Na}) were measured during hypotonic saline infusion by the method of Chaimovitz et al. [10]. Urinary acidification was tested by the method of Wrong and Davies [31], initially, when he had not received spironolactone for eight days and again after administration of the drug was resumed. Urinary ammonium, titratable acid, carbon dioxide content and pH were determined by methods routine to this laboratory [31]. Plasma bicarbonate was calculated from measurements of the arterial blood pH and carbon dioxide tension (pCO_2) performed by routine methods in the hospital pulmonary laboratory.

SPECIAL STUDIES

Angiotensin Infusion Test. The blood pressure response to the infusion of synthetic angiotensin II was performed when the patient was receiving a high (300 meq/24 hours) and a low (10 meq/24 hours) sodium intake (Figure 2). In each instance, marked resistance to blood pressure elevation by the angiotensin was demonstrated.

Response to an Acid Load. Table II illustrates the patient's response to a short ammonium chloride acidification test on two occasions (before and after therapy with spironolactone), and compares the results with the ex-

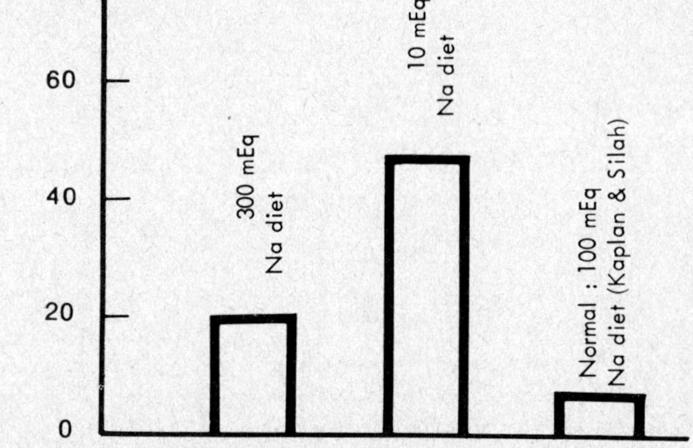

Figure 2. Angiotensin sensitivity of patient on a high and low sodium diet (first two bars) as compared to the normal range established by Kaplan and Silah [28] (last bar).

TABLE II Urinary Acidification Responses at Minimal pH After Administration of Ammonium Chloride (0.1 g/kg). Comparison of Patient's Response Before and After Spironolactone with that of Nine Normal Persons

	Urine					Serum	
	Ammonium (μeq/min)	Titratable Acid (μeq/min)	Bicarbonate (μeq/min)	Total Acid (μeq/min)	pH (units)	Bicarbonate (meq/liter)	Potassium (meq/liter)
No spironolactone	163	27	16	174	6.3	22	2.5
Spironolactone (200 mg/24 hours)	96	67	0.0	163	5.7	14	3.9
Normal + SD*	53 ± 11	38 ± 13	0.0	90.7 ± 21	5.0 ± .2	—	—

* Normal values established in nine persons.

pected normal response. It is apparent that ammonium excretion was greatly enhanced in this patient during both studies, but particularly before the administration of spironolactone. Total acid excretion was also higher than normal in both studies despite inadequate lowering of the urinary pH. In the first study, when the patient was not receiving spironolactone, the serum potassium was low (2.5 meq/liter) and despite a decrease in the serum bicarbonate to 22 meq/liter a significant amount of bicarbonate (16 μeq/min) was leaking into the final urine. When the study was repeated, while the patient was taking spironolactone, a much more severe systemic acidosis was induced, the serum bicarbonate decreasing to 14 meq/liter, and bicarbonate was at last cleared from the urine as the urinary pH fell below 6.0. Calculated bicarbonate reabsorption (T_{HCO_3}) during the first study was 2.04 meq/100

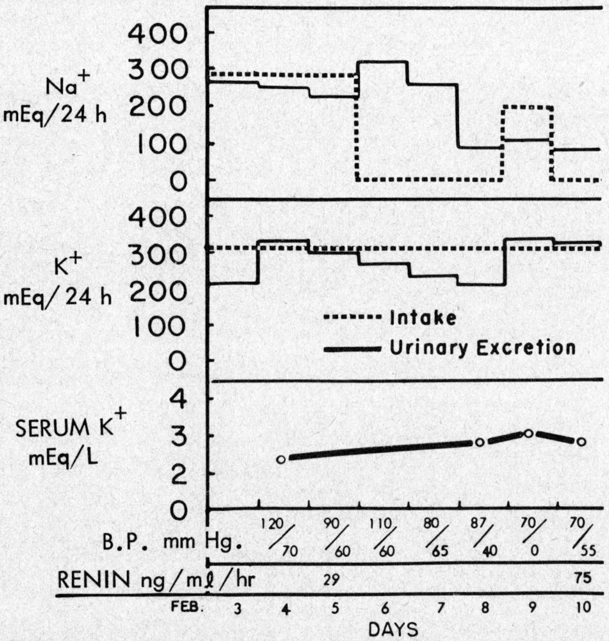

Figure 3. *Response of urinary sodium and potassium excretion to a reduction in sodium intake from 300 to 10 meq/24 hours. The blood pressure determinations were taken on quiet standing after arising from the supine position. Note that the plasma renin activity is measured in ng/ml/hour.*

ml glomerular filtration rate, a value below the expected value for normal man [32].

Influence of Alterations in Dietary Sodium on Urinary Sodium and Potassium Excretion. Figure 3 illustrates the patient's response to the reduction of dietary sodium from 300 meq/24 hours to 10 meq/24 hours. Stool electrolyte concentrations were not measured during this study, but the patient did not experience diarrhea and it is assumed that losses of sodium and potassium in the stool were negligible. A marked negative sodium balance associated with a weight loss of 4 pounds and the development of symptomatic postural hypotension ensued within four days of the dietary change and necessitated the intravenous administration of 155 meq sodium chloride. A slight rise in serum potassium concentration occurred in conjunction with reduced urinary potassium excretion suggesting that potassium retention occurred concomitant with the dietary sodium restriction. Although the tendency to sodium loss was marked, some ability to modulate urinary excretion was retained as indicated by retention of approximately half of the sodium administered on the fourth day of restriction. The plasma renin activity more than doubled from its already markedly elevated state during the course of study.

Influence of Volume Expansion. The striking increase in plasma renin activity noted in the prior study indicated that the renin response to extracellular fluid volume depletion was directionally appropriate although operating at an excessively high level. In order to evaluate further the appropriateness of response to alterations in extracellular fluid volume, the plasma renin activity was measured during the rapid intravenous infusion of 2,000 ml normal saline solution (Figure 4). In association with this maneuver there was a marked decrease in plasma renin activity from 25.4 ng/ml/hour to 9.3 ng/ml/hour indicating a significant suppression of the renin-angiotensin system by acute extracellular fluid volume expansion.

Evaluation of Sodium and Water Reabsorption. An attempt was made to localize the site of sodium reabsorptive defect during infusion of hypotonic saline solution after the serum potassium level had been raised to 3.5 meq/liter. Maximum C_{H_2O} expressed as C_{H_2O}/100 ml glomerular filtration rate was taken as an indicator of the ability to transport sodium in the ascending limb of Henle's loop. The sum of C_{H_2O} and C_{Na} expressed as $C_{H_2O} + C_{Na}$/100 ml glomerular filtration rate was taken as an indicator of fluid delivery out of the proximal tubule. Fractional loop reabsorption ($C_{H_2O}/C_{H_2O} + C_{Na} \times 100$ per cent) was calculated as an indicator of loop function in relation to total distal sodium delivery. Figure 5 demonstrates that the C_{H_2O} was higher than the expected normal and $C_{H_2O}/C_{H_2O} + C_{Na} \times 100$ per cent was at the lower limit of the normal range as established by Chaimovitz et al. [10]. These data suggest intact or supernormal function of the ascending limb for the rate of sodium delivery (vide infra). It is also apparent from Figure 5 that both C_{Na} and $C_{H_2O} + C_{Na}$ were higher than expected, indicating both enhanced delivery of sodium and water out of the proximal tubule into the thick ascending limb and excessive sodium loss into the urine.

Evaluation of the Response to Propranolol Therapy. Figure 6 demonstrates the patient's response to propranolol while receiving a 250 meq sodium diet. Following the administration of 40 mg propranolol daily there was a decrease in sodium excretion, a reduction in standing diastolic blood pressure leading to postural hypotension, and a sharp increase in plasma renin activity to the highest levels recorded in this patient.

COMMENTS

The patient clearly demonstrated the features which have been considered diagnostic of Bartter's syndrome [1–23]: defective urinary concentration (Table I), normal or low blood pressure resistant to the pressor effect of an angiotensin II infusion (Figure 2), increased aldosterone excretion (Table I), increased plasma renin activity (Table I), and hyperplasia of the juxtaglomerular apparatus on renal biopsy (Figure 1).

The time of onset of his illness cannot be precisely determined, but it seems likely that the symptoms of weakness, polyuria and enuresis noted in adolescence were related to unmeasured hypokalemia. However, profound and protracted hypokalemic neuromuscular dysfunction did not occur until later adulthood, a point in life when Bartter's syndrome would seldom be considered in the differential diagnosis of muscle weakness. Thus, this case demonstrates that Bartter's syndrome must be considered along with laxative abuse [33], excessive use of diuretics [24,25] and primary aldosteronism [34] as a cause of hypokalemia in middle-aged adults.

Whether or not the patient's psychiatric difficulties were in any way related to his metabolic disturbance is purely conjectural. Psychiatric problems which improved with correction of hypokalemia have been noted in at least one other adult patient with this syndrome [19], and the fact that his behavior and demeanor were influenced less by large doses of chlorpromazine than by the correction of the serum potassium concentration suggests a relation between his electrolyte disturbance and mental status.

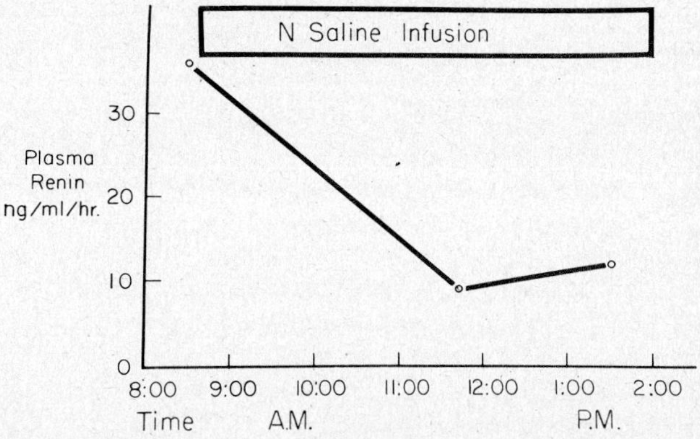

Figure 4. *Response of plasma renin activity to a rapid intravenous infusion of 2,000 ml normal saline solution.*

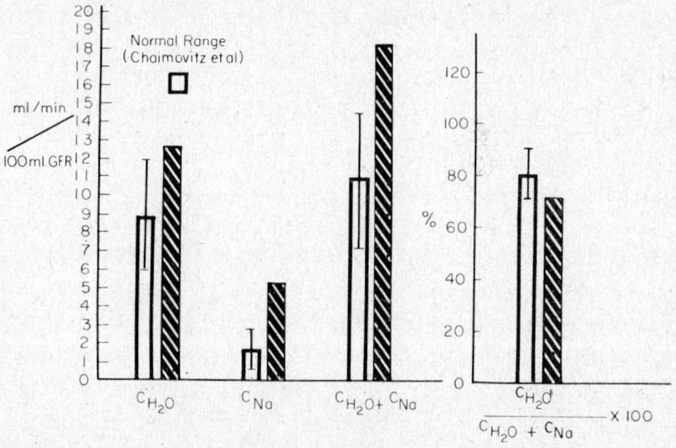

Figure 5. *Comparison of free water clearance (C_{H_2O}), sodium clearance (C_{Na}), distal tubular sodium delivery ($C_{H_2O} + C_{Na}$) and fractional loop reabsorption ($C_{H_2O}/C_{H_2O} + C_{Na} \times 100$ per cent) during infusion of hypotonic saline solution in patient (block bars) with normal values as established by Chaimovitz et al. [10].*

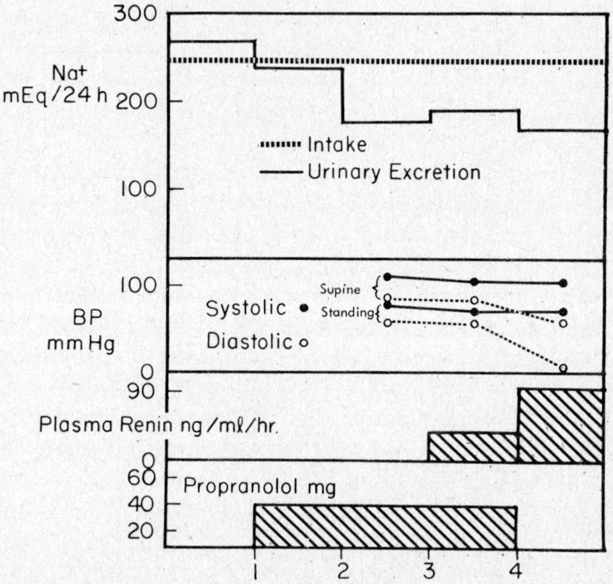

Figure 6. *Response of several parameters to propranolol administration.*

An abnormality in urinary concentration attributed to hypokalemia and leading to polyuria, polydipsia, enuresis and mild hydronephrosis has been frequently encountered in Bartter's syndrome [22]. It is likely that the concentrating defect in the present patient was related, at least in part, to hypokalemia because of the significant improvement in maximum urinary concentration (U_{max}) which occurred after the increase in serum concentration (Table I). Hypokalemia may not offer the entire explanation, however, as pointed out by Proesmans et al. [7] whose patient was unable to produce cyclic AMP in response to antidiuretic hormone stimulation.

The response of our patient to an acid load (Table II) was similar to that of Bartter's original patients [1,2], being characterized by only moderate lowering of the serum bicarbonate concentration, excretion of urine rich in ammonium with very little titratable acid, and less than normal reduction of the urinary pH. As noted in Table II, the magnitude of ammonium excretion when considered in relation to the high urinary pH was strikingly abnormal during the period of testing in a hypokalemic state without aldosterone suppression. It is likely that the enhanced ammonium excretion reflected increased ammonia production induced by a low intracellular potassium concentration [35]. It is also likely that the ready availability of large quantities of ammonia to diffuse into the tubular lumen and buffer secreted hydrogen ions inhibited the patient's ability to maximally acidify the urine. Support for this contention is provided by an analysis of the second acidification test (Table II) which was performed after the serum potassium had been corrected by spironolactone administration. In this circumstance the response in ammonium excretion was considerably less than before therapy; the urine pH fell to 5.7 units; and more hydrogen ion was excreted as titratable acid.

Although this explanation for the abnormal urinary acidification in the patient seems most reasonable, the possibility of a proximal tubular bicarbonate leak must be considered. During the first acidification test, a significant quantity of bicarbonate (16 μeq/min) spilled into the urine at a time when the estimated tubular reabsorption of bicarbonate was 2.04 meq/100 ml glomerular filtration rate. These determinations were made in a nonsteady state but are suggestive of a small leak of bicarbonate from the proximal tubule into the more distal nephron. Such a possibility, although in no way proved by the present study, must be considered in view of the findings relating to sodium reabsorption to be discussed.

The pathogenesis of Bartter's syndrome remains uncertain. Acceptance of Bartter's [1] original thesis of vascular insensitivity to angiotensin as the basic pathogenetic defect in all patients has been difficult for several reasons:

(1) The tendency of many patients [1,3,4,6,10,13,14,16,20,21] to appear volume depleted rather than volume expanded as might be suspected if the hypothesis was correct.

(2) The observation that vascular insensitivity to angiotensin infusion is not unique to Bartter's syndrome but may be seen in many states leading to secondary hyperaldosteronism [36].

(3) The recognition that plasma renin activity and angiotensin sensitivity may vary, at least to some degree, with the state of extracellular fluid volume expansion [3–5,16].

A more plausable explanation of pathogenesis in the patients with a tendency to volume depletion has been advanced recently with the description of several cases in which there appeared to be a primary defect in renal tubular sodium reabsorption [3–5,10,11,13–16,21]. The tendency to renal salt wasting (Figure 3) clearly places the present patient in this category and the directionally appropriate changes in plasma renin activity in response to alterations in extracellular fluid volume (Figures 3 and 4) suggest an intact renin-angiotensin-aldosterone system.

Although tubular sodium reabsorption seems to have been inhibited in many patients, opinion as to the exact site of blockade varies. Several investigators [3,4,13,15] have suggested that the defect in their patients most likely resided in the proximal tubule, and both Chan et al. [14] and Bartter [15] have demonstrated this by finding fractional sodium delivery to the distal nephron ($C_{H_2O} + C_{Na}$) during the infusion of hypotonic saline solution to be elevated. Others [10,16,21] have attributed sodium wasting in their patients to a defect distal to the proximal tubule, probably in the thick ascending limb of Henle's loop. Chaimovitz et al. [10] specifically demonstrated this by finding C_{H_2O} depressed during the infusion of hypotonic saline solution in their patient.

A proximal tubular defect is clearly demonstrated in our patient by the increased delivery of sodium out of the proximal tubule ($C_{H_2O} + C_{Na}$) (Figure 5). In this regard he is similar to the patients of Chan et al. [14] and Bartter [15]. He differs from them, however, in having a fractional loop reabsorption (C_{H_2O}/ $C_{H_2O} + C_{Na} \times 100$ per cent) in the normal range whereas in the other cases this index was markedly reduced. It may be, as implied by Bartter [15], that the patients with both increased distal delivery and decreased fractional loop reabsorption may have defective sodium chloride transport both in the proximal tubule and the ascending limb. If this hypothesis is correct, our patient appears to be unique among patients with Bartter's syndrome studied by the infusion of hypotonic saline solution in demonstrating defective proximal reabsorption and intact loop function. However, our data cannot exclude the possibility of a mild limitation in loop transport which is masked by the overwhelming quantity of solute which is delivered from the proximal tubule to the loop.

A further suggestion of proximal reabsorptive abnormality is provided by the slight increase in urinary alpha amino nitrogen excretion (Table I) and the slight urinary leak of bicarbonate already mentioned. Both of these substances are normally reabsorbed completely in the proximal tubule [37], and their presence is usually interpreted as being indicative of defective reabsorption in that segment.

The conflicting data from different patients as to the proximal or distal tubular site of defective sodium reabsorption suggests that patients with Bartter's syndrome may not represent a homogeneous group. It seems likely that the clinical and laboratory features of the syndrome may well represent only the end result of prolonged stimulation of the renin-angiotensin-aldosterone system induced by one of several pathologic processes including sustained vascular hyporeactivity to angiotensin, as originally postulated by Bartter [1], or by renal sodium wastage from any of the functional reabsorptive sites in the renal tubule.

Accepted therapy for Bartter's syndrome has included the use of potassium chloride supplements and spironolactone or triamterene to inhibit sodium reabsorption and potassium secretion in the distal tubule. Frequently these maneuvers have been only partially successful in maintaining normal serum potassium levels, perhaps because of a tubular defect in potassium reabsorption in some patients [5,17]. Because of its ability to inhibit renin secretion the beta blocking agent, propranolol, has recently been suggested as an effective therapeutic agent in the treatment of Bartter's syndrome [18]. Figure 6 indicates that within three days after initiating therapy with propranolol at a dose of 10 mg four times a day, the patient experienced severe postural hypotension necessitating discontinuation of therapy. It is evident that this adverse drug reaction was related to some effect other than in inhibition of plasma renin activity because the renin activity actually rose in conjunction with the hypotension. The mechanism of action of propranolol in this patient is uncertain but may have been related to a central effect or possibly to a reduction in cardiac output [38]. Thus, our experience would suggest caution in the use of propranolol and other beta blocking agents in patients with the marginal degree of volume expansion frequently seen in Bartter's syndrome. Generalization from experience with one patient are always tenuous; however, the following conclusions seem reasonable from our observations of this patient:

(1) Bartter's syndrome must be considered in the differential diagnosis of hypokalemia in middle-aged and older patients as well as in the young.

(2) The typical findings of Bartter's syndrome may be produced by a heterogeneous group of pathophysiologic disturbances which share the common denominator of marked stimulation of the renin-angiotensin-aldosterone system.

(3) Therapy with beta blocking agents to inhibit renin release should be used with caution in many of these patients because of the possible development of postural hypotension in those whose extracellular fluid volume has been depleted because of renal salt wasting.

ACKNOWLEDGMENT

This work was funded by the Veterans Administration (MRIS 2737-Project 08). We wish to express our deep gratitude to Dr. Frederic B. Westervelt, Jr. (University of Virginia School of Medicine) for his review of the manuscript and to Mrs. Ursula Edmonds who performed the numerous chemical analyses.

REFERENCES

1. Bartter FC, Pronove P, Gill JR Jr, MacCardle RC: Hyperplasia of the juxtaglomerular complex with hyperaldosteronism and hypokalemic alkalosis. Am J Med 33: 811, 1962.
2. Bryan GT, MacCardle RC, Bartter FC: Hyperaldosteronism, hyperplasia of the juxtaglomerular complex, normal blood pressure, and dwarfism: Report of a case. Pediatrics 37: 43, 1966.
3. Cannon PJ, Leeming JM, Sommers SC, et al.: Juxtaglomerular cell hyperplasia and secondary hyperaldosteronism (Bartter's syndrome). A reevaluation of the pathophysiology. Medicine (Baltimore) 47: 107, 1968.
4. Goodman AD, Vagnucci AH, Hartroft PM: Pathogenesis of Bartter's syndrome. N Engl J Med 281: 1435, 1969.
5. Trygstad CW, Mangos JA, Bloodworth JMB Jr, Lobeck CC: A sibship with Bartter's syndrome. Failure of total adrenalectomy to correct the potassium wasting. Pediatrics 44: 234, 1969.
6. Brackett NC Jr, Koppel M, Randall RE Jr, Nixon WP: Hyperplasia of the juxtaglomerular complex with secondary aldosteronism without hypertension (Bartter's syndrome). Am J Med 44: 803, 1968.
7. Proesmans W, Eggermont E, Eeckels R: Antidiuretic therapy in Bartter's syndrome. J Pediatr 82: 538, 1973.

8. Mace JW, Hambidge KM, Gotlin RW, Dubois RS, Solomons CS, Katz FH: Magnesium supplementation in Bartter's syndrome. Arch Dis Child 48: 485, 1973.
9. Greenberg AJ, Arboit JM, New MI, Worthen HG: Normotensive secondary hyperaldosteronism. J Pediatr 69: 719, 1966.
10. Chaimovitz C, Levi J, Better OS, Oslander L, Benderli A: Studies on the site of renal salt loss in a patient with Bartter's syndrome. Pediatr Res 7: 89, 1973.
11. Visser HKA, Degenhart E, Desmit E, Cost WS: Mineralocorticoid excess in two brothers with dwarfism, hypokalaemic alkalosis and normal blood pressure. Acta Endocrinol 55: 661, 1967.
12. Gardner JD, Simopoulos AP, Lapey A, Shibolet S: Altered membrane sodium transport in Bartter's syndrome. J Clin Invest 51: 1565, 1972.
13. Sutherland LE, Hartroft P, Balis JU, Bailey JD, Lynch MJ: Bartter's syndrome. A report of four cases including three in one sibship, with comparative histologic evaluation of the juxtaglomerular apparatuses and glomeruli. Acta Paediatr Scand 201 (Supp): 3, 1970.
14. Chan JCM, Malekzadeh MH, Anand SK: Defect in renal tubular sodium reabsorption in a patient with Bartter's syndrome. Clin Proc Children's Hospital National Medical Center 31: 67, 1975.
15. Bartter FC: The syndrome of juxtaglomerular hyperplasia with aldosteronism, hypokalemic alkalosis and normal blood pressure. Birth Defects 10: 104, 1974.
16. White MG: Bartter's syndrome. A manifestation of renal tubular defects. Arch Intern Med 129: 41, 1972.
17. Takayasu H, Aso Y, Nakauchi K, Kawabe K: A case of Bartter's syndrome with surgical treatment followed for four years. J Clin Endocr 32: 842, 1971.
18. Modlinger RS, Nicolis GL, Krakoff LR, Gabrilove JL: Some observations on the pathogenesis of Bartter's syndrome. N Engl J Med 289: 1022, 1973.
19. Tarm F, Juncos LL, Anderson CF, Donadio JV Jr: Bartter's syndrome. An unusual presentation. Proc Mayo Clin 48: 280, 1973.
20. Beilin LJ, Schiffman N, Crane M, Nelson DH: Hypokalaemic alkalosis and hyperplasia of the juxtaglomerular apparatus without hypertension or oedema. Br Med J 4: 327, 1967.
21. Erkelens DW, Statius Van Eps LW: Bartter's syndrome and erythrocytosis. Am J Med 55: 711, 1973.
22. Dehart HS, Bath NM, Glenn JF, Gunnells JC: Urologic considerations in Bartter's syndrome. J Urol 111: 420, 1974.
23. Heidland A, Kreusser W, Hennemann H, Knauf H, Wigand ME: Excretion of the mono- and divalent ions in relation to flow rate in Bartter's and pseudo Bartter's syndromes in parotid saliva. Comparative studies to the syndrome of Conn. Klin Wochenschr 50: 959, 1972.
24. Ben-Ishay D, Levy M, Birnbaum D: Self-induced secondary hyperaldosteronism simulating Bartter's syndrome. Isr J Med Sci 8: 1835, 1972.
25. Wolff HP, Vecsei P, Kruck F, Roscher S, Brown JJ, Duster-dieck GO, Lever AF, Robertson JIS: Psychiatric disturbance leading to potassium depletion, sodium depletion, raised plasma-renin concentration, and secondary hyperaldosteronism. Lancet 1: 257, 1968.
26. Yeh BPY, Tomko DH, Stacy WK, Bear ES, Haden HT, Falls WF Jr: An analysis of factors influencing sodium and water excretion in uremic man. Kidney Int 7: 103, 1975.
27. Cohen EL, Grim CE, Conn JW, Blough WM Jr, Guyer RB, Kem DC, Lucas CP: Accurate and rapid measurement of plasma renin activity by radioimmunoassay. J Lab Clin Med 77: 1025, 1971.
28. Kaplan NM, Silah JG: The effect of angiotensin II on the blood pressure in humans with hypertensive disease. J Clin Invest 43: 659, 1964.
29. Walser M, Seldin DW, Grollman A: An evaluation of radiosulfate for the determination of the volume of extracellular fluid in man and dogs. J Clin Invest 32: 299, 1953.
30. Wrong O, Davies HEF: The excretion of acid in renal disease. Q J Med 28: 259, 1959.
31. Falls WF: Comparison of urinary acidification and ammonium excretion in normal and gouty subjects. Metabolism 21: 433, 1972.
32. Pitts RF, Ayer JL, Schiess WA: Renal regulation of acid-base balance in man; reabsorption and excretion of bicarbonate. J Clin Invest 28: 35, 1949.
33. Schwartz WB, Relman AS: Metabolic and renal studies in chronic potassium depletion resulting from overuse of laxatives. J Clin Invest 32: 258, 1953.
34. Cain JP, Tuck ML, Williams GH, Dluhy RG, Rosenoff SH: The regulation of aldosterone secretion in primary aldosteronism. Am J Med 53: 627, 1972.
35. Iacobellis M, Muntwyler E, Griffin GE: Kidney glutaminase and carbonic anhydrase activity and tissue electrolyte composition in potassium-deficient dogs. Am J Physiol 183: 395, 1955.
36. Johnston CJ, Jose AD: Reduced vascular response to angiotensin II in secondary hyperaldosteronism. J Clin Invest 42: 1411, 1963.
37. Pitts RF: Physiology of the Kidney and Body Fluids, 3rd ed, Chicago, Year Book Medical Publishers, 1944, p 71; 198.
38. Sowton E, Hamer J: Hemodynamic changes after beta adrenergic blockade. Am J Cardiol 18: 317, 1966.

Hypercalcemia of Acute Renal Failure

Clinical Significance and Pathogenesis

ANTOINE de TORRENTE, M.D.*
TOMAS BERL, M.D.
PETER D. COHN, M.D.
ERNEST KAWAMOTO, M.D.
PHILLIP HERTZ, M.D.
ROBERT W. SCHRIER, M.D.
Denver, Colorado

Hypocalcemia is a frequent accompaniment of acute renal failure, but paradoxically hypercalcemia also has been described in association with acute renal failure. In this paper we describe two patients who provide some insights into both the potential clinical importance and mechanism of the hypercalcemia associated with acute renal failure. The clinical significance is emphasized by the presence of diffuse metastatic calcification observed at postmortem examination in one patient. In both patients the increase in serum calcium concentration was not coincident with a decrease in serum phosphorus concentration; when measured in one patient, serum levels of parathyroid hormone were undetectable. These findings, along with the consistent association with rhabdomyolysis, support the proposal that the hypercalcemia of acute renal failure is caused by dissolution of dystrophic calcifications in traumatized muscle and may lead to severe metastatic calcifications.

Hyperparathyroidism with hypercalcemia is a frequent occurrence in patients with chronic renal failure after kidney transplantation [1]. So-called "tertiary" or "autonomous" hyperparathyroidism also may cause hypercalcemia in some patients with advanced chronic renal failure [2]. The occurrence of hypercalcemia in patients with acute renal failure, however, has been described in only a few patients [3–12]. Moreover, the clinical significance and pathogenesis of this variety of hypercalcemia has not been defined. In this paper we report evidence in two patients with hypercalcemia and acute renal failure which provides some insight into both the clinical significance and pathogenesis of this entity.

CASE REPORTS

Case 1. A 40 year old Caucasian woman was admitted to the psychiatric service of Colorado General Hospital because of depression and symptoms of Parkinson's disease. Prior to admission she had an episode of violent choreiform movements which led to multiple falls. Two days after admission she complained of severe abdominal pain and was noted to have diffuse abdominal tenderness. Her temperature was 38.6°C, blood pressure, 90/0 mm Hg; pulse rate, regular at 120/min; and respirations, 42/min. Laboratory values were sodium, 137 meq/liter; potassium, 7.2 meq/liter; chloride, 90 meq/liter; carbon dioxide, 14 meq/liter; blood urea nitrogen, 60 mg/100 ml; and creatinine, 5.2 mg/100 ml. The serum creatinine phosphokinase level was extremely elevated at 15,000 IU/liter (normal limits: 0 to 50 IU/liter). The patient was anuric and did not respond to the administration of furosemide. Because of the abdominal findings, a laparotomy was performed but revealed

From the Departments of Medicine and Pathology, University of Colorado Medical Center, Denver, Colorado 80220. Requests for reprints should be addressed to Dr. Robert W. Schrier, Division of Renal Diseases, University of Colorado Medical Center, 4200 East Ninth Avenue, Denver, Colorado 80220. Manuscript accepted November 10, 1975.

* Recipient of a Fellowship from Switzerland. Present address: Service de Medicine, Hopital Communal, 2300 La Chaux-de-Fond, Switzerland.

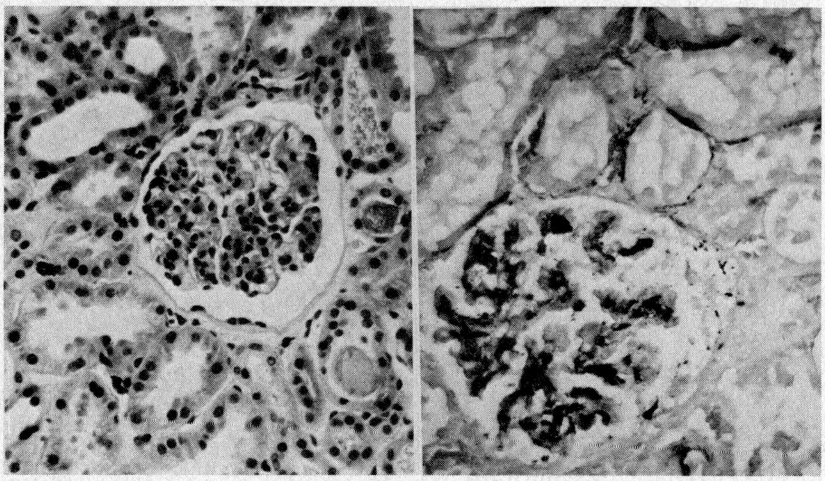

__Figure 1.__ Case 1. Rapid development of renal calcifications in patient. __Left,__ biopsy specimen taken four days after the onset of renal failure reveals a histologic picture compatible with tubular necrosis. __Right,__ the specimen obtained at postmortem examination 20 days later reveals extensive glomerular, peritubular and vascular calcifications. Von Kossa stain was used in both specimens.

no disease. A kidney biopsy specimen obtained at the same time was consistent with the diagnosis of acute tubular necrosis (Figure 1, left). After surgery, the urine output remained below 50 ml/24 hours. The blood urea nitrogen and the creatinine levels rose steadily, and the patient was transferred to the Medical Service at that time. Physical examination revealed a rigid, immobile woman. Her blood pressure was 200/116 mm Hg and the pulse rate was regular at 76/min. The skin showed multiple ecchymoses. Sacral and peripheral edema was also present. The laboratory data were as follows: serum sodium, 137 meq/liter; potassium, 3.6 meq/liter; chloride, 95 meq/liter; carbon dioxide, 13 meq/liter; calcium, 6.0 mg/100 ml; phosphorus, 4.2 mg/100 ml, alkaline phosphatase, 212 IU/liter (normal limits: 56 to 232 IU/liter); and serum albumin, 2.7 g/100 ml. The blood urea nitrogen was 137 mg/100 ml and the serum creatinine 14 mg/100 ml. Urinalysis showed 3+ protein, numerous white blood cells and pigmented casts. Hemodialysis was instituted on an intermittent basis (Table I). The patient remained oliguric throughout her hospital course. On the 16th day of her illness, the serum calcium before dialysis was 11.2 mg/100 ml, the serum phosphorus 6 mg/100 ml; the patient could not tolerate phosphate binding agents. There were no clinical symptoms attributable to the high calcium level which rose to a maximum of 13.8 mg/100 ml with a phosphorus level of 5.8 mg/100 ml at which time the serum albumin was 2.6 g/100 ml. On the 22nd day of her hospitalization, a cough, fever and a right perihilar lung infiltrate developed, no soft calcifications were observed on the chest films. On the 24th day, she had a fatal cardiac arrest. The evolution of the calcium and phosphorus levels during the illness of the patient are summarized in Table I.

TABLE I Occurrence of Hypercalcemia in Acute Renal Failure in the Absence of a Diminishing Serum Phosphate Level

	8/19	8/31*	9/2	9/3	9/6*	9/7
Blood urea nitrogen (mg/100 ml)	128	35	65	89	51	70
Creatinine (mg/100 ml)	11.9	4.9	7.1	8.2	4.5	5.2
Calcium (mg/100 ml)	6.5	13.8	13.4	12.7	12.1	12.4
Phosphorus (mg/100 ml)	4.2	5.8	8.7	10.0	6.8	7.7

*A 6 hour hemodialysis was performed on these days with Dow 4 hollow fiber artifical kidney and a Centry delivery system. The water was treated by reverse osmosis and Renalyte 87 dialysate concentrate (Cobe Laboratories, Lakewood, Colo.); a calcium concentration of 6 mg/100 ml was used.

Autopsy showed that the kidneys were normal in size with a 12 mm cortex and a congested medulla. Light microscopy revealed numerous benzidine positive granular casts in some regenerating tubules. Throughout both kidneys, there were diffuse calcium deposits. These calcifications were noted in the basement membrane of the glomeruli, in Bowman's capsule and in the proximal tubules as well as in the intima of the vessels (Figure 1, right). Three gray and moderately enlarged parathyroid glands were found which showed no microscopic evidence of hyperplasia. The bones were normal without increased osteoclastic resorption. Besides the calcifications in the kidneys, vascular calcifications were found in the myocardium, the lungs, the thyroid gland and in some skeletal muscles (Figure 2). The psoas muscle, among others, had evidence of previous injury with a mononuclear cell infiltrate and scattered fibrosis.

Case 2. A 32 year old carpenter was admitted to the University of California Hospital, San Francisco, because of acute renal failure. Six days before his admission he was found semicomatose after an alcoholic binge. When he was first admitted to a local hospital, a swollen discolored right leg was noticed without an arterial pulse below the popliteal artery. A fasciotomy restored the pulses.Two days later he was noted to have dark brown urine and a decreasing urine output unresponsive to mannitol administration. He was then transferred to the University of California Hospital because of uremia. On admission, physical findings revealed a lethargic and disoriented man. His temperature was 36.8°C, blood pressure, 100/80 mm Hg; pulse rate, regular at

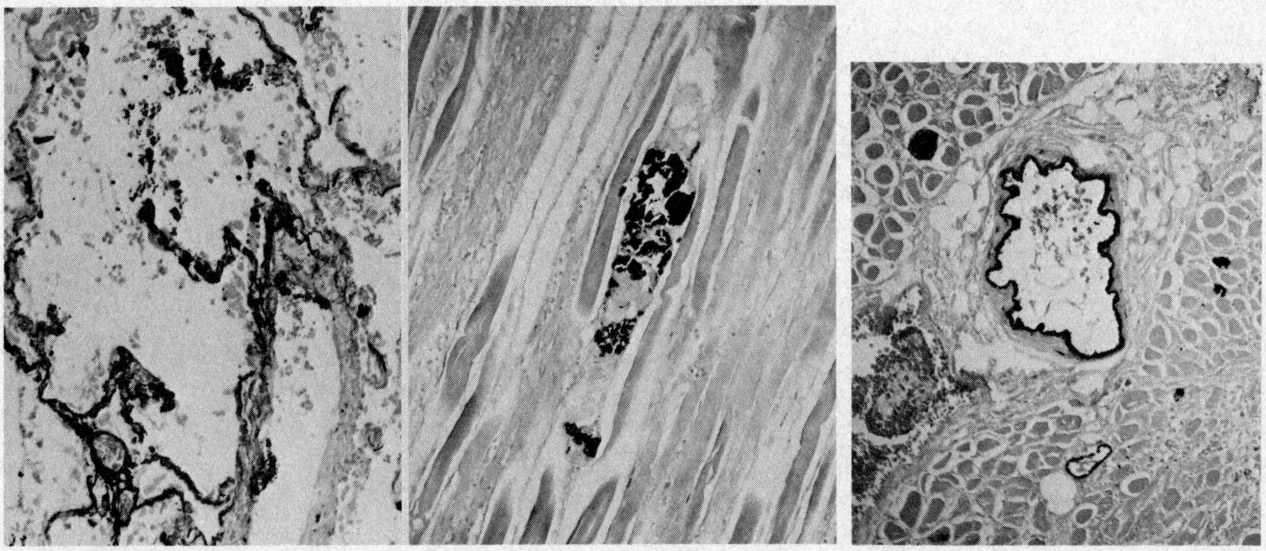

Figure 2. *Case 1. Visceral and vascular calcifications in patient. Metastatic calcifications in the alveolar septums of the lungs* ***(left panel),*** *in injured skeletal muscle* ***(middle panel)*** *and in the intima of a medium size artery* ***(right panel).*** *Von Kossa stain.*

100/min; and respiratory rate, 12/min. Significant physical findings included a grade 2/6 systolic ejection murmur at the left sternal border and a pericardial friction rub. The lower right leg was edematous up to the groin with intact pulses. There was extensive muscle swelling, especially of the right calf. The serum laboratory values on admission were sodium, 120 meq/liter; potassium, 6.3 meq/liter; chloride, 87 meq/liter; carbon dioxide, 18 meq/liter; calcium, 5.9 mg/100 ml; phosphorus, 10.4 mg 100 ml; blood urea nitrogen, 170 mg/100 ml; and creatinine, 25 mg/100 ml. Urinalysis revealed a pH of 6, specific gravity of 1.010, protein 3+ and numerous epithelial cell casts.

Peritoneal and, later, hemodialysis were instituted. The serum calcium level, which had been in the range of 8 to 9 mg/100 ml, was 11.1 mg/100 ml on the 17th day and remained elevated for the next week. At that time the serum was noted to be 11.1 mg/100 ml on the 17th day and remained elevated for the next week. At that time the serum albumin concentration was 3.5 mg/100 ml. As in Case 1, the serum phosphorus level remained elevated throughout this period of hypercalcemia and was in the range of 8.0 to 8.5 mg/100 ml. Immunoassay of parathyroid hormone during the hypercalcemia phase revealed undetectable levels of the hormone (Dr. Betty Roof, University of California, San Francisco). With continued improvement in kidney function, serum calcium levels decreased to normal values. The patient eventually made a full recovery with normal kidney function and no further detectable abnormalities in serum calcium and phosphorus values.

COMMENTS

The histologic evidence of diffuse metastatic calcification in Case 1 emphasizes that the occurrence of hypercalcemia with acute renal failure must be considered as more than a biochemical curiosity. Although clinically significant cutaneous, skeletal and visceral calcifications are known to occur in dialyzed and nondialyzed patients with chronic renal failure, such diffuse metastatic calcification in patients with hypercalcemia and acute renal failure has heretofore not been described. Because of the relatively short duration, it might not seem unreasonable to assume that the hypercalcemia of acute renal failure is of little clinical consequence. Although an occasional mention of calcium deposits in the conjunctivas and kidney tissue has been made [7,8], there has been little emphasis on the potential clinical importance of the hypercalcemia of acute renal failure. The extensive metastatic calcification observed in our patient on postmortem examination was unexpected, but emphasized the potential deleterious consequences of the hypercalcemia associated with acute renal failure.

There are several potential clinical derangements which could result from the degree of metastatic calcification observed in our patient. Myocardial calcification may not only suppress ventricular contractility, but it may also induce various arrythmias [13]. In this regard, it is important to note that our patient's death was associated with cardiac arrest and pulmonary edema, and that diffuse myocardial calcifications were observed at autopsy. The clinical significance of the diffuse alveolar calcifications observed in our patient is difficult to assess, but such pulmonary calcifications in patients with chronic renal failure clearly have been demonstrated to be associated with both restrictive and diffusion defects in ventilatory function [14]. Acute hypercalcemia is also known to cause hypertension [15]. Although our patient was hypertensive during the course of her acute renal failure, the increased blood pressure was present prior to the occurrence of hypercalcemia. A secondary effect of the hypercalcemia to increase blood pressure in such patients with acute renal failure, however, must be considered.

Calcium deposition in the kidneys of patients with hypercalcemia could prolong the duration of the acute renal failure and thus delay the onset of the recovery phase. Such an effect of hypercalcemia is particularly possible in our first patient in whom extensive renal calcification of glomeruli, tubules and vessels was present at postmortem examination. The direct clinical importance of skeletal muscle calcifications would seem to be minimal; however, the potential release of these calcium deposits in the pathogenesis of the hypercalcemia is likely and will be discussed. Calcium phosphate deposits in skin and conjunctivas were not clinically apparent in our patients, but subclinical deposition was demonstrable on histologic examination. Neither patient manifested the physical findings or symptoms of the "red eye" syydrome [16].

As with chronic metastatic calcification, the tissue deposition of calcium salts in patients with hypercalcemia and acute renal failure is probably related at least partially to the level of elevation of the calcium-phosphorus product, as well as to the duration of the elevation. Since hyperphosphatemia is a frequent occurrence in acute renal failure, therapeutic approaches which lower the serum phosphate level including oral administration of phosphate binding antacids and hemodialysis are efficacious in decreasing the calcium-phosphorus product. Obviously, because of the associated hyperphosphatemia, the hypercalcemia of acute renal failure should not be treated by the administration of phosphate salts. Also, other means, such as furosemide and saline solution [17] or sodium sulfate [18] administration, which are dependent on the integrity of renal function are of course ineffective in treating the hypercalcemia of acute renal failure. The use of hemodialysis without calcium in the dialysate is probably the most rapid means of treating the hypercalcemia of acute renal failure. A trial of treatment with glucocorticoid hormone also could be used, but its benefit in patients whose hypercalcemia may be due to release from soft tissues remains to be determined. Taken together these modes of treatment, i.e., antacids, dialysis and perhaps a trial of corticosteroid administration should prevent the widespread metastatic calcification which occurred in our patient with acute renal failure and hypercalcemia.

In addition to emphasizing the potential clinical significance of hypercalcemia associated with acute renal failure, this report also provides some insight into the pathogenesis of the hypercalcemia. The previous finding of "inappropriately" elevated parathyroid hormone levels in association with hypercalcemia and acute renal failure led to the proposal that parathyroid hormone exerts an important causative role in the genesis of the hypercalcemia [810]. More recently, however, it has been established that elevated blood levels of parathyroid hormones are present in patients with acute renal failure who are either hypo- or normocalcemic [19]. Moreover, a resistance to the hypercalcemic effect of parathyroid hormone occurs in patients with acute [20], as well as chronic renal failure [21]. Thus, elevated levels of parathyroid hormone in patients with acute renal failure and hypercalcemia cannot be accepted as solid evidence that the hyperparathyroidism is responsible for the hypercalcemia of acute renal failure. Moreover, in our second patient the parathyroid hormone levels were measured by a sensitive radioimmunoassay and found to be undetectable. This finding not only is consistent with the conclusion that the secondary hyperparathyroidism of acute renal failure is not autonomous [20], but also would seem to exclude the role of parathyroid hormone in the pathogenesis of the hypercalcemia observed in our patient.

The observation that hypercalcemia associated with acute renal failure frequently occurs during the recovery phase of renal failure has led to the suggestion that the falling levels of serum phosphate are responsible for the hypercalcemia [8]. It is known that the movement of calcium and phosphate into bone and soft tissues is interdependent, thus a fall in serum phosphate levels could diminish flux of calcium into bone and thereby result in hypercalcemia [22]. In our patients, however, the serum calcium level rose in the absence of a decrease in serum phosphate concentration or an improvement in renal function. Nevertheless, it is not unreasonable to suggest that a fall in the serum phosphate level during the recovery phase of acute renal failure could contribute to a rise in the serum calcium level, particularly in the presence of persistent hyperparathyroidism and improved skeletal responsiveness to the hormone. This sequence of events, however, occurs in most cases of acute renal failure and, yet, associated hypercalcemia is rare. It would thus seem appropriate to seek another cause for the hypercalcemia of acute renal failure. This is particularly true in our patients in whom hypercalcemia developed in the absence of a fall in serum phosphate levels and prior to the recovery phase of the renal failure.

A common feature existed between our patients, and those previously described with hypercalcemia and acute renal failure. Both of our patients had rhabdomyolysis in association with their acute renal failure; virtually all previously described patients also have had evidence of rhabdomyolysis, either idiopathic, traumatic or toxin-induced [3–8,10–12]. It is, therefore, tempting to postulate that the muscle damage may not only cause myoglobinuria and contribute to the acute renal failure but that it may also be a factor in the hypercalcemia.

Necrotic or devitalized tissues are known to calcify [23]. Experimental work on animals with traumatized muscles has demonstrated that these muscles avidly accumulate calcium, particularly in the presence of renal insufficiency [24]. The profound hypocalcemia sometimes reported in the early course of acute renal failure due to rhabdomyolysis may in part be due to the precipitation of calcium in the necrotic muscles [4,5]. The fate of these dystrophic calcifications is not known precisely, although they have been reported to disappear completely [4]. It therefore seems reasonable to propose that progressive dissolution of these dystrophic calcifications in traumatized skeletal muscle may provide a calcium load which causes an increase in serum calcium concentration. This hypercalcemia may cause diffuse metastatic calcification even as it suppresses the plasma level of parathyroid hormone.

In summary, the hypercalcemia of acute renal failure should be considered as more than a biochemical curiosity and, indeed, may be an event which leads to severe, widespread metastatic calcification. Neither a diminishing serum phosphate level nor an elevated parathyroid hormone level seems to be necessary for the occurrence of the hypercalcemia of acute renal failure. The consistent occurrence of this entity in association with muscle damage suggests a potential causative relationship. It is thus proposed that in the setting of the parathyroid resistance of acute renal failure, dissolution of dystrophic calcifications in traumatized muscle may be an important factor in the hypercalemia of acute renal failure.

ADDENDUM

Since submission of this paper an additional patient with hypercalcemia and acute renal failure has been described by Miach et al. [25]. In this patient also there was no detectable serum level of parathyroid hormone and soft tissue calcifications developed over the five months in which the hypercalcemia persisted.

REFERENCES

1. Hampers CL, Katz AI, Wilson RE, Merril JP: Calcium metabolism and osteodystrophy after renal transplantation. Arch Intern Med 124: 282, 1969.
2. Massry SG, Coburn JW, Popovtzer MM, Shinaberger JH, Maxwell MH, Kleeman CR: Secondary hyperparathyroidism in chronic renal failure. Arch Intern Med 124: 431, 1969.
3. Tavill AS, Evanson JM, DeBaker SB, Hewitt D: Idiopathic paroxysmal myoglobinuria with acute renal failure and hypercalcemia. N Engl J Med 271: 283, 1964.
4. Butikofer E, Molleyres J: Akute ischämische Muskel nekrosen, reversible Muskel verkalkungen und sekundäre Hypercalciämie bei akuter anurie. Schweig Med Wochenschr 98: 961, 1968.
5. Grossmann HH, Lange H: Hypercalcemia in acute renal failure. Ann Intern Med 69: 1332, 1968.
6. Segal AJ, Miller M, Moses AM: Hypercalcemia during the diuretic phase of acute renal failure. Ann Intern Med 68: 1066, 1968.
7. Leonard A, Nelms RJ: Hypercalcemia in diuretic phase of acute renal failure. Ann Intern Med 73: 137, 1970.
8. Leonard CD, Eichner ER: Acute renal failure and transient hypercalcemia in idiopathic rhabdomyolysis. JAMA 211: 1539, 1970.
9. Turkington RW, Delcher HK, Neelon FA, Gitelman HJ: Hypercalcemi following acute renal failure. J Clin Endocrinol 28: 1224, 1968.
10. Wu BC, Pillay VKG, Hawker CD, Armbruster WFW, Shapiro HS, Ing TS: Hypercalcemia in acute renal failure of acute alcoholic rhabdomyolis. S Afr Med J 46: 1631, 1972.
11. Bismuth C, Frejaville JP, Pebay-Peyroula F, Leclerc JP: Rhabdomyolyse diffuse mortelle au lours dùne intoxication par salicylés et nifuroxazide. Nouv Presse Med 1: 397, 1972.
12. Grossman RA, Hamilton RW, Morse BM, Penn AS, Goldberg M: Nontraumatic rhabdomyolysis and acute renal failure. N Engl J Med 291: 807, 1974.
13. Terman DS, Alfrey AC, Hammond WS, Donndelinger T, Ogden DA, Holmes JH: Cardiac calcification in uremia. Am J Med 50: 744, 1971.
14. Conger JD, Hammond WS, Alfrey AC, Contiguglia SR, Stanford RE, Huffer WE: Pulmonary calcification in chronic dialysis patients. Ann Intern Med 83: 330, 1975.
15. Weidmann P, Massry SG, Coburn JW, Maxwell MH, Atteson J, Kleeman CR: Blood pressure effects of acute hypercalcemia. Studies in patients with chronic renal failure. Ann Intern Med 76: 741, 1972.
16. Berlyne GM: Red eyes in renal failure. Lancet 1: 4, 1967.
17. Suki WN, Yium JJ, Von Minden M, Saller-Hebert C, Eknoyan G, Martinez-Maldonado M: Acute treatment of hypercalcemia with furosemide. N Engl J Med 283: 836, 1970.
18. Chakmakjian ZH, Bethune JE: Sodium sulfate treatment of hypercalcemia. N Engl J Med 274: 1, 1966.
19. Kovithavongs T, Becker FO, Ing TS: Parathyroid hyperfunction in acute renal failure. Nephron 9: 349, 1972.
20. Massry SG, Arieff AI, Coburn JW, Palmieri G, Kleeman CR: Divalent ion metabolism in patients with acute renal failure: studies on the mechanism of hypocalcemia. Kidney Int 5: 437, 1974.
21. Massry SG, Coburn JW, Lee DBN, Jowsey J, Kleeman CR: Skeletal resistance to parathyroid hormone in renal failure. Studies in 105 human subjects. Ann Intern Med 78: 357, 1973.
22. Kleeman CR, Massry SG, Coburn JW: The clinical physiology of calcium homeostasis, parathyroid hormone and calcitonin. California Med 114: 16, 1971.
23. Virchow R: Die Cellular pathologie, 4th ed, Berlin, Hirschwald, 1871, p 451.
24. Meroney WH, Arney GK, Segar WE, Balch HH: The acute calcification of traumatized muscle with particular reference to acute post-traumatic renal insufficiency. J Clin Invest 36: 825, 1957.
25. Miach PJ, Dawborn JK, Douglas MC, Jerums-Xipell JM: Prolonged hypercalcemia following acute renal failure. Clin Nephrol 4: 33, 1976.

Primary Empty Sella Syndrome with Visual Field Defects

MAIRE T. BUCKMAN, M.D.
MUHAMMED HUSAIN, M.D.*
THOMAS J. CARLOW, M.D.
GLENN T. PEAKE, M.D.
Albuquerque, New Mexico

A patient with an enlarged, asymmetric sella turcica and visual field defects suggestive of a pituitary or parasellar tumor underwent extensive roentgenographic and pituitary function studies. No abnormalities in pituitary luteinizing hormone, follicle-stimulating hormone, thyroid-stimulating hormone, ACTH, prolactin or vasopressin secretion were detected. Growth hormone secretion was provoked by arginine infusion but not by hypoglycemia. Pneumoencephalography revealed air in the sella turcica, and no evidence of tumor. Thus, an enlarged sella turcica in a patient with visual field defects but normal pituitary function may suggest the presence of an "empty sella syndrome."

A large asymmetric sella turcica in association with a visual field defect suggests the presence of a pituitary or parasellar tumor. Some of these enlarged sellas have been found to be "empty" on pneumoencephalography or during transfrontal or transsphenoidal pituitary surgery. Weiss and Raskind [1] emphasized the need to distinguish between "primary" and "secondary" empty sella syndrome. The secondary syndrome is associated with previous surgical or radiation treatment for pituitary or parapituitary tumor. The primary syndrome, on the other hand, is idiopathic and not associated with such therapeutic maneuvers.

Although visual field defects have regularly been described in the secondary empty sella syndrome, only a few cases of chiasmal defects have been reported in the primary syndrome [2–6]. Pituitary function in the primary empty sella syndrome with visual field impairment has been reported to be (1) compromised by clinical evaluation [2,3], (2) compromised by unspecified pituitary function studies [4], or (3) not evaluated [4,5]. More detailed endocrine studies were carried out in one patient who had diabetes insipidus [6]. In addition to vasopressin deficiency, this patient had modestly impaired growth hormone and cortisol responses to insulin hypoglycemia. The pituitary-thyroidal axis was intact.

We describe here an additional patient with the empty sella syndrome who presented with a large asymmetric sella and bitemporal superior quadrantanopsia. Unlike the previously reported cases of primary empty sella syndrome with visual field impairment in which endocrine status was incompletely evaluated, extensive endocrine studies in our patient revealed normal pituitary function. Since neither irradiation nor surgery, except in the rare instance of progressive visual field loss, is indicated in the empty sella syn-

From the Veterans Administration Hospital and University of New Mexico School of Medicine, Albuquerque, New Mexico 87131. This research was supported by the Veterans Administration (Research and Education Associate Award to Dr. M. Buckman) and by NIH Grant HD05794. Requests for reprints should be addressed to Dr. Maire T. Buckman, Research Service, Veterans Administration Hospital, 2100 Ridgecrest Drive, S.E., Albuquerque, New Mexico 87108. Manuscript accepted November 18, 1975.

* Present address: Veterans Administration Hospital, 1055 Clermont Street, Denver, Colorado 80220.

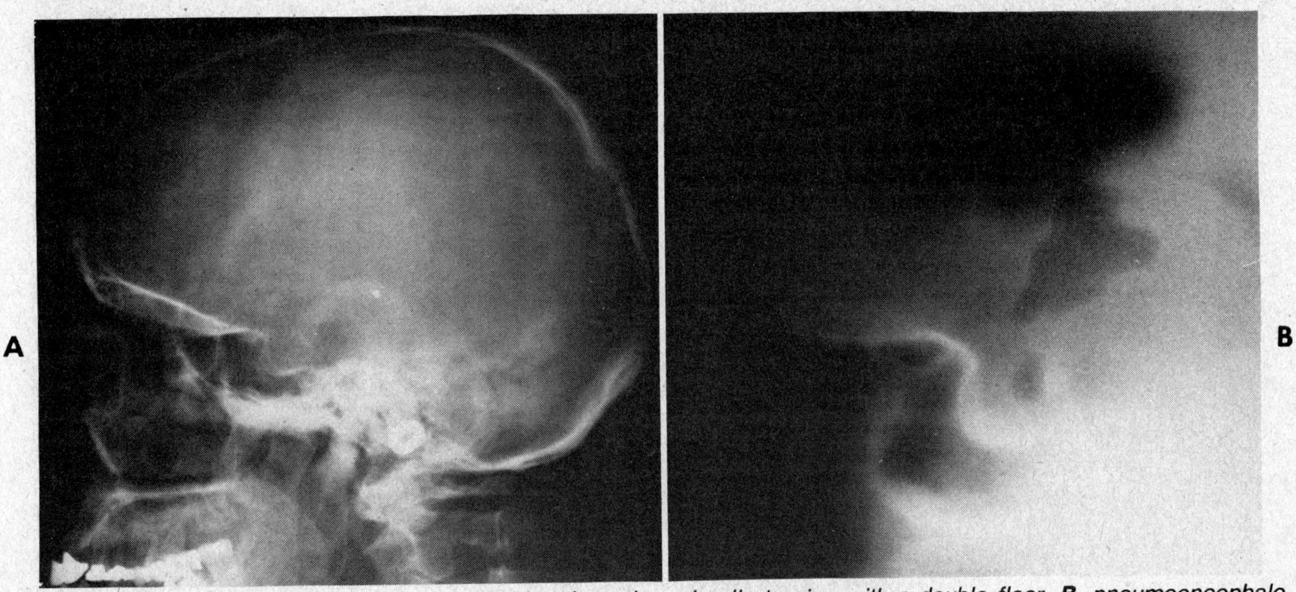

Figure 1. A, lateral skull roentgenogram showing the enlarged sella turcica with a double floor. B, pneumoencephalogram illustrating air in the sella.

drome, pneumoencephalography is an essential diagnostic procedure in any patient presenting with a visual field defect and an enlarged sella turcica.

CASE REPORT

A 47 year old Caucasian man was admitted to the Albuquerque VA Hospital in September 1974 because of impending delirium tremens and blackout spells. The patient admitted to being a heavy alcohol consumer for many years, although the few days prior to admission he had only consumed a few bottles of beer and essentially no other calories. On the morning of admission, the patient stated that he felt dizzy and he lost consciousness for approximately 30 minutes. He described two such prior blackouts, both temporally related to heavy drinking. There was no history suggestive of seizure activity. The patient related a long history of poorly defined headaches in the frontal region and on top of the head, sometimes lasting one to two days. He denied any recent change in the character, location or duration of the headaches. Diminution of visual acuity and occasional diplopia, progressive over the past two years, had forced him to quit his job as a diamond cutter. Three months prior to admission, he had a skull roentgenogram at a local hospital and was told that he had a "brain tumor."

Physical examination revealed a disheveled, tremulous, middle-aged man with a strong odor of alcohol on his breath. Vital signs showed a blood pressure of 160/90 mm Hg, supine; a pulse rate of 104/min; a respiratory rate of 16/min; and an oral temperature of 96.6°F. Habitus was that of a normal man. He had abundant body and facial hair which he had not shaved for several days. Eye examination is subsequently described in detail. His thyroid was normal to palpation. There was no gynecomastia. Genital examination revealed a normal penis and each testicle measured 2 by 4 cm. Neurologic examination, including cranial nerves, motor strength, sensory examination, deep tendon reflexes and cerebellar function, was intact except for a drift of his outstretched right hand and a wide-based gait. Both of the latter abnormalities resolved during the course of his hospitalization. The remainder of the physical examination was unremarkable.

Initial laboratory data revealed normal urinalysis, electrolytes and blood urea nitrogen. Liver function studies showed modestly increased lactic dehydrogenase (LDH), serum glutamic oxaloacetic transaminase (SGOT), alkaline phosphatase and total bilirubin levels consistent with alcoholic liver disease. A random blood sugar level was 126 mg/100 ml. Complete blood count was normal except for a hematocrit value of 55 per cent which reflected a mild state of dehydration. A chest roentgenogram revealed old granulomatous calcifications and old pleural scars, but no acute changes. An electrocardiogram was within normal limits.

A lateral skull roentgenogram showed an enlarged sella turcica with a double floor (Figure 1A). Tomograms of the sella turcica confirmed the presence of a double floor with the anterior portion of the left side depressed compared to the right. Measurements of sellar volume revealed it to be markedly enlarged at 2,040 mm^3 (normal range 240 to 1,092 mm^3) [7]. Carotid artery siphon calcification was seen in the region of the sella. A pneumoencephalogram with polytomography showed extension of subarachnoid air into the posterior portion of the sella turcica, a finding consistent with the empty sella syndrome (Figure 1B). There was no evidence of tumor in the sellar or parasellar region. In addition, there was minimal enlargement of the third and lateral ventricles, and minimal widening of the cerebral sulci, considered consistent with his long history of alcoholic abuse.

Eye Examination. Goldman quantitative perimetry documented a bitemporal quadrantanopsia on three different occasions within an eight month period (Figure 2). There

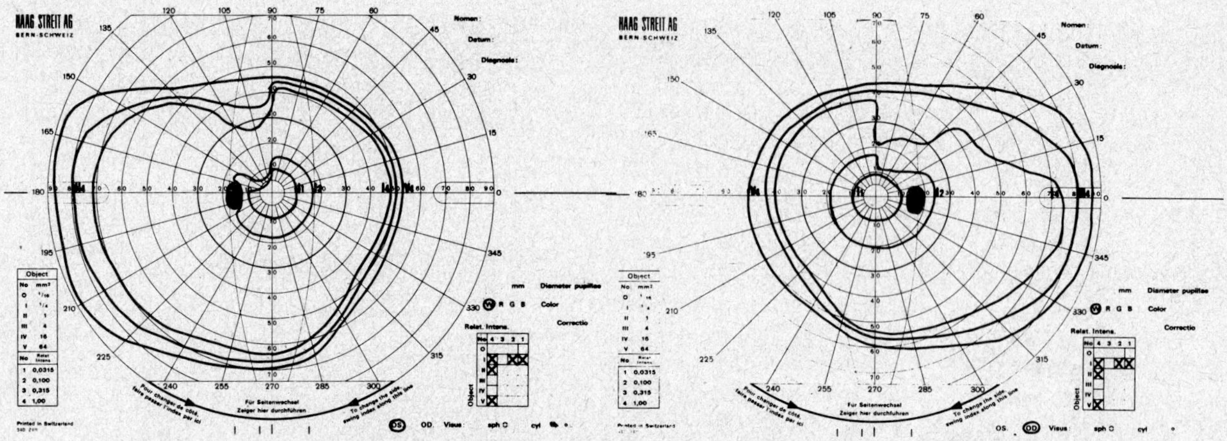

Figure 2. *Goldman quantitative perimetry illustrating the bitemporal superior quadrantanopsia.*

was no progression of the visual field defect during this time span. The visual field defect was more pronounced in the left eye than in the right, being demonstrable with a 1 mm^2 object with unit intensity in the left eye. To demonstrate a temporal defect in the right eye a smaller object of 0.25 mm^2 unit intensity was necessary. Testing of visual acuity revealed a refractile error which could easily be corrected with corrective lenses. Pupillary response to light, ocular motility and ophthalmoscopy were normal.

Endocrine Evaluation. In order to determine the functional reserve of the compressed pituitary gland, an investigation of pituitary function was undertaken. Normal serum thyrosine (T_4), T_3 resin uptake and thyroid stimulating hormone (TSH) (Table I) suggested an intact hypothalamic-pituitary-thyroidal axis. To determine the TSH reserve in this patient more precisely, 500 μg thyrotropin-releasing hormone (TRH) was administered intravenously and TSH levels were determined at timed intervals. Serum TSH rose from a basal level of 1.4 μU/ml to a maximum of 13 μU/ml 45 minutes after the administration of TRH (Figure 3C), indicating adequate pituitary TSH reserve. Hypothalamic-pituitary-testicular function was assessed by serum luteinizing hormone (LH), follicle-stimulating hormone (FSH) and testosterone assay. These were found to be normal (Table I). To assess pituitary-adrenal function, a standard insulin tolerance test was performed; 0.1 unit of regular crystalline insulin per kg body weight was administered intravenously. Blood sugar fell from a basal level of 100 mg/100 ml to a nadir of 45 mg/100 ml 40 minutes after the administration of insulin, resulting in an adequate hypoglycemic stimulus for ACTH secretion. Serum cortisol rose from a basal level of 9 μg/100 ml to a peak level of 24 μg/100 ml 90 minutes after the administration of insulin (Figure 3A). This is considered an adequate cortisol response and suggests an intact pituitary-adrenal axis. Human growth hormone (HGH) was also measured during insulin-induced hypoglycemia, and the response was blunted (Figure 3A). Because hypoglycemia-induced growth hormone response is blunted in some normal subjects [8], a second growth hormone provocative study was performed. Thirty grams of arginine hydrochloride was infused intravenously over a 30 minute period. After this stimulus, HGH rose from a basal level of 6 ng/ml to a peak of 30 ng/ml (Figure 3B), indicating normal pituitary growth hormone reserve to this amino acid stimulus. Pituitary prolactin reserve was studied after the oral administration of a phenothiazine, perphenazine, thought to act primarily via hypothalamic suppression of prolactin inhibitory factor. Radioimmunoassayable serum prolactin increased from 4 ng/ml to a peak of 17 ng/ml (Figure 3D). The normal male response is an increase greater than 8 ng/ml to a value above 15 ng/ml (unpublished data). Prolactin was also measured after direct pituitary stimulation with TRH, and the response to this stimulus was also indicative of normal pituitary prolactin reserve (Figure 3C). Finally, the urine osmolality of 1,063 mOsm/kg following overnight water deprivation was sufficiently high to rule out vasopressin deficiency (Table I). Thus, seven of the nine pituitary hormones were evaluated and no trophic hormone deficiencies or excesses were found to suggest the presence of a functioning pituitary adenoma or significant destruction of pituitary tissue in this patient.

TABLE I Endocrine Studies

Test	Patient	Normal Range
T_4 by RIA (μg/100 ml)	7.8	5–14
T_3 resin uptake (%)	32.7	25–35
TSH (μU/ml)	3.8	<10
LH (mIU/ml)	6.0	<11
FSH (mIU/ml)	8.0	4–25
Testosterone (ng/100 ml)	701.0	300–1,200
Urine osmolality following overnight water deprivation (mOsm/kg)	1,063.0	>600

COMMENT

Busch [9] introduced the term "empty sella" in an investigation of 788 consecutive postmortem specimens to describe the empty appearance of 40 sellas, an incidence of 5.1 per cent. Subsequently, other investigators have confirmed the common occurrence of an empty appearing sella in postmortem studies of subjects without known endocrine disease [10,11]. In addition to the autopsy findings, the term has been used to describe empty appearing sellas on surgical transfrontal or transsphenoidal exposure, and the appearance of air or contrast material in the sella at pneumoencephalography. An incomplete diaphragma sellae appears to be a precondition to the development of this syndrome, permitting extension of the subarachnoid space below the diaphragm [12]. In the primary empty sella syndrome it is postulated that a congenital defect in the diaphragm, coupled with normal and constant pulsations of cerebrospinal fluid, pushes the subarachnoid space farther and farther into the sella, resulting, in time, in compression of the pituitary gland and enlargement of the sella [12]. Alternatively, Sutton and Vezina [13] suggested, in their patients with empty sellas in association with a pituitary tumor, that pituitary tumor apoplexy may result in herniation of the subarachnoid space into the sella through an incompetent diaphragm. Whether primary intrapituitary processes such as cysts can secondarily establish communications with the subarachnoid space in the presence of a competent diaphragm is not known.

Although pituitary function is stated to be normal in most patients with the primary empty sella syndrome [14], thorough and systematic studies of pituitary function have not been reported in these patients. Few studies exist utilizing sensitive and specific radioimmunoassay technics to evaluate not only basal hormone secretion but also pituitary hormone reserve to provocative stimulation. No studies exist in which a complete pituitary evaluation, including TSH, ACTH, FSH, LH, HGH, PRL (prolactin) and AVP (arginine vasopressin) function has been made in the same patient. The status of pituitary function in the primary empty sella syndrome is, therefore, largely unknown.

Despite the conspicuous absence of reports of systematic pituitary evaluation, abnormalities in pituitary function have occasionally been described. The empty sella is known to occur in association with pituitary tumors presenting with acromegaly or the galactorrhea-amenorrhea syndrome [13]. Deficiencies of pituitary LH [15], TSH [16], ACTH [16] and vasopressin [6] have been reported. Abnormalities in growth hormone dynamics have been described by several investigators. Caplan and Dobben [17] reported a blunted growth hormone response to arginine infusion in one patient. Brisman et al. [15] observed a diminished growth hormone response to hypoglycemia in eight of 13 patients. Since the degree of hypoglycemia was not documented in this study,

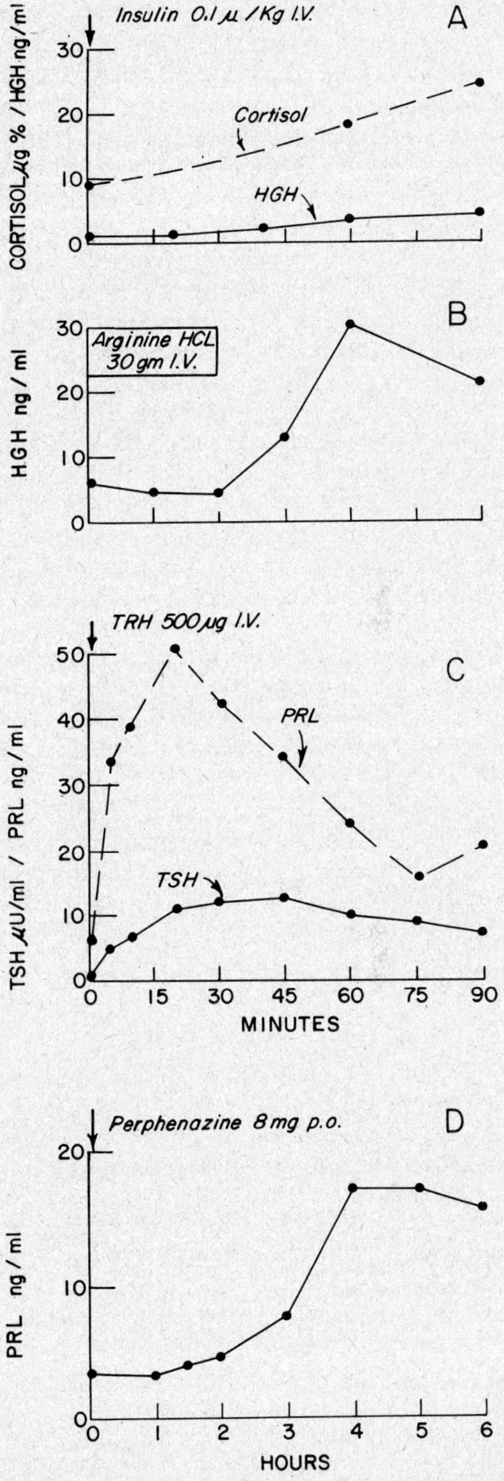

Figure 3. *Dynamic studies of pituitary function. The horizontal axes for panels **A, B** and **C** are depicted in minutes and for panel **D** in hours. **A,** cortisol and growth hormone response to insulin hypoglycemia. **B,** growth hormone response to arginine infusion. **C,** TSH and prolactin response to TRH administration. **D,** prolactin response to perphenazine ingestion.*

these data cannot be interpreted as indicating growth hormone unresponsiveness. Faglia et al. [18] and Neelon et al. [16] described an additional five patients with the primary empty sella syndrome who failed to respond to insulin hypoglycemia. Our patient also failed to show an increase in HGH following insulin hypoglycemia although he had normal HGH dynamics following arginine infusion. Since some normal subjects fail to respond to insulin or to arginine but have a normal response to another stimulus [8], the diagnosis of growth hormone deficiency cannot be established on the basis of only one provocative study.

The most striking abnormality in our patient was the visual field defect manifested by a mild bitemporal superior quadrantanopsia. Although visual field defects are common in secondary empty sella syndrome (secondary to radiotherapy or surgery of the sellar region), they have only rarely been reported in the primary empty sella syndrome. Thorough endocrine evaluation has not been accomplished in the reported cases associated with visual field defects. Robertson [2] described a patient with the primary empty sella syndrome who had clinical evidence of panhypopituitarism and loss of temporal vision. Walsh and Hoyt [3] described a 35 year old man with bitemporal field defects and optic atrophy whose endocrine status was not evaluated although he was stated to be impotent. An additional two patients were described by Mortara et al. [4]: one had an incomplete bitemporal hemianopsia and was stated to be panhypopituitary (no data given); the other patient had a complete bitemporal hemianopsia with incomplete binasal involvement (endocrine function not studied). A fifth patient was described by Metzger and associates [5] with partial binasal and bitemporal field defects whose endocrine status was not described. Matisonn and Pimstone [6] described a sixth patient with diabetes insipidus who had gross visual impairment of the left eye and a temporal field defect in the right.

Surgical exploration of the suprasellar region has been described in three patients with the primary empty sella syndrome. The optic nerves and chiasm dipped into the sella [4] or were in their normal position but thinned [2,4]. These anatomic variations were probably responsible for the visual field defects described.

In summary, we present a patient with a chiasmal visual field defect and an empty sella who was subjected to extensive endocrine evaluation. In contrast to all previously published cases of empty sella syndrome associated with visual field defects, in which there was either evidence of pituitary deficiency or in which the endocrine status was not evaluated, we documented normal pituitary function in our patient. The diagnosis of primary empty sella syndrome should be considered in any patient presenting with an enlarged sella turcica, visual field defects and normal pituitary function.

ACKNOWLEDGMENT

We thank Abbott Laboratories for supplying the TRH and Mr. Vernon Heade, BCMC Clinical Laboratory, for expert technical assistance.

REFERENCES

1. Weiss SR, Raskind R: Non-neoplastic intrasellar cysts. Int Surg 51: 282, 1969.
2. Robertson EG: Pneumoencephalography, 2nd ed. Springfield, Charles C Thomas, 1967, p 314.
3. Walsh FB, Hoyt WF: Clinical Neuro-Ophthalmology, 3rd ed. Baltimore, Williams & Wilkins Co., 1969, p 2098.
4. Mortara R, Norell H: Consequences of a deficient sellar diaphragm. J Neurosurg 32: 565, 1970.
5. Metzger J, Helias A, Messimy R, et al.: Nouveaux cas de selles turciques dites vides avec signes neuro-opthalmologiques ou rhinorrhee. Rev Neurol 123: 435, 1970.
6. Matisonn R, Pimstone B: Diabetes insipidus associated with an empty sella turcica. Postgrad Med J (South Africa) 49: 274, 1973.
7. DiChiro G, Nelson KB: The volume of the sella turcica. Am J Roentgenol 87: 989, 1962.
8. Parker ML, Hammond JM, Daughaday WH: The arginine provocative test: an aid in the diagnosis of hyposomatotropism. J Clin Endocrinol Metab 27: 1129, 1967.
9. Busch W: Die morphologie der sella turcica und ihre beziehungen zur hypophyse. Virchows Arch 320: 437, 1951.
10. Bergland RM, Ray BS, Torack RM: Anatomical variations in the pituitary gland and adjacent structures in 225 human autopsy cases. J Neurosurg 28: 93, 1968.
11. Kaufman B, Chamberlin WB Jr: The ubiquitous "empty" sella turcica. Acta Radiol (Diagn) (Stockh) 13: 413, 1972.
12. Kaufman B: The "empty" sella turcica—a manifestation of the intrasellar subarachnoid space. Radiology 90: 931, 1968.
13. Sutton TG, Vezina JL: Co-existing pituitary adenomas and intrasellar arachnoid invagination. Am J Roentgenol Radium Ther Nucl Med 122: 508, 1974.
14. Hodgson SF, Randall RV, Holman CB, MacCarty CS: Empty sella syndrome: report of 10 cases. Med Clin North Am 56: 897, 1972.
15. Brisman R, Hughes JEO, Holub DA: Endocrine function in nineteen patients with empty sella syndrome. J Clin Endocrinol 34: 570, 1972.
16. Neelon FA, Goree JA, Lebovitz HE: The primary empty sella: clinical and radiographic characteristics and endocrine function. Medicine 52: 73, 1973.
17. Caplan RH, Dobben GD: Endocrine studies in patients with the empty sella syndrome. Arch Intern Med 123: 611, 1969.
18. Faglia G, Ambrosi B, Beck-Peccoz P, Giovanelli M: Disorders of growth hormone and corticotropin regulation in patients with empty sella. J Neurosurg 38: 59, 1973.

The Syndrome of Multiple Endocrine Gland Insufficiency

GERALD B. APPEL, M.D.
DONALD A. HOLUB, M.D.
New York, New York

Addison's disease, when caused by idiopathic atrophy of the adrenal cortex, is frequently associated with other endocrine abnormalities. Primary hypothyroidism and hypogonadism have been reported in association with adrenal insufficiency; understandably, such cases may lead to diagnostic confusion with respect to possible pituitary disease.

This case study concerns a woman who exhibited, in sequence and over a period of 17 years, hypogonadism, hypoadrenalism, diabetes mellitus and, finally, hypothyroidism. Originally misdiagnosed as having Sheehan's syndrome, she eventually became hyperpigmented. The true nature of her illness was then revealed to be primary insufficiency of multiple endocrine glands, with the demonstration of elevated levels of several pituitary hormones.

Because multiple endocrine insufficiencies may coexist or develop with time, we suggest that a patient with a single documented endocrine deficiency be investigated initially and serially for additional glandular deficiencies.

Adrenocortical insufficiency due to idiopathic atrophy of the adrenal cortex is frequently associated with evidence of other endocrine disease. The coexistence of adrenal and thyroid hypofunction has been repeatedly documented since the original report by Schmidt in 1926 [1–3]; coincident Addison's disease and primary gonadal failure have also been reported [4,5]. Whenever the triad of primary adrenal, thyroid and gonadal failure has occurred, it has understandably been confused with disease of the anterior pituitary gland [6,7].

Although increasing numbers of patients with diabetes mellitus and Addison's disease have been described [8–10], the combined occurrence of primary hypoadrenalism, primary hypothyroidism, primary hypogonadism and diabetes in a single patient has been identified only rarely. A review of the literature documents few persons with this tetrad [5,11,12,20]; some of these cases were reported before accurate and sensitive measurements of pituitary trophic hormones were available. Therefore, we describe an additional patient with primary organ failure of the adrenal cortex, thyroid and gonads in conjunction with diabetes mellitus, in whom we have documented thoroughly the adequacy of pituitary function. We will also review briefly the literature on these associations.

CASE REPORT

The patient, a white woman who is now 39 years old, experienced a postpartum hemorrhage for which she required transfusion of 4 units of blood

From the Department of Medicine, Columbia University College of Physicians & Surgeons and The Presbyterian Hospital, New York, New York. Requests for reprints should be addressed to Dr. Donald A. Holub, Department of Medicine, Columbia University College of Physicians & Surgeons, 630 West 165th Street, New York, New York 10032. Manuscript accepted November 20, 1975.

at the age of 20. Although her menses returned and she had an uncomplicated pregnancy one year later, she did not menstruate spontaneously subsequent to this second delivery. She was considered by her family physician to have Sheehan's syndrome and received a variety of sex hormones over the next 12 years with only infrequent withdrawal bleeding. The patient noted some decrease in her pubic hair, but no change in her axillary hair or breast size during this interval, nor did she note any galactorrhea. In 1967, at the age of 26, she complained of weakness, cold intolerance and decreased energy. Her protein-bound iodine level was 7.4 μg/100 ml, T3 (triiodothyronine) resin uptake 0.99, urinary 17-hydroxysteroids 8.3 mg/24 hours and 17-ketosteroids 6.0 mg/ 24 hours. The patient was treated with Cytomel® 5 μg/day with questionable symptomatic improvement. Later the same year, she was hospitalized with dizziness, faintness, abdominal bloating and hypotension. Urinary steroid determinations were reported normal and the urinary follicle-stimulating hormone (FSH) titer was positive at 6 muu (mouse uterine units); however, the urine was collected only a few days after the oral intake of estrogens was discontinued. She was treated with Cytomel 7.5 μg per day, Ovulen® and Dexedrine®, with the diagnosis of amenorrhea secondary to Sheehan's syndrome.

Several months later, in 1968, the patient was seen for the first time at the Columbia-Presbyterian Medical Center with the complaints of positional vertigo, nausea and weakness. Episodes of "being unable to function" secondary to tremulousness, fatigue and mental slowing, each lasting several days, were said to have occurred repeatedly. The results of her physical examination were within normal limits except for a blood pressure of 90/70 mm Hg sitting and supine, and a minimal decrease in pubic hair. Laboratory evaluation revealed a normal urinalysis, complete blood count, erythrocyte sedimentation rate, electrolytes, oral glucose tolerance test, chest roentgenogram, skull films, serum calcium and phosphorus. Endocrine evaluation included an 8 AM plasma cortisol value of 7.2 μg/100 ml (normal 4 to 23 μg/100 ml), urinary ketogenic steroids of 4.7 mg/24 hours (normal 7 to 12 mg/24 hours), and 17-ketosteroids of 1.36 mg/24 hours (normal 6 to 15 mg/24 hours).

The patient underwent an oral Metapyrone® test (750 mg every 4 hours for six doses) with a subnormal response; her ketogenic steroids increased to 8.3 mg/24 hours and 17-ketosteroids to 4.0 mg/24 hours. An intravenous ACTH stimulation test (25 units over 4 hours) demonstrated a subnormal response, the plasma cortisol level rising from 7.2 to 28.8 μg/100 ml (normal rise is to 35 μg/100 ml). Thyroid function tests consisted of T3 resin uptake of 0.61 (normal 0.8 to 1.2), T4 (thyroxine) by column of 5.4 μg/100 ml (normal 3.2 to 6.4) and 24 hour radioiodine uptake of 28 per cent.

Hypoadrenalism secondary to pituitary ACTH insufficiency was thought to explain both her symptoms and the inadequate responses to both exogenous and endogenous ACTH. The patient was treated with cortisone acetate 12.5 mg twice a day with a striking subjective improvement in well being and an increase in her blood pressure to 110/80 mm Hg.

In September 1968 the patient returned for an elective cholecystectomy. Physical examination at this time was normal; blood pressure was 110/70 mm Hg without orthostatic changes. The patient's fasting blood sugar level was 86 mg/100 ml; T4 by column was 5.3 μg/100 ml; T3 resin uptake was 0.83; urinary 17-ketosteroid and ketogenic steroid levels were 7.2 mg/24 hours and 14.5 mg/24 hours, respectively (during continued therapy with cortisone). A urinary gonadotropin bioassay now revealed a level of greater than 50 muu/24 hours. This menopausal level was thought to be incompatible with the longstanding diagnosis of Sheehan's syndrome. However, treatment with cortisone was continued as before.

Over the next two and a half years, the patient's weight increased significantly and the cortisone dose was gradually decreased to 5 mg twice a day. In March 1971, several weeks of diarrhea and abdominal cramps occurred and she noted that her sun tan from the previous summer had not faded as completely as usual. Moreover, her skin became dry, and cold intolerance returned. Physical examination revealed a blood pressure of 95/60 mm Hg supine and 80/60 mm Hg standing. Her skin was now noted to be diffusely hyperpigmented, especially the gums, palate, nipples and areolae, flexion creases and the recent cholecystectomy scar. Thyroid enlargement, loss of axillary hair and sparse pubic hair were also discovered. Skull films and electrolyte levels were normal. The patient's cortisone dose was increased to 15 mg/day. Shortly thereafter, she was hospitalized elsewhere with several days of nausea and vomiting and found to be hypotensive. The patient was discharged on a regimen consisting of 25 mg of cortisone/day and 0.1 mg of Florinef® a day as well as 5 μg of Cytomel twice a day. The patient's Cytomel was later replaced by Thyrolar® 30 mg twice a day and her Florinef dosage was changed to 0.1 mg every second day. When next seen in November 1973, she appeared slightly Cushingoid with rounded facies and a dorsal fat pad; generalized hyperpigmentation was again present. T4 by column was 3.0 μg/100 ml and serum prolactin was 29 ng/ml (normal 0 to 30 ng/ml).

In May 1974, the patient presented to another hospital with five days of polyuria, polydipsia and hazy vision. She had also experienced one week of nausea and vomiting. The patient was found to have a blood sugar level of 642 mg/100 ml and was transferred to Presbyterian Hospital where control of her diabetes mellitus was achieved with 20 units of Lente insulin/day. Further evaluation at this time revealed her serum FSH to be 46 mIU/ml and LH 55 mIU/ml, both values being within the menopausal range. Serum vitamin B_{12} was 1,000 pg/ml, prolactin 10 ng/ml, growth hormone 0.8 ng/ml (normal less than 5 ng/ml), antithyroglobulin antibodies less than 1:16 (normal less than 1:32), free thyroxine 0.9 ng/100 ml (normal 1.0 to 2.4 ng/100 ml), T4 as iodine 2.7 ng/100 ml (normal 3.2 to 6.4 ng/100 ml), T4 as thyroxine 4.1 ng/100 ml (normal 5 to 12), TSH 41 units (normal 0 to 10 units). She was discharged on a regimen of cortisone 12.5 mg twice a day, Florinef 0.1 mg daily, Lente insulin 20 units daily and Synthroid® 0.1 mg daily.

The diagnosis at this time consisted of Addison's disease, primary ovarian failure, primary hypothyroidism and diabetes mellitus. She has done well since as an outpatient.

Subsequent evaluation has demonstrated the presence of antiadrenal antibodies (4+ at 1:4 dilution) and thyroid microsomal antibodies (2+ undiluted).* Thyroid agglutinating antibodies were not present in abnormal titer. Blood obtained 24 hours after the last dose of cortisone revealed an ACTH level of 2,350 pg/ml (normal up to 120 pg/ml), a value consistent with primary adrenal insufficiency. Oral administration of 500 mg of L-dopa elicited the following normal increase in growth hormone levels: 0 minutes 3.0 ng/ml, 20 minutes 3.1 ng/ml, 60 minutes 12.8 ng/ml, 90 minutes 36.0 ng/ml and 120 minutes 16.0 ng/ml.

COMMENTS

When amenorrhea developed in this patient at age 22, it was attributed to Sheehan's syndrome sustained as a consequence of a postpartum hemorrhage one year previously. Many years later, elevated urinary and plasma gonadatrophin levels were demonstrated, making it clear that her amenorrhea was caused by primary ovarian failure. Adrenal insufficiency became symptomatic at age 33. This was initially misdiagnosed as being secondary to her presumed pituitary insufficiency; a definite, although subnormal, response to exogenous ACTH and to Metapyrone-induced endogenous ACTH stimulation seemed to favor this diagnosis. In retrospect, these responses can be interpreted to show that adrenal function was only partially compromised at this time, since subsequent events indicated that her adrenal insufficiency was due to primary adrenal disease. At age 36, when the patient's cortisol dosage was tapered, increased pigmentation developed in a characteristic Addisonian pattern; this, in addition to the necessity for mineralocorticoid replacement therapy, pointed to the true diagnosis of Addison's disease. This has been confirmed by the presence of antiadrenal antibodies, and also by the characteristically high ACTH level. More recently, primary hypothyroidism has been documented, with low thyroxine and elevated TSH levels. Normal prolactin and growth hormone levels, a brisk response of plasma growth hormone levels to L-dopa stimulation, and normal skull films add further support to the concept of an intrinsically normal pituitary gland.

Finally, insulin-dependent diabetes mellitus developed in this patient at the age of 39. She has no family history of diabetes or other endocrine disease. The patient has thus far exhibited no evidence of parathyroid dysfunction, moniliasis or pernicious anemia and vitiligo or alopecia has not developed at any time during her course.

* Usually neither of these antibodies is found in normal plasma.

Abnormalities involving the thyroid are not rare in patients with Addison's disease, particularly when the latter is of the "atrophic," idiopathic type. Since Schmidt's original description [1], numerous patients with this combination of endocrine diseases have been described. A review of over 500 Addisonian patients from the Mayo Clinic from 1913 to 1958 showed 7 per cent with abnormal thyroid glands on palpation and 11 cases of frank myxedema. Atrophy and lymphoid infiltration of the thyroid gland are common in Addisonian patients at autopsy even in the absence of clinical hypothyroidism during life [2]. In a recent series of 174 patients with Addison's disease, evidence of clinical thyroid disease was present in 27 patients [3].

Primary gonadal dysfunction associated with primary adrenal failure is also being reported more frequently. Irvine and Barnes [4] reported that more than 25 per cent of 102 patients with idiopathic Addison's disease had evidence of premature gonadal failure with increased gonadotrophin levels. In another, smaller series, 23 per cent of Addisonian patients exhibited this combination of dysfunction [5].

The association of primary adrenal and gonadal failure can easily be confused with disease of pituitary origin. If primary hypothyroidism is also present, the desire to employ a diagnostic "Law of Parsimony" may lead to the erroneous diagnosis of multiple deficiencies of pituitary trophic hormones [6,7]. The availability of accurate measurement by radioimmunoassay of these trophic hormones should minimize this confusion in the future.

Sixty-three cases of diabetes mellitus associated with Addison's disease were reviewed in 1959 by Beaven et al. [8]. Adrenal failure was noted first in 21 patients, whereas the diabetes was observed first in 37 patients; in five patients both diseases occurred simultaneously. Wehrmacher's review in 1960 confirmed these findings [9]. Solomon et al.'s [10] recent study of 113 patients with coexisting primary adrenal failure and diabetes revealed a greater incidence of this association in patients with idiopathic adrenal failure (67 per cent) than in those with tuberculous origin (14 per cent). The triad of primary adrenal failure, thyroid disease and diabetes mellitus has been noted in several reports [5,8,10].

Addison's disease has also been associated with hypoparathyroidism [13–15], pernicious anemia [16] and vitiligo [17,18].

In contrast to the foregoing associations of multiple glandular failure, the tetrad of primary adrenal failure, primary thyroid failure, primary gonadal failure and diabetes mellitus is rare. In 1952 Crispell and Parson [11] described a 19 year old diabetic girl in whom amenorrhea, primary adrenal failure and subsequently primary thyroid failure developed. Laboratory data confirmed the primary nature of her dysfunctions and on postmortem histologic examination the pituitary gland was normal. In 1962 Christy et al. [12] described a 40 year old woman with amenorrhea in whom hypothyroidism, hypoadrenalism and then diabetes mellitus developed, all of a primary nature. Although initially no antibodies to thyroid and adrenal tissue could be detected, retesting of her serum later revealed these to be present [19]. In 1967 Turkington and Lebovitz [5] described a 51 year old man with primary thyroid failure, followed by Addison's disease, primary gonadal dysfunction and diabetes mellitus. A second patient was noted to have primary failure of the thyroid, adrenals and gonads as well as an abnormal glucose tolerance test. MacCuish et al. [20] mention two female patients in whom oligomenorrhea and amenorrhea developed, then hypothyroidism and eventually Addison's disease and diabetes mellitus. In addition, one of their patients had pernicious anemia. Our patient displayed primary gonadal failure initially, followed by Addison's disease, primary hypothyroidism and finally diabetes mellitus. She is the first of these patients to have thorough documentation of the adequacy of her pituitary status through measurement of all trophic hormone levels and appropriate stimulation tests.

The etiology of multiglandular failure remains unclear. Similarity of pathologic changes in the various organs, consisting of lymphocytic infiltration and fibrosis, lends support to the concept of a common etiologic factor in this syndrome. Patients with "idiopathic" Addison's disease have been shown to have a significant incidence of serum antibodies directed against adrenal tissue [4,21–23]. Such antibodies are not found in patients with tuberculous Addison's disease or in patients with primary adrenal insufficiency due to other specific etiologies. Therefore, some investigators have suggested that these antibodies may play a role in the pathogenesis of the disease rather than representing a nonspecific response to adrenal injury. Antibodies directed against thyroid and gonadal tissues have also been demonstrated in "idiopathic" Addison's disease, but infrequently in patients with primary adrenal failure of other etiologies [4,21,23]. A higher incidence of pluriglandular failure is also present in patients with "idiopathic" or "atrophic" Addison's disease than in those with tuberculous disease. These observations have raised the possibility that idiopathic Addison's disease may be an "autoimmune" disease; certainly, animal models of autoimmune adrenalitis exist, suggesting that this mechanism could be operative in man [24,25]. The possibility of cross autoimmunization between steroid antigens of adrenal and gonadal tissue may account for some aspects of the syndrome of "multiple endocrine glandular insufficiency." Recent workers [20,26] have emphasized the potential role of autoimmunity in diabetes mellitus with documentation of circulating antibodies to pancreatic islet cells in insulin-dependent diabetic patients. These antibodies are found most frequently in diabetic patients who manifest other endocrine gland disorders. The initial forces leading to the postulated immunization still remain unknown for all of these disorders.

The present case report, as well as a review of the literature, leads to several important clinical conclusions: Addison's disease, especially the "idiopathic" variety, is often associated with primary disease of other endocrine organs. This may cause confusion with primary pituitary dysfunction, but measurements of trophic hormones should enable clear differentiation of the two syndromes. Every patient with an idiopathic endocrine deficiency should have a thorough evaluation of other endocrine functions initially. This should be repeated at intervals thereafter because the appearance of disorders of other endocrine glands may be delayed for many years, and there does not seem to be a predictable sequence in the appearance of these endocrine deficiencies.

ACKNOWLEDGMENT

Gratitude is expressed to Dr. David Orth for measurement of ACTH, to Drs. Robert Blizzard and Ann Johansen for measurement of adrenal and thyroid antibodies, and to Dr. Andrew G. Frantz for critical review of the manuscript.

REFERENCES

1. Schmidt MB: Eine Biglandulare Erkrankung (Nebennieren und Schilddruse) bei morbus Addisonii. Verhandlungen der Deutschen Pathologischen. 21: 212, 1926.
2. Gastineau CF, Arnold JW: Thyroid disorders in Addison's disease. Proc Staff Meet Mayo Clin 38: 323, 1963.
3. Carpenter CCJ, Solomon N, Silverberg SG: Schmidt's syndrome. A review of the literature and a report of 15 new cases including 10 instances of coexistent diabetes. Medicine (Baltimore) 43: 153, 1964.
4. Irvine WJ, Barnes EW: Adrenocortical insufficiency. Clin Endocrinol Metab 1: 549, 1972.
5. Turkington RW, Lebovitz ME: Extra-adrenal endocrine deficiencies in Addison's disease. Am J Med 43: 499, 1967.
6. Rupp JJ, Paschkis KE: Pluriglandular insufficiency simulating panhypopituitarium: report of 2 cases. Am J Med 18: 507, 1955.
7. Nicholls MG, Espiner EA, Donald RA: Schmidt's syndrome

presenting as hypopituitarism. Ann Intern Med 80: 505, 1974.

8. Beaven DW, Nelson DM, Renold AE, Thorn GW: Diabetes mellitus and Addison's disease. N Engl J Med 261: 443, 1959.
9. Wehrmacher WH: Addison's disease with diabetes mellitus. Arch Intern Med 108: 114, 1961.
10. Solomon N, Carpenter CCJ, Bennett IL, Marvey AM: Schmidt's syndrome (thyroid and adrenal insufficiency) and coexistent diabetes mellitus. Diabetes 14: 300, 1966.
11. Crispell KR, Parson W: The administration of purified growth hormone to a female with hypoadrenalism, hypothyroidism, diabetes mellitus, and secondary amenorrhea, simulating panhypopituitarism. J Clin Endocrinol Metab 12: 881, 1952.
12. Christy NP, Tomasi TB, Holub DA: Primary ovarian, thyroidal, and adrenocortical deficiencies, simulating pituitary insufficiency, associated with diabetes mellitus. J Clin Endocrinol Metab 22: 155, 1962.
13. Whitaker J, Landing BM, Esselborn VM, Williams RR: The syndrome of familial hypoadrenocorticism, hypoparathyroidism, and superficial moniliasis. J Clin Endocrinol Metab 16: 1374, 1956.
14. Morse WI, Cochrane WA, Landrigan PL: Familial hypoparathyroidism with pernicious anemia, steatorrhea, and adrenocortical insufficiency. N Engl J Med 264: 1021, 1961.
15. Carter AC, Kaplan SA, DeMayo AP, Rosenblum DJ: An unusual case of idiopathic hypoparathyroidism, adrenal insufficiency, hypothyroidism and metastic calcification. J Clin Endocrinol Metab 19: 1633, 1959.
16. Stickland RG: Pernicious anemia and polyendocrine deficiency. Ann Intern Med 70: 1001, 1969.
17. Forcier RJ, McIntyre OR, Frey WG, Andrada JA, Streiff RR: Autoimmunity and multiple endocrine abnormalities. Arch Intern Med 129: 638, 1972.
18. McGregor BC, Katz HI, Doe RP: Vitiligo and multiple glandular insufficiency. JAMA 219: 724, 1972.
19. Blizzard RM, Tomasi TB, Christy NP: Autoantibodies against thyroid and adrenal tissue in a patient with multiple primary endocrine deficiencies. J Clin Endocrinol Metab 23: 1174, 1963.
20. MacCuish AC, Irvine WJ, Barnes EW, Duncan LJP: Antibodies to pancreatic islet cells in insulin-dependent diabetics with coexistent autoimmune disease. Lancet 2: 1529, 1974,
21. Blizzard RM, Chandler AW, Kyle MA, Hung W: Adrenal antibodies in Addison's disease. Lancet 2: 901, 1962.
22. Solomon I, Blizzard RM: Autoimmune disorders of endocrine glands. J Pediatr 63: 1021, 1963.
23. Anderson JR, Goudie RB, Gray KG, Timbury GC: Autoantibodies in Addison's disease. Lancet 1: 1123, 1957.
24. Colover J, Glynn LE: Experimental iso-immune adrenalitis. Immunology 1: 172, 1958.
25. Barnett EV, Dumonde DC, Glynn LE: Induction of autoimmunity to adrenal gland. Immunology 6: 382, 1963.
26. Bottazzo GF, Florin-Christensen A, Doniach D: Islet-cell antibodies in diabetes mellitus with autoimmune polyendocrine deficiencies. Lancet 2: 1279, 1974.

Ectopic Hyperparathyroidism (Pseudohyperparathyroidism) in Esophageal Malignancy

Report of a Case and a Review of the Literature

MARTIN GRAJOWER, M.D.
URIEL S. BARZEL, M.D.
Bronx, New York

Described here is a patient with esophageal carcinoma who had hypercalcemia, an elevated serum level of parathyroid hormone and normal parathyroid glands. A review of the literature reveals that a total of 25 other patients with ectopic hyperparathyroidism in esophageal malignancy have been described, four of whom had documented elevations of serum parathyroid hormone levels. Esophageal neoplasms should be added to the list of tumors associated with ectopic secretion of parathyroid hormone.

The term pseudohyperparathyroidism was first used by Lafferty [1] to describe the occurrence of hypercalcemia in malignant disease without associated bony metastases. The etiology of the elevated serum calcium level in these cases is presumed to be the ectopic secretion of parathyroid hormone by the tumor. We describe here a patient with esophageal epidermoid carcinoma and ectopic hyperparathyroidism, and review the literature for reports of other such cases.

CASE REPORT

This patient was an 80 year old Black man who during the month prior to admission noted poor appetite, some dysphagia, 15 pound weight loss, weakness and a bitter taste in his mouth. He had a vague history of hypertension and reported a moderate consumption of alcohol. On physical examination he was cachectic, with positive findings limited to a hard, tender liver palpable 5 fingerbreadth below the right costal margin. Stool was guaiac positive. The hematocrit value was 36. The blood calcium was 10.8 mg/100 ml, the phosphorus 3.3 mg/100 ml, the chloride 106 meq/liter, and the alkaline phosphatase 205 U (normal less than 85 U). Serum obtained later in the hospital course revealed a calcium of 11.6 mg/100 ml, phosphorus of 2.3 mg/100 ml and a concurrent parathyroid hormone blood level of 48 μleq/ml (as performed by the laboratory of Dr. C. Arnaud [2]).* A urinalysis was normal. The electrocardiogram revealed normal sinus rhythm and a QT interval of 0.32 second with a heart rate of 75. A skeletal survey failed to reveal any bony metastases. The hospital course was complicated by pro-

* The normal blood level of parathyroid hormone at this laboratory [2] is no more than 40 μleq/ml at low normal blood calcium level, and lower at higher blood calcium level. At this patient's calcium blood level, blood parathyroid hormone should be undetectable.

From the Metabolic Endocrine Laboratory, Department of Medicine, Montefiore Hospital and Medical Center; and The Albert Einstein College of Medicine, Bronx, New York. Requests for reprints should be addressed to Dr. U. S. Barzel, Montefiore Hospital and Medical Center, 111 East 210th Street, Bronx, New York 10467. Manuscript accepted October 31, 1975.

gressively increasing hypercalcemia, the development of recurrent seizures, hemiplegia, coma and death. At autopsy he was found to have had an infiltrating epidermoid carcinoma of the middle third of the esophagus with metastases to periesophageal lymph nodes, lungs, liver and brain. No bony metastases were found. The parathyroid glands were normal in size and microscopic appearance.

COMMENTS

The occurrence of hypercalcemia in esophageal neoplasms has gone unrecognized in reviews of esophageal carcinoma [3–5], as well as reviews of hypercalcemia of malignancy [6–9] until recently when Stephens et al. [10] and Benray et al. [11] called attention to it. In addition to their series, and three cases reported by Benson et al. [2] there are only isolated reports of esophageal cancer with ectopic hyperparathyroidism (Table I). All these cases have in common the triad of hypercalcemia, hypophosphatemia and no demonstrable bony metastases which is characteristic of pseudohyperparathyroidism as described by Lafferty [1]. In addition, in some cases normal parathyroid glands are also documented. Other than our case, only Benson et al. [2] reported elevated serum parathyroid hormone levels in their patients. Most recently, Hartman et al. [16] were able to demonstrate in vitro production by squamous cell carcinoma of the esophagus of peptide(s) with properties similar to parathyroid hormone.

TABLE I Esophageal Neoplasms with Ectopic Hyperparathyroidism

Reference	No. of Cases
Ariyan et al. [15]	2
Benray et al. [11]	7
Benson et al. [2]	3*
Hartman et al. [16]	1†
Lafferty [1]	1
Sherwood et al. [13]	1
Snedecor, Baker [12]	1
Stephens et al. [10]	8
Sturgeon [14]	1
Present case	1*

* Parathyroid hormone assay reveals presence of elevated levels in serum.
† In vitro production of parathyroid-like substance by tumor demonstrated.

It thus seems well established that one of the mechanisms of hypercalcemia in esophageal cancer is the ectopic production and secretion of parathyroid hormone. In the growing list of tumors documented to secrete parathyroid hormone, esophageal carcinoma is now definitely included.

REFERENCES

1. Lafferty FW: Pseudohyperparathyroidism. Medicine (Baltimore) 45: 247, 1966.
2. Benson RC, Jr, Riggs BL, Pickard BM, Arnaud CD: Radioimmunoassay of parathyroid hormone in hypercalcemic patients with malignant disease. Am J Med 56: 821, 1974.
3. Burdette WJ: Esophageal carcinoma. Am Fam Physician 5: 88, 1972.
4. Ansari A: Carcinoma of the esophagus: diagnosis and treatment. Geriatrics 26: 98, 1971.
5. Proctor DSC: Oesophageal carcinoma. S Afr Med J 47: 48, 1973.
6. Roof BS: Tumor hypercalcemia (editorial). Calif Med 118: 35, 1973.
7. Mozaffarian G: Hypercalcemia associated with malignancies unexplained by bone metastasis: case reports and review of literature. J Maine Med Assoc 60: 205, 1969.
8. Kessinger A, Lemon HM, Foley JF: Hypercalcemia of malignancy. Geriatrics 27: 97, 1972.
9. Gordan GS: Hyper- and hypocalcemia: pathogenesis and treatments. Ann New York Acad Sci 230: 181, 1974.
10. Stephens RL, Hansen HH, Muggia FM: Hypercalcemia in epidermoid tumors of the head and neck and esophagus. Cancer 31: 1487, 1973.
11. Benrey J, Graham DY, Goyal RK: Hypercalcemia and carcinoma of the esophagus. Ann Intern Med 80: 415, 1974.
12. Snedecor PA, Baker HW: Pseudohyperparathyroidism due to malignant tumors. Cancer 17: 1492, 1964.
13. Sherwood LM, O'Riordan JLH, Aurbach GD, Potts JT Jr: Production of parathyroid hormone by nonparathyroid tumors. J Clin Endocrinol Metab 27: 140, 1967.
14. Sturgeon RR: Hypercalcemia associated with nonparathyroid tumors. Minn Med 52: 1669, 1969.
15. Ariyan S, Farber LR, Hamilton BP, Papac RJ: Pseudohyperparathyroidism in head and neck tumors. Cancer 33: 159, 1974.
16. Hartman CR, MacGregor RR, Chu LLH, McGregor DH, Cohn DV, Hamilton JW: Evidence for the biosynthesis of PTH-like peptides by a human squamous cell carcinoma (abstract). Endocrinology 96: 2, 1975.

Primary Hyperparathyroidism and Breast Cancer

APICHATI VICHAYANRAT, M.D.
AVRAAM AVRAMIDES, M.D.
BERNARD GARDNER, M.D.
STANLEY WALLACH, M.D.*
ANNE C. CARTER, M.D.
Brooklyn, New York

Three cases demonstrating the coexistence of primary hyperparathyroidism and breast carcinoma with the disappearance of hypercalcemia following removal of parathyroid adenomas are presented. In these cases, the patients had the typical diagnostic findings of primary hyperparathyroidism. Reluctance to perform neck explorations in such patients does not appear warranted.

Malignancy is the most common cause of hypercalcemia, and breast cancer is the most common neoplasm causing it [1]. Hypercalcemia is usually caused by osteolytic metastases; however, hypercalcemia may be caused by tumor secretion of parathyroid hormone or other substances which produce osteoclastic activity [2–5]. There is controversy as to what substances produce the hypercalcemia of breast cancer in the absence of skeletal metastases.

Primary hyperparathyroidism is the second most common cause of hypercalcemia and, in women of the same age range as women with breast cancer, the incidence is high. The association of primary hyperparathyroidism with breast cancer has been reported in more than 20 patients [6–10], although detailed data to assist in the differential diagnosis are lacking [9,10].

We describe three patients with breast cancer and hyperparathyroidism in whom hypercalcemia was cured by removal of a parathyroid adenoma. In all three patients, hyperparathyroidism preceded metastatic breast carcinoma. Recurrence of hypercalcemia several years after removal of parathyroid adenomas was associated with osseous metastases in one patient.

CASE REPORTS

Case 1. A 64 year old woman was admitted for evaluation of hypercalcemia in November 1968. Six months previously she had undergone a left radical mastectomy followed by postoperative radiation therapy for an infiltrating ductal carcinoma. A review of the surgical record indicated that preoperative serum calcium levels ranged from 10.4 to 12.0 mg/100 ml; they were 12.0 and 11.0 mg/100 ml, three and five months after the mastectomy. Beginning one month after mastectomy the patient noted polydipsia and nocturia, intermittent frontal headaches, dizziness, nausea and vomiting. She had no history of peptic ulcer or renal calculi. She had undergone subtotal thyroidectomy for an overactive thyroid in 1950.

Physical examination revealed a well developed black woman whose blood pressure was 120/80 mm Hg, temperature 98°F, respiratory rate 20/min and pulse rate 72/min and irregular. There was no band keratopathy, and the optic fundi were normal. No masses were palpable in the neck. The left breast was absent with a well healed scar, and there was no evidence of local recurrence. Auscultation of the heart revealed an irregular rhythm and a grade 2/6 apical systolic murmur. The remainder of the examination was within normal limits.

From the Departments of Medicine and Surgery, State University of New York, Downstate Medical Center and The Kings County Hospital Center, Brooklyn, New York 11203. This study was supported in part by U.S. Public Health Service Research Grant CA 03358; Clinical Research Centers Grant RR 00318, and by a Grant-in-Aid from the Ayerst Laboratories. Requests for reprints should be addressed to Dr. Avraam Avramides, Department of Medicine, State University of New York, Downstate Medical Center—Box 123, 450 Clarkson Avenue, Brooklyn, New York 11203. Manuscript accepted October 28, 1975.

* Present address: Veterans Administration Hospital, Albany, New York 12208.

Laboratory studies revealed a normal blood count and urinalysis. The serum calcium level ranged between 9.9 and 11.2 mg/100 ml, serum phosphate 2.1 and 2.5 mg/100 ml and serum alkaline phosphatase 31 and 51 IU/liter (normal 60 to 110 IU/liter). Roentgenograms of the chest and skeleton revealed no evidence of metastases or subperiosteal bone resorption. An electrocardiogram showed a first degree heart block, wandering atrial pacemaker and occasional premature ventricular contractions.

The hypercalcemia did not decrease during a 10 day prednisone suppression test (10 mg prednisone four times daily). The tubular reabsorption of phosphate (TRP) was 73 per cent on a regular diet (normal 80 to 95 per cent). Creatinine clearance was 73 ml/min. After phosphate supplementation for three days (2 g phosphorus per day as a mixed sodium and potassium phosphate solution) the TRP decreased to 31 per cent. A calcium infusion study, 15 mg/kg infused in 4 hours, resulted in an increase in TRP to 93 per cent. A percutaneous iliac crest bone biopsy specimen revealed normal cancellous bone with no evidence of metastatic cells or of hyperparathyroidism.

As the correct diagnosis of hyperparathyroidism was not certain, a neck exploration was not performed and it was decided to follow the patient for possible recurrence of breast cancer. The patient was lost to follow-up for four years, when she was readmitted in February 1973 because of congestive heart failure and dizziness. An electrocardiogram was compatible with a "sick sinus syndrome" with a ventricular rate of 35/min. A temporary transvenous pacemaker was inserted followed by a permanent one. The serum calcium ranged between 11.7 and 12.7 mg/100 ml, serum immunoreactive parathyroid hormone (iPTH) prior to surgery was 280 μliter equivalents/ml (normal 25 to 100 μliter equivalents), and the serum phosphate was 2.1 mg/100 ml. Skeletal films and a bone scan revealed no evidence of metastases. A neck exploration was performed in November 1973, after her cardiac condition had stabilized. A parathyroid adenoma weighing 320 mg was removed. The serum calcium decreased to 8.6 to 9.1 mg/100 ml. The patient has remained normocalcemic, and she has had no evidence of recurrent breast cancer as of March 1975.

Case 2. A 48 year old woman was admitted in October 1973 for evaluation of hypercalcemia. In January 1971 she underwent a right mastectomy followed by postoperative radiation therapy for an infiltrating ductal adenocarcinoma of the breast with axillary nodes metastases. Her serum calcium preoperatively ranged from 9.9 to 11.6 mg/100 ml and serum phosphate from 2.5 to 3.4 mg/100 ml. In March 1973, a left supraclavicular node metastasis was biopsied and a bilateral oophorectomy performed. The chest film and skeletal survey were negative until July 1973, when a radiolucency was noted in the left ischium. The serum calcium level from May to October 1973 remained elevated in the range of 11.0 to 14.0 mg/100 ml with normal to high levels of serum phosphate. The patient complained of headaches but no nausea, vomiting, polyuria or polydipsia. She lost about 20 pounds during the six months prior to admission. The patient had had mild hypertension for 10 to 15 years for which she had been treated intermittently with chlorothiazide, 500 mg/day. There was no history of peptic ulcer or renal calculi.

Physical examination revealed an alert woman whose blood pressure was 170/100 mm Hg, pulse rate 84/min and regular, respirations 20/min and temperature 96.6°F. There was no band keratopathy. The optic fundi showed a grade 1 retinopathy. A hard, fixed, left supraclavicular lymph node was palpable, measuring 2.5 by 1.5 cm. No other abnormal masses were felt in the neck. The right breast was absent with a healed scar. The remainder of the physical examination was within normal limits.

Laboratory studies revealed a normal blood count, urinalysis, serum electrolyte levels, glucose, blood urea nitrogen and protein. Serum calcium ranged from 10.9 to 13.3 mg/100 ml, serum phosphate from 3.1 to 4.6 mg/100 ml and the serum alkaline phosphatase was 110 IU/liter (normal 35 to 85 IU/liter). Serum protein electrophoresis was normal. A chest film showed infiltration of the upper right lung interpreted as radiation fibrosis. Skeletal roentgenograms revealed a lytic lesion in the left ischium. A percutaneous biopsy specimen of bone from the iliac crest showed no evidence of hyperparathyroidism or metastatic cells.

The serum calcium level remained elevated after the discontinuation of chlorothiazide therapy. Urinary calcium averaged 462 mg/day, range 244 to 587 mg/day, and the TRP on a regular diet was 31 per cent with a creatinine clearance of 119 ml/min. A serum iPTH level, using an antibody directed against the N terminal end of parathyroid hormone, was 103 μliter equivalents/ml (normal 25 to 100 μliter equivalents/ml). A prednisone suppression test did not decrease the serum calcium.

A neck exploration was performed in December 1973, and two parathyroid adenomas weighing 550 and 90 mg were removed. A biopsy specimen of a third parathyroid gland showed normal tissue. The fourth one could not be located. Postoperatively the serum calcium returned to normal. The patient remained normocalcemic and well for almost a year. In November 1974 brain metastases developed and she was given radiation therapy. Generalized metastases to liver, lungs, bones and severe hypercalcemia, 16 mg/100 ml, resulted in death in February 1975. Parathyroid hormone was undetectable at the time of her terminal hypercalcemia.

Case 3. A 74 year old woman was admitted in August 1969 because of nausea, vomiting, epigastric distress, constipation and weight loss. A mass in the right breast was found. The remainder of the physical examination was within normal limits. Serum levels were calcium 11.9 mg/100 ml, phosphate 3.0 mg/100 ml and alkaline phosphatase 13 K.A.U. Other blood studies were within normal limits. Urinary calcium averaged 190 mg/day and the TRP was 76 per cent on a regular diet. A calcium infusion study did not change the TRP. A chest film and skeletal survey disclosed no abnormalities. A series of the upper gastrointestinal tract revealed an active duodenal ulcer; a barium enema was negative. An intravenous pyelogram showed bilateral renal calculi. A percutaneous biopsy of bone from the iliac crest revealed osteoporosis, a few foci of osteoclastic and lacunar resorption suggestive of hyperparathyroidism and no cancer cells. The patient underwent a right simple mastectomy for infiltrating duct cell carcinoma followed by radiation therapy. Five days after mastectomy the serum calcium level was elevated at 11.7 mg/100 ml with a serum phosphate of 2.7 mg/100 ml.

The abdominal symptoms persisted and were poorly controlled with medications. The serum calcium ranged between 10.5 and 11.3 mg/100 ml and the serum phosphate ranged from 2.7 to 3.0 mg/100 ml for the next two years. As there was no evidence of metastatic disease, a neck exploration was performed in July 1971, and a parathyroid adenoma weighing 800 mg was removed. The serum calcium returned to normal with marked diminution in abdominal symptoms.

In November 1973, skin metastases developed followed by liver and osseous metastases. The patient was unsuccessfully treated with an estrogen. She died in March 1974; no autopsy was performed.

Comments: Hypercalcemia occurs at the rate of 23 to 42 per cent of women with breast cancer and is usually associated with demonstrable osseous metastases [11]. However, Gordan et al. [9] reported that in 20 of 80 cases of breast cancer with hypercalcemia skeletal roentgenograms were within normal limits. Gordan and his associates [12,13] identified phytosterols, which produced osteolysis in rats, in the plasma and tumor tissue of hypercalcemic women with breast cancer who did not have osseous metastases. Haddad et al. [14] found circulating levels of phytosterols to be the same in normal and lactating women and in women with breast cancer. High levels of iPTH have been found in tissue obtained at autopsy from two patients with breast cancer [15,16]. Benson et al. [17], using antiserums of varying specificity, reported detectable levels of plasma iPTH in 103 of 108 (95 per cent) patients with hypercalcemia and carcinoma. There were 14 cases of breast carcinoma in this series; osseous metastases were present in 12 and absent in two. Pseudohyperparathyroidism is probably rare in patients with breast cancer.

Powell et al. [18] described 11 patients who had tumors associated with hypercalcemia but who did not have osseous metastases; all had relief of hypercalcemia after removal of the tumors. No iPTH activity was detected in the plasma or tumor tissue suggesting that substances other than parathyroid hormone may cause hypercalcemia. Prostaglandins [19] and osteoclastic activating factor [5] may produce hypercalcemia, although no cases of breast cancer are included in these reports.

When hypercalcemia occurs in patients with breast cancer in the absence of osseous metastases, primary hyperparathyroidism should be considered. Hypophosphatemia, a low TRP, a positive bone biopsy specimen, lack of suppression of the hypercalcemia by adrenocorticosteroids and an elevated or inappropriate serum level of iPTH, suggests primary hyperparathyroidism, but these findings do not distinguish primary from pseudohyperparathyroidism. Pseudohyperparathyroidism is unlikely in patients with breast cancer as already discussed.

Features of pseudohyperparathyroidism which may distinguish it from primary hyperparathyroidism have been reviewed by Lafferty [3]. Rapidly progressive illness, a serum calcium greater than 14 mg/100 ml, absence of renal calculi and subperiosteal bone resorption occur more frequently in pseudohyperparathyroidism. Hyperchloremic acidosis is more characteristic of primary hyperparathyroidism. Adrenocorticosteroids may suppress the hypercalcemia in pseudohyperparathyroidism, whereas suppression of hypercalcemia rarely occurs in primary hyperparathyroidism. These observations are based on comparisons of groups of patients; any single patient may vary widely from the norm.

The presence of hypercalcemia at the time of surgery for primary breast cancer requires diagnostic studies for primary hyperparathyroidism. If the findings are diagnostic for primary hyperparathyroidism, surgical intervention is indicated.

REFERENCES

1. Roof BS, Carpenter B, Fink DJ, Gordan GS: Some thoughts on the nature of ectopic parathyroid hormone. Am J Med 50: 696, 1971.
2. Omenn GS, Roth SI, Baker WH: Hyperparathyroidism associated with malignant tumors of non-parathyroid origin. Cancer 24: 1004, 1969.
3. Lafferty FW: Pseudohyperparathyroidism. Medicine (Baltimore) 45: 247, 1966.
4. Tashjian AH Jr, Levine L, Munson PL: Immunochemical identification of parathyroid hormone in non-parathyroid neoplasms associated with hypercalcemia. J Exp Med 119: 467, 1964.
5. Mundy GR, Luben RA, Raisz LG, Oppenheim JJ, Buell DN: Bone resorbing activity in supernatants from lymphoid cell lines. N Engl J Med 290: 867, 1974.
6. Katz A, Kaplan L, Massey SG, Heller R, Plotkin D, Knight I: Primary hyperparathyroidism in patients with breast carcinoma. Arch Surg 101: 582, 1970.
7. Woolner LW, Keating FR Jr, Black BM: Primary hyperparathyroidism and metastatic breast carcinoma. A case in which breast carcinoma metastasized to a parathyroid adenoma. Cancer 11: 975, 1958.
8. Rockney RE, Kleeman CR, Maxwell MH: Hyperparathyroidism in a patient with Paget's disease and carcinoma of the breast. Arch Intern Med 104: 797, 1959.
9. Gordan GS, Eisenberg E, Loken HF, Gardner B, Hayashida T: Clinical endocrinology of parathyroid hormone excess. Recent Progr Hormone Res 18: 297, 1962.
10. Farr HW, Fahey TJ Jr, Nash AG, Farr CM: Primary hyperparathyroidism and cancer. Am J Surg 126: 539, 1973.

11. Bower BF, Gordan GS: Hormonal effects of non-endocrine tumors. Ann Rev Med 16: 83, 1965.
12. Gordan GS, Cantino TJ, Erhardt L, Hansen J, Lubich WP: Osteolytic sterols in human breast cancer. Science 15: 1226, 1966.
13. Gordan GS, Fitzpatrick ME, Lubich WP: Identification of osteolytic sterols in human breast cancer. Trans Assoc Am Physicians 80: 183, 1967.
14. Haddad JG Jr, Couranz SJ, Avioli LV: Circulating phytosterols in normal females, lactating mothers and breast cancer patients. J Clin Endocrinol Metab 30: 174, 1970.
15. Mavligit GM, Cohen JL, Sherwood LM: Ectopic production of parathyroid hormone by carcinoma of the breast. N Engl J Med 285: 154, 1971.
16. Melick RA, Martin TJ, Hicks JD: Parathyroid hormone production and malignancy. Br Med J 2: 204, 1972.
17. Benson RC Jr, Riggs BL, Richard BM, Arnaud CD: Radioimmunoassay of parathyroid hormone in hypercalcemic patients with malignant disease. Am J Med 56: 821, 1974.
18. Powell D, Singer FR, Murray TM, Minkin C, Potts JT Jr: Nonparathyroid humoral hypercalcemia in patients with neoplastic diseases. N Engl J Med 289: 176, 1973.
19. Raisz LG: Prostaglandins and the hypercalcemia of cancer. N Engl J Med 289: 214, 1973.

Fever with Dissecting Aneurysm of the Aorta

HENRY W. MURRAY, M.D.
JOHN J. MANN, M.D.
ABRAHAM GENECIN, M.D.
VICTOR A. McKUSICK, M.D.
Baltimore, Maryland

Following acute aortic dissection, in two of the four cases we describe the patients experienced a prolonged febrile syndrome which spontaneously resolved five and 11 weeks later. Because of fever and a murmur of aortic regurgitation, the two other patients with aortic dissection were initially treated for acute bacterial endocarditis. These four cases serve to re-emphasize fever as an important clinical manifestation of dissecting aneurysm of the aorta.

The diverse manifestations of dissecting aneurysm of the aorta have been extensively described. Although less well appreciated, fever during the acute phase of aortic dissection is not uncommon [1,2]; however, no cases of prolonged fever have been reported to our knowledge. We describe two such cases in which the patients had prolonged high fever associated with acute dissecting hematoma of the aorta. Furthermore, we report two other cases in which the patients had aortic dissection and whose clinical presentation closely mimicked acute bacterial endocarditis because of fever associated with a regurgitant murmur.

CASE REPORTS

Case 1. A 68 year old white man was referred to The Johns Hopkins Hospital for evaluation of persistent fever. Mild hypertension had been present for seven years, and a chest film taken in June 1973 had shown a "tortuous" aorta. On February 18, 1974, after a night of heavy eating and drinking, the patient awoke with nausea, vomiting, diarrhea, and vague chest and abdominal discomfort. The severity of these symptoms increased over the next hour culminating in a syncopal episode which precipitated his admission to another hospital.

On examination the patient appeared acutely ill and was retching. His blood pressure was 60/0 mm Hg, his pulse 120/min, and he was afebrile. Pertinent findings included peripheral cyanosis, normal chest and heart signs, hypoactive bowel sounds, a minimally enlarged, nontender liver and normal peripheral pulses. Stool guaiac was negative. Initial laboratory data revealed a white blood cell count of 15,000/mm^3, a hematocrit value of 45 per cent, and normal prothrombin time, amylase and blood urea nitrogen. Urinalysis and abdominal flat plate disclosed no abnormalities. An electrocardiogram was within normal limits except for sinus tachycardia, and a portable chest film was interpreted as being unremarkable. The patient's blood pressure was restored with intravenous fluids and methoxamine, which was discontinued 20 hours later without difficulty. The creatinine phosphokinase value remained normal; however, the serum glutamic oxaloacetic transaminase (SGOT) and lactic dehydrogenase (LDH) values rose over two days from 129

From the Department of Medicine, The Johns Hopkins Hospital, Baltimore, Maryland 21205. Requests for reprints should be addressed to Dr. John J. Mann, The Johns Hopkins Hospital, Baltimore, Maryland 21205. Manuscript accepted December 8, 1975.

mIU and 176 mIU to 1,800 mIU and 1,200 mIU, respectively. Bilirubin was 1.4 mg/100 ml, serum glutamic pyruvic transaminase (SGPT) 190 mIU and alkaline phosphatase was normal. A repeat hematocrit value was 35 per cent. On the third hospital day, the patient was stable and had no complaints but fever developed with temperatures to 101°F. The findings on physical examination and the electrocardiogram were unchanged, and intravenous ampicillin therapy was begun. Multiple blood and urine cultures were negative. Over the next four days, temperatures to 102°F persisted as hepatic enzyme and bilirubin levels returned to normal. The hepatitis-associated antigen test (HAA) was negative, the gallbladder was not visualized on oral cholecystogram, and a liver-spleen scan was normal. An x-ray series of the upper gastrointestinal tract revealed duodenal scarring. All medications were discontinued, and the patient was discharged on the 10th day with a temperature of 100.4°F.

During the subsequent four weeks, the patient experienced daily spiking temperatures to 103°F as well as malaise, night sweats, anorexia and a 13 pound weight loss. The hematocrit value decreased to 33 per cent with no evidence of blood loss. He was referred to this hospital on April 14, 1974, for evaluation of this prolonged febrile illness; he was admitted when a large anterior mediastinal mass was found on chest film. On review of available films, it was apparent that marked widening of the ascending aorta had been present at the time of the initial episode in February 1974. The findings on physical examination were unremarkable except for a blood pressure of 200/140 mm Hg. Pertinent laboratory data included a white blood cell count of 6,900/mm^3, a hematocrit value of 36.8 per cent, erythrocyte sedimentation rate of 51 mm/hour, and normal liver function tests and electrocardiogram. Additional studies included several negative blood cultures, a negative serologic test for syphilis (VDRL), negative rheumatoid factor and purified protein derivative skin test.

An aortogram revealed a dissecting aneurysm limited to the aortic arch with no aortic regurgitation. Hypertension was controlled, propranolol therapy was added, and the patient became afebrile during the six-day hospitalization. Over the ensuing 16 months, the patient has remained asymptomatic and afebrile. Because of enlarging size, the aneurysm was resected, successfully, in June 1975.

Comment: Fever prompted the patient's referral and eventual discovery of the aneurysm. The original episode of hypotension and the development of marked anemia suggested that, besides bleeding into the aortic dissection, additional occult leaking perhaps into the pericardium or mediastinum may have occurred. Persistent fever for five weeks accompanied by constitutional symptoms, anemia and an elevated erythrocyte sedimentation rate had raised the question of an underlying systemic disorder.

Case 2. A 27 year old white man with the Marfan syndrome was transferred to The Johns Hopkins Hospital on April 20, 1975, for further management of an acute aortic dissection.

Except for typical Marfan musculoskeletal difficulties, the patient had been in good health until five days before his transfer when he experienced intense back pain and shortness of breath. A chest film and electrocardiogram were interpreted as being within normal limits, but the next morning he was hospitalized because of increased pain. Blood pressure was 150/100 mm Hg, pulse 100/min and temperature 101.6°F. A chest film demonstrated a left pleural effusion as well as a markedly tortuous descending thoracic aorta. The white blood cell count was 14,000/mm^3, hematocrit value 44 per cent, bilirubin level 1.6 mg/100 ml, and urinalysis was normal. A lung scan disclosed no abnormalities and left thoracentesis yielded bloody fluid with a white blood cell count of 860/mm^3 (61 per cent polymorphonuclear leukocytes, 39 per cent mononuclears) and glucose 139 mg/100 ml. Propranolol therapy was begun, but back pain persisted over the next two days, and the patient was transferred.

Physical findings upon admission included typical stigmas of the Marfan syndrome, blood pressure 158/95 mm Hg in both arms, pulse rate 98/min and temperature 102°F. The remainder of the examination was within normal limits except for signs of a left pleural effusion. Peripheral pulses were normal and stool guaiac was negative. Laboratory data revealed a white blood cell count of 11,300/mm^3 with a left shift, a hematocrit value of 42.5 per cent, platelet count 195,000/mm^3 and an erythrocyte sedimentation rate of 55 mm/hour; urinalysis, prothrombin time, serum urea nitrogen, amylase and CPK values were all within normal limits. Liver function tests were abnormal; the bilirubin level was 2.4 mg/100 ml, SGOT 57 mIU, SGPT 32 mIU, alkaline phosphatase 55 mIU and LDH 379 mIU. Chest film demonstrated marked tortuosity and widening of the descending thoracic aorta with a double aortic contour, atelectasis of the lower lobe of the left lung and a small left pleural effusion. Electrocardiogram showed a left ventricular hypertrophy pattern.

The patient was initially managed with parenteral hypotensive agents and oral propranolol. Blood pressure was well-controlled, and the back pain promptly resolved. Aortogram demonstrated a dissecting aortic aneurysm extending from the left subclavian artery to the iliac bifurcation. Multiple cultures of blood, urine and sputum were negative. Left thoracentesis yielded bloody exudative fluid with a white blood cell count of 288/mm^3 (50 per cent polymorphonuclear leukocytes, 50 per cent mononuclears) and sugar 85 mg/100 ml. Smears and cultures of the pleural fluid for bacteria, fungi and acid-fast bacilli were negative.

Daily temperature spikes to 104°F persisted although the patient did not appear clinically septic. Further evaluation included repeatedly negative blood cultures; repeat thoracentesis with similar results; and negative purified protein derivative skin test, serologic test for syphilis (VDRL), rheumatoid factor, antinuclear antibody, lupus erythematosus preparation and febrile agglutinins. An intravenous pyelogram was within normal limits, and serial chest films showed resolution of the pleural effusion and atelectatic changes over the first 10 days. The SGOT level rose to 78 mIU, the SGPT level to 276 mIU, and the alkaline phosphatase level to 63 mIU, but all values including the bilirubin level returned to normal during the next two and a half weeks. The HAA test was negative. The hematocrit value fell to 30 per cent and the stool guaiac remained negative.

The patient was gradually ambulated over the subsequent three weeks, and he experienced no further back pain. Fever with temperatures to 101°–102°F continued throughout this period with no new symptoms or change in physical findings. The white blood cell count was 8,200/mm^3 and the erythrocyte sedimentation rate 55 mm/hour. Fever was suppressed with large doses of acetominophen but recurred promptly whenever therapy was omitted. The administration of aldomet and guanethidine was discontinued because of orthostatic symptoms, and no change in the fever pattern occurred. On the 46th hospital day, the patient was discharged with a temperature of 101°F on a regimen of acetominophen, reserpine and propranolol.

Over the subsequent five weeks he did well at home with intermittent rises in temperature to 101°F. Acetominophen therapy was discontinued during the sixth outpatient week and fever has not recurred.

Comment: Continued fever in this case led to an extensive diagnostic evaluation and prolonged hospital stay. Except for daily fever spikes, the patient was asymptomatic after treatment for the dissection. There was no evidence to suggest progressive dissection, a mycotic aneurysm, or an infected hematoma. Fever became intermittent and finally resolved spontaneously five weeks after discharge.

Case 3. A 33 year old white man was transferred to The Johns Hopkins Hospital on February 22, 1973, because of fever and congestive heart failure. He had been in excellent health until seven days before transfer when he experienced a brief episode of sudden substernal chest pain associated with shortness of breath and blurred vision. The next day, chest pain recurred and later that night headache, nausea, fever and shaking chills developed. These symptoms persisted for two days accompanied by increasing shortness of breath, and tetracycline and aspirin therapy was prescribed. Three days later, he went to a local hospital because of continued fever, chills and breathlessness. There the patient was found to have a temperature of 102°F, a blood pressure of 145/60 mm Hg, signs of severe congestive heart failure and aortic regurgitation; he was transferred to this hospital.

Physical findings on admission included a blood pressure of 120/40 mm Hg, pulse rate 110/min, temperature 101°F; signs of pulmonary edema, murmurs of aortic and mitral regurgitation, a ventricular gallop sound and normal peripheral pulses. Stool guaiac was negative. Laboratory data revealed a white blood cell count of 10,000/mm^3, a hematocrit value of 37 per cent, a platelet count of 230,000/mm^3; serum urea nitrogen, amylase, liver function tests and urinalysis were within normal limits. Chest film demonstrated cardiomegaly, pulmonary vascular congestion and small bilateral pleural effusions. Electrocardiogram showed nonspecific S-T segment and T wave abnormalities. Left thoracentesis yielded exudative serosanguineous fluid with a white blood cell count of 100/mm^3 and a glucose level of 119 mg/100 ml. Lumbar puncture disclosed no abnormalities.

A diagnosis of acute aortic valve endocarditis was made, and therapy with penicillin, methicillin and streptomycin was begun. Fever with temperatures to 102° to 103°F persisted over the next two days. Six blood cultures and cultures of the urine, cerebrospinal and pleural fluids were all negative. Congestive failure was difficult to control despite treatment with digitalis and diuretics, and on the third hospital day the patient underwent aortic valve replacement. At operation, however, a large dissecting aneurysm of the aortic root was discovered and both the aortic valve and ascending aorta were replaced. The mitral valve appeared normal as did the aortic valve leaflets. Smears and cultures of the excised valve were negative. Antimicrobial therapy was discontinued, and postoperatively, low grade fever lasted for four days and did not recur. Propranolol therapy was begun, and the patient was discharged two weeks later. He has remained asymptomatic to the present time.

Case 4. A 37 year old white man was transferred to The Johns Hopkins Hospital on January 20, 1972, because of suspicion of a dissecting aortic aneurysm. The patient had been in good health until seven weeks prior to transfer when he experienced two brief episodes of substernal chest pain. At that time cardiac examination, chest film and electrocardiogram were within normal limits. Nine days before transfer, he experienced 2 hours of substernal chest pain with radiation to the neck and shoulders. The next morming, pain recurred associated with diaphoresis, shortness of breath and generalized weakness; he was admitted to another hospital. Blood pressure was 120/64 mm Hg and temperature 102°F. Except for a grade 2/6 holosystolic apical murmur, the examination was unremarkable. Chest film revealed cardiomegaly, pulmonary vascular congestion and a small right pleural effusion. Electrocardiogram showed sinus tachycardia and S-T segment depression. The white blood cell count was 9,900/mm^3 with a shift to the left, hematocrit value was 44.5 per cent, erythrocyte sedimentation rate 38 mm/hour; urinalysis, liver function tests and cardiac enzymes were all within normal limits.

On the second hospital day fever persisted, an aortic regurgitation murmur was heard, and signs of moderate congestive heart failure were present. Conjunctival petechiae were also noted. Acute bacterial endocarditis was suspected, and penicillin and streptomycin therapy was instituted. Four blood cultures, however, were negative. Over the next week the patient had intermittent episodes of chest pain while remaining mildly febrile. The congestive failure was partially controlled with digitalis and diuretic therapy. Serial electrocardiograms and cardiac enzyme determinations did not document a myocardial infarction. On the seventh day, examination revealed absent pulses in the left arm and decreased pulses in the right arm; the patient was transferred because of suspicion of aortic dissection.

Physical findings included a blood pressure of 100/60 mm Hg (right arm) and 80/60 mm Hg (left arm), temperature 100.8°F, decreased left carotid and barely palpable radial pulses, bibasilar rales, ventricular gallop sound, and murmurs of aortic and mitral regurgitation. Stool guaiac was negative and the hematocrit value was 38 per cent. Aortogram demonstrated a dissecting aneurysm of the aortic root and severe aortic regurgitation. Penicillin and streptomycin therapy was discontinued and prophylactic methicillin was given. At operation on the second hospital day, a large aneurysm of the aortic root with extensive dissection down beneath the coronary ostia was found. The aortic valve and ascending aorta were replaced. The mitral valve appeared normal. Pathologic examination and culture of the aortic valve disclosed no abnormalities, and the excised aorta showed cystic medial necrosis. Postoperatively, the patient was febrile with temperatures to 101°F but after two days remained afebrile. Multiple cultures of blood, urine and sputum were negative. The administration of methicillin was discontinued after seven days and propranolol therapy was begun. Several weeks later the patient was discharged and he has continued asymptomatic to the present time.

Comment: These two cases demonstrate that aortic dissection may closely mimic acute bacterial endocarditis with fever, regurgitant murmurs, abrupt and rapidly progressive congestive heart failure, conjunctival petechiae and anemia. One patient had shaking chills and symptoms of systemic toxicity at the onset of his illness. As illustrated by these patients, several important differential clinical points between these two disorders should be emphasized: (1) chest pain is uncommon and usually not a prominent symptom in patients with endocarditis [3,4]; (2) large vessel occlusion (e.g., bilateral upper extremity and carotid arterial occlusion) is rare in bacterial endocarditis [5]; and (3) when present, a serosanguineous or bloody pleural effusion strongly favors the diagnosis of dissection since such an effusion is distinctly uncommon in left-sided endocarditis.

COMMENTS

In the first two cases, prolonged fever (lasting five and 11 weeks, respectively) followed acute aortic dissection and resolved spontaneously. In both patients, transient hepatic injury manifested by elevated bilirubin and transaminase levels further obscured the cause of the fever. However, despite resolution of the hepatic abnormalities, presumably caused by an ischemic insult associated with acute dissection, the fever persisted. Hyperbilirubinemia may also have been the result of pigment resorption from the aortic hematomas [6]. Consideration was additionally given to dissection associated with a mycotic aneurysm because of the prolonged spiking fever, This complication, however, is rare [7], and the lack of bacteremia and the ultimate outcome in these patients made this possibility extremely remote. Furthermore, antimicrobial therapy in the first case did not affect the fever pattern.

Low grade fever, leukocytosis and increased erythrocyte sedimentation rates are not infrequent during the acute phase of aortic dissection [6–8]. Hirst et al. [2] stated that a temperature higher than 102°F was rare in typical dissections and, if present, should arouse suspicion of a complication or some other disease. However, as illustrated by our first two cases, prolonged and high fever may occur in uncomplicated dissections. McKusick [8] has suggested that fever results from marked tissue destruction associated with the dissecting hematoma. Fever probably occurs through a tissue injury-phagocytosis-pyrogen release mechanism [9]. Similarly, fever may accompany the inflammatory reaction elicited by extravascular sequestration of blood [9]. In our second and third cases, blood was documented in the pleural space, and we suspect similar extravasation of blood occurred at some other site in Case 1. In all cases, of course, hematomas were present in the dissected aortic wall. Resolution of the fever and associated symptoms in Cases 1 and 2 presumably coincided with late resolution of tissue necrosis and resorption of sequestered blood. In patients with previous dissections, recurrence of fever should suggest the possibility of renewed dissection.

Fever in the third and fourth cases was of brief duration. This was probably due to the surgical removal of the pyrogenic aortic hematomas and prevention of formation of a larger hematoma and further tissue destruction by early surgical intervention.

Evaluation of fever in patients who survive acute aortic dissection should be extensive. However, knowledge of the syndrome we describe with prolonged high temperature, which spontaneously remits, may spare other patients long hospitalization and unnecessary diagnostic and therapeutic procedures. Also, as illustrated by the last two cases, dissecting aneurysm may simulate acute bacterial endocarditis. A high index of suspicion as well as the early use of aortography or echocardiography [10,11] would seem appropriate in those patients with atypical histories or physical findings for bacterial endocarditis.

ACKNOWLEDGMENT

We are indebted to Dr. Dean R. Taylor for permission to report Cases 2 and 3.

REFERENCES

1. Baer S, Goldburgh HL: The varied clinical syndromes produced by dissecting aneurysm. Am Heart J 35: 198, 1948.
2. Hirst AE, Johns VJ, Kime SW: Dissecting aneurysm of the aorta: a review of 505 cases. Medicine 37: 217, 1958.
3. Wise JR, Cleland MP, Hallidie-Smith KA, et al.: Urgent aortic-valve replacement for acute aortic regurgitation due to infective endocarditis. Lancet 2: 115, 1971.
4. Hatcher CR, Symbas PN, Logan WD, Abbott OA: Surgical aspects of endocarditis of the aortic root. Am J Cardiol 23: 192, 1969.
5. Weinstein L, Rubin RH: Infective endocarditis—1973. Prog Cardiovasc Dis 16: 239, 1973.

6. Anagnostopoulos CE, Prabhakar MJS, Kittle CF: Aortic dissections and dissecting aneurysms. Am J Cardiol 30: 263, 1972.
7. Sethi GK, Hughes RK, Takaro T: Dissecting aortic aneurysms. Ann Surg 18: 201, 1974.
8. McKusick VA: Dissecting aneurysm of the aorta, Chap 246. Harrison's Principles of Internal Medicine, New York, McGraw-Hill, 1974.
9. Petersdorf RG: Chills and fever, Chap 12. Harrison's Principles of Internal Medicine, New York, McGraw-Hill, 1974.
10. Nanda NC, Gramiak R, Shah PM: Diagnosis of aortic root dissection by echocardiography. Circulation 48: 506, 1973.
11. Dillon JC, Feigenbaum H, Konecke LL, et al: Echocardiographic manifestations of valvular vegetations. Am Heart J 86: 698, 1973.

Thrombocytopenia, Macrothrombocytopathia, Nephritis and Deafness

J. BERNHEIM, M.D.
Kfar Saba, Israel
M. DECHAVANNE, M.D.
P. A. BRYON, M.D.
M. LAGARDE, M.D.
S. COLON, M.D.
N. POZET, M.D.
J. TRAEGER, M.D.
Lyon, France

The association of thrombocytopenia, macrothrombocytopathia, nephritis and deafness is rare. Reported here is a new case of this triple association. The clinical course, the nephropathologic findings and the bilateral neurologic hearing loss were similar to those already reported, with a slowly progressive impairment of renal function accompanied by a persistent proteinuria. The platelet diameters were increased. These macroplatelets contained granules of normal structure but with an irregular distribution in the cytoplasm. In other areas the cytoplasm was rich in surface connected system. The survival of these platelets and their contraction were normal. Their aggregation and excretion in response to collagen, adenosine diphosphate and thrombin, and the values of platelet factor 3 activity were all decreased. The degranulation defect, also present, was observed in the absence of a decrease in intracellular cyclic adenosine 5′-monophosphate (AMP) suggesting a relationship between these two findings.

Alport's syndrome is a well documented hereditary disease with the outstanding pathologic association of nephritis and deafness [1]. The association of nephritis and deafness with thrombocytopenia and macrothrombocytopathia has only been described in one report of two unrelated families [2]. We report here a new case of this triple association without apparent hereditary relationships. The studies of platelet function revealed data, previously unknown to us, concerning cyclic adenosine 5′-monophosphate (AMP) metabolism in platelets. We have studied and present the platelet abnormalities and histopathology of the kidney throughout the course of this patient's disease.

CASE REPORT

This 22 year old Italian man was first seen in 1962, at the age of 10 years, for recurrent epistaxis. Thrombopenic macrothrombocytopathia (platelets ranged between 15,000 and 40,000/mm^3) was detected and, following an unsuccessful trial of corticosteroid therapy, a splenectomy was performed. Postoperatively, although the platelet count remained below 100,000/mm^3, he remained free of bleeding diathesis. Two years later, urinalysis revealed a mild proteinuria of 0.5 g/24 hours without associated microhematuria or hypertension. Duke bleeding time, blood clot retraction, prothrombin consumption and one-stage prothrombin time were all within normal limits. He was next seen in 1968, at the age of 16, when he was presented to our department with persistent nausea, vomiting and vertigo. Investigations showed hypertension (140/110 mm Hg) and proteinuria of 1.2 to 7.1 g/24 hours, but no hematuria. Platelet count at that time ranged from 25,000 to 80,000/mm^3. Creatinine clearance was 54 ml/min, serum uric acid 8.2 mg/100 ml. Blood glucose, blood urea nitrogen, total lipids, serum proteins and immunoglobulins

From the Clinique de Nephrologie et des Maladies Metaboliques and the Clinique d'Hématologie, Hôpital Edouard Herriot, 69374 Lyon, Cedex 2, France. Requests for reprints should be addressed to Dr. J. Bernheim, Renal Unit, Meir General Hospital, affiliated to Tel Aviv University Medical School, Kfar Saba, Israel. Manuscript accepted September 12, 1975.

were all within normal limits. An intravenous pyelogram revealed normal-sized kidneys with no scarring, but decreased visualization of contrast. After control of hypertension with methyldopa a percutaneous biopsy of the left kidney was performed. The biopsy was followed by the development of a perirenal and high periureteral hematoma which progressed in two months to stenosis and hydroephrosis of the left kidney. The stenosis diminished with prednisone therapy. The patient was then followed in our clinic until October 1969, at which time he stopped attending. In December 1973, he was readmitted with headaches and severe uremia (blood urea nitrogen 280 mg/100 ml, serum creatinine 11.3 mg/100 ml), and accelerated hypertension. The glomerular filtration rate was 8 ml/min, uric acid 18.2 mg/100 ml, proteinuria 2.7 to 4.5 g/24 hours with no hematuria or leukocyturia. The hematocrit value was 27 per cent, hemoglobin level 8.7 g/100 ml, C3 was low at 39 mg/100 ml (normal $>$ 65 mg/100 ml) and Australian antigen was found to be positive. Muscle and skin biopsy specimens showed no vasculitis, and immunofluorescence was negative. An audiogram revealed a mild neurologic bilateral hearing loss (55 decibels each side). Activity of hypoxanthine guanine and adenine phosphoribosyl transferase were all within normal limits. Abnormal findings were not detected on karyotype or on phenotypes of haptoglobin and alpha$_1$ antitrypsine. The hypertension was again controlled with alpha methyldopa plus furosemide. On a low protein, high caloric diet, his blood urea nitrogen settled at around 100 mg/100 ml, with blood creatinine 6.5 mg/100 ml. He was discharged in January 1974 but would not attend clinics and discontinued his antihypertensive medication. His last admission, two months later, was for hypertensive encephalopathy. Coma developed and a subdural hematoma was diagnosed by arteriography. He died two days later.

FAMILY HISTORY

Mother: The patient's mother was 60 years old. She had no history of hearing or renal problems. Examination revealed a mild distal tubular dysfunction with inadequate urine concentration ability (Vasopressin test) and low urinary hydrogen ion titer following ammonium chloride administration. The findings on examination for hearing were within normal limits.

Father: The patient's father was 62 years old. Tuberculosis of the left kidney had been treated by nephrectomy in 1947, with no further renal problems. Laboratory examination revealed a decreased glomerular filtration rate (65 ml/min). Para-aminohippurate clearance relative to the glomerular filtration rate was normal, as were the tubular functions. Hearing was normal.

Brother: His brother was 28 years old. He had no history of renal or hearing problems. Glomerular and tubular function tests and hearing were within normal limits.

Sister: His sister had died at age 18 in a car accident. She had no known renal or auditory disease.

Bleeding time, clot retraction, platelet counts and platelet function were normal in all. There was no history of hearing, renal or hematologic disease in any of the relatives still in Italy.

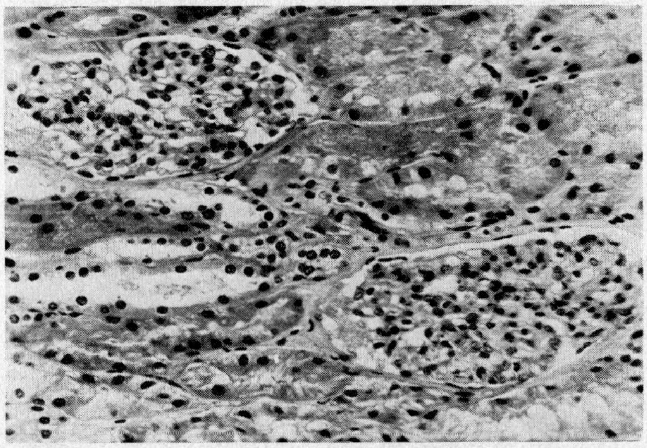

Figure 1. Biopsy specimen obtained during the early phase of renal involvement shows minimal mesangial accentuation but marked thickening of Bowman's capsule.

METHODS

For renal histopathology, all fragments were fixed in Bouin, stained by classic Hemalun phloxine Safran [3], periodic acid-Schiff of MacMannus [4], trichrome of Masson with Weigert hematoxylin and light green [5], and argentic stain of Jones [6]. Examination was by light microscopy with oil immersion at 100, 250, 400 and 1,000 magnifications.

For determination of the platelet diameter, the measurement was made on peripheral blood smears stained with Giemsa. The diameters were measured at 1,000 magnification on a Zeiss double screen mobile glarex. A random count of 500 platelets was made, and the average and standard deviation were calculated from the mean of the log of the diameters.

For the platelet survival study, the method of Aster and Jandl was used [7]. The mean life of newborn platelets was calculated by the tangent to the curve at the time ($t = 0$) and the mean age of circulating platelets was calculated by the area under the curve, measured by planimetry [8].

The aggregation of platelets was measured in platelet rich plasma (PRP) and then in a suspension of washed platelets prepared according to the method of Mustard et al. [9], with a Labintec agregometer. The plasma rich in platelets was obtained by centrifuging venous blood suspended in 3.8 per cent citrate in a 9 to 1 ratio for 10 minutes at 90 g. Aggregation of control platelets was performed at a concentration of 300,000/0.1 μliter and also 50,000/0.1 μliter. The patient was thrombocytopenic and aggregation was carried out on 50,000/0.1 μliter.

The release of platelet serotonin was studied in washed platelets only. Platelets were labeled in the first washing solution by incubation with (^{14}C) 5 hydroxytryptamine creatinine sulfate (54 mCi/ml Amersham) for 20 minutes at 37°C. Release of radioactivity from platelets with the addition of collagen (Sigma), adenosine diphosphate and thrombin to the suspension, was studied concurrently with platelet aggregation. At the maximum aggregation, the mixture was transferred to a plastic tube and centrifuged immediately at 9,000 g for 1 minute in an Eppendorf centrifuge; 0.2 ml aliquots of the supernatant were taken for liquid scintillation counting of radioactivity.

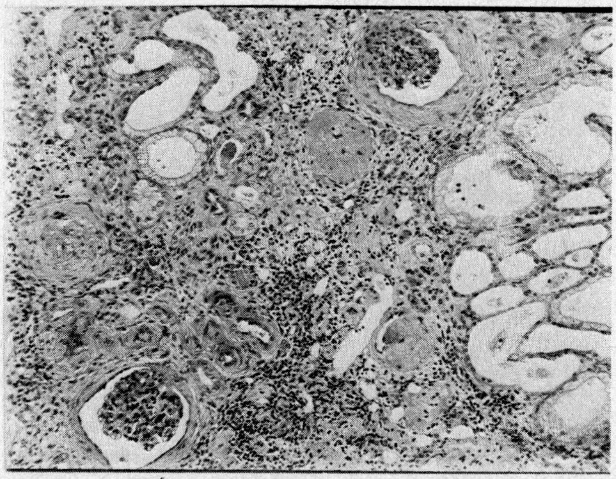

Figure 2. *This renal tissue specimen taken at autopsy shows areas with totally hyalinized glomeruli and other areas of periglomerular fibrosis with contracted glomerular tufts. The tubules are dilated with cellular atrophy and thickening of their basement membranes. Interstitial infiltration with mononuclear cells and interstitial sclerosis is also prominent. There is an absence of lipophage cells in all sections.*

The assay for platelet factor 3 activity used a stypven clotting time based on the method described by Sixma and Nijessen [10]. The total platelet factor 3 activity was measured after double freezing and thawing of the suspension of washed platelets.

The cyclic AMP was measured in washed platelet suspension before, then 1 and 3 minutes after the addition of collagen by the method of Gilman [11]. Proteins were first removed from the platelets by heat precipitation (4 minutes at 100°C) then double freezing and thawing. The cyclic AMP was measured in the supernatant remaining after centrifugation for 1 minute at 9,000 g.

For electron microscopy (EM), megakaryocytes were obtained from a medullary sternal biopsy specimen. The marrow was fixed in 2 per cent glutaraldehyde in phosphate buffer solution pH 7.2, and then stained with 1 per cent osmium tetroxide in the same buffer. Specimens were dehydrated and imbedded in Epon® by the accepted technic. The washed platelets were fixed in 1.5 per cent glutaraldehyde in a plain tyrode buffer. They were secondarily fixed with osmium tetroxide and imbedded in the same manner. The thin sections were stained with uranyl acetate and lead citrate, and examined under the electron microscope by a stereologic method [12]. The volume densities of the platelet granules and of the surface connected system were determined by a point counting method [13].

RESULTS

In the kidney histology (renal biopsy specimen), a slight local axial hypercellularity was evident in 6 of 12 glomerules examined. In all 12 glomerules a small increase of the mesangial matrix and an irregular thickening of Bownan's capsules were noted (Figure 1). The tubules were generally normal, but some thickening of their basement membranes was seen together with

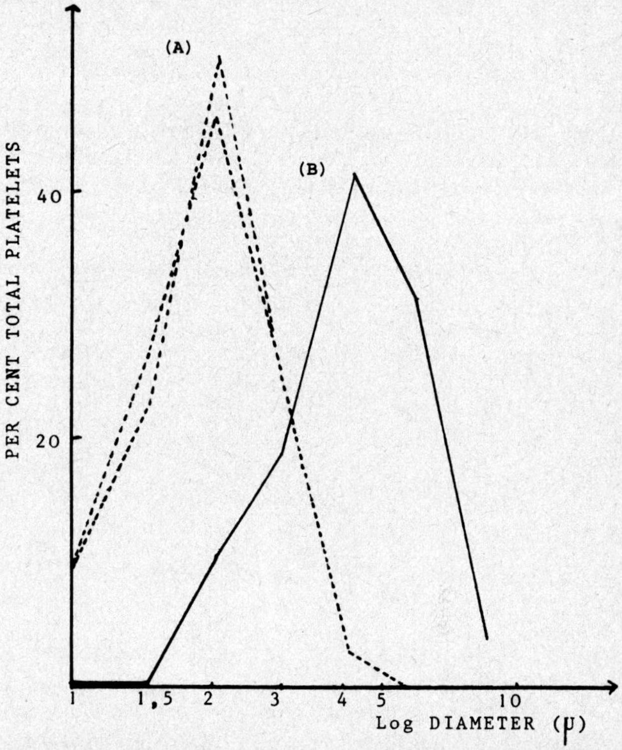

Figure 3. *This graph represents the distribution of the log of the platelet diameters of a control population of platelets (A) and in our patient (B). There is a marked augmentation of the mean of the log diameter of our patient's platelets when compared with the controls.*

some desquamated cells in their lumens. Arterioles showed clarified muscular cells and swollen endothelial nuclei; only one subendothelial hyaline deposit was seen. At autopsy, the kidney showed a few glomeruli with increased mesangial matrix and some local mesangial cell proliferation, but the majority of glomerules were either totally or partially hyalinized. Tubules were atrophic and dilated, interstitial tissue was invaded by inflammatory mononuclear cells, but no lipid cells. Vascular lesions were frequent and characterized by numerous subendothelial hyaline deposits, fibrotic endarteritis and elastic duplication. Over-all, the changes were compatible with chronic interstitial nephritis (Figure 2).

Platelet Diameter and Ultrastructure. Figure 3 shows an augmentation of the platelet diameter. The average diameter of the enlarged platelets was 4.4 μ as compared with an average diameter of 2.1 μ in the control platelets. The distribution of the log of the patient's platelet diameters appears asymmetric; normally, it is symmetric. Electron microscopy revealed macroplatelets containing granules of normal structure, but with an irregular distribution in the cytoplasm. These granules appeared to be concentrated in specific areas in the cytoplasm, whereas in other areas it was rich in

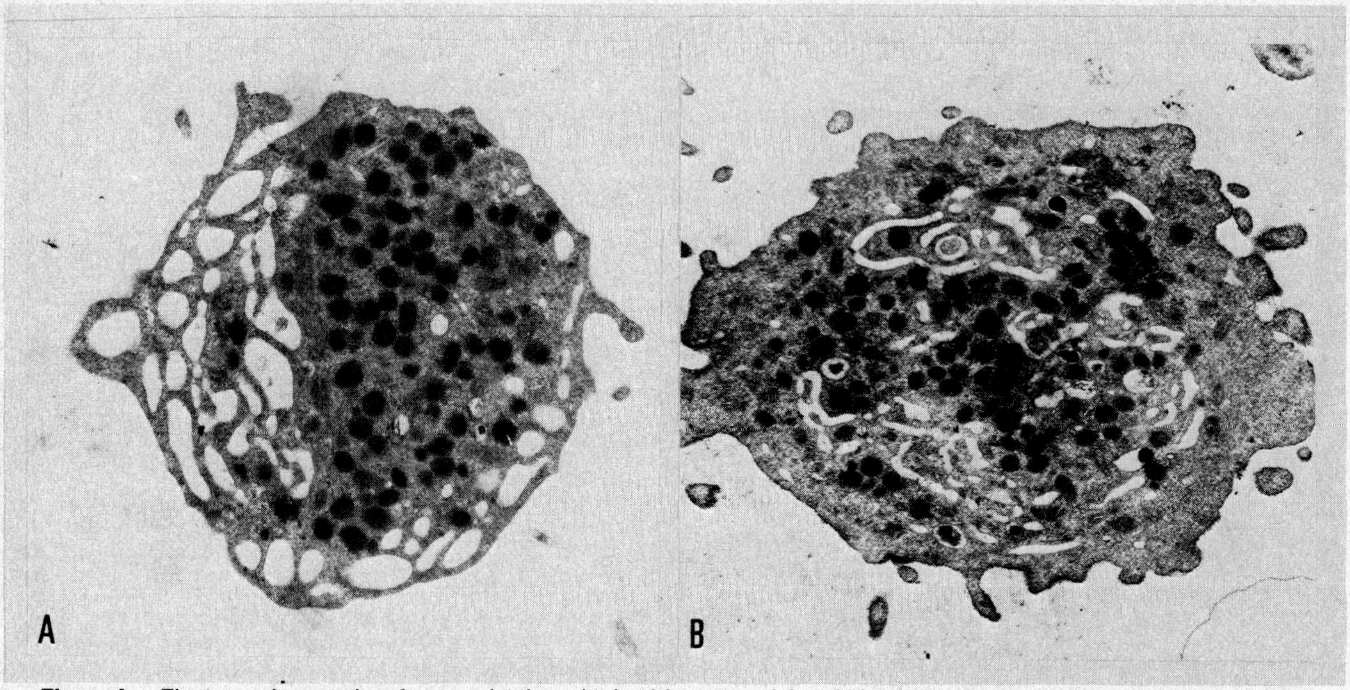

Figure 4. *Electron micrographs of macroplatelets obtained from a peripheral blood sample.* ***A,*** *the platelet granules and the mitochondria are normal but there is a "surface connected system" which appears dilated.* ***B,*** *in presence of collagen there is a reduction in volume of the "surface connected system," but there is no evidence of degranulation.*

"surface connected system" (Figure 4A). The general impression is that there is an overdeveloped membrane system, as if the megakaryocytes were improperly fragmenting.

Platelet Survival. The survival of labeled and reinjected patient's platelets was normal. The mean life span of "newborn" platelets was seven days (normal: 6.1 to 9.3 days), and the mean age of circulating platelets was four days (normal: 3.8 to 4.5 days).

Platelet Function. The value of platelet factor 3 activity in the patient's macroplatelets was decreased to 28 per cent of the value of control platelets adjusted to equivalent amounts of protein. Platelet aggregation and the release of granules were both abnormal. Aggregation induced by either collagen or adenosine diphosphate was decreased, as was the release of C^{14}-labeled serotonin induced by thrombin and collagen. These same abnormalities persisted in suspensions of plasma-rich platelets and in washed platelets (Table I) suggesting an intrinsic platelet defect.

It is also noted that collagen did not induce a decrease of cyclic AMP in the suspension of the patient's washed platelets. In the control subject, cyclic AMP was 115 ± 8.6 pmol/10^9 platelets (or 22 pmol/mg of protein) and decreased to 85 ± 6.8 pmol/10^9 platelets 1 minute after the addition of collagen. This decrease was statistically significant ($p < 0.01$ Mann-Whitney test). At the end of the aggregation test, 3 minutes after adding collagen, cyclic AMP was 100 ± 7.2 pmol/10^9 platelets. In the patient, cyclic AMP was 687 ± 30.2 pmol/10^9 platelets (or 5.4 pmol/mg of protein) prior to aggregation and it did not decrease during aggregation. At maximal aggregation, cyclic AMP was $1{,}210 \pm 38.2$ pmol/10^9 platelets.

The electron microscopic examination of the action of collagen on washed platelets demonstrated the absence of aggregates or microaggregates and degranulation (Figure 4B). Stereologic analysis confirmed that there was no significant diminution in the volume density of granules; this volume, expressed as a percentage of total platelet volume, was 0.200 ± 0.056 prior to the addition of collagen and was unchanged 3 minutes after the addition of collagen (0.183 ± 0.013). But the granular volume of the control platelets decreased significantly ($p < 0.001$) from 0.166 ± 0.011 to 0.037 ± 0.007. Platelet contraction was observed both in the patient and in the control subject.

COMMENTS

Renal Disease. The first kidney biopsy specimen revealed only a few histologic changes; the second was more typical of a chronic interstitial nephritis. This pattern is compatible with the renal findings in Alport's syndrome and with the histologic descriptions by Epstein et al. [2]. The clinical course was also very similar to that in Epstein's cases. One of the surprising findings in our patient was the total lack of macro- or microhematuria during the evolution of his disease.

Platelets. The platelets disorder is characterized by macroplatelets, thrombocytopenia and thrombocytopathia. The abnormal platelets seem to be parts of megakaryocytes that have normal granules, suggesting

TABLE I Results of the Aggregation and Release Response of the Platelets

	Aggregation		(^{14}C) Serotonin-Released (% of lysed platelet)
	Velocity	Maximum	
1—Thrombine 0.1 U*			
Washed platelets (patient) 50,000 μliters/ml	81	86	16
Washed platelets (control) 300,000 μliters/ml	80	87	54
Washed platelets (control) 50,000 μliters/ml	78	75	35
2—Collagen (1/5)*			
PRP (patient) 50,000 μliters/ml	25	30	...
PRP (control) 300,000 μliters/ml	30	62	...
PRP (control) 50,000 μliters/ml	27	30	...
Washed platelets (patient) 50,000 μliters/ml	14	13	2
Washed platelets (control) 300,000 μliters/ml	36	65	50
Washed platelets (control) 50,000 μliters/ml	25	43	28
3—ADP 5 μM*			
PRP (patient) 50,000/0.1 μliter	33	40	...
PRP (control) 300,000/0.1 μliter	92	98	...
PRP (control) 50,000/0.1 μliter	33	38	...

NOTE: PRP = platelet rich plasma. Aggregation was measured by the velocity calculated at the origin of the tangent; this is expressed in percentage of aggregation/min and by the percentage maximum of aggregation.
* Final concentration.

a disorder of fragmentation. The demarcation membrane system of megakaryocytes is found to be irregular and heterogeneous. The increase in diameter with a normal survival time suggests an asynchrony between cytoplasm synthesis and development of demarcation membrane system [14]. An abnormality of megakaryocyte maturation would explain both the thrombocytopenia and the macrocytosis. The alterations in platelet function, characterized by a decrease in platelet aggregation and excretion in response to collagen and thrombin, are associated with an abnormal platelet morphology.

These abnormalities in platelet function are intrinsic to the platelet and not related to the degree or duration of renal failure. This was shown by the platelet dysfunction remaining even after thorough platelet washing. It is interesting to note that the degranulation defect exists with a normal contraction noted by the decrease of the surface connected system [14] in the presence of collagen. The degranulation defect is seen in the absence of a decrease in intracellular cyclic AMP suggesting that platelet contraction is not influenced by cyclic AMP but that the degranulation defect may be related to the absence of a decrease in cyclic AMP.

Association Among Thrombopenia, Macrothrombopathia, Nephritis and Hearing Loss. Thrombocytopenia with or without dysfunction associated with Alport's syndrome was noted by Royer et al. [15] and by Eckstein et al. [16], but without real thrombocytopathia. Gutenberger et al. [17] reported in 1970 an association of familial thrombocytopenia with elevated immunoglobulin A levels and renal disease. In these cases, no thrombopathia or deafness was present, and in our case we did not find any disturbances in the immunoglobulin level, any skin disease or recurrent infections. Skin testing for delayed hypersensitivity was normal in our patient.

The abnormal findings in his family were very few, and only the mild distal tubular disturbance found in his mother may suggest some hereditary basis for his defects. We cannot, here, eliminate or confirm the possibility of a hereditary disorder, but there was no other family history of disease. Karyotyping did not reveal any macroscopic chromosomal abnormalities. Because of the reports of Royer et al. [15], Eckstein et al. [16] and Epstein et al. [2] plus our own case, we must consider that this triple association is not due to chance and that there may be a common inducer of interstitial nephritis, platelet disorder and hearing loss. We were unable to investigate distant relatives, but the absence of uremia, hypertension, bleeding diathesis or deafness in his immediate family suggests that his is an isolated case. These observations lead us to postulate a localized congenital defect in an unknown chromosome or a primary mutation that would be the beginning of a hereditary disease, this patient being the first.

ACKNOWLEDGMENT

We wish to express our thanks to Drs. Neville Pokroy and Robert Morrell for their assistance in editing this paper.

REFERENCES

1. Alport AC: Hereditary familial congenital hemorrhagic nephritis. Br Med J 1: 504, 1927.
2. Epstein MA, Sahed MA, Piel CF, Goodman JR, Berrfield MR, Kushner JH, Ablin RA: Hereditary macrothrombocytopathia, nephritis and deafness. Am J Med 52: 299, 1972.
3. Ganter P, Jolles G: Histochimie normale et pathologique, vol 2, Paris, Gauthier et Villars, 1970, p 1419.
4. Mac Mannus JFA: The periodic acid routine applied to the kidney. Am J Pathol 24: 643, 1948.
5. Ganter P, Jolles G: Histochimie normale et pathologique, vol

2, Paris, Gauthier et Villars, 1970, p 1416.
6. Jones D: Nephrotic glomerulonephritis. Am J Pathol 33: 313, 1957.
7. Aster RH, Jandl JH: Platelet sequestration in man. I. Methods. J Clin Invest 43: 843, 1964.
8. Paulus JM: Platelet Kinetics, Amsterdam, London, North-Holland Publishing Co., 1971, p 357.
9. Mustard JF, Perry DW, Ardlie NG, Packham MA: Preparations of suspensions of washed platelets from humans. Br J Haematol 22: 193, 1972.
10. Sixma JJ, Nijessen JG: Characteristics of platelets factor 3 release during ADP induced aggregation. Comparison with 5 hydroxytryptamine release. Thromb Diath Haemorrh 24: 206, 1970.
11. Gilman AG: A protein binding assay for adenosine 3′–5′ cyclic monophosphate. Proc Natl Acad Sci 67: 305, 1970.
12. Weibel ER, Kistler GS, Scherle WF: Practical stereological methods for morphometric cytology. J Cell Biol 30: 23, 1966.
13. Bryon PA, Lagarde M, Dechavanne M: Analyse stereologique de la concentration et de la degranulation des plaquettes. Application à l'excretion induite par la thrombine. Path Biol (in press).
14. Paulus JM: Production et Destruction des Plaquettes Sanguines. Paris, Masson et Cie, 1974, p 179.
15. Royer P, Habib R, Mathieu R, Broyer M: Nephrologie Pediatrique, Paris, Flammarion Medicine, 1973, p 38.
16. Eckstein JD, Filip DJ, Watts JC: Hereditary thrombocytopenia, deafness and renal disease. Ann Intern Med 82:639,1975.
17. Gutenberger J, Trygstad CW, Stiehm ER, et al.: Familial thrombocytopenia, elevated serum IgA levels and renal disease. Am J Med 49: 729, 1970.

AUGUST 1976

The American Journal of Medicine

VOLUME 61

NUMBER 2

EDITORIALS

Flexible Fiberoptic Bronchoscopy

M. ANEES KHAN, M.D.
MICHAEL E. WHITCOMB, M.D.
GORDON L. SNIDER, M.D.

Since its introduction in 1968, flexible fiberoptic bronchoscopy has had a dramatic impact on the approach to the evaluation and management of patients with a variety of pulmonary disorders. This procedure is easily performed, is associated with few complications and exposes a far greater portion of the tracheobronchial tree to direct visualization than does endoscopy with the rigid bronchoscope. As a result, flexible fiberoptic bronchoscopy has to a great extent replaced rigid bronchoscopy as the procedure of choice for most endoscopic examinations of the tracheobronchial tree. The purpose of this brief review is to emphasize the current role of this procedure in the evaluation and management of patients with pulmonary disease.

PROCEDURE

It should be emphasized at the outset that flexible fiberoptic bronchoscopy should only be performed by persons who have received training in endoscopy. Nevertheless, since one of the major advantages of flexible fiberoptic bronchoscopy is its ease of performance, a few general comments about the technic seem indicated.

Since general anesthesia is never required, flexible fiberoptic bronchoscopy can be easily performed in any clinical setting. In most centers, parenteral premedication is administered to provide mild sedation; however, a thorough examination can be conducted using topical anesthesia alone. Although a permanently equipped endoscopy room is desirable, the procedure can be undertaken at the bedside, in the fluoroscopy suite, emergency room or intensive care unit, as the clinical situation dictates. Flexible fiberoptic bronchoscopy can easily be performed in patients receiving continuous ventilatory assistance by passing the instrument through a side hole of an adapter attached to an endotracheal or tracheostomy tube.

There is some controversy over the method for passing the bronchoscope into the trachea. The transnasal approach popularized by Smiddy is most often employed [1]. Using this technic, most examinations can be performed with the patient sitting comfortably in a chair. Some groups, however, prefer to pass the instrument through a rigid bronchoscope or an endotracheal tube [2,3]. Using this technic, the instrument can be removed and reinserted atraumatically, and adequate control of the airway is guaranteed if a cardiorespiratory complication occurs during the procedure.

From the Pulmonary Disease Section, Department of Medicine, Thorndike Memorial Laboratory, Boston City Hospital and Boston University School of Medicine, Boston, Massachusetts. Requests for reprints should be addressed to Dr. M. Anees Khan, Boston City Hospital, 818 Harrison Avenue, Boston, Massachusetts 02118. Manuscript accepted November 10, 1975.

The experience at this and other centers where the transnasal approach is used almost exclusively does not support the necessity for intubation or rigid bronchoscopy prior to routine flexible fiberoptic bronchoscopy. Removal and reinsertion of the instrument are unnecessary except under unusual circumstances, and life-threatening emergencies are extremely rare if the procedure is performed properly.

DIAGNOSIS

Hemoptysis. The most common indication for endoscopic examination of the tracheobronchial tree is hemoptysis. In the great majority of cases, bleeding occurs at a slow rate so that emergency, life-saving maneuvers are not required, but careful diagnostic evaluation of the site and cause of bleeding is indicated. In these situations flexible fiberoptic bronchoscopy has been demonstrated to be a valuable technic. Because segmental and subsegmental airways can be visualized with the flexible bronchoscope, the diagnostic yield is higher than that obtained when rigid endoscopy is performed. Two studies have carefully assessed the role of flexible fiberoptic bronchoscopy in the evaluation of hemoptysis. Rath et al. established a definite diagnosis in 21 of 31 patients in their series [4] and Smiddy et al. identified a bleeding site in 66 of the 71 patients in their series [5]. Bronchogenic carcinoma was documented as the cause of bleeding in 33 per cent of the patients in the former and 22 per cent of the patients in the latter. Bronchitis was the cause of bleeding in the majority of the patients in each series.

The use of flexible fiberoptic bronchoscopy in the evaluation of patients with massive hemoptysis (>200 cc/24 hours) is controversial. When bleeding is brisk, it is far more difficult to maintain a clear field of vision while using the fiberoptic bronchoscope because of the small aspiration channel of the flexible instrument. However, in Smiddy's series, 12 patients were classified as having massive hemoptysis, and the etiology of the bleeding was identified in all. Nevertheless, many "endoscopists" believe bronchoscopy with the rigid instrument is preferred in the face of massive bleeding.

Bronchogenic Carcinoma. Flexible fiberoptic bronchoscopy is most useful in the evaluation of patients who present symptoms or roentgenographic abnormalities compatible with bronchogenic carcinoma. Patients with hemoptysis comprise a large percentage of those who undergo evaluation for lung cancer despite a normal chest roentgenogram. The role of flexible fiberoptic bronchoscopy in such patients has been discussed. Because of the greatly expanded field of vision, lesions in the more distal airways can be brushed or biopsied under direct vision. Using a 5.2 mm flexible instrument (Olympus BF-5B2), Kovnat et al. demonstrated that all third order, 74 per cent of fourth order and 38 per cent of fifth order bronchi could actually be cannulated with the bronchoscope, whereas all fourth order, 86 per cent of fifth order and 56 per cent of sixth order bronchi could be visualized [6]. Since a far greater area of the tracheobronchial tree can be directly visualized during the endoscopic examination, it is possible to rule out the presence of malignant disease with a high degree of assurance in those clinical settings in which direct roentgenographic manifestations of a lung tumor are absent. Conversely, experience at both Johns Hopkins [7] and the Mayo Clinic [8] has demonstrated the value of flexible fiberoptic bronchoscopy in detecting roentgenographically occult endobronchial tumors in distal airways.

Clinical studies of patients proved to have lung cancer have documented the diagnostic superiority of flexible fiberoptic bronchoscopy over bronchoscopy using the rigid instrument. In a series of 360 cases, Ikeda et al. reported that 140 lesions which could not be seen with the rigid instrument were visualized with the flexible bronchoscope [9]. In a prospective study of 86 patients by Keith et al., the use of the flexible bronchoscope increased the diagnostic yield significantly [10]. Rath et al. judged that of 24 cases of bronchogenic carcinoma diagnosed using the flexible instrument, four would not have been detected by rigid bronchoscopy [4].

The over-all diagnostic value of flexible fiberoptic bronchoscopy in lung cancer is further emphasized by the results of studies in which the flexible bronchoscope alone was used. Marsh and colleagues successfully localized 85 of 94 bronchogenic carcinomas (90 per cent) by direct visualization of the lesion or the results of diagnostic specimens obtained during the procedure [7]. In a series of 130 consecutive cases of lung cancer evaluated by Richardson et al., a specific diagnosis was made by bronchial brushing in 71 of 77 lesions visible through the flexible bronchoscope [11].

The experience with peripheral lesions not visualized during flexible fiberoptic bronchoscopy has also been impressive. Richardson et al. were able to make a positive diagnosis in 78 per cent of the peripheral cancers in which brush biopsy was performed under fluoroscopic control [11]. Similarly, Solomon et al. obtained highly suspicious cytologic specimens in 23 of 25 patients (92 per cent) with peripheral lesions when blind brushing of the suspected subsegment was performed [12]. More recently Goheen et al. [13] and Levin et al. [14] used flexible fiberoptic bronchoscopy to perform transbronchial forceps biopsy of peripheral lung lesions under fluoroscopic control. In patients with lung cancer, a definite diagnosis was made in eight of 12 and six of eight, respectively. The results of these studies make it clear that in the great majority of patients with lung cancer, a specific diagnosis can be made by using the flexible bronchoscope regardless of whether the lesion is visible or not.

Parenchymal Lung Disease. Recent reports have documented that flexible fiberoptic bronchoscopy is also useful in diseases other than lung cancer. This technic is an ideal method for visually cannulating specific subsegmental bronchi in order to obtain secretions or lung tissue for bacteriologic or histopathologic examination.

Fennessy and colleagues demonstrated the value of transbronchial brushing for the diagnosis of peripheral lung lesions [15]. These investigators passed a tip-controlled catheter into the diseased area of the lung under fluoroscopic control. Using the flexible bronchoscope, the brush can more easily be directed into specific areas of the lung. Although this diagnostic approach has not been employed extensively, the previously reported results with the Fennessy technic demonstrate that this is a valuable diagnostic tool for evaluating parenchymal infiltrates. Indeed, the experiences of Repsher et al. and Finley et al. using the flexible bronchoscope in patients having Pneumocystis carinii infections support this contention [16,17].

The technic of transbronchial forceps biopsy of the lung has also been adapted for use with the flexible bronchoscope. Using the rigid instrument, Andersen et al. have clearly demonstrated the value of transbronchial forceps biopsy [18]. The obvious advantage of this technic over transbronchial brushing is the ability to obtain lung tissue for histopathologic examination. Several groups have recently reported their experience with transbronchial forceps biopsy through the flexible bronchoscope [13,14,19–22]. These investigators have demonstrated that parenchymal tissue can be obtained with regularity using this technic, and that despite the small size of the specimen obtained, specific histologic diagnosis can be made.

Koerner et al. recently demonstrated the value of this procedure in patients with sarcoidosis [23]. In their study, 21 of 23 patients with sarcoidosis had a positive biopsy, suggesting that this may be the initial procedure of choice for demonstrating noncaseating granulomas in tissue in this disease. Usual and desquamative interstitial pneumonitis, alveolar proteinosis, lymphangitic carcinomatosis and lymphomatous involvement of the lung are examples of other noninfectious diffuse lung diseases diagnosed using this technic.

Because of the relative ease and safety with which forceps biopsy of the peripheral lung tissue may be performed, this procedure is well suited for gravely ill patients suspected of having an opportunistic pulmonary infection. Several groups have established the value of this diagnostic approach in patients with Pneumocystis carinii infection [14,19,22]. Cytomegalovirus infection [14] and tuberculosis [13,24] have also been diagnosed using this technic.

Because of the small tissue sample obtained, the potential exists for misdiagnosis due to a sampling error. Levin et al. attempted to document the specificity of the procedure. In this study, 15 patients underwent both transbronchial and open lung biopsies [14]. In 11 of these patients, there was a good correlation between the diagnostic tissue obtained by each procedure.

Pneumothorax and hemoptysis are occasional complications of this biopsy procedure [14,23]. A case of fatal pulmonary hemorrhage has been described recently [25].

Therapeutic Considerations. Due to the small size of the aspiration channel of the flexible bronchoscope, a great deal of skepticism has been expressed about the adequacy of managing retained secretions or aspirated foreign bodies with this instrument. Nevertheless, clinical and experimental studies have demonstrated a definite role for flexible fiberoptic bronchoscopy in the management of these clinical states [26–29].

Lindholm et al. have convincingly documented the value of flexible fiberoptic bronchoscopy in the management of atelectasis in patients in respiratory failure, many of whom were receiving ventilatory assistance [26]. In their experience, selective suctioning of involved airways resulted in complete or partial clearing of atelectatic areas in 81 per cent of the patients in whom retained secretions were visible. In addition, in 22 per cent of the patients who had no visible secretions, roentgenographic clearing occurred when selective suctioning of segmental and subsegmental bronchi in the involved areas was performed. The fact that flexible fiberoptic bronchoscopy can be easily performed when an artificial airway is in place makes this an ideal procedure for use in such critically ill patients.

At the present time, rigid bronchoscopy should be considered the procedure of choice for removing aspirated foreign bodies. However, Zavala and Rhodes have investigated the potential role of flexible fiberoptic bronchoscopy in the removal of aspirated foreign objects [29]. These investigators dropped a variety of objects into the tracheobronchial tree of dogs and showed that they could be removed using special extraction instruments with the flexible bronchoscope. In addition, due to the greater field of vision offered by this instrument, objects in smaller bronchi beyond the range of vision of the rigid bronchoscope may be extracted. Refinement in the design of forceps to grasp and hold foreign bodies will undoubtedly expand the number of objects which can be adequately removed with the flexible bronchoscope. To date there are only a few clinical reports of the successful extraction of foreign bodies using flexible fiberoptic bronchoscopy in individual patients [27,30]. As the clinical experience with this technic grows, it is likely that the necessity for rigid bronchoscopy will become an infrequent occurrence.

COMPLICATIONS OF FLEXIBLE FIBEROPTIC BRONCHOSCOPY

One of the remarkable aspects of flexible fiberoptic bronchoscopy is the extraordinarily low complication rate associated with this procedure. In a nationwide survey of people performing flexible fiberoptic bronchoscopy, Credle et al. analyzed almost 25,000 procedures and found the incidence of all complications to be less than 0.1 per cent [31].

Adverse reactions to parenteral premedication or local anesthesia occasionally occur [31]. These reactions are generally not serious. Of more significance is airway obstruction occurring during the procedure. Laryngospasm is the most common etiology and can be prevented with adequate anesthesia of the vocal cords. Obstruction due to the presence of the instrument in the airway is not a problem in most patients due to the small size of the bronchoscope, but it may occur in persons with an artificial airway in place. Difficulty generally occurs only when the airway is less than 8.5 mm in diameter [32,33].

Changes in arterial blood gases are potentially of great significance. A decline in arterial oxygen tension of 15 to 20 mm Hg both during and following the procedure has been documented [34–36]. Although potentially dangerous, significant hypoxemia can be prevented by administering oxygen to patients with borderline hypoxemia. Ventilator patients should routinely receive additional oxygen while undergoing bronchoscopy. Hypercapnia, although distinctly uncommon, may also occur in persons who undergo bronchoscopy while receiving continuous ventilatory assistance [27]. This is avoidable by careful monitoring of the expiratory volume during the procedure and adjusting the tidal volume delivered by the ventilator accordingly.

Premature ventricular contractions, bradycardia and ventricular tachycardia have been reported on occasion [31]. These arrhythmias seem to be related to hypoxemia and can be prevented by ensuring adequate oxygenation and avoidance of indiscriminate suctioning.

Pulmonary infection is another potentially serious complication of flexible fiberoptic bronchoscopy. In Credle's survey this occurred in several patients. In a prospective study of flexible fiberoptic bronchoscopy in 100 consecutive afebrile patients conducted at this institution, pyrexia developed (oral temperature $\geq 101°$ F) in 16 per cent after the procedure [37]. Roentgenographic infiltrates appeared in six; however, bacteremia did not occur in any patient. Kane et al. have also demonstrated that bacteremia does not occur after this procedure [38].

CONCLUSIONS

Flexible fiberoptic bronchoscopy has had a dramatic impact on the practice of pulmonary medicine. The procedure can be easily performed in a variety of clinical situations and is associated with an extraordinarily low complication rate. The role of flexible fiberoptic bronchoscopy in the evaluation of patients suspected of having bronchogenic carcinoma is well established. It seems highly likely that future clinical studies will substantiate the enthusiastic reports of several groups of the role of this technic in the diagnosis of local or diffuse parenchymal lung disease. Similarly, although controversy exists about the role of flexible fiberoptic bronchoscopy in the management of retained secretions or aspirated foreign objects, it is likely that as experience in these areas increases, the value of the routine use of the flexible instrument in the initial evaluation of such patients will be substantiated.

REFERENCES

1. Smiddy JF: Flexible fiberoptic bronchoscope. Ann Intern Med 75: 971, 1971.
2. Tucker GF Jr, Olsen AM, Andrews AH Jr, Pool JL: The flexible fiberscope in bronchoscopic perspective. Chest 64: 149, 1973.
3. Zavala DC, Rhodes ML, Richardson RH, Bedell GN: Fiberoptic and rigid bronchoscopy. The state of the art. Chest 65: 605, 1974.
4. Rath GS, Schaff JT, Snider GL: Flexible fiberoptic bronchoscopy: techniques and review of 100 bronchoscopies. Chest 63: 689, 1973.
5. Smiddy JF, Elliott RC: The evaluation of hemoptysis with fiberoptic bronchoscopy. Chest 64: 158, 1973.
6. Kovnat DM, Rath GS, Anderson WM, Snider GL: Maximal extent of visualization of bronchial tree by flexible fiberoptic bronchoscopy. Am Rev Respir Dis 110: 88, 1974.
7. Marsh BR, Frost JK, Carter D, Erozan YS, Proctor DF: Flexible fiberoptic bronchoscopy; its place in the search for lung cancer. Ann Otol Rhinol Laryngol 82: 757, 1973.
8. Sanderson DR, Fontana RS, Woolner LB, Bernatz PE, Payne WS: Bronchoscopic localization of radiologically occult lung cancer. Chest 65: 608, 1974.
9. Ikeda S, Tsuboi E, Ono R, Ishikawa S: Flexible bronchofiberscope. Jap J Clin Oncol 1: 55, 1971.
10. Keith RG, Taylor GA: Use of the flexible fiberoptic bronchoscope in the diagnosis of malignant tumors of the lung. Can J Surg 16: 118, 1973.
11. Richardson RH, Zavala DC, Mukerjee PK, Bedell GN: The use of fiberoptic bronchoscopy and brush biopsy in the diagnosis of suspected pulmonary malignancy. Am Rev Respir Dis 109: 63, 1974.
12. Solomon DA, Solliday NH, Gracey DR: Cytology in fiberoptic bronchoscopy. Comparison of bronchial brushings, washings and postbronchoscopy sputum. Chest 65: 616,

1974.
13. Goheen J, Gwin E, Hiller C, Henry J, Lampton L, Kerby G, Ruth W: Biopsy of lung nodules and infiltrates beyond visual range of the bronchofiberscope (abstract). Am Rev Respir Dis 109: 690, 1974.
14. Levin DC, Wicks AB, Ellis JH: Transbronchial lung biopsy via the fiberoptic bronchoscope. Am Rev Respir Dis 110: 4, 1974.
15. Fennessy JJ: Transbronchial biopsy of peripheral lung lesions. Radiology 88: 878, 1967.
16. Repsher LH, Schröter G, Hammond WS: Diagnosis of Pneumocystis carinii pneumonitis by means of endobronchial brush biopsy. N Engl J Med 287: 340, 1972.
17. Finley R, Kieff E, Thomsen S, Fennessy J, Beem M, Lerner S, Morello J: Bronchial brushing in the diagnosis of pulmonary disease in patients at risk for opportunistic infection. Am Rev Respir Dis 109: 379, 1974.
18. Andersen HA, Fontana RS: Transbronchoscopic lung biopsy for diffuse pulmonary diseases; techniques and results in 450 cases. Chest 62: 125, 1972.
19. Scheinhorn DJ, Joyner LR, Whitcomb ME: Transbronchial forceps lung biopsy through the fiberoptic bronchoscope in Pneumocystis carinii pneumonia. Chest 66: 294, 1974.
20. Schoenbaum SW, Koerer SK, Ramakrishna B, Goldman ML: Transbronchial biopsy of peripheral lesions with fluoroscopic guidance; use of the fiberoptic bronchoscope. J Can Assoc Radiol 25: 39, 1974.
21. Teirstein AS, Chuang M, Miller A: Application of the flexible bronchoscope. Mt Sinai J Med NY 42: 81, 1975.
22. Joyner LR, Scheinhorn DJ: Transbronchial forceps lung biopsy through fiberoptic bronchoscope. Chest 67: 532, 1975.
23. Koerner SK, Sakowitz AJ, Appelman RI, Becker NH, Schoenbaum SW: Transbronchial lung biopsy for the diagnosis of sarcoidosis. N Engl J Med 293: 268, 1975.
24. Sahn SA, Levin DC: Diagnosis of military tuberculosis by transbronchial lung biopsy. Br Med J 79: 667, 1975.
25. Flick MR, Wasson K, Dunn LJ, Block AJ: Fatal pulmonary hemorrhage after transbronchial lung biopsy through the fiberoptic bronchoscope. Am Rev Respir Dis 111: 853, 1975.
26. Lindholm CE, Ollman B, Snyder J, Millen E, Grenvik A: Flexible fiberoptic bronchoscopy in critical care medicine; diagnosis, therapy and complications. Crit Care Med 2: 250, 1974.
27. Barrett CR, Vecchione JJ, Bell ALL: Flexible fiberoptic bronchoscopy for airway management during acute respiratory failure. Am Rev Respir Dis 109: 429, 1974.
28. Wanner A, Landa J, Neiman RE Jr, Vevaina J, Delgado I: Bedside bronchofiberscopy for atelectasis and lung abscess. JAMA 224: 1281, 1973.
29. Zavala DC, Rhodes ML: Experimental removal of foreign bodies by fiberoptic bronchoscopy. Am Rev Respir Dis 110: 357, 1974.
30. Ikeda S: Atlas of Flexible Bronchofiberscopy, Tokyo, Igaku Shoin Ltd, 1974, p 220.
31. Credle WF, Smiddy JF, Elliott RC: Complications of fiberoptic bronchoscopy. Am Rev Respir Dis 109: 67, 1974.
32. Renz LE, Smiddy JF, Rauscher GR, Kerby GR, Ruth WE: Bronchoscopy in respiratory failure. JAMA 219: 619, 1972.
33. Kovnat DM, Schaff JT, Snider GL: Bronchoscopic perspective (editorial). Chest 65: 606, 1974.
34. Albertini RE, Harrell JH, Kurihara N, Moser KM: Arterial hypoxemia induced by fiberoptic bronchoscopy. JAMA 230: 1666, 1974.
35. Karetzky MS, Garvey JW, Brandstetter RD: Effect of fiberoptic bronchoscopy on arterial oxygen tension. NY State J Med 74: 62, 1974.
36. Pierson DJ, Iseman MD, Sutton FD, Zwillich CW, Creagh CE: Arterial blood gas changes in fiberoptic bronchoscopy during mechanical ventilation. Chest 66: 495, 1974.
37. Pereira W, Kovnat DM, Khan MA, Iacovino JR, Spivak ML, Snider GL: Fever and pneumonia after flexible fiberoptic bronchoscopy. Am Rev Respir Dis 112: 59, 1975.
38. Kane RC, Cohen MH, Fossieck BE Jr, Tvardzik AV: Absence of bacteremia after fiberoptic bronchoscopy. Am Rev Respir Dis 111: 102, 1975.

Primary Medical Care and Training Programs in General Internal Medicine

ROBERT H. CREDE, M.D.
San Francisco, California

Recent comments on available physician manpower, including assessments of the numbers and distribution of various types of physician specialists in the United States, have stressed the need for more physicians who will function as primary care (first contact) practitioners and deliver continuous, comprehensive care [1–3]. Academic medical centers are responsible for exploring the educational implications of such manpower needs and developing residency programs in primary care appropriate to their academic goals and available resources [4,5].

In response to these needs, the Division of Ambulatory and Community Medicine in cooperation with the Departments of Medicine and Pediatrics of the University of California, San Francisco, School of Medicine, assisted by a grant from the Robert Wood Johnson Foundation, has instituted a 36-month primary care residency training program to prepare physicians for practice in general internal medicine or general pediatrics. The two track program (medicine and pediatrics) will provide residents with the skills needed to deliver family-oriented primary care in an ambulatory setting as well as the requisite experience in treating general medical or pediatric patients, who require hospitalization, and will qualify them to take the certification examinations given by the American Boards of Internal Medicine or Pediatrics.

Residency training programs in medicine or pediatrics have traditionally stressed hospital based experience, usually emphasizing subspecialties in the latter part of a two or three year program. Such residencies, when followed by one or two years of subspecialty fellowship, prepare internists and pediatricians whose interests and motivation are usually in the direction of subspecialty practice. It is not surprising that graduates of such traditional programs are much more comfortable in the area of their subspecialty and would be, perhaps, less effective with those patients' problems they considered to be outside their range of expertise. This is to be expected if their previous training has not offered adequate supervised clinical experience in handling a wide range of simple to complicated medical and psychosocial problems on an ambulatory basis. The office practice of general medicine and pediatrics requires an ability to handle such problems, which in many instances constitute the majority of clinical problems confronting such practitioners [6–8]. It is clear that any program designed to train primary care physicians must provide the opportunity to develop skills and attitudes needed for this aspect of patient care while maintaining a high level of basic biomedical knowledge [9]. In the past two years, several articles have appeared which discuss the content of primary care [10,11], outline the philosophy of primary care training programs in internal medicine [12] or describe operating primary care residency training programs [13].

From the Division of Ambulatory and Community Medicine, and the Department of Medicine, University of California, San Francisco, School of Medicine, San Francisco, California. Requests for reprints should be addressed to Dr. Robert H. Crede, Division of Ambulatory and Community Medicine, A 405, University of California, 3rd and Parnassus, San Francisco, California 94143.
Manuscript accepted February 27, 1976.

The thoughtful article by Goroll et al. [14] is the most recent description of a primary care internal medicine training program we have seen.

The University of California, San Francisco, Primary Care Residency Program emphasizes continuous, comprehensive patient care and trains the internal medicine and pediatric residents to work together with a nurse practitioner in the delivery of family-oriented care. Such a model may have a somewhat limited applicability in the "real world" of practice, but it does seem suitable for those medium- to large-sized multispecialty group practices that wish to offer family-oriented care to their patients without operating a family practice unit. Currently, there is a high level of interest in the role of the middle-level practitioners (nurse practitioners, physician assistants) in the delivery of primary health care [15–18]. Such practitioners may assume a greater and more important role in health care delivery in the future, and the experience that general medical or general pediatric residents receive in working effectively with such practitioners may well anticipate a health care delivery pattern for their future practice [19].

The following paragraphs outline several major concepts of the University of California, San Francisco program which are presented from the viewpoint of the internal medicine track but which also apply in general to the pediatric track.

(1) **Sound Base in Parent Discipline.** All housestaff should have a sound base in their parent discipline, either internal medicine or pediatrics, so that both during the period of training and later on in practice they would function as equals with their peers in the scope and depth of their biomedical knowledge and clinical skills. Therefore, approximately the first 18 months of the 36-month training program are essentially indistinguishable from the traditional programs in the two departments. Depending on our experience and the evaluation of our residents, we may expand or contract the period devoted to conventional training in the traditional program. However, housestaff need some identification with the Primary Care Program from the beginning of their internship, and therefore for the first 18 months they spend one-half day a week in the Multispecialty Primary Care Clinic, which is the main base for the ambulatory patient care operations of this training program. In this one-half day a week, each new internal medicine housestaff member gradually accumulates a group of patients and families who look to him, his pediatric housestaff counterpart and the nurse practitioner as the primary source of continuing care.

(2) **Increased Emphasis on Common Problems Seen in Ambulatory Patients.** Primary care housestaff have increased experience in dealing with common medical and psychosocial problems in an ambulatory setting beginning in the first year of training. The formal teaching program for residents in the internal medicine track includes lectures, demonstrations and seminars with emphasis on common problems in general internal medicine. In addition, residents are given the opportunity to develop skills and knowledge that are necessary for the management of common emotional (including "psychosomatic"), dermatologic, neurologic and nonsurgical orthopedic problems seen in general office practice, as well as those skills and technics necessary to diagnose and treat common gynecologic problems.

(3) **A Unique Outpatient Clinic Designed for the Primary Care Training Program.** The Multispecialty Primary Care Clinic has been developed as a separate patient care unit in the University of California, San Francisco Ambulatory Care Center. Because it is contiguous with the General Medical Clinics of the Department of Medicine, faculty and housestaff working in the primary care and in the traditional medicine residency programs have an opportunity to share learning experiences. This clinic is also a major site of medical student teaching where senior medical students are taking a required full-time clerkship in family-oriented primary care. Primary care residents are actively involved in medical student education, as occurs on hospital teaching services.

The Multispecialty Primary Care Clinic is organized as a family-oriented group practice, with an internist, a pediatrician, a psychiatrist and/or clinical psychologist, and a nurse practitioner as the core personnel to provide comprehensive care to family members and individuals. Complete coverage, 24 hours a day, all year long is provided by housestaff (those in the last 18 months of the program) with faculty back up. A full range of medical and allied health specialists are available to this clinic to provide instruction and consultation so that comprehensive health services are available to patients.

(4) **Coordination of Multidisciplinary Activities in Training and Patient Care.** Every effort is made to coordinate the family-oriented patient care activities of the residents in the internal medicine track with those of the residents of the pediatric track, while they are practicing in the Multispecialty Primary Care Clinic. Medical and pediatric residents and nurse practitioners are organized as teams, which facilitates family-centered care, thus improving communication and interpersonal contacts between the families and the members of the team. The nurse practitioners are an integral part of a patient care team and participate in housestaff training sessions thereby enhancing the ability of both to function as team members.

As previously mentioned, housestaff have the opportunity to utilize the services of clinical pharmacists, social workers, dieticians, family counselors and rehabilitation specialists as needed for comprehensive patient care. In addition, such working relationships offer opportunities for interdisciplinary health care team experience.

(5) **Opportunities to Develop Areas of Interest in Depth.** In the last 18 months of the 36-month program, there is increasing experience in the ambulatory setting, predominately in the Multispecialty Primary Care Clinic. However, there is flexibility in the program which allows internal medicine track residents to obtain more in-depth experience by working in subspecialty clinics. Our experience to date has shown that rotations through Cardiac, Gastrointestinal, Rheumatology, Thyroid-Endocrine-Metabolic and Chest Clinics have been very profitable for our advanced primary care housestaff.

Preventive medicine, occupational health, family counseling and rehabilitation are some of the areas emphasized in the training of our primary care residents that are not usually stressed in more traditional programs. In addition, opportunities to work with faculty involved in health services research may stimulate the interest of our housestaff to study the operations of the local unit in some depth. For limited periods, residents may spend one or two half days per week assigned to governmental or private community based agencies that deliver primary care. Such assignments give an added dimension to their clinical experience, and acquaints them with the operation and management of extramural organized patient care programs.

(6) **Continuity of Care.** In order to develop a proper primary care model, residents in the internal medicine track must be able to follow and assume responsibility for the care both in and out of the hospital of those patients to whom they are giving continuing comprehensive care. For this reason, the program permits internal medicine track residents in the Multispecialty Primary Care Clinic to hospitalize their patients on the Adult Primary Care Service. The housestaff assumes responsibility for the day-to-day care of the patient under the supervision of an attending faculty internist from the Primary Care Residency Program. This responsibility for patients, both in the hospital and in the outpatient setting, is an important difference between the internal medicine primary care track and traditional training program. This seems appropriate as part of a supervised learning experience in continuing care of patients because it is consistent with the way the residents will practice as internists on completion of their training.

Every effort is made to achieve an appropriate mix of patients so that the residents' patient care experiences will not be too dissimilar from those they will have in later practice. We anticipate that the University of California, San Francisco campus will soon participate in a privately financed prepaid health plan of limited size and that the residents in the Primary Care Residency Program will serve as the primary care physicians to this group of patients. We believe that the combination of patients seen in the General Medical wards of this academic medical center, plus the patient population of the Multispecialty Primary Care Clinic, gives our primary care internal medicine residents a broad experience in the diagnosis and management of common and esoteric medical problems and will therefore give them the necessary attitudes and skills for the effective practice of general internal medicine.

Our faculty has been impressed by the high calibre of applicants seeking training in this new Primary Care Residency Program, signifying an important shift in the career goals of many outstanding graduates of American medical schools. Such young physicians will form an important resource of skilled primary care physicians, a stated goal of current public policy.

REFERENCES

1. Petersdrof RG: Health manpower: numbers, distribution, quality. Ann Intern Med 82: 694, 1975.
2. Schonfeld HK et al.: Numbers of physicians required for primary medical care. N Engl J Med 286: 571, 1972.
3. Endicott KM: The distribution of physicians geographically and by specialty. Read before the Institute of Medicine, National Academy of Sciences, May 8, 1974.
4. Rogers DE: Medical academe and the problems of health care provision. Arch Intern Med 135: 1364, 1975.
5. Ebert RV: Training of the internist as a primary physician. Arch Intern Med 76: 653, 1972.
6. The National Ambulatory Medical Care Survey 1973 Summary: p 21, 26, 29, 30, National Center for Health Sciences: Vital and Health Statistics Series 13 Number 21, Department of HEW Publication No (HRA) 76-1772.
7. Ebert RV: loc cit.
8. Reitermeier RJ et al.: Participation by internists in primary care. Arch Intern Med 135: 255, 1975.
9. Burnam JF: What one internist does in his practice. Ann Intern Med 78: 437, 1973.
10. Silver HK, McAtee P: A descriptive definition of the scope and content of primary care. Pediatrics 56: 957, 1975.
11. Alpert J, Charney E: The Education of Physicians for Primary Care, Section I: What is Primary Medicine, p 1, Department of HEW Publication No (HRA) 74-3113.
12. Young LE: Changes in the postdoctoral education of internists? Ann Intern Med 83: 728, 1975.
13. Perlman LV et al.: Training for primary care. Arch Intern Med 133: 448, 1974.
14. Goroll AH et al.: Residency training in primary care internal medicine. Ann Intern Med 83: 872, 1975.
15. Sadler AM: New health practitioner education: problems and issues. J Med Educ 50 (suppl): 67, 1975.
16. Lewis CF: The training of new health manpower. J Med Educ 50 (suppl): 75, 1975.
17. Spitzer WO et al.: The Burlington randomized trial of the nurse practitioner. N Engl J Med 290: 251, 1974.
18. Runyan JW Jr: The Memphis chronic disease program. JAMA 231: 264, 1975.
19. Gardner HH, Ouimette R: A nurse-physician team approach in a private internal medicine practice. Arch Intern Med 134: 956, 1974.

Malaria—The Mime

Recent Lessons From a Group of Civilian Travellers

B. H. KEAN, M.D.
PHILIP C. REILLY, Jr., M.D.
New York, New York

Clinical data on 24 civilian patients hospitalized for malaria in The New York Hospital were analyzed. Of 16 patients infected with Plasmodium falciparum, 14 acquired the disease in West Africa.

Only three of the 24 had taken recommended courses of prophylaxis. Diagnosis was invariably, and often dangerously, delayed because physicians often made diagnoses of viral syndromes or used antibiotics; only one patient had a blood smear taken by a personal physician.

Although all patients had fever and chills, classic malarial fever was seen in only seven patients; nausea, vomiting and diarrhea were common. Hepatomegaly and splenomegaly occurred in about half the patients. Blood smears stained in routine fashion by Wright's stain were positive in 23 of 24 patients. A normal leukocyte count was present in 19 of the 24 patients and thrombocytopenia in 16 of 23. The most frequent complications were those of central nervous system involvement.

Therapy consisted mainly of chloroquine phosphate but other drugs, including quinine, pyrimethamine, sulfonamides and primaquine, were used in special situations.

Suggestions for prophylaxis, diagnosis and therapy were made.

In the medical theater of disease mimicry, when a lethal infection masquerades as a "viral syndrome," the virtuoso performer is malaria. Its pernicious nature is most evident while "on the road," where it plays before an audience of unsophisticated physicians.

Thus, despite extensive experience with malaria in Vietnam, the civilian record is embarrassing: one recent study showed a striking 24-fold difference in the case-fatality rate of patients treated in civilian hospitals when compared to those treated in military or Veterans Administration hospitals [1]. Recent mortality figures on Plasmodium falciparum of 7.3 per cent [1] and 10 per cent [2] in civilian hospitals are inordinately high.

It is our purpose here to review our experience with malaria among civilian travellers; to retrace their clinical records exposing pitfalls in diagnosis; and to offer some practical suggestions for physicians in nonendemic areas.

From the Department of Medicine, Division of Infectious Disease, Unit of Tropical Medicine, The New York Hospital-Cornell Medical Center, New York, New York 10021. Requests for reprints should be addressed to Dr. B. H. Kean. Manuscript accepted December 8, 1975.

METHODS AND MATERIALS

We reviewed the charts of all patients with malaria seen at The New York Hospital from January 1968 through May 1975. All diagnoses were confirmed by positive blood smear, and one of us (B.H.K.) saw all the patients during the course of their illness. Of the 27 patients in whom a diagnosis of malaria

TABLE I Types of Malaria Among 24 Civilians Seen at The New York Hospital between January 1968 and May 1975

Species of Plasmodium	No. of Patients
P. falciparum	15
Mixed P. falciparum and P. vivax	1
P. vivax	6
P. malariae	1
P. ovale	1

was made during this period, three were excluded from this series because of special circumstances: one was a Chinese infant with congenital Plasmodium malariae (to be reported elsewhere); another was a Vietnam veteran treated for recurrence of P. vivax; and a third was a scientist with P. falciparum who was treated as an outpatient and his clinical record was incomplete.

The remaining 24 patients were all hospitalized during their illness and these constitute the study group. There were no other cases of malaria among Vietnam veterans; there were no cases of transfusion-induced malaria or malaria associated with intravenous drug abuse. A review of the autopsy records disclosed no deaths due to malaria during the period of study.

Adequate malaria prophylaxis is defined as 500 mg chloroquine (300 mg of chloroquine base) taken weekly one week prior to departure, during the period of stay in the endemic area, and for five or six weeks after departure from the endemic area. (This program is not ideal for Southeast Asia and may be inadequate for other parts of the world—but meets the needs of this study.)

RESULTS

Population. Of the 24 patients in the study group 14 were male (five black and nine white) and ten were female (six black and four white). Their ages ranged from eight years to 68 years, with a mean of 33 years. Three of the patients were native-born Africans; four came from the West Indies; one each was from Burma, Pakistan and New Zealand; 14 were born in the United States (10 white and four black), and all but four of the study group were long-time residents of the United States. The following "occupations" were represented: eight tourists, three students, three government workers, two anthropologists, two children, one pilot, one merchant seaman, one reporter, one stewardess, one nurse and one businessman. Two patients were pregnant. Two returned to the United States by ship, both very ill with symptoms of cerebral malaria. The remainder returned by air.

TABLE II Distribution of Plasmodium Species by Area of Acquisition in 24 Civilians

	Plasmodium Species				
Area	Falciparum	Vivax	Malariae	Ovale	No. of Patients
Africa	14	4	1	1	20
West Africa	14	1	0	1	16
East Africa	0	3	1	0	4
Southeast Asia	1*	3*	0	0	3
Cambodia	1*	1*	0	0	1
Burma	0	1	0	0	1
New Guinea	0	1	0	0	1
Caribbean	1	0	0	0	1
Haiti	1	0	0	0	1

*P. falciparum and P. vivax.

Epidemiology. As shown in Table I, 16 of 24 civilians, or 70 per cent of the study group, had P. falciparum malaria, including all 11 of the black patients. In 14 of 16 patients, P. falciparum malaria was acquired in West Africa (88 per cent) (Table II). The three native Africans and four West Indians all had P. falciparum; the two East Africans acquired the infection while visiting West Africa. In only one case was P. falciparum malaria (mixed) acquired in Southeast Asia. Between September 1974 and May 1975 seven of eight infections seen at this institution were P. falciparum. All six patients who had P. vivax were white.

Timetable. The 16 patients with P. falciparum had been in an endemic area for a period ranging from four days to several years. None of the patients with P. vivax had been in an endemic area for less than three months. Nine patients began to have symptoms of malaria before coming to the United States. Six patients had been in the United States for at least a month before they had any symptoms, and one patient had not been abroad in nine months. Six patients had symptoms for longer than a week before being seen at the hospital. One patient with P. falciparum had been symptomatic in the United States for six weeks and had visited a physician five times before the diagnosis was made at The New York Hospital.

Prophylaxis. Only three of 24 patients took the recommended course of antimalarial prophylaxis. Fifteen patients took no prophylaxis, and 12 of these contracted P. falciparum malaria (80 per cent). Six patients took inadequate malaria prophylaxis: four discontinued the medication while still in an endemic area (three P. falciparum) and two patients discontinued taking antimalarials prematurely on their return to the United States (one P. falciparum). The three remaining patients who took the recommended course of chemoprophylaxis all had P. vivax and had spent at least six months in an endemic area. No patient noted ill effects from antimalarial prophylaxis. No patient took pyrimethamine (Daraprim®) or proguanil prophylaxis.

Diagnosis by Local Physicians. Contact between patients and local physicians before they were seen at The New York Hospital is summarized in Table III.

Eleven of the 14 patients were given antibiotics; at least five of these received tetracycline. One of the two patients referred to this hospital with malaria was initially diagnosed by blood smear as having P. vivax; later, it was shown to be P. falciparum. Thus, nine cases of P. falciparum malaria were missed by local doctors, and in only two of 14 patients (13 per cent) was the correct diagnosis made. There was only an 8 per cent (two of 26) rate of correct diagnosis per physician visit.

Diagnosis by Hospital Physicians. In every case, the first physician to see the patient at this institution elicited a history of travel. Twenty-two of the 24 patients were suspected of having malaria by the first NYH physician who saw them; these were about equally divided between house staff and attending physicians. In one of the remaining two patients, the infection was "picked up" by a laboratory technician examining a routine blood smear; the other patient was suspected of having malaria by the consultation resident in the Emergency Room.

Nineteen of 24 patients had a positive smear diagnosis by the time they were admitted to the ward. In the remaining five, two cases of P. falciparum were diagnosed within 12 hours. The smear diagnosis of P. falciparum malaria was delayed 48 hours in one patient with cerebral symptoms who was the sickest member of the study group. The diagnosis of P. vivax malaria was delayed in two other patients because of negative smears, one of which, on review, contained parasites. On four occasions, the laboratory technician in the Emergency Room alerted the physician to the presence of parasites on routine blood smears.

Malaria Smears. Malaria parasites were seen on both thick and thin smears stained with Giemsa in all 24 patients. In 23 of 24 patients, the parasites were seen on routinely stained (Wright's) blood smears. Among the 14 patients with P. falciparum, ring forms only were seen in 12, and rings and crescents were seen in three. Among the six patients with P. vivax, rings only were seen in two, rings and trophozoites in two, and rings, trophozoites and gametocytes in two.

Clinical Data. Tables IV, V and VI list the clinical symptoms and relevant laboratory data of the 24 patients in the study group. "Classic" malaria fever is defined as a paroxysm of fever which recurs at regular intervals; it occurred in only seven patients. Ten of the 11 patients with nausea and vomiting had P. falciparum malaria as did nine of the ten who complained of diarrhea. The only complaints referable to the central nervous system were confusion or lethargy, and all six patients with these complaints had P. falciparum. None of the patients suffered cardiorespiratory symptoms. Two patients gave a previous history of malaria (both P. vivax); one other patient gave a family history for malaria, and five other patients said that another person in their traveling group had contracted malaria. The physical findings in these patients are summarized in Table V and the laboratory data in Table VI.

TABLE III Analysis of Physician Contact Before Coming to The New York Hospital

Data	No. of Patients
No previous contact with local physician	10
Contact with local physician	14
Patient-visits to local physician	26
Blood smears by local physician	1 (sic!)
Patients referred with diagnosis of malaria	2
Patients referred with diagnosis other than malaria	12
Patients given antibiotics	11 (5 tetracycline)
Patients with P. falciparum seen by local physician*	8

* Of eight patients with undiagnosed P. falciparum malaria, seven had been diagnosed as having "flu" or "viral syndrome," one as having "gastroenteritis."

TABLE IV Symptoms of Malaria in 24 Civilians

Symptoms	Patients No.	Patients %
Fever and chills	24	100
"Classic" malaria fever	7	29
Headache	23	96
Myalgia	11	46
Nausea and vomiting	11	46
Diarrhea	10	42
Abdominal pain	7	29
Weight loss	7	29
Fatigue	6	25
Pharyngitis	4	17
Dysuria	2	8
Darkened urine	1	4
Melena	1	4
Backache	1	4
Lethargy and confusion	6	25

TABLE V Physical Findings in 24 Civilians with Malaria

Physical Findings	No. Patients Positive (Total = 24)	No. P. falciparum (Total = 16)
Temperature		
Less than 38° C	7	4
38¹° to 39⁹°	3	3
39° to 39⁹°	6	2
40° to 49⁹°	6	6
41° to 41⁹°	2	1 mixed
Systolic blood pressure less than 100 mm Hg	6	5
Clinical evidence of shock	3	3
Icterus	5	5
Hepatomegaly	15	10
Splenomegaly	13	7
Central nervous system signs		
Lethargy	4	4
Stupor	2	2
Stupor and meningismus	1	1
Rash	3	1

TABLE VI Laboratory Values in 24 Civilians with Malaria

	Positive/Tested	P. falciparum
Leukopenia (4,000 WBC/mm^3)	3/24	3
Leukocytosis (10,000 WBC/mm^3)	2/24	1
Normal leukocyte count	19/24	12
Anemia (hemoglobin value less than 12%)	8/24	7
Thrombocytopenia	16/23	11
Elevated prothrombin, or partial thromboplastin time	2/18	1
Proteinuria of 1+ or greater	8/24	8
Pyuria (greater than 5 WBC/hpf)	5/24	5
Microscopic hematuria	2/24	1
Elevated blood urea nitrogen level	4/19	4
Elevated creatinine level	4/12	3
Elevated bilirubin level	15/23	11
Elevated SGOT level	13/23	9
Elevated alkaline phosphatase level	7/19	3
Elevated LDH level	13/16	9
Black patients with sickle preparation	7/11 (all neg)	
False-positive VDRL	1/12	0
G-6-PD deficiency-positive	2/14	1
Serology titer for malaria >1/4096	2/2	1
At least 1 stool specimin submitted for ova and parasites	10/24	
Positive stool for ova and parasites	3/10	

NOTE: WBC = white blood cells. SGOT = serum glutamic oxaloacetic transaminase. LDH = lactic dehydrogenase. VDRL = serologic test for syphilis. G-6-PD = glucose-6-phosphate dehydrogenase.

Therapy. All patients were treated initially with chloroquine phosphate. If vomiting was a severe problem, the first dose of the drug was given parenterally. The total dose of chloroquine was 2.5 g for eight patients, 3.0 g for six patients, 3.5 g for five patients, 4.0 g for two patients, 6.5 g for one patient and 1.75 g for the two pediatric patients. Two patients received pyrimethamine and sulfonamide in addition: in one instance because of lack of adequate clinical response to chloroquine and in the other because the disease was acquired in Cambodia where chloroquine resistance is common.* The latter patient was also the only patient to receive quinine. All seven patients with P. vivax malaria were treated with primaquine and nine others, including seven patients with P. falciparum, were given primaquine prophylactically to prevent recurrence of possible occult mixed infection. The dose used was 15 mg daily for 14 days.

Complications of Therapy. In three of the 24 patients, complications developed from therapy with antimalarials. One patient, who was initially being treated as an outpatient for recurrence of P. vivax, took an overdose of chloroquine and experienced lethargy and diplopia; in another, tinnitus developed from quinine, and nystagmus developed in the patient who received 6.5 g of chloroquine. All side effects from the medications were transient. No toxicity developed in the patients who were given primaquine.

Complications of Malaria. Of the seven patients with central nervous system signs and symptoms, four had a severe alteration in state of consciousness but none became comatose. One patient had transient renal failure and the nephrotic syndrome which cleared slowly over several months. Two patients required transfusion. In one patient mild congestive heart failure developed during fluid replacement. Several patients had a "spike" in temperature after chloroquine therapy was begun. No patient showed evidence of disseminated intravascular coagulation, ruptured spleen or cardiopulmonary distress. One patient was shown to be in complete atrioventricular dissociation thought to be on the basis of congenital heart disease. There were no deaths.

Cost of Treatment of Malaria in Civilians. Twenty of the 24 patients were hospitalized for less than a week with a mean hospital duration of 4.8 days. The four with complications were hospitalized for an average of 17.5 days. For the entire study group, the mean duration of hospitalization was 6.9 days.

The hospital bill was available for 16 of the 24 patients: the cost of hospitalization ranged from $502.15 to $7,702.26, with a mean of $1,744.81.

The retail cost for one hundred 500 mg tablets of chloroquine at a pharmacy across the street from this hospital is $5.00. Thus the retail cost of antimalarial prophylaxis is five cents per week. Of the 16 patients whose bill was available, two were foreign visitors who had lived in an endemic area for many years and two contracted vivax malaria even though they ("they said they took") took the recommended chloroquine prophylaxis. The remaining 12 patients' cumulative cost of hospitalization was $22,830.80 and the calculated cost of chloroquine prophylaxis (according to standard recommendations and based on time spent in an endemic area) would have been $20.20 for all 12.

COMMENTS

No one should die of malaria. We believe that the reason no death occurred in this series was mainly because the

* A detailed consideration of the treatment of drug-resistant malaria is beyond the scope of this paper. All patients from Vietnam or neighboring countries in Southeast Asia and those from South America who do not respond promptly in 24 to 36 hours to chloroquine therapy should be treated as though they had resistant malaria. We favor a program that consists of quinine sulfate, 650 mg, three times a day for 10 days, concurrently with pyrimethamine, 50 mg daily for three days, plus sulfadiazine, 500 mg, four times a day for five to 10 days.

hospital staff was alerted almost every July to the dangers of delayed diagnosis. Yet, despite the presence in this institution of a Tropical Medicine Unit and frequent alerts, several of these patients almost "got away." The surest means of increasing mortality in a group of patients with malaria is to entrust their care to physicians who are inexperienced in diagnosing and treating the disease, and yet how many of us see enough malaria to qualify as experts?

As this study shows, most of the problem is in making the diagnosis. What are the mechanics of missing the diagnosis of malaria? James [3] gave an eloquent explanation:

> "It is characteristic of many pernicious symptoms that they tend to prevent the prompt diagnosis of the disease. They may do so either by presenting in a prominent manner a symptom which strongly suggests some other condition than malaria . . . or by presenting in a patient who is obviously very ill, an almost complete absence of what are known to be the usual clinical signs of malaria."

For Osler [4] the clinical problem was to differentiate malaria from typhoid fever; today the practitioner must be wary of assigning to sick travellers a "viral syndrome."

> Hyman [5] reported on "A series of 100 mistaken admission diagnoses of various conditions which subsequently were found to be malaria . . . ."

The clinical features of malaria are well described in standard texts [6,7], and the importance of including a history of travel in the investigation of fever of obscure origin is well documented elsewhere [8]. However, for the amateur malariologist, we offer several practical suggestions derived from our experience.

In any patient who presents with a history of fever and who has travelled to an endemic area, the presumptive diagnosis should not only be "malaria," but also P. falciparum. A standard blood smear should be taken promptly; using a clean slide it may be stained with Giemsa or Wright's stain.* A diligent search under oil immersion power should be made for ring forms since they are the most common and, frequently, the only phase of the parasite encountered. The definitive diagnosis of one of the benign forms of malaria (vivax, malariae, ovale) should only be made by an expert. Degree of parasitemia is an unreliable index of severity of infection, especially in those who have used prophylactic drugs inadequately or who have been treated with antibiotics. If the smear is positive the patient should be given the first dose of chloroquine (1 g) and hospitalized. If the smear is negative, the patient should be hospitalized for serial smears every 4 hours and a specialist's help enlisted. The remaining doses of chloroquine, 500 mg, at 6, 24, 48 and 72 hours (total 3.0 g) should be administered if possible under the supervision of a physician well versed in malaria, and he should make all decisions about using additional therapy such as pyrimethamine, sulfonamide, quinine, etc. Under no circumstances should broad spectrum antibiotics, such as tetracycline, be given before a diagnosis has been ruled out by an expert since these may suppress hematologic evidence of infection.

* We disagree with Wyler [9] who stated recently that the ordinary Wright's stain was inadequate for the diagnosis of malaria. Special stains such as Giemsa are useful for species identification and better detail, but the practical aspect of using a routine blood smear must not be overlooked. Experts, of course, depend upon thick and thin films stained by the Giemsa technic.

TABLE VII Changing Pattern of Imported Malaria in Civilians in the United States of America

	1973	1974
Total cases of imported malaria in civilians in the United States of America	175	302
Total P. falciparum	46	93
Malaria from Africa	80	136
P. falciparum from Africa	28	74
Malaria from West and Central Africa	4	19
P. falciparum from West and Central Africa	1	11
Malaria from Asia	79	113
P. falciparum from Asia	59	86
Malaria from India	10	41

Malaria may cause rapid clinical deterioration; in a matter of hours a patient may progress from seemingly trivial illness to coma and death [10]. Any abnormality of the central nervous system, usually a change in mentation or state of consciousness, is a danger sign and may herald this catastrophe.

The most reliable index of response to therapy is the clinical picture and the central nervous system signs. Fever and hemolysis, after initiating therapy, are not uncommon and should be treated by standard measures according to severity. A useful tool is the bedside "flow sheet" which carries, on a 4 to 6 hour scale, results of serial smears, and determinations of hematocrit, clinical status, temperature and fluid balance. The outpatient treatment of malaria by nonexperts should be discouraged.

Current Situation. Although proper documentation is difficult to obtain, the prevalence of malaria is increasing rather than decreasing in many parts of Africa, Asia and, possibly, South America. During the 10 year period from 1964 through 1973, the number of imported cases of malaria in civilians in the United States of America remained almost constant at 100 to 200 cases per year [11]. However, if one compares figures for 1974 with 1973 (Table VII), there was a striking change in the civilian pattern of malaria imported to this country. This parallels our experience at this hospital. In the nine months from September 1974 [12] to May 1975 there were eight cases of malaria; seven of which were P. falciparum and six of which were from West Africa. On October 28, 1974, two unrelated patients with P. falciparum malaria were in the Emergency Room at the same time.

The total number of foreign visitors to West Africa is estimated at several hundred thousand per year, but no specific figures or trends are available; but in East Africa, the number of tourists to Kenya has not changed significantly over the past four years [13]. We suspect that the recent predominance of malaria imported from West Africa in our series might be due to an increase in travel of black Americans to their ancestral home and possibly to an increase of travel by native Africans to the United States of America.

Since chemoprophylaxis against P. falciparum malaria is effective, inexpensive and virtually harmless, it is distressing that 63 per cent of our study group took no prophylaxis. Whether these persons were properly informed of the danger of malaria is not known. The broad question of the honesty of the malaria warnings given by travel agents, airlines, businesses, organizations and governments is beyond the scope of this paper. Details on malaria for travelers is readily available to physicians from the Center For Disease Control [11] which also will provide clinical assistance on request.

REFERENCES

1. Walzer PD, Gibson JJ, Schultz MG: Malaria fatalities in the United States. Am J Trop Med Hyg 23: 328, 1974.
2. Bruce-Chwatt LJ: Epidemiology of malaria. Br Med J 4: 170, 1971.
3. James WM: 20th Annual Report, Medical Dept., United Fruit Co., p 34, cited from page 1006, Malariology, vol II (Boyd MF, ed), Philadelphia, W. B. Saunders & Co., 1943.
4. Osler W: The diagnosis of malarial fever. Med News 70: 289, 1897.
5. Hyman AS: Clinical masquerades of malaria. Naval Med Bull 45: 287, 1945.
6. Kitchen SF: Malariology, vol II (Boyd MF, ed), Philadelphia, W. B. Saunders & Co., 1943, p 966.
7. Russell PF, West LS, Manwell RD, MacDonald G: Practical Malariology, London, Oxford University Press, 1963, p 365.
8. Maegraith B: Unde venis? The Lancet 1: 401, 1963.
9. Wyler DJ: Southeast Asian refugees and malaria. N Engl J Med 293: 203, 1975.
10. Kean BH, Smith JA: Death due to estivo-autumnal malaria. Am J Trop Med 24: 317, 1944.
11. Center for Disease Control Malaria Surveillance, 1973 Annual Summary. U.S. Public Health Service, Atlanta, Georgia, 1974.
12. Preliminary Reports of Malaria Surveillance, Center for Disease Control, Atlanta, Georgia, 1974. Personal communication.
13. Patterson WD, Waters SR: The Big Picture—Travel '75. Official Annual Report World Travel Trends and Markets 1973–74. Travel Communications Inc., 1975.

The Mechanism of Increase in Total Lung Capacity During Acute Asthma

LEONARD PERESS, M.D.*
GERHART SYBRECHT, M.D.*
PETER T. MACKLEM, M.D.
Montreal, Canada

In order to investigate the mechanism underlying the increased total lung capacity (TLC) observed during an acute asthmatic attack, we measured respiratory mechanics in a specially trained, exercise-induced, asthmatic. During the acute attack his TLC (determined plethysmographically) increased from 7.8 to 9.2 liters. The static pressure-volume curve of the lung shifted to the left and expiratory compliance increased from 0.24 to 0.55 liter/cm H_2O. There was a parallel shift of the static pressure-volume curve of the chest wall resulting in an increase in the outward recoil of this structure. The maximum inspiratory pressure-volume curve of the total respiratory system was shifted so that the inspiratory muscles were able to generate greater pressures at any given lung volume during the attack. The findings indicate that the increase in TLC during acute bronchospasm results from the combination of loss of lung recoil, increased outward recoil of the chest wall and increased strength of contraction of the inspiratory muscles.

During the acute asthmatic attack, a reversible increase in total lung capacity (TLC) has been observed, with changes of up to a 100 per cent [1] increase over reported control values. Studies of pulmonary mechanics in this situation have revealed a loss of lung recoil which, in some cases, has been slowly reversible [2,3]. The marked increase in TLC not only requires loss of lung recoil, but it also requires remarkable alterations in the pressure-volume characteristics of the chest wall. These have not been studied, principally because it takes trained, highly cooperative subjects to obtain reliable, reproducible results.

We have trained and studied a highly cooperative person with asthma induced by exercise whose attacks were characterized by acute reversible loss of elastic recoil, not only to document the rapidly changing pressure-volume characteristics of the lung, but also to determine how the pressure-volume characteristics of the chest wall alter, to account for the observed changes in TLC.

METHODS

Lung volumes were determined with an Emerson Model BP volume displacement plethysmograph, the signal from which was pressure corrected so that its frequency response was adequate to 12 cycles/sec.

Pressure-volume curves of the lung, chest wall and total respiratory system were measured during expiration. The pressure difference across the lung (transpulmonary pressure) was estimated by measuring mouth pressure relative to esophageal pressure, sensed with an esophageal balloon catheter coupled to a Sanborn 267B differential pressure transducer.

From the Meakins-Christie Laboratories, McGill University Clinic, Royal Victoria Hospital, Montreal, Province of Quebec, Canada. Requests for reprints should be addressed to Dr. P. T. Macklem, Meakins-Christie Laboratories, McGill University, 3775 University Street, Montreal H3A 2B4, Canada. Manuscript accepted December 11, 1975.

* Research Fellow—Meakins-Christie Laboratories

TABLE I **Subdivisions of Lung Volume**

Lung Volumes	Control (liters)	Acute Attack (liters)	Predicted (liters)
TLC	7.8	9.2	6.3
FRC	4.2	6.2	3.6
RV	2.8	5.7	2.0
VC	5.0	3.5	4.3

NOTE: TLC = total lung capacity. FRC = functional residual capacity. RV = residual volume. VC = vital capacity.

Esophageal pressure relative to body surface pressure was measured with a second Sanborn 267B transducer and used as an estimate of the pressure across the chest wall (transthoracic pressure). The sum of this pressure and transpulmonary pressure, is mouth pressure relative to body surface pressure and is the pressure difference across the total system (transrespiratory pressure).

All pressure-volume curves were measured under static conditions during expiration. The subject inhaled to TLC and during the subsequent slow expiration, flow was occluded by blocking the mouthpiece to produce periods of zero flow. Prior to the definitive study, the subject underwent a considerable period of training to learn how to relax his respiratory muscles against an occluded mouthpiece in order to obtain reliable pressure-volume curves of the relaxed chest wall at lung volumes greater than functional residual capacity (FRC). He was also trained to perform maximal inspiratory efforts against an occluded airway to obtain reliable maximal inspiratory pressure-volume curves of the chest wall and total respiratory system.

All measurements were made under control conditions when the subject was free of bronchospasm, and they were repeated during a provoked attack which was induced by exercising the subject on an athletic track adjacent to the hospital.

RESULTS

A typical asthmatic attack in this subject was associated with marked wheezing, hyperinflation and an increase in TLC. In one such attack (Table I), TLC increased by 1.4 liters.

The pressure-volume curves of the lung before and during this attack are shown in Figure 1. The data points were collected from at least three expiratory maneuvers. During the attack there was a leftward shift in the curve, with a change in slope towards a more vertical direction. Static compliance measured between FRC and FRC + 500 cc changed from 0.24 liter/cm H_2O to 0.55 liter/cm H_2O. The changes in both lung volumes and in pressure-volume curves were present within minutes of the onset of the provoked asthmatic attack. After bronchodilator therapy, there was a return to near control values in both parameters within an hour.

The pressure-volume curves of the relaxed chest wall are shown in Figure 2. Acute bronchospasm was associated with an upward but parallel shift of the curve. The narrow scatter of the data points indicates that the subject was able to adequately relax his respiratory muscles to obtain reliable pressure-volume curves of the chest wall. In Figure 3, the pressure-volume curves of the total respiratory system are displayed. Since this curve is the summation of the pressure-volume curves

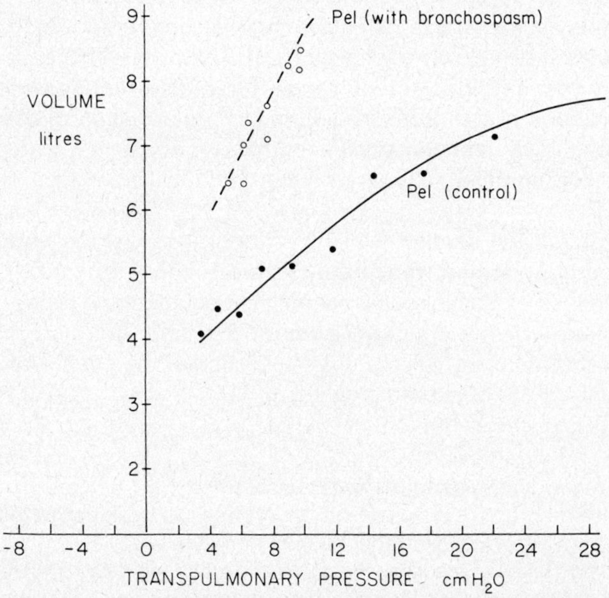

Figure 1. Pressure-volume curves of lung during control conditions and with acute bronchospasm. Volume refers to absolute lung volume.

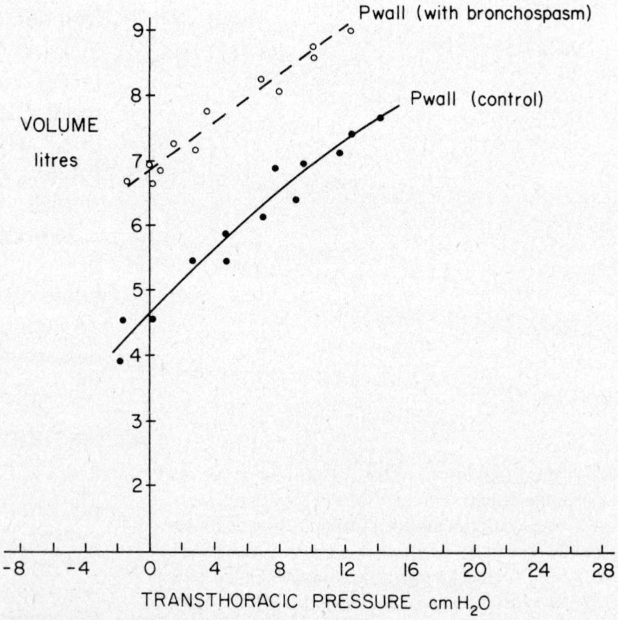

Figure 2. Pressure-volume curves of relaxed chest wall—control and during the acute attack.

of the lung and wall, it is not surprising that there was again a leftward and also a vertical shift of the curve.

Figure 4 illustrates again the relaxed pressure-volume curve of the total respiratory system before and during an attack as shown by the solid lines to the right of the ordinate. When the subject was asked to inspire maximally against an obstructed airway, the relationship between transrespiratory pressure and volume shifted to the curves shown by the dashed line (gas expansion has been ignored). The change in pressure with the maximal inspiratory effort is the horizontal distance between these two curves and is shown by the dotted lines. These curves indicate the maximum pressure the inspiratory muscles can generate at different lung volumes. During the acute attack, there was a leftward shift of this curve, such that, at any given volume, the muscles were able to generate somewhat greater pressures.

In summary, the acute asthmatic attack was accompanied by a striking loss of lung recoil, an upward but parallel shift in the pressure-volume curve of the chest wall and an increase in the strength of the inspiratory muscles.

COMMENTS

The intent of this study was to examine the balance of forces across the thorax in an attempt to understand the remarkable large and rapid changes in TLC which the subject demonstrated during and after the acute asthmatic attack.

TLC is that lung volume at which the maximum inspiratory pressures that can be generated by the chest wall is entirely dissipated across the lungs [4]. As the lungs inflate towards TLC, there is a progressive increase in the elastic recoil pressure, coupled with a decrease in the ability of the inspiratory muscles to generate pressures, presumably due to shortening and diminishing mechanical advantage. The point at which the two become equal and opposite determines TLC. As both the pressure-volume curve of the lung and maximum inspiratory pressure-volume curve of the chest wall progressively flatten as TLC approaches, one would predict that alterations in TLC of the magnitude observed in our patient would necessitate alterations in both curves.

This was the case. With the onset of bronchospasm, there was a remarkable change in the elastic properties. There was a loss of recoil of the lung and an increase in outward recoil of the wall, coupled with enhanced strength of the inspiratory muscles. These changes all favor a new equilibrium at a higher lung volume. In that sense, the changes in TLC are explained, but how the lungs and chest wall alter their elastic properties is not. In particular, the marked and rapid alterations in the pressure-volume curve of the lung is astonishing. In one of Woolcock and Read's cases [1] such rapid changes

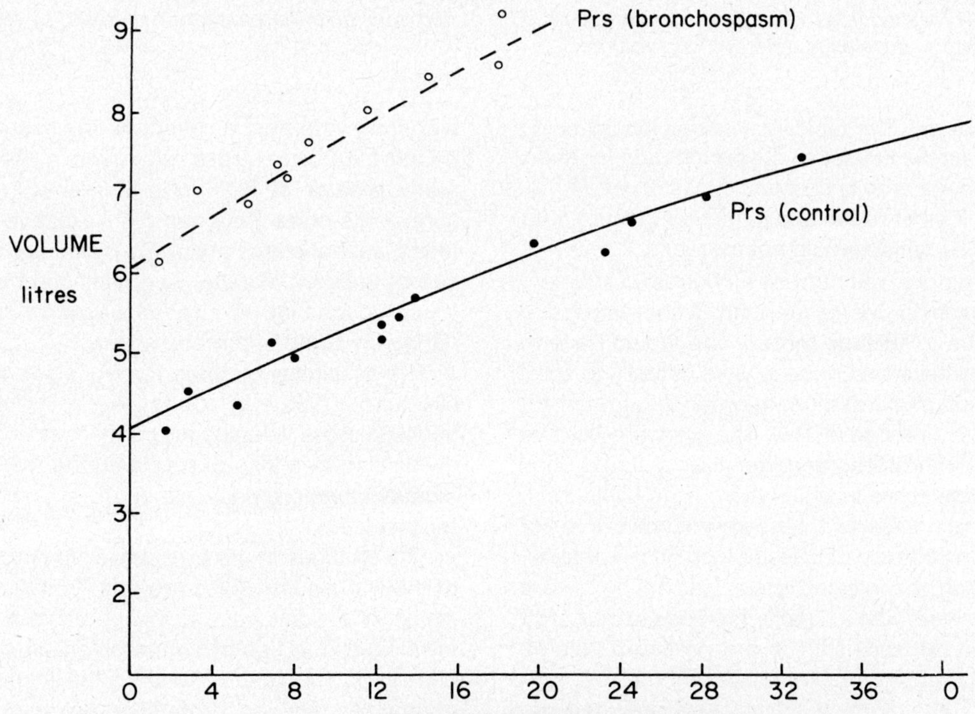

Figure 3. *Pressure-volume curve of the relaxed respiratory system.*

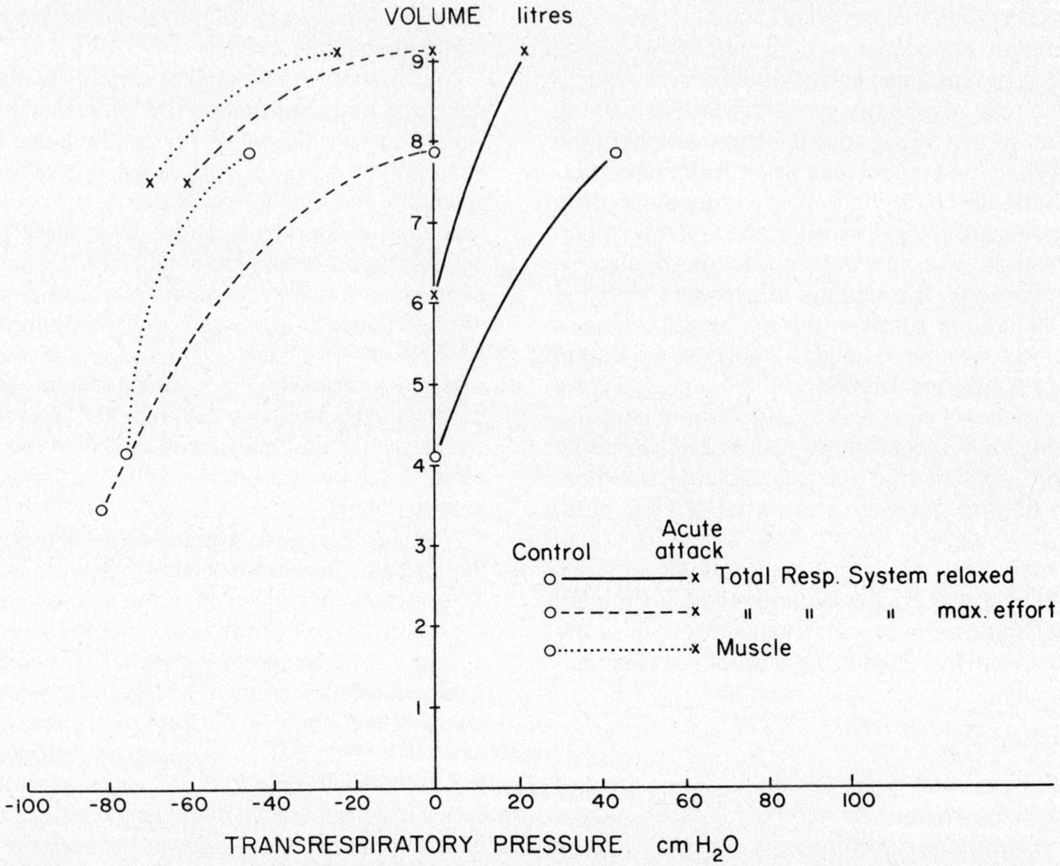

Figure 4. *On right side of ordinate: pressure-volume curves of relaxed total respiratory system. The left side of the ordinate shows the pressure-volume curves of the total system during maximum inspiratory effort (dashed lines which reach the ordinate). The dotted lines give the pressure generated by the inspiratory muscles at different lung volumes.*

were also observed. The rapidity excludes longstanding hyperinflation as the cause, and hyperinflation for short periods of time apparently causes no loss of recoil [3]. Neither is the loss of recoil due to airway closure with gas trapping [5] which would not increase TLC.

It must, therefore, result from a change in inherent surface or tissue forces of the lung. If the change in recoil were due to surface forces, one would have to postulate a decrease in surface tension virtually to zero, both on inflation and deflation, in order to account for the marked loss of recoil at TLC. The pressure-volume curve should, therefore, become like a liquid-filled pressure-volume curve in which there is no hysteresis. To examine this possibility, pressure-volume curves of the lung were repeated during inspiration and expiration. On this occasion, the induced attack was not as severe and was associated with a smaller increase in TLC (400 cc). Despite a leftward shift in the pressure-volume curve (although not as marked as during the first provoked attack), the area of hysteresis remained unchanged.

In view of this, a change in tissue forces would seem more likely. With the hyperinflation and air trapping at high lung volumes, a reduction in tissue forces might be attributable to stress relaxation, a phenomena normally greater at high lung volumes. Pressure measurements were obtained from relatively stable plateaus, so that stress adaptation, although not excluded, seems unlikely. Marshall and Widdicombe [6] however found no change in stress relaxation in one subject during an acute asthmatic attack.

The possibility of some form of acute and reversible structural change in connective tissue such as alterations in cross linkages in collagen and in elastic fibers, giving rise to a loss of recoil during the acute attack, exists but we are unaware of any supporting evidence for this.

The changes in the pressure-volume characteristics of the wall and muscles are equally difficult to explain. Again, one would have to invoke either a change in the intrinsic properties of connective tissue or possibly a change in the resting tone of the inspiratory and/or expiratory muscles, probably reflex in origin. It is conceivable that inspiratory muscle tension is reflexly inhibited as TLC is approached in order to prevent overdistension of the lung and pneumothorax [7]. If such a reflex were stimulated by a critical elastic recoil pressure, then loss of recoil would result in the reflex being initiated at a higher lung volume, thus explaining the shift in the maximum inspiratory pressure-volume curve of the chest wall. Although this is a possibility, the mechanism is purely speculative.

Conventional thinking regarding the elastic properties of lung tissue and the chest wall is that these are fixed, static and virtually immutable properties which do not change rapidly with time. Our studies demonstrate that this may not be the case. Indeed, it appears that the elastic properties of lung and chest wall tissue have the potential of changing rapidly. Before we can understand the nature of the elastic properties of the lungs and chest wall, we will have to understand how these properties can change so dynamically. Our present knowledge is so skimpy in this regard, that such changes fall almost within the realm of the miraculous rather than in the realm of science.

REFERENCES

1. Woolcock AJ, Read J: Lung volumes in exacerbations of asthma. Am J Med 41: 259, 1966.
2. Finucane KE, Colebatch HJH: Elastic behaviour of the lung in patients with airway obstruction. J Appl Physiol 26: 330, 1969.
3. Gold WM, Kaufman HS, Nadel JA: Elastic recoil of the lungs in chronic asthmatic patients before and after therapy. J Appl Physiol 23: 433, 1967.
4. Mead J, Milic-Emili J, Turner JM: Factors limiting the depth of a maximal inspiration in human subjects. J Appl Physiol 18: 295, 1963.
5. Mansell A, Dubrawsky C, Livison M, et al.: Lung mechanics in antigen-induced asthma. J Appl Physiol 37: 297, 1974.
6. Marshall L, Widdicombe JG: Stress relaxation of the human lung. Clin Sci 20: 19, 1960.
7. Campbell ETM, Agnostoni E, Davis JN: The Respiratory Muscles Mechanics and Neural Control. Philadelphia and London, W. B. Saunders Co., 1970, p 70.

Neurologic Involvement in Seven Patients with Behçet's Disease

J. DESMOND O'DUFFY, M.D.
NORMAN P. GOLDSTEIN, M.D.
Rochester, Minnesota

Of 25 patients with Behçet's disease seen in five years at the Mayo Clinic, seven had central nervous system involvement. The mean interval from onset of Behçet's disease to central nervous system involvement was 1.3 years, and the mean period of observation thereafter was 3.8 years. All patients had headache and fever during or preceding exacerbations of the central nervous system disease, and all had cerebrospinal fluid pleocytosis (white cell counts ranged from 6 to 490/mm^3) with predominant lymphocytosis. The mean cerebrospinal fluid protein level was 55 mg/dl, and gamma globulin was less than 15 per cent in six patients. Results of cerebrospinal fluid, lesional and serologic studies for bacterial, fungal and viral agents were negative. Clinical findings included corticospinal tract disease (five patients), cerebellar ataxia (four patients), pseudobulbar palsy (three patients) and transient ocular palsies (three patients). All these occurred in concert with the systemic phases, especially aphthosis. Corticosteroid therapy was used in six patients, cyclophosphamide therapy in two and azathioprine therapy in two. The neurologic manifestations tended to recur when dosages of the drugs were lowered and established central nervous system damage could not be reversed. The case histories suggest that steroids, when used promptly and in sufficient dosage (up to 60 mg prednisone), are effective in reducing or preventing progression of central nervous system disease.

Three patients died, one from Pneumocystis carinii infection, one from neurologic disease and another from presumed myocardial infarction. The central nervous system involvement in Behçet's disease should be diagnosed earlier, and it can be if attention is given to other systemic criteria, that is, aphthous stomatitis, aphthous genital lesions, cutaneous vasculitis, uveitis and synovitis.

Originally described as a triple-symptom complex of oral aphthous ulceration, genital ulceration and hypopyon iritis [1], Behçet's disease is now known to have a wide systemic spectrum [2,3]. Additional features found with varying frequency in this condition include synovitis [4], cutaneous vasculitis resembling erythema nodosum [5], colitis [6], thrombophlebitis [7], large artery aneurysms [8] and encephalopathy [9]. In the absence of a pathognomonic result of a histologic or laboratory test, the diagnosis remains clinical. The appearance of new clinical features months or years after the onset of the illness adds to the diagnostic difficulty. In order to minimize the diagnostic difficulties, new criteria for diagnosis have been proposed [10].

Recurrent oral or genital aphthous ulcers in association with any other two of the following three major criteria are sufficient for diag-

From the Mayo Clinic and Mayo Foundation, Rochester, Minnesota 55901. Requests for reprints should be addressed to Dr. J. Desmond O'Duffy, Section of Publications, Mayo Clinic, Rochester, Minnesota 55901. Manuscript accepted November 12, 1975.

TABLE I Diagnosis of Behçet's Disease

Suggested criteria:
Aphthous stomatitis, aphthous genital ulceration, uveitis, cutaneous vasculitis, synovitis and meningoencephalitis*
Diagnosis:
At least three criteria present, one being recurrent aphthous ulceration
Incomplete form:
Two criteria present, one being recurrent aphthous ulceration
Exclusions:
Inflammatory bowel disease, systemic lupus erythematosus, Reiter's disease and herpetic infections

* Added as a sixth criterion.

nosis [10]: anterior or posterior uveitis, synovitis and cutaneous vasculitis. The incomplete form of Behçet's disease may be suspected if aphthous stomatitis coexists with one other criterion.

In the past, the neurologic complications of Behçet's disease have not received wide recognition. Accordingly, we would like to describe seven patients who were observed during a five year period. Since, with few exceptions [11], previous reports of neurologic involvement were of one or a few cases [12–17] (or a review of a large series of cases from the literature [9,16,17]), we believe that our experience emphasizes the diversity of neurologic manifestations and the limitation of treatment of Behçet's disease involving the central nervous system. In addition, because of the frequency of neurologic disease in our series of patients with Behçet's disease (28 per cent), we suggest that central nervous system involvement be added as a diagnostic criterion (Table I).

OUR SERIES

From March 1970 to February 1975, 25 patients with Behçet's disease were seen by one of us (J.D.O.). Of the 25 patients, 20 fulfilled three or more criteria and five fulfilled two. Patients with granulomatous colitis, systemic lupus erythematosus, local or systemic herpes infections, or Reiter's disease were excluded.

Of the 25 patients, seven had neurologic involvement (Table II). There were five women and two men whose ages at the onset of the disease averaged 29 years (range 19 to 48 years), whose total duration of disease to date or to death averaged 5.1 years (range one to 10 years), and whose duration of disease to first visit averaged 3.7 years (range 0.5 to 7 years). In all seven patients, three or more target organs were affected. The time between the first manifestation and the onset of neurologic disease ranged from 0 to 3 years (mean 1.3 years); in one (Case 7), neurologic manifestations occurred at the onset of disease. In the series, the duration of neurologic disease ranged from 0.50 to 7 years (mean 3.8 years). Three patients have died, one as a result of Pneumocystis carinii pneumonia which occurred during the course of prednisone and cyclophosphamide therapy, another from myocardial infarction and another from the neurologic disease.

Types of Neurologic Disease (Table III). All seven patients had headache and fever during or preceding the central nervous system involvement. Four patients had initial episodes of aseptic meningitis with some neurologic abnormalities, whereas the other three had uncomplicated aseptic meningitis as a predominant neurologic presentation. In two of the three patients (Cases 1 and 3), this pattern preceded other neurologic manifestations by one and four years; in the third patient (Case 5) it was the sole neurologic feature.

The corticospinal tracts were most commonly involved; three patients had hemiparesis and two had quadriparesis. Four patients had cerebellar ataxia and three had pseudobulbar palsy. Three patients (Cases 1, 4 and 7) had transient ocular palsies during neurologic flare-ups. Two patients had documented visual defects. Central nervous system symptoms and signs often occurred in exacerbations that lasted a few days in association with other systemic features of aphthosis, synovitis or fever.

All patients had abnormalities in lumbar cerebrospinal fluid (Table III). White blood cell counts ranged from 6 to 490/mm^3 (mean 117/mm^3), and lymphocytosis was common (range 15 to 100 per cent, mean 74 per cent). In some acute encephalitic flare-ups, polymorphonuclear leukocytes predominated transiently. The total protein content of cerebrospinal fluid ranged from 31 to 96 mg/dl (mean 55 mg/dl). The concentration of cerebrospinal fluid gamma globulin was normal (less than 15 per cent of total protein) in the six patients studied. Cultures of cerebrospinal fluid and oral-genital ulcers for bacteria, fungi and viruses were negative (Table

TABLE II Clinical Features in Seven Cases of Behçet's Disease

Case	Sex and Age (yr) at Onset	Duration (yr) of Disease to First Visit	Age (yr) When Seen	Duration (yr): Of Disease	Duration (yr): Of Neurologic Involvement	Involvement: Oral	Genital	Eye	Skin	Joint	CNS
1	M, 21	7	28	8.5	7	+	+	–	+	+	+
2	F, 27	3	30	5	3	+	+	+	–	+	+
3	F, 27	7	34	10	7	+	+	+	+	+	+
4	F, 19	1/2	20	1	0.5	+	+	–	–	–	+
5	M, 48	1/2	49	1	0.5	+	+	–	–	–	+
6	F, 22	5	27	6.5	5	+	+	+	+	+	+
7	F, 41	3	44	4	4.0	+	–	–	–	+	+

TABLE III Neurologic Features in Seven Cases of Behçet's Disease

		Cerebrospinal Fluid*		
Case	Findings	White Blood Cells (per mm³)	Lymphocytes (%)	Total Protein (mg/dl)
1	Quadriparesis			
	cerebellar	63	100	90
	pseudobulbar	6	100	96
2	Cerebellar	195	60	41
3	Hemiparesis, hemihypesthesia	10	90	31
4	Quadriparesis			
	cerebellar	12	100	44
	pseudobulbar	132	16	50
5	None	52	100	47
6	Hemiparesis	490	15	44
		70	90	35
7	Hemiparesis			
	cerebellar	133	48	
	pseudobulbar	122	100	76

*Values represent single episodes.

TABLE IV Microbiologic Studies on Lesions, Cerebrospinal Fluid (CSF) and Serum in Seven Cases of Behçet's Encephalopathy

	Positive	Negative	Not Performed
Bacterial culture (CSF)			
Routine	0	6	1
Mycobacterium	0	5	2
Fungal culture (CSF)	0	5	2
Fungal serology (serum)	0	4	3
Heterophil agglutination	0	3	4
Viral culture			
Lesion	1*	4	2
CSF	0	5	2
Viral antibody			
Herpes simplex (serum)	†	2	3
Herpes simplex (CSF)	0	2	5
Mumps	‡	1	5
Herpes zoster	§	0	6

* Herpes simplex (penis).
† Antibody titer 1:32 in two patients.
‡ Titer 1:8.
§ Titer 1:16.

IV). A single isolation of herpes simplex virus from a scrotal ulcer was found in an immunosuppressed patient (Case 1). In four patients, serum specimens obtained in the acute phase were tested for antibodies to herpes virus and, in two patients, to other agents known to cause disease of the central nervous system (Table IV); results in all were nondiagnostic.

Six of the seven patients were treated with corticosteroids, alone or in combination with cyclophosphamide (two patients) or azathioprine (two patients) (Table V). Despite generous dosage, such immunosuppression often failed to satisfactorily suppress the neurologic manifestations, which would "break through" as dosages were decreased. However, the only patient who was observed during the entire course of her neurologic disease (Case 2) had a remission with combined prednisone-azathioprine therapy. The few patients in the series obviate statistical analysis of treatment. However, of the three patients in our series who died, two were treated with steroids and cyclophosphamide and the other was untreated.

CASE REPORTS

Case 1. A 28 year old carpenter was examined in June 1974 because of meningitis. Six months previously, he noted episodes of headache, vomiting and fever. Previous study resulted in a diagnosis of aseptic meningitis with cultures of cerebrospinal fluid being negative for bacteria, fungi and viruses; examination of cerebrospinal fluid showed 137 white blood cells/mm³ (90 per cent polymorphonuclear leukocytes). Treatment with various antibiotics failed to diminish his symptoms. During some exacerbations, he had arthralgia of the wrists and ankles, with joint swelling; during others, he had aphthous oral and scrotal ulcers.

Our examination revealed a questionable palsy of the right sixth cranial nerve and an oral temperature of 99.6°F (37.6°C). Because he had suffered shrapnel wounds of the head in Vietnam in 1967, the possibility of intracranial infection was considered. A lumbar puncture showed 30 lymphocytes and 2 polymorphonuclear leukocytes/mm³ and a total protein level of 58 mg/dl, with 12 per cent gamma globulin. An echoencephalogram showed no shift of the midline structures, and an electroencephalogram was normal, as was an EMI-scan (computerized transaxial tomography) of the brain. A repeat lumbar puncture showed an initial pressure of 170 mm water, 140 lymphocytes and 93 polymorphonuclear leukocytes/mm³, and 74 mg of total protein. The sedimentation rate was 42 mm in 1 hour, and the following were within normal limits or negative: serum protein electrophoresis, immunoglobulins, antinuclear antibody, serum hepatitis antigen, rheumatoid factor and mono-spot test. Extensive microbiologic studies were unrewarding and included cerebrospinal fluid cultures for viruses, fungi and

TABLE V Treatment of Neurologic Disease in Seven Cases of Behçet's Disease

Case	Treatment	Daily Dose (mg)	Outcome
1	Prednisone	40–60	Died
	Cyclophosphamide	150–200	
2	Prednisone	60–5	Good suppression
	Azathioprine	150–50	
3	Prednisone	15–30	Partial suppression
	Azathioprine	150–50	
4	Prednisolone	32–16	Partial suppression
5	None	. . .	Died, myocardial infarction
6	Prednisone	60	Died, Pneumocystis pneumonia
	Cyclophosphamide	100	
	Chlorambucil	(?)	
7	Prednisone	20	Persisting episodes

bacteria (including tubercle bacilli); various sites cultured for viruses, Mycoplasma, fungi and yeast were free of pathogens, and serial serum and cerebrospinal fluid agglutination tests for leptospira, mumps (serum 1:8, cerebrospinal fluid less than 1:2), and Mycoplasma were of insignificant titer. A serum titer for herpes simplex antibody was 1:32, and a cerebrospinal fluid titer was less than 1:2. This patient was not treated, and a diagnosis of aseptic meningitis of unknown cause was made. An antistreptolysin O (ASO) titer was 500 Todd units.

The patient's second admission was in August 1974. Two weeks of headaches, diplopia and fever preceded this admission. Neurologic studies performed elsewhere before this admission included an electroencephalogram, which showed "intermittent slowing," and cerebral arteriograms, which were within normal limits. Four days before admission, left hemiparesis developed. The examination revealed an oral temperature of 100.6°F (38.1°C), euphoria, spasticity and weakness of the left upper and lower limbs, bilateral extensor Babinski responses, and incoordination on the left finger-nose and heel-knee tests. The patient had an oral aphtha and a 1 cm scrotal ulcer. The erythrocyte sedimentation rate was 63 mm in 1 hour, and serum immunoglobulin levels were normal. The ASO titer was still elevated at 500 Todd units. A lumbar puncture showed an initial pressure of 192 mm water, 63 lymphocytes/mm^3, no polymorphonuclear leukocytes and a total protein level of 90 mg/dl. Repeated cultures of blood, scrotal ulcer and cerebrospinal fluid for bacteria, viruses and fungi were negative. A repeat cerebrospinal fluid antibody titer for herpes simplex was 1:2, and serologic studies for fungi were negative. Roentgenograms of the small bowel and colon were within normal limits, and a proctoscopic examination showed no ulceration. The diagnosis of Behçet's disease was considered because of the aseptic meningitis with parenchymal disease of the central nervous system, the association of oral and genital ulcers with relapses, and recurrent synovitis. The patient recalled having coexistent oral ulcers and swollen knees (which were aspirated) while in military service in 1967. During the next month, his symptoms and signs worsened, with recrudescence of scrotal ulcers and headache.

The patient's third admission was in September 1974. He had an oral temperature of 101°F (38.3°C), nuchal rigidity, widebased-ataxic gait, spastic-ataxic dysarthria, mild quadriparesis, bilateral extensor Babinski responses, symmetrically increased deep tendon reflexes and increased right palpebral fissure. An examination of the lumbar cerebrospinal fluid yielded 48 lymphocytes and 4 polymorphonuclear leukocytes/mm^3 and a total protein of 144 mg/dl. The erythrocyte sedimentation rate was 64 mm in 1 hour. Again, microbiologic studies of cerebrospinal fluid, blood, urine and scrotal ulcers were unrewarding. The biopsy specimen of the scrotal ulcer showed nonspecific acute and chronic inflammation. The administration of prednisone, in divided doses of 60 mg/day, was started.

The patient's fourth admission was in November 1974. Initially, his condition had improved with prednisone therapy; he was free of headache and ulcers. Inappropriate behavior was attributed to hypersteroidism, and the dose of prednisone was reduced to 40 mg/day. Four days later, nuchal rigidity with fever recurred, and the weakness and ataxia increased. Additional neurologic findings included left hemiplegia, pseudobulbar affect, inability to stand alone and increased ataxia on finger-nose testing, severe dysarthria and horizontal nystagmus on lateral gaze to either side. Cerebrospinal fluid examinations revealed 7 lymphocytes/mm^3 and a total protein level of 96 mg/dl on one occasion, and 17 lymphocytes/mm^3 and a protein level of 71 mg/dl on another. The dose of prednisone was increased to 60 mg/day, and cyclophosphamide (200 mg/day) was added. There was modest diminution in the left hemiplegia, and the patient walked with assistance. Two months later, his neurologic status was unchanged, but episodes of oral and genital ulceration continued. A penile ulcer cultured for virus grew herpes simplex for the first time. A perforated duodenal ulcer complicated treatment in February 1975. Cyclophosphamide therapy was then discontinued. His neurologic status deteriorated, and he died at home in June 1975.

Case 2. A 30 year old housewife presented with aphthous vulvitis and stomatitis in March 1972. She had had recurrent oral aphthae since early childhood, which worsened in 1969, and recurrent crops of vulvar aphthae for one year. In the year preceding the present examination, she had had headaches and cutaneous nodules. Examination showed painful typical superficial canker sores. Viral cultures of both oral and genital ulcers gave no growth. A labial biopsy specimen showed nonspecific abscess formation. An erythrocyte sedimentation rate was 51 mm in 1 hour, and tests for immunoglobulins, antinuclear antibody, rheumatoid factor and serum complement gave normal or negative results.

In November 1972, she experienced right optic papillitis, global headache and nuchal rigidity. Prednisone (60 mg/day) was given, and the optic papillitis lessened. The prednisone therapy was stopped, and nausea, vomiting, vertigo and headache led to her admission. Her oral temperature was 99°F (37.2°C). She had bilateral ataxia on the finger-nose test and tandem gait ataxia. An electroencephalogram was within normal limits. The lumbar puncture revealed an initial pressure of 130 mm water, 195 white blood cells/mm^3 (60 per cent lymphocytes), total protein of 41 mg/dl and 11 per cent gamma globulin. The cerebrospinal fluid grew no bacteria or virus. The use of salicylates relieved her other neurologic symptoms and signs in one week, but the peripheral and central scotomas of optic neuritis in the right visual field persisted. A recurrence of visual blurring in April 1973 was attributed to posterior uveitis and retinal vasculitis; this was successfully treated with 40 mg of prednisone. In May 1973, azathioprine (100 mg daily) was added in the hope of reducing the dose of prednisone to less than 30 mg daily. The uveitis further subsided, and when examined in July 1974, when the patient was not receiving steroid treatment, visual acuity was normal, but there was a small, residual, right central field defect. Azathioprine therapy was continued in a dosage range of 75 to 150 mg daily.

Case 3. A 34 year old housewife presented in April 1972 with chief complaints of headache and ulcers in the mouth and vagina. Seven years previously, she had first noted tender cutaneous nodules and aphthous ulcers in the mouth and vagina. Eighteen months later, headaches began. These would last from hours to days, were bitemporal and sometimes were associated with vomiting. They were aggravated by head movements and often associated with reduced vision. The administration of prednisone, in doses ranging from 15 to 30 mg daily, abolished the headaches and greatly reduced the frequency and severity of the oral and vaginal ulcers. Behçet's disease was diagnosed in 1969 when posterior uveitis was documented. A cerebrospinal fluid examination in 1969 had revealed 142 white blood cells/mm^3 and a total protein level of 52 mg/dl. Attempts to reduce the dose of prednisone below 15 mg daily were not possible because of flares of the mucocutaneous ulcers, blurred vision and headaches. Other complaints included malaise and cramping periumbilical pain.

In 1972, the patient had evidence of hypersteroidism, a normal eye examination and no mucosal ulcers while receiving 30 mg of prednisone/day. The cerebrospinal fluid examination showed an initial pressure of 164 mm water, 2 lymphocytes/mm^3, a protein level of 21 mg/dl and gamma globulin of 12 per cent. Cultures yielded no bacteria, fungi or viruses. As prednisone therapy was withdrawn during a two week period, her headaches and oral ulcers recurred and a temperature of 100°F (37.8°C) was noted. An electroencephalogram, which had been normal on admission, showed nonspecific and mild bitemporal dysrhythmia two weeks after the cessation of prednisone therapy. Subsequently, prednisone in doses from 10 to 15 mg was given because of the headache and ulcerative episodes.

In April 1973, the patient noticed "numbness" in her right hand and forearm associated with intense headache, nausea and vomiting. During the next two to three months, the area of paresthesia involved the entire right upper and lower limbs. Prednisone, in doses of 15 mg daily, was given. Neurologic examination in July 1973 showed right hemiparesis, hypesthesia of the right hand and foot, and slurred speech. There were no visual abnormalities. An electroencephalogram showed the same bitemporal dysrhythmia as was seen in May 1972. An EMI-scan of the brain showed a linear lucency in the right midtemporal region. A roentgenogram of the head was within normal limits, and an echoencephalogram showed no shift of the midline structures. A cerebrospinal fluid examination showed 9 lymphocytes and 1 polymorphonuclear leukocyte/mm^3, a protein content of 31 mg/dl and 12 per cent gamma globulin. Cultures of the cerebrospinal fluid for mycobacteria and viruses were negative. Serologic testing for fungi revealed none. The hemoglobin level was 10.2 g/dl, leukocyte count 4,700/mm^3 and erythrocyte sedimentation rate 13 mm in 1 hour. Prednisone, in a dosage of 60 mg on alternate days, and azathioprine, in 150 mg daily doses, were administered; the doses of these medications were gradually reduced during the next seven months to 10 mg of prednisone and 50 mg of azathioprine daily. The patient's neurologic status was stable initially, but the intermittent headache and oral ulcerations continued. In 1974, she was admitted to her local hospital on 10 occasions because of recurrent meningitis with headache and fever. For each recurrence she was treated with an increase in steroid dose, but relapse would occur as the dosage was lowered below 15 mg daily. When last seen in February 1975, the neurologic status was unchanged but the patient had 5 lymphocytes/mm^3 in the cerebrospinal fluid. Treatment with 100 mg of azathioprine and 20 mg of prednisone daily was reinstituted.

Case 4. A 20 year old woman was examined in August 1974 because of neurologic incapacity from recent encephalitis. The patient had been in normal health until December 1973, when she was ill for three weeks with sore throat, fever, roughening of tongue papillae and aphthous oral ulcers. She was treated with penicillin; although she returned to work in January 1974, she did not feel well. In February 1974, fever with temperatures of 104°F (40.0°C), bilateral hand clumsiness, gait ataxia and vomiting developed. On admission to her local hospital in March 1974, she was lethargic, dysarthric and ataxic, and she had intention tremor and incoordination of the hands. Studies, including carotid arteriograms, pneumoencephalogram and isotope brain scan, revealed no abnormalities. An electroencephalogram showed "minor abnormalities." The lumbar cerebrospinal fluid was under normal pressure and had a total protein content of 58 mg/dl, 24 white blood cells/mm^3, and normal glucose and chloride concentrations. The cerebrospinal fluid test for syphilis was negative. Six days later, the cerebrospinal fluid protein level was 124 mg/dl, and there were 352 white blood cells/mm^3, with negative viral cultures. Dexamethasone therapy was started, and her upper limb incoordination and gait ataxia lessened.

She was referred to another medical center, with a presumptive diagnosis of viral encephalitis. Neurologic abnormalities then included mental dullness, generalized muscle weakness but worse proximally, bilateral ptosis, dysarthria, horizontal and vertical nystagmus, marked gait ataxia, and ataxia and dysmetria of the upper limbs.

The leukocyte count was 18,200/mm^3, with 85 per cent polymorphonuclear leukocytes, and the erythrocyte sedimentation rate was 16 mm in 1 hour. The antinuclear antibody test was negative, as were tests for rheumatoid factor, heterophil agglutination, and blood and throat cultures. The serum IgG level was slightly elevated.

A cerebrospinal fluid examination showed a total protein content of 44 mg/dl, 136 erythrocytes/mm^3, 12 lymphocytes/mm^3 and 11.4 per cent gamma globulin. Steroid therapy was discontinued, and a repeat cerebrospinal fluid examination showed 132 white blood cells/mm^3, total protein 50 mg/dl and 4.5 per cent gamma globulin. An isotope brain scan showed slightly increased uptake of radioactivity in the left hemisphere, which was believed to emanate from within the sigmoid sinus. The computerized transaxial tomography scan showed decreased density in the left inferior temporal lobe and prominence of the left sylvian fissure, suggestive of encephalomalacia. The electroencephalogram was within normal limits. Study of cells from the uterine cervix showed dysplasia, and a biopsy specimen of the cervix demonstrated dysplasia and chronic cervicitis.

When dexamethasone therapy was withdrawn, her fever recurred and the neurologic findings worsened. Partial palsies of the left sixth and seventh cranial nerves were noted. Aphthous stomatitis also recurred. Neither uveitis nor vaginal ulcers was present. Proctoscopic examination and a roentgenographic study of the colon disclosed no abnormalities. Methylprednisolone was given in the dosage of 32 mg daily, orally, and the neurologic and aphthous exacerbations subsided to the status on admission; with the gradual reduction in the dose of methylprednisolone to 16 mg daily, and despite intensive physiotherapy during the next three months, her condition was unchanged.

On our examination in August 1974, she was Cushingoid, in a wheelchair and displayed pathologic emotionality of the pseudobulbar type. The neurologic examination revealed ataxic dysarthria, marked ataxia of gait and all four limbs, resting tremor and reduced alternate motion rate of the hands, and hyperactive deep tendon reflexes in the four extremities. The Babinski response was flexor bilaterally.

Papillary lesions up to 2 cm in size were present on the labia minora and fourchette. The cervical smear showed dysplasia (class III). Biopsy specimens from the vaginal lesions showed epithelial dysplasia and papillary hyperplasia. These lesions were electrocoagulated, and cervical conization was carried out. Histologic study showed cervical dysplasia and an area of grade 3 squamous cell carcinoma in situ. No virus was cultured from the vagina. Studies of serum proteins and antinuclear antibodies were negative.

The neurologic status did not change as a result of a temporary increase in steroid dosage; when the patient was dismissed to her home community, she was receiving 16 mg of methylprednisolone orally each day, with the suggestion that the dose be very gradually reduced as tolerated. By December, her daily dosage was 8 mg and no new neurologic events had occurred.

Case 5. A 49 year old man came to our clinic in April 1974 because of headache and fever. Penile ulcers had developed in October 1973, which lasted a month. Episodes of aphthous stomatitis occurred in November 1973 and again in January 1974, in association with headaches.

The occipital headache was aggravated by coughing and associated with sweating and oral temperature elevations to 100.6°F (38.1°C).

The patient's father had died of "encephalitis" at the age of 39 years. The patient had experienced occasional oral aphthae since the age of 30 years. The results of physical examination were within normal limits except for the oral temperature of 100°F (37.8°C).

However, the lumbar puncture revealed 52 white blood cells/mm^3, all lymphocytes, a total protein level of 47 mg/dl and a glucose concentration of 50 mg/dl. Gram stain of cerebrospinal fluid showed no organisms, and cerebrospinal fluid cultures for fungi, yeasts, bacteria and viruses were negative. The erythrocyte sedimentation rate was 8 mm in 1 hour, and serum protein electrophoresis revealed albumin 4.08 g/dl, alpha$_1$-globulin 0.24 g/dl, alpha$_2$-globulin 0.54 g/dl, beta globulin 0.88 g/dl and gamma globulin 1.14 g/dl. The electroencephalogram was within normal limits. Roentgenograms of the head revealed no abnormalities, but those of the sinuses showed thickened membranes in both antra and ethmoids.

A serum complement fixation titer for herpes simplex virus was 1:32 and for herpes zoster 1:16 (not repeated).

Aspirin was prescribed for headache and fever, and the patient was dismissed with a diagnosis of possible Behçet's disease. He was advised to return for viral culturing of any recurrent mucosal ulcers.

He was seen in May 1974 because of a brief episode of acute pain in the lumbar spine after exercise. At that time, his temperature was normal and the headache was suppressed while he adhered to a regimen of 40 grains of aspirin daily. Neurologic examination showed a slightly reduced right ankle reflex and a hint of left facial weakness. He died suddenly in his local area of a myocardial infarction in September 1974. An autopsy was not performed.

Case 6. A 27 year old housewife was seen in March 1973 because of headache and a five year history of recurring oral aphthous ulcers. In the two years preceding admission, she had experienced cutaneous erythematous nodules and hypersensitivity of the skin from minor trauma, leading to ulceration and healing by scarring, as well as aphthous labial ulcers. In the summer of 1972, she had synovitis of the ankles during a flare of aphthosis, and the first episode of iritis in one eye. Although the acute uveitis responded to an oral prednisone dose of 15 mg daily, the uveitis recurred when the dose was reduced. About the same time, episodic headaches began and each lasted several days. In October 1972, dysphasia and right hemiparesis developed. The cerebrospinal fluid examination showed 200 white blood cells/mm^3. An electroencephalogram and isotope brain scan were within normal limits; carotid arteriograms showed a slight shift of anterior midline structures from left to right, suggestive of edema of the left hemisphere. Large doses of corticosteroids resulted in the clearing of symptoms, but slight reflex asymmetry persisted.

In December 1972, left uveitis developed, both anterior and posterior, for which the patient was treated with low doses of an oral corticosteroid medication. The second episode of neurologic difficulty developed in February 1973 while she was receiving oral steroid therapy. She experienced diplopia, headache, fever, stiff neck and exacerbation of the uveitis. Cerebrospinal fluid examination showed 490 white blood cells/mm^3 and a total protein level of 44 mg/dl. A second cerebral arteriogram was within normal limits. Treatment with prednisone, 100 mg orally in a single dose on alternate days, was added to a short course of intramuscular corticosteroid therapy. A week later, the cerebrospinal fluid contained 70 white blood cells/mm^3. Her vision improved, her cerebral symptoms diminished and the oral prednisone dose was reduced to 75 mg on alternate days.

Our neurologic examination disclosed pallor of the right optic disk, an incomplete right incongruous homonymous defect, hyperreflexia of the right upper and lower limbs, reduced alternate motion rate of the right extremities and an equivocal Babinski sign on the right. Her vision was normal in the right eye and 20/60 in the left. Slit-lamp examination showed inflammatory cells in the vitreous humor of each eye and a few cells on the left anterior lens capsule.

Steroid acne was present. There were no aphthous lesions. An electroencephalogram was within normal limits. The erythrocyte sedimentation rate was 32 mm in 1 hour. Results of the following were within normal limits: serum protein electrophoresis, antinuclear antibody test and rheumatoid factor. Results of cultures for viruses from earlier cerebrospinal fluid specimens were negative, and serial antibodies to herpes virus showed no increase. Behçet's disease was diagnosed; the course of the patient's illness was incompatible with herpes simplex meningoencephalitis, which had been the original diagnosis.

After the patient returned home in March 1973, the steroid dosage was reduced, but meningoencephalitis and uveitis recurred subsequently. Headache and blurred vision and worsening of right hemiparesis responded to combined treatment with an increased dose of prednisone and azathioprine, but the symptoms relapsed as the doses were decreased. The azathioprine therapy was stopped because of its reported lack of efficacy. In July 1974, the patient informed us that she had been given three injections of transfer factor, as well as cyclophosphamide and chlorambucil. At that time, she was receiving 70 mg of oral prednisone daily. She died in August 1974, and an autopsy revealed that death was due to Pneumocystis pneumonia, presumably a complication of the immunosuppressive drugs.

Case 7. A 44 year old housewife was examined in January 1973 because of weakness and slurred speech. The illness had begun in September 1970, when she had generalized paresthesias and headaches one month after her daughter had infectious mononucleosis. Initially, the serum test was positive for mononucleosis, but three months later, the test was negative despite continuing symptoms. Eight separate exacerbations of headache during the following two years were associated with diplopia (cranial nerve involved not known), fever, nuchal stiffness, dysphagia, dysarthria, arthralgia or swollen digital joints. Aphthous oral ulcers often accompanied the neurologic symptoms. Each episode was self-limited, lasting from one to three weeks. In six of the eight episodes of meningoencephalitis, cerebrospinal fluid examinations (Table III) showed pleocytosis with as many as 100 per cent lymphocytes; on one occasion, there were 52 per cent polymorphonuclear leukocytes. A cerebrospinal fluid examination between episodes showed only 14 white blood cells/mm^3 and normal gamma globulin. The serum immunoglobulin levels were normal. A search for viral, bacterial and fungal agents by culture and serology of cerebrospinal fluid had been serially repeated, always with negative results. In the month prior to admission, she experienced a right hemiparesis, gait ataxia, intermittent fever with temperatures to 104°F (40°C) orally and urinary incontinence.

On our examination, she walked with a broad-based spastic-ataxic gait, tending to fall to the left and backward. She displayed pseudobulbar crying, positive sucking reflex and increased jaw reflex. Muscle stretch reflexes were symmetrically increased in the four limbs, and she had a mild spastic right hemiparesis. There was cerebellar incoordination of the four limbs and ataxic dysarthria, and the Babinski responses were extensor bilaterally. There was no uveitis. An electroencephalogram was within normal limits. The lumbar cerebrospinal fluid examination showed a normal initial pressure, total protein 46 mg/dl, 4 lymphocytes/mm^3 and 12 per cent gamma globulin. The following were within normal limits or negative: routine blood studies, serum protein electrophoresis and immunoglobulins, antinuclear antibody, serologic studies for fungi, and cerebrospinal fluid cultures for viruses, fungi and tubercle bacilli. Because the patient's neurologic status was stable, no treatment was given. Subsequently, the patient was given corticosteroids because of recurring episodes. A communication in January 1975 indicated that she had relapses every six to eight weeks and that more difficulty had developed with pseudobulbar palsy and cerebellar dysfunction.

COMMENTS

In 1965, Wolf, Schotland and Phillips [9] reviewed the neurologic manifestations in 64 previously reported cases of Behçet's disease and estimated that manifestations were present in 10 to 25 per cent of them. The mortality rate in the 65 cases (they added one case) was 41 per cent, and death usually occurred within one year after the onset of neurologic manifestations. The clinical features in our cases resembled those reviewed by Wolf et al. and differed only in two respects: the gamma globulin level in the cerebrospinal fluid was normal in our patients and was elevated in two of three patients in their series, and there were more men than women (3:1) in their series. The reasons for the apparent predominance of the disease in men, as suggested by previous reports [3,11], have been reviewed and are unclear [18]. In two large series from North America, women predominated [2,19]. Recently, Chajek and Fainaru [20] observed neurologic complications in 12 of 41 patients with Behçet's disease. Data on spinal fluid and mode of treatment were not given. They stated that all but two patients recovered completely. However, in six of the 12, neurologic manifestations were their "major problem."

Because of the variable course of the disease, the role of corticosteroid or cytostatic treatment (or both) is difficult to evaluate. However, other than neurologic, the manifestations have been controlled with steroid treatment, and review of the published series of "neuro-Behçet" [3,9,12] disease suggests that prevention of neurologic relapses and even death may depend on the administration of large doses of corticosteroids.

The noninfectious disorders from which Behçet's meningoencephalitis needs to be differentiated [21] include (1) Mollaret's meningitis, in which brief episodes of aseptic meningitis without encephalitis recur; (2) sarcoidosis, usually associated with noncaseous granulomas in extracranial sites; and (3) Harada's syndrome (probably synonymous with Vogt-Koyanagi's syndrome) [21], characterized by retinal edema, uveitis and meningoencephalitis, and commonly associated with vitiligo and alopecia. In none of these three disorders does aphthosis occur.

Herpes simplex meningoencephalitis [22,23] is an acute pyrexial illness with a peculiar predilection for the temporal lobes; dementia, seizures and coma are common. Antiherpetic antibody titers in the serum and cerebrospinal fluid usually are elevated after the first week or two, but a definitive diagnosis is based on viral isolation or on microscopic direct immunofluorescence of brain tissue [22,23]. Despite certain clinical clues that Behçet's disease and its associated meningoencephalitis resemble infections by herpes virus hominis, the evidence against implication of this virus in our patient is overwhelming: (1) serum obtained during the acute and convalescent phase from two patients contained no antibody; (2) cerebrospinal fluid titers in two other patients were less than 1:2; and (3) herpes virus was not grown in cultures of ulcerative lesions from four patients. The single positive isolate was from a genital herpetic ulcer of an immunosuppressed patient (Case 1) whose cerebrospinal fluid titer was less than 1:2.

Brain tissue was not obtained for study after any of the three deaths in our series. However, such material has been amply described in other reports [9,14,16] and has revealed meningitis; foci of softening in gray and white matter, often in relation to blood vessels; gliosis with minimal if any demyelination; and cerebral infarction, with infrequently demonstrated frank central nervous system vasculitis.

Whether Behçet's disease is due to a specific virus or whether it is an immune response to an unknown substance has long been debated. In a review of 10 previous cases, we studied the evidence for each [2]. Support for a viral cause was never provided by direct inoculations of pathologic material in cellular laboratory media. Rather it came from inoculations of cerebrospinal fluid into rabbits [24] and of posterior uveal tissue into chorioallantoic membranes, with subsequent passage intracerebrally into mice to cause encephalitis [25]. Further evidence for the presence of a viral agent was provided by Evans, Pallis and Spillane [13], who homogenized the brain of a patient who died, placed the material in chorioallantoic membranes of hen eggs, and passaged a strain that could be neutralized by the serums of six of 11 patients with Behçet's disease but not by the serums of normal control subjects. A critique of the claims for a viral etiology was made by Dowling and associates [26] in 1961, who concluded that it was unproved. However, recent evidence shows that chronic neurologic disease can be caused by "slow viruses," for example, measles virus in subacute sclerosing panencephalitis [27] and unnamed viruses in kuru [28] and Jakob-Creutzfeldt's disease [29]. Because of this recent evidence and because new virologic technics demonstrating slow virus (for example, direct intracerebral inoculation of material from patients with fatal cases of Behçet's disease into monkeys' brains) have not been reported in Behçet's disease, a viral agent may yet be shown to be responsible.

Evidence of altered immunity in Behçet's disease has been provided by several workers [11,30], but a coherent basis for autoimmunity is lacking. The possible immunologic abnormalities include elevated levels of serum alpha$_2$ and gamma globulins [2,11], increased circulating antibodies to human mucosal cells [2,11,30] and lymphocytes that show cytotoxicity to homogenates or cultures of oral epithelium [31]. Studies of T cell function in 15 of our patients with Behçet's disease have not shown any abnormality, as measured by lymphocyte response to phytohemagglutinin or mixed lymphocyte culture [32]. A study of circulating immune complexes in blood and cerebrospinal fluid would be of interest.

Although we [2] and others [7] have written about the unpredictable effect of steroids on the neurologic complications, this aspect requires qualification. There have been no controlled studies using steroids or other therapeutic agents in this disease. Several investigators have concluded that corticosteroids suppress the neurologic manifestations [9,12,33]. These agents do suppress the other systemic findings, including uveitis. Our limited observations suggest that the administration of prednisone in initial doses of 60 mg daily can control or suppress evidence of meningoencephalitis, including pleocytosis and headache, and that such doses are warranted as soon as the diagnosis is made. Too often, diagnosis and treatment are delayed by prolonged microbiologic investigation—after the process has established itself in the central nervous system. At this stage, corticosteroids are only palliative. The single patient in our study (Case 2) who was given prompt treatment (Behçet's disease had been diagnosed before central nervous system involvement), first with prednisone and later with azathioprine plus prednisone, has done well. Uncontrolled observations with the use of such cytotoxic agents as azathioprine [34] and chlorambucil [35] have been made. Each has been reported to be beneficial. Others [2,7] claim favorable response to transfusions of fresh blood or plasma but not when reexamined in a prospective trial [36]. Reports on the use of transfer factor, which was tried because of the initial enthusiasm over blood-component therapy, have suggested temporary improvement in five of seven patients [37,38]. However, future studies of therapy in Behçet's disease should include controlled trials; because of rarity of the disease, these trials probably should be carried out in a collaborative study in many centers. In the meantime, we believe that corticosteroids remain the mainstay of treatment. With prompt diagnosis of Behçet's disease, treatment with corticosteroids possibly might avert the neurologic catastrophies that remain the major cause of disability.

REFERENCES

1. Behçet H: Über rezidivierende, aphthöse, durch ein Virus verursachte Geschwüre am Mund, am Auge und an den Genitalien. Dermatol Monatsschr 105: 1152, 1937.
2. O'Duffy JD, Carney JA, Deodhar S: Behçet's disease: report of 10 cases, 3 with new manifestations. Ann Intern Med 75: 561, 1971.
3. Kalbian VV, Challis MT: Behçet's disease: report of 12 cases with three manifesting as papilledema. Am J Med 49: 823, 1970.
4. Mason RM, Barnes CG: Behçet's syndrome with arthritis. Ann Rheum Dis 28: 95, 1969.
5. Nazzaro P: Cutaneous manifestations of Behçet's disease: clinical and histopathological findings. Symposium on Behçet's Disease, Rome, 1964, (Monacelli M, Nazzaro P, eds), Basel, Switzerland, S. Karger AG, 1966, p 15.
6. Bøe J, Dalgaard JB, Scott D: Mucocutaneous-ocular syndrome with intestinal involvement: a clinical and pathological study of four fatal cases. Am J Med 25: 857, 1958.
7. Haim S, Sherf K: Behcet's disease: presentation of 11 cases and evaluation of treatment. Isr J Med Sci 2: 69, 1966.

8. Enoch BA, Castillo-Olivares JL, Khoo TCL, Grainger RG, Henry L: Major vascular complications in Behçet's syndrome. Postgrad Med J 44: 453, 1968.
9. Wolf SM, Schotland DL, Phillips LL: Involvement of nervous system in Behcet's syndrome. Arch Neurol 12: 315, 1965.
10. O'Duffy JD: Proposes pour le diagnostic de la maladie de Behçet et notes therapeutiques. Revue Méd 36: 2371, 1974.
11. Oshima Y, Shimizu T, Yokohari R, Matsumoto T, Kano K, Kagami T, Nagaya H: Clinical studies on Behçet's syndrome. Ann Rheum Dis 22: 36, 1963.
12. Phillips DL, Scott JS: Recurrent genital and oral ulceration with associated eye lesions: Behçet's syndrome. Lancet 1: 366, 1955.
13. Evans AD, Pallis CA, Spillane JD: Involvement of the nervous system in Behçet's syndrome: report of three cases and isolation of virus. Lancet 2: 349, 1957.
14. Strouth JC, Dyken M: Encephalopathy of Behcet's disease: report of a case. Neurology 14: 794, 1964.
15. Whitty CWM: Neurologic implications of Behcet's syndrome. Neurology 8: 369, 1958.
16. McMenemey WH, Lawrence BJ: Encephalomyelopathy in Behçet's disease: report of necropsy findings in two cases. Lancet 2: 353, 1957.
17. Pallis CA, Fudge BJ: The neurological complications of Behçet's syndrome. Arch Neurol Psychiatr 75: 1, 1956.
18. O'Duffy JD: Behçet's disease (letter to the editor). Ann Intern Med 76: 333, 1972.
19. Cummings N: Personal communication.
20. Chajek T, Fainaru M: Behçet's disease: report of 41 cases and a review of the literature. Medicine (Baltimore) 54: 179, 1975.
21. Hermans PE, Goldstein NP, Wellman WE: Mollaret's meningitis and differential diagnosis of recurrent meningitis: report of case, with review of the literature. Am J Med 52: 128, 1972.
22. Lynch PG, Longson MR: Herpes simplex encephalitis: a report of three further cases. Pathol Eur 8: 149, 1973.
23. Juel-Jensen BE, MacCallum FO: Herpes Simplex Varicella and Zoster: Clinical Manifestations and Treatment. Philadelphia, J. B. Lippincott Co., 1972, p 53.
24. Alm L, Öberg L, Djurförsök Vid SK: Behcet's syndrom: preliminärt meddelande. Nord Med 25: 603, 1945.
25. Sezer FN: The isolation of a virus as the cause of Behçet's disease. Am J Ophthalmol 36: 301, 1953.
26. Dowling GB, Dudgeon JA, Perkins ES: Discussion on Behçet's disease. Proc R Soc Med 54: 101, 1961.
27. Horta-Barbosa L, Fuccilo DA, Sever JL: Subacute sclerosing panencephalitis: isolation of measles virus from a brain biopsy. Nature (Lond) 221: 974, 1969.
28. Peterson DA, Wolfe LG, Deinhardt F, et al.: Transmission of kuru and Creutzfeldt-Jakob disease to marmoset monkeys. Intervirology 2: 14, 1973.
29. Gibbs CJ Jr, Gajdusek DC, Asher DM, et al.: Creutzfeldt-Jakob disease (spongiform encephalopathy): transmission to the chimpanzee. Science 161: 388, 1968.
30. Lehner T: Characterization of mucosal antibodies in recurrent aphthous ulceration and Behçet's syndrome. Arch Oral Biol 14: 843, 1969.
31. Rogers RS, Sams WM Jr, Shorter RG: Lymphocytotoxicity in recurrent aphthous stomatitis: lymphocytotoxicity for oral epithelial cells in recurrent aphthous stomatitis and Behcet syndrome. Arch Dermatol 109: 361, 1974.
32. Taswell H, O'Duffy JD: Unpublished data.
33. Fowler TJ, Humpston DJ, Nussey AM, Small M: Behçet's syndrome with neurological manifestations in two sisters. Br Med J 2: 473, 1968.
34. Rosselet E, Saudan Y, Zenklusen G: Les effets de l'azathioprine ("Imuran") dans la maladie de Behçet: premiers résultats thérapeutiques. Ophthalmologia 156: 218, 1968.
35. Mamo JG, Azzam SA: Treatment of Behçet's disease with chlorambucil. Arch Ophthalmol 84: 446, 1970.
36. O'Duffy JD, Taswell HF: Blood transfusion therapy in Behçet's disease (letter to the editor). Ann Intern Med 80: 279, 1974.
37. Bernhard GC, Heim LR: Transfer factor treatment of Behçet's disease. Proceedings of the VI Pan-American Congress on Rheumatic Diseases, Toronto, 1974, p 18.
38. Wolf RE, Fudenberg HH, Spitler LE, Ziff M: Treatment of Behçet's syndrome with transfer factor. Proceedings of the 39th Annual Meeting of the American Rheumatism Association, New Orleans, 1975, p 32.

Hereditary Antithrombin III Deficiency

Effect of Antithrombin III Deficiency on Platelet Function

ANGELINA CARVALHO, M.D.
LEONARD ELLMAN, M.D.
Boston, Massachusetts

Antithrombin III (AT III) is the main physiologic inhibitor of thrombin, and activated factors X and IX as well. Normal levels of AT III appear to be necessary to maintain blood fluidity and to prevent thrombosis. Four families with AT III deficiency and recurrent venous thromboembolism have been reported on. We present an additional family with AT III deficiency and a high incidence of thromboembolism. AT III levels were determined by both a functional and an immunologic assay. Results of platelet function tests, not previously reported in persons with AT III deficiency, were found to be normal. Following gel filtration, the platelets were very sensitive to thrombin. Thrombin-induced platelet aggregation appears to be dependent on a balance between the amount of thrombin and AT III present.

Despite intensive investigation, hypercoagulable states based on genetic defects have been infrequently identified. In 1965 Egeberg [1] first described a family in which frequent episodes of spontaneous venous thrombosis were associated with a deficiency of antithrombin III (AT III). The defect was inherited as an autosomal dominant trait. Four additional kindreds with AT III deficiency have subsequently been described [2–5]. In this communication we describe another family with AT III deficiency and a high incidence of spontaneous thromboembolism. It is the first family with AT III deficiency in which platelet function tests have been reported.

MATERIALS AND METHODS

Venous blood was collected through siliconized needles into plastic syringes. Nine volumes of blood were added to one volume of 3.8 per cent aqueous sodium citrate in plastic tubes. Control samples were obtained from healthy laboratory personnel.

The prothrombin time [6] and activated partial thromboplastin time [7] were determined according to the methods of Quick [6], and Proctor and Rapaport [7], respectively. The thrombin time was measured by a fibrometer using bovine thrombin (Parke Davis and Co., Detroit, Mich.): 0.2 ml plasma is prewarmed at 37°C for 60 seconds and an equal volume of thrombin-calcium chloride mixture (0.1 M sodium barbital, pH 7.4 in physiologic saline solution and 0.025 M calcium chloride is added leading to a final concentration of thrombin of 1 unit/ml. Fibrinogen was determined by the method of Ratnoff and Menzie [8]. Fibrin(ogen) degradation products were measured using the staphylococcal clumping technic [9]. Plasmin and plasminogen levels were determined on fibrin plates (Enzo-Diffusion Fibrin Plate Test, Hyland Labo-

From the Hematology Unit, Massachusetts General Hospital, Boston, Massachusetts. This study was in part supported by Grant HL-14209-5 from the National Heart and Lung Institute for a Specialized Center of Research in Arteriosclerosis. Requests for reprints should be addressed to Dr. A. Carvalho, Hematology Unit, Massachusetts General Hospital, Boston, Massachusetts 02114. Manuscript accepted December 8, 1975.

TABLE I Coagulation Studies

Group	Platelet Count (per mm³)	Thrombin Time (sec)	Fibrinogen (mg/100 ml)	FDP (μg/ml)	Plasminogen Antigen (mg/100 ml)	Plasminogen Activity (% normal)
Present family						
Case 1	216,000	18.3	410	4.8	12.0	100
Case 2	229,000	17.8	320	2.4	7.8	200
Case 5	245,000	17.0	480	1.2	9.6	90
Case 6	275,000	18.0	250	1.2	4.0	74
Mean	241,250	17.8	365	2.4	8.4	116
Normal subjects (26)						
Mean	250,000	20	250	4.8*	8.4*	160*
(95% range)	(150,000–350,000)	(15–25)	(150–350)	(0–9.6)	(4.76–11.4)	(70–250)

* 18 normal subjects.

ratories, Costa Mesa, Calif.). Plasminogen levels were also determined by radial immunodiffusion, as were alpha$_1$ antitrypsin and alpha$_2$ macroglobulin levels (M-Partigen Immunodiffusion Kits, Behring Diagnostics, Somerville, N.J.).

Determinations of Antithrombin III (AT III). AT III was measured by both a functional and an immunologic assay. The functional assay, based on the progressive neutralization of thrombin by test plasma, was performed according to the method of Howie et al. [10] except that Reptilase, an enzyme obtained from the venom of Bothrops atrox (purchased from Abbott Laboratories, N. Chicago, Ill.), was substituted for ancrod (Arvin®) as the defibrinating agent. The immunologic determination of AT III was performed by the radial immunodiffusion technic [11] using monospecific human AT III antiserum supplied by Behring Diagnostics, Somerville, N.J.

Platelet Function. Platelet aggregation was studied in an aggregometer (Chronolog Corp., Broomall, Pa.) according to a modification of the method of Born [12]. The aggregometer was calibrated so that the per cent transmittance of platelet-rich plasma was recorded as 0 and that of platelet-poor plasma as 100. The difference between 0 and the maximal transmittance produced by a stimulus was defined as the amplitude of response to that stimulus. Each aggregating agent was tested to determine the lowest concentration capable of inducing the same maximum degree of aggregation characteristic of that substance [13].

Aggregating Agents. Adenosine diphosphate (ADP) (Sigma Co., St. Louis, Mo.) was stored frozen at a concentration of 5×10^{-4} M in 0.1 M sodium phosphate buffer, pH 6.8, containing 0.15 M sodium chloride. A fresh solution of 1-epinephrine (Sigma) (2.5×10^{-3} M) in distilled water was prepared daily. Acid-soluble calf skin collagen, at a concentration of 5.5 mg/ml (as determined by measuring the hydroxyproline content and multiplying by 7.1) [14,15] was obtained from Worthington Biochemicals, Freehold, N.J. Collagen was diluted with Tris-hydrochloride pH 7.4. Bovine thrombin (Parke Davis Co., Detroit, Mich.) was purified according to the method of Rosenberg and Waugh [16].

Platelet ^{14}C-Serotonin Release. This was measured according to the method of Jerushalmy and Zucker [17].

Gel-filtered Platelets. Platelets from each person were separated from plasma proteins by gel filtration using a modification of the method of Tangen et al. [18]. Tyrode's buffer, without albumin, was used to suspend the platelets. To 0.5 ml of gel-filtered platelets (130,000 platelets/μl) varying concentrations of purified bovine thrombin and collagen were added, and aggregation was determined in the aggregometer.

TABLE II Antithrombin III Determination (% normal)

Groups	Immunologic Assay	Functional Assay
Present family		
Case 1	40	59
Case 2	40	59
Case 5	50	70
Case 6	35	58
Mean	41	62
Normal subjects (18)		
Mean	104	109
(95% range)	(68–140)	(88–130)

FAMILY HISTORY OF THE FAMILY

Case 1. The propositus, a 46 year old executive, had bilateral thrombophlebitis at age 38 and well-documented pulmonary embolism at age 39 and again at age 42. He has been receiving continuous Coumadin® therapy since the second episode of pulmonary embolism four years ago without recurrence of phlebitis or pulmonary embolism. When seen initially by us, he was also found to have mild hypertriglyceridemia with a type IV pattern on lipoprotein electrophoresis. His triglyceride levels have returned to normal following weight reduction.

Case 2. The wife of the propositus, a healthy 42 year old woman, has no history of thromboembolism. Her AT III level is normal.

Case 3. The older son, a 23 year old laborer, was discharged from the Armed Forces at age 21 because of thrombophlebitis and pulmonary embolism. He has had no recurrence since Coumadin therapy was started two years ago. He was also found to have mild hypertriglyceridemia and type IV hyperlipidemia.

Case 4. The older daughter had an episode of phlebitis at age 16 and died suddenly at age 18. An autopsy demonstrated the cause of death to be massive pulmonary embolism. She was not pregnant and had not been taking oral contraceptives.

TABLE III Platelet Aggregation

Groups	ADP* (μmol) PRP†	EPI* (μmol) PRP	Collagen* (μg/ml) PRP	Collagen* (μg/ml) GFP	Thrombin* (U/ml) PRP	Thrombin* (U/ml) GFP
Present family						
Case 1	1.0	1.25	110	55	0.2	0.01
Case 2	2.0	2.5	110	55	0.4	0.04
Case 5	4.0	2.5	83	58	0.4	0.01
Case 6	1.0	2.5	110	22	0.4	0.02
Mean	2.0	2.19	103	47.5	0.35	0.02
Normal subjects (26)						
Mean	1.7	3.2	88	58‡	0.4‡	0.12‡
(95% range)	(1.0–4.0)	(0.25–10)	(55–220)	(33–83)	(0.16–0.64)	(0.08–0.16)

NOTE: ADP = adenosine diphosphate; EPI = epinephrine; PRP = platelet-rich plasma; GFP = gel filtered platelets.
* Concentration of reagent required for maximal response.
† Platelet-rich plasma.
‡ Eight normal subjects tested.

Case 5. The younger daughter, 13 years old, has not had any thromboembolic episodes. Lipid studies were normal.

Case 6. The younger son, 8 years old, has also been free of thromboembolic complications. Lipoprotein electrophoresis was normal.

The parents of the propositus and his four sibs all enjoy good health; none has a history of thromboembolic complications. Unfortunately, they do not live in the area and were not available for AT III determinations.

RESULTS

Routine Laboratory Evaluation. The propositus (Case 1) and his three living children (Cases 3, 5 and 6) had normal platelet counts, thrombin times, fibrin degradation products, plasmin and plasminogen levels. The fibrinogen level was slightly elevated in the propositus and one child (Case 5) (Table I). Levels of alpha$_1$ antitrypsin and alpha$_2$ macroglobulin were normal in all family members, and agarose gel electrophoresis of serum showed no abnormalities.

Antithrombin III Assays. AT III was measured by both the functional coagulation assay and the immunoassay. Levels of AT III in the propositus and his three offspring were depressed in a parallel and significant manner in both assays (Table II). The wife (Case 2) of the propositus had normal amounts of AT III. An excellent correlation was found between the results of the coagulation and the immunoassay for both normal subjects and the members of this family.

Platelet Function Studies. The minimal concentration to produce full aggregation in platelet-rich plasma was determined for each of four aggregating agents. The subjects with AT III deficiency showed normal aggregation with ADP, l-epinephrine, collagen and thrombin (Table III). In contrast, when their platelets were separated from plasma by gel filtration, there was a marked diminution in the amount of thrombin necessary to induce maximal aggregation; a similar effect was not noted for collagen. Residual AT III was not detectable on intact gel-filtered platelets by the radioimmunodiffusion method.

Serotonin, along with other platelet constituents, is released from platelets during the second wave of aggregation. Serotonin release was normal in the subjects with AT III deficiency although uptake into the storage pool was somewhat decreased (Table IV).

TABLE IV Platelet ^{14}C-Serotonin Release (%)*

Groups	ADP (4 μmol)	EPI (12.5 μmol)	Collagen (110 μg/ml)	Thrombin (0.4 U/ml)	^{14}C-Serotonin Uptake
Present family					
Case 1	64	66	77	48	82
Case 2	38	44	40	—	81
Case 5	31	55	74	31	81
Case 6	29	40	50	39	82
Mean	41	51	60	39	82
Normal subjects (18)					
Mean	48	63	65	65	90
(95% range)	(26–70)	(39–87)	(37–93)	(40–90)	(85–95)

* Per cent released of the total ^{14}C-Serotonin taken up by platelets.

COMMENTS

Thrombin acts at the terminal portion of the coagulation cascade to cleave fibrinopeptides A and B from fibrinogen leading to fibrin polymerization and the development of fibrin clot [19]. Although the action of thrombin is inhibited by $alpha_2$ macroglobulin [20] and $alpha_1$ antitrypsin [21], the main physiologic thrombin inhibitor is AT III, which has been shown to interact stoichiometrically with thrombin [22]. It has recently been demonstrated that the AT III molecule also inhibits activated factors X [23], IX, XI and XII [24] as well as thrombin. It has also become apparent that AT III is identical to the plasma component known as heparin cofactor. The anticoagulant effect of heparin is markedly augmented in the presence of the cofactor [23,25]. AT III thus plays a central role in hemostatic regulation. The binding of AT III to thrombin and other activated coagulation factors appears to be an important biochemical safeguard to maintain blood fluidity and prevent thrombosis.

The existence of people with low levels of AT III, in many of whom deep vein thrombosis and pulmonary embolism develop, supports the biological significance of AT III [1–5]. People homozygous for AT III deficiency have not yet been identified, and this defect may not be compatible with life. The AT III levels of heterozygotes in affected kindreds have ranged from 25 to 50 per cent of normal values. A low AT III level does not invariably lead to thromboembolism and approximately one-third of the people with low levels have been free of thrombosis. Thromboembolic complications have not been reported in affected persons below the age of 10. Acquired deficiency of AT III occurs in women using estrogen-containing contraceptives [26], in people with cirrhosis [27] and in people of advanced age [1,26]. AT III levels are frequently depressed shortly after a thrombotic episode, and this has been attributed to enhanced consumption during clot formation [22,28].

AT III deficiency has been inherited as an autosomal dominant trait in the four kindreds previously reported on [1–5]. Although only a limited number of the members in our family were available for testing, the inheritance also appears to follow an autosomal dominant pattern. It seems very likely that the daughter of the propositus, who had thrombophlebitis at age 16 and died of pulmonary embolism at age 18, was also deficient in AT III. It is perhaps noteworthy that the propositus and his eldest son have type IV hyperlipoproteinemia in addition to AT III deficiency.

Results of platelet function studies have not previously been reported in a family with AT III deficiency. These test results were normal in our family including platelet aggregation in response to the administration of ADP, l-epinephrine, collagen and thrombin, and release of serotonin during the second wave of platelet aggregation. Of interest was the finding that in platelets separated from plasma by gel filtration the amount of thrombin necessary to induce aggregation was markedly reduced. Although we were unable to detect residual AT III on intact gel-filtered platelets because of the relative insensitivity of the immunoassay, we suspect that small amounts remained on their surfaces. AT III-deficient platelets were more reactive to low concentrations of thrombin in the aggregation, probably because less AT III remained on their surfaces. Thrombin-induced platelet aggregation probably involves a balance between the presence of thrombin and platelet bound AT III.

AT III can be measured by both a functional and an immunologic assay. Functional assays of AT III are based on the progressive neutralization of thrombin by test plasma or serum. If serum is used as a source of AT III, levels will be lower than in plasma due to the inactivation of AT III during in vitro clotting [28]. When AT III is measured in plasma, prior removal of the fibrinogen is essential since thrombin is strongly adsorbed to fibrinogen. The defibrination procedure, however, has proved difficult since heat-defibrination may cause loss of AT III activity and thrombin-induced defibrination will lead to variable test results depending on the strength of the thrombin used [10]. In 1973, Howie et al. [10] introduced an AT III assay based on defibrination by ancrod (Arvin), the venom of the Malayan pit viper Agkistrodon rhodostrom. Our functional AT III assay utilizes Howie's method, but substitutes Reptilase, a similar enzyme isolated from the venom of Bothrops atrox, which also induced defibrination without consumption of AT III.

AT III was also assayed by the radial immunodiffusion technic. This assay shows excellent correlation with the functional assay, is simple to perform and the reagents, including the antiserum, are commercially available. Thus, the immunologic assay is well suited as a screening test for AT III deficiency. It should be noted, however, that in one of the previously described kindreds the AT III deficiency was due to the presence of a functionally inactive AT III molecule which gave a normal result in the immunologic test [2]. A similar, but acquired disturbance in AT III synthesis has been reported following l-asparaginase therapy in leukemia [29]. Thus, some subjects with AT III deficiency will be missed if the immunologic test alone is used to screen for AT III deficiency.

In the AT III-deficient kindred described by Marciniak et al. [4], treatment with Coumadin led to a striking rise in AT III levels. This was attributed to either a lower utilization of AT III because of the decrease in levels of vitamin K-dependent coagulation factors, or to a direct effect of Coumadin on AT III synthesis. These findings remain to be confirmed in additional families with AT III deficiency. By whatever mechanism, Coumadin appears to be effective therapy in patients with hereditary AT III deficiency. In our family the two adults with AT III deficiency have not had a recurrence of thromboembolism since Coumadin therapy was started. In view of the high incidence of thromboembolism in the kindreds so far reported on, prophylactic Coumadin therapy should be considered in persons discovered to have hereditary AT III deficiency.

ACKNOWLEDGMENT

We wish to express our appreciation to Reginald Pew, M.D. for calling the family to our attention, and to R. A. Vaillancourt and Rae B. Cabral for their expert technical assistance.

REFERENCES

1. Egeberg O: Inherited antithrombin deficiency causing thrombophilia. Thromb Diath Haemorrh 13: 516, 1965.
2. Van Der Meer J, Stoepman-van Dalen EA, Jensen JMS: Antithrombin III deficiency in a Dutch family. J Clin Pathol 26: 532, 1973.
3. Sas G, Blasko G, Bânhegyi D, et al.: Abnormal antithrombin III (Antithrombin III "Budapest") as a cause of a familial thrombophilia. Thromb Diath Haemorrh 32: 105, 1974.
4. Marciniak E, Farley CH, DeSimone PA: Familial thrombosis due to antithrombin III deficiency. Blood 43: 219, 1974.
5. Shapiro SS, Prager D, Martinez J: Inherited antithrombin III deficiency associated with multiple thromboembolic phenomena (abstract). Blood 42: 1001, 1973.
6. Quick AJ: On quantitative estimation of prothrombin. Am J Clin Pathol 15: 560, 1945.
7. Proctor RR, Rapaport SI: The partial thromboplastin time with kaolin. A simple screening test for first stage plasma clotting factor deficiencies. Am J Clin Pathol 36: 212, 1961.
8. Ratnoff OD, Menzie C: A new method for the determination of fibrinogen in small samples of plasma. J Lab Clin Med 37: 316, 1951.
9. Carvalho AC, Ellman LL, Colman RW: A comparison of the staphylococcal clumping test and an agglutination test for detection of fibrinogen degradation products. Am J Clin Pathol 62: 107, 1974.
10. Howie PW, Prentice CRM, McNicol GP: A method of antithrombin estimation using plasma defibrinated with ancrod. Br J Haematol 25: 101, 1973.
11. Mancini G, Carbonara CO, Heremans JP: Immunochemical quantitation of antigens by single radial immunodiffusion. Immunochemistry 2: 235, 1965.
12. Born GVR: Aggregation of blood platelets by adenosine diphosphate and its reversal. Nature (Lond) 194: 927, 1962.
13. Carvalho AC, Colman RW, Lees RS: Platelet function in hyperlipoproteinemia. N Engl J Med 290: 434, 1974.
14. Gallop PM, Seifter S: Preparation and properties of soluble collagen. Methods Enzymol 6: 635, 1963.
15. Chesney CM, Harper E, Colman RW: Critical role of the carbohydrate side chains of collagen in platelet aggregation. J Clin Invest 51: 2693, 1972.
16. Rosenberg RD, Waugh DP: Multiple bovine thrombin components. J Biol Chem 245: 5049, 1970.
17. Jerushalmy Z, Zucker MB: Some effects of fibrinogen degradation products (FDP) on blood platelets. Thromb Diath Haemorrh 25: 413, 1971.
18. Tangen O, Berman HJ, Marfey P: Gel filtration. A new technique for separation of blood platelets from plasma. Thromb Diath Haemorrh 25: 268, 1971.
19. Blombäck B, Blombäck M, Hessel B, Iwanga S: Structure of N-terminal fragments of fibrinogen and specificity of thrombin. Nature (Lond) 215: 1445, 1967.
20. Lanchantin GF, Plesset ML, Friedmann JA, Hart DW: Dissociation of esterolytic and clotting activities of thrombin by trypsin binding macroglobulin. Proc Soc Exp Biol Med 121: 444, 1966.
21. Rimon A, Shamash Y, Shapiro B: The plasmin inhibitor of human plasma. IV. Its action on plasmin, trypsin, chymotrypsin and thrombin. J Biol Chem 241: 5102, 1966.
22. Abildgaard U: Binding of thrombin to antithrombin III. Scand J Clin Lab Invest 24: 23, 1969.
23. Yin ET, Wessler S, Stoll PJ: Identity of plasma-activated factor X inhibitor with anti-thrombin III and heparin co-factor. J Biol Chem 246: 3712, 1971.
24. Rosenberg RD, Damus PS: The purification and mechanism of action of human anti-thrombin heparin co-factor. J Biol Chem 248: 6490, 1973.
25. Monkhouse FC, France ES, Seegers WH: Studies on the antithrombin and heparin co-factor activities of a fraction adsorbed from plasma by aluminum hydroxide. Circ Res 3: 397, 1955.
26. Fagerhol MK, Abildgaard U: Immunological studies on human antithrombin III. Influence of age, sex and use of oral contraceptives on serum concentration. Scand J Haematol 7: 10, 1970.
27. Abildgaard U, Fagerhol ML, Egeberg O: Comparison of progressive antithrombin activity and the concentrations of three thrombin inhibitors in human plasma. Scand J Clin Lab Invest 26: 349, 1970.
28. Seegers WH, Miller KD, Andrews EB, Murphy RC: Fundamental interactions and the effect of storage, ether, adsorbants and blood clotting on plasma antithrombin activity. Am J Physiol 169: 700, 1952.
29. Conrad J, Durant G, Feger J: Acquired abnormal antithrombin III in l-asparaginase treated patients. IVth International Congress on Thrombosis and Haemastases, Abstracts, Vienna, 1973, p 228.

Renal Responses to PTH in Patients with Hormone-Resistant (Pseudo) Hypoparathyroidism

ARNOLD M. MOSES, M.D.
NEIL BRESLAU, M.D.
RICHARD COULSON, Ph.D.
Syracuse, New York

Five patients with pseudohypoparathyroidism were compared to normal subjects and patients with hypoparathyroidism in their ability to respond to the infusion of parathyroid hormone (PTH) by altering excretion of calcium, sodium, potassium, phosphate and bicarbonate. In patients with pseudohypoparathyroidism, impairment in renal responses to PTH was more generalized than has been recognized. The patterns of responses varied from patient to patient. The most commonly observed abnormality, aside from lack of increase in urinary cyclic adenosine 5′-monophosphate (AMP), was failure to decrease the calcium to sodium clearance ratio, an indication of impaired renal calcium reabsorption. The responses which most closely approximated normal, including a normal decrease in the calcium to sodium clearance ratio, occurred in a patient (Case 1) who had the largest, although impaired, response in cyclic AMP excretion. Conversely, the most abnormal responses occurred in three patients (Cases 2, 4 and 5) who had the smallest increases in cyclic AMP excretion after the administration of PTH. The impaired renal reabsorption of calcium after the administration of PTH (lack of decrease in calcium to sodium clearance ratio) may, when present, be in part responsible for hypocalcemia.

Albright and associates [1] were the first to demonstrate that the chemical abnormalities of pseudohypoparathyroidism were due to resistance to the action of parathyroid hormone (PTH). This was based on the observation that such patients had subnormal phosphaturic responses to the administration of PTH. Because of current usage, we will in this paper refer to this entity as pseudohypoparathyroidism, although we believe that hormone-resistant hypoparathyroidism is a more appropriate term [2]. The markedly impaired urinary excretion of cyclic AMP in response to the administration of PTH in these patients was first demonstrated by Chase et al. [3] and has been found in all but three reported cases [3–5]. The usual explanation for the hypocalcemia in these patients is that it results from insensitivity of skeletal tissue to PTH, or that it is caused by hyperphosphatemia, which in turn results from a diminished phosphaturic response to PTH [6]. Because we were aware of a patient with pseudohypoparathyroidism (Case 2) whose serum phosphate level was normal when she was untreated and hypocalcemic, and since similar cases have been observed [3], and because there is no information on renal tubular responses to the administration of PTH (other than phosphate and cyclic AMP) of patients with pseudohypoparathyroidism, we conducted the present

From the VA Hospital and Departments of Medicine and Pharmacology, State University of New York, Upstate Medical Center, Syracuse, New York 13210. This research was supported by Veterans Administration Research Funds, Grant 5855-01; and Grant RR-229 from the General Clinical Research Centers Program of the Division of Research Resources, National Institutes of Health, Bethesda, Maryland; and U.S. Public Health Service Research Grant 2ROI-AM 14401-04. Requests for reprints should be addressed to Dr. Arnold M. Moses, VA Hospital, 800 Irving Avenue, Syracuse, New York 13210. Manuscript accepted December 5, 1975.

TABLE I Characteristics of Patients with Pseudohypoparathyroidism

Case No.	Age (yr) and Sex	Weight (kg)	Age (yr) at Time of Diagnosis	Pretreatment Serum Calcium (meq/liter)	Pretreatment Phosphate (mg/dl)	Pretreatment Alkaline Phosphatase (K-AU)	Physical Characteristics
1	18,F	77.3	13	2.75	8.1	80	Stocky build, round face, short fingers
2	50,F	90.9	45	2.75	3.3	8.2	Round face, thick, short fingers
3	24,F	63.6	19	2.55	6.4	25	Normal
4	20,F	49.9	20	3.1	5.6	...	Short stature
5	24,F	102.9	10	3.3	8.3	...	Short stature, thick set body build, round face, short neck, shortened fourth metacarpals

NOTE: K-AU = King-Armstrong units.

experiments. We were particularly interested in determining whether or not a defect occurs in renal calcium reabsorption, a mechanism which is important for the maintenance of normal serum calcium concentrations [7,8].

METHODS

Eleven normal, three hypoparathyroid and five pseudohypoparathyroid subjects were studied after obtaining their informed consent. The normal subjects consisted of seven male and four female healthy, nonhospitalized volunteers who ranged in age from 20 to 52 years, and in weight from 56.8 to 73.5 kg. The hypoparathyroid patients included two women (25 and 54 years of age; 68.2 and 61.2 kg) in whom hypoparathyroidism developed after thyroidectomy and one man (53 years of age; 75.2 kg) who had idiopathic hypoparathyroidism. These three patients all appeared normal, had chronic hypocalcemia, hyperphosphatemia, low circulating PTH levels (analyzed by Upjohn Laboratory, Kalamazoo, Michigan, using a radioimmunoassay procedure) and normal urinary excretion of cyclic AMP in response to infused PTH.

The characteristics of the five patients with pseudohypoparathyroidism are presented in Table I. All these patients had chronic hypocalcemia, and four of five had hyperphosphatemia prior to therapy. All had markedly impaired urinary excretion of cyclic AMP in response to the intravenous administration of PTH (Figure 1, Table II). PTH measurements were obtained in two patients (Cases 4 and 5) and levels were elevated. One patient (Case 5) had a value of 1,319 pg/ml (Bio Science Laboratories: normal to 500 pg/ml). Another (Case 4) had two serum PTH assays performed by Dr. Eric Reiss on blood obtained when she was hypocalcemic. The values were 299 and 585 μl eq/ml (normal: 10 to 60 μl eq/ml). Two of the other three patients (Cases 1 and 3) had high serum alkaline phosphatase levels, which decreased to normal after treatment. These two patients also had evidence of subperiosteal bone resorption. Only one patient (Case 5) had the typical features of Albright's osteodystrophy. She was initially evaluated at seven years of age because of short stature and delayed physical and mental growth. At that time she had a normal serum calcium concentration and was reported as having a case of pseudopseudohypoparathyroidism [9]. Subsequently, hypocalcemia and hyperphosphatemia developed. Three of the patients consisted of a mother (Case 2) and two of her daughters (Cases 1 and 3).

All patients continued vitamin D and calcium therapy without interruption, including the day of the study. An intravenous infusion of 250 U PTH (Lilly Parathyroid Injection USP, 100 U/ml, Lot No. 7mm22A, 7mm22D and 8GE52A) was given to each of the subjects in 50 ml of isotonic dextrose over 15 minutes, starting at 9 A.M. The subjects had fasted for at least 9 hours. A large dose of PTH was used because we did not want a failure of response possibly to indicate inadequate stimulation. It is recognized that the dose of PTH used in this experiment is in excess of the amount normally present physiologically, and probably resulted in levels even greater than those present in patients with pseudohypoparathyroidism.

Urine was collected hourly for 2 hours before the infusion and for 3 hours afterward. Each subject was given 200 ml water at the start of the experiment, and an additional 50 ml water after each hourly urine sample was collected, in order to insure adequate urine volume. All urine specimens were analyzed for volume and sodium, potassium, creatinine, calcium, phosphate, cyclic AMP, pH and carbon dioxide content. The bicarbonate concentration was calculated from the last two parameters, using the Henderson-Hasselbalch equation. The pK_a of the bicarbonate was estimated for each urine sample, using the formula $pK_a = 6.33 - 0.5 \times \sqrt{B}$, in which B represents the total cation concentration, estimated in the urine as the sum of the sodium and potassium concentrations [5]. Blood samples were collected just before starting the PTH infusion and hourly thereafter for the next 3 hours, and calcium, phosphate, sodium, potassium and glucose contents were determined. The cyclic AMP content of the urine specimens was assayed by competitive protein binding [10]. Creatinine concentrations were determined by Technicon® Autoanalyzer, and phosphate concentrations were calculated as phosphorus, using a modified Gomori technic [11]. Sodium and potassium content were measured by flame photometry, and calcium by atomic absorption spectrophotometry. Total calcium, not the ultrafilterable fraction, was measured because of preliminary observations that the conditions of this study did not alter the ultrafilterable fraction. The hourly output of each urinary substance was recorded, and for each hour of the study the ratio of the cal-

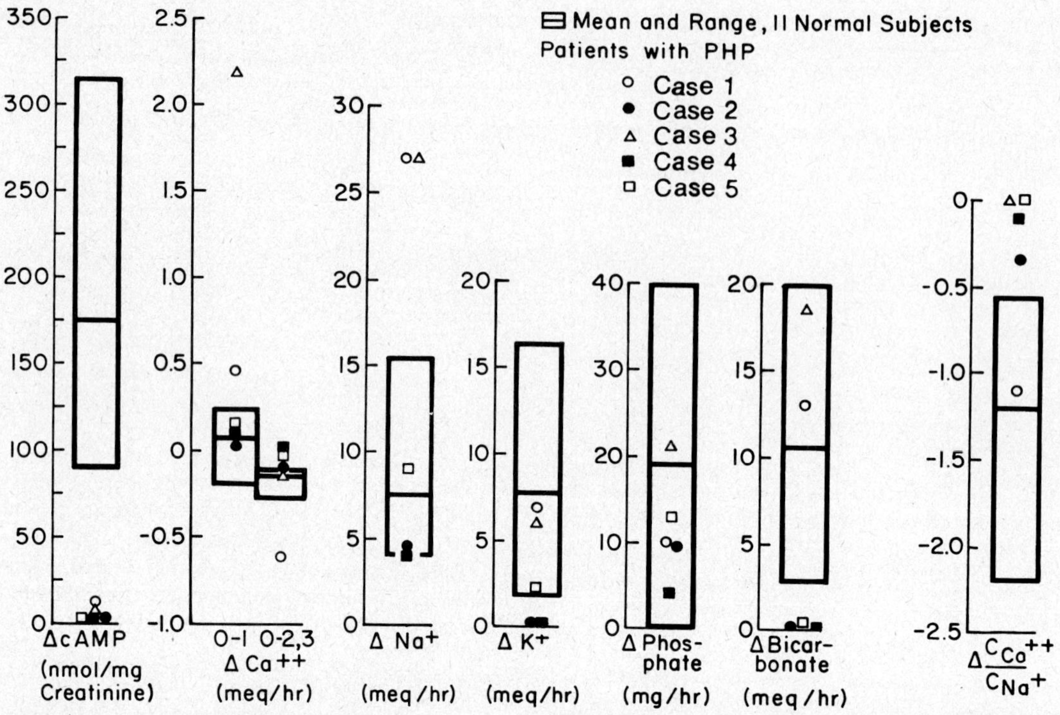

Figure 1. *Changes in the urinary excretion of cyclic AMP, ions and the calcium to sodium clearance ratio following the infusion of 250 U PTH. The rectangles encompass the ranges of responses and the horizontal lines the mean responses in the 11 normal subjects; the symbols represent responses of patients with pseudohypoparathyroidism. With calcium excretion, the first rectangle represents the changes in the first hour after the administration of PTH, and the second rectangle the changes from control to the second or third hours.* $\Delta C_{Ca}:C_{Na}$ *is offset to the right to emphasize that the normal response to PTH is a decrease in ratio.*

cium clearance to the sodium clearance was determined. We used this ratio because it is known that the excretion of calcium is directly proportional to the excretion of sodium [12–14], and that PTH acts to decrease this ratio [15–17]. When possible, comparisons were made by the t test for paired data.

RESULTS

In response to the infusion of PTH, in normal subjects the excretion of cyclic AMP, sodium, potassium, bicarbonate and phosphate was significantly increased (Table II). Calcium excretion was significantly decreased at 2 and 3 hours after the infusion of PTH, and the calcium to sodium clearance ratio was decreased at 1, 2 and 3 hours. Serum calcium was decreased at 1 hour.

The only significant differences between the hypoparathyroid patients and the normal subjects in their responses to PTH were that the former had greater increases in the excretion of cyclic AMP at 1 and 3 hours ($P < 0.02$), and in the excretion of sodium at 2 hours ($P < 0.01$) (Table II).

All the patients with pseudohypoparathyroidism had a markedly impaired excretion of cyclic AMP in response to the infusion of PTH (Table II and Figure 1). Four of the five patients had decreased calcium to sodium clearance ratios in response to PTH, and the response in the entire group was significantly less than normal at 1 and 2 hours after the infusion of PTH. Three of the patients had a clearly abnormal urinary excretion of bicarbonate in response to PTH, and two had an abnormal excretion of potassium in response to PTH, with the response in one additional patient barely falling into the range of normal. The excretion of sodium in response to PTH in the patients with pseudohypoparathyroidism was within the normal or above normal range in all. Four of the five phosphate excretions in these patients were below the mean for normal subjects. The urinary excretion of calcium after the infusion of PTH appears to have a biphasic pattern in normal subjects, there being a slight increase in the first hour and a significant decrease in the second and third hours. In two of the patients with pseudohypoparathyroidism the increases in calcium excretion were greater than in normal subjects in the first hour, and in two others the decrease was less during the second and third hours.

The responses which most closely approximate normal occurred in a patient (Case 1) who had the

TABLE II Response to PTH Infusion at 1, 2 and 3 Hours in 11 Normal Subjects, Three Patients with Hypoparathyroidism and Five Patients with Pseudohypoparathyroidism

	Normal Subjects		Patients with Hypoparathyroidism		Patients with Pseudohypoparathyroidism					P Value
	Mean	SD	Mean	SD	Case 1	Case 2	Case 3	Case 4	Case 5	
Urinary cyclic AMP (nmol/mg creatinine)										
Control	3.36	0.72	2.38	0.35	2.72	3.12	1.73	2.57	2.22	
1 hour	179.25*	67.47	376.53	197.18	15.49	4.16	8.34	4.08	2.88	<0.001
2 hours	8.17	7.32	90.16	136.72	2.79	3.21	1.35	4.04	4.25	NS
3 hours	3.38	1.54	6.90	3.56	3.59	3.44	1.35	2.58	2.47	NS
Urine calcium (meq/hour)										
Control	0.261	0.070	0.165	0.221	0.784	0.231	0.615	0.036	0.192	
1 hour	0.344	0.170	0.085	0.109	1.25	0.258	2.83	0.124	0.376	NS
2 hours	0.150*	0.131	0.085	0.148	0.280	0.138	0.457	0.086	0.173	NS
3 hours	0.159*	0.130	0.073	0.106	0.171	0.183	0.457	0.056	0.167	NS
Urine sodium (meq/hour)										
Control	4.48	1.51	3.33	2.01	10.85	7.15	8.36	1.32	7.55	
1 hour	11.12*	4.28	16.87	12.80	37.52	11.73	35.67	5.25	16.35	NS
2 hours	4.56	3.33	10.20	5.55	7.66	5.49	6.50	3.08	7.74	NS
3 hours	4.70	4.36	4.03	2.88	6.05	9.02	6.50	2.45	7.44	NS
$C_{Ca}:C_{Na}$										
Control	1.82	0.73	1.22	1.05	1.86	0.95	1.81	0.77	0.65	
1 hour	0.91*	0.52	0.54	0.75	0.86	0.65	1.96	0.68	0.65	<0.05
2 hours	0.88*	0.77	0.28	0.49	1.02	0.77	1.79	0.80	0.64	<0.02
3 hours	1.08*	0.96	0.37	0.42	0.76	0.60	1.79	0.65	0.65	NS
Urine potassium (meq/hour)										
Control	3.36	1.65	3.57	1.72	5.40	4.08	3.58	1.54	1.20	
1 hour	11.30*	4.45	10.37	8.00	12.02	4.07	9.28	1.65	3.51	<0.05
2 hours	5.39*	2.25	7.73	5.45	4.09	3.34	3.32	1.32	1.90	NS
3 hours	3.75	0.81	4.76	1.20	2.69	4.30	3.32	1.25	1.82	NS
Urine bicarbonate (meq/hour)										
Control	0.96	2.03	0.65	0.76	0.09	0.00	4.53	0.01	0.06	
1 hour	11.60*	8.17	7.74	4.14	13.13	0.22	23.00	0.15	0.46	NS
2 hours	2.40	2.33	3.39	3.92	3.65	0.35	1.21	0.02	0.46	NS
3 hours	0.73	0.79	0.22	0.36	0.07	0.03	1.21	0.01	0.44	NS
Urine phosphate (mg/hour)										
Control	31.55	13.22	18.01	26.27	3.24	28.15	6.64	4.20	43.32	
1 hour	43.86*	11.62	45.59	26.62	11.06	34.43	27.84	6.00	56.50	NS
2 hours	37.82	18.50	45.79	36.05	13.20	37.76	27.88	7.99	36.41	NS
3 hours	29.34	8.39	20.80	26.85	9.18	37.34	27.88	7.50	32.55	NS
Urine creatinine (mg/hour)										
Control	67.38	11.86	41.47	9.86	63.18	77.32	44.58	37.52	63.59	
1 hour	66.37	15.66	46.33	14.63	56.76	65.92	52.36	36.75	61.09	NS
2 hours	64.61	11.06	44.01	8.70	58.08	72.20	46.74	37.60	63.48	NS
3 hours	64.10	9.94	35.38	6.61	51.68	72.48	46.74	39.50	62.28	NS
Serum calcium (meq/liter)										
Control	5.03	0.33	4.41	0.56	5.20	4.70	5.42	5.05	5.20	
1 hour	4.79*	0.31	4.12	0.17	5.15	4.40	5.28	4.62	4.98	NS
2 hours	4.93	0.29	4.19	0.23	4.95	...	5.12	4.72	4.88	NS
3 hours	4.92	0.34	4.08	0.04	5.05	4.50	5.22	4.68	4.82	NS

* Indicates significant change ($P<0.05$) from pre-PTH (0) to the urines voided at hours 1, 2 or 3 after PTH infusion in normal subjects. Hypoparathyroid subjects had a greater response than the normal subjects in cyclic AMP excretion at 1 and 3 hours and in sodium at 2 hours. The P values refer to a comparison of the changes in the pseudohypoparathyroid patients to the changes in the normal subjects in response to infused PTH. NS indicates $P>0.05$.

largest, although markedly impaired, response in the excretion of cyclic AMP. Conversely, the most abnormal responses occurred in the three patients (Cases 2, 4 and 5) who had the smallest increases in the excretion of cyclic AMP after the infusion of PTH.

COMMENTS

Parathyroid hormone (PTH) acts on the proximal tubule to decrease reabsorption of sodium, calcium, bicarbonate and phosphate [18,19], and on the distal tubule to absorb calcium and decrease the calcium to sodium clearance ratio (C_{Ca}:C_{Na}) [19–21]. With the exception of a calciuretic response, our normal subjects and patients with hypoparathyroidism exhibited these responses and also showed increased potassium excretion (Table II). In contrast, the patients with pseudohypoparathyroidism had significantly impaired responses to PTH in excretion of cyclic AMP, potassium and change in C_{Ca}:C_{Na}. There was, however, great variability in their responses, with the most frequently observed abnormality (four of five patients) being the lack of a decrease in C_{Ca}:C_{Na}. Three patients had subnormal bicarbonate excretion in response to PTH, and two had subnormal potassium excretion, with the response barely falling into the normal range in one patient. The urinary excretion of sodium in response to PTH was extremely variable, being barely normal in two and supranormal in two. One of the normal subjects had no phosphaturic excretion in response to PTH and obviously the patients with pseudohypoparathyroidism could not respond less. However, in four of the five patients the response was less than the mean of the normal subjects. In two patients calcium excretion increased more than in the normal subjects in the first hour after PTH infusion, and in two others calcium excretion decreased less during the second and third hours. Since previous studies in patients with pseudohypoparathyroidism have indicated only abnormal excretion of cyclic AMP [3] and phosphate [1,6] in response to PTH, our patients with pseudohypoparathyroidism have a more generalized impairment in renal response to PTH than has been recognized. It should be remembered that the infusion rate of 250 U PTH over 15 minutes is much greater than the normal secretion rate [22] and therefore the normal responses in the patients with pseudohypoparathyroidism may not usually occur even though the serum PTH levels are increased several fold [3,23,24].

Among the five patients with pseudohypoparathyroidism there appeared to be a correlation between the responses to PTH in excretion of cyclic AMP and the ions measured, since the responses which most closely approximated normal occurred in a patient (Case 1) who had the largest, although still markedly abnormal excretion of cyclic AMP. Conversely, the most abnormal responses occurred in the three patients (Cases 2, 4 and 5) who had the smallest increases in the excretion of cyclic AMP after the administration of PTH.

The proximal tubular effects of PTH are considered to be mediated by cyclic AMP [19]. When normal ion excretion did occur in patients with pseudohypoparathyroidism, other mechanisms may have been involved. Sallis [25] suggested that the phosphaturic excretion in response to PTH may not be due to cyclic AMP. Also, a minimal amount of cyclic AMP may cause a normal ion excretion. We have demonstrated that a minimal excretion of cyclic AMP in response to small amounts of PTH may result in large phosphaturia [26].

PTH influences urinary calcium excretion in two ways: by inhibiting proximal tubular reabsorption [19] and by increasing distal tubular reabsorption [15,19–21]. In our normal subjects a slight calciuresis developed in the first hour after the infusion of PTH (Table II). In the normal subjects and hypoparathyroid patients a significant anticalciuresis developed during the second and third hours after the infusion of PTH. This time course of calcium excretion during and after a brief infusion of PTH has been described previously [27]. In comparison to normal subjects, in two of our patients with pseudohypoparathyroidism an exaggerated calciuric response to PTH developed during the first hour and in two other patients the normal decrease in calcium excretion did not develop at 2 and 3 hours after the PTH (Figure 1).

The infusion of PTH caused marked decreases in C_{Ca}:C_{Na} in normal subjects and patients with hypoparathyroidism (Table II and Figure 1). In contrast, in four of five patients with pseudohypoparathyroidism C_{Ca}:C_{Na} did not change after PTH infusion. These data support the thesis that these four patients have defective mechanisms for renal calcium reabsorption in response to PTH. Bell et al. [28] reported no decrease in urinary calcium excretion after PTH infusion in three patients with pseudohypoparathyroidism. However, no measurements of urinary sodium were made and these investigators could not eliminate the possibility that a natriuresis could have caused the apparent lack of response. Impaired reabsorption of calcium by PTH in patients with pseudohypoparathyroidism may be at least in part responsible for hypocalcemia. Other mechanisms must be involved to explain the hypocalcemia in one patient (Case 1), who had a normal decrease in C_{Ca}:C_{Na} after PTH.

There is no direct evidence that enhancement of calcium reabsorption by PTH in the distal nephron is mediated by cyclic AMP [29]. However, the normal decrease in clearance ratio in the patient with pseudohypoparathyroidism who had the greatest excretion of cyclic AMP in response to PTH would suggest such a mechanism.

The abnormal ion excretion in response to PTH infusion in patients with pseudohypoparathyroidism indicates that vitamin D or normalization of serum calcium does not necessarily restore responsiveness to PTH as has been suggested [5,30,31], and that the abnormal response to infused PTH was probably not related to the elevated blood PTH level, since normalization of serum calcium in these patients suppresses PTH levels to normal [3,24,31].

The decrease in serum calcium at 1 hour was probably due to the hydration technic. Although serum calcium did not increase in any of our groups in the 3 hours following PTH infusion (Table II), in normal subjects given infusions of 2 U PTH/kg body weight/hour an increase in serum calcium would develop beginning at 4 hours [22].

ACKNOWLEDGMENT

We wish to acknowledge the expert technical assistance rendered by Mrs. Bonita Coulson and Miss Karen Tallant, and to thank Dr. K. J. Rao for help with several of the patient studies. We would also like to acknowledge the assistance of Dr. William Bergstrom who brought these patients (Cases 1, 2 and 3) to our attention and made their data available to us.

REFERENCES

1. Albright F, Burnett CH, Smith PH, Parson W: Pseudohypoparathyroidism, an example of Seabright-Bantam syndrome. Endocrinology 30: 922, 1942.
2. Moses AM, Rao KJ, Coulson R, Miller M: Parathyroid hormone deficiency with Albright's hereditary osteodystrophy. J Clin Endocrinol Metab 39: 496, 1974.
3. Chase LR, Melson GL, Aurbach GD: Pseudohypoparathyroidism: defective excretion of 3′,5′-AMP in response to parathyroid hormone. J Clin Invest 48: 1832, 1969.
4. Drezner M, Neelon FA, Lebovitz HE: Pseudohypoparathyroidism type II. A possible defect in the reception of the cyclic AMP signal. N Engl J Med 289: 1056, 1973.
5. Rodriguez HJ, Villarreal H Jr, Klahr S, Slatopolsky E: Pseudohypoparathyroidism type II. Restoration of normal renal responsiveness to parathyroid hormone by calcium administration. J Clin Endocrinol Metab 39: 693, 1974.
6. Rasmussen H: Parathyroid hormone, calcitonin and the calciferols, chap 11. Textbook of Endocrinology (Williams RH, ed), Philadelphia, W. B. Saunders Co., 1974, p 731.
7. Nordin BEC, Peacock M: Role of kidney in regulation of plasma-calcium. Lancet 2: 1280, 1969.
8. Gudmundsson TV, Woodhouse NJY: Regulation of plasma calcium in man. The influence of parathyroid hormone and calcitonin. Hormones 2: 26, 1971.
9. Ray EW: Gardner LI: Pseudo-pseudohypoparathyroidism in a child. Pediatrics 23: 520, 1959.
10. Gilman AG: A protein binding assay for adenosine 3′,5′-cyclic monophosphate. Proc Natl Acad Sci USA 67: 305, 1970.
11. Wolf PL, Williams D, Tsudaka T, Acosta L: Methods and Techniques in Clinical Chemistry, New York, Wiley-Interscience, 1972, p 307.
12. Walser M: Calcium clearance as a function of sodium clearance in the dog. Am J Physiol 200: 1099, 1961.
13. Kleeman CR, Bohaman J, Bernstein D, et al.: Effect of variations in sodium intake on calcium excretion in normal humans. Proc Soc Exp Biol Med 115: 29, 1964.
14. Costanzo LS, Moses AM, Rao KJ, Weiner IM: Dissociation of calcium and sodium clearances in patients with hypoparathyroidism by infusion of chlorothiazide. Metabolism 24: 1367, 1975.
15. Massry SG, Coburn JW, Chapman LW, Kleeman CR: Role of serum Ca, parathyroid hormone, and NaCl infusion in renal Ca and Na clearances. Am J Physiol 214: 1403, 1968.
16. Costanzo LS, Weiner IM: Relationship between clearances of Ca and Na. Effect of distal diuretics and PTH. Am J Physiol 230: 67, 1976.
17. Eisenberg E: Effects of serum calcium level and parathyroid extracts on phosphate and calcium excretion in hypoparathyroid patients. J Clin Invest 44: 942, 1965.
18. Muldowney FP, Carroll DV, Donohoe JF, Freaney R: Correction of renal bicarbonate wastage by parathyroidectomy; implications in acid-base homeostasis. Q J Med 160: 487, 1971.
19. Agus ZS, Gardner LB, Beck LH, Goldberg M: Effects of parathyroid hormone on renal tubular reabsorption of calcium, sodium, and phosphate. Am J Physiol 224: 1143, 1973.
20. Pullman TN, Lavender AR, Aho I, Rasmussen H: Direct renal action of a purified parathyroid extract. Endocrinology 67: 570, 1960.
21. Kleeman CR, Bernstein D, Rockney R, et al.: Studies on the renal clearance of diffusible calcium and the role of the parathyroid glands in its regulation. Yale J Biol Med 34: 1, 1961.
22. Froeling PGAM, Bijovet OLM: Kidney mediated effects of parathyroid hormone on extracellular homeostasis of calcium, phosphate and acid-base balance in man. Neth J Med 17: 174, 1974.
23. Tashjian AH Jr, Frantz AG, Lee JB: Pseudohypoparathyroidism. Assays of parathyroid hormone and thyrocalcitonin. Proc Natl Acad Sci USA 56: 1138, 1966.
24. Birkenhäger JC, Seldenrath HJ, Hackeng WHL, et al.: Calcium and phosphorus metabolism, parathyroid hormone, calcitonin and bone histology in pseudohypoparathyroidism. Eur J Clin Invest 3: 27, 1973.
25. Sallis JD: The mechanism of action of parathyroid hormone. Lack of evidence for the mediation by cyclic adenosine 3′,5′-monophosphate of parathyroid hormone-stimulated phosphaturia. J Endocrinol 46: 185, 1970.
26. Coulson R, Moses AM: Effect of chlorpropamide on renal response to parathyroid hormone in normal subjects and in patients with hypoparathyroidism and pseudohypoparathyroidism. J Pharmacol Exp Ther 194: 603, 1975.
27. Czekalski S, Loreau N, Paillard F, et al.: Effect of bovine parathyroid hormone 1-34 fragment on renal production and excretion of adenosine 3′,5′-monophosphate in man. Eur J Clin Invest 4: 85, 1974.
28. Bell NH, Avery S, Sinha T, et al.: Effects of dibutyryl cyclic adenosine 3′,5′-monophosphate and parathyroid extract on calcium and phosphorus metabolism in hypoparathyroidism and pseudohypoparathyroidism. J Clin Invest 51: 816, 1972.
29. Costanzo LS, Weiner IM: On the hypocalciuric action of chlorothiazide. J Clin Invest 54: 628, 1974.
30. Suh SM, Fraser D, Kooh SW: Pseudohypoparathyroidism. Responsiveness to parathyroid extract induced by vitamin D_2 therapy. J Clin Endocrinol Metab 30: 609, 1970.
31. Stögmann W, Fischer JA: Pseudohypoparathyroidism. Disappearance of the resistance to parathyroid extract during treatment with vitamin D. Am J Med 59: 140, 1975.

Etiology and Prognosis in Acute Post-Transplant Renal Failure

CARL M. KJELLSTRAND, M.D.
ROBERT E. CASALI, M.D.
RICHARD L. SIMMONS, M.D.
JEFFREY R. SHIDEMAN, B.S.
THEODORE J. BUSELMEIER, M.D.
JOHN S. NAJARIAN, M.D.
Minneapolis, Minnesota

During the last seven years we encountered 117 cases of acute renal failure after 492 renal transplants. The affected patients fall into two general groups that can be broadly identified by an ^{131}I-Hippuran renogram: Those in whom low or no uptake is evident on the renogram (group 1) and those in whom good uptake is evident on the renogram (group 2). Fifty per cent of the patients in group 1 have renal arterial thrombosis or hyperacute rejection. These patients should have a renal arteriogram, and immediate nephrectomy may be necessary. The prognosis in these patients is very grave. In group 2, 89 per cent of the patients have acute tubular necrosis, and they do not differ prognostically from patients who experience immediate renal function. Invasive diagnostic procedures should be avoided in this group because they may increase the mortality rate. We believe that repeated renograms, a reduction in azathioprine dosage and careful dialysis is the only treatment necessary.

Failure of a renal allograft to function immediately after transplant is a dismaying complication because continued hemodialysis is necessary. Furthermore, the subtle, early changes in renal function necessary to diagnose ejection are undetectable in face of severe renal failure due to other causes. The medical literature regarding this subject is sparse and confusing. Mowbray [1] reported an extremely high early death rate from this complication apparently caused by azathioprine toxicity. When the azathioprine dosage was decreased in proportion to renal function, the death rate decreased. Sheil et al. [2], Whittaker et al. [3] and Baxby et al. [4] reported high death rates both early and late after transplantation, but Williams et al. [5] report that early kidney malfunction had no adverse consequences for their patients.

During the last seven years a uniform diagnostic and therapeutic approach to this complication has been developed and used in 492 consecutive transplant recipients. To evaluate the importance of post-transplant acute renal failure, all 117 patients who underwent dialysis within the first week after receiving their transplant were evaluated, and the findings in those diagnosed as having acute tubular necrosis were also compared with those in a matched control group of patients who did not require hemodialysis.

From the Dialysis Unit, Departments of Medicine and Surgery, University Hospitals, University of Minnesota, Minneapolis, Minnesota 55455. This study was presented in part to the Fifth Annual Meeting of the American Society of Nephrology, Washington, D.C., 1971, and the NIAMD Conference on Acute Renal Failure, New York, 1973. Requests for reprints should be addressed to Dr. Carl M. Kjellstrand, Box 485, University of Minnesota Hospital, Minneapolis, Minnesota 55455. Manuscript accepted December 8, 1975.

PATIENTS

All patients who received transplants at the University of Minnesota Hospitals between 1968 and June 1974 were reviewed on January 1, 1975. No patient was observed for less than six months and no patient was lost to follow-up.

Of 492 patients, 375 had immediate renal function. In 117 transplant recipients (21 per cent), however, continued dialysis was necessary because of increasing uremia after transplantation.

In 17 (15 per cent) of these 117 patients, problems were caused by hyperacute or accelerated rejections (12 patients), arterial thrombosis (two patients) and ureteral obstruction (three patients). In the remaining 100 patients (85 per cent) the diagnosis was made *by exclusion;* these patients were considered to have ischemic acute renal failure, commonly called acute tubular necrosis. We cannot exclude rejection as a contribution to the renal failure in these 100 patients because renal biopsies were not performed early in the patient's course for reasons discussed herein. Fourteen of these 100 patients had nonoliguric acute tubular necrosis.

The prognostic implications of post-transplant acute tubular necrosis were defined by using a matched control group. If only the prognosis in patients with post-transplant acute tubular necrosis is compared with that in the total group of transplant recipients, no account would be taken of changes in recipient or donor selection, in medical personnel or in immunosuppressive regimens. Therefore the control subjects were chosen by matching each patient with acute tubular necrosis with another patient in whom acute tubular necrosis had not developed by the following criteria: (1) sex of the recipient, (2) the time of transplant (± three months) and (3) the relationship of the donor (related or cadaver). There was no difference in mean age between the group with acute tubular necrosis (mean age 31.8 years) and the control group (mean age 33.5 years). Forty of the 100 in the group with acute tubular necrosis and 42 of the 100 in the control group belonged to groups of patients regarded as being at high risk (below age 15, above age 45, diabetic or ileum bladder [6,7]. In the group with acute tubular necrosis, 16 patients had received a second transplant and one a third transplant; in the control group, two patients had received a second transplant.

METHODS

The transplant recipients underwent a routine of pretransplant work-up procedures [8,9]. Except for a few diabetic patients, each patient underwent bilateral nephrectomy and splenectomy [10]. Transplantation took place two weeks to several months after nephrectomy-splenectomy. Routine immunosuppression consisted of intravenously administered antilymphocyte globulin and 5 mg/day of azathioprine tapered to 2 to 3 mg/kg. When a patient underwent acute renal failure, the azathioprine dose was immediately decreased to 1.5 mg/kg. Except for this, there was no difference in medications between the patients with acute renal failure and the control patients. Prednisone was used in a starting dose of 2 mg/kg for cadaver kidney recipients and 1 mg/kg for donor-related kidney recipients; the dose was tapered to 0.25 to 0.33 mg/kg over several months. For rejection episodes the patients were treated with local radiation, intravenously administered methylprednisolone and an increase in the oral prednisone dosage [8,9].

All kidney donors received renal protective treatment before and during surgery consisting of hydration and intravenously administered mannitol [11]. Only cadaver kidneys from brain dead donors with beating hearts were used. Since 1971, the cadaver kidneys have been preserved by hypothermic bloodless perfusion [12]. Since 1972, most cadaver kidney harvesting has been carried out in hospitals outside the University Hospital utilizing a transportable perfusion unit [12].

Tissue typing is regularly performed but it is the recipients' clinical state, rather than the tissue typing results, that decides which patient receives a particular cadaver kidney. Cross matching for cytotoxic antibodies in prospective recipients against the donor has been performed since mid-1969. Cross matching, using fresh serum obtained only hours before the operation, has been performed since 1970.

When dialysis is necessary, it is performed daily or every other day after transplantation, for only 3 to 4 hours the first week and 6 to 7 hours thereafter. Strict regional heparinization is used in all instances [13] and vigorous ultrafiltration is employed to avoid overhydration.

Diagnostic Procedures in Post-Transplant Oliguria. If there is no immediate diuresis in the adequately hydrated transplant recipient, furosemide in stepwise increasing doses (2 mg/kg, 5 mg/kg, 10 mg/kg) is given. If these measures are not effective within a few hours, an ^{131}I renogram is performed. Twenty microcuries of ^{131}I-Hippuran is given intravenously. A Picker dual rate-meter is used with one probe over the transplanted kidney, that usually is easily localized by palpation. During the first half of the study, the other probe was localized over the contralateral iliac fossa. Later, it was localized over the bladder. The reading of the second probe was used for background measurement. If there is more than 40 per cent of peak activity after a half hour, a gamma camera picture is obtained to try to differentiate between acute tubular necrosis and obstruction. This addition and also ^{99m}Tc pertechnetate studies in patients with poor uptake were available, but not on a routine basis, during the latter part of the study. The results of these technics will therefore not be discussed herein. If good uptake is evident on the renogram, no further diagnostic studies are carried out. If poor uptake is evident, a renal arteriogram is performed to rule out vascular occlusion or evidence of intrarenal thrombosis secondary to hyperacute or accelerated rejection. If the arteriogram shows filling of the kidney and a relatively normal arterial tree with "stretched intrarenal arteries," no further diagnostic studies are performed. If the renal arteriogram shows evidence of thrombosis or hyperacute rejection, a nephrectomy is performed.

Renal biopsies, "second look" operations, routine renal arteriograms or attempts at retrograde pyelography are not used as diagnostic tools for acute renal failure after transplantation. We believe these invasive procedures are dangerous in the newly operated on, immunosuppressed patient who requires dialysis.

Serial radioactive renograms are obtained approximately every four to seven days in these patients. If these show deterioration or if progressive return of renal function is not apparent after three weeks, routine antirejection treatment is instituted [8,9].

Figure 1 illustrates a typical case of acute tubular necrosis after transplantation. Figure 2 shows renograms obtained in the same patient. Figure 3 shows three renal transplant ar-

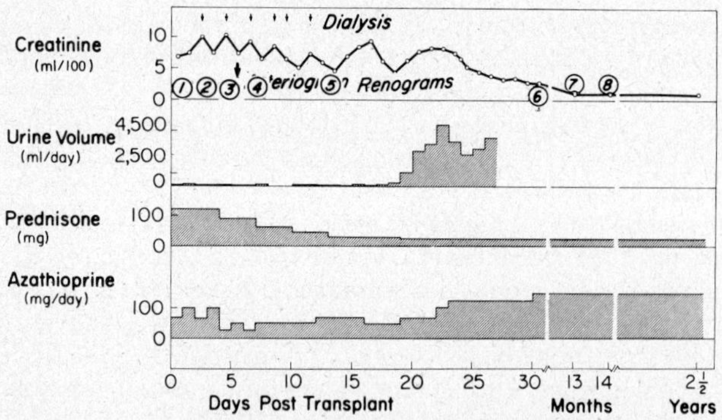

Figure 1. *Course of a patient with acute tubular necrosis after receiving a cadaver transplant. Frequent dialysis under regional heparinization is used after transplantation. The return of urine output is followed by rapid decrease in creatinine towards normal levels after three weeks of dialysis. This patient remains alive with good renal function (creatinine 0.9 mg/100 ml) three years after transplantation.*

teriograms. The upper renal arteriogram (from patient in Figure 1) was interpreted by us as being compatible with acute tubular necrosis. The middle renal arteriogram is interpreted as showing a combination of acute tubular necrosis and severe rejection. The lower renal arteriogram is interpreted as an hyperacute rejection.

For evaluation, we divided the available renograms into two groups, those in which the uptake at 10 minutes was more than or less than twice background measured in the contralateral iliac fossa or over the bladder.

Cumulated survival was calculated according to the life-table method of Merrell and Shuleman [14]. Fisher's exact probability test and Student's t test were used for statistical analysis.

RESULTS

Table I illustrates the over-all results of 492 kidney transplants performed between 1968 and June 1974; 312 (63 per cent) of these are still functioning. The transplants functioned immediately in 375 recipients, but 117 required continued dialysis in the immediate post-transplant period.

Hyperacute Rejection. Twelve kidneys were lost to hyperacute rejection. Four of these were transplanted before routine cross matching utilizing fresh serum. Cytotoxic antibodies directed against the donor were found after transplantation in all cases in which cells were available for later testing. Only three of these 12 recipients are alive, all receiving long-term hemodialysis. Four patients died, within a few days after the transplant, of complications related to the hyperacute rejection; five died later while undergoing long-term dialysis or after retransplantation. Nine of the 12 hyperacute rejections occurred in recipients of second transplants.

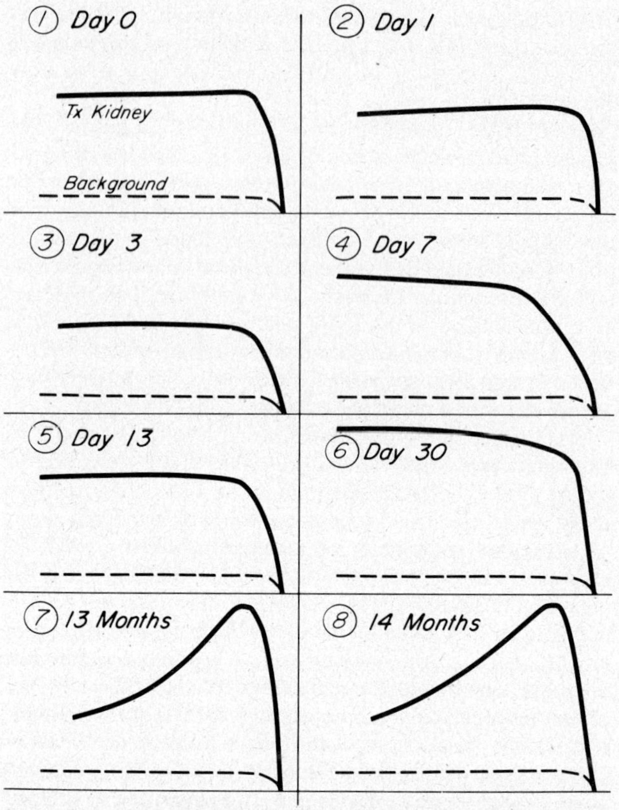

Figure 2. *Renograms of same patient. The numbers refer to the corresponding number on the graph of the patient. Observe the immediate good uptake on the renogram on all examinations. Two renograms obtained 13 and 14 months after transplantation are normal.*

Arterial Thrombosis. Arterial thrombosis occurred in two diabetic patients. Both patients died after receiving a second transplant.

Ureteral Necrosis. Necrosis of the tip of the ureter led to acute renal failure in three cases. For one or two days the renal failures were interpreted as being due to acute tubular necrosis, but urine leaks soon revealed the true cause. All patients underwent reoperation with reimplantation of the ureter; this was successful in two. In one patient local infection developed which necessitated removal of the kidney.

Nonacute tubular necrosis acute renal failure after transplantation is relatively rare in our patients. Arterial thrombosis and hyperacute rejection are extremely dangerous complications. Only three of 14 patients in whom this occurred are alive. The diagnosis is easy to make with a renogram followed by a renal arteriogram. In contrast, obstructive renal failure is much less common and has been diagnosed through urine leaks. We believe that retrograde pyelograms are not justified as a routine procedure as they are technically complicated and potentially traumatic in new transplant re-

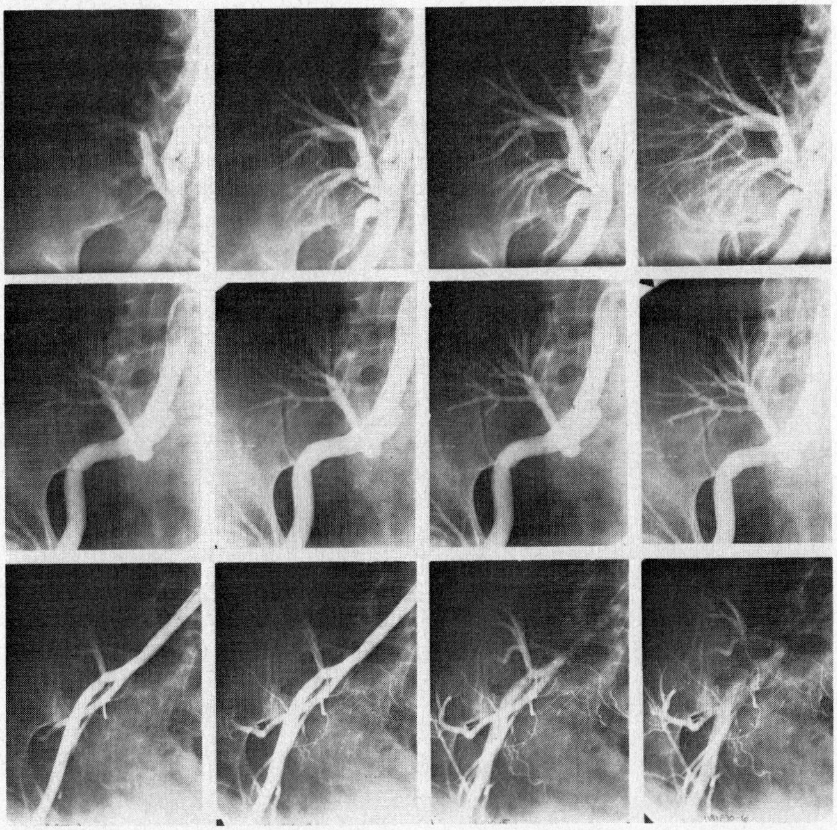

Figure 3. *Top, aortogram of the patient in Figure 1 performed on the fifth day after transplantation. The first picture is taken 6 seconds after injection of contrast media, the following frames are 3 seconds apart. Observe rapid filling of a normal arterial tree.* ***Middle,*** *aortogram, seven days after transplantation in a patient with both acute tubular necrosis and severe rejection. The patient diuresed, but was never able to lower his creatinine below 3 mg/100 ml. He died of infectious complications 11 months after transplantation. Time sequence is the same as in the top frames.* ***Bottom,*** *aortogram of patient with hyperacute rejection one day after transplantation. There is slow filling and absence of small vessels; extremely severe "pruning" is present. This patient underwent nephrectomy and ultimately died of infection. Time sequence is the same as in the top frames.*

TABLE I **Summary of All Kidney Transplants and Acute Post-Transplant Renal Failure at the University of Minnesota (1968—June 1974 as of January 1, 1975)**

	Total Kidneys Transplanted			Donor-Related Kidneys			Cadaver Kidneys		
	Total No.	No. Lost	%	Total No.	No. Lost	%	Total No.	No. Lost	%
Immediate function	375	121	33	238	53	22	137	69	50
Acute post-transplant acute tubular necrosis	100	43	43	32	13	40	68	30	44
Hyperacute rejection	12	12	100	4	4*	100	8	8†	100
Obstruction	3	1	33	3	1	33	—	—	—
Renal arterial thrombosis	2	2	100	2	2‡	100	—	—	—
Sum	492	180	36	279	73	26	213	107	50

* All recipients died, all second transplants.
† Three recipients survived, five second transplants.
‡ Both recipients had diabetes and died.

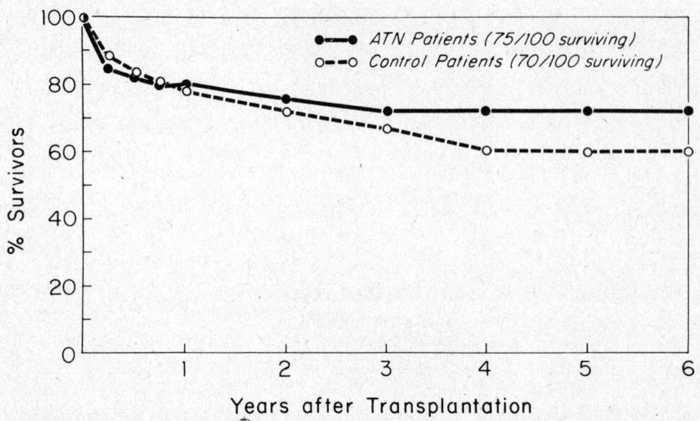

Figure 4. Cumulated survival curves in patients with acute tubular necrosis and matched control. These curves follow each other very closely.

cipients, and only three of 117 such patients (2.6 per cent) had this complication.

Post-Transplant Acute Tubular Necrosis. The remaining 100 patients were *by exclusion* diagnosed as suffering from acute tubular necrosis. Post-transplant acute tubular necrosis occurred in 32 of 279 (11 per cent) patients who received a kidney from a related donor versus 68 of 213 (32 per cent) patients who received a cadaver kidney. It cannot be excluded that mild, transient rejection contributed to the renal failure in these cases.

Survival of Patients with Acute Tubular Necrosis. Of patients with post-transplant acute tubular necrosis, 75 of 100 (75 per cent) survived between six months and seven years after transplantation versus 70 of 100 (70 per cent) of the matched control group. In those who received cadaver kidneys, 49 of 68 (72 per cent) survived compared to 45 of 68 (66 per cent) in the control group without acute tubular necrosis. For recipients of related-donor kidneys, the corresponding figures are 26 of 32 (81 per cent) in the group with acute tubular necrosis and 25 of 32 (78 per cent) in the group without acute tubular necrosis. None of these differences is statistically significant. There is no difference in cumulated survival (Figure 4). The causes of patient death are shown in Table II. Almost 70 per cent of the deaths in both the group with acute tubular necrosis and the control group were due to infections.

TABLE II Comparison of Causes of Death in Patients with Acute Tubular Necrosis (ATN) and Control Patients

Cause of Death	Within 3 Mo After Transplant (no.)	Later than 3 Mo After Transplant (no.)	Total (no.)
Infection			
ATN	8	6	14
Control	7	12	19
Technical			
ATN	3	0	3
Control	2	0	2
Cardiovascular			
ATN	2	2	4
Control	2	4	6
Other			
ATN	1	3	4
Control	1	2	3
Sum			
ATN	14	11	25
Control	12	18	30

NOTE: Causes of patient death divided into early and late deaths. Neither early nor late total deaths are significantly different at the 10 per cent level between the patients with acute tubular necrosis and the control group.

Survival of Kidneys. Figures 5 and 6 present cumulative functional survival of related-donor and cadaver kidneys and compares patients with acute tubular necrosis to matched controls. Presently, of cadaver kidneys, 38 of 68 (55 per cent) function in the group with acute tubular necrosis versus 35 of 68 (52 per cent) in

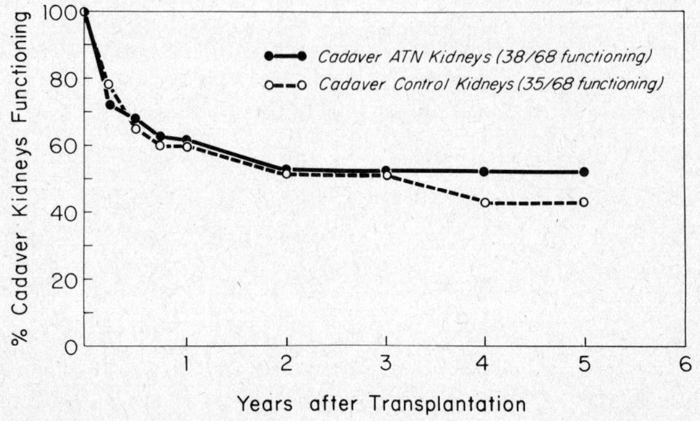

Figure 5. Cumulated functional survival of cadaver kidneys. There is no difference between acute tubular necrosis and control kidneys.

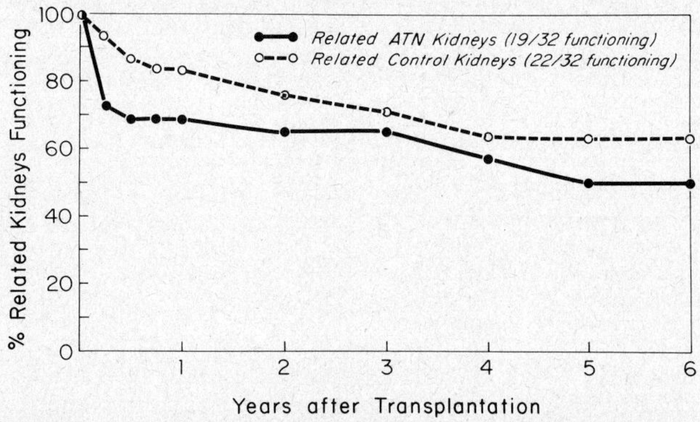

Figure 6. Cumulated functional survival of donor-related kidneys. There is a significantly better early survival in control kidneys when compared to kidneys with acute tubular necrosis.

TABLE III Comparison of Causes of Loss of Cadaver Kidneys in Patients with Acute Tubular Necrosis (ATN) and Control Patients

	Within 3 Mo After Transplant (no.)	Later than 3 Mo After Transplant (no.)	Total (no.)
Death of Patient			
ATN	9	4	13
Control	6	10	16
Rejection			
ATN	4	7	11
Control	6	7	13
Urologic			
ATN	3	0	3
Control	2	0	2
Other			
ATN	3	0	3
Control	2	0	2
Sum			
ATN	19	11	30
Control	16	17	33

NOTE: Neither the kidney loss occurring early, late nor the total loss is significantly different between the groups at the 10 per cent level.

TABLE IV Comparison of Causes of Loss of Donor-Related Kidneys in Patients with Acute Tubular Necrosis (ATN) and Control Patients

	Within 3 Mo After Transplant (no.)	Later than 3 Mo After Transplant (no.)	Total (no.)
Death of Patient			
ATN	4	1	5
Control	2	3	5
Rejection			
ATN	4	2	6
Control	1	3	4
Urologic			
ATN	2	0	2
Control	0	1	1
Sum			
ATN	10	3	13
Control	3	7	10

NOTE: There is a statistically significant tendency for the kidneys with acute tubular necrosis to be lost early ($p < 0.05$). However, the late and the total loss rate are no different between patients with acute tubular necrosis and control patients.

the control group without acute tubular necrosis. Of 32 related-donor kidneys in patients with acute tubular necrosis, 19 (60 per cent) are still functioning versus 22 (69 per cent) in the control group. None of these differences is statistically significant. Table III outlines the causes of kidney loss in recipients who received cadaver kidneys and compares them in the group with acute tubular necrosis and the control group. Most losses of kidneys occurred because the patient died with a functioning kidney. Rejection is the second most common cause. There is no statistical difference in cumulated functional survival of the cadaver kidneys (Figure 5) between the kidneys with acute tubular necrosis and the control kidneys without acute tubular necrosis.

However, there is a significant difference between the patients with acute tubular necrosis and those in the control group who received donor-related kidneys (Table IV, Figure 6). The losses of kidneys tend to occur early in the group with acute tubular necrosis and late in the control group. The total results, however, are not significantly different, nor can one discern a difference in causes of kidney loss (Table IV) due to the small number in each category.

The incidence of acute tubular necrosis in donor-related kidneys has remained at approximately 10 per cent during the entire seven year period under study. Contrary, the incidence of acute tubular necrosis in cadaver transplants has more than doubled from 15 per cent before 1971 (the year perfusion was instituted) to approximately 36 per cent since then. It is difficult, however, to know if this is related to the perfusion itself or to a more liberal acceptance of cadaver kidneys even from donors in shock and with moderate elevations in creatinine levels.

Renal Functional Recovery. Twelve patients with acute tubular necrosis never achieved a serum creatinine level of less than 2 mg/100 ml after transplantation versus only one patient in the control group. Four of these patients with post-transplant acute tubular necrosis died before renal function became normal. All four had hemorrhagic complications. In three of the 12 patients, the kidneys were removed before renal function ensued, in one because of a bladder leak, in one because of bleeding and infection around the transplanted kidneys, and in the third because of sudden arterial thrombosis at the beginning of the diuresis. The remaining five patients diuresed over 1,000 cc; one, however, had to continue receiving long-term hemodialysis and ultimately died. In two of these five, recovery from acute tubular necrosis was complicated by rejection that ultimately led to kidney loss and a return to dialysis. One patient has had repeated rejection episodes but does not need dialysis, although she has severe chronic renal failure with a serum creatinine of 5 mg/100 ml seven months after transplantation. The fifth patient died of cytomegalovirus disease two months after receiving the transplant, with a creatinine level of 2.5 mg/100 ml. The one control patient, in whom the creatinine level never went below 2 mg/100 ml, died of infection six months after receiving the transplant.

TABLE V Comparison of Renal Function, Rejections and Blood Pressure in Transplant Recipients with Acute Tubular Necrosis and Control Patients

	Acute Tubular Necrosis	Matched Control
Creatinine (mg/100 ml)	1.43 ± 0.72	1.39 ± 0.55
Blood urea nitrogen (mg/100 ml)	27.9 ± 18.9	27.4 ± 18.3
Rejection episodes	0.44 ± 0.63	0.50 ± 0.7
Blood pressure (mm Hg)	123/78	122/73

NOTE: There is no statistical difference in either creatinine or blood urea nitrogen levels or in rejection episodes or blood pressure.

TABLE VI Results of 89 Renograms, Obtained Within Four Days of Transplantation, in Patients with Acute Renal Failure After Transplantation

	No. Available Renograms	Good Renal Uptake (>2 × Background)		Low Renal Uptake (<2 × Background)	
Acute tubular necrosis	72	63	(89%)	9	(50%)
Hyperacute rejection	12 } 14	5 }	5 (7%)	7 }	9 (50%)
Renal arterial thrombosis	2	0		2	
Obstruction	3	3	(4%)	0	...
Sum	89	71	(100%)	18	(100%)

In the remaining 88 patients with acute tubular necrosis and in the 99 control patients, the creatinine level was less than 2 mg/100 ml. At present, 56 and 57 kidneys, respectively, are functioning. Four patients with acute tubular necrosis have chronic renal failure, as defined by a serum creatinine of more than 2 mg/100 ml, as do three patients in the control group without acute tubular necrosis.

The renal function, blood pressure and the number of rejections in these patients are compared in Table V. There is no statistical difference between the two groups. The patients with acute tubular necrosis do not require more antihypertensive medications than those in the control group without acute tubular necrosis.

The mean duration of anuria (<50 ml/day) was 1.5 days (range 0 to 17 days). Diuresis of more than 300 ml/day was achieved after a mean of 11 days (1 to 35 days), and the serum creatinine level was less than 2 mg/100 ml after a mean of 23 days (range 10 to 77 days) in the patients who experienced acute tubular necrosis.

Prolonged Acute Tubular Necrosis After Transplantation. To investigate the prognostic implications of prolonged acute tubular necrosis, we did a special analysis of all patients who had a period of anuria or oliguria, or a creatinine level of more than 2 mg/100 ml, more than twice that of the mean for the patients in the group with acute tubular necrosis. One such patient with acute tubular necrosis and one control patient lost their kidney grafts. The mean serum creatinine, blood urea nitrogen and blood pressure levels do not differ between the patients with prolonged acute tubular necrosis and the control group. Therefore, even prolonged acute tubular necrosis is compatible with a successful outcome.

Diagnostic Accuracy and Prognostic Implications of Early Renograms in Patients with Renal Failure. Eighty-nine renograms were available for analysis; they were obtained within four days after transplantation in the 117 patients who expérienced acute renal failure. The result of these renograms is summarized in Table VI.

Of 72 renograms in the patients with acute tubular necrosis, 63 (88 per cent) showed an uptake of more than twice that of background. Usually this uptake was four to ten times that of background. Nine (12 per cent) of the patients with acute tubular necrosis had an uptake of less than twice that of background. One of these patients never had a creatinine level of less than 2 mg/100 ml and ultimately lost his kidney. The other eight patients still have functioning kidneys and creatinine levels of less than 2 mg/100 ml. Six of these patients have had prolonged acute tubular necrosis with a serum creatinine of more than 2 mg/100 ml over 23 days (the mean for the entire group).

Five (42 per cent) of twelve renograms obtained in patients with hyperacute or accelerated rejections showed an uptake of more than twice that of the background. But four of these patients showed rapid deterioration, and one patient had a rupture of the kidney which required its removal. Both patients with renal arterial occlusion showed no uptake on renogram. All three patients with ureteral tip necrosis showed good uptake in their renograms.

We thus find early renograms to be a valuable tool in patients with acute renal failure after transplantation because they identify the majority of patients who require no further diagnostic invasive tests as those with good uptake. Only a minority of these patients, five of 71 (7 per cent) had accelerated or hyperacute rejection that made nephrectomy necessary. A minority of patients, 18 of 89 (24 per cent), had an uptake of less than twice that of the background. Nine (50 per cent) of these patients lost their kidneys because of irreversible ischemic damage secondary to arterial thrombosis or hyperacute rejection.

We believe that the radioactive renogram is the single

most important diagnostic procedure in post-transplant patients with acute renal failure. It is not dangerous and yields valuable information for the patient's further management.

Only seven of the 100 patients with acute tubular necrosis underwent an arteriogram, and six of these arteriograms were performed on the 61 patients who received transplants before 1973. Sixteen of the 100 patients with acute tubular necrosis were treated for rejection when they underwent dialysis. Only one of these patients was among the 39 patients with acute tubular necrosis who received transplants in 1973–1974. No patient with acute tubular necrosis underwent retrograde pyelography, renal biopsy or an operation for renal diagnostic purposes while undergoing dialysis.

COMMENTS

The patients with post-transplant renal failure will fall into two groups. In the majority of these patients, those undergoing acute tubular necrosis, post-transplant renal failure is of no prognostic consequence and is therefore a benign complication. The smaller number of patients, however, who undergo rapid necrosis of the transplanted kidney secondary to hyperacute rejection or arterial thrombosis, have an extremely grave prognosis. Fortunately, a single noninvasive benign diagnostic procedure, ^{131}I-Hippuran renogram, will establish the correct diagnosis in the majority of these cases, making it necessary to proceed to a renal arteriogram in only a few patients. Postrenal acute renal failure was rare. Although these patients survived, the prognosis of urologic complications after renal transplantation is serious [15].

Our findings are in agreement with the experience of Williams et al. [5] and Mowbray [1] who concluded that post-transplant acute renal failure was usually of no serious consequence for the patients. Our findings are contrary to those of Sheil et al., Whittacker et al. and Baxby et al. [2–4], but the studies are not directly comparable. (1) When studying prognosis, we excluded the patients with hyperacute rejection, arterial thrombosis or obstruction. (2) We have much more data and used a matched control group. (3) We avoided invasive diagnostic procedures. None of our patients underwent biopsies, retrograde pyelographies or "second look" operations during acute renal failure, and in only seven of the patients with acute tubular necrosis was an arteriogram obtained. Whittacker et al. [3] used repeated invasive diagnostic tests in 59 per cent of the patients with acute renal failure but in only 30 per cent of the recipients with good immediate renal function. They believe this is one of the reasons for the high death rate of their patients with acute renal failure. If uptake is evident on the renogram, we believe one should not proceed to further diagnostic tests but should only repeat renograms at regular intervals and expect return of renal function.

We also decrease the dosage of azathioprine, although some studies suggest that this drug is not metabolized through the kidney [16]. However, one cannot rule out that the "immunosuppressive effect of renal failure and surgery" [1,17–19] is additive to the toxicity of azathioprine. We treated only 16 of 100 patients with acute tubular necrosis for rejection because the renogram showed deterioration or because the oliguric period extended beyond three weeks, the mean time it took the creatinine level to reach less than 2 mg/100 ml. It is possible that more frequent use of ^{131}I-Hippuran renogram, or the use of ^{99m}Tc pertechnetate or ^{99m}Tc sulfur colloid with sequential scintigraphy, may improve on the diagnosis of rejection in patients with acute tubular necrosis [20–22]. This may result in even greater safety by reducing the unnecessary use of prednisone in those erroneously suspected of having a rejection. Large dose prednisone therapy is associated with an increased morbidity and mortality [23–25].

The reason for the difference between our material and that of Baxby et al. [4] is partially due to other factors. One of these is probably that cadaver transplants in England frequently are obtained from patients whose heart has been stopped for a prolonged period of time; thus, "dead kidneys" may be used in up to 20 per cent [26], as brain death is not recognized in that country. Secondly, Baxby and co-workers encountered an inordinate amount of dialysis-related problems. In their report of 16 cases there were four dialysis-related deaths: one cerebral vascular accident, one episode of heart failure and two episodes of bleeding. Strict fluid limitation and adherence to strict regional heparinization [13] during dialysis should prevent heart failure and bleeding due to dialysis.

The reason for the difference between our material and that of Sheil et al. [2] is difficult to analyze because their material concerning patients with acute renal failure is summarized. Our incidence of post-transplant renal failure, 21 per cent, is similar to theirs and lower than that reported by several other groups [3–5].

The influence of kidney perfusion on acute tubular necrosis is difficult to evaluate. Since the introduction of perfusion, our incidence of acute tubular necrosis in cadaver kidneys had doubled. However, more liberal criteria in accepting these kidneys have also been applied. Cadaver kidney transplantation now takes place at a much more leisurely rate. While the kidney is being perfused, one can tissue type, cross match and dialyze the potential recipient. As the prognosis in the patient with acute tubular necrosis does not seem to differ from that in the patient with immediate function, we believe cadaver kidneys should not be discarded for fear of encountering acute tubular necrosis.

Delayed recovery of renal function after transplantation removes the most valuable index of rejection, decline in renal function. However, with our simple set of diagnostic tests and routine treatment, undetected rejection during these first three weeks does not seem a major problem. In twelve patients with acute tubular necrosis, the kidneys were lost before the creatinine level was below 2 mg/100 ml. Seven of these losses seem to be related to technical problems rather than to the acute tubular necrosis itself. Of the remaining five patients, rejection was diagnosed by a sudden, renewed increase in falling serum creatinine levels. Despite treatment, there was progression to irreversible renal failure in three of these patients and severe chronic renal failure in two. The relative importance of acute tubular necrosis and rejection in these latter five patients cannot be definitely elucidated. Williams et al. interpreted acute tubular necrosis as being protective against rejection [5]. In our study, the mean number of rejection episodes was somewhat lower in those with acute tubular necrosis when compared to the matched controls, but this difference was not significant. It is also possible that more sophisticated *diagnostic radionuclide* technics may lessen this early loss rate [20–22].

The ultimate survival and renal function, as estimated by creatinine levels and blood pressure levels in our patients with acute tubular necrosis did not differ from that in the matched control group. This finding agrees with previous follow-up studies of acute renal failure [27,28] that have shown that most survivors of episodes of acute tubular necrosis usually have a minimal or no clinical defect in renal function. It is in variance, however, with our finding of a 10 per cent incidence of severe chronic renal failure following nontransplant acute postsurgical renal failure [29]. Any conclusions in this regard remain futile, however, as the materials cannot be directly compared. This study suggests that the persistent renal functional defect, if any, after post-transplant acute tubular necrosis is negligible compared to the other factors influencing long-term function in the renal graft. Obviously all transplanted kidneys undergo a period of ischemia. The difference in degree between the kidneys with acute tubular necrosis and those without may thus be only a small matter.

This study may also answer one question of great concern to nephrologists: What is the cause of the high mortality rate of patients with postsurgical acute tubular necrosis [30–33]? As all our patients underwent an equivalent type of surgery, renal transplantation, and as the patients with acute tubular necrosis did no worse than the ones with immediate function, the high mortality rate in postsurgical acute tubular necrosis is probably mainly due to the basic disease. Thus in patients with postsurgical acute tubular necrosis the mortality rate would probably be similar even if they had not experienced acute tubular necrosis as a consequence of the catastrophe that led to it.

REFERENCES

1. Mowbray JF: Peritoneal dialysis for pre- and postoperative management in a cadaveric transplantation program. Trans Am Soc Artif Intern Organs 13: 46, 1967.
2. Sheil AGR, Stewart JH, Johnson JR, et al.: Evaluation of cadaver-donor renal transplantation. Transplantation Proc 3: 347, 1971.
3. Whittaker JR, Veith FJ, Soberman R, et al.: The fate of the renal transplant with delayed function. Surg Gynecol Obstet 136: 919, 1973.
4. Baxby K, Taylor RMR, Anderson M, et al.: Assessment of cadaveric kidneys for transplantation. Lancet 2: 977, 1974.
5. Williams OM, White HJO, Hume DM: Factors influencing the long term functional success rate of human renal allografts. Transplantation 5: 837, 1967.
6. Kjellstrand CM: Renal transplantation versus chronic hemodialysis, indications and contraindications. Tissue Typing and Organ Transplantation (Yunis E, Gatti RA, Amos B, eds), New York, Academic Press, 1973, p 143.
7. Simmons RL, Kjellstrand CM, Buselmeier TJ, Najarian JS: Renal transplantation in high risk patients. Arch Surg 103: 290, 1971.
8. Kjellstrand CM, Simmons RL, Buselmeier TJ, Najarian JS: Recipient selection, medical management and dialysis (in renal transplantation). Transplantation (Najarian JS, Simmons, RL, eds), Philadelphia, Lea & Febiger, 1972, p 418.
9. Simmons RL, Kjellstrand CM, Najarian JS: Technique, complications and results (in renal transplantation). Transplantation (Najarian JS, Simmons RL, eds), Philadelphia, Lea & Febiger, 1972, p 445.
10. Kjellstrand CM, Shideman JR, Simmons RL, et al.: Renal transplantation in insulin-dependent diabetic patients. Kidney Int 6: S15, 1974.
11. Najarian JS, Gulyassy PP, Stoney RJ, et al.: Protection of the donor kidney during homotransplantation. Ann Surg 164: 398, 1966.
12. Moberg AW, Santiago EA, Mason RV, et al.: Transportable organ-perfusion system for kidney preservation. Lancet 2: 1403, 1971.
13. Kjellstrand CM, Buselmeier TJ: A simple method for anticoagulation during pre- and postoperative hemodialysis, avoiding rebound phenomenon. Surgery 72: 630, 1972.
14. Merrell M, Shulman LE: Determination of prognosis in chronic disease illustrated by systemic lupus erythematosus. J Chronic Dis 1: 12, 1955.
15. Weil R, Simmons RL, Tallent MB, et al.: Prevention of urological complications after kidney transplantation. Ann Surg 174: 154, 1971.
16. Bach JF, Dardenne M: The metabolism of azathioprine in renal failure. Transplantation 12: 253, 1971.
17. Howard RJ, Simmons RL: Acquired immunological deficiencies after trauma and surgery. Surg Gynecol Obstet 139: 771, 1974.
18. Mannick JA, Powers JH, Mithoefer J, Ferrebee JW: Renal transplantation in azotemic dogs. Surgery 47: 340, 1960.

19. Wilson WEC, Kirkpatrick CH, Talmage DW: Suppression of immunologic responsiveness in uremia. Ann Intern Med 62: 1, 1965.
20. Solaric-George EA, Anderson CB, Codd JE, et al.: Differentiation of acute tubular necrosis and rejection by dual radionuclide transplant renography. Proceedings of the Clinical Dialysis and Transplant Forum 3: 77, 1973.
21. Zum Winkel K, Harlest H, Das KB, Newiger T: Applications of radionuclides in renal transplantation. Semin Nucl Med 4: 169, 1974.
22. Codd JE, Mohapatra RN, George EA, et al.: Diagnosis of renal allograft rejection by 99^m Tc sulfur colloid visualization. Proceedings of the Clinical Dialysis and Transplant Forum 4: 131, 1974.
23. Simmons RL, Tallent MB, Kjellstrand CM, Najarian JS: Prevention of death following renal transplantation. 1. Recognizable patterns leading to death in long-term survivors. Am J Surg 119: 553, 1970.
24. Simmons RL, Weil R, Tallent MB, et al.: Do mild infections trigger the rejection of renal allografts? Transplant Proc 2: 419, 1970.
25. Black HR, Finkelstein FO: Risk factors in renal transplantation (abstract). American Society of Nephrology, 1973, p 12.
26. Festenstein H, Sachs JA, Oliver RTD, et al.: Multicentre collaboration in 162 tissue-typed renal transplants. Lancet 2: 225, 1971.
27. Lewers DT, Mathew TH, Maher JF, Schreiner GE: Long-term follow up of renal function and histology after acute tubular necrosis. Ann Intern Med 73: 523, 1970.
28. Hall JW, Johnson WH, Maher FT, Hunt JC: Immediate and long-term prognosis in acute renal failure. Ann Intern Med 73: 515, 1970.
29. Merino GE, Buselmeier TJ, Kjellstrand CM: Postoperative chronic renal failure—a new syndrome? Ann Surg 182: 37, 1975.
30. Alwall N; Kjellstrand CM: Acute renal failure—A study of 639 cases involving 1073 treatment with the artificial kidney over the period 1946–1961, chap 16. Therapeutic and Diagnostic Problems in Severe Renal Failure (Alwall N, ed), Stockholm, Scandinavian University Books, Bonniers, 1963.
31. Kornhall S: Acute renal failure in surgical diseases with special regard to neglected complications. Acta Chir Scand 419 (suppl): 1, 1971.
32. Stott RB, Ogg CS, Cameron JS, Bewick M: Why the persistently high mortality in acute renal failure? Lancet 2: 75, 1972.
33. Kleinknecht D, Jungers P, Chanard J, et al.: Uremic and nonuremic complications in acute renal failure; evaluation of early and frequent dialysis on prognosis. Kidney Int 1: 190, 1972.

Recurrent Nephrolithiasis: Natural History and Effect of Phosphate Therapy

A Double-Blind Controlled Study

BRUCE ETTINGER, M.D.
San Francisco, California

In a double-blind controlled clinical study, 71 patients with recurrent calcium oxalate stones were divided into three treatment groups: those who received potassium acid phosphate, those who received an inert placebo, and those who received a low calcium diet only. Follow-up periods averaged 2.9 years. Although the mean urinary calcium level of the patients who received phosphate was reduced 33 per cent, their renal stone disease did not diminish. Mean urinary phosphorus increased 88 per cent with phosphate treatment but did not correlate with the decrease in urinary calcium, or with treatment success. The data did not suggest that phosphorus and its metabolites retard calcium oxalate crystallization in urine. No evidence appeared for an association of hypercalciuria with severe stone disease, or with a specific clinical or chemical response to phosphate therapy. Patients whose urinary calcium level fell more than 25 per cent when dietary calcium was reduced may have excessive gastrointestinal calcium absorption, which appears to be associated with improved chemical response to phosphate therapy.

Within the last two decades, more than a score of investigators have published results of drug prophylaxis for recurrent kidney stones. In none of those studies was the double-blind control method used; hence all suffered the many biases inherent in uncontrolled drug evaluation. Reported here are clinical and laboratory observations after therapy with inorganic phosphate, an inert placebo or a low calcium diet in 71 patients who participated in a double-blind study for a mean period of 2.9 years.

PATIENTS AND METHODS

The patients were members of the prepaid Kaiser Foundation Health Plan, served by physicians of The Permanente Medical Group in San Francisco, California. Referral of patients from the departments of urology and medicine of this medical center was solicited by me. Patients with recurrent calcium oxalate stones were admitted to the study if they (1) showed active stone disease, having passed at least two stones during the immediately preceding five years, at least one of which had been passed within the most recent two years, (2) were free of urinary infection, (3) had normal renal function and normal levels of serum calcium, urine oxalate and uric acid, and (4) gave consent after having been informed of the study design. Each patient had previously been advised by another physician to restrict dairy food intake so that the diet would contain approximately 600 mg of calcium daily.

From the Department of Internal Medicine, Kaiser-Permanente Medical Center, San Francisco, California. This study was supported by the Community Service Program of the Kaiser Foundation Hospitals. Requests for reprints should be addressed to Dr. Bruce Ettinger, Department of Internal Medicine, Kaiser-Permanente Medical Center, 2200 O'Farrell Street, San Francisco, California 94115. Manuscript accepted December 8, 1975.

TABLE I Initial Clinical Findings in the Three Treatment Groups

	Group 1	Group 2	Group 3
Patients (no.)	25	20	26
Mean age (yr)	41.4	46.9	43.3
Years of stone passage, median (yr)	10	7	6
Males (%)	84	75	89
Patients with hypercalciuria (%)	24	25	19
Pretreatment stone passage rate*	0.67	0.78	0.57
Pretreatment lithotomy rate*	0.055	0.092	0.024
Patients with roentgenographic evidence of stones (%)	48	35	38

NOTE: Group 1 = patients treated with phosphate. Group 2 = patients treated with a placebo. Group 3 = patients treated with diet alone.

* See text for derivation of rate.

TABLE II Initial Mean Serum and Urine Chemical Values in the Three Groups

	Group 1	Group 2	Group 3	Normal Values
Patients (no.)	25	20	26	
Serum				
Calcium (mg/100 ml)	9.5	9.7	9.6	9.5 ± 0.8
Phosphorus (mg/100 ml)	3.4	3.3	3.2	4.0 ± 0.6
Alkaline phosphatase (K-A U)	9.3	8.3	7.6	3–13
Uric acid (mg/100 ml)	5.7	5.6	5.7	5.3 ± 1.2
Urine				
Calcium (mg/24 hr)				
Low dairy diet	238	237	214	<300
Low calcium diet	202	234	181	<250
Phosphorus (mg/100 ml)	907	877	905	780–1,100
Uric acid (mg/24 hr)	729	660	684	400–800

NOTE: Group 1 = 25 patients treated with phosphate. Group 2 = 20 patients treated with a placebo. Group 3 = 26 patients treated with diet alone.

Random assignment provided 25 patients in a phosphate-treated group (group 1) and 20 patients in a placebo-treated group (group 2). A third group of 26 patients satisfied the same entry criteria, but these patients either refused phosphate/placebo therapy (seven patients), stopped phosphate/placebo treatment after a few weeks (five patients) or were referred after 1971 when this study was closed to new entrants (14 patients); these 26 patients are termed the "diet therapy group" (group 3). The patients in three groups were similar in age and sex distribution, in the clinical expression of their kidney stone disease (Table I) and in mean base line serum and urine chemistry values (Table II). Urinary calcium levels were measured while the patients were adhering to a diet restricted to approximately 600 mg of calcium daily; then after reduction of calcium intake to approximately 300 mg daily. Under these conditions, hypercalciuria was defined by the generally accepted criteria: $\geq$300 mg/24 hours in men; $\geq$250 mg/24 hours in women. Hypercalciuria was noted in 24 per cent of the patients in group 1, in 25 per cent of the patients in group 2 and in 19 per cent of the patients in group 3.

Potassium acid phosphate (K-Phos®, Beach Pharmaceuticals) was administered in four divided doses daily. The initial dose of 11 tablets daily provided 1.4 g of elemental phosphorus. Each placebo tablet, identical in appearance to the phosphate tablets, contained 0.5 g of lactose; the same number of tablets/day was given, similarly divided. If stone formation continued, the dose of phosphate or placebo was increased by 1 to 5 tablets daily, depending on the patient's clinical response. Gastrointestinal intolerance frequently limited the total dose to 12 tablets daily.

Each patient in all three groups was instructed on entry into the study to maintain a diet low in dairy foods, providing approximately 600 mg of calcium daily.

Serum levels of calcium, phosphorus, creatinine, alkaline phosphatase and uric acid; and 24-hour urinary excretion of calcium, phosphorus, creatinine, uric acid and oxalate were measured three, six and 12 months after admission to the study, and yearly thereafter. Patients were examined for eye calcification by an ophthalmologist using a slit lamp, before therapy and yearly after the start of therapy.

Rates of stone passage and stone removal in the years before treatment were compared with those during treatment. For this comparison, the pretreatment period was defined as the number of years, up to 10, between passage of the first stone and the beginning of treatment in this study. The pre-

TABLE III Stone Events per Patient per Year Before and During Therapy with Phosphate, Placebo or Diet Alone

	Group 1		Group 2		Group 3	
	Before	During	Before	During	Before	During
Patient years	183	77	120	60	123	71
Stone passage rate						
Over-all	0.67	0.54	0.78	0.33	0.57	0.32
Patients with hypercalciuria	0.48 (N = 6)	0.44	0.58 (N = 5)	0.54	0.84 (N = 5)	0.72
Patients stone-free at start of study	0.58 (N = 12)	0.28	0.75 (N = 12)	0.05	0.57 (N = 15)	0.28
Lithotomy rate	0.055	0.013	0.092	0.000	0.024	0.028
Stones per patient seen on roentgenogram	1.56	1.68	1.00	0.80	0.62	0.73

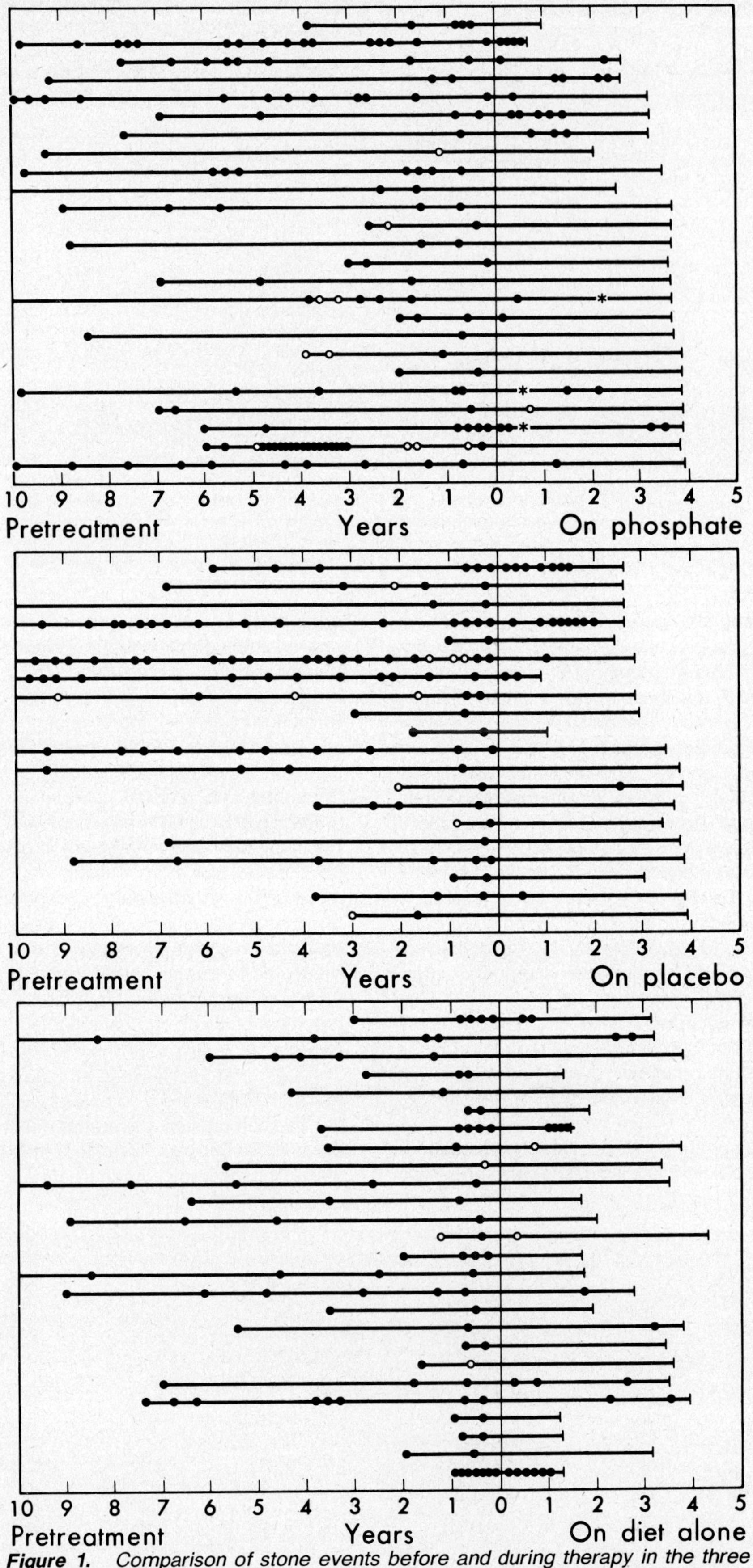

Figure 1. *Comparison of stone events before and during therapy in the three treatment groups. • Stone passage. * Multiple small stone passage. ○ Lithotomy.*

treatment rate of stone events was defined as the total number of stones less the index stone, divided by the number of years in the pretreatment period. The pretreatment lithotomy rate was defined as the total number of lithotomies divided by the number of years in the pretreatment period. The number of stones seen on an anteroposterior roentgenogram of the abdomen or on an excretory urogram at the time of entry into the study was compared with the number observed at last follow-up examination.

RESULTS

Patients' cooperation was excellent as judged by pill counts in groups 1 and 2, and by diet review performed at each clinic visit in all patients.

Stone Passage and Lithotomy. The mean rates of stone passage and lithotomy, and the number of stones per patient seen on roentgenograms during therapy are summarized in Table III. No significant intergroup differences were observed. The mean number of stones per patient seen on abdominal roentgenogram remained constant, precluding "washout" of stones or their dissolution in response to therapy. Patients with no roentgenographic evidence of stones at the start of the study showed a much lower rate of stone passage subsequently. In each treatment group, stone passage rates decreased sharply during therapy: that in group 2 fell to 7 per cent of the prestudy rate; that in group 3 to 49 per cent; and that in group 1 to 48 per cent of the prestudy rate.

The considerable individual variation in stone passage is displayed in Figure 1. The apparent cessation of stone passage during the first months of study contrasts with the highest rate of stone passage just before study, which prompted the patients' referral. Similar bursts of stone passage followed by quiescent periods are noted in the histories of most patients with nephrolithiasis seen in our medical center. A remission artifact would be introduced by any study using short-term pretreatment and follow-up periods.

Although the average frequency of stone passage for the patients in this series was once every two years, a large number of patients remained stone-free during the follow-up period. A life-table analysis of the relapse rates for the three study groups appears in Figure 2. On the average, 25 per cent of the patients had a relapse

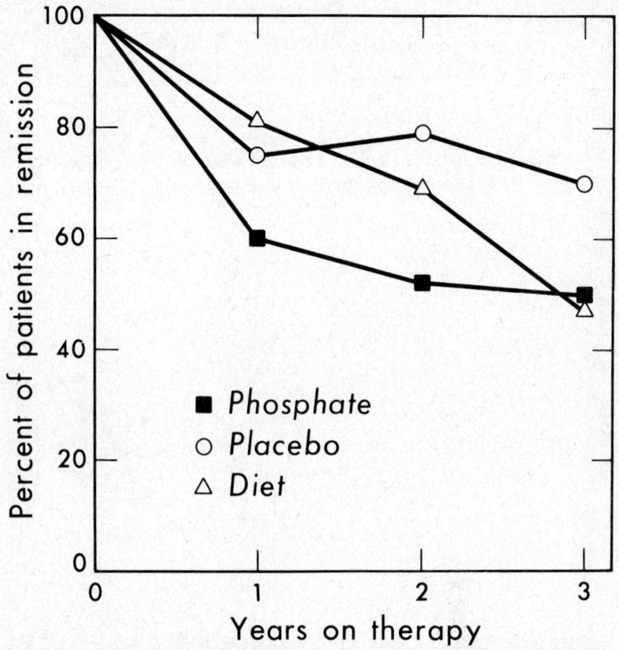

Figure 2. Life table analysis: per cent of patients remaining in remission (no passage of new stones; no new stones on roentgenogram) in the three treatment groups.

during the first year; a smaller percentage of the remainder had a relapse during the second year. After three years' experience, 70 per cent of the patients in group 2, 50 per cent of those in group 1 and 47 per cent of those in group 3 are in remission.

Urinary Chemical Changes. Restriction of dietary calcium, from 600 mg to 300 mg daily, resulted in a greater than 25 per cent reduction in urinary calcium excretion in 38 per cent of the patients in group 1, 25 per cent of those in group 2 and 43 per cent of those in group 3. Hypercalciuric patients were no more likely than normocalciuric patients to respond to dietary calcium restriction in this way. Regardless of their response to a low calcium diet, all patients were directed to maintain a diet low in dairy products throughout the study period.

In group 1 (Table IV), mean phosphorus excretion nearly doubled during the treatment period, whereas mean calcium excretion decreased to 33 per cent of base line values and remained stable thereafter.

TABLE IV Mean Urinary Calcium and Phosphorus Values During Phosphate Therapy in 25 Patients

	Base Line (Low Dairy Food Intake)	Duration of Treatment				
		3 mo	6 mo	1 yr	2 yr	3 yr
Subjects (no.)	25	18	14	21	20	10
Calcium (mg/100 ml)	238 ± 21*	173 ± 17	168 ± 17	146 ± 14	150 ± 13	183 ± 43
Phosphorus (mg/100 ml)	907 ± 69	1,712 ± 67	1,718 ± 126	1,720 ± 97	1,678 ± 102	2,126 ± 200

* Standard error of the mean.

TABLE V Reported Effects of Various Therapies on Stone Passage and Lithotomy Rates in Patients with Nephrolithiasis

Reference	Type of Therapy	No. of Patients	Mean No. of Years of Treatment	Stone Passage Rate		Lithotomy Rate	
				Before Treatment	During Treatment	Before Treatment	During Treatment
Coe, Kavalach [15]	None	17	2.4	0.32	0.51	. . .	. . .
Melnick et al. [11]	None	68	4.0	1.52	0.75	. . .	. . .
Ettinger, Kolb [13]	Inorganic phosphate	47	5.5	1.1	0.70	0.12	0.04
Pak et al. [16]	Cellulose phosphate	16	2.6	3.8	0.27	0.10	0.00
Pietrek, Kokot [14]	Cellulose phosphate	7	0.6	2.4	0.72	. . .	. . .
Coe, Kavalach [15]	Trichlor-methiazide	96	0.6	0.25	0.07	. . .	. . .
Prien, Gershoff [17]	Magnesium oxide-pyridoxine	149	4.1	1.3	0.10	. . .	. . .
Melnick et al. [11]	Magnesium oxide	142	3.0	1.43	0.32	. . .	. . .

Side Effects. Each of the three forms of treatment was well tolerated. The most frequently noted and persistent symptom was an increase in stool softness, but the percentages of patients in whom this occurred were similar in groups 1 (16 per cent) and 2 (20 per cent). No patient in group 2 gave a history of lactose intolerance; it is most unlikely that so small a dose could cause that phenomenon.

COMMENTS

In two independent studies of the natural history of kidney stone events [1,2], recurrence rates were found to increase from 14 per cent in the first year to 42 to 50 per cent at five years. The findings herein conform to those reported rates, regardless of the therapeutic regimen used in these patients.

Several investigators have remarked on the capricious nature of stone events [1–4]; yet many have ascribed beneficial effects to various forms of therapy although they have not performed objective, long-term, controlled studies [5–17], necessitating critical review of the bases upon which these treatments have been recommended. Table V summarizes the data in several recent studies that provide figures for comparison of the effects of drug regimens. In collaboration with Dr. F. O. Kolb, of the University of California San Francisco, I studied 47 patients with recurrent stone formation, who received inorganic phosphate therapy for more than five years [13]. A significant reduction in the lithotomy rate, but no decrease in stone passage, was noted. In the patients in group 2, there is an equally impressive reduction in lithotomy rate.

Cellulose phosphate was used by Pak et al. [16] in a group of patients with a remarkably high pretreatment stone passage rate: 3.8 stones per patient per year. **During treatment,** the stone passage rate for the same patients was similar to that noted herein in groups 2 and 3. Pietrek and Kokot [14], using cellulose phosphate in a study that must be criticized for its small number (seven) of subjects and the brevity of follow-up, noted high stone passage rates before treatment, and during treatment rates similar to those in the group 2 of the present study. Prien and Gershoff [17] reported that treatment with magnesium and pyridoxine could prevent recurrence of kidney stones; but a significant bias was introduced into their study by excluding from analysis 44 per cent of the patients in whom treatment was begun: one-third of the excluded patients appear to have represented treatment failure; they had episodes of colic, and therapy was discontinued because it was not efficacious. Treating 142 patients with magnesium oxide, Melnick et al. [11] used as controls retrospective chart analysis of another 68 patients. The groups may not have been comparable, since different bases for selection were used for the two groups. Magnesium oxide treatment was associated with a 78 per cent reduction in stone passage, whereas those who received no treatment showed a 49 per cent reduction in stone passage. These investigators reported that magnesium oxide induced complete remission of stone passage for two years in only 63 per cent of the patients, a rate that is similar to that which occurs during the natural course of untreated nephrolithiasis. Coe and Kavalach [15] used trichlormethiazide therapy in hypercalciuric patients whose stone passage rates appeared to be lower than reported in previously mentioned studies. No control group was analyzed; and the average duration of treatment was 20 months; approximately 20 per cent of the patients were followed for less than one year.

The development of extraskeletal calcification has

been reported in patients receiving inorganic phosphate therapy [18], but eye examinations in the patients of the present series disclosed no increase in preexisting calcifications in four patients and no new calcifications in any. Occasional loose stools were noted with equal frequency in groups 1 and 2. Diarrhea, however, has been found to occur more frequently in patients with recurrent kidney stones than in normal subjects [19].

The data from this study were examined for variables that might predict successful response to therapy. Hypercalciuria does not appear to be associated with more severe stone disease; nor does its presence affect the clinical or chemical response to phosphate therapy. Those patients who responded to a change from a low dairy product diet (approximately 600 mg of calcium) to a low calcium (300 mg) diet by having a greater than 25 per cent reduction in urinary calcium could be considered to be a subgroup with excessive gastrointestinal absorption of calcium, rather than excessive renal calcium wastage. Hyperabsorption of calcium appears to be associated with an improved chemical response to phosphate treatment. Patients showing a hyperabsorption pattern responded with a 49 per cent reduction in urinary calcium; whereas the remainder of the patients in group 1 showed a 24 per cent reduction in urinary calcium excretion. Mean urine phosphorus increased 88 per cent with phosphate treatment, but no correlation was seen between the degree of the increase in urinary phosphorus and the degree of the decrease in urinary calcium. Similarly, there was no difference in urinary phosphorus levels between patients who continued to pass stones and those who did not. Our data do not support the view of Howard et al. [5] that phosphorus and its metabolic products retard calcium oxalate crystallization in urine. In patients whose roentgenograms showed no stones at the start of the study, the subsequent clinical course appeared to be less severe than in those whose initial roentgenograms revealed stones, regardless of the type of treatment given. I noted similar results in a previous study with Kolb [13].

A short-term study of drug therapy of recurrent kidney stone disease is likely to disclose beneficial effects if one simply compares the stone passage events in each patient before treatment, with those during treatment. The effects of any form of therapy must be compared with the approximately 50 per cent reduction in stone passage that is seen during two to three years' observation with placebo or diet therapy alone. The present study showed that patients with recurrent calcium oxalate kidney stones derived no benefit from phosphate therapy. The data suggest that patients whose urine calcium levels fell as oral calcium intake was reduced are more responsive than others to the hypocalciuric effects of phosphate treatment. Whereas hypercalciuria does not correlate with increased severity of urolithiasis, a reduction of urinary calcium may afford some protection against calcium stones. It is possible that other factors such as brushite crystal formation or subclinical dehydration secondary to loose stools, could diminish the effect of lowered urinary calcium excretion induced by phosphate treatment.

It is recommended, on the basis of these observations, that patients be spared the cost, inconvenience and possible side effects of aggressive medical treatment for this disorder, particularly if they are free of renal calcification. Until it becomes possible to identify those subgroups of stone-forming patients who have need for and who will benefit from any of a variety of therapies, the results of only adequately controlled studies in which patients have been observed for a minimum of three years should be accepted for consideration.

ACKNOWLEDGMENT

I express my gratitude to Mr. Richard Jenkins, Beach Pharmaceutical Company, for providing phosphate (K-Phos®) and placebo tablets.

REFERENCES

1. Blacklock NJ: The pattern of urolithiasis in the Royal Navy. Proceedings of the Renal Stone Research Symposium, Leeds, England, April 1968 (Hodgkinson A, Nordin BEC, eds), London, Churchill, 1969, p 33.
2. Williams RE: The natural history of renal lithiasis. Proceedings of the Renal Stone Research Symposium, Leeds, England, April 1968 (Hodgkinson A, Nordin BEC, eds), London, Churchill, 1969, p 65.
3. Kolb FO: General approach to the treatment of the patient with renal stones. Mod Treat 4: 464, 1967.
4. Hockaday TDR, Smith LH Jr: Renal calculi. DM November, 1963.
5. Howard JE, Thomas WC Jr, Mukai T, et al.: The calcification of cartilage by urine, and a suggestion for therapy in patients with certain kinds of calculi. Trans Assoc Am Physicians 75: 301, 1962.
6. Dent CE, Harper CM, Parfitt AM: The effect of cellulose phosphate on calcium metabolism in patients with hypercalciuria. Clin Sci 27: 417, 1964.
7. Edwards NA, Russell RGG, Hodgkinson A: The effect of oral phosphate in patients with recurrent renal calculus. Br J Urol 37: 390, 1965.
8. Bernstein DS, Newton R: The effect of oral sodium phosphate on the formation of renal calculi and on idiopathic hypercalciuria. Lancet 2: 1105, 1966.
9. Thomas WC Jr, Miller GH Jr: Inorganic phosphates in the treatment of renal calculi. Mod Treat 4: 494, 1967.
10. Pak CYC, Wortsman J, Bennett JE, et al.: Control of hypercalcemia with cellulose phosphate. J Clin Endocrinol Metab 28: 1829, 1968.
11. Melnick I, Landes RR, Hoffman AA, Burch JF: Magnesium therapy for recurring calcium oxalate urinary calculi. J Urol 105: 119, 1971.
12. Smith LH, Thomas WC Jr, Arnaud CD: Orthophosphate therapy

in calcium renal lithiasis. International Symposium on Renal Stone Research, Madrid, 1972 (Cifuentes Delatte L, Rapado A, Hodgkinson A, eds), Basel, S. Karger, 1973, p 188.
13. Ettinger B, Kolb FO: Inorganic phosphate treatment of nephrolithiasis. Am J Med 55: 32, 1973.
14. Pietrek J, Kokot F: Treatment of patients with calcium-containing renal stones with cellulose phosphate. Br J Urol 45: 136, 1973.
15. Coe L, Kavalach AG: Hypercalciuria and hyperuricosuria in patients with calcium nephrolithiasis. N Engl J Med 291: 1344, 1974.
16. Pak CYC, Delea CS, Bartter FC: Successful treatment of recurrent nephrolithiasis (calcium stones) with cellulose phosphate. N Engl J Med 290: 175, 1974.
17. Prien EL Sr, Gershoff SF: Magnesium oxide-pyridoxine therapy for recurrent calcium oxalate calculi. J Urol 112: 509, 1974.
18. Dudley FJ, Blackburn CRB: Extraskeletal calcification complicating oral neutral-phosphate therapy. Lancet 2: 628, 1970.
19. Lavan JN, Neale FC, Posen S: Urinary calculi. Clinical, biochemical and radiological studies in 619 patients. Med J Aust 2: 1049, 1971.

Irreversible Acute Renal Failure in Idiopathic Nephrotic Syndrome

LEOPOLDO RAIJ, M.D.
WILLIAM F. KEANE, M.D.
ARTHUR LEONARD, M.D.
FRED L. SHAPIRO, M.D.
Minneapolis, Minnesota

In five adult patients (aged 44 to 74 years) with idiopathic nephrotic syndrome, irreversible acute renal failure developed. Prior renal disease, associated systemic illness or occlusion of major renal vasculature was not present. All patients continued to excrete large amounts of proteins (8.6 to 15 g/24 hours) despite a minimal glomerular filtration rate and severe oliguria. One patient died after five months without recovering renal function. Four patients have required hemodialysis for a period of 12 to 58 months. The failure to recover renal function could not be explained by the light microscopic findings. It is suggested that the irreversibility of the renal failure may be related to either permanent alterations in renal blood flow or ultrastructural changes, or to both. Clinically, adult patients in whom acute renal failure develops during the course of idiopathic nephrotic syndrome seem to have a grave prognosis. Protracted oliguria or irreversible renal failure can be expected to occur.

The prognosis in patients with the nephrotic syndrome depends upon its etiology and histopathology, usually ascertainable by renal biopsy. In patients in whom acute renal failure develops the outcome is determined by a multitude of factors including age, etiology and nonrenal complications. However, patients who survive acute renal failure have been reported to recover renal function and not to require chronic hemodialysis [1, 2]. In the present study, we describe five patients in whom irreversible acute renal failure developed during the course of idiopathic nephrotic syndrome and who have required dialysis for periods up to 58 months.

Case 1. This 68 year old retired farmer consulted his physician because of pedal and periorbital edema with an associated 35 pound weight gain in the last week of December 1973. He had no history of prior renal disease, systemic illness or exposure to known nephrotoxins. Physical examination revealed generalized edema but was otherwise noncontributory. Blood pressure was 240/110 mm Hg. The hematocrit value was 40 per cent and the white blood cell count was 6,300/mm^3 with a normal differential. Urinalysis revealed a specific gravity of 1.023, 4+ protein, multiple granular casts, 3 to 4 red blood cells/hpf and 12 to 15 white blood cells/hpf. The serum electrolytes were normal; blood urea nitrogen was 101 mg/dl and serum creatinine 4.8 mg/dl. Serum total protein was 4.1 g/dl and serum albumin was 1.8 g/dl. Antistreptolysin O (ASO) titer was within normal limits. Urine volumes varied between 800 and 1,000 cc/24 hours. An intravenous pyelogram revealed diminished function bilaterally but normal-sized kidneys. The patient was treated with methyldopa, 250 mg given twice a day, and fu-

From the Regional Kidney Disease Program and the Department of Medicine, Hennepin County Medical Center and the University of Minnesota, Minneapolis, Minnesota. Requests for reprints should be addressed to Dr. Leopoldo Raij, Regional Kidney Disease Program, 701 Park Avenue South, Minneapolis, Minnesota 55415. Manuscript accepted December 11, 1975.

TABLE I Clinical and Laboratory Data Preceding Institution of Hemodialysis

Case No.	Age (yr) and Sex	Blood Pressure (mm Hg)	Blood Urea Nitrogen/Serum Creatinine (mg/dl)	Creatinine Clearance (cc/min)	Serum Total Protein (g/dl)	Serum Albumin (g/dl)	Maximum 24-Hour Urine Output (cc)	24-Hour Urine (g)	$C_{Alb}:C_{Cr}$*
1	68, M	145/85	199/12.5	4.6	3.9	1.3	600	15	0.11
2	66, M	160/90	185/10.5	2	4.6	2.4	200	14	0.15
3	74, M	170/90	105/5.9	7	4.2	1.2	400	8.6	...
4	44, M	150/90	115/8	7	4.0	1.4	600	13	0.06
5	63, M	140/90	107/10	2	4.3	1.1	600	15	...

* C_{Alb} = clearance of albumin. C_{Cr} = clearance of creatinine.

rosemide, 80 mg given twice a day. There was no response to diuretic therapy and generalized edema persisted. His renal function deteriorated further and he was referred to the Regional Kidney Disease Program (RKDP) in the second week of February 1974. On admission he was disoriented. Physical examination revealed generalized edema but the findings were otherwise unremarkable. The blood pressure was 145/85 mm Hg. The hematocrit value was 27.6 per cent with a normal white blood cell count and differential. Urinalysis revealed a specific gravity of 1.014, 4+ protein and occasional white blood cells/hpf and red blood cells/hpf. Blood urea nitrogen was 199 mg/dl and serum creatinine 12.5 mg/dl. Creatinine clearance was 4.6 cc/min; the 24-hour protein excretion was 15 g with urine volumes not exceeding 600 cc/24 hours. Serum total protein was 3.9 g/dl; the serum albumin was 1.3 g/dl. Serum electrophoresis did not show evidence of a myeloma protein. Urine electrophoresis revealed that the urine protein was mainly albumin with variable quantities of different globulin fractions. The ratio of the clearance of albumin to the clearance of creatinine ($C_{Alb}:C_{Cr}$) was 0.11. Fluorescent antinuclear antibody was negative. Total hemolytic complement, C3 and C4 were normal. Selective renal arteriograms and an inferior venacavogram with selective renal vein studies were within normal limits. A retrograde pyelogram revealed no obstruction. Hemodialysis was instituted with progressive improvement in the patient's sensorium. A summary of the laboratory data preceding institution of hemodialysis is shown in Table I. A renal biopsy was performed 10 weeks after the onset of symptoms. Multiple intravenous infusions of salt poor albumin were also given, and, although the serum albumin level rose to 3.6 g/dl, the patient remained oliguric with urine outputs consistently below 600 cc/day and continued to excrete approximately 7 g of protein/24 hours. He failed to recover renal function and has been treated with thrice weekly hemodialysis for over 14 months.

Case 2. This 66 year old man was well until December 1973 when malaise, peripheral edema and weight gain developed. He was seen by his private physician and in the second week of January 1974 was referred to the RKDP for evaluation. He had no history of previous renal disease, systemic illness or exposure to known nephrotoxins. Physical examination was within normal limits except for the presence of anasarca. The blood pressure was 160/90 mm Hg. The hematocrit value was 37 per cent with a normal white blood cell count and differential. Urinalysis showed a specific gravity of 1.016; 4+ protein, 0 to 2 white blood cells/hpf, 0 to 2 red blood cells/hpf and an occasional granular cast. Serum electrolytes were normal; blood urea nitrogen was 156 mg/dl,

TABLE II Summary of Light Microscopic Changes

	Case 1	Case 2	Case 3		Case 4		Case 5	
Biopsy number	1	1	1	PM*	1	2†	1	2‡
Glomeruli								
Number of glomeruli	12	5	7	>100	6	15	17	8
Basement membrane thickening	0	0	0	0	0	0	0	0
Focal segmental sclerosis	+ JM	0	±	± to +	0	+ JM	± FL	± FL
Complete hyalinization	0	0	+	+	0	0	0	0
Mesangial proliferation	± FL	±	±	± to +	0	0	± FL	± FL
Increased mesangial matrix	± to +	+ FL	+	+	± FL	+ FL	+ FL	+ FL
Endothelial cell proliferation	0	0	0		0	0	0	0
Interstitium								
Fibrosis	± to +	±	+ to ++	+ to ++	±	±	±	± to +
Edema	++	+	±	±	+	+	±	+
Tubular changes	++ FL	+ to ++	+ to ++	+ to ++	+	+	+	+
Vascular changes	+	+	+	+ to ++	—	±	+	+

NOTE: 0 = not present; ± mild or rare; + = moderate, ++ marked; FL = focal and local; JM = juxtamedullary.
* Postmortem, five months after initial biopsy.
† Three months after initial biopsy.
‡ Five months after initial biopsy.

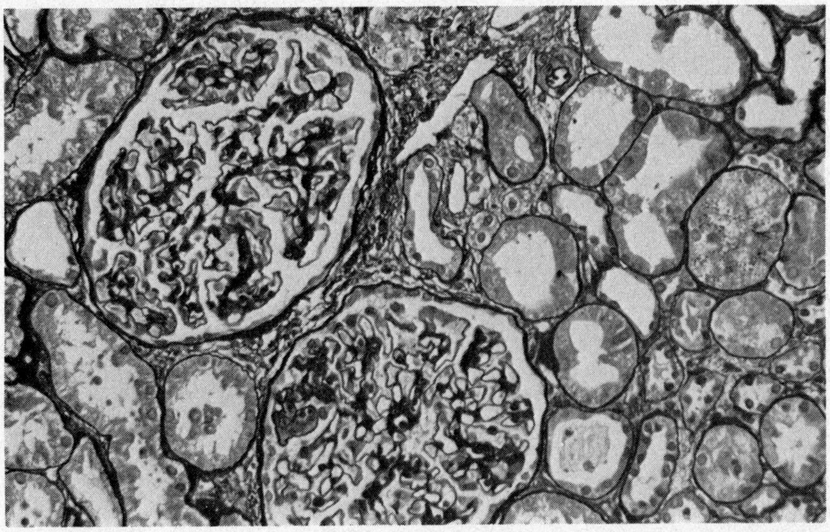

Figure 1. *Glomeruli and associated tubules from patient (Case 2) exhibiting minimal increase in mesangial matrix. The tubules show slight dilatation, occasional flattened epithelium and degenerating cells. Jones' silver stain; original magnification × 277, reduced by 20 per cent.*

serum creatinine 5.8 mg/dl, serum total protein 4.6 g/dl and serum albumin 2.4 g/dl. Serum electrophoresis did not show evidence of a myeloma protein. The urinary excretion of sodium and potassium was 16 meq/liter and 47 meq/liter, respectively. Urinary protein excretion was 14 g/24 hours. The proteinuria consisted primarily of albumin with variable quantities of different globulin fractions consistent with a nonselective proteinuria. The C_{Alb}:C_{Cr} was 0.15. Total hemolytic complement, C3 and C4 were within normal limits. Fluorescent antinuclear antibody was negative; ASO titer was within normal limits. Roentgenologic studies, including selective renal arteriograms, selective renal vein studies and retrograde pyelogram, were all within normal limits. Both kidneys were of normal size. Despite intravenous infusions of salt poor albumin and furosemide, the urine output was approximately 200 cc/24 hours. The blood urea nitrogen increased to 185 mg/dl and the serum creatinine to 10.5 mg/dl; creatinine clearance was 2 cc/min, and hemodialysis was instituted. A summary of the laboratory data preceding institution of hemodialysis is shown in Table I. During the last week of January a percutaneous renal biopsy was performed (Table II and Figure 1). Treatment with high protein diet and prednisone, 60 mg/day, was begun. The administration of prednisone was discontinued after one month because of lack of response. While receiving dialysis, the serum albumin level progressively rose to 3.4 g/dl but the patient remained oliguric with urine outputs not exceeding 200 cc/24 hours. Urine protein excretion continued at approximately 5 g/24 hours. Renal function continues to be minimal and he has been treated with regular hemodialysis for the past 16 months.

Case 3. This 74 year old retired minister underwent a transurethral resection of an enlarged prostate in March 1973. At that time, the blood urea nitrogen was 16 mg/dl. In January 1974 he noted progressive pedal edema and a 25 pound weight gain over a three week period. During the first week of February, he was admitted to another hospital where he was noted to be oliguric. The blood urea nitrogen was 105

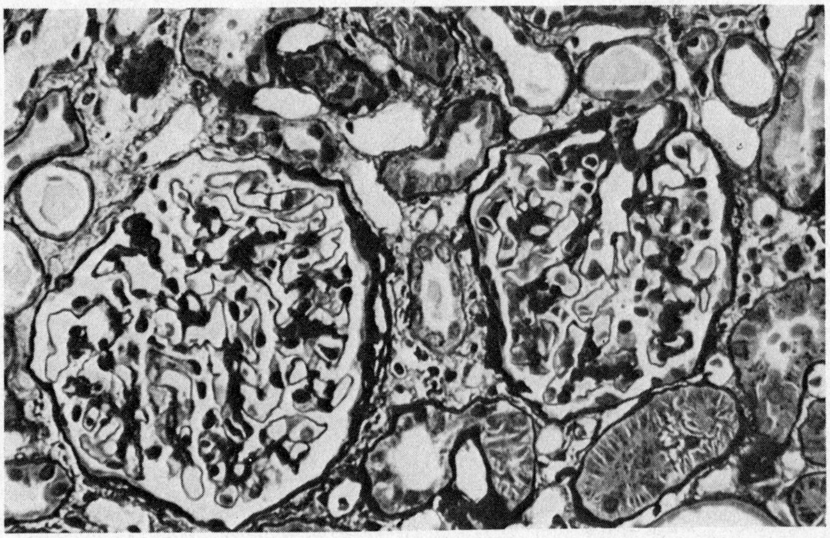

Figure 2. *Biopsy specimen from patient (Case 3) demonstrating glomeruli with minimal mesangial increase and normal glomerular basement membrane. Jones' silver stain; original magnification × 400, reduced by 20 per cent.*

mg/dl and serum creatinine 3.9 mg/dl. Urinalysis revealed a specific gravity of 1.014, 4+ protein, 0 to 2 white blood cells/hpf, 1 to 2 red blood cells/hpf and an occasional cast. He was treated with intravenous infusions of salt poor albumin and with furosemide without clinical improvement. Renal biopsy was performed (Table II, Figures 2 and 3). Two weeks later he was referred to the RKDP for further evaluation. He had no history of prior systemic illness or exposure to known nephrotoxins. Physical examination revealed generalized edema but was otherwise noncontributory. His blood pressure was 170/90 mm Hg. Initial laboratory data revealed a serum sodium of 126 meq/liter; serum potassium of 4.5 meq/liter, blood urea nitrogen of 105 mg/dl and a serum creatinine of 5.9 mg/dl. The creatinine clearance was 7 cc/min. Urinary protein excretion was 8.6 g/24 hours. Serum electrophoresis did not reveal a myeloma protein; Bence-Jones proteinuria was absent. Urinary sodium was 129 meq/liter and urinary potassium 38 meq/liter while he was receiving furosemide. Serum total protein was 4.2 g/dl and serum albumin 1.2 g/dl. Fluorescent antinuclear antibody was negative; ASO titer was normal. Total hemolytic complement, C3 and C4 were within normal limits. An intravenous pyelogram revealed normal-sized kidneys. Selective renal arteriograms and selective renal vein studies were within normal limits. Retrograde pyelograms revealed no obstruction. The patient was treated with intravenous infusions of salt poor albumin and furosemide but failed to respond. He remained oliguric with urine outputs of approximately 400 cc/day. Because of severe anorexia, nausea and vomiting, hemodialysis was begun. During the hospital course the patient became febrile (102°F) and hypotensive (blood pressure 70/0 mm). Urine culture revealed 10^5 colonies/ml of Escherichia coli. He was treated with intravenous albumin and saline solutions. Gentamicin was given in a dosage appropriate for his degree of renal

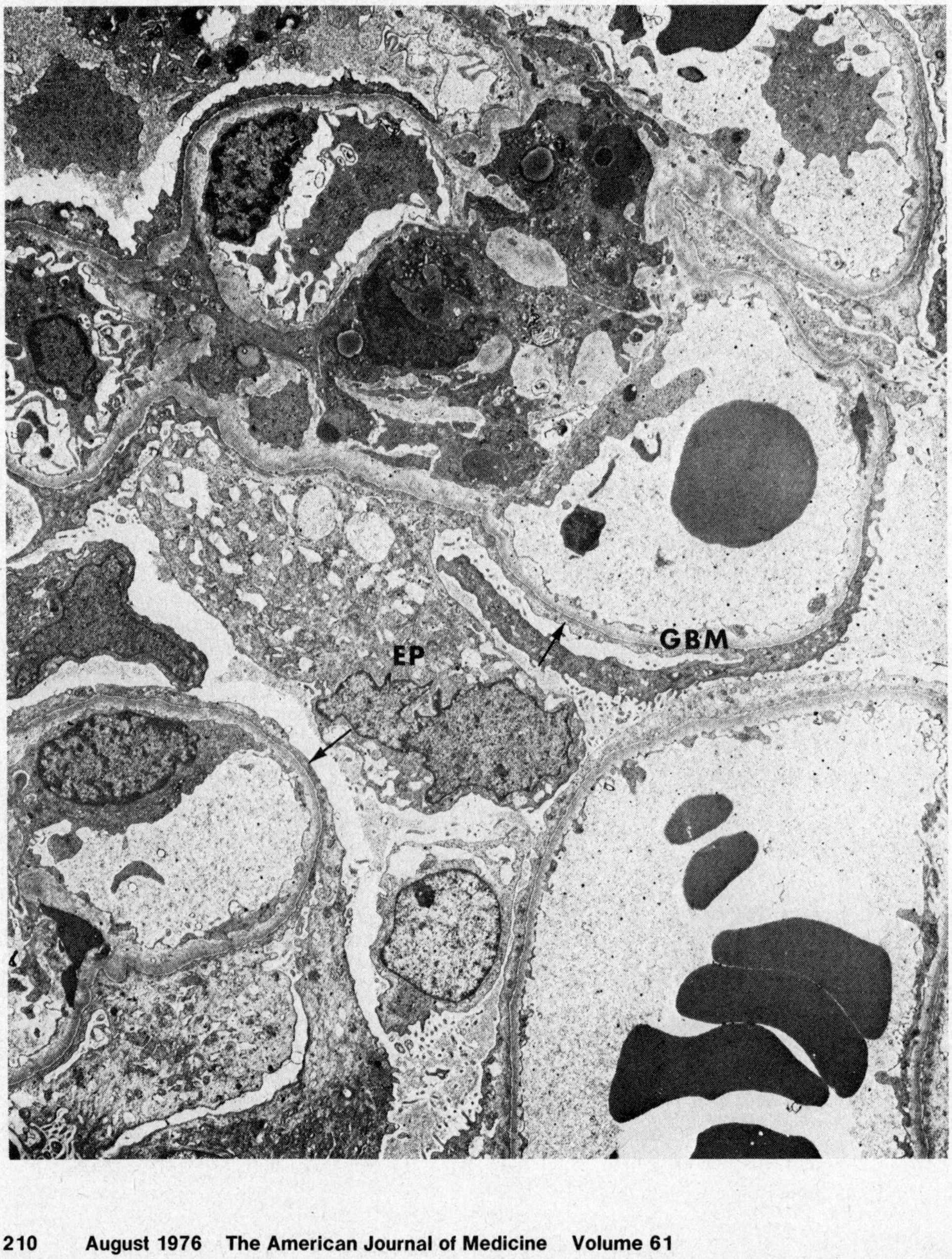

Figure 3. *Electron micrograph from the biopsy specimen of patient (Case 3) demonstrating glomerular basement membranes of normal thickness and lack of electron dense deposits. Note extensive fusion of epithelial cell (EP) foot processes* ***(arrows).*** *Original magnification × 6,100, reduced by 30 per cent.*

insufficiency [3]. His blood pressure promptly stabilized and he became afebrile within 24 hours. He continued to be oliguric necessitating hemodialysis three times a week. The serum albumin level progressively rose to 3.8 g/24 hours, but he remained oliguric excreting approximately 100 cc/24 hours of urine containing 5 to 8 g of protein. Maintenance hemodialysis was continued for four months but he manifested poor emotional adaptation to treatment; in June 1974, he refused long-term hemodialysis. He died three weeks later and a postmortem examination confined to the kidneys demonstrated patent renal vasculature. Microscopic examination revealed changes similar to those seen in the original biopsy specimen (Table II, Figure 4).

Case 4. This 44 year old migrant farm worker consulted his physician because of progressive peripheral edema and a decrease in urine output at the end of January 1974. Physical examination was noncontributory except for peripheral edema. Blood pressure was 140/85 mm Hg. Laboratory data revealed a blood urea nitrogen of 52 mg/dl; serum creatinine of 1.5 mg/dl, and a urinary protein excretion of 20 g/24 hours. Urinalysis revealed a specific gravity of 1.020, 4+ protein and a negative microscopic examination. The first renal biopsy was performed three weeks after the onset of illness and a diagnosis of idiopathic nephrotic syndrome was made (Table II). Prednisone, 40 mg twice a day, was given for 10 days. Because of deterioration of renal function he was transferred to the RKDP at the beginning of April 1974. There was no history of exposure to known nephrotoxins or systemic illness. Physical examination was noncontributory except for peripheral edema. Blood pressure was 150/90 mm Hg. Initial laboratory data revealed a blood urea nitrogen of 115 mg/dl and a serum creatinine of 8 mg/dl. The creatinine clearance was 7 cc/min. The 24 hour urine protein excretion was 13 g. Serum total protein was 4.0 g/dl and the serum albumin was 1.4 g/dl. Total hemolytic complement, C3 and C4 were within normal limits. Fluorescent antinuclear antibody was negative. Serum electrophoresis did not reveal the presence of a myeloma protein. Urine electrophoresis revealed predominately albumin with variable quantities of different globulin fractions consistent with a nonselective proteinuria. C_{Alb}:C_{Cr} was 0.06. An intravenous pyelogram revealed normal-sized kidneys. Selective renal arteriograms and renal vein studies were within normal limits. Due to uremic symptoms, anasarca and severe oliguria, unresponsiveness to furosemide therapy and intravenous infusions of salt poor albumin, hemodialysis was instituted. The summary of the laboratory values before dialysis is shown in Table I. The administration of prednisone was continued for one month and then discontinued because of lack of response. A second renal biopsy was performed three months after the initial one (Table II). While receiving dialysis, the serum albumin level rose to 3.2 g/dl but the patient remained oliguric, excreting approximately 200 cc/day of urine; proteinuria continued in the range of 15 g/24 hours. Because of the persistent renal impairment, he has been treated with hemodialysis three times a week for the past 12 months.

Case 5. This 63 year old farmer was well until the end of May 1970 when periorbital edema and progressive swelling of the legs developed. There was no history of systemic illness or exposure to known nephrotoxins. Physical examination revealed generalized edema. Blood pressure was 140/90 mg Hg. Initial laboratory studies in June 1970 included a blood urea nitrogen of 41 mg/dl, serum creatinine of 1.7 mg/dl, serum albumin of 1.3 g/dl and a 24-hour urine protein excretion of 15.9 g. The urinalysis revealed a specific gravity of 1.024, 4+ protein, occasional white blood cells/hpf and granular casts. Serum electrophoresis did not reveal a myeloma protein. Total hemolytic complement was normal. An intravenous pyelogram revealed normal-sized kidneys. A percutaneous renal biopsy was performed in June 1970 (Table II). A diagnosis of idiopathic nephrotic syndrome was made and prednisone, 80 mg every other day, and furosemide were given. He was readmitted during August 1970 because of persistent proteinuria and deterioration of renal function accompanied by oliguria. Laboratory studies showed a blood urea nitrogen of 95 mg/dl, serum creatinine of 3.8 mg/dl and serum albumin of 1.1 g/dl. Urinalysis revealed a specific gravity of 1.015, 4+ protein, occasional white blood cells/hpf

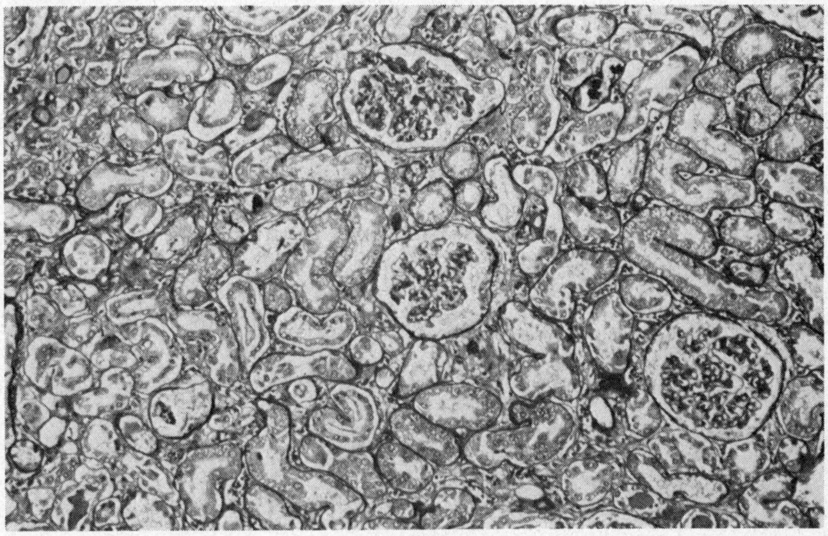

Figure 4. *Postmortem specimen from patient (Case 3) showing good preservation of the glomeruli and the interstitium. Slight dilatation of tubules can be seen. Jones' silver stain; original magnification × 134, reduced by 20 per cent.*

and an occasional cast. Creatinine clearance was 2 cc/min. Because of anasarca, oliguria and failure to respond to the administration of furosemide and intravenous infusions of salt poor albumin, peritoneal dialysis was instituted. After 24 hours of uncomplicated peritoneal dialysis, abdominal pain, hypotension (80/50 mm Hg) and fever (101°F) developed. Volume expanders, hydrocortisone and sodium colistimethate (1.5 mg/kg/24 hours) were administered and his condition stabilized promptly. An exploratory laparotomy was performed which revealed no evidence of peritonitis or perforated viscus. Hypotension did not recur, and the patient recovered uneventfully. However, renal function did not improve; blood urea nitrogen was 107 mg/dl and serum creatinine 10 mg/dl. He was referred to the RKDP where hemodialysis was instituted at the end of August 1970. Selective renal arteriograms and renal vein studies were within normal limits. Retrograde pyelography revealed patent ureters. A second renal biopsy was performed five months after the initial one (Table II). The serum albumin level subsequently rose to 3.8 g/dl, but he remained oliguric with 24-hour urine outputs not exceeding 600 cc and containing approximately 15 g of protein. He has required regular hemodialysis for the last 58 months.

RENAL BIOPSIES

Methods. Portions of the kidney biopsy specimen were fixed in 10 per cent buffered formalin. Paraffin-embedded sections were stained with hematoxylin and eosin, Mallory's trichrome, periodic acid-Schiff and Jones' silver methenamine for light microscopy. Portions of the biopsy specimens were frozen in isopentane prechilled in liquid nitrogen and stained with fluorescein-labeled specific antiserums to human immunoglobulins G (IgG), A (IgA), M (IgM), fibrinogen and C3 by methods previously described [4,5]. Electron microscopic studies were performed on tissue prepared by double fixation using 3 per cent glutaraldehyde and 2 per cent osmic acid. The tissue was dehydrated in alcohol and embedded in epoxy resin (Epon® 812). Thin sections were cut with LKB ultratome and stained with uranyl acetate and lead citrate.

Histopathology. Examination of glomeruli in renal biopsy specimens revealed minimal mesangial proliferation in a focal and segmental distribution in all but one patient (Case 4). The Jones' silver stain demonstrated normal thickness of the glomerular basement membranes with no evidence of spikes (Figure 2). Distinct focal segmental glomerulosclerosis was seen in one juxtamedullary glomeruli in Case 1 and in two glomeruli in Case 4. Complete hyalinization of one of seven glomeruli was noted in Case 3. The interstitium did not show cellular infiltrates and the degree of interstitial fibrosis was variable. It was moderately severe in Case 3 (Figures 2 and 4) and minimal in Cases 1 and 5. Variable degrees of interstitial edema were present in all patients. In Cases 1, 2, 3 and 5 (Figures 1 and 4) many tubules were dilated; some presented a flat epithelium with areas of regeneration. In the other case the proximal tubular cells had a foamy appearance, but were otherwise normal. Arterioles and arteries demonstrated fibrous thickening of the intima and some increase of the media, changes similar to those seen in patients of the same age without renal disease.

Immunofluorescent studies were negative for immunoglobulin and complement components in frozen sections of kidney biopsy specimens in all patients. Electron microscopic studies performed on tissue obtained in Cases 3 and 4 revealed diffuse fusion of the epithelial cell foot processes, with abscence of electron dense deposits or thickening of the glomerular basement membrane (Figure 3). (The electron microscopic studies were kindly performed by Drs. Robert Anderson and Nancy Staley.)

COMMENTS

In five patients with idiopathic nephrotic syndrome acute renal failure developed during the course of their disease. Neither renal vascular occlusion nor marked histologic alterations in the glomeruli or interstitium could adequately explain the severity of the renal impairment.

No patient was exposed to recognized nephrotoxins prior to the onset of acute renal failure. Although all patients received diuretics, the interstitial nephritis occasionally induced by these drugs [6] was not found in the study of the biopsy specimens. The immunofluorescent studies gave no evidence of immunologically mediated injury. Cases 1 through 4 were referred to the RKDP within a two month period. However, neither environmental nor occupational factors could be defined that would establish a relationship between the etiology of the disease and its temporal appearance. Nosologically, our patients would be classified within the group of patients with idiopathic nephrotic syndrome. In two of them, light microscopic studies revealed focal glomerulosclerosis whereas the other three patients showed a focal and segmental increase in the mesangial matrix with minimal degrees of proliferation. The tubular changes observed in some biopsy specimens were compatible with those seen in acute tubular necrosis [7].

Hypovolemia, occasionally leading to hypotension and shock, has been documented in patients with the nephrotic syndrome [8]. A marked reduction in blood pressure did not precede the onset of acute renal failure in any of our patients, but a brief episode of hypotension complicated the clinical course of two of them.

The pathophysiology of acute renal failure remains unclear, although alterations in renal hemodynamics are believed important. Hollenberg et al. [9,10] observed a two thirds reduction in renal blood flow in patients with acute renal failure, independent of the etiology. They also found that the decrease in blood flow was preferentially cortical and probably induced by an increase in vascular resistance. Utilizing renal micropuncture technics, many investigators have documented a marked decrease or complete lack of glomerular filtration in different experimental models of acute renal failure [11,12]. The mechanisms of these changes have not been elucidated but recent observations tend to incriminate the renin-angiotensin system [13]. Experimentally, chronic volume expansion protects against [14], whereas volume depletion predisposes to, the development of acute renal failure [15]. Patients with the nephrotic syndrome are subjected to a persistent decrease in plasma volume which may lead to renal underperfusion. Under these circumstances further insults, however minimal, may upset the precariously balanced renal perfusion and contribute to the development of acute renal failure. Included in this category of insults may be a sudden worsening of the nephrotic syndrome with or without clinically evident episodes of hypotension.

Three patients were treated with corticosteroids but none responded. It is interesting to note that all patients continued to excrete large amounts of protein despite severe oliguria (Table I). The C_{Alb}:C_{Cr} in our patients was 0.06 to 0.15 (Table I). The similar ratio in a hypothetical nephrotic patient with a creatinine clearance of 80 cc/min, serum albumin of 1.5 g/dl, urine output of 1,200 cc/24 hours and with a 24-hour albumin excretion of 9 g, would be 0.005. The heavy, nonselective proteinuria in our oliguric patients may be due to a marked increase in glomerular permeability to large molecules despite a low glomerular filtration rate [16]. A concomitant decrease in the reabsorptive capacity of injured tubules cannot be excluded, particularly since patients with acute tubular necrosis are known to excrete small amounts of low molecular weight proteins that are normally reabsorbed by the tubules [17].

The permeability characteristics of the glomerulus continue to be controversial. Current evidence supports the existence of a two stage barrier to filtration of large molecules, involving both the glomerular basement membrane and the epithelial cells [18]. The glomerular epithelial cell foot processes line the outer surface of the glomerular basement membrane; between the foot processes epithelial slit pores have been demonstrated. Studies utilizing ultrastructural tracers indicate that the final barrier for small molecules may be at the level of the epithelial slit pores [19]. Increased permeability of the glomerular basement membrane and proteinuria are regularly associated with diffuse fusion of the foot processes; this is considered to be a nonspecific reaction to the increased passage of protein [20].

Robson et al. [16] found that children with lipoid nephrosis have a marked decrease in the clearance of polyvinylpyrrolidone molecules with a radius less than 35 Å. Remission of the nephrotic syndrome after steroid therapy results in normalization of the clearance of these small molecules. These investigators suggested that the selective reduction in the clearance of small molecules, including inulin, may be due to the severe swelling and fusion of the foot processes with obliteration of the slit pores.

Cox et al. [21] studied the mechanisms of oliguria in a model of unilateral acute renal failure induced by the intrarenal infusion of norepinephrine. After measuring different physiologic parameters, they concluded that a marked reduction in glomerular permeability was an important factor in the decreased formation of filtrate observed in that model. Transmission and scanning electron microscopic studies revealed loss of the foot process structure, a finding similar to but more severe than that present in the nephrotic syndrome. These investigators hypothesized that the decrease in glomerular permeability may be related to the changes observed in the epithelial cells by electron microscopy.

Based on the reports of Robson et al. [17] and Cox et al. [21], it is tempting to speculate that the severe impairment in glomerular filtration rate noted in our patients could in part be secondary to a similar structural change. This concept is supported by the electron microscopic studies of the biopsy specimens obtained from two patients which showed extensive fusion of the foot processes and otherwise normal glomerular basement membranes.

Although, histologically, the tubular changes observed in our patients were similar to those occasionally seen in patients with acute renal failure of diverse etiologies, their clinical outcome was different. The majority of investigators agree that most patients with "classic" acute renal failure recover renal function but not necessarily to normal levels. Lewers et al. [1] studied a group of 30 patients two to 15 years after they had had acute renal failure; they found that 40 per cent did not regain normal renal function but only three had creatinine clearances below 80 cc/min. Hall et al. [2] studied the immediate and long-term prognosis in 186 patients with acute renal failure. In 22 of 87 survivors studied an average of 45 months after the onset of acute renal failure, recovery of renal function was incomplete. Although patients over 40 years of age rarely achieved normal clearance values, clinical recovery was good and none required long-term hemodialysis.

In the present study, in no patient did renal function recover and all required regular hemodialysis in order to sustain life. One patient (Case 3) died after 150 days of oliguria when he refused long-term dialysis. The other four patients have been managed by long-term hemodialysis for periods of 12 to 58 months.

Acute renal failure complicating the course of the idiopathic nephrotic syndrome was the subject of two previous reports [22,23] that included a total of five adult patients (aged 44 to 60 years). Although all these patients regained renal function, the average duration of oliguria was 43 days. This greatly exceeds the 10 to 16 days of oliguria encountered in most patients with acute renal failure secondary to diverse etiologies [2,24]. We have also observed a 65 year old patient (not included in this report) with idiopathic nephrotic syndrome and acute renal failure in whom, however, renal function did recover, but after 30 days of oliguria. The protracted oliguria, reported in this study, and irreversible renal failure, are not explained by the pathologic findings seen by light microscopy. It remains to be determined whether the failure to recover renal function can be explained by permanent alterations in intrarenal blood flow, the ultrastructural changes or both.

From the clinical point of view, it becomes evident that acute renal failure in adult patients with the idiopathic nephrotic syndrome carries a grave prognosis with a high incidence of either prolonged oliguria or irreversible renal failure.

ACKNOWLEDGMENT

We wish to thank Drs. Robert Vernier, Alfred F. Michael and Alfred J. Fish for their constructive criticism of the manuscript. We are also thankful to Dr. John Crosson for his cooperation with the histopathology.

REFERENCES

1. Lewers DT, Matthew TH, Maher JF, Schreiner GE: Long-term follow-up of renal function and histology after acute tubular necrosis. Ann Intern Med 73: 523, 1970.
2. Hall JW, Johnson WJ, Maher FT, Hunt JC: Immediate and long-term prognosis in acute renal failure. Ann Intern Med 73: 515, 1970.
3. Chan RA, Benner EJ, Hoeprich PD: Gentamicin therapy in renal failure. A nomogram for dosage. Ann Intern Med 76: 773, 1972.
4. Raij L, Hoyer JR, Michael AF: Steroid resistant nephrotic syndrome. Recurrence after transplantation. Ann Intern Med 77: 581, 1972.
5. Michael AF, Drummond KN, Good RA, Vernier RL: Acute poststreptococcal glomerulonephritis: immune deposit disease. J Clin Invest 45: 237, 1966.
6. Lyons H, Pinn VW, Cortell S, et al.: Allergic interstitial nephritis causing reversible renal failure in four patients with idiopathic nephrotic syndrome. N Engl J Med 288: 124, 1973.
7. Heptinstall RH: Pathology of the Kidney, 2nd ed, Boston, Little, Brown & Co., 1974, p 781.
8. Yamauchi H, Hopper J: Hypovolemic shock and hypotension as a complication in the nephrotic syndrome. Ann Intern Med 60: 242, 1964.
9. Hollenberg NK, Epstein M, Rosen SM, et al.: Acute oliguric renal failure in man. Evidence for preferential renal cortical ischemia. Medicine (Balt) 47: 455, 1968.
10. Hollenberg NK, Adams DF, Oken DE, et al.: Acute renal failure due to nephrotoxins. N Engl J Med 282: 1329, 1970.
11. Flamenbaum W, McDonald FD, DiBona GF, Oken DE: Micropuncture study of renal tubule factors in low dose mercury poisoning. Nephron 8: 221, 1971.
12. Oken DE, DiBona GF, McDonald FD: Micropuncture studies of the recovery phase of myohemoglobinuric acute renal failure in the rat. J Clin Invest 49: 730, 1970.
13. Oken D: An overview of the pathophysiology of vasomotor nephropathy. Proceedings of Conference on Acute Renal Failure (Friedman EA, Eliahou HE, eds), Department of Health, Education and Welfare, Publication no. (NIH) 74-608, 1973, p 89.
14. Thiel G, McDonald FD, Oken DE: Micropuncture studies of the basis for protection of renin depleted rats from glycerol induced acute renal failure. Nephron 7: 67, 1970.
15. Thiel G, Wilson DR, Arce ML, Oken DE: Glycerol induced hemoglobinuric acute renal failure in the rat. Nephron 4: 276, 1967.
16. Robson AM, Giangiacomo J, Kienstra RA, et al.: Normal glomerular permeability and its modification by minimal change nephrotic syndrome. J Clin Invest 54: 1190, 1974.
17. Dillard MG, Pesce AJ, Pollak VE, Boreisha I: Proteinuria and renal protein clearances in patients with renal tubular disorders. J Lab Clin Med 78: 203, 1971.
18. Caulfield JP, Farquhar MG: The permeability of glomerular capillaries to graded dextrans. Identification of the basement membrane as the primary filtration barrier. J Cell Biol 63: 883, 1974.
19. Karnovsky MJ, Ainsworth SK: The structural basis of glomerular filtration. Advances in Nephrology, vol 2 (Hamburger J, Crosnier J, Maxwell M, eds), Chicago, Year Book Medical Publishers, 1972, p 35.
20. Vernier RL, Papermaster BW, Olness K, et al.: Morphologic studies of the mechanism of proteinuria. Am J Dis Child 100: 476, 1960.
21. Cox JW, Bachler RW, Sharma H, et al.: Studies on the mechanism of oliguria in a model of unilateral acute renal failure. J Clin Invest 53: 1546, 1974.
22. Chamberlain MJ, Pringle A, Wrong OM: Oliguric renal failure in the nephrotic syndrome. Q J Med 138: 215, 1966.
23. Conolly NE, Wrong OM, Jones NF: Reversible renal failure in idiopathic nephrotic syndrome with minimal glomerular changes. Lancet 1: 665, 1968.
24. Swann RC, Merrill JP: The clinical course of acute renal failure. Medicine (Balt) 32: 215, 1953.

Comparative Effects of Lidocaine and Procainamide on Acutely Impaired Hemodynamics

JEFFREY R. BURTON, M.D.
M. THOMAS MATHEW, M.D.
PAUL W. ARMSTRONG, M.D.*
Kingston, Ontario, Canada

Controversy exists regarding the relative safety of intravenously administered lidocaine and procainamide to patients with acutely impaired hemodynamics. Accordingly, their effects were studied in 15 such patients, 14 with acute myocardial infarction and one with cardiomyopathy and severe congestive heart failure. All had elevated levels of pulmonary capillary wedge pressure (>15 mm Hg) and/or low cardiac index (<2.5 liters/min/m^2). Patients were given lidocaine, a 100 mg bolus followed by a 3 mg/min infusion and, after at least a 30 minute recovery period, procainamide, a 100 mg bolus over 2 minutes followed by a 20 mg/min infusion for 20 to 25 minutes. Hemodynamic measurements were compared early and late in the infusion of each drug. Small, clinically insignificant differences were observed in the hemodynamic responses to the drugs, and no clinically significant deterioration occurred with either. Conventional therapeutic doses of intravenous procainamide can be administered by this regimen, to patients with acute myocardial infarction complicated by cardiac failure or low cardiac output, without producing deleterious hemodynamic effects.

Lidocaine and procainamide are agents with proved antiarrhythmic efficacy which are currently in widespread use for the treatment of important ventricular arrhythmias following acute myocardial infarction. Controversy exists, however, regarding their relative safety in patients with acutely impaired hemodynamics. Traditionally, intravenously administered lidocaine has been considered to have a wide margin of safety and little deleterious hemodynamic effect, whereas intravenously administered procainamide has been used with greater caution because of its potential negative inotropic and hypotensive effects.

Although lidocaine is a useful initial antiarrhythmic drug, there is frequently a need for an alternative drug in patients with acute myocardial infarction complicated by important ventricular arrhythmia and impaired hemodynamics.

Miller et al. [1] have demonstrated, in a group of patients with acute myocardial infarction, that similar hemodynamic effects were seen with both drugs and that no deterioration occurred with either. These patients did not have important hemodynamic impairment and the investigators emphasized the need for further investigation in patients with severely deranged ventricular function.

From the Department of Medicine, Queen's University and Kingston General Hospital, Kingston, Ontario, Canada. Requests for reprints should be addressed to Dr. P. W. Armstrong, Department of Medicine, Queen's University, Kingston, Ontario, Canada. Manuscript accepted January 23, 1976.
* Recipient of a Senior Research Fellowship from the Ontario Heart Foundation.

Accordingly, the purpose of this investigation was to compare the hemodynamic effects of these drugs in patients with severely deranged ventricular function.

SUBJECTS AND METHODS

Fifteen male patients, aged 38 to 74 years (mean 58 years), were studied soon after their admission to the Connell Coronary Care Unit at the Kingston General Hospital. Fourteen had clinical, enzyme and electrocardiographic evidence of acute transmural myocardial infarction (eight inferior and six anterior), and one had severe congestive heart failure secondary to cardiomyopathy. All had had important ventricular arrhythmias within the 24 hours prior to this study. These consisted of ventricular tachycardia, ventricular fibrillation or both in 11 patients, and either frequent (greater than 6/minute) ventricular premature contractions or "R on T" ventricular premature contractions in the remainder.

The hemodynamic criteria for admission to the study were a mean pulmonary capillary wedge pressure greater than 15 mm Hg (11 patients), and/or a cardiac index of less than 2.5 liters/min/m^2 (nine patients). None was in cardiogenic shock.

Informed consent was obtained from all patients. Instrumentation was performed in the following manner. A thermistor Swan-Ganz catheter was passed to the pulmonary artery with the aid of electrocardiographic and pressure monitoring. A Teflon® cannula was placed in the radial artery. Pulmonary arterial pressure, pulmonary capillary wedge pressure obtained by balloon occlusion, and systemic arterial pressure were monitored using Statham P23DB or Ailtech MS 10-S pressure transducers. Cardiac outputs were measured, at least in duplicate, by the thermal dilution technic. Pressures and cardiac output curves were displayed on a VR-6 Electronics for Medicine oscilloscopic recorder, and cardiac outputs were computed electronically using an Edwards cardiac output computer.

Of the 15 patients, 12 had been previously instrumented for the purpose of monitoring vasodilator therapy (intravenous nitroglycerin or sodium nitroprusside), but in all cases, administration of these drugs had been terminated for at least 40 minutes prior to this study. In addition, three patients had received intravenous digoxin but none within 6 hours of this investigation. No other drugs were administered immediately before or during the study.

In four patients evidence of impaired renal function was manifested by small elevations in serum creatinine levels (1.58 to 2.54 mg/100 ml). Although most patients had elevation of SGOT and LDH levels related to their myocardial infarction, none had significant elevations of serum alkaline phosphatase or bilirubin levels to suggest important hepatic impairment.

As indicated, the purpose of this study was to compare the hemodynamic effects of the drugs. Several of these patients had no ventricular arrhythmia at the time of this study but were thought to be candidates for antiarrhythmic prophylaxis because of the serious nature of the arrhythmias which had occurred in the previous 24 hours. For this reason, it is difficult to make any statistically valid conclusions regarding the comparative antiarrhythmic effects of the doses of lidocaine and procainamide employed. In those patients who had ventricular arrhythmia at the time of the study, diminution in the arrhythmia was noted during infusion of both drugs. No patient was experiencing hemodynamically important ventricular arrhythmia at the time of the study, and hence its correction was not a factor in the hemodynamic responses observed.

The study was performed as follows. Control observations were made over a period of 15 to 20 minutes, and hemodynamic parameters were observed continuously during the drug infusions. Lidocaine, 100 mg, was administered intravenously over 30 seconds, followed by an infusion of 3 mg/min for 20 minutes using a Harvard infusion pump. After at least a 30 minute recovery period, during which parameters returned to control levels, 100 mg of procainamide was given intravenously over 2 minutes followed by a constant infusion of 20 mg/min for 20 to 25 minutes. These drug doses were used in an attempt to simulate conventional clinical usage.

Derived data were calculated using the following formulas: SI = CI/HR, LVSWI = (MAP − PCW) (SI) (1.36)/100, TPR = MAP/CO, where SI is stroke index in ml/m^2, CI is cardiac index in liters/min/m^2, HR is heart rate, LVSWI is left ventricular stroke work index in g-m/m^2, MAP is mean arterial pressure in mm Hg, PCW is mean pulmonary capillary wedge pressure in mm Hg, TPR is total peripheral resistance in units, and CO is cardiac output in liters/min.

Statistical analysis was performed using Student's t test with paired and unpaired comparisons when appropriate.

RESULTS

No clinically important prolongation of Q-T interval or QRS duration and no A-V block or other conduction disturbance developed during the administration of either drug. No significant ill effects were experienced by any patient during the infusions. It should be mentioned, however, that one patient had a fall in cardiac index from 1.83 to 1.34 liters/min/m^2 and another an increase in pulmonary capillary wedge pressure from 24 to 30 mm Hg, both during lidocaine infusions. Neither occurrence was associated with objective clinical evidence of deterioration.

Hemodynamic comparisons have been made between lidocaine and procainamide early (5 to 7 minutes) in the infusions and late (20 to 25 minutes). Table I displays the mean and standard error of the mean for each of the parameters measured during the control period, early and late during the infusion of each drug.

Small increases in heart rate, pulmonary capillary wedge pressure, mean arterial pressure and total peripheral resistance, and small decreases in cardiac index, stroke index and left ventricular stroke work index were observed early during the lidocaine infusion. Only the small increments in heart rate and total peripheral resistance were demonstrated late during the lidocaine infusion. Early during procainamide infusion, a statistically significant but small decrease in mean arterial

TABLE I Hemodynamic Effects of Lidocaine and Procainamide*

Event	Heart Rate	PCW (mm Hg)	MAP (mm Hg)	PA (mm Hg)	RA (mm Hg)	CI (liters/min/m²)	SI (ml/m²)	LVSWI (g-m/m²)	TPR (units)
Control (lidocaine)	79 ± 5	20 ± 2	87 ± 5	30 ± 3	8 ± 1	2.6 ± 0.2	34 ± 3	33 ± 4	18 ± 1
Early lidocaine	81 ± 5†	21 ± 2‡	89 ± 5‡	30 ± 2	8 ± 1	2.5 ± 0.2‡	32 ± 3†	30 ± 4‡	20 ± 1†
Late lidocaine	80 ± 5†	21 ± 2	89 ± 5	29 ± 2	9 ± 1	2.5 ± 0.1	32 ± 2	31 ± 4	20 ± 1†
Control (procainamide)	79 ± 4	19 ± 2	86 ± 5	28 ± 3	9 ± 1	2.5 ± 0.2	34 ± 3	32 ± 4	18 ± 1
Early procainamide	79 ± 4	19 ± 2	83 ± 3§	27 ± 2	8 ± 1‖	2.5 ± 0.2	34 ± 3	31 ± 4	18 ± 1
Late procainamide	81 ± 5	19 ± 2	83 ± 4	27 ± 2‡	8 ± 1	2.5 ± 0.2	32 ± 3‡	29 ± 4†	18 ± 1

NOTE: CI = cardiac index. LVSWI = left ventricular stroke work index. MAP = mean arterial pressure. PA = mean pulmonary artery pressure. PCW = mean pulmonary capillary wedge pressure. RA = mean right atrial pressure. SI = stroke index. TPR = total peripheral resistance.

*Means ± standard errors of the mean.

†P < 0.025 ‡P < 0.05 §P < 0.005 ‖P < 0.001.

pressure (3 mm Hg) and a small decrease in right atrial pressure were observed. Late during the infusion, small decreases in mean pulmonary artery pressure, stroke index and left ventricular stroke work index were demonstrated.

Once these hemodynamic changes from control produced by each drug were examined, the data were analyzed to determine whether the hemodynamic response observed with lidocaine differed from that observed with procainamide.

Table II compares the mean changes from control with each drug, both early and late during the infusions. No significant differences between the two drugs were observed in the response of heart rate, pulmonary capillary wedge pressure, cardiac index, mean pulmonary artery pressure or left ventricular stroke work index. There were small differences in the responses of right atrial pressure, early and late, and of stroke index early in the infusion only.

Figure 1 displays the changes from control in mean arterial pressure and total peripheral resistance seen with the two drugs early during the infusions. Mean arterial pressure and total peripheral resistance increased slightly with lidocaine and decreased slightly with procainamide; the differences, although small, were statistically significant. Changes of similar direction and magnitude were seen late during the infusions but did not achieve statistical significance.

COMMENTS

In summary, the hemodynamic effects of lidocaine were characterized by small increments in heart rate, pulmonary capillary wedge pressure, arterial pressure and total peripheral resistance, and small decreases in cardiac index, stroke index and left ventricular stroke work index. Procainamide produced small falls in arterial pressure, right atrial pressure, pulmonary artery pressure, stroke index and left ventricular stroke work

TABLE II Comparison of Changes Produced by Lidocaine and Procainamide*

Event	△ Heart Rate	△ PCW (mm Hg)	△ MAP (mm Hg)	△ PA (mm Hg)	△ RA (mm Hg)	△ CI (liters/min/m²)	△ SI (ml/m²)	△ LVSWI (g-m/m²)	△ TPR (units)
Early lidocaine	2.6 ± 1.0	1.7 ± 0.7	1.7 ± 0.7	0.5 ± 1.3	0.4 ± 0.5	−0.1 ± 0.1	−2.4 ± 0.9	−2.5 ± 1.1	1.5 ± 0.5
Early procainamide	0.1 ± 0.9	0.1 ± 0.5	−2.9 ± 0.7	−0.9 ± 0.6	−1.2 ± 0.3	0 ± 0	0.1 ± 0.7	−1.4 ± 0.7	−0.7 ± 0.4
P	NS	NS	<0.001	NS	<0.01	NS	<0.05	NS	<0.005
Late lidocaine	2.0 ± 0.7	0.9 ± 0.8	1.9 ± 1.6	−0.7 ± 1.2	0.8 ± 0.5	−0.1 ± 0.1	−2.3 ± 1.2	−1.8 ± 1.4	1.2 ± 0.5
Late procainamide	2.1 ± 1.6	−0.1 ± 0.6	−2.8 ± 1.8	−1.1 ± 0.5	−0.6 ± 0.3	−0.1 ± 0.1	−1.9 ± 0.8	−3.1 ± 1.1	−0.1 ± 0.8
P	NS	NS	NS	NS	<0.05	NS	NS	NS	NS

NOTE: CI = cardiac index. LVSWI = left ventricular stroke work index. MAP = mean arterial pressure. NS = not significant. P = confidence level. PA = mean pulmonary artery pressure. PCW = mean pulmonary capillary wedge pressure. RA = mean right atrial pressure. SI = stroke index. TPR = total peripheral resistance.

* Changes from control (△)—compared by Student's t test.

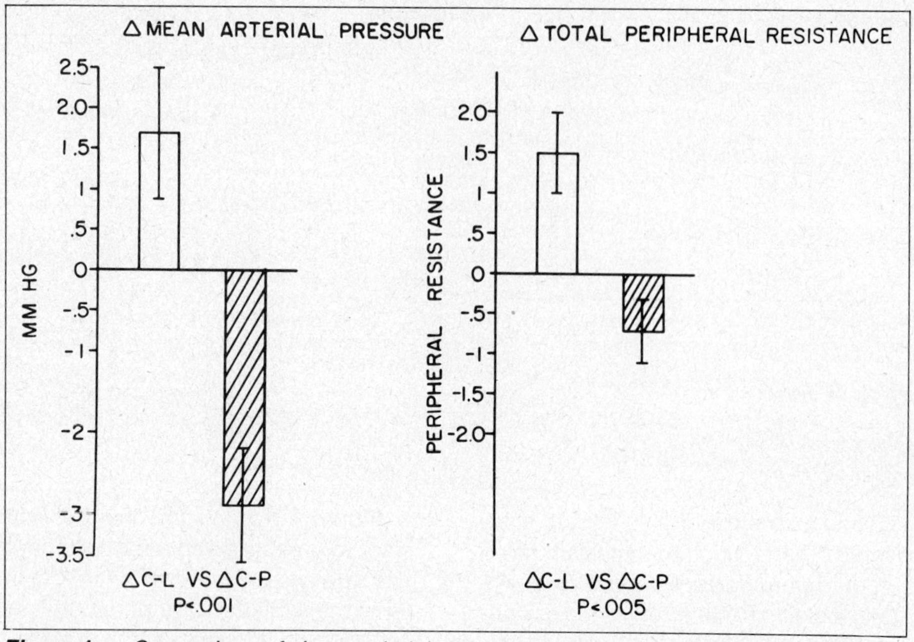

Figure 1. *Comparison of changes (Δ) in mean arterial pressure (left panel) and total peripheral resistance in units (right panel) 5 to 7 minutes after the administration of lidocaine and procainamide. Δ C − L = change from control with lidocaine. Δ C − P = change from control with procainamide. Open bar = lidocaine. Hatched bar = procainamide.*

index. It should be emphasized that, although many of these changes achieved statistical significance, they were very small and of little or no clinical importance.

Although blood levels of lidocaine and procainamide were not measured, the doses employed are those frequently used clinically and would be expected to produce blood levels within the therapeutic range [2–8].

A large body of literature supports the thesis that in therapeutic doses, lidocaine has only infrequent and minor extracardiac toxic effects, and produces little deleterious hemodynamic effect [9–16]. However, a few investigators have suggested a need for caution in its use, especially in patients with congestive heart failure or hepatic disease [5,17]. Relatively little attention has been paid to its negative inotropic effect [7,18,19].

In contrast, many studies have emphasized the negative inotropic and hypotensive effects of procainamide [20–23]. In most of these studies, the drug has been given either as a bolus injection or at very rapid infusion rates. We believe that this may help to explain the difference between their results and ours.

Of considerable interest is the work of Austen et al. who studied the effects of procainamide and lidocaine in a variety of dose ranges at different rates of administration. These investigators demonstrated that rapid administration of procainamide to dogs was associated with hypotension and decreased contractility, which was dose-related. However, similar doses given more slowly produced a small increase in contractile force. In the same experiment, a comparable decrease in contractile force was demonstrated with lidocaine; this was not influenced by the rate of administration.

In the light of Austen's work and this study, the rate of administration of these antiarrhythmic drugs merits further comment. This study demonstrates that the hemodynamic changes seen with lidocaine were more apparent early than late during the infusion, suggesting that these changes were in part due to the rapid administration of the bolus injection. On the basis of these observations, it would seem more prudent to administer the loading dose more slowly.

Much of the cardiac depressant effects noted previously with procainamide may be related to the rapidity with which it was administered. A safer alternative mode of administration, as employed in this study, is the administration of a 100 mg bolus over 2 minutes followed by an infusion of 20 mg/min for 20 to 25 minutes. This dose schedule provided 500 to 600 mg of procainamide to patients with severe myocardial dysfunction without deleterious hemodynamic effect.

The patient with acute myocardial infarction complicated by important ventricular arrhythmia and cardiac failure or low cardiac output poses a difficult therapeutic challenge. In this situation, when lidocaine has been ineffective or has produced toxic effects, and rapid results are desired, what pharmacologic alternatives are available? Quinidine, although possessing antiarrhythmic efficacy similar to procainamide, is generally considered unsafe for intravenous administration because of its potential for producing serious arrhythmias, hypotension, syncope and even death [24–26]. All these complications have been reported to be more frequent with quinidine than with procainamide [27]. Although diphenylhydantoin has been reported to have cardiac depressant effects [28], they are probably less than those of any of the alternative agents [29,30]. Sometimes diphenylhydantoin is a useful antiarrhythmic agent [31], but it is frequently ineffective in preventing important ventricular arrhythmias [32]. Digitalis may improve certain ventricular arrhythmias by ameliorating cardiac function in the setting of heart failure or low cardiac output. Its use in acute myocardial infarction is not without hazard [33–35]. Propranolol is relatively contraindicated in patients who already have important myocardial dysfunction, because of its negative inotropic effects which would further depress cardiac output and increase left ventricular filling pressure [36,37].

Intravenous procainamide is an effective alternative to lidocaine, and this study has demonstrated that it can be administered safely over a 20 minute period in conventional clinical doses, in the presence of impaired hemodynamics following myocardial infarction. This agent provides the best and safest alternative to lidocaine in a common and difficult clinical situation.

ACKNOWLEDGMENT

It is a pleasure to acknowledge the invaluable help of Mrs. Sheila Dee, R.N., Miss Marlene Adam, B.Sc.N. and the nurses of the Coronary Care Unit, as well as the expert technical assistance of Mr. James McKinven.

REFERENCES

1. Miller RR, Hilliard G, Lies JE, Massumi RA, Zelis R, Mason DT, Amsterdam EA: Hemodynamic effects of procainamide in patients with acute myocardial infarction and comparison with lidocaine. Am J Med 55: 161, 1973.
2. Bigger JT, Heissenbuttel RH: The use of procainamide and lidocaine in the treatment of cardiac arrhythmias. Prog Cardiovasc Dis 11: 515, 1969.
3. Giardina EV, Heissenbuttel RH, Bigger JT: Intermittent intravenous procainamide to treat ventricular arrhythmias. Correlation of plasma concentration with effect on arrhythmia, electrocardiogram, and blood pressure. Ann Intern Med 78: 183, 1973.
4. Koch-Weser J, Klein SW: Procainamide dosage schedules, plasma concentrations and clinical effects. JAMA 215: 1454, 1971.
5. Thomson PD, Melmon KL, Richardson JA, Cohn PK, Steinbrunn W., Cudihee R, Rowland M: Lidocaine pharmacokinetics in advanced heart failure, liver disease, and renal failure in humans. Ann Intern Med 78: 499, 1973.
6. Wyman MG: Prevention of primary ventricular fibrillation in acute myocardial infarction (abstract). Am J Cardiol 29: 298, 1972.
7. Raftery EB, Rehman MF, Manks DC, Oram S: Incidence and management of ventricular arrhythmias after acute myocardial infarction. Br Heart J 31: 273, 1969.
8. Bellet S: Clinical Disorders of the Heart Beat, 3rd ed, Philadelphia, Lea & Febiger, 1971, p 1036.
9. Grossman JI, Cooper JA, Frieden J: Cardiovascular effects of infusion of lidocaine on patients with heart disease. Am J Cardiol 24: 191, 1969.
10. Kimball JY, Killip T: Aggressive treatment of arrhythmias in acute myocardial infarction: procedures and results. Prog Cardiovasc Dis 10: 483, 1968.
11. Cullhead, I: Hemodynamic effects of lidocaine. Acta Med Scand 186: 53, 1969.
12. Spracklen FHN, Kimerling JJ, Besterman EMM, Litchfield JW: Use of lignocaine in treatment of cardiac arrhythmias. Br Med J 1: 89, 1968.
13. Stannard M, Sloman G, Sangster L: Haemodynamic effects of lignocaine in acute myocardial infarction. Br Med J 2: 468, 1968.
14. Klein SW, Sutherland RIL, Morch JE: Hemodynamic effects of intravenous lidocaine in man. Can Med Ass J 99: 472, 1968.
15. Mason DT, Spann JF, Zelis R, Amsterdam EA: Effects of antiarrhythmic drugs on myocardial performance in man: assessment by the maximal velocity of contractile element shortening (abstract). Am J Cardiol 25: 114, 1970.
16. Harrison DC, Sprouse JH, Morrow AG: The antiarrhythmic properties of lidocaine and procainamide. Circulation 28: 486, 1963.
17. Stenson RE, Constantino RT, Harrison DC: Interrelationships of hepatic blood flow, cardiac output, and blood levels of lidocaine in man. Circulation 43: 205, 1971.
18. Austen WG, Moran JM: Cardiac and peripheral vascular effects of lidocaine and procainamide. Am J Cardiol 16: 701, 1965.
19. Schumacher RR, Lieberson AD, Childress RH, Williams JF Jr: Hemodynamic effects of lidocaine in patients with heart disease. Circulation 37: 965, 1968.
20. McClendon RL, Hansen WR, Kinsman JM: Hemodynamic changes following procainamide administered intravenously. Am J Med Sci 222: 375, 1951.
21. Folle LE, Aviado DM: The cardiopulmonary effects of quinidine and procainamide. J Pharmacol Exp Ther 154: 92, 1966.
22. Berry K, Garrett EL, Bellet S, Gefter WI: The use of pronestyl in treatment of ectopic rhythms: 98 episodes in 78 patients. Am J Med 11: 431, 1951.
23. McCord MC, Taguchi JT: A study of the effect of procainamide hydrochloride in supraventricular arrhythmias. Circulation 4: 387, 1951.
24. Acierno LJ, Gubner R: Utility and limitations of intravenous quinidine in arrhythmias. Am Heart J 41: 733, 1951.
25. Gold H: Quinidine in Disorders of the Heart, New York, Harper & Bros., 1950.
26. Hoffman B, Bigger JT: Antiarrhythmic Drugs in Drill's Phar-

macology in Medicine, 4th ed, New York, McGraw Hill, 1971, p 844.
27. Bellet S: Clinical Disorders of the Heart Beat, 3rd ed, Philadelphia, Lea & Febiger, 1971, p 1022.
28. Puri PS: The effect of diphenylhydantoin sodium (Dilantin) on myocardial contractility and hemodynamics. Am Heart J 82: 62, 1967.
29. Nayler WG, McInnes I, Swann JB, Race D, Carson V, Lowe TE: Some effects of diphenylhydantoin and propranolol on the cardiovascular system. Am Heart J 75: 83, 1968.
30. Conn RD, Kennedy JW, Blackman JR: The hemodynamic effects of diphenylhydantoin. Am Heart J 73: 500, 1967.
31. Mercer EN, Osborne JA: The current status of diphenylhydantoin in heart disease. Ann Intern Med 67: 1084, 1967.
32. Stone N, Klein MD, Lown B: Diphenylhydantoin in the prevention of recurring ventricular tachycardia. Circulation 43: 420, 1971.
33. Morris JJ Jr, Taft CV, Whalen RE, McIntosh HD: Digitalis and experimental myocardial infarction. Am Heart J 77: 342, 1969.
34. Kumar R, Hood WB Jr, Joison J, Gilmour DP, Norman JC, Abelmann WH: Experimental myocardial infarction. VI. Efficacy and toxicity of digitalis in acute and healing phase in intact conscious dogs. J Clin Invest 49: 358, 1970.
35. Smith TW, Haber E: Digitalis (second of four parts). N Engl J Med 289: 1010, 1973.
36. Stephen SA: Unwanted effects of propranolol. Am J Cardiol 18: 463, 1966.
37. Sowton E, Hamer J: Hemodynamic changes after beta adrenergic blockade. Am J Cardiol 18: 317, 1966.

Idiopathic Late-Onset Immunoglobulin Deficiency

Clinical Observations in 50 Patients

PAUL E. HERMANS, M.D.
JOSE A. DIAZ-BUXO, M.D.
JOHN D. STOBO, M.D.
Rochester, Minnesota

Fifty patients with late-onset idiopathic immunoglobulin deficiency were studied and the frequency of various clinical associations and complications was observed. Men and women were equally affected, although the age at onset in men peaked in the third decade whereas it was more uniformly distributed in women. Sinobronchopulmonary infections were common and were caused by Haemophilus influenzae. Diplococcus pneumoniae, Streptococcus pyogenes and Staphylococcus aureus: bronchiectasis occurred in 28 per cent. Thirty patients (60 per cent) had diarrhea, which was often associated with steatorrhea, giardiasis, achlorhydria, abnormal Schilling tests and morphologic abnormalities on small bowel biopsy specimens, including nodular lymphoid hyperplasia; three patients had pernicious anemia. In the 20 patients without diarrhea these abnormalities were not observed except for giardiasis in one patient and achlorhydria in two patients. Cholelithiasis occurred in both groups in about a third of the patients tested.

A high degree of susceptibility to neoplasia was noted. Thyroid abnormalities, including primary hypothyroidism and Graves' disease, were observed in six patients. Additional occasional findings were vitiligo, keratoconjunctivitis sicca and arthritis. Splenomegaly occurred in 14 (28 per cent) patients.

The percentage of B lymphocytes in the blood was determined in 10 patients; it was normal or slightly decreased in eight patients and low in two patients.

In 1952 Bruton [1] described the entity of congenital agammaglobulinemia in a young boy who had severe recurrent bacterial infections. Two years later the first reports of hypogammaglobulinemia acquired in adolescence or in adulthood appeared [2–5]. Reports of a large number of patients with acquired idiopathic hypogammaglobulinemia appeared subsequently and served to illustrate different features of this disease. Well documented have been its variable association with diarrhea and malabsorption [2,6–19], thymoma [9,19–28], nodular lymphoid hyperplasia of the small intestine [15,17,29–39], achlorhydria [14,15,40,41] and pernicious anemia [14,15,41–45], and its complications of giardiasis [14,15,17,18,37,39], bronchiectasis [14,17,40], gastric carcinoma [45–47], lymphoreticular malignancy [48,49] and cholelithiasis [50]. In several reviews the various aspects of the clinical syndrome, based on observations and the composite information derived from the literature [51,52], have been described.

The proceedings of two workshops on the primary immunodefi-

From the Division of Infectious Diseases, Department of Internal Medicine, and the Department of Immunology, Mayo Clinic and Mayo Foundation, Rochester, Minnesota. Requests for reprints should be addressed to Dr. P. E. Hermans, Mayo Clinic, 200 First Street SW, Rochester, Minnesota 55901. Manuscript accepted November 19, 1975.

TABLE I Idiopathic Late-Onset Immunoglobulin Deficiency: Distribution of Immunoglobulin Levels (44 Patients Studied)

IgG (normal, 6.4–14.3 mg/ml)		IgA (normal, 0.5–3.0 mg/ml)		IgM (normal, 0.4–1.4 mg/ml)	
Values (mg/ml)	Patients (no.)	Values (mg/ml)	Patients (no.)	Values (mg/ml)	Patients (no.)
0–0.00	1	0–0.00	24	0–0.00	16
0–0.39	9	0–0.09	0	0–0.09	4
0.4–0.59	2	0.1–0.19	3	0.1–0.19	8
0.6–0.79	4	0.2–0.29	10	0.2–0.29	8
0.8–0.89	2	0.3–0.39	2	0.3–0.39	0
0.9–0.99	2	0.4–0.49	3	0.4–0.49	2
1.0–1.19	3	0.5–0.59	1	0.5–0.59	2
1.2–1.39	2	0.6–0.69	1	0.6–0.69	3
1.4–1.99	8			0.7–0.79	1
2.0–3.00	9				
3.0–3.75	2				

ciency diseases of man, held in 1967 and 1973, also include studies of several problems related to idiopathic late-onset immunoglobulin deficiency [53,54].

The patients with late-onset immunoglobulin deficiency included in this study are also referred to as having "common variable immunodeficiency," according to the World Health Organization classification of primary immunodeficiencies [55].

Fifty patients with idiopathic late-onset immunoglobulin deficiency were seen at the Mayo Clinic between 1960 and 1973. The clinical observations in this consecutive series of cases made it possible to establish, with some degree of accuracy, the relative frequency with which various clinical features occurred. In addition, new observations were made on the development of malignancy of lymphoreticular and epithelial origin and of thyroid disorders. The clinical features of idiopathic late-onset immunoglobulin deficiency and the various associations and complications observed over an aggregate period of 2,500 patient-months form the basis of this report.

MATERIAL AND METHODS

Idiopathic late-onset immunoglobulin deficiency is defined as a condition characterized by abnormally low immunoglobulin levels and recurrent infections in patients with no clinical evidence of increased susceptibility to infections for several years after birth. The earliest onset of an unusual susceptibility to infections in this series was at seven years of age. (Three patients in whom the age at onset of clinical illness was difficult to determine, and probably occurred in the first few years of life, were excluded.) Conditions leading to secondary immunoglobulin deficiency, such as chronic lymphocytic leukemia, lymphocytic lymphoma, multiple myeloma and nephrosis, were ruled out by conventional methods and by adequate periods of observation (average of 51 months per patient).

This study encompasses 50 consecutive patients fulfilling these criteria. These patients first came to our attention primarily because of recurrent respiratory tract infections or gastrointestinal symptoms, or both.

In all patients the total gamma globulin fraction of the serum was determined by paper protein electrophoresis until 1971, when this method was replaced by cellulose acetate protein electrophoresis (normal values 0.8 to 1.6 g/dl). In three patients, who subsequently died or were lost to follow-up, the diagnosis of hypogammaglobulinemia was made by paper protein electrophoresis alone because they were seen in the early period of the study when quantitative methods to measure immunoglobulins were not yet available. For the same reasons, in another three patients only immunoelectrophoresis was used besides paper protein electrophoresis. Quantitative determination of serum immunoglobulins G (IgG), M (IgM) and A (IgA), according to the method of Mancini and associates [56], has been carried out in 44 patients since 1965. Investigation of patients with decreased serum immunoglobulin concentration disclosed that in those with unusual susceptibility to infections IgG levels were 3.75 mg/ml or less. Table I shows the distribution of the serum concentration of IgG, IgA and IgM in this group of patients. The various patterns of immunoglobulin levels will be discussed under "General Findings."

Quantitation of thymus-derived lymphocytes (T cells) was carried out by means of the sheep red blood cell (SRBC) rosette technic [57]. The frequency of small round cells binding three or more SRBCs was enumerated by light microscopy. The frequency of B cells was determined with anti-immunoglobulin, which contained specificities for human kappa and lambda chains [58]. T and B cells were enumerated in the peripheral blood of 10 patients, seven of whom are included in the current series of 50 patients. Three additional patients were included after compilation of the clinical data on the first 50 patients was completed.

During the years of observation, various clinical associations were detected in these patients by means of history, physical examination, and conventional laboratory tests and diagnostic roentgenologic methods, according to the patient's medical needs. In a number of patients, additional observations were made during surgical procedures and at autopsy.

(In the tables that list individual patients, a numerical designation is used to identify patients for convenience because the same patients may be listed in more than one table.)

GENERAL FINDINGS

Sex Distribution and Racial Background. There were 27 males and 23 females. All were Caucasian except for one black female. The course of illness, the various complications and the associated clinical findings to be discussed occurred without any particular predilection for either sex. Exceptions to this rule were the development of lymphoreticular malignancy in two males, three of four thymomas in males and four of six thyroid disorders in females.

Age at Onset. The age at onset of idiopathic late-onset

TABLE II Age at Onset

Age (yr)	Males (no.)	Females (no.)	Total (no.)
7–9	1	2	3
10–19	5	3	8
20–29	14	3	17
30–39	2	5	7
40–49	2	4	6
50–59	3	6	9
Totals	27	23	50

TABLE III Age at Diagnosis

Age (yr)	Males (no.)	Females (no.)	Total (no.)
10–19	1	2	3
20–29	6	2	8
30–39	10	3	13
40–49	4	6	10
50–59	4	6	10
60–69	2	3	5
≥70	0	1	1
Totals	27	23	50

immunoglobulin deficiency (Table II) was sometimes difficult to determine precisely, because the onset was often insidious. (As mentioned, three cases in which the immune deficiency may have been mildly manifested in the first few years of life were not included in the study.) For practical reasons, the age at onset was taken as the approximate age at which significant and recurrent symptoms (infections and gastrointestinal dysfunction) first became evident and subsequently persisted or recurred. The mean age at onset for the group was 30.7 years, being 26.9 years for males and 35.2 years for females. The males showed a definite peak incidence in the third decade, whereas females followed a more uniform distribution between the first and sixth decades. The earliest age at onset was seven years and the latest, 67 years.

Age at Time of Diagnosis. The age at the time of diagnosis is the age at which the diagnosis of idiopathic late-onset immunoglobulin deficiency was confirmed for the first time by objective criteria.

Decreased serum gamma globulin levels as determined by electrophoresis and decreased serum IgG, IgM and IgA were noted in 44 patients. In six additional patients, studied between 1960 and 1964, the diagnosis was made by electrophoresis only. The patient's age at the time of diagnosis is listed in Table III. The mean age at which the diagnosis was confirmed was 41.9 years (38.6 years for males and 45.7 for females).

Observation Period and Duration of Disease. The mean observation period for our patients was 50.7 months, which represents approximately 2,500 patient-months of observation. The distribution of the observation period is given in Table IV. Duration of illness was determined from the patient's age at onset of symptoms until the patient's age at the last observation or at death (Table V).

Distribution Patterns of Serum IgG, IgM and IgA. All 44 patients whose serum IgG, IgM and IgA were measured had reduced concentrations of IgG, ranging from 0.00 to 3.75 mg/ml. Measurements of IgA and IgM serum levels revealed seven patterns, as shown in Table VI. In 35 patients (groups 1 through 4) IgA and IgM values were below the lower limits of normal. Of these 35 patients, 11 had undetectable amounts of IgA and IgM with the method used, 11 had undetectable amounts of IgA and subnormal levels of IgM, five had subnormal but detectable amounts of IgA with undetectable IgM, and eight patients had subnormal levels of IgA and IgM. Nine patients had normal levels of IgM (groups 5 through 7); of these, two had undetectable levels of IgA, five had subnormal levels of IgA, and two had normal levels of IgA. Thus, 42 patients had subnormal levels of IgA, undetectable in 24, and 35 patients had subnormal levels of IgM, undetectable in 16. The two patients in whom levels of both IgA and IgM were within the normal

TABLE IV Period of Observation*

Period	Males (no.)	Females (no.)	Total (no.)
<1 mo	4	4	8
1 mo–5 mo	4	5	9
6 mo–11 mo	1	0	1
1–4 yr	10	5	15
5–9 yr	4	6	10
10–14 yr	3	1	4
15–19 yr	1	2	3
Totals	27	23	50

*Total of 2,500 patient-months; mean observation period--50.7 months/patient.

TABLE V Duration of Illness

Duration	Males (no.)	Females (no.)	Total (no.)
<5 mo	1	2	3
6 mo–1 yr	0	1	1
1–4 yr	4	4	8
5–9 yr	5	4	9
10–19 yr	7	7	14
20–29 yr	7	4	11
30–39 yr	3	0	3
40–49 yr	0	1	1
Totals	27	23	50

TABLE VI Patterns of Immunoglobulin Deficiency (in 44 Patients)*

Group	IgG	IgA	IgM	No. of Patients
1	D	A	A	11
2	D	A	D	11
3	D	D	A	5
4	D	D	D	8
5	D	A	N	2
6	D	D	N	5
7	D	N	N	2

*D = below lower limit of normal range; A = absent; N = normal.

range had the following concentrations of serum immunoglobulins: IgG 0.54, IgA 0.54 and IgM 0.50 mg/ml; and IgG 0.25, IgA 0.52 and IgM 0.64 mg/ml. The five patients with normal levels of IgM and decreased but detectable levels of IgA had the following values for IgG, IgA and IgM: 2.10, 0.25 and 0.41; 2.00, 0.20 and 0.57; 1.25, 0.16 and 0.67; 0.53, 0.46 and 0.62; and 0.29, 0.29 and 0.78 mg/ml, respectively. Of the 24 patients who had undetectable amounts of IgA, 12 had IgG levels between 1.05 and 3.75 mg/ml, and 12 had IgG levels between 0.00 and 1.00 mg/ml. The patients in whom neither IgA nor IgM was detectable were similarly distributed with regard to IgG levels. In a number of patients, IgG levels partially reflected prophylactically administered pooled human gamma globulin. Since the interval between the last dose of gamma globulin and the determination of serum immunoglobulins was variable, and most patients lived a great distance from this medical center, this variable could not be controlled. Of the 13 patients with IgG levels of more than 1.50 mg/ml, three had undetectable levels of IgA and IgM, five had undetectable levels of IgA only, and the remaining five had subnormal levels of IgA. All but three of the 13 had subnormal levels of IgM, and in these three, levels were in the low normal range measuring 0.41, 0.41 and 0.57 mg/ml.

Additional Immunologic Observations. Because of the chronicity of bronchopulmonary infections in a number of patients, they were skin-tested with tuberculin and histoplasmin. Four of 28 patients reacted to the administration of 5 tuberculin units (TU) and four of 21 reacted to 250 TU; thus, eight of 28 patients reacted to first- or second-strength tuberculin skin tests. Four of 11 patients reacted to histoplasmin skin tests. Two of these patients had positive skin tests to both tuberculin and histoplasmin. Thus, 10 of 28 patients reacted to either or both antigens. Studies are in progress on the frequency of circulating T and B lymphocytes and in vitro stimulation of lymphocytes with mitogens (see "Comments").

Preliminary results showed a normal or near-normal percentage of circulating B cells in eight of 10 patients studied. Two patients (Cases 51 and 52) had less than 3 per cent and 5 per cent B cells, respectively (Table VII). One patient (Case 23) had an increased percentage of T cells, and two patients (Cases 19 and 51) had a decreased percentage of T cells—44 per cent and 33 per cent, respectively (Table VII).

One patient (Case 19) was being treated with therapeutic doses of prednisone to control an extremely severe malabsorption problem when the determination of T and B cells were made.

In several patients an unusually large percentage of

TABLE VII Determination of T and B Cells

Case No.	Sex	Age (yr) At Onset of LID	Age (yr) At Time of Test	T Cells (%)	B Cells (%)	Gap* (%)	Associated Abnormalities
4	F	50	60	61	14	25	Achlorhydria; pernicious anemia; cholelithiasis; chronic pancreatitis; diarrhea; steatorrhea; nodular lymphoid hyperplasia
19	M	21	29	44	16	40	Cleft palate; achlorhydria; diarrhea; steatorrhea; cholelithiasis
21	M	20	44	71	23	6	Achlorhydria; diarrhea; steatorrhea; nodular lymphoid hyperplasia
23	M	29	31	82	10	8	Diarrhea; giardiasis; nodular lymphoid hyperplasia
29	M	21	42	76	12	12	Achlorhydria; diarrhea; steatorrhea; cholelithiasis
36	M	26	46	68	15	17	Diarrhea; giardiasis; cholelithiasis
47	M	18	35	75	13	12	None
51†	M	7	26	34	<3	64	Diarrhea
52†	M	20	44	78	5	17	None
53†	F	14	22	65	21	14	Diarrhea
Normal				72 ± 4	17 ± 4	3–19	

*Cells unaccounted for after enumeration of T and B cells.
†Three patients who were seen after compilation of clinical data on the first 50 patients was completed.

lymphocytes remained unaccounted for after the percentages of T and B cells had been totalled. Preliminary results also revealed a subnormal, but usually not absent, capability of reacting by delayed hypersensitvity to streptokinase-streptodornase, Candida, mumps and trichophyton antigens. Seven of nine patients did not respond with antibody formation to typhoid vaccination (three injections at weekly intervals); two responded but failed to show a reaction to a booster injection several months after the initial immunization procedures.

CLINICAL MANIFESTATIONS

Infections. The great majority of patients with idiopathic late-onset immunoglobulin deficiency first came to the attention of the clinician because of recurrent infections, particularly of the respiratory tract. The frequency and severity of the infections were variable; they often increased with the duration of the immunoglobulin deficiency. The patients suffered from repeated respiratory tract infections, including pneumonia in 86 per cent of them; however, some patients had only intermittent or chronic otitis and purulent sinusitis. As shown in Table VIII, more than half of the patients had repeated and severe upper respiratory tract infections and sinusitis, and almost one-third had episodes of otitis media. In those with the most severe and frequent infections, tenacious chronic bronchitis culminated in bronchiectasis in about one third of them. The diagnosis of bronchiectasis was based on a typical history of chronic, copious expectoration of purulent sputum and on characteristic roentgenologic findings including bronchography when needed for diagnosis. In eight cases histologic examination of lung tissue obtained during lobectomy further confirmed the diagnosis of bronchiectasis. Haemophilus influenzae, Diplococcus pneumoniae, Streptococcus pyogenes and Staphylococcus aureus were the predominant organisms in the secretions during active episodes of respiratory tract infections.

Nonrespiratory tract infections were less frequent and included meningitis in two patients, bacteremia in five, intra-abdominal abscesses in one, a hematogenously acquired perinephric abscess in one and urinary tract infections in four.

The two instances of meningitis occurred elsewhere rather early in the course of the disease and information about the causative organisms was not available.

Only four episodes of bacteremia in four patients were documented by us. The responsible organisms were H. influenzae, Escherichia coli, Bacteroides fragilis and Staph. aureus. The source of Esch. coli as a bloodstream invader was the respiratory tract. It was a complication of pneumonia caused by Esch. coli in a patient who had been receiving penicillin and tetracycline intermittently and prednisone daily, the latter given to control a severe malabsorption syndrome. The portal of entry in the case of B. fragilis bacteremia was the biliary tract, and this was a sequela of cholecystectomy in a patient with acute cholecystitis complicated by cholelithiasis. The bacteremia due to Staph. aureus occurred as a complication of a furuncle leading to a perinephritic abscess from which the same microorganism was cultured. Although hospitalization for pneumonia was common for these patients, and blood cultures were obtained routinely, no additional instances of bacteremia were documented. Pseudomonas bacteremia occurred as a terminal event elsewhere in a patient with a thymoma who experienced bone marrow aplasia with pancytopenia.

TABLE VIII Associated Infections

Infection	Per Cent of Patients
Sinusitis	66
Otitis media	32
Pneumonia	86
1–10 episodes	68
10 or more episodes	18
Bronchiectasis	28
Empyema	4
Meningitis	4
Bacteremia	5
Cholecystitis (acute)	4
Urinary tract infection	8
Giardiasis	34
Staphylococcal enterocolitis	4

Only four patients had confirmed urinary tract infections, and only one of these recurred while the patient was under our care. The microorganisms recovered from the urine were Esch. coli, Pseudomonas aeruginosa, Aerobacter aerogenes and Proteus mirabilis. One of these patients had concomitant nephrolithiasis, which was also detected in two additional patients.

One episode of staphylococcal enterocolitis was well documented in one patient, and an episode probably occurred in a second patient.

In no instance were fungal infections considered of clinical importance. Candida albicans was cultured from the urine in one patient and from bronchopulmonary secretions in six others, but these isolates were not considered significant. The syndrome of chronic mucocutaneous candidiasis was not encountered in any of the 50 patients.

Among the parasitic infections, Giardia lamblia requires emphasis and will be discussed in the section on gastrointestinal abnormalities. In three patients Trichomonas hominis was detected in stool specimens.

Gastrointestinal Abnormalities. Diarrhea: Thirty of the 50 patients had chronic or frequently recurring diarrhea. The mean age at onset and at objective diagnosis by means of immunoglobulin determination, and the mean

TABLE IX Summary of Chief Gastrointestinal Abnormalities*

Abnormalities	30 Patients With Diarrhea	20 Patients Without Diarrhea	Total No. of Patients
Decreased serum carotene	18/28 (64)	3/11 (27)	21/39 (54)
Decreased serum calcium	12/27 (44)	3/12 (25)	15/39 (38)
Prolonged prothrombin time	8/24 (33)	4/12 (33)	12/36 (33)
Fecal fat increased†	16/26 (61)	0/7 (0)	16/33 (48)
Giardia lamblia, in feces	16/25 (64)	1/10 (10)	17/35 (49)
Achlorhydria	9/17 (53)	2/8 (25)	11/25 (44)
Hypochlorhydria‡	4/17 (23)	2/8 (25)	6/25 (24)
Normal gastric HCl	4/17 (23)	4/8 (50)	8/25 (32)
Abnormal Schilling test§	9/14 (64)	0/2 (0)	9/16 (56)
Stage I and II abnormal	6/14 (43)	0/2 (0)	6/16 (37)
Pernicious anemia	3/14 (21)	0/2 (0)	3/16 (19)
Small bowel x-ray studies			
Abnormal	16/28 (57)	0/14 (0)	16/42 (38)
Malabsorption with NLH‖	8/28 (28)	0/14 (0)	8/42 (19)
Malabsorption only	8/28 (28)	0/14 (0)	8/42 (19)
Small bowel biopsies			
Abnormal	18/21 (86)	0/30 (0)	18/24 (75)
Triad (lymphocytic infiltration, atrophy, blunting)	5/21 (24)	0/3 (0)	5/24 (21)
Triad with NLH	13/21 (62)	0/3 (0)	13/24 (54)
Cholelithiasis	8/23 (35)	4/14 (28)	12/37 (32)
Rectal NLH	2/18 (11)	2/10 (20)	4/28 (14)

*Numerator indicates number of patients with abnormality, denominator indicates total number of patients tested for abnormality, figure in parentheses is percentage.
†Quantitative method on 48- or 72-hour specimen.
‡Hydrochloric acid present only after stimulation with histamine or Histalog.
§Without and after administration of intrinsic factor.
‖NLH = nodular lymphoid hyperplasia.

number of years of duration of illness and of observation, did not differ significantly in the two groups of patients. There was no significant difference in the mean total serum gamma globulin or in the mean concentration of IgG, IgA and IgM between the two groups. The susceptibility to infections as determined by the average number of pneumonic episodes, which was 5.5 per patient, was identical in the patients with and without diarrhea; and the percentage of patients who experienced bronchiectasis was 28 per cent and 21 per cent, respectively. The chief gastrointestinal abnormalities detected in patients with and without diarrhea and in the total group of patients are listed in Table IX.

Malabsorption: Patients with diarrhea often had decreased serum levels of carotene and calcium, prolonged prothrombin time and steatorrhea. None of the seven patients without diarrhea who were tested for steatorrhea had increased fecal fat excretion. A few patients without diarrhea had abnormal serum levels of carotene, calcium and prothrombin. Two-stage Schilling tests were performed in almost half of the patients with diarrhea, and results were abnormal in 64 per cent; they were consistent with pernicious anemia in three patients (21 per cent of those tested), and consistent with malabsorption without and with intrinsic factor in 43 per cent of 14 patients tested. Only two patients without diarrhea who had Schilling tests had normal results.

One patient had pancreatic lithiasis and another had had several mild episodes of pancreatitis without coexistent cholelithiasis. Two patients had evidence of pancreatic exocrine hypofunction when amino acid mixtures were given by intraduodenal intubation, but they showed normal pancreatic excretory function when pancreozymin was administered parenterally. Two brothers, 27 and 19 years old, whose susceptibility to infections began at the age of 11 and 7 years, respectively, had acquired extensive bronchiectasis and experienced diarrhea only when ingesting dairy products. This was confirmed by positive challenge tests.

Giardiasis: G. lamblia was detected in 64 per cent of 25 patients tested among the group with diarrhea and in only one of 10 patients without diarrhea. A search for Giardia in duodenal contents was unrewarding in three patients with diarrhea and negative stool specimens. A systematic search for Giardia in small bowel specimens of patients with negative stool specimens was not carried out. The percentage of patients with giardiasis could therefore have been even higher than 64 per cent. However, therapy with metronidazole (Flagyl®) in several patients with severe diarrhea and steatorrhea in whom giardiasis was not detected (up to 60 g of fat excreted in the feces/24 hours) did not control the diarrhea.

Gastrointestinal Studies (Table IX). Small bowel roentgenologic studies: These studies were made in all but two of the 30 patients with diarrhea; 28 per cent had a malabsorption pattern with nodular lymphoid hyperplasia of various degree, and 28 per cent had a malabsorption pattern only. Almost half of the patients without diarrhea had such studies and the results were normal.

Small bowel biopsies (Figure 1): In the group of patients with diarrhea, tissue was obtained perorally for biopsy in 21 of them, and biopsies were repeated during subsequent visits in a number of patients. In 24 per cent of the patients who underwent biopsy, a triad was seen

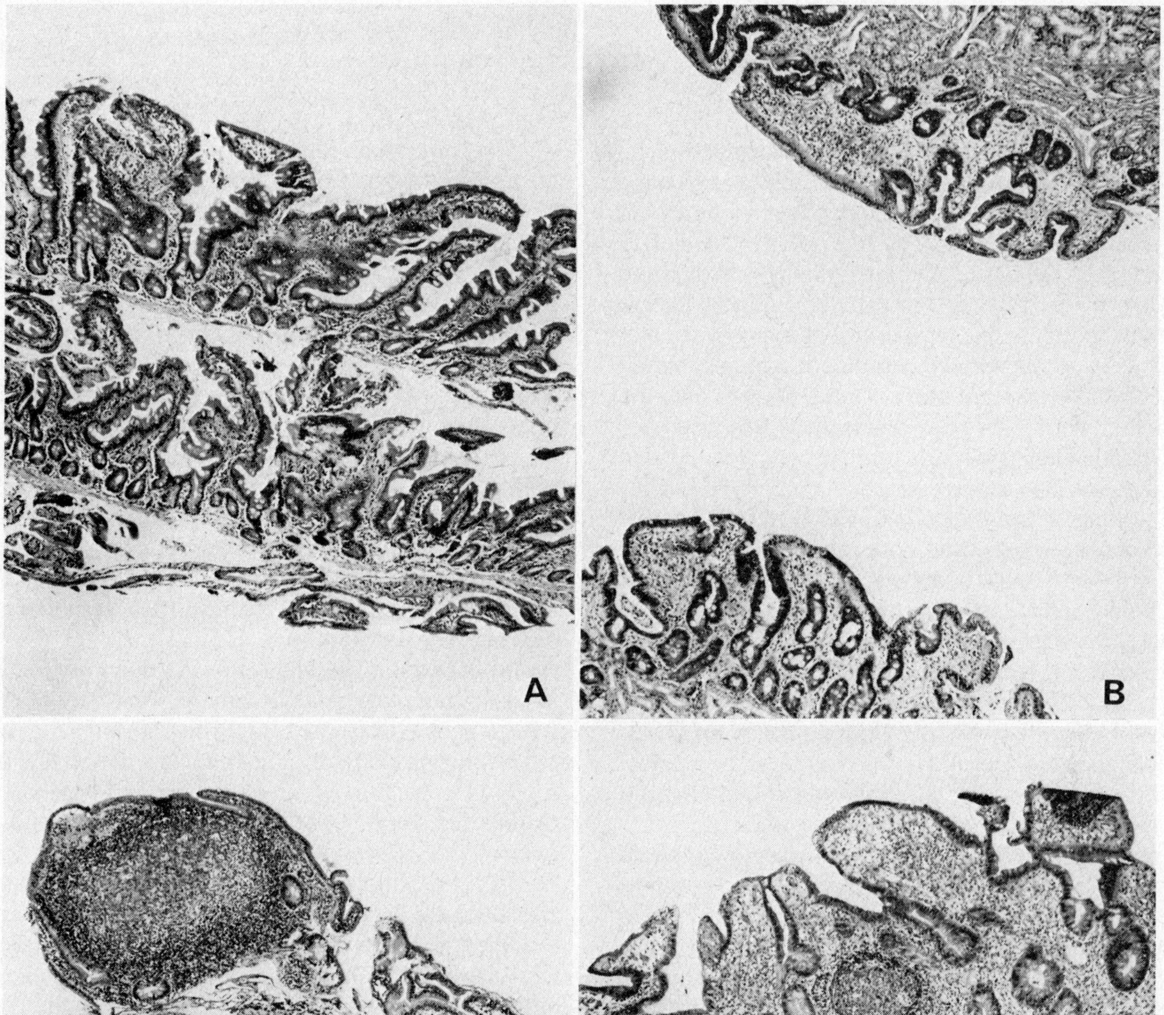

*Figure 1. Morphology of small intestine in enteropathic idiopathic immunoglobulin deficiency of late onset. Original magnification ×64. **A,** minor changes consisting of slight blunting of some villi without epithelial atrophy. There is mild cellular infiltration. **B,** considerable blunting of villi, minimal epithelial atrophy. Cellular infiltration. **C,** nodular lymphoid hyperplasia. Fairly normal villi in area adjacent to the lymphoid nodules that project into the lumen. **D,** mixed lesions. Blunting of villi, cellular infiltration and small lymphoid nodules that do not project into the lumen.*

TABLE X Correlation Between Type of Diarrhea and Status of Gastric Hydrochloric Acid Production

Status	30 Patients with Diarrhea: Steatorrhea (16 patients)	No Steatorrhea (10 patients)	Not Tested (4 patients)	20 Patients Without Diarrhea	Total No. of Patients
Achlorhydria	8	1	...	2	11
Hypochlorhydria	3	1	...	2	6
Normal hydrochloride	2	2	...	4	8
Not tested	3	6	4	12	25

consisting of a variable degree of lymphocytic infiltration of the lamina propria, epithelial atrophy and blunting of villi. In 62 per cent of the patients, nodular lymphoid hyperplasia of various degrees was noted in addition to the triad. Thus, 86 per cent of the patients with diarrhea who underwent biopsy had morphologic abnormalities. Only three patients had an extreme degree of nodular lymphoid hyperplasia with prominent nodules. When nodules were prominent, the villi were effaced over the nodules but were present in areas away from the nodules. The blunting of villi was often present focally, and normal appearing villi were present in other areas. Only three patients without diarrhea underwent biopsy; their specimens showed a normal morphology. In all 13 patients who had nodular lymphoid hyperplasia on biopsy, roentgenographic studies of the small intestine were made. The x-ray pattern was diagnostic of nodular lymphoid hyperplasia in six patients and suggestive in two; no abnormality was found in five patients. Of the five patients in whom biopsy specimens did not reveal lymphoid nodular hyperplasia, one had no x-ray studies, two had changes on roentgenograms suggesting the abnormality and two had normal x-ray findings.

Proctoscopic Studies. Rectal hyperplastic lymphoid nodules were observed in only four of 28 patients (14 per cent) who underwent proctoscopy. Two of these patients had diarrhea and two did not. One of the patients with rectal nodules had nodular lymphoid hyperplasia of the small intestine and two did not, as demonstrated by biopsies; the fourth patient did not undergo biopsy. Eleven of the 13 patients with nodular lymphoid hyperplasia underwent proctoscopic examinations; in 10 the mucosa appeared normal, and one had hyperplastic lymphoid nodules.

TABLE XI Correlation Between Status of Gastric Hydrochloric Acid Production and Presence or Absence of Giardia lamblia in Feces

Status	G. lamblia: Present (17 patients)	Absent (18 patients)	Not Tested, (15 patients)	Total No. of Patients
Achlorhydria	4	6	1	11
Hypochlorhydria	3	3		6
Normal hydrochloride	1	3	4	8
Not tested	9	6	10	25

Gastric Acid Production. Achlorhydria after maximal stimulation with betazole (Histalog®) was detected in 53 per cent of 17 patients who had diarrhea and in 25 per cent of eight patients who did not. Thus, achlorhydria was present in 44 per cent of the total of 25 patients tested. Hypochlorhydria, defined as the production of hydrochloric acid only after stimulation, was present with equal frequency in both groups of patients. Hydrochloric acid was present without stimulation twice as often in the patients without diarrhea as in those with diarrhea.

Cholelithiasis. Cholelithiasis was documented in 12 patients, six male and six female. The diagnosis was arrived at by gallbladder roentgenograms in 10, a history of cholecystectomy for cholelithiasis in one and at autopsy in one. Thirty-four of the 50 patients had gallbladder films or other adequate observations. Thus, the over-all prevalence was 24 per cent, although 35 per cent of the patients with adequate observations had cholelithiasis. We have previously established that the prevalence of cholelithiasis in patients with idiopathic late-onset immunoglobulin deficiency is significantly higher than in those without such a deficiency [50].

Gastrointestinal Neoplasia. The development of gastrointestinal neoplasia, which occurred in seven patients, is discussed in a separate section on neoplasia.

Correlations. Table X shows a rather strong correlation between achlorhydria and diarrhea, especially with steatorrheal diarrhea. Eight of 13 patients, with steatorrhea who were tested for gastric acid, had achlorhydria. The total number of patients with achlorhydria was 11. Only two of the patients with steatorrhea had gastric acid without betazole stimulation. There was no particular correlation between the presence of achlorhydria and the detection of G. lamblia in stool specimens, as shown in Table XI. The correlation between the presence of diarrhea and the finding of G. lamblia in stool specimens is shown in Table XII. The

TABLE XII Correlation Between Diagnosis of Nodular Lymphoid Hyperplasia (NLH) by Biopsy and Presence or Absence of Giardia lamblia in Feces

	Nodular Lymphoid Hyperplasia		
	Present	Absent	No. of Patients
G. lamblia present	8	2	17
G. lamblia absent	4	6	18
Not tested	1	3	15

TABLE XIII Miscellaneous Associated Conditions

Condition	No.	%
Splenomegaly	14	28
Clubbing of fingers	6	12
Keratoconjunctivitis sicca	3	6
Arthritis	4	8
Hay fever (past history)	5	10
Penicillin allergy (past history)	9	18
Nephrolithiasis	3	6
Eczema	6	12
Vitiligo	3	6
Psoriasis	1	2

correlation seems strongest in patients with nonsteatorrheal diarrhea. Of the 13 patients in whom nodular lymphoid hyperplasia was diagnosed by small bowel biopsies, seven had steatorrhea.

Miscellaneous Abnormalities. Table XIII lists the frequency with which certain other abnormalities were noted such as splenomegaly, clubbing of the fingers, keratoconjunctivitis sicca, rheumatoid-like arthritis, nephrolithiasis, eczema, vitiligo and psoriasis. A past history consistent with immediate-type allergies, including hay fever and hives, was not uncommon in patients with idiopathic late-onset immunoglobulin deficiency, but as the immunoglobulin deficiency developed, the tendency to experience allergic reactions disappeared. Three patients had an anaphylactoid reaction to intramuscularly administered gamma globulin but tolerated the same therapy well subsequently. It is assumed that these patients had a reaction to small amounts of gamma globulin which were inadvertently introduced into a blood vessel directly.

The only allergic problems observed after the immunoglobulin deficiency had been well established were in an occasional patient who experienced a late skin eruption while receiving ampicillin.

A history of tonsillectomy was obtained in 17 patients (34 per cent) and of appendectomy in 23 patients (46 per cent).

Malignant Neoplasia. Neoplasia occurred in 12 patients (24 per cent) with late-onset immunoglobulin deficiency (Table XIV); in eight patients (16 per cent) the neoplasia was malignant, as verified by pathologic-anatomic examination. Six of the malignant lesions were of the epithelial type and two of lymphoreticular origin.

Epithelial Malignant Disease (Table XIV). Three patients in whom gastric carcinoma developed were

TABLE XIV Neoplasia Associated With Late-Onset Immunoglobulin Deficiency (LID)

Case No.	Sex	Age (yr) At Onset of LID	Age (yr) At Diagnosis of Neoplasia	Type of Neoplasia	Associated Abnormalities*
18	M	26	59	Carcinoma of stomach	Diarrhea; steatorrhea; primary myxedema
26	F	31	56	Carcinoma of stomach	Diarrhea; steatorrhea; NLH; pernicious anemia
49	M	21	31	Carcinoma of stomach	Diarrhea; NLH
14	F	39	54	Carcinoma of stomach	Diarrhea; steatorrhea; NLH
25	F	27	48	Carcinoma of sigmoid	Diarrhea; NLH; toxic thyroid nodule
45	M	52	59	Squamous cell carcinoma of lung	Diabetes mellitus
17	M	35	67	Lymphoma of rectum and sigmoid	Diarrhea; NLH; goiter of unknown type
34	M	45	45 49	Thymoma; lymphoma (disseminated)	None
1	M	57	62 52	Thymoma; polyposis of colon	Nephrolithiasis; diarrhea; keratoconjunctivitis sicca
39	M	56	59	Thymoma	None
13	F	67	73	Thymoma	Keratoconjunctivitis sicca; aplastic anemia
6	F	30	48	Agnogenic myeloid metaplasia	None

*NLH = nodular lymphoid hyperplasia of small intestine.

TABLE XV Associated Thyroid Abnormalities (6 Patients) in Late-Onset Immunoglobulin Deficiency (LID)

Case No.	Sex	Age (yr) At Onset of LID	Age (yr) At Diagnosis of Thyroid Abnormality	Type of Thyroid Disorder	Associated Abnormalities*
12	F	30	35	Graves' disease (thyroidectomy)	Keratoconjunctivitis sicca; eczematoid dermatitis; diarrhea; NLH
22	F	67	67	Graves' disease	None
25	F	27	49	Toxic thyroid nodule	Diarrhea; NLH; carcinoma of sigmoid
17	M	35	32	Goiter (type?) (thyroidectomy)	Diarrhea; NLH; lymphoma of rectum and cecum
18	M	26	58	Spontaneous primary myxedema	Diarrhea; steatorrhea; carcinoma of stomach
42	F	34	46 50	Iodide goiter† Spontaneous primary myxedema	Granulomatosis; ovalocytosis

*NLH = nodular lymphoid hyperplasia of small intestine.
†One sister had Graves' disease.

previously described by our group and a fourth patient has been observed since. The age at which carcinoma of the stomach was diagnosed was 31, 54, 56 and 59 years, occurring 10, 15, 25 and 33 years after the onset of clinical evidence of immunoglobulin deficiency. Two patients were men and two were women. In three of the four patients nodular lymphoid hyperplasia of the small intestine was associated with diarrhea before the development of the malignant lesion, in two with mild and in one with moderately severe steatorrhea. G. lamblia was detected in stool specimens of the three patients with steatorrhea and T. hominis in the fourth patient. Achlorhydria and pernicious anemia were noted in one of the patients, but in two patients histologic examination did not reveal atrophic gastritis. Two patients also had mild splenomegaly and another patient had primary myxedema with increased serum levels of thyroid-stimulating hormone.

A fifth patient had carcinoma of the sigmoid colon. This patient also had nodular lymphoid hyperplasia and a history of a toxic thyroid nodule for which she had been treated with radioactive iodine. Thus, all but one of the five patients with an epithelial malignant lesion of the gastrointestinal tract had associated nodular lymphoid hyperplasia. A sixth patient, a heavy cigarette smoker, had squamous cell carcinoma of the lung and no associated abnormalities except diabetes mellitus.

Lymphoreticular Malignancy (Table XIV). One patient had a bifocal lymphoblastic lymphoma of the rectum and cecum. The rectal lesion was diagnosed and treated with radiation, but the cecal lesion remained undiagnosed until the patient died from peritonitis that complicated perforation of the cecum. At autopsy (which was performed elsewhere) there was no evidence of lymphoma outside these two areas of the lower intestinal tract. This patient also had associated nodular lymphoid hyperplasia of the small intestine and a history of a thyroidectomy for a goiter of unknown type.

The second patient with a lymphoreticular malignant lesion had a lymphocytic lymphoma that had invaded multiple organs. In this patient a thymoma was diagnosed four years before the lymphoma became clinically manifest.

The mean period between the onset of idiopathic late-onset immunoglobulin deficiency and the appearance of neoplasia in the patients who did not have thymoma was 20.9 years. Of the six patients in whom epithelial or lymphoreticular malignant disease originated in the gastrointestinal tract, five had associated nodular lymphoid hyperplasia and three had a thyroid abnormality.

Benign Neoplasia. Thymoma (Table XIV): Four patients had a thymoma (Good's syndrome). One of these patients also had polyposis of the colon, an adenoma of the gallbladder, episodes of watery diarrhea, a history of nephrolithiasis and keratoconjunctivitis sicca. One patient, already mentioned earlier, had a lymphocytic lymphoma that was disseminated widely, and another patient had associated hypochlorhydria. A fourth patient had red cell aplasia that progressed to bone marrow aplasia; the patient died of pneumonia complicated by bacteremia due to P. aeruginosa.

Three thymomas were well encapsulated; two of these were of the spindle cell type and one was predominantly lymphocytic in type mixed with spindling reticuloepithelial elements. The presence of a thymoma in a fourth patient was noted elsewhere, and no information was obtainable about the type of thymoma.

Others: Polyposis of the colon, which occurred in a

TABLE XVI Mortality in Idiopathic Late-Onset Immunoglobulin Deficiency (LID)

Case No.	Sex	Duration of LID (yr)	Cause of Death	Age at Death (yr)	Associated Conditions*
18	M	28	Carcinoma of stomach	62	Diarrhea; steatorrhea; primary myxedema
26	F	26	Carcinoma of stomach	57	Diarrhea; steatorrhea; pernicious anemia; NLH
49	M	10	Carcinoma of stomach	31	Diarrhea; NLH
14	F	26	Carcinoma of stomach	54	Diarrhea; steatorrhea; NLH
17	M	32	Lymphoma of rectum and cecum	67	Diarrhea; NLH; goiter of unknown type
34	M	4	Disseminated lymphoma	50	Thymoma
45	M	8	Carcinoma of lung	60	Diabetes mellitus
30	F	18	Bacteroides fragilis bacteremia	73	Cholecystitis with intra-abdominal abscess
13	F	6	Pseudomonas aeruginosa pneumonia and bacteremia	63	Thymoma bone marrow aplasia; pancytopenia; kerato-conjunctivitis sicca
41	F	<1	Unknown	54	None
48	F	15	Unknown	25	Diarrhea
25	F	30	Unknown	57	Diarrhea; NLH; toxic thyroid nodule; carcinoma of sigmoid at age 49

*NLH = nodular lymphoid hyperplasia of small intestine.

patient in whom a thymoma subsequently developed, has been mentioned. Agnogenic myeloid metaplasia was diagnosed in one patient with no other associated conditions. None of the four patients with thymoma had associated nodular lymphoid hyperplasia or a thyroid disorder.

Thyroid Abnormalities. Six patients (12 per cent) had thyroid abnormalities of various types (Table XV). Two patients had Graves' disease. In one patient this began concomitantly with the first clinical evidence of immunoglobulin deficiency, and in the other patient it began five years after the onset of immunoglobulin deficiency. Both of these patients also had a malabsorption syndrome. Two other patients had myxedema and in both the serum concentration of thyroid-stimulating hormone was significantly increased. Myxedema developed spontaneously in one patient 22 years after the clinical onset of immunoglobulin deficiency; carcinoma of the stomach occurred in this patient. In the second patient, myxedema was associated with an iodide goiter [59], which regressed as the patient became euthyroid again when use of iodide expectorants was stopped. Four years later, spontaneous primary hypothyroidism developed. This patient is of additional interest in that she had pulmonary lesions resembling those of rheumatoid lung disease and cholelithiasis, whereas a sister had been treated at this institution for Graves' disease and cholelithiasis but had normal serum levels of immunoglobulins. A fifth patient had a history of thyroidectomy for a goiter of unknown origin two years before the first clinical evidence of immunoglobulin deficiency. He experienced bifocal lymphoma limited to the rectum and cecum. A sixth patient had been treated with radioactive iodine for a toxic thyroid nodule 22 years after the first clinical manifestations of the immunoglobulin deficiency. This patient had adenocarcinoma of the rectosigmoid area. Thus, in three, or half, of the patients who had thyroid abnormalities, a malignant lesion developed in the gastrointestinal tract, namely, carcinoma of the stomach, carcinoma of the sigmoid and lymphoma of the rectum and cecum. Three of the patients had concomitant nodular lymphoid hyperplasia of the small intestine; in two of these, malignant disease of the intestinal tract complicated the course of illness.

MORTALITY

Twelve patients in this series died (Table XVI). In three patients who died elsewhere, the cause of death could not be ascertained. In nine patients, the cause could be determined at autopsy carried out at this institution or elsewhere. One patient died of peritonitis and bacteremia due to B. fragilis which complicated acute cholecystitis at the age of 73 years, 18 years after the first clinical manifestation of the immunoglobulin deficiency. A second patient died of pneumonia with bacteremia due to P. aeruginosa. This patient had a thymoma and experienced red cell aplasia that progressed to bone marrow aplasia with pancytopenia. Death occurred at the age of 63 years, six years after the clinical onset of the immunoglobulin deficiency. In seven patients, death was related directly to the development of malignant neoplasms—in four, adenocarcinoma of the stomach; in one (who had a thymoma), disseminated lymphoblastic lymphoma; in one, lymphoblastic lymphoma (involving only the rectum and cecum and leading to perforation of the cecum and death from peritonitis); and in one patient, squamous cell carcinoma of the lung.

Thus of the nine patients in whom the cause of death is known, only two succumbed to a primary infection. The seven others died of the consequences of malignant neoplasia, which was of epithelial origin in five and of lymphoreticular origin in two patients.

ILLNESSES IN RELATIVES OF PATIENTS

Although family histories obtained from patients are not always reliable, we do have the following information. There was a strikingly low frequency of increased susceptibility to infections among relatives. Two brothers in the study group itself had hypogammaglobulinemia, and one additional patient had a brother with a history of hypogammaglobulinemia. One patient's son was found to have an isolated deficiency of IgA, and he had a history of meningitis. Seven patients stated that their fathers had had carcinoma, and two that their mothers had had a malignant disease. A 10th patient stated that both parents had had a carcinoma and a sister, leukemia. Five patients had one or more siblings who had died in early infancy. Six patients gave a history of at least one immediate relative having a disease suggesting rheumatoid arthritis. One patient stated that a sister had pernicious anemia. A history of toxic goiter was obtained affecting a mother of one patient and a sister of another. Seven patients had at least one parent or sibling who suffered from asthma.

THERAPY

It is difficult to evaluate the efficacy of therapy in patients with idiopathic late-onset immunoglobulin deficiency. Antimicrobial agents are given to combat implicated bacterial agents and pooled human gamma globulin is given for partial replacement, at best, of the deficiency in gamma globulins. For evaluation of the adequacy of these therapeutic measures, an untreated control group would be required, preferably in a double-blind study. However, in such a study, the control group may be at risk.

Major infections, such as bacterial pneumonias, respond satisfactorily to appropriate parenteral antibiotic therapy. In the current series only one patient died from the sequela of pneumonia. This patient was the only one who had experienced pancytopenia secondary to bone marrow aplasia in association with a thymoma, the infectious agent being P. aeruginosa. Because most episodes of respiratory tract infections in immunoglobulin-deficient patients are caused by D. pneumoniae, H. influenzae and, more rarely, Staph. aureus, antibiotic therapy is begun with a combination of ampicillin, 1 g every 4 hours, and methicillin or a comparable penicillinase-resistant penicillin, 1 g every 4 hours. Both are given by intravenous infusion over a period of about 30 minutes in order to achieve high serum levels. If the causative microorganism is identified in sputum or blood cultures, treatment is changed or restricted to penicillin G, 10 million units/24 hours for D. pneumoniae, ampicillin for H. influenzae or methicillin for Staph. aureus in the doses mentioned. The recent emergence of ampicillin-resistant strains of H. influenzae causing meningitis in young children [60] is of concern and should suggest substituting chloramphenicol, at a dose of 1 g every 6 hours intravenously, for ampicillin.

For the patient in whom pneumonia develops during the intermittent or continuous use of orally administered ampicillin or tetracycline, the possibility of a superinfection due to gram-negative bacilli should be considered. Gentamicin is recommended, at a dose of 1.7 mg/kg body weight every 8 hours intramuscularly or intravenously, in addition to ampicillin and methicillin, until clinical and bacteriologic data warrant change to more specific antimicrobial therapy. All patients seem to benefit from the intermittent use of oral ampicillin, 0.5 g four times a day, or tetracycline, 0.5 four times daily, for the prevention or control of minor sinorespiratory tract infections. Alternating between one week of antibiotic therapy and one week of no therapy is recommended to prevent superinfection.

Treatment of the patient who has bronchiectasis poses a special challenge. The alternating program of oral ampicillin or tetracycline mentioned seems helpful. It does not obviate periodic hospitalization for treatment with parenteral antibiotics. Empirically, a program has been developed that combines ampicillin, 1 g every 4 hours, with clindamycin, 600 mg every 6 hours, and gentamicin, 1.7 mg/kg body weight every 8 hours given intravenously (although gentamicin can be given intramuscularly as well), for a period of about one week. Malaise and anorexia will invariably disappear and purulent sputum will be converted to small amounts of mucoid secretions. Postural drainage and physiotherapeutic measures for the chest are used, and the patient is instructed in both methods. When bronchiectasis is localized, lobectomy should be considered. The Caldwell-Luc surgical procedure seems to have been of benefit in patients with chronic purulent sinusitis who did not respond satisfactorily to oral antibiotic therapy.

Pooled human gamma globulin appears to be beneficial in most patients. At best, it is only a partial replacement—quantitatively because the amounts that can be given are limited, and qualitatively because the preparations available contain virtually no IgA and IgM. In the adult of average weight, a loading dose of 60 ml is given intramuscularly over a period of three to four days; this is followed by 20 to 30 ml every three weeks. A number of patients with immunoglobulin deficiency have a history of severe allergic reactions of the immediate type, including penicillin reactions. In our experience, skin testing reveals that if such allergy was indeed present, the capacity to develop an allergic reaction to penicillin and its derivatives ceases when the immunoglobulin deficiency is well developed. This is an important consideration in the antibiotic treatment of patients with immunoglobulin deficiency, although prior skin testing must still be carried out.

The problems of diarrhea and steatorrhea are particularly difficult from a therapeutic point of view. Metronidazole should be used in all patients who have giardiasis. Patients with severe diarrhea, with or without malabsorption, in whom a search for G. lamblia has been unrewarding may nonetheless be given one course of metronidazole empirically. Many patients will continue to complain about significant diarrhea after G. lamblia has been eradicated. Tetracycline given orally has been beneficial in some cases. Stool cultures should be obtained to determine whether salmonellosis, shigellosis or staphylococcosis is present, to be followed by specific therapy when indicated.

An occasional patient has responded to the administration of cholestyramine, of gamma globulin and of intravenous fresh plasma. Some patients are refractory to all these measures. A gluten-free diet has been advocated for the management of diarrhea, but it has not been helpful in this series. In one patient with an extremely severe malabsorption syndrome, remission was nearly complete after therapy with moderately large doses of oral prednisone, but relapse occurred after the dose was decreased to maintenance levels.

An awareness of the propensity of patients with late-onset idiopathic immunoglobulin deficiency to experience cholelithiasis and gastrointestinal malignancy should lead to appropriate diagnostic tests and surgical therapy.

COMMENTS

Since the original description of idiopathic late-onset immunoglobulin deficiency [2–8], it has been realized that the late-onset form of the disease varies from the congenital form in several important ways. In the congenital form, diarrhea and malabsorption are rare, and arthritis is relatively common [52]. Children with congenital agammaglobulinemia have poorly developed tonsillar lymphoidal tissue and no Peyer's patches [61]. In the late-onset form, tonsillar hyperplasia and nodular lymphoid hyperplasia of the small intestine are often present [15,17,18,29–39]; 46 per cent of our patients had a history of tonsillectomy.

In considering the cause of the diarrhea, secondary mechanisms such as bacterial overgrowth of the normal enteric flora [39], salmonellosis [14], shigellosis [14], and giardiasis [14,15,17,18,39] are thought to be factors. It is not known why such mechanisms do not operate more commonly in the congenital form of the disease, since humoral host defense mechanisms are similarly affected and even more seriously so. Our observations that 40 per cent of the patients did not have diarrhea and 34 per cent had no evidence of malabsorption, and that these problems did not develop during years of follow-up, suggest an essential difference between the two forms. Also, several of our patients with severe diarrhea and malabsorption did not have giardiasis, did not respond to therapy with metronidazole and responded only partially to therapy with tetracycline and other antimicrobial agents. This suggests that other mechanisms, such as an intrinsic epithelial defect or an inflammatory process of unknown origin, are important.

The rather strong correlation noted between achlorhydria and diarrhea, especially steatorrheal diarrhea, is of interest. The lack of gastric acid may add to the patient's vulnerability to bacterial colonization of the small intestine [62]. Alternatively, atrophic gastritis and intestinal malabsorption may be causally related by the operation of a common pathogen mechanism at both sites—the stomach and the small intestine. Observations on the effect of large doses of prednisone in combination with tetracycline are of interest. This form of therapy was resorted to in a patient with the most severe malabsorption problem in this series. In this patient, who was achlorhydric, there was simultaneous resumption of hydrochloric acid production and partial remission of intestinal dysfunction [63].

An additional factor that may occasionally contribute to the development of diarrhea and malabsorption is pancreatitis [17,64]. It was observed in one of our patients. Evidence was obtained in two patients of secondary exocrine pancreatic insufficiency due to a defect of secretion of pancreozymin by the epithelium of the small intestine. Disaccharidase deficiency has also been described in immunoglobulin deficiency [65]; two brothers in the current series had diarrhea only when ingesting lactose-containing food.

The initial interest in the lesion termed "nodular lymphoid hyperplasia" of the small intestine in idiopathic late-onset immunoglobulin deficiency [15,29–31] was due to its sharp contrast with the paucity or absence of Peyer's plaques, and appendiceal and tonsillar lymphoid tissue in congenital X-linked agammaglobulinemia. Similar lesions have been observed in the rectum and sigmoid in a few patients [37]. Rectal lesions were detected in four of our patients, but they could not be correlated with the presence of the lesions in the small intestine. Nodular lymphoid hyperplasia of the small intestine has also been described in selective immunoglobulin A deficiency [36] and in immunoglobulin deficiency associated with noncaseating granulomatosis of lymph nodes [38]. The lesions must be differentiated from benign lymphoid polyposis of the ileum [66,67], malignant melanoma [68] and benign lymphoid polyposis of the colon [69]. Recently, the concept has been revived that gut-associated lymphoid tissue may represent the mammalian bursa-equivalent [70].

In our series there was a propensity for the development of gastrointestinal malignancy in association with nodular lymphoid hyperplasia of the small intestine. Nodular lymphoid hyperplasia was detected in 62 per cent of 21 patients who had diarrhea and whose small bowel was studied by biopsy. Steatorrhea was present in just over half of the 13 patients with nodular lymphoid hyperplasia.

Hughes and associates [17] have suggested, on the basis of five cases, that all patients with idiopathic late-onset immunoglobulin deficiency and intestinal dysfunction have nodular lymphoid hyperplasia and that these lesions may disappear. Our studies do not support this conclusion; we have never observed the disappearance of nodular lymphoid hyperplasia once it was detected. The extensive studies of Ament and Rubin [39], utilizing 384 biopsy specimens of the small intestine from eight patients with "gastrointestinal immunodeficiency," have shown three different types of morphologic changes: nodular lymphoid hyperplasia, hypogammaglobulinemic sprue and mixed lesions. Eradication of giardiasis often leads to clinical diminution of intestinal symptoms and mucosal morphology except for the lesion of nodular lymphoid hyperplasia [39].

Recent studies in several laboratories revealed that most patients with late-onset immunoglobulin deficiency have normal numbers of circulating type B lymphocytes in contrast to children with congenital disease, who have very low counts or absent B cells [71–76]. Preliminary studies at this institution in 10 patients have shown that eight had normal or slightly decreased numbers of B cells and two had low counts of circulating B cells (5 per cent or less). It is noteworthy that, in several of our patients, after the percentages of T and B cells had been totalled, a significant percentage of cells remained unaccounted for. It is conceivable, but it was not demonstrated, that the functions of the cells that could not be accounted for, or a fraction thereof, differ from those of T or B cells or that they lack the receptors needed for their detection by the methods that were used.

These findings have been interpreted as reflecting an inability of B cells to mature to immunoglobulin-secreting plasma cells [71]. Waldmann and associates [77] provided evidence that, in a group of patients with late-onset immunoglobulin deficiency, a suppressor population of T cells interferes with B-cell function of immunoglobulin secretion. There is additional evidence of T-cell dysfunction in some patients with late-onset immunoglobulin deficiency in that delayed hypersensitivity is not entirely normal as shown by skin testing and in vitro stimulation of lymphocytes with the mitogen phytohemagglutinin [74,75a]. Similar findings have been obtained at this institution in current studies [75b].

It remains to be determined whether such functional abnormalities of T cells are a result of intercurrent infectious episodes [76].

These newer concepts about the cause of the disease and aberrations in the T-cell system are of considerable potential interest with regard to several clinical problems that occur in patients with late-onset immunoglobulin deficiency.

The pathogenesis of pernicious anemia had rather generally been understood to be autoimmune and to be mediated by humoral mechanisms. The development of pernicious anemia and achlorhydria in patients with an antibody deficiency syndrome [14,41–46] requires an explanation that extends beyond this traditional concept. Twomey and associates [41,45] showed that, indeed, autoantibodies are not detectable in either the serum or the gastric secretions of patients with late-onset immunoglobulin deficiency in whom pernicious anemia develops. Recently, several investigators obtained evidence suggesting that cellular (lymphocytic) mechanisms are involved in the autoimmune process [78–80].

The propensity of patients with late-onset immunoglobulin deficiency disease for thyroid abnormalities is also of interest. The occurrence of pernicious anemia with hypogammaglobulinemia in a patient, pernicious anemia and myxedema in her mother, and latent pernicious anemia in a sister of the mother was described by Lee and associates [43]. Ammann and Hong [81] recorded the frequent occurrence of autoimmune disorders, including pernicious anemia and thyroiditis, in patients with selective IgA deficiency.

The results of observations in patients with idiopathic late-onset immunoglobulin deficiency further emphasize the vulnerability of the gastric and intestinal epithelium and of the thyroid gland in this immune deficiency.

In chronic mucocutaneous candidiasis, in which an abnormality of delayed hypersensitivity is common, there is a propensity for the production of autoantibodies. It is of interest that in this immune deficiency, achlorhydria, pernicious anemia and primary endocrine insufficiency of the parathyroids, thyroid, adrenals and ovaries are often present [82–85].

Increased susceptibility to tumorigenesis has been well documented in a number of immune deficiencies [46,48,49], especially those that involve the T-cell system. The finding of 14 tumors in 12 of our patients (or 24 per cent) with late-onset immunoglobulin deficiency is striking and suggests that immunologic surveillance in such patients is also affected. The recent finding of T-cell aberrations in patients with late-onset disease in contrast to those with congenital agammaglobulinemia may have a bearing on the high frequency with which neoplasia develops [74,75,77]. In the current series of patients, 16 per cent had malignant neoplasia; the ratio of epithelial to lymphoreticular malignancy was 3 to 1. This is twice the estimated risk of malignancy (8 per cent) in a study by Kersey and associates [49] based on information accumulated from the literature and by correspondence. It appears from our observation that the risk of development of malignant neoplasia is among the highest of any immunodeficiency in man [48,49] and that malignant disease of epithelial origin predominates. These observations differ from the results of the data collected by Kersey and associates [49], which showed a predominance of lymphoreticular types of malignancy, and probably reflect the advantage of continued observation of a large group of patients in one single medical center.

On clinical grounds, we have been impressed by the contrast between two major groups of patients with idiopathic late-onset immunoglobulin deficiency. One group of patients suffers from the direct consequences of an antibody deficiency state; they have recurrent and severe upper and lower respiratory tract infections, mainly of bacterial origin. This group appears to be resistant to intestinal disorders. The other group consists of patients with diarrhea, malabsorption and weight loss, a syndrome that is superimposed on the clinical manifestations of an antibody deficiency syndrome. Further refinement in the clinical classification of patients with late-onset immunoglobulin deficiency can be introduced by taking into account the presence or absence of a thymoma, nodular lymphoid hyperplasia of the intestine and atrophic gastritis. In addition, the morphologic alterations of the mucosa of the small intestine in patients with the enteropathic variety of the disease can be used.

Ultimately, however, the classification of these patients will depend on inclusion of the results of newer knowledge that takes into account aberrations of T and B lymphocytes, the regulatory mechanisms that limit or enhance their function, and enzymatic defects that may exist in either or both cell lines, or subpopulations of T and B cells that may cause immune incompetence. Genetic abnormalities demonstrated in some patients with immunoglobulin deficiency and their relatives [86–91] require further elucidation and should be incorporated into a more definitive classification of the disease.

REFERENCES

1. Bruton OC: Agammaglobulinemia. Pediatrics 9: 722, 1952.
2. Sanford JP, Favour CB, Tribeman MS: Absence of serum gamma globulins in an adult. N Engl J Med 250: 1027, 1954.
3. Zinneman HH, Hall WH, Heller BI: Acquired agammaglobulinemia: report of three cases. JAMA 156: 1390, 1954.
4. Prasad AS, Koza DW: Agammaglobulinemia. Ann Intern Med 41: 629, 1954.
5. Grant GH, Wallace WD: Agammaglobulinaemia. Lancet 2: 671, 1954.
6. Barandun S, Büchler H, Hässig A: Das Antikörpermangelsyndrom. Agammaglobulinämie. Schweiz Med Wochenschr 86: 33, 1956.
7. Wall RL, Saslaw S: Adult agammaglobulinemia. Arch Intern Med 95: 33, 1955.
8. Rosecan M, Trobaugh FE Jr, Danforth WH: Agammaglobulinemia in the adult. Am J Med 19: 303, 1955.
9. Ramos AJ: Diagnostic problem: presentation of case. JAMA 160: 1317, 1956.
10. Barandun S, Huser HJ, Hässig A: Klinische Erscheinungsformen des Antikörpermangelsyndroms. Schweiz Med Wochenschr 88: 78, 1958.
11. Vesin P, Cattan R: Antibody deficiencies and intestinal disorders. Plasma Proteins and Gastrointestinal Tract in Health and Disease, Proceedings of the International Symposium, Paris, August 1961 (Schartz M, Vesin P, eds), Baltimore, Williams & Wilkins Co., 1963, p 214.
12. Huizenga KA, Wollaeger EE, Green PA, McKenzie BF: Serum globulin deficiencies in non-tropical sprue, with report of two cases of acquired agammaglobulinemia. Am J Med 31: 572, 1961.
13. Pelkonen R, Siurala M, Vuopio P: Inherited agammaglobulinemia with malabsorption and marked alterations in the gastrointestinal mucosa. Acta Med Scand 173: 549, 1963.
14. Waldmann TA, Laster L: Abnormalities of albumin metabolism in patients with hypogammaglobulinemia. J Clin Invest 43: 1025, 1964.
15. Hermans PE, Huizenga KA, Hoffman HN II, et al.: Dysgammaglobulinemia associated with nodular lymphoid hyperplasia of the small intestine. Am J Med 40: 78, 1966.
16. Gelzayd EA, McCleery JL, Melnyk CS, Kraft SC: Intestinal malabsorption and immunoglobulin deficiency. Arch Intern Med 127: 141, 1971.
17. Hughes WS, Cerda JJ, Holtzapple P, Brooks FP: Primary hypogammaglobulinemia and malabsorption. Ann Intern Med 74: 903, 1971.
18. Ament ME, Ochs HD, Davis SD: Structure and function of the gastrointestinal tract in primary immunodeficiency syndromes: a study of 39 patients. Medicine (Baltimore) 52: 227, 1973.
19. Conn HO, Quintiliani R: Severe diarrhea controlled by gamma globulin in a patient with agammaglobulinemia, amyloidosis, and thymoma. Ann Intern Med 65: 528, 1966.
20. Martin CM, Gordon RS, McCullough NB: Acquired hypogammaglobulinemia in an adult: report of a case, with clinical and experimental studies. N Engl J Med 254: 449, 1956.
21. MacLean LD, Zak SJ, Varco RL, Good RA: Thymic tumor and acquired agammaglobulinemia: a clinical and experimental study of the immune response. Surgery 40: 1010, 1956.
22. Lambie AT, Burrows BA, Sommers SC: Clinicopathologic conference; refractory anemia, agammaglobulinemia, and mediastinal tumor. Am J Clin Pathol 27: 444, 1957.
23. Gafni J, Michaeli D, Heller H: Idiopathic acquired agammaglobulinemia associated with thymoma: report of two cases and review of the literature. N Engl J Med 263: 536, 1960.
24. Godfrey S: Thymoma with hypogammaglobulinaemia in an identical twin. Br Med J 1: 1159, 1964.
25. Jacox RF, Mongan ES, Hanshaw JB, Leddy JP: Hypogamma-

globulinemia with thymoma and probable pulmonary infection with cytomegalovirus. N Engl J Med 271: 1091, 1964.
26. Chapin MA: Benign thymoma, refractory anemia and hypogammaglobulinemia: case report. J Maine Med Assoc 56: 83, 1965.
27. Gehrmann G, Engstfeld G: Thymoma and agammaglobulinaemia. Ger Med Mon 10: 381, 1965.
28. Kirk BW, Freedman SO: Hypogammaglobulinemia, thymoma and ulcerative colitis. Can Med Assoc J 96: 1272, 1967.
29. Firkin BG, Blackburn CRB: Congenital and acquired agammaglobulinaemia: a report of four cases. Q J Med ns 27: 187, 1958.
30. Frik W, Heinkel K, Zeitler G: Vermehrung und Hyperplasie von Lymphfollikeln als Ursache granulärer Füllungsdefekte im Röntgenbild des gesamten Dünndarms. Fortschr Geb Roentgenstr Nuklearmed 99: 65, 1963.
31. Hermans PE: Nodular lymphoid hyperplasia of the small intestine and hypogammaglobulinemia: theoretical and practical considerations. Fed Proc 26: 1606, 1967.
32. Hodgson JR, Hoffman HN II, Huizenga KA: Roentgenologic features of lymphoid hyperplasia of the small intestine associated with dysgammaglobulinemia. Radiology 88: 883, 1967.
33. Goulston K, Stephen D: Nodular lymphoid hyperplasia of the small intestine associated with hypogammaglobulinaemia. Australas Radiol 12: 225, 1968.
34. Kirkpatrick CH, Waxman D, Smith OD, Schimke RN: Hypogammaglobulinemia with nodular lymphoid hyperplasia of the small bowel. Arch Intern Med 121: 273, 1968.
35. Grise JW: Dysgammaglobulinemia with nodular lymphoid hyperplasia of the small intestine: a case report. Radiology 90: 579, 1968.
36. Gryboski JD, Self TW, Clemett A, Herskovic T: Selective immunoglobulin A deficiency and intestinal nodular lymphoid hyperplasia: correction of diarrhea with antibiotics and plasma. Pediatrics 42: 833, 1968.
37. Bird DC, Jacobs JB, Silbiger M, Wolff SM: Hypogammaglobulinemia with nodular lymphoid hyperplasia of the small intestine: report of a case with rectosigmoid involvement. Radiology 92: 1535, 1969.
38. Davis SD, Eidelman S, Loop JW: Nodular lymphoid hyperplasia of the small intestine and sarcoidosis. Arch Intern Med 126: 668, 1970.
39. Ament ME, Rubin CE: Relation of giardiasis to abnormal intestinal structure and function in gastrointestinal immunodeficiency syndromes. Gastroenterology 62: 216, 1972.
40. Van Leeuwen L, Van Dommelen CKV: Agammaglobulinemie. Ned Tijdschr Geneeskd 100: 1303, 1956.
41. Twomey JJ, Jordan PH Jr, Laughter AH, et al.: The gastric disorder in immunoglobulin-deficient patients. Ann Intern Med 72: 499, 1970.
42. Larsson SO, Hagelquist E, Cöster C: Hypogammaglobulinaemia and pernicious anaemia. Acta Haematol (Basel) 26: 50, 1961.
43. Lee FI, Jenkins GC, Hughes DTD, Kazantzis G: Pernicious anaemia, myxoedema, and hypogammaglobulinaemia: a family study. Br Med J 1: 598, 1964.
44. Conn HO, Binder H, Burns B: Pernicious anemia and immunologic deficiency. Ann Intern Med 68: 603, 1968.
45. Twomey JJ, Jordan PH, Jarrold T, et al.: The syndrome of immunoglobulin deficiency and pernicious anemia. Am J Med 47: 340, 1969.
46. Hermans PE, Huizenga KA: Association of gastric carcinoma with idiopathic late-onset immunoglobulin deficiency. Ann Intern Med 76: 605, 1972.
47. Forssman O, Herner B: Acquired agammaglobulinaemia and malabsorption. Acta Med Scand 176: 779, 1964.
48. Waldmann TA, Strober W, Blaese RM: Immunodeficiency disease and malignancy: various immunologic deficiencies of man and the role of immune processes in the control of malignant disease. Ann Intern Med 77: 605, 1972.
49. Kersey JH, Spector BD, Good RA: Primary immunodeficiency diseases and cancer: the immunodeficiency-cancer registry. Int J Cancer 12: 333, 1973.
50. Diaz-Buxo JA, Hermans PE, Elveback LR: Prevalence of cholelithiasis in idiopathic late-onset immunoglobulin deficiency. Ann Intern Med 82: 213, 1975.
51. Gitlin D, Janeway CA, Apt L, Craig JM: Agammaglobulinemia. Cellular and Humoral Aspects of the Hypersensitive States: A Symposium Held at the New York Academy of Medicine (Lawrence HS, ed), New York, Hoeber Medical Division, Harper & Bros, 1959, p 375.
52. Rosen FS, Janeway CA: The gamma globulins. III. The antibody deficiency syndromes. N Engl J Med 275: 709, 1966.
53. Bergsma D (editor): Immunologic deficiency diseases in man. Birth Defects 4: 1, 1968.
54. Gergsma D (editor): Immunodeficiency in man and animals. Birth Defects 11: 1, 1975.
55. Fudenberg H, Good RA, Goodman HC, et al.: Primary immunodeficiencies: report of a World Health Organization committee. Pediatrics 47: 927, 1971.
56. Mancini G, Carbonara AO, Heremans JF: Immunochemical quantitation of antigens by single radial immunodiffusion. Immunochemistry 2: 235, 1965.
57. Jondal M, Holm G, Wigzell H: Surface markers on human T and B lymphocytes. I. A large population of lymphocytes forming nonimmune rosettes with sheep red blood cells. J Exp Med 136: 207, 1972.
58. Stobo JD, Rosenthal AS, Paul WE: Functional heterogeneity of murine lymphoid cells. V. Lymphocytes lacking detectable surface θ or immunoglobulin determinants. J Exp Med 138: 71, 1973.
59. Paris J, McConahey WM, Owen CA Jr, et al.: Iodide goiter. J Clin Endocrinol Metab 20: 57, 1960.
60. Schiffer MS, MacLowry J, Schneerson R, Robbins JB: Clinical, bacteriological, and immunological characterisation of ampicillin-resistant Haemophilus influenzae type B. Lancet 2: 257, 1974.
61. Peterson RDA, Cooper MD, Good RA: The pathogenesis of immunologic deficiency diseases. Am J Med 38: 579, 1965.
62. Giannella RA, Broitman SA, Zamcheck N: Influence of gastric acidity on bacterial and parasitic enteric infections: a perspective. Ann Intern Med 78: 271, 1973.
63. Diaz-Buxo JA, Hermans PE, Huizenga KA: Gastrointestinal dysfunction in immunoglobulin deficiency: effect of corticosteroids and tetracycline. JAMA. 233: 1189, 1975.
64. Cooke WT, Weiner W, Shinton NK: Agammaglobulinaemia: report of two adult cases. Br Med J 1: 1151, 1957.
65. Dubois RS, Roy CC, Fulginiti VA, et al.: Disaccharidase deficiency in children with immunologic deficits. J Pediatr 76: 377, 1970.
66. Cosens CG: Gastro-intestinal pseudoleukemia: a case report. Ann Surg 148: 129, 1958.
67. Patel VK, Awen CF: Benign lymphoid polyposis of ileum: three cases and a review of the literature. Can J Surg 14: 402, 1971.
68. Haskin BJ: Multiple nodules of the small bowel. JAMA 200: 634, 1967.
69. Collins JO, Falk M, Guibone R: Benign lymphoid polyposis of the colon: a case report. Pediatrics 38: 897, 1966.
70. Chapman HA, Johnson JS, Cooper MD: Ontogeny of Peyer's patches and immunoglobulin-containing cells in pigs. J Immunol 112: 555, 1974.
71. Cooper MD, Lawton AR, Bockman DE: Agammaglobulinaemia with B lymphocytes: specific defect of plasma-cell differentiation. Lancet 2: 791, 1971.
72. Siegel FP, Pernis B, Kunkel HG: Lymphocytes in human immunodeficiency states: a study of membrane-associated

immunoglobulins. Eur J Immunol 1: 482, 1971.

73. Abdou NI, Casella SR, Abdou NL, Abrahamsohn IA: Comparative study of bone marrow and blood B cells in infantile and acquired agammaglobulinemia. J Clin Invest 52: 2218, 1973.
74. Preud'Homme JL, Griscelli C, Seligmann M: Immunoglobulins on the surface of lymphocytes in fifty patients with primary immunodeficiency diseases. Clin Immunol Immunopathol 1: 241, 1973.
75. (a) Gajl-Peczalska KJ, Park BH, Biggar WD, Good RA: B and T lymphocytes in primary immunodeficiency disease in man. J Clin Invest 52: 919, 1973.
    (b) Paul S, Stabo J, Hermans PE, Tomasi TB: Unpublished data.
76. Schiff RI, Buckley RH, Gilbertsen RB, Metzgar RS: Membrane receptors and in vitro responsiveness of lymphocytes in human immunodeficiency. J Immunol 112: 376, 1974.
77. Waldmann TA, Durm M, Broder S, et al.: Role of suppressor T cells in pathogenesis of common variable hypogammaglobulinaemia. Lancet 2: 609, 1974.
78. Rose MS, Chanarin I, Doniach D, et al.: Intrinsic-factor antibodies in absence of pernicious anaemia: 3–7-year follow-up. Lancet 2: 9, 1970.
79. Goldstone AH, Calder EA, Barnes EW, Irvine WJ: The effect of gastric antigens on the in vitro migration of leucocytes from patients with atrophic gastritis and pernicious anaemia. Clin Exp Immunol 14: 501, 1973.
80. Chanarin I, James D: Humoral and cell-mediated intrinsic-factor antibody in pernicious anaemia. Lancet 1: 1078, 1974.
81. Ammann AJ, Hong R: Selective IgA deficiency: presentation of 30 cases and a review of the literature. Medicine (Baltimore) 50: 223, 1971.
82. Chilgren RA, Meuwissen HJ, Quie PG, Hong R: Chronic mucocutaneous candidiasis, deficiency of delayed hypersensitivity, and selective local antibody defect. Lancet 2: 688, 1967.
83. Wuepper KD, Fudenberg HH: Moniliasis, "autoimmune" polyendocrinopathy, and immunologic family study. Clin Exp Immunol 2: 71, 1967.
84. Hermans PE, Ulrich JA, Markowitz H: Chronic mucocutaneous candidiasis as a surface expression of deep-seated abnormalities: report of a syndrome of superficial candidiasis, absence of delayed hypersensitivity and aminoaciduria. Am J Med 47: 503, 1969.
85. Kirkpatrick CH, Rich RR, Bennett JE: Chronic mucocutaneous candidiasis; model-building in cellular immunology. Ann Intern Med 74: 955, 1971.
86. Fudenberg H, German JL III, Kunkel HG: The occurrence of rheumatoid factor and other gamma globulin abnormalities in the families of patients with agammaglobulinemia (abstract). J Clin Invest 39: 987, 1960.
87. Wollheim F: Inherited "acquired" hypogammaglobulinaemia. Lancet 1: 316, 1961.
88. Wolf JK, Gokcen M, Good RA: The relationship of acquired agammaglobulinemia to other mesenchymal diseases: a family study (abstract). Proc Cent Soc Clin Res 34: 90, 1961.
89. Buckley RH, Sidbury JB Jr: Hereditary alterations in the immune response: coexistence of "agammaglobulinemia," acquired hypogammaglobulinemia and selective immunoglobulin deficiency in a sibship. Pediatr Res 2: 72, 1968.
90. Schwartz RH, Schenk EA, Berman J, Ellis BA: Hereditary nonlymphopenic agammaglobulinemia with splenomegaly: a family study. J Lab Clin Med 74: 203, 1969.
91. Nell PA, Ammann AJ, Hong R, Stiehm ER: Familial selective IgA deficiency. Pediatrics 49: 71, 1972.

INFORMATION FOR AUTHORS

PREPARATION OF MANUSCRIPTS

Manuscripts should be typed on one side of the sheet, doublespaced, on white bond paper, 8½ by 11 inches, with margins of 1 inch. Two copies of the manuscript and illustrations should be sent to the Editor at 666 Fifth Avenue, New York, New York 10019. Title page should include full name, degrees and affiliation of all authors, the source from which the article emanates, and the name and address of the person to whom requests for reprints should be addressed.

All manuscript pages including tables and legends should be numbered consecutively in the upper right hand corner.

The number of manuscript pages, the number of illustrations and the number of tables should be indicated at the bottom of the covering letter.

Every article must be preceded by an abstract (not to exceed 350 words). This obviates the need for a summary. In addition, for the convenience of our readers, we require a brief abstract (not exceeding 100 to 125 words) and key words for indexing purposes. These brief abstracts appear in the back of the *Journal* in the same issue in which the paper appears.

Since all manuscripts submitted for publication in the *Journal* are sent out for review before a final decision is made, there is generally a lapse of three to six weeks before contributors are notified. If you have received an acknowledgment of receipt, there is no need to call the *Journal* office; your manuscript has not gone astray. The decision will be forthcoming shortly.

PREPARATION OF ILLUSTRATIONS AND TABLES

Illustrations must be black and white glossy prints or professional drawings in india ink; they should be unmounted. The name of the lead author and the title of the article should be typed on a label and affixed to the back of each illustration; the top should be indicated.

Reference to all illustrations should be inserted in the text in consecutive order. Legends for the illustrations should be typed, double spaced, on a separate sheet with numbers corresponding to those on the photographs or drawings. They should not be attached to the pictures.

Tables should be typed on separate sheets and should be set up in accordance with the style of the Journal. Units of measure should be confined to column headings. Abbreviations should be kept to a minimum and should conform with those used by the *Journal* or listed as acceptable in the Council of Biology Editors Style Manual. Any variations should be explained. All vertical rules should be omitted.

The publisher allows a fixed amount towards the reproduction of illustrations and tables. Charges in excess of this amount must be assumed by the authors. The Editor reserves the right to limit the number of illustrations and/or tables.

PREPARATION OF BIBLIOGRAPHY

Bibliographic references should be listed chronologically on a separate sheet (not in footnotes) as referred to in the text and should be typed (double-spaced) in accordance with the style and abbreviations (open punctuation) used by Index Medicus; only the first page of the journal citation is necessary. Examples follow:

For periodical references:

22. Theologides A, Kennedy BJ: Toxoplasmic myocarditis and pericarditis. Am J Med 47: 169, 1969.

For book references (with chapter):

18. Schiebler GL, Van Mieron LHS, Krovetz LJ: Diseases of the tricuspid valve, chap 2. Heart Disease in Infants, Children and Adolescents (Moss AJ, Adams F, eds), Baltimore, Williams & Wilkins, 1968.

For book references (without chapter):

13. Berne E: Principles of Group Treatment, New York, Oxford University Press, 1966, p 26.

Authors are responsible for the accuracy of all references.

REPRINTS

Price schedules and order cards for reprints are mailed to the person so listed in the footnote on the title page.

The American Journal of Medicine, **666 Fifth Avenue, New York, New York 10019**

Hodgkin's Disease with Nervous System Manifestations

Stenographic reports, edited by Philip E. Cryer, M.D. and John M. Kissane, M.D., of weekly clinicopathologic conferences held in Barnes and Wohl Hospitals, are published in each issue of the Journal. These conferences are participated in jointly by members of the Departments of Internal Medicine and Pathology of Washington University School of Medicine.

A 22 year old woman was admitted to Barnes Hospital on August 1, 1975, with fever and a productive cough. She died two weeks later.

A right supraclavicular mass was biopsied and revealed Hodgkin's disease, mixed cellularity type in early December 1971. On admission to Barnes Hospital on December 17, 1971, the patient was asymptomatic but 1.5 cm left supraclavicular and 2.0 cm left axillary lymph nodes were palpable. There was no evidence of Hodgkin's disease on chest films. Because the patient was seven and a half months pregnant, further diagnostic studies were deferred. Radiation (4,000 rads) was administered to the neck, axillae and upper mediastinum, and the enlarged lymph nodes regressed. Vaginal delivery of a normal infant on February 3, 1972, was uncomplicated.

On readmission on March 12, 1972, chest films showed widening of the mediastinum. Intravenous urograms and lymphangiograms were within normal limits as were routine serum chemistry studies. During performance of the lymphangiograms, 8 to 10 ml of Ethiodol® was inadvertently injected intravenously with subsequent acute but transient pulmonary symptoms. On April 4, there was persistent widening of the mediastinum. The vital capacity was 3.2 liters (80 per cent of predicted) and the forced expiratory volume 3.0 liters at 1 second (87 per cent of predicted). A staging laparotomy, with splenectomy and biopsies of the liver, multiple lymph nodes and the sternal bone marrow, was performed on April 6, 1972. There was no evidence of Hodgkin's disease in any of the tissues removed. Radiation (4,000 rads) to the lower mediastinum and abdomen was administered.

The patient felt well until night sweats, low grade fever, nonproductive cough and pleuritic right chest pain prompted her readmission on November 14, 1972. There was a confluent density in the lower lobe of the right lung on chest roentgenograms. This was biopsied at thoracotomy and found to be Hodgkin's disease, mixed cellularity type.

Treatment with cyclophosphamide, vincristine, procarbazine and prednisone was begun and continued over the next five months; the administration of procarbazine and prednisone was continued until December 1973.

Fever and jaundice led to the patient's readmission on December 26, 1973. The liver was not enlarged. The total serum bilirubin level rose to 9.7 mg/100 ml and the serum glutamic oxaloacetic transaminase level (SGOT) to 1,075 mIU/ml. The serum alkaline phosphatase was 215 mIU/ml. The serum was positive for HBsAg. A liver biopsy specimen was consistent with viral hepatitis; there was no evidence of Hodgkin's disease. Without therapy (aside from an increase in the prednisone dose to 50 mg daily) the patient's condition improved, and the serum bilirubin and SGOT levels were normal two weeks later. The vital capacity was 2.0 liters and the forced expiratory volume 1.9 liters at 1 second. Weekly therapy with vinblastine, 5 mg intravenously, was begun.

The patient was hospitalized on June 9, 1974, with fever, pustular skin lesions, painful knees and ankles with effusion, erythema and warmth of the knees and a vaginal discharge. A clinical diagnosis of gonococcemia was made, and the patient responded to therapy with large doses of penicillin. Cultures of the blood, vaginal discharge, pustule contents, throat and rectum were all negative.

Roentgenographic evidence of progression of the lesion in the lower lobe of the right lung and the appearance of nodular lesions in the lower lobe of the left lung led to discontinuation of vinblastine therapy and institution of a regimen consisting of bleomycin, vincristine, prednisone, adriamycin and imadazole carboxamide in February 1975.

The patient was readmitted on May 8 with increasingly severe headaches, weakness of the lower extremities, difficulty in walking and incontinence of urine. The cerebrospinal fluid contained 235 cells/mm^3 (95 per cent eosinophils); a Reed-Sternberg cell was seen in the spinal fluid. Computerized axial tomography of the brain demonstrated an area of diminished density in the region of the right temporal lobe. A myelogram showed no block. Radiation therapy was given to the whole head, and treatment with intrathecal methotrexate and cytosine arabinoside was begun. The intrathecal treatment was repeated on July 18.

Fever, with temperatures to 104°F, and a productive cough led to the patient's final admission to Barnes Hospital on August 1, 1975. Physical findings included ptosis of the left upper lid, bilateral Babinski's sign and diminished vibratory and position sense in the lower extremities. There were increased breath sounds and rales at the base of the right lung. The liver extended 4 cm below the right costal margin. The white blood cell count was 1,800/mm^3, the hematocrit value 34 per cent. The prothrombin time was 16.2 seconds (62 per cent). The cerebrospinal fluid was normal. Gram-positive diplococci were seen in the sputum. Chest roentgenograms showed an increase in the infiltrates in the lower lobe of the right lung and interval appearance of a cavity in the lower lobe of the right lung. Culture of material obtained during attempted brush biopsy of the cavity grew Staphylococcus aureus. Fungal cultures were negative. Therapy with penicillin and gentamicin, and subsequently oxacillin, was followed by defervescence. However, on August 14 increased shortness of breath and anxiety occurred, the blood pressure was unobtainable and the patient died.

CLINICAL DISCUSSION

Dr. Edward Reinhard: This young woman was 17 years old and six and a half months pregnant when she discovered a right supraclavicular mass on November 10, 1971. Biopsy of this mass in December 1971 revealed Hodgkin's disease, mixed cell type. She had no "B" symptoms (i.e., chills, fever, sweats or weight loss) at that time. She was admitted to Barnes Hospital on December 17, 1971. Examination at that time revealed a 1.5 cm lymph node on the left side of the neck and a 2 cm left axillary lymph node. There were no other abnormal findings. Roentgenograms of the chest were said to be within normal limits. Further work-up was delayed until after delivery. The patient was given 4,000 rads to the neck, axillas and the upper mediastinum. The usual mantle port was abbreviated at the mid-sternum because the patient was pregnant. After this treatment, the palpable nodes disappeared. Five and a half weeks after delivery of a normal baby, the patient was admitted to Barnes Hospital for staging. Roentgenograms of the chest showed mediastinal widening. Staging procedures, including a laparotomy, revealed no involvement below the diaphragm and the condition was therefore staged as 2A. She was then given 4,000 rads to the lower mediastinum and the para-aortic nodes down to the pelvic rim. No chemotherapy was given at that time.

The patient was readmitted in November 1972 with fever, sweats, cough and vague chest pain on the right side. Chest films showed a density in the lower lobe of the right lung. Thoracotomy with biopsy of a pleural nodule and biopsy of the infiltrate in the middle lobe of the right lung revealed Hodgkin's disease, mixed cellularity type. The patient's condition therefore was at that time in stage 4B. She was given COPP (cyclophosphamide, vincristine, procarbazine and prednisone) therapy for five months and was then maintained on prednisone and procarbazine for another eight months. While on this therapy, her symptoms were well controlled and she remained asymptomatic until December 26, 1973, when she was readmitted with fever, jaundice and increased hepatic enzymes. Hodgkin's disease of the liver was suspected, but a liver biopsy specimen showed no Hodgkin's disease and there were changes thought to be consistent with viral hepatitis. HBsAg was present in the serum. She was discharged taking prednisone, 50 mg daily. Two weeks later she had gained 14 pounds, the jaundice had cleared, and the serum levels of the hepatic enzymes had returned to normal. Vinblastine therapy was started at that time.

Five months later she was readmitted with fever, sweats, bilateral ankle pain, hot, red knees, pustular skin lesions on the thorax and lower abdomen, and a white vaginal discharge. Despite the fact that all cultures of blood, pustular fluid, vaginal secretions and urine were negative; she was presumed to have gonococcemia and was given intensive penicillin treatment to which she responded.

There was progression of her lung lesion while she was receiving maintenance vinblastine therapy. In February 1975 she was readmitted and therapy was started with bleomycin, vincristine, prednisone, adriamycin and imadazole carboxamide. An episode of pneumonia in the lower lobe of the right lung three months later responded promptly to penicillin and gentamicin therapy.

On May 8, 1975, she was readmitted with severe headaches, weakness of the legs, difficulty in walking and bladder dysfunction. The spinal fluid cell count was $235/mm^3$; most of the cells were eosinophils, although there were also lymphocytes and monocytes, and one Dorothy Reed cell was seen. Computerized axial tomography (EMI scan) of the brain showed a lesion thought to be Hodgkin's disease of the meninges. The patient was then given intrathecal methotrexate and cytosine arabinoside, and radiation therapy to the head. The intrathecal injection of methotrexate and cytosine arabinoside was repeated several times later on. The patient was readmitted a month later with fever and moniliasis, both of which cleared up following treatment with amphotericin B, ampicillin and gentamicin. Another EMI scan of the brain again showed the same lesion. On her final admission, August 1, 1975, the patient had fever, a productive cough, ptosis of the left upper lid, decreased breath sounds and rales at the base of the right lung. Babinski's sign was present bilaterally, and there was decreased pin prick, vibratory and proprioceptive sensation in both lower extremities. The spinal fluid was normal. There were gram-positive diplococci in the sputum. Chest films revealed parenchymal and pleural disease, and a cavity with a fluid level in the lower lobe of the right lung. Culture of a specimen obtained by brush biopsy revealed Staph. aureus. The patient was given gentamicin and massive doses of penicillin; two days later oxacillin therapy was added to the therapeutic regimen. The patient became afebrile by August 7, 1975, but a week later she had shortness of breath and rather shortly thereafter she had a cardiac arrest. She was resuscitated but died 2 hours later.

Dr. Stuart Sagel will now show us the roentgenograms.

Dr. Stuart Sagel: The first film available, obtained in March 1972, demonstrated a lobulated mass within the right paratracheal area and anterior mediastinum (Figure 1), consistent with the diagnosis of Hodgkin's disease. By November 1972 there was complete disappearance of the mediastinal mass. Some tethering of the vessels medially within the upper mediastinum consistent with radiation fibrosis was noted (Figure 2). In addition, extensive consolidation of the middle and lower lobes of the right lung was present. A lung biopsy specimen obtained shortly after this film was made disclosed parenchymal Hodgkin's disease.

A film obtained in July 1973 following chemotherapy demonstrated almost complete resolution of the disease in the middle and lower lobes of the right lung. Several subsequent interval films obtained over the next nine months demonstrated that the infiltration within the middle and lower lobes on the right side appeared and disappeared, probably in conjunction with changes of chemotherapy. It is certainly not atypical for Hodgkin's disease to recur in the identical location within the lung following prior treatment with chemotherapy.

In 1974, in addition to recurrent nodular densities in the lower lobe of the right lung and a small right pleural effusion, multiple subpleural nodular densities were present in the upper lobe of the left lung, again a typical pattern of pulmonary parenchymal Hodgkin's disease [1]. A repeat film in June 1975 demonstrated marked resolution of the infiltrate in the lower lobe of the right lung with some minimal residual changes and complete clearing of the disease in the left lung.

The chest film on the final admission showed recurrence of disease within the lower lobe of the right lung. A large cavitary lesion with an air fluid level (Figure 3) was present. A few nodular densities were also noted within the lower lobe of the left lung. All the parenchymal changes, including the cavity, are most consistent with Hodgkin's disease involving the lung. Conceivably, some superimposed infection was occurring in the lower lobe of the right lung. However, a point against this is that during the final admission there was no change in the chest film over a 14 day period. Certainly one would have expected a staphylococcal pneumonia to have progressed in this time interval. I might add that in a recent review of fluoroscopically assisted biopsy technics we found that transthoracic needle aspiration biopsy has a significantly higher diagnostic yield (90 per cent) than transbronchial brush biopsy (33 per cent) in the definitive diagnosis of parenchymal Hodgkin's disease.

A computerized transaxial tomographic study of the head (EMI scan) performed in June demonstrated an area of low absorption density in the right temporal lobe extending quite deep into the brain parenchyma. However, no evidence of ventricular dilatation or mid-line shift was present. The area of diminished density is nonspecific, but in this patient, who almost certainly had meningeal involvement with Hodgkin's disease, it probably represents contiguous invasion of the brain substance. Conceivably, it may simply represent some

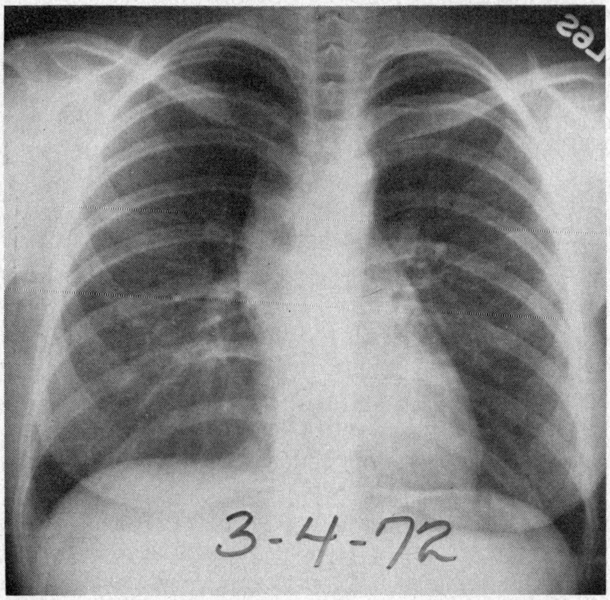

Figure 1. *Chest film obtained in March 1972 demonstrating a lobulated right paratracheal mass.*

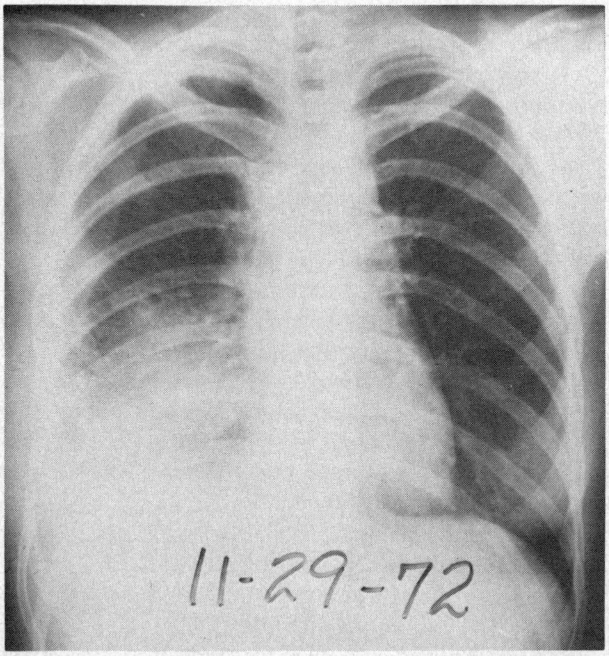

Figure 2. *Chest film obtained in November 1972 demonstrating disappearance of the paratracheal mass and extensive consolidation of the lower lobe and middle lobe of the right lung.*

edema surrounding the meningeal involvement. Much less likely would be a cerebral infarct or infection.

Dr. Reinhard: Dr. Tuteur, as far as I can tell from the hospital records, this patient had no dsypnea, cough or any other respiratory symptoms prior to the time she was found to have Hodgkin's disease in December 1971, and chest films on that original admission were said to be within normal limits. She then received radiation therapy to the neck, axillas and mediastinum. In February 1972, during a performance of lymphangiograms, 10 ml of Ethiodol was inadvertently injected intravenously. At this time she undoubtedly had rather massive oil embolization of the lungs and this was actually documented on the films. Two months later roentgenograms of the chest showed clearing of the Ethiodol microemboli, and pulmonary function studies at this time were fairly normal. Do you think that this accident resulted in any permanent injury to the lung?

Dr. Peter Tuteur: I surely doubt oil embolization would result in persistent findings three and a half years later. If this were blood clot embolization, one might expect to have some remnants of organization of the emboli and "webs" might be seen in the pulmonary circulation.

Dr. Reinhard: Dr. Sagel, would you comment on the hazards of Ethiodol lymphangiography and the dangers of doing this procedure in patients who have chronic lung disease?

Dr. Sagel: All patients in whom Ethiodol is used as the contrast medium for lymphangiography have oil embolization to the lung. Studies have shown that following lymphangiography there is a diminution in pulmonary function of approximately 30 per cent for the subse-

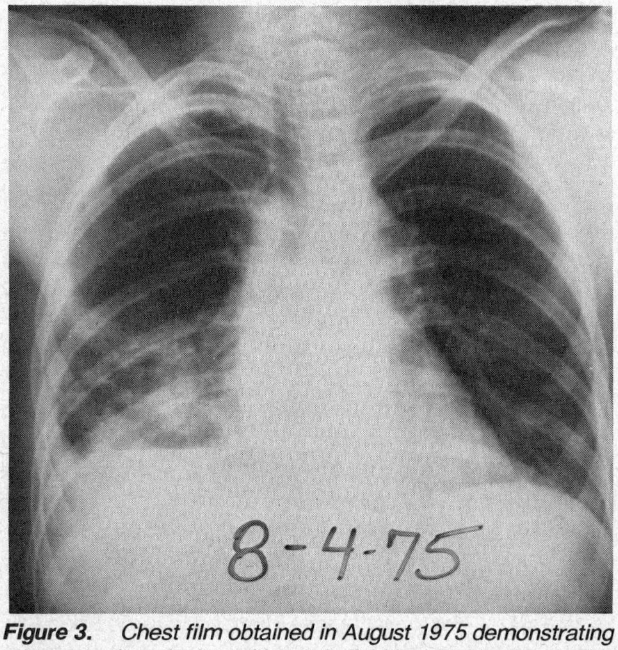

Figure 3. *Chest film obtained in August 1975 demonstrating a large cavitary lesion with an air-fluid level in the lower lobe of the right lung.*

quent 24 to 48 hours [2,3]. Obviously, in a patient who has underlying lung disease, a 30 per cent decrease in pulmonary function could produce dire results. In patients with otherwise healthy lungs, this diminution in pulmonary function is rarely accompanied by any but minimal symptoms. A complication in this particular case is that a large volume of the oily contrast media was inadvertently injected into a peripheral vein, but I would expect the effects of oil embolization to the lung to have been minimal in his young patient and to have entirely resolved within several days.

Dr. Reinhard: I think it needs to be emphasized, however, that obtaining a lymphangiogram in a patient who has severe lung disease is very hazardous. I remember in the early days when we were just starting to perform lymphangiograms in this hospital, I was called urgently to see a patient in whom lymphangiograms had been performed. She was an elderly woman with severe restrictive lung disease in whom very profound dsypnea developed right after the procedure, and she died a half an hour later.

Dr. Mill, would you comment on the problem of treating a pregnant woman with Hodgkin's disease? How much spray radiation do you get to the uterus when you treat down to the mid-mediastinum?

Dr. William Mill: In order to minimize the scattered radiation to the uterus, we treated the cervical and axillary nodes but not the uninvolved mediastinum. The problem of treating a pregnant patient with Hodgkin's disease has occurred only once before in my experience in the past 10 years. Estimates of the dose to the uterus are approximately 0.5 per cent of the tumor dose to a "mantle" port. We have not calculated the dose to the uterus in this patient with a "modified mantle" port, but it would be less than that. There are no data available to determine the risk of injury to the fetus with this dose. After the staging laparotomy, this patient received radiation to the mediastinal and para-aortic regions. The mediastinal portion of the port allowed a margin for the mass which had appeared in the right paratracheal region. The treatment port margin appears adequate in retrospect.

Dr. Reinhard: Will you comment on the hazards of taking a chest roentgenogram in the first trimester of pregnancy. I am aware that in the department of Radiology great efforts are made to avoid taking x-ray films of any kind on pregnant women. But obviously some women come in who are only a week or so pregnant and do not know it, and certainly x-ray films are inadvertently taken of women in the very early stages of pregnancy. What dosage would be delivered to the uterus in a normal pregnant woman if plain chest films were taken?

Dr. Mill: On a standard posteroanterior chest film the dose to the ovaries is approximately 0.3 mR. It is difficult to determine the significance of this dose. Any radiation should be avoided if possible, but if medically indicated, it may be necessary to take the risk. The data we have available with regard to the effects of radiation on the human embryo and fetus are minimal. Griem, Meier and Dobben [4] described a group of women who received routine diagnostic pelvimetry early in pregnancy. The estimated dose to the fetus was between 1.5 and 3 rads. Follow-up questionnaires and examinations revealed no increase in congenital malformations of the eye or central nervous system. There was, however, a significant increase in the number of hemangiomas.

Dr. Reinhard: Dr. Herzig, how about the dangers of Hodgkin's disease in pregnancy. Does pregnancy adversely affect Hodgkin's disease, and do you think that a woman who has Hodgkin's disease should be advised not to have further children?

Dr. Geoffrey Herzig: Generally, it is said, Hodgkin's disease occurring during pregnancy does have a worse prognosis, but I have not reviewed the original case material personally. It seems likely that these patients are inadequately staged and treated because of the pregnancy, as opposed to any other biologic phenomenon.

Dr. Reinhard: I looked this up some time ago, and the data indicate that the incidence of recurrence of the disease is not increased in patients with Hodgkin's disease if the disease is not active when they become pregnant. Such a woman is no more likely to have a recurrence of the disease during pregnancy than if she were not pregnant. I had a patient about 20 years ago with Hodgkin's disease. She received a much lower dose of radiation to much more limited fields of her neck and mediastinum only. I was younger and more naive then, than I am now. I knew she was a very devout Catholic and I advised her that it probably would be wise not to have any more children. She said she thought I was a fine doctor but to please keep my nose out of her other business. She subsequently had six more pregnancies. All the children are well, she is now entirely free of her Hodgkin's disease but totally exhausted from raising her large family.

Dr. Herzig, this patient had Hodgkin's disease, mixed cell type, stage 2A in April 1972. She received 4,000 rads to this modified mantle port. She was treated after delivery by radiation therapy delivered to fields that completed what we now call an "extended mantle port." That is, she ended up receiving radiation therapy to a complete mantle and to the para-aortic nodes. No chemotherapy was given at the completion of the radiation therapy. Do you think that the patient should have been started on chemotherapy at this time or do you think there is any evidence that this would have decreased the likelihood of her having the recurrence that she obviously had four or five months later?

Dr. Herzig: That is a hard question to answer. I think that chemotherapy given after irradiation would have decreased the likelihood of an early relapse, but whether it would have had any beneficial effect on her ultimate survival, in comparison to chemotherapy given at the time of documented recurrence, is the question that really remains. The most recent compilation of data from Stanford for patients with stage 1 and 2 disease (mixed cellularity) randomized to extended field radiation therapy or to extended field radiation therapy plus MOP (nitrogen mustard, vincristine and procarbazine) reveals a two year disease free survival of 50 per cent with radiation alone, and 100 per cent with radiation plus MOP. However there was no difference in the over-all survival of patients after five years [5].

Dr. Reinhard: Apparently when patients who received no chemotherapy have a recurrence, they can be treated effectively with chemotherapy and they possibly would be as well off as if they had been given the chemotherapy early.

Dr. Herzig: Right. Although there is some conflict in the published data, several reports indicate that patients who received extensive radiation therapy before they presented with disseminated disease respond equally as well to combination chemotherapy as patients who presented with stage 3B or stage 4 disease without prior therapy [6,7]. I think in this patient the difficulty when she presented in December was what to do with her being seven and a half months pregnant. As an alternative to delaying staging and therapy until after her delivery, it might have been possible to deliver her within a few weeks by Cesarean section and to do a staging laparotomy in conjunction with that procedure. Her disease would still have been in stage 2A, but she could probably have received radiation to an extended mantle port which would have included the area in which mediastinal disease subsequently developed and which was excluded from the actual treatment port. It is certainly easier to suggest that this would have been the thing to do in retrospect than it was at the time.

Dr. Reinhard: Well, it is something one should consider in a case like this, particulary when the patient has mixed cell type Hodgkin's disease. If it were the nodular sclerosing type, we would be more inclined to wait. Now, will you comment on the subsequent chemotherapy that this patient received? I am particularly interested in the rather prolonged maintenance therapy with procarbazine and prednisone. Do you have any experience with this?

Dr. Herzig: In terms of the selection of COPP instead of MOP, the response rates are equivalent. So, I think that was a perfectly good choice of therapy for someone with extranodal disease [7]. In terms of maintenance therapy, there is no really good evidence that maintenance prolongs the duration of remission, if patients have really been treated to complete remission. I think that is the difference between the National Cancer Institute series in which they found no benefit in a randomized trial of maintenance chemotherapy following MOP-induced remissions, as opposed to some of the cooperative group trials. It appears to be a question of giving really adequate therapy in your initial induction and, in that setting, there does not seem to be any benefit from maintenance [8].

Dr. Reinhard: Dr. Loeb, would you care to comment on this patient's therapy?

Dr. Virgil Loeb: This patient received seven courses of intensive combination chemotherapy between December and July 1973. Each monthly course consisted of two intravenous injections of cyclophosphamide and vincristine given one week apart along with two weeks of oral procarbazine and prednisone; this was followed by 14 days with no medication. At the completion of the seven month treatment period, there was no subjective or objective evidence of lymphoma and the chest film showed no suggestion of parenchymal involvement of the lung. Because of compelling socioemotional factors, as well as logistical considerations, it was elected to change the treatment strategy to an orally administered program of combination chemotherapy. Accordingly, intermittent courses of procarbazine, prednisone and cyclophosphamide were started; these drugs were taken for 10 consecutive days of each month. This was continued until December 1973 when jaundice developed and she entered the hospital with a presumptive diagnosis of hepatitis.

Dr. Reinhard: The next development was the occurrence of fever, night sweats, cough and right pleural chest pain which, on biopsy, turned out to be due to Hodgkin's disease involving the lung and the pleura cavity. At this time the patient was started on COPP therapy. You will note that subsequently a fairly large cavity developed with a fluid level in the lower right lung and, as Dr. Sagel has already emphasized, this is certainly compatible with Hodgkin's disease. What is the mechanism of this, Dr. Mill? Do you think the cavity results from necrosis in the center of a mass of Hodgkin's disease, and does one see this more frequently in patients who are intensively treated or can it occur without therapy?

Dr. Mill: I have seen cavitation infrequently in Hodgkin's disease. It does occur, particularly when there is a large mass, and then usually after treatment. There is usually some degree of superimposed infection.

Dr. Reinhard: I remember one patient in whom a large cavity developed. An autopsy was performed and the cavity was in a mass of Hodgkin's tissue. The patient had not received any therapy during the preceding year. The patient we are discussing today received COPP therapy which resulted in marked diminution in the lung lesions, and the patient got along reasonably well until March 1973, when she was readmitted to the hospital with fever, jaundice, and elevated SGOT, SGPT and alkaline phosphatase levels. Dr. Alpers, certainly the first thing that one would think of in this situation would be Hodgkin's disease of the liver. Short of a liver biopsy, how do you go about differentiating between infiltrative disease of the liver and hepatitis? This patient had not had any transfusions.

Dr. David Alpers: First of all, there are no good prospective studies to answer the question you asked. All the studies on liver disease and Hodgkin's disease are from autopsy series in which the predominant hepatic lesion is Hodgkin's disease [9–11]. That does not tell you too much when the patient is not terminally ill. Secondly, one can say that when Hodgkin's disease involves the liver and jaundice is present, hepatomegaly is usually present. Thus, in the absence of hepatomegaly the jaundice probably was not due to Hodgkin's disease. The larger the liver, the more likely the involvement with Hodgkin's disease [12]. Another clue clinically that is helpful is that Hodgkin's disease, when it is present in the liver, is usually associated with splenomegaly [12]. But, this patient's spleen had already been taken out. It is worthwhile to remember that about 3 per cent of all patients who have negative liver biopsies at laparotomy and a normal looking liver still may have Hodgkin's disease of the liver. However, the biopsy in 1973 showed viral hepatitis, not just normal liver. The one laboratory test that may be helpful is that the transaminase levels tend not to be very elevated in Hodgkin's disease of the liver itself. The data on this are very poor. Levitan [9] made this statement in 1961, but he did not give the transaminase data. I think that a SGOT of 1,075 mIU/ml would really make Hodgkin's disease of the liver unlikely. And I think that the thinking must have been just that, because her physicians did a liver biopsy. Since the diagnosis of Hodgkin's disease is so infrequently based on the findings of a liver biopsy, they probably were looking for hepatitis rather than Hodgkin's disease on the biopsy.

Dr. Reinhard: This patient received prednisone, 50 mg daily, and showed rapid improvement. Do you think that prednisone caused the improvement?

Dr. Alpers: Well, it probably played a role. You can decrease the level of bilirubin to some extent with prednisone even with extrahepatic obstruction. However, her condition improved because her hepatitis resolved.

Dr. Reinhard: Under what circumstances do you use prednisone in treating ordinary viral hepatitis?

Dr. Alpers: Never, if you are certain of your diagnosis.

Dr. Reinhard: Do you think this patient would have gotten along just as well then if we had not given it to her?

Dr. Alpers: If you did not think she needed her prednisone for her Hodgkin's disease, I would not have given it to her.

Dr. Reinhard: Six months later the patient was admitted to the hospital with fever, sweats, ankle pain, red, hot knee joints, a sticky white vaginal discharge and pustular skin lesions. Dr. Gelb, five blood cultures were negative; cultures of the pustules, the throat, the vaginal secretions and the rectal secretions were all negative. Despite this, the diagnosis of gonococcemia was made, and the patient was treated accordingly. Does this seem to be a reasonable diagnosis to you under these circumstances?

Dr. Lawrence Gelb: Yes, it does. There are several points that can be made about this particular presentation. First, is the differential diagnosis of the illness itself. There is considerable evidence to suggest that this was probably a case of infectious arthritis rather than some other form of acute arthritis. And second, having made that distinction, that the probable etiologic agent was the gonococcus. Several things point to gonorrhea in this particular patient. One is her age. If you look at studies of infectious arthritis, you will find that the majority of patients 15 to 39 years old had gonorrhea. In one study [13], 27 of 31 in this age range had gonorrhea. Another point is the patient's sex. Eighty-six per cent of the women in this study had gonorrhea as opposed to another form of infectious arthritis. Together this meant that 96 per cent of women 15 to 39 years of age presenting with infectious arthritis had gonorrhea. Additional support for this position can be obtained by looking at the characteristics of the clinical presentation. Only 35 per cent of the gonococcal arthritis in this study by Garcia-Kutzbach was monoarticular, whereas 92 per cent of the arthritis caused by other agents presented in this fashion. Our patient apparently had disease in both knees and both ankles with frank arthritis at least in the knees. Also, she had genitourinary findings which are present in about 65 per cent of the cases due to gonococcus but only in 6 per cent of other infectious arthritities. Laboratory tests like the white blood cell count, the sedimentation rate or the characteristics of the joint fluid do not distinguish among the various infectious etiologies. So, I think that the clinical diagnosis was correct and this patient did have gonococcal septicemia and arthritis.

Dr. Reinhard: Are you at all surprised that all the cultures were negative?

Dr. Gelb: No. This raises the question, and I think an important one, of whether there is any difference between culture positive and culture negative gonococcal arthritis. Many studies suggest that there is not [14,15]. If you divide the patients with apparent gonococcal sepsis into three groups–definite with positive joint or blood cultures, probable with positive cultures only from primary areas of infection, and possible with only the clinical presentation and therapeutic response to suggest gonorrhea—and compare them with respect to the clinical characteristics of the disease, the presentation, the response to therapy, the joints involved and the presence of skin lesions, there is no difference. All have a uniformly rapid response to penicillin therapy. This again suggests that the diagnosis of gonorrhea in this case was reasonable, even though the cultures were negative. Were any of the lesions or the vaginal exudate gram stained?

Dr. Reinhard: Not to my knowledge.

Dr. Gelb: There are many reasons why the cultures can be negative. Gonococci are extremely fastidious organisms, they are often rare in joint fluid, blood and skin lesions and therefore are not cultured in almost half the cases of disseminated disease [14]. Organisms can often be seen, however, and gram stains of lesions and exudates can be helpful. In addition, strains of gonococci which disseminate have been found to be extremely sensitive to antibiotics [16] and, thus, prior treatment may also reduce the probability of positive cultures but not necessarily positive gram stains. The lack of positive cultures in this case is, therefore, not especially bothersome.

Dr. Reinhard: Thank you very much. Eleven months later the patient was readmitted to the hospital with increasingly severe headaches, weakness of the legs, difficulty in walking and bladder dysfunction. The spinal fluid white cell count at this time was 235/mm^3; most of the cells were eosinophils, although monocytes and lymphocytes were also seen and a Dorothy Reed cell was identified. Dr. Rogers, will you discuss the involvement of the central nervous system by Hodgkin's disease. Actually this is not very common, and I wonder if you will tell us the various types of involvement that can occur and talk about the spinal fluid findings in Hodgkin's disease.

Dr. John Rogers: This patient's course is representative of reports concerning Hodgkin's disease involving the central nervous system. We have two problems that are interrelated here. One, as you pointed out, concerns her presentation with headaches, weakness, pleocytosis in her cerebrospinal fluid and, presumably, a meningeal mass on her EMI scan. This was almost certainly intracranial Hodgkin's disease. The second problem concerns the occurrence of bilateral Babinski's signs with decreased lower extremity proprioception and vibratory sensation; at that time her cerebrospinal fluid was clear. A myelogram was negative. The reason for the latter problem is less clear, but I want to approach it also.

In discussing central nervous system Hodgkin's disease, I will consider spinal involvement first, and then intracranial involvement. Spinal involvement is not infrequent [17]. Involvement of the spine is generally thought to occur by contiguous extension from adjacent lymphoid tissue. For instance, in a book on bone changes in hematologic disorders by Mosley [18], it is stated that the spine is the most common site of bony involvement in this disease; roentgenographically, when this occurs, one first sees anterior erosion of the affected vertebrae, then later a paravertebral mass and obliteration of the disc space. A similar mechanism pertains, then, to involvement of the spinal cord itself. The disease extends into the intervertebral foramina and can be silent for a long time until a nerve or the cord itself becomes compressed; at that time the patient may have pain, paresthesias or weakness. It is interesting that roentgenographic evidence of bony lesions in the spine is seen less frequently when epidural cord compression is caused by Hodgkin's disease, in contrast to cord compression complicating other malignancies such as carcinoma or myeloma [19].

I have chosen a representative series of 21 patients reported on from Johns Hopkins in whom epidural lymphoma developed [20]. The report summarizes their experience from 1952 to 1969. Sixteen patients with Hodgkin's disease, or 4 per cent of the total patients with that disease seen, had epidural cord compression. It was rather unusual for other types of lymphoma to cause this complication. Their experience is similar to that of other series in the literature; in the past, in 4 to 5 per cent of patients with Hodgkin's disease cord compression developed sometime during the course. Whether modern therapy will alter these figures is not known.

Intracranial epidural involvement is less common than cord involvement, as one might expect, since there is less lymphoid tissue adjacent to the bone involved, but intracranial involvement is thought to occur by the same mechanism. The disease extends through the foramina of the skull, first involving the epidural space and then, rarely, involving the meninges and the brain itself. As you might expect, cranial nerve dysfunction and symptoms of increased intracranial pressure are the usual presenting features. This, of course, fits with our patient's course. True meningeal invasion by Hodgkin's disease is much less common. In a series from Stanford [21], for instance, 21 patients with lymphoma had lymphomatous meningitis; this diagnosis was made by either seeing lymphoma cells in the cerebrospinal fluid or demonstrating them at autopsy. It is interesting that only two of these 21 patients had Hodgkin's disease, and 15 of the 21 had histiocytic lymphoma. In these cases, almost universally, the cerebrospinal fluid protein level was elevated; pleocytosis and increased cerebrospinal fluid pressure were variably present. Actual invasion of the brain by Hodgkin's disease is rare, but it can occur by infiltration along the perivascular and perilymphatic Virchow-Robin spaces [22].

Now, to focus on the patient's cerebrospinal fluid eosinophilia, I will mention a case report in which the findings were similar [23]. A young woman with Hodgkin's disease of one year's duration presented with peripheral blood eosinophilia, and persistent cerebrospinal fluid eosinophilia developed, sometimes to quite striking levels. Shortly before death she was noted to have 60 "malignant reticulum cells" in her cerebrospinal fluid. At autopsy she had diffuse meningeal involvement with Hodgkin's disease. In another case report [24], in a patient with epidural intracranial involvement with Hodgkin's disease, a subdural effusion developed and the effusion fluid contained large numbers of eosinophils. To my knowledge, cerebrospinal fluid eosinophilia has not been reported to occur in cryptococcal meningitis.

Dr. Reinhard: Dr. Tuteur, would you comment on the ultimate cause of death in this patient. What happened terminally?

Dr. Tuteur: I think anytime a patient with a chronic illness experiences sudden death, particularly after being at bed rest or near bed rest for 14 or 15 days as was the case here, pulmonary embolism has to be considered strongly. One intriguing thought, which probably will not turn out to be the case, is that the Candida known to be present in her mouth for months disseminated and that the Candida as well as the Hodgkin's disease infiltrated the central nervous system and contributed to her sudden death.

Dr. Reinhard: Our final diagnosis is Hodgkin's disease, mixed cell type, very widespread with involvement of the lungs, pleura and meninges. I think it will be very surprising if there is not extensive involvement intraabdominally, although we do not have good documentation of that. I think that terminally the patient had superimposed infection of the lungs and I also think she had pulmonary emboli.

PATHOLOGIC DISCUSSION

Dr. Joseph Williamson: The major organ systems involved with Hodgkin's disease at autopsy included lymph nodes, lung, liver and the nervous system. The para-aortic, parapancreatic and mediastinal lymph nodes were extensively involved. They were 2 to 3 cm in diameter and contained multiple areas of necrosis. The histologic appearance of the tumor infiltrate was quite characteristic of mixed cell Hodgkin's disease—in addition to many large neoplastic reticulocytes and Reed-Sternberg cells, there were eosinophils, neutrophilic polymorphonuclear granulocytes, plasma cells and lymphocytes. Compared to its appearance in the original biopsy, the tumor at autopsy contained fewer eosinophils and considerably more Reed-Sternberg cells, changes consistent with progression to a more malignant stage.

The lower lobe of the right lung was essentially replaced by fibrous tissue and contained two cavities, one about 2 cm in diameter and another about 5 cm in diameter (Figure 4). The lumen of the larger cavity contained necrotic tumor (Figure 5). The right hemidiaphragm was bound to the lower lobe of the right lung by dense fibrous adhesions. Numerous large and small thromboemboli, some of which were very recent and some of which were partially organized, were considered to be the immediate cause of death. There was generalized interstitial pneumonitis and fibrosis and multiple foci of organizing pneumonia.

Numerous nodules of Hodgkin's tumor were present on lumbar nerve roots and meninges (Figure 6). On microscopic examination, tumor was found to infiltrate the nerve roots extensively (Figure 7). Examination of

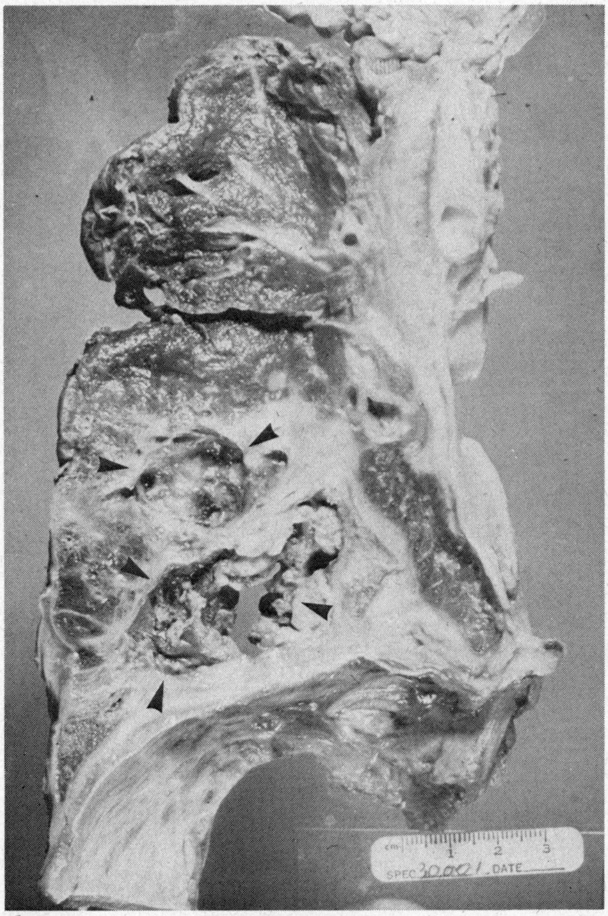

__Figure 4.__ Section through the right lung demonstrating two cavities (__arrows__) in the lower lobe and adhesion of the right hemidiaphragm to the pleura.

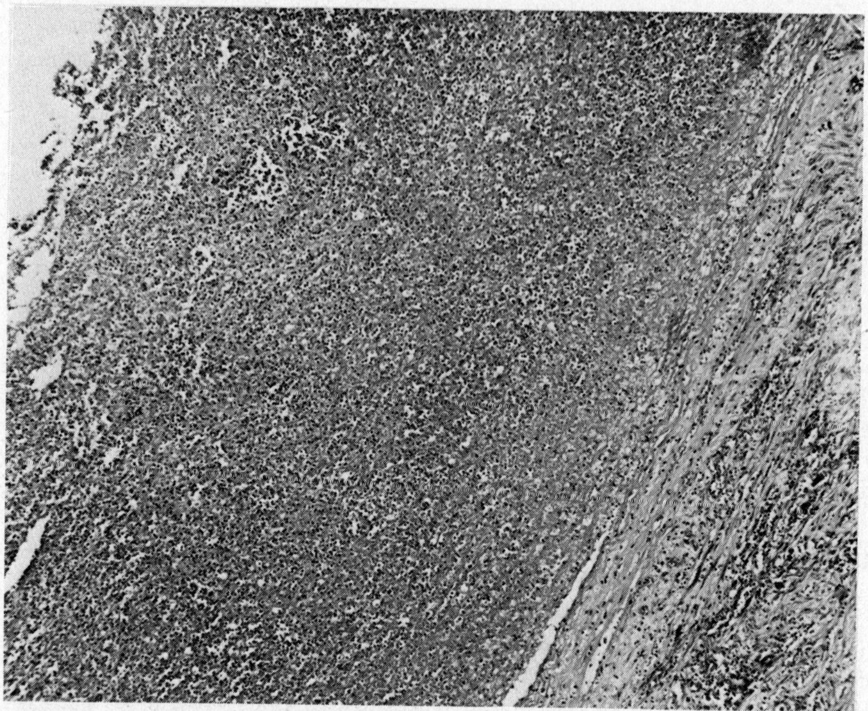

Figure 5. Photomicrograph of the wall of the larger cavity in the lower lobe. The cavity lumen is in the upper left corner, the fibrous wall at the lower right. Necrotic tumor is present in between. Hematoxylin and eosin stain; original magnification X 63.

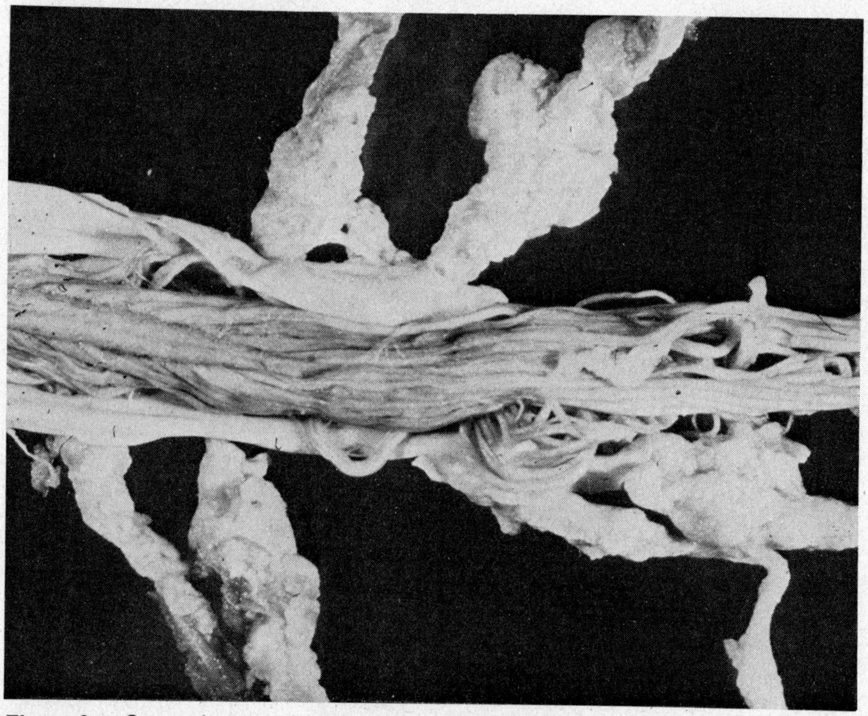

Figure 6. Gross photograph of the cauda equina with large tumor nodules on lumbar nerve roots.

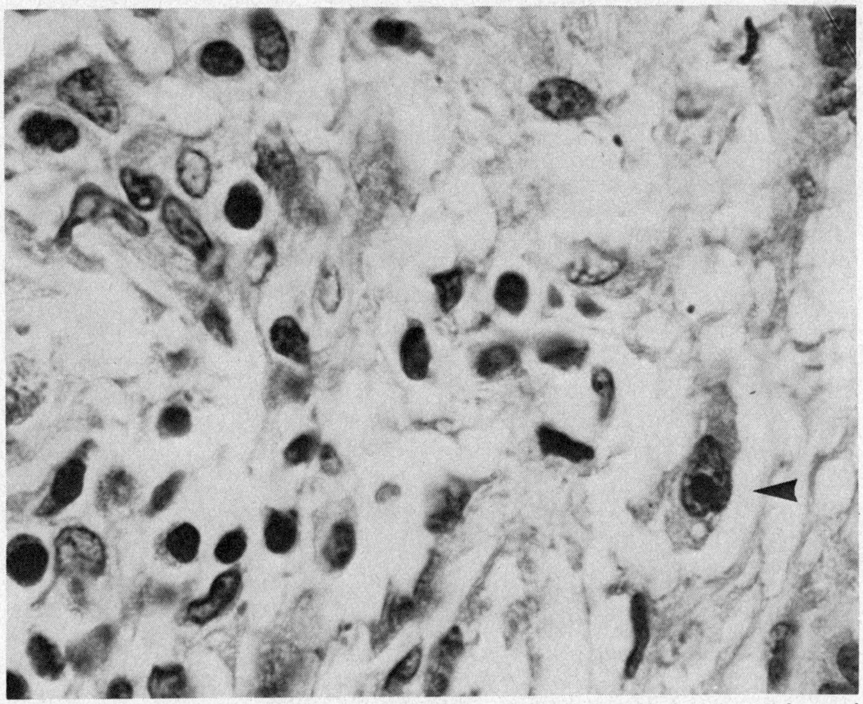

Figure 7. *Photomicrograph demonstrating tumor infiltrate and Hodgkin's cell (**arrow**) in lumbar nerve root. Hematoxylin and eosin stain; original magnification X 400.*

the brain revealed only a 1 cm area of thinned cortex in the right temporal lobe. The microscopic correlate of this lesion was loss of neurons and gliosis.

There was superficial ulceration of the esophageal mucosa overlying focal tumor infiltrates. The liver was quite congested and involved with Hodgkin's disease by direct extension of tumor from contiguous peripancreatic lymph nodes. Consistent with the steroid therapy the patient received, Crook's hyaline change was demonstrable in pituitary basophils and the adrenal cortex was atrophic.

In conclusion, although central nervous system involvement in Hodgkin's disease is unusual, this patient's course and the pathologic changes observed were characteristic of Hodgkin's disease, mixed cell type [25]. The immediate cause of death was pulmonary thromboembolism, the source of which was not apparent at autopsy.

REFERENCES

1. Stolberg HO, et al.: Hodgkin's disease of the lung. Roentgenologic-pathologic correlation. Am J Roentgenol 92: 96, 1964.
2. Gold WM, et al.: Pulmonary-function abnormalities after lymphangiography. N Engl J Med 273: 519, 1965.
3. Koehler PR: Complications of lymphography. Lymphology 1: 116, 1968.
4. Griem ML, Meier P, Dobben MD: Analysis of the morbidity and mortality of children irradiated in fetal life. Radiology 88: 347, 1967.
5. Rosenberg SA, Kaplan HS: The management of stages I, II and III Hodgkin's disease with combined radiotherapy and chemotherapy. Cancer 35: 55, 1975.
6. DeVita VI Jr, Canellos GP, Moxley JH: A decade of combination chemotherapy of advanced Hodgkin's disease. Cancer 30: 1495, 1972.
7. Goldsmith MA, Carter SK: Combination chemotherapy of advanced Hodgkin's disease. Cancer 33: 1, 1974.
8. Young RC, Canellos GP, Chabner BA, et al.: Maintenance chemotherapy for advanced Hodgkin's disease in remission. Lancet 1: 1339, 1973.
9. Levitan R, Diamond HD, Craver LF: Jaundice in Hodgkin's disease. Am J Med 30: 99, 1961.
10. Bouronche BA, Old JW, Vasquez AG: Pathogenesis of jaundice in Hodgkin's disease. Arch Intern Med 110: 872, 1962.
11. Davey FR, Doyle WF: Hepatic alteratives in Hodgkin's disease. NY State J Med 73: 1981, 1973.
12. Ultmann JE, Moren EM: Clinical cough and complications of Hodgkin's disease. Arch Intern Med 131: 332, 1973.
13. Garcia-Kutzbach A, Masi AT: Acute infectious agent arthritis (IAA). A detailed comparison of proved gonococcal and other blood-borne bacterial arthritis. J Rheumatol 1: 93, 1974.
14. Garcia-Kutzbach A, Dismuke SE, Masi AT: Gonococcal arthritis. Clinical features and results of penicillin therapy. J Rheumatol 1: 210, 1974.
15. Blankenship RM, Holmes RK, Sanford JP: Treatment of disseminated gonococcal infection. N Engl J Med 290: 267, 1974.
16. Wiesner PJ, Handsfield HH, Holmes KK: Low antibiotic resistance of gonococci causing disseminated infection. N Engl J Med 288: 1221, 1973.

17. Jackson M Jr, Parker F Jr: Hodgkin's disease. V. Involvement of certain other organs. N Engl J Med 233: 369, 1945.
18. Moseley JF: Bone Changes In Hematological Disorders (Roentgen Aspects). New York, Grune & Stratton, 1963, p 203.
19. Botterell EH, Fitzgerald GW: Spinal cord compression produced by extradural malignant tumors. Early recognition, treatment and results. Can Med Assoc J 80: 791, 1959.
20. Mullins GM, Flynn JPG, El-Mahdi AM, et al.: Malignant lymphoma of the spinal epidural space. Ann Intern Med 74: 416, 1971.
21. Griffin JW, Thompson RW, Mitchinson MJ, de Kiewiet JC, et al.: Lymphomatous leptomeningitis. Am J Med 51: 200, 1971.
22. Marshall G, Roessmann U, van den Noort S: Invasive Hodgkin's disease of brain. Cancer 22: 621, 1968.
23. Evans RJC, McElwain TJ: Eosinophilic meningitis in Hodgkin's disease. Br J Clin Pract 23: 382, 1969.
24. McDonald JV, Burton R: Subdural effusion in Hodgkin's disease. Arch Neurol 15: 649, 1966.
25. Ioachim HL: New vistas in Hodgkin's disease. Pathol Ann 10: 419, 1975.

Selected and edited by Richard T. Silver, M.D. and Alexander G. Bearn, M.D.
Department of Medicine, The New York Hospital-Cornell Medical Center, New York, New York

Male Pseudohermaphroditism: The Complexities of Male Phenotypic Development

Lecturers

JULIANNE IMPERATO-McGINLEY, M.D.
RALPH E. PETERSON, M.D.*
New York, New York

Dr. Ralph Peterson: A pseudohermaphrodite is a person with ambiguity of the internal or external genitalia but not of the gonads. A male pseudohermaphrodite has only testicular tissue and the genital ambiguity involves an error of sex differentiation. The testes may be rudimentary or quite normal in development.

In mammals, male phenotypic sexual development is a process mediated by the synthesis and action of several fetal hormones. In this review we will discuss the hormonal processes that regulate male sexual differentiation in the fetus, outline the genetic and biochemical mechanisms causing the many varieties of male pseudohermaphroditism and finally describe biochemical studies from our laboratory defining a new form of male pseudohermaphroditism—5α reductase deficiency.

Dr. Julianne Imperato-McGinley: The fetus is bipotential as far as sexual differentiation is concerned, and the bipotentiality includes the gonad, the internal sex structures and the external genitalia. An undifferentiated or biopotential gonad is present briefly in every fetus, male or female, and its development begins during the fifth week of fetal life, when a thickened area of coelomic epithelium (germinal epithelium) appears on the medial aspect of the mesonephros (Figure 1). The proliferation of cells of the germinal epithelium and of the underlying mesenchyme produce a prominence on the medial side of each mesonephros known as the gonadal ridge. Following this, cords of cells (primary sex cords) proliferate from the epithelium into the mesenchyme, and the gonad at this stage consists essentially of mesodermal cells of coelomic epithelial origin [1,2].

During the sixth week of fetal life the primordial germ cells migrate into the underlying mesenchyme and the undifferentiated or bipotential gonad is formed. The primordial germ cells, however, are visible early in the fourth week among the endodermal cells of the wall of the yolk sac near the origin of the allantois [3–5]. During folding of the embryo, part of the yolk sac is incorporated into the embryo and the primordial germ cells migrate along the dorsal mesentery to the gonadal ridges (Figure 2). The germ cells are spherical and larger than the mesenchymal cells, with large vesicular nuclei and abundant cytoplasm.

From the Division of Endocrinology, Department of Medicine, The New York Hospital-Cornell University Medical College, New York, New York. Requests for reprints should be addressed to Dr. Julianne Imperato-McGinley, The New York Hospital-Cornell Medical Center, 525 East 68th Street, New York, New York 10021.
Manuscript accepted October 31, 1975.
* NIH Research Career Awardee K6-AM-14241-13.

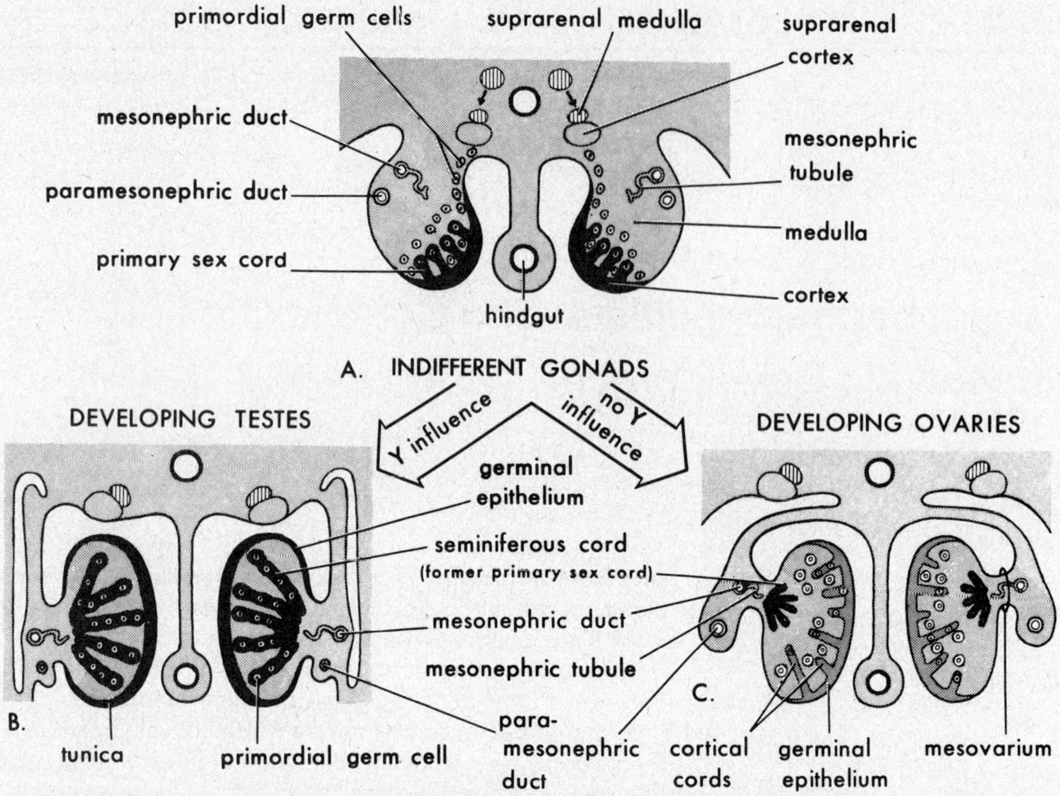

Figure 1. Development of the bipotential gonad from the coelomic epithelium (primary sex cords), underlying mesenchymal tissue (medulla), and primordial germ cells ([2], p 209).

The undifferentiated gonad, therefore, is formed from three sources, the coelomic epithelium, the underlying mesenchyme and the primordial germ cells. The primordial germ cells become spermatogonia in the male and the ova in the female; the sex cords form the seminiferous tubules in the male and the primary ovarian follicles in the female; and the mesenchymal cells form the Leydig cells in the male and the theca and stromal cells in the female [6].

Development of the Testes and Ovaries. The testes develop from the bipotential gonad at approximately the seventh week of gestation. Ovarian development, however, does not begin until the 13th week, when the first meiotic prophases appear in some of the germ cells located deepest in the outer cellular layer. True ovarian organogenesis, however, does not begin until after the 16th week, when the first follicles appear near the center of the ovary [7] (Figure 1).

Ductal Development. Both Mullerian and Wolffian ducts are present in the fetus early in gestation. In the female, the Mullerian ducts differentiate to form the fallopian tubes, uterus and upper portion of the vagina, and the Wolffian anlage disappear. In the male, the Wolffian ducts differentiate to form the epididymis, vas deferens and seminal vesicles, and there is inhibition of the Mullerian anlage [8] (Figure 3).

Development of the External Genitalia. The external genitalia, like the gonad, develop from common primordia; the urogenital tubercle, urogenital swellings and urogenital folds. In the female, the urogenital tubercle becomes the clitoris, the urogenital swellings the labia majora and the urogenital folds the labia minora. In the male, the urogenital tubercle becomes the glans penis, the urogenital folds the shaft of the penis and the urogenital swellings the scrotum [9] (Figure 4).

Control of Female and Male Phenotypic Development. Since the fetus is bipotential, what determines male or female phenotypic appearance? Neither the 46 XX complement nor the ovaries is necessary for development of the female accessory sex organs [7]. In addition, if male rabbit fetuses are castrated before differentiation of the genitalia, a female phenotype will develop. Testicular influence is therefore necessary to alter the natural tendency of the fetus toward the development of the female phenotype. Consequently, in the absence of the testes, regardless of whether or not the ovaries are present,

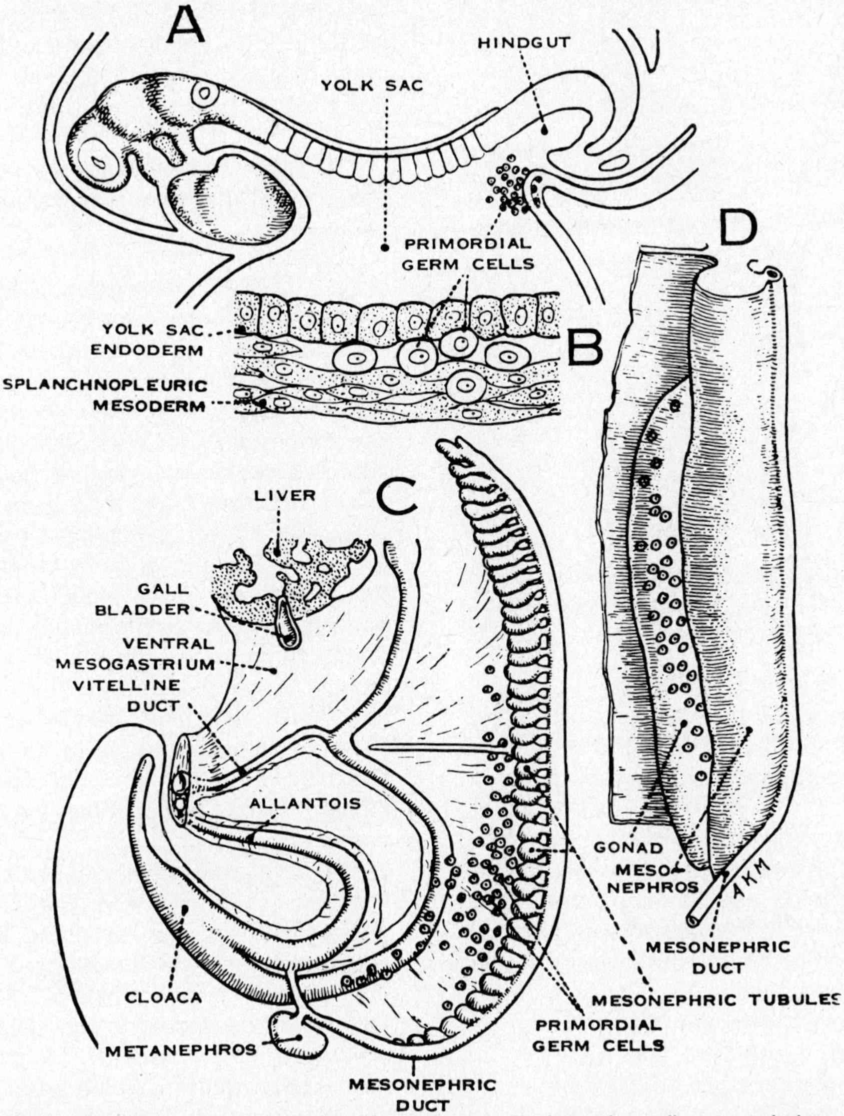

Figure 2. *Migration of the primordial germ cells from the yolk sac endoderm ([6], p 402).*

there is inhibition of the Wolffian anlage, with Mullerian ductal differentiation to the uterus, fallopian tubes and upper portion of the vagina, and female differentiation of the external genitalia. Thus, femaleness represents the innate tendency of the fetus, and does not require gonadal influence [7] (Figure 5).

A 46 XX complement, however, is necessary to maintain normal ovarian development in the female. Singh et al. [10] studied abortuses with a 45 XO complement, and found that the ovarian tissue contained primary follicles. In adults with a 45 XO complement, however, the follicles are no longer present; only streaked gonads containing whorls of connective tissue remain [11]. The 46 XX complement, therefore, appears to be necessary for the maintenance of ovarian follicules; however, its absolute role in normal ovarian development has not been established. Of course, at puberty, normal ovarian function regulates the development of female secondary sexual characteristics.

Since a complete 46 XX chromosome complement is critical for the presence of normal ovaries at birth, the deletion of any portion of an X chromosome will result in streaked gonads. Deletion of the short arm of the X is associated with streaked gonads, and with the skeletal and somatic anomalies of Turner's syndrome found in 45 XO subjects. Long arm deletions, however, are usually associated with streaked gonads and none of the stigmata of Turner's syndrome. Thus, although an intact 46 XX com-

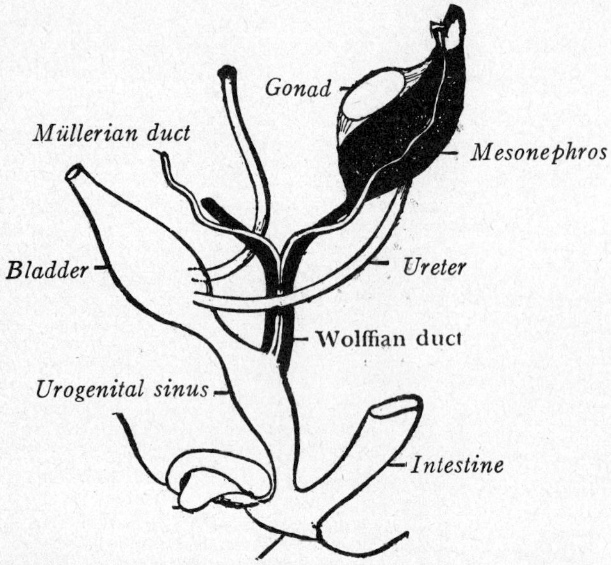

Figure 3. *Anlage of the internal accessory sex organs present in the male and female fetus early in gestation—Mullerian and Wolffian ducts ([1], p 340).*

plement is necessary for the presence of normal ovaries at birth, the other skeletal and somatic anomalies are due to monosomy of loci on the short arm of the X [12].

The development of the male phenotype is more complex and, as stated earlier, to initiate the process the testes must develop and function normally. In man, testicular differentiation appears to be controlled by the Y chromosome, in particular, the short arm of the Y. Support for the hypothesis of the Y chromosome control of testicular differentiation and development in man arises from the fact that if an XY normal male is compared to an XO female, and an XXY Klinefelter male is compared to the XX female, then it appears that the addition of the Y chromosome is associated with testes and a male phenotype [9]. Deletions of the short arm of the Y chromosome with resultant streaked gonads and a female phenotype have been reported—evidence for the importance of the short arm of the Y in controlling testicular differentiation [13].

The enigma of 46 (XX) subjects with testes and a male phenotype is seemingly contradictory to the evidence for Y chromosomal control of testicular differentiation. In these subjects, there may be a hidden or undetected Y chromosome (XX/XY), or Y chromosomal material may be translocated to the paternal X chromosome or to an autosome [14,15]. The ability to identify Y chromosomal material on the X chromosome or autosome in 46 XX males has heretofore been impossible for methodologic reasons [16]; although it has been found that the distal portion of the long arm of the Y has a zone of bright fluorescence when stained with quinicrine mustard [17]. With this technic Y chromosome material has not been detected thus far in XX males [18,19]. The technic, however, yields no information about the short arm of the Y, in which the testes determining loci are thought to be present, and the area which presumably would be translocated to a paternal X chromosome or autosome in an 46 XX subject with testes. The discovery of a H-Y histocompatibility antigen, thought to be located near the testes determining genes on the Y chromosome, if found to be present in XX males, may ultimately settle the problem of the necessity of the Y chromosome in testicular differentiation [20–22]. In certain 46 XX males, a mutant autosomal gene which overrides the sex determining effect of the normal female (46 XX) may be present. This would be similar to the situation in the goat in which the mutant gene, P (for polled) induces male sexual differentiation in the homozygous state in the 46 XX animal [23]. However, this would be a distinctly abnormal situation and not related to normal control of sexual differentiation.

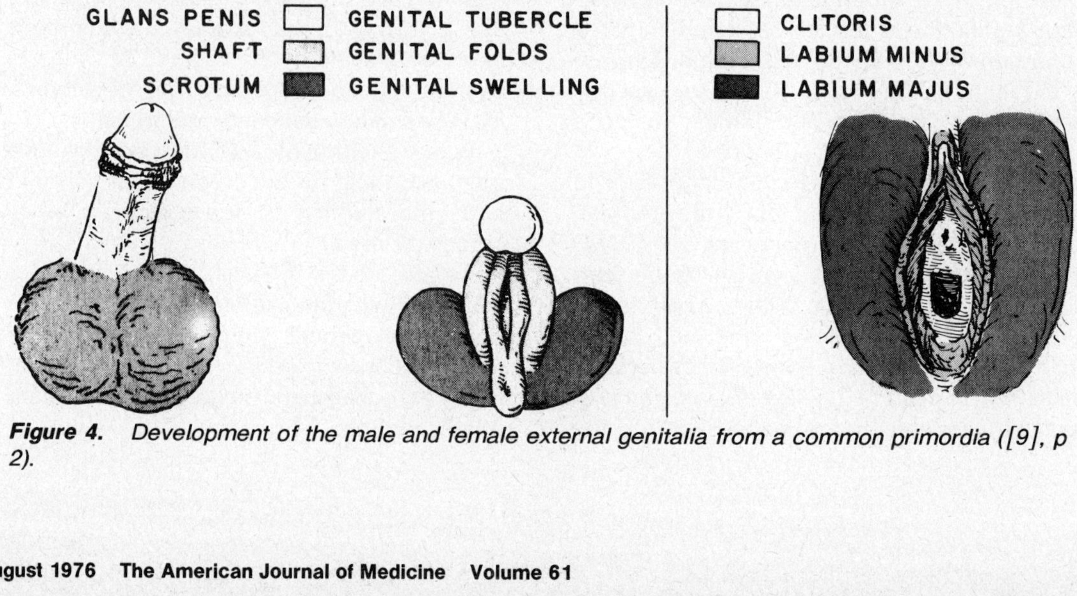

Figure 4. *Development of the male and female external genitalia from a common primordia ([9], p 2).*

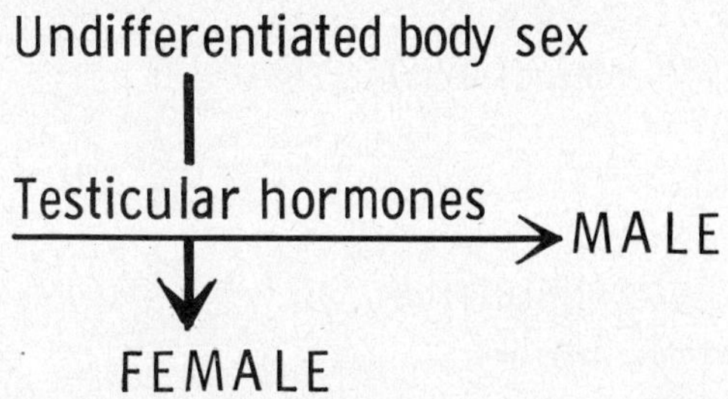

Figure 5. *The female phenotype develops independently of the gonads whereas the male phenotype requires the hormonal influence of the testes.*

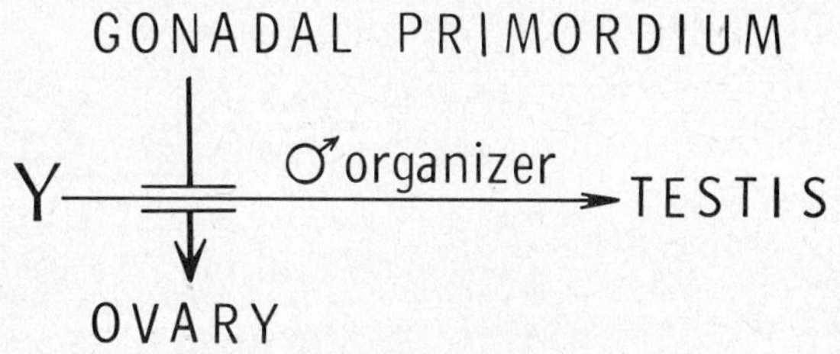

Figure 6. *Testicular organizer (inducer) substance under Y chromosome control causes development of the testis on a gonadal primordium which would otherwise develop as an ovary.*

The mechanism by which the Y chromosome controls testicular differentiation has not been ascertained. Witschi [24–26] in 1951 proposed the concept of corticomedullary antagonism and revived the notion of gonadal hermaphroditism. He assumed that the undifferentiated gonad is made up of two morphologically distinct and physiologically antagonistic components, a cortical inducer stimulating development of the ovarian cortex and inhibiting the medulla, and a medullary inducer inhibiting the cortex and stimulating testicular development. Genetic sex factors are responsible for the prevalence of either the medulla or the cortex. The theory, however, does not take into account the chronologic asymmetry of gonadal differentiation in the two sexes. Testes differentiate early and the ovaries later.

Because of the chronologic asymmetry in gonadal development Jost et al. [27] theorized, on the basis of his experiments with freemartins,* that the undifferentiated gonad will develop as an ovary, but that some local mechanism working under the influence of the genes for maleness, an "inducer substance," imposes testicular organogenesis at an early age on the gonadal primordium. From the freemartin experiments, he postulated that testicular differentiation is probably controlled by a testicular organizer (not an androgen) produced by cells within the gonad, which influence the other cells of the gonad, and impose male organogenesis. Thus, in the normal male, the Y chromosome may control the production of this inducer or organizer substance present locally in the gonadal primordia to cause testicular differentiation. Jost et al. [27] postulated that the gonad will develop as an ovary unless influenced by the testicular inducer substance which is under genetic control. Therefore, testicular organization may be actively imposed on a primordium which would otherwise eventually acquire an ovarian structure (Figure 6).

Testicular differentiation occurs between the seventh and the eighth week of intrauterine life. The seminiferous tubules form, and from approximately the eighth week of gestation, the Leydig cells differentiate, increase in number and secrete testosterone. At the beginning of the third month they completely fill the interstitial spaces between the seminiferous cords. This Leydig cell hyperplasia corresponds in time to the peak levels of human chorionic gonadotropin (hCG) in the fetal and maternal circulation, and in the maternal urine [28]. Concomitant with the peak levels of hCG in the mother and fetus there is a peak in testosterone production by the testes at the time of Wolffian ductal differentiation to the vas deferens, epididymis and seminal vesicles, and differentiation of the male external genitalia [29]. Inhibition of the Mullerian anlage also occurs at this time [8].

Studies on fetal rabbits have shown that when testosterone was implanted into the peritoneal cavity of castrated animals (male and female), Wolffian differentiation, as well as masculinization of the external genitalia occurred, demonstrating these events to be androgen-mediated. Testosterone implantation,* however, did not produce inhibition of the Mullerian ducts [7]. The use of the antiandrogen cyproterone acetate which inhibits androgen action, results in a lack of differentiation of the Wolffian system and severe ambiguity of the external genitalia in some animals. However, inhibition of the Mullerian anlage always proceeds normally and is not under androgen control [30]. Thus, it appears that the testes, in addition to testosterone secretion by the Leydig cells, secrete during the critical period of sexual differentiation another substance, called the Mullerian inhibiting

* A freemartin is a female twin who becomes a female pseudohermaphrodite as a result of sharing a common blood supply with a male co-twin. At birth ovarian development is impaired, and within the gonadal tissue there are seminiferous tubes. There is complete regression of the Mullerian ducts, with slight masculinization of internal and external sex structures (seminal vesicles and sometimes clitoral enlargement) [27].

* Testosterone implantation alone does not cause complete Wolffian differentiation. The testes are needed to produce a "stabilizing factor," which acts with testosterone to cause normal Wolffian differentiation [7].

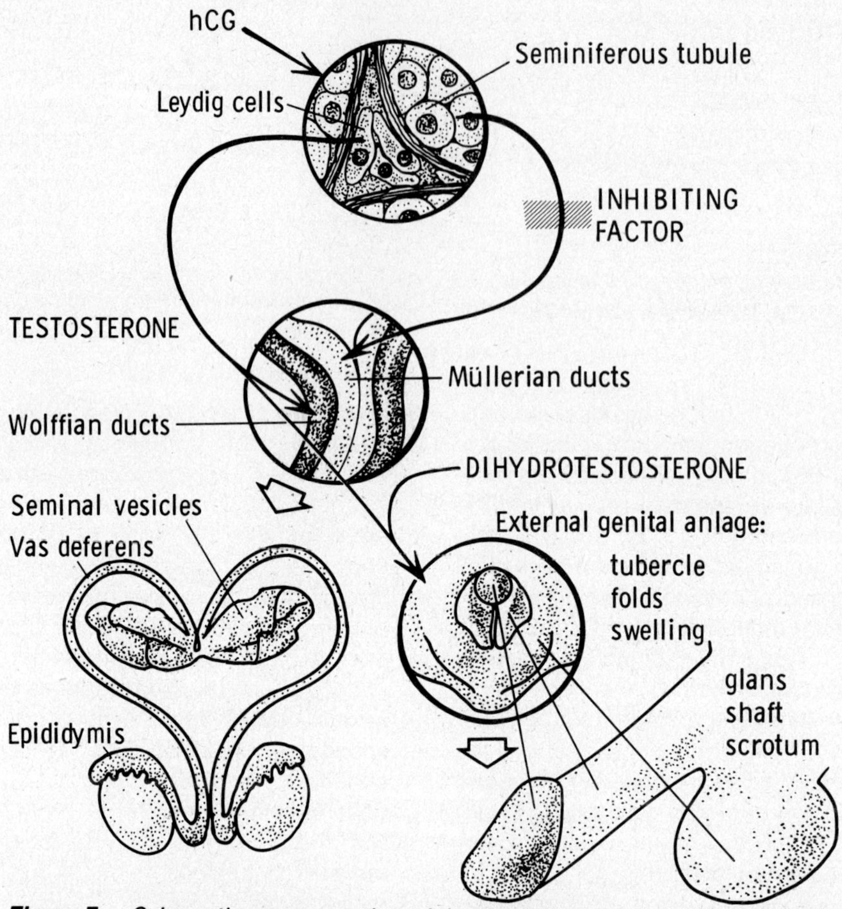

Figure 7. *Schematic representation of the three hormones necessary for development of the male phenotype—testosterone and Mullerian inhibiting factor from the testes, and dihydrotesterone from the periphery.*

factor, which specifically inhibits the Mullerian anlage. The action of this substance, cannot be duplicated by androgens, it is not affected by congenital or drug-induced insensitivity to androgens, and it is restricted to the Mullerian duct in direct contact with the fetal testis. It appears to be secreted by the Sertoli cells of the seminiferous tubules and is probably a high molecular weight polypeptide [31,32]. Thus, both testosterone and the Mullerian inhibiting factor must be secreted by the testes at a critical period in utero for development of the male phenotype.

Nevertheless, abnormalities in phenotypic development can still occur despite normal testicular development with adequate secretion of both testosterone and the Mullerian inhibiting factor at the critical period during gestation. Within the last 10 years investigators have shown that testosterone may act as a prehormone in certain androgen-dependent target areas. In specific target areas, testosterone is converted to 5α dihydrotestosterone by the microsomal enzyme, steroid Δ^4 5α reductase. In addition, in rabbit, rat [33] and human [34] fetuses, the capacity to convert testosterone to dihydrotestosterone in the urogenital sinus and urogenital tubercle, is present prior to differentiation of these tissues to the prostate and external genitalia. In the Wolffian duct, however, synthesis of dihydrotestosterone does not occur until after its differentiation to the epididymis, vas deferens and seminal vesicles. The data suggest that two androgens, testosterone and its metabolite dihydrotestosterone, are involved in sexual differentiation in the male fetus, with selective roles for each hormone during embryogenesis. The male pseudohermaphrodites with 5α reductase deficiency and decreased dihydrotestosterone production, to be discussed later, have defined the necessity for dihydrotestosterone in the formation of the external genitalia and have delineated specific actions for the two androgens in utero.

Finally, androgen action must be initiated at the target areas. Testosterone enters the cell and either binds to a cytoplasmic receptor or, depending upon the target tissue, is converted to dihydrotestosterone, which binds to the cytoplasmic receptor. Following this, the androgen-receptor complex gains access to the nucleus, in which it binds to the chromatin and initiates transcription of messenger ribonucleic acid RNA resulting, ultimately, in the complex metabolic processes of androgen action [35,36].

Thus, for the normal development of the male phenotype in utero, the testes must differentiate and function normally, so that at a critical period the Mullerian inhibiting factor, probably secreted by the Sertoli cells, and testosterone, secreted by the Leydig cells, and produced in sufficient amounts. The Mullerian inhibiting factor, acting locally, suppresses the Mullerian anlage, whereas testosterone, acting systemically, causes differentiation of the Wolffian anlage. At the urogenital tubercle, urogenital sinus and urogenital folds testosterone enters the cells, in which it is converted by the enzyme 5α reductase to dihydrotestosterone, which results in differentiation of the male external genitalia (Figure 7). Depending upon the specific target tissue, either testosterone or dihydrotestosterone complexes with the cytoplasmic receptor, and this receptor-hormone complex is transferred to the nucleus to initiate androgen action.

This multifactorial process is under complex genetic control. As mentioned previously, the Y chromosome is involved in testicular differentiation from the bipotential gonad. From human subjects in whom inherited deficiencies of one or another substance occur, it appears that the enzymes involved in testosterone biosynthesis, and the enzyme 5α reductase, are regulated by genes located on the autosomes. Inherited forms of Mullerian inhibiting factor deficiency (either synthesis or action) are transmitted as a recessive trait, either autosomal or X-linked. From the linkage studies in (Tfm/y) mice, it has also been shown that genes (either structural or regulatory) located on the X chromosome control the cytoplasmic receptor at the androgen dependent target area [37]. Thus, normal male phenotypic development is regulated by gene loci on the autosomes as well as both X and Y chromosomes (Figure 8).

CAUSES OF MALE PSEUDOHERMAPHRODITISM

Having covered the evolution of the male phenotype, we can now outline the known etiologic causes for male pseudohermaphroditism or incomplete masculinization (Table I). They can be divided into three basic categories: (1) disorders of testicular differentiation and development, (2) disorders of testicular function, and (3) disorders of function at the androgen dependent target areas.

GENETIC CONTROL OF MALE PHENOTYPE

• Y chromosome	Testicular differentiation
• X chromosome	End organ sensitivity - cytoplasmic receptor
• Autosome	Enzymatic control of testosterone biosynthesis Conversion of testosterone to dihydrotestosterone
• Recessive trait (autosomal or X-linked)	Control of mullerian inhibitor factor biosynthesis or action

Figure 8. *Regulation of male phenotypic development by gene loci on the autosomes and sex chromosomes.*

Disorders of Testicular Differentiation and Development. Disorders of testicular differentiation and development could theoretically involve at least two types of developmental dysfunction. The first would be an abnormality in the formation of the bipotential gonad. As previously mentioned, the germ cells migrate from the endoderm of the yolk sac to the germinal ridge. This migration may be necessary to induce formation of the indifferent gonad; any abnormality in this step might result in agonadia or a streaked or dysgenetic gonad [3].

The second would be an abnormality in the formation or development of a testis from the bipotential gonad. This involves an abnormality of the testes determining genes or testicular inducer genes on the short arm of the Y chromosome. In this situation, the absence, abnormal formation or delayed secretion of the testicular inducer substance may result in

TABLE I **Classification of Male Pseudohermaphroditism**

Disorders of testicular differentiation
Chromosome or gene deletions involving the Y chromosome
Disorders of testicular function
Gonadotropin unresponsiveness
Abnormalities of Mullerian Inhibiting factor synthesis or action
Testosterone biosynthetic deficiencies
cholesterol 20α, 22 hydroxylase and/or 20, 22 desmolase
17α hydroxylase
17, 20 desmolase
3β-ol dehydrogenase: Δ5 isomerase
17β hydroxysteroid dehydrogenase
Disorders of function at the androgen dependent target areas
Androgen receptor defects
Enzyme deficiencies in testosterone metabolism
5α reductase deficiency

streaked gonads or in varying degrees of testicular dysgenesis.

With abnormal or poorly developed testes (dysgenetic testes), secondary functional defects result, with impairment in the secretion of Mullerian inhibiting factor and testosterone at a critical period in utero. Therefore, depending upon the timing and extent of the functional defects, a female phenotype or an incomplete masculinization of the internal and external sex structures will result.

Complete deletion of the Y chromosome results in a 45 XO chromosome complement, with streaked gonads and Turner's syndrome as mentioned earlier. As a result of the Y chromosome deletion there is loss of the testicular inducer substance and, in its absence, testicular differentiation does not occur and the gonad develops as an ovary [27]. In the presence of the 45 XO complement, however, ovarian development will not be maintained and streaked gonads with a resultant female phenotype develop.

Two cases of deletion of the short arm of the Y with a female phenotype have been reported [13], supporting the same concept and pointing to the short arm of the Y as the region specifically involved in testicular differentiation.

If there is a partial deletion in some cell lines, mosaicism (XO/XY) occurs and this results in the syndrome of mixed gonadal dysgenesis. The condition is characterized by a testis on one side and a streaked gonad on the other. In this clinical situation there appears to be a more severe loss of testicular inducing substance on the side of the streak, perhaps related to the preponderance of the XO cell line in the streaked gonad at the time of sexual differentiation. The testes is also functionally dysgenetic as evidenced by diminished virilization of the external genitalia and the presence of fallopian tubes and a uterus. The affected subjects invariably have a uterus, and most have bilateral fallopain tubes. When the vas deferens is present it is almost always on the side of the testes. The external genitalia demonstrate substantial degrees of ambiguity, since two-thirds of the affected subjects have been raised as girls. Turner's stigmata occur in approximately one-third of the affected [38,39]. Thus, although one testis is present, it obviously is incapable of adequate function at the time of male sexual differentiation.

There are at least two reports of subjects with a XO/XY complement and bilateral streaked gonads [40], as well as patients with the (XO/XY) complement and bilateral testes [41,42]. Therefore, the clinical syndrome of mixed gonadal dysgenesis with the mosaic XO/XY complement may be just one entity in a spectrum ranging from streaked gonads and a female phenotype to varied abnormalities of testicular development (symmetrical or asymmetrical) and genital ambiguity, perhaps depending upon the preponderance of a particular cell line, either XO or XY, within the gonad at the time of sexual differentiation [43,44].

Theoretically nonvisible damage can occur to the testes determining gene(s) on the short arm of the Y resulting in male pseudohermaphroditism and this may be the situation in testicular dysgenesis syndromes in which mosaicism has not been found. However, every attempt should be made to rule out mosaicism by culturing different cell lines in affected subjects. With the complete absence of the testicular inducing substance, the syndrome of XY gonadal dysgenesis with bilateral streaks and a totally female phenotype results [45]. With an incomplete defect, variable degrees of testicular dysgenesis with ambiguous genitalia can occur, and may even resemble the syndrome of mixed gonadal dysgenesis with an XO/XY complement [38,46–48] and dysgenetic testes on one side and a streak on the other (Figure 9). If the genes on the Y chromosome preventing Turner's somatic stigmata are also affected, the entire spectrum with the features of Turner's syndrome can also be observed.

Familial cases of XY gonadal dysgenesis have been described [49–52] and there are at least two cases in which the mode of inheritance appears to be X linked recessive or autosomal dominant sex limited [53,54]. In these cases the abnormality does not appear to be secondary to gene defect(s) regulating testicular differentiation located on the Y chromosome but may be secondary to an abnormality of the gene(s) regulating the formation of the bipotential gonad which might be located on an X chromosome or an autosome. Thus, one could have genotypic heterogeneity resulting in the syndrome of XY gonadal dysgenesis with its typical phenotypic, histologic and gonadal appearance.

Disorders of Testicular Function. Gonadotropin unresponsiveness: In utero, Leydig cell differentiation and secretion is under the control of placental hCG. The absence of abnormality of the receptor for hCG-LH could, in theory, result in an absent or inadequate production of testosterone and varying degrees of genital ambiguity. Although this defect has not been demonstrated in man, there may be an animal model [55].

Mullerian inhibiting factor deficiency: Abnormalities affecting either synthesis or action of Mullerian inhibiting factor (some inherited) have been described [56–60]. The affected males have bilateral testes with normal male Wolffian differentiation and male external genitalia. However, Mullerian suppression does not occur, and they have a uterus and fal-

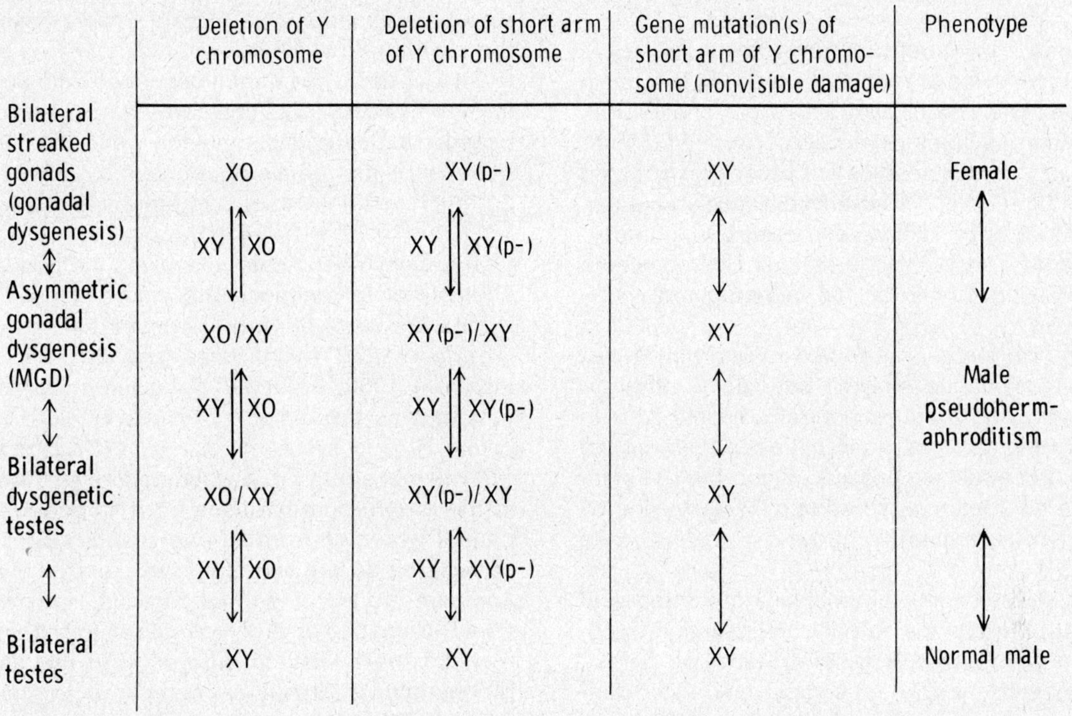

Figure 9. *Spectrum of testicular differentiation and incomplete masculinization secondary to Y chromosome abnormalities.*

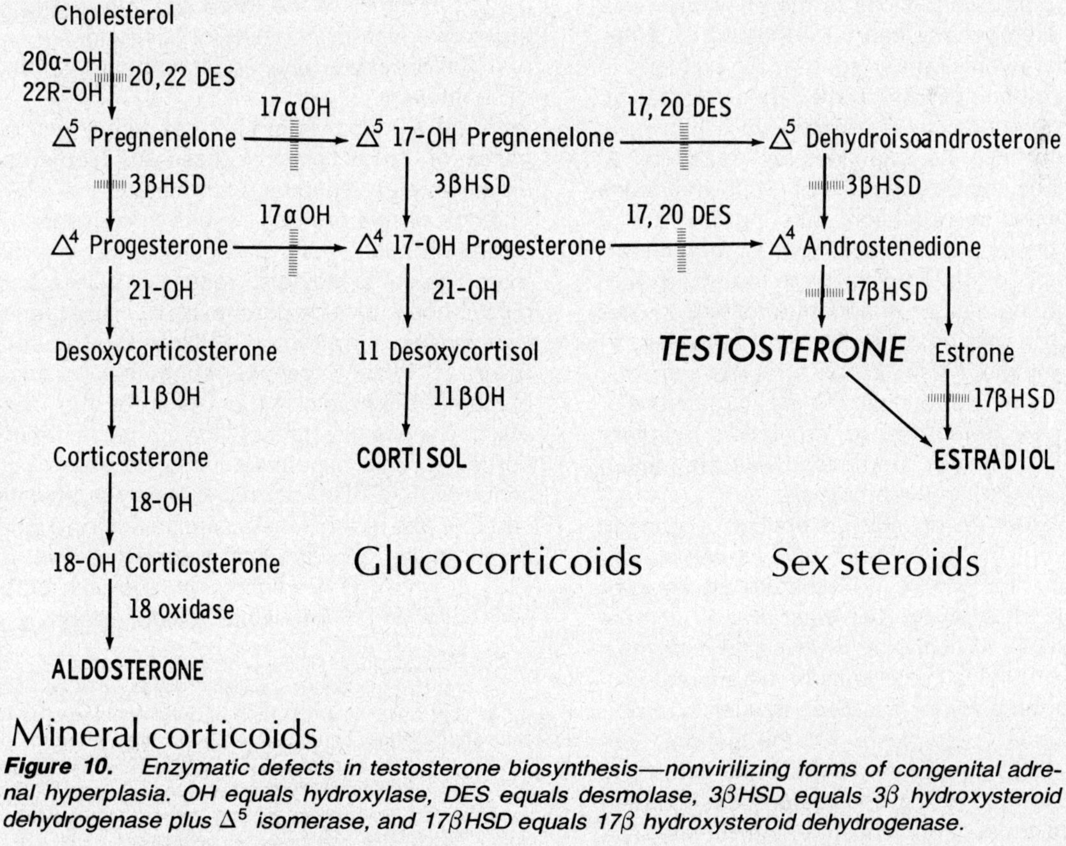

Figure 10. *Enzymatic defects in testosterone biosynthesis—nonvirilizing forms of congenital adrenal hyperplasia. OH equals hydroxylase, DES equals desmolase, 3βHSD equals 3β hydroxysteroid dehydrogenase plus Δ^5 isomerase, and 17βHSD equals 17β hydroxysteroid dehydrogenase.*

lopian tubes which may present as an inguinal hernia (hernia inguinalis).

Testosterone biosynthetic deficiencies: There are eight known enzymatic reactions involving five basic steps in testosterone biosynthesis from cholesterol, and defects in all steps have been described (Figure 10). The enzyme deficiencies are present in both the gonads and the adrenals, and inheritance is autosomal recessive with clinical expression in homozygous subjects. These enzyme deficiencies constitute the nonvirilizing forms of the adrenogenital syndrome.

In utero, the testes in affected males with a testosterone biosynthetic enzyme deficiency, differentiate normally and produce normal amounts of Mullerian inhibiting factor at a critical period, so that no Mullerian structures are present. Since the deficiencies cause an impaired secretion of testosterone by the Leydig cells, ambiguity of the external genitalia results.

In general, the degree of ambiguity of the external genitalia at birth and the amount of virilization at puberty will reflect the severity of the enzyme defect; therefore, each enzyme deficiency may show considerable phenotypic heterogeneity. Since the genes responsible for the abnormalities of enzymatic function may be mutants at the structural loci that code for the amino acid sequences of the enzymes [61], phenotype heterogeneity can be attributed to different mutational events which bring about changes in the structure of the enzyme, thus altering its catalytic efficiency. Phenotypic heterogeneity in some subjects could also be explained by mutations at sites other then the structural loci. Such mutations can be classified as regulatory (altering the rate of synthesis or degradation of the enzyme), architectural (affecting incorporation of enzyme molecules into active sites in the cell) or temporal (affecting the development of the tissue, or the time of activation of regulatory systems). Also, in the affected subjects, the mutations may be identical but the penetrance or expression may differ due to regulation by other gene loci. Direct studies are needed with the mutant enzymes to help define the problem.

In 1957 Prader et al. [62] described a genetic male with Wolffian differentiation but with female external genitalia. No urinary 17-ketosteroids were detected. At six days of age the child died in adrenal crisis. At autopsy the adrenals showed an enormous accumulation of lipids in the cells of the adrenal cortex; and thus the disorder has been labeled congenital lipoid adrenal hyperplasia. Of the patients described [63–72], most have died in early infancy in adrenal crisis due to decreased glucorticoid and mineralocorticoid production. The affected males have male gonaducts, with either female external genitalia or severe ambiguity of the external genitalia. As would be expected the female infants have normal female internal and external accessory sex organs.

Two children have been described who survived to early childhood. One child was a six year old male pseudohermaphrodite, and the other an eight year old phenotypic female but genetic male, with severe adrenal insufficiency in whom testes were found [72].

The biosynthetic defect involves the conversion of cholesterol to pregnenolone, and at least three enzymes are involved in this transformation—20α hydroxylase, 22R hydroxylase and 20α-22R desmolase.* In 1962, a genetic defect in cholesterol desmolase was postulated by Prader et al. [76] as the cause of this syndrome. In 1971 Degenhart et al. [71] demonstrated that when cholesterol was added to the enzyme preparations from adrenal tissue of a patient who died from adrenal lipoid hyperplasia, its conversion to pregnenolone was extremely low as compared to that in normal controls. However, when 20α hydroxycholesterol was added to the incubation medium there was no difference in the amount of pregnenolone formed as compared to that in the controls, thus demonstrating a possible deficiency of 20α cholesterol hydroxylase as the cause for the lipoid adrenal hyperplasia [71]. Theoretically, a deficiency of either of the three enzymes necessary for the conversion of cholesterol to pregnenolone could result in the same phenotypic appearance and adrenal pathology.

In 1961 Bongiovanni [77] described the first three cases of 3β-ol dehydrogenase-$\Delta 5$ isomerase deficiency in both males and females. In the male, a deficiency of this enzyme results in decreased testosterone production and ambiguity of the external genitalia. The deficiency also results in a decrease in the biosynthesis of aldosterone and cortisol, and in severe cases the affected children died in salt-losing crisis in infancy despite seemingly adequate replacement therapy. As a result of the decreased plasma levels of cortisol, the negative feedback of cortisol on the hypothalamus is decreased, causing increased ACTH secretion which stimulates the adrenal, and results in elevated levels of $\Delta 5$ steroids; in particular dehydroisoandrosterone. The females [78] are normal or slightly virilized with clitoral hypertrophy and slight labial fusion, probably secon-

* From careful kinetic analysis, Burstein et al. [73] have shown that a significant portion of pregnenolone produced from cholesterol cannot be accounted for by the sum of the reactions involving hydroxylations at C-20 and C-22. Thus the traditional side chain compounds hydroxylated at C-20 and C-22 may not be obligatory intermediates, but rather by-products resulting from competitive reactions of short-lived, reactive species [74,75].

dary to increased amounts of dehydroisoandrosterone which in large amounts is slightly androgenic. In males, however, dehydroisoandrosterone is not sufficient to cause masculinization of the external genitalia, and ambiguity results because of decreased testosterone biosynthesis.

Three males described in the literature reached puberty; interestingly, gynecomastia developed in all [79–81]. It is theorized that inadequate testosterone production in utero by the male fetus fails to suppress the breast anlage so that a puberty gynecomastia occurs [82,83]. Long-term survivals have been reported in a number of other cases thought to represent less severe enzyme deficiency states [78–87].

In 1966 Bigileri et al. [88] described the first case of 17α hydroxylase deficiency in a genetic and phenotypic female who presented, at age 35, with sexual infantilism. Since then five females [89–91] and three males [92–94] with this condition have been reported. With 17α hydroxylase deficiency there is a decrease in glucocorticoid (cortisol) production and a decrease in androgen production. The decrease in plasma cortisol causes increased ACTH secretion which results in a compensatory increase in the C21, 17 desoxysteroids; corticosterone, and desoxycorticosterone. The hypertension and hypokalemia frequently present in affected individuals are attributed to the excess desoxycorticosterone secretion. Plasma renin activity and aldosterone secretion are suppressed. The mechanism for the suppression is thought to be secondary to excess desoxycorticosterone secretion causing increased tubular reabsorption of sodium resulting in increased plasma volume. The hypoaldosteronism has also been attributed to defective 18-hydroxylation [88,92]. It is, however, difficult to conceive of an inherited disorder effecting two steroid biosynthetic enzymes unless it is theorized that the deficiency of one enzyme somehow affects the activity of the second.

In 1972 Zachman et al. [94] described a child with male pseudohermaphroditism, and suggested that the defect was secondary to 17, 20 desmolase deficiency. Unfortunately, no plasma steroid data were reported, and the results of the testicular incubation studies were not compared to those of normal testicular tissue. Although a well documented case has yet to be described, another possible case has been reported in an abstract [96].

In 1971 Saez [97,98] described the first case of 17β-hydroxysteroid dehydrogenase deficiency. Since then three additional cases (including two in siblings) have been described. All subjects were genetic and gonadal males with such marked ambiguity of the external genitalia at birth (labia majora, minora, enlarged clitoris and blind vaginal pouch) that they were raised as girls [99,100]. In two subjects mild virilism and breast development occurred at puberty. With 17β-hydroxysteroid dehydrogenase deficiency, there is a marked increase in plasma androstenedione, and in the affected individuals with breast development, the androstenedione was converted to estrone and then to estradiol with resulting gynecomastia. However, in the two siblings described by Givens et al. [100] virilization occurred, but gynecomastia did not develop. In these subjects the androstenedione levels were as high as in the other cases, but the conversion of androstenedione to estrone was markedly decreased. In one sibling, the estrone was normal and the estradiol slightly above normal, whereas in the other the estrone was three times normal and the estradiol was normal for males.

The affected sibling with 17β-hydroxysteroid dehydrogenase deficiency, without breast development, had been assigned to the phenotypic category pseudovaginal perineoscrotal hypospadias [101]. This is the same category that the individuals with 5α reductase deficiency, to be described later, would have been assigned to if categorized by phenotypic appearance alone. Since the same phenotype may occur as the result of different biochemical defects, classifications based on phenotype alone are no longer valid. They are extremely misleading and are to be avoided.

Disorders of Function at the Androgen Dependent Target Area. Androgen receptor deficiency: *Complete Testicular Feminization.* This clinical condition is an inherited form of male pseudohermaphroditism in which the affected subjects present with a female phenotype and totally female psychosexual orientation [102,103]. They are genetic (46 XY) and gonadal males. The testes differentiate normally and secrete adequate amounts of Mullerian inhibiting factor and testosterone. Mullerian inhibiting factor suppresses the Mullerian anlage and consequently the fallopian tubes, uterus and upper portion of the vagina are absent. However, despite the normal to high normal plasma levels of testosterone, there is no masculinization of the androgen dependent sex organs or the brain, at birth or postpubertally. Consequently there is no differentiation of the Wolffian anlage (an occasional remnant has been reported) and the external genitalia are totally female with a clitoris, labia majora, labia minora and a short vagina ending blindly.

Because of the totally female appearance of the external genitalia at birth, the affected subjects are raised as girls. The condition, therefore, is rarely diagnosed before puberty. Occasionally, a prepubertal diagnosis is made when inguinal or labial masses are palpated in a female child and are found to be testes.

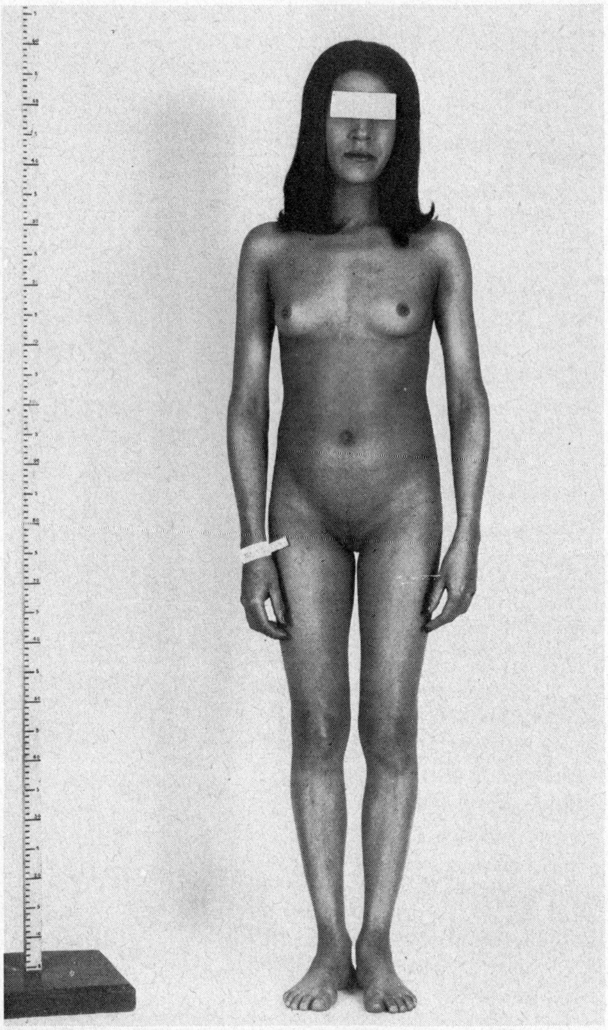

Figure 11. *Postpubertal phenotypic female with the syndrome of testicular feminization.*

At puberty, breast development occurs. There is scant to absent pubic and axillary hair, and medical attention is sought because of primary amenorrhea. A presumptive diagnosis of testicular feminization can be considered in a phenotypic female presenting with primary amenorrhea, good breast development, and scant to absent pubic and axillary hair, who on pelvic examination has a short vagina with an absent cervix and uterus (Figure 11).

The histology of the testes cannot be distinguished from that of normal males prepubertally. Postpubertally, the gross appearance is similar to cryptorchid testes except for its nodular appearance. Histologic sections of the testes reveal immature tubular development with sertoli cells and spermatogonia but no spermatogenesis. Clumps of tubules forming tubular adenomas are frequently found. The Leydig cells are hyperplastic, and electron microscopic studies reveal abundant smooth endoplasmic reticulum and mitochondria with tubular cristae—the classic structures associated with steroid production and correlating well with the normal plasma testosterone levels. In some respects, however, the Leydig cells on electron microscopy resemble fetal Leydig cells [104,105].

In human subjects, the mode of inheritance is not definitely known. From pedigree studies, however, the defect has been found to be maternally transmitted with only males expressing the condition, suggesting inheritance as X-linked recessive or autosomal dominant-sex limited (males) (Figure 12). Attempts to determine X-linked inheritance in man by demonstrating linkage to known X borne markers such as color blindness [106], hemophilia [107] and the Xg immunoglobulin [108] have been unsuccessful. Linkage studies involving autosomally linked blood groups ABO, MNs, Rh, Duffy and Kidd, P, Lutheran, Kell, Dombrock have also been negative [108]. In the Tfm/y mouse, however, the condition is clearly inherited as X-linked recessive, as determined by linkage to tabby and blotchy fur whose loci are known to be on the X chromosome [109]. Ohno [110] has postulated that the X chromosomes of all mammals are homologous and that genes X-linked in one species are X-linked in all, including man.

In 1957 Wilkins [111] suggested that the syndrome of testicular feminization was secondary to androgen insensitivity at the target area. He administered testosterone intramuscularly and failed to note nitrogen retention or virilization.

In 1968, however, Mauvais-Jarvis et al. [112] indicated that a deficiency of the enzyme 5α reductase resulted in decreased conversion of testosterone to dihydrotestosterone, and was the cause of the syndrome. They administered radioactive testosterone by the intravenous, percutaneous and oral route to normal males, and to patients with testicular feminization. When testosterone was given orally, patients with testicular feminization showed a decrease in the 5α metabolite, 3α, 5α androstanediol, as compared to normal males. When testosterone was administered by the intravenous or percutaneous route to normal males, the percentage of urinary 3α, 5α androstanediol was three to six times higher than that arising from an oral dose indicating extrahepatic 5α reduction in the peripheral tissue. However, in patients with feminizing testes the percentage of androstanediol remained the same regardless of the route of administration of radioactive testosterone.

In 1969 Wilson and Walker [113] found a decreased rate of conversion of testosterone to 5α dihydrotestosterone in skin slices obtained from the labia majora of the affected subjects as compared to slices from the labia and scrota in normal subjects. These findings were confirmed by others [114,115].

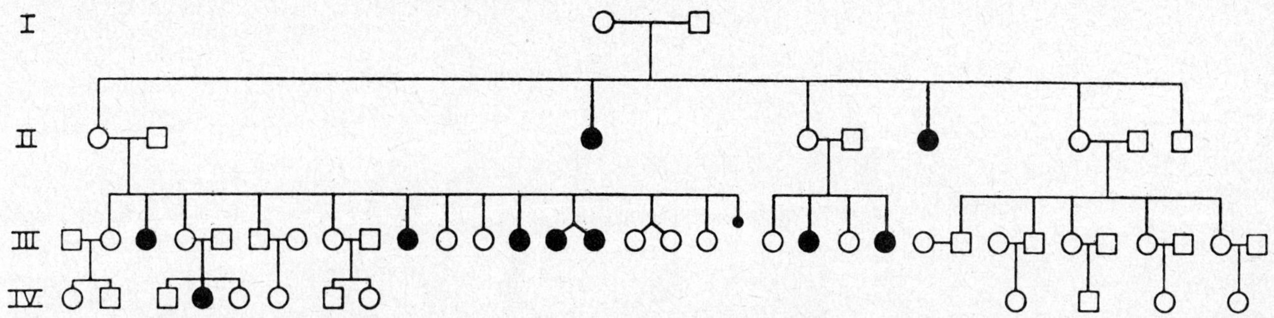

Figure 12. Pedigree of a family with testicular feminization showing maternal transmission of the defect with expression limited to males [163]. ○ = normal (46/XX), ● = testicular feminization (46/XY).

More recent studies have demonstrated that 5α reductase deficiency is not the primary defect and support Wilkin's original theory that the defect is secondary to androgen insensitivity at the target area. Jenkins and Ash [116], and Kelch et al. [117], found no difference in 5α reduction in the sex skin of normal subjects versus those with testicular feminization. Plasma levels of dihydrotestosterone in testicular feminization are normal or elevated as compared to eugonadal males [118] (Figure 13). Testicular venous plasma dihydrotestosterone levels indicate gonadal secretion of this steroid [119], and in vitro studies show formation of 5α reduced steroids by the testis [120]. In addition the mean blood production rate of dihydrotestosterone is within the normal range for males [121]. The conversion of testosterone to dihydrotestosterone, and the metabolic clearance rates for testosterone and dihydrotestosterone are in the range for females [121,122]. Since patients with testicular feminization have plasma sex binding globulin values similar to those of normal women, the resulant increased steroid protein binding may account for the decreased clearances and conversion ratios [123]. Administration of testosterone or dihydrotestosterone intramuscularly fails to evoke positive nitrogen, calcium or citrate balance and no virilization occurs [124–127]. If a deficiency of dihydrotestosterone were the primary defect, as

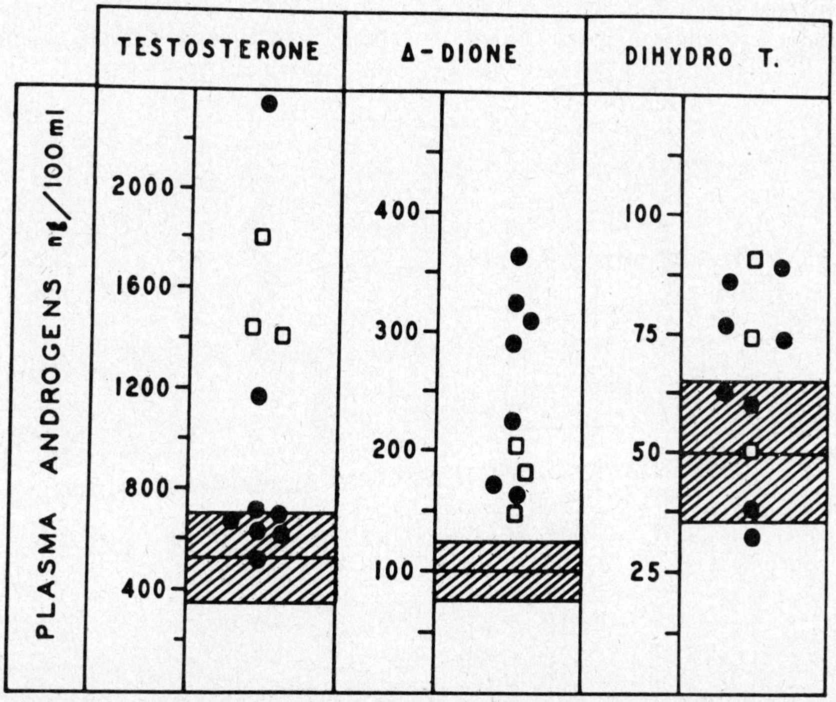

Figure 13. Plasma levels of testosterone, androstenedione and dihydrotestosterone in testicular feminization [118]. ● = female external genitalia, □ = partial masculinization.

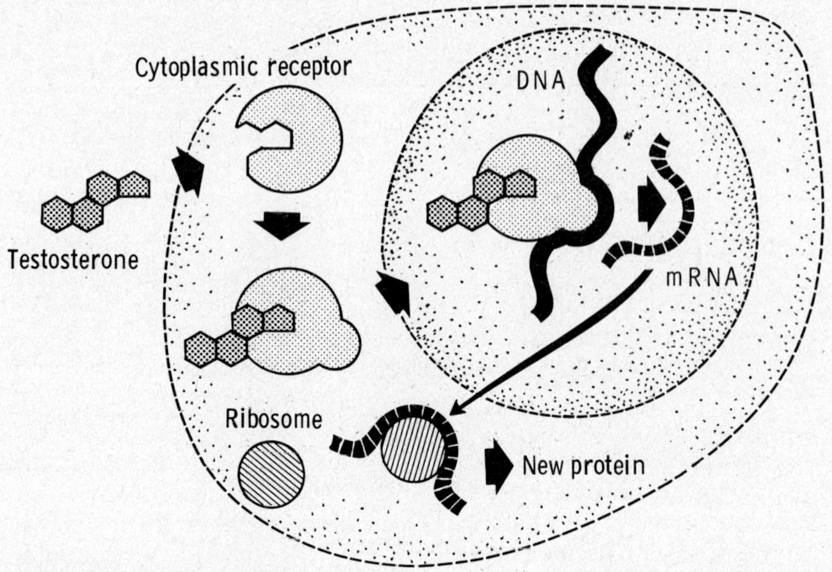

Figure 14. Diagrammatic representation of the mechanism of action of testosterone at the cellular site of action.

had been postulated, one would expect a metabolic or clinical response during its administration.

Animal studies using the Tfm/y rat and Tfm/y mouse have shown that the defect is either secondary to absent binding of the androgen to the cytosol receptor at the target area [55,128], or to absent binding of the androgen cytosol receptor complex to the nucleus [129], thereby preventing initiation of androgen action. In human subjects a defect in the binding of androgen to the cytosol was demonstrated by Keenan et al. [130] in cultured fibroblasts from subjects with testicular feminization.

The primary defect in human subjects, therefore, appears to be the inability of testosterone and dihydrotestosterone to bind to the cytoplasmic receptor at the target area, thereby preventing transfer of the androgen receptor complex to the nucleus to initiate androgen action (Figures 14 and 15).

In the Tfm/y mouse Ohno [131] has described another mutant gene on the X chromosome which

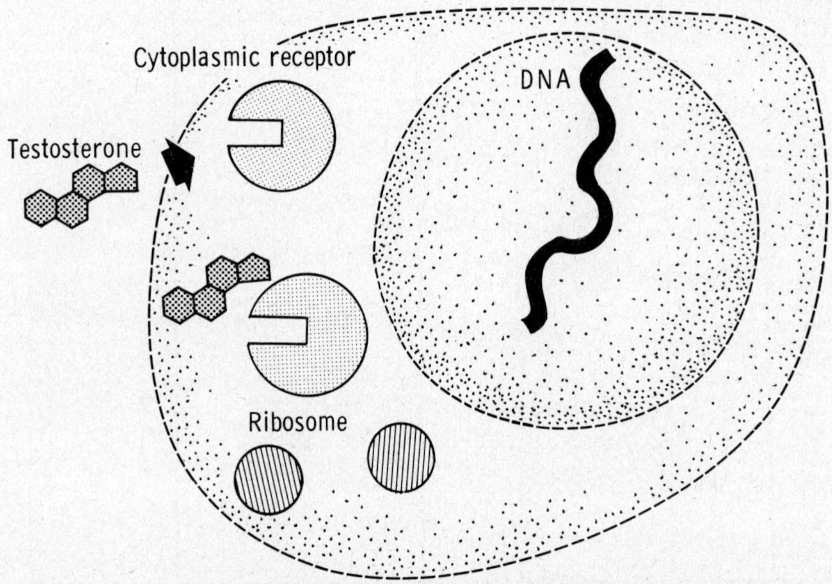

Figure 15. Diagrammatic representation of the lack of initiation of testosterone action in testicular feminization when adequate formation of the testosterone or dihydrotestosterone cytoplasmic receptor complex is impaired.

modifies the expression of the Tfm gene and restores a measure of androgen responsiveness, indicating that the Tfm mutation may not represent a gene deletion. Therefore, one might expect to find in Tfm cells an altered receptor rather than its absence. However, whether the Tfm loci alters the structure of the androgen receptor or regulates its activity is not known.

Plasma levels of luteinizing hormone (LH) are elevated in testicular feminization despite normal to high normal male levels of testosterone and dihydrotesterone [118,132]. Follicle-stimulating hormone (FSH) levels are normal to slightly elevated [118,132]. The high concentrations of sex binding globulin may alter the concentration of unbound plasma testosterone resulting in the high LH values [123]. Another possible explanation is relative androgen insensitivity at the hypothalamus, resulting in the negative feedback control being set at a higher level. The administration of androgen [133] or estrogens, however, suppresses gonadotrophin levels as it does in normal males and castration results in a further elevation of LH and FSH levels [132].

Urinary estrogens are in the high male to low female range. The testes in this condition make substantial amounts of estradiol [98,117], and an increased production rate of estrone and estradiol has been described [134]. However, normal male plasma levels of estradiol have been reported [132]. How then can breast development at puberty be explained? It has been theorized that the androgen insensitivity causes lack of suppression of the breast anlage in utero and, therefore, at puberty, in the continuing setting of androgen unresponsiveness even normal male levels of estrogen can result in gynecomastia [82,83].

Incomplete Testicular Feminization. Incomplete forms of testicular feminization have been described, and are presumably due to a partial defect at the cytoplasmic receptor level. The affected subjects have varying degrees of masculinization of the internal and external male accessory sex organs, and at puberty have some degree of virilization and almost invariably breast development [134]. At one end of the spectrum is the family of Lubs et al. [135] in which four or five affected family members were raised as females. They differ from complete testicular feminization in that there was partial Wolffian development, pubic and axillary hair, an android build and labioscrotal fusion. The patient of Gilbert-Dreyfus et al. [136] was more masculine, and was raised as a male; at puberty partial virilization occurred and the patient was capable of a male coital role although significant gynecomastia was present. The major abnormality was failure of posterior migration of the labioscrotal folds, with incomplete mid-line fusion. At the most masculine end of the spectrum is the syndrome of Reifenstein [137] in which the affected have a male phenotype but varying degrees of hypospadias. All were raised as males. Breast enlargement occurred at puberty with deficient virilization, a feminine fat distribution and azoospermia [138,139].

Recently Wilson et al. [134] described a family with incomplete testicular feminization, in which the phenotype in the 11 affected members ranged from a severe defect in virilization with breast development to a minimal defect in virilization with a microphallus and a bifid scrotum, but with no hypospadias or gynecomastia. Because of the phenotypic variability within the family, they postulate that all forms of incomplete testicular feminization result from a single mutant gene that is variably expressed.

To make a diagnosis of incomplete testicular feminization a testosterone biosynthetic defect must be excluded since many of these enzyme deficiencies result in ambiguity of the external genitalia at birth, with incomplete virilization and gynecomastia at puberty. Regardless of the phenotype, therefore, the diagnosis should be considered in affected subjects who have bilateral functional testes with normal to high plasma levels of testosterone and no evidence of an abnormality in testosterone biosynthesis.

Dr. Peterson will discuss the results of our investigation of a new form of male pseudohermaphroditism—5α reductase deficiency. This entity demonstrates for the first time an inherited abnormality of steroid metabolism, in which the basic defect resides in the hormone responsive tissues. It is also the first inherited disorder of steroid metabolism in which carriers or heterozygotes can be detected.

With the collaboration of Dr. Teofilo Gautier, Universidad Nacional Pedro Henriquez Urena, Department of Pediatrics, Santo Domingo, Dominican Republic, we are continuing to obtain pedigree information and are discovering an increasing number of affected subjects, making this the largest known pedigree for any form of male pseudohermaphroditism.

Dr. Ralph E. Peterson: I will now discuss a disorder of function at the enzyme-dependent target area secondary to an enzyme deficiency in testosterone metabolism.

5α Reductase Deficiency. Recently we have described an inherited form of male pseudohermaphroditism secondary to steroid 5α reductase deficiency in man [140,141] (Figure 16). This description has defined the necessity for dihydrotestosterone in the differentiation of male external genitalia in utero in man and confirms the experimental data described earlier.

In the southwestern section of the Dominican Republic, within four villages, there are 17 known fami-

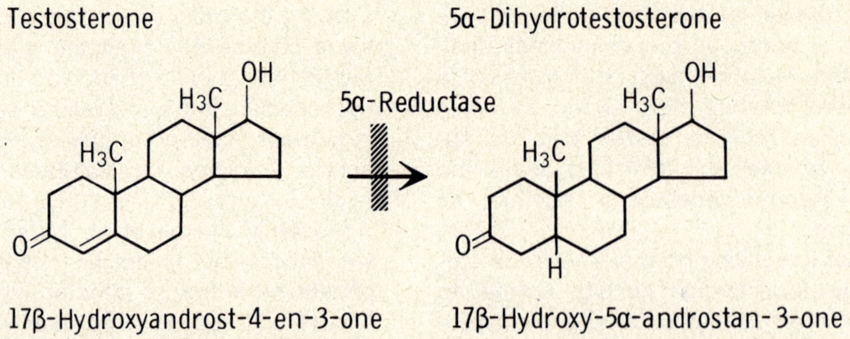

Figure 16. *Decreased dihydrotestosterone formation secondary to deficient steroid 5α reductase activity.*

lies with 30 male pseudohermaphrodites. Interrelationships between most of the families have been established and in 13 of the 17 families at least one line of descent can be traced to a common ancestor, demonstrating a founder effect. The parents are phenotypically normal, but, as will be mentioned later, most have an abnormal ratio of urinary C19 steroid 5β:5α metabolites in an intermediate or carrier range. Thus, the increased incidence of consanguinity in phenotypically normal parents, together with the biochemical abnormality demonstrated in both parents, support an autosomal mode of inheritance.

At birth, the defect in the affected males is limited to the external genitalia. The phallus is small and clitoral-like, with no urethral orifice. In 29 of the 30 subjects examined, a urogenital sinus opens on the perineum, and within the urogenital sinus there are two orifices. The anterior opening leads to the urethra and the posterior one to a blind vaginal pouch. In one subject, however, the urethra opens directly on the perineum with the vaginal pouch opening into the urethra. Internally, there is complete Mullerian inhibition and Wolffian differentiation to the vas deferens, epididymis and seminal vesicles. The testes are located in the inguinal canal or labia.

At puberty the affected males show virilization, their voices deepen and there is a significant increase in muscle mass (Figure 17). The penis grows to adult proportions, the bifid scrotum elongates and becomes rugated and hyperpigmented, and the testes enlarge and descend (if not already in the scrotum). The affected males have erections and with orgasm there is an ejaculate. Semen analysis in one patient revealed a sperm count of 40 million per cc, with 80 per cent motility and no abnormal forms. Although they are capable of intromission, insemination is not possible because of the position of the urethra. Regardless of the sex of rearing, all postpubertal males appear to have a male gender identity and all except one have assumed the male role.

The marked ambiguity of the external genitalia at birth and the contrasting male puberty, precluded a deficiency of testosterone production. Also, the virilization without breast development at puberty made it unlikely that this was a form of the testicular feminization syndrome.

The initial data confirmed our impression. In the postpubertal affected males, the plasma FSH, LH and testosterone levels in four affected subjects were within normal limits as were plasma cortisol concentration, urinary 17-hydroxycorticosteroid excretion and urinary 17-ketosteroid excretion. Urinary estrogen excretion was also in the normal range for adult males.

In four males, the plasma dihydrotestosterone ranged from 16 to 20 ng/100 ml (female range) with testosterone values ranging from 470 to 960 ng/100 ml. In normal males, the ratio of testosterone to dihydrotestosterone is approximately 10–14:1 whereas in the affected males, it was 40:1.

In two affected males the per cent conversion of testosterone to 5α dihydrotestosterone was measured during the constant infusion of radioactive testosterone. The per cent conversion was 0.48 and 0.85 and was significantly lower than the reported normal range of 2.5 to 7.0 [142–144].

The rate of metabolism of testosterone was measured in skin fibroblast cultures. In two homozygous males the rate of disappearance of testosterone was markedly decreased as compared to that in three normal controls, as was the rate of formation of the 5α metabolites androstanedione, dihydrotestosterone, androsterone and androstanediol* [141].

* Walsh et al. [145] described two siblings with an inherited form of male pseudohermaphroditism, and in one incubations of skin slices showed a decreased conversion of testosterone to dihydrotestosterone, indicating 5α reductase deficiency as the probable etiology.

Testosterone is metabolized in the liver via reduction of the double bond at the A:B ring junction by Δ^4 5β reductase(s) of the cytosol and Δ^4-5α reductase(s) of the membranes of the endoplasmic reticulum [146]. However, a substantial fraction of testosterone is metabolized extrahepatically and most, if not all, proceeds to the 5α configuration [147,148]. These metabolites are excreted in the urine as conjugates. In the presence of decreased 5α reductase activity, the rate of excretion of urinary 5α C19 steroids would be decreased and therefore, the ratio of 5β:5α steroids increased.

The urinary ratios of etiocholanolone (3α, 5β) to androsterone (3α, 5α) were measured following glucuronidase hydrolysis. In the affected, the mean ratio was 8.5 with a range of 7.3 to 11.8, and in the normal subjects the mean ratio was 1.2 with a range of 0.5 to 2.0. Urinary etiocholanediol (3α, 5β) to androstanediol (3α, 5α) ratios were also measured. In affected males, the ratio was 6.0 to 11.8, whereas the normal male range was 0.8 to 3.0. Confirmation of the abnormal urinary 5β:5α C19 steroid ratios was also obtained after the infusion of tracer doses of radioactive testosterone.

The urinary C19 5β:5α steroid ratios (endogenous and radioactive) were also determined in the parents (obligate carriers) and in female siblings of the affected. In many of the carriers, the ratios were abnormal and in an intermediate range between affected and normal.

While screening the families of the affected, seven females were found to have 5β:5α C19 steroid ratios similar to the affected males and thus are homozygous for the condition. One homozygous female is the mother of an affected male, and five females are siblings of affected males. Therefore, the homozygous females are phenotypic females with a normal menstrual history and fertility. Thus, as might be predicted, in females there does not appear to be any role for dihydrotestosterone either in sexual differentiation in utero, or ovarian function including fertility at puberty.

Prepubertal affected males also have an abnormal urinary steroid ratio when compared to normal male children or subjects with other forms of prepubertal male pseudohermaphroditism [149]. This is of some importance in newborn male pseudohermaphrodites with this degree of ambiguity of the external genitalia since the inclination of pediatricians would be to raise the child as a girl, perform castration and then corrective surgery at the appropriate time. Therefore, screening new born male pseudohermaphrodites by determining the endogenous 5β:5α C19 urinary steroid ratios might be of value in identifying those infants with 5α reductase deficiency. Because of the definite male puberty (including the growth of the phallus, erections and semen) appropriate masculinizing reconstructive surgery of the external genitalia could be carried out so that at puberty normal sexual activity and fertility would be possible. It should be remembered, however, that we have not seen the entire spectrum of the disorder, and that there may be situations in which the deficiency is so severe that dihydrotestosterone is virtually absent during the period of sexual differentiation. In these cases the males would be born with normal female external genitalia or with slight clitoral hypertrophy, and obviously the sex of rearing should be female.

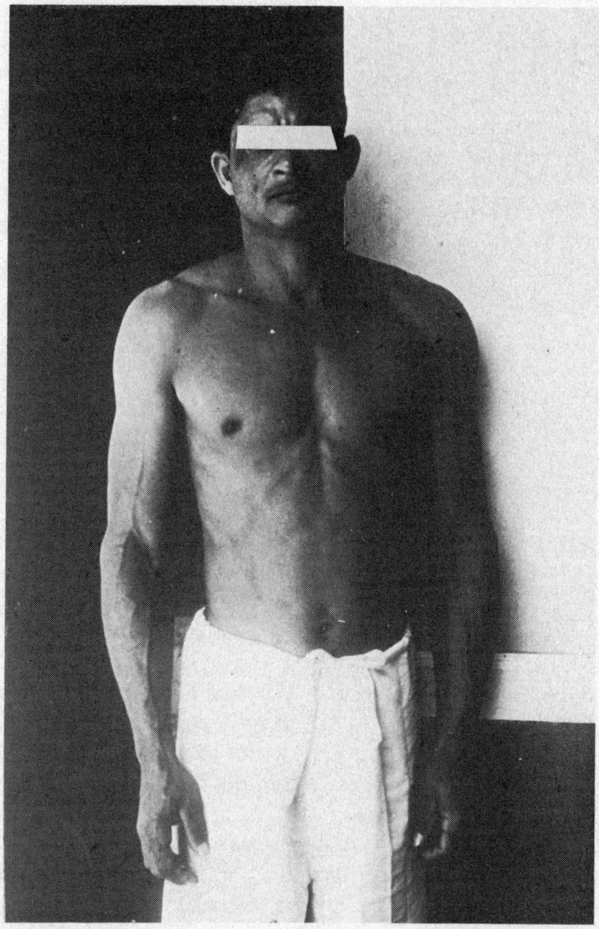

Figure 17. *Postpubertal male with 5α-reductase deficiency. Note the pubertal development in this patient in contrast to patient with testicular feminization (Figure 11)—both disorders of androgen function at the target areas.*

What factors other than 5α reductase deficiency can alter the urinary 5β:5α C19 steroid ratios? In both men and women the ratio increases slightly with age [150]. Abnormal ratios can also occur in

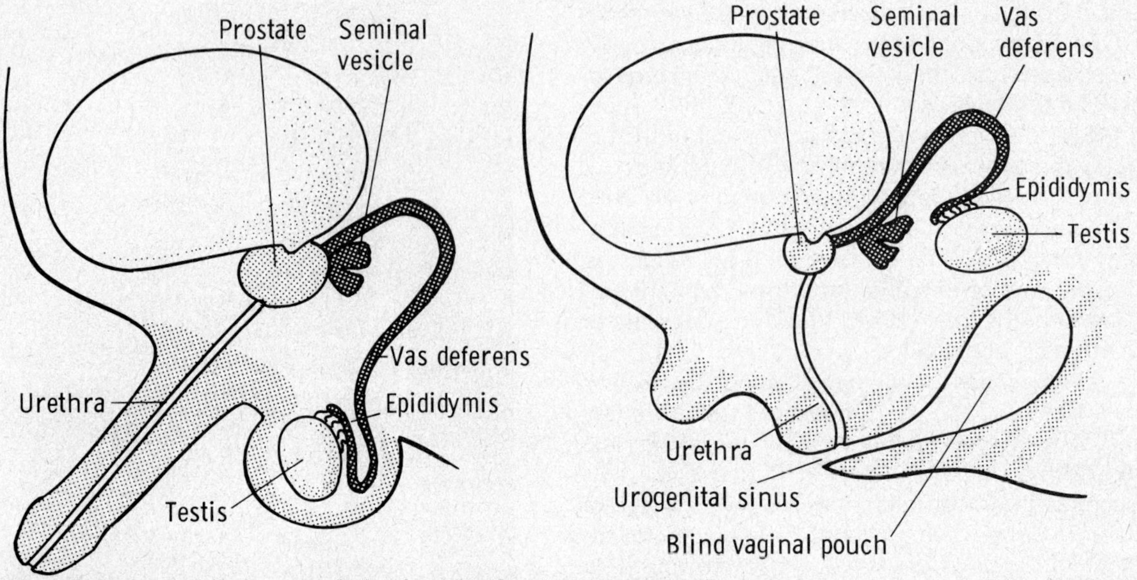

Figure 18. *Illustration of the hypothesis for the role of testosterone and dihydrotesterone in sexual differentiation in utero. Dark stippled area = testosterone-dependent. Light stippled area = dihydrotestosterone-dependent.*

some patients with chronic illness [151], hypothyroidism [152], acute intermittant porphyria [153] and in conditions of glucocorticoid excess [154,155]. Phenobarbital will also alter the 5β:5α ratio by decreasing the excretion of the urinary 5α androgen metabolites [156]. In all these conditions, with the exception of hypothyroidism, and a few patients with acute intermittent porphyria, the ratios are in the 5α reductase deficiency carrier range.

The biochemical data demonstrate a deficiency of 5α reductase activity. However, it is not known whether the deficient formation of 5α steroid metabolites is due to a defect in the gene coding for enzyme synthesis, regulation, availability of cofactors, or inhibitors of 5α reductase. Irrespective of the nature of the defect, however, the result is decreased production of 5α dihydrotestosterone.

This unique clinical entity in man, characterized by normal plasma levels of testosterone with decreased plasma levels of dihydrotestosterone, provides an opportunity to delineate the major actions of these two hormones in the male, both in utero and after birth (Figure 18).

Dihydrotestosterone is the mediator of male differentiation of the external genitalia, since the affected males have ambiguous genitalia with normal testosterone and decreased dihydrotestosterone plasma levels. However, in this entity Wolffian differentiation proceeds normally and, therefore, is a testosterone- and not a dihydrotestosterone-mediated event. Puberty is unambiguously male, with the major anabolic events mediated by testosterone. There is an increase in muscle mass together with growth of the phallus and scrotum and deepening of the voice. Although in utero dihydrotestosterone induces differentiation of the external genitalia, at puberty the anabolic steroid testosterone causes growth of the genitalia [157]. Concomitant with puberty, there is a male sex drive with normal male sexual activity and this too must be controlled by testosterone irrespective of its conversion to dihydrotestosterone [158,159]. Breast development does not occur at puberty and it appears that testosterone is the major androgen suppressing the breast anlage in utero, so that at puberty no gynecomastia occurs [82,83].

Complete spermatogenesis is present in the affected males and it is likely, therefore, that the testosterone rather than dihydrotestosterone regulates spermatogenesis [160].

Prostate enlargement [161], facial and male pattern body hair, acne [162], and temporal recession of the hairline do not occur in the affected males and appear to be dihydrotestosterone-mediated events.

In summary, we have reviewed the classic morphologic and experimental data showing the important role of chromosome constitution in sex differentiation (testicular organogenesis), and the decisive hormonal role of the embryonic testes in the development of the male phenotype. In addition, we have reviewed the important role of androgen action at the responsive (dependent) target sites in the expression of maleness. Thus the ontogeny for maleness is a complex and precarious process—a continuing struggle against the basic trend toward femaleness.

REFERENCES

1. Arey L: Development Anatomy: A Textbook and Laboratory Manual of Embryology. Philadelphia, W. B. Saunders Co., 1965.
2. Moore KL: The Developing Human: Clinically Oriented Embryology. Philadelphia, W. B. Saunders Co., 1973.
3. Everett WB: Observational and experimental evidences relating to the origin and differentiation of the definitive germ cells in mice. J Exp Zool 92: 49, 1943.
4. Mintz B, Russell ES: Developmental modifications of primordial germ cells induced by the w-series genes in the mouse embryo. Anat Rec 122: 443, 1955.
5. Mintz B, Russell ES: Gene induced embryological modifications of primordial germ cells in the mouse. J Exp Zool 134: 207, 1957.
6. Hamilton WJ, Boyd JD, Mossman HW: Human Embryology, Baltimore, The Williams & Wilkins Co., 1972.
7. Jost A: Problems of fetal endocrinology. The gonadal and hypophyseal hormones. Recent Prog Horm Res 8: 379, 1953.
8. Jirasek JE: Development of the Genital System and Male Pseudohermaphroditism, Baltimore & London, Johns Hopkins Press, 1971.
9. Federman DD: Abnormal Sexual Development. A Genetic and Endocrine Approach to Differential Diagnosis. Philadelphia, W. B. Saunders Co., 1967.
10. Singh RP, Carr DH: The anatomy and histology of XO human embryos and fetuses. Anat Rec 155: 369, 1966.
11. Jones HW, Ferguson-Smith MA, Heller RH: The pathology and cytogenetics of gonadal agenesis. Am J Obstet Gynec 87: 578, 1963.
12. Ferguson-Smith MA: Karotype-phenotype correlations in gonadal dysgenesis and their bearing on the pathogenesis of malformations. J Med Genet 2: 142, 1965.
13. Jacobs PA, Ross A: Structural abnormalities of the Y chromosome in man. Nature (Lond) 210: 352, 1966.
14. Ferguson-Smith MA: Hypothesis: X-Y chromosomal interchange in the aetiology of true hermaphrodites and of XX Klinefelter's syndrome. Lancet 2: 475, 1966.
15. de la Chapelle A: Analytic review. Nature and origin of males with XX sex chromosomes. Am J Hum Genet 24: 71, 1972.
16. Jacobs PA: Structural abnormalities of the sex chromosomes. Br Med Bull 25: 94, 1969.
17. Cervenka J, Jacobson DE, Gorlin RJ: Fluorescing structures of human metaphase chromosomes. Detection of "Y body." Am J Hum Genet 23: 317, 1917.
18. Philip J, Nielsen H, Skakkeback NE, Boczkowski K: Testing the hypothesis of Y translocation in XX males by fluorescence microscopy after quinacrine dihydrochloride staining. Lancet 1: 858, 1971.
19. Fraccaro MZ, Tiepolo O, Zuffardi C, Barigozzi A, Dolfini S: Fluorescence and Y translocation in XX males. Lancet 1: 858, 1971.
20. Wachtel SS, Koo GC, Zuckermann EE, Hammerling U, Schneid MP, Boyse EA: Serological crossreactivity between H-Y (male) antigens of mouse and man. Proc Natl Acad Sci 71: 1215, 1974.
21. Wachtel SS, Koo GC, Boyse EA: Evolutionary conservation of H-Y (male) antigen. Nature (Lond) 254: 270, 1975.
22. Koo GC, Stackpole CW, Boyse EA, Hammerling U, Lardis MP: Topographical location of H-Y antigen on mouse spermatozoa by immunoelectromicroscopy. Proc Natl Acad Sci 70: 1502, 1973.
23. Hamerton JL, Dickson JM, Pollard CE, Grieves SA, Short RV: Genetic intersexuality in goats. J Reprod Fert 7: 25, 1969.
24. Witschi E: Embryogenesis of the adrenal and the reproductive glands. Recent Prog Horm Res 6: 1, 1951.
25. Witchi E: Development of Vertebrates. Philadelphia, W. B. Saunders Co., 1956.
26. Witschi E: Biochemistry of sex differentiation in vertebrate embryos. The Biochemistry of Animal Development, vol 2, (Weber R, ed), New York, Academic Press Inc., 1967, p 193.
27. Jost A, Vigier B, Prepin J, Perchelle JP: Studies on sex differentiation in mammals. Recent Prog Hormone Res 29: 1, 1973.
28. Reyes FI, Winter JSD, Faiman C: Studies on human sexual development. I. Fetal gonadal and adrenal sex steroids. J Clin Endocrinol 37: 74, 1973.
29. Reyes FI, Boroditsky RS, Winter JSD, Faiman C: Studies on human sexual development. II. Fetal and maternal serum gonadotropin and sex steroid concentrations. J Clin Endocrinol 38: 612, 1974.
30. Neumann F, von Berswordt-Wallrabe R, Elger W, Steinbeck H, Hahn JD, Kramer M: Aspects of androgen-dependent events as studied by antiandrogens. Recent Prog Hormone Res 26: 337, 1970.
31. Josso N: Permeability of membranes to the Mullerian-inhibiting substance synthesized by the human fetal testis in vitro. A clue to its biochemical nature. J Clin Endocrinol Metab 34: 265, 1972.
32. Blanchard M-G, Josso N: Source of the anti-Mullerian hormone synthesized by the fetal testis. Mullerian-inhibiting activity of fetal bovine sertoli cells in tissue culture. Pediat Res 8: 968, 1974.
33. Wilson JD, Lasnitzki I: Dihydrotestosterone formation in fetal tissues of the rabbit and rat. Endocrinology 89: 659, 1971.
34. Siiteri P, Wilson JD: Testosterone formation and metabolism during male sexual differentiation in the human embryo. J Clin Endocrinol 38: 113, 1974.
35. O'Malley BW, Means AR: Female steroid hormones and target cell nuclei. Science 183: 610, 1974.
36. King RJB, Mainwaring WIP: Steroid-Cell Interactions. London, Butterworths, 1974.
37. Lyon MF, Hawkes SG: X-linked gene for testicular feminization in the mouse. Natuure (Lond) 227: 1217, 1970.
38. Davidoff F, Federmann DD: Mixed gonadal dysgenesis. Pediatrics 52: 727, 1973.
39. Zah W, Kalderon AE, Tucci JR: Mixed gonadal dysgenesis. Acta Endocrinol 79: 3, 1975.
40. Jacobs PA, Bucktow KE, King MJ, Harnden DC, Court-Brown WM, McBride JA, MacGregor TN, Maclean N: Cytogenetic studies in primary amenorrhea. Lancet 1: 1183, 1961.
41. Ferrier P, Ferrier S, Klein D, Fernex C: XY/XO mosaicism. Lancet 1: 54, 1963.
42. Ross GT, Holland JM, Kiser WS, Douglas GW: XO/XY chromosomal mosaicism and extragenital stigmata of Turner's syndrome in a phenotypic male. J Clin Endocrinol Metab 25: 141, 1965.
43. O'Riordan ML, Berry EW, Tough IM: Chromosome studies on bone marrow from a male control population. Br J Haematol 19: 83, 1970.
44. Pierre RV, Hoagland HC: 45,X cell lines in adult men: loss of Y chromosome, a normal aging phenomenon? Mayo Clin Proc 46: 52, 1971.
45. Simpson JL, Christakos AC, Horwith M, Silverman FS: Gonadal dysgenesis in individuals with apparently normal chromosomal complements. Tabulation of cases and compilation of genetic data. Birth Defects—The Second Conference on the Clinical Delineation of Birth

Defects, Baltimore, The Williams & Wilkins Co., 1971, p 215.
46. Barr ML, Carr DH, Plunkett ER, Soltan HC, Wiens RG: Male pseudohermaphroditism and pure gonadal dysgenesis in sisters. Am J Obstet Gynecol 99: 1047, 1967.
47. Bergada C, Cleveland WW, Jones HW Jr, Wilkins L: Gonadal histology in patients with male pseudohermaphroditism and atypical gonadal dysgenesis; relation to theories of sex differentiation. Acta Endocrinol 40: 493, 1962.
48. Alexander DS, Ferguson-Smith MA: Chromosomal studies in some variants of male pseudohermaphroditism. Pediatrics 28: 759, 1961.
49. Frasier SD, Bashore RA, Mosier HD: Gonadoblastoma associated with pure gonadal dysgenesis in monozygous twins. J Pediatr 64: 740, 1964.
50. Cohen MM, Shaw MW: Two XY siblings with gonadal dysgenesis and a female phenotype. N Engl J Med 272: 1083, 1965.
51. Brogger A, Strand A: Contributions to the study of the so called pure gonadal dysgenesis. Acta Endocrinol (Kbh) 48: 490, 1965.
52. Sternberg WH, Barclay DL, Kloepfer HW: Familial XY gonadal dysgenesis. N Engl J Med 278: 695, 1968.
53. Espiner EA, Veale AMO, Sands VE, Fitzgerald PH: Familial syndrome of streak gonads and normal male karyotype in five phenotypic females. N Engl J Med 283: 6, 1970.
54. Chemke J, Carmichael R, Stewart JM, Geer RH, Robinson A: Familial XY gonadal dysgenesis. J Med Genet 7: 105, 1970.
55. Bardin CW, Bullock LP, Sherins RJ, Mowszowicz I, Blackburn WR: Androgen metabolism and mechanism of action in male pseudohermaphroditism. A study of testicular feminization. Recent Prog Horm Res 29: 65, 1973.
56. Guell-Gonzalez JR, Paramio-Ruibal A, Delgado-Morales B: Male pseudohermaphroditism with internal bisexual genitals (a report on two brothers). Rev Roum Endocrinol 7: 343, 1970.
57. Morillo-Cucci G, German J: Males with a uterus and fallopian tubes, a rare disorder of sexual development. Birth Defects 7: 229, 1971.
58. David L, Saez JM, Francois R: Male pseudohermaphroditism in brothers. Acta Paediatr Scand 61: 249, 1972.
59. Brook CGD, Wagner H, Zachmann M, Prader A, Armendares S, Frenk S, Aleman P, Najjar SS, Slim MS, Genton N, Bozic C: Familial occurrence of persistent Mullerian structures in otherwise normal males. Br Med J 1: 771, 1973.
60. Armendares S, Buentello L, Frenk S: Two male sibs with uterus and fallopian tubes: a rare, probably inherited disorder. Clin Genet 4: 291, 1973.
61. Paigen K: The genetics of enzyme regulation. Enzyme Synthesis and Degradation in Mammalian Systems, Baltimore and London, University Park Press, 1971, p 1.
62. Prader A, Siebenmann RE: Nebenniereninsuffizienz bei kongenitaler lipoid Hyperplasie der Nebennieren. Helv Paediat Acta 12: 569, 1957.
63. Tilp A: Hochgradige Verfettung der Nebennieren eines Sauglings. Verh Deutsch Ges Pathol 16: 305, 1913.
64. Brutschy P: Hochgradige Lipoid Hyperplasie beider Nebennieren mit herdformigen Kalkablagerungen bei enem Fall von Hypospadiasis penis-scrotalis und doppelseitigem Kryptorchismus mit unecter akzessorischer Nebenniere am rechten Hoden (Pseudohermaphroditismus masculinus externus). Frankfurt Z Pathol 24: 203, 1921.
65. Zahn J: Ueber Intersexualitat und Nebennierenrindenhyperplasie. Schweiz Med Wochenschr 78: 480, 1948.
66. Sandison AT: A form of lipoidosis of the adrenal cortex in an infant. Arch Dis Child 30: 538, 1955.
67. Dhom G: Zur Morphologie und Genese der kongenitalen Nebennierenrinden-Hyperplasie beim mannlichen Scheinzwitter. Zentralbl Allg Pathol 97: 23, 1958.
68. O'Doherty NJ: Lipoid adrenal hyperplasia. Guy's Hosp Rep 113: 368, 1964.
69. Camacho AM, Kowarski A, Migeon CJ, Brough AJ: Congenital adrenal hyperplasia due to a deficiency of one of the enzymes involved in the biosynthesis of pregnenolone. J Clin Endocrinol Metab 28: 153, 1968.
70. Grumbach MM, Van Wyk JJ: Textbook of Endocrinology (Williams RH, ed), Philadelphia, W. B. Saunders Co., 1974, p. 423.
71. Degenhart HJ, Visser HKA, Boon H, O'Doherty NJ: Evidence for deficient 20α-cholesterol-hydroxylase activity in adrenal tissue of a patient with lipoid adrenal hyperplasia. Acta Endocrinol 71: 512, 1972.
72. Kirkland RT, Kirkland JL, Johnson CM, Horning M, Librik L, Clayton GW: Congenital lipoid adrenal hyperplasia in an eight-year-old phenotypic female. J Clin Endocrinol Metab 36: 488, 1973.
73. Burstein S, Kendall HL, Gut M: Transformation of labelled cholesterol, 20α hydroxycholesterol, (22R)-22-hydroxycholesterol, and (22R)-20α,22 dihydroxycholesterol by adrenal acetone-dried preparation from guinea pigs, cattle and man. Steroids 15: 809, 1970.
74. Luttrell B, Hochberg RB, Dixon WR, McDonald PD, Lieberman S: Studies on the biosynthetic conversion of cholesterol into pregnenolone. J Biol Chem 247: 1462, 1972.
75. Hochberg RB, McDonald PD, Feldman M, Lieberman S: Studies on the biosynthetic conversion of cholesterol into pregnenolone. J Biol Chem 249: 1277, 1974.
76. Prader A, Gurtner HP: Zur Genetik de Kongenitalen Lipoidhyperplasie der Nebennieren. Helv Paediatr Acta 17: 285, 1962.
77. Bongiovanni AM: Unusual steroid pattern in congenital adrenal hyperplasia: deficiency of 3β-hydroxy-dehydrogenase. J Clin Endocrinol Metab 21: 860, 1961.
78. Zachmann M, Vollmin JA, Murset G, Curtius H-Ch, Prader A: Unusual type of congenital adrenal hyperplasia probably due to deficiency of 3β-hydroxysteroid dehydrogenase. Case report of a surviving girl and steroid studies. J Clin Endocrinol Metab 30: 719, 1970.
79. Parks GA, Bermudez JA, Anast CS, Bongiovanni AM, New MI: Pubertal boy with the 3β-hydroxysteroid dehydrogenase defect. J Clin Endocrinol Metab 39: 206, 1974.
80. Janne O, Perheentupa J, Viinikka L, Vihko R: Testicular endocrine function in a pubertal boy with 3β-hydroxysteroid dehydrogenase deficiency. J Clin Endocrinol Metab 39: 206, 1974.
81. Schneider G, Genel M, Bongiovanni AM, Goldman AS, Rosenfield RL: Persistent testicular Δ^5-isomerase-3β-hydroxysteroid dehydrogenase (Δ^5-3β-HSD) deficiency in the Δ^5-3β-HSD form of congenital adrenal hyperplasia. J Clin Invest 55: 681, 1975.
82. Raynaud A: Morphogenesis in the mammary gland. Milk: The Mammary Gland and its Secretions (Kon SK, Cowie AT, eds), New York, Academic Press, Inc., 1961, p 3.
83. Neumann F, Elger W: The effect of the anti-androgen 1,2α-methylene-6-chloro-$\Delta^{4,6}$-pregnadiene-17-α-ol-3,20-dione-17α-acetate (cyproterone acetate) on the development of the mammary glands of male foetal rats. J Endocrinol 36: 347, 1966.
84. Hamilton W, Brush MG: Four clinical variants of congenital adrenal hyperplasia. Arch Dis Child 39: 66, 1964.
85. Rivarola MA, Saez JM, Migeon CJ: Studies of androgens in patients with congenital adrenal hyperplasia. J Clin Endocrinol Metab 27: 624, 1967.
86. Kenny FM, Reynolds JW, Green OC: Partial 3β-hydroxysteroid dehydrogenase (3β-HSD) deficiency in a family with congenital adrenal hyperplasia: evidence for in-

creasing 3β-HSD activity with age. Pediatrics 48: 756, 1971.
87. Cathro DM, Birchall K, Mitchell FL, Forsyth CC: 3β-21-dihydroxypregn-5-ene-20-one in urine of normal newborn infants and in third day urine of child with deficiency of 3β-hydroxysteroid-dehydrogenase. Arch Dis Child 40: 251, 1965.
88. Biglieri EG, Herron MA, Brust N: 17-hydroxylation deficiency in man. J Clin Invest 45: 1946, 1966.
89. Goldsmith O, Solomon DH, Horton R: Hypogonadism and mineralocorticoid excess: the 17-hydroxylase syndrome. N Engl J Med 277: 673, 1967.
90. Linquette M, Dupont A, Racadot A, Lefebvre J, May JP, Cappoen JP: Deficit en 17-hydroxylase. Ann d'Endocrinol 32: 574, 1971.
91. Mallin SR: Congenital adrenal hyperplasia secondary to 17-hydroxylase deficiency: two sisters with amenorrhea, hypokalemia, hypertension, and cystic ovaries. Ann Intern Med 70: 69, 1969.
92. New MI: Male pseudohermaphroditism due to 17α-hydroxylase deficiency. J Clin Invest 49: 1930, 1970.
93. Mantero F, Busnardo B, Riondel A, Veyrat R, Austoni M: Hypertension arterielle, alcalose hypokaliemique et pseudohermaphrodisme male par deficit en 17α-hydroxylase. Schweiz Med Wochenschr 101: 38, 1971.
94. Bricaire H, Luton JP, Laudat P, Legrand JC, Turpin G, Corvol P, Lemmer M: A new male pseudohermaphroditism associated with hypertension due to a block of 17α-hydroxylation. J Clin Endocrinol Metab 35: 67, 1972.
95. Zachmann M, Vollmin JA, Hamilton W, Prader A: Steroid 17,20-desmolase deficiency. A new cause of male pseudohermaphroditism. Clin Endocrinol 1: 369, 1972.
96. Goebelsmann U, Davajan V, Israel R, Mestman JH, Mishell DR Jr, Zachmann M: Male pseudohermaphroditism consistent with 17,20-desmolase deficiency. Endocrine Society 56th Annual Meeting, 1974.
97. Saez JM, DePeretti E, Morera AM, et al.: Familial male pseudohermaphroditism with gynecomastia due to a testicular 17-ketosteroid reductase defect. I. Studies in vivo. J Clin Endocrinol Metab 32: 604, 1971.
98. Saez JM, Morera AM, DePeretti E, Bertrand J: Further in vivo studies in male pseudohermaphroditism with gynecomastia due to a testicular 17-steroid reductase defect (compared to a case of testicular feminization). J Clin Endocrinol Metab 34: 598, 1972.
99. Goebelsmann U, Horton R, Mestman JH, Arce JJ, Nagata Y, Nakamura RM, Thorneycroft IH, Mishell DR Jr: Male pseudohermaphroditism due to testicular 17β-hydroxysteroid dehydrogenase deficiency. J Clin Endocrinol Metab 36: 867, 1973.
100. Givens JR, Wiser WL, Summitt RL, Kerber IJ, Andersen RN, Pittaway DE, Fish SA: Familial male pseudohermaphroditism without gynecomastia due to deficient testicular 17-ketosteroid reductase activity. N Engl J Med 291: 938, 1974.
101. Opitz JM, Simpson JL, Sario GE, Summitt RL, German J, New M: Pseudovaginal preineoscrotal hypospadias. Clin Genet 3: 1, 1972.
102. Morris JM: The syndrome of testicular feminization in male pseudohermaphrodites. Am J Obstet Gynec 65: 1192, 1953.
103. Morris JM, Mahesh VB: Further observations on the syndrome, "testicular feminization." Am J Obstet Gynec 87: 731, 1963.
104. Ferenczy A, Richart RM: The fine structure of the gonads in the complete form of testicular feminization syndrome. Am J Obstet Gynec 113: 399, 1972.
105. Gordon GB, Miller LR, Bensch KG: Electron microscopic observations of the gonad in the testicular feminization syndrome. Lab Invest 13: 152, 1964.
106. Steward JSS: Testicular feminisation and colour-blindness. Lancet 2: 592, 1959.
107. Nilsson IM, Bergman S, Reitalu J, Waldenström J: Haemophilia A in a "girl" with male sex-chromatin pattern. Lancet 2: 264, 1959.
108. Sanger R, Tippett P, Gavin J, Gooch A, Race R: Inheritance of testicular feminization syndrome: Some negative linkage findings. J Med Genet 6: 26, 1969.
109. Lyon MF, Hawkes SG: X-linked gene for testicular feminization in the mouse. Nature (Lond) 227: 1217, 1970.
110. Ohno S: Sex Chromosomes and Sex-Linked Genes, Berlin, Springer-Verlag, 1967.
111. Wilkins L: The Diagnosis and Treatment of Endocrine Disorders in Childhood and Adolescence, Springfield, Ill., Charles C Thomas, 1957, p 276.
112. Mauvais-Jarvis P, Bercovici JP, Crepy O, Gauthier F: Studies on testosterone metabolism in subjects with testicular feminization syndrome. J Clin Invest 49: 31, 1970.
113. Wilson JD, Walker JD: The conversion of testosterone to 5α-andro-stan-17β-ol-3 one (dihydrotestosterone) by skin slices of man. J Clin Invest 48: 371, 1969.
114. Northcutt RC, Island DP, Liddle GW: An explanation for target organ unresponsiveness in the testicular feminization syndrome. J Clin Endocrinol Metab 29: 422, 1969.
115. Karsznia R, Wyss RH, Heinrichs WL, Herrmann WL: Testicular feminization. An apparent enzyme defect. Gynaecologia 167: 197, 1969.
116. Jenkins JS, Ash S: The metabolism of testosterone by skin in normal subjects and in testicular feminization. J Endocrinol 49: 515, 1971.
117. Kelch RP, Jenner MR, Weinstein R, Kaplan SL, Grumbach MM: Estradiol and testosterone secretion by human, simian, and canine testes, in males with hypogonadism and in male pseudohermaphrodites with the feminizing testes syndrome. J Clin Invest 51: 824, 1972.
118. Tremblay RR, Foley TP Jr, Corvol P, Park I, Kowarski A, Blizzard RM, Jones HW Jr, Migeon CJ: Plasma concentration of testosterone, dihydrotestosterone, testosterone-oestradiol binding globulin, and pituitary gonadotropins in the syndrome of male pseudo-hermaphroditism with testicular feminization. Acta Endocrinol 70: 331, 1972.
119. Wieland RG, Chen JC, Zorn EM, Webster KD, Tang PH: Gonadal and peripheral venous levels of dihydrotestosterone in a patient with testicular feminization. J Lab Clin Med 78: 825, 1971.
120. Richards G, Neville AM: Formation and metabolism of 5α-reduced steroids by gonadal tissue in testicular feminization. J Endocrinol 62: 405, 1974.
121. Tremblay RR, Kowarski A, Park I, Migeon CJ: Blood production rate of dihydrotestosterone in the syndrome of male pseudohermaphroditism. J Clin Endocrinol Metab 35: 101, 1972.
122. Judd HL, Hamiltin CR, Barlow JJ, et al.: Androgen and gonadotropin dynamics in testicular feminization syndrome. J Clin Endocrinol Metab 34: 229, 1972.
123. Mauvais-Jarvis P, Crepy O, Bercovici JP: Further studies on the pathophysiology of testicular feminization syndrome. J Clin Endocrinol Metab 32: 568, 1971.
124. French FS, Van Wyk JJ, Baggett B, Easterling WE, Talbert LM, Johnston FR, Forchielli E, Dey AC: Further evidence of a target organ defect in the syndrome of testicular feminization. J Clin Endocrinol Metab 26: 493, 1966.
125. Rosenfield RL, Lawrence AM, Liao S, Landau RL: Androgens and androgen responsiveness in the feminizing testis syndrome. Comparison of complete and "incomplete" forms. J Clin Endocrinol Metab 32: 625, 1971.
126. Strickland AL, French FS: Absence of response to dihydrotestosterone in the syndrome of testicular feminization. J Clin Endocrinol 29: 1284, 1969.
127. Castaneda E, Perez AE, Guillen MA, Ramirez-Robles S,

Gual C, Perez-Palacios G: Metabolic studies in a patient with testicular feminization syndrome. Am J Obstet Gynec 110: 1002, 1971.
128. Gehring U, Tomkins G: Characterization of a hormone receptor defect in the androgen-insensitivity mutant. Cell 3: 59, 1974.
129. Goldstein JL, Wilson JD: Studies on the pathogenesis of pseudohermaphroditism in the mouse with testicular feminization. J Clin Invest 51: 1647, 1972.
130. Keenan BS, Meyer WJ III, Hadjian AJ, Jones HW, Migeon CJ: Syndrome of androgen insensitivity in man. Absence of 5α-dihydrotestosterone binding protein in skin fibroblast. J Clin Endocrinol Metab 38: 1143, 1974.
131. Ohno S, Christian L, Attardi BJ, Kan J: Modification of expression of the testicular feminization (Tfm) gene of the mouse by a "controlling agent" gene. Nature (New Biol) 245: 92, 1973.
132. Faiman C, Winter JSD: The control of gonadotropin secretion in complete testicular feminization. J Clin Endocrinol Metab 39: 631, 1974.
133. Rivarola MA, Saez JM, Meyer WJ, Kenny FM, Migeon CJ: Studies of androgens in the syndrome of male pseudohermaphroditism with testicular feminization. J Clin Endocrinol Metab 27: 371, 1967.
134. Wilson JD, Harrod MJ, Goldstein JL, Hemsell DL, MacDonald PC: Familial incomplete male pseudohermaphroditism, type I. Evidence of androgen resistance and variable clinical manifestations in a family with the Reifenstein syndrome. N Engl J Med 290: 1097, 1974.
135. Lubs HA Jr, Vilar O, Bergenstal DM: Familial male pseudohermaphroditism with labial testes and partial feminization: endocrine studies and genetic aspects. J Clin Endocrinol Metab 19: 1110, 1959.
136. Gilbert-Dreyfus S, Sebaoun CA, Belaisch J: Étude d'un cas familial d'androgynoidisme avec hypospadias grave, gynecomastie et hypoestrogenie. Ann Endocrinol 18: 93, 1957.
137. Reifenstein EC Jr: Hereditary familial hypogonadism. Proc Am Fed Clin Res 3: 86, 1947.
138. Bowen P, Lee CSN, Migeon CJ, Kaplan NM, Whalley PJ, McKusick VA, Reifenstein EC Jr: Hereditary male pseudohermaphroditism with hypogonadism, hypospadias, and gynecomastia (Reifenstein's syndrome). Ann Intern Med 62: 252, 1965.
139. Bremner WJ, Ott J, Moore DJ, Paulsen CA: Reifenstein's syndrome: Investigation of linkage to X-chromosomal loci. Clin Genet 6: 216, 1974.
140. Imperato-McGinley J, Guerrero L, Gautier T, Peterson RE: Steroid 5α-reductase deficiency in man. An inherited form of male pseudohermaphroditism. Science 186: 1213, 1974.
141. Imperato-McGinley J, Guerrero L, Gautier T, German JL, Peterson RE: Steroid 5α-reductase deficiency in man. An inherited form of male pseudohermaphroditism. Genetic Forms of Hypogonadism (Bergsma D, ed), New York, Stratton Intercontinental Medical Book Corporation, 1975, p 91.
142. Ito T, Horton R: The source of plasma dihydrotestosterone in man. J Clin Invest 50: 1621, 1971.
143. Mahoudeau J, Bardin WC, Lipsett MB: The metabolic clearance rate and origin of plasma dihydrotestosterone in man and its conversion to the 5α-androstanediols. J Clin Invest 50: 1338, 1971.
144. Saez JM, Forest MG, Morera AM, Bertrand J: Metabolic clearance rate and blood production rate of testosterone and dihydrotestosterone in normal subjects, during pregnancy and in hyperthyroidism. J Clin Invest 51: 1226, 1972.
145. Walsh PC, Madden JD, Harrod MJ, Goldstein JL, MacDonald PD, Wilson JD: Familial incomplete male pseudohermaphroditism, type 2. Decreased dihydrotestosterone formation in pseudovaginal perineoscrotal hypospadias. N Engl J Med 291: 944, 1974.
146. Peterson RE: Metabolism of Adrenal Cortical Steroids (Christy N, ed), New York, Harper & Row, 1971, p 87.
147. Rivarola MA, Singleton RT, Migeon CJ: Splanchnic extraction and interconversion of testosterone and androstenedione in man. J Clin Invest 46: 2095, 1967.
148. Gomez E, Frost P: Testosterone metabolism and androgenic effect. Adv Biol Skin 12: 367, 1972.
149. Peterson RE et al: Male pseudohermaphroditism due to steroid 5α-reductase deficiency. Am J Med (in press).
150. Pincus G, Dorfman RI, Romanoff LP, Rubin BL, Bloch E, Carlo J, Freeman, H: Steroid metabolism in aging men and women. Recent Prog Horm Res 11: 307, 1955.
151. Zumoff B, Bradlow HL, Gallagher TF, Hellman L: Decreased conversion of androgens to normal 17-ketosteroid metabolites: a non-specific consequence of illness. J Clin Endocrinol Metab 32: 824, 1971.
152. Hellman L, Bradlow HL, Zumoff B, Fukushima DK, Gallagher TF: Thyroid-androgen interrelations and the hypocholesterolemic effect of androsterone. J Clin Endocrinol Metab 19: 936, 1959.
153. Kappas A, Bradlow HL, Gillette PN, Gallagher T: Studies in porphyria: A defect in the reductive transformation of natural steroid hormones in the hereditary liver disease, acute intermittent porphyria. J Exp Med 136: 1043, 1972.
154. James VHT: The excretion of individual 17-oxosteroids in Cushing's syndrome. J Endocrinol 23: 119, 1961.
155. Wilson H, Schenker S: Effect of corticosteroids on urinary 5β and 5α C19 steroids in man. Acta Endocrinol 46: 197, 1964.
156. Bradlow HL, Zumoff B, Fukushima DK, Hellman L, Bickers DR, Alvares AP, Kappas A: Drug induced alteration of steroid hormone metabolism in man. Ann NY Acad Sci 212: 148, 1973.
157. Jung I, Baulieu E-E: Testosterone cytosol "receptor" in the rat levator ani muscle. Nature (New Biol) 237: 24, 1972.
158. McDonald P, Beyer C, Newton F, Brien B, Baker R, Tan HS, Sampson C, Kitching P, Greenhill R, Pritchard D: Failure of 5α-dihydrotestosterone to initiate sexual behaviour in the castrated male rat. Nature (Lond) 227: 964, 1970.
159. Baum ML, Vreeburg JTM: Copulation in castrated male rats following combined treatment with estradiol and dihydrotestosterone. Science 182: 283, 1973.
160. Ryan KJ, Naftolin F, Reddy V, Flores F, Petro Z: Estrogen formation in the brain. Am J Obstet Gynec 114: 454, 1972.
161. Flores F, Naftolin F, Ryan KJ, White RJ: Estrogen formation by the isolated perfused Rhesus monkey brain. Science 180: 1074, 1973.
162. Sherins RJ, Loriaux DL: Studies on the role of sex steroids in the feedback control of FSH concentrations in men. J Clin Endocrinol Metab 36: 886, 1973.
163. Stewart-Bentley M, Odell W, Horton R: Feedback control of luteinizing hormone in normal adult men. J Clin Endocrinol Metab 38: 545, 1974.
164. Steinberger E: Hormonal control of mammalian spermatogenesis. Physiol Rev 51: 1, 1971.
165. Sitteri PK, Wilson JD, Mayfield JA: Dihydrotestosterone in prostatic hypertrophy. J Clin Invest 49: 1737, 1970.
166. Sansone G, Reisner RM: Differential rates of conversion of testosterone to dihydrotestosterone in acne and in normal human skin—a possible pathogenic factor in acne. J Invest Dermatol 56: 366, 1971.
167. Stenchever MA, Ng ABP, Jones GK, Jarvis JA: Testicular feminization syndrome. Chromosomal, histologic, and genetic studies in a large kindred. Obstet Gynecol 33: 649, 1969.

Echocardiographic Detection of Fungal Vegetations in Candida Parasilopsis Endocarditis

JOSEPH A. C. GOMES, M.D.*
JAIME CALDERON, M.D.†
FOUAD LAJAM, M.D.
HIDEKI SAKURAI, M.D.
HOWARD S. FRIEDMAN, M.D.
With the technical assistance of
JOSEPH S. TATZ, C.B.S.
New York, New York

A case of primary Candida parasilopsis endocarditis in a heroin addict involving the aortic valve is presented. Abnormal echoes in the aortic root during diastole and in the aortic valve during systole and diastole produced by fungal vegetations were found. The demonstration of fungal vegetations by echocardiography in the absence of positive blood cultures and systemic embolization is a useful diagnostic tool which should be utilized when fungal endocarditis is suspected.

Since its original description by Friedman and Donaldson in 1939 [1], the incidence of Candida endocarditis has been increasing. Prior to the era of surgical therapy, this condition had a mortality of 89 per cent [2]. Because fungal endocarditis is frequently associated with negative blood cultures and because of the reported observation that positive cultures for Candida may not be associated with valvular involvement [3], recognition of this disorder by noninvasive technics has become important. The hallmark of Candida endocarditis is the production of bulky exophytic vegetations. Recognition of these vegetations in patients with Candida endocarditis might therefore be critical in the absence of other clues for the prompt institution of effective and aggressive therapy. Our purpose here is to report on the echocardiographic identification of such vegetations found prior to surgery in a patient with C. parasilopsis endocarditis, whose blood cultures were negative prior to surgery.

CASE REPORT

A 55 year old black man, a known heroin addict for 30 years, was admitted to the medical service of the Bronx VA Hospital because of generalized weakness and malaise of three months' duration, a fleeting rash over the lower extremities and trunk, and progressive dyspnea on exertion for three weeks. He denied experiencing fever or rigors. There was no past history of cardiac murmurs, diabetes mellitus or hypertension.

On physical examination the pulse rate was 110/min, the blood pressure 120/70 mm Hg and the temperature 103°F. There was a purpuric rash over the lower extremities and the lower trunk. All peripheral pulses were palpable. Examination of the heart revealed a grade 2/6 ejection systolic murmur and a grade 2/6 decrescendo diastolic murmur over the aortic area. Auscultation of the lungs revealed few bilateral basilar rales. The liver and spleen were palpable and enlarged. Laboratory data showed a hemoglobin level of 11 g/100 ml, and a white blood cell count of 4,400/mm^3 with a differential count of 3 per cent stab forms, 49 per cent segmented neutrophils, 45 per cent lymphocytes and 3 per cent monocytes. Other laboratory findings were within

From the Veterans Administration Hospital, Bronx, New York 10468, and the Departments of Medicine and Surgery, the Mount Sinai School of Medicine, New York, New York 10029. Requests for reprints should be addressed to Dr. Howard S. Friedman, Cardiac Section, V.A. Hospital, 130 W. Kingsbridge Road, Bronx, New York 10468.
Manuscript accepted October 1, 1975.

* Present address: Cardiopulmonary Laboratory, USPHS Hospital, Staten Island, New York 10304.

† Present address: Medical Practice P.A., 8100 Marty, Overland Park, Kansas 66204.

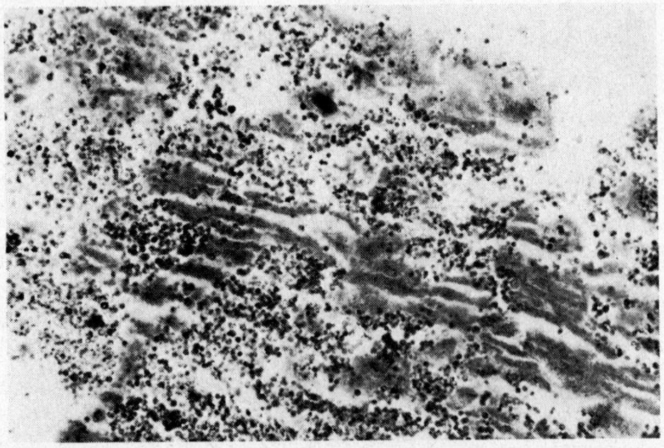

Figure 1. Microscopic section of the resected aortic valve shows dense infiltration with yeast cells.

normal limits. An electrocardiogram showed sinus tachycardia at a rate of 115/min, abnormal left axis deviation, and nonspecific S-T segment and T wave changes. A chest film showed a slight increase in the transverse diameter of the heart. After obtaining blood for several cultures, therapy with cephalothin, gentamycin and methadone was instituted. The patient became afebrile on the third hospital day, and blood cultures previously obtained were reported to be negative. On the fourth hospital day, a right pleural effusion and evidence of left ventricular failure developed. The patient was promptly treated with digoxin and diuretics.

On the eighth hospital day the patient became febrile and tachypneic, with a pulse rate of 120/min and a blood pressure of 180/60 mm Hg. Cardiac auscultation revealed a grade 4/6 diastolic murmur at the aortic area and apex. A holosystolic murmur was also heard along the left sternal border with radiation towards the apex. A chest film showed pulmonary congestion and increased heart size. Echocardiography was performed using a Unirad Ultrasonoscope, Model 175B and an unfocused transducer, employing piezoelectric crystal 0.5 of an inch in diameter with a resonant frequency of 2.5 MHz. The echocardiograms were recorded on a Cambridge phonocardiogram recorder coupled to the Unirad Ultrasonoscope. Because of the patient's worsening hemodynamic status and the appearance of a distinct holosystolic murmur, he underwent cardiac catheterization and emergency open heart surgery.

At surgery all three cusps of the aortic valve were found to be involved and covered on the aortic as well as the ventricular surface by polypoid vegetations which extended into the ventricular cavity simulating finger-like projections. A microscopic section obtained from the resected valve is shown in Figure 1. There was no direct invasion of the ventricular endocardium or the aortic root. There was a 2 mm hole in the right coronary cusp of the aortic valve. The aortic valve was replaced with a Björk-Shiley prosthesis. The administration of amphotericin B, 5 mg/kg/day intravenously, and 5-fluorocytosine, 2 g orally every 6 hours, was started immediately after surgery.

ECHOCARDIOGRAPHIC FINDINGS

Figure 2 shows the aortic root and aortic valve echograms from a normal subject. Aortic leaflet echoes are sharp, free of any thickening and there are no abnormal echoes. Figure 3 shows the aortic root and aortic valve echoes found in the patient. An abnormal cluster of echoes are seen in the aortic root (Figure 3A). The mobility and the high intensity of these abnormal echoes is evident. Abnormal echoes are also visualized on the aortic valve in systole and diastole (Figure 3B). After reduction of gain setting, abnormal echoes are still visible on the aortic valve in systole and diastole (Figure 4). The aortic valve excursion was normal. There was premature closure of the mitral valve and diastolic fluttering of the anterior mitral valve leaflet.

CARDIAC CATHETERIZATION DATA

Right atrial pressure was normal. Pulmonary artery pressure was 57/30 mm Hg with a mean of 30 mm Hg. Aortic pressure was 152/46 mm Hg with a mean of 106

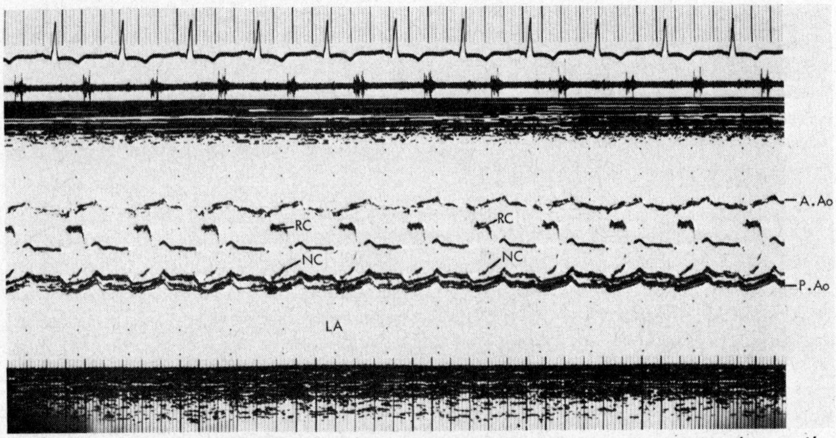

Figure 2. Normal aortic root and aortic valve echogram. A.Ao = anterior aortic root. P.Ao = posterior aortic root. RC = right coronary cusp of the aortic valve. NC = noncoronary cusp of the aortic valve. The echoes are sharp and free of any thickening, and there are no abnormal echoes on the aortic valve.

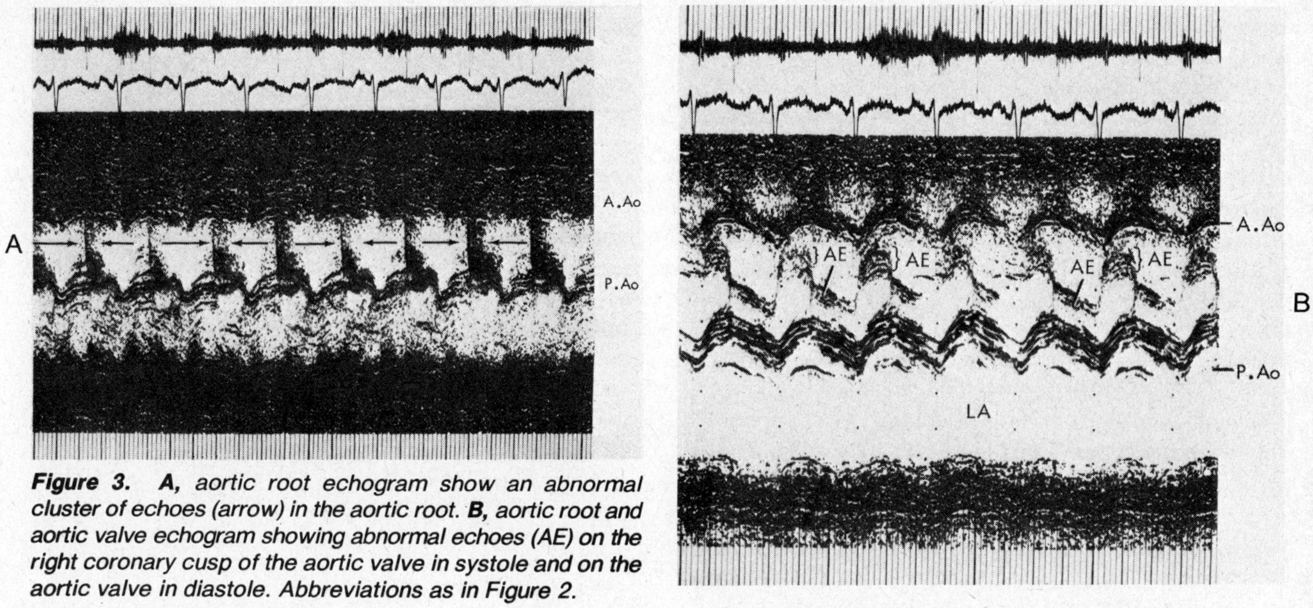

Figure 3. ***A,*** *aortic root echogram show an abnormal cluster of echoes (arrow) in the aortic root.* ***B,*** *aortic root and aortic valve echogram showing abnormal echoes (AE) on the right coronary cusp of the aortic valve in systole and on the aortic valve in diastole. Abbreviations as in Figure 2.*

mm Hg. Left ventricular pressure was 152/46 mm Hg. The pulmonary artery wedge mean pressure was 25 mm Hg. There was no gradient across the aortic or pulmonary valves. Cardiac index was 3.36 liters/min. Ejection fraction was 56 per cent. There was no oxygen step-up in the right-sided cardiac chambers.

A high supra-aortic angiogram revealed 4+ aortic regurgitation. The left ventriculogram showed a dilated left ventricle but no mitral insufficiency.

COMMENTS

The diagnosis of Candida endocarditis is frequently difficult, particularly in the absence of positive blood cultures and systemic embolization. The accepted methods of diagnosis are blood cultures and Candida serology [4–6]. However, the organism may be only sporadically recovered despite multiple blood cultures and requires prolonged incubation [2]. Frequently, when the Candida organism is recovered, particularly from a single culture, the tendency has been to regard it as a contaminant [2]. In our patient, not until the 10th hospital day were the blood cultures diagnostic of C. parasilopsis, a common organism in heroin addicts [7,8].

The use of echocardiography in assessing the location and size of bacterial and fungal vegetations has not been fully established. Dillon et al. [9] undertook a study to visualize vegetations by echocardiography and to determine what size these vegetations had to be in order to be seen on echograms. In eight patients with autopsy or surgically proved bacterial endocarditis, they found nonuniform thickening of the valve but unrestricted motion of the involved leaflets. The ability to recognize these echoes depended on the size of the vegetations being at least 2 mm in diameter. Their observations were recently confirmed by De Maria et al. [10]. Since fungal vegetations are large and bulky, then, theoretically, they would more likely be detected by echocardiography than bacterial vegetations. In our patient, abnormal echoes were found in the aortic root in dias-

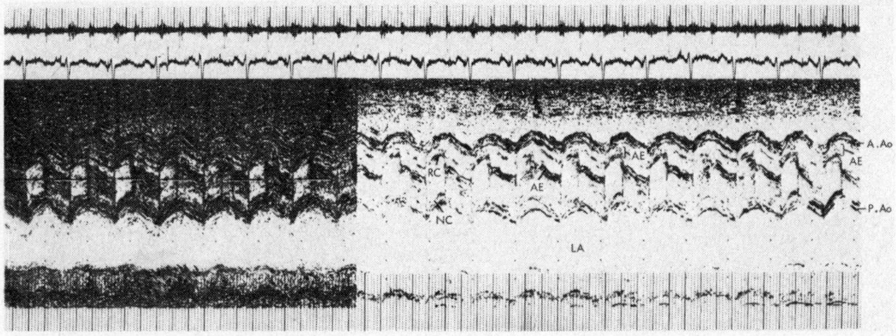

Figure 4. *Aortic root and aortic valve echograms at high (left panel) and low gains (right panel) showing abnormal echoes (AE) at both gain settings.*

tole and in the aortic valve in both systole and diastole. At surgery, bulky vegetations were found that would explain these findings.

Recently, Gotlieb et al. [11] reported two cases of Candida endocarditis in which abnormal "shaggy" echoes were demonstrated in the aortic root only in diastole. They, however, were unable to visualize the location of these echoes in systole. Shelbert and Muller [12] also detected fungal vegetations on a Starr-Edwards mitral prosthesis. Thus, these studies and our findings show that there are echocardiographic features that suggest primary fungal endocarditis: (1) Abnormal echo clusters are visible intermittently in the aortic root; (2) valve leaflets are thickened with abnormal "shaggy" echoes that may be visible in both systole and diastole; (3) leaflet excursion itself is generally normal, except, perhaps, in those cases in which the valve leaflets are extensively damaged. The presence of normal leaflet mobility would distinguish the echocardiographic findings of primary endocarditis from those of calcific aortic stenosis, a disorder in which abnormal echoes are also present but leaflet excursion is reduced.

Thus, echocardiography appears to be a sensitive noninvasive technic for detecting fungal vegetations in endocarditis. Use of this diagnostic tool in the absence of systemic emboli and negative blood cultures may provide enough information so that early diagnosis can be made. It is recommended that drug addicts, patients receiving multiple antibiotics and immunosuppressive therapy, and those undergoing hyperalimentation should be screened by echocardiography when endocarditis is suspected.

REFERENCES

1. Friedman NB, Donaldson L: Chicago Pathologic Society; systemic mycosis with mycotic endocarditis. Arch Pathol 27: 394, 1939.
2. Kay JH, Bernstein S, Tsuji HK, Redington JV, Milgram M, Brem T: Surgical treatment of Candida endocarditis. JAMA 203: 105, 1968.
3. Ellis CA, Spivack ML: The significance of Candidemia. Ann Intern Med 67: 511, 1967.
4. Harris PD, Yeoh CB, Breault J, Meltzer J, Katz S: Fungal endocarditis secondary to drug addiction—recent concepts in diagnosis and surgery. J Thorac Cardiovasc Surg 63: 980, 1972.
5. Seelig MS, Speth CP, Kozinn PJ, Toni EF, Taschdjian CL: Candida endocarditis after cardiac surgery—clued to earlier detection. J Thoracic Cardiovasc Surg 65: 583, 1973.
6. Seelig MS, Speth CP, Kozinn PJ, Taschdjian CL, Toni EF, Goldberg J: Patterns of Candida endocarditis following cardiac surgery. Importance of early diagnosis and therapy (an analysis of 91 cases). Prog Cardiovasc Dis 42: 125, 1974.
7. Louria DB, Hensle T, Rose J: The major medical complications of heroin addiction. Ann Intern Med 67: 1, 1967.
8. Hoeprich PD, Ingraham JL, Kleker E, Jay Winship M: Development of resistance to 5-fluorocytosine in Candida parasilopsis during therapy. J Infect Dis 130: 112, 1974.
9. Dillon JC, Feigenbaum H, Konecke LH, Davis RH, Chang S: Echocardiographic manifestations of valvular vegetations. Am Heart J 86: 698, 1973.
10. DeMaria AN, Ding JF, Sabel AF, Candel CC, Millar RR, Mason DT: Echography and phonography of acute aortic regurgitation in bacterial endocarditis. Ann Intern Med 82: 329, 1975.
11. Gotlieb S, Khuddus SA, Balooki H, Dominguez RT, Myerburg RJ: Echocardiographic diagnosis of aortic valve vegetations in Candida endocarditis. Circulation 50: 826, 1974.
12. Shelbert HR, Mueller OR: Detection of fungal vegetations involving a Starr-Edward mitral prosthesis by means of ultrasound. Vasc Surg 6: 20, 1972.

Tuberculous Arthritis

A Report of Two Cases with Review of Biopsy and Synovial Fluid Findings

RICHARD WALLACE, M.D.*
ALAN S. COHEN, M.D.
Boston, Massachusetts

Two cases of tuberculous arthritis with synovial fluid findings are presented, and the major series with culture results and synovial fluid analyses are reviewed. Synovial fluid cultures are positive for tuberculosis in almost 80 per cent of proved cases. Specimens obtained by open synovial biopsy are positive by histology or culture in over 90 per cent of proved cases. Little experience with closed needle biopsy has been published. About one-fifth of the patients with tuberculous arthritis will have a positive synovial fluid acid-fast smear for tubercle bacilli. The tuberculous synovial effusion invariably has an elevated protein level, fair to poor mucin clot formation and usually a low joint fluid sugar level. The synovial fluid white cell count is usually in the range of 10,000 to 20,000 cells/mm^3, but it varies widely. Most fluids exhibited a predominance of polymorphonuclear leukocytes. The importance of bacteriologic or histologic study of synovial fluid and membrane in establishing the diagnosis is emphasized. In general, this disease is different from tuberculous involvement of serous membranes both in the frequency of positive cultures and in the difference in cellular response.

Tuberculosis remains a significant public health and general medical problem despite improved technics of diagnosis and treatment over the last decade. Involvement of joints with the tubercle bacillus is an uncommon but treatable type of arthritis. Diagnosis involves an awareness of the problem and clinical setting, and the utilization of synovial biopsy, synovial fluid analysis and culture. Tuberculous arthritis often is an enigmatic disease [1], and as many as 50 per cent of current cases occur in the absence of signs of pulmonary tuberculosis [2]. The joint symptoms may not be significant and often are present for months or years before the diagnosis is considered. In Walker's review [3] of 18 cases of skeletal tuberculosis, the average duration of symptoms before the clinical diagnosis of tuberculosis was made was 19 months, with a range of from two months to 12 years. As a result, the disease often has a chronic course, and the diagnosis is not made or considered until cartilage or bone destruction is present and joint function compromised.

In recent clinical reviews of tuberculous arthritis [2,4,5], there has been little or no mention of synovial fluid findings, an important diagnostic analysis. It is our purpose herein to present two cases of tuberculous arthritis with synovial fluid analyses and to review the previously published cases in which synovial fluid analyses and synovial biopsy have been performed.

From the Thorndike Memorial Laboratory, The Channing Laboratory, and the Department of Medicine, Boston City Hospital, Boston University School of Medicine, Boston, Massachusetts. Grants in support of these studies have been received from the USPHS, NIAMDD, NIH (AM-04599, TI-AM-5285 and RR-533), the Massachusetts Chapter of the Arthritis Foundation and the Arthritis Foundation. Requests for reprints should be addressed to Dr. Alan S. Cohen, Thorndike 314, Thorndike Memorial Laboratory, Boston City Hospital, Boston, Massachusetts 02118. Manuscript accepted October 16, 1975.

* Present address: Baylor University College of Medicine, Texas Medical Center, Houston, Texas 77025.

CASE REPORTS

Case 1. A 47 year old white woman with chronic alcoholism was admitted complaining of chronic pain in the right knee. Three months before her admission she fell, and since that time noted gradually increasing pain and discomfort in the right knee. She denied any history of fever, weight loss or sputum production. A previous liver biopsy specimen had shown fatty nutritional cirrhosis. One year previously the patient had had a negative old tuberculin (OT) test, but a positive second strength test (250 TU). A chest roentgenogram at that time showed bilateral apical scarring.

Physical examination on admission revealed a swollen, warm and boggy right knee with an obvious effusion. There was a slightly diminished range of motion with pain on flexion and extension. All other joints were normal.

Complete blood count and differential count, urinalysis and electrolyte levels were within normal limits. Chest roentgenogram revealed numerous right apical calcifications and bilateral apical thickening. Arthrocentesis of the right knee yielded 30 ml of serosanguineous fluid with a red cell count of 12,000/mm^3; a white cell count of 40 cells/mm^3 (no differential count was reported); and a total protein content of 4.4 g/100 ml. Synovial fluid sugar was 40 mg/100 ml with a simultaneous blood sugar of 90 mg/100 ml. The mucin was poor. No crystals were seen. Gram stain and bacterial cultures were negative. An acid-fast bacilli smear was not made, but fluid was sent for culture. The patient was discharged with a diagnosis of post-traumatic arthritis of the right knee and was treated symptomatically. Her knee continued to be swollen and slightly painful on walking. Culture of the synovial fluid grew M. tuberculosis, and the patient was readmitted.

The findings on physical examination were unchanged from the previous admission. A roentgenogram of the right knee revealed an effusion without cartilage or bony lesions. A repeat arthrocentesis and a closed needle biopsy of the right knee were performed. Synovial fluid analysis revealed no red cells with a white cell count of 1,100 cells/mm^3 with 20 per cent polymorphonuclear leukocytes and 80 per cent mononuclear cells. The synovial fluid sugar content was 50 mg/100 ml with a simultaneous fasting blood sugar level of 90 mg/100 ml. An acid-fast bacilli smear was negative. The synovial membrane biopsy specimen was reported as showing noncaseating granuloma compatible with tuberculosis. The patient was treated with isoniazid, ethambutol and streptomycin, knee casts (while awake) and physiotherapy. By the end of three months she was ambulating freely without pain, and following hospital discharge has remained asymptomatic for six years.

Comment: The low white cell count in the synovial fluid was against the clinical diagnosis of infectious arthritis, despite the high protein level, poor mucin and blood synovial glucose difference of 50 mg/100 ml. The routine culture grew M. tuberculosis and the subsequent synovial biopsy specimen confirmed the diagnosis.

Case 2. A 20 year old Portuguese man, born in the Cape Verde Islands, was admitted complaining of a mass on his right chest wall. The patient had been in good health until one and a half months prior to admission when he noticed a small lump on the right side of his chest, which had gradually increased in size. There was no history of tuberculosis, fever or back pain.

Physical examination revealed only a 5 by 5 cm cystic, nontender mass which was fixed to the chest wall in the area of the eighth and ninth ribs in the right posterior clavicular line. A chest roentgenogram, urinalysis, complete blood count and differential count, blood urea nitrogen and electrolyte levels were within normal limits. Surgical exploration revealed a necrotic cyst-like mass involving the chest wall. Pathologic sections showed caseating granulomas with positive smears for acid-fast bacilli. The patient was started on isoniazid and ethambutol therapy. A thoraco-lumbar spine film showed destruction of the inferior aspect of the second lumbar vertebrae and the superior aspect of the third lumbar vertebrae with loss of the intervertebral space. An intermediate strength purified protein derivative test was positive. The patient was discharged with the diagnosis of probable Pott's disease and a tuberculous abscess of the right costal margin. Ten days after his hospital discharge, the patient noted the onset of pain in his left hip and was readmitted. The findings on physical examination were unchanged except for the presence of tenderness around the left hip and a limited range of motion in both internal and external rotation. An antero-posterior film of the pelvis revealed bulging of the left hip capsule without bone changes. An intravenous pyelogram revealed marked displacement of the lower pole of the left kidney with anterior displacement of both ureters.

The patient underwent closed arthrocentesis of the left hip and 20 ml of cloudy fluid were obtained. The white cell count was 95,000 cells/mm^3 with 99 per cent polymorphonuclear leukocytes and 1 per cent mononuclear cells. Gram stain and acid-fast bacilli stain were negative; mucin was poor. A repeat aspiration several days later revealed a white cell count of 42,000 cells/mm^3 with a differential count of 80 per cent polymorphonuclear cells, 12 per cent lymphocytes and 8 per cent mononuclear cells. Gram stain, aerobic and anaerobic bacterial cultures were negative. Chemistry studies revealed a sugar level of 50 mg/100 ml with a blood sugar content of 108 mg/100 ml; the total protein content was 6.0 g/100 ml. A closed biopsy attempt was unsuccessful. The clinical impression was that the patient had tuberculosis of the spine with subsequent development of a large paraspinal and psoas abscess. This had dissected around the chest wall to produce the previously noted cold abscess and now had dissected into the area of the left hip joint. Acid-fast bacilli cultures of both synovial fluids were negative; however, culture of the chest wall abscess was positive for M. tuberculosis. The patient was treated with bed rest, isoniazid, ethambutol and streptomycin with gradual improvement. When last seen one year later, he had gained 20 pounds and was asymptomatic.

Comment: The diagnosis was fairly obvious with the presence of a huge psoas abscess which was tuberculous in origin. Despite the high white cell count in the synovial fluid, cultures of acid-fast bacilli were negative.

COMMENTS

Synovial fluid analysis has become a valuable tool for the diagnosis and evaluation of the rheumatic diseases.

TABLE I Synovial Fluid Culture and Biopsy Results in Tuberculous Arthritis

Series	Frequency Positive Synovial Fluid Culture	Laboratory Method	Frequency of Positive Synovial Histology	Frequency of Positive Synovial Biopsy Culture	Frequency of Positive AFB Smears of Synovial Fluid
Kling (1939) [6]	34/44	Guinea pig culture	10*	Unknown	9/44
Holmdahl (1950) [7]	19/22	Guinea pig	50/51	Unknown	Unknown
Ropes, Bauer (1953) [8]	22/29	Guinea pig culture	13/13	Unknown	Unknown
Hald (1964) [9]	Unknown	Unknown	85/90†	137/141†	Unknown
Razdan et al. (1966) [10]	Unknown	Unknown	33/39	Unknown	Unknown
Friedman (1970) [11]	13*	Culture	9/9	Unknown	1/13
Berney et al. (1972) [4]	15/18	Culture	19/20	3/8	4/15
Present 2 cases (1975)	1/2	Culture	1/1	Not done	0/2
Totals	91/115 (79%)		210/223 (94%)	140/149 (94%)	14/74 (19%)

NOTE: AFB = acid-fact bacilli.
* Not included in totals, as denominator is not known.
† Included only cases in which biopsy was obtained prior to therapy; also includes small number of specimens from patients with vertebral tuberculosis.

Despite the large numbers of patients with tuberculous arthritis in the prechemotherapeutic era, very few were analyzed in this fashion.

The general appearance of the joint fluid in tuberculous arthritis depends on the stage of the disease. In tuberculous synovitis (without bone or cartilage involvement), the synovial fluid has the general appearance of any chronic effusion. It is xanthochromic, and (unlike that in Case 1) typically is not hemorrhagic. As the disease progresses with bone and joint destruction, the synovial fluid may develop a yellowish-white, almost gelatinous appearance that does not settle out into layers even with centrifugation [6]. This may represent degenerated cartilage or soft tissue debris.

The most sensitive method of clinical diagnosis of tuberculous arthritis has been the open joint biopsy. The incidence of pyogenic complications or sinus tract formation with this technic was very low even before good tuberculosis chemotherapy [7,10]. Seven of the most detailed series of biopsy and culture results from the literature are listed in Table I. Only those series in which it was possible to determine the relative frequency of positive biopsy or culture results have been included. The combined series were all open biopsies, and except for one of Berney's cases [4] and our Case 1, no detailed experience with closed needle biopsy has been published.

Of 223 cases of subsequently proved tuberculous arthritis in which synovial biopsies were performed, joint histology was positive in 210 (94 per cent). This was defined as caseating or noncaseating granulomas, with or without positive acid-fast smears or culture. Hence, even with open surgical biopsy, 6 per cent of cases will be missed if one relies on histopathology alone. It is also well known that other diseases may produce synovial granulomas. Any of the fungal joint diseases may produce a histologic picture indistinguishable from tuberculosis. There have been several reports of atypical mycobacteria producing a destructive arthritis, some with granulomatous inflammation [12,13]. Sarcoidosis and, on occasion, erythema nodosum may produce noncaseating granulomas of the synovium [14]. Traumatic fat necrosis, brucellosis, Crohn's disease and foreign body giant cell reaction are other possible causes of granulomatous synovitis. It is possible that some of the diagnoses in the past which depended on histopathology alone were inaccurate. The value of acid-fast smears of synovial biopsy specimen seems limited. In the two small series in which it was reported [4,11], histologic sections were positive in only three of 29 cases (10 per cent).

Little emphasis, except for Hald's series [9], was placed on culture results of the biopsy tissue, and most biopsy specimens reported as positive were based on histology alone. In the 149 cases in which synovial tissue was cultured, cultures or guinea pig inoculations for tuberculosis were positive in 94 per cent. This is higher than the culture returns of biopsy material for pleural tuberculosis, which is positive in only 60 to 80 per cent of proved cases [15,16]. The higher incidence of both biopsy and culture results may be explained in part because all synovial biopsies were open surgical biopsies in which both selection and size of the biopsy specimens were better. The current experience with pleural tuberculosis has been with closed needle biopsy, with no selection and smaller tissue samples.

The incidence of positive synovial fluid cultures in patients with proved tuberculous arthritis was 79 per

TABLE II Synovial Fluid Total Protein in Tuberculous Arthritis

Series	Fluids (no.)	Range (g/100 ml)	Mean Value (g/100 ml)
Keefer et al. (1934) [22]	6	4.3–5.5	5.0
Ropes, Bauer (1953) [8]	9	4.1–6.3	5.3
Walczak, Stonawski (1972) [23]	8	3.5–4.7	4.1
This series (1975)	2	4.4 and 6.0	5.2
Totals	25	3.5–6.3	4.8

cent (Table I). The incidence seemed comparable in the older studies using guinea pig inoculation [6,7] and modern culture methods [4]. There were no attempts in any of the series to correlate frequency of positive cultures with duration of infection, white cell count or quantity of fluid cultured. With both pleural and peritoneal tuberculosis it has been suggested that the incidence of positive cultures is significantly increased by culture of larger quantities of fluid [17,18]. Thus, although there is a high yield from culture of synovial fluid, in about 20 per cent of the cases biopsy will be required to make the diagnosis of tuberculous arthritis. In many instances a wait of four to six weeks for synovial culture results is inappropriate; these patients should undergo a synovial biopsy when tuberculosis is suspected.

Acid-fast smears of the synovial fluid were reported as positive in 14 of 74 cases (19 per cent). This incidence of positive smears is higher than is usually seen with effusions secondary to pleural, pericardial or peritoneal tuberculosis. Despite the fact that these latter serous membranes are often diffusely involved by tuberculous inflammation with viable organisms, in only 5 to 10 per cent of effusions will the acid-fast smear be positive [18,19], and generally in less than 50 per cent

TABLE III Synovial Fluid Glucose Values in Tuberculous Arthritis

Series	Joint Fluid Sugar <50 mg/100 ml	Blood-Synovial Fluid Glucose Difference ≥40 mg/100 ml
Keefer et al. (1934) [22]	0/10	0/10
Ropes, Bauer (1953) [8]	19/24	19/24
Garg et al. (1972) [24]	11/15	11/15
Present cases (1975)	1/2	2/2
Totals	31/51 (61%)	32/51 (63%)

of effusions are cultures positive [16,19,20]. The mechanism of production of the effusion in tuberculous involvement of these serous membranes is thought to be in part a hypersensitivity reaction to tuberculoprotein which leaks into the serous space. This would explain why large quantities of fluid are often present in the absence of clinically detectable infection. The synovial membrane is different histologically and functionally from the serous membranes [21]. It also appears from this review to behave somewhat differently from other tuberculous infections in that the incidence of positive acid-fast smears (19 per cent) and joint fluid culture (79 per cent) of the effusions are much higher. This would also suggest that performance of the acid-fast smear is useful in tuberculous arthritis and may allow an early diagnosis.

The cumulative cases in which synovial fluid protein was analyzed is small, i.e., 25 cases (Table II). The protein content of normal synovial fluid is under 2.0 g/100 ml and usually represents 25 to 30 per cent of the total serum protein. Any protein level of over 2.5 g/100 ml can be regarded as abnormal [21]. Elevated protein levels in tuberculous arthritis seem to be a uniform finding. No measured protein level in this series was under 3.5 g/100 ml and the majority were in the range of 4 to 6 g/100 ml. It is of interest in Case 1 that despite the very low white cell count, the protein level was still elevated. Walczak and Stonawski [23] studied the electrophoresis of joint fluid in eight cases of proved tuberculous arthritis and found the results comparable to those of simultaneous studies of serum in relative concentrations. The levels of complement were not reported.

Most of the current series of synovial fluid analysis in the rheumatic diseases have utilized the mucin clot formation to evaluate synovial fluid mucin. This involves grading the mucin clot formed by the addition of 2 per cent acetic acid as "good," "fair," "poor" and "very poor." Garg et al.'s [24] is the only known series that evaluated mucin clot formation in tuberculous arthritis. These investigators reported that in five of 15 cases mucin was "fair" and in 10 of 15 it was "poor." In our two cases, mucin clot formation was "poor." This may be a clue to suspect inflammatory or infectious disease in those cases in which the white cell count are in a noninflammatory range. This has previously been utilized to help in diagnosing early rheumatoid arthritis in the presence of low white cell counts in the synovial fluid.

The joint fluid sugar level has been accepted as "low" in tuberculosis by many investigators, although it is striking that only slightly more than 50 cases could be found (Table III). The normal glucose level in synovial fluid is usually within 10 to 20 mg/100 ml of the blood sugar level in the fasting state [8,21,30]. In 61 per cent

TABLE IV Synovial Fluid White Cell Counts and Differential Counts in Tuberculous Arthritis

Series	No. of Fluids	White Blood Cell Range (per mm³)	Polymorphonuclears (%)	Average White Blood Cell (per mm³)	Average Polymorphonuclears (%)	Cases with Polymorphonuclear Predominance (no.)
Keefer et al. (1934) [22]	10	6,500–110,000	59–93	28,258	73	9/10
Kling (1939) [6]	16	1,500–136,000	10–84	16,200	51	—
Ropes, Bauer (1953) [8]	28	2,500–105,000	18–96	19,470	60	—
Garg et al. (1972) [24]	15	1,000–20,000	—	—	—	12/15
Present 2 cases (1975)	2	40–95,000	20–99	—	—	1/2
Totals	71	40–136,000	10–99	—	—	22/27

(31 of 51) of cases of tuberculous arthritis, the joint fluid sugar level was less than 50 mg/100 ml, and in 63 per cent (32 of 51) of cases, a blood-synovial glucose difference of 40 mg/100 ml or more was demonstrated. In Ropes and Bauer's series [8] of comparative blood-synovial glucose differences in all the common rheumatic diseases, only septic joints due to bacterial infection and rheumatoid arthritis showed more than an isolated case with this glucose difference. Keefer et al. [22] attempted to correlate the synovial glucose level with the cell count, and in a small series was able to show that high synovial white cell counts tended to be associated with lower joint fluid sugar levels in the absence of infection. Ropes and Bauer [8] also demonstrated that after a meal, the synovial fluid demonstrates the same increase of glucose as serum. There is a lag period of several hours, however, so that the level in synovial fluid initially is lower than that in blood, and then for several hours may remain elevated after the blood sugar level has returned to normal. In Keefer et al.'s series [22] of tuberculous arthritis in which no attempt was made to keep the patients fasting, many of the synovial fluid sugar levels were higher than the blood sugar levels. It raises the possibility that a higher percentage of blood-synovial glucose differences might have been observed if the patients were fasting.

The range of synovial white cell counts in the reported series was extremely wide. Counts were as low as 1,000 and as high as 136,000 cells/mm³ (Table IV). Our first case is interesting in that the white cell count was the lowest (40 cells) reported in tuberculous arthritis. The average white cell count ranged from 10,000 to 20,000 cells, but on occasion it rose to the range usually regarded as "septic," "bacterial," with counts of greater than 50,000 to 100,000 cells/mm³. The differential counts were surprising. In all four major series (totaling 69 cases) in which differential white cell counts were examined, polymorphonuclear leukocytes predominated. In the specific cases in which it was looked for, there was a majority of polymorphonuclear leukocytes in 22 of 27 cases (82 per cent). However, in very few cases were polymorphonuclear leukocytes over 90 per cent, the usual differential finding in septic joints secondary to pyogenic bacterial infection. Several investigators [8,26] commented that early in the disease with only "synovial" involvement, the synovial white cell counts were low and tended to be lymphocytic, but as the disease became more chronic (often with cartilage and bone involvement) the white cell count and percentage of polymorphonuclear leukocytes rose dramatically. There was no clinical documentation of this impression, and in the series reviewed (Table IV) no attempt was made to correlate the white cell count and differential count with chronicity or extent of the disease. This polymorphonuclear predominance is different from tuberculous involvement of the serous membranes, as chronic tuberculosis is almost always associated with a predominance of lymphocytes. This, in part, may reflect the generally higher white cell counts and more advanced disease often seen with tuberculous arthritis, for patients with clinical "empyema" of the serous membranes with obviously much higher white cell counts also tend to have a predominance of polymorphonuclear leukocytes. In summary, the white cell count and differential count were not helpful in making a specific diagnosis, but more importantly, one could not exclude tuberculosis on the basis of synovial white cell count or numbers of polymorphonuclear leukocytes present.

No single test of synovial fluid was diagnostic of tuberculosis except for a positive acid-fast bacilli smear or culture. The findings of a chronic inflammatory joint fluid with a high white cell count, poor mucin clot formation and a low joint fluid sugar level in the absence of bacterial infection or rheumatoid arthritis were highly suggestive of tuberculosis. It should be pointed out that all these findings, including monoarticular arthritis, are consistent with rheumatoid arthritis as well. For these reasons, synovial fluid culture and biopsy (with culture) are essential diagnostic procedures. Synovial biopsy remains the single most effective means of diagnosis of this disease.

REFERENCES

1. Hunt DD: Problems in diagnosing osteoarticular tuberculosis. JAMA 190: 95, 1964.
2. Davidson PT, Horowitz I: Skeletal tuberculosis. A review with patient presentations and discussion. Am J Med 48: 77, 1970.
3. Walker GF: Failure of early recognition of skeletal tuberculosis. Br Med J 1: 682, 1968.
4. Berney S, Goldstein M, Bishko F: Clinical and diagnostic features of tuberculous arthritis. Am J Med 53: 36, 1972.
5. LaFond EM: Analysis of adult skeletal tuberculosis. J Bone Joint Surg 40A: 346, 1958.
6. Kling DH: The Synovial Membrane and the Synovial Fluid, Los Angeles, Med Press, 1938.
7. Holmdahl HC: Tuberculosis of the knee. Acta Orthop Scand 20: 19, 1950.
8. Ropes MW, Bauer W: Synovial Fluid Changes in Joint Disease, Cambridge, Mass., Harvard University Press, 1953.
9. Hald J: The value of histological and bacteriological examination in tuberculosis of bones and joints. Acta Orthop Scand 35: 91, 1964.
10. Razdan AN, Bhargava KS, Ram A: Synovial biopsy in osteoarticular tuberculosis. J Indian Medical Assoc 46: 422, 1966.
11. Friedman B, Kapur VN: The management of tuberculosis of the knee joint. Am Rev Respir Dis 101: 265, 1970.
12. Klinenberg JR, Grimley PM, Seegmiller JE: Destructive polyarthritis due to a photochromogenic mycobacterium. N Engl J Med 272: 190, 1965.
13. Karlson AG, Bickel WH, Soule EH: Destructive arthritis of the knee associated with a skotochromogenic acid-fast organism. Surgery 51: 334, 1962.
14. Spilberg I, Siltzbach LE, McEwen C: The arthritis of sarcoidosis. Arthritis Rheumat 12: 126, 1969.
15. Levine H, Metzger W, Lacera D, Kay L: Diagnosis of tuberculous pleurisy by culture of pleural biopsy specimen, Arch Int Med 126: 269, 1970.
16. Berger HW: Tuberculous pleurisy. Chest 63: 88, 1973.
17. Barber LM, Mazzadi L, Deakins DD: Glucose level in pleural fluid as a diagnostic aid. Dis Chest 31: 680, 1957.
18. Singh MM, Bhargava AN, Jain KP: Tuberculous peritonitis. N Engl J Med 281: 1091, 1969.
19. Schepers GWH: Tuberculous pericarditis. Am J Cardiol 9: 248, 1962.
20. Sochocky S: Tuberculous peritonitis. A review of 100 Cases. Am Rev Respir Dis 95: 398, 1967.
21. Cohen AS, Brandt K, Krey PR: Synovial fluid. Laboratory Diagnostic Procedures of the Rheumatic Diseases (Cohen AS, ed), Boston, Little Brown & Co., 1975 p 1.
22. Keefer CS, Myers WK, Holmes WF Jr: Characteristics of the synovial fluid in various types of arthritis. Arch Intern Med 54: 872, 1934.
23. Walczak Z, Stonawski Z: Phosphatase activity and protein content in the articular exudate and in blood serum. Polish Med J 9: 815, 1972.
24. Garg ML, Kumar R, Chugh TD, Maini PS: Value of synovial fluid analysis as a diagnostic tool in arthritis. Ind J Med Res 60: 233, 1972.
25. Hollander JL, McCarty DJ Jr: Arthritis and Allied Conditions, 8th ed, Philadelphia, Lea & Febiger, 1972.

Therapy for Disseminated Coccidioidomycosis with Transfer Factor from a Related Donor

RUSSELL W. STEELE, M.D.
BARRY E. SIEGER, M.D.
THEODORE R. McNITT, M.D.
LAYNE O. GENTRY, M.D.
WILLIAM L. MOORE, Jr., M.D.
Fort Sam Houston, Texas

A 17 year old caucasian woman in whom disseminated coccidioidomycosis developed with culture positive meningitis during her third trimester of pregnancy was treated with amphotericin B and subsequently with transfer factor prepared from her father's peripheral lymphocytes. Clinical response and in vivo and in vitro immunologic data indicated that this transfer factor afforded a significant contribution to her survival whereas previous therapy with transfer factor from an unrelated donor provided only transient immunologic reactivity. This experience suggests that transfer factor prepared from a related donor with positive responses to C. immitis may be more efficacious than that prepared from an unrelated donor.

Coccidioidomycosis, if contracted during pregnancy, is associated with a much higher risk of dissemination and a more severe prognosis than the disease in a nonpregnant patient [1–3]. Moreover, both the incidence of dissemination and mortality increase with increasing gestation [1,2]. Prior to the use of amphotericin B, mortality approached 100 per cent when disseminated coccidioidomycosis developed during the third trimester of pregnancy; and even with the introduction of amphotericin B mortality has remained high [1–4].

In the patient we describe disseminated coccidioidomycosis developed with culture positive meningitis during her last trimester of pregnancy, and therefore she presented with a minimal chance of survival. The patient was treated with amphotericin B, transfer factor from an unrelated donor, and later transfer factor prepared from her father. Sustained remission has been achieved with 15 months post-treatment follow-up now available. It was believed both by clinical response and by in vivo and in vitro laboratory data that the transfer factor prepared from her father afforded a significant contribution to her survival.

From the Section of Infectious Diseases, Departments of Medicine and Pediatrics, Brooke Army Medical Center, Fort Sam Houston, Texas. This work was supported in part by research grant No. C-42-74 from the Clinical Investigation Unit of Brooke Army Medical Center. The opinions or assertions contained herein are the private ones of the authors and are not to be interpreted as official or reflecting the view of the Department of the Army. Requests for reprints should be addressed to Dr. Russell W. Steele, Infectious Diseases and Immunology, Department of Pediatrics, Brooke Army Medical Center, Fort Sam Houston, Texas 78234. Manuscript accepted October 22, 1975.

MATERIALS AND METHODS

Lymphocyte Blastogenesis. In vitro determination of cellular immunity to coccidioidin, as well as other control antigens, was accomplished by measuring lymphocyte blastogenesis following incubation with the antigens under investigation. Coccidioidin was obtained as a commercial lot from Cutter Laboratories and this preparation was dialyzed six times against 200 volumes of 0.15 M sodium chloride for 48 hours to remove preservatives. The material was stored at −20°C until used. Maximum in vitro stimulation of lymphocytes was obtained with a 1:5000 dilution; sensitivity of this material was examined in a previous communication [5]. Lymphocytes were separated from 5 ml of peripheral whole blood by a modification of the Hypaque-Ficoll gradient technic. The cell suspension was washed twice in culture medium and the lymphocytes were adjusted to a concentration of 2×10^6 ml in RPMI 1640 medium with Hepes buffer containing 100 units of penicillin/ml, 100 μg of streptomycin/ml and 20 per cent autologous plasma. Using a biopipet, 0.1 ml of the lymphocyte suspension (2×10^5 lymphocytes) was mixed with an equal volume of antigenic material in one well of sterile flat-bottomed microtest plates. All cultures were prepared in triplicate along with control cultures containing lymphocytes incubated with medium alone. The plates were covered with sterile plastic lids, and cultures were incubated for five days. Twenty-four hours prior to harvest, 0.05 ml of RPMI 1640 medium containing 1 μCi of tritiated(^{3}H)-thymidine was added to each well. A harvesting apparatus previously described [6] was employed for the separation of reacting cells on glass fiber filters, for washing of these cells and for recovery of the radioactive material incorporated by stimulated lymphocytes. The glass fiber discs were then dried in an oven, and transferred to vials containing 5 ml of scintillation fluid for counting in a Beckman liquid scintillation spectrometer. The average counts/minute (cpm) of triplicate samples were determined and results were expressed as a blastogenic index: cpm of ^{3}H-thymidine uptake for lymphocytes incubated with antigen divided by uptake following incubation with medium alone:

$$\text{blastogenic index} = \frac{\text{cpm for lymphocytes + coccidioidin}}{\text{cpm for lymphocytes + medium}}$$

Based on previous studies, a blastogenic index ≥ 3.0 was considered a positive response.

Transfer Factor. Dialyzable transfer factor was prepared and purified by the methods of Lawrence and Al-Askari [7]. Approximately 500 cc of whole blood were obtained by venipuncture, and lymphocytes were separated from the cell pack using a Hypaque-Ficoll gradient, centrifuging at 4°C to maintain optimal recovery of transfer factor. The lymphocytes were freeze-thawed in the presence of DNase 10 times, and subsequently dialyzed and concentrated by lyophilization. Potency was confirmed by passive transfer of 0.1 ml intradermally into negative human recipients followed in 72 hours by skin testing in the same site as the transfer factor injection. By this method, multiple antigens were examined with only those which showed positive skin reactivity in the donor being positive in the recipients. Induration in a previously negative recipient was greater than 5 mm to a 1:10 dilution of coccidioidin for both transfer factor preparations.

CASE REPORT

Our patient was a 17 year old caucasian housewife, living in North Carolina. One week prior to delivery of her first child, she experienced fever, malaise and shortness of breath which spontaneously remitted. She had an uncomplicated labor and delivered a normal infant. On the first postpartum day, fever developed with temperature to 103.8°F. The clinical impression was endometritis, and sodium ampicillin therapy was instituted followed by a reported defervescence of fever. One week later, she again became febrile and at this time was noted to have bilateral pulmonary parenchymal nodular infiltrates and splenomegaly. She was treated with sodium cephalothin without response. Because of persistence of fever and headache, a lumbar puncture was performed. The cerebrospinal fluid contained 49 white blood cells, 39 neutrophils and 100 lymphocytes; protein and glucose were normal. On historic review, it was found that during her second trimester she had traveled by car to California, during which time she had spent 2 hours in the San Joaquin Valley area. During the third trimester of pregnancy, she had received a package of clothing with several articles wrapped in dusty newspaper sent from relatives in the San Joaquin Valley. Either incident might have represented fomite transmission of C. immitis. A repeat lumbar puncture two weeks postpartum revealed 833 white blood cells, 71 per cent neutrophils, 29 per cent lymphocytes, glucose of 24 mg/100 ml, and protein 89 mg/100 ml. Complement fixation titers to C. immitis were positive in this cerebrospinal fluid at titers of 1:20 with a concomitant serum titer of 1:320. C. immitis was also cultured from this sample of spinal fluid. The patient was transferred to Brooke Army Medical Center for further evaluation and treatment. On arrival, examination documented the findings of intermittent disorientation, papilledema, pupillary asymmetry, right-sided central facial weakness, right ninth cranial nerve palsy, weakness of the lower right extremity and clonus of the lower left extremity. A four vessel cerebral arteriogram revealed dilatation of the lateral ventricles. Skin tests to monilia, mumps and tetanus toxoid demonstrated greater than 10 mm induration but a skin test for C. immitis (coccidioidin U.S.P., 1:10, Cutter Laboratories, Berkely, Calif.) was negative. In vitro lymphocyte blastogenic responses to the mitogens, phytohemagglutinin, pokeweed, concanavalin A were positive as were the responses to the antigens, monilia, mumps and tetanus toxoid. In vitro lymphocyte blastogenic responses to coccidioidin were negative.

The patient was started on amphotericin B intravenously, increasing the dose to 30 mg three times per week. Large doses were associated with marked idiosyncratic reactions, especially hypotension. Intravenous therapy was continued for 10 months at which time she had received a total dose of 4,500 mg. The administration of amphotericin B was also started intracisternally, and the dose was gradually increased to 0.3 mg twice weekly. She received a total of 6.7 mg over four months by this route. Attempts to use an Ommya reservoir for intraventricular therapy failed because of infection of one reservoir with Staphylococcus epidermidis and malfunction of a second apparatus. Despite the schedule of amphotericin B therapy, the patient's condition progressively deteriorated. Although her cerebrospinal fluid cultures of C. immitis became negative following institution of amphotericin B therapy, her complement fixation titers in serum stabilized at 1:128 and in the cerebrospinal fluid at 1:8. Because of this poor clinical response and the persistent antibody titers, it was elected to treat the patient with human dialyzable transfer factor. The donor of the transfer factor had had pulmonary

TABLE I In Vivo and In Vitro Evaluation of Cellular Immunity During Two Courses of Transfer Factor Therapy

	1973				1974								
	Nov. 2–Dec. 15	Dec. 15	Dec. 22	Dec. 29	Jan. 5	Jan. 8–Feb. 1	Feb. 1	Feb. 7	Feb. 14	Mar.	Apr.	May–Aug.	Sept.
Therapy													
Transfer factor	–	+	+	+	+	–	+	+	+	–	–	–	–
Amphotericin B		Unrelated donor					Related donor						
intravenous	←	—	—	—	—	—	—	—	—	—	—	—	→
intracisternal	←	—	—	—	—	—	—	→					
Skin tests*													
Cocci	0	7	4	0	0	0	3	8	17	>15	>15	>15	>15
Monilia	13	17	ND	11	ND	12	15	ND	12	>15	>15	>15	>15
Blastogenesis†													
Cocci	0.6–1.1	13.7	5.3	2.6	1.9	0.9–1.5	8.9	11.2	5.5	5.7–11.4	13.3	9.0–15.1	10.9
Monilia	3.8–10.7	8.1	8.5	11.8	7.4	6.7–9.9	12.0	17.7	10.8	9.4–16.8	15.2	8.5–14.7	17.2
Antibody													
Serum	1:320–1:160	1:128	1:128	ND	1:128	ND	1:128	ND	ND	1:32	1:16	1:16	1:8
Cerebrospinal fluid	1:20	1:8	1:8	ND	1:8	ND	1:8	ND	ND	0	0	0	0
Cerebrospinal culture	+	–	–	ND	–	ND	–	ND	ND	–	–	–	–

NOTE: Rules indicate duration of therapy. ND = not done. Skin test reactions to coccidioidin 1:10 for the donors were: unrelated donor 37 mm induration, related donor 43 mm and to monilia 1:100 were: unrelated donor 21 mm, related donor 17 mm.

* Skin tests were applied 72 hours after the dose of transfer factor was given and were measured as millimeters of induration at 48 hours.

† Expressed as a blastogenic index: cpm of ^{3}H-thymidine uptake for lymphocytes incubated with antigen divided by uptake following incubation with medium alone.

coccidioidomycosis at age 13. He had remained skin test positive and when intradermally tested with soluble coccidioidin reacted with 8 mm of induration using a 1:1000 dilution and 37 mm of induration with a 1:10 dilution. These skin tests were recorded at 48 hours.

The patient was given 1 unit (equivalent to 1 × 10^9 lymphocytes) of transfer factor subcutaneously at weekly intervals for four consecutive weeks (Table I). Three days after receiving the first unit she was retested, at which time the skin test response to 1:10 coccidioidin demonstrated induration of 6 by 7 mm. In vitro lymphocyte blastogenic responses increased from a blastogenic index of 1.07 to 13.7 at this time. These responses, however, were transient, and both in vivo and in vitro measurements reverted to negative despite the administration of additional transfer .actor. The patient deteriorated neurologically as a result of obstructive hydrocephalus and a ventriculoperitoneal shunt was placed.

Three months after her admission, it was learned that her father had had pulmonary coccidioidomycosis at age 13. He was strongly positive to a 1:10 dilution of coccidioidin intradermally reacting with 43 mm of induration. Dialyzable transfer factor was prepared from the patient's father as previously described and the patient was given 1 unit subcutaneously each week for three consecutive weeks. The coccidioidin skin tests after the first unit were positive at 8 mm of induration and following the third unit increased to 17 mm of induration. Her blastogenic index after administration of the first unit increased from 1.45 to 8.9. Both the skin test and the blastogenic index remained positive over the eight months they were followed. Following therapy with transfer factor from her father, the patient experienced gradual but progressive improvement over four months. Her condition then stabilized and no further significant improvement occurred over an additional 15 months of observation.

COMMENTS

The more severe prognosis for coccidioidomycosis in the pregnant patient is most likely attributable to the known transient depression of cell mediated immunity demonstrated during gestation [8]; the risk of dissemination then increases to an estimated 20 per cent, 100 times that of the nonpregnant white woman and three times that of the nonpregnant black [2]. A majority of reported cases have occurred during the third trimester [1–3]. The exact mechanism of this maternal response remains poorly understood but is apparently directed to protect the developing fetus from rejection. Such tolerance during pregnancy may carry over to newly introduced foreign antigens such as fungal antigens with resultant proliferation of suppressor T cells and subsequent depression of cell mediated immune reactions to the invading organisms [9]. Accepting this hypothesis, the role of immunotherapeutic products like transfer factor can better be explained. Another suggested mechanism is the elaboration of an inhibitory factor into the serum during gestation which depresses cellular immunity [10]; in the present studies, no such factor could be demonstrated since C. immitis blastogenic assays for known positive controls were not decreased in the presence of the patient's serum, nor were her responses any different when comparing AB positive serum or fetal calf serum to autologous serum as the medium supplement.

The present case illustrates the associations between pregnancy, disseminated coccidioidomycosis and defects in cellular immunity. In this patient the defect appeared specific to C. immitis since in vivo and in vitro reactivity to other fungal, viral and bacterial antigens as well as nonspecific in vitro stimulation with mitogens was normal.

A therapeutic effect was achieved when cocci-positive transfer factor from a related donor was combined with amphotericin B. No apparent clinical response and only transient conversion of cellular immune responses was seen with amphotericin B and cocci-positive transfer factor from the unrelated donor during a four month period of observation.

It is of course not certain that the clinical benefit was related primarily to the second series of transfer factor but most evidence, as observed, suggests this. This question then remains whether the fact that the transfer factor donor was related to the recipient was a significant factor in success of therapy. The skin test and in vitro responses of the two transfer factor donors were comparable and therefore indicate that potency of transfer factor as judged by donor responses alone could not account for the differences in efficacy.

A number of clinical reports have attested to the efficacy of transfer factor for severe coccidioidomycosis as well as for other infectious processes such as chronic mucocutaneous candidiasis, and available information for transfer factor therapy has been summarized previously [11]. A recent review from the Coccidioidomycosis Cooperative Treatment Group (CCTG) represents the largest series of patients, 42, treated with transfer factor for coccidioidomycosis [12] and the present case was included in this study. Clinical and immunologic responses were variable for the 42 patients, but data did suggest clinical efficacy of transfer factor. More definitive information hopefully will be obtained by the CCTG in a controlled prospective trial of placebo transfer factor versus coccidioidomycosis positive transfer factor currently in progress.

Finally, in studies employing transfer factor as immunotherapy for patients with osteogenic sarcoma, donors with similar environmental exposure appear preferable, and these are often relatives [13]. The present report suggests that both the environmental exposure to the agent, in this case C. immitis, as well as the donor being related to the recipient of transfer factor may be of importance for efficacy of transfer factor therapy.

REFERENCES

1. Smale LE, Waechter KG: Dissemination of coccidioidomycosis in pregnancy. Am J Obstet Gynecol 107: 356, 1970.
2. Harris RE: Coccidioidomycosis complicating pregnancy. Report of 3 cases and review of the literature. Obstet Gynecol 28: 401, 1966.
3. Hadsall FJ, Acquarelli MJ: Disseminated coccidioidomycosis presenting as facial granulomas in pregnancy: a report of two cases and a review of the literature. The Laryngoscope 83: 51, 1973.
4. Pappagianis D: Personal communication, 1975.
5. Steele RW, Cannady PB Jr, Moore WC Jr, Gentry LO: Skin test and blastogenic responses to sporothrix schenckii. J Clin Invest 57: 156, 1976.
6. Steele RW, Hensen SA, Vincent MM, Fuccillo DA, Bellanti JA: A ^{51}Cr microassay technique for cell-mediated immunity to viruses. J Immunol 110: 1502, 1973.
7. Lawrence HS: Transfer factor. Adv Immunol 11: 195, 1969.
8. Thong YH, Steele RW, Vincent MM, Hensen SA, Bellanti JA: Impaired in-vitro cell-mediated immunity to rubella virus during pregnancy. N Engl J Med 289: 604, 1973.
9. Kantor FS: Infection, anergy and cell-mediated immunity. N Engl J Med 292: 629, 1975.
10. Ceppellini R, Bonnard GD, Coppo F: Mixed leukocyte cultures and HL-A antigens. I. Reactivity of young fetuses, newborns and mothers at delivery. Transplant Proc 3: 58, 1971.
11. Kirkpatrick CH, Gallin JI: Treatment of infectious and neoplastic diseases with transfer factor. Oncology 29: 46, 1974.
12. Graybill JR: Transfer factor in coccidioidomycosis. Clin Res 23: 304, 1975.
13. Levin AS, Byers VS, Fudenberg HH, Wybran J, Hackett AJ, Johnston JO, Spitler LE: Osteogenic sarcoma: immunologic parameters before and during immunotherapy with tumor-specific transfer factor. J Clin Invest 55: 487, 1975.

Allopurinol Hypersensitivity

Granular Deposition of IgM at the Dermal-Epidermal Junction

PETER D. UTSINGER, M.D.
WILLIAM J. YOUNT, M.D.
Chapel Hill, North Carolina

A patient with allopurinol hypersensitivity, manifested by fever, lymphadenopathy and a severe erythematous, morbilliform, maculopapular rash was studied. On immunofluorescent staining of the patient's skin, heavy granular deposits of immunoglobulin M (IgM) were found at the dermal-epidermal junction. Transformation of the patient's lymphocytes could not be effected by a variety of combinations of allopurinol, allopurinol metabolites and serum. These data suggested that the hypersensitivity reaction caused by allopurinol had immune complex deposition as the central feature in pathogenesis. The predominance of IgM may provide a distinctive feature from the deposits generally seen in systemic and discoid lupus erythematosus.

In the 12 years since its introduction, allopurinol has become the most commonly employed drug for the control of hyperuricemia. In about 10 per cent of the patients who receive allopurinol untoward reactions develop, most commonly diarrhea, abdominal pain or skin rash [1,2]. In most cases, these complications are short-lived and of little clinical importance. In a small number of patients, however, a severe clinical syndrome develops, consisting of dermatitis, fever, eosinophilia, renal insufficiency and hepatitis, suggestive of a hypersensitivity reaction [3–5]. The mechanism of the suspected hypersensitivity reaction is unknown. Herein, we report our immunologic studies on a patient with severe allopurinol hypersensitivity, and document the presence of granular cutaneous deposits of immunoglobulin M (IgM) and, to a lesser degree, immunoglobulin G (IgG) at the dermal-epidermal junction. The predominance of IgM may provide a distinguishing feature from the deposits characteristic of systemic lupus erythematosus (SLE). An attempt to elute deposits with excess antigen was unsuccessful but may provide an approach to immunochemical diagnosis.

CASE REPORT

The patient is a 57 year old white woman. In 1952, she was found to be hypertensive, but she received no consistent treatment until 1969. At that time, congestive heart failure, glycosuria and an elevated fasting blood sugar level were noted. She was treated with a low-salt, diabetic diet, chlorthiazide (500 mg twice a day) and digoxin (0.5 mg orally every day). She did well until March 1975, when she stopped taking her digoxin and chlorthiazide. Five days later, she noted shortness of breath and came to the hospital. On physical examination, the blood pressure was 180/70 mm Hg. There were inspiratory rales, bilateral pretibial edema to the knees, and the liver edge was palpable 5 cm below the right costal margin. No tophi were palpable. The white blood cell

From the Division of Clinical Immunology and Rheumatology, Department of Medicine and Bacteriology (Immunology), University of North Carolina, School of Medicine, Chapel Hill, North Carolina 27514. This study was supported in part by Grants AI 10327, AM 15866, HL 03650 from the U.S. Public Health Service, a Grant from The Arthritis Foundation, The Regional Medical Program and The Jefferson-Pilot Foundation. Requests for reprints should be addressed to Dr. Peter D. Utsinger, Division of Clinical Immunology and Rheumatology, Department of Medicine, University of North Carolina, Chapel Hill, North Carolina 27514. Manuscript accepted October 16, 1975.

count was 9,000/mm^3, 78 per cent were polymorphonuclear leukocytes, 20 per cent lymphocytes, and 2 per cent monocytes. The hematocrit value was 31 per cent. The serum blood urea nitrogen was 34 mg/100 ml, serum creatinine 1.4 mg/100 ml and creatinine clearance 62 ml/min. The uric acid level was 12.1 mg/100 ml. The patient was digitalized and discharged on a daily regimen of digoxin, 0.125 mg, and furosemide, 80 mg. Despite the absence of a history of gout, the administration of allopurinol, 300 mg daily, was started on March 26, 1975. On April 4, 1975, there were no signs of congestive heart failure and the serum uric acid was 2.9 mg/100 ml. On April 25, she noted a pruritic rash and fever. On physical examination, the temperature was 103°F orally, blood pressure 120/50 mm Hg, pulse rate 82 beats/min and regular, and respirations 12. There was an erythematous, morbilliform, maculopapular rash over the trunk and extremities, and cervical, axillary and inguinal lymphadenopathy. There was no hepatomegaly, no rales and no edema. Allopurinol hypersensitivity was suspected, and the administration of both allopurinol and furosemide was discontinued. The white blood cell count was 13,700/mm^3 (36 per cent polymorphonuclear leukocytes, 38 per cent eosinophils, 2 per cent basophils, 14 per cent lymphocytes, 8 per cent monocytes and 1 per cent atypical lymphocytes). The serum glutamic oxaloacetic transaminase (SGOT) was 80 (normal 8 to 40 U/ml), serum glutamic pyruvic transaminase (SGPT) 77 (normal 8 to 35 U/ml), lactic dehydrogenase (LDH) 676 (normal 100 to 350 U/ml), alkaline phosphatase 5.4 (normal 2 to 6 U/ml) and creatinine phosphokinase 1.2 U/ml. A lupus erythematosus cell preparation and tests for antinuclear antibodies were negative. The patient was treated with 1 per cent hydrocortisone cream, Tylenol® and Benadryl®, 50 mg every 4 hours. Six days later, she was afebrile, and the rash was subjectively and objectively improved. The administration of furosemide was restarted. Two months later, she was doing well, and the rash had healed.

MATERIALS AND METHODS

Patients. Skin biopsy specimens from 11 patients with definite systemic lupus erythematosus (SLE) by American Rheumatism Association Criteria [6], and two patients with discoid lupus erythematosus (DLE) were studied by direct immunofluorescence. The results were compared to the findings in our patient with allopurinol hypersensitivity.

Preparation of Fluorescent Antiserums. Procedures for isolation of myeloma proteins, Bence Jones proteins and IgM macroglobulins, and for preparation of heavy and light chains, and papain and pepsin digestion fragments, have been reported [7,8]. Antiserums polyvalent for human immunoglobulins and antiserums specific for human immunoglobulin classes, IgG subclasses and light chain types were prepared by immunization of rabbits, goats, cynomolgus and rhesus monkeys, and baboons, and their specificity was ascertained. Antiserums to human complement components C3 and C4 were obtained from Hyland Laboratories. Antiserum to C1q was prepared by immunization of a goat with purified C1q [9]. The antiserum was rendered specific by absorption with sepharose-conjugated globulin prepared by precipitation with half-saturated ammonium sulfate and removal of C1q from the redissolved material by precipitation at 56°C for 30 minutes.

Specificity of each antiserum was established by the following criteria: (1) Ouchterlony double diffusion, (2) hemagglutination by the fluorescent conjugate of human type O, Rh-positive erythrocytes to which purified myeloma proteins were coupled with bis-diazotized benzidine, (3) blockage of fluorescence by prior incubation with unconjugated antiserum, and (4) blockage of fluorescence only by purified proteins of the designated specificity. Tissue was stained as previously described [7]. The preparations were examined in a Leitz Orthoplan fluorescent microscope with an Osram HBO-200 mercury vapor lamp, Plöem vertical illuminator with the appropriate combinations of excitor filters, dichroic mirrors and barrier filters for either fluorescein or rhodamine. For each experiment, antiserum absorbed with purified immunoglobulins of the designated specificity was used as a control.

Attempted Elution of Immunoglobulins in Antigen Excess. Tissue sections were washed in phosphate buffered saline solution (pH 7.4) and then washed in solutions of excess antigen, including allopurinol 17 mg/ml, its primary metabolite oxypurinol 12 mg/ml, and furosemide 40 mg/ml at pH 8.0 for time intervals of 2 to 72 hours at 37°C. Sections were then evaluated by staining with polyvalent antiserum with specificity for gamma, mu, kappa and lambda chains and by staining with antiserum specific for IgM and compared with appropriate controls.

C1q Precipitin Test. A search for circulating immune complexes was carried out by Ouchterlony double diffusion experiments of serum versus the purified C1q component of complement according to the method of Agnello et al. [9]. The precipitin test was capable of detecting 60 μg/ml of purified aggregated IgG.

Mononuclear Cell Isolation. Peripheral blood was drawn into a heparinized syringe and sedimented at room temperature. The leukocyte-rich supernatant was centrifuged and the cells were washed in 10 per cent fetal calf serum–Roswell Park Memorial Institute (FCS-RPMI) 1640. Washed cells were recentrifuged and suspended in 5 cc of cold 10 per cent FCS-RPMI 1640, layered over 3 cc of Ficoll-Hypaque solution [10] and centrifuged at 300 g at room temperature for 25 minutes. For the T- and B-cell enumerations, only preparations with a mononuclear cell yield of greater than 70 per cent were used. Cells from the interface were then washed three times in cold 10 per cent FCS-RPMI at 200 g at 4°C for 5 minutes and were finally resuspended in 10 per cent FCS-RPMI at a concentration of 1×10^6/ml.

T-Cell Enumeration. Spontaneous cold sheep erythrocyte rosettes (E) were assayed as previously described by a variation of the method of Ross [11,12]. Sheep red blood cells (SRBC) stored less than two weeks were washed twice with phosphate buffered saline solution (pH 7.2) at 4°C at 200 g. Then equal volumes of 1×10^6 lymphocytes in 25 per cent FCS-RPMI and 100 to 200 $\times$ 10^6 SRBC/ml were incubated in 10 mm by 75 mm glass tubes at 37°C for 5 minutes, centrifuged at room temperature at 200 g for 5 minutes, and incubated at 4°C for 12 hours. An 8 to 10 mm column of cells was withdrawn from the sedimented red cells and lymphocytes with a long Pasteur pipette, and gently agitated. A drop was expressed onto a glass slide, overlaid with a coverslip, and 500 cells were counted. A mononuclear cell with more than two adherent SRBC was considered to be a T-rosette.

B-Cell Enumeration. Lymphocytes in a concentration of 1 to 2 × 10^6 in 0.05 cc of 10 per cent FCS-RPMI 1640 were incubated with 0.05 to 0.10 cc of fluorescein-conjugated polyvalent antihuman immunoglobulin and antiserums specific for human gamma, mu, alpha and delta heavy chains, and kappa and lambda light chains, in 10 mm by 75 mm glass tubes for 1 hour at 4°C, washed three times with 10 cc of cold FCS-RPMI and mounted on glass slides. The cells were overlayered with a coverslip, and 1,000 cells were counted with a Leitz ultraviolet microscope equipped with a mercury arc HBO-200 lamp using BG 38 and 490 nm (FITC) exciter filters and a K510 nm barrier filter, by epi-illumination and simultaneous phase contrast to identify all nonstaining cells as previously described [12]. Antiserums were ultracentrifuged at 100,000 g for 2 hours immediately before use.

Monocyte Identification. Monocytes were identified by their ability to phagocytose 0.81 μ polystyrene beads and by their histology utilizing alpha-naphthyl acetate staining, as previously described [12]. Monocytes were eliminated from the subsequent enumeration of T- and B-lymphocyte percentages.

Lymphocyte Cultures. RPMI 1640 with 10 per cent FCS supplemented with 300 mmol glutamine, 100 U/ml penicillin and 100 μg/ml streptomycin was the medium used in all cell cultures. In all experiments, lymphocyte viability by trypan blue exclusion was greater than 90 per cent.

Duplicate cultures of 0.5 × 10^6 lymphocytes in 1 ml medium were made in 10 by 75 mm sterile capped tissue culture tubes (Falcon) for each concentration of mitogen (PHA* [Burroughs Wellcome] 1 μg, and PWM* [Grand Island Biological] 10 μg), antigen (Candida [Hollister-Stier] 10 μg), and drug (allopurinol and oxypurinol 0.5 μg, 1 μg, 10 μg, 50 μg, 100 μg and 500 μg). Cultures were incubated at 37°C in a 5 per cent carbon dioxide atmosphere for three days, five days and seven days in every experiment. One microcurie of tritiated thymidine (New England Nuclear, Boston, Massachusetts) was added to each tube for the last 5 hours of culture. The trichloracetic acid insoluble radioactivity of cells collected on millipore filters (HAMK) was measured in a liquid scintillation counter. All data are expressed as the maximal stimulation index (counts per minute in stimulation culture/counts per minute in control culture). To determine the maximal stimulation index, the stimulation index for each day of culture and each concentration of drug was determined, and the highest (maximal) stimulation index was then recorded. There was close approximation of the background incorporation of tritiated thymidine within each group; consequently, differences in the stimulation index result solely from differences in the incorporation of tritiated thymidine by the stimulated lymphocytes.

* PHA = phytohemagglutinin. PWM = pokeweed mitogen.

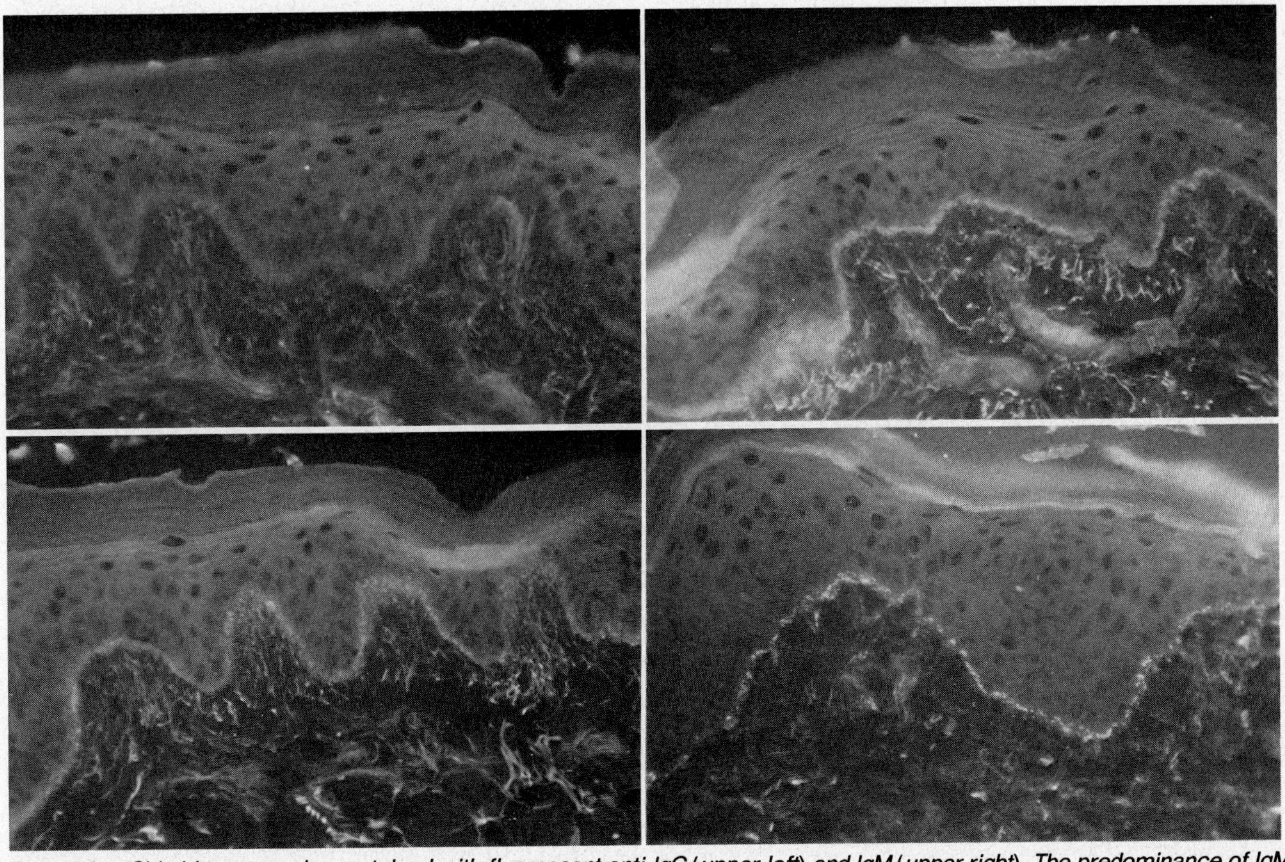

Figure 1. *Skin biopsy specimen stained with fluorescent anti-IgG (upper left) and IgM (upper right). The predominance of IgM staining is apparent. Staining with anti-IgA, IgD and IgE was negative. For the purposes of comparison, granular deposits of IgG (lower left) and IgM (lower right) are shown from a patient with SLE. Heavy granular deposits of both IgG and IgM are present.*

Serum Inhibitors. To study the effects of autologous or allogeneic serum on the transformation response of the patient's lymphocytes, 0.5 ml of the respective serum was added to each culture tube, as previously described [12].

Mixed Lymphocyte Cultures. The technic used was a variation of the method of Hartzman [13]. Lymphocytes were purified as described herein (referred to as responding lymphocytes). A 1×10^7 aliquot of these lymphocytes was incubated with 25 μg/ml mitomycin C for 20 minutes, washed thrice with RPMI and resuspended in 25 per cent plasma (referred to as stimulator lymphocytes). 5×10^5 stimulator cells/cc were mixed with 3×10^5 responder lymphocytes in quadruplicate in a total volume of 0.2 cc in microtiter plates (Linbro). The cultures were incubated for five days at 37°C in 5 per cent carbon dioxide and pulsed with tritiated thymidine (1 μc/well) for 18 hours, and the trichloracetic acid insoluble radioactivity of cells was collected on millipore filters (HAMK) and measured in a liquid scintillation counter.

Drug Preparation. Allopurinol and oxypurinol were partially dissolved in sterile water at a concentration of 25 mg/cc; complete solubilization was effected by stirring the resultant suspension over heat while adding 1 M sodium hydroxide to a final pH of 8.0.

RESULTS

Immunopathologic Findings. Four millimeter punch biopsy specimens taken from involved skin revealed heavy granular deposits at the dermal-epidermal junction with two antiserums polyvalent for human immunoglobulins and with a monospecific antiserum for IgM (Figure 1). Trace deposits were found with an antiserum specific for IgG and the C3 of component of complement. There was no staining with antiserums specific for IgA, IgD, IgE, C1q, C4 or fibrin-fibrinogen. In a control group of patients with SLE or DLE, staining was found with antiserums to both IgM and IgG (Table I). In no instance was a predominance of IgM found in the patients with SLE or DLE.

Attempted elution of immunoglobulins was carried out using solutions of allopurinol 17 mg/ml, oxypurinol 12 mg/ml, lasix 40 mg/ml or buffer alone at pH 8.0. Tissue sections were washed with gentle shaking for time intervals of 2, 16 and 72 hours at 25°C and 37°C, and then stained with polyvalent and IgM antiserums to assess for elution of deposited immunoglobulins. No elution of immunoglobulins was observed.

Since some features of the clinical syndrome resembled serum sickness and other "immune complex" disorders, a search for immune complexes in the serum was made using the C1q precipitin assay. No precipitation was noted in Ouchterlony double diffusion experiments of the patient's serum versus purified C1q. Control preparations of purified aggregated IgG precipitated at a minimum concentration of 60 μg/ml.

Since a disproportion of lymphocyte subpopulations might imply an imbalance in immunoregulation, the percentage of peripheral blood T- and B-lymphocytes was determined. The percentage of T-lymphocytes was 84 per cent and of B-lymphocytes 14 per cent, within the normal range of our laboratory.

As can be seen in Table II, lymphocytes cultured for three, five and seven days in the presence of 0.5 μg to 500 μg of allopurinol and 0.5 μg to 500 μg of oxypurinol failed to increase the incorporation of tritiated thymidine over background. These same lymphocytes had a marked transformation response to the mitogens PHA and PWM, the antigen Candida, and allogeneic cells in a unidirectional mixed lymphocyte response. Consequently, it seems unlikely that the failure to respond was due to an inherent defect in the ability of the lymphocyte to transform. To examine the possibility that the allopurinol or oxypurinol solution was toxic to the lymphocytes, patient lymphocytes were incubated with varying concentrations of allopurinol and oxypurinol and then stimulated with PHA; there was an increase in the incorporation of tritiated thymidine similar to that when patient lymphocytes were incubated with PHA alone.

Since serum factors have been implicated in hypersensitivity responses to drugs, patient lymphocytes were incubated with serum obtained from selected

TABLE I Immunopathology of Skin in Patient with Allopurinol Sensitivity versus 11 Patients with SLE or DLE

Case	Diagnosis	Polyvalent	IgG	IgA	IgM	IgD	IgE	C1q	C3	C4	Fibrin-Fibrinogen
Present	AH	3+	tr	. . .	3+	. . .	. . .	. . .	. . .	. . .	. . .
1	SLE	2+	2+	. . .	2+	. . .	. . .	2+	1+	. . .	. . .
2	SLE	2+	3+	. . .	2+	2+	2+	. . .	. . .	. . .	. . .
3	SLE	2+	2+	. . .	2+	. . .	. . .	. . .	. . .	. . .	. . .
4	SLE	1+	1+	. . .	tr	. . .	. . .	. . .	1+	tr	. . .
5	SLE	1+	. . .	. . .	. . .	. . .	. . .	. . .	. . .	. . .	. . .
6	SLE	4+	3+	2+	1+	. . .	. . .	. . .	2+	2+	. . .
7	SLE	2+	2+	. . .	. . .	. . .	. . .		1+	. . .	. . .
8	SLE	2+	. . .	. . .	. . .	. . .	. . .	1+	2+	. . .	. . .
9	SLE	1+	1+	. . .	. . .	. . .	. . .	. . .	tr	. . .	. . .
10	SLE	3+	2+	. . .	2+	. . .	. . .	tr	tr	. . .	. . .
11	DLE	3+	3+	. . .	1+	1+	. . .	2+	. . .	. . .	. . .

NOTE: AH = allopurinol hypersensitivity.

points of the hospitalization including samples prior to and at the peak of clinical toxicity. No change in the transformation of lymphocytes was noted (Table III). Since it has been reported that lymphocytes from patients with fixed drug eruption may transform in the presence of autologous serum and drug, appropriate experiments were performed. Lymphocytes were incubated with serum (taken at the acme of clinical toxicity) and drug (oxypurinol 10 μg, or allopurinol 10 μg) in combination. Again, as seen in Table III, no increase in thymidine incorporation was noted.

In an attempt to detect a response of patient lymphocytes to a nonoxypurinol metabolite such as allopurinol 1-N-ribonucleoside or allopurinol 1-N-ribonucleotide, lymphocytes were cultured in the presence of allogeneic serum alone, allogeneic serum plus allopurinol (10 μg), and allogeneic serum plus oxypurinol (10 μg) taken from two patients with allopurinol treated gout. Again, no increase in the incorporation of tritiated thymidine was noted.

COMMENTS

Most rheumatologists would not advocate the use of allopurinol in patients with asymptomatic hyperuricemia, particularly when a thiazide diuretic is a contributing factor. A more conservative approach to this patient, and one which we would advocate, would have been to discontinue the use of hydrochlorthiazide and to treat the patient's hypertension with another drug.

This patient manifests a number of features commonly present in allopurinol hypersensitivity as described by Young et al. [5] including (1) a history of hypertension and renal insufficiency, (2) no history of gouty arthritis, (3) prior treatment with thiazide diuretics, (4) commencement of illness four to six weeks after the administration of allopurinol was started, (5) abnormal liver function studies and/or hepatomegaly, (6) generalized desquamative maculopapular pruritic eruption and (7) eosinophilia. Rapid loss of renal function, oliguria, gastrointestinal bleeding and a prolonged illness are also commonly found. The short course of our patient's illness may have been related to the maintenance of her renal function since both allopurinol and oxypurinol are excreted by the kidney. Other patients with a similar prompt recovery after allopurinol hypersensitivity have been studied.*

The principal disorders in the differential diagnosis of granular deposition of immunoglobulin at the dermal-epidermal junction are SLE, mixed connective tissue disease syndrome and DLE. The absence of suggestive clinical features and the repeatedly negative antinuclear antibodies render SLE and the mixed connective disease syndrome highly unlikely. In addition, the skin lesions bore no resemblance to DLE, grossly or microscopically. Current evidence indicates that lupus nephritis results from deposition of immune complexes in renal glomeruli [14]. Koffler et al. [15] used acid elution or DNAase to elute antibodies, and Krishman and Kaplan [16] studied acid eluates from isolated glomeruli. Analysis of the specificity of such eluates has revealed antibody to nucleoprotein, double-stranded deoxyribonucleic acid (DNA) and phosphate buffer extractable antigen. A small percentage of patients with SLE nephritis manifest linear staining in glomeruli, and the patient described by Kantor [3] with allopurinol hypersensitivity had linear deposition of IgG on the glomerular basement membrane.

Landry and Sams [17] characterized acid eluates from skin of patients with SLE. They observed such eluates to be rich in antinuclear antibodies and some eluates to contain antibodies to double-stranded DNA,

* Tabulation of serious skin reactions associated with zyloprim, Medical Division, Burroughs Wellcome, Research Triangle Park, N.C.

TABLE II Response of Patient Lymphocytes to Drugs, Mitogens, Antigens and Allogeneic Cells

	SI*	CPM†
Oxypurinol	1.6	1,331
Allopurinol	1.3	1,116
PHA	50	40,597
PWM	36	29,199
Candida	10	8,261
Allogeneic cells (MLR)	6.6	6,297
Oxypurinol + PHA	48	39,241
Allopurinol + PHA	47	38,453

NOTE: PHA = phytohemagglutinin; PWM = pokeweed mitogen; MLR = mixed lymphocyte reaction.
* Maximal stimulation index (SI) as defined in "Materials and Methods."
† Counts per minute in stimulated culture.

TABLE III Response of Patient Lymphocytes to Autologous Serum, Autologous Serum and Drug, Allogeneic Serum, Allogeneic Serum and Drug

	SI*	CPM†
Autologous serum	0.98	742
Autologous serum + 10 μg oxypurinol	1.11	841
Autologous serum + 10 μg allopurinol	0.81	613
Allogeneic serum no. 1‡	0.93	706
Allogeneic serum no. 1‡ + 10 μg oxypurinol	1.03	783
Allogeneic serum no. 1‡ + 10 μg allopurinol	1.09	824
Allogeneic serum no. 2‡	1.07	804
Allogeneic serum no. 2‡ + 10 μg oxypurinol	1.05	795
Allogeneic serum no. 2‡ + 10 μg allopurinol	0.99	752

*Maximal stimulation index (SI) as defined in "Materials and Methods."
†Counts per minute in stimulated culture.
‡ From a patient with gouty arthritis treated with daily allopurinol, 300 mg, orally.

and extractable nuclear antigens as well. Levitin et al. [18] described granular deposits of immunoglobulins at the dermal-epidermal junction in three of six patients with the mixed connective tissue disease syndrome and high titers of antibody to RNAase labile extractable nuclear antigen. In SLE, the presence of cutaneous deposits in uninvolved, nonlight exposed skin correlates well with the presence of immune complex nephritis [21]. In the mixed connective tissue disease syndrome, renal disease is uncommon and may not correlate with cutaneous deposits [18–20].

Antibodies to basement membrane have also been identified in eluates from skin in two patients with SLE [17]. Wierzchowiecki et al. [22] also found basement membrane antibodies reacting with human skin and rabbit esophagus, but not with rat kidney. The antigen in skin was destroyed by sodium metaperiodate suggesting a carbohydrate moiety as the principal antigenic constituent. In all reported series of immune deposition in skin in SLE, IgG has been the predominant immunoglobulin with lesser deposition of IgM and IgA [22–25]. The predominance of IgM with only trace amounts of IgG, as seen in this patient, is very uncommon in SLE and should raise the suspicion of another pathogenetic process. In this regard, Caperton [27] recently reported deposits of IgM at the dermal-epidermal junction in a patient with eosinophilic fasciitis. The predominance of IgG deposits in SLE and DLE is in good agreement with the characterization of antinuclear antibodies, the principal constituents of glomerular and cutaneous eluates. In all reported series, IgG predominates in antinuclear antibodies with lesser numbers of serums and generally lower titers of IgM antinuclear antibodies, with IgA even less common [7,27–30]. In our own experience characterizing antinuclear antibodies as to immunoglobulin class and IgG subclass, only one instance of antinuclear antibody restricted to the IgM class was found [7]. The predominance of IgM in immune deposits might suggest a correlation with a primary response, and perhaps patients with a more protracted exposure to an offending drug will manifest a greater predisposition to IgG deposition. The deposition of complement components has indicated both the activation of the classic and alternate pathways in the complement cascade [31]. In the present instance, only trace deposits of C3 were found.

Using a variety of culture technics, we were unable to demonstrate in this patient cellular hypersensitivity as evidenced by an absence of lymphocyte transformation. The absence of an increased background incorporation of tritiated thymidine makes it very unlikely that in vivo transformation had occurred, rendering the lymphocyte unable to divide in vitro, as has previously been described in penicillin drug allergy [32]. Evidence for a serum transforming factor could not be obtained in experiments utilizing allogeneic lymphocytes cultured in the patient's plasma, autologous lymphocytes cultured in autologous plasma, and autologous lymphocytes cultured in autologous plasma with solubilized allopurinol or oxypurinol added. Nor could the patient's lymphocytes be transformed in the presence of media and allopurinol, media and oxypurinol; or media and donor serum presumed to contain allopurinol metabolites, or media and donor serum and allopurinol or oxypurinol. Thus, transformation of the lymphocytes could not be effected by the drug itself, a drug metabolite, a serum factor, or a combination of these, as has been documented by others in reference to chlorpropamide, penicillin, streptomycin, phenolphthalein, aminopyrine, acetylsalicylic acid and other drugs [33–35]. It is very unlikely that an inherent defect was present in the patient's lymphocytes, since they responded well to plant lectins, antigen and allogeneic cells. The studies on this patient thus indicate a more purely humoral immunopathogenesis, and are somewhat against the presence of concomitant or helper T-cell sensitization.

We were unable to find evidence of serum immune complexes by the C1q precipitin method. The C1q component of complement is known to precipitate soluble immune complexes in gel diffusion [9]. It is possible that immune complexes were present in a size not readily precipitable by C1q or present in a concentration less than 60 μg/ml, a concentration too small to precipitate with C1q in agar.

A variety of diseases are associated with dermal-epidermal immunofluorescence, including pemphigus, bullous pemphigoid, cicatricial pemphigoid, dermatitis herpetiformis, DLE, SLE and mixed connective tissue disease syndrome. In patients with pemphigus and bullous pemphigoid, circulating epithelial autoantibodies are found.

In patients with pemphigus, intercellular antibodies are found with deposits in the intercellular regions of the epidermis. In patients with bullous and cicatrical pemphigoid, basement membrane antibodies produce linear deposits at the dermal-epidermal junction. In patients with dermatitis herpetiformis, skin biopsy specimens show deposits of immunoglobulins, mainly IgA, usually within the dermal papillae but also at the basement membrane. In patients with SLE, direct immunofluorescence of skin biopsy specimens reveals granular deposits of primarily IgG and complement at the dermal-epidermal junction and in some patients linear deposits as well which may be masked by the heavier granular deposition. In dermatitis herpetiformis and SLE, there is strong evidence for the presence of immune complexes circulating in serum [14,37]. The granular type of staining found by immunofluorescence is consistent with the hypothesis that the circulating immune complexes are "trapped" in the skin. In SLE the restriction in specificity of eluates to nuclear antigens in both kidney and skin lends considerable further support to this hypothesis [15,16].

A variety of mechanisms may be found to explain "allergic" reactions to drugs. The most common mechanism involves the development of antibodies towards antigenic determinants on the drug. Resultant reactions occur when antibody-stimulated amplification systems damage organs or cells in which the drug has lodged. Alternatively, the drug may act as a hapten enabling the production of antibody with specificity for both the drug and for the patient's own tissue. Such a mechanism has been shown to result in linear staining of glomerular basement membrane in methicillin nephritis with the dimethoxyphenylpenicilloyl metabolite coupling to basement membrane protein and serving as a hapten [38]. This break in tolerance then results in true autoimmunity. Both mechanisms could result in the production of circulating immune complexes. The resultant damage depends greatly on the size and solubility of the complexes formed and local tissue factors such as hydrostatic pressure and vascular permeability. Following deposition of the complex, tissue damage results from attraction of lymphocytes and production of cytotoxic factors, activation of complement, attraction of polymorphonuclear leukocytes and release of their lyzosomal enzymes, and deposition of fibrin [39,40].

In the present instance, this chain of events was thought to have been initiated by allopurinol; it subsided after administration of the drug was stopped. The reaction was of sufficient severity that rechallenge was not attempted. The pathogenesis appears to have been primarily on the basis of immune complex deposition rather than via the chemical coupling of allopurinol to anatomic structures in the skin or via the development of sensitized T-cells. The predominance of granular deposits of IgM in the basement membrane zone, a finding which is highly unusual in SLE, suggested the possibility of another pathogenetic process.

ACKNOWLEDGMENT

The skilled assistance of Mr. C. Randall Fuller, Ms. Helen Tillotson and Ms. Janet Fallon in these studies is gratefully acknowledged.

ADDENUM

Immune complexes were found in serum taken at the acme of clinical toxicity by the Raji cell technic.

REFERENCES

1. Rundles RW, Metz EN, Silberman HR: Allopurinol in the treatment of gout. Ann Intern Med 64: 229, 1966.
2. Gutman AB: Hyperuricemia and its management. Drug Therap 5: 29, 1971.
3. Kantor GI: Toxic epidermal necrolysis, azotemia, and death after allopurinol therapy. JAMA 212: 478, 1970.
4. Mills RM Jr: Severe hypersensitivity reactions associated with allopurinol. JAMA 216: 799, 1971.
5. Young JL, Boswell RB, Nies AS: Severe allopurinol hypersensitivity. Arch Intern Med 134: 553, 1974.
6. Cohen AS, Reynolds WE, Franklin EC, Kukla JP, Ropes MW, Shulman LE, Wallace SL: Preliminary criteria for the classification of systemic lupus erythematosus. Bull Rheum Dis 21: 643, 1971.
7. Puritz EM, Yount WJ, Newell M, Utsinger PD: Immunoglobulin classes and IgG subclasses of human antinuclear antibodies. Clin Immunol Immunopathol 2: 98, 1973.
8. Yount WJ, Kunkel HG, Litwin SD: Studies of the Vi(γ_{2c}) subgroup of γ-globulin. A relationship between concentration and genetic type among normal individuals. J Exp Med 125: 177, 1967.
9. Agnello V, Koffler D, Eisenberg JW, Winchester RJ, Kunkel HG: C1q precipitins in the sera of patients with systemic lupus erythematosus and other hypocomplementemic states. Characterization of high and low molecular weight types. J Exp Med 134: 228s, 1971.
10. Boyum A: Isolation of mononuclear cells and granulocytes from human blood. Scand J Clin Lab Invest 21 (suppl 97): 51, 1968.
11. Ross GD, Rabellino EM, Folley MJ, Grey HM: Combined studies of complement receptor and surface immunoglobulin-bearing cells and sheep erythrocyte rosette-forming cells in normal and leukemic human lymphocytes. J Clin Invest 52: 377, 1973.
12. Utsinger PD: Impaired T-cell transformation in chronic lymphocytic leukemia (CLL). Demonstration of a blastogenesis inhibitory factor. Blood 46: 883, 1975.
13. Hartzman RJ, Segall M, Bach ML, Bach FM: Histocompatibility matching. VI. Miniaturization of the mixed lymphocyte culture test: a preliminary report. Transplantation 11: 268, 1971.
14. Koffler D, Angello V, Thoburn R, Kunkel HG: Systemic lupus erythematosus. Prototype of immune complex nephritis in man. J Exp Med 134s: 1695, 1971.
15. Koffler D, Schur PH, Kunkel HG: Immunological studies concerning the nephritis of systemic lupus erythematosus. J Exp Med 126: 607, 1967.
16. Krishman C, Kaplan MH: Immunopathologic studies of systemic lupus erythematosus. II. Antinuclear reaction of gamma-globulin eluted from homogenates and isolated glomeruli of kidneys from patients with lupus nephritis. J Clin Invest 46: 569, 1967.
17. Landry M, Sams WM Jr: Systemic lupus erythematosus. Studies of the antibodies bound to skin. J Clin Invest 52: 1967, 1973.
18. Levitin PM, Weary PE, Giuliano VJ: The immunofluorescent "band" test for mixed connective tissue disease. Ann Intern Med 83: 53, 1975.
19. Sharp GC, Irvin WS, LaRoque RL: Association of autoantibodies to different nuclear antigens with clinical patterns of rheumatic disease and responsiveness to therapy. J Clin Invest 50: 350, 1971.
20. Sharp GC, Irvin WS, Tan EM: Mixed connective tissue disease—an apparently distinct rheumatic disease syndrome associated with a specific antibody to an extractable nuclear antigen (ENA). Am J Med 52: 148, 1972.
21. Gilliam JN, Cheatum DE, Hurd ER: Immunoglobulin in clinically uninvolved skin in systemic lupus erythematosus. Association with renal disease. J Clin Invest 53: 1434, 1974.
22. Wierzchowieki MO, Quismorio FP, Friou GJ: Immunoglobulin

deposits of skin in systemic lupus erythematosus. Arthritis Rheum 18: 77, 1975.
23. Burnham TK, Neblet TR, Fine G: The application of the fluorescent antibody technique to the investigation of lupus erythematosus and various dermatoses. J Invest Derm 41: 451, 1963.
24. Tan EM, Kunkel HG: An immunofluorescent study of the skin lesions in systemic lupus erythematosus. Arthritis Rheum 9: 37, 1966.
25. Cormane RH, Ballieux RE, Kalsbeck GL, Hijmans W: Classification of immunoglobulins in the dermo-epidermal junction in lupus erythematosus. Clin Exp Immunol 1: 207, 1966.
26. Burnham TK, Fine G: The immunofluorescent "band" test for lupus erythematosus. Arch Derm 99: 413, 1969.
27. Caperton EM, Hathaway DE: Scleroderma with eosinophilia and hypergammaglobulinemia: the Shulman syndrome (abstract 54a). Program of the 39th Annual Meeting of the ARA Section of the Arthritis Foundation, 1975.
28. Rothfield NF, Stoller BD: The relation of immunoglobulin class, pattern of antinuclear antibody, and complement-fixing antibodies to DNA in sera from patients with systemic lupus erythematosus. J Clin Invest 46: 1785, 1967.
29. Kacaki JN, Callerame ML, Blomgren SE, Vaughn JH: Immunoglobulin G subclasses of antinuclear antibodies and renal deposits. Arthritis Rheum 14: 276, 1971.
30. Schur PH, Monroe M, Rothfield N: The γG subclass of antinuclear and antinucleic acid antibodies. Arthritis Rheum 15: 174, 1972.
31. Rothfield N, Ross HA, Minta JO, Lepow IH: Glomerular and dermal deposition of properdin in systemic lupus erythematosus. N Engl J Med 287: 681, 1972.
32. Gill FA: The association of increased spontaneous lymphocyte transformation in vitro with clinical manifestations of drug hypersensitivity. J Immunol 98: 778, 1967.
33. Sarkany I: Lymphocyte transformation in drug hypersensitivity. Lancet 1: 743, 1967.
34. Wyatt E, Greaves M, Søndergaard J: Fixed drug eruption (phenolphthalein). Arch Derm 106: 671, 1972.
35. Gimenez-Camarasa JM, Garcia-Calderon P, De Moragas JM: Lymphocyte transformation test in fixed drug eruption. N Engl J Med 16: 819, 1975.
36. Beutner EH, Chorzelski TP, Bean SF, Jordan RE: Immunopathology of the Skin: Labeled Antibody Studies, Pennsylvania, Dowden Hutchinson & Ross, Inc., 1973, p 1.
37. Mowbray JF, Holborow EJ, Hoffbrand AV, Seah PP, Fry L: Circulating immune complexes in dermatitis herpetiformis. Lancet 1: 400, 1973.
38. Baldwin DS, Levin BB, McCluskey RT, Gallo GR: Renal failure and interstitial nephritis due to penicillin and methicillin. N Engl J Med 279: 1245, 1968.
39. Ward PA: Complement-derived leukotactic factors in pathological fluids. J Exp Med 134: 109s, 1971.
40. Weissman G, Zurier RB, Speiler PJ, Goldstein IM: Mechanisms of lysosomal enzyme release from leukocytes exposed to immune complexes and other particles. J Exp Med 134: 1495, 1971.

A Case of Bilateral Escherichia coli Endogenous Endophthalmitis

W. LEE FANNING, M.D.
JAMES STUBBERT, M.D.
E. S. IRWIN, M.D.
MARK D. ARONSON, M.D.*
Burlington, Vermont

The first reported case of bilateral endogenous endophthalmitis is presented and discussed with reference to pertinent literature. Diagnostic and therapeutic recommendations for suspected gram-negative endophthalmitis are presented and include: immediate paracentesis of the eye for gram stain and culture, systemic therapy with an antibiotic such as gentamicin and either subconjunctival, subtenon or intraocular injection of antibiotics. Despite these measures vision may be lost and, as in this case, enucleation necessary.

Endogenous or metastatic purulent endophthalmitis is a rare complication of microbial septicemia. It has been associated with pneumonia and endocarditis [1], meningococcal meningitis [2], pyelonephritis [3] and prostatic surgery [4]. With the advent of specific and broad spectrum antimicrobials, the incidence of this devastating complication has become distinctly unusual with few cases appearing in the modern English literature [1–4]. Bilateral endogenous endophthalmitis has not been reported previously.

The following case is presented to highlight the need for the internist and ophthalmologist to act aggressively, both diagnostically and therapeutically, in patients with proved or suspected endophthalmitis.

CASE REPORT

A 56 year old white housewife from Vermont had been well all her life until six months prior to admission when she began to notice fatigue, weight loss and increased urinary output. Two weeks prior to admission she suffered minor trauma to her right toe. Unexpectedly, skin breakdown and discoloration ensued over the next week. Four days prior to admission the onset of marked bilateral eye tenderness and photophobia were noted, followed in rapid succession by scotoma, blurred vision and, finally, only light perception and severe persistent global eye pain. On presentation to a local hospital, clouding of eye chambers bilaterally, a gangrenous right great toe, and hyperglycemia were noted. She was transferred to the Medical Center Hospital of Vermont and on admission she was noted to be an afebrile, frail, chronically ill appearing white woman. The eyes showed conjunctival purulence and edema, normal sclera and sluggishly reacting pupils. Funduscopic examination was not possible due to a hazy opacification of the vitreous bilaterally (slit lamp as well as ophthalmoscopic examination). Tonometry revealed a tension of R28 and L20 initially. The ears, nose and mouth were normal, lymphadenopathy was not present, the lungs were clear and a grade 2/4 systolic ejection murmur was heard along the left sternal border. The extremity examination revealed symmetric and full pulsation throughout, without bruits. A necrotic gangrenous great toe on the right was noted.

From the Department of Medicine, University of Vermont College of Medicine, Burlington, Vermont. Requests for reprints should be addressed to Dr. Lee Fanning, Given C315, University of Vermont College of Medicine, Department of Medicine, Burlington, Vermont 05401. Manuscript accepted November 6, 1975.

* Present address: Internal Medicine Department, Beth Israel Hospital, Boston, Massachusetts 02115.

The hematocrit value was 35 per cent, the white blood cell count 11,300/mm^3 with 69 per cent neutrophils, 10 per cent band forms, 17 per cent lymphocytes, 3 per cent monocytes and 1 per cent eosinophil. The urinalysis showed 1+ glucose, many white blood cells and bacteria. The creatinine and glucose were 0.6 mg/dl and 150 mg/dl, respectively. Cultures of her urine, right and left eye vitreous (obtained by paracentesis of the posterior chamber), and gangrenous toe all yielded an Escherichia coli with identical sensitivity patterns. All were sensitive to chloramphenicol, cephalothin, tetracycline, colistin, gentamicin and kanamycin, and resistant to ampicillin and carbenicillin. Subsequent serologic identification (kindly performed for us by C. Riddle, Enteric Section, Center for Disease Control, Atlanta, Georgia) revealed isolates in both the right and left eye, and three subsequent cultures from a draining ankle wound to be 016:HNM.

Antibiotic therapy consisted of parenterally administered chloramphenicol (1 g every 6 hours) and gentamicin (120 mg every 8 hours), and subconjunctival gentamicin (40 mg every 24 hours). Additionally, large doses of prednisone were administered. Despite therapy, the patient's vision deteriorated with loss of all light perception bilaterally, and sclerosing of the vitreous opacifications. After two weeks of therapy, paracentesis of the right vitreous chamber was repeated and again yielded an identical Esch. coli. Bilateral evisceration of the eyes was performed, and follow-up antibiotic therapy with chloramphenicol and then tetracycline was administered for a total of 10 days. No further orbital infection occurred and rehabilitation therapy was begun.

Early in her hospital course, diabetes mellitus was diagnosed, and therapy with insulin was begun. The gangrenous toe, which had been debrided, healed well, but two months after discharge an abscess developed on the right ankle and an identical Esch. coli was isolated. A roentgenogram confirmed the presence of osteomyelitis, and therapy was begun with cephalexin for a three month period. Healing occurred and a six months follow-up examination revealed no evidence of infection.

COMMENTS

Purulent intraocular infections are severe, often lead to loss of vision and require prompt intervention. They may be either exogenous or endogenous in origin. Exogenous infections generally occur after trauma or eye surgery. Serious intraocular infection following clean eye surgery is extremely rare, ranging from 0.1 to 0.3 per cent in most series [5]. The principal organisms involved in this form of intraocular infection are Staphylococcus aureus and gram-negative bacilli including Proteus [6], Pseudomonas [7], Esch. coli [8], Pasteurella septica [9] and Vibrio [10].

Endogenous eye infections are much less frequent, and have been reported to be secondary to infections such as pyelonephritis [3], sepsis following prostatic resection [4], ureteral obstruction [11], endocarditis [1] and meningitis [2]. Fungal endogenous endophthalmitis has been reported in immunosuppressed persons [12,13].

Endogenous intraocular infections can be further classified as either panophthalmitis—a fulminant inflammation of the intraocular contents with accompanying necrosis of the sclera or cornea with extension to the orbit, or endophthalmitis—a suppurative inflammation of the intraocular contents but without extension through all layers of the eye. Endophthalmitis is regarded as a less fulminant infection, but it may lead to rapid blindness despite aggressive therapy as witnessed in this patient.

Most cases of endogenous intraocular infections reported in the preantibiotic era did not include culture results of material from the suspected primary source in conjunction with the eye culture. However, in 1930 Levine [14] reported a case of panophthalmitis with Esch. coli cultured from urine, blood and the right eye. This patient like ours, was diabetic. More recent cases have included culture results from possible sites of infection other than the eye including blood, urine, sputum and spinal fluid, and the organisms from these sites have had the same sensitivity patterns as the organisms cultured from the eye [3,4,11]. Similarly our patient had an identical organism isolated from the urine, both eyes, the gangrenous toe and from a draining ankle lesion. A literature search did not reveal other reports of endogenous bilateral gram-negative endophthalmitis or panophthalmitis in the English literature.

Because endogenous eye infections can be so rapidly devastating, patients with suspected or proved systemic infections, in whom pain in the eye or blurred vision develop, should immediately be evaluated for this complication. Our experience and the literature suggest that this include immediate paracentesis for cultures and gram stain, in addition to cultures of any other sites of possible infection including blood cultures [5]. Therapy, even when begun immediately, has in large part been unsuccessful in preventing blindness once the infection is established. Only one report of vision being saved in a person with endophthalmitis could be found, and this infection was exogenous in origin [15].

Parenteral administration of most antibiotics does not achieve consistently adequate intraocular bacterial minimal inhibitory levels. This is true even for a drug like chloramphenicol which penetrates well into most body areas. A useful review of antibiotic use in intraocular infection is available [5].

Gentamicin is currently regarded as the drug of choice for most unknown systemic gram-negative infections. However, even at maximally recommended systemic doses, inadequate levels in eye tissue and aqueous fluid may result [16]. Subconjunctival injection of 20 mg of gentamicin in rabbits has been reported to yield results exceeding the minimal inhibitory concentration of Pseudomonas and most Staph. aureus isolates [16]. Gentamicin concentrations between 0.8 and 14.5

μg/ml in aqueous fluid have been achieved using 10 mg subconjunctivally in preoperative patients undergoing cataract removal [17]. Subtenon injection plus intramuscular gentamicin appears to give higher gentamicin levels in the aqueous of inflamed rabbit eyes then either used alone [15]. The subtenon route was employed successfully in a person who had an exogenously introduced Pseudomonas infection [15]. Recently Payman et al. [18] suggested that intravitreal injection of 500 μg of gentamicin yields extremely high vitreous levels in rabbits without ill effects, and much higher gentamicin levels in the vitreous than when given via any other route. This study also suggests that vitreous gentamicin levels of 4 μg/ml will persist for 96 hours using this method. Unfortunately, the proper local dosage, route or interval of antibiotics is not clearly established. Antibiotic levels in the serum and ocular fluid may be helpful in making these decisions.

It would seem, based on the literature, that for suspected or proved gram-negative intraocular infections, systemic and either subconjunctival, subtenon or intraocular injection of gentamicin be employed. Paracentesis should be utilized to help establish the original bacteriologic diagnosis and to confirm the effectiveness of therapy in eradicating the organisms.

Despite these efforts, once intraocular infection has developed, blindness may ensue and enucleation may become necessary.

REFERENCES

1. Johnson A: Metastatic septic endophthalmitis. Southern Med J 62: 879, 1969.
2. Williams DN, Geddes AM: Meningococcal meningitis complicated by pericarditis, panophthalmitis and arthritis. Br Med J 2: 93, 1970.
3. Weil VJ, Laval I, Sturman RM: Escherichia coli panophthalmitis from pyelonephritis. Arch Ophthalmol (Paris) 57: 58, 1957.
4. Ellenberger C, Sturgill BC: Endogenous Pseudomonas panophthalmitis. Am J Ophthalmol 65: 607, 1968.
5. Garrod LP, Lambert H, O'Grady F: Antibiotic and Chemotherapy, Edinburgh & London, Churchill Livingstone 1973, p 429.
6. Crabb AM, Fielding IL, Urmsby HL: Bacillus proteus endophthalmitis. Am J Ophthalmol 43: 86, 1957.
7. Cassady JV: Pseudomonas corneal ulcerations. Am J Ophthalmol 48: 741, 1959.
8. Grayson MC: Pneumato-ophthalmitis. A case of E. coli panophthalmitis. Br J Ophthalmol 56: 68, 1972.
9. Galloway NR, Robinson GE: Panophthalmitis due to Pasteurella septica. Br J Ophthalmol 57: 153, 1973.
10. Wahl JW: Vibrio endophthalmitis. Arch Ophthalmol 91: 423, 1974.
11. Laffers Z, Bolsoky S: Endogenous Proteus panophthalmitis. Am J Ophthalmol 54: 83, 1962.
12. Meyers BR, Licherman TW, Ferry AP: Candida endophthalmitis complicating candidemia. Ann Intern Med 79: 647, 1973.
13. Edwards J, Foos R, Montgomerie J, Guze L: Ocular manifestations of Candida septicemia: review of 26 cases of hematogenous Candida endophthalmitis. Medicine 53: 47, 1974.
14. Levine I: Metastatic Bacillus coli panophthalmitis from calculus pyonephrosis. Arch Ophthalmol 3: 410, 1930.
15. Golden B: Sub-tenon injection of gentamicin for bacterial infections of the eye. J Infect Dis 124: S271, 1971.
16. Litwack KD, Pettit T, Johnson BL: Penetration of gentamicin. Arch Ophthalmol 82: 687, 1969.
17. Furgiuele F: Penetration of gentamicin into the aqueous humor of human eyes. Am J Ophthalmol 69: 481, 1970.
18. Peyman GA, May D, Erickson E, Apple D: Intraocular injection of gentamicin. Arch Ophthalmol 92: 42, 1974.

Malignant External Otitis: A Severe Form of Otitis in Diabetic Patients

DAWLAT A. ZAKY, M.D.
DAVID W. BENTLEY, M.D.
KARL LOWY, M.D.
ROBERT F. BETTS, M.D.
R. GORDON DOUGLAS, Jr., M.D.
Rochester, New York

Two cases of malignant external otitis are presented and the literature is reviewed. The disease seems to occur exclusively in elderly diabetic patients. Diagnosis is mostly a clinical one, and requires a high index of suspicion. The characteristic clinical manifestations are pain and severe tenderness of the tissues around the ear and mastoid, persistent drainage and the presence of granulation tissue at the junction of the osseus and cartilagenous portions of the external ear. Roentgenographic findings are not helpful in the early stages. The pathogenesis of this disease depends on the presence of clefts in the cartilage forming the floor of the external auditory canal at its junction with the osseus portion through which infection can spread from the external ear to the deep soft tissues. Serious and often fatal complications may ensue. The most common and earliest symptom to appear is facial nerve palsy. Pseudomonas aeruginosa has been isolated uniformly, in pure or mixed cultures. This entity, therefore, should be borne in mind whenever an elderly diabetic patient presents with external otitis not amenable to the usual methods of therapy. Ps. aeruginosa should be strongly suspected, and its isolation should prompt vigorous systemic treatment with gentamicin and carbenicillin before extensive necrosis of cartilage and bone takes place. Any delay in diagnosis and management will lead to serious and often fatal complications.

Malignant external otitis is a severe form of external otitis occurring in elderly diabetic patients; it is caused by Pseudomonas aeruginosa. If unrecognized it can progress to serious complications including invasion of cartilage, bone, nerves and soft tissues, resulting in osteomyelitis of the skull, multiple cranial nerve palsies and death. Although this entity has been previously described in the otolaryngologic literature [1–6], there are few reports [7] in the general medical literature. In one year we observed two cases, and for the first time became aware of the seriousness of this condition. We describe these two cases and review the literature to stress the seriousness of external otitis when it occurs in the elderly diabetic patient.

CASE REPORTS

Case 1. A 75 year old white male patient was first seen by us on January 5, 1972, with a three week history of severe persistent pain in and discharge from the right external ear. He was a diabetic of six years' duration, well controlled with chlorpropamide therapy. He also suffered from chronic otitis media of the right ear, with perforation of the tympanic membrane and re-

From the Infectious Disease Unit, Department of Medicine and the Division of Otology, Department of Surgery, University of Rochester School of Medicine and Dentistry, 601 Elmwood Avenue, Rochester, New York 14642. Requests for reprints should be addressed to Dr. Dawlat A. Zaky, University of Rochester School of Medicine and Dentistry, Box 695, Rochester, New York 14642.
Manuscript accepted November 24, 1975.

curring intermittent discharge. On examination he had edema and tenderness of the external ear. Initial culture of the purulent discharge grew enterococcus, Candida albicans and Ps. aeruginosa. He was treated with 5 per cent silver nitrate local drops and oral ampicillin.

Because of a poor response, he was admitted to the hospital on January 21, 1972, and underwent a simple mastoidectomy. At surgery, a small polyp was removed from the floor of the canal, and the tissue around the cartilagenous portion of the external ear was found to be infected. Cultures from the deep pus grew Ps. aeruginosa and C. albicans. He was treated locally with Cortisporin® (polymyxin B-neomycin-hydrocortisone) drops, continued on ampicillin, and discharged on January 28, 1972.

On February 9, 1972, he was readmitted with severe pain in his right ear and a persistent purulent discharge from the inferior pole of the mastoidectomy incision. Culture of the discharge again grew Ps. aeruginosa. Systemic treatment was begun with carbenicillin, 5 g intravenously every 6 hours, and gentamicin, 2.5 mg/kg/day intramuscularly in divided doses. On the fourth day of treatment renal function deteriorated with an increase in serum blood urea nitrogen and creatinine to 60 mg/100 ml and 3.1 mg/100 ml, respectively. This was thought to be due to a toxic nephropathy from phenanthrene anesthesia. By this time the pain had ceased, and the wound appeared to heal without drainage. Because of the deterioration in renal function and the uncertain role of Pseudomonas, the administration of all antimicrobials was discontinued.

The patient was readmitted on February 23, 1972, with a sudden onset of severe right temporal pain with no discharge from the ear canal. The area of the posterior auricular drain was opened demonstrating a purulent exudate which grew Ps. aeruginosa. The minimum inhibitory concentration for gentamicin, carbenicillin and the combination was measured by the "checkerboard" technic adapted to the microtiter system [8]. End points were determined by noting which wells with the lowest concentration of antimicrobial alone and in combination contained no visible growth after incubation at 37°C overnight. Synergy was defined as occurring when the minimal inhibitory concentration of each of the drugs in the combination was one-quarter or less of the minimal inhibitory concentrations of each drug alone. The minimal inhibitory concentration for gentamicin was 3.12 μg/ml and for carbenicillin 125 μg/ml. In combination, synergy was demonstrated with a minimal inhibitory concentration for gentamicin of 0.195 μg/ml and for carbenicillin 3.12 μg/ml.

Early in the hospitalization the patient was afebrile with a leukocyte count of 14,200/mm^3 with 77 per cent neutrophils, and his sedimentation rate was 52 mm/hour. Blood urea nitrogen was 52 mg/100 ml and serum creatinine was 2.8 mg/100 ml. Shortly thereafer, a sudden right facial paralysis developed. Therapy with carbenicillin, 5 g intravenously every 8 hours, and gentamicin, in a dose of 1 mg/kg/day, was started immediately; doses were reduced for his degree of renal failure. On March 10, 1972, he underwent a complete simple mastoidectomy with decompression of the facial nerve, and the antimicrobial therapy was continued for four weeks. The pain and discharge diminished, but the paralysis persisted and he was discharged on April 10, 1972.

He was readmitted on May 27, 1972, with recurrence of right temporoparietal pain, and he underwent evaluation to exclude a brain abscess or tumor. A cerebrovascular accident developed and he had a cardiopulmonary arrest on June 10, 1972, from which he could not be resuscitated. At autopsy, the brain, the right sphenoid ridge, and the right seventh and eighth cranial nerve roots demonstrated no abnormality. There was no indication of sinus thrombosis or meningitis.

Comment: Because this patient suffered from chronic otitis media, his symptoms were attributed partly to complicating mastoiditis. The importance of vigorous treatment of the Ps. aeruginosa isolated was not at first fully appreciated. The finding at surgery of extensive infection around the cartilagenous portion of the external ear, and the subsequent development of facial palsy alerted us to the danger of malignant external otitis, hence more extensive debridement was carried out and specific therapy directed against Ps. aeruginosa was instituted.

Case 2. A 57 year old white female patient first complained of severe pain and swelling of her right external ear on October 20, 1972. She was a diabetic of 16 years' duration, receiving oral chlorpropamide therapy. Her diabetes was complicated by ophthalmopathy and blindness, peripheral neuropathy, diabetic gangrene necessitating below knee amputation of the right leg, and impaired renal function secondary to presumed Kimmelstiel Wilson disease. She also had complete deafness of her left ear of eight years' duration, the etiology of which was never defined but which had been attributed to diabetes. She was treated locally with Burrow's solution and colistin drops plus oral erythromycin. No cultures were obtained. Ear, nose and throat evaluation was obtained on November 4, 1972, for persistent ear pain and marked decrease in hearing. Examination revealed an edematous canal and meatus, with cellulitis around the external ear, and much flaky debris in the meatus. Local treatment with Neo-Delta-Cortef® (neomycin sulfate-prednisolone acetate) drops was started.

On November 14, 1972, a polypoid swelling of the external ear was first observed, and she was treated locally with Cortisporin® (polymyxin B-neomycin-hydrocortisone) and Chloromycetin® (chloramphenicol) drops on a wick. This was removed after 48 hours and a large amount of purulent exudate drained which on culture grew Proteus mirabilis and Enterococcus. She was again treated locally with colistin drops and systemically with oral Chloromycetin for five days with no apparent response. On December 8, 1972, the polypoid mass was removed, and the tympanic membrane was found to be intact. Biopsy revealed chronic granulation tissue; local treatment was continued with colistin drops.

Pain over the mastoid and upper part of the neck prompted another evaluation on January 24, 1973. Objectively she had warmth, tenderness and pain on deep pressure over her mastoid area, and the external canal was still edematous. Roentgenograms showed increased density of the tip of the right mastoid. The impression at that time was otitis media with mastoiditis. Cultures from the external ear again grew Enterococcus, and she was treated with oral ampicillin for two weeks.

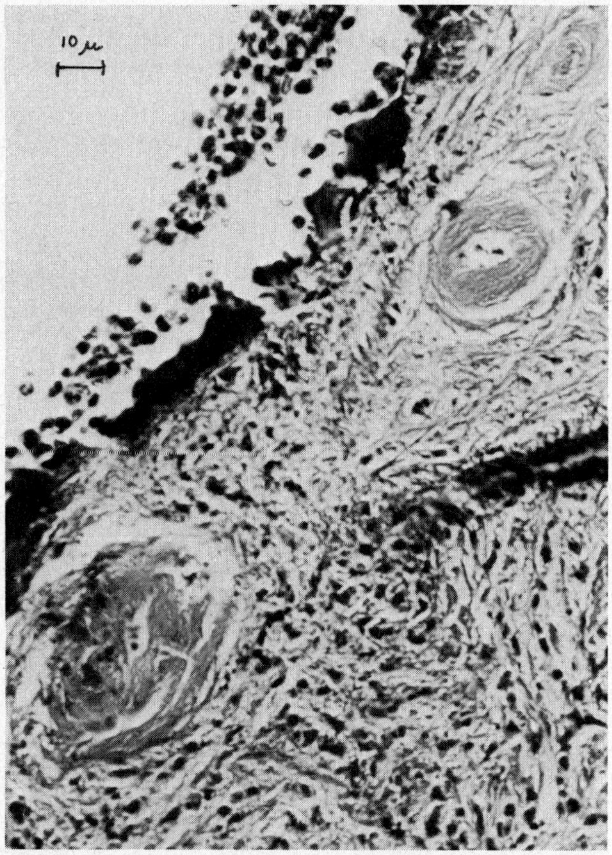

Figure 1. *Section through subcutaneous tissues of the ear canal. Hyalin deposition and thickening of the intima of blood vessels are clearly seen.*

On February 15, 1973, the mastoid pain became very severe and there was warmth overlying the mastoid, but the drainage from the external ear had ceased. She was treated with codeine, hot packs and oral cephalexin for two weeks. However, the pain over the mastoid continued to be very severe and radiated to the temporal area and down the head and neck. Ear, nose and throat examination showed little evidence for acute ear disease, with a clear external canal, a normal tympanic membrane and no drainage. Skull films did not demonstrate sinusitis. The pain was considered to have a large functional component, and a tranquilizer was prescribed.

On March 5, 1973, there was a sudden onset of right facial nerve palsy. The impression at that time was Bell's palsy of diabetic neuropathy, because there was no evidence for acute ear disease and no evidence of bone necrosis secondary to osteomyelitis. On March 8, 1973, evidence developed of involvement of the right 12th cranial nerve with fasciculation and deviation to the right of the tongue. A lumbar puncture and brain scan were negative. Repeat roentgenograms showed no evidence for cholesteatoma or coalescent mastoiditis. Myringotomy was performed on March 12, 1973, with the production of serous fluid which grew only one colony of Staphylococcus aureus on culture. On March 18 evidence developed of extension of cranial nerve involvement to the ninth, 10th and 11th cranial nerves manifested by right palatal asymmetry and right sternomastoid weakness. A repeat lumbar puncture was performed on March 19, which was normal. Throughout her course she remained afebrile but had a persistently elevated sedimentation rate, ranging from 67 to 146 mm/hour on repeated determinations.

At this time the diagnosis of malignant external otitis was considered despite the absence of Pseudomonas on repeated cultures. She underwent surgery on March 29, 1973; when the periosteum of the external ear was elevated, pus issued from a deep abscess, and a sinus tract could be followed to the stylomastoid foramen. The mastoid and tegmen were found to be normal. Necrotic tissue was excised and examined histopathologically. Figure 1 shows hyaline degeneration of the subcutaneous tissue as well as thickening of the intima of blood vessels. Culture of the pus yielded a pure growth of Ps. aeruginosa.

Systemic antibiotic therapy was started on March 30, 1973: gentamicin 2 mg/kg/day in divided doses intravenously, and carbenicillin 4 g intravenously every 6 hours. The minimal inhibitory concentration for gentamicin was 0.39 μg/ml, for carbenicillin 62.5 μg/ml and for tobramycin 0.195 μg/ml. Checkerboard studies did not reveal synergy between gentamicin and carbenicillin. Serum levels of gentamicin were 11.5 μg/ml 2 hours after a dose and 3.13 μg/ml 1 hour before the next dose was given. The dose of gentamicin was then reduced to 1.5 mg/kg/day in divided doses, and carbenicillin was increased to 5 g every 6 hours.

Despite careful monitoring with antimicrobial levels and audiograms, her hearing decreased on the right side. Gentamicin therapy was discontinued, and tobramycin therapy was instituted on April 10, 1973, at a lower dose of 50 mg intravenously every 12 hours in hopes of avoiding further eighth nerve toxicity. This regimen was continued until May 22, 1973, with close monitoring of her renal function. Serum dilution studies were made frequently and consistently demonstrated inhibition in the range of 1:8 to 1:16.

After surgery, the pain in the ear and mastoid diminished, and she had no discharge or tinnitus. But she continued to have recurring occipital headaches which finally subsided during the last weeks of antibiotic therapy. The ninth and tenth cranial nerve involvement diminished, but there was no change in her seventh cranial nerve function. Her sedimentation rate remained elevated.

She was followed with serial audiograms until August 1973. At that time some hearing was still present, and the patient could make use of a hearing aid. On March 20, 1974, one year after her operation, hearing had disappeared completely and no caloric response could be elicited. No vestibular tests were made before that date, but the patient never had any vestibular signs or symptoms.

Comment: There are two interesting features about this case. First, the external otitis seemed initially to heal completely with conservative therapy despite increasing pain and successive involvement of the cranial nerves. And secondly, Pseudomonas was never cultured at any time from her external ear discharge; the local use of colistin drops may have inhibited recovery of the organism. Only when pus was obtained surgically from the deep abscess cavity was Ps. aeruginosa detected.

The cause of the unrelenting, progressive loss of hearing in this patient is hard to establish. Although it is true that there was increasing deafness during antibiotic treatment, complete loss was observed only many months after discontinuation of the treatment. It also needs to be stressed that this patient had a total hearing loss in the left ear many years before which had been attributed to diabetes.

COMMENTS

In 1968 Chandler [1] first described this entity. Several case reports were subsequently published primarily in the otolaryngologic literature [2–5,7]. A summary of the salient features of these cases is given in Table I. In 1972 Chandler [6] summarized his experience in treating a total of 38 patients which included the 13 he had described previously. He did not give detailed descriptions of all these patients so they are not included in Table I, information from this series will, however, be included in the discussion when appropriate. To date, a total of 59 cases (including the two in this communication) have been reported in the English literature.

This disease occurs mainly in the elderly, with 31 (91 per cent) of 34 cases occurring in patients 55 years of age or older. Males and females are equally affected. A history of precipitating factors, such as swimming or wearing a hearing aid may be elicited but is often absent. Diabetes was present in 55 (93 per cent) of the 59 and varied from severe cases to clinical diabetes. It is not clear what features of the diabetic patient predispose him to this devastating infection. It has been suggested [5] that the pathologic changes in the ears and temporal bones of patients with malignant external otitis constitute the otologic equivalent of the diabetic gangrene occurring in the limbs. Biopsy specimens in one of Chandler's cases [7] and both of ours demonstrated the marked intimal proliferation in blood vessels, which would support this concept.

The pathology and pathogenesis of the disease have been described [1]. Histologically, there are clefts in the cartilage forming the floor of the external auditory canal at its junction with the osseous portion through which infection can spread from the external ear to the deep soft tissues, the parotid gland and the temporomandibular joint. The periosteum and cortical bone at first are resistant to spread of infection but later the bone itself becomes involved, and infection extends to the mastoid air cells and bone marrow. Once osteomyelitis of the temporal bone has developed it spreads to the bone marrow of the base of the skull. The tympanic membrane remains intact, but it may be difficult to visualize due to the presence of granulation tissue in the external ear or the edema of the external ear canal.

The most common complication (occurring in nearly 50 per cent of the cases reported) is facial nerve palsy which is usually the first sign of neurologic involvement. This generally is due to soft tissue infection at its exit from the stylomastoid foramen, but occasionally occurs as a result of osteomyelitis in the bony canal itself. It is a serious prognostic sign, eight of Chandler's 16 patients with this sign died [6]. The onset of hoarseness, dysphagia, aspiration and choking signal involvement of the 10th, 11th and 12th cranial nerves as a result of osteomyelitis of the base of the skull. In the later stages of the disease, infection can spread to involve the third, fifth, sixth and eighth cranial nerves as well. The cerebrospinal fluid, as noted in our two cases and those reported by Dinapoli and Thomas [7], is normal despite multiple cranial nerve involvement. Meningitis is usually a very rare and late complication [3]. A high mortality is associated with malignant external otitis. As noted in Table I, 18 (53 per cent) of 34 patients reported on have died. Most were elderly diabetic patients in poor health with generalized arteriosclerosis and cardiovascular disease in whom infection and repeated surgical procedures led to a rapid downhill course.

TABLE I **Clinical Features in 34* Cases of Malignant External Otitis**

Data	No.	Per Cent
Patient population		
Male/Female, 19/15		
Elderly (55 years or >)	31	91
Diabetic	30	82
Signs and symptoms		
Pain	34	100
Purulent discharge	33	97
Bilateral involvement	7	21
Polyp in external ear	30	88
Complications		
Cranial nerve involvement		
VII	16	47
Other	9	27
Meningitis	4	11
Mortality	18	53
Culture		
Pseudomonas (pure)	32	100†
Pseudomonas (mixed)	5	16†

*Information from [1-5,7] and the present study.
†Culture reports available in 32 cases only.

Ps. aeruginosa has been isolated in all cases reported in the literature in which culture results are available. It is isolated generally in pure culture, but in a few cases, mixed cultures with Proteus species, Staphylococcus aureus or Enterococcus were noted [1,2,5]. In one case described by Evans and Richards [5], and in our second case, Pseudomonas was never cultured from the external ear drainage. Pseudomonas species have been found only rarely in normal ears. In a study by Singer and co-workers [9] members of the Pseudomonas group (unidentified species) were found frequently in external otitis, following trauma and swimming. Thus, this organism may be encountered in external otitis and otitis media, but it does not seem to cause malignant external otitis except in elderly diabetic patients. The predisposition of Pseudomonas to invade blood vessels and soft tissues [10,11], coupled with the already diseased blood vessels of the diabetic patient, may explain the relentless progression of this disease.

Diagnosis of malignant external otitis in early cases is mostly a clinical one and requires a high index of suspicion and a knowledge of this entity. The typical history is that of a persistent otitis externa due to Pseudomonas aeruginosa in an elderly diabetic patient that does not respond to topical therapy. The principle symptom is persistent pain which is constant and severe. The characteristic local findings are a persistent drainage, swelling and severe tenderness of the tissues around the ear and mastoid, and granulation tissue at the junction of the osseous and cartilagenous portions of the external ear. Roentgenographic findings [2], best appreciated by tomography, are not helpful in the early stages of the disease when involvement is limited to the soft tissues, but later they allow an accurate evaluation of the extent and progression of the disease. The disease is not usually associated with general manifestations of infection. The patients are generally afebrile, and the leukocyte count is either normal or mildly increased. The sedimentation rate may prove helpful in the diagnosis; it was persistently increased in our two cases as well as in the cases described by Dinapoli and Thomas [7] and Shanon et al. [4].

Successful treatment of this condition depends on early diagnosis. We believe that, when a diabetic patient presents with external otitis due to Ps. aeruginosa and has not responded to the usual treatment, he should be hospitalized and treated with systemic antibiotics for four to six weeks. Because of the poor vascularity of the involved area there is a need for high antibiotic levels in blood. Carbenicillin may be superior to gentamicin in its ability to penetrate into tissues; its disadvantage, however, is the development of resistance during treatment. Therefore, it is preferable to use full doses of both carbenicillin (24 g/day) and gentamicin (3 mg/kg/day) in the presence of normal renal function. If synergy [8] can be demonstrated, this may permit some reduction in dosage of the more toxic gentamicin which would be of value especially in the elderly diabetic patient with varying degrees of renal failure [12,13]. Otologic and renal function must be carefully monitored during therapy because large doses are required to penetrate the bone and halt infection. Tobramycin, a recently FDA-approved aminoglycoside, is similar to gentamicin but is two to four times more active in vitro [14]. In the second case presented, we chose tobramycin (minimal inhibitory concentration 0.195 μg/ml versus 0.39 μg/ml for gentamicin) when signs of eighth nerve toxicity developed to allow a lower dose of the potent aminoglycoside in the hopes of avoiding further toxicity. Further experience is needed to know whether this type of maneuver will be beneficial.

Locally, the existing granulation tissue should be removed and any abscess cavity curetted. If, however, granulation tissue continues to recur, adequate surgical debridement of all infected tissues is necessary. Chandler [1], initially stressed the importance of complete surgical debridement of all infected tissues and stated that limited surgery invariably leads to recurrence. In 1972 [6], following the introduction of carbenicillin, he suggested that local debridgement together with systemic antibiotics may be sufficient for cure.

REFERENCES

1. Chandler J: Malignant external otitis. Laryngoscope 78: 1257, 1968.
2. Kim BH: Roentgenographic findings of malignant external otitis. Am J Roentgenol Radium Ther Nucl Med 112: 366, 1971.
3. Wilson DF, Pulec JL: Malignant external otitis. Arch Otolaryngol 93: 419, 1971.
4. Shanon E, Bialystock G, Schujman E, Loewenthal H: Pseudomonal granulomatous external otitis. Acta Otolaryngol 73: 374, 1972.
5. Evans ITG, Richards SH: Malignant (necrotising) otitis externa. J Laryngol Otol 87: 13, 1973.
6. Chandler JR: Pathogenesis and treatment of facial paralysis due to malignant external otitis. Ann Otol Rhinol Laryngol 81: 648, 1972.
7. Dinapoli RP, Thomas JE: Neurologic aspects of malignant external otitis. Report of three cases. Mayo Clin Proc 46: 339, 1971.
8. Smith CB, Dans PE, Wilfert JN, Finland M: Use of gentamicin in combinations with other antibiotics. J Infect Dis 119: 370, 1969.
9. Singer DE, Freeman E, Hoffert WR, Keys RJ, Mitchell RB, Hardy AV: Otitis externa. Bacteriological and mycological studies. Ann Otol Rhinol Laryngol 61: 317, 1952.
10. Hubbard JD, King H, Beamer PR: The pathogenicity of Pseudomonas aeruginosa (Bacillus Pyocyaneous): Experimental studies and report of a case. Am J Clin Pathol 28: 243, 1957.
11. Rabin ER, Graber CD, Vogel EH: Fatal pseudomonas infection in burned patients. A clinical, bacteriological and anatomic study. N Engl J Med 265: 1225, 1961.
12. Eickhoff TC: In vitro effects of carbenicillin combined with gentamicin or polymyxin B against Pseudomonas aeruginosa. Appl Microbiol 18: 469, 1969.
13. Phair JP, Watanakunakorn C, Bannister T: In vitro susceptibility of Pseudomonas aeruginosa to carbenicillin and the combination of carbenicillin and gentamicin. Appl Microbiol 18: 303, 1969.
14. Kluge RM, Standiford HC, Tatem B, et al.: Comparative activity of tobramycin, amikacin, and gentamicin alone and with carbenicillin against Pseudomonas aeruginosa. Antimicrob Agents Chemother 6: 442, 1974.

SEPTEMBER 1976

The American Journal of Medicine

VOLUME 61

NUMBER 3

EDITORIALS

Cellular Origins of Autoantibody—A Perplexing Question

A. D. BANKHURST, M.D.*
R. C. WILLIAMS, Jr., M.D.
Albuquerque, New Mexico

During the past several years, autoantigen-binding cells have been detected in the peripheral blood of normal subjects and patients with autoimmune disease. Such autoradiographic methods which identify specific antigen-sensitive lymphocytes have provided us with a probe to investigate some of the basic cellular mechanisms controlling the regulation of the autoimmune response. Studies of autoantigen-binding cells have been performed using radiolabeled thyroglobulin and native-DNA (n-DNA) in normal subjects and patients with thyroiditis or systemic lupus erythematosus (SLE). In the case of both autoantigens, it became apparent that a low number of thyroglobulin-binding cells (216 per 10^6 lymphocytes) and n-DNA-binding lymphocytes (49 per 10^5 lymphocytes) were present in normal people. Increased numbers of n-DNA-binding cells were found in patients with active SLE (416 per 10^5 lymphocytes). Furthermore, the vast majority of autoantigen-binding cells were predominantly B lymphocytes in either normal subjects or patients with SLE. Such data on autoantigen-binding cells would argue against the possibility that autoimmunity is due to the emergence of autoantigen-specific helper T cells which would syngeristically enable programmed B lymphocytes to proliferate into autoantibody-producing plasma cells. Several hypothetic mechanisms are proposed which bypass the requirement for T cells reactive with autoantigens which would trigger the proliferation of autoantigen specific B lymphocytes.

A considerable effort has been expended during the past 20 years in studies related to definition, molecular characterization and specificity of various autoantibodies. Thus, initial reports describing rheumatoid factors in the serum of patients with rheumatoid arthritis [1–3] were followed over the ensuing years by a multitude of studies relating to the details of reactivity, autospecificity and the possible role of such antibodies. In like manner, the first reports and characterization of antinuclear and specific anti-DNA antibody in the serum of pa-

From the Department of Medicine, University of New Mexico, School of Medicine, Bernalillo County Medical Center, Stanford and Lomas, Albuquerque, New Mexico 87131. This study was supported in part by grants 13824-05 and TO1AI 00353-5 from the U.S. Public Health Service and in part by the Arthritis Foundation. Requests for reprints should be addressed to Dr. A. D. Bankhurst. Manuscript accepted January 9, 1976.

* Senior Investigator of the Arthritis Foundation.

tients with systemic lupus erythematosus (SLE) [4–7] once again were followed by an avalanche of careful and increasingly sophisticated studies regarding the immunoglobulin class, discrete molecular specificity and possible physiologic importance of antibodies to nuclear components, particularly to native DNA (n-DNA). In the case of antibodies to n-DNA, it appears that their appearance is fundamental to the development of immune complex disease in lupus glomeruli [8–10]. Whether or not rheumatoid factors or anti-n-DNA antibody represent examples of true autoantibodies to autologous tissue components, or the response of the body to altered self components, has never been finally answered; there is considerable evidence that such antibodies do indeed show a remarkable degree of specificity for unaltered native immunoglobulin or preparations of autologous n-DNA.

One of the most puzzling aspects of so-called autoimmune responses is linked to the enigma as to exactly how such a process is initiated. During the past several years, a great deal of new information bearing on fundamental processes controlling or influencing the initiation of the immune response has accumulated. If one attempts to focus on the precise mechanisms by which antibodies to such potential autoantigens as thyroglobulin or n-DNA are generated, some fascinating data are now available.

For some time, it has been recognized that there exists in the body a heterogeneous population of antigen-binding cells which appear somehow to be preset or preprogrammed to proliferate into cells forming an antibody product or an immune response specific for the diverse antigens which a person will be presented with during his lifetime. The potential fundamental importance of antigen-binding cells to the success of any immune response was clearly identified by antigen suicide or kamikaze-type experiments conducted by several groups of investigators [11–13]. Thus, it was shown that if an immunocompetent cell was exposed to a specific antigen to which it had never been previously exposed, and if the antigen were so highly labeled (high specific radioactivity) as to be able to kill cells to which it bound, then after such treatment the animal reconstituted with such a treated cell suspension would no longer be capable of mounting an immune response to that particular antigen. The kamikaze antigen had forever eliminated antigen-binding cells specific for that particular antigen. In many of these studies antigen-binding cells were identified as cells with apparent bone marrow-derived (B) cell characteristics, namely, possessing cell surface immunoglobulin markers. On the other hand, antigen-binding thymus-derived (T) cells were also repeatedly identified [14,15]. Of interest are recent reports which appear to show antigen-binding cells in both so-called responder and nonresponder strains of experimental animals [16,17]. In this context, nonresponder strains—so-named because they appear to harbor immune response genes which somehow turn off their immune responses to certain well-defined synthetic antigens—nonetheless, have a normal complement of antigen-binding cells for these synthetic antigens. Recently, the lack of an immune response in nonresponder strains was linked to an active postantigen binding process related to activation of specific suppressor T cell populations [18,19]. With these guidelines clearly in mind, it is of considerable interest to examine what is known about certain kinds of antigen-binding cells in normal man and in those with disease states.

The question was first approached using thyroglobulin, a high molecular weight protein present in normal thyroid glands. Patients with a wide variety of thyroid disorders often have been noted to show high titers of antibody to thyroglobulin, presumably induced by the initial proliferation and division of virgin autoantigen-binding cells specific for antigens on thyroglobulin. When the numbers of cells binding thyroglobulin were enumerated in normal subjects, the surprising finding became apparent that a significant number of thyroglobulin-binding antigen-binding cells (216 per 10^6 lymphocytes) were present in normal people [20]. Admittedly, the actual numbers of thyroglobulin-binding cells were considerably lower in normal subjects than in subjects with so-called autoimmune thyroid disorders [21]; however, the fact remained that a low, but relatively constant number of thyroglobulin-binding cells was consistently found in normal people.

As a corollary to these enigmatic findings, recent studies appear to indicate an analogous situation if one examines n-DNA-binding cells in both normal subjects and subjects with SLE [22]. Here, as was noted with thyroglobulin-binding cells, normal asymptomatic subjects, without SLE, showed a low but significant number of autoantigen-binding cells with apparent primary specificity for n-DNA [22]. The n-DNA-antigen-binding cells in both normal subjects (49 ± 40 per 10^5 lymphocytes, mean ± SD) and patients with active SLE (416 ± 270 per 10^5 lymphocytes) appeared to be B cells, since radioautographic studies combined with immunofluorescent studies showed concordance of surface immunoglobulin and labeled n-DNA in approximately 80 to 90 per cent of antigen-binding cells. Moreover, removal of B cells bearing surface immunoglobulin receptors by immunoglobulin-anti-immunoglobulin insolubilized columns virtually eliminated n-DNA-antigen-binding cells in most instances. If a significant difference existed in relative cell types functioning as n-DNA-antigen-binding cells in normal persons and in patients with SLE, one would have expected to have detected differences in ratios of T or B autoantigen-binding cells in the two populations. One feature conceivably influencing these results is the possibility that the autoradiographic technics used for the detection of n-DNA-antigen-binding cells may somehow preferentially slant the assay towards detection of B-type autoantigen-binding cells. However, the data now available relative to two types of potential autoimmune reactions appear to coincide in that the difference between normal subjects and patients is essentially one of numbers of detectable autoantigen-binding cells, rather than proportions of T or B autoantigen-binding cells.

Thus, part of the original clonal selection theory of Burnet may need to be adjusted to fit with these experimental data. The surveillance mechanisms of the body may not periodically eliminate autoantigen-binding cells as was put forward in the concept of the forbidden clones [23]. Somehow, nevertheless, the normal person is capable of containing the potentially self-reactive proliferation of thyroglobulin or n-DNA-antigen-binding cells. The real vexing question now seems to be what basic control mechanism has gone awry in progressive and often eventually lethal conditions such as SLE in which an unbridled proliferation of n-DNA-antigen-binding cells is allowed to continue generation of circulating anti-DNA antibodies, subsequent immune complexes, progressive lupus nephritis and finally death?

A great deal of hypothesizing has been done recently about conditions such as SLE being linked to a lack of effective suppressor T cell function [24–27]. Moreover, there is now some experimental data which appear to support the concept that lack of suppressor T cell activity is related to clinical deterioration in NZB mice [28–32]. Our data showing approximately equal proportions of B cell n-DNA-antigen-binding cells in both normal persons and patients with SLE do not fit with the idea of decreased suppressor T cell activity in SLE, since if this were true, one would have perhaps expected higher proportions of T n-DNA-antigen-binding cells in normal healthy adults than in those with SLE. The basic problem with testing of the suppresor cell hypothesis, of course, remains in the assay systems since as yet no direct identification, and thus enumeration, of suppressor T cells is possible. Nevertheless, it is reasonable to anticipate perhaps that antigen-specific receptors on T cells, whether the cells have a suppressor or helper functional role, could be identified by a similar autoradiographic technic.

The data on autoantigen-binding cells would also argue against the possibility that autoimmunity is simply the emergence of autoantigen-specific helper T cells to synergistically enable preexisting autoantigen-specific B lymphocytes to proliferate into autoantibody-producing plasma cells. In other words, we are confronted with the possibility that the initiation of an autoimmune response may involve a mechanism which

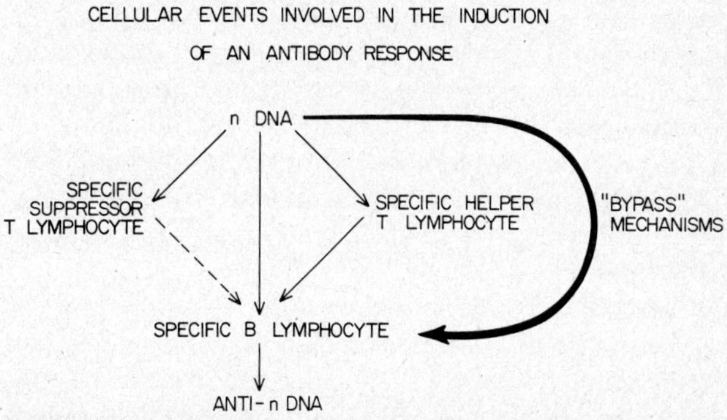

Figure 1. *Hypothetical scheme for the initiation of anti-n-DNA antibody in patients with SLE. Stimulation by antigen or lymphocyte is indicated by a solid line; inhibition is shown by a dotted line. The bypass mechanisms include the following: (1) a virus infection which provides a carrier for the hapten-like n-DNA; (2) an adjuvant or mitogen stimulation nonspecifically of the n-DNA-specific B lymphocyte; (3) a modification of n-DNA which provides a crossreacting antigen reactive with T lymphocytes and n-DNA specific B lymphocytes.*

bypasses the participation of autoantigen-specific T lymphocytes. These bypass mechanisms could provide the necessary stimulation to the autoantigen-specific B lymphocytes analogous to the T helper effect which occurs in the usual immune response to thymic-dependent antigens [27].

What are these mechanisms which bypass the requirement for T cells responsive against autoantigens and enable autoantibody formation to ensue? Some hypothetical bypass mechanisms leading to the triggering of autoantigen-sensitive B lymphocytes, in this case B cells reactive with n-DNA, are schematically outlined in Figure 1. First, this might be achieved by a virus infection. Since host antigens may be found in the envelope of some viruses, it follows that viruses and autoantigens could form common immunogenic units similar to a hapten-carrier system. In support of this hypothesis is the work of Schoyen and co-workers [33] who showed that infection of adult chickens with influenza virus coated with allantoic antigens after their propagation in chick eggs will produce autoantibody against the same fetal antigen found only in the bile of adult birds. Likewise, Tonetti and co-workers [34], have shown that infection of New Zealand strain mice with lymphocytic choriomeningitis virus accelerates the onset of spontaneous autoimmunity in these mice. Certainly the existence of virus-like particles in the tissues of patients with SLE [35] makes the possibility of a viral carrier a tantalyzing possibility. This concept of a self-antigen complexing with a carrier, and the subsequent emergence of autoantibodies directed against the self antigen, can be extended to other types of carriers. For example, the formation of antinuclear factors in patients treated with hydralazine, procainamide and other drugs [36] could be an analogous hapten-carrier stimulation of autoimmunity. In this case, the drug would be forming a complex with nucleoprotein and could be functioning as a carrier, stimulating drug reactive T cells which provide a helper stimulus and bypass the requirement for autoantigen reactive T cells. Some recent experimental data supporting this concept have been presented by Yamauchi et al. [37].

Second, an autoantigen-specific B cell may be triggered by a nonspecific stimulation such as a mitogen or adjuvant. This nonspecific stimulation could be mediated via a direct interaction with the specific B cell or indirectly via interaction with T cells which somehow indirectly activate the autoantigen-specific B cell. The former possibility is supported by the work of Fournie and co-workers [38], who found that endotoxin, a B cell mitogen in mice, can stimulate the formation of anti-DNA antibodies in a wide variety of mouse strains. Likewise, it is known that several adjuvants increase the proliferation of T lymphocytes and that the augmentation of antibody formation attributed to these adjuvants is dependent on the presence of T lymphocytes [39]. It is conceivable, however, that some adjuvants may exert a carrier effect also, as in the case of the mycobacteria present in complete Freund's adjuvant which could form complexes with host antigens.

Third, it is possible that a crossreacting, modified antigen could stimulate the autoantigen-specific B cell. In this light, one might envision one antigenic determinant on the altered host antigen reacting with a T cell which, in turn, supplies a stimulatory effect on the autoantigen-specific B cell. Such a mechanism is supported by the work of Weigle and Nakamura [40], who found that antithyroglobulin antibodies could be induced in rabbits only with heterologous and modified thyroglobulin under conditions in which autologous thyroglobulin was ineffective. One can only speculate how such an alteration of host antigens could arise, but possibly any site of inflammation with attendent release of proteolytic and other degradative enzymes could lead to the formation of altered self components. The possibility of such a modification of self-antigens by inflammatory states is supported by the presence of antibodies against altered human serum albumin in patients with alcoholic liver disease [41].

In summary, the potential for the emergence of autoimmunity presumably exists within all normal subjects. The B lymphocytes reactive with self-components may be held in abeyance only by the absence of stimulation from a T cell helper consort. In this view, the unleashing of autoimmunity could arise by the intercession of a B cell stimulant by one of several bypass mechanisms which circumvent the need for autoantigen specific T lymphocytes.

REFERENCES

1. Franklin EC, Holman MR, Muller-Eberhard, et al.: An unusual protein component of high molecular weight in the serum of certain patients with rheumatoid arthritis. J Exp Med 105: 425, 1957.
2. Franklin EC, Kunkel HG, Muller-Eberhard, et al.: Relation of high molecular weight proteins to the serological reactions in rheumatoid arthritis. Ann Rheum Dis 16: 315, 1957.
3. Kunkel HG, Franklin EC, Muller-Eberhard HJ: Studies on the isolation and characterization of the "rheumatoid factor." J Clin Invest 38: 424, 1959.
4. Seligmann M: Mise en évidence dans le sérum de malades atteints de lupus érythemateux disséminé d'une substance determinant une réaction de précipitation avec l'acid désoxyribonucleique. Comptes Rendus de L'Academie des Sciences (Paris) 245: 243, 1957.
5. Cepellini R, Polli E, Celada F: A DNA-reacting factor in serum of a patient with lupus erythematosus diffusus. Proc Soc Exp Biol Med 96: 575, 1957.
6. Robbins WC, Holman HR, Diecher H, et al.: Complement fixation with cell nuclei and DNA in lupus erythematosus. Proc Soc Exp Biol Med 96: 575, 1957.
7. Deicher HRB, Holman HR, Kunkel HG: The precipitin reaction between DNA and a serum factor in systemic lupus erythematosus. J Exp Med 109: 97, 1959.
8. Krishman C, Kaplan MH: Immunopathologic studies of systemic lupus erythematosus. II. Antinuclear reaction of - globulin eluted from homogenates and isolated glomeruli of kidneys from patients with lupus nephritis. J Clin Invest 46: 569, 1967.
9. Koffler D, Schur PH, Kunkel HG: Immunological studies concerning the nephritis of systemic lupus erythematosus. J Exp Med 126: 607, 1967.
10. Koffler D. Agnello V, Thoburn R, et al.: Systemic lupus erythematosus: prototype of immune complex nephritis in man. J Exp Med 134: 169S, 1971.
11. Ada FL, Byrt P: Specific inactivation of antigen-reactive cells with ^{125}I-labelled antigen. Nature (Lond) 222: 1291, 1969.
12. Basten A. Miller JFAP, Warner WL, et al.: Specific inactivation of thymus-derived (T) lymphocytes and non-thymus-derived (B) lymphocytes by ^{125}I-labelled antigen. Nature (New Biol) 231: 104, 1971.
13. Ada GL: Antigen-binding cells in tolerance and immunity. Transplant Rev 5: 105, 1970.
14. Dwyer JM, Warner NL, MacKay IR: Specificity and nature of the antigen combining site on fetal and mature thymus lymphocytes. J Immunol 108: 1439, 1972.
15. Hammerling GT, McDevitt HO: Antigen binding T and B Lymphocytes. I. Differences in cellular specificity and influence of metabolic activity on interaction of antigen with B and T cells. J Immunol 112: 1726, 1974.
16. Hammerling GJ, McDevitt HO: Comparative analysis of antigen-binding T cells in genetic high and low responder mice. J Exp Med 140: 1180, 1974.
17. Kennedy JL, Dorf ME, Unanue ER, et al.: Binding of poly ($Glu^{60}Ala^{30}Tyr^{10}$) by thymic lymphocytes from genetic responder and non-responder mice: effect of antihistocompatibility serum. J Immunol 114: 1670, 1975.
18. Kapp JA, Pierce CW, Schlossman S, et al.: Genetic control of immune responses in vitro. V. Stimulation of suppressor T cells in non-responder mice by the terpolymer L-glutamic acid (^{60}L-alanine^{30}-L-tyrosine^{10} (GAT). J Exp Med 140: 648, 1974.
19. Kapp JA, Pierce CW, Benacerraf B: Genetic control of immune

responses in vitro. VI. Experimental conditions for the development of helper T cell activity specific for the terpolymer L-glutamic acid (^{60}L-alanine^{30}-L-tyrosine^{10} (GAT) in nonresponder mice. J Exp Med 142: 50, 1975.
20. Bankhurst AD, Torrigiani G, Allison AC: Lymphocytes binding human thyroglobulin in healthy people and its relevance to tolerance for autoantigens. Lancet 1: 226, 1973.
21. Roberts IM. Whittingham S, MacKay IR: Tolerance to an autoantigen thyroglobulin. Lancet 2: 936, 1973.
22. Bankhurst AD, Williams RC Jr: Identification of DNA-binding lymphocytes in patients with systemic lupus erythematosus. J Clin Invest 56: 1378, 1975.
23. Burnet F: The clonal selection theory of acquired immunity. (Burnet F, ed), Cambridge, Massachusetts, Cambridge University Press, 1969.
24. Allison AC: Heberden oration: mechanisms of tolerance and autoimmunity. Ann Rheum Dis 32: 283, 1973.
25. Allison AC, Denman AM, Barnes RD: Cooperating and controlling functions of thymus-derived lymphocytes in relation to autoimmunity. Lancet 2: 135, 1971.
26. Messner RP, Lindstrom FD, Williams RC Jr: Peripheral blood lymphocytes cell surface markers during the course of systemic lupus erythematosus. J Clin Invest 52: 3046, 1973.
27. Katz DH, Benacerraf B: The regulatory influence of activated T cells on B cell response to antigen. Advances in Immunology, vol. 15 (Dixon F, Kunkel HG, eds), New York, Academic Press, 1972, p 1.
28. Morse HC III, Steinberg AD, Schur PH, et al.: Spontaneous "autoimmune disease" in nude mice. J Immunol 113: 688, 1974.
29. Barhold DR, Kysela S, Steinberg AD: Decline in suppressor T cell function with age in female NZB mice. J Immunol 112: 9, 1974.
30. Stutman O, Yunis EJ, Good RA: Deficient immunologic functions of NZB mice. Proc Soc Exp Biol Med 127: 1204, 1968.
31. Steinberg AD, Law LD, Talal N: The role of NZB/NZW F_1 Thymus in experimental tolerance and autoimmunity. Arthritis Rheum 13: 369, 1970.
32. Gershwin ME, Steinberg AD: Suppression of autoimmune hemolytic anemia in New Zealand (NZB) mice by syngeneic young thymocytes. Clin Immunol Immunopathol 4: 38, 1975.
33. Schoyen R, Hargoe A, Wang L: Influenza virus HI-antibody combining with normal chick material and produced in hens immunized with chick grown influenza virus. Acta Pathol Microbiol Scand 68: 1103, 1966.
34. Tonietti G, Oldstone MBA, Dixon FJ: The effect of induced chronic viral infections on the immunologic diseases of New Zealand Mice. J Exp Med 132: 89, 1970.
35. Klippel JH, Grimley PM, Decker JL: Lymphocyte tubuloreticular structures in lupus erythematosus. Ann Intern Med 81: 355, 1974.
36. Lee SL, Rivero I, Siegel M: Activation of systemic lupus erythematosus by drugs. Arch Intern Med 117: 620, 1966.
37. Yamauchi Y, Litwin A, Adams L, et al.: Induction of antibodies to nuclear antigens in rabbits by immunization with hydralazine-human serum albumin conjugates. J Clin Invest 56: 958, 1975.
38. Fournie GJ, Lambert PH, Miescher PA: Release of DNA in circulating blood and induction of anti-DNA antibodies after infection of bacterial lipo polysaccharides. J Exp Med 140: 1189, 1974.
39. Allison AC: "Effects of adjuvants on different cell types and their interactions," Ciba Foundation Symposium on Immunopotentiation, London, Church, 1973.
40. Weigle WO, Nakamura RM: The development of autoimmune thyroiditis in rabbits following injection of aqueous preparations of heterologous thyroglobulins. J Immunol 99: 223, 1967.
41. Hauptman S, Tomasi TB Jr: Antibodies to human albumin in cirrhotic sera. J Clin Invest 54: 122, 1974.

Acute Renal Success

The Unexpected Logic of Oliguria in Acute Renal Failure*

KLAUS THURAU, M.D.
Munich, West Germany
JOHN W. BOYLAN, M.D.†
Buffalo, New York

The clinical condition known as acute renal failure is recognized by the onset of oliguria, its course is marked by the persistence of oliguria, and recovery is heralded by the advent of diuresis. The dramatic character of oliguria has made it the focus of attention for the physician. Oliguria was viewed as the primary event and therapy was directed to measures to restore urine flow rate to normal. Little thought has been given to the concept that the kidney may be acting appropriately in making a small volume of urine or that oliguria may be the necessary consequence of a functional adaptation protecting the patient from a graver danger.

A PARTICULAR POINT OF VIEW

Experimental research during the last decade [1–9] has provided new insight into the functional alterations and adaptations in the kidney during acute renal failure; we would like to discuss the condition from a rather particular point of view. Our thesis is that the oliguria of acute *reversible* renal failure results from the operation of an intrarenal regulating mechanism present in the normal kidney and working, in the case of acute renal failure, to the immediate benefit of the patient. The immediate benefit is life-saving, as will be shown; certain long-term effects are less desirable.

THE INHERENT DANGER OF OUR HIGH FILTRATION RATE

The kidney has a reputation for sensible behavior. As the exacting guardian of our internal environment, it has been credited with discriminatory activity in the selection of filtered plasma constituents for reabsorption or excretion. The large glomerular filtration rate, a heritage from our aquatic ancestors, has been retained in the mammalian kidney because it serves its important function of continuously reprocessing the plasma. In this reprocessing, the entire circulating plasma volume is filtered and reabsorbed twice an hour. As a means of adjusting the body fluid composition, the function is effective but it contains an inherent danger—that of severe fluid loss if the reabsorptive mechanism should fail.

DISTINCTIVE FEATURE OF TUBULAR REABSORPTION

The coupled events of filtration and reabsorption occur at the capillary end of all vascular beds and are accomplished in most regions by purely physical forces, the balance between hydrostatic and colloid oncotic pressures first described by Starling. By and large, the composition of filtrate and reabsorbate is the same, and no discrimination

From the Department of Physiology, University of Munich, West Germany; and the Department of Medicine, State University of New York at Buffalo. Requests for reprints should be addressed to Prof. Klaus Thurau, Department of Physiology, 8 Munich 2, Pettenkoferstr 12 West Germany, or to Dr. John W. Boylan, Veterans Administration Hospital, Buffalo, New York 14215. Manuscript accepted February 27, 1976.

*This paper is dedicated to Prof. Kurt Kramer.

†Written during the tenure of an Alexander von Humboldt Senior Scientist Award.

is exercised (Figure 1). In the kidney, however, a layer of epithelial cells (the tubular wall) is interposed between the site of filtration and that of re-entry of the filtrate to the blood stream. This distinctive addition to the system refines the reabsorptive process and enables a degree of selectivity in solute excretion (Figure 1). Salt and water are reabsorbed in large volumes, creatinine and urea for the most part are excreted. Tubular cell activity defines the composition of both reabsorbate and final urine. Selectivity ends at the basal surface of tubular cells, and re-entry into the vascular compartment is accomplished, as in the peripheral circulation, by Starling forces, without further discrimination as to composition.

GLOMERULAR FILTRATION RATE AND TUBULAR REABSORPTION ARE SEPARATELY POWERED

The energy source for glomerular filtration, the left ventricle, is distinct from the metabolic energy of reabsorption, generated locally by the tubular epithelial cells. It is this locally-produced energy that brings to the blind force of filtration the refinement of differential selectivity in the reabsorptive process. Although the energies of these two basic renal operations are independently derived, they must be adaptively coupled to one another. The adaptive coupling is described phenomenologically as tubuloglomerular balance [12–15], a process by which the rate of tubular reabsorption sets the filtration rate. This setting is imperative since failure of reabsorptive function in the presence of continued filtration would result in a devastating loss of body fluids.

A LINK BETWEEN FILTRATION AND REABSORPTION

In most systemic capillaries, filtration and reabsorption are intrinsically joined. The hydrostatic force that results in filtration at the arterial end of a capillary provides the energy for reabsorption by concentrating colloids. The opposing filtration pressure is dissipated by the high resistance of the capillaries, and colloid oncotic pressure becomes increasingly effective, favoring reabsorption.

What mechanism exists to adjust filtration rate to reabsorptive capacity in the nephron? To be effective it should comprise monitoring and reacting components by which some sensing device reads a signal reflecting the adequacy of reabsorption and initiates a response at the glomerular level. The structural basis for such a system has been found in every mammalian nephron examined [16–19] and is embodied in the juxtaglomerular apparatus (Figure 2). The juxtaglomerular apparatus joins a late segment of each nephron to the vascular pole of its own glomerulus. At the end of the thick ascending limb of Henle's loop, where the nephron returns to its glomerulus, the cells of the tubular wall are differentiated into the *macula densa* cells and lie in

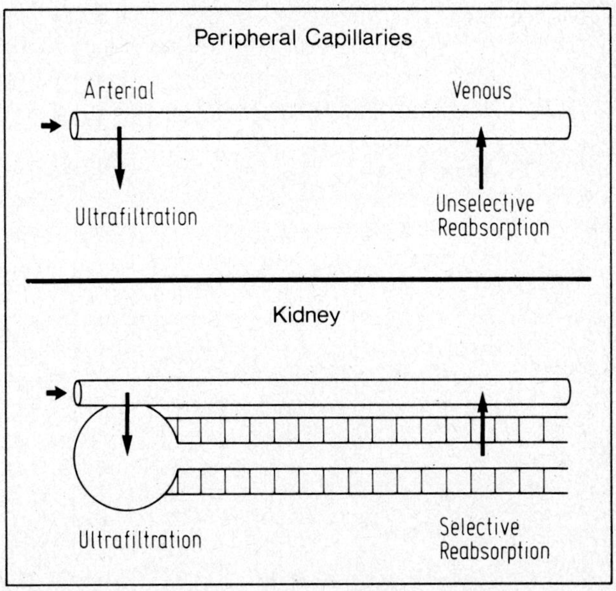

Figure 1. *Schematic representation of fluid movement across the capillaries in the peripheral circulation and in the kidney. The extravascular fluid movement is determined in peripheral capillaries by physical forces (Starling mechanism) and, hence, is unselective, whereas, in the kidney, energy for a discriminating reabsorptive process is supplied by an interposed cell layer (tubular cells).*

intimate apposition to the walls of the glomerular arterioles. Here the cells of the media are transformed to large secretory-type cells filled with electron-dense granules (renin). This anatomic arrangement is ideally suited to monitor an intratubular event (reabsorption) and to initiate a response (filtration).

FEEDBACK CONTROL OF GLOMERULAR FILTRATION RATE—THE SIGNAL

The signal that is read by the tubular component (macula densa) of the juxtaglomerular apparatus is the sodium chloride concentration of tubular fluid at that site [10,11,14,21]. Present evidence more specifically favors chloride ion concentration as the definitive signal [22], and the concentration of this ion here is related to the reabsorptive activity of the entire nephron. The largest volume of filtrate is reabsorbed proximally, at a chloride concentration close to the plasma value. Filtrate arriving at the site of the *macula densa* has, under normal conditions, lost over 80 per cent of its original volume and its sodium chloride concentration is, for the first time along the nephron, below plasma value—about one-seventh in fact [1,23,25]. This low chloride concentration is established by the thick ascending limb of Henle's loop, the cells of which actively transport chloride [26] without equivalent water.

An increased signal, reporting imbalance between filtration and reabsorption, can be induced experi-

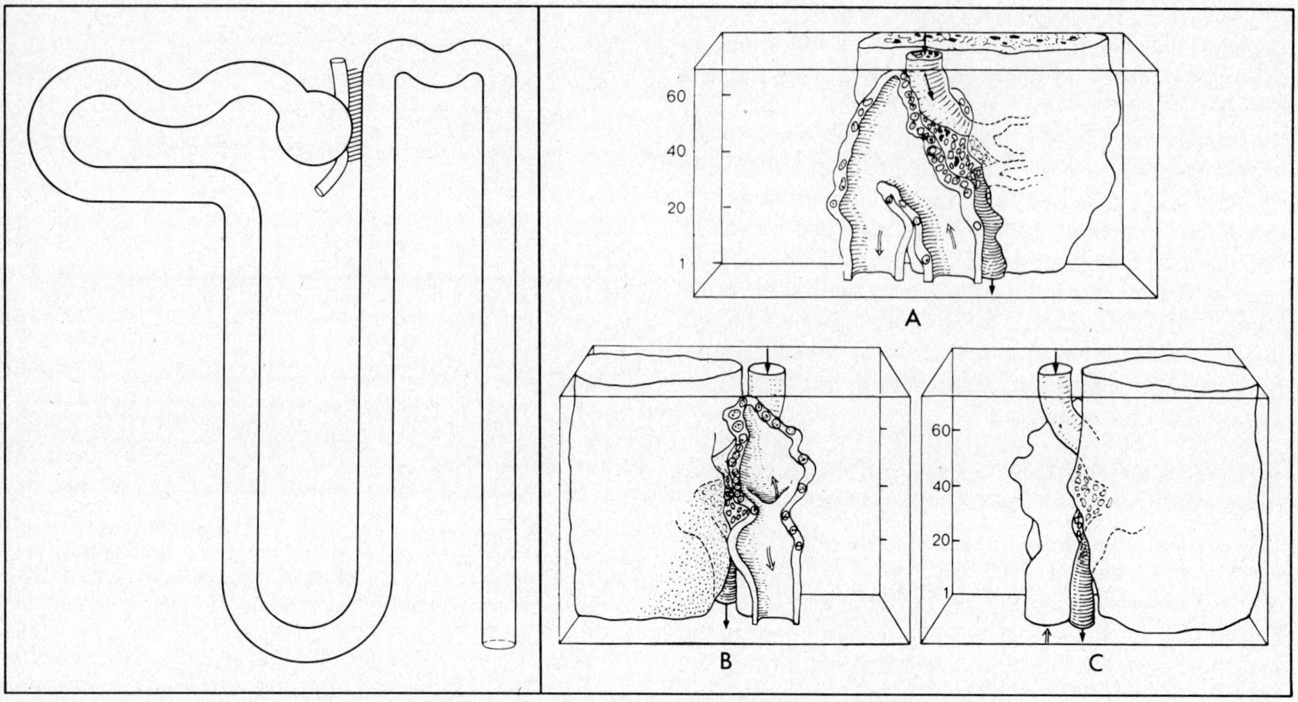

Figure 2. ***Left,*** *schematic representation of the anatomic relationship of the juxtaglomerular apparatus (hatched area) within the single nephron unit. The juxtaglomerular apparatus forms a functional link between the end of Henle's loop and the vascular pole of the glomerulus of the same nephron.* ***Right,*** *scale reconstruction (190:1) of the vascular pole of a human glomerulus with juxtaglomerular apparatus from 1.9 μ thick, Giemsa-stained serial sections.* ***A,*** *from above,* ***B,*** *from the left,* ***C,*** *from the right. The flow direction of blood* ***(closed arrows)*** *and urine* ***(open arrows)*** *is indicated. The Goormaghtigh cells in the angle between the two arterioles, the cell nuclei of the macula densa and in the remaining part of the tubule are shown. The arteriolar component of the apparatus is not shown. In the background (A) of the vascular pole and to its left and right (B and C) is the outer surface of Bowman's capsule [20].*

mentally in two ways: (1) One is by augmenting the perfusion rate through the nephron, a condition simulating increased glomerular filtration rate. This leads to an increase in sodium chloride concentration at the *macula densa* [14,23,24] since tubular reabsorptive activity does not increase in proportion to the increased tubular flow rate. (2) Another is by reducing the tubular reabsorptive capacity. Here, the increased sodium chloride concentration at the *macula densa* reflects the failure of the tubular epithelium to reabsorb [1,11]. Either maneuver causes an imbalance between solute load to the nephron and reabsorptive capacity of tubular cells.

FEEDBACK CONTROL OF GLOMERULAR FILTRATION RATE—THE RESPONSE

The appropriate response to a signal reporting reabsorptive failure is reduction in filtration rate; this has been found in experimental animals with induced acute renal failure [5] and in the clinical condition in man [27]. Filtration rate is reduced by vasoconstriction of the glomerular arterioles and, possibly, by retraction of the glomerular tuft [28,29], activities that simultaneously reduce renal blood flow [30–32]. Evidence is accumulating that the vasoactive material is angiotensin II, locally formed at the site of the juxtaglomerular apparatus and acting in situ. It has been shown that the juxtaglomerular apparatus is supplied with all the components necessary to manufacture and to degrade angiotensin II [35]. Converting enzyme inhibitors reduce the intensity of the response [36] as does depletion of renal renin [10,34–39].

Data have been furnished recently to confirm the intrarenal formation of angiotensin II [40] and its release primarily into the renal interstitium rather than into the blood [41]. Experimentally, when tubular fluid sodium chloride concentration of a single nephron is increased at the macula densa (Figure 3), the renin activity of the attached juxtaglomerular apparatus increases proportionately [21] and the filtration rate of that nephron decreases [14,42]. These findings together demonstrate the existence of a tubuloglomerular feedback mechanism whereby single nephron (and in the aggregate, whole kidney) glomerular filtration rate is regulated according to the efficiency of reabsorption. Brandt-Rehberg [12], who introduced creatinine as a marker for the measurement of glomerular filtration rate, was to our knowledge, the first to point out the relationship between tubular reabsorptive capacity and the glomerular filtration rate when he wrote in 1929: "Es bedeutet hier, daβ jede Schädigung der Tubuli, die eine Einschränkung in der Resorptionsfähigkeit dieser Gebilde bewirkt, auch eine sofortige Herabsetzung der Glomerulifunktion mit sich bringt." (Translation: This means that any damage to the tubules, which leads to a curtailment of their ability to reabsorb, will also lead to an immediate reduction in the function of the glomeruli.)

SEQUENCE LEADING TO OLIGURIA

Whatever the initiating cause of acute renal failure (toxic, ischemic, etc.), the injury affects tubular transport activity, that function of the kidney that depends on locally generated energy [3,33,34,43,44]. When tubular reabsorptive capacity and net volume reabsorption have been examined in animal models of acute renal failure they have been found to be significantly depressed [2,3,5,45–47]. The result is an increase in sodium chloride concentration of tubular fluid arriving at the *macula densa*. In addition, these experimental animals have been found to have increased renin activity in their juxtaglomerular apparatus [9,48–50] just as the renin activity in the single juxtaglomerular apparatus of normal kidneys increased when their macula densa segments were perfused with fluid of high sodium chloride concentration [21,35].

In acute renal failure, therefore, the feedback mechanism described and schematically illustrated in Figure 4, provides a means to maintain tubuloglomerular balance by reducing the glomerular filtration rate to a level compatible with the attenuated reabsorptive capacity. Both the sensing and response elements of the feedback mechanism have been found to be functionally intact in various models of acute renal failure [9].

GLOMERULAR DEFENSE OF VOLUME

Reduction in glomerular filtration rate to conform to diminished reabsorptive capacity means that the glomeruli have taken over the volume-conserving function normally exercised by the tubules. The importance of this reduction in glomerular filtration rate is made clearer by considering what might happen if the glomerular filtration rate remained normal and the tubular reabsorption were reduced by 50 per cent. Urinary volume and sodium excretion would be half the filtered load. In man, the result would be a urinary volume loss of approximately 60 ml/min and, unless salt and water loss could be replaced, the organism would lose its last sodium ion within a few hours. Volume conservation by reversible glomerular shutdown is immediately effective

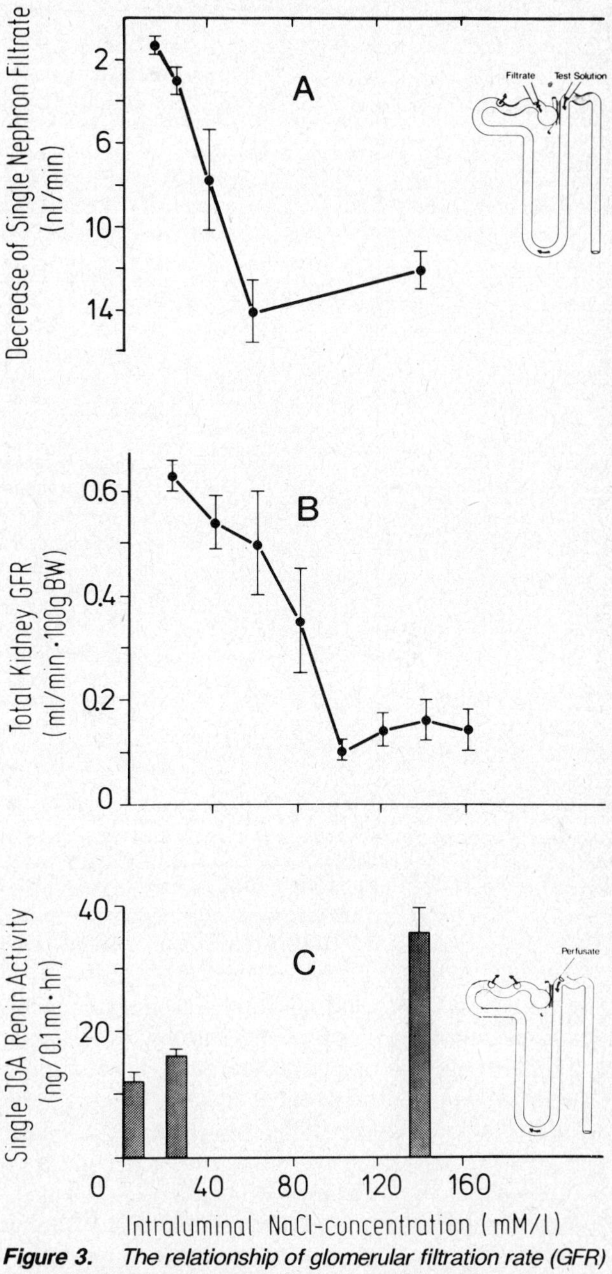

Figure 3. *The relationship of glomerular filtration rate (GFR) (solid line) and renin activity in the juxtaglomerular apparatus (JGA) (solid bars) to the sodium chloride concentration in tubular fluid of early distal tubule.* ***A,*** *in the normal rat kidney, retrograde perfusion of a macula densa segment with increasing sodium chloride concentration is associated with a progressive fall in simultaneously measured single nephron filtration rate (after 22).* ***B,*** *in the normal and postischemic rat kidney, total kidney filtration rate correlates closely with sodium*$^{+}$ *concentration in the early distal tubular fluid (after 1).* ***C,*** *in the normal rat kidney, retrogade perfusion of the macula densa segment with sodium chloride-free mannitol or with 140 mmol sodium chloride and determination of renin activity in the attached juxtaglomerular cell complex. Renin activity associated with 25 mmol sodium chloride (middle bar) was obtained from juxtaglomerular apparatus of nephrons naturally perfused from the glomerulus [21].*

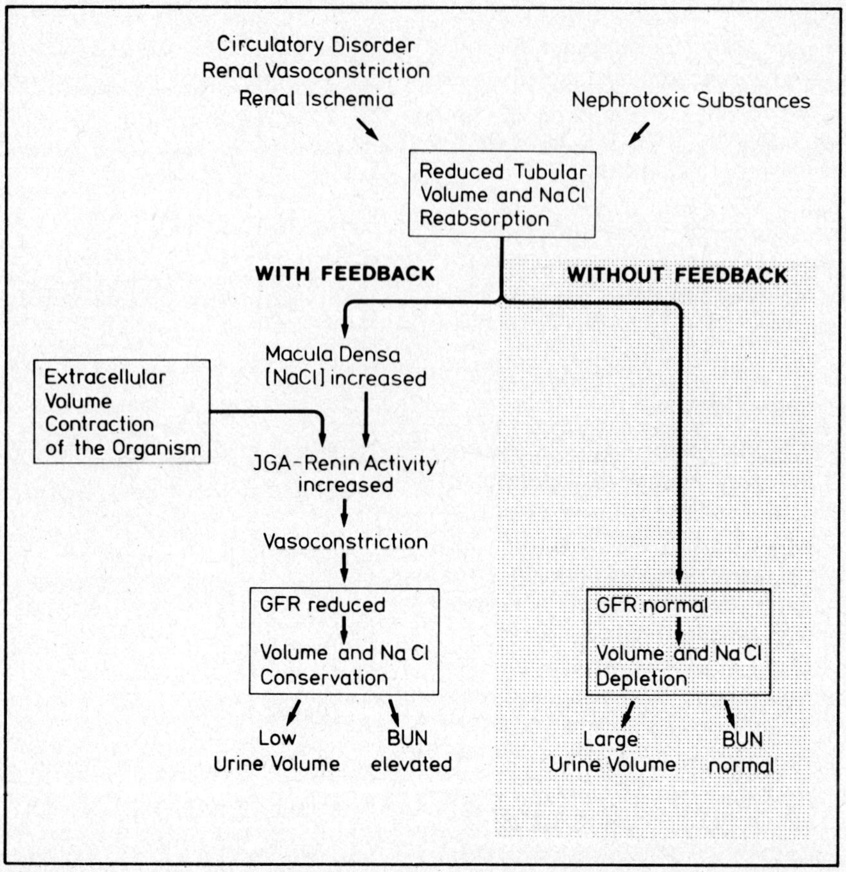

Figure 4. *Diagram illustrating the postulated effect of the presence or absence of tubuloglomerular feedback on urine volume and blood urea nitrogen in the inadequately reabsorbing tubules of an acute renal failure kidney.*

and therefore life-saving. It has the disadvantage of being indiscriminate; consequently nitrogenous wastes and other materials regularly cleared by filtration are retained. The immediate threat of death by hypovolemia is averted at the expense of the regulation of body fluid composition. This decision allows the organism time to repair structure and function of the damaged tubules.

Nephron damage in acute renal failure is of quite variable severity. Many instances of tubular injury undoubtedly occur in which the reduction in glomerular filtration rate is moderate and retention insufficient to come to the clinician's attention. It is only when reabsorptive function is severely reduced that depression of the glomerular filtration rate leads to a degree of retention that is clinically relevant. The degree of retention in some measure, therefore, reflects the extent of tubular reabsorptive insufficiency.

LOSS OF CONCENTRATING ABILITY AND HIGH URINARY SODIUM

The distinctive defect in tubular sodium chloride reabsorption, here presented as the determinant of oliguria, has other effects on renal function, and these have provided diagnostic guides to the recognition of acute renal failure. Diminished urinary concentrating ability is characteristic [51]. For maximum efficiency, the concentrating process requires a filtration rate large enough to insure adequate delivery of solute to the countercurrent system and an intact function of loop transport of sodium chloride [52]. Both activities are prerequisite for the establishment of a medullary osmotic gradient, the basis of urinary concentration, and both activities are impaired in acute renal failure. The result is a small volume of isosmotic urine with a high sodium concentration, a combination found only in acute renal failure or end-stage renal disease. In balance studies of patients in acute renal failure, the mean urinary sodium concentration during the oliguric phase is often in excess of 85 meq/liter [53,63]. Values greater than 25 meq/liter during oliguria are considered diagnostic [54]. In contrast, prerenal oliguria, usually the result of dehydration or volume loss, is associated with avid sodium retention.

THE SIGNAL PERSISTS UNTIL HEALING

The persistence of oliguria long after removal of the precipitating cause of acute renal failure has always troubled the thoughtful physician as has the unexplained appearance of diuresis. Both findings are readily accounted for in the present concept when we consider that as long as tubular reabsorptive capacity is interfered with, so long will sodium chloride concentration remain increased in tubular fluid and be monitored at the *macula densa*. The signal for reduced glomerular filtration rate and its correlated renal blood flow will persist until tubular function is restored. This is reflected in a decrease in urinary sodium concentration from high values in the first days of oliguria to lower values when urine flow is approaching normal (Figure 5). Healing of tubular cell injury requires from a few days to two or more weeks, depending on the severity of the lesion, and it is not surprising that the period of glomerular shutdown reflects this variability of time. As each nephron regains its reabsorptive function, the sodium chloride concentration of tubular fluid arriving at its *macula densa* is reduced and filtration to that nephron increases. Not uncommonly, in the restoration of tubular function, the glomerular filtration rate is not perfectly matched to reabsorptive capacity and a period of imbalance intervenes, manifested by polyuria. Salt wasting is characteristic of this phase [63] and replacement must be carefully matched to urinary loss. During functional maturation of regenerating tubules, small increases in the glomerular filtration rate result in large increments in urine flow and, until the capacity for maximum sodium salvage is restored, a period of negative balance is likely.

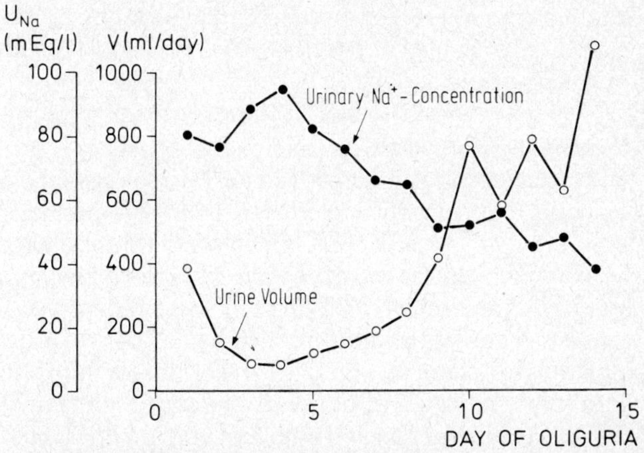

Figure 5. *Urinary sodium concentration and urine volume during the oliguric and recovery phases of acute renal failure in man (redrawn from data of [53]).*

ACUTE RENAL FAILURE REDEFINED

So the accusation implied in the term "acute renal failure" is only partially just. Due to injury, the tubules have failed in their reabsorptive function but immediate massive volume loss has been prevented by the feedback mechanism of the juxtaglomerular apparatus, a fail-safe device that guards volume by indiscriminate retention. The system continues to operate, like a finger in the dike, until tubular function is reestablished. The scope and efficiency of this volume-conserving mechanism, the normal operation of which is scarcely discernible, are revealed only in the extraordinary condition of tubular failure.

A MODULATOR OF THE JUXTAGLOMERULAR APPARATUS SYSTEM

The system has another input in addition to the signal to the *macula densa* and that is the "state of fullness" of the extracellular space, i.e., the volume reserve of the organism. Volume expansion decreases renin activity in the juxtaglomerular apparatus [55] and this is coincident with a reduced gain of the feedback control system thereby reset to a lower level of responsiveness [10,37–39]. Hence reduction in glomerular filtration rate is less pronounced when the stimulus impinges on a system made less sensitive by volume expansion.

In contrast, during volume depletion, renin activity in the juxtaglomerular apparatus is increased and a given increase in sodium chloride concentration at the *macula densa* results in a greater depression in the glomerular filtration rate than would occur in the normal or expanded state (Figure 4). The afferent pathway of this input is unknown but is thought by some to originate from baroreceptors in the walls of the glomerular arterioles [56] or from changes in ionic composition of juxtaglomerular apparatus cells associated with volume expansion or contraction [38].

THE LOGIC OF PROTECTION FROM GLOMERULAR SHUTDOWN

It follows that the likelihood of acute renal failure developing in a given situation is best minimized by a state of volume expansion. The consequent lowering of renin activity in the juxtaglomerular system prevents the kidney from reacting too intensely to tubular injury, that is, by too drastic a reduction in glomerular filtration rate and renal blood flow thus exacerbating the ischemic condition. The common clinical impression that patients whose extracellular volume is contracted are more prone to the development of acute renal failure was borne out by experiments in which volume expanded rats were significantly protected [57,58]. The efficacy of loop diuretics in some cases of acute renal failure is consistent with the ability of these diuretics to interfere with the perception and/or transmission of the signal at the *macula densa* [9,59].

POLYURIC ACUTE RENAL FAILURE

No system is infallible and we should expect cases of acute renal failure to occur in which the volume-preserving function of the feedback system does not properly respond. Whatever the cause (failure of *macula densa* to read the signal, enzyme defect, substrate inadequacy, etc.), reduced reabsorptive capacity in the presence of an uncontrolled filtration rate should result in massive volume loss.

A literature search in fact discovers cases of massive polyuria (45 to 70 liters/day approximating half or more of simultaneously measured filtration rate), in instances of tubular injury in which glomerular filtration rate was *not* curtailed [44,60]. *This* is complete renal failure wherein both tubular and glomerular volume-conserving mechanisms are bankrupt. It is of interest that one of these is a case of postobstructive nephropathy [60], a salt-losing state, in which the major defect in reabsorption is thought to occur in the proximal tubule [61,62]. Some ascending limb function is apparently spared since a dilute urine can be formed [61]; whether this fact or a direct compressive injury to the juxtaglomerular apparatus is responsible for failure of the feedback mechanism is presently speculative.

SUMMARY AND CONCLUSION

The magnitude of glomerular filtration imposes the necessity of a safety mechanism to protect the body from serious fluid loss if tubular reabsorption should fail. This need appears to be met by the juxtaglomerular apparatus which contains a sensing element to recognize tubular reabsorptive activity and a response component to adjust the glomerular filtration rate proportionately. The system is operating in acute renal failure and preserves body fluids by glomerular shutdown, with resulting oliguria. Once acute renal failure is manifest, rational therapy might be directed to an attempt to moderate the renal response, i.e., the degree of glomerular shutdown either at the level of signal perception or juxtaglomerular apparatus enzyme activity. Such methods are conjectural, but it may be possible in this way to adjust renal perfusion to a rate that is adequate to promote healing and a degree of excretory function without jeopardizing volume conservation. Dialysis and careful fluid balance will support the patient until healing is complete.

The basic pattern of the tubuloglomerular feedback system has been defined by experimental analysis. Many intricacies, especially details of signal transmission and the pathway leading to angiotensin II formation, remain as subjects for future investigation.

ACKNOWLEDGMENT

We take pleasure in acknowledging the assistance of Martha Manning, Research Librarian, Health Science Library, State University of New York at Buffalo.

REFERENCES

1. Schnermann J, Nagel W, Thurau K: Die frühdistale Natriumkozentration in Rattennieren nach renaler Ischämie und hämorrhagischer Hypotension. Pflüegers Arch 287: 296, 1966.
2. Henry LN, Lane CE, Kashgarian M: Micropuncture studies of the pathophysiology of acute renal failure in the rat. Lab Invest 19: 309, 1968.
3. Thurau K: Pathophysiologie des akuten Nierenversagens. Anaesthesiologie und Wiederbelebung 49, Berlin-Heidelberg, Springer-Verlag, 1970.
4. Oken DE: Modern concepts of the role of nephrotoxic agents in the pathogenesis of acute renal failure. Prog Biochem Pharmacol 7: 1, 1971.
5. Flamenbaum W: Pathophysiology of acute renal failure. Arch Intern Med 131: 911, 1973.
6. Bohle A, Thurau K: Funktion und Morphologie der Niere im akuten Nierenversagen. Verh Dtsch Ges Inn Med 80: 565, 1974.
7. Symposium on Experimental Models and Pathophysiology of Acute Renal Failure, Rottach-Egern 1975. Kidney Int Supplement (in preparation).
8. Finn WF, Arendshort WJ, Gottschalk CW: Pathogenesis of oliguria in acute renal failure. Circ Res 36: 675, 1975.
9. Mason J, Thurau K: The physiological mechanisms responsible for the adjustment of renal function during acute renal failure. Proceedings of the Sixth International Congress on Nephrology, Florence, 1975. Basel, S. Karger, 1976.
10. Thurau K, Schnermann J: Die Natriumkonzentration an den macula densa-Zellen als regulierender Faktor für das Glomerulumfiltrat. Klin Wochenschr 43: 410, 1965.
11. Thurau K, Schnermann J, Nagel W, et al.: Composition of tubular fluid in the macula densa segment as a factor regulating the function of the juxtaglomerular apparatus. Circ Res 20/21 (suppl 2): 79, 1, 1967.
12. Brandt-Rehberg P: Über die Bestimmung der Menges des Glomerulumfitrates mittel Kreatinin als Nierenfunktionsprüfung, nebst einigen Theorien über die Harnbereitung. Zentralbl Inn Med 50: 367, 1929.
13. Bojesen E: The renal mechanism of 'dilution diuresis' and salt excretion in dogs. Acta Physiol Scand 32: 129, 1954.
14. Schnermann J, Wright FS, Davis JM, et al.: Regulation of superficial nephron filtration rate by tubulo-glomerular feedback. Pflüegers Arch Ges Physiol 318: 147, 1970.
15. Thurau K: The juxtaglomerular apparatus; its role in the function of the single nephron unit. Modern Diuretic Therapy, Amsterdam, Excerpta Medica, 1973.
16. Ruyter JH: Über einen merkwürdigen Abschnitt der vasa afferentia der Mäuseniere. Z Zellforsch 2: 242, 1925.
17. Oberling C: L'existence d'une housse neuro-musculaire au niveau des arterès glomerulaires de l'homme. C R Acad Sci (D) Paris 184: 1200, 1927.
18. Goormaghtigh N: Les segments neuromyo-artériels, juxtaglomerulaires du rein. Arch Biol (Liege) 43: 575, 1932.
19. Zimmermann KW: Über den Bau des Glomerulus der Säugerniere. Z Mikrosk Anat Forsch 32: 176, 1933.
20. Christensen JA, Meyer DS, Bohle A: The structure of the human juxtaglomerular apparatus. Virchows Arch [Pathol Anat] 367: 83, 1975.
21. Thurau K, Dahlheim H, Grüner A, et al.: Activation of renin in the single juxtaglomerular apparatus by sodium chloride in the tubular fluid at the macula densa. Circ Res 31 (suppl 2): 182, 1972.
22. Schnermann J: Regulation of single nephron filtration rate by feedback: facts and theories. Clin Nephrol 3: 75, 1975.
23. Cortney MA, Nagel W, Thurau K: A micropuncture study of the relationship between flow-rate through the loop of Henle and sodium concentration in the distal tubule. Arch Ges Physiol 287: 286, 1966.

24. Morgan T, Berliner RW: A study by continuous microperfusion of water and electrolyte movements in the loop of Henle and distal tubule of the rat. Nephron 6: 388, 1969.
25. Malnic G, Klose RM, Giebisch G: Micropuncture study of distal tubular potassium and sodium transport in rat nephron. Am J Physiol 211: 529, 1966.
26. Burg M, Green N: Function of the thick ascending limb of Henle's loop. Am J Physiol 224: 659, 1973.
27. Acute Renal Failure (Flynn CT, ed), Lancaster, England, Medical and Technical Publishing Co., 1974.
28. Thurau K: Influence of sodium concentration at macula densa cells on tubular sodium load. Ann NY Acad Sci 139: 388, 1966.
29. Osborne MJ, Droz B, Meyer P, Morel F: Angiotensin II. Renal localization in glomerular mesangial cells by autoradiography. Kidney Int 8: 245, 1975.
30. Munck O: Renal circulation in acute renal failure. Oxford, Blackwell Scientific Publications, 1958.
31. Reubi FC, Grossweiler N, Gürtler R: A dye dilution method of measuring renal blood flow in man with special reference to the anuric subject. Proc Soc Exp Biol 111: 760, 1962.
32. Hollenberg NK, Epstein M, Rosen SM, et al.: Acute oliguric renal failure in man: evidence for preferential renal cortical ischemia. Medicine (Baltimore) 47: 455, 1968.
33. Bohle A, Jahnecke J, Rauscher A: Vergleichende histometrische Untersuchungen an bioptisch und autoptisch gewonnenem Nierengewebe mit normaler Funktion und bei akutem Nierenversagen. Klin Wochenschr 42: 1, 1964.
34. Bohle A: Renal morphology of acute renal failure in man. Proceedings of the Sixth International Congress of Nephrology, Florence, 1975. Basel, S. Karger, 1976.
35. Thurau K, Mason J: The intrarenal function of the juxtaglomerular apparatus. Physiology of the Kidneys and Urinary Tract, Intern Review of Science, Intern Review of Physiology, London, Medical and Technical Publishing Co., 1974, p 357.
36. Stowe NT, Schnermann J: Renin angiotensin mediation of tubuloglomerular feedback control of filtration rate. Fed Proc 33: 347, 1974.
37. Dev B, Drescher C, Schnermann J: Resetting of tubuloglomerular feedback sensitivity by dietary salt intake. Pflüegers Arch 346: 263, 1974.
38. Thurau K: Modification of angiotensin mediated tubulo-glomerular feedback by extracellular volume. Kidney Int 8: 202, 1975.
39. Schnermann J, Hermle M, Schmidmeier E, Dahlheim H: Impaired potency for feedback regulation of glomerular filtration rate in DOCA escaped rat. Pflüegers Arch 358: 325, 1975.
40. Mendelsohn FAO: Direct evidence for local formation of angiotensin II in kidney. Proceedings of the Sixth International Congress on Nephrology, Florence, 1975.
41. Morgan T, Davis JM: Renin secretion at the individual nephron level. Pflüegers Arch 359: 23, 1975.
42. Hierholzer K, Muller-Suur R, Gutsc HU, et al.: Filtration in surface glomeruli as regulated by flow rate through the loop of Henle. Pflüegers Arch 352: 315, 1974.
43. Wolheim E: Tubuläre Insuffizienz und sogen. akutes Nierenversagen. Münchener Med Wochenschr 14: 597, 1959.
44. Hsu CH, Preuss HG, Argy WP, Schreiner GE: Prolonged tubular malfunction following acute oliguric renal failure. Nephron 13: 342, 1974.
45. Biber TUL, Mylle MMA, Baines AD, et al.: A study by micropuncture and microdissection of acute renal damage in rats. Am J Med 44: 664, 1968.
46. Tanner GA, Sloan KL, Sophasan S: Effects of renal artery occlusion on kidney function in the rat. Kidney Int 4: 377, 1973.
47. Flamenbaum W, Huddleston ML, McNeil JS, Hamburger RJ: Uranyl nitrate-induced acute renal failure in the rat. Micropuncture and renal hemodynamic studies. Kidney Int 6: 408, 1974.
48. Vogt Ch, Stowe N, Dahlheim H, et al.: Mechanisms determining GFR after renal ischemia. Pflüegers Arch 343: R 42, 1973.
49. Flamenbaum W, Hamburger RJ: The role of the renin angiotensin system (RAS) in the initiating phase of uranyl nitrate induced acute renal failure in the rat (abstract). American Society of Nephrologists, 7th Annual Meeting, p 27, 1974.
50. Weber PC, Held E, Uhlich E, Eigler J: Reaction constants of renin in juxtaglomerular apparatus and plasma renin activity after renal ischemia and hemorrhage. Kidney Int 7: 331, 1975.
51. Buckhorn E: (I) Störungen der Harnkonzentrierung. (II) Akutes Nierenversagen, Handbuch Inn Med 5. Aufl. VIII/1, Heidelberg, Berlin, Springer-Verlag, 1968, pp 491, 942.
52. Ullrich KJ, Kramer K, Boylan JW: Present knowledge of the countercurrent system in the mammalian kidney. Progr Cardiovasc Dis 3: 395, 1961.
53. Meroney WH, Rubini ME: Kidney function during acute tubular necrosis: clinical studies and a theory. Metabolism 8: 2, 1959.
54. Porter GA, Starr A: Management of postoperative renal failure following cardiovascular surgery. Surgery 65: 390, 1969.
55. Granger P, Dahlheim H, Thurau K: Enzyme activities of single juxtaglomerular apparatuses in the rat kidney. Kidney Int 1: 78, 1972.
56. Tobian L: Sodium, renal arterial distension and the juxtaglomerular apparatus. Can Med Assoc J 90: 160, 1964.
57. Thiel G, Wilson DR, Arce ML, Oken DE: Glycerol induced hemoglobinuric acute renal failure in the rat. Nephron 4: 276, 1967.
58. DiBona GF, McDonald FD, Flamengaum W, et al.: Maintenance of renal function in salt loaded rats despite severe tubular necrosis, induced by $HgCl_2$. Nephron 8: 205, 1971.
59. Wright FS, Schnermann J: Interference with feedback control of glomerular filtration rate by furosemide, triflocin and cyanide. J Clin Invest 53: 1695, 1974.
60. Witte MH, Short FA, Hollander W: Massive polyuria and natriuresis following relief of urinary tract obstruction. Am J Med 37: 320, 1964.
61. Bricker NS, Shwayri ED, Reardan JB, et al.: An abnormality in renal function resulting from urinary tract obstruction. Am J Med 23: 554, 1957.
62. Bricker NS, Klahr S: Obstructive nephropathy. Diseases of the Kidney (Straus MB, Welt LG, eds), Boston, Little, Brown & Co., 1971.
63. Bluemle LW, Potter HP, Elkinton JR: Changes in body composition in acute renal failure. J Clin Invest 35: 1094, 1956.

IgM Pyroglobulinemia with Erythrocytosis Presenting as Hyperviscosity Syndrome

I. Clinical Features and Viscometric Studies

SHAUN R. McCANN, M.B., B.Ch.*
HORACE H. ZINNEMAN, M.D.
MARTIN M. OKEN, M.D.
MICHAEL C. LEARY, M.S.†
WILLIAM R. SWAIM, M.D.
MARK MOORE, M.D.
Minneapolis, Minnesota

The hyperviscosity syndrome is described in a patient with erythrocytosis and an immunoglobulin M with kappa light chain (IgMK) macroglobulinemia. Viscometric studies were carried out on whole blood and demonstrated the contribution of both the increased hematocrit value and the macroglobulinemia to the whole blood viscosity. Clinical improvement followed phlebotomy and was accompanied by a decrease in whole blood viscosity. Continued treatment with chlorambucil has been associated with a long symptom-free period. The macroglobulin was characterized as a monoclonal IgMK pyroglobulin which retained its thermoprecipitability when reduced to 7S monomers. The presence of IgMK aggregates in the serum may have contributed to the increase in blood viscosity.

The hyperviscosity syndrome may occur in patients with macroglobulinemia [1] or erythrocytosis [2]. The occurrence of both macroglobulinemia and erythrocytosis in the same patient can be expected to produce hyperviscosity at a relatively low level of each as their effect on blood viscosity is synergistic [3,4]. Measurement of whole blood viscosity in these circumstances is clinically relevant.

We describe a patient with macroglobulinemia, erythrocytosis and the hyperviscosity syndrome. Clinical improvement followed reduction in the hematocrit value and immunoglobulin M with kappa light chains (IgMK) level by phlebotomy. Protein studies showed that the macroglobulin was an IgMK pyroglobulin which retained its thermoprecipitability when reduced to 7S monomers.

CASE REPORT

A 65 year old man was hospitalized for evaluation of a five month history of increasing fatigue and a single episode of transient cerebral ischemia manifested by arm and facial paresthesias three days before his admission. He had a two month history of pruritus following hot shower baths. Six weeks before his admission he was noted to have an aortic diastolic murmur, congestive heart failure and a hemoglobin level of 19.8 g/100 ml. Digoxin therapy was instituted without symptomatic improvement. The physical findings on admission were those of a thin, well-muscled man with a ruddy facies. His blood pressure was 110/65 mm Hg and his pulse rate was 60/min. The optic fundi were normal. Bibasilar rales were heard. The point of maximal impulse was in the sixth intercostal space in the anterior axillary line, and a blowing diastolic murmur was audible at the left sternal border. The liver was not

From the Section of Hematology, Infectious Diseases and Department of Laboratory Medicine and Pathology, Veterans Administration Hospital, and University of Minnesota School of Medicine, Minneapolis, Minnesota. Requests for reprints should be addressed to Dr. Horace H. Zinneman, Veterans Administration Hospital, 54th Street and 48th Avenue South, Minneapolis, Minnesota 55417. Manuscript accepted January 12, 1976.

* Present address: Department of Clinical Haematology, Meath Hospital, Dublin 8, Ireland.

† Present address: Chevron Research Company, Standard Avenue, Richmond, California 94800.

enlarged, but a firm, nontender spleen was palpable 7 cm below the left costal margin. The remainder of the physical examination, including a detailed neurologic evaluation, was within normal limits.

Laboratory examination revealed a hemoglobin level of 17.7 g/100 ml; a microhematocrit value of 58 per cent, a reticulocyte count of 1.4 per cent; and 15,300/mm^3 white blood cells, with 77 per cent neutrophils, 6 per cent band forms, 14 per cent lymphocytes, 2 per cent monocytes and 1 per cent eosinophils. The platelet count was 142,000/mm^3. Blood urea nitrogen was 25 mg/100 ml and serum uric acid was 9.0 mg/100 ml. Serum total protein was 7.8 g/100 ml, and serum protein electrophoresis revealed a sharp peak migrating in the gamma region (Figure 1A). This protein was subsequently characterized as a monoclonal IgMK pyroglobulin. Quantitative determination of serum immunoglobulins revealed IgM 4,000 mg, IgG 850 mg and IgA 85 mg/100 ml. Urinalysis was normal and there was less than 10 mg of urinary light chain excretion per 24 hours. Serum vitamin B_{12} by an Euglena gracilis method [5] was 486 pg/ml (normal range 155 to 550 pg/ml), and the leukocyte alkaline phosphatase score was 289 (normal range 30 to 100). Serum iron was 41 μg/100 ml (normal range 75 to 175 μg/100 ml), and total iron-binding capacity was 321 μg/100 ml (normal range 250 to 410 μg/100 ml).

A chest roentgenogram revealed cardiac enlargement and an electrocardiogram showed left ventricular hypertrophy. An intravenous pyelogram was normal.

Scanning with 4 mCi ^{99M}Tc sulfur colloid, intravenously, confirmed the clinical findings of a normal-sized liver and an enlarged spleen. The oxygen tension at which the hemoglobin was 50 per cent saturated (P_{50}) as measured using a Radiometer Dissociation Curve Analyzer I was normal at 27 mm Hg.

The peripheral blood smear showed a leukoerythroblastic picture with occasional giant platelets and rouleaux formation. Occasional plasmacytoid lymphocytes were seen in the blood and bone marrow, but in small numbers, and therefore were not considered diagnostic. The bone marrow was solidly hypercellular with evidence of myeloid and megakaryocyte hyperplasia and reduced iron stores.

Coagulation screening tests (Table I) revealed a prolonged prothrombin time (PT) and partial thromboplastin time (PTT).

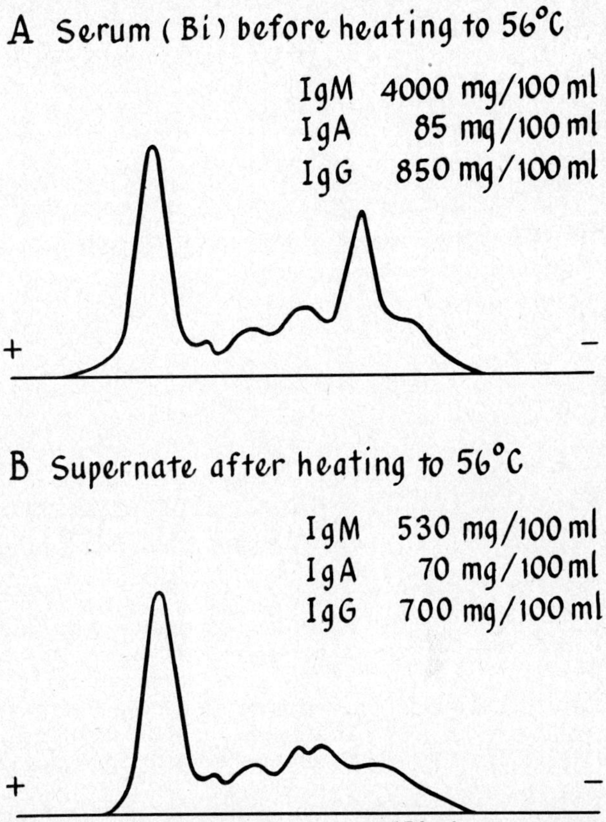

Figure 1. *Electrophoresis of serum (Bi) shows a monoclonal peak* ***(A)****. After gelling at 56° C and centrifugation the monoclonal peak has disappeared from the supernate* ***(B)****.*

Further evaluation showed a decrease in the activity of factors V, VIII and XI. Normal values were consistently found for the thrombin time (TT) as well as for factor II, VII, IX and X activity. There was no increase in circulating fibrin split products (FSP) as assayed by the staphylococcal clumping test [6]. The bleeding time (Ivy method), glass bead platelet adhesion and aggregation response to ADP were normal. Further platelet aggregation studies showed a delayed response to collagen and no response to epinephrine. Serotonin produced a biphasic response.

TABLE I **Coagulation Results**

Date	PT (sec)	PTT (sec)	TT (sec)	Factor V (%)	Factor VIII (%)	Factor XI (%)	HCT (%)
Normal values	10.5–12.5	26–41	13–19	50–150	50–150	65–135	42 ± 5
9/23/74	15.0	68.3	16.9	23	33	42	58
9/24/74	15.0	51.0	13.3	45	29	65	58
9/27/74	14.9	48.1	12.7	29	38	26	56
11/4/74	13.8	45.9	14.0	56	86	. . .	43
2/11/75	12.6	42.4	14.6	66	48	. . .	42
4/9/75	12.0	43.6	14.4	62	37	. . .	42
6/18/75	11.5	41.5	13.6	75	51	. . .	42
7/23/75	11.6	38.7	12.9	60	62	47	42

NOTE: PT = prothrombin time. PTT = partial thromboplastin time. TT = thrombin time. HCT = hematocrit.

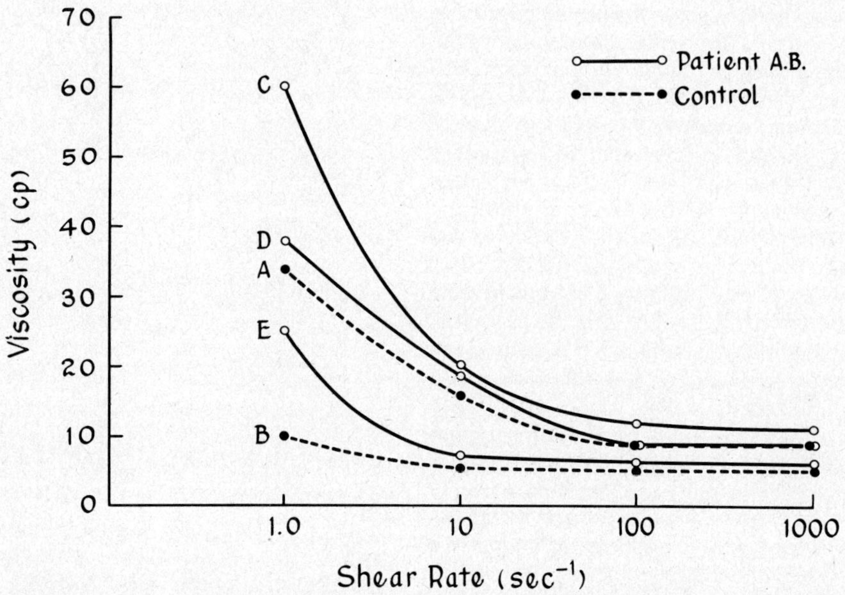

Figure 2. *Plot of whole blood viscosity (cP) measured at varying shear rates.* ***Line A*** *represents normal blood with the hematocrit value (HCT) adjusted to 58 per cent, and* ***line B*** *normal blood with a HCT of 43 per cent.* ***Line C*** *represents the patient's blood on admission,* ***line D*** *after the first phlebotomy when the HCT was 43 per cent and the IgM was 3,200 mg/100 ml, and* ***line E,*** *the patient's blood after further reduction of the IgM to 2,500 mg/100 ml.*

Whole blood viscosity was elevated (Figure 2C), and a diagnosis of hyperviscosity syndrome was made. Because of the significant erythrocytosis, phlebotomy was elected rather than plasmapheresis, and 500 ml of blood was removed. Thereafter a total of 1,500 cc of blood was removed during a 12 day period. The patient noted marked symptomatic improvement within 24 hours after the initial phlebotomy.

Treatment with chlorambucil, 10 mg/day, was then initiated. Following discharge, treatment was continued with chlorambucil, 6 mg/day. Eleven months after presentation, the patient is still asymptomatic and fully active (as a farmer) with no signs of congestive heart failure despite the discontinuance of digoxin.

METHODS AND RESULTS OF SPECIAL STUDIES

Viscosity Studies. All measurements of whole blood viscosity were made with a Model R.18 Weissenberg Rheogoniometer [7] which had been modified to measure blood viscosity at low shear rates. The instrument used in this study is described in detail elsewhere [8,9].

The R.18 Weissenberg Rheogoniometer is a rotational viscosimeter incorporating a cone-plate geometry. In this study the cone-plate geometry was replaced with a biconicylinder geometry which resulted in a uniform shear field. All air-blood contact was eliminated during operation.

In principle, the viscosimeter measures torque developed within a fluid at various shear rates. An inner bob is suspended in a metal cup. The blood sample is placed in the cup and is sheared by rotating the cup at various speeds with a geared motor. The resultant torque produced on the inner bob is subsequently detected with a torsion wire system. Viscosity is then calculated from the following equation: $n = KM/S$ where n = viscosity (centipoise), K = constant of conversion, M = torque on bob (dynes/cm) and S = rotation rate of cup (rpm).

All viscosity measurements were performed at 25° ± 2°C on fresh heparinized blood. Microhematocrit measurements were made on all samples. Control samples were taken from volunteer donors and the hematocrit value was adjusted to the desired value by removing plasma as required. The samples were injected at the rate of 5 ml/min into the sample chamber. The cup was then rotated at several speeds, and the subsequent torque on the bob was measured permitting calculation of viscosity. Viscosity values were obtained at shear rates of 1, 10, 100 and 1,000 sec^{-1} for all samples tested.

The whole blood viscosity of this patient with a hematocrit value of 58 per cent was 20 centipoise when measured at a shear rate of 10 sec^{-1}. Normal blood with a hematocrit value of 43 per cent had a viscosity of 5.5 centipoise at this shear rate. This increased to 16 centipoise when the hematocrit value was adjusted to 58 per cent by removing plasma. After phlebotomy with reduction of the patient's hematocrit value to 43 per cent and IgM to 2,500 mg/100 ml, blood viscosity decreased to 6.8 centipoise at a shear rate of 10 sec^{-1} (Figure 2E).

Coagulation Studies. Assays of coagulation factor activity were carried out utilizing standard methods [10] (Table I). Platelet aggregation studies were carried out using concentrations of 1.2 μg ADP, 0.8 mg collagen, 6.875×10^{-6} M epinephrine and 1×10^{-5} M serotonin, respectively, per ml of platelet rich plasma.

Assays for inhibitor to factors V and VIII were negative. In these studies, the patient's plasma was incubated for 30 and 60 minutes with control plasma and a modified PT and PTT was performed to assay factors V and VIII, respectively, on the postincubation mixture [10]. Similar assays for inhibitors to factors VIII and XI, utilizing the patient's purified IgM and IgG, were also negative.

Immunochemical Studies. The presence of a pyroglobulin was detected when serum was heated to 56°C for 30 minutes in preparation for complement fixation tests. Further increases or reductions of temperature failed to solubilize the pyrogel. Serum protein electrophoresis, using cellulose acetate, revealed a monoclonal peak migrating in the gamma region (Figure 1A). A quantitative determination of immunoglobulin revealed the concentration of IgM to be 4,000 mg/100 ml. Centrifugation of the pyrogel at 1,500 G, using an International Centrifuge Universal Model UV for 30 minutes, made the collection of a supernate possible. Comparison of the electrophoretic patterns of serum and supernate (Figure 1A and 1B) showed that the monoclonal peak had virtually disappeared in the supernate. Measurements by single radial immunodiffusion showed that the serum concentration of 4,000 mg/100 ml had been reduced to 530 mg/100 ml in the supernate, whereas levels of IgG and IgA were essentially unchanged (Figure 1), indicating that the pyroglobulin was contained in the IgM peak. There was no evidence of cryoglobulins.

The pyroglobulin was separated from other serum components by starch block electrophoresis. IgM was then separated from other immunoglobulins by passage through a Sephadex® G-200 (Pharmacia) column, and its purity was confirmed by immunoelectrophoresis against heavy and light chain specific antiserums. This showed the pyroglobulin to be a monoclonal IgM hereafter referred to as IgMK(Bi). Ultracentrifugation of the IgMK(Bi) at 60,000 rpm in a Spinco (Model E) analytical ultracentrifuge revealed two peaks (Figure 3), a major of 18S (65 per cent) and a minor one of 22S (35 per cent) indicating the presence of aggregates of IgMK(Bi). Aliquots of pure IgMK(Bi) and of a monomer preparation IgM_sK(Bi) did form a gel when similarly treated. Further details of this work along with additional immunochemical studies of the pyroglobulin are the subject of a separate report [11].

COMMENTS

This patient was admitted to the hospital with extreme fatigue, refractory congestive heart failure and a history of a recent transient ischemic attack, all of which were thought to be manifestations of the hyperviscosity syndrome [1]. Splenomegaly, erythrocytosis and macroglobulinemia were evident. Bone marrow examination revealed occasional plasmacytoid lymphocytes, and the serum macroglobulin was found to be a monoclonal IgMK. Although the magnitude of the monoclonal IgM spike (Figure 1A) suggests Waldenström's macroglobulinemia, the morphologic picture does not permit a definite diagnosis at this point.

Immediate phlebotomy was indicated because of a combination of erythrocytosis and macroglobulinemia.

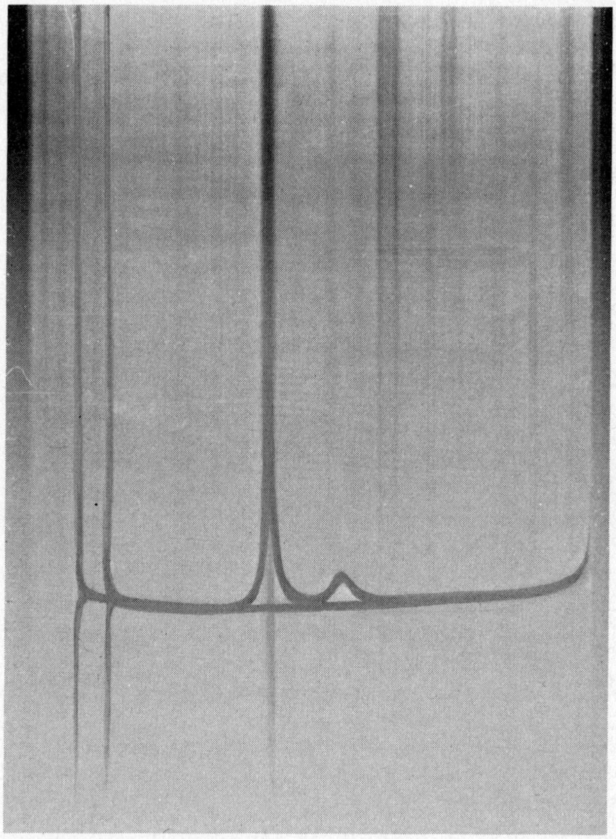

Figure 3. *Ultracentrifugation of IgMK(Bi) at 60,000 rpm after 16 minutes shows two peaks, one of 18S (65 per cent) and the other of 22S (35 per cent).*

Consequently, pretreatment measurement of red cell mass was precluded and the etiology of the erythrocytosis remains obscure. The coagulation abnormalities are in agreement with those described by Perkins et al. [12] in patients with macroglobulinemia. Prolongation of the thrombin time due to interference of fibrin polymerization has been described in patients with multiple myeloma [13,14] and in one patient with multiple myeloma and IgA pyroglobulinemia [15]. This abnormality was not present in this patient.

The plasma proteins and erythrocytes are two major factors contributing to the viscosity of whole blood, and their effects on whole blood viscosity are synergistic. Dysproteinemias, however, are commonly associated with anemia and the associated hyperviscosity syndromes which result from elevation of serum globulin levels are mitigated by the decreased hematocrit value. Thus, measurements of serum viscosity alone may not reflect the true clinical situation, if the contribution of the hematocrit to the blood viscosity is overlooked. Rosenblum and Asofski [16] showed that in macroglobulinemic mice blood viscosity was normal at low hematocrit values but that it markedly increased as the hematocrit value was increased. The danger of blood transfusions in patients with dysproteinemias has been referred to by Tuddenham et al. [17].

The measurement of whole blood viscosity poses a problem as blood behaves as a non-Newtonian fluid [18]. Therefore, defined shear rates must be used as it is known that blood viscosity increases markedly at low rates of shear [18]. The clinically applicable shear rate is difficult to determine because of the wide range of shear rates found throughout the vascular system [19]. The shear rate of blood in arterioles is about 10 sec^{-1} [19], and our results would suggest that whole blood viscosity measurements at this and lower rates of shear may correlate well with signs and symptoms of hyperviscosity. The clinical response in the patient corresponded best with changes in blood viscosity at shear rates of 1.0 and 10 sec^{-1}. At shear rates of greater than 100 sec^{-1} whole blood behaves as expected as a Newtonian fluid (Figure 2).

The viscosity relative to water [1] of a purified solution of IgMK(Bi) at a concentration of 1,040 mg/100 ml was 1.7. The relative viscosity of a solution of pooled purified IgM from patients with hepatic cirrhosis was 1.0 when measured at a similar concentration. This difference in relative viscosity of IgMK(Bi) may be due to the presence of 22S polymers of IgMK(Bi) which were demonstrated by ultracentrifugation.

Pyroglobulins are immunoglobulins which form an irreversible precipitate when serum is heated to 56° to 60°C [20]. They are not associated with a symptom complex as are cryoglobulins and are usually discovered during the performance of a complement fixation test. They are commonly associated with multiple myeloma and were first reported in patients with macroglobulinemia by Stefanini et al. [21] in 1970. Pyroglobulins have been reported in the immunoglobulin classes IgG, IgA and IgM [22]. The interesting combination of cryo- and pyroprecipitation of some pathologic immunoglobulins has been noted by Meltzer and Franklin [23], Invernizzi et al. [22] and Watanabe et al. [24].

Previous studies of the mechanism of pyrogel formation yielded conflicting results. In this case, however, the macroglobulin clearly retained its thermoprecipitability when reduced to monomers, but this property was lost following further reduction to heavy and light chains. Further studies of IgMK(Bi) [11] implicate hydrophobic bonding and participation of IgMK(Bi) pentamers in the pyrogel formation.

REFERENCES

1. Fahey JL, Barth WF, Soloman A: Serum hyperviscosity syndrome. JAMA 192: 464, 1965.
2. Wells R: Syndromes of hyperviscosity. N Engl J Med 283: 183, 1970.
3. Chien S, Usami S, Taylor HN: Effects of hematocrit and plasma proteins on human blood rheology at low shear rates. J Appl Physiol 21: 81, 1966.
4. Wells R, Gaurouski TH, Cox PJ: Influence of fibrinogen on flow properties of erythrocyte suspensions. Am J Physiol 207: 1035, 1964.
5. Mollin DL, Ross GIM: Vitamin B_{12} concentrations of serum and urine of normals and of patients with megaloblastic anemias and other diseases. J Clin Pathol 5: 129, 1952.
6. Hawiger I, Niewjarowski S, Gurewich V, Thomas DP: Measurement of fibrinogen and fibrin degradation products by staphylococcal clumping test. J Clin Lab Med 75: 93, 1970.
7. Weissenberg K: Manual for R.18 Weissenberg Rheogoniometer. Farol Research Engineers Ltd, Bognor Regis, England, 1963.
8. Leary MC, Keller KH, Macosko CW: Modification of the Rheogoniometer for viscosity and elasticity of blood (abstract). Rheol Bull 44: 6, 1975.
9. Leary MC: On the design and testing of a new Rheogoniometer for viscosity and elasticity measurements of blood. MS Thesis. Department of Chemical Engineering and Material Science, University of Minnesota, 1975.
10. Owen CA, Bowie EJW, Didisheim P, Thompson JH: Tests of hemostasis and blood coagulation, chap 2. The diagnosis of bleeding disorders, Boston, Little, Brown & Co., 1969.
11. McCann SR, Zinneman HH, Oken MM, Sinha AA: IgM pyroglobulinemia with erythrocytosis presenting as hyperviscosity syndrome. II. Biochemical properties and mechanisms of pyrogel formation. Am J Med 61: 321, 1976.
12. Perkins HA, MacKenzie MR, Fudenberg HH: Hemostatic defects in dysproteinemias. Blood 35: 695, 1970.
13. Coleman M, Vigliano EM, Weksler ME, Nachman RL: Inhibition of fibrin monomer polymerization by lambda myeloma globulins. Blood 39: 210, 1972.
14. Sanchez-Avalos J, Soong BCF, Miller SP: Coagulation disorders in cancer. II. Multiple myeloma. Cancer 23: 1388, 1966.
15. Sugai S: IgA pyroglobulin, hyperviscosity syndrome and coagulation abnormalities in a patient with multiple myeloma. Blood 39: 224, 1972.
16. Rosenblum WI, Asofski RM: Factors affecting the blood viscosity in macroglobulinemic mice. J Lab Clin Med 71: 201, 1968.
17. Tuddenham EGD, Whittaker JA, Bradley J, Lilleyman JS, James DR: Hyperviscosity syndrome in IgA multiple myeloma. Br J Haematol 27: 65, 1974.
18. Merrill EW: Rheology of blood. Physiol Rev 49: 863, 1969.
19. Wells RE, Merrill EW: Influence of flow properties of blood upon viscosity-hematocrit relationships. J Clin Invest 41: 1591, 1962.
20. Martin WJ, Matheson DR: Pyroglobulinemia. Heat coagulable globulin in the blood. Proc Mayo Clin 28: 545, 1953.
21. Stefanini M, McConnell EE, Andracki EG, Swanstro WJ, Durr P: Macropyroglobulinemia. Am J Clin Pathol 54: 94, 1970.
22. Invernizzi F, Cattaneo R, Rossodi SAN, Secondo V, Balestritti G, Zanussi C: Pyroglobulinemia. Acta Haematol 50: 65, 1973.
23. Meltzer M, Franklin EC: Cryoglobulinemia. A clinical and laboratory study. Am J Med 40: 837, 1966.
24. Watanabe A, Kitamura M, Shimizu M: Immunoglobulin A (IgA) with properties of both cryoglobulin and pyroglobulin. Clin Chim Acta 52: 231, 1974.

IgM Pyroglobulinemia with Erythrocytosis Presenting as Hyperviscosity Syndrome

II. Biochemical Properties and Mechanisms of Pyrogel Formation

SHAUN R. McCANN, M.B., B.Ch.*
HORACE H. ZINNEMAN, M.D.
MARTIN M. OKEN, M.D.
AKHOURI A. SINHA, Ph.D.
Minneapolis, Minnesota

An immunoglobulin M with kappa light chains (IgMK) pyroglobulin from a patient with hyperviscosity syndrome, erythrocytosis and coagulation defects has been studied for its immunochemical properties. At physiologic temperatures the purified macropyroglobulin showed a striking tendency to aggregate in the pentamer as well as in the monomer form. This property was also observed in its H chains. Aggregate formation of the pentamers may have contributed to the blood viscosity and coagulation defects. Formation of pyrogel at 56°C was observed with pentamers as well as monomers, but not with separated H or L chains. Amino acid analysis showed quantitative abnormalities of aspartic acid, glycine, cystine and leucine within the H chains. Solubility of the pyrogel in sodium dodecyl sulfate, the pyroglobulin's tendency to aggregate and the cystine deficit of H chains implicate conformational changes leading to hydrophobic bonding at 56°C in the formation of pyrogel.

The study of a patient with macropyroglobulinemia and erythrocytosis, presenting as hyperviscosity syndrome [1], has been extended to additional biochemical and immunochemical inquiries. Previous reports of IgM pyroglobulins have differed in respect to thermoprecipitability of monomers (IgM_s) and the mechanisms of pyrogel formation. Previously Zinneman and Seal [2] presented evidence that hydrophobic bonding was essential in the formation of pyrogel in an IgG pyroglobulin. This study investigates the biochemical properties of IgMK(Bi) [1] and provides further evidence for hydrophobic bonding in the formation of pyrogels.

MATERIALS AND METHODS

The first steps toward isolation and purification of the pyroglobulin consisted of the separation of immunoglobulins from other serum components by starch block electrophoresis. IgM could then be separated from immunoglobulins of lesser molecular weight by passage through a 2.5 by 100 cm column of Sephadex® G-200 (Pharmacia), using 0.1 M phosphate buffer of pH 7.8. The purity of the frontally eluted IgM was confirmed by immunoelectrophoresis against specific heavy and light chain antiserums.

Ultracentrifugation was carried out at 60,000 rpm in a Spinco (Model E) analytical centrifuge. Reduction of IgMK(Bi) to monomers (IgM_sK) was obtained by reduction with 0.03M 2-mercaptoethanol and alkylation by iodoacetamide. Ultracentrifugation of this product showed one 8S peak, confirming the reduction to monomers. Heavy and light chains were prepared

From the Section of Infectious Diseases, Hematology, and Department of Laboratory Medicine and Pathology, Veterans Administration Hospital and University of Minnesota School of Medicine, Minneapolis, Minnesota. Requests for reprints should be addressed to Dr. Horace H. Zinneman, Veterans Administration Hospital, 54th Street and 48th Avenue South, Minneapolis, Minnesota 55417. Manuscript accepted January 12, 1976.

* Present address: Department of Clinical Haematology, Meath Hospital, Dublin 8, Ireland.

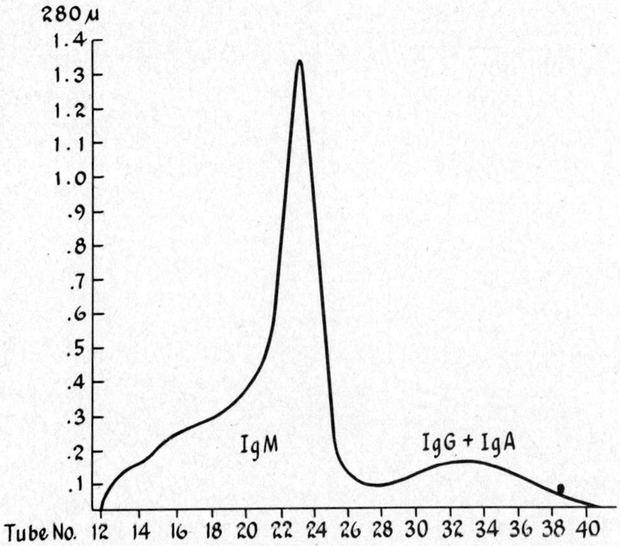

Figure 1. *Gel filtration of immunoglobulins on a column of Sephadex G-200. The frontal eluate of IgM has a shoulder of polymerization.*

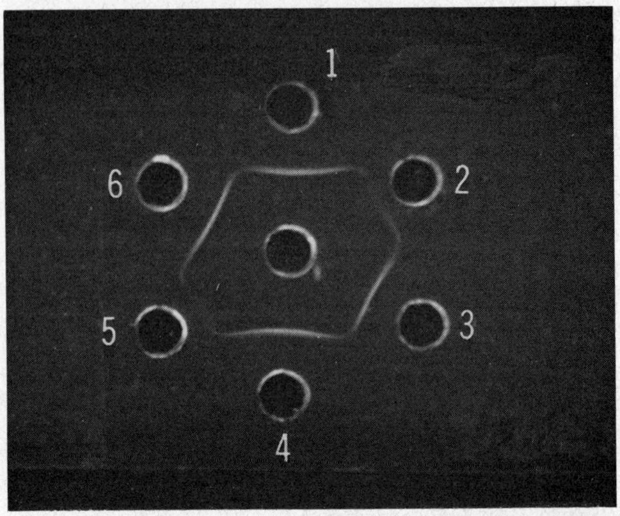

Figure 2. *Comparison of IgMK(Bi) with five IgM's of cirrhotic subjects. Anti-μ rabbit serum in center well. IgMK(Bi) in well Number 1, and wells Number 2–6 contain purified IgM from five cirrhotic subjects. IgMK(Bi) forms lines of identity with normal IgM.*

by reduction of 30 mg IgMK(Bi) in 0.312 ml of 1.0M 2-mercaptoethanol and alkylation with 920 mg of iodoacetamide. Separation of heavy from light chains was obtained by passage through a column of Sephadex G-75 (Pharmacia) in a medium of 0.5 N propionic acid. The purity of these preparations was verified by immunoelectrophoresis against specific antiserums as well as by ultracentrifugation. IgMK(Bi) as well as its heavy and light chains were subjected to acid hydrolysis and measured for amino acid content by means of ion exchange chromatography on columns of amberlite resin, in a Spinco, Model 120 automatic amino acid analyzer.

IgMK(Bi) was assayed for sialic acid content by the method of Warren [3]. Fucose, hexose and hexosamine were quantified according to Winzler [4].

In order to study the pyrogel's ultrastructure, IgMK(Bi) was heated to 56°C for 30 minutes, and the resulting gel centrifuged to remove some of the trapped physiologic sodium chloride solution. The resulting pyroglobulin pellet was then fixed for 2 hours in cold 3 per cent glutaraldehyde in 0.1M phosphate buffer and post-fixed in buffered 1 per cent osmium tetroxide for 1 hour. The pellet was then dehydrated in graded ethyl alcohol and embedded in Epon® 812 [5]. Thin sections were stained with a combination of uranyl acetate and lead citrate, and examined with an RCA-EMU-4 electron microscope. Unstained sections were also examined.

RESULTS

After separation of immunoglobulins from other serum components by starch block electrophoresis, IgMK(Bi) could be obtained in pure form by gel filtration on columns of Sephadex G-200. On elution, the frontal IgM peak had a "shoulder" of heavier weight molecules, indicating a tendency to aggregation (Figure 1). The purity of the frontal peak as well as of its "shoulder" (as IgM) was confirmed by immunoelectrophoresis, which also established the monoclonal character of this IgM macropyroglobulin, which had neither euglobulin nor antiglobulin activity. IgMK(Bi) was found by double immunodiffusion to be antigenically identical with IgM from five patients with Laennec's cirrhosis (Figure 2). As described in part I of this study [1], ultracentrifugation showed peaks of 19S and 22S, confirming the presence of aggregates of IgMK(Bi). Monomers of this macropyroglobulin, with sedimentation constants of 8S retained their thermoprecipitability at 56°C, but heavy and light chains did not. However, ultracentrifugation of H chains did not show the usual symmetrical peak, but one which extended from 3S to 6S, indicating the formation of H chain aggregates (Figure 3).

Amino acid analysis of IgMK(Bi) showed an abnormal number of aspartic acid, glycine, cystine and leucine residues, compared to studies of normal IgM in this laboratory (Table I). The nonpolar residues of glycine and leucine were increased. The aspartic acid content was increased, whereas the cystine content was decreased. These abnormalities were noted in the heavy chains only. The carbohydrate components of IgMK(Bi) were within the normal range (Table II).

Treatment of the pyrogel with 6 M urea broke it up into strands, but failed to bring it into solution. Concentrated sodium hydroxide seemed to solubilize the pyrogel, but electrophoresis showed that the pyrogel had been hydrolyzed. Heating of the patient's IgA and IgG failed to produce precipitates or gels, confirming that IgMK(Bi) alone was the pyroglobulin. Addition of

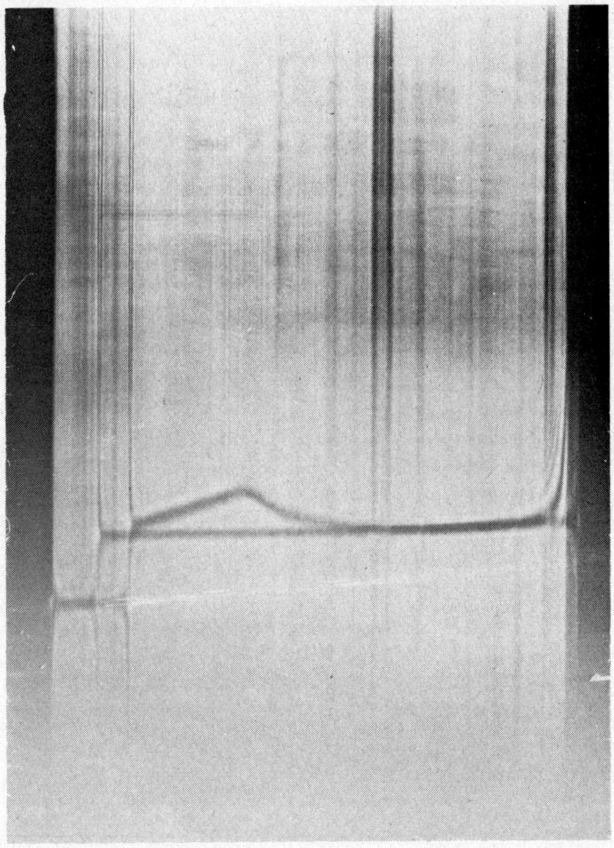

Figure 3. *Polymerization of H chains from 3S to 6S observed at ultracentrifugation at 60,000 rpm after 32 minutes.*

TABLE I Amino Acid Composition of $IgM_SK(Bi)$ and Its Heavy and Light Chains

Amino Acid	IgM_SK-(Bi)*	Normal Range*	μ Chain*	Normal Range*	K Chain*	Normal Range*
Lysine	66	64–86	24	21–30	9	9–10
Histidine	20	18–24	8	8–10	2	2–3
Arginine	46	34–46	19	16–19	4	4–6
Aspartic acid†	160	108–118	54	39–44	22	15–20
Threonine	136	124–148	48	45–56	19	16–20
Serine	190	188–208	68	65–69	25	25–30
Glutamic acid	132	126–138	44	42–48	21	19–22
Proline	122	83–130	47	44–51	14	12–14
Glycine†	220	198–212	75	68–72	32	29–32
Alanine	158	126–160	55	46–56	23	21–23
Cystine/2†	26	30–34	8	12–15	4	4–6
Valine	148	138–156	54	46–62	16	14–17
Methionine	10	12–14	4	3–6	0	0
Isoleucine	46	36–50	16	15–20	6	5–7
Leucine†	120	110–112	39	35–38	20	16–19
Tyrosine	34	34–42	10	10–12	6	5–7
Phenylalanine	40	38–48	14	14–18	6	6–9

* Calculated as moles of amino acid per mole of protein.
† Denotes amino acids with quantitative μ chain abnormalities.

TABLE II Carbohydrate Components of the Pyroglobulin Calculated as Mol/Mol of IgM_s

	$IgM_SK(Bi)$	Normal Range
Sialic acid	2.0	2.0–3.0
Fucose	4.0	2.0–5.0
Hexose	28.0	10.0–42.0
Hexosamine	20.0	14.0–26.0

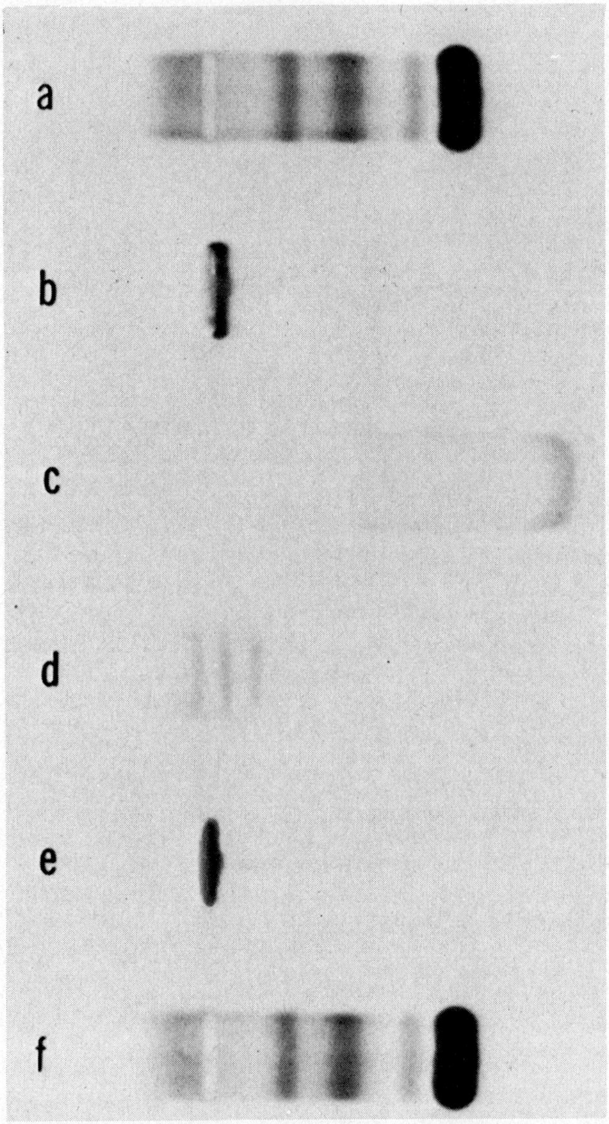

Figure 4. *Electrophoresis on a supporting medium of cellulose acetate, comparing the mobility of normal serum (**a** and **f**) with IgMK(Bi) (**b**), the SDS-IgMK-complex (**c**), H and L chains of IgMK(Bi) (**d**) and IgMK(Bi) in 6 M urea (**e**). When complexed with SDS, IgMK(Bi) has acquired additional negative charges, which impart anodal mobility exceeding that of albumin.*

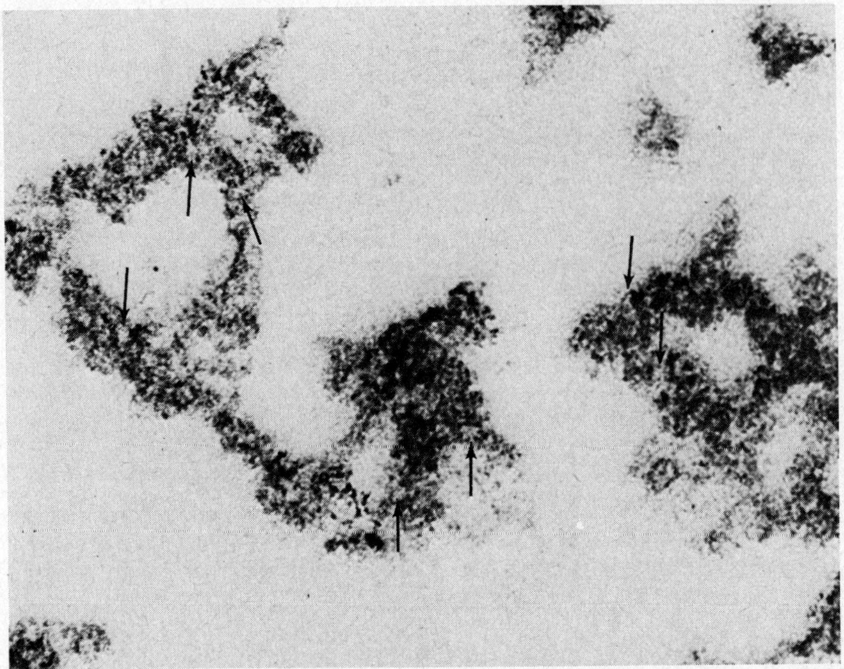

Figure 5. *An electron micrograph, original magnification × 103,300, reduced by 14 per cent; shows a meshwork of IgM molecules which appear translucent and are outlined by the darker counter stain (uranyl acetate and lead citrate).* ***Arrows*** *indicate some of the pentamer forms of IgMK(Bi) which lie within the plane of the cut.*

these immunoglobulins to IgMK(Bi) did not result in coprecipitation upon heating to 56°C. Alteration of pH by appropriate buffers within a pH range from 3 to 9 failed to inhibit pyroprecipitation, although the gel appeared to be maximal at pH 7.3. Variations of ionic strength using sodium chloride in concentrations between 3 and 10 per cent failed to inhibit pyrogel formation.

The pyrogel could be brought completely into solution by addition of sodium dodecyl sulfate (SDS) at a ratio of 30 mol of SDS to 1 mol of IgMK(Bi). Electrophoresis of the SDS-IgMK(Bi) complex showed that it had acquired a considerably greater electrophoretic mobility than the original IgMK(Bi) (Figure 4). Electron microscopy was helpful in providing additional information concerning the structure of the pyrogel. Figure 5 shows a section of the gel which appears to consist of a mesh of IgM pentamers.

COMMENTS

Previous studies designed to elucidate the nature of pyrogel formation have yielded conflicting results. Patterson and co-workers [6] described a patient with IgM pyroglobulinemia and lymphoma. This pyroglobulin lost thermoprecipitability when broken into 7S monomers. Stefanini et al. [7] described six patients with Waldenström's disease and IgM pyroglobulinemia. Treatment with 2-mercaptoethanol and iodoacetamide partially inhibited thermoprecipitability. However, the degree of reduction by 2-mercaptoethanol was not documented by sedimentation coefficients. Our findings concerning the thermoprecipitability of the 7S monomers are in agreement with those of Invernizzi et al [8]. The decreased number of cystine residues and the increase in the glycine and leucine residues in the H chains of IgMK(Bi) may be of significance, since they may represent a relative excess of nonpolar residues.

Whereas carbohydrate components and their abnormalities have been shown to influence the solubility of cryoglobulins [9–12], they have been found to be normal in one IgG pyroglobulin studied by Zinneman and Seal [2] as well as in IgMK(Bi) of the present study.

IgMK(Bi) was solubilized with sodium dodecyl sulfate (SDS), as was the IgG pyroglobulin previously reported by Zinneman and Seal. Solubility with SDS leading to SDS-IgM complexes implicates hydrophobic bonding in the pyrogel formation. The tendency of IgMK(Bi) and its H chains to aggregate is compatible with cystine and methionine deficit and loss of polarity under physiological conditions.

The cited abnormalities of amino acid composition, particularly the low number of cystine residues, may be responsible for abnormal secondary and tertiary conformation, resulting in loss of surface polarity of

IgMK(Bi) to a point where solubility can be maintained only by means of aggregation. Further conformational changes, due to heating, expose additional nonpolar residues of the molecule's hydrophobic interior. Whereas the abnormal H chains alone do not form pyrogels, they do so together with L chains which normally show a change of solubility at 56°C, and strong hydrophobic bonds, involving both H and L chains, result in pyrogel.

A basic difference between cryoglobulins and pyroglobulins is the appearance of reversible noncovalent bonds and solubility changes on cooling of the former. Pyroglobulins, however, have a temperature-dependent instability, which leads to irreversible hydrophobic bonding at 56°C. The occasional combination of cryoprecipitation and pyrogel formation [13,14] would presume the presence of both defects in the same molecule.

ACKNOWLEDGMENT

We thank Mrs. Marilyn G. Goodsell for valuable technical assistance.

REFERENCES

1. McCann SR, Zinneman HH, Oken MM, Leary MC, Swaim WR, Moore M: IgM pyroglobulinemia with erythrocytosis presenting as hyperviscosity syndrome. I. Clinical features and viscometric studies. Am J Med 61: 316, 1976.
2. Zinneman HH, Seal US: The role of hydrophobic bonding in the thermoprecipitation of a pyroglobulin. Rev Europ Étud Clin Biol 6: 668, 1971.
3. Warren L: The thiobarbituric acid assay of sialic acids. J Biol Chem 234: 1971, 1959.
4. Winzler RJ: Methods of biochemical analysis, chap 2. Determination of Glycoproteins, vol 2 (Glick D, ed), New York, Interscience, 1955.
5. Luft JH: Improvements in epoxy resin embedding methods. J Biophys Biochem Cytol 9: 409, 1961.
6. Patterson R, Roberts M, Rambach W, Falleroni A: An IgM pyroglobulin associated with lymphosarcoma. Am J Med 48: 503, 1970.
7. Stefanini M, McConnell EE, Andracki EG, Swanstro WJ, Durr P: Macropyroglobulinemia. Am J Clin Pathol 54: 94, 1970.
8. Invernizzi F, Cattaneo R, Rossodi SAN, et al.: Pyroglobulinemia. Acta Haematol 50: 65, 1973.
9. Zinneman HH, Levi D, Seal US: On the nature of cryoglobulins. J Immunol 100: 594, 1968.
10. McIntosh RM, Kaufman DB, Kulvinskas C, Grossman BJ: Cryoglobulins. I. Studies on the nature, incidence and clinical significance of serum cryoproteins in glomerulonephritis. J Lab Clin Med 75: 566, 1970.
11. McIntosh RM, Kulvinskas C, Kaufman DB: Cryoglobulins. II. The biological and chemical properties of cryoproteins to acute post streptococcal glomerulonephritis. Int Arch Allergy Appl Immunol 41: 700, 1971.
12. Zlotnick A, Slaim S, Eliakim M: Mixed cryoglobulinemia with a monoclonal IgM component associated with chronic liver disease. Israel J Med Sci 8: 1068, 1972.
13. Meltzer M, Franklin EC, Elias K, et al.: Cryoglobulinemia—a clinical and laboratory study. II. Cryoglobulins with rheumatoid factor activity. Am J Med 40: 837, 1966.
14. Watanabe A, Kitamura M, Shimizu M: Immunoglobulin A (IgA) with properties of both cryoglobulin and pyroglobulin. Clin Chim Acta 52: 231, 1974.

Diagnosis of Cytomegalovirus Pneumonia in Compromised Hosts

PAUL S. ABDALLAH, M.D.
JAMES B. D. MARK, M.D.
THOMAS C. MERIGAN, M.D.
Stanford, California

Sixteen patients with cytomegalovirus pulmonary infection are described. In 11 the diagnosis was made antemortem by lung aspirate or biopsy, and in five the diagnosis was made at postmortem by typical lung histology and positive viral lung cultures. All patients were immunosuppressed by both their underlying diseases and treatment with corticosteroids and other chemotherapy. Although other pathogens were identified at lung biopsy in most patients (73 per cent), primarily Pneumocystis carinii, evidence is offered to demonstrate that cytomegalovirus can cause significant pulmonary disease alone, leading to respiratory failure and death.

Cytomegalovirus (CMV) has been implicated in pulmonary disease in compromised hosts [1–4] based on autopsy findings or serologic evidence for viral infection without support for specific pulmonary involvement for the virus [5,6]. The incidence of CMV infection, as demonstrated by viral shedding and serologic response, has approached 80 to 90 per cent in leukemic patients and transplant recipients [7–9]. Various clinical syndromes have been attributed to CMV (such as postperfusion or mononucleosis-like syndromes, hepatitis, hemolytic anemia and pneumonitis) [10], but the true incidence of lung involvement by CMV in compromised hosts is not known. In addition, its real significance as a pulmonary pathogen is not clear, since it is often associated with other infectious agents, particularly Pneumocystis carinii [11–13]. Postmortem studies have documented lung involvement with CMV in up to 50 per cent of patients with leukemia and transplant recipients [14,15], yet the diagnosis is seldom made antemortem and usually without confirmatory evidence of actual tissue involvement, either by lung biopsy or aspirate. In fact, only five cases have been documented antemortem by lung aspirate or biopsy [16–19], and these are scattered in the literature.

In this paper, we describe a series of 16 patients from Stanford University Hospital with CMV pulmonary infection. In 11 the diagnosis was made antemortem by lung aspirate or biopsy, and in five the diagnosis was made postmortem by typical lung histology and positive viral lung cultures. Evidence is offered to demonstrate that on occasion CMV can cause significant pulmonary disease without other agents being demonstrated, and an attempt is made to describe the clinical characteristics of this group of patients and to define a population at risk.

From the Division of Infectious Diseases, Department of Medicine and Department of Surgery, Stanford University School of Medicine, Stanford, California 94305. This study was supported by a grant (AI-05629) from the U.S. Public Health Service. Requests for reprints should be addressed to Dr. Thomas C. Merigan, Division of Infectious Diseases, Stanford University Medical Center, Stanford, California. Manuscript accepted January 9, 1976.

METHODS

An analysis was undertaken of the records of the Diagnostic Virology Laboratory at Stanford from May 1970 to September 1974 of all patients in whom lung biopsy specimens, aspirates and necropsy specimens were positive

TABLE I Characteristics of 16 Patients with CMV Pulmonary Infection

Data	No.	Data	No.
Presenting Findings		Laboratory data	
Types of underlying disease		Granulocytopenia (<1500)	4/16
Heart transplant	5	Atypical lymphocytes	0/12
Renal transplant	4	Evidence of acute hepatitis	1/15
Lymphoma	4	CMV serology (fourfold rise in titer or single elevated titer ≥1:16)	7/12
Leukemia	2		
Solid tumor	1	Positive CMV cultures at peripheral sites	
Prior therapy			
Current steroids	16/16*	Throat/sputum	1/6
Current chemotherapy	16/16	Transtracheal aspirate	0/1
Irradiation (within last 6 mo)	5/16	Urine	2/6
		Bronchial washings	0/1
Prior antibiotics (within last mo)	7/14	Cerebrospinal fluid	0/2
		Blood	2/3
Duration of respiratory symptoms (prior to biopsy):		Clinical course	
		Duration of respiratory illness (in 16 patients, in weeks)	
< week	2/8		
1 to 2 weeks	5/8	Survivors 3, 3, 7, 3	
> 2 weeks	1/8	Fatal cases 6, 3, 4, 3, 6, 2, 1, 6, 2, 1	
Dyspnea	11/15		
Sputum production		Mortality: 6 of 11 died within one to three weeks of lung biopsy or aspirate.	
Scanty	7/10		
Productive	3/10	Patients who had CMV alone: 2 of 2 died within two to three weeks of biopsy or aspirate	
Fever (temperature >38.5°C)	16/16		
Hypoxia (PO_2 < 60)			
Initial finding	6/15	Cause of death (if known)	
Later finding	6/15	Progressive respiratory insufficiency	9/11
Chest roentgenogram			
Predominant interstitial	9/16		
Predominant alveolar	4/16		
Other (cavity, nodule)	3/16		

NOTE: PO_2 = oxygen tension.
* Number with given characteristic/total number of patients in whom information is available.

for CMV, and then the hospital records of these patients were analyzed for certain characteristics. This was a retrospective study and involved patients only at Stanford affiliated teaching hospitals (Palo Alto Veterans Administration Hospital, Children's Hospital at Stanford and Stanford University Hospital). Viral cultures were obtained on lung aspirates and biopsy specimens from 55 patients, and 11 of these were positive for CMV. No other viruses were found except in one patient's biopsy specimen which demonstrated both CMV and Herpes zoster. Five additional patients had positive CMV lung cultures at autopsy; together these form the series of 16 patients.

Lung aspirate specimens were usually placed in viral holding medium and immediately brought to the Diagnostic Virology Laboratory where they were inoculated into human foreskin fibroblast monolayers. Lung biopsy and necropsy specimens were handled similarly, except that holding medium was not used and tissue was either immediately inoculated or frozen at −70°C

RESULTS

The characteristics of the 16 patients with CMV pulmonary infections are described in Table I. All were either transplant recipients or else had underlying neoplastic disorders, and all received suppressive doses of corticosteroids and chemotherapy for their underlying diseases. Hence, all were severely immunocompromised hosts, and opportunistic infections were considered in their diagnostic evaluation. Respiratory symptoms, usually dyspnea and cough, had only been present for a short duration (less than two weeks) before lung biopsy or aspiration was carried out in this group of patients. The most consistent clinical findings were fever, nonproductive cough and dyspnea associated with marked hypoxemia. In six of 15 patients the arterial oxygen tension was less than 60 on admission to the hospital; in an additional six patients this finding developed during hospitalization. This was an important prognostic indicator as 11 of the 12 patients with hypoxemia died, and all three patients without hypoxemia survived hospitalization.

Chest x-ray findings in 13 of the 16 patients were predominantly diffuse interstitial or alveolar infiltrates, other x-ray patterns (nodule, cavity) were present in the remaining three patients. All three patients in whom CMV alone was isolated from lung tissue had a chest x-ray pattern of diffuse interstitial or alveolar infiltrates. The total duration of respiratory symptoms varied from a relatively rapid course of one week to a chronic progressive process of seven weeks. The hospital course

TABLE II Other Pulmonary Infections Associated with CMV in This Series

Infection	No. of Patients
Pneumocystis carinii	6
Aspergillus	2*
Gram-negative bacteria	2*
Nocardiosis	1
Tuberculosis	1
Herpes zoster	1

* One patient had both a gram-negative bacteria and an Aspergillus infection.

varied from gradual pulmonary improvement, with slow resolution of the chest x-ray findings over several weeks in the survivors, to rapidly progressive respiratory failure in the survivors, to rapidly progressive respiratory failure and death in other patients. Of the 11 patients in whom the diagnosis was made by lung biopsy or aspiration, six died within one to three weeks of the procedure. Of the remaining five, one died of progressive lymphoma, unresponsive to chemotherapy, and four are still living. In three of these four compromised hosts P. carinii was identified at lung biopsy; the fourth had Nocardia asteroides. Both patients in whom CMV alone was found in the lung biopsy specimen died of progressive respiratory failure within two to three weeks of biopsy.

Laboratory data revealed that no patients had atypical lymphocytes on peripheral blood smears and only one patient had evidence of acute hepatitis. Thus, in no patients did their conditions fit previously described syndromes of systemic CMV infection, such as "postperfusion hepatitis" or "mononucleosis-like syndrome" despite the fact that this virus was isolated from lung biopsy or aspirate specimens in 11 of the patients and from lung necropsy specimens in the remaining five. Granulocytopenia did not appear to be a predisposing factor to CMV infections, and CMV complement fixation serology was only positive in seven of twelve patients. Absence of a serologic response to infecting organisms [20] may occur in patients with these underlying disorders, and titers may rise for inexplicable reasons in immunosuppressed and normal patients, hence serology alone is not particularly helpful in the diagnosis of pulmonary CMV infection.

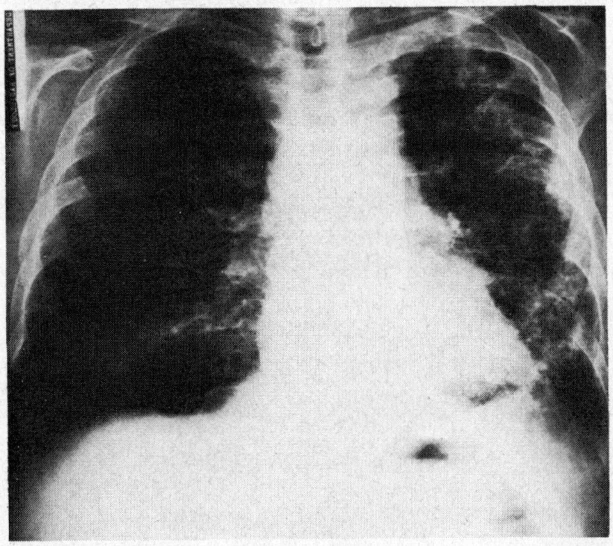

Figure 1. Initial chest roentgenogram demonstrating diffuse bilateral pulmonary infiltrates in Case 5.

The presence of CMV in peripheral sites (oropharynx, urine) was difficult to assess since specimens for viral cultures were not taken from multiple sites in all patients. Only one of the six patients in whom cultures were obtained had CMV in their oropharynx and two of six in their urine. The two isolates of CMV from blood indicate that this may be a useful diagnostic aid in the future.

Table II indicates that the other pulmonary infections associated with CMV in our series of 16 patients. All such pathogens were documented by lung biopsy, aspirate and/or autopsy. Mixed pulmonary infections were common with Pneumocystis carinii being found in six patients, indicating an incidence of approximately 35 per cent. This associaion of CMV and Pneumocystis pulmonary infections has been noted before [21] and the mechanism remains unclear. Other pathogens were Aspergillus [2], gram-negative bacteria [2], Nocardia [1], tuberculosis [1] and Herpes zoster [1]. In three patients no infectious agents were isolated from lung tissue other than CMV (Table III), and these are considered to represent isolated cases of CMV pneumonia with CMV appearing as the only pathogen. In two of the three patients the diagnosis was made by antemortem lung biopsy specimens whereas in the third the diagnosis was made at autopsy. The two patients in whom the diagnosis was made antemortem are discussed in detail to illustrate some of the clinical features of their illness.

One patient (Case 4) was a 45 year old white woman with stage IV B histiocytic lymphoma, taking Cytoxan®, Velban®, Procarbazine® and prednisone, who was admitted with two weeks of dyspnea, nonproductive cough and fever. Her initial chest film revealed a lingular alveolar infiltrate with progression over a week to a diffuse bilateral alveolar pattern. Her course was characterized by daily spikes in temperature to 40°C for five weeks, with progressive dyspnea and hypoxemia (arterial oxygen tension was 40 on 40 per cent oxygen); cultures of blood, urine, sputum and transtracheal specimens were negative, and therapeutic trials of multiple antibiotics and amphoterocin B resulted in no improvement. Ten days after admission, she underwent an open lung biopsy which revealed interstitial pneumonitis. Special stains for fungi, acid-fast bacilli and P. carinii were all negative as well as bacterial and fungal cultures. CMV was isolated from her lung biopsy specimen and blood, and an esophageal biopsy per-

TABLE III Comparison of Lung Biopsy and Aspirates with Postmortem Results

	Lung Biopsy Specimens or Aspirates		Lung Necropsy	
Case No.	Histology or Cytology	CMV Culture	Histology	CMV Culture
1	Nocardia	3+	Alive	
2*	Typical eosinophilic intranuclear inclusion bodies	2+	Aspergillosis, extensive interstitial pneumonitis with inclusion bodies	2+
3*	N.D.	3+	Abscess in upper right lung, extensive interstitial pneumonitis with inclusion bodies	N.D.
4	Interstitial pneumonitis	3+	Interstitial pneumonitis	2+
5	Interstitial pneumonitis	3+	Interstitial pneumonitis	1+
6	P. carinii interstitial pneumonitis with inclusion bodies	3+	Alive	
7	Lymphoma	2+	Lymphoma	N.D.
8	P. carinii	1+	Alive	
9	Tuberculosis	2+	Tuberculosis, interstitial pneumonitis with inclusion bodies	N.D.
10	P. carinii, interstitial pneumonitis with inclusion bodies	1+	P. carinii, interstitial pneumonitis with inclusion bodies	N.D.
11	P. carinii interstitial pneumonitis	3+	Alive	

NOTE: N.D. = not done. 3+ = heavy (growth at 7–14 days), 2+ = moderate (growth at 15–21 days), 1+ = light (growth at 22–28 days).
* Lung aspirate only.

formed 17 days after admission because of severe esophagitis revealed intranuclear inclusion bodies compatible with CMV infection; unfortunately, no viral cultures were obtained from the specimen. Subsequent clinical course was one of progressive respiratory failure and death five weeks after admission. Autopsy revealed bilateral bronchopneumonia with interstitial fibrosis and pneumonitis on histologic analysis, and no evidence of lymphoma or other organisms despite careful study with appropriate stains. Postmortem cultures of material from her lungs revealed CMV with no other organisms identified.

Another patient (Case 5) was a 78 year old white man with chronic myelogeneous leukemia who was admitted with two weeks of fever, tachypnea and dyspnea. He had been taking Myleran®, 4 to 6 mg/day, intermittently for four months, and corticosteroids for two months. The initial chest film (Figure 1) revealed a diffuse bilateral interstitial infiltrate; his arterial oxygen tension was 41 on admission. Sputum and urine cytology, and viral cultures were negative as were bronchial washings. The patient had daily spikes in temperature to 39° or 40°C, and an empiric trial of Pentamidine® and antibiotics resulted in no improvement. A single CMV complement-fixation antibody assay on serum revealed a titer of 1:1,024, and on the sixth hospital day an open lung biopsy demonstrated interstitial pneumonitis with nuclear atypicalities. Special stains for acid-fast organisms, fungi, and P. carinii were all negative as were bacteriologic and fungal cultures. CMV was reported growing from the lung biopsy specimen 14 days after thoracotomy, and the subsequent clinical course was one of respiratory failure and death two and a half weeks after admission. Autopsy revealed pulmonary consolidation with interstitial pneumonitis, and CMV was isolated from lung tissue. No other organisms were identified at postmortem.

It is reasonable to assume that these two cases, with good pathologic, bacteriologic and virologic examinations, represent true CMV pneumonia with this agent acting as a pathogen. In both cases, no organisms other than CMV were isolated from either lung biopsy or necropsy specimens, and the histology of interstitial pneumonitis is compatible with viral pneumonia. In addition, the positive viral cultures of blood and urine in Case 4 and the high CMV titers in Case 5 are supportive evidence for CMV infection.

Table III compares the results of antemortem examination of lung tissue in the seven patients who eventually died. At least seven of the 10 patients in whom histology was available had a histologic process compatible with CMV infection (i.e., inclusion bodies, interstitial pneumonitis); of the seven patients who came to autopsy, six had a compatible histologic picture of interstitial pneumonitis with inclusion bodies and/or positive viral cultures consistent with CMV. Viral lung cultures in all three patients in this series, in whom specimens were taken at autopsy, were positive for CMV. Only one patient (Case 7) lacked histologic evidence of CMV infection postmortem, and he died of extensive lymphoma. Unfortunately, no viral cultures were obtained on his autopsy material. An attempt was

TABLE IV Comparison of Patients Who had Pulmonary Aspirate or Biopsy Specimen with Positive Cultures for CMV Compared to Those with Negative Cultures

	Positive Viral Culture (11 patients)		Negative Viral Culture (44 patients)
Underlying disease			
Transplant	46%	p<0.01	11%
Lymphoma	27%	N.S.	41%
Other Tumor	27%	N.S.	20%
Connective tissue diseases, etc.	0%	p<0.05	27%
Chest roentgenogram			
Predominant interstitial	64%	0.10	33%
Predominant alveolar	18%	N.S.	40%
Other	18%	N.S.	26%
Lung biopsy/aspirate pathology			
Intranuclear inclusion bodies*	30%†	p<0.025	5%
Interstitial pneumonitis	60%	p<0.10	31%
Other	30%	p<0.05	64%
Other pulmonary infections‡			
Pneumocystis	37%	N.S.	18%§
Aspergillus	9%	N.S.	9%
Gram-negative bacteria	9%	N.S.	0%
Nocardia	9%	N.S.	2%
Tuberculosis	9%	N.S.	0%
Staphylococcal	0%	N.S.	2%
Total with any infection	72%	0.10	22%
Hospital mortality	55%	N.S.	30%

NOTE: N.S. = not significant.
* Two patients had both intranuclear inclusion bodies and interstitial pneumonitis.
† Pathologic study results of biopsy specimen only available for 10 of these 11 patients.
‡ Confirmed by lung biopsy or aspirate and/or autopsy.
§ Two patients had both P. carinii and Aspergillus.

also made to correlate the length of time for lung cultures to become positive with the severity of pulmonary illness, but no trend could be detected.

Table IV is a comparison of the 11 patients with positive lung aspirates or biopsy specimens for CMV, with 44 patients studied during the same period of time with negative lung aspirates or biopsy specimens. The latter were analyzed similarly as a control and demonstrate several differences from the group with positive cultures. A significantly higher percentage of patients with CMV had received organ transplants (46 per cent versus 11 per cent), and 27 per cent of patients with negative viral cultures had other forms of underlying disease, primarily connective tissue disorders, as compared to none in the group whose cultures were positive, with its heavy incidence of transplant recipients and lymphoma patients. Chest films usually showed an interstitial or alveolar pattern in both groups with patients in the CMV group being twice as likely to show an interstitial process, and an alveolar pattern being twice as common in the negative culture group whose cultures were negative. Lung histology was more helpful in predicting the presence or absence of CMV, especially when intranuclear inclusion bodies were seen. Thirty per cent of patients with CMV had intranuclear inclusion bodies as opposed to 5 per cent of the control group ($p > 0.025$). Interestingly, eight of 11 (73 per cent) patients in the CMV culture positive group had other pulmonary infections identified at lung biopsy whereas only 12 of 44 (27 per cent) in the control group had other pathogens identified. This again demonstrates the striking association of CMV with other infectious agents, particularly P. carinii.

This study demonstrates the ability of CMV to produce a spectrum of disease ranging from asymptomatic viral shedding to rapidly progressive fatal pneumonitis. Host factors, such as presence of tumor and immunosuppression, would seem to play a major role in determining pathogenicity of the virus. The literature is replete with reports of transplant recipients or leukemic patients shedding CMV in urine or oropharynx with no apparent disease [5–9]. One patient (Case 1) in our series, who had a lung nodule and in whom both CMV and Nocardia were isolated from lung aspirate, may represent an early phase of pulmonary viral parenchymal involvement. Sputum cultures were positive and a CMV seroconversion was documented. This heart transplant patient recovered completely after treatment for Nocardia and is still living.

Other patients had mixed pulmonary infections, particularly Pneumocystis carinii, which may represent some type of unique symbiotic relationship between the two organisms or just reflect the fact that both organisms are ubiquitous and their latent state is activated by similar sorts of immunosuppression. Of the four patients with P. carinii and CMV diagnosed antemortem, three recovered and are still living after Pentamidine treatment for P. carinii, demonstrating the apparently trivial role of CMV as a pathogen in these patients. Although, it is possible that CMV infection may even in this group have acted as a predisposing factor for infection by other pathogens.

Finally, the most severe form of CMV pulmonary infection was rapidly progressive interstitial pneumonitis. At least three patients had this particular form of pneumonia with no evidence for other underlying pulmonary pathogens. Other groups have reported similar cases of rapidly fatal interstitial pneumonitis, mainly diagnosed at autopsy, and in a recent report of bone marrow transplant recipients it is suggested that this infection threatens to compromise the usefulness of this innovative form of cancer therapy [22].

Another major point raised by our series is the need for rapid diagnosis and viral isolation technics in this group of patients. A recent autopsy study [23] suggests that viral isolation from lung tissue is approximately six times more sensitive than histologic detection of CMV. Vigorous diagnostic evaluation, including lung aspirate or biopsy material, is necessary for definitive therapy, especially as antiviral chemotherapy of the herpes viruses becomes more feasible. There were no deaths or major complications from lung aspirate or biopsy in our group, and a report [24] from our institution describes the experience with this technic in compromised hosts.

Although viral culture is a more sensitive technic than histologic detection of CMV in lung tissue, the major difficulty with viral isolation is the time required; that is seven to 25 days. Histologic and cytological technics are important adjuncts in the diagnosis of CMV infection, available shortly after biopsy, but often the "typical" histology of intranuclear inclusion bodies is not seen or may be confused with other viruses, particularly other herpes viruses. Rapid viral diagnosis is needed, especially with the rapid progression of pneumonia in some patients. One method which holds promise is that of specific immunofluorescent stains with anti-CMV serums [25], similar to the fluorescent-antibody stains which we currently utilize for diagnosis of herpes simplex and varicella-zoster infections of the skin [26]. This can give an accurate diagnosis within 1 to 2 hours of obtaining tissue.

Recently some investigators have stressed diagnosis of CMV pneumonia by noninvasive technics, particularly bronchoscopy [17]. Since many compromised hosts may shed CMV from their oropharynx [5], we believe that the usefulness of this procedure is limited by the possibility of contamination from above and thus the inability to document parenchymal pulmonary infection. Valuable time may be lost trying to interpret the significance of CMV isolated from bronchial washings, and even immunofluorescent staining cells from this site may not allow one to differentiate significant infection from asymptomatic virus infections concomitant with other pulmonary pathogens.

Finally, our series indicates a certain population at risk for complications of CMV infection, at least in our particular institution. Of 55 lung aspirates and biopsy specimens obtained over four years which were cultured for virus, 11 were positive for CMV, an incidence of 20 per cent, and these were strictly confined to compromised hosts with transplants or tumor. All 11 patients were currently receiving corticosteroids and chemotherapy, and most (82 per cent) had an x-ray pattern of interstitial or alveolar infiltrates. Our current approach to these patients is a vigorous early diagnostic effort, which includes lung aspirate or biopsy. In view of the severity of CMV pneumonitis in our patient population, we believe that this approach is justified. With ongoing clinical trials of antiviral agents for other herpes viral infections, a controlled study of antiviral chemotherapy in early well studied cases of CMV pneumonia would soon seem to be useful.

ACKNOWLEDGMENT

We are grateful to Miss Ann Schwartzkopf for her aid in data collection and analysis.

REFERENCES

1. Craighead JE: Pulmonary cytomegalovirus infection in the adult. Am J Pathol 63: 487, 1971.
2. Evans DJ, Williams ED: Cytomegalic inclusion disease in the adult. J Clin Pathol 21: 311, 1968.
3. Hill RB, Jr, Rowlands DT, Jr, Rifkind D: Infectious pulmonary disease in patients receiving immunosuppressive therapy for organ transplantation. N Engl J Med 271: 1021, 1964.
4. Bodey GP, Wertlake PT, Douglas G, Levin RH: Cytomegalic inclusion disease in patients with acute leukemia. Ann Intern Med 62: 899, 1965.
5. Henson D, Siegal SE, Fuccillo DA, et al.: Cytomegalovirus infections during acute childhood leukemia. J Infect Dis 126: 469, 1972.
6. Duvall CP, Casazza AR, Grimley PM, et al.: Recovery of cytomegaloviruses from adults with neoplastic disease. Ann Intern Med 64: 531, 1966.
7. Pien FD, Smith TF, Anderson CF, et al.: Herpesviruses in renal transplant patients. Transplantation 16: 489, 1973.
8. Lopez C, Simmons RL, Mauer M, et al.: Role of virus infections in immunosuppressed renal transplant patients. Trans Proc 5: 803, 1973.
9. Weller TH: The cytomegaloviruses. N Engl J Med 285: 203, 1971.
10. Klemola E, Stenström R, von Essen R: Pneumonia as a clinical manifestation of cytomegalovirus in previously healthy adults. Scand J Infect Dis 4: 7, 1972.
11. Rifkind D, Faris TD, Hill RB: Pneumocystis carinii pneumonia. Ann Intern Med 65: 943, 1966.
12. Rosen P, Armstrong D, Ramos C: Pneumocystis carinii pneumonia. Am J Med 53: 428, 1972.
13. Goodell B, Jacobs JB, Powell RD, DeVita VT: Pneumocystis carinii. The spectrum of diffuse interstitial pneumonia in patients with neoplastic disease. Ann Intern Med 72: 337, 1970.
14. Hill RB, Dahrling BE, Starzl TE, Rifkind D: Death after transplantation. Am J Med 42: 327, 1967.
15. Nieman P, Wasserman PB, Wentworth BB, et al.: Interstitial pneumonia and cytomegalovirus infection as complications of human marrow transplantation. Transplantation 15: 478, 1973.
16. Jeffery JR, Guttman RD, Becklake MR, et al.: Recovery from severe cytomegalovirus pneumonia in a renal transplant patient. Am Rev Respir Dis 109: 129, 1974.
17. Behrens HW, Quick CA: Bronchoscopic diagnosis of cytomegalovirus infection. J Infect Dis 130: 174, 1974.
18. Simmons RL, Uranga VM, La Plante ES, et al.: Pulmonary

complications in transplant recipients. Arch Surg 105: 260, 1972.
19. Case records of Massachusetts general hospital (case 15-1973). N Engl J Med 288: 780, 1973.
20. Roth JA, Siegel SE, Levine AS, Bernard CW: Fatal recurrent toxoplasmosis in a patient initially infected via a leukocyte transfusion. Am J Clin Pathol 56: 601, 1971.
21. Wang, N-S, Huang S-N, Thurlbeck WM: Combined pneumocystis carinii and cytomegalovirus infection. Arch Pathol 90: 529, 1970.
22. Myers JD, Spencer HC, Watts JC, et al.: Cytomegalovirus pneumonia after human marrow transplantation. Ann Intern Med 82: 181, 1975.
23. Smith TF, Holley KE, Keys TF, Macasaet FF: Cytomegalovirus studies on autopsy tissue. Am J Clin Pathol 63: 854, 1975.
24. Greenman RL, Goodall PT, King D: Lung biopsy in immunocompromised hosts. Am J Med 59: 488, 1975.
25. Huang Y-T, Huang E-S, Pagano JS: Antisera to human cytomegalovirus prepared in the guinea pig. Specific immunofluorescence and complement fixation tests. J Immunol 112: 528, 1974.
26. Schmidt NJ, Lennette EH, Woodie JD, Ho, H: Immunofluorescent staining in the laboratory diagnosis of varicella—zoster virus infection. J Lab Clin Med 66: 403, 1965.

Clinical and Laboratory Evaluation of Elderly Patients with Heterophil-Antibody Positive Infectious Mononucleosis

Report of Seven Patients, Ages 40 to 78

CHARLES A. HORWITZ, M.D.
Minneapolis, Minnesota

WERNER HENLE, M.D.
GERTRUDE HENLE, M.D.
Philadelphia, Pennsylvania

MARVIN SEGAL, M.D.
THOMAS ARNOLD, M.D.
Minneapolis, Minnesota

F. BRUCE LEWIS, M.D.
DAVID ZANICK, M.D.
St. Paul, Minnesota

PATRICK C. J. WARD, M.D.
Minneapolis, Minnesota

Clinical, hematologic, biochemical and serologic data are recorded in seven patients aged 40 to 78 years with heterophil-antibody positive infectious mononucleosis (HA+ IM). Clinical observations included fever of 22 to 30 days' duration (five of seven patients), sore throat (six of seven patients), myalgia (five of seven patients) and prominent lymph adenopathy (two of seven patients). Initial blood smears revealed significant numbers of atypical lymphocytes in only five of seven patients; however, on serial testing, in the remaining two patients Downey cells developed to a degree seen in most young adult patients with infectious mononucleosis. Comparison of liver function data from these and younger patients suggests that abnormalities tend to be more marked in those in the older than in those in the younger age range.

Serologic tests confirmed primary Epstein-Barr virus (EBV) infections in all seven patients based on detection of IgM antibodies to EB viral capsid antigen in specimens obtained early, but not late, in the course of the infection, transitory antibody responses to the D (diffuse) component of the EBV-induced early antigen complex, and the initial absence and later development of antibodies to the EBV-associated nuclear antigen. Thus, the serologic data did not differ from those seen in younger patients. These results show that infectious mononucleosis should be included in the differential diagnosis of fever, sore throat and myalgia with or without significant cervical adenopathy in elderly persons.

From the Departments of Pathology and Medicine, Mount Sinai and Northwestern Hospitals and the University of Minnesota Medical School, Minneapolis, Minnesota; Bethesda and St. Luke's Hospitals, St. Paul, Minnesota; and the Division of Virology, Children's Hospital of Philadelphia, and the School of Medicine, University of Pennsylvania, Philadelphia, Pennsylvania. This laboratory investigation was supported by Laboratory Development Fund 380-10-27, Mount Sinai Hospital Laboratory and Research Grant No. CA 04568 and Contract "N01"-CP-33272 within the Virus Cancer Program, National Cancer Program, National Cancer Institute, U.S. Public Health Service. Requests for reprints should be addressed to Dr. Charles A. Horwitz, Mount Sinai Hospital, 2215 Park Avenue, Minneapolis, Minnesota 55404. Manuscript accepted January 12, 1976.

Heterophil-antibody positive infectious mononucleosis (HA+ IM), now known to be caused by primary Epstein-Barr virus (EBV) infections [1,2] occurs mainly in young adults, 15 to 25 years of age [3]. Although primary EBV infections in childhood are often heterophil-antibody negative (HA−) [4,5] and frequently atypical or even occult clinically, typical HA+ IM does occur in infants and children [6,7]. The majority of persons over age 40 have had past contact with the EBV and, thus, are immune to subsequent re-infection [8–10]. A minority of such patients, however, have never been exposed to the virus and, hence, are susceptible to HA+ IM [11–16]. Such cases, satisfying clinical, hematologic and serologic criteria of infectious mononucleosis have been reported in elderly patients ($\geq$ 40)

[17–19]. In a recent study [3], 23 of 3,043 (0.76 per cent) cases of HA+ IM, were in patients over 40. This group included five patients aged 50 to 59 years and three aged 60 to 69 years. HA+ IM due to EBV has also been reported following blood transfusion in an 86 year old patient [20].

Over a 36 month interval, we received HA+ serums from seven patients, aged 40 to 78 years. In the majority of these, factors such as age, febrile presentation, absence of significant adenopathy or significant numbers of atypical lymphocytes had caused some uncertainty as to diagnosis, and further studies were requested. In this report, we record clinical, hematologic, biochemical and serologic data from these patients.

METHODS

Heterophil Antibodies. The presence of heterophil antibodies was determined by standard methods [21,22] following differential absorption of the serums with guinea pig kidney and beef red blood cell suspensions, using either horse or sheep red blood cells. When horse cells were used, the data were interpreted as positive if the guinea pig kidney absorbed titer was greater than the simultaneously performed beef cell absorbed titer [21]. Sheep red cell agglutinin data were interpreted by standard methods [22].

Serum bilirubin, alkaline phosphatase (AP) and glutamic oxaloacetic transaminase (SGOT) levels were determined on the SMA-12 multichannel Autoanalyzer® (Technicon, Inc.). Normal values are bilirubin <1.0 mg/100 ml, AP <90 mU/ml (<125 in those over 20 years of age) and SGOT <40 mU/ml. Serum gamma glutamyl transpeptidase (GGT) was determined on the Gilford 2400 by a standard method. Upper limits of normal in our laboratory as derived from healthy pre-employees and students, are 25 mU/ml (age 1 to 25 years) and 36 mU/ml (age >25 years). **Cold agglutinins** (CA's) were measured following overnight incubation (4°C) with 2 per cent human group O red blood cells. The specificity of CA's was determined by parallel titrations against both adult and cord red blood cells. Cold agglutinins with maximal reactivity against adult cells were considered anti-"I" whereas those with preferential reactivity against cord cells were anti-"i." **Hepatitis B antigen** (HBAg) was detected by either isoprecipitin or radioimmunoassay (RIA) technics.

Epstein-Barr Virus (EBV)-Related Serology. Antibodies to EBV-related antigens were detected by indirect immunofluorescence tests [10,23–27]. IgG antibodies to viral capsid antigens (VCA) were determined by routine procedures [23] using smears of EB-3 cells of Burkitt's lymphoma origin of which 5 to 10 per cent produce virus particles (producer line). Antibodies to the early antigen (EA) complex were determined [24], using the Raji line of cultured Burkitt's tumor cells which are normally free of VCA or EA-positive cells (nonproducer), but carry EBV genomes. These cells were superinfected with EBV from a producer line to induce EA synthesis in about 10 per cent at 48 hours. Fixation of the cell smears with either acetone or methanol allowed detection of antibodies to the D and R or only the D components of the EA complex, respectively. Antibodies to EBV-associated nuclear antigen (EBNA) were determined on Raji cell smears using a modification of the anticomplement immunofluorescence method of Reedman and Klein [25,26]. IgM antibodies to VCA were determined by indirect immunofluorescence using smears of HR-1 cells of Burkitt's lymphoma origin which had been maintained at 32°C for 10 days without refeeding and fluorescein conjugated goat antibodies to human IgM (Dakopatts A/S).

Interpretation of EBV-specific Serologic Data. As reviewed earlier [10], evidence for a concurrent or recent primary EBV infection can be obtained with initial serum specimens by one or more of the following results: detection of VCA-specific IgM antibodies, high titers of IgG antibodies to VCA (≧ 1:320), presence of anti-D and absence of anti-EBNA (<1:2). Confirmation is provided when subsequent serums show increases in anti-VCA and anti-D titers (relatively rarely) and later disappearance of IgM antibodies and anti-D, and development of anti-EBNA. Constant VCA-specific IgG and anti-EBNA titers (usually between 1:10 and 1:160) and absence of VCA-specific IgM and of anti-D denotes, as a rule, long past primary EBV infections. Absence of all antibodies in initial and late serums excludes past as well as recent primary EBV infections.

Antibodies to Cytomegalovirus. These were determined by standard complement fixation technic using antigen prepared from the AD-169 strain of virus (Flow Laboratories, Rockville, Maryland). Fourfold rises in titer are usually taken to indicate concurrent infections.

RESULTS

The pertinent clinical, hematologic, biochemical and serologic data from the seven patients with HA+ IM, aged 40 to 78 years, are recorded in Tables I, II and III. Most patients presented with fever and malaise with or without myalgia (Table I). These symptoms had been present for a minimum of 12 days in four of seven patients and four to eight days in three of seven patients prior to medical consultation. Three patients received antibiotics without clinical improvement prior to subsequent hospitalization. Significant cervical adenopathy was present in no more than two of seven patients (in marked contrast to young adults in whom significant adenopathy is seen in over 80 per cent of those with infectious mononucleosis [28,29]. Sore throat, a common (85 per cent) feature of infectious mononucleosis in younger persons, was also present in six of our seven patients. In two patients (Cases 3 and 4), significant numbers of atypical lymphocytes were absent on initial smears but evolved on serial testing (Table II). One patient (Case 4), age 46, presenting with mainly respiratory symptoms, fever, interstitial pneumonitis and cold agglutinin titers (1:224), was initially considered to have primary atypical pneumonia. Only when atypical lymphocytes were seen one week after admission were heterophil studies performed and reported as positive. Even this laboratory result was questioned by the clinician because repeated subsequent examinations failed to reveal significant cervical adenopathy. Etiologic

TABLE I Significant Clinical Data from Seven Patients with HA+ IM (40 to 78 years of age)

Case No.	Sex and Age (yr)	Duration of Fever (days)	Myalgia	Sore Throat	Anti-biotic Rx	Throat Culture	Cough Coryza	Pharyngeal Injection/ Exudate	Cervical Adenopathy (1–4+)	Hepatomegaly	Splenomegaly	Jaundice	Severity of Illness (1–4+)	Additional Comments
1	M, 40	(4–5)	+	+	–	ND	+	?	Present (1+) "few shotty nodes"	+	+	–	(2+)	Persistent malaise (60–99 days)
2	F, 43	(11–12)	–	+	–	–	–	+	Present (2+)	+	+	–	(1–2+)	
3	M, 45	24	+	+	+	–	+	+	Present (1+) "small submandibular nodes"	+	+	+	(4+)	Penicillin, Keflex® treatment; intense myalgia, jaundice, arthritis, liver biopsy—"mono-hepatitis," erythematous macular rash
4	F, 46	(28–30)	+	+	+	ND	+	+	Present (1+) "one small posterior node"	–	–	–	(2+)	Mainly upper respiratory presentation, associated interstitial pneumonitis, Keflex treatment, morbilliform rash
5	F, 55	(24–28)	+	+	+	+	–	+	Prominent (4+) (posterior and anterior)	–	–	–	(2+)	Associated beta streptococcal pharyngitis, penicillin treatment, lymph node biopsy: "reactive"; bone marrow aspiration: no granulomas, late (30 days post-onset)—isolated transient VII cranial nerve paresis
6	M, 60	22	–	–	+	–	–	–	Not detected	–	–	–	(2+)	Clinical presentation: **fever;** Terramycin® treatment, one small axillary node
7	M, 78	23	+	+	–	–	–	+	Not detected	–	–	–	(3+)	Clinical presentation: **fever**, intense myalgia and sore throat; associated paroxysmal atrial tachycardia; digoxin, fluids and salicylate therapy

TABLE II Laboratory Findings in Seven Patients with HA+ IM (40 to 78 years of age)

Case No.	Sex and Age (yr)	Days after Onset	Mononuclears* Atypical Lymphocytes per 100 WBC's	HA† (Horse Cells) GP	HA† (Sheep Cells) GP	HA† (Sheep Cells) B	Bilirubin (mg/100 ml)	AP (mU/ml)	SGOT (mU/ml)	GGT (mU/ml)	Cold Agglutinins i	Cold Agglutinins I
1	M, 40	12	78 (49)	114,688	7,168	28	0.4‡	100	104	51	28	14
		22	58 (30)	57,344	3,584	28	0.5	103	115	45	56	28
		33	33 (17)	14,336	1,792	7	0.6	74	33	21	14	28
		67	40 (13)	3,584	224	14	ND	ND	ND	13	7	28
		119	26 (8)	448	28	7	ND	ND	ND	12	<7	28
		435	27 (<2)	14	<14	14	ND	ND	ND	10	7	28
2	F, 43	4	87 (58)	7,168	ND	ND	1.0	50	90	ND	14	<7
		24	ND (>10)	896	56	<7	0.5	ND	ND	ND	14	<7
3	M, 45	8	24 (<2)	ND	ND	ND	7.2‡	600	207	ND	ND	ND
		11	47 (<5)	ND	ND	ND	11.2	610	230	ND	ND	ND
		14	51 (>10)	ND	ND	ND	8.4	820	280	ND	ND	ND
		17	70 (18)	14,336	112	7	5.7	810	220	600	448	224
		28	80 (>20)	3,584	112	<7	1.6	456	88	209	56	224
		37	72 (>20)	ND	ND	ND	1.0	197	64	ND	ND	ND
		59	58 (?)	ND	ND	ND	0.6	191	57	ND	ND	ND
		87	ND	ND	ND	ND	0.4	136	36	ND	ND	ND
4	F, 46	21	25 (<2)	112	28	<7	0.7‡	67	30	ND	14	448
		28	79 (>20)	896	224	<7	0.5	123	82	44	14	112
		32	65 (>20)	ND	ND	ND	0.4	104	64	ND	ND	ND
		39	ND ND	3,584	ND	ND	ND	ND	ND	36	<7	56
		873	42 (<5)	<7	<7	<7	ND	ND	ND	11	<7	7
5	F, 55	15	>90 (>20)	ND	ND	ND	0.2‡	375	340	ND	ND	ND
		21	84 (42)	3,584	896	<7	0.2	247	102	238	<7	7
		63	75 (12)	1,792	224	<7	ND	ND	ND	18	<7	14
6	M, 60	6	ND ND	ND	ND	ND	0.4‡	55	25	ND	ND	ND
		16	85 (47)	3,584	448	<7	0.5	161	168	345	56	28
		25	ND ND	ND	ND	ND	0.4	102	60	ND	ND	ND
		51	ND ND	ND	ND	ND	0.4	55	30	ND	ND	ND
7	M, 78	16	48 (10)	3,584	896	7	0.8‡	345	120	258	7	<7
		21	ND ND	1,792	112	7	0.5	182	73	66	28	<7
		28	79 (>50)	448	112	<7	0.6	165	61	150	14	<7
		35	52 (26)	896	56	<7	0.8	110	42	81	14	<7
		155	55 (<10)	56	7	7	0.8	174	25	18	7	<7

NOTE: Normal values: Bilirubin (<1.0 mg/100 ml); alkaline phosphatase, AP (<90 mU/ml); serum glutamic oxaloacetic transaminase, SGOT (<40 mU/ml); and gamma glutamyl transpeptidase, GGT (<37 mU/ml). ND = not done.

* Mononuclear cells including lymphocytes and monocytes per 100 WBC's. Numbers in parentheses refer to number of atypical lymphocytes per 100 WBC's.

† HA refers to heterophil antibody titers following serum absorption with a guinea pig kidney (GP) or beef red cell (B) suspensions.

‡ No HBAg detected by isoprecipitation or radioimmunoassay technic.

studies excluded mycoplasma pneumonia as the causative agent and confirmed a concurrent primary EBV infection (Table III).

Two patients (one age 60 [Case 6] and one age 78 [Case 7]) had febrile presentations without significant (Case 6) or detectable (Case 7) adenopathy. In both patients, the detection of atypical lymphocytosis led to heterophil-antibody studies. In both, repeated examinations by several observers over several days failed to reveal significant adenopathy. One (Case 7) had been seen initially as an outpatient with an apparent viral illness and was hospitalized because profound malaise and paroxysmal atrial tachycardia developed. The latter was controlled by digoxin and his condition improved after four or five days of bed rest.

Another patient, age 55 (Case 5), presented with fever and very prominent cervical adenopathy. Despite atypical lymphocytosis and heterophil-positivity, lymph node excision was performed to exclude malignant lymphoma. Sections confirmed the benign nature of the lesion. She was subsequently discharged, afebrile, and clinically improved. Two to three weeks later, a unilateral seventh cranial nerve palsy developed. There were no other neurologic defects and the palsy slowly resolved over the next several months. Because of the temporal association, the late cranial palsy was thought to be a sequelae of infectious mononucleosis, as observed in other cases [30].

Two nonhospitalized patients (Cases 1 and 2) were also initially febrile but without prominent adenopathy. Blood smears revealed many Downey cells and led to diagnostic heterophil studies.

TABLE III EBV/CMV-Related Serologic Data in Seven Patients with HA+ IM (40 to 78 years of age)*

Case No.	Sex and Age (yr)	Days after Onset	VCA IgM	VCA IgG	D	R	EBNA	CMV
1	M, 40	12	80–160	320–640	40	?	<2	ND
		33	20–40	320	40	?	<2	<1:8
		67	<10	320	20–40	?	10	ND
		119	<10	160	20-	?	20	<1:8
		435	<10	160	<10	<10	40	ND
2	F, 43	4	80	20–40	10	?	<2	ND
		11	40	160	40	?	<2	ND
		24	ND	80	40	?	<2	ND
3	M, 45	17	20	160	<10	<10	<2	1:128
		29	80	80	<10	<10	<2	1:64
4	F, 46	21	40	<2	<2	<2	<2	1:16
		23	20–40	80	40	?	<2	ND
		26	10	80	40	?	<2	ND
		28	<10	80	80	?	<2	ND
		39	ND	80	20–40	?	<2	1:16
		873	ND	40	<10	<10	10	ND
5	F, 55	21	40	160	20	?	<2	<1:8
		63	10	40	5	?	<2	<1:8
6	M, 60	17	40	160	40	?	<2	ND†
7	M, 78	16	20	80–160	10	?	<2	1:8
		21	10	80	<10	20	<2	ND
		28	<10	80–160	<10	10	<2	ND
		35	<10	40–80	<10	20	<2	1:8
		155	<10	80	<10	10	20	ND

* Antibody titers to Epstein-Barr viral capsid antigens (VCA), including both IgM and IgG antibodies, to the "D" and "R" components of the early antigen complex and to EBV-associated nuclear antigen (EBNA). ND = not done. Cytomegalovirus (CMV) titers were performed by complement fixation technic.

† Urine cultures for cytomegalovirus (CMV)—negative.

The most difficult diagnostic problem occurred in a 45 year old man (Case 3) who presented with a one week history of fever, myalgia and pharyngitis. The Monospot® test was negative, and blood smears showed 27 per cent lymphocytes without atypical forms. Penicillin was administered without effect and he was later hospitalized because of persistent fever and jaundice (bilirubin 7.2 mg/100 ml). Physical examination revealed a few small unimpressive submandibular lymph nodes, right upper quadrant tenderness and hepatomegaly. Heterophil studies were positive early in his hospital course. However, because of minimal adenopathy, the initial absence of lymphocyte atypia and deteriorating liver function studies (bilirubin rising to peak levels of 11.2 mg/100 ml), diagnostic uncertainty remained and a liver biopsy was performed. The biopsy specimen showed a moderate portal mononuclear cell infiltrate without significant hepatocellular alterations. The changes were more consistent with infectious mononucleosis than with viral hepatitis. Although fever persisted for the initial 17 days of his 23 day hospitalization, jaundice cleared and liver function eventually returned toward normal. Subsequent follow-up studies failed to reveal any sequelae to this illness. Despite the very striking bilirubin levels, peak SGOT levels were only 280 mU/ml, a feature strongly favoring acute infectious mononucleosis over hepatitis A or B.

The biochemical profiles in six of the seven patients (Table II) revealed peak bilirubin levels of 1.0 mg/100 ml in association with moderately elevated AP, SGOT and GGT levels. This bilirubin-enzyme dissociation is considered useful in supporting the diagnosis of infectious mononucleosis [31–34], especially in heterophil negative (HA−) patients whose smears show characteristic atypical lymphocytes. This type of biochemical profile has been encountered in approximately 75 per cent of our serially studied cases of infectious mononucleosis.

The EBV-related serology confirmed these cases as primary EBV infections (Table III) as evident from the early presence of VCA-specific IgM antibodies and initial absence of anti-EBNA. In two cases, additional confirmatory data were provided by peak levels (1:320) of VCA-specific IgG (Case 1) and observed seroconversion in serial specimens (Case 4). In the five other cases, peak anti-VCA IgG levels were 1:160, which per se are nondiagnostic of current EBV infection, since such levels are also seen in patients with long past (months or years) EBV infections [10]. However, in four of these five patients, the anti-VCA titers were accompanied by anti-D which is diagnostic of primary EBV

TABLE IV Mean Peak Levels of Serum Bilirubin, SGOT, AP and GGT in HA+ IM in Different Age Groups

Ages (yr)	Cases (no.)	Bilirubin* (mg/ 100 ml)	AP* (mU/ml)	SGOT* (mU/ml)	GGT* (mU/ml)
9–15	7	0.69	179.71	88.00	56.71
16–25	42	1.25	225.43	197.17	107.74
26–39	9	2.11	353.77	204.67	366.44
40–78	6	2.33	321.16	184.17	256.00

NOTE: Normal values: Bilirubin (<1 mg/100 ml); glutamic oxaloacetic transaminase, SGOT (<40 mU/ml); alkaline phosphatase, AP (<90 mU/ml); and gamma glutamyl transpeptidase, GGT (<37 mU/ml, age >25 and <26 mY/ml, ages 1–25).
* Mean values calculated from peak levels derived from at least three serial specimens collected from each of 64 patients with acute HA+ IM.

infection as a rule, since this antibody is found only occasionally in healthy donors. One patient (Case 3), with a peak anti-VCA IgG level of 1:160 without detectable anti-D or anti-R, was confirmed as having primary EBV infection on the basis of anti-VCA IgM and initial absence of anti-EBNA. Serial specimens from another patient (Case 7) were of interest in that with the decline of the transient anti-D response, anti-R became the predominant and then sole antibody to the EA complex in late convalescence. Anti-R was still detectable in the final specimen received 155 days after onset. The persistent detection of anti-R is thought to be related to an unusually brisk EBV carrier state which is normally established in the lymphoreticular system following primary EBV infections [1]. Anti-R was detected either initially or in late convalescence in 14 of our 90 previously described patients with HA+ IM [10,27]. In summary, the EBV-related serologic data from these seven patients are no different from those of young adults with HA+ IM.

COMMENTS

The seven elderly patients in this study were clearly experiencing primary EBV infections. Most initially presented with fever, sore throat and myalgia, and infectious mononucleosis was not an initial consideration either because of their age (all patients), relative absence of cervical adenopathy (five patients), initial absence of atypical lymphocytes (two patients) [35] or intense jaundice (one patient). Heterophil, biochemical and EBV serologic data eventually confirmed the diagnosis of infectious mononucleosis in all cases.

Evans noted that elderly people with infectious mononucleosis often have more severe illnesses and complications (e.g., jaundice) [3]. In five of our seven patients, the duration of fever varied from 22 to 30 days, time intervals considerably in excess of those seen in most young adults with infectious mononucleosis. Illnesses of marked severity were clearly recorded in Case 3 (intense jaundice, protracted fever) and Case 7 (prolonged fever, severe prostration and paroxysmal atrial tachycardia). The illnesses in our other five patients were retrospectively judged to be of only moderate severity. Steroid therapy, usually reserved for more severe cases, was not administered to any of our patients. However, steroids were considered but never administered in Case 3 during the phase of rapidly rising serum bilirubin levels.

In an attempt to gauge the severity of illness (versus younger patients) more objectively, we compared peak biochemical abnormalities in the present series with those of younger patients with infectious mononucleosis. Only cases in which at least three serial biochemical profiles were available were included. These acute specimens covered at least a 14 day interval. However, in some cases, further profiles were available through an additional six weeks of illness. *Peak* acute levels of bilirubin, AP, SGOT and GGT were tabulated in order to derive mean values for the different age groups (Table IV). Despite the small numbers of patients in several of these groups, the results, in general, suggest more marked abnormalities in older patients (ages 26 to 78 years), thus, supporting Evans' claim that HA+ IM may be more severe with advancing age [3]. Whereas it is well known that in individual cases, liver function studies may not correlate with clinical findings, in general, there appears to be some relationship between the impairment of liver function and the severity of illness [36].

The incidence of HA+ IM in older persons is difficult to determine. Twenty-three cases were confirmed as infectious mononucleosis from a total of 701 specimens received from patients 40 to 69 years of age at the Wisconsin State Board of Health, 1965–1967 [3]. These 23 cases represented 0.76 per cent of a total of 3,043 confirmed cases during this interval. Four cases in our present series were derived from 300 cases of HA+ IM representing 1.3 per cent. The three other cases (Cases 3, 5 and 6) in this study were obtained from other hospitals.

Over several years, serums from 13 cases of suspected HA+ IM from older patients ($\geqq$ age 41) were submitted to one of us (W.H.) for serologic confirmation of primary EBV infections. Although from most patients only single serum specimens became available, a definite diagnosis could be established in eight (41 to 81 years of age), a probable diagnosis in three (41 to 59 years of age) and a questionable diagnosis in two (52 to 62 years of age). Although detailed histories from these patients were not available, adenopathy was mentioned in only three of seven in whom some details were submitted.

REFERENCES

1. Henle W, Henle G: Epstein-Barr virus. The cause of infectious mononucleosis. A review. Oncogenesis and herpes-viruses (Biggs PM, de-The G, Payne LN, eds), Lyon, International Agency of Research on Cancer, 1972, p 269.
2. Henle W, Henle G: Epstein-Barr virus and infectious mononucleosis. N Engl J Med 288: 263, 1973.
3. Evans AS: Infectious mononucleosis: recent developments. GP 40: 128, 1969.
4. Henle G, Henle W: Observations on childhood infections with the Epstein-Barr virus. J Infect Dis 121: 303, 1970.
5. Joncas J, Mintyan C: Serological response of the EBV antibodies in pediatric cases of infectious mononucleosis and in their contacts. Can Med Assoc J 102: 1260, 1970.
6. Baehner RL, Shuler SE: Infectious mononucleosis in childhood—clinical expressions, serologic findings, complications, prognosis. Clin Pediatr 6: 393, 1967.
7. Starling KA, Fernback DJ: Infectious mononucleosis in the preschool child (letter to editor). JAMA 203: 810, 1968.
8. Sumaya CV, Henle W, Henle G, Smith M, LeBlanc D: Seroepidemiologic study of Epstein-Barr virus infections in a rural community. J Infect Dis 131: 403, 1975.
9. Hewetson JF, Rocchi G, Henle W, Henle G: Neutralizing antibodies to Epstein-Barr virus in healthy populations and patients with infectious mononucleosis. J Infect Dis 128: 283, 1973.
10. Henle W, Henle G, Horwitz CA: Epstein-Barr virus specific diagnostic tests in infectious mononucleosis. Hum Pathol 5: 551, 1974.
11. Henle G, Henle W, Diehl V: Relation of Burkitt's tumor-associated herpes-type virus to infectious mononucleosis. Proc Natl Acad Sci (USA) 59: 94, 1968.
12. Niederman JC, McCollum RW, Henle G, Henle W: Infectious mononucleosis. Clinical manifestations in relation to EB virus antibodies. JAMA 203: 205, 1968.
13. Evans AS, Niederman JC, McCollum RW: Sero-epidemiologic studies of infectious mononucleosis with EB virus. N Engl J Med 279: 1121, 1968.
14. Hirshaut Y, Christenson WN, Perimutter JC: Prospective study of herpes-like virus role in infectious mononucleosis. Clin Res 19: 459, 1971.
15. University Health Physicians and Public Health Laboratory Service Laboratories. Infectious mononucleosis and its relationship to EB virus antibody. Br Med J 4: 643, 1971.
16. Hallee TJ, Evans AS, Niederman JC, Brooks CM, Voegtly JH: Infectious mononucleosis at the United States Military Academy. A prospective study of a single class over 4 years. Yale J Biol Med 3: 182, 1974.
17. Dunnett WN: Infectious mononucleosis. Br Med J 1: 1187, 1963.
18. Schultz AL, Hall WH: Clinical observations in 100 cases of infectious mononucleosis and the results of treatment with penicillin and aureomycin. Ann Intern Med 36: 1498, 1952.
19. Belfrage S: Infectious mononucleosis—an epidemiological and clinical study. Acta Med Scand 171: 531, 1962.
20. Blacklow NR, Watson BK, Miller G, Jacobson BM: Mononucleosis with heterophil antibodies and EB virus infection. Am J Med 51: 549, 1971.
21. Davidsohn I, Nelson DA: The Blood, chap 5, Todd-Sanford's Clinical Diagnosis by Laboratory Methods, 14th ed (Davidsohn I, Henry JB, eds), Philadelphia, W.B. Saunders Co., 1969.
22. Lee CL, Zandrew F, Davidsohn I: Horse agglutinins in infectious mononucleosis. III. Criterion for differential diagnosis. J Clin Pathol 21: 631, 1968.
23. Henle G, Henle W: Immunofluorescence in cells derived from Burkitt's lymphoma. J Bacteriol 91: 1248, 1966.
24. Henle G, Henle W, Klein G: Demonstration of two distinct components in the early antigen complex of Epstein-Barr virus-infected cells. Int J Cancer 8: 272, 1971.
25. Reedman BM, Klein G: Cellular localization of an Epstein-Barr virus (EBV)-associated component-fixing antigen in producer and non-producer lymphoblastoid cell lines. Int J Cancer 11: 499, 1973.
26. Henle G, Henle W, Horwitz CA: Antibodies to Epstein-Barr virus-associated nuclear antigen in infectious mononucleosis. J Infect Dis 130: 231, 1974.
27. Horwitz CA, Henle W, Henle G, Schmitz H: Clinical evaluation of patients with infectious mononucleosis and development of antibodies to the R component of the Epstein-Barr virus-induced early antigen complex. Am J Med 58: 330, 1975.
28. Hoagland RJ: The clinical manifestations of infectious mononucleosis—a report of 200 cases. Am J Med Sci 240: 21, 1960.
29. Finch SC: Clinical symptoms and signs of infectious mononucleosis, chap 2. Infectious Mononucleosis (Carter RL, Penman HC, eds), Oxford, Blackwell Scientific Publications, 1969.
30. Grose C, Henle W, Henle G, Feorino PM: Primary Epstein-Barr virus infections in acute neurologic diseases. N Engl J Med 292: 392, 1975.
31. Barondess JA, Erle H: Serum alkaline phosphatase activity in hepatitis of infectious mononucleosis. Am J Med 29: 43, 1960.
32. Futterweit W: Serum alkaline phosphatase activity in infectious mononucleosis. A clinical study of fifty-five cases. Arch Intern Med 108: 253, 1961.
33. Rosalki SB, Jones TG, Verney AF: Transaminase and liver function studies in infectious mononucleosis. Br Med J 1: 929, 1960.
34. Shuster F, Ognibene AJ: Dissociation of serum bilirubin and alkaline phosphatase in infectious mononucleosis. JAMA 209: 267, 1969.
35. Bernstein A: Infectious mononucleosis. Medicine (Baltimore) 19: 85, 1940.
36. Finch SC: Laboratory findings in infectious mononucleosis, chap 3. Infectious Mononucleosis (Carter RL, Penman HC, eds), Oxford, Blackwell Scientific Publications, 1969.

Clinical, Epidemiologic and Bacteriologic Observations of an Outbreak of Methicillin-Resistant Staphylococcus aureus at a Large Community Hospital

JOSEPH J. KLIMEK, M.D.
FREDERICK J. MARSIK, Ph.D.*
RAYMOND C. BARTLETT, M.D.
BARBARA WEIR, R.N.
PATRICIA SHEA, R.N.
RICHARD QUINTILIANI, M.D.
Hartford, Connecticut

Over a 12 month period, 61 isolates of methicillin-resistant Staphylococcus aureus (MR-SA) were obtained in 23 hospitalized patients. Eighty-six per cent of the patients were over 50 years of age, and 91 per cent were in the postoperative period. In 10 patients (43 per cent), MR-SA was the major pathogen, producing either pneumonia, empyema, osteomyelitis, lung abscess, enterocolitis, wound infection or bacteremia with sepsis. Three patients in this group died despite therapy with antibiotics with in vitro activity against these organisms. All the patients probably acquired their MR-SA in the hospital, and five carriers of the organism were identified among hospital personnel. This outbreak demonstrates the ability of MR-SA not only to colonize many patients in a relatively brief period of time, but also to produce serious disease.

Only two years after the introduction of methicillin in 1959, strains of Staphylococcus aureus appeared that were resistant to this antibiotic [1–3]. Although they were initially detected in England, similar methicillin-resistant strains of Staph. aureus (MR-SA) have subsequently been isolated in many other parts of the world [4–10].

Although sporadic cases of infection due to MR-SA were reported in the early 1960's, it was not until 1968 that Barrett described the first outbreak of a large number (18) of cases in the United States [11].

We recently observed a similar large outbreak at Hartford Hospital between April 1974 and April 1975 in which 61 isolates of MR-SA were recovered in 23 patients. Clinical, bacteriologic and epidemiologic observations in these 23 cases are the subject of this communication. Of additional clinical importance was the fact that in 10 patients the MR-SA was the definitive pathogen, producing bacteremia, empyema, osteomyelitis, enterocolitis, pneumonia, wound infection and a lung abscess.

MATERIALS AND METHODS

Bacterial Isolates and Antimicrobial Susceptibility Testing. Isolation of staphylococci from clinical specimens was carried out in the microbiology laboratory of Hartford Hospital. Initial identification of Staph. aureus was based on colonial morphology in sheep blood agar and a positive slide and tube coagulase test.

From the Department of Medicine, Hartford Hospital, Hartford, Connecticut 06115. Requests for reprints should be addressed to Dr. Richard Quintiliani, Hartford Hospital, Hartford, Connecticut 06115. Manuscript accepted January 29, 1976.

* Present address: Division of Microbiology, University of Virginia Medical School, Charlottesville, Virginia 22901.

All isolates of Staph. aureus were tested by the Kirby-Bauer method [12] with plates incubated at 35°C. The initial isolates (34) of MR-SA from various body sites were tested for their susceptibility to chloramphenicol, gentamicin, tetracycline, cephalothin, clindamycin, erythromycin, methicillin and penicillin. In subsequent isolates from the same sites, antimicrobial susceptibility patterns were determined against cephalothin, clindamycin, erythromycin, methicillin and penicillin.

Minimal inhibitory concentrations (MIC) for the initial isolates were determined by tube dilution and agar dilution technics at Bristol Laboratories (Division of Bristol-Myers Co., Syracuse, N.Y.) with an inoculum of 100,000 organisms. Staphylococci were considered resistant if the MIC of methicillin was 12.5 μg/ml or greater after 24 hours incubation at 37°C [13].

Biochemical tests were performed on the 34 initial isolates of MR-SA by the microbiology laboratory of Hartford Hospital according to the methods described by Baird-Parker [14] and Bentley [15]. The MR-SA isolate was considered the definitive pathogen if it was recovered either as a pure culture from an obvious site of infection or from an area of the body normally totally devoid of microorganisms.

Bacteriophage Typing. Bacteriophage typing was performed by the Connecticut State Department of Health, Laboratory Division, and was confirmed by the Bacteriology Section, Bureau of Laboratories, Communicable Disease Center, Atlanta, Georgia. Phages tested include the following: Group 1—29, 52, 52A, 79, 80; Group 2—3A, 3C, 55, 71; Group 3—6, 42E, 47, 53, 54, 75, 77, 83A, 84, 85; Miscellaneous—81, 91 (WH1), 95, 96.

Patients. The 23 patients in this report were admitted to the surgical or medical services of Hartford Hospital, Hartford, Connecticut between March 14, 1974, and January 10, 1975.

There were seven (30 per cent) women and 16 (70 per cent) men. They ranged in age from 23 to 84 years; 86 per cent were over age 50 and 36 per cent were over age 70. Twenty-one (91 per cent) patients were in the postoperative period (two with multiple trauma, two with burns and the remaining 17 for various surgical procedures), one patient had lactic acidosis and shock, and one was an otherwise healthy nurse who had worked in close contact with infected patients. Six (26 per cent) of the surgical patients also had a neoplasm.

Environmental Studies. The surgical service is located on a single floor and is divided into five geographically separate wards: A is the surgical intensive care unit, and B, C, D and E are general surgical wards. The medical service is similarly planned and is located three floors above surgery. All nurses and aides carry out their primary duties within the confines of a single ward, but there is extensive movement of physicians and ancillary personnel (respiratory therapists, laboratory personnel) between wards. Most of the patients in this study occupied single rooms, but, at times during their stay in the hospital, some were in four-bed rooms. All patients were isolated within 48 hours after the first positive culture for MR-SA was obtained. The patients were placed in a single room and strict isolation was observed, including gowns, gloves, hand washing and masks.

TABLE I Patients with Definite Infection from Methicillin-Resistant Staph. aureus (MR-SA)

Age (yr)	Admitting Diagnosis	Sites MR-SA Recovered	Infection	Prior Antibiotic Treatment	Therapy	Outcome
62	Multiple trauma	Stool (5)	Enterocolitis	Cefazolin	Clindamycin	Home
84	Cancer of the esophagus	Chest tube (1)	Empyema	Gentamicin, cefazolin, cephalothin	Gentamicin, cefazolin	Died
58	Chronic obstructive pulmonary disease	Chest tube (2)	Empyema	None	Cefazolin	Home
23	Osteomyelitis	Thumb	Osteomyelitis	None	Cefazolin	Home
54	Aortic valve replacement	Wound, blood, gastrostomy tube	Bacteremia	Cefazolin, ampicillin, cephalothin	Cephalothin, gentamicin, vancomycin	Died
69	Cancer of the pancreas, chronic obstructive pulmonary disease	Sputum (2)	Pneumonia	Cephalothin, gentamicin, clindamycin, ampicillin	Gentamicin, cephalothin	Died
62	Burns	Wound (5)	Wound infection	Penicillin	Cefazolin	Died
42	Elephantiasis	Blood (1), wound	Bacteremia	Cephalothin	Cefazolin	Home
35	Regional enteritis	Blood (5), neck abscess, central venous pressure catheter, central venous pressure wound	Bacteremia	None	Clindamycin	Home
65	Bowel obstruction	Sputum (3), lung aspirate	Lung abscess	Cefazolin, gentamicin, clindamycin, chloramphenicol	Vancomycin	Home

NOTE: Number in parentheses indicate the number of positive cultures.

TABLE II Hartford Hospital Screening for Methicillin-Resistant Staph. aureus (May to October 1974)

Personnel	No.	Positive Cultures of Staph. aureus: Methicillin-Sensitive	Methicillin-Resistant
Interns	9	3	0
Nurses (A)*	52	4	3
Nurses (B)†	47	7	2
Staff doctors	3	3	0
Respiratory therapists	48	12	0
Recovery room technicians	19	1	0
Operating room scrub nurses	24	6	0
Totals	202	36	5

* A = Surgical Intensive Care Unit.
† B = Intermediate Surgical Care Unit.

Five months after the initial isolate, MR-SA continued to be a problem despite isolation of infected or colonized patients and identification of carriers. In order to determine whether the hospital environment could be a source of contamination, sampling of the nursing units where most of the MR-SA were recovered was begun on October 2, 1974. Air samples were obtained on two successive days in rooms with patients who harbored MR-SA and in rooms (or intensive care unit cubicles) where infected or colonized patients had been previously located. A TDL Slit Air Sampler was used with a setting of 1 cubic foot/min for 20 minutes. Rodac plates containing standard methods agar were used to sample the surfaces of floors, drapes, counter tops and air vents.

RESULTS

Of the initial 34 MR-SA isolates from various body sites, all were found to be resistant to erythromycin, penicillin and tetracycline, and sensitive to cephalothin and gentamicin; 12 isolates were resistant to both chloramphenicol and clindamycin; 13 isolates were resistant to chloramphenicol and sensitive to clindamycin; eight isolates were sensitive to chloramphenicol and resistant to clindamycin; and one isolate was sensitive to both chloramphenicol and clindamycin. The MIC of methicillin for the 61 MR-SA ranged from 2 to 128 μg/ml after 24 hours of incubation, whereas, after 48 hours, all the isolates were resistant to at least 28 μg/ml. The MIC for cephalothin ranged from 0.25 to 32 μg/ml after 24 hours, and from 1 to 64 μg/ml after 48 hours. None of the MR-SA isolates was phage typable.

None of the 34 isolates tested produced acid from the following sugars: arabinose, cellobiose, dextrin, galactose, inositol, zylose, rhamnose, salicin, alpha-methyl glucoside and raffinose. All 34 isolates produced acid from maltose, mannitol and glycerin. All isolates produced phosphatase and lipase. All isolates hydrolyzed hippurate and DNA. None of the MR-SA hydrolyzed either gelatin or hemoglobin.

Nineteen (82 per cent) of the 23 patients had received one or more antibiotics before acquiring MR-SA: sixteen had received a cephalosporin derivative and three had received either clindamycin or lincomycin. No one received a penicillinase-resistant penicillin.

In 21 (91 per cent) patients MR-SA were definitely acquired in the hospital, with an interval of four to 56 days between their admission and the first positive culture.

The major sources for the 61 MR-SA were sputum, wounds, blood, stools and chest tube drains where 18, 16, 7, 6 and 4 isolates were recovered. Two isolates were grown from central venous catheter tips and leg ulcers while a single isolate was recovered from each of the following sites: tracheostomy, excised tissue, skin graft, bone, abscess in the neck and a lung aspirate. MR-SA was isolated in pure culture in 10 patients (43 per cent) in whom these organisms were considered to be the definitive pathogen. MR-SA was isolated for the first time between the fourth and 54th hospital day in these patients. In the patients in whom MR-SA was the definitive pathogen (Table I), the infections included pneumonia (one patient), empyema (two patients), osteomyelitis (one patient), lung abscess (one patient), enterocolitis (one patient), burn infection (one patient) and bacteremia with sepsis (three patients). In eight of these patients, the organism was recovered from body sites normally totally devoid of microorganisms. Of the four patients who died, three were receiving antibiotics that had in vitro activity against these organisms for at least seven days. Two had malignancies (pancreas, esophagus) and one had extensive complications following aortic valve replacement, including an intraoperative cerebrovascular accident, massive postoperative gastrointestinal bleeding, pneumonia and empyema. The fourth patient died with Pseudomonas bacteremia. Whether nurse carriers of MR-SA were the source of these organisms in their patients or vice versa cannot be established with certainty, since the nurses cared for different patients on a daily basis.

Fifty-seven per cent of the cases (13 patients) probably represented colonization in that MR-SA were recovered in mixed culture from sputum or surgical wounds in the absence of any obvious evidence of infection. Treatment with cephalosporins alone, cephalosporins in combination with gentamicin, clindamycin or vancomycin was successful in eliminating MR-SA in six of these patients. In the remaining seven patients, no specific attempt was made to eradicate the staphylococci.

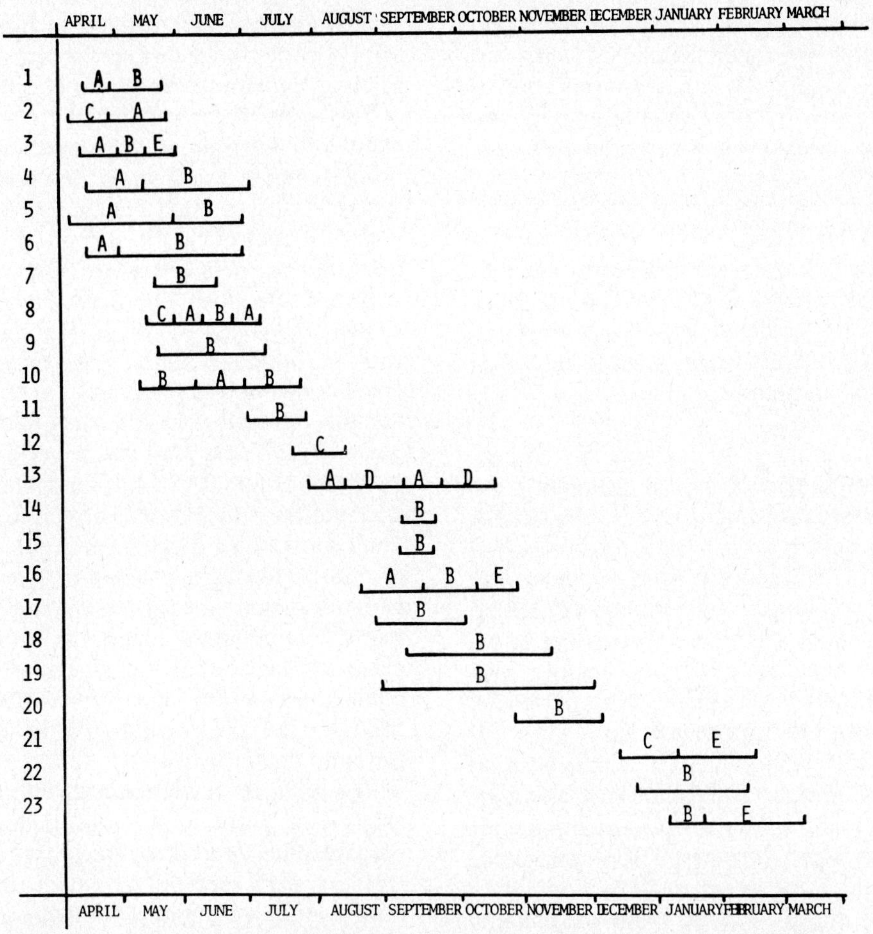

Figure 1. Location and length of hospitalization of patients from whom methicillin-resistant Staphylococcus aureus was isolated. A = surgical intensive care unit; B = intermediate surgical unit; C = general surgical ward; D = general surgical ward; E = isolated surgical ward.

Nares cultures were obtained at several intervals between May and October, 1974, on all personnel who came in close contact with patients with MR-SA. These carrier data are depicted in Table II and show that five nurses were identified as possible sources for these organisms and that all worked in the same side of the same floor. All had taken care of infected or colonized patients before being identified as carriers.

Two of these carriers were found in the initial screening cultures of surgical intensive care personnel (A) and were removed from that area and treated. Carriers were removed from any direct patient contact, instructed to take hexachlorophene showers daily for one week and to apply local bacitracin ointment three times daily for one week. Follow-up cultures were taken weekly and, if negative for three consecutive weeks, the nurse was allowed to return to her unit. The problem of MR-SA continued into June 1974, so additional screening cultures were obtained in personnel in the surgical intensive care unit (A) and intermediate surgical unit (B), as well as operating and recovery room personnel; two additional carriers were detected on B. After removal and treatment of these second two carriers, the number of MR-SA isolated declined until another outbreak occurred in the surgical intensive care units in August and September. Material for cultures was again taken, and a nurse from A who previously had been colonized with methicillin-sensitive staphylococci, now harbored MR-SA in her nares.

Figure 1 indicates the length of stay and the location of the patients with MR-SA while in the hospital. The initial isolates were recovered from a patient, 23 days after being admitted to A (surgical intensive care unit) with multiple trauma. The patient was transferred to B, which routinely accepts patients from the intensive care unit. All the subsequent isolates of MR-SA were from patients who had sometime during their hospitalization been on one of these two wards (A or B), with four exceptions: two patients (Cases 14 and 15), on the medical floor, were cared for by a surgical nurse (later identified as a carrier) who usually worked on B but who had been transferred to the medical floor for a day; and two patients (Cases 12 and 21) who were on C during their entire hospital stay but may have been exposed to nurses who were occasionally transferred from A or B to C.

Environmental sampling yielded no MR-SA. All air samples contained Bacillus species, Staphylococcus epidermidis and yeast. Surface samples were found to contain the same contaminants found in the air. Environmental cultures were obtained only once (over a two day period) since no MR-SA were found in the environment in the initial samples.

COMMENTS

This outbreak of MR-SA involving 23 patients is the largest reported so far in the United States. The MR-SA strains isolated in this study are similar to those reported by others [16–20], for they displayed multiple drug resistance, including penicillin, and required incubation at 37°C for recognition of methicillin-resistance. Although none of the isolates was phage typable, biochemical testing indicated that a single strain of MR-SA was probably responsible for the outbreak.

Because of the multiplicity of antibiotics administered to these patients, it is not possible to draw any conclusions regarding the correlation between the use of antibiotics and the incidence of methicillin-resistance. Although most patients received multiple antibiotics prior to the recovery of MR-SA, there were four patients in whom this was not true. Thus, our experience supports the impression of Parker and Hewitt [13] that prior antibiotic exposure is not essential to acquire MR-SA. Of further interest in our series is the observation that no patient received a penicillinase-resistant penicillin.

Although all isolates were sensitive to cephalosporins in vitro, these antibiotics were not very successful either in eradicating them from a patient or in preventing colonization, as indicated by the observation that 16 patients (69 per cent) received a cephalosporin antibiotic in the interim between admissions to the hospital and isolation of the MR-SA and that three patients died while being treated with a cephalosporin alone or in combination with an aminoglycoside. This disappointing result with cephalosporins against MR-SA is consistent with the view of Acar et al. [21] who concluded that cephalosporins alone failed in many cases to clear MR-SA bacteremia, despite reports of in vitro sensitivity of the organism to this group of antibiotics.

The epidemiologic data in this study demonstrate the ability of this strain of Staphylococcus not only to colonize patients but also to produce serious disease. When it became apparent that isolation technics alone were not controlling the spread of MR-SA (13 isolates from four patients in the first 30 days), an attempt was undertaken to identify carriers of the organism. Hospital employees and "common denominator" physicians were screened by culturing the nares, conjunctiva and any wounds on the fingers or hands. The findings of a number of carriers in this study dispel the notion suggested by O'Toole [22] that the poor carrier colonizing potential of MR-SA is an explanation for its failure to become an established problem in the United States. The probable transfer of the organism from the nares of one carrier to two patients (Cases 14 and 15) for whom she cared for only an 8 hour period demonstrates the serious potential for spread when dealing with this strain of Staphylococcus. However, our environmental studies agree with the observation of O'Toole that MR-SA exhibits poor potential for colonization of the physical environment.

The patients in whom MR-SA were recovered were recovering from major intra-abdominal or thoracic surgery, multiple trauma, burns or malignancy. Although isolates from sputum and wounds were the most common (55 per cent of all isolates), bacteremia occurred in three patients; in all instances, the bacteremia was a sequel to wound infection with this organism. Isolation from empyema fluid or blood was associated with greatest morbidity. The four deaths occurred in patients with other debilitating problems, of whom two had underlying malignancy, whereas one had numerous postoperative complications of major surgery and in one with severe burns Pseudomonas sepsis developed.

Detailed epidemiologic surveillance, prompt isolation of patients with infection from MR-SA and removal of carriers of this organism from patient care areas were sufficient to control this outbreak.

ACKNOWLEDGMENT

The technical assistance of Janice Tetreault is gratefully acknowledged.

REFERENCES

1. Jevons MP: Celbenin-resistant staphylococci. Br Med J 1: 124, 1961.
2. Barber M: Methicillin-resistant staphylococci. J Clin Pathol 14: 385, 1961.
3. Knox R, Smith JT: Nature of penicillin resistance in staphylococci. Lancet 2: 520, 1961.
4. Barber M, Waterworth PM: Antibacterial activity of penicillins. Br Med J 1: 1159, 1962.
5. Beck A, Evans IL: Resistance to newer penicillins. Br Med J 1: 887, 1963.
6. Jevons MP, Coe AW, Parker MT: Methicillin resistance in staphylococci. Lancet 1: 904, 1963.
7. Stewart GT, Holt RJ: Evaluation of natural resistance to newer penicillins. Br Med J 1: 308, 1963.
8. Dyke KGH, Jevons MP, Parker MT: Penicillinase production and intrinsic resistance to penicillins in Staphylococcus

aureus. Lancet 1: 835, 1966.
9. Colley EW, McNichol MW, Bracken PM: Methicillin-resistant staphylococci in a general hospital. Lancet 1: 595, 1965.
10. Gill FA, Hook EW: Changing patterns of bacterial resistance to antimicrobial drugs. Am J Med 39: 780, 1965.
11. Barrett FF, Read FM, Finland M: Methicillin-resistant Staphylococcus aureus at Boston City Hospital. N Engl J Med 279: 441, 1968.
12. Bauer AW, Kirby WMM, Sherris JC: Antibiotic susceptibility testing by a standardized single disk method. Am J Clin Pathol 45: 493, 1966.
13. Parker MT, Hewitt JG: Methicillin resistance in Staphylococcus aureus. Lancet 1: 800, 1970.
14. Baird-Parker AC: A classification of micrococci and staphylococci based on physiological and biochemical tests. J Gen Microbiol 30: 409, 1963.
15. Bentley DW, Hague RV, Murphy RA, et al.: Biotyping, an epidemiological tool for coagulase-negative staphylococci. Antimicrob Agents Chemother p 54, 1967.
16. Bulger RJ: Methicillin-resistant strain of Staphylococcus aureus. Ann Intern Med 67: 81, 1967.
17. Benner EJ, Morthland V: Methicillin-resistant Staphylococcus aureus. Antimicrobial susceptibility. N Engl J Med 277: 678, 1967.
18. Finland M: Hospital acquired infection: the problems of methicillin-resistant Staphylococcus aureus and infections with Klebsiella pneumoniae. Am J Med Sci 264: 207, 1972.
19. Hoeprich PD, Benner EJ, Kayser FH: Susceptibility of methicillin-resistant Staphylococcus aureus to twelve antimicrobial agents. Antimicrob Agents Chemother p 104, 1969.
20. Sabath LD, Barrett RF, Wilcox C, et al.: Methicillin resistance of Staphylococcus aureus and Staphylococcus epidermidis. Antimicrob Agents Chemother p 302, 1968.
21. Acar JF, Chabbert YA: Methicillin-resistant staphylococcemia: failure of treatment with cephalosporins. Antimicrob Agents Chemother p 280, 1971.
22. O'Toole RD, Drew WL, Dattlegren BJ, et al.: An outbreak of methicillin-resistant Staphylococcus aureus infection. JAMA 213: 257, 1970.

Sepsis Associated with Decubitus Ulcers

JEFFREY E. GALPIN, M.D.
ANTHONY W. CHOW, M.D.
ARNOLD S. BAYER, M.D.
LUCIEN B. GUZE, M.D.
Los Angeles, California

Among 21 patients with sepsis attributed solely to decubitus ulcers, bacteremia was documented in 16 (76 per cent). Bacteremia involved obligate anaerobes in eight patients (50 per cent) and was polymicrobial in eight patients (50 per cent). Twelve of 17 patients who received appropriate antibiotics had persistent bacteremia; in five patients, bacteremia was terminated only after surgical debridement. Ten of these 21 patients died, eight despite appropriate antibiotics. Among 14 patients who underwent surgical debridement, only four patients died. Surgical debridement and antibiotics effective against aerobic as well as anaerobic bacteria are both important in the treatment of this serious complication.

The bacteriology of decubitus ulcers associated with sepsis has been poorly defined. Several investigators have suggested the predominance of Staphylococcus aureus, Streptococcus faecalis and coliforms as the causative organisms [1–3]. Appropriate anaerobic culture technics were not utilized in these studies. Our experience with 21 patients with sepsis solely attributed to decubitus ulcers is presented. Fastidious aerobic and anaerobic culture technics were employed. The high incidence of anaerobic bacteremia, exceedingly high mortality and necessity of surgical debridement for radical cure of this infection are emphasized.

MATERIALS AND METHODS

Medical records of all patients with sepsis associated with decubitus ulcers admitted to Harbor General Hospital between 1970 and 1974 were reviewed. Twenty-one patients in whom sepsis could be attributed solely to decubitus ulcers by clinical, roentgenographic and microbiologic criteria are included in this report. Cultures of the decubiti were obtained by needle aspiration, surgical drainage or cotton swab. Specimens were collected in gassed containers flushed with carbon dioxide to preclude aeration during transport, and inoculated on routine as well as prereduced anaerobically sterilized (PRAS) media using the Virginia Polytechnic Institute roll-tube technic [4]. Blood cultures were obtained and inoculated at the bedside into aerobic brain heart infusion broth (Difco Laboratories) as well as thioglycollate broth (Difco Laboratories) or PRAS brain heart infusion broth supplemented with yeast extract, cysteine, menadione and hemin (Scott Laboratories). Aerobic isolates were identified by standard procedures; obligate anaerobes and microaerophilic organisms were identified and speciated according to Holdeman and Moore [4]. A Beckman pH-meter was used for recording carbohydrate fermentation reactions, and the Dohrmann AnaBac chromatograph was used for fatty acid analysis. Antibiotic susceptibility testing of aerobic blood isolates was determined by the Kirby-Bauer disc diffusion method [5]. Susceptibility of anaerobic blood isolates was performed by an agar dilution technic [6].

From the Department of Medicine, Harbor General Hospital, Torrance; Research and Medical Services, Veterans Administration, Wadsworth Hospital Center, Los Angeles; and UCLA School of Medicine, Los Angeles, California. Requests for reprints should be addressed to Dr. Jeffrey E. Galpin, Division of Infectious Disease, Harbor General Hospital, 1000 West Carson Street, Torrance, California 90509. Manuscript accepted January 28, 1976.

TABLE I Clinical and Microbiologic Summary of 21 Patients with Decubitus Ulcers and Evidence of Sepsis

Case No.	Age (yr) and Sex	Persistent or Recurrent Fever	Persistent (+) Blood Cultures	Number of (+) Blood Cultures	Osteomyelitis	Predisposing Illness	Number of Decubitus Ulcers and Location
1	20,M	+	+	4 for anaerobic streptococcus; 5 for Bacteroides fragilis; 5 for Proteus, mirabilis	–	Paraplegia	Single large, sacral
2	22,M	+	+	7 for Staph. aureus	–	Bedridden with endocarditis	Sacral
3	23,M	+	+	2 for anaerobic streptococcus; 2 for Bacteroides fragilis	+	Paraplegia	Sacral
4	25,M	–	+	2 for Eubacterium, Bacteroides fragilis, Proteus mirabilis	–	Paraplegia	Sacral, knees
5	28,M	–	+	1 for Staphylococcus aureus; 1 for Proteus mirabilis; Staph. aureus	–	Quadriplegia	Scaral, bilateral, trochanteric
6	29,M	+	+	4 for Bacteroides fragilis	–	Quadriplegia	Sacral, shoulder, patella, heels, knees, trochanteric
7	30,M	+	–	None	–	Chronic arachnoiditis	Trochanteric
8	34,M	+	–	None	+	Paraplegia	Buttock, deep to ischium
9	38,F	+	+	3 for Bacteroides fragilis; 2 for Peptostreptococcus	–	Multiple sclerosis	Sacral
10	41,F	+	+	2 for Proteus mirabilis	–	Paraplegia	Heels, ischial
11	52,M	+	+	2 for anaerobic streptococcus	+	Paraplegia	Buttocks, ischial, trochanteric, pretibial
12	53,M	+	+	2 for Bacteroides fragilis	+	Multiple sclerosis	Bilateral ischial, bilateral malleoli, trochanteric
13	54,M	+	–	None	+	Transverse myelitis	Bilateral heels, sacral, ankle
14	57,F	–	+	2 for Bacteroides fragilis; 2 for Escherichia coli	–	Mental retardation, chronic debilitation	Buttock
15	63,M	–	–	None	–	Cerebrovascular disease; quadriplegia	Bilateral peritibial, buttock, scalp
16	77,F	–	–	None	–	Cerebrovascular disease	Coccyx, ischial
17	78,F	+	+	2 for Bacteroides fragilis, anaerobic streptococcus	+	Diabetes mellitus	Sacral, buttock, bilateral ankles
18	78,F	–	+	2 for Bacteroides fragilis	–	Atherosclerosis, amputee	Buttock
19	82, F	+	+	7 for group A streptococcus; 1 for group D streptococcus	+	Cerebrovascular disease; hemiplegia	Many lower extremity, sacral, finger, trochanteric, knee
20	86,M	–	+	4 for Staphylococcus aureus	+	Cerebrovascular disease, chronic brain syndrome	Heels, bilateral buttocks, sacral
21	90,M	–	+	6 for Proteus mirabilis	–	Atherosclerosis	Sacral, ankles, trochanteric, ischial

TABLE II Decubitus Ulcers in 21 Patients with Sepsis

Location and Extent of Lesions	No. of Patients
Single ulcer	8
Multiple ulcers	13
Location of ulcers	
Sacral	12
Buttocks	7
Trochanteric	7
Ischial	5
Heels	4
Knees	3
Ankles	3
Pretibial	2
Finger	1
Scalp	1
Coccyx	1
Malleoli	1
Osteomyelitis of underlying bone	8
Putrid discharge	13

TABLE III Microbiology of Decubitus Ulcers in 21 Patients (Including 16 with Bacteremia)

	No. of Patients	
Microbial Isolates	Decubitus	Blood
Aerobic Isolates		
Proteus mirabilis	14	5
vulgaris	1	0
Escherichia coli	9	1
Pseudomonas	5	0
Klebsiella	4	0
Enterobacter	3	0
Providencia	1	0
Staph. aureus	6	3
epidermidis	5	0
Streptococci		
Group A	2	1
Group D	11	1
Not Group A or D	1	0
Diphtheroids	3	0
Candida	1	0
Anaerobic Isolates		
Bacteroides fragilis	4	8
corrodans	1	0
Peptococcus and Peptostreptococcus	3	5
Microaerophilic streptococcus	1	0
Clostridium	3	0
Eubacterium	0	1

RESULTS

Clinical and Laboratory Features. Table I summarizes the clinical and microbiologic data from each of the 21 patients. All but three of the patients had a neurologic disease leading to severe motor and/or sensory deficit. Almost one half of these patients presented with generalized vascular disease.

All patients presented with high fever, chills, hypotension, tachycardia and/or tachypnea. The clinical presentation in 13 patients (62 per cent), was distinctive because of recurrent or persistent fever in the face of antibiotic therapy. Multiple, noncontiguous ulcers were noted in 13 patients (Tables I and II). Most ulcers were more extensive than described during initial assessment. Osteomyelitis was documented roentgenographically or surgically in eight patients (40 per cent) (Table I). The largest and most frequent ulcers were found on the sacrum, buttocks or trochanteric areas. Lesions were foul-smelling in 13 patients, and marked tissue necrosis was observed in 18 of 21 patients.

Microbiology of Decubitus Ulcers and Associated Bacteremia. Sixteen of 21 patients (76 per cent) had documented bacteremia which was persistent in all cases (Table I). The predominant blood isolates included Bacteroides fragilis, Peptococcus, Peptostreptococcus, Proteus mirabilis and Staph. aureus (Table III). In eight patients, bacteremia was polymicrobial. Anaerobes were exclusively isolated in seven patients; aerobes were exclusively isolated in six patients; and mixed aerobic and anaerobic organisms were isolated in three patients. The predominant organisms cultured from decubiti included Proteus mirabilis, Group D streptococci, Escherichia coli, staphylococci and Pseudomonas species (Table III). Although six times as many aerobes as anaerobes were isolated from decubitus ulcers, more anaerobes than aerobes were recovered from blood.

Therapy and Outcome (Table IV). Ten of the 21 patients died with an over-all mortality of 48 per cent. Mortality was highest in patients over the age of 60 (seven of seven) and in patients with multiple lesions (eight of 13). All patients were treated with antibiotics for suspected sepsis. Sixteen patients received gentamicin or kanamycin in combination with clindamycin or chloramphenicol; eight patients died. From the subsequent in vitro susceptibility data, this regimen was chosen appropriately in all 16 patients. Five patients received gentamicin or kanamycin in combination with penicillin, ampicillin or cephalothin. From the subsequent in vitro data, this regimen was "inappropriately" chosen in four patients, two of whom died with Bacteroides fragilis bacteremia, which would not be expected to respond to the antibiotics administered. Fourteen patients underwent surgical debridement of the decubitus lesions and only four patients died. Among five patients, bacteremia was persistent despite the administration of appropriate antibiotics, but it was terminated after surgical debridement.

COMMENTS

Our experience underscores the serious nature of sepsis associated with decubitus ulcers. Bacteremia was documented in 16 of 21 patients and was persistent

TABLE IV Therapy and Outcome in 21 Patients with Decubitus Ulcers and Sepsis

Case No.	Antibiotic Therapy		Surgical Intervention	Outcome
1*	Cephalothin, Kanamycin	–	Yes	Survived
2*	Methicillin, Gentamicin, Chloramphenicol	+	Yes†	Survived
3*	Gentamicin, Cephalothin	–	Yes	Survived
4*	Gentamicin, Clindamycin	+	No	Died
5*	Gentamicin, Cephalothin	+	No	Survived
6*	Gentamicin, Ampicillin, Clindamycin	+	Yes†	Survived
7	Gentamicin, Clindamycin	+	Yes	Survived
8	Gentamicin, Cephalothin, Clindamycin	+	Yes	Survived
9*	Gentamicin, Cephalothin, Clindamycin	+	Yes	Died
10*	Gentamicin, Clindamycin	+	Yes†	Survived
11*	Gentamicin, Clindamycin	+	Yes†	Survived
12*	Ampicillin, Cephalothin, Kanamycin,	–	Yes	Died
13	Gentamicin, Ampicillin, Clindamycin	+	Yes	Survived
14*	Gentamicin, Clindamycin	+	Yes†	Survived
15	Gentamicin, Clindamycin	+	No	Died
16	Gentamicin, Clindamycin	+	No	Died
17*	Gentamicin, Cephalothin, Kanamycin, Clindamycin	+	No	Died
18*	Kanamycin, Cephalothin	–	No	Died
19*	Gentamicin, Clindamycin	+	Yes	Died
20*	Gentamicin, Clindamycin, Methicillin	+	Yes	Died
21*	Gentamicin, Clindamycin	+	No	Died

NOTE: + = appropriate therapy; — = inappropriate therapy.
*Patients with documented bacteremia.
†Patients whose bacteremia was terminated only after surgical debridement and grafting.

in all. Mortality was 48 per cent despite appropriate antibiotic therapy. Moreover, the importance of obligate anaerobes, particularly Bacteroides fragilis, in bacteremia associated with decubitus ulcers is confirmed [7–11]. These findings suggest that in the absence of other obvious foci of infection, the decubitus ulcer should be considered an important cause of sepsis. Since anaerobic and polymicrobial isolates are frequently recovered from blood, initial therapy in such patients should include either clindamycin or chloramphenicol for coverage of anaerobic bacteria, particularly Bacteroides fragilis. These agents are also effective against staphylococci and non-group D streptococci. In addition, an aminoglycoside should be administered to provide coverage for coliform organisms which may also play an important role in these infections. Group D streptococci would not be covered by such a combination. However, despite frequent isolation in decubitus ulcers, this organism was isolated from blood cultures in only one of our patients. There is no convincing evidence that group D streptococci play a significant role in sepsis associated with decubitus ulcers.

The most important treatment of sepsis associated with decubitus ulcers is surgical debridement. The common finding of persistent bacteremia despite appropriate antibiotic therapy in our patients, and its termination with surgical debridement, further attests to the importance of this procedure. It is apparent, however, that despite all appropriate therapeutic measures, prognosis remains poor, and aggressive preventative measures offer the only hope of effective reduction in both incidence and mortality of this serious complication.

REFERENCES

1. Vasile J, Chaitin H: Prognostic factors in decubitus ulcers of the aged. Geriatrics 27: 126, 1972.
2. Bendy RH Jr, Nuccio PA, Wolfe E, Collins B, Tamburro C, Glass W, Martin CM: Relationship of quantitative wound bacterial counts of healing of decubiti: effect of topical gentamicin. Antimicrobial Agents and Chemotherapy—1964. (Sylvester JC, ed), Ann Arbor, American Society of Microbiology, 1965, p 147.
3. Alder VG, Gillespie WA: Pressure sores and staphylococcal cross-infection: detection of sources by means of settleplates. Lancet 2: 1356, 1964.
4. Virginia Polytechnic Institute and State University Anaerobe

Laboratory: Anaerobe Laboratory Manual (Holdeman LV, Moore WEC, eds), Blacksburg, Virginia, Virginia Polytechnic Institute and State University Anaerobe Laboratory, 1972.

5. Bauer AW, Kirby WMM, Sherris JC, Turck M: Antibiotic susceptibility testing by a standardized single disc method. Am J Clin Pathol 45: 493, 1966.
6. Chow AW, Montgomerie JZ, Guze LB: Parenteral clindamycin for severe anaerobic infections. Arch Intern Med 134: 78, 1974.
7. Tynes BS, Frommeyer WB Jr: Bacteroides septicemia—cultural, clinical and therapeutic features in a series of 25 patients. Ann Intern Med 56: 12, 1962.
8. Gelb AF, Seligman SJ: Bacteroidaceae bacteremia—effects of age and focus of infection upon clinical course. JAMA 212: 1038, 1970.
9. Peromet M, Labbe M, Yourassowsky E, Schoutens E: Anaerobic bacteria isolated from decubitus ulcers. Infection 1: 205, 1973.
10. Rissing JP, Crowder JG, Dunfee T, White A: Bacteroides bacteremia from decubitus ulcers. S Med J 67: 1179, 1974.
11. Chow AW, Guze LB: Bacteroidaceae bacteremia—clinical experience with 112 patients. Medicine (Baltimore) 53: 93, 1974.

Metastatic Infection Secondary to Genitourinary Tract Sepsis

MIKE B. SIROKY, M.D.
ROBERT A. MOYLAN, M.D.
GEORGE AUSTEN, Jr., M.D.
CARL A. OLSSON, M.D.
Boston, Massachusetts

Metastatic infections arising from sepsis in the genitourinary tract are reviewed in 175 cases, including five in which we treated the patients. The skeleton was the most common site of metastasis (59 per cent). The endocardium was next most frequently involved (28 per cent). Gram-negative organisms were implicated in less than two-thirds of the cases (59 per cent). Impaired host defense mechanisms were noted in 25 per cent of the patients experiencing metastatic infections.

The lower urinary tract was the source of metastasis in 75 per cent of the patients, particularly after urologic manipulation in men. Women were more likely to experience metastatic infection from the upper urinary tract. Anatomic and pathologic considerations explaining these sex differences are presented.

The genitourinary tract is well recognized as a portal through which bacteria may gain access to the blood stream. Under most circumstances, the resulting bacteremia is of short duration due to rapid clearance of the bacteria by the reticuloendothelial system. Occasionally, however, metastatic infections are established in distant organs. Having recently encountered several examples of metastatic sepsis, we undertook a review of our own and others' experience with this relatively rare condition.

MATERIALS AND METHODS

Five instances of distant infection resulting from genitourinary tract sepsis seen in our participating institutions during the past decade are summarized in Table I and discussed in detail herein. Data on metastatic infection related to a genitourinary tract source discovered in an extensive search of the literature [1–78] were combined with our own experience, resulting in a total of 179 examples in 175 patients.

In each case, the following aspects were of particular interest and recorded for analysis: (1) microorganisms responsible for metastatic infection, (2) site of access to the blood stream by bacteria, (3) site of metastatic infection, (4) causal relationship of urologic instrumentation, (5) host susceptibility factors and (6) morbidity and mortality. In many instances, pertinent facts were missing from the cases reported in the literature, resulting in variations in the data base employed for calculating percentages.

Reports of metastatic infection in the literature which did not contain sufficient documentation or appropriate data were not included in our analysis. Nevertheless, they are listed in the bibliography as they may be of interest to some readers [79–91].

From the Department of Urology, Boston University Medical Center, Boston, Massachusetts. Requests for reprints should be addressed to Dr. Carl A. Olsson, Urology Department, University Hospital, 75 E. Newton Street, Boston, Massachusetts 02118. Manuscript accepted January 20, 1976.

TABLE I **Metastatic Infection Secondary to Genitourinary Sepsis Seen at Boston University Medical Center, 1963–1973**

Case No.	Age (yr) and Sex	Urinary Tract Source	Organism	Metastatic Infection	Debilitating Disease	Outcome
1	73,M	Bladder, kidney	Esch. coli	Septic arthritis	Cirrhosis, malnutrition	Died
2	74,M	Prostate	Esch. coli	Osteomyelitis	None	Cured
3	48,M	Urethra	Esch. coli	Mediastinal abscess	Malnutrition	Cured
4	56,M	Urethra, prostate	Esch. coli	Osteomyelitis	Anemia, cirrhosis	Cured
5	70,M	Urethra, prostate	Pseudomonas aeruginosa	Osteomyelitis	Diabetes, cancer	Cured

CASE REPORTS

Case 1. A 73 year old white man (VA 028094327) with a past history of alcoholism, Laennec's cirrhosis and chronic diarrhea was admitted with lethargy, confusion and a temperature of 104°F. On physical examination the liver was palpable 5 cm below the right costal margin, the spleen was enlarged, the bladder was distended and the prostate was 2+ enlarged. Pertinent laboratory findings included a white blood cell count of 23,000/mm^3 with a shift to the left, creatinine 3.0 mg/100 ml, serum bicarbonate 10.5 meq/liter, bromsulfalein retention 28.6 per cent. Following admission, the bladder was catheterized and drained of purulent urine growing Escherichia coli. The left elbow became swollen, and joint tap revealed pus filled with gram-negative rods which later grew Esch. coli. Treatment for gram-negative septicemia was instituted immediately with intravenous kanamycin. The kidneys were only faintly outlined by an emergency excretory urogram. Despite antibiotic and fluid therapy, refractory hypotension rapidly developed and the patient died at the end of the second hospital day. Postmortem examination revealed bilateral acute pyelonephritis, hemorrhagic cystitis, benign prostatic hypertrophy, Laennec's cirrhosis and bilateral bronchopneumonia. Culture of the heart blood grew Esch. coli.

This is an example of metastatic Esch. coli infection arising from the genitourinary tract to the elbow joint in the context of an obviously debilitated alcoholic patient.

Case 2. A 74 year old man (VA U49284) was admitted because of urinary burning and frequency. The patient had a five year history of recurrent prostatitis and partial bladder outlet obstruction. Physical examination revealed an absent right testicle, atrophic left testicle and a tender 20 g prostate. Urinalysis showed large numbers of white cells, and urine culture grew a few colonies of Esch. coli. At cystoscopy, a moderately trabeculated bladder and prominent bladder neck

A

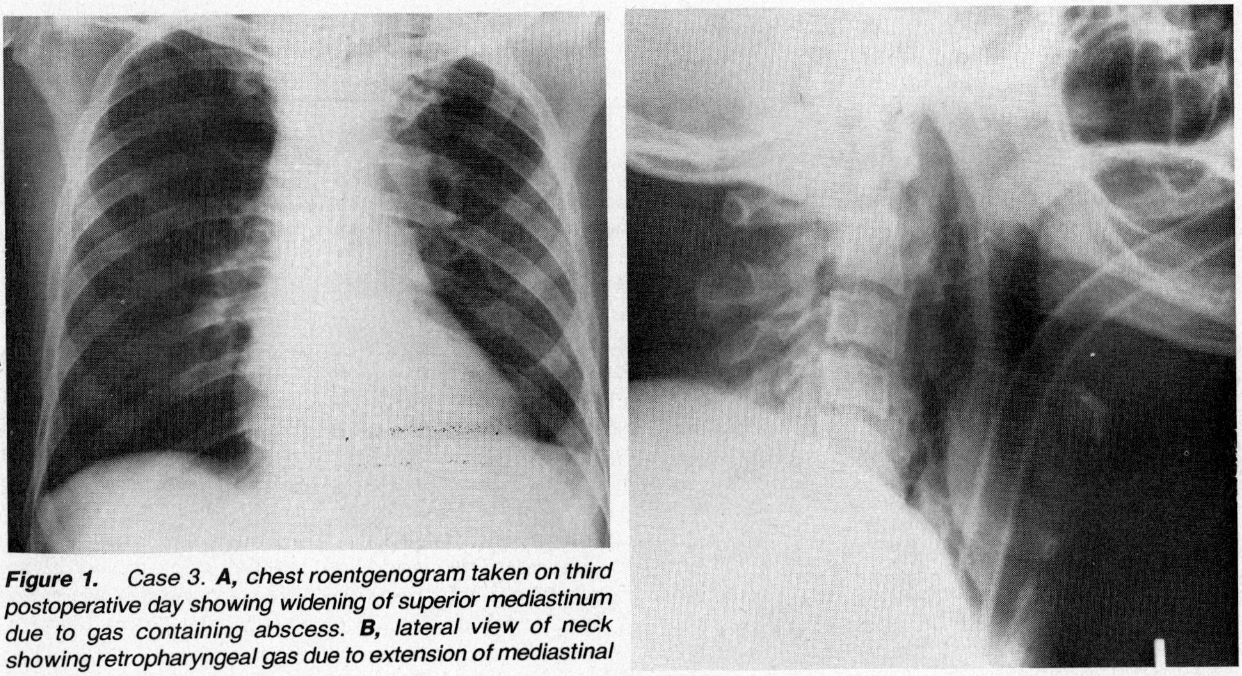

B

*Figure 1. Case 3. **A,** chest roentgenogram taken on third postoperative day showing widening of superior mediastinum due to gas containing abscess. **B,** lateral view of neck showing retropharyngeal gas due to extension of mediastinal abscess.*

were noted. Two days after instrumentation the patient experienced severe back pain, fever (with a temperature to 104°F), nausea and vomiting. A presumptive diagnosis of pyelonephritis was made, and chloramphenicol was given. Blood cultures grew Esch. coli sensitive to all antibiotics tested. The next day the patient became febrile again (temperature 106°F) and kanamycin was substituted for the antibiotics being given. However, complaints of back pain persisted and daily fever continued. An intravenous pyelogram and lumbar spine films were within normal limits. Two weeks after cystoscopy, the administration of all antibiotics was stopped and the patient was observed for further signs. One month after cystoscopy, tenderness over the second and third lumbar vertebrae was noted, and lumbar spine films showed collapse of the disc space between the second and third lumbar vertebrae. Bone scan showed increased uptake of radioisotope in the same area. Blood cultures again became positive for Esch. coli; cure was achieved by a regimen of antibiotics and bed rest for six weeks.

Culture of material from disc spaces was not available in this case, but the temporal sequence of urinary tract instrumentation in the presence of infection, positive blood cultures and skeletal infection strongly suggests metastatic infection. Metastatic osteomyelitis of the spine may be easily mistaken for pyelonephritis after instrumentation.

Case 3. A 48 year old black man (BCH 2268381) with a past history of alcoholism and malnutrition entered with a painful perineal mass of several days' duration. Physical examination revealed a fluctuant mass in the perineum. Laboratory findings were total protein 5.5 g/100 ml, albumin 2.0 g/100 ml, blood urea nitrogen 70 mg/100 ml and hematocrit value 38 per cent. The patient was taken to the operating room for drainage of a large periurethral abscess and suprapubic diversion of urine. Cultures of the abscess grew Esch. coli sensitive to the antibiotics used. The patient remained febrile postoperatively, however, and blood cultures grew Esch. coli. Four days postoperatively a tender mass was noted in the left side of the neck. A chest film showed a widened superior mediastinum (Figure 1A). Barium swallow showed an intact esophagus with a retropharyngeal collection of air (Figure 1B). Mediastinal exploration revealed a large abscess cavity extending from the retropharyngeal space to the superior mediastinum. Esch. coli was grown from this material. Drainage of this cavity was established and antibiotic therapy for two more weeks was given; the patient recovered uneventfully.

This case demonstrates rapid development of metastatic infection in a debilitated host following manipulation of a large abscess. A febrile course following drainage of an abscess should suggest inadequate drainage, inappropriate antibiotic therapy or, rarely, metastatic focus.

Case 4. In a 56 year old man (BCH 210699422) admitted for elective gastrectomy, urinary retention, fever and left flank pain developed. One month before admission, he had undergone closure of a perforated duodenal ulcer. Past medical history included alcoholism, mild liver dysfunction and poor

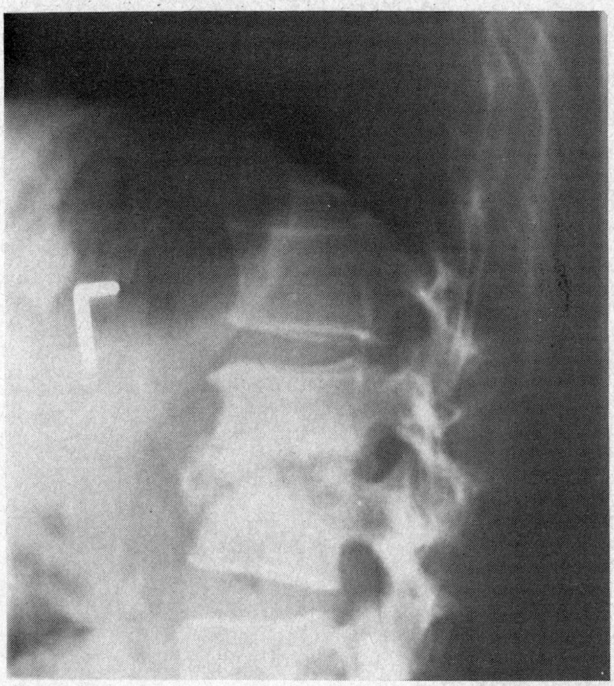

Figure 2. *Case 4. Lateral view of lumbar spine showing second and third lumbar vertebrae involved by osteomyelitis.*

nutrition. Physical examination revealed a thin man with left costovertebral angle tenderness, a distended bladder and a small, benign prostate. Bladder catheterization produced a large quantity of urine growing Esch. coli. He was given ampicillin and his condition improved rapidly. Six weeks later, with sterile urine culture, he underwent transurethral bladder neck resection. Postoperatively, he began to complain of severe, persistent lumbar back pain. Roentgenograms showed destruction and partial collapse of the second and third lumbar vertebrae (Figure 2). Bone aspirate grew Esch. coli with sensitivities identical to the previous urinary organism. Immobilization and the administration of antibiotics for six weeks resulted in marked improvement.

In this case it is difficult to determine whether seeding of the lumbar spine occurred during the initial episode involving bladder catheterization or during the later transurethral operation. However, isolation of the same organism from both original and secondary focus seems strong evidence of metastatic infection.

Case 5. A 70 year old diabetic man (UH 511485) was admitted because of hematuria and a prostatic nodule. Cystoscopy revealed a superficial bladder tumor which was resected transurethrally. A needle biopsy specimen of the prostate was negative for malignancy. Postoperative urine culture grew greater than 100,000 colonies of Pseudomonas aeruginosa. Ten days later fever and right flank pain developed which responded rapidly to the administration of sodium colistimethate. Seven months later he was readmitted with radicular cervical pain. There were findings of hypesthesia of the right thumb, upper forearm and biceps weakness. Cervical spine films showed disc space infection at the fifth and sixth cervical vertebrae with partial collapse and sub-

TABLE II Sites of Metastatic Infection from Genitourinary Sources*

Metastatic Site	Examples No.	Examples %
Skeletal	106	59
Endocarditis	51	29
Chest	8	4
Central nervous system	5	3
Eye	4	2
Miscellaneous	5	3

*179 examples in 175 patients.

luxation; cervical myelogram showed incomplete block at the level of the fifth and sixth cervical vertebrae. Antibiotic therapy with nafcillin and gentamicin was instituted prior to a decompression cervical laminectomy. Material for culture taken at surgery by the neurosurgeon was negative. Antibiotic therapy was continued for four weeks postoperatively, with marked improvement at discharge.

Although bacteriologic evidence is lacking in this case, it is reasonable to assume a relationship between the prior urinary tract infection, urinary tract manipulation and subsequent disc space infection. An interval of seven months is well within the reported range of observation.

RESULTS

Combining our five cases (Table I) with those encountered in a literature survey [1–78] produced a total of 179 examples of metastatic infection resulting from urinary tract sepsis in 175 patients. Data regarding both patient age and sex were available in 173 cases [1–58,60,62–78, present report]. There were 149 males (86 per cent) and 24 females (14 per cent), who ranged in age from one month to 89 years. The mean age was slightly higher for males (57.8 years) than for females (52.3 years).

The sites affected by metastatic infection from genitourinary sources in the total series of 175 patients are summarized in Table II. The majority of metastatic infections involved the bones and joints, totalling 106 cases [1–41] and accounting for 59 per cent of the series. Endocarditis was noted in 51 cases (28 per cent) [39,40,42–65]. Metastatic ophthalmitis [65–68], various chest infections [48,69–73], infections of the central nervous system [63,74–77] and other miscellaneous sites [73,78] accounted for the remaining 22 cases (12 per cent).

Organisms responsible for the development of metastatic infection from urinary tract sepsis are outlined in Table III. In only 148 patients was sufficient information available to allow the recording of one or more organisms found both in the genitourinary tract and in a metastatic focus. In the 27 remaining patients who had clinical evidence of metastatic infection, an organism was mentioned in one focus only. These were primarily cases of metastatic osteomyelitis in which bacteriologic evidence is difficult to obtain. A total of 159 different organisms was recovered from the 148 patients [1,3,4,9–17,19,27,29–78, present report]. As might be expected, the majority of the organisms were gram-negative (59 per cent) [3,4,9–28,30–32,34–78, present report].

TABLE III Organisms Isolated from Patients with Metastatic Infection*

Organisms	No.
Gram-positive	
Streptococcus fecalis	32
Staphylococcus aureus	31
Group B Streptococcus	2
Gram-negative	
Escherichia coli	41
Pseudomonas aeruginosa	19
Klebsiella-Aerobacter	10
Proteus mirabilis	9
Serratia marcescens	5
"Paracolon" bacilli	4
Providence species	2
Bacteroides species	2
Alcaligenes fecalis	2
Salmonella species	1
Gram-negative rod	1

*159 isolates in 148 patients.

TABLE IV Urologic Diagnoses in Patients with Metastatic Infections*

Diagnosis	No.
Upper Urinary Tract (46 diagnoses)	
Pyelonephritis	16
Nephrolithiasis	16
Perinephric abscess	3
Hydronephrosis	6
Ureteral stone	2
Renal abscess	1
Polycystic kidneys	1
Renal adenoma	1
Lower Urinary Tract (136 diagnoses)	
Benign prostatic hypertrophy	62
Urethral stricture	24
Prostatitis/abscess	12
Bladder neck contracture	6
Bladder stone	5
Bladder cancer	5
Cystitis	3
Periurethral abscess	4
Prostatic nodule	3
Neurogenic bladder	3
Urinary retention	2
Prostate cancer	2
Bladder diverticulum	2
Seminal vesiculitis	1
Ruptured urethra	1
Urethral valve	1

*182 diagnoses in 142 patients.

A primary urologic diagnosis suggesting localization of sepsis to a particular genitourinary organ was available in 142 patients with 182 diagnoses (Table IV). Sepsis involving the upper urinary tract could be presumed in 46 instances (25 per cent) [3–5,19,20,28,33–35,39,40,44,46,48,50,56,57,60,66–69,73,75, present report] most commonly resulting from pyelonephritis or nephrolithiasis (infected). Localization of infection to the lower genitourinary tract was presumed in 136 cases (75 per cent) [1,2,4,7,9,11–46,48–71,73–78, present report] in which the common diagnoses were benign prostatic hypertrophy, urethral stricture and prostatitis or prostatic abscess.

Many patients with metastatic infection related to urinary tract sepsis had undergone some form of urologic manipulation (Table V). Data regarding urologic manipulation were available in 173 patients [1–6,9–78, present report]. No urologic procedure could be implicated in the development of metastatic infection in 36 patients (21 per cent) [6,13,19,20,23–35,37,40,46–48,52–56,66,67,69,70,73,76, present report]. However, 137 patients (79 per cent) had undergone a total of 165 urologic manipulations at some time prior to the development of metastatic sepsis. Only 15 procedures (9 per cent) had been performed on the upper urinary tract [4,5,19,20,28,34,35,49,50,68, 73,75]. On the other hand, 150 manipulations were performed on the lower urinary tract (91 per cent) [1,4,9–12,14–27, 29–33,35–45,49–51,53,55,57–69, 71–78, present report]. It should be noted that, in deriving these figures, simple procedures such as prostatic massage and urethral catheterization were included as urologic manipulations. The most common lower urinary tract manipulations were cystoscopy or urethral dilatation, transurethral prostatic resection and open prostatectomy. Table V shows that the male prostate and urethra can be implicated in about 70 per cent of the patients in whom metastatic infection developed secondary to genitourinary manipulation.

TABLE V Urologic Manipulations in Patients with Metastatic Infection*

Procedure	No.
Upper Urinary Tract (15 Procedures)	
Pyelolithotomy	4
Nephrectomy	4
Drain perinephric abscess	2
Ureterolithotomy	2
Nephrostomy	1
Drain renal cyst	1
Open renal biopsy	1
Lower Urinary Tract (150 Procedures)	
Transurethral prostatic resection	32
Open prostatectomy	24
Cystoscopy	23
Urethral dilatation	22
Ureteral catheterization	13
Cystostomy	13
Prostatectomy, unspecified	4
Drainage prostatic abscess	4
Prostate message	3
Needle biopsy prostate	3
Drain periurethral abscess	2
Partial cystectomy	1
Bladder diverticulectomy	1
Cystolithotomy	1
Bladder biopsy	1
Ureteral stone extraction	1
Perineal prostatectomy	1
External urethrotomy	1

*165 procedures in 137 patients.

TABLE VI Impaired Host Defenses Noted in Patients with Metastatic Infections

Underlying Disease	No. of Examples
Diabetes mellitus	16
Malignancy	8
Cirrhosis	5
Uremia	4
Malnutrition	2
Anemia	1
Collagen disease	1

*Data base: 130 patients of whom 32 patients were found to have the 37 diagnoses listed.

The possibility that impaired host defenses against infection contributed to the development of metastatic sepsis was investigated in 130 patients in whom sufficient data were available. Of these, 32 patients (24.6 per cent) had underlying disease which may have contributed to impairment of host defenses against infection [24–26,37–41,43,48–50,54–56,58,63,67, 68,70–72,76, present report] (Table VI). A total of 37 diseases was noted in these 32 patients, with diabetes and malignancy most prominent. On the other hand, about 75 per cent of patients in whom metastatic infections developed from urinary tract sources had no detrimental systemic host factor recognized.

Skeletal Metastases. Bony structures were the most frequent site of infective metastases from urinary tract sources, being documented in 106 cases [1–41, present report] (Table VII). Osteomyelitis of the spine

TABLE VII Skeletal Metastases in Patients with Metastatic Infection

	Patients	
Metastatic Site	No.	%
Spine	88	83
Lumbar	39	...
Thoracic	35	...
Cervical	13	...
Unspecified	1	...
Joints	14	13.2
Long bones	4	3.8

TABLE VIII Endocarditis in Patients with Metastatic Infection*

	Patients	
	No.	%
Sex distribution		
Males	41	84
Females	8	16
Prior heart disease	31/41	76
Lower urinary tract diagnosis	47/59	80
Organisms		
Gram-positive	32	65.3
Streptococcus fecalis	28	
Group B Streptococcus	2	
Staphylococcus aureus	2	
Gram-negative	17	34.7

*51 patients with 59 urologic diagnoses.

constituted the major portion of these, occurring in 88 patients (83 per cent) [2–28,33,35,36,38–40, present report]. The lower vertebrae were most frequently involved as noted by other investigators [23]. Septic arthritis occurred in 14 patients [4,23,29–31,33,37,41, present report] and osteomyelitis of long bones in four patients [1,4,32,34].

A remarkable latency period may separate the events of urinary sepsis and the onset of symptoms due to osteomyelitis. In 48 cases in which information was available, a mean latency period of 54 days was noted [23–36,38–40, present report]. The morbidity and mortality of metastatic skeletal infections were considerable. In 60 cases in which data were available, the average period from onset of disease to resolution or stabilization was in excess of seven months [3–6,10,11,13,14,16–18,20–25,27, 29–31, 34,35,37,38, 40,41, present report]; in 50 cases in which the outcome was described, there were five deaths (mortality rate of 10 per cent) [35,40, present report].

In about 80 per cent of cases of metastatic skeletal infection, the presumed focus of origin was in the lower genitourinary tract. Access to the spine by organisms via Batson's plexus may explain this observation [92]. The type of organism causing metastatic osteomyelitis or septic arthritis varied only slightly from the figures presented for all metastatic infections. For example, in reviewing 81 cases in which information was available, 68 per cent of the isolates were gram-negative bacteria [3,4,9–17,19–27,30–32,34,41, present report]. Gram-positive bacteria were largely limited to Staphylococcus aureus [1,4,11,19,20,23,24,29,33, 35,39,40].

Endocarditis. Fifty-one patients in whom bacterial endocarditis developed (Table VIII) represent the second largest group of patients with metastatic infections resulting from urinary tract sepsis [39,40,43–65]. With regard to features such as underlying debilitating disease and genitourinary tract sources of sepsis, no significant differences exist between this group and the total series of patients. The presence of prior endocardial damage predisposing to bacterial colonization was reviewed in 41 cases in which data were available [42–46,48–50,52–65]. In 31 of these cases (76 per cent), the patients had evidence of prior heart disease; in 10 cases (24 per cent), the patients [43–45,49,50,52–54] had no prior cardiac abnormality. Organisms responsible for bacterial endocarditis differed considerably from those responsible for metastatic infections in general. For example, in this group, 65 per cent of isolates were gram-positive bacteria of which Streptococcus faecalis comprised the majority (87 per cent) [42,44,49,51,52,55,64]. In assessing the mortality of this condition, five cases in which the patients were treated during the preantibiotic era, all of whom died, were omitted from review [60–64]. A case reported as part of an autopsy survey was also excluded [59]. The over-all mortality rate was 62 per cent in the 47 remaining cases.

Chest Infections. This group of eight patients included three cases of septic pulmonary emboli [69,71], two examples of lung abscess [48,72] and single episodes of infective pneumonitis [73], empyema [70] and mediastinal abscess (present report). A high incidence of underlying debilitating disease was noted in this group (five of eight patients) [48,70–72, present report]. Perhaps related to the latter feature was the remarkable mortality, as seven of the eight patients died. The unusual organisms isolated from these patients included Pseudomonas species [69,70], Bacteroides species [71], Providence species [72] and Serratia marcescens [48].

Central Nervous System Infection. Four examples of meningitis and one of subdural empyema comprised this group of five patients [63,74–77]. Two patients had underlying debilitating disease [63,76] and mortality was high (three patients died) [75–77]. Similar to the group with metastatic chest infections, unusual organisms were isolated including Pseudomonas aeruginosa [63,75], Klebsiella species [74,77] and Aerobacter aerogenes [76]. Due to anastomoses between the veins of the vertebral column and the skull, these central nervous system infections may represent the most distant metastases possible via Batson's plexus [23,92].

Eye. In four patients secondary endophthalmitis developed [65–68]. Diabetes mellitus was present in two patients [67,68]. Two of the patients died, and the other two had a permanent loss of vision in the affected eye.

Miscellaneous Infections. Five patients had miscellaneous infections secondary to genitourinary tract sepsis including three cases of subcutaneous abscess [73], one retroperitoneal abscess [78] and one prostatic abscess following drainage of a perinephric abscess [79]. Three cases involved Staphylococcus aureus [73]. There was one mortality in this group.

COMMENTS

In view of the remarkable ease with which bacteria in the genitourinary tract may enter the blood stream [93–108], it is striking that development of metastatic infections is not more common. It is a tribute to natural host defenses that only 179 reported instances of metastatic infection from the genitourinary tract were encountered in this review. In various reviews of gram-negative septicemia, a genitourinary portal of entry has been implicated in from 11 per cent to 75 per cent of the cases [109–120], most reviews citing a figure near 40 per cent. Cases of septicemia resulting from the genitourinary tract had prior urologic manipulation in 21 per cent to 90 per cent of cases [110–112,114,117,120].

Certain characteristics of metastatic infections, noted in this review, may be of importance in their pathogenesis. Anatomic considerations appear to have a significant role in the development of skeletal metastatic foci [23,92]; local host factors, such as damaged endocardium, may contribute in cases of metastatic endocarditis [53,122–126], and systemic host influences, such as debilitating disease, may be important determinants in other cases, e.g., chest infections [111–113,115,119,127,128].

Batson's vertebral plexus, receiving blood from the pelvic organs, surrounds the spine and communicates with intracranial venous sinuses at the base of the skull [23]. Thus, an anatomic pathway exists to explain the prominence of skeletal (primarily vertebral) infections metastatic from genitourinary organs (primarily lower tract). The role of Batson's plexus in the development of metastatic infections may be clarified by examining the different pathogenetic characteristics in males and females in this series (Table IX). Although urinary tract infections in general are more common in females, males constitute a decided majority of patients with metastatic infection from the septic urinary tract (86 per cent versus 14 per cent). In males, sepsis originated in a lower urinary tract organ in 75 per cent of the cases; the condition developed almost equally from upper and lower urinary tract sources in females. Finally, urologic manipulation (especially of the lower tract) much more commonly preceded the development of metastatic infection in males than in females. Pathogenetic mechanisms which may explain these observations are (1) male anatomic characteristics, such as the long urethra invested within the vascular corpus spongiosum and the abundant plexus of periprostatic veins, result in easy access to the blood stream for lower urinary tract bacteria; (2) blood from the pelvic organs may bypass both hepatic and pulmonary reticuloendothelial systems via Batson's plexus. Thus, bacterial seeding of blood from the pelvic organs which can circumvent the primary reticuloendothelial organs may be of importance in the pathogenesis of metastatic infection. This mechanism may explain the preponderance of males as well as the distinctive distribution of these lesions.

TABLE IX **Pathogenetic Characteristics in Males and Females with Metastatic Infections**

	Males		Females	
	No.	%	No.	%
Incidence of metastatic infection	149	86	24	14
Lower urinary tract source	112	75	13	52
Urologic manipulation	125	84	8	32
Lower tract manipulation	106	71	4	20

Furthermore, it is instructive to examine those patients in whom only an upper tract source of sepsis was present, e.g., a diagnosis of infection or procedure limited to the upper tract with no evidence of lower tract sepsis. There were 28 such patients in this series of which 16 could be classified as to side of lesion (Table X). Fourteen of the sixteen patients had left-sided sepsis as a source (87.5 per cent). Of these 14 patients, eight suffered metastases to skeletal structures, primarily vertebral. Of the two patients with right-sided sources, there was one case of endocarditis and one of meningitis. Anatomic dissections show that the left renal vein communicates in 70 per cent of the cases with lumbar or vertebral veins whereas the right renal vein empties directly into the vena cava [129–131]. This fact may be of importance in the pathogenesis of metastatic infection from the upper urinary tract, explaining the large proportion of metastases arising from left-sided renal sources (87.5 per cent) as well as their predilection for the vertebral column (57 per cent).

SUMMARY

An extensive review of metastatic infections resulting from urinary tract sepsis is presented, combining our experience with that in previously reported cases.

TABLE X **Metastatic Infection from Upper Urinary Tract Sepsis***

	Upper Tract Source	
Metastatic Site	Right Side	Left Side
Skeletal	0	8
Endocarditis	1	3
Ophthalmitis	0	3
Central nervous system	1	0

*Data base: 16 patients of whom 11 had procedure on side indicated and 5 had diagnosis of sepsis on side indicated.

Special attention was paid to organisms implicated in metastatic infection, site of blood stream invasion by organisms, site of metastatic infection, relationship to urologic manipulation, host susceptibility factors, and morbidity and mortality features. Osteomyelitis and endocarditis were the most common metastatic infections. The possible pathogenesis of metastatic infections is considered in the light of anatomic as well local and systemic host factors. A mechanism is proposed to explain the development as well as characteristic distribution of metastatic infection from the genitourinary tract.

REFERENCES

1. Pedersen J: A case of prostatic infection complicated by osteomyelitis. J Urol 7: 405, 1922.
2. Carson HW: Acute osteomyelitis of the spine. Br J Surg 18: 400, 1931.
3. Selig S: Bacillus proteus osteomyelitis of the spine. J Bone Joint Surg (Am) 16: 189, 1934.
4. Kretschmer JL, Ockuly EA: Osteomyelitis secondary to infection of the genitourinary tract. J Urol 34: 142, 1935.
5. Flemming C: Chronic staphylococcal osteomyelitis of the spine. Proc R Soc Med 28: 897, 1935.
6. Wilson TH: Acute osteomyelitis of atlas and axis with recovery. Proc R Soc Med 28: 902, 1935.
7. Kulowski J: Pyogenic osteomyelitis of the spine: an analysis and discussion of 102 cases. J Bone Joint Surg (Am) 18: 343, 1936.
8. Stotz: Wirbelosteomyelitis. Zentralbl Chir 65: 53, 1938.
9. Kusunoki T: Uber einen Fall Von Pyocyaneus-osteomyelitis der Wirbelstinule un Anschuluss an Pyelonephritis. Z Urol 32: 699, 1938.
10. Schein AJ: Bacillus pyocyaneus osteomyelitis of the spine. Arch Surg 41: 750, 1940.
11. Deming CL, Zaff F: Metastatic vertebral osteomyelitis complicating prostatic surgery. Trans Am Assoc Genitourin Surg 35: 287, 1943.
12. Donahue CD: Osteitis of the spine. J Urol 61: 405, 1949.
13. Hurwitz A, Albertson HA: Cervical osteomyelitis and urinary tract infection caused by Escherichia coli. N Engl J Med 243: 562, 1950.
14. Adlerman EJ, Duff J: Osteomyelitis of the cervical vertebras as a complication of urinary tract disease. JAMA 148: 283, 1952.
15. Chrichton EP, Hamman HA: Typhoid osteomyelitis of spine treated with Chloromycetin. Can Med Assoc J 69: 529, 1953.
16. Wood HLC: Some problems on the borderline of orthopaedics. Proc R Soc Med 47: 927, 1954.
17. Mussey RD: Osteomyelitis of the spine from urinary infections. Ill Med J 105: 253, 1954.
18. DeFeo E: Osteomyelitis of the spine following prostatic surgery. Radiology 62: 396, 1954.
19. Leigh TF, Kelly RP, Weens HS: Spinal osteomyelitis associated with urinary tract infections. Radiology 65: 334, 1954.
20. Henson SW, Covetry MB: Osteomyelitis of the vertebrae as the result of infection of the urinary tract. Surg Gynecol Obstet 102: 207, 1956.
21. Lame EL: Vertebral osteomyelitis following operation on the urinary tract or sigmoid. Am J Roentgenol Radium Ther Nucl Med 75: 938, 1956.
22. Liming RW, Youngs FJ: Metastatic vertebral osteomyelitis following prostatic surgery. Radiology 67: 92, 1956.
23. Henriques CQ: Osteomyelitis as a complication in urology. Br J Surg 46: 19, 1958.
24. Bruno MS, Silverberg TN, Goldstein DH: Embolic osteomyelitis of the spine as a complication of infection of the urinary tract. Am J Med 29: 865, 1960.
25. Waisbren BA: Pyogenic osteomyelitis and arthritis of the spine treated with combinations of antibiotics and gamma globulin. J Bone Joint Surg (Am) 42A: 414, 1960.
26. Stone DB, Bonfiglio M: Pyogenic vertebral osteomyelitis. Arch Intern Med 112: 491, 1963.
27. Sierra MA, Luparello FJ, Lewin JR: Vertebral osteomyelitis and urinary tract infections. Arch Intern Med 108: 196, 1961.
28. Skalkea G, Georgoulis B, Rowntree T: Vertebral osteomyelitis complicating operations of abdominal viscera. NY State J Med 67: 1323, 1967.
29. Bulmer JH: Septic arthritis of the hip in adults. J Bone Joint Surg (AM) 48B: 289, 1966.
30. Lame EL: Arthritis of the hip following urinary tract operations. Radiology 65: 194, 1955.
31. Friedenberg ZB: Osteitis pubis with involvement of the hip joint. J Bone Joint Surg (Am) 32A: 924, 1950.
32. Kormins C, Skapinker S, Kay S: Osteomyelitis of long bones caused by Friedländer's bacillus. Br J Radiol 23: 168, 1950.
33. Bedow FH, Weisl H: Skeletal infection as a complication of general surgery. Lancet 2: 743, 1961.
34. Smith AG: Hematogenous Friedländer's bacillus osteomyelitis. JAMA 195: 1060, 1966.
35. Robinson BHB, Lessof MH: Osteomyelitis of the spine. Guys Hosp Rep 110: 303, 1961.
36. Eliason O, Dunlop D: Osteomyelitis of the spine following needle biopsy of the prostate. J Urol 94: 271, 1965.
37. Atlas E, Belding ME: Serratia marcescens arthritis requiring amputation. JAMA 204: 167, 1968.
38. Stuppler SA, Kandzari SJ, Milam DF: Transrectal needle biopsy of prostate. Urology 3: 82, 1974.
39. Wiley AM, Trueta J: The vascular anatomy of the spine and its relationship to pyogenic vertebral osteomyelitis. J Bone Joint Surg (Am) 41B: 796, 1959.
40. Genster HG, Andersen MJF: Spinal osteomyelitis complicating urinary tract infection. J Urol 107: 109, 1972.
41. Yosowitz GM: Serratia arthritis of the hip. Clin Orthop 85: 122, 1972.
42. Meneely JK: Bacterial endocarditis following urethral manipulation. N Engl J Med 239: 708, 1948.
43. Merritt WA: Bacterial endocarditis as a complication of transurethral prostatic resection. J Urol 65: 100, 1951.
44. Finn JJ Jr, Kane LW: Enterococcal endocarditis as a complication of urologic instrumentation. J Urol 68: 933, 1952.
45. Wheat RP, Zucherman A, Rantz LA: Infection due to chromobacteria. Arch Intern Med 88: 461, 1951.
46. Smith AG: Endocarditis due to E. coli. N Engl J Med 243: 129, 1950.
47. Hawe AJ, Hughes MH: Bacterial endocarditis due to Chromobacterium prodigiosum. Br Med J 1: 968, 1954.
48. Harris JA, Cobbs CG: Persistent gram-negative bacteremia. Am J Surg 125: 705, 1973.
49. Lloyd-Still JD: Bacterial endocarditis and urology. Br Med J 1: 768, 1965.
50. Robertson T: Paracolon Bacillus endocarditis of the pulmonic valve secondary to infected polycystic kidneys. Arch Pathol 43: 318, 1947.
51. Harvard CWH, Garrod LP, Waterworth PM: Deaf or dead? A case of subacute bacterial endocarditis treated with penicillin and neomycin. Br Med J 1: 688, 1959.
52. Reyes MP, Palutke WA, Wylin RF: Pseudomonas endocarditis

at the Detroit Medical Center, 1969–1972. Medicine (Baltimore) 52: 173, 1973.
53. Koeing MG, Kaye D: Enterococcal endocarditis. N Engl J Med 264: 257, 1961.
54. Duma RJ, Weinberg AN, Medrek TF, et al.: Streptococcal infections. Medicine (Baltimore) 48: 87, 1969.
55. Geraci JE: The antibiotic therapy of bacterial endocarditis. Med Clin North Am 42: 1101, 1958.
56. Friedman IA, Goldin M: Paracolon endocarditis. Am J Clin Pathol 19: 840, 1949.
57. Waisbren WA, Hastings EV: Bacterial endocarditis due to Pseudomonas aeruginosa. Arch Pathol 55: 218, 1953.
58. Sussman N, Cohen I, Freund AJ: Acute Aerobacter aerogenes endocarditis complicating genitourinary tract infection. NY State J Med 50: 583, 1950.
59. McLaughlin WL, Bowler JP: The causes of death following transurethral resection of prostate. J Urol 59: 1233, 1948.
60. Duhig JV: Septicemia and acute infective endocarditis due to Bacterium coli. Med J Aust 1: 435, 1933.
61. Dickar L: Acute bacterial endocarditis due to Bacterium acid-lactici. Arch Intern Med 19: 146, 1943.
62. Fish GW, Hamd MD, Kern WF Jr: Acute bacterial endocarditis due to Pseudomonas aeruginosa. Am J Pathol 13: 212, 1937.
63. Moragues V, Hendersen WAD: Endocarditis due to Pseudomonas aeruginosa. Arch Intern Med 19: 145, 1943.
64. Skinner D, Edwards JE: Enterococcal endocarditis. N Engl J Med 226: 8, 1942.
65. Ellenburger C, Sturgill BC: Endogenous Pseudomonas panopthalmitis. Am J Ophthalmol 65: 607, 1968.
66. Levine J: Metastatic Bacillus coli panopthalmitis from calculous pyonephrosis. Arch Ophthalmol 3: 410, 1930.
67. Laffers Z, Bozsoky S: Endogenous Proteus panopthalmitis. Am J Ophthalmol 54: 83, 1962.
68. Weil UJ, Laval J, Sturman RM: Escherichia coli panopthalmitis from pyelonephritis. Arch Ophthalmol 57: 58, 1957.
69. Kline BS, Maschke AS: Three fatal cases of Bacillus pyocyaneus infection. JAMA 98: 528, 1932.
70. Stanley MM: Bacillus pyocyaneus infections. Am J Med 2: 253, 347, 1947.
71. Thompson H, Beaver DC: Bacteremia due to organisms of the genus Bacteroides. Med Clin North Am 15: 1611, 1932.
72. Solberg CO, Matsen JM: Infections with Providence bacilli. Am J Med 50: 241, 1971.
73. Hyman A, Edelman L: Medical and surgical aspects of hematogenous infections in urology. J Urol 28: 173, 1932.
74. Genert AS, Brigham WG, Hamilton RD: Bilateral subdural empyema. J Neurosurg 20: 524, 1963.
75. Slutsky W, Martin P: Pyocyaneus meningitis. JAMA 113: 1400, 1939.
76. Hough PT, Adelson L: Meningitis caused by Friedländer's bacillus or Aerobacter aerogenes. J Clin Pathol 17: 534, 1947.
77. Macky F, Morris EA: Bacillus Friedländer meningitis secondary to prostatic suppuration. N Engl Med J 42: 258, 1943.
78. James B, Evans RG, Hoeprich PD: Providence bacillus bacteremia and septicopyemia. Am J Med 45: 943, 1968.
79. Clark A: Remarks on catheter fever. Lancet 1: 161, 1884.
80. Crabtree EG: Observations on the etiology of renal infections. Lancet Clin Cincinnati 115: 96, 1916.
81. Silver CM: Pelvic bone changes following suprapubic prostatectomy. Bull Hosp Joint Dis 2: 10, 1941.
82. Tunick IS, Stone JR: Friedländer's bacillus osteomyelitis. Bull Hosp Joint Dis 2: 55, 1941.
83. Kendrick JI, Hartman JT: Infections metastatic to the vertebral column. JAMA 186: 1093, 1963.
84. Lenhartz H: Uber Die Septische Endocarditis. Munch Med Wochenschr 48: 1123, 1901.
85. Bertelsmann R, Man: Das Eindungen Bokterrin in die Blutbehn als eime Ursache des Urethralfiebers. Munch Med Wochenschr 49: 521, 1902.
86. Thayer WS: Studies on bacterial (infective) endocarditis. Johns Hopkins Hosp Rep 22: 1, 1926.
87. Blumer G: Subacute bacterial endocarditis. Medicine (Baltimore) 2: 105, 1923.
88. Middleton WS, Burke M: Streptococcus viridans endocarditis lenta; a clinicopathological analysis of experiences in the Wisconsin General Hospital. Am J Med Sci 198: 301, 1939.
89. Lichtman P, Master AM: The incidence of valvular heart disease in people over fifty and penicillin prophylaxis of bacterial endocarditis. NY State J Med 49: 1693, 1949.
90. Davies DL: Iridocyclitis of obscure origin. Trans Ophthalmol Soc UK 37: 220, 1912.
91. Brown AL: Chronic uveitis. Arch Ophthalmol 12: 730, 1934.
92. Batson OV: The function of the vertebral veins and their role in the spread of metastases. Ann Surg 112: 138, 1940.
93. Scott WW: Blood stream infections in urology. J Urol 21: 527, 1929.
94. Barrington FJF, Wright HD: Bacteremia following operations on the urethra. J Path Bact 33: 871, 1930.
95. Powers JH: Bacteremia following instrumentation of the infected urinary tract. NY State J Med 36: 323, 1936.
96. Richards JH: Bacteremia following irritation of foci of infection. JAMA 99: 1496, 1932.
97. Brown CL, Browning WH, Thompson L: Transient bacteremia following TURP. J Urol 63: 155, 1950.
98. Creevey CD, Feeney MJ: Routine use of antibiotics in transurethral prostatic resection. A clinical investigation. J Urol 71: 615, 1954.
99. Kidd EE, Burnside K: Bacteremia septicemia and intravascular hemolysis during transurethral resection of the prostate. Br J Urol 37: 551, 1965.
100. Marshall H: Bacteremia following retropubic prostatectomy. Br J Urol 33: 25, 1961.
101. Grey DN: The incidence and type of bacteremia at the time of various prostatectomy procedures. J Urol 73: 709, 1955.
102. Hewitt CB, Overholt EL, Finde RJ: Gram-negative septicemia in urology. J Urol 93: 299, 1965.
103. Mitchell JP, Slade N, Linton KB: Instrumental bacteremia and its prevention. Br J Urol 34: 454, 1962.
104. Steyn JH, Logie WJ: Bacteremia following prostatectomy. Br J Urol 34: 459, 1962.
105. Miller A, Gillespie WA, Linton KB, et al.: Postoperative infection in urology. Lancet 1: 608, 1958.
106. Ives JCJ, Brown AK, Jones WW, et al.: Bacteremia following urological surgery. Br J Surg 58: 449, 1971.
107. Last PM, Harbison PA, Marsh JA: Bacteremia after urological instrumentation. Lancet 1: 74, 1966.
108. Slade N: Bacteremia and septicemia after urological operations. Proc R Soc Med 51: 331, 1958.
109. Hodgin UC, Sanford JP: Gram-negative rod bacteremia. Am J Med 39: 952, 1965.
110. McCabe WR, Jackson G: Gram-negative bacteremia. Arch Intern Med 110: 847, 1962.
111. Spittel JA, Martin WJ, Wellman WE, et al.: Bacteremia owing to Escherichia coli. Mayo Clin Proc 29: 447, 1954.
112. Curtin JA, Petersdorf RG, Bennett K: Pseudomonas bacteremia: review of ninety-one cases. Ann Intern Med 54: 1077, 1961.
113. Fishman LS, Armstrong D: Pseudomonas aeruginosa bacteremia in patients with neoplastic disease. Cancer 30: 764, 1972.
114. Hall WH, Gold D: Shock associated with bacteremia. Arch Intern Med 96: 403, 1955.
115. Wiffert JN, Barrett FF, Kass EH: Bacteremia due to Serratia

marcescens. N Engl J Med 279: 286, 1968.
116. Marztegui JI, Beigelersen JZ, Cheng WB, et al.: Bacteremia due to gram-negative rods. N Engl J Med 272: 222, 1965.
117. Martin WJ, Spittel JA, Nichols DR, et al.: Bacteremia caused by Aerobacter aerogenes. Mayo Clin Proc 29: 541, 1954.
118. Skinner D, Keefer CS: Significance of bacteremia caused by Staphylococcus aureus. Arch Intern Med 68: 851, 1941.
119. Faber V, Jessen O, Rosendal K, et al.: Staphylococcal bacteremia. Br Med J 2: 1832, 1960.
120. Martin WJ, Spittel JA, Wellmein WE, et al.: Bacteremia owing to Pseudomonas aeruginosa: review of ten cases. Mayo Clin Proc 29: 562, 1954.
121. Sullivan NM, Suttes VL, Carter WT, et al.: Bacteremia after genitourinary tract manipulation. Bacteriologic aspect and evaluation of various blood culture systems. Appl Microbiol 23: 1101, 1972.
122. Dowling HF, Lippen M, Caldwell ER, et al.: Staphylococcal endocarditis. An analysis of twenty-five cases treated with antibiotics, together with a review of the recent literature. Medicine (Baltimore) 31: 155, 1952.
123. Geraci JE, Martin WJ: Antibiotic therapy of bacterial endocarditis. Circulation 10: 173, 1954.
124. Vogler WR, Dorney ER, Budger HA: Bacterial endocarditis. Am J Med 32: 910, 1962.
125. Pankey GA: Acute bacterial endocarditis at the University of Minnesota Hospital, 1939–1959. Am Heart J 64: 583, 1962.
126. Pankey GA: Subacute bacterial endocarditis at the University of Minnesota Hospital, 1939–1959. Ann Intern Med 55: 550, 1961.
127. Fried MA, Vort KL: The importance of underlying disease in patients with gram-negative bacteremia. Arch Intern Med 121: 145, 1968.
128. Dodson WH: Serratia marcescens septicemia. Arch Intern Med 121: 145, 1968.
129. Anson BJ, Cauldwell EW: Pararenal vascular system; study of 425 anatomical specimens. Q Bull Northwest Univ Med School 21: 320, 1947.
130. Anson BJ, Cauldwell EW, Pich JW, et al.: Anatomy of pararenal system of veins with comments on renal arteries. J Urol 60: 714, 1948.
131. Wohl GT: Vertebral metastases in renal carcinoma. Am J Roentgenol Radium Ther Nucl Med 75: 930, 1956.

The Cardiac Conduction System in Progressive Systemic Sclerosis

Clinical and Pathologic Features of 35 Patients

REN L. RIDOLFI, M.D.
BERNADINE H. BULKLEY, M.D.
GROVER M. HUTCHINS, M.D.
Baltimore, Maryland

Progressive systemic sclerosis may be associated with focal myocardial fibrosis. Electrocardiographic abnormalities including conduction block are common in progressive systemic sclerosis but whether they are due to direct destruction of the specialized conduction tissue of the heart is uncertain. The conduction systems of 35 patients with progressive systemic sclerosis were studied. Of these 35 patients, 17 (50 per cent) had myocardial fibrosis of the type seen in progressive systemic sclerosis. In 10 of the 17, it was severe. Sinus node fibrosis was present in 13 patients and was nearly as frequent in those with as in those without the progressive systemic sclerosis myocardial lesion. Overlying pericarditis may have contributed to the fibrotic changes within the sinoatrial nodes in seven of the 13 patients. The atrioventricular node and main His bundles were normal. However, fibrotic changes were found in the proximal bundle systems in six patients. In three of the six, severe myocardial progressive systemic sclerosis was present; two had focal fibrous atrophy of the left bundle, and one had complete interruption of the right bundle. In only the latter patient was this reflected in the electrocardiogram which showed a right bundle branch block. Three patients without progressive systemic sclerosis myocardial lesions also had fibrous atrophy of a portion of the proximal left bundle branch, and in one the electrocardiogram showed an isolated left anterior hemiblock. Thus, morphologic abnormalities within the conduction system in our patients are difficult to attribute to progressive systemic sclerosis per se. Furthermore, although conduction abnormalities were more frequent in patients with myocardial disease, specific conduction system disease was not the cause in most patients. As has been noted in ischemic heart disease, the conduction system appears to be relatively spared from the myocardial changes of progressive systemic sclerosis, and the high incidence of conduction disturbances in this condition may be a consequence, rather, of damage to working myocardium.

Progressive systemic sclerosis may lead to a peculiar form of myocardial fibrosis unassociated with coronary artery disease [1–7] which has been proposed to be secondary to a "Raynaud's phenomenon" of intramyocardial vessels [8]. Arrhythmias and electrocardiographic conduction disturbances are frequent [9–11], but whether these disturbances are a consequence of direct damage to the specialized

From the Departments of Pathology and Medicine, The Johns Hopkins University School of Medicine and Hospital, Baltimore, Maryland. This study was supported by Contract PN43-67-1444, Grant P17-H1,17655-01, and Training Grant 5T01 HLO 5735 with the National Institutes of Health, Public Health Service, Department of Health, Education and Welfare. Requests for reprints should be addressed to Dr. Grover M. Hutchins, Department of Pathology, The Johns Hopkins Hospital, Baltimore, Maryland 21205. Manuscript accepted January 30, 1976.

TABLE I The Conduction System in Progressive Systemic Sclerosis: Clinical and Pathologic Features of 35 Patients

	Severity of PSS Myocardial Lesion		
	Severe	Mild	Absent
Clinical			
Number of patients	10	7	18
Age range (average)	17–69 (43)	35–64 (34)	25–74 (43)
Men:women	5:5	3:4	4:14
Congestive heart failure	5 (50%)	3 (43%)	8 (44%)
Systemic hypertension	1 (10%)	4 (57%)	13 (72%)
Electrocardiogram			
Left anterior hemiblock	0	0	1 (6%)
Left bundle branch block	0	1 (14%)	0
Right bundle branch block	3 (30%)	1 (14%)	3 (17%)
Complete heart block	1 (10%)	0	0
Left ventricular hypertrophy	1 (10%)	1 (14%)	4 (22%)
Right ventricular hypertrophy	1 (10%)	0	2 (11%)
Premature atrial contractions	0	0	3 (17%)
Premature ventricular contractions	4 (40%)	0	2 (11%)
1st degree heart block plus left anterior hemiblock	0 (0)	2 (29%)	1 (6%)
Nonspecific ST-T wave changes	5 (50%)	2 (29%)	3 (17%)
Normal	0	1 (14%)	2 (11%)
Conduction system pathology			
Sinoatrial node fibrosis	4 (40%)	3 (43%)	6 (33%)
Mild	3 (30%)	2 (29%)	5 (26%)
Severe	1 (10%)	1 (14%)	1 (6%)
Bundle branch fibrosis			
Left	2 (20%)	0	3 (17%)
Right	1 (10%)	0	0

cardiac conducting tissues [12,13] is unclear. Clinical and pathologic features of 35 patients with progressive systemic sclerosis from the autopsy files of The Johns Hopkins Hospital were reviewed, and their conduction systems studied in detail.

Pathologic changes within the cardiac conducting system were infrequent, despite the presence of focal myocardial contraction band necrosis and fibrosis elsewhere in the heart, and rarely accounted for rhythm and conduction abnormalities.

MATERIALS AND METHODS

The records of all patients with progressive systemic sclerosis in the autopsy files of The Johns Hopkins Hospital were reviewed. There was a total of 52 cases in which a clinical diagnosis of progressive systemic sclerosis had been made, with pathologic confirmation. In 35 of the 52 cases, specialized conducting tissues of the heart were available for study. In all cases clinical histories were reviewed, the gross hearts examined and histologic sections from atrial and ventricular myocardium studied. Twelve hearts had been examined after postmortem angiography and fixation in distention [14], and they were also studied by micro-angiographic technic.

In 31 of 35 hearts the atrioventricular node and bundle branch networks were removed in a single block [14]. The blocks were serially sectioned at 8 μ intervals and every fifteenth section was retained; two of every three retained sections were stained with hematoxylin and eosin or aldehyde fuchsin-elastic stain, respectively, and every third section was stained as indicated with either Verhoeff-Van Gieson elastic, Masson's trichrome or phosphotungstic acid-hematoxylin stain. In 32 of 35 hearts the sinoatrial node was present and was removed in a single block as described by Hudson [15], and further sectioned as previously described herein.

RESULTS

Clinical Findings. Clinical and pathologic findings are summarized in Table I. The 35 patients ranged in age from 17 to 74 years (average 44 years); 12 were male and 23 were female. There were changes consistent with progressive systemic sclerosis involvement of the skin in all patients. Nineteen patients had known hypertension and 19 were in some degree of clinically evident congestive heart failure. Electrocardiographic abnormalities included right axis deviation in eight patients, right bundle branch block in seven patients, left anterior hemiblock in four, left ventricular hypertrophy in six and right ventricular hypertrophy in three patients. Complete heart block was present in one patient. Five of seven patients with right bundle branch block were in congestive heart failure, and four of the seven had myocardial scarring (Table I). Six patients had documented premature ventricular contractions; four of whom had progressive systemic sclerosis type myocardial lesions. Three patients had premature atrial contractions.

Morphologic Findings. Of the 35 patients, 17 had moderate to severe patchy scarring and focal necroses of the progressive systemic sclerosis type unassociated with extramural coronary artery disease [8]. Fifteen hearts had an associated fibrous or fibrinous pericarditis. Eleven of these 15 patients had severe renal disease or were uremic during life; one had a severe constrictive pericarditis unassociated with renal disease.

Thirteen of 32 sinoatrial nodes showed fibrotic changes. The fibrosis was mild in six, moderate in four and marked in three (see Figure 1). These fibrotic changes were associated with an overlying pericarditis in seven of the 13 patients. In all patients the artery to the sinoatrial node and its approaches were normal. Mild fibrotic changes were unassociated with corresponding electrocardiographic abnormalities.

The atrioventricular nodes, main His bundles and small intramyocardial coronary branches directly serving these structures were free of pathologic change in all 31 patients examined (Figure 2). Abnormalities within the *distal* bundle branch systems, however, were present in six patients. Five had idiopathic atrophy and fibrosis of the proximal left bundle branch network. In two, these changes were severe and in three, mild to moderate in degree. In a sixth patient, there was interruption of the proximal right bundle by fibrosis (Figure 3). Despite the fibrosis, small intramyocardial vessels were unremarkable in these regions of the conduction network. Bundle branch fibrosis was associated with severe progressive systemic sclerosis myocardial lesions in three patients, and with no myocardial lesions in three.

Extramural coronary arteriosclerosis was minimal in all but three patients, in whom moderate to severe changes were present. Pathologic changes within smaller intramyocardial branches were negligible in all. The three patients with significant epicardial coronary artery disease did not show myocardial lesions of the progressive systemic sclerosis type, and except for mild fibrosis of the sinoatrial node in one case, these patients did not have conduction system lesions. Thus, morphologic changes in the coronary arterial tree did not correlate with clinical or pathologic disturbances of the conduction system.

COMMENTS

Findings from this study indicate that focal fibrotic changes may be present within the sinoatrial node or proximal portions of the bundle branch systems but that they are unrelated to the presence of progressive systemic sclerosis type myocardial fibrosis, and that they are infrequently of clinical significance. In 13 of 32 sinoatrial nodes there was some degree of fibrotic replacement of node tissue, but in only three were these changes severe, and in no instance was a documented electrocardiographic abnormality attributable to these changes. Sinus node fibrosis was associated with an overlying uremic pericarditis in eight nodes; this has been implicated as a cause of nodal fibrosis [16,17]. In all nodes examined the vessels distributing to these specialized structures were patent.

The atrioventricular node and distal conducting tissues were abnormal in six patients, and in two of them there was a corresponding electrocardiographic conducting disturbance. One patient had idiopathic atrophy and fibrosis of the proximal left bundle and associated left anterior hemiblock but no other areas of scarring or abnormality in the heart. The second patient had fibrous obliteration of the proximal right bundle associated with severe progressive systemic sclerosis type scarring throughout the myocardium, and the electrocardiogram showed right bundle branch block. In the other four patients with idiopathic atrophy and fibrosis of the proximal left bundle branches, in only one of whom the changes were severe, the electrocardiograms were normal. Idiopathic bundle branch fibrosis is a well recognized but poorly understood entity [18–21], and in these patients did not appear to bear any direct relationship to their underlying progressive systemic sclerosis.

Electrocardiographic evidence of bundle branch block was as often *unassociated* with morphologic changes in the conduction system: three patients had left anterior hemiblock, and six had right bundle branch block and normal conduction tissue morphologically. Associated severe pulmonary disease may have accounted for the right bundle branch block in at least five of the six patients.

Few studies of the conducting system in progressive systemic sclerosis have been undertaken. James [13] examined the cardiac conducting systems in eight patients with progressive systemic sclerosis and described sclerotic changes particularly in the sinoatrial nodes and, to a lesser degree, in the His-bundle portions of the conduction system. Lev [12] described a single patient with scleroderma and complete heart block, and noted both focal scarring and degenerative fibroelastotic changes within the conducting tissues. One patient in our series had permanent complete heart block; fibrotic changes were present in the sinoatrial node but the atrioventricular conduction tissue was intact. Myocardial scarring was clearly responsible for disruption of the conduction system leading to electrocardiographic conduction disturbances in one of our patients, and in that patient extensive myocardial scarring caused right bundle branch block. Of the other five patients with mild fibrotic changes in the bundle systems, two had scarring elsewhere in the heart suggestive of progressive sys-

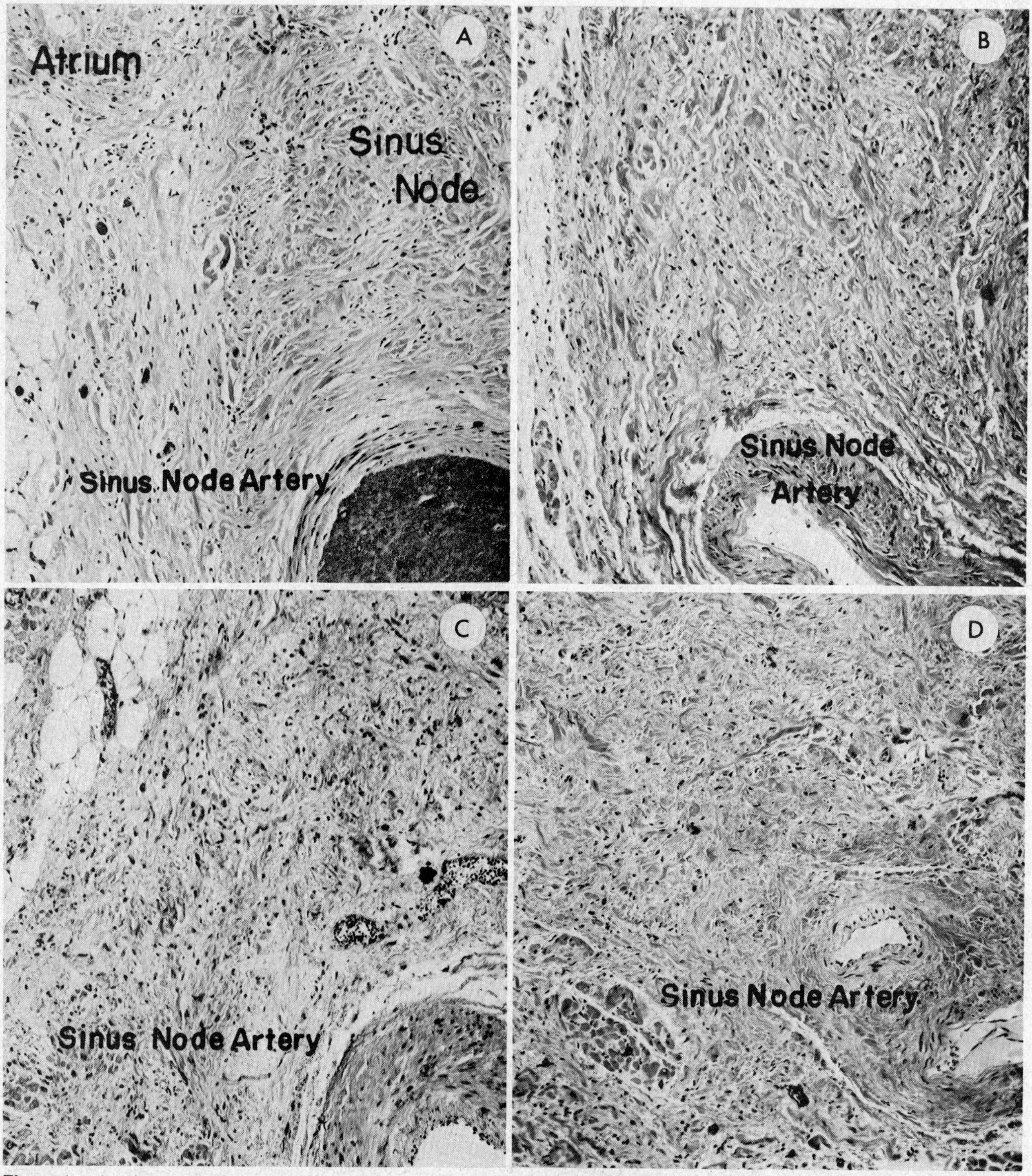

Figure 1. ***A,*** *normal sinoatrial node from a patient with scleroderma. Nodal fibers are seen above the sinus node artery which is filled with dark staining injection mass in the lower right. Normal atrial myocardium is seen at the left.* ***B,*** *mildly fibrotic sinoatrial node with sinus node artery below. There is mild replacement of nodal fibers by fibrous tissue. Electrocardiogram showed no abnormality.* ***C,*** *portion of sinoatrial node with moderate fibrosis. Electrocardiogram was normal.* ***D,*** *severely fibrotic sinoatrial node with patent sinus node artery at the lower right. There is prominent fibrous replacement with only scattered residual nodal fibers. Electrocardiogram showed left anterior hemiblock but no atrial rhythm abnormality. All hematoxylin and eosin stain; original magnification × 90, reduced by 5 per cent.*

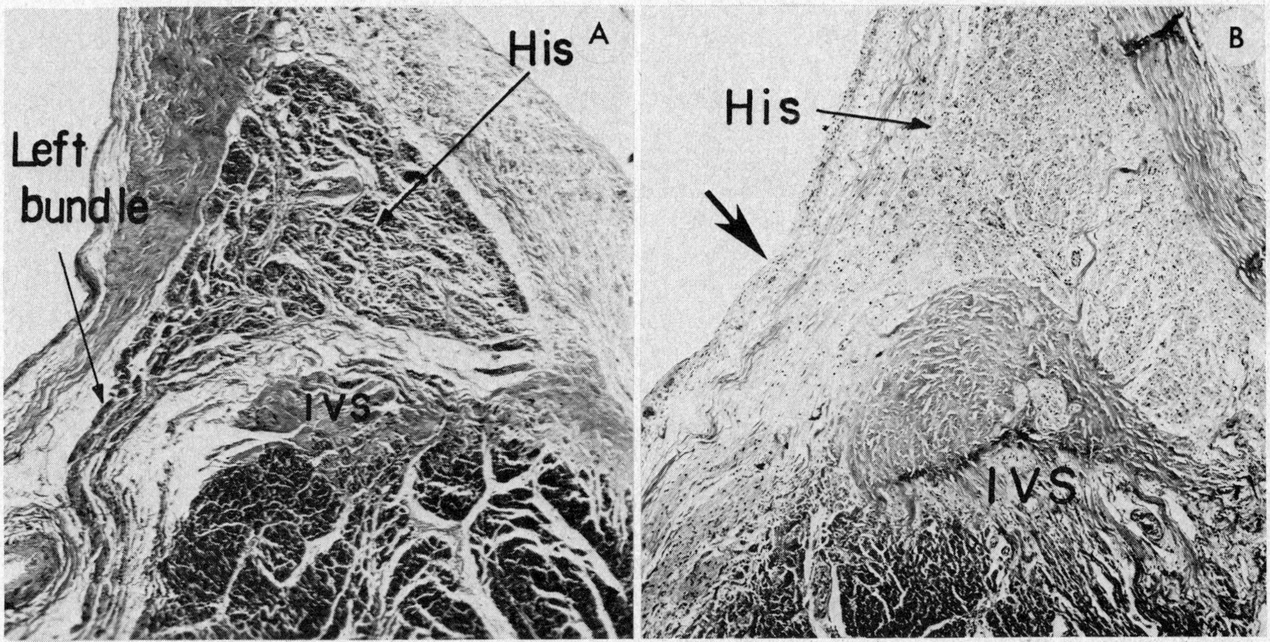

Figure 2. ***A,*** *histologic section through high ventricular septum showing normal portion of His bundle (center) and proximal left bundle branch on the left.* ***B,*** *similar section in another patient with scleroderma showing His bundle and idiopathic atrophy and fibrosis of the proximal left bundle branch* ***(arrow).*** *The distal fibers of the left bundle were intact. Electrocardiogram showed first degree heart block and left anterior hemiblock. IVS = interventricular septum. Hematoxylin and eosin stain; original magnification ×45, reduced by 5 per cent*

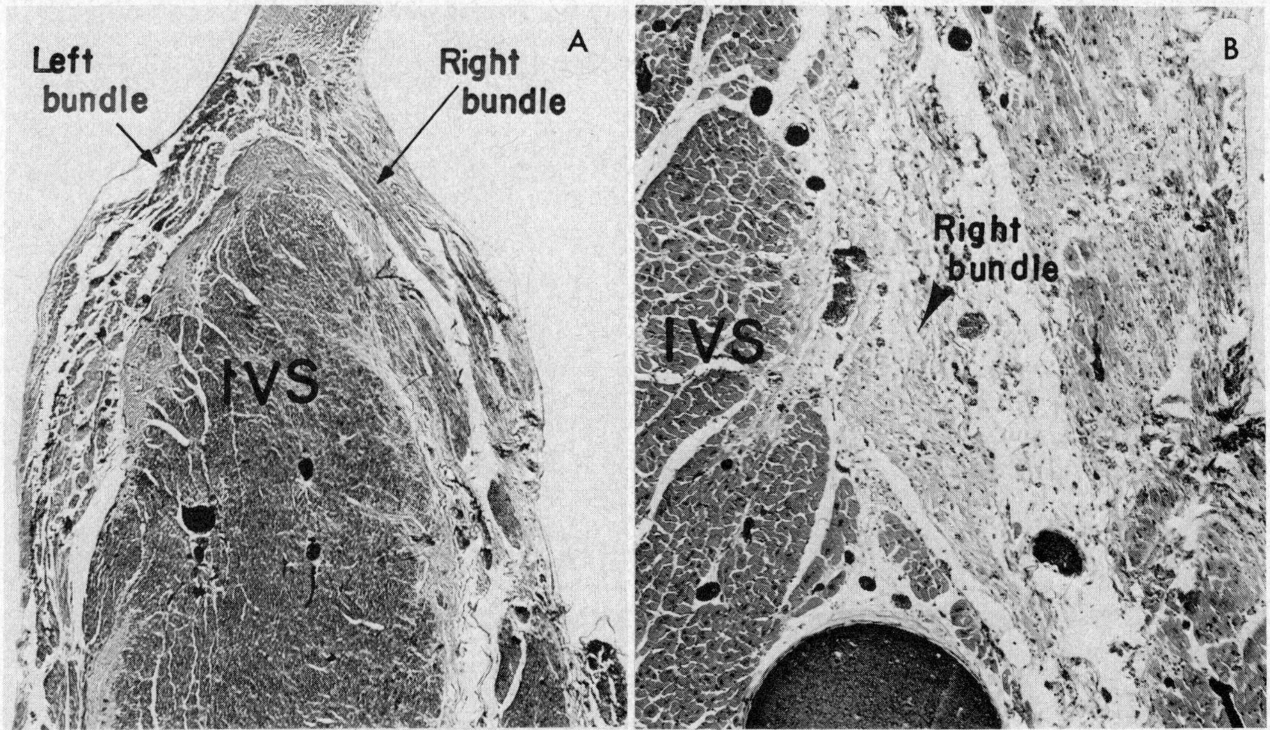

Figure 3. ***A,*** *histologic section through the anterior portion of the conduction system in a patient with scleroderma and severe myocardial fibrosis. Anterior fascicles of the proximal left bundle are seen subendocardially on the left and the proximal portion of the right bundle on the right. Note the focal myocardial fibrosis, particularly in the subendocardial region near the right bundle.* ***B,*** *subendocardial region in the same case several step-sections away from that seen at left. The right bundle branch was traced into the region of fibrosis seen centrally. Electrocardiogram showed right bundle branch block. IVS = interventricular septum. Hematoxylin and eosin stain; original magnification ×30* ***(A)*** *and ×60* ***(B),*** *reduced by 5 per cent.*

temic sclerosis type change and three did not. Thus, focal fibrotic changes within the sinoatrial nodes and bundle systems were generally present with equal frequency in the groups of patients with and without scleroderma heart disease. Although progressive systemic sclerosis scarring may be extensive, interruption of the specialized conduction tissue was present in only one of our 10 patients with severe generalized myocardial fibrosis. Despite the greater frequency of electrocardiographic abnormalities in patients with progressive systemic sclerosis heart disease, conduction system disease per se was rarely the cause. The majority of conduction disturbances present in this latter group with severe progressive systemic sclerosis myocardial disease appear to be a consequence of damaged myocardium rather than a specific damage to the proximal portion of the specialized conduction tissue.

In a recent study [8] the focal replacement fibrosis characteristic of progressive systemic sclerosis heart disease was shown to evolve from foci of contraction band necrosis. In the absence of demonstrable morphologic changes in intramyocardial vessels it was suggested that the focal contraction band necrosis was caused by an intermittent spasm (Raynaud's phenomenon) of the supplying vessels. The idea is supported by the demonstration that contraction band necrosis is the characteristic injury found following reperfusion of transiently unperfused myocardium [22,23]. In the present study the conduction tissue of the heart was relatively spared of injury by the progressive systemic sclerosis disease process when compared to changes noted within the working myocardium. The relative rarity of injury in the specialized conduction tissue in the heart with severe progressive systemic sclerosis lesions may be similar to the sparing of these tissues noted in patients with ischemic heart disease [18]. Compared to the working myocardium, the specialized conduction tissue of the heart appears to be less sensitive to ischemic injury; this may account for the relatively infrequent involvement of the specialized conduction of the heart by the sclerodermatous process.

REFERENCES

1. East T, Oram S: The heart in scleroderma. Br Heart J 9: 167, 1947.
2. Barritt DW, O'Brien W: Heart disease in scleroderma. Br Heart J 14: 421, 1952.
3. Conner PK, Bashour FA: Cardiopulmonary changes in scleroderma. A physiologic study. Am Heart J 61: 494, 1961.
4. Sackner MA, Heinz ER, Steinberg AJ: The heart in scleroderma. Am J Cardiol 17: 542, 1966.
5. Weiss S, Stead EA Jr, Warren JV, Bailey OT: Scleroderma heart disease with a consideration of certain other visceral manifestations of scleroderma. Arch Intern Med 71: 749, 1943.
6. D'Angelo WA, Fries JF, Masi AT, Shulman LE: Pathologic observations in systemic sclerosis (scleroderma). A study of 58 autopsy cases and 58 matched controls. Am J Med 46: 428, 1968.
7. Hurly J, Coe J, Weber L: Scleroderma heart disease. Am Heart J 42: 758, 1951.
8. Bulkley BH, Ridolfi RL, Salyer WR, Hutchins GM: Myocardial lesions of progressive systemic sclerosis. A cause of cardiac dysfunction. Circulation 53: 483, 1976.
9. Escudero J, McDevitt E: The electrocardiogram in scleroderma. Am Heart J 56: 846, 1958.
10. Windesheim JH, Parkin TW: Electrocardiograms of 90 patients with acrosclerosis and progressive diffuse sclerosis (scleroderma). Circulation 17: 874, 1958.
11. Barr IM, Abramov A, Dreyfuss F, Yahini JH, Neufeld HN: Progressive heart block in a case of scleroderma. Isr J Med Sci 6: 373, 1970.
12. Lev M, Landowne M, Matchar JC, Wagner JA: Systemic scleroderma with complete heart block. Report of a case with comprehensive study of the conducting system. Am Heart J 72: 13, 1966.
13. James TN: De subitaneis mortibus. VIII. Coronary arteries and conduction system in scleroderma heart disease. Circulation 50: 844, 1974.
14. Hutchins GM, Anaya OA: Measurements of cardiac size, chamber volumes and valve orifices at autopsy. Johns Hopkins Med J 133: 96, 1973.
15. Hudson REB: The human pacemaker and its pathology. Br Heart J 22: 153, 1960.
16. James TN: Pericarditis and the sinus node. Arch Intern Med 110: 305, 1962.
17. Terman DS, Alfrey AC, Hammond WS, Donndelinger T, Ogden DA, Holmes JH: Cardiac calcification in uremia. A clinical biochemical and pathologic study. Am J Med 50: 744, 1971.
18. Davies MJ: Pathology of Conducting Tissue of the Heart, London, Butterworth & Co., 1971.
19. Harris A, Davies M, Redwood D, Leatham A, Siddons H: Aetiology of chronic heart block. A clinicopathological correlation in 65 cases. Br Heart J 31: 206, 1969.
20. Lev M, Unger PN, Rosen KM, Bharati S: The anatomic substrate of complete left bundle branch block. Circulation 50: 479, 1974.
21. Lenègre J: Les blocs auriculo-ventriculaires complets chroniques. Étude des causes et des lésions à propos de 37 cas. Malattie Cardiovascolari 3: 311, 1962.
22. Jennings RB, Sommers HM, Herdson PB, Kaltenbach JP: Ischemic injury of myocardium. Ann NY Acad Sci 156: 61, 1969.
23. Reichenbach DC, Benditt EP: Myofibrillar degeneration. A response of the myocardial cell to injury. Arch Pathol 85: 189, 1968.

Jaundice in Pregnancy—1976

R. THOMAS HOLZBACH, M.D.
Cleveland, Ohio

An integrative survey is given of three disease processes, in which recent progress of a fundamental nature has been made, primarily affecting the liver, either coincident with or caused by the gravid state. The three conditions considered include (1) recurrent cholestasis of pregnancy (RCP), (2) viral hepatitis coincident with pregnancy, and (3) acute fatty liver of pregnancy (AFLP). In addition to an assessment of our present knowledge with respect to RCP and AFLP, new genetic hypotheses are proposed. In the latter, the proposal of an ornithine transcarbamylase deficiency, similar to that seen in Reye's syndrome, has potential therapeutic implications that are explored. In light of the currently available information on the interaction between maternal viral hepatitis and the variant forms of vertical maternal-fetal transmission, tentative recommendations regarding management of the newborn are suggested.

The purpose of this survey is to present a highly selective overview of three disease entities that account for the vast majority of instances of jaundice associated with pregnancy. The criteria for selection, besides frequency of occurrence include (1) fundamental biologic importance by reason of broader pathophysiologic or epidemiologic implications, (2) impact of the underlying disease process upon the liver as the primary target organ, and (3) steady progress in understanding the processes involved, as a result of continued investigation. A survey of recently published work indicates that three conditions fulfill these criteria: (1) recurrent cholestasis of pregnancy, (2) viral hepatitis coincident with pregnancy, and (3) acute fatty liver of pregnancy. Within this limited scope and perspective, main emphasis will be placed on an extensive body of biologically important and clinically useful information which has been accumulating. Except for landmark observations, previous reviews [1,2] of the subject have obviated the need to include all published work of the past 20 years.

PHYSIOLOGIC ALTERATIONS IN HEPATIC FUNCTION DURING PREGNANCY

Although biochemical alterations occur in association with pregnancy [1], it is not known whether these changes predispose to an increased susceptibility to hepatic disease. Such changes include increases in specific binding proteins for multiple hormones, e.g., transcortin, thyroxine-binding globulin and testosterone-binding protein, concomitant with decreased levels of haptoglobin and albu-

From the Gastrointestinal Research Unit, Department of Gastroenterology, The Cleveland Clinic Foundation, 9500 Euclid Avenue, Cleveland, Ohio 44106. This study was supported in part by U.S. Public Health Service Grant AM 17562. Requests for reprints should be addressed to Dr. R. Thomas Holzbach. Manuscript accepted November 18, 1975.

min. In contrast, total globulin concentration can increase by as much as 1 g during gestation. The cause, pattern and significance of these changes are poorly understood and in many cases, may not be due to a definable hepatic alteration. Also, of the many functional changes in liver-specific metabolism peculiar to pregnancy, none have any known relevance to an increased risk or propensity to viral hepatitis or acute fatty liver of pregnancy.

The clinical form of this latter disorder appears dependent upon the interaction of undernutrition and exposure to certain potentiating drugs which inhibit lipid transport or mobilization or both. In any case, the physiologic determinants inducing deviations from the nongravid state seem to be attributable to two factors: (1) exposure to sustained high levels of endogenous gonadal and placentally-derived steroids, and (2) increased metabolic activity of the maternal liver when the fetus enlarges to an appreciable size, related to the known fact that the fetal liver is considerably less than a mature functioning unit until several weeks postpartum.

In contrast to the foregoing, one aspect of liver function consistently altered in late pregnancy has attracted considerable attention because of its probable relevance to the syndrome of recurrent cholestasis of pregnancy. This refers to a clinically covert, mild form of bile secretory impairment manifest as a transient, reduced ability to clear at a normal rate, certain infused anions exemplified by sulfobromophthalein sodium (BSP) when the maximal clearance threshold is challenged [3,4]. Although significant hyperbilirubinemia is not seen in normal pregnancy, despite the fact that its clearance pathway appears identical to that for BSP, such impaired clearance can be considered a mild form of "functional" cholestasis without detectable morphologic or histologic features. The explanation for the secretory or clearance alteration has been attributed through several lines of direct and circumstantial evidence to raised levels of circulating endogenous gonadal and placental hormones.

RECURRENT CHOLESTASIS OF PREGNANCY

In normal pregnant women, alterations of liver function occur, which are similar qualitatively to those observed in patients with recurrent jaundice of pregnancy and its clinical and biochemical [5,6] formé fruste, pruritis gravidarum. In general, it seems reasonable to consider that recurrent jaundice of pregnancy results from an exaggeration of "physiologic" alterations in liver function, as suggested by Adlercreutz and associates [7–9]. The clinical syndrome, biochemical abnormalities and histologic picture show the typical features of intrahepatic cholestasis classically related to the administration of certain anabolic steroids, especially 17-alpha alkyl-substituted ones, recognized soon after these were first introduced for clinical therapeutic use, and subsequently systematically evaluated [10–14]. In accordance with this view, the features typically occur in the third trimester of pregnancy, although in 20 to 30 per cent of the cases it is believed that the earliest symptoms (e.g., pruritis) appear as early as the late first trimester or in mid-gestation [15,16]. Occasionally, patients predisposed to this syndrome even have the same milder clinical analog of transient generalized pruritis intramenstrually, usually on a predictable regular basis. Pruritis gravidarum, unassociated with clinical jaundice, is now widely accepted as merely a mild analog of the recurrent cholestasis of pregnancy syndrome for three reasons: (1) usual confinement to late pregnancy with puerperal subsidence, (2) severe generalized pruritis is the most distressing symptom of the cholestatic jaundice syndrome in pregnancy, and (3) patients with known susceptibility to cholestatic jaundice in one pregnancy may have this milder clinical picture in a subsequent or an antecedent pregnancy. In fact, one of the more puzzling aspects of the recurrent cholestasis of pregnancy syndrome is this clinical unpredictability. In successive pregnancies, for example, (1) the patient may exhibit progressively severe and earlier symptoms and biochemical manifestations, (2) the severity may be variable, (3) intervening pregnancies may be accompanied by pruritis gravidum alone, or by no manifestations of the overt cholestatic syndrome, with only the clinically inapparent "physiologic" excretory defect previously outlined as a "normal" accompaniment of late pregnancy.

For practical purposes, although this disorder is not likely of recent vintage, it was not separated from other causes of jaundice in pregnancy, notably hepatitis, until reports from Scandinavia, some 20 years ago, by Svanborg [17], Thorling [18], and Svanborg and Ohlsson [19]. This advance in recognition was made possible not only by astute clinical observation, but also by the development of the percutaneous needle liver biopsy technic. The latter permitted clinicopathologic correlations to be made for the first time in this nonfatal hepatic disorder in which information was seldom, if ever, available at autopsy.

Anabolic steroid-induced cholestatic jaundice had recently been defined with biopsy correlations, and the new pregnancy-associated syndrome emphasized by Thorling differed from hepatitis, not only histologically but also by a striking nonrandom distribution mainly in the third trimester of pregnancy. It was, therefore, a logical conjecture that the recurrent cholestasis of pregnancy form of cholestasis was produced in the susceptible patient by the known striking increase in endogenous gonadal and placentally-derived hormones characteristic of late pregnancy.

Chance prompted the next advance in defining the syndrome by verifying the steroid-induction hypothesis. Approximately 10 years after the initial identification of recurrent cholestasis of pregnancy, well into a new era of the oral administration and testing of a series of combined synthetic estrogenic and progestational hormones for contraceptive purposes, there were a series of reports of occasional instances of cholestatic jaundice associated with their use. Between 1964 and 1966 a number of reports [20–22] documented, for the first time, the now well accepted unusual sensitivity of patients with recurrent cholestasis of pregnancy to this complication. Paradoxically, the patients receiving this oral contraceptive therapy were so treated, with the well-intentioned aim of preventing pregnancy-associated recurrences of the distressing recurrent cholestasis of pregnancy syndrome. There was evidence to suggest that more than 50 per cent of the women manifesting the cholestatic syndrome associated with oral contraceptive administration had a previous history of pruritis gravidarum and/or cholestatic jaundice in earlier pregnancies [23,24]. The next obvious problem was to determine which of the two types of synthetic steroids was the more likely responsible for inducing the cholestasis process. Kreek and associates [25–27] provided data from a series of clinical challenge studies which indicated that the estrogenic component was the essential determinant. Not all prior or subsequent studies were in agreement that the progestin component was unessential [9,13,14,28–30], and some suggested a dominant role for the latter. The point is difficult to dissect with certainty [31], since as concluded by Adlercreutz and Tenhunen [9], it is highly probable that the two components act synergistically. This interaction appears to be complex for several reasons: (1) impairment of BSP disposal by 17-alpha substituted 19-norsteroids, although less potent than that associated with both natural and synthetic estrogens, may be due to their biotransformation to estrogens [32,33], especially ethinyl estradiol; (2) as a result of the ethinyl group in the 17-alpha position, the progestins may have an inherent BSP-retaining effect on the basis of a structural analogy of this component to anabolic steroids; (3) although the estrogenic compounds in general have a profound inhibiting effect on secretory mechanisms, this alone seldom seems sufficient to explain elevated transaminase levels. Some investigators have suggested [29] that the progestin component may, in fact, be the primary cause of increased serum enzyme activities; (4) estrogens may potentiate a progestin effect on serum enzymes by inhibiting the progestin component metabolizing enzyme in hepatocytes.

In addition to these difficulties, in attempting to sort out and distinguish the normal pharmacologic effects of the estrogen and progestin classes of steroidal compounds on liver metabolism, there is another complicating host factor that may further confound attempts to define the interactions of these steroids with and upon the liver. There is as yet, incomplete but suggestive evidence for a genetically determined hypersensitivity of host response to these compounds in certain sibships [20,24,34–36]. This has been invoked to explain the unusual propensity for certain patients in such sibships who have also previously experienced the recurrent cholestasis of pregnancy syndrome, to have jaundice and cholestatic symptoms when taking the oral contraceptives.

Information to suggest this has been available for the past decade, but the degree of apparent penetrance of the putative genetic gonadal steroid hypersensitivity appears small, and it remains unclear whether this would be more likely sex-linked or autosomal. Critical testing of this genetic hypothesis is obviously needed. Experimental evidence to support inferentially the genetically-determined hypersensitivity hypothesis was given by Arias [37] who showed in connection with the oral administration of contraceptives either jaundice developing in previously anicteric patients or an accentuation of preexisting hyperbilirubinemia. The patients observed in these studies, all of whom were known to have such suspected genetically-determined preexisting abnormalities as the Dubin-Johnson syndrome [38,39], the recurrent cholestasis of pregnancy syndrome and the syndrome of benign familial recurrent cholestasis [40,41], experienced new or heightened jaundice and cholestatic symptoms upon taking the oral contraceptive steroids.

Ethyl estradiol administration in animal experiments is well known to diminish not only the rate and volume of bile flow [42–46], but also the secretion rates of BSP, bilirubin, estradiol itself and its main conjugates [27,42,44] as well as taurocholate conjugation and secretion. The mechanism in most of these studies appeared to be primarily an enhancement of canalicular fluid back-diffusion from bile to plasma. Evidence favoring a more direct inhibition of secretion into the canaliculus has included an estrone-mediated reduction of bile flow in association with a diminished choleretic response to dehydrocholate infusion in treated animals [43]. Further, recent studies have emphasized the importance of this mechanism by demonstrating not only an estrogen impairment of the bile salt nondependent (BSND) fraction of canalicular water but also the prevention and partial reversal of this effect following the administration of phenobarbital [47,48], a known inducer of BSND bile flow. Thus, there is convincing evidence that at least two physiologic mechanisms may be operative in estrogen-induced impairment of bile flow.

A precise mechanistic explanation of the actual process of cholestasis is not yet available. Clearly, the recent work has been aimed more at a physiologic understanding of the process as opposed to the previous preoccupation with interpretations based solely on detailed morphologic studies [49]. The present state of work aims at a better structure-function definition of the intracellular secretory apparatus [50–59] which, at least in the case of bile acids, has definitely been shown to be the rate-limiting step in the removal process [60].

Several studies strongly suggest, compared to appropriate controls, an increased incidence and predisposition to gallstone formation in women subject to prolonged exposure to oral contraceptives or who in long-term follow-up studies have previously experienced the recurrent cholestasis of pregnancy syndrome [61–64]. At the present time, the mechanism mediating this association in either circumstance has not yet been elucidated.

VIRAL HEPATITIS AND PREGNANCY

Since the establishment of a relationship between the serologic "Australia antigen" (presently designated HBsAg = surface antigen for B virus) and acute viral hepatitis B [65–68], many uses of this immunologic marker have been made to elucidate the role of a primary viral etiology in a variety of the more chronic forms of liver disease. Another application of this technic that has been the focus of considerable attention has been the establishment of the existence of the antigen carrier state, and its biologic and clinicopathologic consequences.

In the case of these developments with relationship to pregnancy, clinical studies reported over the past 20 years have not indicated that pregnant women are especially at risk for either more frequent attacks of viral hepatitis, or to episodes of greater severity with more frequent complications. There has been no doubt that, as with most cases of viral hepatitis occurring in adults, the preponderance is properly designated B virus hepatitis, in view of the high association of HBsAg seropositivity. Special attention has therefore focused on two main areas of interest in connection with maternal-fetal relationships, otherwise termed the question of vertical transmission. These have been evaluated from the standpoint of two forms of maternal interaction with the B hepatitis virus: (1) typical maternal viral hepatitis and (2) existence of a maternal chronic carrier state without overt clinical hepatitis. The issues deal with the possibility of such fetal complications as persistent B virus antigenemia, (HBsAg), chronic and possibly severe and rapidly fatal hepatitis, milder forms of persistent neonatal hepatitis with or without cirrhosis [69–77] and fetal malformation [78,79].

The possible modes of vertical transmission have included at least four routes by which HBsAg may be transmitted from mother to infant: (1) transplacental transmission in utero; (2) transmission by blood contamination during the delivery process; (3) fecal-oral transmission in the puerperium or early postpartum period; and (4) transcolostral transmission. The clinical implications of these different routes may be of significant practical importance, in view of the fact that transplacental transmission is not preventable, whereas transmission via the other routes is preventable. Implications regarding immediate separation of mother and fetus after birth (with its obvious disadvantageous psychologic effects) would be of little benefit, if transplacental transmission were the operative or predominant route.

The earlier papers [80–85] on this subject were severely limited by insufficient numbers of mother-infant pairs and by the availability of only relatively insensitive antigen detection methods. Thus, in retrospect, the almost total lack of positive findings supporting any evidence for transmission in the earlier work is not surprising. Sweitzer's group [86–88] in Los Angeles, however, using the more sensitive radioimmunoassay method, established several major points: (1) the frequency of HBsAg transmission from mother to infant is more than 75 per cent when acute type B hepatitis occurs in the third trimester of pregnancy or early in the postpartum period; (2) conversely, when such maternal hepatitis occurs in the first two trimesters of pregnancy in their population (about 10 per cent), the incidence of transmission is comparatively low; (3) the incidence of vertical transmission by any definition, is similarly low in fetuses of mothers exhibiting the chronic asymptomatic carrier state; (4) the most common response of neonates to third trimester maternal B virus hepatitis exposure is chronic, hepatitis B, with persistent antigenemia (HBsAg), and biochemical as well as histologic features of unresolved hepatitis. Several smaller studies by independent groups have recently provided further evidence to support the findings of Schweitzer et al., that transmission of HBsAg from mother to infant occurs in association with peripartum maternal hepatitis leading to chronic fetal antigenemia with hepatitis [89–92], and that children of asymptomatic chronic HBsAg carrier mothers generally do not become infected with hepatitis B virus before or at birth, despite the known intense exposure to HBsAg from the mother.

Somewhat at variance with this are additional recent studies. One from Taiwan [93] concurred with the general consensus that virus transmission occurs nearly exclusively about the time of labor and delivery. Findings differed from the Los Angeles studies, as well and from those of several other geographic regions, in that approximately one third of the infants born on Taiwan to mothers exhibiting the chronic carrier state became persistently seropositive for HBsAg. Similar findings were recently reported from Bougainville [94]. In another study, the generally held concept that viral hepatitis in the neonate is mild, with a benign course, was challenged. It has been suggested that this possibly incorrect view was based on the premise of the dominance of the characteristic clinical features of childhood hepatitis caused by the short incubation, IH or "A" hepatitis virus (HBsAg negative), although follow-up in most series of HBsAg positive infants suggests that this may not necessarily be the case. Dupuy et al. [95] in a selected series of HBsAg-associated neonatal hepatitis patients have also shown that, with an as yet unknown frequency in such patients under the age of six months, hepatitis can be manifest in the severe or fulminant form with a high mortality. In their series, five of the affected infants appeared to derive the HBsAg from asymptomatic maternal chronic carriers. Several of the previously cited recent studies have also provided persuasive evidence for the development of severe chronic cirrhosis in childhood, in association with persistent HBs antigenemia.

In all these studies on vertical transmission, the question of frequency of transplacental transmission could never be satisfactorily resolved. In the most recent summary of Sweitzer's experience [88] with 17 HBsAg positive infants, only four could be judged to have been infected via this route based on the observation of cord blood positivity using radioimmunoassay and subsequent persistent fetal antigenemia following a transient period of fetal seronegativity. That this could represent a serious underestimate of the true incidence of the infectivity of cord blood is suggested by previous work, demonstrating unequivocally the inadequate sensitivity of *all* existing HBsAg serologic detection methods for serum possessing virus transmission capability [96]. Since transcolostral transmission was excluded in a recent large series [88], and since the frequency of transplacental transmission is probably an underestimate, a reasonable conjecture is that in approximately half the instances, the fecal-oral transmission route is responsible, and in the remaining half the infection occurs transplacentally. There are, however, no firm data to support these estimates. The difficulty of demonstrating fetal cord seropositivity, in the presence of easily demonstrable maternal HBs antigenemia, provides evidence that the placenta represents at least a partial barrier to the passage of HBsAg and the virus.

Given the obvious limitations of current information regarding the fetal consequences of maternal HBsAg hepatitis or the carrier state, the following recommendations seem reasonable: (1) the occurrence of hepatitis in the first and second trimester does not constitute reasonable justification for terminating the pregnancy; indeed, in the usual benign course of such maternal hepatitis, only routine therapeutic measures are indicated; (2) in third trimester prepartum, intrapartum, early puerperal maternal hepatitis, or the maternal chronic carrier state, the fetus, upon recognition of this state by serologic testing of all mothers at delivery and after fetal serologic testing, should at present be passively immunized with hyperimmune serum globulin, whether or not the fetus is seropositive [97,98]. Follow-up serial HBsAg measurements in the infant should be made, and in the case of seropositivity that is resistant, recurrent or of delayed onset, the passive immunity approach should be repeated. Evidence to date suggests that such passive immunization, although not completely preventive of either acute hepatitis or the chronic carrier state, is sufficiently effective that the known potential consequences of persistent seropositivity clearly justify this recommendation. Schweitzer et al. [87] have reported two cases of overt acute icteric HBsAg hepatitis that occurred within the first six months postpartum. In these instances, the illness was brief and mild, antigenemia (HBsAg) transient, and significant titers of HBsAb (antibody to HBsAg) developed after recovery. More such observations and follow-up are needed in similar situations, but this appears to represent a subgroup with a different host-agent interaction suggesting an effective role for some form of active immunization. That such will be forthcoming and available within the next several years has become virtually assured [99,100]. When available, there seems little doubt that regardless of the duration of protection that is eventually demonstrated by use of the vaccine, a superiority over the use of passive immunization in the circumstances outlined here can reasonably be expected; and in these instances, it will probably supplant the passive immunization approach.

ACUTE FATTY LIVER OF PREGNANCY

This is the least common and most lethal of the three conditions discussed here. Its actual incidence is difficult to determine, as there is a high probability that it is frequently misdiagnosed and categorized vaguely as some form or variant of "toxemia of pregnancy." This is not too surprising, because of its onset in late pregnancy and the production of multisystem manifestations. For these reasons, the available publications, probably less than 60 in the English language [101], may be unrelated to the true incidence. The clinical features have been described in detail, and are mainly characterized by third trimester jaundice in association with headache, severe nausea, abdominal pain, hematemesis, stupor, and progressive hepatic and renal failure. There is an extremely high maternal and fetal mortality, stillbirth with maternal death occurring a few days postpartum [102–106]. The liver biopsy specimen during recovery or at autopsy usually shows characteristic lesions different from that seen in hepatitis. Instead of necrosis and fibrosis, there is no loss of lobular structure, but instead a nearly panlobular with centrilobular dominance of microvacuolar fatty infiltration of the cytosol which, in contrast to the large fatty cysts in the hepatocyte associated with alcoholic toxicity, leaves undisturbed the central position of the nucleus.

The similarity between the histologic lesions produced and those associated with tetracycline and related antibiotic compounds has long been noted [107–110]. In fact, a potentiating effect has been suggested by more than one series of observations in which the use of tetracycline was prompted by the identification of a septic problem, often pyelonephritis, in a previously somewhat undernourished gravid woman [111–113]. Since tetracycline or related compounds had previously been shown by fluorescence microscopy to localize primarily in mitochondria [114], and also since tetracycline has been demonstrated to impair activity of mitochondrial oxidative phosphorylating enzymes [115], this was initially believed its primary mode of hepatotoxicity. Such explanations, however, failed to explain the almost unique propensity of this form of hepatotoxin (with the exception of alcohol), to produce extensive and rapid, widespread intracellular fat accumulation. Other major hepatoxic drug effects are primarily manifest by cholestasis or hepatocyte necrosis similar to viral hepatitis. The mode of action of the necrosis-producing class of drugs is primarily a consequence of covalent binding of an activated metabolite to intracellular macromolecules, exemplified by compounds such as acetaminophen, furosemide and the isoniazid cogeners as recently summarized by Daly and co-workers [116] and by Mitchell and Jollows [117]. Since fatty liver does not play a prominent role in drugs with this form of hepatotoxicity, unlike that of tetracycline, the applicability of these new concepts to the clinical syndrome constituting acute fatty liver of pregnancy seems unlikely.

There have been two recent developments which may begin to shed some light on this heretofore enigmatic, and virtually untreatable disease. The histologic lesions and clinical picture of acute fatty liver of pregnancy have been observed to show a striking similarity to those seen in Reye's syndrome, a condition virtually exclusively confined to children. Recent work has identified a new inborn error of metabolism, ornithine transcarbamylase deficiency—highly lethal in male neonates [118,119]. This genetic condition features, among other characteristics, encephalopathy, severe acidosis and hyperuricemia—all likewise characteristic of Reye's syndrome, with the exception of chronic protein intolerance in the genetic disorder. Thaler and associates [120,121] have recently provided direct evidence of a previously unrecognized, protein tolerant variant of ornithine-transcarbamylase deficiency affecting both sexes in association with Reye's syndrome. According to this concept, accumulation of fat in hepatocytes and elsewhere, primarily in the form of triglycerides, in the smooth endoplasmic reticulum is explained by accumulation of orotic acid consequent to the urea cycle enzyme disturbance. Orotic acid-induced fatty liver has long been recognized [122] and there is presumptive evidence that the associated striking accumulation of triglyceride is caused by defective protein, and hence lipoprotein synthesis, producing impaired lipid mobilization or transport [123]. Further evidence for a genetic enzymatic effect in Reye's syndrome arises from its identification in siblings [121].

In any case, the similarities, besides the previously indicated clinicopathologic features between Reye's syndrome and the acute fatty liver of pregnancy include (1) sudden onset in a previously well subject; (2) precipitation by external (infection) or metabolic (pregnancy) stress in association with at least short-term undernutrition; and (3) the triad of hepatic and renal failure with encephalopathy manifested by stupor and high mortality. The suggested role of either a genetically covert or an acute urea cycle enzyme deficiency in Reye's syndrome is recent. But already available is persuasive albeit preliminary biochemical evidence to support the postulate [124]. Recent and isolated reports of moderate therapeutic success by parenteral infusion of ornithine or citrulline in Reye's syndrome also support the validity of these observations [120,124]. Critical testing of the hypothesis for the analogy offered here between Reye's syndrome and the acute fatty liver of pregnancy is needed in the form of biochemical measurements in identified cases, for the presence of high levels of serum orotic acid, serum ammonia and from assays of hepatic tissue of the postulated deficient enzymes, especially of ornithine transcarbamylase [120]. In addition, therapeutic trials of parenterally administered ornithine or citrulline in the acute fatty liver of pregnancy seem warranted. Acute fatty liver of pregnancy is known to be usually severe, with a mortality rate estimated as high as 75 per cent, but the true figure may be considerably lower. The only therapy shown to have any reasonable certainty of effect is early termination of pregnancy. If the postulated metabolic defect can be corrected and the patient's nutritional state improved, perhaps this extreme measure would not necessarily be perceived as compulsory for maternal salvage.

Briefly, the other phenomenon recently observed with acute fatty liver of pregnancy is an association with disseminated intravascular coagulation which, although probably secondary, may explain some of the diverse clinical manifestations, including the high incidence of gastrointestinal hemorrhage and the deposition of fibrin in renal glomeruli leading to anuria. Two recent reports have documented this complication [125,126] which, in all future cases when present, should be identified and treated appropriately [127]. In view of the present lack of therapeutic options, this integrative summary may prove useful by presenting some new approaches, which could lead to improved maternal and fetal survival.

REFERENCES

1. Song C, Rifkind AB, Gillette PN, Kappas A: Hormones and the liver. The effect of estrogens, progestins and pregnancy on hepatic function. Am J Obstet Gynecol 105: 813, 1969.
2. Iber FL: Jaundice in pregnancy—a review. Am J Obstet Gynecol 91: 725, 1965.
3. Combes B, Shibata H, Adams R, Mitchell BD, Trammel V: Alterations in sulfobromophthalein sodium removal mechanisms from blood during normal pregnancy. J Clin Invest 42: 1431, 1963.
4. Kater RMH, Harrison DD, Mistilis SP: Alterations in sulfobromophthalein sodium removal from blood in patients with pruritis of pregnancy. Gastroenterology 53: 941, 1967.
5. Sjövall K, Sjövall J: Serum bile acid levels pregnancy with pruritis. Clin Chim Acta 13: 207, 1966.
6. Sjövall K, Sjövall J: Steroid sulfates in plasma from pregnant women with pruritis and elevated serum bile acid levels. Ann Clin Res 2: 321, 1970.
7. Adlercreutz H, Svanborg A, Ånberg Å: Recurrent jaundice in pregnancy. II. A study of estrogens and their conjugation in late pregnancy. Am J Med 42: 341, 1967.
8. Tikkanen MJ, Adlercreutz H: Recurrent jaundice in pregnancy. III. Quantitative determination of urinary estriol conjugates, including studies in pruritis gravidarum. Am J Med 54: 600, 1973.
9. Adlercreutz H, Tenhunen R: Some aspects of the interaction between natural and synthetic female sex hormones and the liver. Am J Med 49: 631, 1970.
10. Mueller MN, Kappas A: Estrogen pharmacology. I. Influence of estradiol and estriol on hepatic disposal of sulfobromophthalein (BSP) in man. J Clin Invest 43: 1905, 1964.
11. Kottra LL, Kappas A: Estrogen pharmcology. III. Effect of estradiol on plasma disappearance rate of sulfobromophthalein in man. Arch Intern Med 117: 373, 1966.
12. Gallagher TF Jr, Mueller MN, Kappas A: Estrogen pharmacology. IV. Studies on the structural basis for estrogen-induced impairment of liver function. Medicine (Baltimore) 45: 471, 1966.
13. Scherb J, Kirschner M, Arias IM: Studies of hepatic excretory function. The effect of 17-alpha-19-nortestosterone on sulfobromophthalein sodium (BSP) metabolism in man. J Clin Invest 42: 404, 1963.
14. Kleiner GJ, Dresch L, Arias IM: Studies of hepatic excretory function. II. The effect of norethynodrel and mestranol on bromosulfalein sodium metabolism in women of childbearing age. N Engl J Med 723: 420, 1965.
15. Haemmerli UP, Wyss HI: Recurrent intrahepatic cholestasis of pregnancy. Report of six cases, and review of the literature. Medicine (Baltimore) 46: 299, 1967.
16. Haemmerli UP: Jaundice during pregnancy. With special emphasis on recurrent jaundice during pregnancy and its differential diagnosis. Acta Med Scand 179 (suppl 444): 1, 1966.
17. Svanborg A: A study of recurrent jaundice in pregnancy. Acta Obstet Gynecol Scand 33: 434, 1954.
18. Thorling L: Jaundice in pregnancy. A clinical study. Acta Med Scand 302 (suppl 151): 1, 1955.
19. Svanborg A, Ohlsson S: Recurrent jaundice of pregnancy. A clinical study of twenty-two cases. Am J Med 27: 40, 1959.
20. Holzbach RT, Sanders JH: Recurrent intrahepatic cholestasis of pregnancy: observations on pathogenesis. JAMA 193: 542, 1965.
21. Boake WC, Schade SG, Morrisey JF, Schaffner F: Intrahepatic cholestatic jaundice of pregnancy followed by Enovid-induced cholestatic jaundice: report of a case. Ann Intern Med 63: 302, 1965.
22. Orrellana-alcade JM, Dominguez JP: Jaundice and oral contraceptive drugs. Lancet 2: 1278, 1966.
23. Ockner RK, Davidson CS: Hepatic effects of oral contraceptives. N Engl J Med 276: 331, 1967.
24. Kappas A: Estrogens and the liver. Gastroenterology 52: 113, 1967.
25. Kreek MJ, Weser E, Sleisenger MH, Jeffries GH: Idiopathic cholestasis of pregnancy–the response to challenge with synthetic estrogen, ethinyl estradiol. N Engl J Med 277: 1391, 1967.
26. Kreek MJ, Sleisenger MH, Jefferies GH: Recurrent cholestatic jaundice of pregnancy with demonstrated estrogen sensitivity. Am J Med 43: 795, 1967.

27. Kreek MJ: Cholestasis of pregnancy and during ethinyl estradiol administration in the human and rat. Metabolic Effects of Gonadal Hormones and Contraceptive Steroids (Salhanick HA, Kipnis DM, VandeWiele RL, eds), New York, Plenum Press, 1969, p 40.
28. Drill VA: Benign cholestatic jaundice of pregnancy and benign cholestatic jaundice from oral contraceptives. Am J Obstet Gynecol 119: 165, 1974.
29. Adlercreutz H, Eisalo A, Heino A, Luukkainen T, Penttilä I, Saukkonen H: Investigations on the effect of an oral contraceptive and its components on liver function, serum proteins, copper, ceruloplasmin and alpha-glutamyl peptidase in post-menopausal women. Scand J Gastroenterol 3: 273, 1968.
30. Delorimer AA, Gordan GS, Lowe RC, Carbone JV: Methyltestosterone, related steroids and liver function. Arch Intern Med 116: 289, 1965.
31. Urban E, Frank BW, Kern F Jr: Liver dysfunction with mestranol but not with norethynodrel in a patient with Enovid®-induced jaundice. Ann Intern Med 68: 598, 1968.
32. Marver HS, Schmidt R: Biotransformation in the liver. Implications for human disease. Gastroenterology 55: 282, 1968.
33. Paulsen CA: Progestin metabolism. Special reference to estrogenic pathways. Metabolism 14: 313, 1965.
34. Somayaji BN, Price JH, Harris AW, Flewett TH: Norethisterone jaundice in two sisters. Br Med J 2: 281, 1968.
35. Furhoff A-K, Hellstrom K: Jaundice in pregnancy. A follow-up study of the series of women originally reported by L Thorling. I. The pregnancies. Acta Med Scand 193: 259, 1973.
36. Dalen E, Westerholm B: Occurrence of hepatic impairment in women jaundiced by oral contraceptives and in their mothers and sisters. Acta Med Scand 195: 459, 1974.
37. Arias IM: Some effects of contraceptive steroids on hepatic function in normal women and in patients with acquired and inheritable defects in hepatic excretory function. Metabolic Effects of Gonadal Hormones and Contraceptive Steroids (Salhanick HA, Kipnis DM, VandeWiele RL, eds), New York, Plenum Press, 1969 p 30.
38. Dubin IN: Chronic idiopathic jaundice. Am J Med 24: 268, 1958.
39. Fleischner G, Arias IM: Recent advances in bilirubin formation, transport, metabolism and excretion. Am J Med 49: 576, 1970.
40. Summerskill WHJ: The syndrome of benign recurrent cholestasis. Am J Med 38: 298, 1965.
41. Tygstrup N, Jensen B: Intermittent intrahepatic cholestasis of unknown etiology in five young males from the Faroe Islands. Acta Med Scand 185: 523, 1969.
42. Kreek MJ, Peterson RE, Sleisenger MH, Jefferies GH: Effects of ethinyl estradiol-induced cholestasis on bile flow and biliary excretion of estradiol and estradiol glucuronide by the rat. Proc Soc Exp Biol Med 131: 646, 1969.
43. Forker EL: The effect of estrogen on bile formation in the rat. J Clin Invest 48: 654, 1969.
44. Harkavy M, Javitt NB: Effect of ethinyl estradiol on hepatic excretory function of the rat. Metabolic Effects of Gonadal Hormones and Contraceptive Steroids (Salhanick HA, Kipnis DM, VandeWiele RL, eds), New York, Plenum Press, 1969, p 11.
45. Palmer RH, Gallagher TF Jr, Mueller MN, Kappas A: The effect of natural and synthetic estrogens on the excretion of BSP by the liver. Metabolic Effects of Gonadal Hormones and Contraceptive Steroids (Salhanick HA, Kipnis DM, VandeWiele RL, eds), New York, Plenum Press, 1969, p 19.
46. Kern F Jr, Eriksson H, Sjövall J: Effect of ethinyl estradiol on conjugation of cholic acid. Gastroenterology 67: 802, 1974a.
47. Gumucio JJ, Valdivieso D: Studies on the mechanism of the ethinyl-estradiol impairment of bile flow and bile salt excretion in the rat. Gastroenterology 61: 339, 1971.
48. Gumucio JJ, Accatino L, Macho AM, Contreras A: Effect of phenobarbital on the ethinyl estradiol-induced cholestasis in the rat. Gastroenterology 65: 651, 1973.
49. Popper H: Cholestasis. Ann Rev Med 19: 39, 1968.
50. Javitt NB, Arias IM: Intrahepatic cholestasis. A functional approach to pathogenesis. Gastroenterology 53: 171, 1967.
51. Ritt DJ, Schenker S, Combes B: Taurocholic acid stimulation of apparent maximal biliary excretion of sulfobromophthalein sodium (BSP). Gastroenterology 52: 322, 1967a.
52. Javitt NB: Cholestasis in rats induced by taurolithocholate. Nature (Lond) 210: 1262, 1966.
53. Javitt NB, Emerman S: Effect of sodium taurolithocholate on bile flow and bile acid excretion. J Clin Invest 47: 1002, 1968.
54. Berthelot P, Erlanger S, Dhumeaux D, Preaux A: Mechanism of phenobarbital-induced hypercholeresis in the rat. Am J Physiol 219: 809, 1970.
55. Erlinger S, Dhumeaux D, Berthelot P, Dumont M: Effect of inhibitors of sodium transport on bile formation in the rabbit. Am J Physiol 219: 416, 1970.
56. Scherstén T, Nilsson S, Cahlin E, Filipson M, Brodin-Persson G: Relationship between the biliary excretion of bile acids and the excretion of water, lecithin, and cholesterol in man. Eur J Clin Invest 1: 242, 1971.
57. Javitt NB: The cholestatic syndrome—1971. Am J Med 51: 637, 1971.
58. Carey MC, Hirom PC, Small DM: Precipitation of bile salts by chlorpromazine; the protective effect of lecithin (abstract). Gastroenterology 66: 671, 1974.
59. Ros ER, Small DM, Carey MC: The effects of chlorpromazine hydrochloride on bile formation and biliary lipid secretion in the primate (abstract). Gastroenterology 68: 975, 1975.
60. Glasinovic J-C, Dumont M, Erlinger S: Hepatocellular uptake of taurocholate in the dog. J Clin Invest 55: 419, 1975.
61. Gallstones and estrogens (editorial). N Engl J Med 290: 51, 1974.
62. Howat JMT, Jones CB, Schonfield PF: Gallstones and oral contraceptives. J Int Med Res 3: 59, 1975.
63. Furhoff A-K: Itching in pregnancy. A fifteen year follow-up study. Acta Med Scand 196: 403, 1974.
64. Furhoff A-K, Hellström K: Jaundice in pregnancy—a follow-up study of the series of women originally reported by L. Thorling. II. Present health of the women. Acta Med Scand 196: 181, 1974.
65. Blumberg BS, Sutnick AI, London WT: Hepatitis and leukemia. Their relation to Australia antigen. Bull NY Acad Med 44: 1566, 1968.
66. Prince AM: An antigen detected in the blood during the incubation period of serum hepatitis. Proc Natl Acad Sci USA 60: 814, 1968.
67. Giles JP, McCollum RW, Berndtson LW Jr, Krugman S: Viral hepatitis. Relation to Austrialia/SH antigen to the Willowbrook MS-2 strain. N Engl J Med 281: 119, 1969.
68. Blumberg BS, Friedlander JS, Woodside A, Sutnick AI, London WT: Australia antigen and hepatitis. Autosomal recessive inheritance to infection in humans. Proc Natl Acad Sci USA 62: 1108, 1969.
69. Stokes J, Berk JE, Malamut LL, Drake ME, Barondess JA, Bashe JA, Wolman WJ, Farquhar JD, Bevan B, Drum-

mond RJ, Maycock Wd'A, Capps RB, Bennett AM: The carrier state in viral hepatitis. JAMA 154: 1059, 1954.
70. Alagille D: Clinical aspects of neonatal hepatitis. Am J Dis Child 123: 287, 1972.
71. Kattamis CA, Demetrios D, Matsanoitis NS: Australia antigen and neonatal hepatitis syndrome. Pediatrics 54: 157, 1974.
72. Chandra RK: Immunological picture in Indian childhood cirrhosis. Lancet 1: 537, 1970.
73. Chandra RK, Chawla V, Verma IC, Ghai OP, Malik GK: Hepatitis-associated antigen and depressed cellular immunity in Indian childhood cirrhosis. Am J Dis Child 123: 408, 1972.
74. Wright R, Perkins JR, Bower BD, Jerrome DW: Cirrhosis associated with the Australia antigen in an infant who acquired hepatitis from her mother. Br Med J 4: 719, 1970.
75. Gillespie A, Dorman D, Walker-Smith JA, Yu JS: Neonatal hepatitis and Australia antigen. Lancet 2: 1081, 1970.
76. Garty R, Bar-Schany S, Gordin A: Possible transplacental transmission of serum hepatitis. Lancet 2: 434, 1971.
77. Bancroft WH, Warkel RL, Talbert AA, Russell PK: Family with hepatitis-associated antigen. JAMA 217: 1817, 1971.
78. Mansell RV: Infectious hepatitis in the first trimester of pregnancy and its effect on the fetus. Am J Obstet Gynecol 69: 1136, 1955.
79. Marshall WC, Dudgeon JA; Australia antigen in a child with congenital transformations and in his mother. Am J Dis Child 123: 378, 1972.
80. London WT, Difigilia M, Rodgers J: Failure of transplacental transmission of Australia antigen. Lancet 2: 900, 1969.
81. Smithwick EM, Go SC: Hepatitis-associated antigen in cord and maternal sera. Lancet 2: 1080, 1970.
82. Sweitzer IL, Spears RL: Hepatitis-associated antigen (Australia antigen) in mother and infant. N Engl J Med 283: 570, 1970.
83. Lyons KP, Guze LB: Australia antigen associated hepatitis. Radioimmunoassay in mother and infant. JAMA 215: 981, 1971.
84. Cherubin CE: Risk of post-transfusion hepatitis in recipients of blood containing SH antigen at Harlem Hospital. Lancet 1: 627, 1971.
85. Holzbach RT: Australia antigen hepatitis in pregnancy. Evidence against transplacental transmission of Australia antigen in early and late pregnancy. Arch Intern Med 130: 234, 1972.
86. Schweitzer IL, Wing A, McPeak C, Spears RL: Hepatitis and hepatitis-associated antigen in 56 mother-infant pairs. JAMA 220: 1092, 1972.
87. Schweitzer IL, Mosley JW, Ashcavai M, Edwards VM, Overby LB: Factors influencing neonatal infection B by hepatitis B virus. Gastroenterology 65: 277, 1973.
88. Schweitzer IL, Dunn AEG, Peters RL, Spears RL: Viral hepatitis B in neonates and infants. Am J Med 55: 762, 1973.
89. Skinhøj P, Sardemann H, Cohen J, Mikkelsen M, Olesen H: Hepatitis associated antigen (HAA) in pregnant women and their newborn infants. Am J Dis Child i23: 380, 1972.
90. Skinhøj P, Olesen H, Cohen J, Mikkelsen M: Hepatitis associated antigen in pregnant women. Acta Pathol Microbiol Scand (B) 80: 362, 1972.
91. Merrill DA, Dubois RS, Kohler PF: Neonatal onset of the hepatitis-associated antigen carrier state. N Engl J Med 287: 1280, 1972.
92. Papaevangelou G, Hoofnagle J, Kremastinou J: Transplacental transmission of hepatitis B virus by symptom-free chronic carrier mothers. Lancet 2: 746, 1974.
93. Stevens CE, Beasley RP, Tsui J, Lee W-C: Vertical transmission of hepatitis B antigen in Taiwan. N Engl J Med 292: 771, 1975.
94. Muzzur S, Blumberg BS, Friedlander JS: Silent maternal transmission of Australia antigen. Nature (Lond) 247: 41, 1974.
95. Dupuy JM, Frommel D, Alagille D: Severe viral hepatitis type B in infancy. Lancet 1: 191, 1975.
96. Barker LF, Schulman NR, Murray R, Hirschman RJ, Ratner F, Diefenbach WCL, Geller HM: Transmission of serum hepatitis. JAMA 211: 1509, 1970.
97. Szmuness W, Prince AM, Goodman M, Ehrich C, Pick R, Ansari M: Hepatitis B immune serum globulin in prevention of non-parenterally transmitted hepatitis B. N Engl J Med 290: 701, 1974.
98. Kohler PF, Dubois RS, Merrill DA, Bowes WA: Prevention of chronic neonatal hepatitis B virus infection with antibody to the hepatitis B surface antigen. N Engl J Med 291: 1378, 1974.
99. Krugman S, Giles JP, Hammond J: Viral hepatitis, type B (MS-2 strain). Studies on active immunization. JAMA 217: 41, 1971.
100. Maugh TH II: Hepatitis B: A new vaccine ready for human testing. Science 188: 137, 1975.
101. Hatfield AK, Stein JH, Greenberger NJ, Abernathy RW, Ferris TF: Idiopathic acute fatty liver of pregnancy—death from extrahepatic manifestations. Am J Dig Dis 17: 167, 1972.
102. Sheehan HL: The pathology of acute yellow atrophy and delayed chloroform poisoning. J Obstet Gynaecol Br Commonw 47: 49, 1940.
103. Ober WB, Lecompte PM: Acute fatty metamorphosis of the liver associated with pregnancy. A distinctive lesion. Am J Med 19: 743, 1955.
104. Czernobilsky B, Bergnes MA: Acute fatty metamorphosis of the liver in pregnancy with associated liver cell necrosis. Obstet Gynecol 26: 792, 1965.
105. Duma RJ, Dowling EA, Alexander HC, Sibrans D, Dempsey H: Acute fatty liver of pregnancy. Report of a surviving patient studies with serial liver biopsies. Ann Intern Med 63: 851, 1965.
106. Morrin PAF, Homta SP, Valberg LS, Benscome SA, Kipke GF, Wyllie JC: Acute renal failure in association with fatty liver of pregnancy. Recovery after 14 days of complete anuria. Am J Med 42: 844, 1967.
107. Tickton HE, Robinson MM: Effects of some antimicrobial agents on the liver. Ann NY Acad Sci 104: 1080, 1963.
108. Schultz JC, Adamson JS Jr, Workman WW, Norman TD: Fatal liver disease after intravenous administration of tetracycline in high dosage. N Engl J Med 269: 999, 1963.
109. Dowling HF, Lepper MH: Hepatic reactions to tetracycline. JAMA 188: 307, 1964.
110. Wruble LD, Ladman AJ, Britt IG, Cummins AJ: Hepatotoxicity produced by tetracycline overdosage. JAMA 192: 6, 1965.
111. Whalley PJ, Adams RH, Combes B: Tetracycline toxicity in pregnancy. Liver and pancreatic dysfunction. JAMA 189: 357, 1964.
112. Kunelis CT, Peter JL, Edmondson HA: Fatty liver of pregnancy and its relationship to tetracycline therapy. Am J Med 38: 359, 1965.
113. Schiffer MA: Fatty liver associated with administration of tetracycline in pregnant and nonpregnant women. Am J Obstet Gynecol 96: 326, 1966.
114. Dubuy HG, Shownacre JL: Selective localization of tetracycline in mitochondria of liver cells. Science 133: 196, 1961.
115. VanMeter JC, Spector A, Oleson JJ, Williams JH: In vitro action of aureomycin on oxidative phosphorylation in

animal tissues. Proc Soc Exp Biol Med 81: 215, 1952.
116. Daly JW, Jerina DM, Witkop B: Arene oxides and the NIH shift. The metabolism, toxicity, and carcinogenicity of aromatic compounds. Experientia 28: 1129, 1972.
117. Mitchell JR, Jollows DJ: Metabolic activation of drugs to toxic substances. Gastroenterology 68: 392, 1975.
118. Alexander AGM, Rosenberg LE, Snodgrass PJ, Nuzum CT: Ornithine transcarbamylase deficiency—a cause of lethal neonatal hyperammonemia in males. N Engl J Med 288: 1, 1973.
119. Short EM, Conn HO, Snodgrass PJ, Campbell AGM, Rosenberg LE: Evidence for x-linked dominant inheritance of ornithine transcarbamylase deficiency. N Engl J Med 288: 7, 1973.
120. Thaler MM, Hoogenraad NJ, Boswell M: Reye's syndrome due to a novel protein tolerant variant of ornithine-transcarbamylase deficiency. Lancet 2: 438, 1974.
121. Thaler MM: Reye's syndrome. View Dig Dis 6: 3, 1974.
122. Windmiller HG: An orotic acid-induced adenine-reversed inhibition of hepatic lipoprotein secretion in man. J Biol Chem 239: 530, 1964.
123. Jatlow P, Adams WR, Handschumacher RE: Pathogenesis of orotic acid-induced fatty change in the rat liver. Am J Pathol 47: 125, 1965.
124. Snodgrass PJ, Delong GR: Ornithine transcarbamylase deficiency in Reye's syndrome. Gastroenterology 68: 1085, 1975.
125. Holzbach RT: Actue fatty liver of pregnancy with disseminated intravascular coagulation. Obstet Gynecol 43: 740, 1974.
126. Cano RI, Delman MR, Pitchumoni CS, Lev R, Rosenthal WS: Acute fatty liver of pregnancy. Complication by disseminated intravascular coagulation. JAMA 231: 159, 1975.
127. Rake MO, Shilkin KB, Winch J, Flute PT, Lewis ML, Williams R: Early and intensive therapy of intravascular coagulation in acute liver failure. Lancet 2: 1215, 1971.

American Burkitt's Lymphoma

Stenographic reports, edited by Philip E. Cryer, M.D. and John M. Kissane, M.D., of weekly clinicopathologic conferences held in Barnes and Wohl Hospitals, are published in each issue of the Journal. These conferences are participated in jointly by members of the Departments of Internal Medicine and Pathology of Washington University School of Medicine.

A 17 year old boy was admitted to Barnes Hospital on December 23, 1975, because of increasing jaundice and weight loss of four weeks' duration.

Aside from a transient episode of low back pain in mid-November, the patient was in apparent good health until late November 1975 when numbness of the lower lip and chin, pain in the right upper abdominal quadrant and nausea with episodic vomiting developed, and jaundice was noted. The serum bilirubin concentration was 5.0 mg/100 ml. HB_sAg was not demonstrable. An episode of upper gastrointestinal hemorrhage, for which he required blood transfusions, occurred in early December. An x-ray series of the upper gastrointestinal tract was reportedly within normal limits. Diplopia on left lateral gaze was noted. Abdominal pain and episodic vomiting continued, and jaundice intensified. Prednisone, 30 mg daily, was administered. A mass in the anterior portion of the neck was noted approximately two weeks prior to admission. Over the week before admission a nonproductive cough, night sweats and a low grade fever developed. The serum bilirubin concentration was 20 mg/100 ml. The patient had lost 30 pounds in weight over approximately one month.

On admission the patient was deeply icteric and appeared chronically ill. The blood pressure was 130/80 mm Hg, the pulse rate 100/minute and the temperature 37.5°C. Positive findings included a 2 cm, firm nodule in the left lobe of the thyroid and tender hepatomegaly with a 14 cm percussion span. The spleen was not palpable and there was no lymphadenopathy. Aside from a left lateral rectus palsy, the neurologic examination was within normal limits. A 1 cm nodule along the left spermatic cord was found to transilluminate; the testes were normal. The rectal examination was within normal limits and the stool quaiac was negative.

Initial laboratory data included a hemoglobin level of 10.1 g/100 ml and a hematocrit value of 28 per cent with normal red blood cell indices. Three nucleated red blood cells/100 white blood cells were seen on the peripheral smear. The white blood cell count was 7,100/mm^3 with 2 per cent basophils, 8 per cent eosinophils, 1 per cent myeloblasts, 7 per cent myelocytes, 7 per cent metamyelocytes, 16 per cent band forms, 18 per cent segmented neutrophils, 34 per cent lymphocytes and 11 per cent monocytes. The platelet count was 130,000/mm^3. The serum total bilirubin was 21.5 mg/100 ml (the direct bilirubin 9.8 mg/100 ml), the serum alkaline phosphatase 645 mIU/ml, the serum glutamic-oxaloacetic transaminase (SGOT) 84 mIU/ml, the serum cholesterol 660 mg/100 ml and the serum albumin 3.1 g/100 ml. The prothrombin time was normal. There was 4+ bilirubinuria and moderate urinary urobilinogen.

Chest films were within normal limits aside from showing a mass in the left side of the neck impinging on the trachea. The serum thyroxine concentration was 3.2 μg/100 ml. The thyroid nodule did not concentrate isotope on scans. Films of the upper gastrointestinal tract demonstrated thickened mucosal folds in the stomach and constant defects in the duodenum. Several hepatic filling defects, hepatic enlargement and mild splenic enlargement were noted on liver-spleen scans. Brain scans were within normal limits.

An operation was performed on the third hospital day.

CLINICAL DISCUSSION

Dr. Stuart Kornfeld: We are presented with a 17 year old boy who had a rapidly progressive disease involving multiple organ systems, including the gastrointestinal tract, liver, bone marrow, central nervous system and thyroid. We have evidence for the rapid appearance of a mass lesion in the thyroid, the presence of space occupying lesions in the liver and the suggestion of an infiltrative process in the bone marrow. That is, the patient had a classic leukoerythroblastic peripheral blood picture with nucleated red blood cells and a shift to the left in the white blood cell series associated with only a mild anemia. Although acute leukemia may occasionally present with this peripheral blood picture (the so-called aleukemic leukemic state), these findings are most often seen when the bone marrow is infiltrated with malignant cells. So, based on several lines of information, it is reasonable to conclude that the patient has some type of neoplastic disorder involving many organ systems.

In terms of the various neoplastic disorders which must be considered in the differential diagnosis, I think it is helpful to review the relative incidence of different cancers in teenagers. In the age group 15 to 19 years, there are four major cancers: leukemia, brain tumors, lymphomas and bone cancer. The incidence of neuroblastoma and Wilm's tumor in this age group is markedly lower than in younger patients. Of the four common tumors, we can readily rule out three. The type of acute leukemia seen in this age group is usually acute lymphoblastic leukemia in which the bone marrow is infiltrated with lymphoblasts, and almost always lymphoblasts are present in the peripheral blood. In addition, these patients usually have generalized lymphadenopathy and splenomegaly, and they often have mediastinal masses. None of these findings was present in our patient. Furthermore, although tissue infiltration with leukemic cells is very common, it would be unusual to have liver infiltration to the extent that this patient apparently has. Therefore, we can rule out acute lymphoblastic leukemia. A brain tumor or a bone tumor such as osteogenic sarcoma can be excluded on the basis of the clinical presentation. Statistically, then, we are left with a malignant lymphoma as the most likely diagnosis.

Now let us mention a few of the other tumors which, although rare in this age group, should be considered in the differential diagnosis. Wilm's tumor usually presents as a hard, defined abdominal mass of gradual onset. It metastasizes to the lungs most commonly whereas bone marrow and liver metastases are unusual. Neuroblastoma may also present with abdominal involvement, but usually with a firm, smooth, palpable defined mass. This tumor may metastasize to the bone marrow and the liver. As in Wilm's tumor, the onset tends to be gradual. Therefore, we can rule out these two tumors. Embryonal rhabdomyosarcoma of childhood most frequently arises in the head and neck region, but it may originate in the pelvis, particularly in the bladder and prostate in boys. Less frequently, in this age group, it involves the paravertebral and flank muscles, and the extremities. It may metastasize regionally, especially to lymph nodes, or distally to the lungs, the bone marrow and the bones. So, again, without evidence of bladder or prostate involvement, and with evidence of gastrointestinal tract and central nervous system involvement, this tumor becomes unlikely. About 10 to 15 per cent of childhood tumors are teratomas, but 90 per cent of these are benign. In addition, they mostly involve the gonads, although they may be retroperitoneal and occasionally involve the abdominal viscera. Usually they are asymptomatic masses that are picked up incidently, but if they involve the gastrointestinal tract, they may lead to local symptoms. Finally, the clinical picture is compatible with a highly malignant, poorly differentiated or undifferentiated carcinoma that has metastasized widely, although such a rapid course would be unusual.

Having eliminated most of the neoplasms, I would like to consider malignant lymphoma of childhood. This patient's clinical presentation is most compatible with this diagnosis; in fact, it is rather typical of childhood non-Hodgkin's lymphoma. In children, Hodgkin's disease presents very much as it does in adults, with involvement primarily of the lymph nodes and a relatively low frequency of extralymphatic involvement. Therefore, the diagnosis of Hodgkin's disease in this patient is not likely. On the other hand, non-Hodgkin's lymphoma tends to be a much more aggressive disease in children than in adults, with a higher incidence of major abdominal and extranodal involvement at the time of initial presentation. For example, in a series of 405 adult patients with various types of non-Hodgkin's lymphoma studied at Stanford [1], more than 98 per cent had lymph node involvement. That is, only six of 405 patients presented with involvement confined to extralymphatic organs. Over-all, however, 39 per cent of the patients had evidence of extranodal disease in addition to nodal disease at the time of presentation. The two most frequent sites of extranodal involvement were the bone marrow and the gastrointestinal tract, with 16 per cent of patients having involvement of each of these organs. There was a lower incidence of involvement of the skin, thyroid, ovaries and other areas. The point is, that over 98 per cent of the adult patients did have clinically detectable lymph node involvement. In non-Hodgkin's lymphoma in children, on the other hand, abdominal involvement, particularly of the lymphoid tissues of the gastrointestinal tract, and extra-lymphatic involvement without significant peripheral node involvement are very common. In a recent series of 31 patients from the Children's Hospital of Philadelphia [2], 32 per cent presented with primary gastrointestinal tract involvement, another 23 per cent with primary extralymphatic involvement; only 45 per cent of the patients had primary lymph node involvement. In a larger series of children with non-Hodgkin's lymphoma from the Sloan-Kettering Cancer Center [3], only 25 per cent of them had peripheral lymphadenopathy whereas 19 per cent presented with primary bowel involvement. In most series of non-Hodgkin's lymphoma in children there is also a high incidence of central nervous system involvement, usually consisting of meningeal infiltration. This usually can be diagnosed by performing a lumbar puncture and demonstrating the presence of lymphoma cells in the cerebrospinal fluid. Such a procedure would have been useful in evaluating the patient under discussion. There is also a high incidence of bone marrow involvement in children with non-Hodgkin's lymphoma and, in fact, in approximately 20 per cent of the patients with this disease a leukemic peripheral blood picture will develop. The diagnosis of non-Hodgkin's lymphoma of the childhood type is compatible with the abdominal, bone marrow, central nervous system and thyroid involvement seen in the patient under discussion. Liver involvement to the degree present in this patient is unusual as a presenting sign of the disease, but it can occur and massive liver infiltration is commonly seen later in the course of the disease. At this point I would like to ask Dr. Jost to present the films.

Dr. R. Gilbert Jost: The chest film obtained at the time of admission was completely within normal limits, except that the trachea deviated slightly to the right, suggesting the possibility of a small thyroid mass. In fact, a pertechnitate scan of the thyroid confirmed the presence of a cold nodule in the lower pole of the left lobe. There was no evidence of mediastinal or hilar adenopathy on the chest films.

We were told that an upper gastrointestinal study made in early December was interpreted as being within normal limits. It is therefore clear that we are dealing with a very aggressive lesion, for only a few weeks later the folds of the fundus and body of the stomach were markedly thickened. Thickened folds of this type can be associated with a number of entities including giant hypertrophic gastritis, the Zollinger-Ellison syndrome, peptic disease and infiltrating carcinoma as well as lymphoma. However, there were some additional findings. There was a nodular filling defect in the duodenal bulb, and some persistent irregular filling defects were present in the second portion of the duodenum. A lateral view of the stomach demonstrated that the duodenal bulb and sweep were pushed forward by a large retroperitoneal mass. This mass effect was in the region of the common duct and could explain the patient's clinical presentation of obstructive jaundice. The liver-spleen scans showed definite evidence of hepatosplenomegaly. In addition, the liver was inhomogeneous and there were several nodular filling defects, particularly in the left lobe.

The findings suggest then that we are dealing with a highly aggressive tumor thrusting itself into the region of the duodenum and retroperitoneum. It is difficult to be certain about the exact etiology of this tumor. It is unlikely, in view of the normal motility of the stomach, that this organ was infiltrated by carcinoma. It would be possible, however, for a large retroperitoneal neoplasm to invade the splenic vein, creating gastric varices which could appear as thickened gastric folds. Nevertheless, the most attractive diagnosis that would explain this rather widespread constellation of findings would be an aggressive lymphoma, invading the stomach, duodenum, liver, spleen and retroperitoneum.

Dr. Kornfeld: Thank you. I have mentioned that non-Hodgkin's lymphoma in children is a more aggressive disease than non-Hodgkin's lymphoma in adults. This is reflected in the histologic types observed in the two age groups. In the Stanford series [1], 44 per cent of adults had a nodular type of lymphoma whereas 56 per cent had a diffuse type. In contrast, in most series of childhood non-Hodgkin's lymphoma, over 95 per cent of the children are classified as having a diffuse type of histology. This is important because the prognosis in patients with nodular lymphomas is better than in patients with diffuse lymphomas of the same cell type. Thus, the difference in the histologic patterns seen in the two age groups correlate well with the difference in the clinical picture.

The fulminant nature of this patient's disease brings to mind a particular type of childhood lymphoma termed Burkitt's lymphoma. Burkitt's lymphoma is the most common tumor in children of tropical Africa and it is now being recognized with increasing frequency in the United States. It is characterized by a very rapid onset and a rapidly fatal course if untreated. In the African patients, there is a predilection for involvement of the jaw, the abdomen and the gonads with a relative sparing of peripheral lymph nodes. Although only 7 per cent of the African patients had documented central nervous system involvement, paraplegia was the criteria for diagnosis rather than an abnormal lumbar puncture, so this is probably a minimal estimate. Thyroid involvement occurs in about 4 per cent of the patients, whereas bone marrow involvement was reported in 8 to 17 per cent. When the marrow is infiltrated with Burkitt's cells, a leukoerythroblastic peripheral blood picture may develop as seen in the patient under discussion. However transformation to acute leukemia is rare. In the cases reported from the United States [4], there is a lower incidence of jaw involvement although it is still frequent. Abdominal involvement is very common, occurring in about 60 per cent of patients. This high incidence, in comparison to the African patients, probably reflects the fact that many of the American patients underwent staging laparotomies for diagnostic purposes. The American patients also have a high incidence of gonadal involvement and 40 per cent have peripheral lymphadenopathy. In the African patients, jaw involvement is age related. Thus, in patients under age 3 years there is virtually a 100 per cent incidence of jaw involvement whereas in patients over age 15 years only 15 per cent have jaw involvement. Therefore, the lack of jaw involvement in our 17 year old patient is compatible with the data from both countries. In Africa, Burkitt's lymphoma is primarily a disease of children 12 years of age and younger. However, in the United States, although the peak incidence is also in that same age group, the disease has been diagnosed in many patients considerably older, including several in the 16 to 18 year age group.

One reason for the great interest in Burkitt's lymphoma is that in the African cases there is epidemiologic evidence to suggest that the Epstein-Barr (EB) virus may have an etiologic role. I have asked Dr. Rogers to review for us the association between the EB virus and Burkitt's lymphoma.

Dr. John Rogers: Let me summarize two important points which are fundamental to understanding this association. First, Burkitt's is the only lymphoma known to carry the EB virus. It is important to point out that in Africa, where by age 3 years 80 per cent of the children have serologic evidence of previous infection by EB virus, other lymphomas do not carry the virus. This is a fairly specific association between a virus and a lymphoid malignancy. Second, EB virus is known to have dramatic lymphocyte transforming properties. For instance, as a general rule, normal human peripheral blood lymphocytes will not grow in long-term culture; the only way to obtain a long-term lymphocyte cell line is to infect the cells first with the EB virus. In fact, virtually all the long-term human lymphocyte cell lines available now carry EB virus for that reason. This ability to transform lymphocytes is manifested in a common benign disease. It is now thought that the syndrome of infectious mononucleosis is a result of a sort of "war" between B lymphocytes that are transformed by EB virus and T lymphocytes that have specific killer recognition for these transformed B lymphocytes. Many of the atypical lymphocytes in infectious mononucleosis are T lymphocytes responding to the transformed B cells. In addition, EB virus has been shown to cause lymphomas in certain new world monkeys, both by directly injecting the monkeys with EB virus and by removing the monkey's lymphocytes, exposing them to the virus in vitro, and then returning them to the monkey.

Superficially, these two facts support the idea that Burkitt's lymphoma is, in fact, caused by EB virus. But, a comparison between African and American Burkitt's lymphoma makes this a very complex issue. First, in both African and American cases of Burkitt's lymphoma there is monoclonal proliferation of malignant B lymphocytes. These cells carry the usual B lymphocyte surface markers such as cell surface immunoglobulin and complement receptors. Lymphocytes from both types of Burkitt's lymphoma carry a specific EB virus receptor; Klein [5] showed that this is a marker for B lymphocytes and may be either identical to the complement receptor or very close to it. Most cell lines established from either type of Burkitt's lymphoma can be superinfected with EB virus. In short, there appears to be no fundamental biologic difference between the B lymphocytes in African cases and the B lymphocytes in cases occurring outside that region. However, the two diseases differ dramatically in their association with EB virus. In 97 per cent of the African Burkitt's cases, EB virus deoxyribonucleic acid (DNA) is carried within the lymphoma cells; this analysis has been made both on long-term cell culture lines derived from such tumors, and on fresh tumor cells directly. In distinction, a small number, probably less than 10 per cent of the cells in non-African cases carry the EB virus DNA. This is a most important difference. It clearly shows that Burkitt's lymphoma cannot be caused exclusively by EB virus. One would be tempted to conclude that African Burkitt's lymphoma just passively carries the virus, and that the virus has no causative role at all, but we cannot dismiss the information I summarized initially and we cannot dismiss the fact that in regions in which Burkitt's lymphomas carry the virus, such as in Africa, the incidence of this lymphoma is much higher than elsewhere. Klein [6] has recently proposed a solution to this complex question; his solution involves an hypothesis that the virus is an important co-factor that can interact with some other factor in causing Burkitt's lymphoma. We obviously do not know what the other factor is. We do know, for instance, that genetic factors can influence whether or not cells will undergo malignant transformation; in patients with Fanconi's anemia, ataxia telangiectasia or xeroderma pigmentosum the probability of cancer developing is high. Cultured cells from these patients frequently show chromosome aberrations, such as broken chromosomes and translocations, and have a much higher incidence of chromosome breakage when exposed to agents such as ultraviolet light. In addition, cells from these persons are much more readily transformed by an animal DNA tumor virus, the SV40 virus. This implies that a normal cell has some mechanism for suppressing a malignant urge; in cases such as Fanconi's anemia the mechanism for suppressing malignancy is defective. When an oncogenic stimulus, such as the SV40 virus, is added the cell capitulates and is readily transformed into malignancy. Klein's theory is that the factor that may cause Burkitt's lymphoma may be widespread, and may be banging on B lymphocytes everywhere. Theoretically, normal B lymphocytes can suppress this malignant stimulus and continue on their way in all but very rare cases. When you superimpose upon this unknown factor the EB virus, which is oncogenic at least in monkeys, you may generate an oncogenic punch that a B lymphocyte has difficulty resisting. Just as an addendum, it is interesting to note that a very specific chromosome 14 aberration has been reported to occur in most cases of African Burkitt's lymphoma [7]. It is reported in a paper in press (cited by Klein [6]) that a similar chromosomal abnormality exists in American cases.

Dr. Kornfeld: We should mention that although the EB virus is associated almost exclusively with Burkitt's lymphoma among the lymphomas, it is also associated with nasopharyngeal carcinoma.

I would like now to consider the therapy of non-Hodgkin's lymphoma of childhood. In the field of chemotherapy, some of the most spectacular advances have been made in the treatment of children with acute lymphoblastic leukemia, with current protocols resulting in long-term remissions and possibly cures in about 50 per cent of the patients. However, until recently, the results have been much poorer in children with non-Hodgkin's lymphoma with the exception of certain patients with Burkitt's lymphoma. I have asked Dr. Hillinger to discuss the current status of the treatment of children with non-Hodgkin's lymphoma.

Dr. Stephen Hillinger: As Dr. Kornfeld mentioned, the lymphomas in children are very aggressive. Although in the adult we generally treat stage I or II lymphoma principally with radiation therapy, and more advanced lymphomas with moderate doses of chemotherapy, this approach has not been utilized with much success in lymphomas in children. Because of the high incidence of central nervous system involvement and leukemic transformation, more aggressive, leukemia-types of regimens are being used to treat lymphomas in children. The validity of this approach is supported by statistical evidence. A series from the M.D. Anderson Hospital showed that the median survival in children with stage I lymphoma was only six months as compared to adults with stage I lymphomas who have a 60 to 75 per cent 5 year survival. The over-all median survival for children with stage I lymphoma, as compared to children with all the stages of lymphoma, shows only about a 1 month difference (six months for those with stage I and five months for those with all other stages). Thus, the change in approach has been toward treating this disorder with very aggressive chemotherapy.

The first major protocol that addressed itself to lymphoma in children came out of St. Judes Hospital [8]. That group used a modification of their acute lymphoblastic leukemia regimen. They described eight children with lymphoma, all of whom had early stages, either stage I or II. In other words, their patients did not have significant organ infiltration, and only one side of the diaphragm was involved. They had an over-all 88 per cent complete remission rate. Although their follow-up was short, six of these eight patients were free of disease at 16 to 27 months.

Another major protocol came from Memorial Hospital [9,10]. That group studied several different protocols in children with lymphoma. Their first protocol consisted of moderate doses of cyclophosphamide. With this, they treated 18 patients. Although the complete remission rate was not noted, they did have 22 per cent disease-free survivors, with a 33 per cent over-all survival. This latter figure included two additional patients who went on to be treated with their second protocol. The median survival for those treated with cyclophosphamide alone was 11 1/2 months, which was only twice the survival of historical controls. However, their most recent protocol involved a complicated 10 drug regimen, radiation therapy to sites of bulk disease and intrathecal methotrexate. In 43 children with lymphoma they achieved a 93 per cent complete remission rate. At the median observation time of 21+ months, there was an 81 per cent disease-free survival rate. The survival rate of patients presenting initially with extranodal disease was poorer than in those presenting with nodal disease [10]. As compared to other protocols, the presence of bone marrow involvement at presentation was not a poor prognostic sign, although infiltration of the central nervous system was. Histologically, only patients with diffuse, undifferentiated histology did poorly on this protocol.

The leading diagnosis in today's patient is Burkitt's lymphoma. I would like to review the special chemotherapeutic protocols that have been used in that entity. Burkitt's lymphoma is a subcategory of lymphoma that would be classified as a diffuse, undifferentiated lymphoma and identified specifically by certain cytologic characteristics. Most of the early treatment experience in this disorder was obtained, for obvious reasons, in Uganda, with the collaboration of the National Cancer Institute. Using cyclophosphamide, complete remission was achieved in 90 per cent of the patients [11]. However, there was a high relapse rate and at two years the over-all survival was approximately 33 per cent. However, those who remained disease-free after two years were apparently cured of their disease. The remission and survival rates for Burkitt's lymphoma, using large doses of cyclophosphamide, as seen in the United States are similar to those reported from Uganda. Because of the high incidence of tumor relapse, Ziegler's group at the National Cancer Institute has used several new protocols to see if they could improve upon on these statistics. Their first protocol involved the use of cyclophosphamide, vincristine, methotrexate (systemic and intrathecal) local irradiation and immunotherapy with BCG and Raji (a Burkitt cell line) cell vaccine [12]. Of 15 patients entered on this protocol, there was an 86 per cent complete remission rate, but the over-all survival rate was 38 per cent, which was not statistically different from that obtained with the use of cyclophosphamide alone. Both the use of prophylactic intrathecal chemotherapy and the use of immunotherapy provided no discernible improvement. Their latest protocol includes cyclophosphamide, vincristine, methotrexate and prednisone given in larger doses. They achieved a 100 per cent complete remission rate in 12 patients. However, after six months, three of these had a relapse.* Lastly, four patients have received bone marrow autografts at the National Cancer Institute.† Although these patients were in complete remission, they had their bone marrow aspirated, frozen and stored. After clinical relapse, they were treated with a bone marrow transplantation type of drug regimen, followed by the infusion of autologous stored marrow. Of four patients with Burkitt's lymphoma treated with autografting regimens, an unmaintained complete remission, lasting 3 and 10 months, has occurred in two. Two of the four died from cyclophosphamide-induced cardiac toxicity.

Dr. Kornfeld: Finally, we need to discuss the operation which was performed. To establish the diagnosis, it is necessary to obtain a biopsy specimen of the tumor and, suspecting that the bone marrow is involved with the malignant process, I think the simplest place to start would be with a bone marrow biopsy and a touch preparation which should show the typical vacuolated, undifferentiated lymphoblasts of Burkitt's lymphoma or possibly the lymphoblasts or the histiocytes indicative of one of the other forms of childhood non-Hodgkin's lymphoma. Regardless of what type of lymphoma we are dealing with, the bone marrow would be likely to give a diagnosis. If this procedure was unsuccessful or if the pathologist said that more tissue was required, then an exploratory laparotomy would have to have been performed. Dr. Franssila will present the pathology.

PATHOLOGIC DISCUSSION

Dr. Kaarle Franssila: At laparotomy a large tumor was found in the region of the head of the pancreas. There were many nodules in the liver, and the gallbaldder and the duodenum was also grossly involved.

Histologic sections of the liver, gallbladder and duodenal wall all revealed tumor tissue. The tumor was composed of sheets of closely packed cells with round nuclei and scant cytoplasm (Figure 1). There was little variation in the size of the nuclei. The cytoplasm of the tumor cells stained with methyl-green-pyronin, but not with periodic acid-Schiff. Intermixed with the tumor cells were numerous histiocytes with abundant clear cytoplasm containing nuclear fragments and producing the so-called "starry-sky" pattern. The nuclei of the tumor cells and of the histiocytes were of about the same size. The bone marrow biopsy specimen taken 1 month later showed total replacement of the marrow elements by the tumor tissue mentioned. In a touch specimen, mononuclear cells with vacuolated deeply basophilic cytoplasm were seen (Figure 2).

The histologic picture corresponds to a malignant lymphoma, undifferentiated, Burkitt's type. This diagnosis can be regarded as justified since the clinical

* Ziegler JC, personal communication.

† Herzig GP, personal communication.

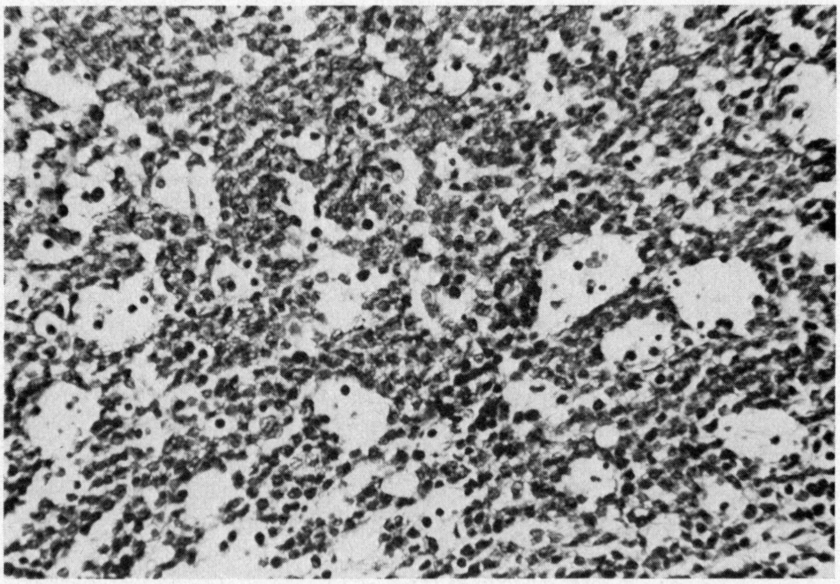

Figure 1. *The tumor is composed of monotonous mononuclear cells intermixed with histiocytes containing nuclear debris and producing the so-called "starry-sky" pattern. Hematoxylin and eosin stain; original magnification × 350, reduced by 30 per cent.*

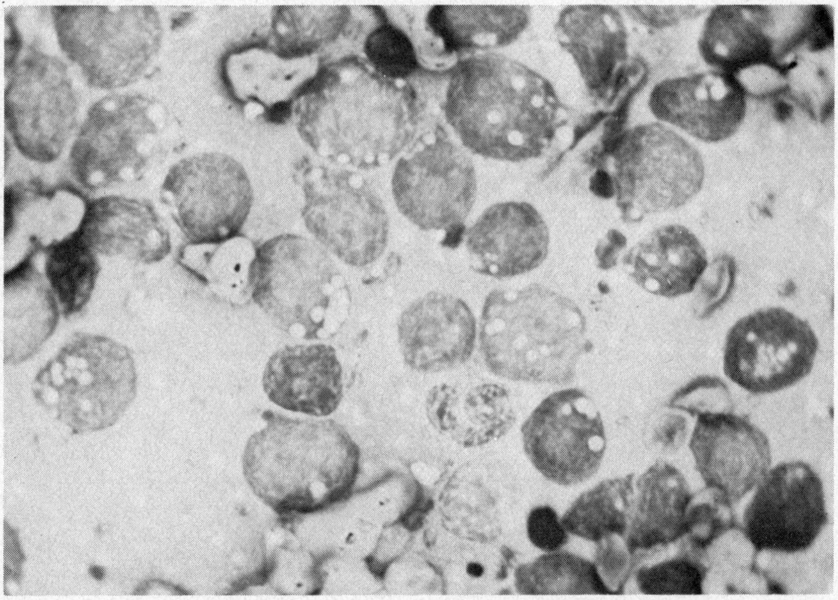

Figure 2. *Touch specimen of the bone marrow core shows mononuclear cells with scant vacuolated cytoplasm. Wright's stain; original magnification × 1,500, reduced by 17 per cent.*

picture of a young patient with extra-nodal disease involving the abdominal and retroperitoneal organs is also typical for Burkitt's lymphoma.

Dr. Kornfeld: Do we have a follow-up on this patient?

Dr. John Burch: The patient is being treated with a modification of the National Cancer Institute COMP protocol (cyclophosphamide, vincristine, methotrexate, prednisone) mentioned by Dr. Hillinger. To date, he has shown an excellent response. Results of his thyroid scan and liver function tests are now within normal limits, and his most recent bone marrow biopsy specimen showed no evidence of residual disease.

Dr. Kornfeld: I might stress that the atypical feature in this patient is the severe liver involvement.

REFERENCES

1. Jones S, Fuks Z, Bull M, et al.: Non-Hodgkin's lymphoma. IV. Clinicopathologic correlation in 405 cases. Cancer 31: 806, 1973.
2. Murphy S, Frizzera G, Evans A: A study of childhood non-Hodgkin's lymphoma. Cancer 36: 2121, 1975.
3. Wollner N, Burchenal JH, Lieberman PH, et al.: Non-Hodgkin's lymphoma in children. A comparative study of two modes of therapy. Cancer 37: 123, 1976.
4. Levine PH, Connelly RR, Berard CW, et al.: The American Burkitt Lymphoma registry. A progress report. Ann Intern Med 83: 31, 1975.
5. Jondal M, Klein G: Surface markers on human band T lymphocytes. II. Presence of Epstein-Barr virus receptors on B lymphocytes. J Exp Med 138: 1365, 1973.
6. Klein G: The Epstein-Barr virus and neoplasia. N Engl J Med 293: 1353, 1975.
7. Manolov G, Manolova Y: Marker band in one chromosome 14 from Burkitt lymphomas. Nature (Lond) 237: 33, 1972.
8. Aur JA, Hustu HO, Simone JV, et al.: Therapy of localized and regional lymphosarcoma of childhood. Cancer 27: 1328, 1971.
9. Wollner N, Burchenal JH, Lieberman PH, et al.: Non-Hodgkin's lymphoma in children. Med Pediatr Oncol 1: 235, 1975.
10. Wollner N, Burchenal JH, Lieberman PH, et al.: Non-Hodgkin's lymphoma in children. Cancer 37: 123, 1976.
11. Ziegler JL, Morrow RH, Fass L, et al.: Treatment of Burkitt's lymphoma with cyclophosphamide. Comparative Leukemia Research 1969. Bibl Haematol 36: 701, 1970.
12. Ziegler JL, Young RC, Pomeroy TC: Combined modality treatment of American Burkitt's lymphoma (abstract). Am Soc Clin Oncol 16: 249, 1975.

Selected and edited by Richard T. Silver, M.D. and Alexander G. Bearn, M.D.
Department of Medicine, The New York Hospital-Cornell Medical Center, New York, New York

Vasculitis Syndromes: Clinical and Experimental Models

Lecturers:

CHARLES L. CHRISTIAN, M.D.
JOHN S. SERGENT, M.D.
New York, New York

Dr. Charles L. Christian: The subject of this Symposium began a little more than 100 years ago with the description of periarteritis nodosa by two German physicians, Kussmaul and Maier [1]. They encountered a 27 year old man with an acute illness characterized by fever, productive cough, proteinuria, urine casts, profound muscle weakness, peripheral neuritis and abdominal pain. They were puzzled. Their preliminary clinical diagnosis was "chlorotic marasmus"; tuberculosis and trichiniasis were considered. The patient was unique in their experience. They stated, "it is understandable that we looked forward to autopsy with the greatest eagerness" [1]. In this regard they were nearly frustrated, for their surgical colleagues obtained the deceased and proceeded to practice surgical procedures. Sufficient parts were retrieved, however, for histologic studies. These revealed widespread vasculitis. The degree of inflammation and exudation of the vessel walls was focal, giving rise to nodular excrescences along the course of arteries.

The next historic development in the light of this Symposium was the recognition of an experimental model of arteritis: acute serum sickness. The related topics of serum sickness and immune complex disease have been subjects of recent and comprehensive reviews [2,3]. It is my intention now to briefly summarize some of the concepts derived from experimental studies that appear to have relevance to the pathogenesis of human vasculitis syndromes.

Figure 1 illustrates schematically the relationships between antigen concentration and lesions in acute serum sickness. Studies by numerous laboratories have established that the rapid disappearance in circulating antigen, seven to 10 days after administration of a single large dose of heterologous serum albumin, corresponds to the presence of circulating immune complexes and the development of lesions and hypocomplementemia. Although glomerulonephritis and diffuse arteritis may be severe, these lesions heal in the majority of animals without chronic residue. When daily smaller doses of antigen are administered, the results (summarized in Figure 2) are quite different. The host response is variable: some animals are immunologically tolerant; the majority manifest very rapid clearance of each dose of antigen and a minority of animals (10 to 20 per cent) form complexes which are slowly cleared from circulation over a period of several hours or more. Only the latter group, with slow elimination of immune complexes, manifest chronic glomerulonephritis. Arteritis, which is conspicuous in acute serum sickness, is not a feature of the chronic model. Two host variables, one relating to the quantity of the immune response and the other relating to the quality of antibodies produced, have been suggested as bases for the two patterns of immune complex elimination [4,5]. In high antibody responders, the daily dose of antigen forms large complexes in antibody excess that are rapidly and efficiently removed by reticuloendothelial organs. With a modest immune response, the same dose of antigen can form intermediate size complexes, in relative antigen excess, that are less efficiently removed from the circulation. With regard to the quality of the immune response, there is evidence that animals manifesting slow complex elimination produce antibodies against a limited number of antigenic determinants on the complex antigen. If only a few of the several antigenic determinants on bovine serum albumin provoke an immune response, there are limitations in the size of lattice work formed by antigen and antibody, and these smaller complexes are relatively inefficiently removed by reticuloendothelial organs. Aside from the effects of antibody quantity and quality, there are other variables that may influence the pathogenicity of immune complexes. Blockade of the reticuloendothelial organs might alter the clearance rate of immune complexes, allowing their deposition in glomerular capillaries. Accessory factors in serum, such as complement and rheumatoid factors, theoretically could have a protective effect by facilitating clearance of complexes, and the liberation of vasoactive substances from platelets and mast cells can promote the localization of immune complexes [6].

As noted, a contrast between acute and chronic serum sickness is the absence of arteritis in the latter model. Figure 3 is a schematic representation of an hypothesis that might account for this difference. For several days after a single large dose of antigen, prior to the development of antibody, the antigen equilibrates with extravascular sites. Following immune response, antigen which persists in the intravascular space is rapidly eliminated but, in addition, extravascular sites, e.g. arterial walls, which contain antigen are targets of immunologic attack. In such a scheme there are both tissue-directed immunologic injury and the formation of circulating complexes. In chronic serum sickness, the smaller doses of antigen administered daily form complexes that are largely limited to the intravascular space; and overt immunologic injury, for a variety of reasons, is relatively restricted to renal glomeruli.

Studies of classic serum sickness, noted herein, have contributed enormously to our understanding of the immunologic events involved in the pathogenesis of arteritis, but there are other experimental models that probably have a greater relevance to arteritis in man. These are induced by microbial stimuli. The best characterized model of virus-induced vasculitis involves

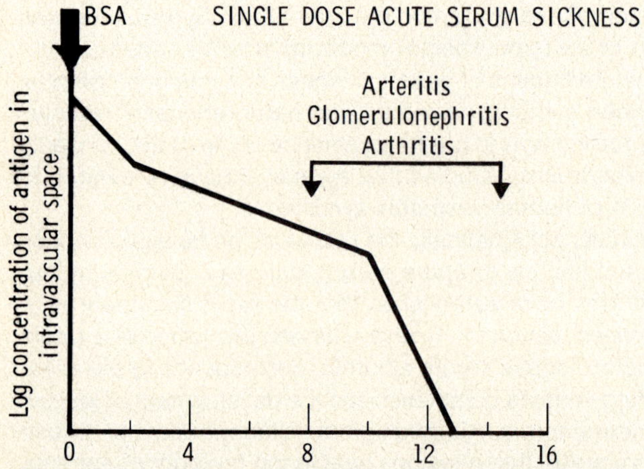

Figure 1. Summary of the relationship of circulating antigen concentration to the development of acute serum sickness, following the administration of a single large dose of heterologous serum albumin. The occurrence of lesions corresponds to the rapid phase of antigen elimination (dependent on the host immune response) during which time circulating immune complexes are demonstrable.

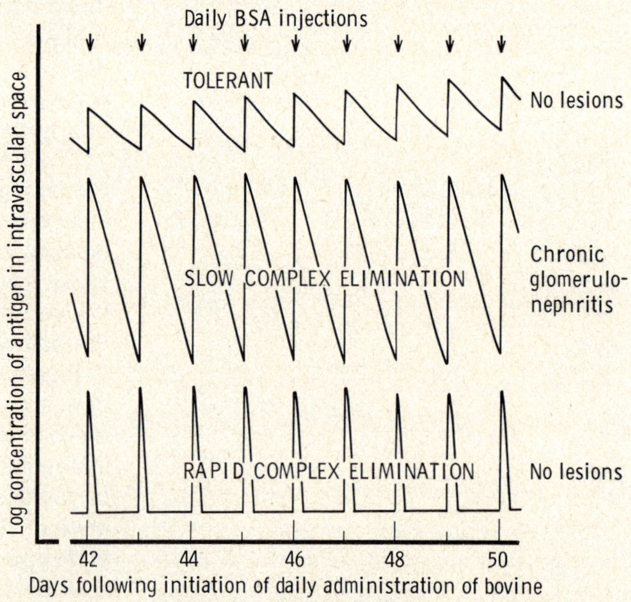

Figure 2. Schematic representation of three patterns of host response to chronic immunization with heterologous serum albumin. The level and persistence of circulating antigen (in the form of immune complexes), influenced by qualitative and quantitative variables of the immune response, correlate with presence or absence of chronic glomerulitis (see text).

lymphochoriomeningitis (LCM) virus [7]. Infection acquired early in life, either in utero or neonatally, does not result in the characteristic meningoencephalitis. Such animals gradually manifest chronic vascular lesions in the face of persistent high levels of virus in blood and tissues. The lesions have been shown to result from deposition of immune complexes, involving LCM virus, that form in the presence of excess viral antigen, a state which may be analogous to HB_s associated arteritis in man [8,9]. There are notable mouse strain differences in susceptibility to chronic LCM disease which have been correlated with the H-2 histocompatibility system [10].

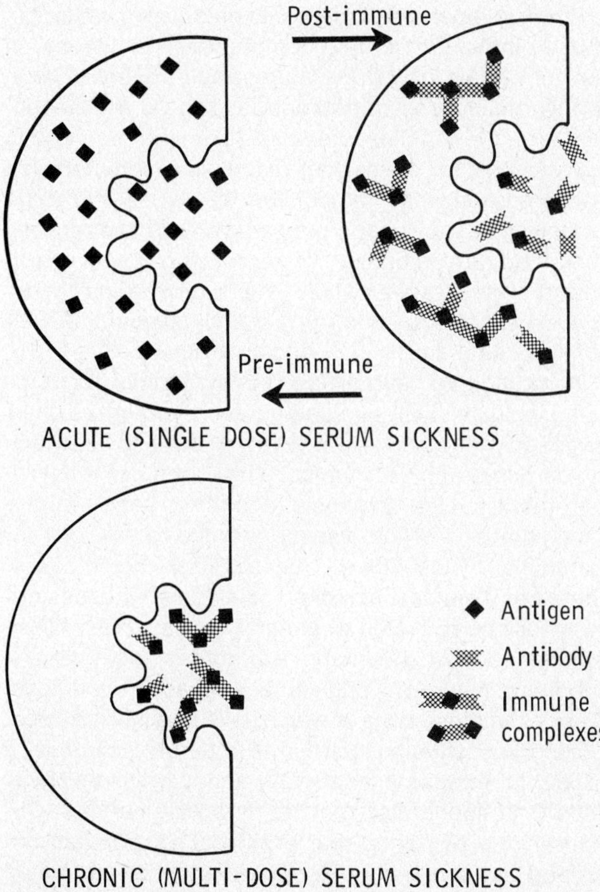

Figure 3. *Schematic hypothesis regarding different immunologic mechanisms involved in acute versus chronic serum sickness. With the acute model there is equilibration of the large dose of antigen with extravascular spaces, including arterial walls, prior to the immune response. (The illustration represents a cross section of an artery.) Following the development of the immune response, antibody forms complexes with residual circulating antigen and initiates immunologic injury in extravascular tissues containing antigen. In the model of chronic serum sickness, it is postulated that the smaller doses of antigen (administered daily) form complexes that are relatively restricted to the intravascular space. The fate of such complexes, and whether or not chronic glomerulonephritis develops, depend on multiple host variables (see text).*

Although most of the viral-induced models of vasculitis, such as chronic LCM infection and Aleutian disease of mink, appear to involve the host immune response in pathogenesis, there are some possible exceptions. A naturally occurring disease in horses, equine viral arteritis, reaches its peak expression approximately one week following infection, but lesions begin to occur by the fifth day and correlate in time with the demonstration of virus in vessel walls [11]. These observations suggest that virus may initiate arteritis without the mediation of the immune response. A more convincing demonstration of direct microbial mediation of arteritis derives from studies of Dr. Lewis Thomas approximately a decade ago. Dr. Thomas studied a model of central nervous system arteritis in turkeys infected with Mycoplasma gallisepticum [12]. In turkeys inoculated with a dose of 10^7 organisms clinical illness and lesions developed within seven to 14 days, quite consistent with immunologic mediation. However, with larger doses (10^{11} organisms) clinical evidence of disease occurred within 1 hour and arteritic lesions were identifiable as early as 24 hours.

To summarize the subject of experimental vasculitis, most studies suggest that the host immune response is involved in pathogenesis and that the immunologic stimulus in syndromes of man and experimental species may result from atypical infection. Additionally, some infectious agents may have the capacity to induce vasculitis without immunologic mediation. The remainder of this Symposium will relate to vasculitis syndromes in man and possible analogies between clinical and experimental models.

For most of the past century, the diagnosis of diffuse vasculitis has been, like Kussmaul and Maier's experience, based on necropsy studies. With the advent of diagnostic biopsies, a relatively recent development, a broader spectrum of vasculitis syndromes has been recognized, some of them clinically and pathologically distinct from periarteritis nodosa. Dr. John Sergent, who has reviewed the experience with arteritis syndromes at this Center, will review some of the clinical and pathologic associations of vasculitis.

Dr. John Sergent: In this discussion, the term "vasculitis" denotes pathologically demonstrable inflammation and necrosis of vessels, in association with clinical syndromes in which the predominant manifestations may be explained on the basis of vascular inflammation. Thus, we are excluding such conditions as scleroderma, in which the vascular involvement is primarily obliterative and noninflammatory, and malignant hypertension, in which the vascular necrosis is clearly secondary to the blood pressure elevation, and not the primary problem.

As the clinical syndromes associated with inflammatory vasculitis are enumerated, it is important to remember that the diagnosis of vasculitis is no more specific than is pneumonitis or nephritis. In some patients, evidence of vasculitis may be the only finding demonstrable, whereas in others, vascular inflammation may have occurred in the setting of another, more complex, illness.

Following the initial description of vasculitis as a distinct pathologic entity by Kussmaul and Maier in 1866 [13], the terms "periarteritis nodosa" and "polyarteritis nodosa" were used to describe a variety of diseases associated with vasculitis, without much effort to differentiate one disease from another.

Realizing that necrotizing vasculitis as a pathologic finding was associated with a variety of different syndromes, Zeek [14] proposed a classification which is still widely used. Dr. Zeek believed that most patients with generalized vasculitis should be classified into one of five types. *Hypersensitivity angiitis* was an acute fulminant illness associated with necrotizing glomerulitis and inflammatory vasculitis of the small vessels of the kidneys, heart and lungs. *Allergic granulomatous arteritis,* frequently associated with asthma and other allergic diseases, involved inflammation in arteries of variable sizes associated with granuloma formation. *Rheumatic arteritis,* complicating fulminant rheumatic fever, involved small vessels, especially in the heart, and was associated with Aschoff bodies. Classic *periarteritis nodosa* conformed to the syndrome described by Kussmaul and Maier, with inflammation of medium-sized arteries, especially prominent at major bifurcations. *Temporal arteritis* was recognized as a distinct clinical syndrome, with multinucleated giant cells and cellulitis as well as vasculitis in the cranial arteries. This classification, with elaboration by other pathologists and clinicians, has proved useful, especially for comparisons among large series of patients. Unfortunately, such classifications are more important in retrospective reviews of large numbers of patients than in the clinical evaluation of individual patients. In this discussion, therefore, we will concentrate on clinical syndromes associated with necrotizing vasculitis and not attempt rigid classification according to pathologic criteria.

Table I summarizes some of the clinical syndromes which have been associated with necrotizing vasculitis. This compilation is not comprehensive; indeed, a careful review of the literature would reveal a large variety of illnesses sometimes associated with vasculitis, e.g., the localized vasculitis sometimes found in the appendix, or the dermal vasculitis associated with erythema nodosum. In addition, the list seems to be expanding year by year. For example, we have recently described an "epidemic" of necrotizing vasculitis following serous otitis media. Others have recently described the association of necrotizing vasculitis with amphetamine abuse [28] and ulcerative colitis [33].

As noted, we have divided the syndrome of necrotizing vasculitis into two categories. Syndromes characterized by vasculitis include those diseases in which the demonstration of the vasculitis is the essential requirement for the diagnosis, and all or nearly all the manifestations of the disease are due to vascular inflammation. These are all diseases of unknown cause. The other diseases, listed in Table II, are illnesses occasionally complicated by generalized vasculitis. These include several rheumatic syndromes, asthma and Loeffler's syndrome, and some neoplastic conditions. Other examples, some of which have been well studied, include vasculitis associated with serum sickness, a variety of infections (especially endocarditis and hepatitis B antigenemia) and the paraproteinemias. Obviously, the evidence that a clinical association described is real and not coincidental must be examined carefully. For example, Rich and others reported cases

TABLE I Clinical Classification of Vasculitis Syndromes

Characterized by Necrotizing Vasculitis	
Temporal arteritis	Henoch-Schonlein purpura
Wegener's granulomatosis	"Classic" polyarteritis nodosa
Aortic arch arteritis	
Occasionally Complicated by Necrotizing Vasculitis	
Rheumatic diseases	**Hypersensitivity**
Rheumatoid arthritis [15]	Serum sickness [24, 25]
Systemic lupus erythematosus [16]	Drug allergy [26, 27]
Dermatomyositis [17]	Amphetamine abuse [28]
Rheumatic fever [14]	**Paraproteinemias**
Infections	Essential cryoglobulinemia [29]
Hepatitis B [8]	Multiple myeloma [30]
Acute respiratory infections [18]	Macroglobulinemia [31]
Streptococcal infections [19]	**Others**
Poststreptococcal glomerulonephritis [20]	Dermal vasculitis [32]
Bacterial endocarditis [21]	Ulcerative colitis [33]
Respiratory diseases	Cogan's syndrome [34]
Loeffler's syndrome [22]	Colon carcinoma [35]
Asthma [22]	
Serous otitis media [23]	

TABLE II Presenting Manifestations of Vasculitis

	HB_s Positive (9 patients)		HB_s Negative (13 patients)	
	No.	Per Cent	No.	Per Cent
Arthralgias	9	100	7	54
Mononeuritis	7	77	7	54
Fever	6	66	9	69
Abdominal pain	5	55	4	31
Renal disease	4	44	8	62
Central nervous system	3	33	5	38

of vasculitis secondary to sulfonamides, yet, as Zeek pointed out, in that era it was unusual for any patient to come to autopsy without at least a trial of sulfonamide therapy; hence, the association may have been fortuitous.

Because of its importance in our current understanding of the mechanisms of induction of vascular injury, serum sickness deserves special comment. Serum sickness as a cause of necrotizing vasculitis was first described in 1937 by Clark and Kaplan [24]. They described pathologic findings in two patients who died of acute serum sickness reactions as part of their therapy for severe pneumococcal infections. Both patients had histiocytic infiltration around arteries, and one had necrotizing arteritis and periarteritis of the coronary arteries. Arnold Rich [25], in 1942, described five similar cases which he attributed to serum, sulfonamides or both, and he emphasized the importance of searching for the inciting antigen in all cases of periarteritis nodosa. The following year, Rich and Gregory [36] produced vasculitis in rabbits by intravenous injections of horse serum.

In the search for possible causes of necrotizing vasculitis, these experiments and observations marked the end of the era searching for infectious agents or their toxic products which could cause vasculitis. The succeeding era began. It was marked by the recognition that immunologic factors may be involved in many, or perhaps most, of these cases. Currently, we are in yet another era, in which the source of immunologic stimulation is being sought in the sphere of chronic infection.

Clinically, serum sickness in the previously nonimmunized patient usually begins about 10 days after injection, and is characterized by fever, urticaria and arthralgias. Most cases resolve in a few days; however, in more severely affected patients, frank arthritis, glomerulonephritis and occasional necrotizing vasculitis develop. The importance of serum sickness is far out of proportion to its frequency, because today true serum sickness is rare. However, the clinical and laboratory models of serum sickness have provided much of the impetus for research into the causes of other vascular, renal and rheumatic disorders over the past 30 years.

Of the various diseases associated with vasculitis which are listed in Table I, there is some evidence in several of them that immune complexes may mediate the vasculitis, in a manner analogous to serum sickness. Although we do not have time now to review the available evidence in each of these syndromes or diseases, we will discuss selected conditions for which the immune complex model is a reasonable explanation for vasculitis.

In several of the diseases listed, notably rheumatoid arthritis, systemic lupus erythematosus (SLE), essential cryoglobulinemia and bacterial endocarditis, vasculitic manifestations are usually accompanied by striking serologic abnormalities, supporting the concept that active immune phenomena are taking place. For example, active vasculitis in these diseases is often accompanied by hypocomplementemia, the formation of antibodies or rheumatoid factors, and by the presence in the serum of cryoglobulins. These cryoglobulins are usually composed of immunoglobulins G (IgG) and M (IgM), rheumatoid factor and complement components [37]. In the conditions noted herein the activity of the vascular inflammation tends to wax and wane proportional to the degree of serologic abnormalities. A tenable hypothesis is that the vasculitis is induced by circulating immune complexes, including complement-fixing cryoglobulins. Although the evidence that these complexes actually induce the vascular injury is not conclusive, the reason for the hypothesis can be easily understood by a brief review of the vasculitis associated with rheumatoid arthritis. Vasculitis is an essential part of the early phase of development of the subcutaneous nodule, and some believe that vascular injury may be the primary lesion in all manifestations of rheumatoid arthritis [38]. As a clinically important problem distinct from other manifestations, however, vasculitis takes two forms. The first, and most common, is a low grade vasculitis, primarily in the skin, which leads to areas of skin necrosis and ulceration. Patients with indolent skin ulcers frequently manifest peripheral neuropathy of the stocking-glove type, thought to be due to vasculitis in the vasa vasorum, but the majority do not have signs of necrotizing vasculitis elsewhere. The second, much less common, form of vasculitis in rheumatoid arthritis is a clinical syndrome similar to polyarteritis nodosa, with fever, mononeuropathy, extensive digital gangrene and death due to infarction of vital organs, such as the gastrointestinal tract. An earlier view that this syndrome is a consequence of corticosteroid therapy has not been substantiated; rather it seems more likely that diffuse vasculitis is an expression of *very severe* rheumatoid arthritis and that such patients are more likely to receive corticosteroid drugs. In addition to cryoglobulins, patients with rheumatoid vasculitis often have intermediate and high molecular weight immune complexes demonstrable by ultracentrifugation of serum. Various laboratories, notably that of Kunkel, Winchester and their associates [39], have demonstrated that these complexes, like the cryoglobulins, contain IgM, or IgG rheumatoid factors complexed with IgG. Although the amount of these complexes usually increases with the severity of the rheumatoid disease, the fact that such complexes are demonstrable in many patients with no evidence of vasculitis suggests that their mere presence is not sufficient, per se, to cause vasculitis. Other factors, not yet understood, may influence the pathogenetic expression of complexes.

Systemic lupus erythematosus, in which there is abundant evidence for circulating immune complexes, is also associated occasionally with vasculitis: chronic skin ulcers, digital gangrene, mononeuritis multiplex and, rarely, involvement of medium- or larger-sized vessels, such as mesenteric and coronary arteries.

In contrast to the cryoglobulinemia associated with rheumatoid arthritis, SLE or bacterial endocarditis, primary or essential cryoglobulinemia (Meltzer-Franklin syndrome) [40] appears to result from autonomous paraprotein production. This syndrome is associated with large amounts of cryoglobulins which, like those seen in rheumatoid arthritis, or SLE, usually contain IgM rheumatoid factor, IgG and complement components. However, in essential cryoglobulinemia the IgM rheumatoid factor is homogeneous and monoclonal, i.e., contains only one type of light chain. Thus, these patients have a disorder of B lymphocytes in which the physical-chemical nature of the paraprotein appears to determine the clinical pattern of disease. Although other B lymphocyte disorders may present as myeloma, lymphomas or amyloidosis, the paraprotein in these patients presumably mediates vasculitis and glomerulonephritis via the formation of complement fixing complexes.

After reviewing serum sickness (explicitly immunologic in origin) and cryoglobulinema, rheumatoid arthritis and SLE, which are syndromes wherein immune complexes appear to play roles in inducing vasculitis, I would like to discuss the only chronic sustained form of vasculitis in man which is known to be associated with viral infection. This type of vasculitis is associated with hepatitis B (HB_s) antigenemia. HB_s antigenemia is an important cause of generalized necrotizing vasculitis, and may account for the largest identifiable subgroup of such patients. Of the 22 patients with generalized necrotizing vasculitis we studied, nine were HB_s positive. Although a frequency of 41 per cent is undoubtedly related in part to selective referral patterns, others have reported as many as 20 to 30 per cent of patients with vasculitis in unselected series to be HB_s positive. HB_s associated vasculitis was described simultaneously in 1970 by Gocke et al. [8] and by Trepo and Thivolet [9]. The clinical features of nine patients with HB_s associated vasculitis and those of the 13 patients with vasculitis who were HB_s antigen and antibody negative are summarized in Table II. The clinical manifestations noted were common in both groups, the incidences of arthralgia and mononeuritis were higher in HB_s positive patients, and renal disease was slightly more frequent in HB_s negative subjects.

The clinical courses in the nine HB_s positive patients have been extremely variable. Pre-existing liver disease was present in some, but not all, before the development of vasculitis. Two had biopsy-proved chronic active hepatitis. Three patients have died of complications of vasculitis, and one died of chronic liver disease. Of the survivors, one is clinically well but has mild elevations of serum transaminase. The other four all have residual manifestations of vasculitis, including neuropathy, azotemia, hypertension and residual central nervous system damage.

The pathologic findings in this group were varied: primarily small vessel occlusion in some, involvement of small muscular arteries in others, and involvement of larger vessels in still others. Although the exact mechanism of induction of the vasculitis is unclear, there is evidence implicating immune phenomena [8].

Management. Excluding cases in which the cause of vasculitis is known, i.e., bacterial endocarditis or drug hypersensitivity, therapy is based on our ability to nonspecifically modify the inflammatory response and the host immune system. In two of the vasculitis syndromes, an empirical approach has been quite successful. These are Wegener's granulomatosis, in which excellent results have been reported with cyclophosphamide [41], and temporal arteritis, in which corticosteroid therapy usually results in dramatic symptomatic and objective benefits [42]. Interestingly, in both of these conditions the evidence that immunologic events are important is meager, yet therapy is relatively successful.

With the other vasculitis syndromes, management decisions are influenced by organ patterns of involvement. If there is evidence of significant renal disease, ischemia of the gastrointestinal tract or major neurologic disability, corticosteroid therapy with relatively large doses (prednisone, approximately 1/mg/kg/day) is usually instituted. If the patient improves immediately, the dose is reduced slowly after a few weeks, while observing closely for evidence of recurrent activity of vasculitis. If the patient does not respond satisfactorily, or if the disease worsens as the dose of corticosteroid drug is reduced, it is common practice to initiate additional drug therapy, usually cyclophosphamide or azathioprine. This approach is based on the fact that many patients enter periods of prolonged or permanent remission; such patients are not necessarily committed to a lifetime of corticosteroid and/or immunosuppressive therapy. The six surviving patients with vasculitis associated with HB_s antigenemia were successfully withdrawn from both corticosteroid and immunosuppressive agents, without recurrence of active vasculitis.

In summary, it should be emphasized that generalized vasculitis is not a disease, but a syndrome. As such, it may be only part of a much broader clinical picture, as in rheumatoid arthritis or hepatitis B infection, or it may dominate the clinical picture, as in Wegener's granulomatosis. It is well to remember that, in the past, patients with HB_s associated arteritis or essential cryoglobulinemia (now classed as diseases sometimes associated with vasculitis) have been included in series of patients diagnosed as having "polyarteritis nodosa." As more specific causes of vasculitis are identified in the future, the term "periarteritis nodosa" will have no more clinical importance than "chlorotic marasmus."

SUMMARY

Dr. Christian: Dr. Sergent has emphasized that diffuse vasculitis is not a disease but rather a manifestation of what may be a variety of etiologic stimuli. There are a few syndromes, such as Wegener's granulomatosis and giant cell arteritis, in which clinical and pathologic features are unique, but the majority of patients with vasculitis do not have distinguishing pathologic expressions. Immunologic mediation of disease is explicit in most animal models of vasculitis and is suspect in the human syndromes. HB virus infection, which may be associated with as many as one-third of the patients with diffuse vasculitis, may play a role analogous to viral infection in chronic LCM disease of mice. The recognition of HB_s associated vasculitis adds to speculations that other viral agents may be implicated in arteritis syndromes of man.

DISCUSSION

Dr. Robert Lightfoot: Is there anything distinctive about the hepatitis B antigen in patients with vasculitis in comparison with other chronic carriers?

Dr. Sergent: No. Dr. George LeBouvier performed HB_s antigen subtyping on our patients and found a subtype distribution similar to that in the general clinic carrier population. We have not found any consistent variations in titer of this HB_s antigen in patients followed serially, which raises the possibility that the HB_s antigen is only a marker for the disease and may not be the antigen responsible for the vasculitis. We are planning to look for hepatitis B core (HB_c) antigen and antibody in our serums.

Dr. Richard Silver: You have described the potpourri of symptoms assigned to the general category of necrotizing vasculitis. Assuming that we have excluded all the diseases with which arteritis may be associated, we are still left with a number of patients without any recognized associated illness. Would you use the term polyarteritis nodosa to describe these patients?

Dr. Sergent: Personally, I prefer to avoid that term because it means different things to different people. Some use it as a generic term to describe most cases of necrotizing vasculitis; others restrict the term to the classic disease as described by Kussmaul and Maier. I might add that if used in this latter, strict sense, polyarteritis nodosa is a very rare disease. Of our last 23 patients, only one fills these requirements.

To avoid confusion, I would use necrotizing vasculitis as the generic term to include all patients with this pathologic finding, and then categorize according to the presence (or absence) of any clinical associations.

Dr. Christian: Dr. Christian Trepo, who has worked in the area of vasculitis associated with HB_s antigenemia, is in the audience. Dr. Trepo, do you have any comments?

Dr. Christian Trepo: In our experience, chronic carriers of the HB_s antigen always have free antibody to the hepatitis B core in their serum, so I doubt that this approach will be informative. I am also interested in the results of therapy in your HB_s patients. Have you been able to withdraw therapy in all patients without a recurrence of disease?

Dr. Sergent: Yes. Three of our patients died of complications of their vasculitis within the first few months of illness. The remainder were treated for periods of several months to a year or so; all have subsequently had therapy withdrawn without recurrence of vasculitis, despite persistent HB_s antigenemia.

Dr. Christian: To close on an optimistic note, I would like to emphasize that many patients with necrotizing vasculitis appear to have self-limited courses—a finite period of active disease. If the phase of active disease can be suppressed with adrenocortical steroid or cytotoxic drugs, and if there has not been irreparable damage to vital organs, the prognosis is much better than the literature suggests.

REFERENCES

1. Bloomfield AL: Periarteritis nodosa. A Bibliography of Internal Medicine, Selected Diseases, Chicago, University of Chicago Press, 1960, p 53.
2. Unanue ER, Dixon FJ: Experimental glomerulonephritis. Immunological events and pathogenetic mechanisms. Adv Immunol 6: 1, 1967.
3. Cochrane CG, Koffler D: Immune complex disease. Adv Immunol 16: 185, 1973.
4. Dixon FJ, Feldman JD, Vasquez JJ: Experimental glomerulonephritis. J Exp Med 113: 899, 1961.
5. Pincus T, Haberkern R, Christian CL: Experimental chronic glomerulitis. J Exp Med 127: 819, 1968.
6. Henson PM, Cochrane CG: Acute immune complex disease in rabbits. The role of complement and of a leukocyte-dependent release of vasoactive amines from platelets. J Exp Med 133: 554, 1971.
7. Oldstone MBA, Dixon FJ: Pathogenesis of chronic disease associated with persistent lymphocytic choriomeningitis viral infection. II. Relationship of the antilymphocytic choriomeningitis immune response to tissue injury in chronic lymphocytic choriomeningitis disease. J Exp Med 131: 1, 1970.
8. Gocke DJ, Hsu K, Morgan G, et al.: Association between polyarteritis and Australia antigen. Lancet 2: 1149, 1970.
9. Trepo C, Thivolet J: Hepatitis associated antigen and periarteritis nodosa (PAN). Vox Sang 19: 410, 1970.
10. Oldstone MBA, Dixon FJ, Mitchell GF, McDevitt HO: Histocompatibility-linked genetic control of disease suscepti-

bility. Murine lymphocytic choriomeningitis virus infection. J Exp Med 137: 1201, 1973.
11. Estes PC, Cheville NF: The ultrastructure of vascular lesions in equine viral arteritis. Am J Pathol 58: 235, 1970.
12. Thomas L, Davidson M, McCluskey RT: Studies of PPLO infection. I. The production of cerebral polyarteritis by Mycoplasma gallisepticum in turkeys: the neurotoxic property of the Mycoplasma. J Exp Med 123: 897, 1966.
13. Kussmaul A, Maier R: Ueber eine bisher nicht beschreibene eigenthümliche arterienerkrankung die mit morbus brightii und rapid furtschreitender allgemeiner muskellähmung einhegeht. Deutsches Arch Klin Med 1: 484, 1866.
14. Zeek P: Periarteritis: a critical review. Am J Clin Pathol 22: 777, 1952.
15. Bywaters EGL: Peripheral vascular obstruction in rheumatoid arthritis and its relationship to other vascular lesions. Ann Rheum Dis 16: 84, 1957.
16. Cruickshank B: Lupus Erythematosus, 2nd ed (Dubois EL, ed), Los Angeles, University of Southern California Press, 1974, p 28.
17. Banker BQ, Victor M: Dermatomyositis (systemic angiopathy) of childhood. Medicine (Baltimore) 45: 261, 1966.
18. Rose G: The natural history of polyarteritis. Br Med J 2: 1148, 1957.
19. Rose GA, Spencer H: Polyarteritis nodosa. Q J Med 26: 43, 1957.
20. Fordham CC, Epstein FH, Huffiner WD, Harrington JT: Polyarteritis and acute post-streptococcal glomerulonephritis. Ann Intern Med 61: 89, 1964.
21. Kerr A: Subacute Bacterial Endocarditis, Springfield, Charles C Thomas, 1955.
22. Churg J, Strauss L: Allergic granulomatosis, allergic angiitis, and periarteritis nodosa. Am J Pathol 27: 277, 1951.
23. Sergent JS, Christian CL: Necrotizing vasculitis after acute serous otitis media. Ann Intern Med 81: 195, 1974.
24. Clark E, Kaplan BI: Endocardial, arterial, and other mesenchymal alterations associated with serum disease in man. Arch Pathol 24: 458, 1937.
25. Rich AR: The role of hypersensitivity in periarteritis nodosa. Bull Johns Hopkins Hosp 71: 123, 1942.
26. Young JL, Boswell RB, Nies AS: Severe allopurinol hypersensitivity. Arch Intern Med 134: 553, 1974.
27. Mowrey FH, Lundley EA: The clinical manifestations of essential polyangiitis (periarteritis nodosa), with emphasis on the hepatic manifestations. Ann Intern Med 40: 1145, 1954.
28. Citron BP, Halpern M, McCarron M, et al.: Necrotizing angiitis associated with drug abuse. N Engl J Med 283: 1003, 1970.
29. Reza MJ, Roth BE, Pops MA, Goldberg LS: Intestinal vasculitis in essential, mixed cryoglobulinemia. Ann Intern Med 81: 632, 1974.
30. Brout J-C, Clauvel J-P, Danon F, et al.: Biologic and clinical significance of cryoglobulins. Am J Med 57: 775, 1974.
31. Grey H, Kohler P: Cryoimmunoglobulins. Sem Hematol 10: 87, 1973.
32. Winkelmann RK, Schroeter AL, Kierland RR, Ryan TR: Clinical studies of livedoid vasculitis (segmental hyalinizing vasculitis). Mayo Clin Proc 49: 746, 1974.
33. Wackers F, Tytgat G, Vreeken J: Necrotizing vasculitis and ulcerative colitis. Br Med J 4: 83, 1974.
34. Cody D, Williams H: Cogan's syndrome. Laryngoscope 70: 447, 1960.
35. Posner J: Personal communication.
36. Rich AR, Gregory JE: The experimental demonstration that periarteritis nodosa is a manifestation of hypersensitivity. Bull Johns Hopkins Hosp 72: 65, 1943.
37. Hanauer L, Christian C: Studies of cryoproteins in systemic lupus erythematosus. J Clin Invest 46: 400, 1967.
38. Sokoloff L: The Peripheral Blood Vessels (Orbison JL, Smith DE, eds), Baltimore, Williams & Wilkins Co., 1963, p 297.
39. Winchester R, Kunkel H, Agnello V: Occurrence of γ-globulin complexes in serum and joint fluid of rheumatoid arthritis patients: use of monoclonal rheumatoid factors as reagents for their demonstration. J Exp Med 134: 286s, 1971.
40. Meltzer M, Franklin EC: Cryoglobulinemia—a study of 29 patients. I. IgG and IgM cryoglobulins and factors affecting cryoprecipitability. Am J Med 40: 837, 1966.
41. Fauci AS, Wolff SM: Wegener's granulomatosis: studies in eighteen patients and a review of the literature. Medicine (Baltimore) 52: 535, 1973.
42. Russell RWR: Giant cell arteritis. Q J Med 28: 471, 1959.

Immunodeficiency, Xanthomas and Obstructive Liver Disease

J. NEVIN ISENBERG, M.D., Ph.D.*
RUSSELL F. HANSON, M.D., Ph.D.
GAIL C. WILLIAMS, M.S.
JAMES ZAVORAL, M.D.
ARTHUR R. PAGE, M.D.
HARVEY L. SHARP, M.D.
Minneapolis, Minnesota

Chronic obstructive liver disease and secondary hyperlipidemia developed in an immunodeficient boy. Sequential addition of cholestyramine and phenobarbital to his medical regimen, following an initial response to bile drainage, resulted in the disappearance of xanthomas and pruritus, and the restoration of normal serum concentrations of lipids and bile acids. This improvement may result from shifting the bile acid pool from the peripheral blood compartment to the enterohepatic circulation.

The prevalence of liver disease in immunodeficiency syndromes is low compared to disorders of the gastrointestinal tract [1,2]. Initial reports emphasized the fatal outcome of patients who had findings compatible with viral hepatitis [3,4]. Subsequent case reports have dealt with chronic liver diseases in persons with a variety of immunodeficiencies [5,6]. We wish to report the clinical, pathologic and bile acid alterations before and after therapy in a young immunodeficient man with striking hyperlipidemia.

CASE REPORT

During his first eight years of life, this patient experienced multiple recurrent pyogenic infections of the lung and soft tissues for which he required prolonged hospitalizations for parenteral antibiotic therapy and local treatment. He was the fifth child and only male in a family that had no other history of increased susceptibility to infections or liver diseases. The childhood viral illnesses, mumps and varicella, were handled without complication.

At eight years and eight months of age, his serum electrophoretic pattern showed a very low gamma globulin peak (0.24 g/100 ml). The quantitative immunoglobulin analysis confirmed a deficiency in immunoglobulin G (IgG) (11 mg/100 ml) and immunoglobulin A (IgA) (0 mg/100 ml) with normal immunoglobulin M (IgM) (120 mg/100 ml). Despite the administration of intramuscular gamma globulin, inadequate levels of IgG were obtained, his pulmonary status deteriorated and he was referred to this hospital.

Admitted with moderate respiratory distress and hepatosplenomegaly attributed to cor pulmonale, he progressed to respiratory failure and required mechanical support. With vigorous respiratory care, antibiotic therapy and infusion of maternal plasma, he recovered. He was discharged on 20 cc gamma globulin every other week and a prophylactic pulmonary regimen including mist tent and bronchial drainage.

The patient first came to the attention of the Pediatric Gastroenterology Section on his fourth admission at eleven and a half years of age. Four months prior to admission (after an extended period free of illness) he had abdominal pain and a fever. Laboratory tests, performed at his local hospital, were

From the Departments of Pediatrics and Medicine, University of Minnesota Hospitals, Minneapolis, Minnesota. This study was supported in part by the Beckman Liver Research Fund, the Lutzi Memorial Fund, Grant AM 15077 (R.F.H.), by a grant (RR-400) from the General Clinical Research Centers Program of the Division of Research Resources, National Institutes of Health, U.S. Public Health Service Grant 5T01-HD-0053-14 (J.N.I.) and The National Foundation. Requests for reprints should be addressed to Dr. Harvey L. Sharp, Box 279, Mayo, University of Minnesota Hospitals, Minneapolis, Minnesota 55455. Manuscript accepted November 20, 1975.

* Present address: UCLA School of Medicine, Department of Pediatrics, Los Angeles, California 90024.

TABLE I Liver Function Studies and Serum Lipid Levels

Laboratory Tests*	Normal Values	a†	b	c	d†	e†	f
Bilirubin (mg/100 ml)	<0.3	2.0	3.2	0.9	0.7	0.6	0.5
Direct /total	1.6	4.0	5.9	1.9	2.5	0.8	0.9
Bile acids (μg/ml)							
Dihydroxy	<2	15	1.8	2.9	5.0	1.6	3.2
Trihydroxy	<3	103	3.5	5.7	19.0	2.6	3.3
OCT (IU/liter)	<45	323‡	. . .	729‡	595‡	724	513
SGOT (IU/liter)	<26.5	95‡	38	102‡	127‡	138	84
AP (IU/liter)	<500	2,003‡	841	1,587‡	1,380	2,022	2,286
γGT (U/liter)	<25	1,835	328‡	. . .	383‡	1,710	1,660
Cholesterol (mg/100 ml)	<283	2,100	948	154	238	214	
(% esters)	(70–78)	. . .	(69)	. . .	. . .	(63)	. . .
Triglycerides (mg/100 ml)	<233	165	1,008	142	197	223	. . .
Phospholipids (mg/100 ml)	<250	2,193	. . .	. . .	404	437	. . .

NOTE: a = On admission. b = Two weeks after operation with complete biliary diversion. c = At time of T tube removal on 12 g cholestyramine daily (7 wk postop). d = Cholestyramine—24 g daily (5 mo postop). e = Same dose cholestyramine (24 g) with phenobarbital blood level >20 μg/ml (11 mo postop). f = Same dose of cholestyramine with phenobarbital blood level 17 μg/ml (17 mo postop).
*OCT = ornithine carbamoyl transferase. SGOT = serum glutamate-oxalacetic transaminase. AP = alkaline phosphatase. γGT = gamma glutamyl transpeptidase.
†Corresponds with a bile acid metabolic study (Table III).
‡Average of two or more values during admission.

consistent with cholestatic liver disease with an elevated serum bilirubin level (2.5 mg/100 ml direct; 4.4 mg/100 ml total) and a serum alkaline phosphatase level proportionately more elevated than were the serum transaminase concentrations. He returned to normal activities despite persistent mild jaundice and noted only mild fatigue until three weeks before admission when he began to have pruritus, and raised yellowish lesions appeared on his palms, soles and buttocks.

Exposures to hepatitis, injections and blood products other than his biweekly gamma globulin shots, and potentially toxic compounds or medications were denied. On physical examination he had scleral icterus, xanthomatous lesions in the palmar and planter creases, and over the buttocks, evidence of excoriation, an enlarged nodular liver, a spleen palpable 4 cm below the costal margin but, surprisingly, no clubbing. Diffuse lymphadenopathy, most evident in the anterior cervical area, was present. Slit-lamp examination of the cornea disclosed no abnormalities.

Liver function studies, serum lipid levels and bile acid concentrations are summarized in Table I, column a. A per-

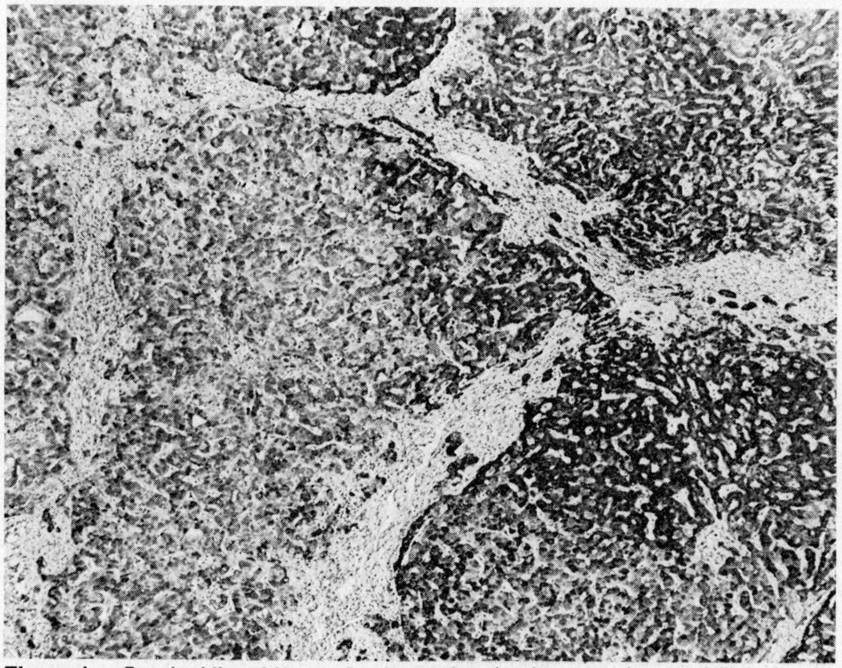

Figure 1. Surgical liver biopsy specimen showing increase in portal fibrosis with extension to adjacent portal areas. The limiting plate remains intact. Periodic acid-Schiff stain; original magnification × 60, reduced by 7 per cent.

cutaneous liver biopsy was performed after the demonstration of normal coagulation parameters. Pathologic changes were noted in the portal areas and parenchymal architecture (Figure 1). Portal areas were more prominent because of the increase in loose connective tissue which contained a variety of inflammatory cells and bile duct proliferation (Figure 2). The limiting plate was intact except for scattered areas in which proliferating bile ducts and inflammatory cells extended into the parenchyma. The hepatocytes, Kupffer cells and bile duct epithelial cells contained lipid-laden vacuoles of varied sizes. Some hepatocytes were arranged in acinar formation around a dilated canaliculus. Both intracellular and extracellular cholestasis were noted. No inclusion bodies were seen at the light or ultrastructural level. A reticulin stain confirmed the impression of cirrhosis. Viral cultures of urine, stool and throat showed no growth. The blood was negative for hepatitis B antigen as well as for viral particles after processing for examination by negative staining under the electron microscope. Alpha feto protein, $alpha_1$ antitrypsin, serum ceruloplasmin, and serum and urine copper levels did not identify an etiology for the hepatic disease. Rheumatoid factor, lupus erythematosus preparation, heterophil titer, plus antismooth muscle and antinuclear antibodies were negative. Antimitochondrial antibodies were positive at the 1:30 dilution. X-ray examination of the entire small bowel and colon was within normal limits as was proctosigmoidoscopy.

When the external biliary tree failed to visualize with a large dose intravenous cholangiogram, a retrograde cholangiographic study was made by Dr. Jack Vennes, Minneapolis Veterans Administration Hospital (Figure 3). The patency of the system was established, but the intrahepatic ducts and the gallbladder could not be visualized. Multiple irregular filling defects were observed along the length of the biliary tree. An exploratory laparotomy was carried out to distinguish between malignancy, an inflammatory process like sclerosing cholangitis, or sludged bile.

At surgery, an enlarged gallbladder was punctured, and watery pale green bile was aspirated. When no outflow of contrast medium from the gallbladder could be demonstrated, the common duct was punctured for dye injection (Figure 4). This study showed patency of the entire biliary system including the gallbladder, but marginal irregularities were prominent. Frozen section of a lymph node showed reactive hyperplasia with histiocytes. A further exploration of the common duct to differentiate between thick tenacious bile and an inflammatory process was undertaken via the cystic duct after cholecystectomy. On palpation, the common duct was described as thickened but not hard. No plaques or stones were identified. Thick bile was aspirated and a T tube was placed for irrigation, drainage and a final cholangiogram which no longer showed marginal irregularities. No inflammatory or malignant changes were noted on histologic examination of specimens from the cystic duct and common duct, but the wall of the gallbladder contained prominent fibrosis and chronic inflammatory cells.

Liver, lymph node, gallbladder and bile specimens obtained at surgery were cultured for aerobic and anaerobic bacteria and viral agents. Hemophilus influenzae was grown in a broth culture of the bile taken from the gallbladder. In the next three weeks, intermittent cultures of bile draining from the T tube also grew out H. influenzae at a time when the patient's pharynx was heavily colonized with the same species. A

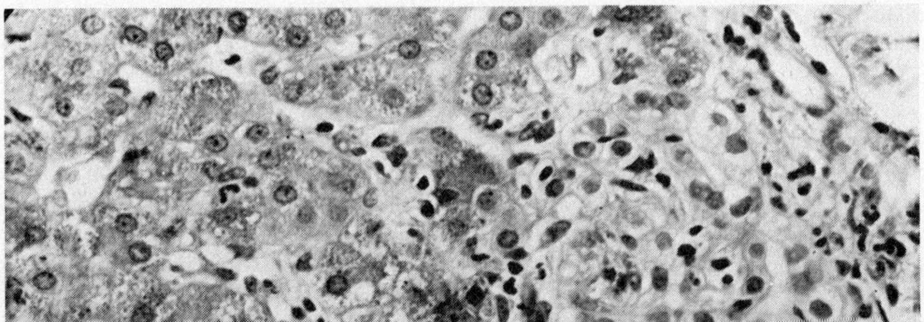

Figure 2. *Percutaneous liver biopsy specimen showing marked bile duct proliferation extending into the parenchyma at the edge of a portal area. Mixed inflammatory cells are present without piecemeal necrosis. Periodic acid-Schiff stain; original magnification × 375, reduced by 7 per cent.*

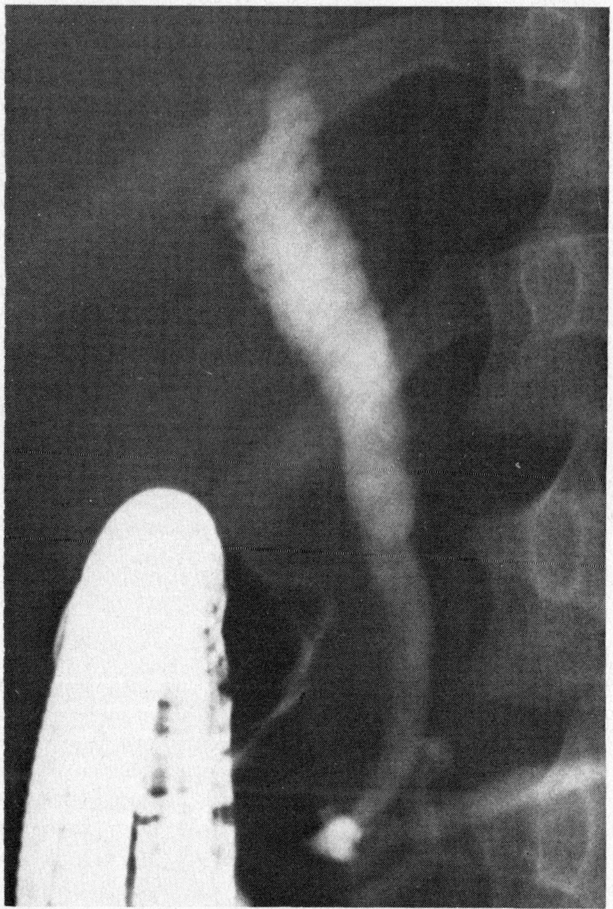

Figure 3. *Retrograde cholangiogram showing mural irregularities without visualization of the gallbladder or intrahepatic bile ducts (courtesy of Dr. Vennes, VA Hospital, Minneapolis, Minnesota).*

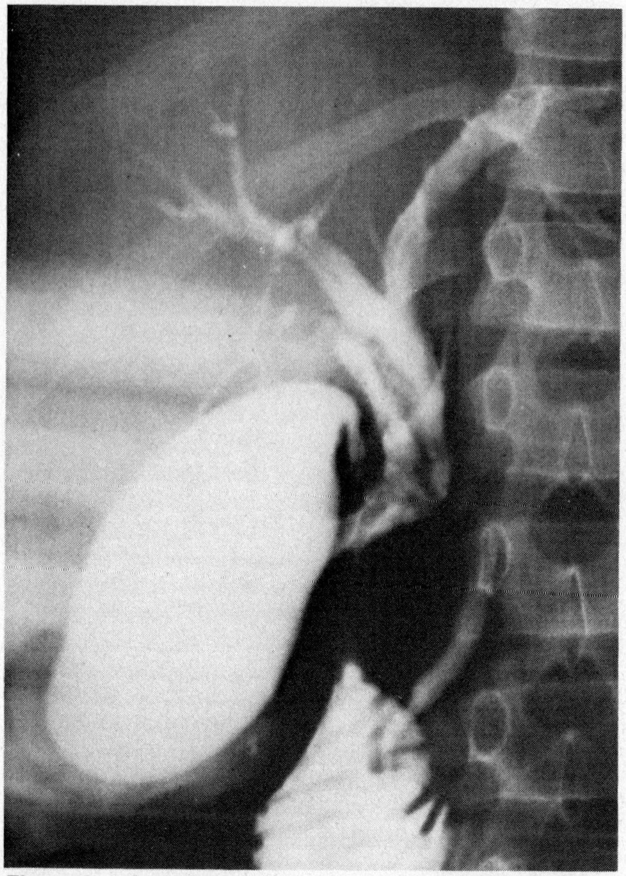

Figure 4. *Operative cholangiogram obtained after puncture of common bile duct demonstrating "pruned-tree silhouette" of intrahepatic bile ducts and normal appearing gallbladder. Free flow of contrast medium into the duodenum is demonstrated.*

percutaneous liver biopsy specimen obtained during this period did not grow out the organism. Counterimmunoelectrophoresis of a bile specimen did not demonstrate Hemophilus antigens (courtesy of Dr. Harry Hill). Various strains of H. influenzae demonstrated little or no growth in the patient's bile. Despite equivocal evidence for the role played by this organism in the patient's biliary tract disease, a three month course of large dose ampicillin therapy was initiated. No recrudescence of symptoms occurred when administration of the antibiotic was stopped, but the patient was rapidly recolonized by Hemophilus species.

During the period of T tube diversion, the patient's liver function studies and hyperlipidemia improved (Table I, column b). Cholestyramine therapy was introduced prior to removal of the T tube and increased to a daily dose of 24 g when the tube was withdrawn. Subsequently, phenobarbital was added to stimulate bile flow and augment the net excretion of cholesterol in the form of its bile acid derivatives. A blood phenobarbital level greater than 20 μg/ml was considered adequate. Laboratory results for these periods are included in Table I, columns c, d and e. Bile acid pool size, production rate and half-life were assessed at each phase of the medical management (see "Special Studies").

Serum concentrations of liver enzymes remained elevated while the bilirubin, bile acid and lipid concentrations were within normal limits (Table I, column e). At the time of his most recent evaluation, his immunologic status was once again assessed (Table II). The lymphadenopathy noted at the outset of his liver disease was now more prominent and included the axillary and inguinal regions. A lymph node was excised from the left axilla for histologic examination and aerobic, anaerobic, fungal and Mycobacterial culture. No organisms were cultured and serum tests for Toxoplasmosis antibodies, histoplasmosis, blastomycosis, coccidiomycosis and febrile agglutinins were negative. Under the microscope, noncaseating granulomas of the epithelioid type were seen without any evidence of lymphomatous change. Special stains failed to demonstrate any organisms. No hilar adenopathy and no granulomatous lesions were seen on the chest film. Furthermore, no granulomas were seen in the percutaneous liver biopsy specimen which demonstrated marked portal fibrosis with reduced inflammatory cell infiltrate.

SPECIAL STUDIES—METHODS AND RESULTS

In order to assess the influences of cholestyramine and phenobarbital therapy on the bile acid pool size and

TABLE II Immunologic Status

I. Humoral system
 A. Immunoglobulins (before a supplemental gamma globulin dose) IgA = 0 mg/100 ml, IgG = 287 mg/100 ml, IgM = 55 mg/100 ml, IgE = 5 IU/ml.
 B. B cells by EAC rosettes = 36 per cent (normal mean 12 per cent).
 C. IgM "B" cells by immunoglobulin staining = 24 per cent (normal range 4.4 to 13 per cent).
 D. Isohemagglutinin titers: Anti A (saline) 1:32, (Coombs) 1:64
 Anti B (saline) 1:4, (Coombs) 1:8
II. Cell-mediated system
 A. Weakly positive skin test — SKSD.
 B. Normal numbers of "T" cells — 1,200 (SR BC binding).
 C. 41 per cent "T" cells (normal 50 to 78 per cent).
 D. Response of lymphocytes to PHA, Con A, mixed lymphocyte culture = 50 per cent of normal.
III. Phagocytic system
 A. Normal white blood count and differential.
 B. Chemotaxis normal.
 C. Hexose monophosphate shunt activity normal.

production rate in this patient with acquired obstructive liver disease and hyperlipidemia, he was given radioisotopically labelled cholic acid and chenodeoxycholic acid on three occasions. After obtaining the informed consent of the patient and his family, 3 to 6 μc of uniformly labelled tritiated (^{3}H)-cholic acid and 24-^{14}C-chenodeoxycholic acid (New England Nuclear) were given orally as the sodium salts for each study. During the second and third studies, cholestyramine was withheld on the initial day to avoid binding of label and fecal loss prior to entry into the pool. All three studies were carried out in the Clinical Research Center while the patient was receiving a low cholesterol diet appropriate for his age.

For each study the bile pool was sampled on five consecutive days by aspiration of 1 to 3 ml of fluid from the duodenum. The bile samples were diluted with ethanol, filtered and evaporated. Hydrolysis was carried out with cholyl glycine hydrolase [7]. After acidification and extraction, the bile acids were methylated, acetylated [8] and quantitated by gas liquid chromatography. Gas liquid chromatography was carried out on a Barber-Colman gas chromatograph (Searle Analytic Corp.), equipped with a hydrogen flame detector and a 1.8 m by 4 mm (ID) U-shaped glass column packed with 0.5 per cent QF-1 on Gas Chrom Q (Applied Science Laboratories). The column and injector were heated to 240°C, and the detector was heated to 260°C. Liquid scintillation counting was used to measure radioactivity. A fluoralloy TLA counting mixture (Beckman Instruments) was used in the counting vials, and quenching and spillover were estimated by adding an internal standard of ^{3}H-toluene and ^{14}C-toluene to the counting vials. The specific activity for each specimen was calculated and computer analysis, employing the method of least squares [9], was used to determine the best fit of the specific activity data to the equation of Linstedt [10], from which pool size and synthesis rate were obtained.

The results of these determinations and the conditions which they reflect are shown in Table III. Cholestyramine reduced the chenodeoxycholic acid pool but the cholate pool doubled. The addition of phenobarbital markedly increased the production rate of chenodeoxycholate and restored the pool size without much effect on cholate metabolism.

COMMENTS

Our patient is classified as having a form of common variable immunodeficiency with reduced "T" cell function and an increased number of "B" cells with reduced or absent ability to synthesize IgA, IgG and IgE, but normal synthesis of IgM antibodies. Whether these patients have an intrinsic "B" cell defect which prohibits maturation to immunoglobin-producing plasma cells or an overactive "T" cell production of a suppressor substance which inhibits this transformation has not been evaluated in sufficient numbers of patients to permit deeper understanding of this phenomenon.

A more complete deficiency of immunoglobulin synthesis was apparently present in the initial four immunodeficient patients who succumbed to hepatitis [3,4]. The cytoplasmic and intranuclear inclusion bodies implicated a viral etiology in two of these patients [4]. Since then, one patient with agammaglobulinemia,

TABLE III Bile Acid Pool Size, Production Rate, Half-Life and Serum Concentration During Sequential Phases of Medical Management

	Cholic Acid				Chenodeoxycholic Acid			
Treatment	Pool Size (mg/m²)	Production Rate (mg/m²/day)	Half-Life (days)	Serum Concentration (μg/ml)	Pool Size (mg/m²)	Production Rate (mg/m²/day)	Half-Life (days)	Serum Concentration (μg/ml)
Base line	144	20	5	103	72	13	3.75	15
Cholestyramine (24 g/day)	329	152	1.5	19	21	30	0.5	5
Cholestyramine plus phenobarbital	375	144	1.8	2.6	79	78	0.7	0.6

persistent hepatitis B antigen and mild liver function has been described. Therefore, viral hepatitis is not uniformly fatal in agammaglobulinemia. In our patient, no viruses have been cultured, serum antiviral antibody titers were not elevated, hepatitis B antigen was not present and neither inclusion bodies nor viral-like particles have been identified at the light or ultrastructural level.

Obstructive jaundice was reported in an eight year old girl with combined immunodeficiency and lymphopenia [6]. An operative cholangiogram demonstrated a stricture of the common bile duct with dilatation of the hepatic ducts and poor filling of their smaller radicals. In contrast, the cholangiograms from our patient and the one described by Williams and co-workers [5] both show a generalized narrowing of the intrahepatic biliary system or "pruned-tree silhouette." This pattern may be found in intrahepatic sclerosing cholangitis and biliary cirrhosis not associated with extrahepatic obstruction [11]. Neither patient was very jaundiced, but both had a marked increase in serum alkaline phosphatase. Our patient had pruritus and hyperlipidemia which were not reported in the patient of Williams et al. [5]. In contrast to our patient's immunoglobulin profile, their patient had increased IgG, low IgA, no detectable IgM and serum isohemagglutinin levels less than 1:4. No antimitochondrial antibodies were detected in her serum, but a high titer of smooth muscle antibody was present. This finding, once thought specific for chronic active hepatitis has since been observed in several entities [12]. Williams et al. concluded that her liver lesion was an intrahepatic sclerosing cholangitis but could find no evidence for the systemic conditions with which this lesion is usually associated [6].

We believe that the lesion in our patient is likewise predominantly the result of an intrahepatic process and that the mural irregularities noted on the cholangiogram were not sufficient to result in partial obstruction and a secondary biliary cirrhosis. Thus, the increased portal fibrosis, marked ductular proliferation and mixed inflammatory cell infiltrate noted must be otherwise explained. Neutrophils, readily found, were never noted within the lumen of a bile duct, and microabscesses were absent. In addition, the lack of fever and the pain in the right upper quadrant present strong evidence against ascending cholangitis. Lymphocytes and plasma cells were seen, but there was no suggestion of germinal center formation. No multinucleated giant cells or epithelioid granulomas have been identified despite the findings in the lymph node removed from our patient. The parenchyma was well preserved except where the limiting plate was invaded by proliferating bile ducts and, very rarely, inflammatory cells.

The biochemical findings of an elevated alkaline phosphatase level, hyperbileacidemia, hyperlipidemia with preserved hepatic synthetic function and only a mildly elevated bilirubin level suggest primary biliary cirrhosis. Yet the age and sex of the patient, and the onset of jaundice several months prior to pruritus, are atypical. Initially, the serum antimitochondrial antibody was elevated to 1:30. All subsequent determinations using the same rat kidney tissue as the in vitro antigen source were negative. Furthermore, despite the normal levels of serum IgM in our patient, the isohemagglutinin titers in saline were low, suggesting that even this immunoglobulin has limited functional significance. Although the evidence for intrinsic biliary cirrhosis was appreciable, the process was not primary biliary cirrhosis in the classic sense. We remain open to the possibility that the changes in the liver and the lymph node were related and that they were the result of this immunodeficient patient's unique response to an infectious agent which has not been identified.

The hyperlipidemia attributed to his obstructive liver disease simulated hyperlipoproteinemia type II. No other members of his family have an abnormal lipid profile. Cholesterol and phospholipids were increased while fasting serum triglyceride concentrations have been within the normal range which is like type IIa. No protein comparable to lipoprotein-X was identified on polyacrylamide electrophoresis.

With a low cholesterol diet and medical management, lipid levels have returned to normal. Lipoprotein electrophoresis has not been repeated. Throughout the course of his disease, our patient has continued to esterify two thirds of the cholesterol levels so that both free and esterified cholesterol levels have been elevated. This pattern has been noted previously in obstructive jaundice in which measurements have shown increased lecithin-cholesterol acyltransferase activity [13].

The use of cholestyramine in the treatment of hypercholesterolemia and its action by interruption of the enterohepatic circulation of bile acids is well known [14]. Cholestyramine relieves pruritus in patients with intrahepatic obstructive liver disease [15]. Phenobarbital enhances the secretion of bile in some of these same patients [16]. Others have noted decreases in serum cholesterol levels in patients with hyperlipidemia and obstructive liver disease [17].

In anticipation that no surgically correctable cause for obstruction would be found and that our patient's pruritus and xanthomatosis would be treated medically, we obtained base line measurements of bile acid pool size and turnover to assess in a step-by-step fashion the effects these agents might have on the metabolism of these excretory products of cholesterol metabolism.

The data for the pool sizes and production rates of the primary bile acids of our patient are shown in Table III. Unfortunately, control values for normal 12 year old subjects have not been reported. However, the bile acid kinetic data observed in our patient are much lower than those reported by Vlahcevic et al. for normal adult men [18], adjusted to a meter squared basis. Our patient's cholic acid (C) pool size (144 mg/m^2) was 25 per cent of that reported for normal adults (600 mg/m^2) and the production rate only 11 per cent, which is consistent with the longer half-life determined (five days) in our patient, in contrast to the 2.2 days noted in normal subjects [18]. The chenodeoxycholic acid (CD) pool size and production rate were both 15 per cent of normal, however, the half-life of 3.75 days is comparable to that seen in normal subjects [18].

Cirrhosis [19] and hyperlipoproteinemia [20,21] have both been shown to alter bile acid metabolism. In 10 patients with alcoholic cirrhosis, Vlahcevic et al. [19] found a 50 per cent reduction in the cholic acid pool, a 75 per cent reduction in the production rate and doubling of the half-life. No significant reduction was noted in the chenodeoxycholic acid pool size, but the production rate was decreased by about 30 per cent and the half-life remained the same when compared to that in normal subjects [19]. The serum bile acid levels and the presence or absence of pruritus was not reported for this group.

Einarrson et al. [20] investigated the bile acid metabolism in patients with various types of hyperlipoproteinemias and demonstrated a reduction in pool size and production rate of cholic acid in persons with type IIa hyperlipoproteinemia. However, the chenodeoxycholic acid pool size and production rate were greater than those in their normal controls. Smaller pool sizes of both primary bile acids were found in the type IIa subgroup with gallbladder disease. When these data are adjusted for surface area differences, they further emphasize the small pool sizes (225 versus 144 mg C/m^2; 308 versus 72 mg CD/m^2) and production rates (185 versus 20 mg C/m^2/day; 108 versus 13 mg CD/m^2/day) of the primary bile acids seen in patients with type II hyperlipoproteinemia with gallbladder disease and our patient, respectively.

The predominance of cholic acid in the serum has previously been noted in obstructive liver disease [15–17,22]. Normal persons have a cholic acid pool size that is slightly larger than that of the chenodeoxycholic acid pool giving a C:CD ratio of approximately 1:0.8 [18]. However, patients with cirrhosis have a pool size ratio of approximately 0.77 [19] and in patients with type IIa hyperlipoproteinemia with gallbladder disease the ratio is approximately 0.73 [20]. Therefore, our patient's serum bile acid pattern and pool size C:CD ratio of 2.0 are consistent with that seen in patients with obstructive liver disease.

Interruption of the enterohepatic circulation of bile acids with cholestyramine in healthy volunteer subjects increases the cholic acid pool size and reduces the chenodeoxycholic acid pool size with a resultant C:CD ratio of 5.6 [23]. Similar changes take place in patients with hyperlipoproteinemia (type II) given cholestyramine [21]. The magnitude of increase in the cholic acid pool size and decrease in chenodeoxycholic acid pool size changes the pretreatment C:CD ratio of less than one to a ratio of 3.4 with treatment [21]. In our patient, the cholic acid predominance became more pronounced with cholestyramine as the pool size doubled while the chenodeoxycholic acid pool size was reduced giving a C:CD ratio of 15. Thus, these three clinical situations, the changes induced by cholestyramine, are consistent irrespective of the clinical state.

The effects of phenobarbital on bile acid metabolism are less predictable. In four healthy human subjects treated with phenobarbital, three demonstrated an increase in cholic acid pool size and production rate and an over-all increase in fecal bile acid loss [24]. Similar increases in chenodeoxycholic acid kinetics were noted in the one patient investigated. The fourth subject did not show any changes in bile acid metabolism and also failed to demonstrate an increase in plasma antipyrine clearance, a technic used to monitor microsomal enzyme induction. Therefore, the changes observed in bile acid kinetics in the three subjects who responded to phenobarbital were attributed to an increase in cholesterol synthesis and induction of enzymes involved in cholesterol catabolism [24].

Watkins et al. [25] have recently published bile acid kinetic data on the human premature infants. The average pool sizes and synthetic rates were only 13.1 mg and 5.6 mg/day, respectively, for cholic acid, and 6.4 mg and 2.6 mg/day, respectively, for chenodeoxycholic acid calculated on a meter square basis. In contrast, the values of a smaller premature infant whose mother had been receiving 120 mg of phenobarbital for the entire pregnancy were 85.8 mg and 26.3 mg/day, respectively, for cholic acid and, 51.4 mg and 15.1 mg/day, respectively, for chenodeoxycholic acid. Thus, phenobarbital increased the pool size and synthesis rates of both primary bile acids.

The reduction of serum bilirubin and bile acid concentrations with relief of pruritus in patients with intrahepatic cholestasis treated with phenobarbital has been reported [16,22]. This observation plus the enhanced bile flow and biliary excretion of bile salts noted in primates treated with phenobarbital [26] would suggest that bile salt pool sizes are reduced or that shifts between a serum compartment and other compartments occur as the result of phenobarbital treatment. Since bile salt synthesis rates and pool sizes are increased despite the increased biliary secretion in the treated monkeys [20], the former hypothesis is not substantiated.

Previous reports of children with cholestasis secondary to intrahepatic paucity of bile ducts or benign recurrent cholestasis has provided evidence that phenobarbital treatment results in a shift of the bile acid pools from the serum to the enterohepatic circulation [16,22,27]. The pool sizes of both primary bile acids in one of these patients were reduced with the phenobarbital therapy [22], in contrast to the other reports [24–26]. However, the proportionate decrease in the serum concentrations of cholic acid and chenodeoxycholic acid was greater than the pool size reductions so that with phenobarbital therapy smaller fractions of both bile acid pools were present in the peripheral blood compartment. In addition, the administration of phenobarbital resulted in an increased fecal excretion of bile acids [22]. The control investigation in this child was 14 days after stopping phenobarbital. Thus, these changes were toward restoration of the normal situation in which 99+ per cent of the bile acids are present in the enterohepatic circulation [22]. The liver lesion in these patients is functionally comparable to that of our patient as it represents an intrahepatic obstruction to bile secretion with preservation of parenchymal function.

Increased production and pool size were measured for both bile acids when phenobarbital was added to the medical regimen of our patient and the serum bile acid concentrations returned to normal (Table III). The C:CD ratio (4.7) was reduced and reflects the greater influence of phenobarbital on chenodeoxycholic acid production in this patient. Prior to treatment, nearly 100 per cent of the cholic acid pool was present in peripheral blood. When the patient was receiving cholestyramine, that proportion was reduced to 8.5 per cent and restored to normal (1 per cent) with the addition of phenobarbital. The effect of phenobarbital on the chenodeoxycholic acid pool size and synthesis rate was less dramatic as noted in the earlier report [22].

REFERENCES

1. Brown WR, Butterfield D, Savage D, Tada T: Clinical microbiological and immunological studies in patients with immunoglobulin deficiencies and gastrointestinal disorders. Gut 13: 441, 1972.
2. Ament ME, Ochs HD, Davis SD: Structure and function of the gastrointestinal tract in primary immunodeficiency syndromes—a study of 39 patients. Medicine (Baltmore) 52: 227, 1973.
3. Janeway CA, Gitlin D: The gamma globulins. Advances in Pediatrics, vol 9 (Levine SZ, ed). Chicago, Year Book Publishers, Inc., 1957, p 105.
4. Good RA, Page AR: Fatal complications of virus hepatitis in two patients with agammaglobulinemia. Am J Med 29: 804, 1960.
5. Record CO, Eddleston ALWF, Shilkin KB, Williams R: Intrahepatic sclerosing cholangitis associated with familial immunodeficiency syndrome. Lancet 2: 18, 1973.
6. Thomas IT, Ochs KD, Wedgwood RJ: Liver disease and immunodeficiency syndromes. Lancet 1: 311, 1974.
7. Nair PP, Gordon M, Rebach J: The enzymatic clearance of the carbon nitrogen bond in 3α, 7α, 12α-trihydroxy-5 β-cholan-24-oylglycine. J Biol Chem 242: 7, 1967.
8. Roovers S, Evrard E, Vanderhaeghe H: An improved method for measuring human blood bile acids. Clin Chim Acta 19: 449, 1968.
9. Brevington PR: Least squares fit to an arbitrary function. Data Reduction and Error Analysis for the Physical Sciences, New York, McGraw-Hill, 1969, p 204.
10. Lindstedt S: The turnover of cholic acid in man. Acta Physiol Scand 40: 1, 1957.
11. Lefton HB, Winkelman EI: Endoscopic retrograde cholangiographic evaluation of sclerosing cholangitis. Clev Clin Quart 41: 143, 1974.
12. Doniach D, Walker G: Immunopathology of liver disease. Progress in Liver Diseases, vol 4 (Popper H, Schaffner F, eds). New York, Grune & Stratton, Inc., 1972, p. 387.
13. Kepkay DL, Poon R, Simon JB: Lecithin-cholesterol acyltransferase and serum cholesterol esterification in obstructive jaundice. J Lab Clin Med 81: 172, 1973.
14. Grundy SM: Treatment of hypercholesterolemia by interference with bile acid metabolism. Arch Intern Med 130: 638, 1972.
15. Sharp HL, Carey JB Jr, White JG, Krivit W: Cholestyramine therapy in patients with a paucity of intrahepatic bile ducts. J Pediatr 71: 723, 1967.
16. Sharp HL, Mirkin BL: Effect of phenobarbital on hyperbilirubinemia, bile acid metabolism and microsomal enzyme activity in chronic intrahepatic cholestasis of childhood. J Pediatr 81: 116, 1972.
17. Linarelli LG, Hengstenberg FH, Drash AL: Effect of phenobarbital on hyperlipemia in patients with intrahepatic and extrahepatic cholestasis. J Pediatr 83: 291, 1973.
18. Vlahcevic ZR, Miller SR, Farrar JT, Swell L: Kinetics and pool size of primary bile acids in man. Gastroenterology 61: 85, 1971.
19. Vlahcevic ZR, Juttijudata P, Bell CC Jr, Swell L: Bile acid metabolism in patients with cirrhosis. II. Cholic and chenodeoxycholic acid metabolism. Gastroenterology 62: 1174, 1972.
20. Einarrson K, Hellstrom K, Kallner M: Bile acid kinetics in relation to sex, serum lipids, body weights and gallbladder disease in patients with various types of hyperlipoproteinemia. J Clin Invest 54: 1301, 1974.
21. Einarrson K, Hellstrom K, Kallner M: The effect of cholestyramine on the elimination of cholesterol as bile acids in patients with hyperlipoproteinemia type II and type IV. Europ J Clin Invest 4: 405, 1974.
22. Stiehl A, Thaler MM, Admirand WH: Effects of phenobarbital on bile salt metabolism in cholestasis due to intrahepatic bile duct hypoplasia. Pediatrics 51: 992, 1973.
23. Garbutt JT, Kenney TJ: Effect of cholestyramine on bile acid metabolism in normal man. J Clin Invest 51: 2781, 1972.
24. Miller NE, Nestel PJ: Altered bile acid metabolism during treatment with phenobarbitone. Clin Sci Molec Med 45: 257, 1973.
25. Watkins JB, Szczepanik P, Gould JB: Bile salt metabolism in the human premature infant. Preliminary observations of pool size and synthesis rate following prenatal administration of dexamethasone and phenobarbital. Gastroenterology 69: 706, 1975.
26. Redinger RN, Small DM: The effect of phenobarbital upon bile salt synthesis and pool size, biliary lipid secretion and bile composition. J Clin Invest 52: 161, 1973.
27. Stiehl A, Thaler MM, Admirand WH: The effects of phenobarbital on bile salts and bilirubin in patients with intrahepatic and extrahepatic cholestasis. N Engl J Med 286: 858, 1972.

Goodpasture's Syndrome in a Patient with the Nail-Patella Syndrome

JOHN J. CURTIS, M.D.
DINYAR BHATHENA, M.D.
RICHARD P. LEACH, M.D.
JOHN H. GALLA, M.D.
BRUCE A. LUCAS, M.D.
ROBERT G. LUKE, M.B., ChB.
Lexington, Kentucky

A patient with the nail-patella syndrome in whom end-stage renal failure developed as the result of Goodpasture's syndrome is described. Lesions characteristic of both rare diseases were seen on renal morphology. It is postulated that the glomerular membrane alteration of the nail-patella syndrome predisposed to the development of antiglomerular basement membrane antibody and hence Goodpasture's syndrome. A review of the incidence of renal failure in the nail-patella syndrome suggests that renal involvement can no longer be regarded as benign and that immune mechanisms may be related to progressive renal disease in some cases.

The glomerular basement membrane (GBM) is the primary site of injury in the renal disease associated both with Goodpasture's syndrome and with the nail-patella syndrome. We have observed a patient in whom Goodpasture's syndrome, with the classic clinical, immunologic and histologic findings, developed in a setting of the nail-patella syndrome. Despite widespread and severe glomerular destruction we were able to demonstrate the recently described characteristic renal lesion of the nail-patella syndrome [1] in this patient's GBM.

Considerable evidence [2,3] exists that anti-GBM antibody plays an important pathogenetic role in the glomerular and pulmonary alveolar damage characteristic of Goodpasture's syndrome, but the events leading to development of this antibody remain unknown. We postulate that an abnormal basement membrane, associated with the nail-patella syndrome, predisposed to development of anti-GBM antibody and Goodpasture's syndrome.

CASE REPORT

The patient is a 17 year old white male janitor from Eastern Kentucky. Since birth, he and his family had noted dysplastic fingernails and unusual-looking knees (Figure 1). Several of his cousins have similar abnormalities. He was otherwise in good health until two months before admission to the University of Kentucky Medical Center (UKMC). At that time he had a febrile illness with sore throat and malaise. One week later he noted increasing weakness and ankle edema. Over the next week, the edema increased and he noted "Coke-colored" urine. One week before his UKMC admission he saw a physician in his hometown who admitted him to the local hospital. During the hospitalization slight hemoptysis developed. He was told that he had "kidney failure" and was referred to us.

On admission to UKMC, physical examination revealed a pale, slightly agitated, young man in moderate respiratory distress. Vital signs included a blood pressure of 150/80 mm Hg, pulse rate of 110/min, respiratory rate

From the Nephrology Division of the Department of Medicine, the Urology Division of the Department of Surgery and the Department of Pathology of the University of Kentucky Medical Center, Lexington, Kentucky. Requests for reprints should be addressed to Dr. John Curtis, Department of Medicine, University of Kentucky Medical Center, 800 Rose Street, Lexington, Kentucky 40506.
Manuscript accepted November 20, 1975.

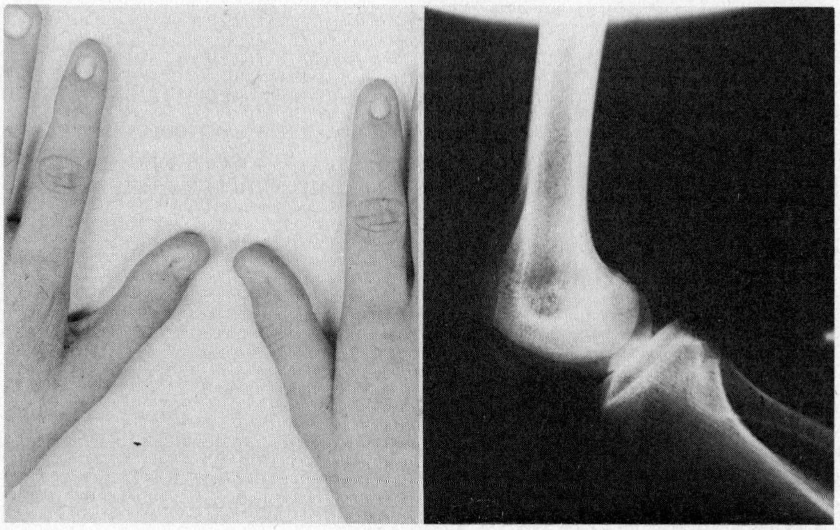

Figure 1. *The characteristic fingernail (anonychia) and patella (dysplastic or absent) lesions of the nail-patella syndrome are demonstrated in our case.*

of 25/min and temperature of 36.7°C. Rales were heard at the bases of both lungs. A 2/6 systolic ejection murmur was heard at the cardiac apex. Four plus edema of the extremities, anonychia of the fingernails and dysplasia of patellas were present.

On admission the hemoglobin level was 5.9 g/100 mg, red blood cell indices were normal, and the total white blood cell count was 14,000/mm^3. Reticulocyte count, platelet count, prothrombin time and partial thromboplastin time were all within normal limits. Stool guaiac test was trace positive. Blood urea nitrogen was 186 mg/dl and serum creatinine 7.2

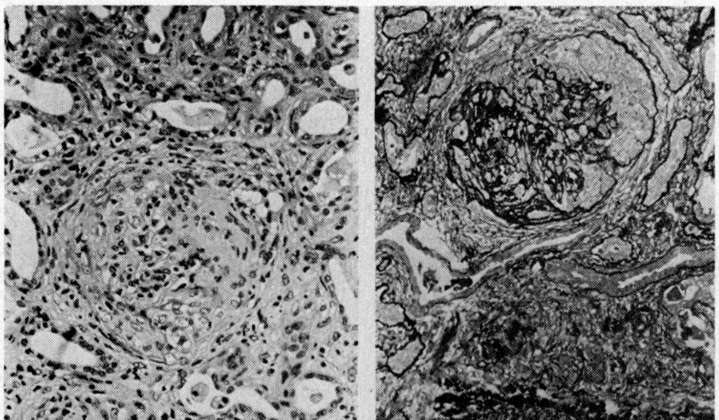

Figure 2. ***A,*** *photomicrograph of a typical glomerulus showing crescent formation. Note the tubular atrophy. Hematoxylin and eosin stain; magnification ×200, from an original color (Ektachrome) transparency, reduced by 11 per cent.* ***B,*** *photomicrograph of silver-stained renal tissue to illustrate the "skeleton morphology" of altered glomerular structure. Below is an unaltered artery. Periodic acid-silver methenamine methods stain; magnification ×200, from an original color (Ektachrome) transparency, reduced by 11 per cent.*

mg/dl. Serum sodium was 141 meq/liter, potassium 9.0 meq/liter, bicarbonate 14 meq/liter and chloride 111 meq/liter. Urinalysis demonstrated a specific gravity of 1.010, pH of 6, 4+ protein, and too numerous to count red blood cells, white blood cells and granular casts per high power field. An electrocardiogram demonstrated sinus tachycardia with tall, peaked T waves in the precordial leads and small, nearly absent, P waves. A chest film demonstrated bilateral hilar infiltrates.

Emergency treatment of hyperkalemia was instituted and peritoneal dialysis was begun. Over the next 12 hours the dialysis ran smoothly and more than 2 liters of fluid were removed. Serum potassium returned to normal. Nevertheless, several hours later marked hemoptysis developed and the arterial oxygen tension (PO_2) fell to 34 mm Hg. A chest film showed marked increase of the bilateral infiltrates. Examination of the sputum revealed hemosiderin-laden macrophages. An endotracheal tube was inserted and assisted respiration was begun. Intravenous methylprednisone (1,000 mg) was given. A Swan-Ganz catheter was inserted and left atrial pressure was not increased. An emergency kidney biopsy was performed which disclosed diffuse proliferative extracapillary glomerulonephritis (Figure 2). Immunofluorescent studies revealed strongly positive linear staining of all GBMs for immunoglobulin G (IgG) and beta$_1$C along with fibrin in the epithelial crescents (Figure 3). Despite assisted respiration with 100 per cent oxygen, steroid therapy and further volume depletion via hypertonic dialysate, arterial PO_2 could not be maintained above 40 mm Hg and brisk hemoptysis continued. An emergency bilateral nephrectomy was performed, following which an immediate improvement in respiratory function was noted. Hemoptysis ceased and the endotracheal tube was removed 24 hours later.

Serum anti-GBM antibody was present in high titer. A roentgenogram of the hips was characteristic of the nail-patella syndrome (Figure 4). Antinuclear antibody, anti-DNA antibody and lupus erythematosus preparations were all negative. A test for Australia antigen was negative. Serum

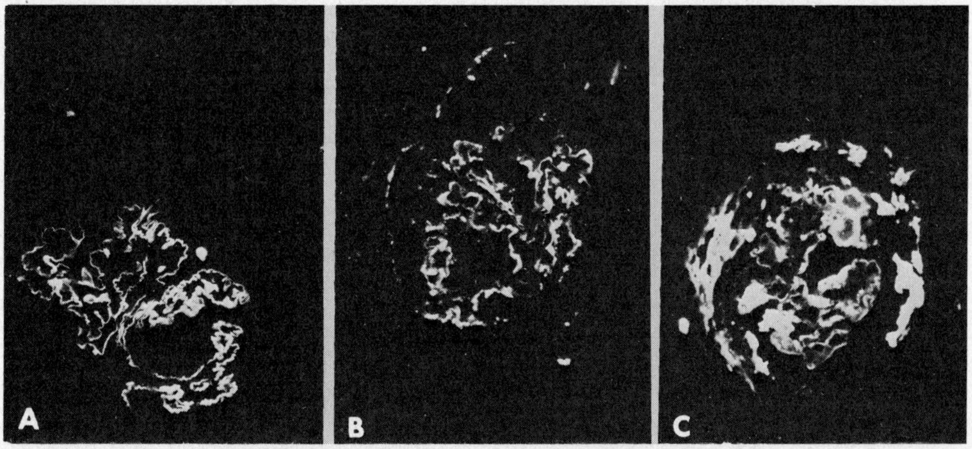

Figure 3. *A, immunofluorescence photomicrograph depicting bright linear fluorescence for IgG along peripheral GBM. Note the discontinuities in the GBM. Portions of GBM show "wrinkling collapse." Magnification ×200, from an original color (Ektachrome, tungsten) transparency, reduced by 11 per cent.* ***B,*** *immunofluorescence photomicrograph depicting predominantly linear fluorescence for beta$_1$C along peripheral GBM. A portion of Bowman's capsule also stains, with an intervening unstained zone representing a crescent. Magnification ×200, from an original color (Ektachrome, tungsten) transparencey, reduced by 11 per cent.* ***C,*** *immunofluorescence photomicrograph depicting fibrin deposition in a glomerulus. Much of the fibrin lies in the crescent, but some is also seen in the glomerular tuft. Magnification ×200, from an original color (Ektachrome, tungsten) transparency, reduced by 11 per cent.*

iron level was 45 μg/dl and total iron-binding capacity was 180 μg/dl. Electron microscopy of renal biopsy material revealed abnormal collagen-like fibers in the GBM consistent with the lesion characteristic of the nail-patella syndrome [1] (Figure 5).

The patient had an uneventful recovery from surgery and is currently receiving long-term hemodialysis awaiting a cadaver kidney transplant. He has had no further episodes of hemoptysis, and pulmonary function studies are within normal limits.

METHODS

For study by immunofluorescence technics, frozen sections 2 to 4 μ thick were cut from freshly collected, snap-frozen (−70°C) tissue blocks embedded in optimum cutting temperature compound (Ames). Staining was performed by the direct method using commercially-prepared, fluorescein-conjugated (Meloy) goat antiserums each of human IgG, beta$_1$C, IgA, IgM and fibrin, and whose individual optimum staining dilutions were predetermined and specificities tested by immunoelectrophoretic and Ouchterlony double diffusion procedures.

Histologic slides included 1 to 2 μ thick sections stained by hematoxylin and eosin, periodic acid-Schiff and periodic acid-silver methenamine methods, the last having the Masson trichrome counterstain.

Thin sections for electron microscopic studies were prepared from Epon-embedded, glutaraldehyde-fixed, osmium post-fixed fresh tissue cubes and double stained with lead citrate-uranyl acetate by standard procedures. Additionally, staining with phosphotungstic acid was performed on selected grids according to the method of Marinozzi [4].

Serum anti-GBM antibody was determined by indirect immunofluorescence assay [3] in the laboratory of Dr. Richard J. Glassock. Serum was 4+ positive for anti-GBM antibody undiluted, and 3+ positive at a 1 to 4 dilution.

COMMENT

This patient demonstrated all the characteristic features of Goodpasture's syndrome as detailed by Benoit et al. [5] and Bach et al. [6]. The dramatic resolution of the pulmonary infiltrates and increase in arterial oxygen saturation after bilateral nephrectomy have been previously documented [7–10].

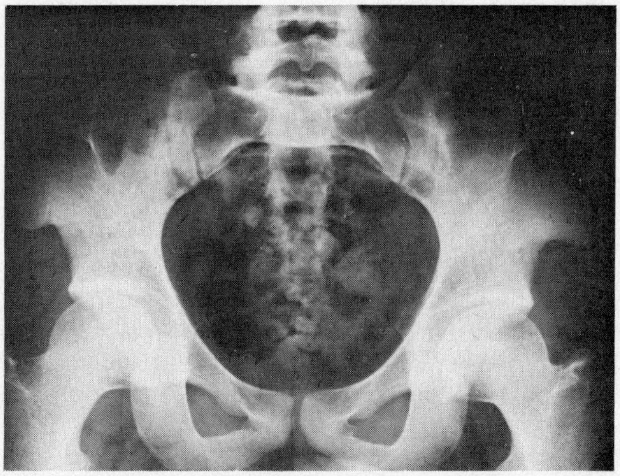

Figure 4. *Roentgenogram of patient's pelvis—note iliac horns.*

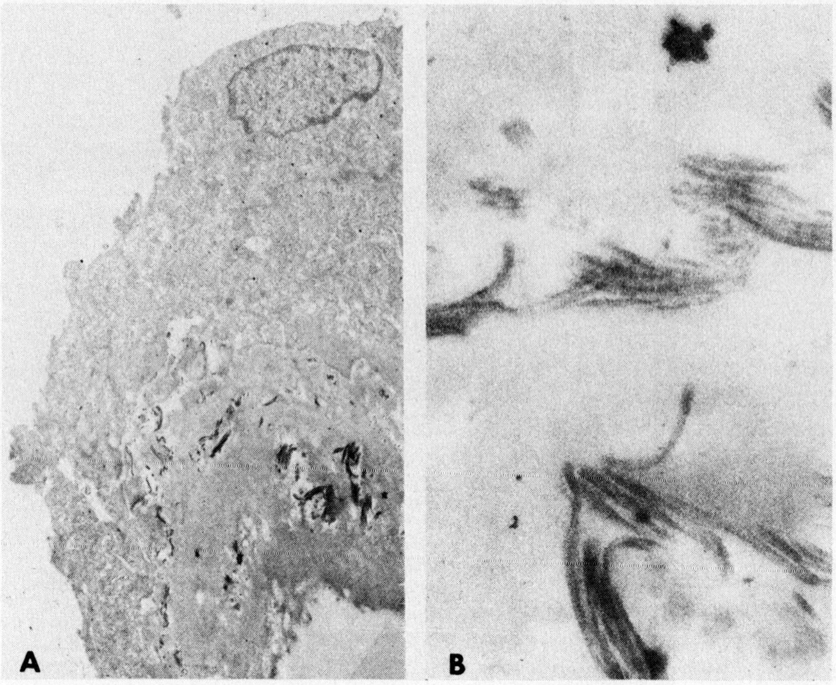

***Figure 5.** **A,** electronmicrograph showing phosphotungstic acid-positive (darkly stained) fibers within the peripheral basement membrane of a patent glomerular capillary loop. Many fiber-bundles lie in electron-lucent pockets within the lamina densa of the somewhat irregular peripheral GBM. These findings were not visible in the regular (lead citrate-uranyl acetate) stained sections. **B,** electronmicrograph depicting, at high magnification, detailed ultrastructure of the phosphotungstic acid-positive fibers shown in A. Note the cross striations whose periodicity was distinct from that of fibrin, which, however, was seen in other locations in lead citrate-uranyl acetate stained sections of glomeruli. Phosphotungstic acid stain; magnification × 6,600 approx. (A), × 5,600 approx. (B), reduced by 25 per cent.*

Considerable evidence has been accumulated that the pathogenic mechanism responsible for the necrotizing inflammation in glomeruli and hemorrhage in the lung is related to the deposition of anti-GBM antibody with linear staining of IgG and complement in glomeruli. This antibody may also attack the lung because of a similarity in the antigenicity of glomerular and alveolar basement membrane [2,11]. An etiologic relationship between the antibody and glomerular damage has been suggested by elution of anti-GBM antibody and reproduction of glomerulonephritis in animals given injections of the eluted antibody [3,12].

Although the deposition of complement-fixing antibody appears to be an important mechanism in producing glomerular necrosis, the factors influencing the development of such an antibody are unknown [13]. In many cases hemoptysis antedates the development of the renal lesion by considerable periods of time, up to seven years [14], suggesting that development of the antibody may be related to primary events in the lung. Indeed Duncan et al. [15] speculated that influenza may be an important etiologic factor in some cases, perhaps releasing alveolar basement membrane into the circulation. In a recently reported case [16], classic membranous glomerulonephritis, which had been followed for several years and documented by renal biopsy, was complicated by the development of rapidly progressive glomerulonephritis. Although linear fluorescence to IgG was not demonstrated, as it is in our case, serum anti-GBM antibody was present. These investigators speculated that with the constant deposition of immune complexes on the basement membrane, GBM antigen was released into the circulation leading to the development of anti-GBM antibody and the secondary complication of rapidly progressive glomerulonephritis. Sternlieb and co-workers [17] suggested that d-penicillamine may have been the agent that induced anti-GBM antibody formation in three patients with Wilson's disease. Lewis et al. [13] discuss four possible mechanisms for the development of anti-GBM antibody: (1) altered native GBM antigen, (2) altered immune system access to normal GBM antigen, (3) antibody capable of cross reacting with normal GBM antigen formed via immune system exposure to nonrenal endogenous antigen (e.g., lung alveolar basement membrane antigen), (4) antibody capable of cross reacting with normal GBM antigen formed via immune system exposure to antigens in the cell walls of bacteria. Thus, although the mechanisms for development of anti-GBM antibody are unknown, investigators have suggested viruses, bacteria, drugs, diseased GBM, abnormal GBM exposure to the immune system and various immune system cross reaction models as possible explanations.

The nail-patella syndrome, first described by Little in 1897 [18], is rare and in a recent review of the literature by Simila there were only 52 cases with renal involvement [19]. In early reports the renal lesion was considered to be relatively benign and usually manifested only by asymptomatic proteinuria. However, end-stage renal failure has developed in at least 21 patients with the nail-patella syndrome [1,18–28]; four others have required kidney transplants [28,30,31]. Thus, this form of renal disease can no longer be considered benign. Our patient fulfulls the diagnostic criteria for the nail-patella syndrome, including the presence of iliac horns which are pathognomonic [32].

The presence of fibrillar collagen-like material in the GBM is considered specific for the nail-patella syndrome by several investigators [1,23,33,34]. Hoyer et al. [1] have postulated that the renal involvement may occur as a result of an abnormality of connective tissue metabolism with abnormal collagen fibers trapped in the GBM or, perhaps, the basement membrane itself is metabolized abnormally. Both Hoyer et al. [1] and Bennett et al. [23] have reported results of immunofluorescent studies of renal tissue from patients with the nail-patella syndrome. Although these investigators demonstrated positive immunofluorescent staining (usually trace positive focal and local beta$_1$C in differing locations and patterns), none thought there was strong evidence for immunologic mediation of this disease. In our case, unlike those of Hoyer and Bennett, strongly positive linear fluorescence of both IgG and beta$_1$C was associated with a high titer of anti-GBM antibody. Unfortunately, in most of the previously reported cases of nail-patella syndrome that have progressed to end-stage kidney disease, there is no record of immunofluorescent renal studies. What role, if any, the immune system plays in those cases in which renal function is deteriorating is not known.

Our case demonstrates the occurrence of two rare syndromes in the same patient. Even though the site of injury to the kidney is the same for both of these disease processes, it is possible that this represents only coincidence. The other possibility is that in some way the two processes are related. Current theories concerning Goodpasture's syndrome do not explain how the GBM triggers an attack via the immune system. Moreover theories as to the cause of the nail-patella syndrome do not explain the presence of the immunofluorescent findings noted. It is attractive to speculate that the diffuse connective tissue disorder in our patient resulted in either disturbed antigenicity or abnormal exposure of the GBM and thus eventually led to the development of Goodpasture's syndrome.

ACKNOWLEDGMENT

We are indebted to Mrs. Bernadine Jones and Mrs. Merle Wekstein for their technical assistance.

ADDENDUM

Since submission of the original manuscript, we have followed the patient's serum anti-GBM antibody. Four months after bilateral nephrectomy his antibody titer fell to only 1+ positive (undiluted) and he received a cadaver kidney transplant. His serum creatinine is currently 1.4 mg/dl and his 24 hour urine protein is less than 200 mg. Based on the case report of Uranga et al. [31] we have rapidly reduced the steroid dosage in our patient in hopes of avoiding aseptic necrosis of his hips. At present, he has no evidence of that complication, any further respiratory difficulties or recurrence of either renal disease.

REFERENCES

1. Hoyer JR, Michael AF, Vernier RL: Renal disease in nail-patella syndrome: clinical and morphologic studies. Kidney Int 2: 231, 1972.
2. McPhaul JJ, Dixon FJ: Characterization of human anti-glomerular basement membrane antibodies eluted from glomerulonephritic kidneys. J Clin Invest 491: 308, 1970.
3. Lerner RA, Glassock RJ, Dixon FJ: The role of anti-glomerular basement membrane antibody in the pathogenesis of human glomerulonephritis. J Exp Med 126: 989, 1967.
4. Marinozzi V: The role of fixation in electron staining. J Roy Microscopical Soc 81: 141, 1963.
5. Benoit FL, Rulon DB, Theil GB, Doolan PD, Watten RH: Goodpasture's syndrome. A clinicopathologic enity. Am J Med 37: 424, 1964.
6. Bach J, Dardenne M, Hinglais N, Mahieu P: Role of anti-basement membrane immunity in human glomerulonephritis, Chap 5. Advances in Nephrology (Hamburger J, Crosnier J, Maxwell MH, eds), Chicago, Year Book Medical Publishers, 1972.
7. Maddack RK, Stevens LE, Reemtsma K, Bloomer HA: Goodpasture's syndrome: cessation of pulmonary hemorrhage after bilateral nephrectomy. Ann Intern Med 67: 1258, 1967.
8. Nowokowski A, Grove RB, Kind LH, Antonovych TT, Fortner RW, Kniesser MR, Carter CB, Knepshield JH: Goodpasture's syndrome: recovery from severe pulmonary hemorrhage after bilateral nephrectomy. Ann Intern Med 75: 243, 1971.
9. Siegel RR: The basis of pulmonary disease resolution after

nephrectomy in Goodpasture's syndrome. Am J Med Sci 259: 201, 1970.
10. Halgrimson CG, Wilson CB, Dixon FJ, Penn I, Anderson JT, Ogden DA, Starzl TE: Goodpasture's syndrome, treatment with nephrectomy and renal transplantation. Arch Surg 103: 283, 1971.
11. Koffler D, Sandson J, Carr R, Kunkel HG: Immunologic studies concerning the pulmonary lesions in Goodpasture's syndrome. Am J Pathol 54: 293, 1969.
12. Unanue ER, Dixon FJ: Experimental allergic glomerulonephritis induced in the rabbit with heterologous renal antigens. J Exp Med 125: 149, 1967.
13. Lewis EJ, Cavallo T, Harrington JT, Cotran RS: An immunopathologic study of rapidly progressive glomerulonephritis in the adult. Human Pathol 2: 185, 1971.
14. Scheer RL, Grossman MA: Immune aspects of the glomerulonephritis associated with pulmonary hemorrhage. Ann Intern Med 60: 1009, 1964.
15. Duncan DA, Drummond KM, Michael AF, Vernier RL: Pulmonary hemorrhage and glomerulonephritis. Ann Intern Med 62: 920, 1965.
16. Klassen J, Elwood C, Grossberg AL, Milgrom F, Montes M, Sepulveda M, Andres GA: evolution of membranous nephropathy into anti-glomerular basement membrane glomerulonephritis. N Engl J Med 290: 1340, 1974.
17. Sternlieb I, Bennett B, Scheinburg IH: D-Penicillamine induced Goodpasture's syndrome in Wilson's disease. Ann Intern Med 82: 773, 1975.
18. Little EM: Congenital absence or delayed development of the patella. Lancet 2: 78, 1897.
19. Simila S, Vesa L, Wasz-Hockert O: Hereditary onycho-osteodysplasia (the nail-patella syndrome) with nephrosis-like renal disease in a newborn boy. Pediatrics 46: 61, 1970.
20. Hawkins CF, Smith OE: Renal dysplasia in a family with multiple hereditary abnormalities including iliac horns. Lancet 1: 803, 1950.
21. Baixey AM, Burke RM: Arthro onychodysplasia. Am J Med 8: 738, 1950.
22. Wright LA, Herbert FL: Fatal renal disease associated with hereditary osteo-onychodysplasia. Southern Med J 62: 833, 1969.
23. Bennett WM, Musgrave JE, Campbell RA, Elliot D, Cox R, Brooks RE, Lovrien EW, Beals RK, Porter GA: The nephropathy of the nail-patella syndrome. Am J Med 54: 304, 1973.
24. Darlington D, Hawkins CF: Nail-patella syndrome with iliac horns and hereditary nephropathy. J Bone Joint Surg 49: 164, 1967.
25. Leahy MS: The hereditary nephropathy of osteo-onychodysplasia. Am J Dis Child 112: 237, 1966.
26. Jameson RJ, Lawher SD, Renwick JH: Nail-patella syndrome: clinical and linkage data on family G. Ann Hum Genet 20: 348, 1956.
27. Hakosolo J, Simila S, Vesa L, Jarvi J: Renal abnormalities in hereditary onycho-osteodysplasia. Ann Paediat Fenn 14: 55, 1968.
28. Eisenberg KS, Potter DE, Bovill EG: Osteo-onychodystrophy with nephropathy and renal osteodystrophy. A case report. J Bone Joint Surg 54-A: 1301, 1972.
29. Schroeder G: Osteo-onychodysplasia Heredtaria Z. Menschl Vererb Konstitutional 36: 42, 1961.
30. Organ Transplant Registry, Personal communication, Chicago, August 8, 1975.
31. Uranga VM, Simmons RL, Hoyer JR, Kjellstrand CM, Buselmeier TJ, Najarian TS: Renal transplantation for the nail-patella syndrome. Am J Surg 125: 777, 1973.
32. Carbonara P, Alpert M: Hereditary osteo-onychodysplasia. Am J Med Sci 248: 138, 1964.
33. Morita T, Laughlin LO, Kawano K, Kimmelstiel P, Suzuki Y, Churg J: Nail-patella syndrome. Arch Intern Med 131: 271, 1973.
34. Ben-Bassat M, Cohen L, Rosenfelt J: The glomerular basement membrane in the nail-patella syndrome. Arch Pathol 92: 350, 1971.

The Appearance of Nonlinear Deposits of Immunoglobulins in Goodpasture's Syndrome

LAWRENCE C. Y. AGODOA, M.D.
GARY E. STRIKER, M.D.
Seattle, Washington

C. R. P. GEORGE, M.D.*
Seattle, Washington

RICHARD GLASSOCK, M.D.
Los Angeles, California

LEONARD J. QUADRACCI, M.D.
Seattle, Washington

A twenty year old woman presented with pulmonary hemorrhage and glomerulonephritis with linear deposition of IgG on the glomerular capillary basement membrane, and high titer of antiglomerular basement membrane antibody in her serum. Without treatment, renal function, which was transiently impaired, has improved, pulmonary hemorrhage subsided, and repeat renal biopsies have revealed the appearance of nonlinear in addition to the linear deposition of IgG on the glomerular capillary basement membrane in the face of diminished serum antiglomerular basement membrane antibody titer.

The poor prognosis of glomerulonephritis with pulmonary hemorrhage and antiglomerular basement membrane antibodies (Goodpasture's syndrome) has often been recorded in the literature. However, spontaneous remission [1–5] or apparent response to steroids or immunosuppressive agents has been reported [6–9]. The diagnosis of the syndrome has been based on the clinical presentation of pulmonary hemorrhage, with antiglomerular basement membrane antibody glomerulonephritis, with linear deposition of immunoglobulin G (IgG) (and C3) on the glomerular capillary basement membrane. We present a case of Goodpasture's syndrome with spontaneous remission, and the development of nonlinear deposition of IgG in addition to the linear IgG deposition on the glomerular capillary basement membrane.

CASE REPORT

A twenty year old Caucasian woman was well until December 1972 when she presented at another hospital with complaints of cough, weakness and an episode of syncope. She did not have hemoptysis, but was found to have a pulmonary infiltrate, iron deficiency anemia, hematuria with red cell casts and proteinuria. Pulmonary hemosiderosis was found by lung biopsy (the lung biopsy specimen was not processed for immunofluorescence). She was referred to UWSM hospital in March 1973, at which time the urinary sediment findings were confirmed. Electrolytes and hemogram were within normal limits, serum creatinine was 1.2 mg/dl, creatinine clearance was 85 ml/min, 24 hour urine protein was 1.5 g and serum antiglomerular basement membrane antibody titer was positive in 1:64 dilution. The antistreptolysin O titer, antinuclear antibody and total complement were normal. A renal biopsy was performed. Light microscopy findings were as follows: 19 glomeruli were present, 1 of which was completely obsolescent; 2 of the remaining 18 glomeruli showed epithelial cell proliferation with crescent formation; and all the 18 nonobsolescent

From the Departments of Pathology and Medicine, University of Washington, Seattle, Washington; and the Department of Medicine, Harbor General Hospital and University of California, Los Angeles, California. This study was supported in part by Grants HL-03174, AM-05383 and AM-15857 from the National Institute of Health. Requests for reprints should be addressed to Dr. Lawrence Agodoa, Department of Pathology, University of Washington, Seattle, Washington 98195. Manuscript accepted October 10, 1975.

* Present address: 408 Monna Vale Road, St. Ives, NSW 2075, Australia.

TABLE I Summary of Laboratory Data and Glomerular Changes

Date	C_{cr} (ml/min)	24 hr Urine Protein (g)	Serum AntiGBL Antibody Titer	Light Microscopy		Immunofluorescence IgG	Immunofluorescence C_3	Immunofluorescence IgA	Immunofluorescence IgM	Electron Microscopy
March 1973	85	1.5	1:64	Obsolescence:	1/19 glomeruli	4+ linear	2+ linear	Neg	Neg	Endothelial cells—mild increase in cytoplasm
				Crescents:	2/18 glomeruli					GBL—irregular thickening, with irregularity epithelial surface of the lamina rara externa
				Mesangial sclerosis:	mild, all glomeruli					Mesangium—focal areas of sclerosis present
Aug. 1973	143	1.3	Positive in undiluted	Obsolescence:	1/43 glomeruli	4+ linear	Neg	Neg	Neg	Endothelial cells—increase in cytoplasm
				Crescents:	5/42 glomeruli					GBL—irregular thickening, large electron dense granules on the subepithelial surface
				Synechiae:	10/42 glomeruli	2+ irregular granular				
				Mesangial sclerosis:	moderate, all glomeruli					Mesangium—focal areas of sclerosis
July 1974	146	0.04	Negative	Obsolescence:	3/20 glomeruli	4+ linear	Neg	Neg	Neg	Endothelial cells—increase in cytoplasm
				Crescents:	none seen	3–4+				GBL—irregular thickening, many large, electron dense granules on the subepithelial surface
				Mesangial sclerosis:	mild, all glomeruli	granular				Mesangium—focal areas of sclerosis

NOTE: C_{cr} = creatinine clearance. GBL = glomerular basal lomina.

glomeruli showed mild to moderate mesangial sclerosis. Five per cent of the tubules were atrophic and many of them contained red blood cells and red blood cell casts. The interstitium was diffusely edematous and infiltrated with mononuclear (predominantly plasma) cells, and occasional polymorphonuclear leukocytes and eosinophils. The vessels appeared normal. Immunofluorescence microscopy (Figure 1A) showed 4+ linear deposition of IgG and 2+ linear deposits of β_1C globulins on the glomerular capillary basal lamina of all glomeruli; staining was negative for IgA and IgM. Electron microscopy (Figure 1B) revealed irregularly thickened glomerular capillary basal lamina of all glomeruli; staining was negative for IgA and IgM. Electron microscopy (Figure 1B) revealed irregularly thickened glomerular capillary basal lamina with irregular expansion of the lamina rara interna. The lamina densa contained scattered electron dense particles, and the lamina rara externa showed irregularity with small electron dense material irregularly distributed in it. The glomerular capillary endothelial cells showed mild increase in cytoplasm, and occasional myxovirus-like particles. Mild mesangial sclerosis was present (Table I).

The patient had a rapid recovery in symptoms without treatment, but the urinary sediment continued to show red blood cells and red blood casts.

She was readmitted to the UWSM in August 1973 for follow-up evaluation. She was symptom-free except for easy fatigability. Complete blood count and electrolytes were within normal limits. Urinalysis revealed many red blood cells, red blood cell casts, oval fat bodies and granular casts. The 24 hour urinary protein was 1.3 g. Serum creatinine was 0.8, creatinine clearance was 143 cc/min. Serum antiglomerular basement membrane antibody titer was positive only in the undiluted specimen. No antibodies reactive with tubular brush border were found. Light microscopic examination of a repeat renal biopsy specimen revealed that 1 of 43 glomeruli was completely obsolescent, 5 of 42 showed epithelial cell proliferation with crescents, and synechiae were noted in 10 of 42 glomeruli. Immunofluorescence microscopy (Figure 2A) showed 4+ linear, as well as (2+) irregular granular deposition of IgG on the glomerular capillary basal lamina. IgA, IgM and β_1C were not detected. Electron microscopic findings were similar to the first biopsy except for the appearance of large electron dense granules on the subepithelial surface of the glomerular capillary basal lamina (Figure 2B). There was an increase in mesangial matrix. Moderate interstitial fibrosis and edema were present. The vessels remained normal.

In July 1974, she was readmitted for reevaluation. She had remained symptom-free. Complete blood count and electrolytes were within normal limits; blood urea nitrogen was 14 mg/dl; serum creatinine 0.7 mg/dl; creatinine clearance 145 cc/min; urinalysis: no red blood cells or red blood cell casts, but a few white blood cells; 24 hour urinary protein 40 mg. Serum antiglomerular basement membrane antibody level was negative.

Light microscopic examination of a third renal biopsy specimen revealed that 3 of 20 glomeruli present were completely obsolescent. All the nonobsolescent glomeruli showed mild diffuse mesangial sclerosis, and there was

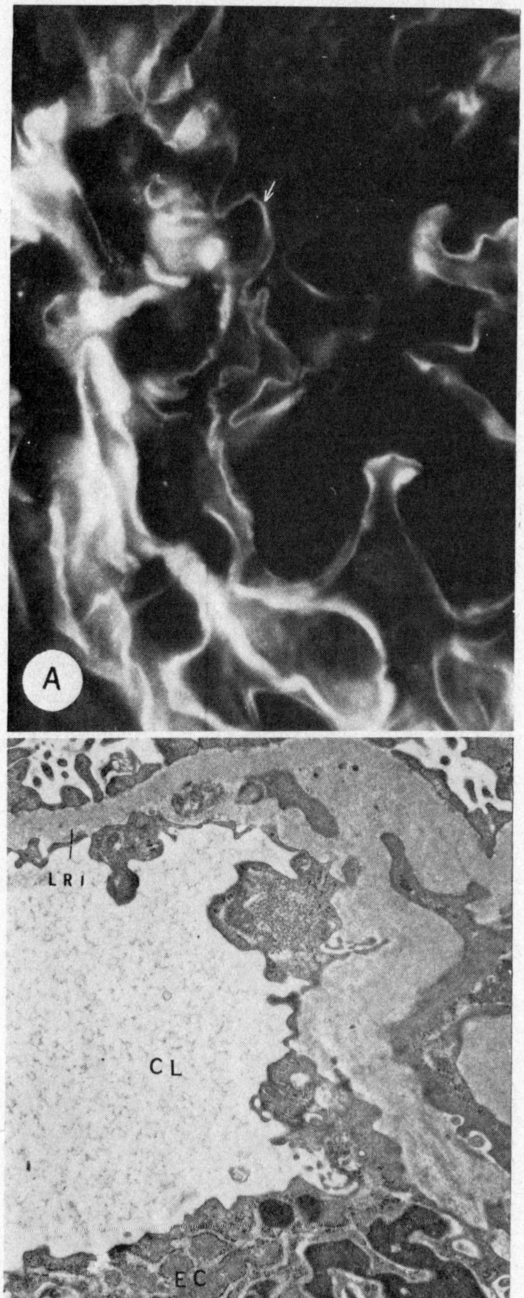

Figure 1. ***A,*** *immunofluorescence of the glomerulus in the first renal biopsy specimen showing linear deposition of IgG on the glomerular capillary basement membrane* ***(arrow).*** *Magnification × 410.* ***B,*** *electron micrograph of the glomerulus in the first renal biopsy specimen showing irregularly expanded lamina rara interna (LRI) and irregular lamina rara externa (LRE). CL = capillary lumen, ED = endothelial cell, EpC = epithelial cell. Magnification × 11,340, reduced by 17 per cent.*

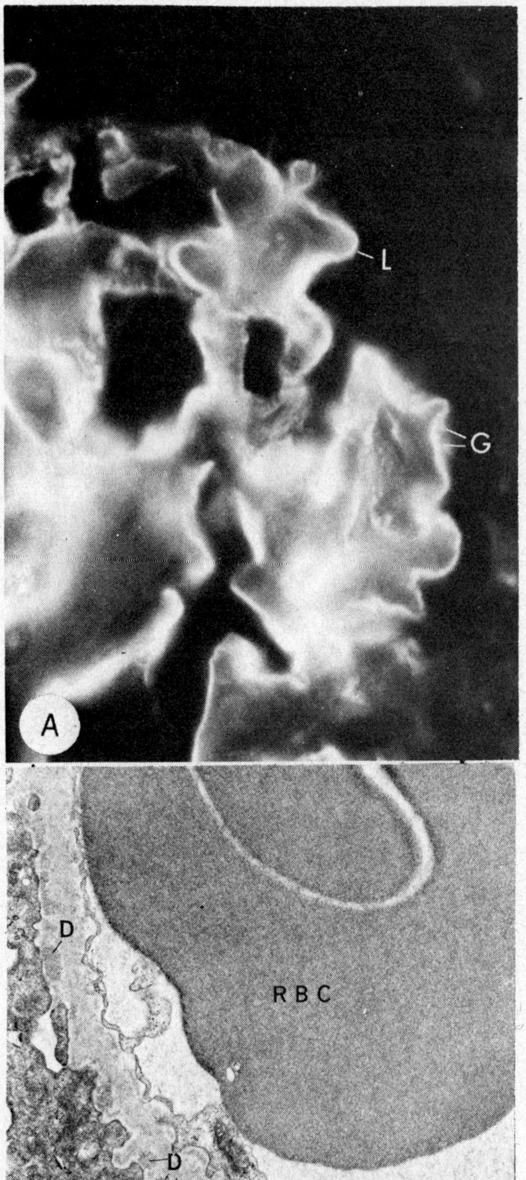

Figure 2. ***A,*** *immunofluorescence of the glomerulus in the second renal biopsy specimen showing linear (L) and granular (G) deposition of IgG on the glomerular capillary basement membrane. Magnification × 410.* ***B,*** *electron micrograph of the glomerulus in the second renal biopsy specimen showing subepithelial electron dense granules (D). CL = capillary lumen, EpC = epithelial cell, RBC = red blood cell. Magnification × 9,000, reduced by 5 per cent.*

patchy fibrosis involving approximately 5 per cent interstitium. Immunofluorescence microscopy revealed 4+ linear deposition of IgG and many granules of IgG on the glomerular capillary basal lamina (Figure 3A). Staining was negative for IgA, IgM and β_1C. Electron microscopic findings were similar to those observed on the second biopsy specimen except for more numerous electron dense deposits on the subepithelial surface of the glomerular capillary basal lamina (Figure 3B). Despite a reduction in degree of staining with antihuman IgG, no distinct reaction of antiglomerular basal lamina antiserum with the granular deposits could be visualized before or after elution. She has remained symptom-free except for one episode of Escherichia coli cystitis which responded to ampicillin, three months after the third biopsy. At that time, serum creatinine was 0.7 mg/dl and creatinine clearance was 160 cc/min and the 24 hour urine protein was 0.02 mg. Repeat serologic tests of complement antinuclear antibody, serologic test for syphilis and lupus erythematosus preparations have been negative. There is no history of serum sickness or exposure to drugs.

MATERIALS AND METHODS

Two pieces of renal tissue were obtained by percutaneous needle biopsy; one pièce was frozen for immunofluorescence, and the other was fixed in 6.25 per cent cold buffered glutaraldehyde. The frozen piece was sectioned and stained with fluoresceinated antiserum for IgG, C_3, IgA and IgM [10]. The specimen fixed in gluteraldehyde was longitudinally bisected; one-half was embedded in paraffin and stained with hematoxylin and eosin, periodic acid-Schiff, methenamine silver and Gomori's trichrome. The second half was postfixed in 1 per cent buffered osmium tetraoxide and embedded in epoxy resin. Thin sections were cut on the LKB III ultratome, stained for 2 hours with uranyl acetate, then with lead citrate for 5 minutes. The sections were examined with an electron microscope (AEI 801). Serum specimens were frozen immediately and used for the determination of serum antiglomerular basement membrane antibody titer. Antiglomerular basement membrane antibody titer was determined by an indirect immunofluorescent assay using serial dilutions of serum in buffered saline solution and a normal human kidney prefixed in acetone as substrate.

An attempt was made to identify and localize glomerular basement membrane antigen in the granular deposits seen in the third biopsy specimen. The patient's IgG was isolated from an early serum sample by DEAE chromatography and conjugated to fluorescein using the dialysis method of Clark and Shepard [11]. This conjugated antiserum stained normal human kidney glomerular basement membrane in a linear fashion. Unfixed frozen sections of one biopsy specimen were reacted with conjugated antiglomerular basement membrane derived with fluorescein-conjugated antihuman IgG from the patient with and without elution at room temperature for 30 to 45 minutes with 0.02 M citrate solution at pH 3.2 and 1.0 M sodium chloride. Inadequate material was available for testing for renal tubular antigen deposits.

COMMENTS

The clinical course of this patient was that of spontaneous remission of Goodpasture's syndrome. The course of Goodpasture's syndrome has been generally considered to be quite aggressive, but some patients have responded favorably to steroids and/or immunosuppressive agents. Seaton et al. [5] described a patient who had spontaneous remission, and a second who failed to respond to corticosteroid administration but responded favorably to the administration of azathioprine.

The renal biopsy specimen from this patient had the typical crescent formation in only a few glomeruli, but diffuse linear deposition of IgG and C_3 on the glomerular basement membrane. The serum antiglomerular basement membrane antibody titer was initially elevated (1:16 to 1:64) but subsequently decreased to positive in an undiluted serum only. At the time of the lower titer, the immunofluorescent microscopy revealed granular deposition of IgG on the glomerular capillary basement membrane, as well as the persistent linear staining. Other than two episodes of urinary tract infection with Esch. coli in the past, she has had none of the usual diseases associated with the development of nonlinear, immune complex type deposition in the glomeruli. Nor has she had any clinical or serologic evidence for endogenous antigenic stimuli such as in systemic lupus erythematosus or tumor.

The sequence of events leading to the development of antiglomerular basement membrane antibodies, with the subsequent deposition of immunoglobulins on the glomerular capillary basement membrane and the lung basement membrane in Goodpasture's syndrome is poorly understood. By injecting heterologous glomerular basement membrane and Freund's adjuvant in sheep, Steblay induced glomerulonephritis with crescent formation, and circulating serum antiglomerular basement membrane antibodies in these animals [12,13]. In human subjects, the possible explanations suggested for the development of antiglomerular basement membrane antibodies include an antibody response to (1) antigenic transformation of the glomerular basement membrane, (2) immunization with a cross-

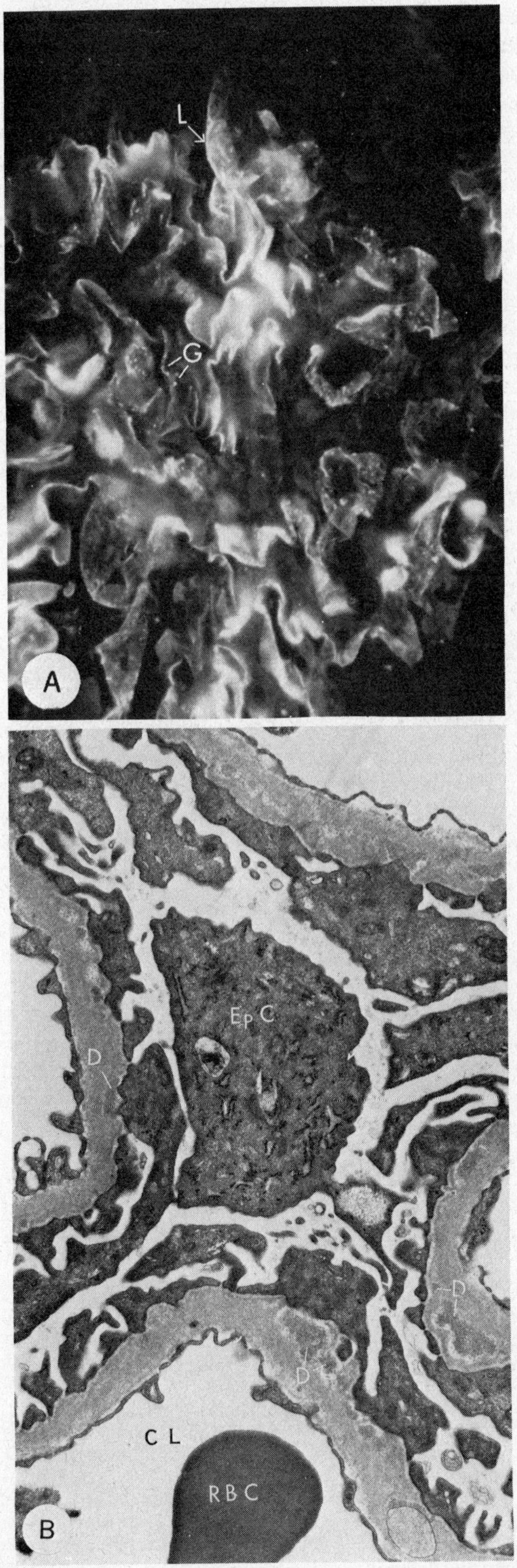

Figure 3. ***A,*** *immunofluorescence of the glomerulus in the third renal biopsy specimen showing linear (L) and granular (G) deposition of IgG on the glomerular capillary basement membrane. Magnification × 258.* ***B,*** *electron micrograph of the glomerulus in the third renal biopsy specimen showing many large subepithelial electron dense deposits (D). CL = capillary lumen, EpC = epithelial cell, RBC = red blood cell. Magnification × 11,340, reduced by 11 per cent.*

reacting glomerular basement membrane-like antigen, and (3) the breaking of tolerance to the individual's own glomerular basement membrane. The antibody formed then combines with the glomerular basement membrane antigen(s), and therefore deposits in a regular, linear fashion on the glomerular capillary basement membrane [14–16].

Nonlinear deposits are thought to arise from antigen-antibody complexes that become trapped in the glomerular capillary basement membrane. The antigen may be demonstrable in the deposits, or specific antibody may be eluted from the kidney [17]. Therefore, the presence of nonlinear deposits in this patient indicates that antibodies are reacting with an antigen (solubilized glomerular basement membrane or from other sources) and that antigen-antibody complexes are present in the circulation, which then become trapped in the glomerular capillary basement membrane.

Several possible explanations could be given for the nonlinear deposition of the immunoglobulin and complement C_3 on the glomerular capillary basement membrane in this patient. It is conceivable that she had occult bacterial infection (streptococcal, or staphylococcal) or viral infections capable of producing antigen-antibody complexes. The immune complex deposits present in poststreptococcal glomerulonephritis are of the nonlinear (lumpy-bumpy) type, and it has been reported that streptococcal cell wall has antigenic determinants that cross react with the glomerular basement membrane [18]. It is therefore conceivable that streptococcal infection may have triggered the development of the antiglomerular basement membrane antibody nephritis. However, this patient did not initially present with the typical immune complex deposits one would expect in poststreptococcal glomerulonephritis. Furthermore, the nonlinear deposits were present in a "regular" fashion, as characteristically seen in early membranous glomerulonephritis. It has been shown that patients with poststreptococcal glomerulonephritis may progress from the lumpy-bumpy type deposits to linear deposition of IgG on the glomerular capillary basement membrane [19]. Similarly, an occasional patient has been shown to progress from membranous glomerulonephritis to rapidly progressive renal disease characterized by extensive crescent formation (but without demonstration of the typically linear deposition of IgG) [20]. Granular deposition of IgG on the glomerular capillary basement membrane has also been described in patients presenting with hemoptysis and hematuria with or without renal failure [21]. This patient presented with the typical clinical picture of Goodpasture's syndrome, but with linear deposition of IgG preceding the development of granular type deposition. Alternatively, the nonlinear deposition of the complexes could represent a continuum of the disease. One could speculate that [IgG]—[anti-IgG] complexes could be deposited on the glomerular capillary basement membrane; or, antiglomerular basement membrane antibody plus glomerular basement membrane antigen in circulation or locally in the capillary wall may be of the right proportion to lead to deposition. It is also possible (although not proved) that tubular damage may have released renal tubular antigen, leading to formation of antibodies of IgG variety against the tubular antigen. The presence of complexes IgG-antitubular basement membrane antigen in circulation may then lead to deposition in the glomerular capillary basement membrane.

The genesis of the nonlinear deposits may be explained by further studies to elucidate the nature of the antigen in the complex.

ACKNOWLEDGMENT

The expert technical assistance of Denise Larsen is gratefully acknowledged. Dr. Lawrence Agodoa is the recipient of the NIH Fellowship 5 F 22 AM00101-02.

REFERENCES

1. Scheer RL, Grossman MA: Immune aspects of the glomerulonephritis Associated with pulmonary hemorrhage. Ann Intern Med 60: 1009, 1964.
2. Solberg CO: Glomerulonephritis with lung purpura (Goodpasture's syndrome). Acta Med Scand 186: 401, 1969.
3. Elder JL, Kirk GM, Smith WG: Idiopathic pulmonary hemosiderosis and the Goodpasture's syndrome. Br Med J 2: 1152, 1965.
4. McCall CB, Ham's TR, Hatch FE: Nonfatal pulmonary hemorrhage and glomerulonephritis. Am Rev Respir Dis 91: 424, 1965.
5. Seaton A, Meland JM, Lapp NL: Remission of Goodpasture's syndrome: report of two patients treated by immunosuppression and review of the literature. Thorax 26: 683, 1971.
6. Lehman JD, Cross KR: Pulmonary hemosiderosis and glomerulonephritis. Iowa St Med Soc 51: 279, 1961.
7. Area EA, Clanoff DV: Prolonged survival of Goodpasture's syndrome. Arch Intern Med 114: 453, 1964.
8. Walker JM, Jockes AM: Survival after haemoptysis and nephritis. Lancet 2: 1199, 1963.
9. Proskey AJ, Weatherbee L, Easterling RE, Greene JA, Weller JM: Goodpasture's syndrome. A report of five cases and review of the literature. Am J Med 48: 162, 1970.
10. Coons AH, Kaplan MH: Localization of antigen in tissue cells. II. Improvements in a method for detection of antigens by means of fluorescent antibody. J Exp Med 91: 1, 1950.
11. Clarke HF, Shepard CC: A dialysis technique for preparing fluorescent antibody. Virology 20: 642, 1963.

12. Steblay RW: Glomerulonephritis induced in sheep by injections of human lung and Freund's adjuvant. J Exp Med 116: 253, 1962.
13. Steblay RW, Rudolfsky U: Autoimmune glomerulonephritis induced in sheep by injections of human lung and Freund's adjuvant. Science 160: 204, 1968.
14. Wilson CB: Immunologic glomerular injury. Postgrad Med 54: 157, 1973.
15. Dixon FJ: The pathogenesis of glomerulonephritis. Am J Med 44: 493, 1968.
16. Vernier RL, Tinglof B, Urizar R, Litman N, Smith F Jr: Immunofluorescence studies in renal disease. Proceedings of Third International Congress of Nephrology 3: 83, 1966.
17. Lerner RA, Glassock RJ, Dixon FJ: The role of antiglomerular basement membrane antibody in the pathogenesis of human glomerulonephritis. J Exp Med 126: 989, 1967.
18. Lange CF: Chemistry of cross reactive fragments of streptococcal cell membrane and human glomerular basement membrane. Transpl Proc 1: 959, 1969.
19. Baldwin DS, Gluck MC, Schacht RG, Gallo G: The longterm course of post streptococcal glomerulonephritis. Ann Int Med 80: 342, 1974.
20. Klassen J, Elwood C, Grossberg AL, Milgrom F, Montes M, Sepulveda M, Andres GA: Evolution of membranous glomerulonephritis into anti-glomerular-basement-membrane glomerulonephritis. N Engl J Med 290: 1340, 1974.
21. Beirne GJ, Kopp WL, Zimmerman SW: Goodpasture syndrome. Dissociation from antibodies to glomerular basement membrane. Arch Intern Med 132: 261, 1973.

Splenosis: Autotransplantation of Splenic Tissue

C. RICHARD FLEMING, M.D.
E. ROLLAND DICKSON, M.D.
EDGAR G. HARRISON, Jr., M.D.*
Rochester, Minnesota

Splenosis is the autotransplantation of splenic tissue that usually follows traumatic rupture of the spleen. Generally, the splenic implants are numerous and are located within the peritoneal cavity; however, extra-abdominal splenosis does occur. The implants are rarely clinically significant and are incidental findings at autopsy or at abdominal operation, unrelated to and distant from the splenic trauma and splenectomy. Splenic implants retain their ability to function, and recurrence of a hematologic disease for which the spleen was previously removed should alert the clinician to the possibility of splenosis. The differential diagnosis includes accessory spleens, endometriosis, hemangiomas and metastatic cancer. We report three cases, two of which represent unusual complications of splenosis: a twisted pedicle of a splenic implant, which apparently caused abdominal pain, and recurrent Felty's syndrome associated with splenosis and an accessory spleen.

Splenosis is the autotransplantation of splenic tissue which is usually subsequent to traumatic rupture of the spleen. Characteristically, the disrupted splenic pulp implants appear as multiple reddish blue nodules on the parietal peritoneum, omentum, mesentery or serosal surfaces of the small or large bowel. They are rarely of clinical significance, and they are usually incidental findings at autopsy or at abdominal surgery many years after splenectomy for traumatic rupture. The true prevalence of splenosis must be greater than the world literature review of 75 cases in 1973 [1], because many patients who undergo splenectomy after splenic rupture never have another abdominal operation or never undergo postmortem examination. There are probably others with splenosis who may have experienced minor splenic rupture and recovered spontaneously without surgical intervention.

We report three additional cases. Two of the cases represent unusual complications associated with splenosis: recurrent Felty's syndrome after splenectomy and a twisted pedicle of a splenic implant, which apparently caused abdominal pain.

From the Mayo Clinic and Mayo Foundation, Rochester, Minnesota. Requests for reprints should be addressed to Dr. C. R. Fleming, c/o Section of Publications, Mayo Clinic, 200 First Street SW, Rochester, MN 55901. Manuscript accepted October 28, 1975.

* Deceased, July 5, 1975.

CASE REPORTS

Case 1. In 1966, a 12 year old girl fell and struck her left flank, rupturing her spleen. Thirty-six hours later, splenectomy was performed. Pathologically, there was a recent transcapsular hematoma irregularly extending into the splenic red pulp, which was otherwise not unusual in appearance (Figure 1A). Follicles had moderate germinal activity.

In September 1972, she was examined by her local physician because, for one month she had had daily lower abdominal pain that occasionally extended into her left flank. Results of routine blood tests were within normal limits except for a hemoglobin level of 5.2 g/dl. The serum iron level was 24 mg/dl, with a total iron-binding capacity of 506 mg/dl. There was no history of melena, hematemesis or hematochezia, and the patient's menstrual blood flows had never been excessive. Roentgenograms of the stomach, small intestine and colon showed no abnormalities. The patient was given oral ferrous sulfate and there was a prompt reticulocyte response; by December 1972, the hemoglobin level was 14 g/dl.

The patient was first evaluated at the Mayo Clinic in March 1973. She had continued to experience daily lower abdominal cramping pain, which was unrelated to eating and was unrelieved by antacids. The patient had no diarrhea, no fever and no loss of weight. The findings on physical examination were unremarkable. Pertinent laboratory data included a hemoglobin level of 13.8 g/dl, a leukocyte count of 6,100/mm^3, with a normal differential count, and a peripheral blood smear showing Howell-Jolly bodies. The following were normal: serum and urine amylase levels; serum lipase level; reticulocyte count; platelet count; roentgenograms of the stomach, small bowel and colon; and results of proctoscopy, excretory urography, an ear, nose, and throat examination (searching for telangiectasia), esophagogastroduodenoscopy, selective celiac and superior mesenteric arteriography and abdominal radioisotope scanning using sodium pertechnetate in search of Meckel's diverticulum.

The patient was dismissed with instructions to return at the first evidence of gastrointestinal bleeding. She continued to have abdominal pain daily and underwent exploratory laparotomy in her local community in June 1973. At laparotomy, a 4 by 1.5 cm piece of splenic tissue attached to a long twisted pedicle popped into the wound. Further examination of the abdomen revealed numerous splenic implants on the greater omentum. No splenic implants were seen on the viscera of the abdomen, and no other abnormalities were noted. The entire greater omentum was resected.

Pathologically, the splenic implants had thin fibrous capsules and occasional lymph follicles, some of which projected through the capsule (Figure 1B). Trabecular structures, including the usual trabecular vessels of the spleen, were lacking. Some follicles had germinal activity with adjacent sheathed small arteries, and the pulp sinuses and cords were well formed and similar to those seen at the time of the original splenectomy.

The patient has remained asymptomatic during the six month postoperative follow-up period. Specifically, abdominal pain has not recurred and the hemoglobin level has remained normal. The previous iron-deficiency anemia remains unexplained, however.

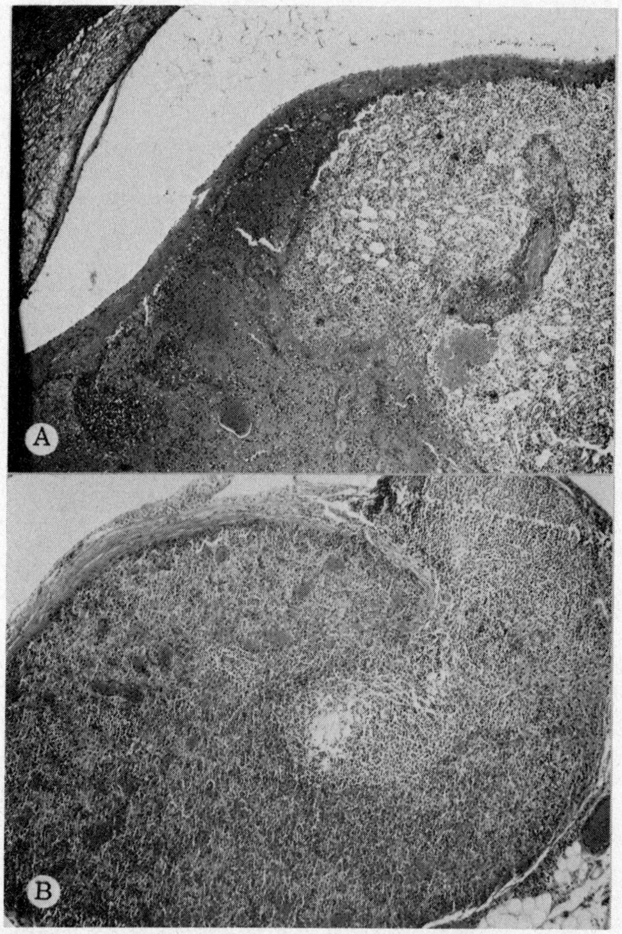

Figure 1. *Case 1.* ***A****, spleen. Splenic transcapsular hematoma also involves red pulp; note trabeculum on right.* ***B****, typical splenic implant in which trabecular structure or associated vessels are lacking. Hematoxylin and eosin stain; magnification × 64* ***(A)****, × 80* ***(B)****, reduced by 20 per cent.*

Case 2. A 49 year old man was referred to the Mayo Clinic in February 1973 because of pneumonia. The patient's history included disabling rheumatoid arthritis for 11 years and chronic asthmatic bronchitis for several years. In 1941, he "injured his spleen" in an automobile accident; however, no surgery was performed.

From 1968 to 1971, he experienced recurrent episodes of pneumonia and recurrent infections of his toes and fingers. Associated with these infections were leukocyte counts of 1,000/mm^3, with only 2 per cent neutrophils. Because of the recurrent life-threatening infections and a diagnosis of Felty's syndrome, splenectomy was performed at another institution in 1971. The spleen weighed 380 g and contained an accessory spleen that appeared to be cut in half. No other splenic tissue was noted at surgery. After surgery, the patient was free of infection for two years despite leukocyte counts of less than 2,800/mm^3.

At the patient's first admission to our clinic in February 1973, a cavitating lesion was found in the upper lobe of his left lung. Sputum cultures grew Pseudomonas aeruginosa,

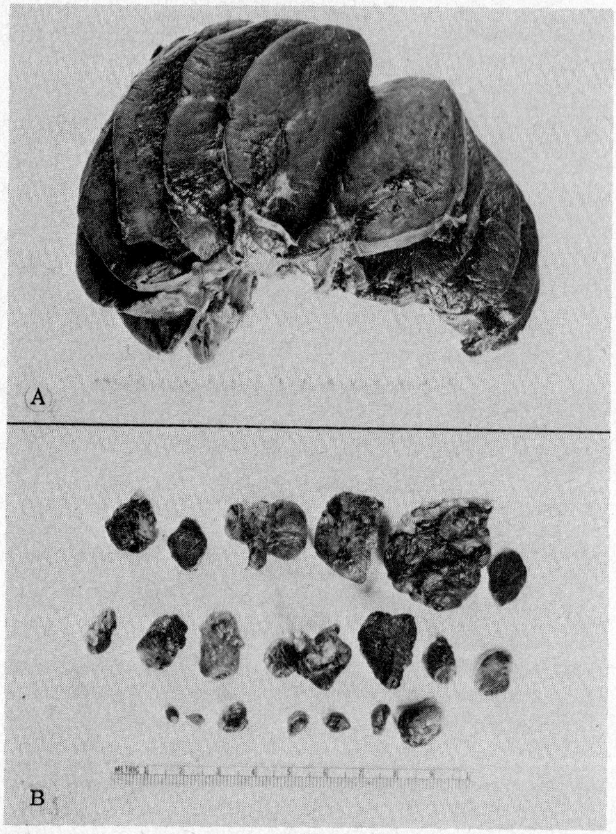

Figure 2. *Case 2.* ***A****, massive accessory splenomegaly seen in gross surgical specimen in Felty's syndrome.* ***B****, splenosis due to multiple splenic implants of variable size removed at surgery.*

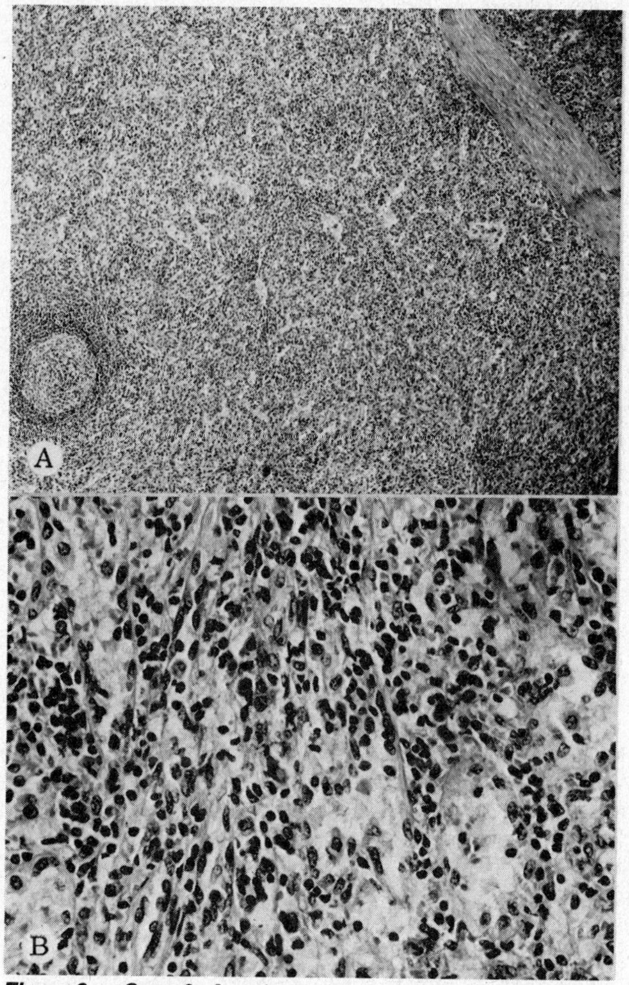

Figure 3. *Case 2.* ***A****, splenic pulp showing germinal activity of follicles of white pulp and widening of cords of Billroth due to increased mononuclear cells. Note trabeculum of accessory spleen.* ***B****, prominent lymphoid cells in pulp cords, including lymphocytes and plasma cells with histiocytes, which are also seen in sinuses. Hematoxylin and eosin stain; magnification* × *64* ***(A)****,* × *400* ***(B)****, reduced by 15 per cent.*

and therapy with gentamicin and carbenicillin was begun. A peripheral blood smear showed no Howell-Jolly bodies or other evidence of a postsplenectomy state; neutropenia and marked rouleau formation were noted. The hemoglobin level was 11.0 g/dl, platelets 203,000/mm^3 and leukocytes 2,000/mm^3, with a differential count of 29 per cent segmented neutrophils, 39 per cent lymphocytes, 23 per cent monocytes and 9 per cent eosinophils. A scan of the liver and spleen showed an enlarged liver and a large mass in the left upper quadrant.

Because of the life-threatening pulmonary infection and evidence suggestive of a residual spleen, laparotomy was performed. A 17 by 9 cm accessory spleen weighing 1,040 g (Figure 2A) was removed from the left upper quadrant. Approximately 40 splenic implants (Figure 2B) in the omentum, ranging in diameter from 0.3 to 3.0 cm, also were removed. A liver biopsy specimen obtained at surgery was essentially normal microscopically.

Histopathologic review of the spleen (removed in 1971) revealed slight germinal activity of malpighian follicles and moderate plasmacytosis in the cords of Billroth. There was moderate widening of the cords due to increased plasma cells, lymphocytes and some histiocytes, which were also noted in the sinuses. The appearance of the sinusoidal lining cells was not unusual, and phagocytosis was not prominent. Moderate deposition of hemosiderin and focal recent hemorrhages were noted in the red pulp.

Findings in the massive accessory spleen (noted in 1973) were similar to those of the spleen (removed in 1971) (Figure 3A). Slight germinal activity of follicles and moderate plasmacytosis in association with lymphocytes and histiocytes had widened the cords of Billroth (Figure 3B). There was focal deposition of hemosiderin in the pulp. The splenic implants had no germinal activity of follicles, and plasma cell infiltration of cords was moderate. The vascular and trabecular structures seen in the spleen and accessory spleen were lacking, whereas occasional follicles were noted, some of which were outside the thin fibrous capsule. No significant phagocytic activity was detected, and polymorphonuclear leukocytes were infrequent.

The patient's pulmonary infection cleared during a three-week postoperative period in the hospital. On the day after splenectomy, a peripheral blood smear showed a typical postsplenectomy erythrocyte pattern, including Howell-Jolly bodies. During a nine month follow-up period, there were no infections, and a leukocyte count eight months after removal of the accessory spleen and splenic implants was 5,200/mm^3, with 81 per cent lymphocytes, 9 per cent monocytes, 6 per cent segmented neutrophils and 4 per cent band neutrophils.

Case 3. A 14 year old boy was crushed beneath his motor scooter in 1952. He was admitted in a state of shock, with a left pneumothorax and multiple rib fractures. When signs of generalized peritonitis developed, surgery was advised. Surgery revealed that the abdomen was filled with approximately 1,500 ml of old blood; the spleen had been ruptured and torn off its pedicle, and the dome of the right lobe of the liver had been severely contused. Splenectomy was performed, and the peritoneal cavity was sponged free of blood. The patient was dismissed on the 14th postoperative day.

The patient was seen in the emergency room in July 1954 with a 12 hour history of epigastric and periumbilical cramping abdominal pain; he had vomited much yellow-green liquid. Findings on physical examination and a roentgenogram of the abdomen were suggestive of partial small bowel obstruction. When attempts at decompression by a Miller-Abbott tube and intravenous fluids did not relieve the boy's symptoms in 48 hours, the patient underwent laparotomy. Surgery revealed multiple fibrous adhesions in the left upper quadrant. Dilated loops of jejunum were present above an obstructing fibrous band across the mid-jejunum. Multiple, small, reddish blue nodules also were noted on the mesentery and the serosal surface of the intestines. Microscopically, these were confirmed as being typical splenic implants.

During the next two and a half months, the patient experienced three additional episodes of cramping abdominal pain associated with nausea and vomiting. In October 1954, he was rehospitalized after 18 hours of upper abdominal colic and vomiting, which began 1 hour after his evening meal. Abdominal exploration revealed a firm fibrous band obstructing the jejunum. The splenic implants were again noted but were not near the intestinal obstruction.

COMMENTS

One of our three patients had findings that have not been previously described in association with splenic implants. It seems likely that the abdominal pain of our first patient was caused by the twisting of the long pedicle attached to the splenic nodule. After surgical resection of the splenic implants and greater omentum, the patient was relieved of her abdominal pain. Our second patient has been described by Perry and Bayrd [2] as being the first with recurrent Felty's syndrome. Resection of splenic tissue on two occasions improved the patient's clinical status but did not sustain the neutrophil response. The fact that the accessory spleen was the only splenic tissue showing uptake of ^{99m}Tc was suggestive evidence that this tissue was related to the recurrent problems. Our third patient had the characteristic features of splenosis [3,4], in which splenic implants are noted incidentally during exploration for intestinal obstruction secondary to adhesions years after splenectomy for traumatic rupture of the spleen. Splenosis was an incidental finding at two operations subsequent to splenectomy, and the location of the implants did not suggest that they were related to the intestinal obstruction.

Pathogenesis. Splenosis has been shown to arise from the transplantation of splenic pulp in dogs [5], rats [6], rabbits [7], monkeys [8] and mice [9]. Splenosis resulted when a partial splenectomy was performed in monkeys, presumably from leakage of pulp from the cut surface of the spleen. However, if the monkey underwent a nontraumatic total splenectomy, splenic implants were prevented [8]. Our second patient had partial removal of an accessory spleen during the original splenectomy, and splenosis may have resulted from the seeding of splenic pulp from the transected remnant of accessory spleen.

Other theories about the pathogenesis of splenosis exist. Von Stubenrauch [10] performed splenectomy in dogs and seeded the crushed splenic pulp throughout the peritoneal cavity. He misinterpreted the viable splenic implants to be compensatory "splenoids" arising anew from the peritoneum. Splenic vein emboli of splenic pulp resulted in viable liver implants in dogs [10]. A hematogeneous spread of splenic pulp may be the basis for the implants [11] when splenic trauma did not precede the diagnosis of splenosis.

Perla [6] described the histologic sequence in the regeneration of autoplastic splenic transplants in albino rats. Within 24 hours after transplantation, the splenic implants underwent degeneration. Only reticulum cells at the periphery of spleen tissue survived and proliferated to penetrate to the necrotic center by day 3. Regeneration of transplants was complete between days 12 and 21. Perla believed that the reticulum cell of the splenic implants served as the precursor of structural elements by retaining its potentiality for differentiation.

Description and Locations. The splenic implants are described as reddish blue nodules that may be sessile or pedunculated. Their numbers vary from only a few to 400, and their sizes range from a few millimeters to 7 cm. Because the blood supply to the nodules is by small arteries penetrating the capsule and not by a major hilar artery, the nodules may outgrow their blood supply; this may be the reason that implants rarely have a diameter greater than 3 cm [12]. The implants may be located anywhere within the peritoneal cavity, but they are more commonly located on the serosal surfaces of the small intestine, greater omentum, parietal peritoneum, large intestine, mesentery and undersurface of the diaphragm [1]. In two reported cases, patients with surgically diagnosed splenosis presented clinically with stomach masses [13,14].

Splenic implants within the pleural cavity [15–17] or pericardium [18] can be traced to penetrating abdominal trauma, in which a rent in the left hemidiaphragm was associated with splenic rupture. Patients with splenosis within the pleural cavity have undergone thoracotomy because of suspected bronchogenic carcinoma; some of them have had nodules that enlarged on serial roentgenograms of the chest [15]. Subcutaneous nodules, proved to be splenosis, have resulted from splenic pulp being seeded in the surgical scar [12,19].

Clinical Features. It is impossible to predict in which patients who undergo splenectomy for ruptured spleen splenosis will develop. The time delay from splenic rupture to splenectomy and the amount of blood described in the peritoneal cavity at surgery are not related to an increased incidence of splenosis [20]. The time interval between rupture and diagnosis of splenosis has varied from five months to 32 years. Seventy per cent of the patients have been teen-agers at the time of splenic injury, which probably reflects only an increased likelihood for trauma in the younger person [1].

Splenosis rarely causes symptoms. Usually, the patient undergoes abdominal operation for a disease unrelated to and far from the splenic trauma, and the implants are noted incidentally. Patients with intestinal obstruction in whom the splenic implants have appeared to be causally related to the obstruction have been described [21,22]. However, most patients with small bowel obstruction and splenosis have had adhesions that were not related anatomically to the implants [3,4]. Of 55 patients with splenosis described in the literature by 1972 [21], 14 had exploratory laparotomy for vague abdominal complaints, "possibly caused" by splenosis. Brewster [1] emphasized that most patients with splenosis at surgery have not had further abdominal pain, whether or not the nodules have been removed. Our patient (Case 1) probably represents the first patient in whom a twisted pedicle of a splenic implant seemed to be responsible for abdominal pain.

Splenic implants have retained their ability to function. Williams [23] placed a splenic autograft into a microscopic chamber in a rabbit's ear and demonstated red cells being ingested by splenic macrophages. Uptake of chromium-labeled red blood cells into peritoneal implants has been documented in man [11]. A subcutaneous splenic implant in the chest wall resulting from a previous gunshot wound enlarged during a malarial relapse [19]. Recurrent congenital hemolytic anemia has been considered to be secondary to splenosis; however, the cause of the jaundice was unclear since choledocholithiasis and hepatic duct stricture also were present [24]. Uptake of ^{99m}Tc-sulfur colloid by splenosis is further evidence of functioning tissue. Nodules that were 3 cm in diameter have shown uptake on ^{99m}Tc-sulfur colloid scans [25]; however, in our Case 2, there was no uptake in the nodules, which were as large as 3 cm in diameter. The marked concentration of isotope in the enlarged liver and huge accessory spleen may have prevented detection of uptake in the splenic implants. As in our Case 2, the absence of Howell-Jolly bodies, siderocytes and other postsplenectomy abnormalities on peripheral blood smear in a patient who has had a splenectomy should raise the possibility of functioning splenic tissue [2]. In our Case 1, a peripheral blood smear was suggestive of hyposplenism, and in Case 3 a smear was not obtained.

Differential Diagnosis. The differential diagnosis of the nodules includes metastatic carcinoma, endometriosis, hemangiomas and accessory spleens. Metastatic nodules are usually white and plaque-like, as compared to the reddish blue nodules of splenosis. Color cannot be used to differentiate splenosis from endometriosis, but in endometriosis, the nodules are usually embedded in the serosal surface of the intestinal wall and are not sessile or pedunculated, as in splenosis. Hemangiomas may have similar appearances, but, in general, there are fewer nodules and they are easily compressible and refill after the pressure has been released.

Splenosis is easily distinguished from the accessory spleen. Compared to the rarity of splenosis, accessory spleens have been found in 10 to 44 per cent of cases at autopsy [12]. There are usually many splenic implants in splenosis, but rarely are there more than six accessory spleens. Accessory spleens are located near the principal spleen and correspond to the embryologic development of the spleen to the left side of the dorsal mesogastrium, but the nodules in splenosis can be found anywhere in and beyond the peritoneal cavity. Even when the accessory spleens are far removed from the left upper quadrant, they are supplied by branches of the splenic artery. Accessory spleens resemble in miniature the principal spleen. In contrast, the splenic implants possess no hilus and derive their blood supplies from new arteries that penetrate the capsule. The capsule of the splenosis nodules is derived from surrounding reactive granulation and fibrous tissues, and is usually devoid of smooth muscle and elastic tissue components—components that are seen in the capsules and trabeculae of accessory spleens. The capsule of splenic implants may be relatively thicker than that of accessory spleens and has been reported to be due to the "enormous proliferation of connective tissue" [7]. The trabeculae of the implants are deficient or absent. Difference of opinion exists about splenic pulp in splenosis. Some investigators have described the pulp as being indistinguishable from that of the normal spleen, whereas others have commented on the irregular and poorly defined follicles [3], the decrease in the number of germinal centers [20] and the absence of ellipsoids [4]. Shaw and Shafi [26] described scattered foci of plasmocytes, macrophages and hemosiderin deposits. In our three cases, the fibrous capsule was devoid of smooth muscle and elastic tissues, and lacked trabeculae and associated vessels. However, the number of lymph follicles per low power field and structure of the red pulp were similar to the parent spleen, whether the spleen was previously normal (Cases 1 and 3) or abnormal (Case 2) in Felty's syndrome.

Diagnosis and Management. Splenosis should be suspected in a patient who has had splenectomy for splenic trauma and who later presents with abdominal pain or in a patient who has recurrence of a hematologic disease for which the spleen was previously removed. A peripheral blood smear may show evidence of functioning splenic tissue. Radioisotope scanning may show uptake by the nodules, and laparoscopy, with a biopsy specimen taken under direct vision, may help in making the diagnosis. The surgeon must recognize the entity and avoid unnecessary resection. There is a difference of opinion regarding what should be done when the implants are unexpectedly encountered, but if multiple nodules can be removed easily, as by omentectomy [1], this should be done. Otherwise, resection should be reserved for implants that may be a source of future intestinal obstruction. Iatrogenic splenosis can be avoided if great care is taken not to tear the splenic capsule during splenectomy.

REFERENCES

1. Brewster DC: Splenosis: report of two cases and review of the literature. Am J Surg 126: 14, 1973.
2. Perry MC, Bayrd ED: Recurrent Felty's syndrome associated with splenosis and probable splenic regeneration. Mayo Clin Proc 49: 875, 1974.
3. Storsteen KA, ReMine WH: Rupture of the spleen with splenic implants: splenosis; review of the literature and report of a case. Ann Surg 137: 551, 1953.
4. Mackie WJ, Miller DF: Splenosis: a case report and some considerations on the function of splenotic tissue. Br J Surg 60: 56, 1973.
5. Von Stubenrauch: Milzregeneration und Milzersatz. Verh Dtsch Ges Chir 41: 213, 1912.
6. Perla D: The regeneration of autoplastic splenic transplants. Am J Pathol 12: 665, 1936.
7. Manley OT, Marine D: The transplantation of splenic tissue into the subcutaneous fascia of the abdomen in rabbits. J Exp Med 25: 619, 1917.
8. Kreuter E: Experimentelle Untersuchungen über die Entstehung der sogenannten Nebenmilzen, insbesondere nach Milzverletzungen. Bruns Beitr Klin Chir 118: 76, 1920.
9. Calder RM: Autoplastic splenic grafts: their use in the study of the growth of splenic tissue. J Pathol 49: 351, 1939.
10. Von Stubenrauch: Experimentelle Untersuchungen über die Entstehung der sogenannten Nebenmilzen, insbesondere nach Milzverletzungen. Bruns Beitr Klin Chir 119: 710, 1920.
11. Koumans RKJ: Splenosis peritonei. Ned Tijdschr Geneeskd 111: 1028, 1967.
12. Cohen EA: Splenosis: review and report of subcutaneous splenic implant. Arch Surg 69: 777, 1954.
13. Otteman MG, Wise JK, Henson SW: Splenosis as lesion of the stomach: splenosis secondary to old trauma with autotransplantation of splenic tissue into the wall of the stomach presented as an intramural fundal lesion. Rocky Mt Med J 69: 53, 1972.
14. Gammill SL, VanCraig H: Splenosis:autotransplantation of splenic tissue following trauma. JAMA 208: 1387, 1969.
15. Dalton ML Jr, Strange WH, Downs EA: Intrathoracic splenosis: case report and review of the literature. Am Rev Respir Dis 103: 827, 1971.
16. Skinner EF, Hurteau WW: Autotransplantation of spleen into thorax. J Thorac Surg 33: 807, 1957.
17. Ahmadi A, Faber LP, Milloy F, Jensik RJ: Intrathoracic splenosis. J Thorac Cardiovasc Surg 55: 677, 1968.
18. Ovnatanyan KT: Splenosis of the pericardium. Vestn Khir 97: 59, 1966.
19. Gill AJ: Traumatic autograft of splenic tissue in the body wall. J Lab Clin Med 29: 247, 1944.
20. Widmann WD, Laubscher FA: Splenosis: a disease or a beneficial condition? Arch Surg 102: 152, 1971.
21. Trimble C, Eason FJ: A complication of splenosis. J Trauma 12: 358, 1972.
22. Prasad C, Beck R: Unusual problems in surgery: splenosis and intestinal obstruction. Mt Sinai J Med NY 35: 534, 1968.
23. Williams RG: Microscopic structure and behavior of spleen autografts in rabbits. Am J Anat 87: 459, 1950.
24. Stobie GH: Splenosis. Can Med Assoc J 56: 374, 1947.
25. Jacobson SJ, DeNardo GL: Case report: splenosis demonstrated by splenic scan. J Nucl Med 12: 570, 1971.
26. Shaw AFB, Shafi A: Traumatic autoplastic transplantation of splenic tissue in man with observations on the late results of splenectomy in six cases. J Pathol 45: 215, 1937.

Regression of Atherosclerotic Stenosing Lesions of the Renal Arteries and Spontaneous Cure of Systemic Hypertension Through Control of Hyperlipidemia

LOTFY L. BASTA, M.D.*
CHAD WILLIAMS, M.D.†
J. MICHAEL KIOSCHOS, M.D.
ARTHUR A. SPECTOR, M.D.
Iowa City, Iowa

We describe a 49 year old woman with impressive regression of renal artery stenosing atherosclerotic lesions in response to sustained excellent control of hyperlipidemia.

Initially, she had high blood pressure necessitating combined drug therapy with chlorothiazide, methyldopa and propranolol, with only moderately satisfactory control. Renal arteriography revealed a 90 per cent stenosing lesion of the right renal artery and 75 per cent narrowing of the left renal artery. Peripheral vein plasma renin was markedly increased at 32 ng/ml. With a combination of cholestyramine and clofibrate, serum lipids were maintained at normal values for several years. Increased blood pressure diminished spontaneously, and the patient has maintained normal blood pressures after discontinuation of antihypertensive therapy. Repeat renal arteriograms showed almost complete regression of the right renal artery lesion and a possible decrease in left renal artery disease. Peripheral vein plasma renin became normal at 3 ng/ml.

This case illustrates that sustained control of hyperlipidemia could lead to regression of atherosclerotic nodules and impressive clinical improvement in certain patients.

In experimental atherosclerosis in animals, regression of atherosclerotic lesions has been demonstrated in response to measures that lower serum cholesterol [1–5]. The lipid content of such lesions was observed to decrease in parallel with the decrease in serum lipids [6–8].

By contrast, studies in human subjects have generally failed to show significant regression in nodular atherosclerosis in response to control of hyperlipidemia.

We have followed a patient with hyperlipidemia and generalized atherosclerosis manifest by symptomatic coronary artery disease and systemic hypertension presumably secondary to renal artery atherosclerotic stenosing lesions. Regression of the renal artery stenosis was demonstrated with adequate rigorous control of hyperlipidemia. Simultaneously, systemic hypertension regressed spontaneously after it had been difficult to control with medications. Normal blood pressures were maintained for two years without medications thereafter.

From the Cardiovascular Division, University of Iowa Hospital, Iowa City, Iowa 52242. Requests for reprints should be addressed to Dr. L. L. Basta. Manuscript accepted October 31, 1975.

* Present address: The University of Oklahoma, Health Sciences Center, P.O. Box 26901, Oklahoma City, Oklahoma 73190.

† Present address: Methodist Hospital, Des Moines, Iowa.

TABLE I Cholesterol and Triglyceride Levels Before Treatment and In Response to Various Drug Regimens

Date	Drug Treatment (g) Choles-tyramine	Drug Treatment (g) Clofibrate	Choles-terol (mg/dl)	Triglyc-eride (mg/dl)
1/25/71	None	None	340	157
1/26/71	12	—	—	—
2/25/71	—	—	196	535
2/26/71	24	—	—	—
4/22/71	—	—	172	1,132
4/23/71	24	2	—	—
6/3/71	24	2	167	207
8/5/71	24	2	142	147
8/6/71	16	2	—	—
1/27/72	16	2	158	74
8/17/72	16	2	164	80
2/15/73	16	2	179	110
8/30/73	16	2	154	114
12/27/73	16	2	165	95
1/24/74	16	2	167	119
5/16/74	16	2	151	121

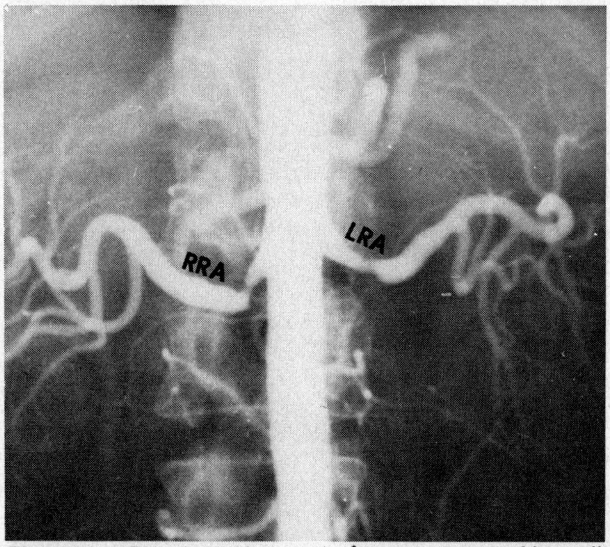

Figure 1. *Renal arteriogram before treatment of hyperlipidemia showing 90 per cent occlusion of right renal artery (RRA) and 75 per cent occlusion of left renal artery (LRA).*

CASE REPORT

A 49 year old white woman was referred to the University of Iowa Hospital in July 1970 because of angina pectoris that recurred frequently on mild exertion, during sleep and occasionally at rest. She gave a history of systemic hypertension, for which she had received intermittent antihypertensive therapy during the previous 15 years. There was no adequate record of the blood pressure measurements during those years, but the blood pressure was reportedly 230/132 mm Hg six months prior to referral, at which time she was receiving methyldopa and chlorothiazide therapy. The patient also related that, for two years, she had had elevated blood sugar levels that did not require specific treatment. She had smoked one pack of cigarettes a day for over 20 years.

Family history revealed that the father died at age 42 years from congestive cardiac failure, the mother died at age 62 years with a "large heart" and diabetes mellitus, the patient's brother sustained a myocardial infarction at age 60, one sister had been under treatment for angina pectoris and diabetes mellitus at age 65, and the remaining sister aged 42 was apparently healthy.

Clinical examination revealed a slender woman who weighed 43 kg and who was in no apparent distress. The pulse rate was 72 beats/min and regular, and the blood pressure, from the right arm, was 165/95 mm Hg with the patient in the sitting position and 160/100 mm Hg with the patient standing.

There were no clinical features suggesting hyperlipidemia, and the clinical cardiovascular examination revealed no abnormality other than a questionably audible fourth heart sound.

The rest of clinical examination was essentially normal. The urinalysis, blood picture and serum electrolytes were normal. The 2 hour postprandial blood sugar level was 147 mg/100 ml. The urine vanillylmandelic acid was normal at 5 mg/24 hours collection. Serum cholesterol was 340 mg/100 ml, serum triglyceride 154 mg/100 ml (Table I); serum lipoprotein electrophoresis was interpreted as showing a probable type II abnormality.

An electrocardiogram showed flat T waves over the inferior cardiac surface. A Master 2-step exercise test resulted in a 1 mm S-T depression in the electrocardiogram, and the test was interpreted as positive for myocardial ischemia. Roentgenograms of the chest revealed a normal cardiac size.

Intravenous pyelograms showed delayed visualization of the right caliceal system, with the longitudinal axis of the right kidney measuring 12.6 cm and that of the left kidney 14.4 cm.

Peripheral vein plasma renin was grossly increased at 32 ng/ml (normal 0.8 to 4 ng/ml).

The renal arteriograms showed severe bilateral atherosclerotic disease with 90 per cent occlusion of the right renal artery and 75 per cent narrowing of the left artery (Figure 1).

Coronary arteriograms revealed 95 per cent occlusion of the left main circumflex coronary artery and significant disease in the other vessels.

The patient was instructed in a 200 mg/day low-cholesterol diet and the administration of cholestyramine, 4 g three times daily, was started. In an attempt to achieve a greater reduction in the serum cholesterol concentration, the dose was increased to 8 g three times daily one month later. Subsequently, the serum cholesterol was found to decrease to 196 mg/100 ml, but serum triglycerides showed a marked increase (Table I), presumably due to the replacement of dietary fat with carbohydrates and/or possibly due to cholestyramine therapy [9,10]. The administration of clofibrate was started in a dose of 1 g

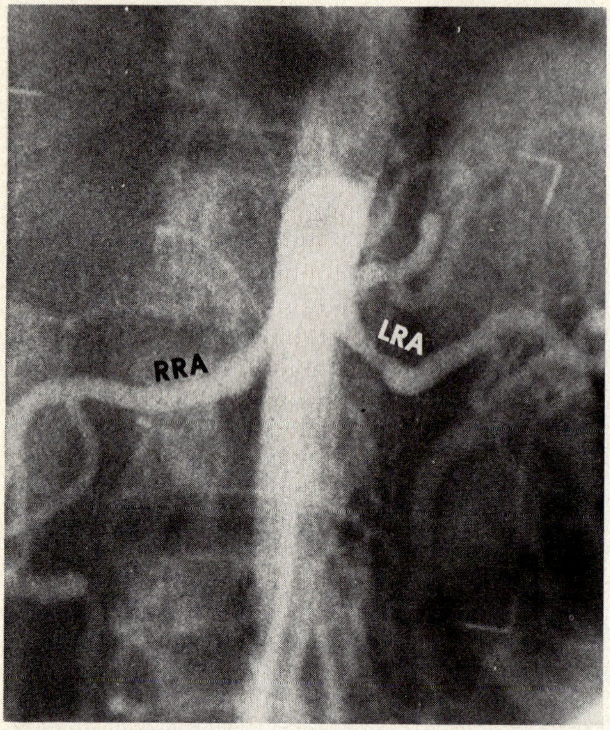

Figure. 2. Renal arteriograms performed nearly three years after sustained control of serum lipids. Note the almost complete resolution of right renal artery (RRA) lesion and possible regression in left renal artery (LRA) lesion.

twice daily, in addition to cholestyramine. Serum lipids were well controlled thereafter. One year later the dose of cholestyramine was reduced to 16 g daily, and clofibrate was maintained at 1 g twice daily with sustained excellent control of serum lipids.

For the high blood pressure, the patient was initially given methyldopa, 250 mg three times daily, and chlorothiazide, 500 mg daily. Drug doses had to be increased two months later to 1 g methyldopa and 1 g chlorothiazide daily. Later, propranolol was added in a dose of 20 mg every 6 hours while chlorothiazide was maintained.

In addition to the previous medications, the patient was advised to use Nitroglycerine sublingually to abort attacks of angina pectoris. Also, isosorbide dinitrate was given 10 mg sublingually every 6 hours. Because of a lack of improvement in exercise tolerance, the patient underwent saphenous vein bypass surgery in June 1971 with subsequent amelioration of angina pectoris. Propranolol therapy was discontinued. The patient was maintained on the rest of the medications in the same dosage, as already outlined, for the following year.

In June 1972 the blood pressure was 125/75 mm Hg, and methyldopa was decreased to 250 mg twice daily and chlorothiazide to 500 mg/day. The patient remained normotensive, and all antihypertensive medications were discontinued in the following few months.

In January 1974 she underwent a repeat routine coronary angiographic study which revealed patent aortocoronary saphenous vein grafts and suggested some regression in the underlying coronary artery disease. Renal arteriograms (Figure 2), viewed from various angles, revealed marked regression of the right renal artery lesion and some regression of left renal artery disease. A treadmill exercise test showed no limitation in exercise tolerance, normal blood pressure response to exercise and no ischemic changes in the electrocardiogram.

Peripheral vein plasma renin was normal at 3 ng/ml.

The patient was maintained on an 1,800 calorie low-cholesterol diet, and a combination of cholestyramine 16 g/day and clofibrate 2 g/day. She has continued to do well.

COMMENTS

This case shows that adequate control of hyperlipidemia can occasionally lead to regression of atherosclerotic lesions. Our patient had longstanding hypertension requiring multiple drug therapy with only a moderately satisfactory response. The hypertensive state was believed to be due to the atherosclerotic renal artery stenosis demonstrated in the renal arteriograms. This was further suggested by the markedly elevated plasma renin level in the peripheral vein blood. Spontaneous regression of hypertension to normal blood pressure levels, allowing discontinuation of antihypertensive therapy, followed sustained excellent control of the hyperlipidemic state. Simultaneously, the plasma renin level became normal, and renal artery stenosis (by repeat renal arteriography) regressed significantly.

There is ample evidence that animals in which atherosclerosis is induced often show impressive regression of the atherosclerotic lesions when maintained on regression diets [1–5], or in response to other measures that lower serum cholesterol [11–15]. Such regression involves reduction of the intracellular content of cholesterol but not of the other components of the atherosclerotic lesion [1]. Therefore, it has been questioned whether findings in animal experiments apply to lesions in human subjects which are often complicated by hemorrhage, extensive accretion of scleroprotein, necrosis and calcification [1]. Furthermore, it is not clear whether extracellular lipid within a plaque could be mobilized as a result of a reduced serum lipid concentration.

Attempts to induce regression of atherosclerosis in man through the control of hyperlipidemia, have been generally disappointing. Rowe and co-workers [16] reported on seven patients in whom coronary arteriography was repeated one year or longer after adequate control of hyperlipidemia with ileal bypass and, when required, additional drug therapy. The coronary angiograms revealed no resolution of arterial obstruction, and in several of their patients there was a progression of the coronary artery obstruction. Cohn and Langston [17] reported similar results in a prospective study on 40 patients in whom coronary angiograms were obtained before they were treated double-blind with placebo or clofibrate. These investigators noted that clofibrate did not influence significantly the rate of progression of coronary artery disease as assessed by repeat angiography after one year of therapy. However, this study included 31 patients who were subjected to aortocoronary bypass surgery which could have biased the results adversely. There is ample recent evidence that this type of surgery tends to accelerate the rate of progression of the underlying coronary artery disease [18].

In an angiographic study of pelvic and coronary arteries before and two years after partial ileal bypass for the treatment of hyperlipidemia, Knight and co-workers [19] encountered no instance of improvement in pelvic arteriograms in nine patients studied. In twenty-two coronary artery studies, these investigators encountered no change in the disease in 12 patients and progression of the disease in five. However, there was questionable improvement in two, and true arteriographic evidence of disease regression in three patients (13.6 per cent).

The question of whether proper control of hyperlipidemia for several years will ultimately cause a regression of atherosclerotic disease in a substantial number of patients remains unanswered. As is evidenced by the present case, however, regression of at least certain types of atherosclerosis through control of hyperlipidemia appears to be feasible. It is possible that our patient represents a rare example in which the atheromas were structurally more like lesions induced experimentally in animals in response to atherogenic diet, and therefore the lesions were composed primarily of masses of intimal fat rather than connective tissue elements [1]. On the other hand, even severe atheromas in human subjects equilibrate with labelled plasma cholesterol [20,21]. Therefore, it is conceivable that a significant decrease in the atheroma lipid content could be achieved even in sclerotic lesions through sustained lowering of serum lipid levels.

Although the clinical course in our patient suggests strongly that the regression of hypertension resulted from regression of renal artery atherosclerosis through the control of hyperlipidemia, a cause and effect relationship cannot be firmly established. It is possible that cessation of smoking, alterations in life style or other unidentified factors might have contributed to this patient's improvement.

REFERENCES

1. Armstrong ML, Warner ED, Connor WE: Regression of coronary atheromatosis in rhesus monkeys. Circ Res 27: 59, 1970.
2. Horlick L, Katz LN: Retrogression of atherosclerotic lesions on cessation of cholesterol feeding in the chick. J Lab Clin Med 34: 1427, 1949.
3. Peterson JE, Hirst AE: Studies on the relation of diet, cholesterol and atheroma in chickens. Circulation 3: 116, 1951.
4. Bevins M, Davison JD, Kendall FE: Regression of lesions in canine atherosclerosis. Arch Pathol 70: 712, 1960.
5. Friedman M, Byers SO: Observations concerning the evolution of atherosclerosis in the rabbit after cessation of cholesterol feeding. Am J Path 43: 349, 1963.
6. Armstrong ML, Megan MB: Lipid depletion in atheromatous coronary arteries in rhesus monkeys after regression diets. Circ Res 30: 675, 1972.
7. Dayton S, Hashimoto S: Recent advances in molecular pathology. A review. Cholesterol flux and metabolism in arterial tissue and in atheromata. Exp Molec Pathol 13: 253, 1970.
8. Lofland HB, Clarkson TB: Bi-directional transfer of cholesterol in normal aorta, fatty streaks and atheromatous plaques. Proc Soc Exp Biol Med 133: 1, 1970.
9. Jepson EM, Fahmy MFI, Torrens PE, Billimoria JD: Treatment of essential hyperlipidaemia. Lancet 2: 1315, 1969.
10. Grundy SM, Ahrens EH Jr, Salen G: Interruption of the enterohepatic circulation of bile acids in man. Comparative effects of cholestyramine and ileal exclusion on cholesterol metabolism. J Lab Clin Med 78: 94, 1971.
11. Frost JW, Finch WT, Younger R, Butts WH, Scott HW Jr: Pilot study of the therapeutic effects of ileal bypass in dogs with experimentally established hypercholesterolemia and atherosclerosis. Surg Forum 21: 398, 1970.
12. Shepard GH, Wimberly JE, Younger RK, Stephenson SE Jr, Scott HW Jr: Effects of bypass of the distal third of the small intestine on experimental hypercholesterolemia and atherosclerosis in rhesus monkeys. Surg Forum 19: 302, 1968.
13. Scott HW Jr, Stephenson SE Jr, Hayes CW, Younger RK: Effects of bypass of the distal fourth of small intestine on experimental hypercholesterolemia and atherosclerosis in rhesus monkeys. Surg Gynecol Obstet 125: 3, 1967.
14. Younger RK, Shepard GH, Butts WH, Scott HW Jr: Comparison of the protective effects of cholestyramine and ileal bypass in rhesus monkeys on an atherogenic regimen. Surg Forum 20: 101, 1969.
15. Gomes MM, Kottke BA, Bernatz P, Titus JL: Effect of ileal bypass on aortic atherosclerosis of white carneau pigeons. Surgery 70: 353, 1971.
16. Rowe GG, Young WP, Wasserburger RH: The effects of reduced serum cholesterol on human coronary atherosclerosis. Circulation 39 (suppl 3): 22, 1969.
17. Cohn K, Langston M: Effect of clofibrate on progression of coronary disease. A prospective, angiographic study in man. Circulation 47, 48 (suppl 4): 55, 1973.
18. Glassman E, Spencer FC, Krauss KR, Weisinger B, Isom OW: Changes in the underlying coronary circulation secondary to bypass grafting. Circulation 49, 50 (suppl 2): 80, 1974.
19. Knight L, Scheibel R, Amplatz K, Varco RL, Buchwald H: Radiographic appraisal of the Minnesota partial ileal bypass study. Surg Forum 23: 141, 1972.
20. Gould RG, Jones RJ, Wissler RW: Lability of cholesterol in human atherosclerotic plaques. Circulation 20: 967, 1959.
21. Field H Jr, Swell L, Schools PE Jr, Treadwell CR: Dynamic aspects of cholesterol metabolism in different areas of the aorta and other tissues in man and their relationship to atherosclerosis. Circulation 22: 547, 1960.

Arthritis with an Inflammatory Dermatosis Resembling Sweet's Syndrome

Report of a Unique Case and Review of the Literature on Arthritis Associated with Inflammatory Dermatoses

DAVID E. TRENTHAM, M.D.*
ALFONSE T. MASI, M.D., D.P.H.
GEORGE F. BALE, M.D.

A patient with a unique case of chronic episodic arthritis coincident with flares of acneform, pustular, nodular and ulcerating skin lesions was observed over a five-year period. This patient and a review of the literature on arthritis associated with the inflammatory dermatoses provide evidence which may interrelate several of these nosologically confusing skin conditions, e.g., the family of leukocytoclastic angiitides with the newly posited acute febrile neutrophilic dermatosis of Sweet. Systemic manifestations and a variety of acneform, pustular, nodular and ulcerating cutaneous lesions in the inflammatory dermatoses are best explained by small vessel involvement, with individual syndromes being determined by the type and degree of vascular change. Perivascular neutrophilic infiltration is the unifying histologic feature of these small vessel diseases. Neutrophil infiltration differentiates these entities, and our patient, from the histologically nonspecific inflammations of the skin, e.g., Behçet's disease and pyoderma gangrenosum, which, although capable of causing identically appearing skin lesions, consist predominantly of lymphocytic dermal infiltrates even in the earlier stages. It appears important to recognize these morphologically varied acute inflammatory dermatoses with perivascular neutrophilic infiltration in view of their systemic features and the dramatic efficacy of corticosteroid therapy.

From the Department of Medicine, Division of Connective Tissue Diseases, Section of Rheumatology, University of Tennessee Center for the Health Sciences; and the Department of Pathology, Baptist Memorial Hospital, Memphis, Tennessee. This study was supported in part by Grants AM-12049 and AM-05055 of the National Institute of Arthritis, Metabolism, and Digestive Diseases, Bethesda, Maryland. Requests for reprints should be addressed to Dr. A. T. Masi, Division of Connective Tissue Diseases, University of Tennessee Center for the Health Sciences, 858 Madison Avenue, Memphis, Tennessee 38163. Manuscript accepted December 5, 1975.

* Present address: Department of Medicine, Robert Breck Brigham Hospital, 125 Parker Hill Avenue, Boston, Massachusetts 02120.

Arthritis concurring with a variety of acneform, pustular, nodular or ulcerating inflammatory skin lesions is an intriguing but relatively undefined association. For example, arthritis can be found in association with these skin lesions in diseases generally believed to have a vasculitic basis, e.g., leukocytoclastic angiitis [1], erythema elevatum diutinum [2–4] and dermatitis nodularis necrotica [5]. On the other hand, identical joint symptoms and skin lesions can occur in entities in which vascular involvement is implicated but in which typical histologic features of vasculitis are not always identified, e.g., Behçet's syndrome [6–9], erythema nodosum [10,11], pyoderma gangrenosum [12–16] and, as most recently described, acute febrile neutrophilic dermatosis (Sweet's syndrome) [17–29].

Sweet's syndrome, first described in 1964 and now reported in 44 cases, consists of four cardinal features [29]: (1) An acute or episodic course with fever and neutrophilic leukocytosis. (2) A composite of raised painful plaques, nodules or pustules in an acral or truncal distribution with complete resolution of lesions without scarring. (3) Histologically, a dense inflammatory infiltrate in a perivascular distribution in the mid- and upper dermis consisting of a predominance of neutrophils with a variable proportion of lymphocytes and other inflammatory cells. There are no overtly vasculitic vessel wall changes. (4) Failure of antibiotics to alter the course of the disease but a prompt and dramatic response to systemic corticosteroid therapy.

Longitudinal observations were made over a five-year period on a unique patient with a chronic intermittent polyarthritis associated with flares of acneform, pustular, nodular and, occasionally, ulcerating skin lesions. Histologically, these lesions were characterized by a dense neutrophilic infiltration at all stages studied. Although many aspects of this case closely resemble Sweet's syndrome, the lack of plaque formation and occasional ulcerating lesions are important deterrents to this diagnosis. Analogously, this patient demonstrates features of other inflammatory dermatoses, but, nevertheless, the syndrome does not fit into the accepted diagnostic criteria of any currently recognized disease entity. A comparison of this patient's manifestations with those described in the various inflammatory dermatoses has revealed important interrelationships among them suggesting a spectrum of diseases. Finally, his dramatic response to corticosteroid therapy, typical of inflammatory dermatoses with neutrophilic infiltration, further unifies them and underscores their therapeutic efficacy in these nosologically confusing syndromes.

CASE REPORT

The patient, a 31 year old black male nurse's aide, was admitted to the Memphis VA Hospital in July 1974 with a history of chronic episodic polyarthritis synchronous with flares of nodular and pustular skin lesions of five-years' duration. Previously healthy, he had the sudden onset in 1969 of pain in the right hip which abated with the self-administration of aspirin. Over the ensuing 14 months he experienced episodes of asymmetric arthralgia of the left hip and right knee and ankle. These episodes would recur at one to four month intervals and persist for two to four weeks. Simultaneous with his cyclical arthralgia, he would have an explosive painful skin eruption consisting of papules and nodules on his face, neck, trunk and all extremities, including the dorsum of his hands. The lesions over his shins and calves would initially appear as 1 to 5 cm nodules clinically indistinguishable from erythema nodosum. Crops of these superficial skin lesions would evolve in various stages of development for a one to three week period, gradually assuming a more raised acneform appearance. The epithelium over many of the nodules would thin, become mammilated, and pustules would form which occasionally drained a nonpurulent serous discharge. The lesions (Figure 1) would heal with occasional scarring and residual hyper- and hypopigmentation. During these episodes of arthralgias and skin eruptions, the patient would feel markedly ill, remain in bed for at least the initial two weeks

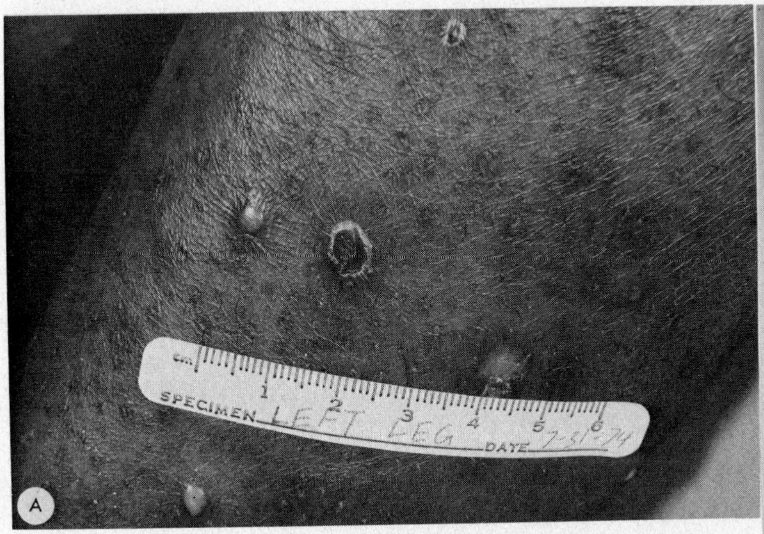

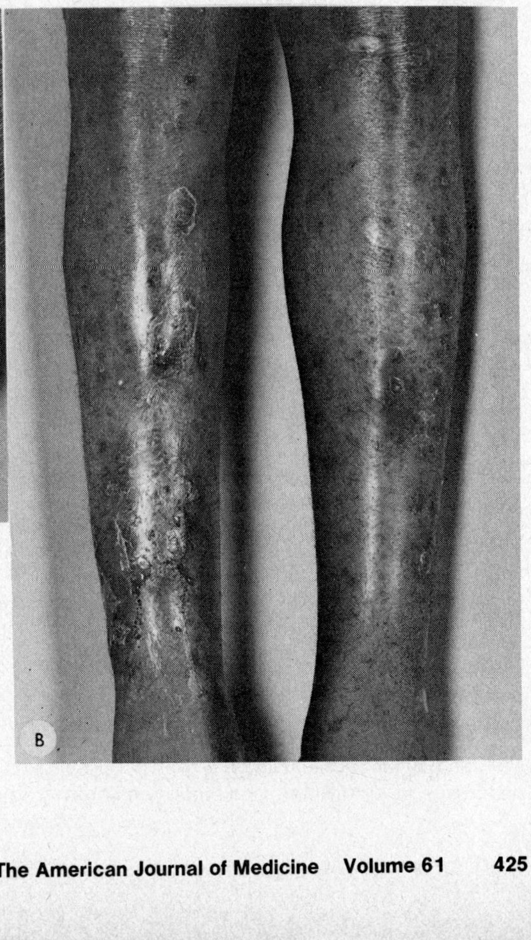

Figure 1. ***A,*** *acral distribution of pustules and papules.* ***B,*** *along with ulcerating nodules. Residual hyper- and hypopigmentation is evident.*

of illness, and experience a low grade fever without chills, night sweats or weight loss. He never experienced conjunctivitis, urethritis, lesions on his mucous membranes or genitalia, or neurologic symptoms. Except for the intake of salicylates for joint pains, drug use, heavy alcohol ingestion, family history of arthritis or allergies were denied.

Persistence of the cyclical arthralgia and painful eruptive lesions prompted him to stop work and seek medical attention in February 1971. Physical examination on admission at that time showed a temperature of 99.4°F orally, tenderness on active and passive movement of the left wrist and right ankle, and multiple nontender 1 cm lymph nodes in the supraclavicular, axillary and inguinal areas. No oral or genital ulcers, seborrhea or nail changes were observed. The optic discs were sharp, and the previously described nodular and pustular facial, truncal and acral lesions were present.

All roentgenograms were within normal limits except for views of the right ankle which showed a periosteal reaction involving the medial malleolus as well as the base of the fifth metatarsal with a mild degree of osteoporosis. Minced synovial and bone biopsy specimens from his right ankle and from skin lesions grew out only Staphylococcus epidermidis and an anaerobic gram-positive rod which was reported to be possibly a Corynebacterium species. All other cultures for acid-fast bacteria, pyogens and fungi were negative. The only laboratory abnormalities were a minimally elevated serum alkaline phosphatase level of 17.5 King-Armstrong Units (normal 8 to 14), serum glutamic oxaloacetic transaminase (SGOT) level of 84 mU/ml (normal less than 50 mU/ml), a bromosulfalein retention of 18 per cent at 45 minutes (normal less than 5 per cent) and a hemoglobin electrophoresis showing AS hemoglobin. Glucose 6-phosphate dehydrogenase (G 6-PD) deficiency screen was negative. Serum immunoglobulins and dinitrochlorobenzene (DNCB) delayed hypersensitivity skin challenge were normal. A liver biopsy specimen was interpreted as showing a minimal focal reactive hepatitis; no granulomas were seen. Rheumatoid factor and antinuclear antibody tests were negative.

Because of the possibility that the patient had Corynebacterium osteomyelitis of the right ankle, therapy with clindamycin, 600 mg daily, was begun in April 1971. The polyarthralgia concurrent with the acneform skin lesions continued during four months of clindamycin therapy. The patient returned to work for only a short time, since he was unable to remain on his feet.

On two subsequent prolonged hospitalizations, in September 1972 and July to December 1974, both the clinical and laboratory features remained unchanged. He continued to experience simultaneous exacerbations of his arthritis and skin lesions, and to feel markedly ill with a low grade fever and leukocytosis at the onset of his eruptions. Serum screen for bromide or iodides, uric acid, serologic tests for syphilis (VDRL and FTA-ABS), antinuclear antibodies, latex agglutination for rheumatoid factor, creatinine, 17-hydroxycorticosteroid and 17-ketosteroid excretions, antistreptolysin, antiDNase B, antihyaluronidase, streptozyme, hepatitis-associated antigen (HB_sAg), intermediate and second-strength purified protein derivative and histoplasmin skin tests, fungal serology, sacroiliac roentgenograms, studies of the upper gastrointestinal tract and small bowel, barium enema studies, sigmoidoscopy, slit-lamp and otolaryngologic examinations for oral lesions, complement (C3), cryoglobulins and blood cultures were all negative or within normal limits. Creatinine clearance was 101 ml/min. Serum protein electrophoresis showed a total protein of 7.0 g (normal 6.4 to 7.9 g), albumin 43 per cent (53.5 to 66.3 per cent), $alpha_1$ globulin 4.8 per cent (2.2 to 5.0 per cent), $alpha_2$ globulin 12.5 per cent (6.6 to 12.9 per cent), beta globulin 13.7 per cent (7.3 to 14.5 per cent) and gamma globulins 26.0 per cent (10.4 to 19.4 per cent). Serum radial immunodiffusion showed an immunoglobulin G (IgG) level of 1,870 mg/100 ml (normal 300 to 1,700 mg/100 ml), an immunoglobulin A (IgA) level of 249 mg/100 ml (70 to 350 mg/100 ml) and an immunoglobulin M (IgM) level of 139 mg/100 ml (70 to 210 mg/100 ml).

Positive findings on his admission in July 1974 included pain, swelling and mild heat of the ankles, knees and left elbow. There was pain on external rotation of the left hip, and a minimal effusion and limitation of inversion and eversion of the right ankle. Aspiration of the ankle showed a poor mucin clot, 250 white blood cells/mm^3 (5 per cent segmented, 95 per cent monocytic) and a total protein of 4.7 g/100 ml. Cultures and examination for crystals were negative. A roentgenogram of this ankle again showed a periosteal reaction of the os calcis, medial malleolus and base of the fifth metatarsal. Multiple cultures of the blood, nasal septum, os calcis and skin lesions for acid-fast, fungal, aerobic or anaerobic bacterial organisms were negative.

A liver scan showed homogeneous uptake in a slightly enlarged liver. A spleen scan was within normal limits. The alkaline phosphatase level remained mildly elevated (244 IU, normal 30 to 85 IU). A liver biopsy specimen obtained three years after his first biopsy again showed a nonspecific focal reactive hepatitis with moderate dilatation of the sinusoids and a mild mononuclear cell infiltration of the periportal spaces. The bile ducts were normal, and no granulomas were seen.

Four skin biopsy specimens (Figures 2 and 3) of the papules, pustules, nodules and ulcers in various stages of development have shown either a normal or a mildly edematous squamous epithelium with sharply demarcated areas of dense neutrophilic infiltration in the mid and upper dermis. Eosinophils and lymphocytes were occasionally seen. Capillary and venular dilatation was seen in the superficial areas with occasional swelling of endothelial cells of deeper arterioles and perivascular round cell infiltration but no fibrinoid changes, basement membrane thickening or evidence of an acute vasculitis. A mild degree of dermal edema and nuclear dust was present with a few areas of erythrocyte extravasation. One small intra-epithelial pustule was seen filled with neutrophils. Gram stains of the tissue showed no organisms.

The patient's ankle, knee and elbow synovitis and skin lesions did not respond to three-week trials of aspirin (6 g daily), indomethacin (150 mg daily), oral penicillin (phenoxymethylpenicillin 1 g daily), tetracycline (2 g daily) and salicylazosulfapyridine (Azulfidine® 9 g daily). During these trials his temperature ranged between 98.6° and 100.2°F orally, his Westergren sedimentation rate between 23 and 56 mm/hour, and white cell count between 10,300 and 14,200/mm^3 (56 to 75 per cent polymorphonuclear leukocytes). During three months of continuously active arthritis and evolving skin eruptions, at least three pustules rapidly enlarged and formed ulcerating 4 to 6 cm lesions with a ne-

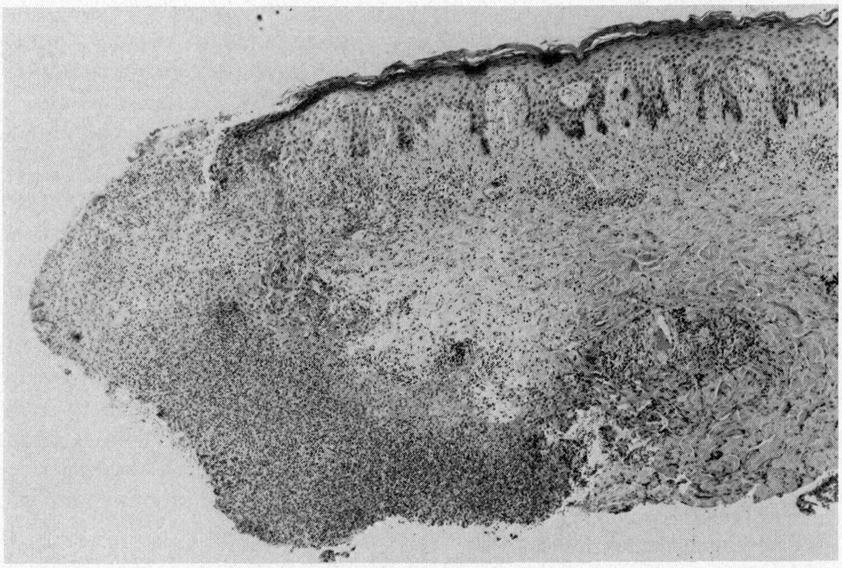

Figure 2. *Skin biopsy specimen showing areas of intense cellular infiltration of the dermis with normal epithelium adjacent to lesion. Hematoxylin and eosin stain; original magnification ×85, reduced by 32 per cent.*

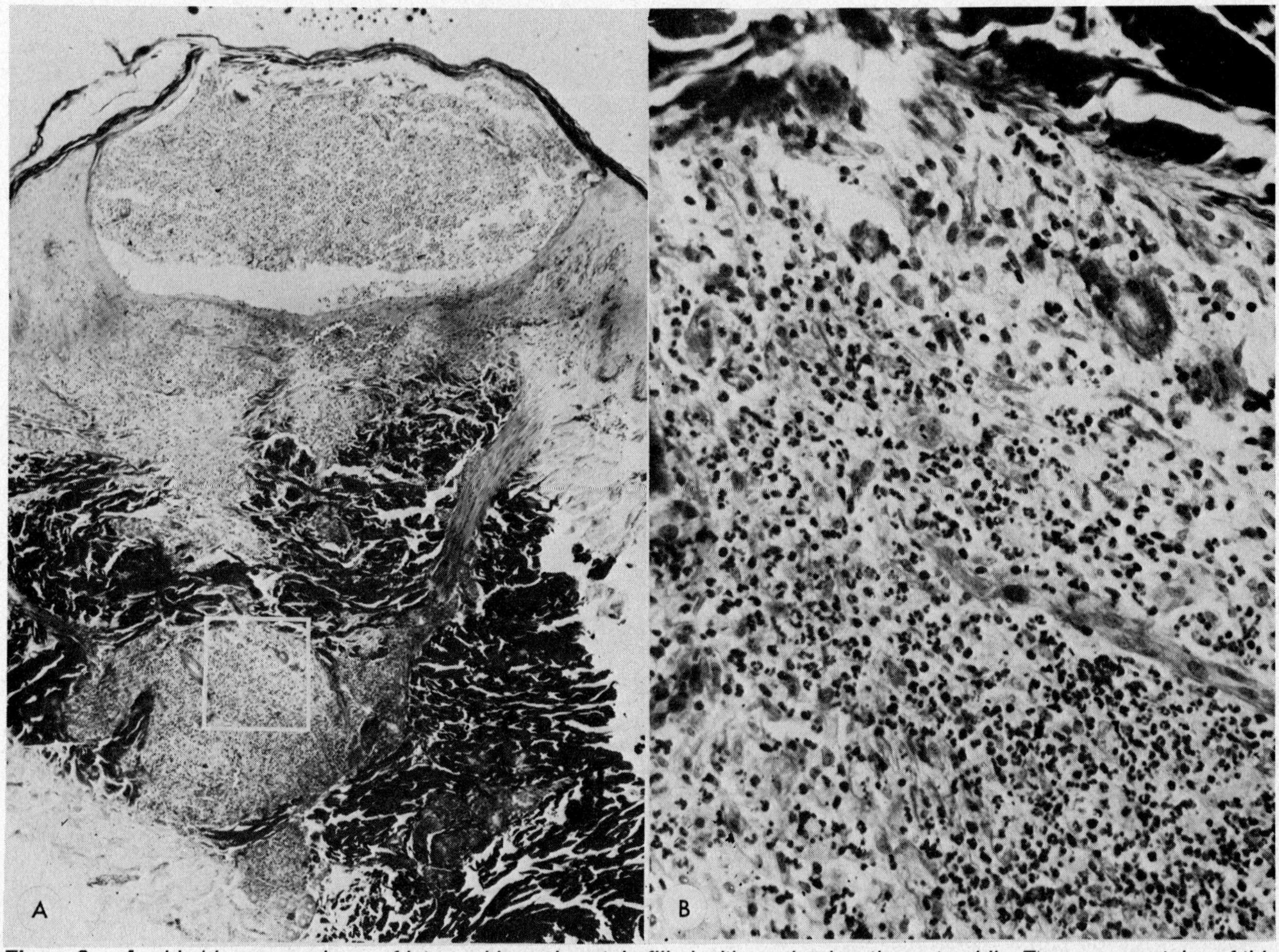

Figure 3. ***A,*** *skin biopsy specimen of intra-epidermal pustule filled with predominantly neutrophils. Tissue gram stains of this lesion were negative.* ***B,*** *enlargement of the dermal area enclosed in A showing the neutrophil infiltrate and occasional neutrophil fragmentation. Hematoxylin and eosin stain, original magnification × 100 (A) and × 450 (B), reduced by 25 per cent.*

crotic base and dark undermined margins over a two- to four-day period. These lesions (Figure 4) were present on the anterior tibial surface and calves, and were morphologically consistent with pyoderma gangrenosum. Biopsy showed again only dermal inflammation with mainly neutrophil infiltration.

A trial of prednisone therapy, 40 mg daily, was begun, and dramatic improvement in his arthritis and acneform skin lesions was noted within two to three days. His skin lesions healed completely over a three-week period, and he remained symptom free while the dose of steroids was gradually tapered over a four month period. He remained well, after cessation of these agents in January 1975, and left our community in March of that year. However, in May, his arthritis and pustular skin lesions abruptly recurred, and his condition failed to improve with tetracycline and indomethacin therapy, while under another physician's care. In spite of the patient relating a previous good response to corticosteroids, the physician was reluctant to restart use of these agents. At present, however, we have communicated details of the patient's course and anticipate reinstitution of prednisone therapy.

SPECIAL STUDIES

Total hemolytic complement activity (CH 50) was 67.6 units/ml, the normal range in this laboratory being 29 to 45 units/ml [30]. Serum undiluted and in 1/10 dilutions was negative for antinuclear factor activity. A nitroblue tetrazolium test showed no impairment of neutrophil phagocytic function. The patient's HL-A type [31] was A_2 in the first and A_8 and A_{12} in the second segregant series.

Direct immunofluorescence of involved and uninvolved skin, including the pyodermatous lesions, was negative for IgG, IgM, and C3. A threefold rise in antibody titer was noted two weeks after immunization with 0.5 ml of monovalent typhoid vaccine.

Cellular immunity was assayed by intradermal skin tests with 0.1 ml Candida, mumps and streptokinase-streptodornase (SK-SD) antigens. Normal sensitization with 2,4-dinitrochlorobenzene (DNCB) [32] had been previously achieved. The patient was nonreactive to mumps but showed 5 mm induration to Candida and 8 mm to SK-SD at 48 and 72 hours. Results of in vitro lymphocyte transformation revealed a modest impairment in response to phytohemagglutinin (PHA) and values for antigen stimulation which were within the lower normal range for this laboratory [33].

COMMENTS

Polyarthralgia or arthritis has frequently been reported in association with a variety of inflammatory acneform, pustular, nodular or ulcerating skin lesions [1–28,34–46]. Arthritis and inflammatory cutaneous lesions can occur with pustular psoriasis [34], Reiter's disease [35], Behçet's syndrome [6–9], erythema nodosum [10,11], the nodose skin lesions of pancreatic disease [36], hypersensitivity angiitis [1], pyoderma gangrenosum [12–16], dermatitis nodularis necrotica [5], erythema elevatum diutinum [3,4], acne conglobata [37–40], allergic cutaneous arteriolitis (Ruiter's disease) [41–43], the nodular dermal allergides of Gougerot and Duperrat [44], polyarteritis nodosa [45,46] and, as more recently reported, with an acute febrile neutrophilic dermatosis (Sweet's syndrome) [17–29].

The peripheral nondeforming arthritis associated with these inflammatory dermal lesions is remarkably similar. The tendency to an episodic, pauciarticular, asymmetric, large joint and lower extremity involvement also conforms to the pattern of arthritis associated with inflammatory bowel disease. Features shared by all of these dermal and intestinal arthritides are a more acute and shorter duration of exacerbations, a tendency for complete recovery without residual disability, and a lack of cortical erosions, ankylosis, morning stiffness or muscle wasting. These are distinctly dissimilar from rheumatoid arthritis [47,48].

Unlike the uniform pattern of arthritis in these in-

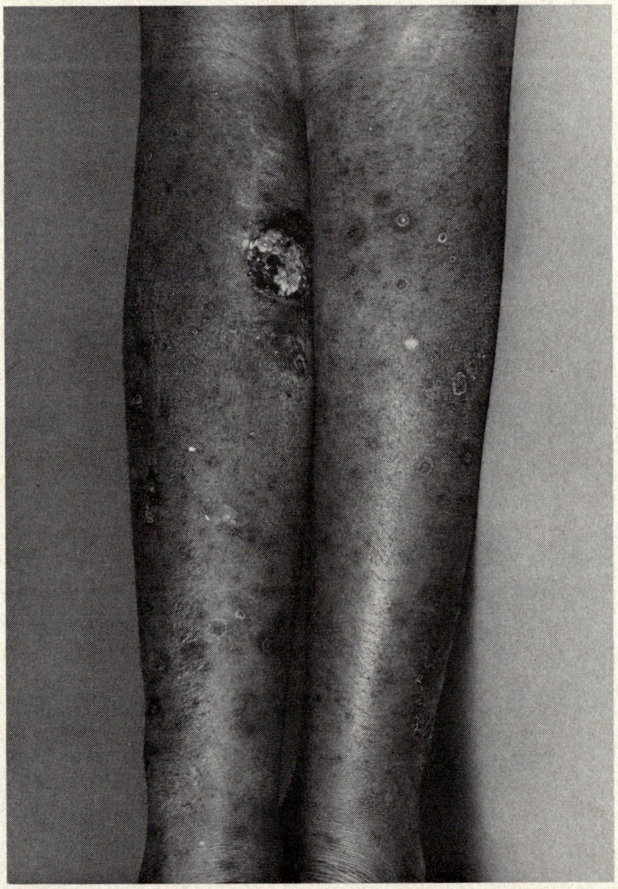

Figure 4. Five centimeter necrotic ulcerated area on left calf. Although this lesion grossly resembles pyoderma gangrenosum, the underlying dermal infiltrate was neutrophilic.

flammatory skin diseases, the cutaneous lesions have varied clinical, gross and microscopic features with a confusing nosology. Concerning the vasculitic skin diseases, Sams and Logan [49] recently commented that "One major obstacle to significant progress in the past has been the tiresome preoccupation with addition to and subtraction from the already inscrutable morass of clinical syndromes. It is hoped, as further clinical and experimental data accrue, that a more reasonable classification on the basis of pathogenesis may be feasible."

Winkelmann and Ditto [1] performed a major service by classifying the cutaneous and visceral lesions of Gougerot, Ruiter, erythema elevatum diutinum and dermatitis nodularis necrotica into a family of leukocytoclastic angiitides on the basis of a common histologic feature of small vessel vasculitis with necrosis, fibrinoid change and cellular infiltration, predominantly neutrophils, of the vessel walls and periadventitial region. More recently Braverman [50] has stressed the breadth of the clinical spectrum and the interrelationship of the cutaneous and systemic features of leukocytoclastic angiitis. The longitudinal observations of our patient provide evidence that other types of inflammatory dermatoses may belong to a still further expanded disease spectrum, extending beyond the leukocytoclastic angiitides.

Many features of our patient are typical of the acute febrile neutrophilic dermatosis of Sweet [17–29], such as the numerous episodes of an explosive eruption of raised painful nodules on the face, neck, trunk and limbs. Later the nodules would form pustules, and fever would develop with marked systemic toxicity, blood neutrophilic leukocytosis and, histologically, a dense dermal neutrophilic infiltration but, importantly, without histologic evidence of acute vasculitis. Furthermore, the mainly superficial nature of our patient's skin lesions, lack of response to antibiotic therapy or to nonsteroidal antiinflammatory agents, and dramatic response to the administration of steroids were all striking features and consistent with the acute neutrophilic dermatosis of Sweet. However, his lack of plaque formation, which is considered to be the prototypical lesion of Sweet's syndrome [17], and the occasional pyoderma gangrenosum-like ulcers, which have not been previously reported in Sweet's syndrome, argue against this diagnosis.

Similarly, our patient's dramatic response to steroid therapy and neutrophilic infiltration might simulate a leukocytoclastic angiitis; however, the lack of necrotizing vasculitis, purpuric skin lesions and only minimal scarring exclude this particular syndrome. Likewise, a primary diagnosis of pyoderma gangrenosum would only poorly explain his multiple other skin lesions and the neutrophilic infiltration would be distinctly unusual [56].

His episodic polyarthritis, which monotonously coincided with flares of his various types of skin lesions, was characteristic of many of these acute inflammatory dermatoses. This recurring feature further unifies his dermal lesions and makes us reluctant to partition his lesions into separate nosologic entities. Behçet's disease, the full features of which our patient did not have, e.g., oral or genital ulcers or neurologic involvement, is another example of a disease with a similar arthritis in which a multitude of skin lesions, including acne, pyoderma gangrenosum, erythema nodosum and thrombophlebitis can occur [7,8].

Clinical differentiation among the acute inflammatory dermatoses associated with arthritis, such as conglobate acne [38,40], Behçet's syndrome [7–9], pyoderma gangrenosum [13–16,51], leukocytoclastic angiitides [5,52,53], and the acute febrile neutrophilic dermatosis of Sweet [17–29], is difficult since all can appear as explosive painful crops of acneform lesions, nodules or papules which later can become pustular or, as previously reported in all except Sweet's syndrome, ulcerate. Systemic manifestations such as malaise, fever or arthralgia are commonly shared features. Kierland [54], Brunsting [55] and, more recently, Montgomery [56] have noted similarities among many of these inflammatory pustular or pyodermatous lesions. Thus, these acute inflammatory dermatoses, often with similar and significant systemic features, such as arthritis, may clinically be better considered as a spectrum rather than as nosologically confusing diseases sui generis (Table I).

One can better differentiate these entities histologically than clinically. Our patient's dense perivascular neutrophil infiltration of the dermis without necrotizing vasculitis clearly separates his disease, on the one hand, from leukocytoclastic angiitis and, on the other, from the non-neutrophilic inflammatory skin conditions, such as Behçet's disease [8] and pyoderma gangrenosum, considered histologically nonspecific [51,56]. Even in the earliest lesions, lymphocytes are the predominant infiltrating cells in Behçet's disease [57] and pyoderma gangrenosum [51]. Our patient's biopsy specimens showed changes typical of the histopathologic features of the newly posited syndrome of Sweet, which is, again, a dense dermal infiltrate in a perivascular distribution composed predominantly of neutrophils with a variable number of lymphocytes and eosinophils, but without vessel wall necrosis or fibrinoid change [17,29]. The minor degree of intrinsic microvascular change in this painful eruption separates it histologically from leukocytoclastic angiitis, but these entities may, nevertheless, belong to a common disease spectrum since capillary and venular vasodilatation and endothelial swelling are present in both disorders [1,17,21].

TABLE I Features of Acute Inflammatory Dermatoses Associated with Arthritis

	Leukocytoclastic Angiitis	Acute Febrile Neutrophilic Dermatosis	Our Patient	Pyoderma Gangrenosum	Behçet's Disease
Systemic Features					
Preceding upper respiratory infection	V	+	–	–	–
Acute occurrence	+	+	+	+	+
Tendency to recur	+	+	+	+	+
Fever with attacks	+	+	+	V	+
Leukocytosis	V	+	+	V	V
Systemic toxicity	+	+	+	V	+
Peripheral arthritis*	+	+	+	+	+
Response to steroids	+	+	+	V	V
Cutaneous Features					
Necrotic	+	–	+	+	+
Purpuric, raised	+	–	–	–	–
Acneform	+	+	+	+	+
Pustular, vesicular	+	+	+	+	+
Nodular	+	+	+	+	+
Ulcerating	+	–	+	+	+
Scar producing	+	–	+	+	+
Histology					
Small vessel necrosis and hemorrhage	+	–	–	–	–
Primary fibrinoid vessel wall change	+	–	–	–	–
Endothelial proliferation and swelling	+	+	+	+	+
Neutrophilic perivascular infiltrate	+	+	+	–	–

NOTE: V = variable.
*Nondeforming, asymmetric, large joints usually

The favorable response to steroid therapy is shared by the acute neutrophilic dermatosis of Sweet [17,21,24] and leukocytoclastic angiitis [1]. This further favors a grouped taxonomy for these small vessel neutrophilic, cutaneous and systemic syndromes, and tends to separate them from pyoderma gangrenosum [14,16,58,59] and Behçet's disease [6,7] in which the response to steroid therapy is more variable.

Pathogenetically, it also appears reasonable to regard our patient's synovitis and focal hepatitis as manifestations of an ongoing systemic process including an inflammatory dermatosis. Just as erythema nodosum can demonstrate a varied histologic spectrum from thrombophlebitis to leukocytoclastic angiitis to no evidence of vasculitis [11], so these inflammatory dermatosis syndromes may also be considered to belong to an overlapping disease spectrum in which arthritis is linked to a variety of skin lesions, perhaps by an underlying vascular involvement of varied types and severity. Again, Behçet's disease would be an obvious parallel in which a process strongly suspected of involving the vasculature [57] causes a variety of systemic and previously mentioned dermatologic features, often with little histologic evidence of acute vasculitis per se [9]. Likewise, skin involvement by acute vasculitis can produce a continuum of urticaria, erythema, purpura, vesiculation, pustulation to infarction [60]. Another feature, perhaps implicating vascular involvement in our patient, is the periosteal reaction around his ankle, which is intriguingly similar to that reported in cases of lower extremity periostitis with joint swelling but no clubbing and biopsy proved evidence of arteritis. Generally these patients also had a dramatic response to steroid therapy [61–63].

CONCLUSION

Although the etiology and pathogenesis are unknown, available data suggest that the leukocytoclastic angiitides and the neutrophilic dermatosis of Sweet may belong to a common disease spectrum. A patient was carefully studied over five years who, in terms of a clinical composite, appears unique. However, many of his clinical and histologic features, such as an episodic nondeforming arthritis, are shared with this group of dermatoses. This patient and a review of the literature suggest that leukocytoclastic angiitis and the acute febrile neutrophilic dermatosis of Sweet are interrelated histologically by a dense neutrophilic infiltrate around small vessels, and are characterized by systemic and cutaneous manifestations. The diagnostic difficulty in categorizing this patient may indicate that the particular clinical syndrome is determined by the type and intensity of vasculitis, indicated by features such as the presence or absence of fibrinoid change, necrosis and luminal occlusion. These neutrophilic small vessel syndromes can be differentiated from the histologically nonspecific inflammatory diseases, such as Behçet's disease and pyoderma gangrenosum, but clinically all can cause skin lesions with similar appearance and systemic features. Further longitudinal investigations of such patients may provide additional evidence for interrelationships among these entities. Despite the varied morphologic presentations of the neutrophilic dermatoses, their severe systemic symptoms and their favorable response to corticosteroid therapy demand diagnostic awareness.

ACKNOWLEDGMENT

We gratefully acknowledge the excellent technical help of Margarett Key.

REFERENCES

1. Winkelmann RK, Ditto WB: Cutaneous and visceral syndromes of necrotizing or "allergic" angiitis. Medicine 43: 59, 1964.
2. Beer WE: Erythema elevatum diutinum. Proc R Soc Med 56: 909, 1963.
3. Mraz JP, Newcomer VD: Erythema elevatum diutinum. Arch Dermatol 96: 235, 1967.
4. Weidman FD, Besancon JH: Erythema elevatum diutinum. Arch Dermatol 20: 593, 1929.
5. Duemling WW: Dermatitis nodularis necrotica. Arch Dermatol 21: 229, 1930.
6. Mason RM, Barnes CG: Behçet's syndrome with arthritis. Ann Rheum Dis 28: 95, 1969.
7. Kalbian VV, Challis MT: Behçet's disease. Report of 12 cases with three manifesting as papilledema. Am J Med 49: 823, 1970.
8. Cummings NA: The oral-mucosal manifestations of rheumatic diseases. Rheumatology 4: 60, 1973.
9. Graykowski EA, Barile MF, Lee WB, Stanley HR: Recurrent aphthous stomatitis. JAMA 196: 637, 1966.
10. Truelove LH: Articular manifestations of erythema nodosum. Ann Rheum Dis 19: 174, 1960.
11. Blomgren SE: Erythema nodosum. Semin Arthritis Rheum 4: 1, 1974.
12. Ricketts WE, Kirsner JB, Rothmer S: Pyoderma gangrenosum in chronic nonspecific ulcerative colitis. Am J Med 5: 69, 1948.
13. Perry HO, Brunsting LA: Pyoderma gangrenosum. Arch Dermatol 75: 380, 1957.
14. Ayers S Jr, Ayers S III: Pyoderma gangrenosum with an unusual syndrome of ulcers, vesicles and arthritis. Arch Dermatol 77: 270, 1958.
15. Perry HO: Pyoderma gangrenosum. South Med J 62: 899, 1969.
16. Lazarus GS, Goldsmith LA, Rocklin RE, et al.: Pyoderma gangrenosum, altered delayed hypersensitivity, and polyarthritis. Arch Dermatol 105: 46, 1972.
17. Sweet RD: An acute febrile neutrophilic dermatosis. Br J Dermatol 76: 394, 1964.
18. Robinson BHB: New dermatosis. Br Med J 1: 190, 1965.
19. Fuld H: New dermatosis. Br Med J 1: 382, 1965.
20. Sweet RD: Further observations on acute febrile neutrophilic dermatosis. Br J Dermatol 80: 800, 1968.
21. Crow KD, Kerdel-Vegas F, Rook A: Acute febrile neutrophilic dermatosis: Sweet's syndrome. Dermatologica 139: 123, 1969.
22. Brenan JA: Acute febrile neutrophilic dermatosis (Sweet). Australas J Dermatol 10: 186, 1969.
23. Evans S, Evans CC: Acute febrile neutrophilic dermatosis—two cases. Dermatologica 143: 153, 1971.
24. Goldman GC, Moschella SL: Acute febrile neutrophilic dermatosis (Sweet's syndrome). Arch Dermatol 103: 654, 1971.
25. Shapiro L, Baraf CS, Richheimer LL: Sweet's syndrome (acute febrile neutrophilic dermatosis). Arch Dermatol 103: 81, 1971.
26. Frayha R, Matta M, Kurban A: Sweet's syndrome simulating systemic lupus erythematosus. Dermatologica 144: 321, 1972.
27. Raff M, Santler R: Akute febrile neutrophile Dermatose (Sweet syndrom). Hautarzt 23: 415, 1972.
28. Krauser RE, Schumacher HR: The arthritis of Sweet's syndrome. Arthritis Rheum 18: 35, 1975.
29. Gunawardena DA, Gunawardena KA, Ratnayaka RMRS, Vasanthanathan NS: The clinical spectrum of Sweet's syndrome (acute febrile neutrophilic dermatosis)—a report of 18 cases. Br J Dermatol 92: 363, 1975.
30. Townes AS: Complement levels in disease. Johns Hopkins Med J 120: 337, 1967.
31. Mittal KK, Mickey MR, Singal DP, Terasaki P: Serotyping for homotransplantation. XVIII. Refinement of microdroplet lymphocyte cytotoxicity test. Transplantation 6: 913, 1968.
32. Waldorf DS, Wilkins RF, Decker JL: Impaired delayed hypersensitivity in an aging population. JAMA 203: 831, 1968.
33. Paty JG, Sienknecht CW, Townes AS, et al.: Impaired cell-mediated immunity in systemic lupus erythematosus (SLE): a controlled study of 23 untreated patients. Am J Med 59: 769, 1975.
34. Perry HO, Mayne JG: Psoriasis and Reiter's syndrome. Arch Dermatol 92: 129, 1965.
35. Montgomery MM, Poske RM, Barton EM, et al.: The mucocutaneous lesions of Reiter's syndrome. Ann Intern Med 51: 99, 1959.
36. Mullin GT, Caperton EM, Crespin SR, Williams RC: Arthritis and skin lesions resembling erythema nodosum in pancreatic disease. Ann Intern Med 68: 75, 1968.
37. Burnes RE, Colville JM: Acne conglobata with septicemia (?). Arch Dermatol 79: 361, 1959.
38. Windon RE, Sanford JP, Ziff M: Acne conglobata and arthritis. Arthritis Rheum 4: 632, 1961.
39. Moschella SL: Report of a case of acne conglobata and arthritis. Bull Assoc Milit Dermatologists 13: 15, 1964.
40. Kelly AP, Burns RE: Acute febrile ulcerative conglobate acne with polyarthralgia. Arch Dermatol 104: 182, 1971.
41. Ruiter M: A case of allergic cutaneous vasculitis (arteriolitis allergica). Br J Dermatol 65: 77, 1953.
42. Ruiter M: Some further observations on allergic cutaneous arteriolitis. Br J Dermatol 66: 174, 1954.
43. Ruiter M: Purpura rheumatica: allergic cutaneous arteriolitis. A type of. Br J Dermatol 68: 16, 1956.
44. Gougerot H, Duperrat B: The nodular dermal allergides of Gougerot. Br J Dermatol 66: 283, 1954.
45. Lyell A, Church R: The cutaneous manifestations of polyarteritis nodosa. Br J Dermatol 66: 335, 1954.
46. Borrie P: Cutaneous polyarteritis nodosa. Br J Dermatol 87: 87, 1972.
47. Wright V, Watkinson G: The arthritis of ulcerative colitis. Medicine (Baltimore) 38: 243, 1959.
48. Moll JMH, Haslock I, Macrae IF, Wright V: Associations between ankylosing spondylitis, psoriatic arthritis, Reiter's disease, the intestinal arthropathies, and Behçet's syn-

drome. Medicine (Baltimore) 53: 343, 1974.
49. Sams WM Jr, Logan WS: The skin as a reflector of immunologic change. Rheumatology 4: 129, 1973.
50. Braverman IM: The angiitides, chap 8. Skin Signs of Systemic Disease, Philadelphia, W. B. Saunders, 1970, p 330.
51. Dantzig PL: Pyoderma gangrenosum. N Engl J Med 292: 47, 1974.
52. Marshall J, Pepler WJ: Dermatitis nodularis necroticans—variant of vasculitis. S Afr Med J 27: 160, 1953.
53. Brinkley GW: Dermatitis nodularis necrotica. Arch Dermatol 75: 387, 1957.
54. Kierland RR: Unusual pyodermas. Minn Med 34: 319, 1951.
55. Brunsting HA: Hydradenitis and other variants of acne. Arch Dermatol 65: 303, 1952.
56. Montgomery H: Acute inflammatory dermatoses and pyodermas, chap 18. Dermatopathology, New York, Harper & Row, 1967, p 463.
57. Lehner T: Pathology of recurrent oral ulceration in Behçet's syndrome: light, electron, and fluorescence microscopy. J Pathol 97: 481, 1969.
58. Wright ET, Greco PJ: Pyoderma gangrenosum: report of a case controlled by cortisone. Arch Dermatol 74: 543, 1956.
59. Delescluse J, de Bast C, Achten G: Pyoderma gangrenosum with altered cellular immunity and dermonecrotic factor. Br J Dermatol 87: 529, 1972.
60. Ryan TJ: Inflammation, fibrin, and fibrinolysis, chap 20. The Physiology and Pathophysiology of the Skin (Jarrett A, ed), New York, Academic Press, 1973, p 745.
61. Saville PD: Polyarteritis nodosa with new bone formation. J Bone Joint Surg 38B: 327, 1956.
62. Ball J, Grayzel AL: Arteritis and localized periosteal new bone formation. J Bone Joint Surg 46B: 244, 1964.
63. Woodward AH, Andreine PH: Periosteal new bone formation in polyarteritis nodosa. Arthritis Rheum 17: 1017, 1974.

Absence of Immune Deficiencies in a Case of Progressive Multifocal Leukoencephalopathy

DAVID ROCKWELL, M.D.
FREDERICK L. RUBEN, M.D.
ALAN WINKELSTEIN, M.D.
HARVEY MENDELOW, M.D.
Pittsburgh, Pennsylvania

Progressive multifocal leukoencephalopathy (PML) is a rare disease related to a slow virus infection of the central nervous system; it is usually seen in patients who have impaired immunologic function. The present patient with biopsy-proved PML was found to have no demonstrable defects in either cellular or humoral immunity as assessed by multiple parameters. Thus, it appears that PML may occur in the presence of intact immune responses.

Progressive multifocal leukoencephalopathy (PML) is described as a rare demyelinating neurologic disorder commonly associated with diseases in which defects of immunologic competence are seen [1]. In this report we describe an unusual patient with PML in whom extensive immunologic testing failed to reveal any deficits in either the humoral or cell-mediated systems.

CASE REPORT

This patient was a 45 year old black housewife who was admitted to Montefiore Hospital in June 1973, because of progressive mental deterioration and motor abnormalities. She had a two-year history of vague neurologic complaints including paresthesias, weakness, syncopal episodes and difficulty with articulation. No neurologic diagnosis had been made despite repeated evaluations. Past history included inactive pulmonary tuberculosis diagnosed in 1960 and treated with isoniazid, para-aminosalicylic acid and streptomycin. One month prior to admission, the patient demonstrated markedly garbled speech; neurologic evaluation revealed a right hemiparesis, right facial weakness, deviation of the tongue to the right, exaggerated deep-tendon reflexes on the right, and positive Babinski and Hoffman's tests. These abnormalities persisted until the patient's admission. Skull films, an echo encephalogram and a lumbar puncture revealed no abnormalities. An electroencephalogram displayed a delta-wave focus in the left hemisphere. A left carotid arteriogram revealed slight shift of the anterior cerebral artery to the left. The patient showed improvement with intensive physiotherapy, and no further diagnostic procedures were undertaken. All studies for active tuberculosis were negative.

Five days after discharge, she was readmitted with a history of several grand mal seizures. The neurologic findings described were unchanged. She was treated with diphenylhydantoin and phenobarbital without recurrence of convulsions. This time a lumbar puncture revealed slight elevation of the cerebrospinal fluid protein (51 mg/100 ml). A Technetium-99m brain scan suggested slightly increased uptake over the left hemisphere; a pneumoencephalogram revealed deviation of the septum pellucidum to the right with absence of free air over the left convexity. A repeat carotid arteriogram

From the Department of Medicine and Pathology, Montefiore Hospital, University of Pittsburgh School of Medicine, Pittsburgh, Pennsylvania. Requests for reprints should be addressed to Dr. Frederick L. Ruben, Montefiore Hospital, 3459 Fifth Avenue, Pittsburgh, Pennsylvania 15213.
Manuscript accepted November 10, 1975.

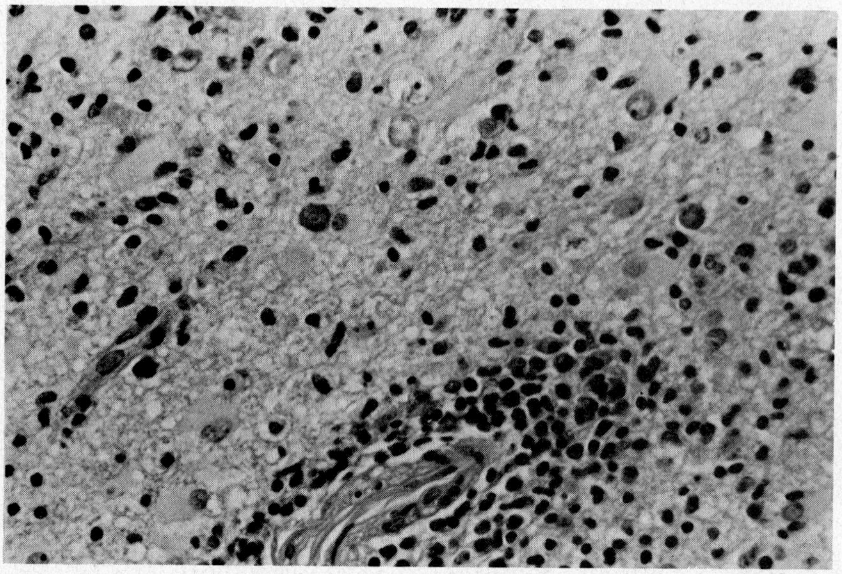

Figure 1. *Perivascular cuffing by mononuclear inflammatory cells is seen in the lower part of the field. Numerous atypical protoplasmic astrocytes and enlarged oligodendroglial nuclei are present in the demyelinated white matter. Hematoxylin and eosin stain; magnification × 480, reduced by 3 per cent.*

again revealed subtle changes suggesting a left temporal lesion. A left temporal lobe brain biopsy was performed on September 5, 1973, and the diagnosis of PML was established (see "laboratory results"). After the immunologic evaluation (to be described), informed consent was obtained from the patient's husband and treatment was begun with cytosine arabinoside, 60 mg/m^2/day given intravenously over six days, with 10 mg/m^2 given intrathecally on days 3 and 4. There was an equivocal response to this treatment as judged by a decrease in her aphasia and modest improvement in her ability to perform simple motor functions.

Following discharge, she has remained in a nursing home for 20 months. Her degree of aphasia is unchanged, and she has demonstrated a gradual deterioration of motor function.

LABORATORY RESULTS

Brain Biopsy. Histologic examination of the tissue from the left temporal lobe biopsy revealed a minimal leptomeningeal mononuclear inflammatory cell infiltrate. The cortical architecture was intact and unremarkable; however, at the junction of cortex and white matter, a zone of demyelination was encountered. This extended into the underlying white matter to the depth of the biopsy and was sharply demarcated by a border of mononuclear inflammatory cell infiltration, predominantly perivascular in location (Figure 1). Within this zone, extensive demyelination was present with numerous lipid-laden macrophages identified. Some interruption of axis cylinders was evident, but frank necrosis was not observed. Bizarre astrocytes with visible cytoplasm and prominent enlarged nuclei, occasionally binucleate or showing mitoses could be identified, particularly at the periphery of the demyelinated area and in the adjacent cortex and white matter (Figure 2). The oligoendrocytes were also markedly altered with enlargement of their nuclei and homogenization of the chromatin. Occasional eosinophilic intranuclear inclusion bodies with a peripheral rim of condensed chromatin were found among these cells (Figure 3).

Immunologic Studies. Tests for competence of humoral immunity included a normal serum immunoelectrophoresis. Quantitative immunoglobulins were: immunoglobulin G (IgG) 1,278 ± 69, immunoglobulin A (IgA) 366 ± 34 and immunoglobulin M (IgM) 125 ± 7 (all within normal limits). Isohemagglutinins were present. The serum complement level was C′3-220 mg/100 ml (normal 145 ± 22 mg/100 ml). Plasma cells constituted a normal proportion of a bone marrow aspirate. Viral challenge with a commercial bivalent influenza vaccine demonstrated a greater than fourfold rise in the hemagglutination-inhibition antibody titers to both viruses. The number of peripheral blood B-type lymphocytes as determined by surface immunoglobulins, using fluorescein-conjugated monovalent antiserum, were within the normal range.

Tests primarily of cellular immunity included blood lymphocyte counts which were normal (1,600 to 2,300 cells/mm^3), skin tests which were positive for tuberculin and Candida antigens, and dinitrochlorobenzene (DNCB) skin test response which was demonstrated 10 days after initial sensitization. Challenge with DNCB three months later showed a positive recall reaction. The patient's lymphocytes transformed normally in response to pokeweed and phytohemagglutinin as well as purified protein derivative tuberculin antigen. T-cell lymphocytes, determined by sheep erythrocyte rosette test, were normal.

Other studies performed to suggest a specific viral etiology (courtesy of Dr. B. Padgett, Madison, Wisc.) included specific antiviral antibodies against JC virus (reciprocal titer was 8192 on three samples collected

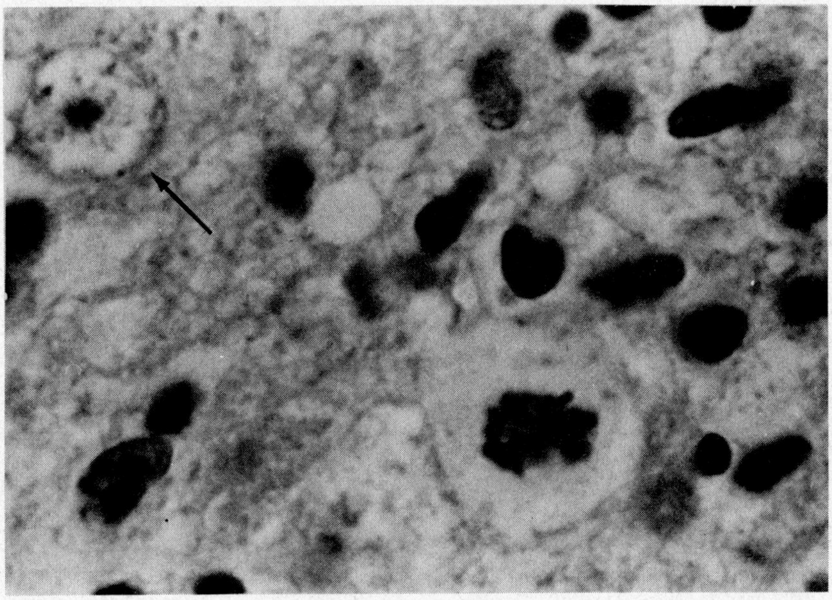

Figure 2. *Bizarre enlarged astrocyte nucleus **(arrow)** upper left, and astrocyte in mitosis, lower right. Hematoxylin and eosin stain; magnification × 2,000, reduced by 3 per cent.*

on separate dates) and BK virus (reciprocal titer was 64 on the three separate samples). Electron microscopic immunoagglutination [11] studies performed on a small portion of the biopsy sample were inconclusive due to the lack of viral particles present (courtesy of Dr. L.P. Weiner at Johns Hopkins Hospital).

COMMENTS

In most previously reported cases of PML, the affected persons have had a second disease classically associated with impairment of immune defense systems. PML is usually observed as a terminal event in a number of chronic disorders characterized by immunologic impairment including Hodgkin's disease, chronic lymphocytic leukemia, multiple myeloma, Whipple's disease, tuberculosis and sarcoidosis [1]. It has been suspected that these abnormalities could limit a host's ability to respond appropriately to a slow virus infection of the central nervous system with demyelinization as the end result [2,3]. In most reports of PML, including cases arising in apparently normal persons, the immunologic status of the patients was not determined; however, in two patients in whom such studies were performed, there was documented impairment of cellular and humoral responses [4,5]. The present case is, therefore, unusual in that this disease occurred in the absence of demonstrable defects in either humoral or cell-mediated immunity.

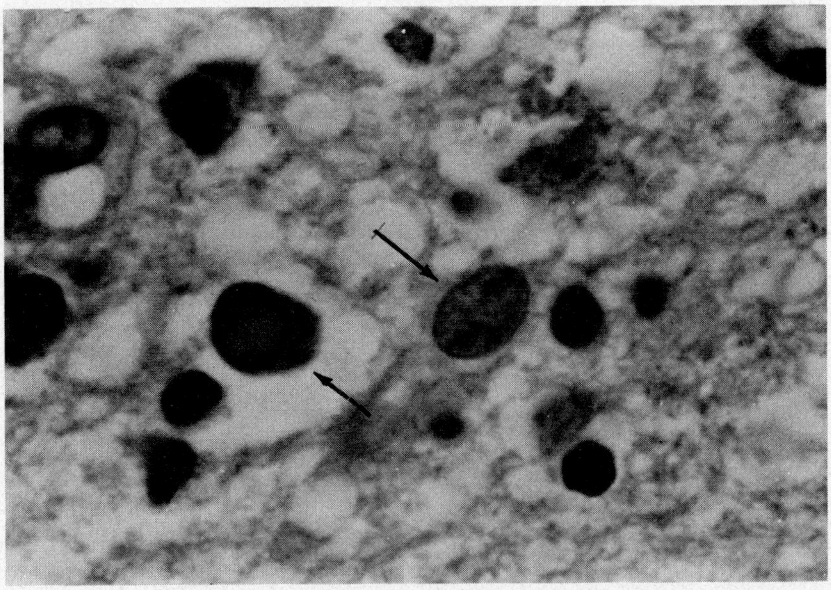

Figure 3. *Atypical enlarged oligodendrocyte nuclei, one of which contains an inclusion body **(arrows)**. Hematoxylin and eosin stain; magnification × 2,000, reduced by 3 per cent.*

The diagnosis of PML was made by finding the characteristic demyelinated lesions in the white matter on brain biopsy. This specimen was somewhat unique in that a perivascular mononuclear cellular infiltration was readily apparent; these infiltrates have either been absent or scattered and minimal in most reported cases, and their presence in this case may correlate with the demonstration of an intact immune system. It is also of interest that this perivascular inflammatory cell response was noted in the case recorded by Hedley-White et al. [6] in which the patient had a remission and a five-year survival.

Accumulating evidence suggests that PML is a slow virus disease [7]. By histopathologic criteria, the lesions are characteristic of viral cytopathology. Electron microscopic studies of biopsy material have demonstrated intranuclear inclusion bodies having the appearance of a papovavirus [4,5,8–17]; these inclusion bodies can also be shown in glial cell tissue cultures inoculated with biopsy material [9]. Immunologic assays and virus isolation suggest that the pathogenic viruses are the SV-40 or the JC agents [9–11,16,18]. Our studies showed no rises in antibody titer to the JC or BK agents. Studies related to the SV-40 virus were not available, but the long survival of our patient is similar to that in other cases related to SV-40 [10].

In summary, this case demonstrates that PML, although usually occurring in patients with active chronic diseases and possible immune deficiencies, can develop in an immunologically competent host. This further suggests that factors other than immunologic competence must be considered in the genesis of this disease.

ACKNOWLEDGMENT

We thank Dr. Richard T. Johnson for advice in the evaluation of this patient.

REFERENCES

1. Fermaglich J, Hardman JM, Earle KM: Spontaneous progressive multifocal leukoencephalopathy. Neurology (Minn) 20: 479, 1970.
2. Richardson EP: Progressive multifocal leukoencephalopathy. N Engl J Med 265: 815, 1961.
3. Cavanagh JB, Greenbaum D, Marshall AHE, Rubinstein LJ: Cerebral demyelination associated with diseases of the reticuloendothelial system. Lancet 2: 524, 1959.
4. Ellison GW: Progressive multifocal leukoencephalopathy. Investigation of the immunologic status of a patient with lymphosarcoma and PML. J Neuropathol Exp Neurol 28: 501, 1969.
5. Knight A, O'Brien P, Osoba D: Spontaneous progressive multifocal leukoencephalopathy. Immunologic aspects. Ann Intern Med 77: 229, 1972.
6. Hedley-White ET, Smith BP, Tyler HR, Peterson WP: Multifocal leukoencephalopathy with remission and five year survival. J Neuropathol Exp Neurol 25: 107, 1966.
7. Weiner LP, Johnson RT, Herdon RM: Viral infections and demyelinating diseases. N Engl J Med 288: 1103, 1973.
8. Davies JA, Hughes JT, Oppenheimer DR: Richardson's disease (Progressive multifocal leukoencephalopathy). Q J Med 42: 481, 1973.
9. Padgett BL, Walker DL, ZuRhein GM, Eckroade RJ: Cultivation of papova-like virus from human brain with progressive multifocal leucoencephalopathy. Lancet 1: 1257, 1971.
10. Weiner LP, Herndon RM, Narayan O, Johnson RT, Shah K, Rubinstein LJ, Preziosi TJ, Conley FK: Isolation of virus related to SV-40 from patients with progressive multifocal leukoencephalopathy. N Engl J Med 286: 385, 1972.
11. Penney JB, Weiner LP, Herndon RM, Narayan O, Johnson RT: Virions from progressive multifocal leukoencephalopathy. Rapid serologic identification by electron microscopy. Science 178: 60, 1972.
12. Bolton CF, Rozdilsky B: Primary progressive multifocal leukoencephalopathy. A case report. Neurology (Minn) 21: 72, 1971.
13. Silverman L, Rubinstein LJ: Electron microscopic observations on a case of progressive multifocal leukoencephalopathy. Acta Neuropathol 5: 215, 1965.
14. Manz HJ, Dinsdale HB, Morrin PAF: Progressive multifocal leukoencephalopathy after renal transplantation. Ann Intern Med 75: 77, 1971.
15. Howatson AF, Nagai M, ZuRhein GM: Polyoma-like virions in human demyelinating brain disease. Can Med Assoc J 93: 379, 1965.
16. Narayan O, Penney JB, Johnson RT, Herndon RM, Weiner LP: Etiology of progressive multifocal leukoencephalopathy. Identification of papovavirus. N Engl J Med 289: 1278, 1973.
17. Conomy JP, Beard NS, Matsumoto H, Roessmann U: Cytarabine treatment of progressive multifocal leukoencephalopathy. JAMA 229: 1313, 1974.
18. Bauer WR, Turel AP, Johnson KP: Progressive multifocal leukoencephalopathy and cytarabine. Remission with treatment. JAMA 226: 174, 1973.

Sickle Cell–β^0 Thalassemia Variant with High Hemoglobin F and Mild Clinical Course

JOSEPH R. SHAEFFER, Ph.D.
JOEL L. MOAKE, M.D.
WITH THE TECHNICAL ASSISTANCE OF
LOIS KLEVE
Houston, Texas

A 70 year old Black woman had chronic hemolytic anemia without recurrent painful crises. Hemoglobin pattern by electrophoresis was hemoglobin S (69 to 71 per cent), hemoglobin A_2 (4.6 per cent) and hemoglobin F (24 to 27 per cent). No hemoglobin A was detected, and the hemoglobin F was distributed heterogeneously in the red cells. Reticulocyte alpha/nonalpha globin chain synthetic ratios were 1.44 to 1.62. Thus, the patient had a high hemoglobin F variant of S-beta zero (β^0) thalassemia which has not been described previously. Her clinical course has been mild in comparison with S-β^0 thalassemia patients who do not have extremely elevated hemoglobin F levels.

Fetal hemoglobin (hemoglobin F) concentrations are increased in many adult patients with chronic anemia [1], including sickle cell disease. In sickle cell-beta thalassemia (S-β thalassemia), hemoglobin F levels may be 3 to 13 per cent [2]. However, higher concentrations of hemoglobin F have been observed rarely in this syndrome [3].

Two types of S-β thalassemia have been recognized: (1) S-β^+ thalassemia associated with incomplete suppression of beta globin chain synthesis and the presence of hemoglobin A; and (2) S-β^0 thalassemia in which beta globin chain synthesis and hemoglobin A formation are absent. Mean hemoglobin F values (3.8 to 7.3 per cent) [2] have not been found to differ significantly in these two types of S-β thalassemia. However, it has been suggested [2,3] that the clinical course of S-β^0 thalassemia is more severe than S-β^+ thalassemia.

We describe an elderly Black woman with clinically mild S-β^0 thalassemia and very high hemoglobin F levels (24 to 27 per cent). This high F variant of S-β^0 thalassemia is, heretofore, undescribed.

CASE REPORT

This 70 year old Black woman had chronic hemolytic anemia (hemoglobin 10 to 11 g/100 ml, reticulocytes 5 to 15 per cent, unconjugated bilirubin 2 to 3 mg/100 ml) unassociated with recurrent painful crises. Sickled, targeted and teardrop red cells, as well as normoblasts, were present on blood films. Leukocytes and platelets were normal, and the spleen was not palpable. There was marrow erythroid hyperplasia and sideroblastosis with many ringed forms.

Standard technics were used for cellulose acetate hemoglobin electrophoresis [4], quantification of hemoglobin F by alkali denaturation of red cell lysates [5], and acid elution [5] for the evaluation of red cell hemoglobin F distribution. Globin chain synthesis studies using tritiated (^3H) leucine incorporation into reticulocyte protein were performed as described elsewhere

From the Department of Biology, M.D. Anderson Hospital and Tumor Institute and the Division of Hematology, University of Texas Medical School, Houston, Texas. This study was supported in part by Medical Genetics Center Grant GM 19513 from the National Institute of General Medical Sciences. Requests for reprints should be addressed to Dr. Joel L. Moake, Division of Hematology, University of Texas Medical School, 6400 West Cullen Street, Houston, Texas 77025. Manuscript accepted November 6, 1975.

TABLE I Hemoglobin Values in S-β^0 Thalassemia with High Hemoglobin F

Hemoglobin electrophoresis:	
Hemoglobin S	= 69–71%
Hemoglobin A	= 0
Hemoglobin A_2	= 4.6%
Hemoglobin F	= 24–27%
Hemoglobin F (alkali denaturation)	= 21–25%
Hemoglobin F distribution	= heterogeneous
Reticulocyte globin chain synthesis:	
alpha/nonalpha*	= 1.62
alpha/nonalpha†	= 1.44

*Incubation of reticulocytes with ^{3}H-leucine for 20 minutes.
†Incubation of reticulocytes with ^{3}H-leucine for 60 minutes.

[6,7]. Results are shown in Table I. This patient has one asymptomatic son (age 42) with hemoglobin AS (hemoglobin A 60 per cent, hemoglobin S 40 per cent).

COMMENTS

When the patient's reticulocytes were incubated with ^{3}H-leucine for 20 and 60 minutes in a medium supporting protein synthesis [6,7], the alpha/nonalpha globin chain synthetic ratios (α/nonα) were 1.62 and 1.44, respectively. These values, which indicate unbalanced globin chain synthesis, are similar to α/non-α synthetic ratios in heterozygous beta thalassemia [8–10], and are unlike the balanced globin chain synthesis in homozygous sickle cell anemia [11]. Moreover, balanced α/non-α globin chain synthetic ratios are observed in heterozygous hereditary persistence of hemoglobin F (HPFH) [12]. The unbalanced α/non-α globin chain ratios and the heterogeneous distribution of hemoglobin F in the red cells of this patient are evidence against homozygosity for the sickle cell gene or heterozygosity for the HPFH gene as the cause of her unusually elevated hemoglobin F levels.

The thalassemia gene in this patient is associated with total suppression of normal β^A globin chain synthesis. Although hemoglobin A_2 is increased, hemoglobin A has not been detected. The quantity of hemoglobin F determined by electrophoresis (24 to 27 per cent) differs only slightly from the hemoglobin F concentrations obtained by alkali denaturation (21 to 25 per cent), suggesting that hemoglobin F bands were not contaminated by hemoglobin A. Moreover, when ^{3}H-leucine-labeled lysates from the patient's reticulocytes were mixed with nonradiolabeled hemoglobin A, no radioactivity migrated with hemoglobin A or with the β^A chain on electrophoresis [4,7].

These data distinguish this patient from other persons with S-β^0 thalassemia. Levels of hemoglobin F exceeding 15 per cent are unusual in adults with S-β thalassemia [13]. Weatherall [3] described an 18 year old man with mild S-β^+ thalassemia and high hemoglobin F (26.1 per cent), and Pearson [14] reported on a healthy middle aged woman with probable S-δ^0 β^0 thalassemia and a hemoglobin F of 37.1 per cent. However, this patient is unique in that her high hemoglobin F (24 to 27 per cent) is associated with total suppression of β^A globin chain synthesis and S-β^0 thalassemia. Her advanced age and mild clinical course are, presumably, related to the very high hemoglobin F levels.

REFERENCES

1. Kazazian HH: Regulation of fetal hemoglobin production. Sem Hematol 11: 525, 1974.
2. Serjeant GR, Ashcroft MT, Serjeant BE, Milner PF: The clinical features of sickle-cell/β thalassaemia in Jamaica. Br J Haematol 24: 19, 1973.
3. Weatherall DJ: Biochemical phenotypes of thalassemia in the American Negro population. Ann NY Acad Sci 119: 450, 1964.
4. Shaeffer JR: Structure and synthesis of the unstable hemoglobin Sabine (α_2 β_2 91 Leu → Pro). J. Biol Chem 248: 7473, 1973.
5. Efremov GD, Huisman THJ: The laboratory diagnosis of the hemoglobinopathies. Clin Haematol 3: 527, 1974.
6. Shaeffer JR, Longley MA, DeSimone J, Kleve LJ: Patterns of hemoglobin assembly in reticulocytes of sickle cell trait individuals. J Biol Chem 250: 8630, 1975.
7. DeSimone J, Kleve L, Longley MA, Shaeffer J: Unbalanced globin chain synthesis in reticulocytes of sickle cell trait individuals with low concentrations of hemoglobin S. Biochem Biophys Res Commun 59: 564, 1974.
8. Weatherall DJ, Clegg JB, Na-Nakorn S, Wasi P: The pattern of disordered hemoglobin synthesis in homozygous and heterozygous β-thalassaemia. Br J Haematol 16: 251, 1969.
9. Bank A, Dow LW, Farace MG, O'Donnell JV, Ford S, Natta C: Changes in globin synthesis with erythroid cell maturation in sickle thalassemia. Blood 41: 353, 1973.
10. Gill FM, Schwartz E: Synthesis of globin chains in sickle β-thalassemia. J Clin Invest 52: 709, 1973.
11. Sarup BM, White JM: The synthesis of globin peptide chains in sickle-cell disease. Br J Haematol 27: 153, 1974.
12. Natta CL, Niazi GA, Ford S, Bank A: Balanced globin chain synthesis in hereditary persistence of fetal hemoglobin. J Clin Invest 54: 433, 1974.
13. Weatherall DJ, Clegg JB: The Thalassaemia Syndromes, 2nd ed, Oxford, Blackwell Scientific Publications, 1972, p 146.
14. Pearson HA: Hemoglobin S-thalassemia syndrome in Negro children. Ann NY Acad Sci 165: 83, 1969.

Thrombotic Thrombocytopenic Purpura—Remission Following Splenectomy

Report of a Case and Review of the Literature

PATRICIA M. REYNOLDS, M.B., B.S.
JOHN M. JACKSON, B.Sc., M.B., Ch.B.
JOHN A. S. BRINE, M.B., B.S.
A. BRIAN VIVIAN, F.R.A.C.S.
Perth, Western Australia

A case of thrombotic thrombocytopenic purpura in which sustained remission followed splenectomy is described. Strong serologic evidence of concurrent infection with Mycoplasma pneumoniae was found in this case. Previously reported cases in which thrombotic thrombocytopenic purpura has been associated with infections are reviewed. An approach to management of this unusual and frequently fatal condition, is suggested, based on a detailed review of the recent literature.

Thrombotic thrombocytopenic purpura is a rare disease from which recovery is still sufficiently uncommon to warrant publication. Since a number of different lines of management have been advocated, analysis of the care of the survivors might provide clues to the optimal therapy. A review of the treatment of survivors suggests that antiplatelet agents, aspirin and dipyridamole, and splenectomy are beneficial in this condition. We describe here a patient with thrombotic thrombocytopenic purpura whose condition improved after splenectomy; complete remission was eventually achieved. This patient also had disseminated intravascular coagulation, a relatively infrequent complication of thrombotic thrombocytopenic purpura. The cause of thrombotic thrombocytopenic purpura remains unknown and, although an infectious agent has frequently been suspected, in only one case has a microorganism been isolated, a microtatobiote [1]. In our case there was serologic evidence of infection by Mycoplasma pneumoniae.

CASE REPORT

A 17 year old white woman was admitted to the hospital because of the acute onset of confusion and disorientation. Four days earlier, she had begun treatment with ampicillin and prochloperazine for symptoms of an upper respiratory tract infection associated with vomiting. She had previously been in good health.

On physical examination she was a plump, very pale, slightly icteric young woman, agitated, confused and disorientated, with a temperature of 39°C. Blood pressure was 130/90 mm Hg. There was generalized petechial purpura and slight dark blood loss per vaginam, the cervical os being closed. A provisional diagnosis of septic abortion was made, and treatment was begun with lincomycin, penicillin, gentamicin, hydrocortisone and red cell and platelet transfusions. Her condition improved gradually over 48 hours. The

From the Department of Haematology, Royal Perth Hospital, Perth, Western Australia. Requests for reprints should be directed to Dr. John M. Jackson. Manuscript accepted November 26, 1975.

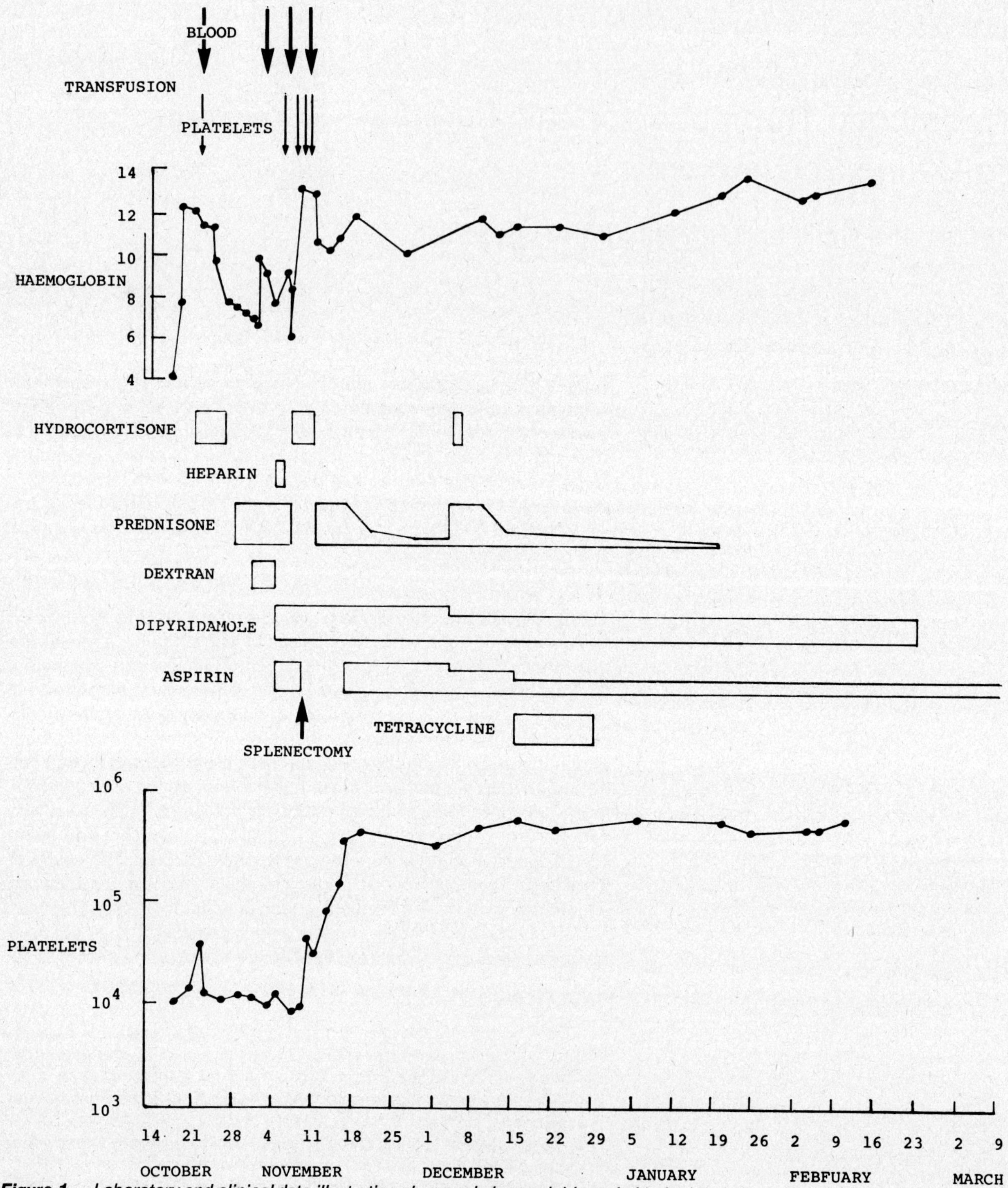

Figure 1. *Laboratory and clinical data illustrating changes in hemoglobin and platelet levels in relation to the various treatment modalities.*

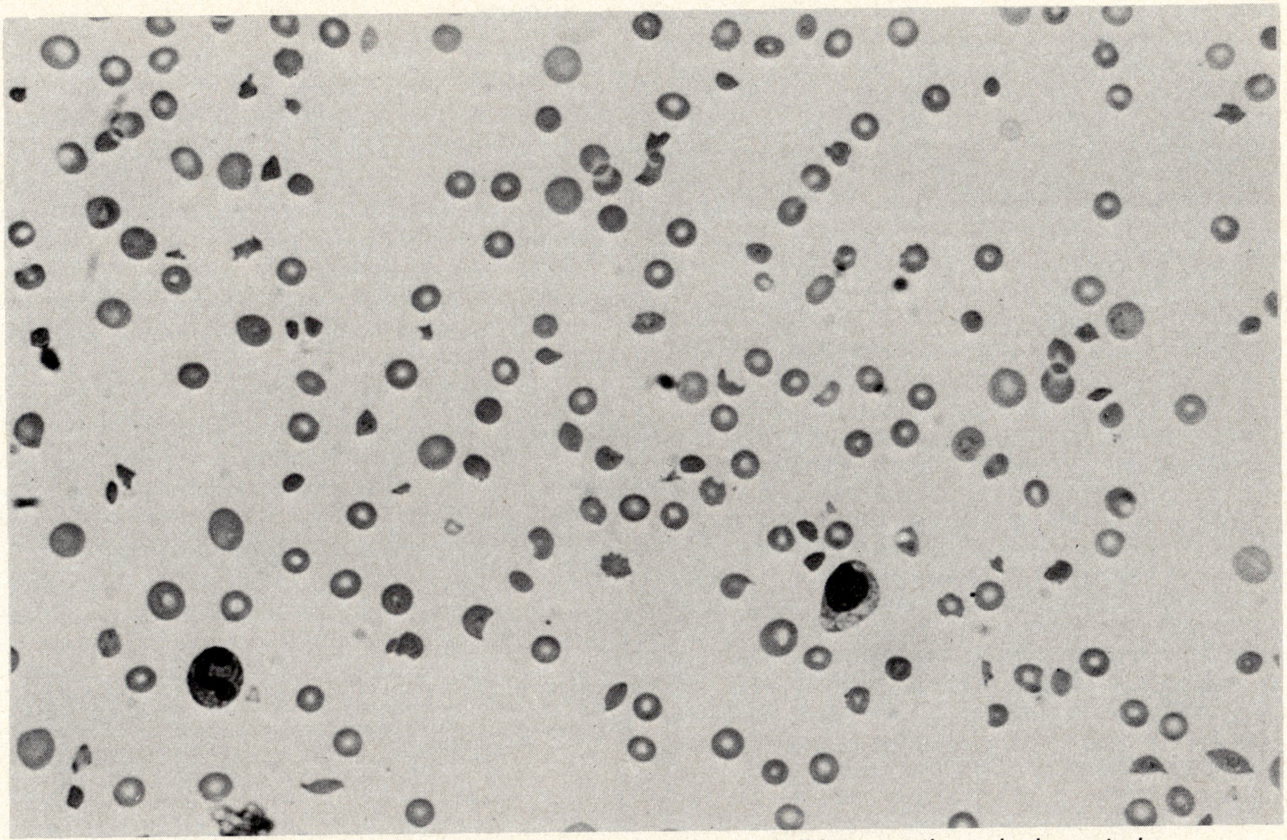

Figure 2. *Blood film shortly after admission illustrating red cell fragmentation and spherocytosis.*

findings were then reviewed, and a diagnosis of thrombotic thrombocytopenic purpura (Moschcowitz's syndrome) was made on the basis of the clinical presentation and investigations to be detailed.

Details of treatment are shown in Figure 1. The administration of prednisone, 60 mg daily, was followed by the administration of 10 per cent dextran (molecular weight 40,000), 250 ml twice daily, without benefit. Heparin, 10,000 units twice daily, together with supplemental coagulation factors in the form of cryoprecipitate and concentrated factors II-VII-IX-X was substituted for dextran but it was discontinued after 10 hours because of massive gastrointestinal hemorrhage. Treatment with dipyridamole, 100 mg given four times daily, and aspirin, 300 mg given four times daily, was then commenced and three days later, there still being no improvement, splenectomy was performed (19th day after admission). Throughout the patient had been drowsy, irritable and confused but without localizing neurologic signs. However, one day postoperatively, two episodes of severe expressive dysphasia were observed, each lasted about 2 hours. Subsequently, her general condition and alertness rapidly improved, and 14 days postoperatively she was discharged with no abnormal signs or symptoms. Three weeks after discharge, a two week course of tetracycline, 250 mg four times daily, was given because of serologic evidence of infection with Mycoplasma pneumoniae.

Since discharge there has been no evidence of recurrence and she remains well six months after diagnosis.

INVESTIGATIONS

Hematologic. On admission the hemoglobin concentration was 5.4 g per cent, hematocrit value 17 per cent, white blood cell count 15,300/μl with 77 per cent polymorphonuclear leukocytes, 15 per cent lymphocytes, 6 per cent monocytes and 2 per cent myelocytes; platelets were less than 10,000/μl. The blood film (Figure 2) showed anisocytosis, polychromasia, many red cell fragments, including helmet forms, microspherocytes and leukoerythroblastosis (erythroblasts less than 1 per cent of total nucleated cell count). The blood film appearances persisted until after splenectomy when numbers of fragments and microspherocytes gradually decreased and by three months after discharge the film was within normal limits, apart from the usual postsplenectomy changes.

Reticulocyte counts varied between 17 and 34 per cent over the first three weeks. Ten days after splenectomy they were 12 per cent, falling gradually to normal levels by three months after discharge. The hemolytic nature of the anemia was supported by the findings of plasma hemoglobin 15.5 mg per cent, haptoglobins less than 10 mg per cent, plasma bilirubin 2.2 mg/100 ml, lactic dehydrogenase 1,720 U/liter (normal 130 to 230 U/liter) and a bone marrow biopsy specimen showing normoblastic erythroid hyperplasia. Granulocyte precursors (normal maturation sequence) and the megakaryocytic series were also hyperplastic. The direct Coombs test on the day of admission was negative, but when tested again four days later it was weakly positive using a broad spectrum antiserum. With specific antiserums the red cells appeared to be coated with the beta$_1$C component of complement. The test was still positive and of the same character six days later, but it reverted to negative on the 17th day after admission.

There was evidence of disseminated intravascular coagulation, the prothrombin time being prolonged between 16 and 48 seconds (control 12 to 13 seconds), the thrombin clotting time between 12 and 15 seconds (normal control 10 to 11 seconds), and fibrin degradation products were variously increased from 20 to 320 μg/ml. The plasma fibrinogen level however was consistently within the normal range (150 to 345 mg/ml), and repeated dilute plasma clot lysis tests showed no evidence of abnormal fibrinolytic activity. All coagulation parameters returned to normal within one week of splenectomy and have remained so to date.

Microbiologic. The initial provisional diagnosis of septic abortion was excluded by finding a negative pregnancy test (Gravindex) result, failure to isolate pathogens from high vaginal swabs and sterile blood cultures. From a wide range of serologic investigations performed 10 days after admission (adenovirus, influenza A, B and C, parainfluenza 1, 2 and 3, respiratory syncytial virus, psittacosis/lymphogranuloma venereum, Coxiella burneti, mumps, rubella, Coxsackie B1-5 and Mycoplasma pneumoniae), the only significant finding was the presence of complement fixing antibody to M. pneumoniae in a titer of 1:320. Twenty six days after admission, the titer was 1:160 and 45 days after admission 1:80. Tetracycline was given for two weeks at this time. The titer was 1:40, 20 weeks after presentation. Serum cold hemagglutinins, first searched for 12 days after admission, were present only at a titer of 1:8.

Splenic Histology. The resected spleen weighed 200 g. Histologic examination showed eccentric subintimal eosinophilic thickening in many of the small arterioles causing subtotal to total obstruction. Some of the occlusive masses had a positive staining reaction for fibrin. There was no evidence of vasculitis. The appearances were characteristic of vascular changes in thrombotic thrombocytopenic purpura.

Others. Electroencephalogram performed on two occasions showed a mild excess of slow activity with no focal or epileptiform features.

Urine sediment contained an occasional hyaline, and coarsely and finely granular casts. Her urine sediment was normal on discharge. Blood urea varied between 41 and 116 mg/100 ml (normal range 18 to 48 mg/100 ml) during admission; it was normal when last checked two months after discharge.

Chest roentgenograms performed on six occasions during hospitalization were all within normal limits.

MATERIALS AND METHODS

Standard hematological methods were used [2]. Platelet counts were performed using the Coulter model B [3]. Fibrinogen degradation products were assayed by Thrombo-Wellcotest, utilizing sensitized latex particles. Biochemical analysis was performed on Technicon® 1260 using standard methods. Complement fixation test for M. pneumoniae was performed by the method of Bradstreet and Taylor [4].

COMMENTS

The diagnosis of thrombotic thrombocytopenic purpura, or Moschcowitz's syndrome, was made in our patient on the basis of the classic findings of thrombocytopenia, microangiopathic hemolytic anemia, fluctuating neurologic signs, impaired renal function and fever, and was confirmed by the presence of typical histologic features in the surgically removed spleen.

It has been argued that thrombotic thrombocytopenic purpura is a syndrome, rather than a specific disease entity [5]. Among the inciting factors, various infections have been implicated although much less frequently than in the closely related hemolytic-uremic syndrome [6]. Berberich et al. [7] reported a fourfold increase in neutralizing antibody titers to Coxsackie B viruses in two patients diagnosed as having thrombotic thrombocytopenic purpura. However, one of these patients, a six year old boy, is probably better classified as an example of the hemolytic-uremic syndrome because of his age, absence of definite neurologic features, lack of histologic diagnosis and rapid recovery without treatment. A case of probable thrombotic thrombocytopenic purpura occurring in a 23 year old nurse, two weeks after influenza vaccination, has been reported [8]. This also took a benign course, the patient recovered completely with prednisolone alone. Thrombotic thrombocytopenic purpura has also been described occurring within 24 hours of combined triple antigen and typhoid A and B vaccination [9]. This was a fatal case in an infant, confirmed by autopsy findings of typical subendothelial and intravascular fibrinoid deposits in the capillaries and arterioles of virtually all organs. A particularly convincing association with infection was described by Mettler [1] who reported the isolation of a microtatobiote (a rickettsia-like organism) from the blood of a patient with typical fatal thrombotic thrombocytopenic purpura. The same organism was also isolated from two children with the hemolytic-uremic syndrome.

Syndromes closely resembling thrombotic thrombocytopenic purpura have also been described in association with generalized aspergillosis and in a case of probable meningococcemia [5]. Paz et al. [10] described simultaneous occurrence of rapidly fatal thrombotic thrombocytopenic purpura in siblings, raising the possibility of an infectious etiology. Watson and Cooper [11] also described a fatal case of thrombotic thrombocytopenic purpura in a man whose wife died six months later of a very similar illness. In none of these cases was an infectious agent isolated. In a further instance of a syndrome diagnosed as thrombotic thrombocytopenic purpura occurring in two sisters [12], the disease ran a chronic course and was probably better categorized as systemic lupus erythematosus. The time sequence is not indicated.

In the present case the evidence for infection with M. pneumoniae rests on the changing titers of complement fixing antibodies to Mycoplasma. This antibody reaches peak levels three to four weeks after infection, remains near there for four to six months, then falls gradually to minimal levels over two to three years [13]. The absence of lower respiratory tract disease is compatible with the diagnosis, as the majority of M. pneumoniae infections are upper respiratory illnesses [13]. The association of thrombotic thrombocytopenic purpura with M. pneumoniae infection has not previously been reported.

Hemolytic anemia occurs in a small proportion of cases of M. pneumoniae infection and is characteristically associated with high titers of cold hemagglutinins [14], which in the present case was only 1:8. The presence of β_1C complement on the surface of the red blood cells most probably represents the fixing of antibody-antigen combination to the surface of innocent "by-stander" erythrocytes rather than an autoimmune mechanism [15]. In one series [16], the majority of patients with recent M. pneumoniae infection showed weak positive direct Coombs' tests, which also gave a positive result with anticomplement (anti β_1C). Such a reaction was not specific for M. pneumoniae as it was also observed, although less frequently, among patients with other respiratory tract infections.

The presence of disseminated intravascular coagulation (DIC) was searched for systematically in 12 patients with thrombotic thrombocytopenic purpura by Jaffe et al. [17], who found no coagulation abnormalities in six cases, minimal abnormalities in three and definite DIC in three. In our case, DIC was present and was an important factor in prompting heparin therapy which was given together with coagulation factor supplementation. Heparin therapy was withdrawn after massive gastrointestinal bleeding which occurred 10 hours after its initiation. All signs of DIC resolved within one week of splenectomy.

It is of interest that the gross degree of red cell fragmentation at the beginning of the illness in our case prevented accurate platelet counting with the Coulter model B. Some fragments were of the same order of size as platelets, and false high counts were recorded. Counting by hand, using the formal-citrate dilution technic, avoided this problem.

Over 340 cases of thrombotic thrombocytopenic purpura have now been reported including at least 62 cases in which the patients have survived for three months or longer. We have reviewed the literature in detail since 1968, separating cases into those in which the illness proved fatal within a three month period and those in which the patients were alive at the date of publication or who survived for more than three months (Tables I and II). Results of treatment were reviewed in 1972 by Schwartz et al. [33] who tabulated the treatment of a total of 32 long-term survivors described prior to 1972. The most successful treatment seemed to be a combination of large dose corticosteroids and splenectomy, this being used in 21 of the 32 patients and in an additional two who received heparin in addition. Since 1968, 18 additional cases have been published in which the use of the combination of steroids and splenectomy has been successful [17–19, 22,28,29,33,34,36,38] including two cases detailed by Schwartz et al. [33].

In some of these cases other agents were also used: heparin [19,28,29,36], dextran [38], dextran and heparin [38], aspirin and dipyridamole [17,36], and heparin, aspirin and dipyridamole [34]. During the same period, eight fatal cases of thrombotic thrombocytopenic purpura in which the patients were treated with this combination, that is corticosteroids and splenectomy, were also reported [17,36,38,51].

Antiplatelet agents, usually aspirin and dipyridamole, were first used by Zacharski et al. in 1971 [30]. A total of at least eight cases have now been published [7,17,30,31,34,36,37,51] and it is remarkable that in only one of these was there a fatal outcome [51], but all had also been given corticosteroids and some heparin therapy, and/or been subjected to splenectomy. Only four cases were histologically confirmed, and in each this was done by examination of the resected spleen [17,34,36,51]. In the other cases, histologic confirmation was not sought. Aspirin without the concurrent dipyridamole seems to have been less successful, there being only one survivor [27] (also receiving corticosteroids), whereas four fatal cases have been described [17,46]. In one of the fatal cases the patient received aspirin alone, in the others the patients also received steroids, dextran and heparin in various combinations. Although the number of cases in which antiplatelet agents were used is so far small, the proportion of survivors in those reported (eight of 13, i.e., about 60 per cent) is very high; this seems to be a promising form of treatment deserving further trial.

In comparison, of the 39 patients reported on since 1968 who underwent splenectomy, there were 28 survivors (about 70 per cent). It is, of course, probable that the literature is biased in favor of successfully treated patients, making it difficult to draw definite conclusions from these figures.

In our case, clinical and hematologic improvement dates from splenectomy (Figure 1), and it is impossible to assess the precise contribution of aspirin and dipyridamole, which were introduced only three days prior to splenectomy.

In conclusion, it would seem that a trial of a combination of dipyridamole and aspirin should probably be the first line of specific therapy, followed by splenectomy if improvement is not obtained. The place of corticosteroid therapy is impossible to assess as these drugs have been used in almost every reported case of thrombotic thrombocytopenic purpura.

TABLE I **Thrombotic Thrombocytopenia Purpura Survivors (patients who were alive at date of publication or who survived for more than three months from diagnosis)**

Sex, Age (yr)	CS	Splen	Dex	Hep	Asp	Dip	Survival (mo)	Diagnostic Criteria	Comment	Reference
F, 19	+	+	...	...	...	...	38	HTARN	Death due to thrombotic thrombocytopenia purpura	[18]
F, 31	+	+	...	+	...	...	6	TARN	Spleen histology negative	[19]
M, 11	+	...	...	...	...	...	36	TARNF	No histology	[20]
F, 22	+	+	...	...	...	...	120	HTA N	...	[21]
F, 33	+	+	...	...	...	...	60	HTA N	...	[21]
F, 34	+	+	...	...	...	...	24	HTARNF	...	[21]
F, 3	+	+	...	...	...	...	36	TA	Death due to thrombotic thrombocytopenic, purpura HT(A)RNF	[22]
F, 6	+	+	...	...	...	...	84	HTARN	Death due to thrombotic thrombocytopenia purpura	[23]
F, 38	+	+	...	+	...	...	72	HTAR(N)F	...	[23]
F, 43	+	+	...	...	...	...	38	HT(A)RNF	...	[23]
F, 48	+	+	...	...	...	...	20	T(A)RNF	Spleen histology negative	[23]
F, 45	+	+	...	...	...	...	10	TARNF	Negative histology spleen; death believed due to thrombotic thrombocytopenia purpura	[23]
F, 33	+	...	+	+	...	...	12	HTARNF	Histology on marrow biopsy	[24]
F, 21	+	+	...	...	...	...	36	HTARN	...	[25]
M, 68	+	...		+	...	...	6	TARNF	Lymph node biopsy negative; no other histology	[26]
F, 38	+	...	...	...	+	...	2	TARN	No histology	[27]
F, 45	+	+	...	+	...	...	7	HTARNF	...	[28]
F, 48	+	+	...	+	...	...	36	HTARN	...	[29]
F, 67	+	...	...	...	+	+	1	TARN	No histology	[30]
M, 26	+	...	...	+	+	+	8	TAR	No histology	[31]
F, 29	+	...	...	+	...	...	6	HTARN	Death due to thrombotic thrombocytopenia purpura	[32]
F, 52	+	+	...	...	...	...	36	HTARNF	Histology on gum biopsy	[33]
F, 18	+	+	...	...	...	...	24	HTARNF	Histology on gum biopsy	[33]
F, 17	+	+	...	+	+	+	12	HTARNF	...	[34]
F, 39	+	+	...	...	+	+	Not stated	HTAR(N)F	...	[17]
M, 45	+	...	...	+	...	...	3	TARNF	No histology	[35]
M, 28	+	+	...	...	+	+	12	HTARNF	Histology on gum biopsy	[36]
F, 40	+	+	...	+	...	...	120	HTARNF	Continued active disease	[36]
F, 41	+	...	...	...	...	...	30	H	Death due to thrombotic thrombocytopenia purpura	[36]
F, 22	+	+	...	...	...	...	84	H	→ Diagnostic criteria not detailed (applies to bracketed H rows)	[36]
F, 22	+	+	...	...	...	...	78	H		[36]
M, 33	+	+	...	...	...	...	18	H		[36]
F, 23	+	...	...	+	...	...	Not stated	TAR(N)	No histology	[8]
M, 14	+	...	...	...	+	+	18	TARNF	No histology	[37]
M, 35	+	+	+	...	...	...	48	HTARN	...	[38]
M, 17	+	+	+	...	...	...	48	HTA NF	...	[38]
F, 52	+	+	+	...	...	...	16	HTARNF	...	[38]
F, 29	+	+	+	...	...	...	12	HTA NF	...	[38]
M, 68	+	+	+	+	...	...	4	TARNF	Spleen histology negative	[38]

(Continued)

TABLE I (Contd) **Thrombotic Thrombocytopenia Purpura Survivors (patients who were alive at date of publication or who survived for more than three months from diagnosis)**

Sex, Age (yr)	CS	Splen	Dex	Hep	Asp	Dip	Survival (mo)	Diagnostic Criteria	Comment	Reference
F, 14	+	...	...	+	+	+	4	TARNF	No histology	[7]
F, 15	+	...	...	+	...	...	Not stated	TARNF	No histology	[7]
M, 6	...	...	...	...	...	...	Not stated	TAR(N)F	No histology	[7]
F, 41	...	...	...	...	...	...	192	T(A)(N)F	Death due to thrombotic thrombocytopenia purpura	[39]

NOTE: H = typical histology (in spleen unless otherwise stated). T = thrombocytopenia. A = anemia, ( ) indicates not stated to be microangiopathic in type. R = renal manifestations. N = neurologic manifestations, ( ) indicates only altered conscious state or doubtful findings. F = fever. CS = corticosteroids. Splen = splenectomy. Dex = dextran. Hep = heparin. Asp = aspirin. Dip = dipyridamole.

TABLE II **Fatal Cases of Thrombotic Thrombocytopenia Purpura (patients who died within three months of diagnosis)**

No. of Cases	CS	Splen	Dex	Hep	Asp	Dip	Diagnostic Criteria	Comment	Reference
1	...	...	...	...	...	...	H (A)R	...	(40)
1	+	...	...	...	...	...	HTARN	Histology adrenals only positive (full autopsy)	(41)
1	...	...	...	...	...	...	HT(A)	...	(18)
1	+	...	...	...	...	...	HTARNF	...	(42)
1	+	...	...	...	...	...	HT(A)RNF	...	(43)
2	+	+	...	...	...	...	HT(A)RNF	...	(23)
1	+	...	...	+	...	...	HTARNF	...	(44)
1	...	+	...	...	...	...	HT(A)RN	Isolation of microtatobiote	(1)
2	+	...	...	...	...	...	HTAR(N)F HT(A)RNF	Sisters, simultaneous disease	(10)
1	+	...	...	+	...	...	HTA N	...	(45)
1	...	...	...	...	+	...	HT(A) NF	...	(46)
1	+	...	...	...	...	...	HT(A)RN	...	(47)
1	+	...	...	...	...	...	HTAR(N)	...	(48)
1	+	...	...	...	...	...	HT(A)(N)F	...	(49)
2	...	...	...	...	...	...	HT(A)R F HTA NF	...	(49)
2	+	+	...	+	...	...	HTAR HT(A) N	Husband and wife	(11)
1	+	...	...	...	...	...	HTARNF	...	(50)
3	+	...	...	...	...	...	All HTARNF	In one case, positive histology kidneys only	(17)
1	+	...	+	...	...	...	HTAR(N)F	...	(17)
1	+	...	+	+	+	...	HTARNF	...	(17)
1	+	+	+	...	...	...	HTARNF	...	(17)
1	+	...	...	+	...	...	HTARNF	...	(17)
1	+	+	...	+	...	...	HTARNF	...	(17)
1	+	+	...	...	...	...	HTARNF	...	(17)
1	+	...	...	+	+	...	HTAR(N)F	...	(17)
1	+	...	...	...	+	...	HTAR(N)F	...	(17)
1	+	+	...	...	+	+	HTARNF	...	(51)
3	+	...	...	...	...	...	All HTA NF		(52)
1	+	+	...	...	...	...	H	Diagnostic criteria not detailed	(36)
1	+	...	+	...	...	...	HTARN	...	(53)
1	+	+	+	...	...	...	HTA NF	...	(38)
1	+	...	...	+	...	...	HTARNF	...	(54)
1	+	...	+	+	...	...	HTA (N)F	...	(54)

NOTE: H = typical histology in organs (other than kidney) at autopsy. T = thrombocytopenia. A = anemia, ( ) indicates not stated to be microangiopathic in type. R = renal manifestations. N = neurologic manifestations, ( ) indicates only altered conscious state or doubtful findings. F = fever. CS = corticosteroids. Splen = splenectomy. Dex = dextran. Hep = heparin. Asp = aspirin. Dip = dipyridamole.

ACKNOWLEDGMENT

We thank Dr L. R. Matz, Pathologist, for help with the histopathologic findings and constructive comments on this paper.

ADDENDUM

As of June 1976, the patient has required no further therapy and remains well with no evidence of recurrent disease.

REFERENCES

1. Mettler NE: Isolation of a microtatobiote from patients with haemolytic-uraemic syndrome and thrombotic thrombocytopenic purpura and from mites in the United States. N Engl J Med 281: 1023, 1969.
2. Dacie JV, Lewis SM: Practical Haematology, London, J & A Churchill, 1970.
3. Davis RE, Green R: Automatic platelet counting with the Coulter particle counter. J Clin Pathol 20: 777, 1967.
4. Bradstreet CMP, Taylor CED: Technique of complement-fixation test applicable to the diagnosis of virus diseases. Monthly Bulletin G.B. Ministry of Health 21: 96, 1962.
5. Umlas J, Kaiser J: Thrombohemolytic thrombocytopenic purpura (TTP)—a disease or a syndrome? Am J Med 49: 723, 1970.
6. Brain MC: The haemolytic-uraemic syndrome. Sem Haematol 6: 162, 1969.
7. Berberich F, Cuene SA, Chard RL, Hartmann JR: Thrombotic thrombocytopenic purpura. Three cases with platelet and fibrinogen survival studies. J Pediatr 84: 503, 1974.
8. Brown RC, Blecher TE, French EA, Toghill PJ: Thrombotic thrombocytopenic purpura after influenza vaccination. Br Med J 2: 303, 1973.
9. Frick PG, Hitzig WH: Simultaneous thrombotic thrombocytopenic purpura and agammaglobulinaemia. Lancet 2: 1401, 1960.
10. Paz RA, Elijovich F, Barcat JA, Sanchez-Avalos JG: Fatal simultaneous thrombocytopenic purpura in siblings. Br Med J 4: 727, 1969.
11. Watson CG, Cooper WM: Thrombotic thrombocytopenic purpura—concomitant occurrence in husband and wife. JAMA 215: 1821, 1971.
12. Norkin SA, Freedman HH, Evans GW: Thrombotic thrombocytopenic purpura in siblings. Am J Med 43: 294, 1967.
13. Murray HW, Masur H, Senterfit LB, Roberts RB: The protean manifestations of Mycoplasma pneumoniae infection in adults. Am J Med 58: 229, 1975.
14. Barrett-Connor E: Anemia and infection. Am J Med 52: 242, 1972.
15. Pirofsky B: General clinical concepts, chap 2. Autoimmunization and the Autoimmune Haemolytic Anaemias, Baltimore, Williams & Wilkins, 1969.
16. Feizi T: Cold agglutinins, the direct Coombs test and serum immunoglobulins in Mycoplasma pneumoniae infections. Ann NY Acad Sci 143: 800, 1967.
17. Jaffe EA, Nachman RL, Merskey C: Thrombotic thrombocytopenic purpura—coagulation parameters in twelve patients. Blood 42: 499, 1973.
18. Pirer MS: Thrombotic thrombocytopenic purpura during pregnancy. Am J Obstet Gynecol 100: 302, 1968.
19. Richardson JH, Smith BT: Thrombotic thrombocytopenic purpura—survival in pregnancy with heparin therapy. JAMA 203: 518, 1968.
20. Rivero I, Ritz ND: Abnormal fibrinogen in thrombotic thrombocytopenic purpura. Blood 32: 140, 1968.
21. Hill JB, Cooper WM: Thrombotic thrombocytopenic purpura—treatment with corticosteroids and splenectomy. Arch Intern Med 122: 353, 1968.
22. Clinico Pathological Conference. Texas Children's Hospital. J Pediatr 73: 788, 1968.
23. Bernard RP, Bauman AW, Schwartz SI: Splenectomy for thrombotic thrombocytopenic purpura. Ann Surg 169: 616, 1969.
24. Van Slyck EJ, Jurgensen JG, Cargill JW: Diabetes insipidus in thrombotic thrombocytopenic purpura. JAMA 209: 768, 1969.
25. Scharoff JR, Serlin N, Atamer MA: Thrombotic thrombocytopenic purpura—report of a case treated with splenectomy and steroids. Acta Haematol 41: 180, 1969.
26. Fiddes PJ, Penny R: Fibrin degradation products in thrombotic thrombocytopenic purpura. Aust Ann Med 4: 350, 1970.
27. Jobin F, Delage JM: Aspirin and prednisone in microangiopathic haemolytic anaemia. Lancet 2: 208, 1970.
28. Tartaglia AP, Burkart PT: Thrombotic thrombocytopenic purpura—remission following haemodialysis. JAMA 218: 999, 1971.
29. Kutell MA, Alfrey CP, Hettig RA: T.T.P. treatment. N Engl J Med 285: 971, 1971.
30. Zacharski LR, Walworth C, McIntyre OR: Antiplatelet therapy for thrombotic thrombocytopenic purpura. N Engl J Med 285: 408, 1971.
31. Giromini M, Bouvier CA, Dami R, Denizot M, Jeannet M: Effect of dipyridamole and aspirin in thrombotic microangiopathy. Br Med J 1: 545, 1972.
32. Perel ID: Thrombotic thrombocytopenic purpura presenting as eclampsia. Aust NZ J Obstet Gynecol 12: 257, 1972.
33. Schwartz J, Rosenberg A, Cooperberg AA: Thrombotic thrombocytopenic purpura. Successful treatment of two cases. Can Med Assoc J 106: 1200, 1972.
34. Amir J, Krauss S: Treatment of thrombotic thrombocytopenic purpura with anti platelet drugs. Blood 42: 27, 1973.
35. Burr WA: Thrombotic thrombocytopenic purpura. Proc Roy Soc Med 66: 650, 1973.
36. Goldenfarb PB, Finch SC: Thrombotic thrombocytopenic purpura. A 10 year survey. JAMA 226: 644, 1973.
37. Rossi EC, Redondo D, Borges WH: Thrombotic thrombocytopenic purpura—survival following treatment with aspirin, dipyridamole, and prednisone. JAMA 228: 1141, 1974.
38. Cuttner J: Splenectomy, steroids and dextran 70 in thrombotic thrombocytopenic purpura. JAMA 227: 397, 1974.
39. Boswell DC, Sierra G: Probable 16 year course in a patient with thrombotic thrombocytopenic purpura. Ill Med J 145: 29, 1974.
40. McCutcheon SA: Case of renal thrombotic thrombocytopenic purpura with comments on coagulation and immunofluorescent studies. Henry Ford Hosp Med J 16: 239, 1968.
41. Hinton P: Haemolytic-uraemic syndrome. Report of two cases. Can Med Assoc J 98: 819, 1968.
42. Castleman B, McNeely BV: Case records of the Massachusetts General Hospital. N Engl J Med 278: 1336, 1968.
43. Castleman B, McNeely BV: Case records of the Massachusetts General Hospital. N Engl J Med 278: 36, 1968.
44. Christoffersen P, Henriksen H, Larsen NA, Nielsen B, Willumsen J: The haemolytic-uraemic syndrome. Thrombotic thrombocytopenic purpura in an eight-year-old boy. Danish Med Bull 16: 252, 1969.
45. Tapp E, Geary CG, Dawson DW: Thrombotic thrombocytopenic purpura with macroscopic infarction. J Pathol 97: 711, 1969.
46. Aronson SM: Clinico Neuropathological Conference. Dis Nerv Syst 30: 493, 1969.
47. Percival SP: Ocular findings in thrombotic thrombocytopenic purpura. Br J Ophthal 54: 73, 1970.
48. Popescu ER: Thrombotic thrombocytopenic purpura—its classification. Rom Med Rev 14: 30, 1970.

49. Steinberg AD, Green WT, Talal N: Thrombotic thrombocytopenic purpura complicating Sjögren's syndrome. JAMA 215: 757, 1971.
50. Mant MJ, Cauchi MN, Medley G: Thrombotic thrombocytopenic purpura. Report of a case with possible immune etiology. Blood 40: 416, 1972.
51. Neame PB, Lechago J, Ling ET, Koval A: Thrombotic thrombocytopenic purpura. Report of a case with disseminated intravascular platelet aggregation. Blood 42: 805, 1973.
52. Mitch WE, Spivak JL, Spangler DB, Bell WR: Thrombotic thrombocytopenic purpura presenting with gynecological manifestations. Lancet 1: 850, 1973.
53. Olsen H: Thrombotic thrombocytopenic purpura as a cause of pancreatitis—report of a case and review of the literature. Am J Dig Dis 18: 238, 1973.
54. Schuette PT, Brabham AM, Eurenius K: Thrombotic thrombocytopenic purpura—a re-evaluation. South Med J 67: 915, 1974.

INFORMATION FOR AUTHORS

PREPARATION OF MANUSCRIPTS

Manuscripts should be typed on one side of the sheet, doublespaced, on white bond paper, 8½ by 11 inches, with margins of 1 inch. Two copies of the manuscript and illustrations should be sent to the Editor at 666 Fifth Avenue, New York, New York 10019. Title page should include full name, degrees and affiliation of all authors, the source from which the article emanates, and the name and address of the person to whom requests for reprints should be addressed.

All manuscript pages including tables and legends should be numbered consecutively in the upper right hand corner.

The number of manuscript pages, the number of illustrations and the number of tables should be indicated at the bottom of the covering letter.

Every article must be preceded by an abstract (not to exceed 350 words). This obviates the need for a summary. In addition, for the convenience of our readers, we require a brief abstract (not exceeding 100 to 125 words) and key words for indexing purposes. These brief abstracts appear in the back of the *Journal* in the same issue in which the paper appears.

Since all manuscripts submitted for publication in the *Journal* are sent out for review before a final decision is made, there is generally a lapse of three to six weeks before contributors are notified. If you have received an acknowledgment of receipt, there is no need to call the *Journal* office; your manuscript has not gone astray. The decision will be forthcoming shortly.

PREPARATION OF ILLUSTRATIONS AND TABLES

Illustrations must be black and white glossy prints or professional drawings in india ink; they should be unmounted. The name of the lead author and the title of the article should be typed on a label and affixed to the back of each illustration; the top should be indicated.

Reference to all illustrations should be inserted in the text in consecutive order. Legends for the illustrations should be typed, double spaced, on a separate sheet with numbers corresponding to those on the photographs or drawings. They should not be attached to the pictures.

Tables should be typed on separate sheets and should be set up in accordance with the style of the Journal. Units of measure should be confined to column headings. Abbreviations should be kept to a minimum and should conform with those used by the *Journal* or listed as acceptable in the Council of Biology Editors Style Manual. Any variations should be explained. All vertical rules should be omitted.

The publisher allows a fixed amount towards the reproduction of illustrations and tables. Charges in excess of this amount must be assumed by the authors. The Editor reserves the right to limit the number of illustrations and/or tables.

PREPARATION OF BIBLIOGRAPHY

Bibliographic references should be listed chronologically on a separate sheet (not in footnotes) as referred to in the text and should be typed (double-spaced) in accordance with the style and abbreviations (open punctuation) used by Index Medicus; only the first page of the journal citation is necessary. Examples follow:

For periodical references:

22. Theologides A, Kennedy BJ: Toxoplasmic myocarditis and pericarditis. Am J Med 47: 169, 1969.

For book references (with chapter):

18. Schiebler GL, Van Mieron LHS, Krovetz LJ: Diseases of the tricuspid valve, chap 2. Heart Disease in Infants, Children and Adolescents (Moss AJ, Adams F, eds), Baltimore, Williams & Wilkins, 1968.

For book references (without chapter):

13. Berne E: Principles of Group Treatment, New York, Oxford University Press, 1966, p 26.

Authors are responsible for the accuracy of all references.

REPRINTS

Price schedules and order cards for reprints are mailed to the person so listed in the footnote on the title page.

The American Journal of Medicine, **666 Fifth Avenue, New York, New York 10019**

OCTOBER 1976

The American Journal of Medicine

VOLUME 61

NUMBER 4

EDITORIAL

Ventricular Rhythm Disorders and Sudden Cardiac Death

B. LEVITT, M.D.*
N. A. CAGIN, M.D.
J. C. SOMBERG, M.D.
J. J. KLEID, M.D.
New York, New York

The management of ventricular rhythm disorders in patients with chronic ischemic heart disease and the prophylaxis of sudden cardiac death is perhaps one of the most challenging problems facing the physician today. A rational approach to this problem includes (1) identification of the patients with disorders of ventricular rhythm who are at risk; (2) an assessment of the efficacy of the antiarrhythmic agents currently available for the prophylaxis or treatment of ventricular rhythm disorders associated with sudden death and (3) an exploration of novel approaches to antiarrhythmic prophylaxis and therapy in an effort to resolve this difficult clinical problem.

Sudden cardiac death is generally thought to result from lethal ventricular rhythm disorders. The identification of patients with disorders of ventricular rhythm who are subject to sudden cardiac death depends upon the technics utilized to detect the rhythm disorders. The use of the routine electrocardiogram has provided important insight into this problem. Approximately 3.6 per cent of the subjects in the general population exhibit ventricular rhythm disorders on routine electrocardiographic study, and a sixfold increase in the incidence of sudden cardiac death has been reported in these subjects [1]. Similar data have been derived from the analysis of hospital outpatient records [2]. Ventricular ectopic activity was considered most malignant in patients with ischemic heart disease, and benign in the absence of clinical evidence of organic heart disease [2–4].

The introduction of ambulatory electrocardiographic monitoring has provided a major addition to the technical armamentarium for the identification and clinical assessment of disorders of rhythm and conduction. Although the ordinary electrocardiogram may provide from 70 to 100 beats for review, the 24 hour continuous electrocardiographic tape provides between 80,000 and 120,000 beats for review, permitting the identification of ventricular ectopic rhythms. These were significantly associated with ischemic heart disease and an increased risk of sudden cardiac death [5].

Patients who have survived a myocardial infarction constitute a special population of patients with chronic ischemic heart disease.

From the Division of Cardiology and Clinical Pharmacology, Department of Medicine, New York Medical College, New York, New York. Requests for reprints should be addressed to Dr. Barrie Levitt, New York Medical College, 1249 Fifth Avenue, New York, New York 10029. Manuscript accepted April 5, 1976.

* Irma Hirschl Career Scientist.

In this subgroup, 60 to 75 per cent of subjects have demonstrable ventricular ectopy [6–9] and an almost fivefold increase in the risk of sudden cardiac death [9,10]. It is noteworthy that ventricular arrhythmias observed early in the hospital phase of acute myocardial infarction appear to bear no relationship to the occurrence of sudden death after discharge; ventricular arrhythmias observed in the later phases of the disease carry more grave prognostic significance [8]. Stress electrocardiographic studies have been successfully employed in the identification of patients with ventricular rhythm disorders [9]. In patients with ischemic heart disease, more than 60 per cent exhibit ectopic activity when subjected to such stress [9].

If we accept that patients with chronic ischemic heart disease who manifest ventricular rhythm disorders are at special risk, we must next examine the options available to improve their outlook. We can attempt to abolish the ambulatory ventricular arrhythmia or reduce its intensity; we can attempt antiarrhythmic prophylaxis of ventricular ectopy associated with a future ischemic insult or we may attempt therapy of ventricular ectopy after the new ischemic insult has occurred.

The first approach to the problem is usually an attempt to suppress ventricular rhythm disorders in the ambulatory patient with ischemic heart disease. There is, however, no proof that suppression of the rhythm disorder will protect against sudden death. Moreover, suppression of ventricular ectopy is difficult to achieve and involves a serious risk of drug toxicity. The reported over-all success rate of antiarrhythmic drug therapy in the ambulatory patient is between 20 and 35 per cent [10–12]. Although this number is not terribly encouraging we can expect that at least one-third of the patients at risk may respond to antiarrhythmic suppression with quinidine, procainamide or a combination of these agents.

A second approach to the prevention of sudden death is the prophylaxis of the arrhythmias resulting from new ischemic injury in the prehospital phase. The studies of Fowler's group with quinidine [13] and Koch Weser's group with procainamide [14] appear to hold promise of some success in this area. Both groups of investigators found that quinidine and procainamide, respectively, were effective in suppressing ventricular rhythm disorders associated with acute myocardial infarction in the Coronary Care Unit; mortality was not influenced in either study however. The question remains whether ventricular arrhythmias seen in the early hospital phase are analogous to arrhythmias seen in the prehospital phase. Recent work by Wellens and Durrer [15] would seem to indicate that ventricular tachycardia in the early hospital phase may be a disorder of automaticity whereas prehospital and late hospital phase ventricular rhythm disorders may be re-entrant as well as automatic in origin. The capacity to extrapolate from arrhythmias observed in the hospital to those observed in the prehospital phase of myocardial infarction continues to be an open question at this time. The efficacy of antiarrhythmic prophylaxis in the prehospital phase of the disease is equally unresolved.

A third approach to sudden cardiac death, especially in patients in whom death is not instantaneous, is the treatment of the arrhythmia by the patient himself or by an emergency medical team after the patient begins to experience the symptoms of acute myocardial infarction. Lidocaine has been prepared as an auto injector, the Lidopen, by Sarnoff and his group [16]. These workers propose that the patient, equipped with an electrocardiographic transmitter the size of a cigarette case, can transmit his electrocardiogram to an appropriate center. On command from the center, the patient can self-administer 300 mg of lidocaine intramuscularly. Such an injection might result in effective blood levels of lidocaine for as long as 2 hours, and thereby diminish the incidence of ventricular fibrillation. Valentine's [17] recent study with lidocaine appears to support this view. A similar approach has been suggested with procainamide [18]. The use of both drugs has been reported to reduce the incidence of primary ventricular fibrillation in those with acute myocardial infarction [19].

Finally, we must develop new and better antiarrhythmic drugs which will prevent rhythm disorders associated with acute myocardial ischemia without massive myocardial depression. Both experimental and clinical evidence indicate that rhythm disorders in the early phase of acute myocardial infarction result in large measure from disordered neural discharge [20,21]. Adrenergic influence has been associated experimentally and clinically with anterior wall ischemia [20,22].

In the experimental animal, drugs and maneuvers which depress the nervous system but spare the heart have been effective in controlling neurally induced arrhythmias [23,24]. It may be that by directing our attention to what Lown et al. [25] have called the neurophysiologic trigger as opposed to the cardiac target, it may be possible to substantially influence the number of deaths in the prehospital phase of acute myocardial infarction.

REFERENCES

1. Chiang BN, Perlman LV, Ostrander LD Jr, et al.: Heart disease and sudden death in the Tecumseh epidemiologic study. Ann Intern Med 70: 1159, 1969.
2. Desai DC, Hershberg PI, Alexander S: Clinical significance of ventricular premature beats in an outpatient population. Chest 64: 564, 1973.

3. Fisher FD, Tyroler HA: Relationship between ventricular premature contractions on routine electrocardiography and subsequent sudden death from coronary heart disease. Circulation 47: 712, 1973.
4. Tominaga S, Blackburn H: Prognostic importance of premature beats following myocardial infarction. JAMA 223: 1116, 1973.
5. Hinkle LE Jr, Carver ST, Stevens M: The frequency of asymptomatic disturbances of cardiac rhythm and conduction in middle-aged men. Am J Cardiol 24: 629, 1969.
6. Moss AJ, Schnitzler R, Green R, et al.: Ventricular arrhythmias three weeks after acute myocardial infarction. Ann Intern Med 75: 837, 1971.
7. Kotler MN, Tabatznik B, Mower MM, et al.: Prognostic significance of ventricular ectopic beats with respect to sudden death in the late postinfarction period. Circulation 47: 959, 1973.
8. Vismara LA, Amsterdam EA, Mason DT: Relation of ventricular arrhythmias in the late hospital phase of acute myocardial infarction to sudden death after hospital discharge. Am J Med 59: 6, 1975.
9. Jelinek MV, Lown B: Exercise stress testing for exposure of cardiac arrhythmia. Prog Cardiovasc Dis 16: 497, 1974.
10. Gey GO, Levy RH, Pettet G, et al.: Quinidine plasma concentration and exertional arrhythmia. Am Heart J 90: 19, 1975.
11. Jelinek MV, Lohrbauer L, Lown B: Antiarrhythmic drug therapy for sporadic ventricular ectopic arrhythmias. Circulation 49: 659, 1974.
12. Gey GO, Levy RH, Fisher LD, et al.: Plasma concentration of procainamide and prevalence of exertional arrhythmias. Ann Intern Med 80: 718, 1974.
13. Bloomfield SS, Romhilt DW, Chou Te-Chiuan, et al.: Quinidine for prophylaxis or arrhythmias in acute myocardial infarction. N Engl J Med 285: 979, 1971.
14. Koch-Weser J, Klein SW, Foo-Canto L, et al.: Antiarrhythmic prophylaxis with procainamide in acute myocardial infarction. N Engl J Med 281: 1253, 1969.
15. Wellens HJJ, Lie KI, Durrer D: Further observations on ventricular tachycardia as studied by electrical stimulation of the heart (chronic recurrent ventricular tachycardia and ventricular tachycardia during acute myocardial infarction). Circulation 49: 647, 1974.
16. Sarnoff SJ: A plan for reducing the prehospital mortality due to acute myocardial infarction. Carl J. Wiggers Award Lecture, Circulation Group, American Physiological Society, April 14, 1970.
17. Valentine PA, Freu JL, Mashford ML, et al.: Lidocaine in the prevention of sudden death in the prehospital phase of acute infarction. N Engl J Med 291: 1327, 1974.
18. Koch-Weser J: Antiarrhythmic prophylaxis in ambulatory patients with coronary heart disease. Arch Intern Med 129: 763, 1972.
19. Wyman MG, Hammersmith L: Comprehensive treatment plan for the prevention of primary ventricular fibrillation in acute myocardial infarction. Am J Cardiol 33: 661, 1974.
20. Webb SW, Adgey AAJ, Pantridge JF: Preliminary communications—autonomic disturbance at onset of acute myocardial infarction, Brit Med J 3: 89, 1972.
21. Gillis RA: Role of the nervous system in the arrhythmias produced by coronary occlusion in the cat. Am Heart J 81: 677, 1971.
22. Pearle DL, Carr PB, Gillis RA: Influence of site of occlusion on the cardiovascular changes induced by coronary ligation. Fed Proc 33: 518, 1974.
23. Levitt B, Raines A, Sohn YJ, et al.: The nervous system as a site of action for digitalis and antiarrhythmic drugs. J Mt Sinai Hospital 37: 227, 1970.
24. Levitt B, Cagin NA, Somberg JC, et al.: Alteration of the effects and distribution of ouabain by spinal cord transection in the cat. J Pharmacol Exp Therap 185: 24, 1973.
25. Lown B, Tykocinski M, Garfein A, et al.: Sleep and ventricular premature beats. Circulation 48: 691, 1973.

The Short- and Long-Term Prognosis of Patients with Transmural and Nontransmural Myocardial Infarction

DAVID S. CANNOM, M.D.
WILLIAM LEVY, B.A.
LAWRENCE S. COHEN, M.D.
New Haven, Connecticut

To compare the long-term prognosis in patients surviving transmural with patients surviving nontransmural myocardial infarctions, the records of 188 consecutive patients with clinical histories and enzyme elevations consistent with acute infarction were reviewed. According to standard electrocardiographic criteria the patients were divided into two groups: 148 with transmural myocardial infarction (group 1) and 40 with nontransmural myocardial infarction (group 2). Of the patients who survived hospitalization, follow-up data were obtained on 119 of 124 patients in group 1 and 36 of 37 patients in group 2 at a mean follow-up period of 36 months. In group 2, the patients had a high incidence of sudden death after discharge (33 per cent in group 2 versus 15 per cent in group 1, $p < 0.02$) as well as a significantly higher incidence of death from all cardiac causes (41.6 per cent in group 2 versus 24.3 per cent in group 1, $p < 0.05$). Furthermore, the patients in group 2 still alive at the end of the follow-up period had an increased incidence of angina pectoris and of recurrent infarction. The data suggest that patients with nontransmural myocardial infarction carry a particularly guarded prognosis.

Sudden death is a major unsolved problem in ischemic heart disease and has prompted investigators to identify subgroups at high risk (for sudden death) and to design appropriate pharmacologic or surgical preventive measures. Survivors of acute myocardial infarction represent one high risk group with an annual mortality due to sudden death estimated at 5 per cent [1]. The present study was undertaken to analyze subsets within this group who may be at particularly high risk.

Recent studies comparing the clinical course of patients with transmural myocardial infarctions and nontransmural (or subendocardial) myocardial infarctions have found little difference in in-hospital morbidity and mortality [2–4]. Few studies, however, have adequately compared the course of these patients after discharge. Although it has been postulated that patients who survive nontransmural myocardial infarction are prone to fatal arrhythmias and sudden death [5–7], supporting clinical studies have not proved this thesis. In this study we summarize the experience of one institution in treating patients during the calendar year 1971 and provide new data regarding the long-term prognosis in the patients who survived their initial infarction.

From the Cardiology Section, Yale University School of Medicine, New Haven, Connecticut. Requests for reprints should be addressed to Dr. Cannom, 87 LMP, 333 Cedar Street, New Haven, Connecticut 06510. Manuscript accepted March 19, 1976.

MATERIALS AND METHODS

The hospital records of 418 consecutive patients admitted to Yale-New Haven Hospital between January 1 and December 31, 1971, with a diagnosis of possible or definite myocardial infarction were reviewed by one or more of us. Of these patients, 219 were determined to have sustained an acute myocardial infarction by the following criteria: (1) A history of chest pain thought to be ischemic in etiology occurring within 48 hours prior to admission. (2) Serum enzyme elevations consistent with an acute myocardial infarction, specifically, an increase in serum glutamic oxaloacetic transaminase (SGOT) to a level above normal limits (10 to 35 units) with a peak value at least 100 per cent greater than the lowest recorded initial value. Patients with associated medical conditions that might explain an elevated SGOT level were excluded. All patients also had a parallel increase in creatine phosphokinase (CPK) and in lactic dehydrogenase (LDH) levels, although less rigid criteria were applied to the interpretation of these values.

Patients meeting the criteria for acute myocardial infarction were divided into two groups according to electrocardiographic changes noted during hospitalization: **Group1. Transmural myocardial infarction:** This group consisted of 148 patients whose serial electrocardiograms showed acute S-T segment elevations >1 mm with subsequent evolution of pathologic Q waves >1 mm in depth and at least 0.04 second in duration. **Group 2. Nontransmural myocardial infarction:** In this group were 40 patients whose serial electrocardiograms showed only persistent ischemic changes, either S-T segment depression ≥1 mm (with or without symmetrical T wave inversion) or symmetrical T wave inversion alone. Q waves did not evolve in these patients [8–12]. These changes were considered secondary to acute ischemia and not explained by digitalis effect, left ventricular hypertrophy, electrolyte disturbance or any other condition similarly causing ST-T wave changes [13,14]. The remaining 31 patients were excluded from the study for the following reasons: three patients had nonatherosclerotic heart disease and 28 patients presented with serial electrocardiograms which could not be classified with *certainty* into either group because of either equivocable changes not consistent with the strict criteria for either group or because of conduction disturbances at the time of admission.

Daily enzyme determinations were available for all patients as were daily electrocardiograms and recording of dysrhythmias detected during monitoring in the coronary care unit. The patient records were reviewed to document preinfarction clinical status, in-hospital complications and cause of death.

To examine the course after discharge of the 161 patients who survived their hospitalization, intensive effort was made to contact each patient's private physician. Information sought included clinical course after discharge and circumstances of death if the patient had died. For those patients who had not been followed by a physician, telephone contact was made directly with the patient, or with his family if the patient had died. Follow-up information was obtained on 155 of the 161 patients: 119 of 124 (96 per cent) in group 1 and 36 of 37 (97 per cent) in group 2. The mean follow-up period for all patients was 36 months but this was extended to at least 40 months for patients still alive at the end of the follow-up period. Patients discharged who died during the follow-up period were classified into three groups according to the cause of death: (1) **Sudden death:** Death occurring within 1 hour after onset of cardiac symptoms and before hospital admission. (2) **Other cardiac death:** Death known to occur after hospital admission for subsequent acute infarction or for intractable congestive heart failure. (3) **Death from noncardiac causes:** The Chi-square method was used for statistical analysis of the data; p values of less than 0.05 were considered significant.

RESULTS

Preadmission History. A comparison of the preinfarction clinical histories of the patients in groups 1 and 2 is shown in Table I. The average patient age and male-to-female ratio were similar in the two groups. There was also no significant difference between the two groups in the incidence of a history of previous infarction, congestive heart failure, hypertension or diabetes. In group 2, the patients had a significantly higher incidence of previous angina (85 per cent versus 61.5 per cent in group 1, $p < 0.01$).

In-Hospital Course. As noted previously the electrocardiographic changes manifested by the patients in group 2 were S-T segment depression and/or T wave inversions. The relative frequency of these changes and their localization are shown in Table II. The most common pattern was S-T segment depression in the anterior-lateral precordial leads with or without accompanying T wave inversion. This pattern was noted in 22 patients or 55 per cent of the patients in group 2 (second column, Table II).

Other changes in this group are outlined in Table II. Of note is that only seven patients (17.5 per cent) had electrocardiograms which demonstrated only T wave inversions in the anterior and/or inferior leads.

The electrocardiographic changes of the patients in group 2 persisted for at least 24 hours in all 40 patients and for at least four days in 38 (95 per cent) of them. These changes tended to resolve gradually during hospitalization, with the S-T segments generally reverting to normal before the T waves, if both were present. However, in only four patients did the electrocardiogram show a complete return to their preinfarction status by the time of discharge. Of the 33 patients with S-T segment depression on the electrocardiogram obtained on admission, 12 had resolution of this change by the time of discharge. In only four of 33 patients with abnormal T wave inversions on their electrocardiogram did these T waves return to an upright status by discharge.

The electrocardiographic changes accepted as diagnostic for acute transmural infarction were classic S-T segment elevations with Q wave evolution. An approximately equal number of the patients in group 1 showed these changes in the anterior leads alone and

TABLE I History Before Admission

Data	Group 1 No.	Group 1 %	Group 2 No.	Group 2 %	p
Number of patients	148		40		
Average age (yr)	60.1		63		NS
Sex (no. of males)	117	72	28	70	NS
History of previous angina	91	61.5	34	85	<0.01
History of previous myocardial infarction	37	25	13	32.5	NS
History of congestive heart failure	34	23	15	37.5	NS
History of hypertension	47	31.8	9	22.5	NS
History of diabetes	25	16.9	7	17.5	NS

NOTE: NS = not significant.

TABLE II Site of Infarction

	Anterior-Lateral Leads Only* No.	%	Inferior Leads Only† No.	%	Both No.	%	Total No.	%
Electrocardiographic Localization of Transmural Myocardial Infarction (148 Cases)	66	45	68	46	14	9		
Electrocardiographic Manifestations of Nontransmural Myocardial Infarction (40 Cases)								
S-T segment depression with T wave inversion	16		1		9		26	65
S-T segment depression only	6		0		1		7	17.5
T wave inversion only	3		2		2		7	17.5
S-T segment elevation aVR	. . .		. . .		. . .		18	45

* Leads V_1 through V_6, I and aVL.
† Leads II, III and aVF.

TABLE III Complications After Myocardial Infarction

Complications	Group 1 No.	Group 1 %	Group 2 No.	Group 2 %	p
Ventricular premature contractions	82	55.4	24	60	NS
Atrial fibrillation	19	12.8	3	7.3	NS
Atrial flutter	9	6.0	2	4.9	NS
Accelerated idioventricular tachycardia	26	18	2	5	<0.02
Ventricular tachycardia	25	17.5	1	2.5	<0.02
Ventricular fibrillation	10	6.8	0	0	NS
Asystole	4	3.0	1	2.5	NS
Atrioventricular block:					
First-degree	24	16.2	3	7.5	. . .
Second-degree	4	2.7	0	0	. . .
Third-degree	10	6.8	1	2.5	. . .
Total	38	25.7	4	10	<0.05
Distal conduction defects:					
Right bundle branch block	16	10.8	0	0	. . .
Left bundle branch block	11	7.4	2	5.0	. . .
Left anterior hemiblock	22	14.8	5	12.5	. . .
Left posterior hemiblock	2	1.3	0	0	. . .
Total no. of patients with defects	36	24.3	7	17.5	NS

TABLE IV Complications After Myocardial Infarction

Complications	Group 1 No.	Group 1 %	Group 2 No.	Group 2 %	p
Congestive heart failure*	106	71.6	26	65.0	NS
Moderate to severe congestive heart failure†	68	45.9	13	32.5	NS
Cardiogenic shock‡	12	8.1	1	2.5	NS
Mortality	24	16.8	3	7.5	NS

* Rales at lung bases, S_3, or x-ray findings of vascular redistribution or Kerley B lines.
† Persistent failure or pulmonary edema requiring digitalis and/or diuretic therapy.
‡ Drop in blood pressure to <90 mm Hg systolic with decrease in mental status and/or cyanosis, requiring pressor therapy.

in the inferior leads alone. Fourteen patients (9 per cent) showed new Q waves in both the anterior and inferior leads.

Cardiac enzyme elevations were on the average significantly higher (p <0.01) in group 1 than in group 2. Peak levels for the two groups were as follows: in group 1, patients had an average SGOT of 222 units, a CPK of 297 units and an LDH of 1,663 units; in contrast, in group 2, patients had an average SGOT of 119 units, a CPK of 157 units and an LDH of 980 units. The upper limit of normal for these values at our institution are SGOT 40 units, CPK 80 units and LDH 600 units.

The two groups were also compared for the usual complications of infarction: congestive heart failure, dysrhythmias, atrioventricular block, distal conduction defects, cardiogenic shock and mortality. As shown in Tables III and IV, all these complications tended to be more common in group 1; however, statistical significance was achieved only in the difference in the incidence of in-hospital ventricular tachycardia (17.5 per cent in group 1 versus 2.5 per cent in group 2, p <0.02), in the incidence of accelerated idioventricular tachycardia (18 per cent in group 1 versus 5 per cent in group 2, p <0.02) and in the incidence of one or more forms of atrioventricular block (25.7 per cent in group 1 versus 10 per cent in group 2, p <0.05). Of the patients in group 1, 6.8 per cent experienced primary ventricular fibrillation as compared to none of those in group 2. Cardiogenic shock occurred in 8 per cent of the patients in group 1 and 2.5 per cent of the patients in group 2.

TABLE V Course After Discharge

Data	Group 1 No.	Group 1 %	Group 2 No.	Group 2 %	p
Discharged from hospital	124		37		
Contacted for follow-up	119		36		
Alive	83	69.8	19	52.8	<0.05
Sudden death	18	15.1	12	33.3	<0.02
Other cardiac death	11	9.2	3	8.3	NS
Death noncardiac cause	7	5.9	2	5.6	NS
Cumulative mortality (includes in-hospital deaths)	60/143	42	20/39	51.3	NS

TABLE VI Cardiovascular Status of Patients Alive at the End of the Follow-Up Period

	Group 1 No.	Group 1 %	Group 2 No.	Group 2 %	p
Patients alive	83		19*		
Angina present at least occasionally	53	63.8	15	83	<0.05
Angina Class II†	30	36.2	11	61	<0.05
Congestive heart failure	39	47.6	7	39	NS
Recurrent myocardial infarction	10	12	5	26	NS

* One patient was known to be alive and without recurrent myocardial infarction; however, other information about angina, congestive heart failure could not be obtained.

† New York Heart Association Classification—angina occurring regularly with strenuous exertion. Criteria added in this study for Class II angina was that it occur at least once a month.

Neither of these differences achieved statistical significance. In-hospital mortality was 16.8 per cent for group 1 and 7.5 per cent for group 2, also a statistically insignificant difference. The most common causes of death were cardiogenic shock and lethal dysrhythmias which accounted for two thirds of the mortality in both groups.

Course After Discharge. Of the 161 patients who survived the index 1971 infarction and were discharged from the hospital, follow-up information was obtained on 119 in group 1 and 36 in group 2. The patient's course after discharge is shown in Tables V and VI. Only 53 per cent of the discharged patients in group 2 were still alive at the end of the follow-up period which extended for at least 40 months after the infarction for all patients. This survival rate is in contrast to the 70 per cent survival shown by the patients in group 1 discharged during the same period. This difference achieved statistical significance with a p value of <0.05.

Careful analysis of the causes of death in both groups showed that the apparent reason for this poor long-term survival in group 2 was the high incidence of sudden death occurring in these patients. Sudden death was the most common cause of death after discharge in both groups, accounting for 80 per cent of the cardiac deaths after discharge (12 of 15) in group 2 and for 62 per cent of the deaths (18 of 29) in group 1 (Table V). The incidence of death from other cardiac causes, including intractable heart failure and documented re-infarction, was similar in the two groups (9.2 per cent in group 1 and 8.3 per cent in group 2), as was the incidence of death from noncardiac causes (5.9 per cent in group 1 and 5.6 per cent in group 2). The cumulative mortality, a figure including both in-hospital deaths immediately after the index infarction as well as deaths occurring in the follow-up period, was 51 per cent in group 2 and 42 per cent in group 1, a difference which was not statistically significant (Table V).

Figure 1 shows in actuarial form the survival curves for the two groups after discharge after the 1971 infarction. Patients who died from noncardiac causes were excluded from this graph; therefore, if one assumes that the sudden deaths in both groups were cardiac in etiology, then the decline in slope of the survival curves on this graph is secondary solely to cardiac-related mortality. As noted, the two populations followed a comparable course through 24 months; however, by 40 months the patients in group 2 showed a cardiac-related mortality of 41 per cent versus 23 per cent for patients in group 1, a statistically significant difference with $p < 0.05$. The average interval between discharge and death for those patients who died during this period after discharge was 15.8 months in group 1 and 21.6 months in group 2.

A comparison of the cardiovascular status of the 83 patients in group 1 and of the 19 in group 2 still alive at the end of the follow-up period is shown in Table VI. There was no significant difference between the two groups in terms of incidence of congestive heart failure or of recurrent infarction; however, the incidence of recurrent angina was significantly higher in group 2.

An attempt was made to identify those factors in the patients' clinical history and hospital course that were associated with an unfavorable prognosis after discharge. As shown in Table VII, each factor was examined independently for its effect on the mortality of patients who presented with or in whom the stated factor developed in contrast to patients who lacked the factor. For the patients in group 1, the following seemed to be statistically correlated with an increase in cardiac mortality after discharge: a history of congestive heart failure prior to admission, a history of cardiac symptoms prior to admission of greater than five years, the presence of persistent congestive heart failure in the hospital after infarction, and, finally, involvement of the anterior myocardial wall as indicated by diagnostic changes in the anterior precordial leads on the elec-

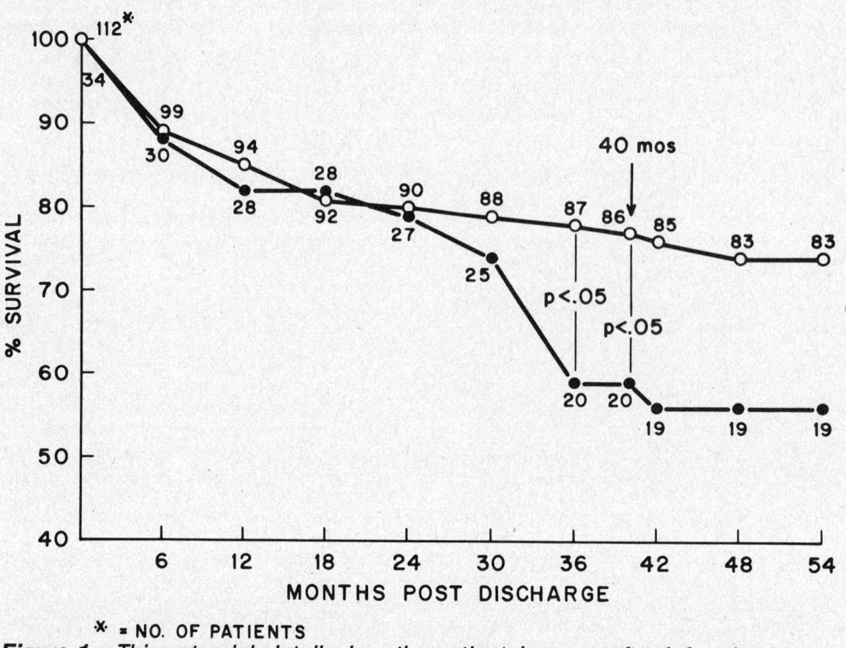

Figure 1. *This actuarial plot displays the patients' course after infarction (group 1, open circles; group 2, closed circles). Shown on the ordinate is the per cent of patients alive and on the abscissa the number of months after index infarction in 1971. The two populations follow a comparable course through 24 months; marked differences in survival are noted at 36 months (mean follow-up period) achieving statistical significance at the p <0.05 level.*

TABLE VII Relationship of Historical Data and In-Hospital Course to Cardiac Mortality After Discharge

	Group 1					Group 2				
	Present		Not Present			Present		Not Present		
	No.	%*	No.	%	p	No.	%	No.	%	p
Historical data										
Age (60 yr)	4/14	29	11/22	50	NS	15/47	32	14/72	19	NS
Previous angina Class II	10/24	42	5/12	42	NS	16/50	32	14/69	19	NS
Previous myocardial infarction	5/13	39	10/23	43	NS	9/27	33	27/92	22	NS
Previous congestive heart failure	6/14	43	9/32	28	NS	11/20	55	18/99	18	<0.01
Previous hypertension	4/9	44	11/27	41	NS	11/41	27	18/78	23	NS
More than 5 year history of cardiac symptoms prior to myocardial infarction	6/16	38	9/20	45	NS	8/17	47	21/102	20	<0.05
In-hospital course										
Persistent congestive heart failure after myocardial infarction	6/9	67	9/27	33	<0.1	19/45	42	10/74	14	<0.01
Peak SGOT 100	8/16	50	7/20	35	NS	...	...	...	...	...
Peak SGOT 200	...	...	...	...	...	13/48	22	16/61	26	NS
Ventricular premature contractions	9/21	43	6/15	40	NS	17/60	28	12/59	20	NS
Primary S-T segment changes in anterior leads on EKG (depression for nontransmural myocardial infarction and elevation for transmural myocardial infarction)	14/28	50	1/8	12.5	<0.1	20/62	32	9/57	16	<0.05

NOTE: Denominator represents number of patients with (or without) stated factor. Numerator indicates number of deaths after discharge among these patients.

* Calculated mortality rate is given under per cent.

trocardiogram. For the patients in group 2, these factors could not be shown to have a statistically significant effect on the prognosis after discharge, partially because of the smaller number of patients involved.

The mortality after discharge of the patients in group 2 whose electrocardiograms demonstrated S-T segment depression in the anterior precordial leads was 50 per cent as compared to 12.5 per cent of those patients whose electrocardiograms showed only T wave inversions or S-T depression limited to the inferior leads. This difference did not achieve significance when analyzed statistically. However, when one examines the entire group of patients including the three who died in the hospital, the cumulative mortality, including deaths after discharge and in the hospital, is 54.8 per cent for the patients with anterior precordial S-T segment depression on the electrocardiogram as compared to a cumulative mortality of 12.5 per cent for the patients with T wave inversions or S-T depression in inferior leads. This difference achieves statistical significance with a p value of <0.05.

The following factors could not be demonstrated in this study to be associated with a significantly poorer course after discharge for any of the patients: history of previous angina, history of previous infarction, history of hypertension, high enzyme elevations during infarction or the occurrence of ventricular premature contractions recorded in the CCU.

COMMENTS

The results of this study suggest that patients sustaining nontransmural infarctions have a generally guarded prognosis after discharge. The only other investigator to examine specifically the after discharge course of patients with nontransmural infarction versus that of patients with post-transmural infarctions was Rigo et al. [4] in a study of 49 patients with nontransmural myocardial infarction and 111 patients with transmural myocardial infarction. They found a 19 per cent mortality for the 41 discharged patients with nontransmural myocardial infarction during a follow-up period of 20 months. This was comparable to the 18 per cent mortality demonstrated by the 81 discharged patients with transmural myocardial infarction. These investigators suggest that patients with nontransmural infarction may have a high incidence of fatal arrhythmias after discharge although the causes of death of their patients are not specified. Interestingly, our study also showed a 19 per cent mortality over the first 20 months for the discharged patients with nontransmural myocardial infarction (group 2). The patients with transmural myocardial infarction also had a 19 per cent mortality during this period. However, by 40 months after the index infarction the mortality after discharge of our patients in group 2 was 47 per cent versus 30 per cent for the patients in group 1. The number of patients in group 2 of this study was relatively small, making definitive interpretation difficult; however, these data strongly imply that the prognosis in patients with nontransmural infarction after discharge is at least the same if not less favorable than that of patients with transmural myocardial infarction.

An attempt was made to identify those factors in the history before infarction and the hospital course after infarction that might be predictive of prognosis after discharge. For the patients in group 1 several general factors such as duration of cardiovascular disease prior to admission, congestive heart failure either historically or in the hospital after infarction and involvement of the anterior wall in the infarction, did prove to be associated with a poorer prognosis after discharge (Table VII). For group 2 these and other factors listed could not be shown to have a statistical effect on the course after discharge.

It is of note, however, that patients with nontransmural myocardial infarction and S-T segment depression in the anterior leads on their admission electrocardiogram appeared to have a poorer prognosis than those patients with either T wave inversions only or S-T segment changes limited to the inferior leads. In a study of 300 patients admitted to a coronary care unit, Lown [15] found a similar discrepancy between the in-hospital prognosis of patients with nontransmural infarction and S-T segment depression and those with only T wave inversion. The patients with T wave inversion had an in-hospital mortality of 0 per cent versus that of 28 per cent for the patients with S-T segment depression.

It was somewhat surprising that in light of the high incidence of sudden death after discharge in both groups, especially in group 2 (33 per cent, see "Results"), no correlation could be demonstrated between the occurrence of ventricular ectopy during infarction and sudden death after discharge. Vismara et al. [16] have shown that ventricular arrhythmias recorded late in the hospital course after infarction are more predictive of sudden death after discharge than those recorded in the CCU. The ventricular ectopy of the patients in this study after their stay in the CCU and after discharge was not examined. Thus the finding of no obvious relationship between ectopy in the CCU and sudden death after discharge does not rule out an association between late in-hospital ventricular ectopy and later sudden death in the patients with nontransmural myocardial infarction.

One likely hypothesis for the apparent disparity in clinical course between the two groups is that many of the patients with transmural myocardial infarction who survived the period immediately after infarction have likely had an isolated occlusion of a coronary artery with acute infarction and subsequent scar formation with the elimination of ischemic tissue. Conversely, the patients with nontransmural myocardial infarction without transmural scar may well be more prone to recurrent ischemic events with electrophysiologic subendocardial instability resulting in lethal arrhythmias and sudden death. Certainly the high incidence of sudden death and recurrent angina that the patients with nontransmural myocardial infarction demonstrated after discharge is in support of this hypothesis. However, only a study analyzing the occurrence of arrhythmias after infarction in both groups will definitively resolve this hypothesis.

An alternative, although related hypothesis is based on recent studies by Reeves et al. [17] and Burggraf et al. [18] who suggested that the prognosis of patients with coronary artery disease is best correlated with the degree of coronary stenosis and number of vessels involved as documented by angiography rather than with the clinical manifestations of coronary disease such as angina, infarction or acute coronary insufficiency. Therefore, it may be that the poor prognosis of patients after a nontransmural myocardial infarction indicates that these patients have more advanced underlying coronary artery disease than the patient with transmural myocardial infarction. Little angiographic data were available concerning the coronary anatomy of the patients in this study; however, Madigan et al. [19] performed early coronary angiography on 32 patients with nontransmural infarction and demonstrated that 97 per cent had greater than 75 per cent stenosis in at least one major artery and that 67 per cent had significant involvement of two or more vessels. Furthermore, 70 per cent of these patients with two to three vessel disease were considered to be potentially suitable candidates for bypass surgery.

This study suggests two therapeutic interventions for this high risk group. Even in the absence of a documented increased incidence of ventricular ectopy in those patients with nontransmural myocardial infarction who die suddenly, the question of the prophylactic efficacy of antiarrhythmic treatment arises. Koch-Weser [1] suggests that long-term antiarrhythmic treatment should be considered in any group of patients with an annual dysrhythmic mortality of 10 per cent or greater, and according to the results of this study, the patients with nontransmural myocardial infarction fulfill this criteria. The efficacy and relative benefit of presently available antiarrhythmic agents used to prevent sudden death is an area of controversy. With new, less toxic antiarrhythmic drugs becoming available, a randomized study appears indicated to examine the use of antiarrhythmic prophylaxis in patients with nontransmural myocardial infarction.

The poor prognosis of the patients with nontransmural myocardial infarction as well as the possibility that they have areas of viable, yet ischemic-prone myocardium adjacent to infarcted areas suggests that these patients may be suitable candidates for early angiographic studies and for surgical revascularization if appropriate. Although the effect of coronary artery bypass grafting on prolongation of life and prevention of infarction is still unclear [20], a well controlled, prospective study seems indicated to determine its effect on the long-term prognosis of patients with nontransmural myocardial infarction.

REFERENCES

1. Koch-Weser J: Antiarrhythmic prophylaxis in ambulatory patients with coronary heart disease. Arch Intern Med 129: 763, 1972.
2. Scheinman NM, Abbott JA: Clinical significance of transmural versus nontransmural electrocardiographic changes in patients with acute myocardial infarction. Am J Med 55: 602, 1973.
3. Madias JE, Chahine RA, Gorlin R, et al.: A comparison of transmural and nontransmural acute myocardial infarction. Circulation 49: 498, 1974.
4. Rigo P, Murray M, Taylor DR, et al.: Hemodynamic and prognostic findings in patients with transmural and nontransmural infarction. Circulation 51: 1064, 1975.
5. Salisbury PF, Cross CE, Rieben PA: Acute ischemia of inner layers of ventricular wall. Am Heart J 66: 650, 1963.
6. Eliot RS, Holsinger JW: A unified concept of the pathophysiology of myocardial infarction and sudden death. Chest 62: 469, 1972.
7. Stimmel B, Katz AM, Donoso E: Q-wave development in acute subendocardial infarction. Arch Intern Med 131: 676, 1973.
8. Levine HD, Ford RV: Subendocardial infarction. Circulation 1: 246, 1950.
9. Myers GB, Sears CH, Hiratzka T: Correlation of electrocardiographic and pathologic findings in ring-like subendocardial infarction of the left ventricle. Am J Med Sci 222: 417, 1951.
10. Yu PNG, Stewart JM: Subendocardial myocardial infarction with special reference to the electrocardiographic changes. Am Heart J 39: 862, 1950.
11. Cook RW, Edwards JE, Pruitt RD: Electrocardiographic changes in acute subendocardial infarcts: 11 small subendocardial infarcts. Circulation 18: 613, 1958.
12. Georas CS, Dahlquist D, Cutts FB: Subendocardial infarction. Arch Intern Med 111: 488, 1963.
13. Caskey TD, Estes EH: Deviation of the S-T segment: a review. Am J Med 36: 424, 1964.
14. Pruitt RD, Klakeg CH, Chapin LE: Certain clinical states and pathologic changes associated with deeply inverted T waves in the precordial electrocardiogram. Circulation 11: 517, 1955.
15. Lown B, Vassaux C, Hood WB, et al.: Unresolved problems in coronary care. Am J Cardiol 20: 494, 1967.
16. Vismara LA, Amsterdam EA, Mason DT: Relation of ventricular arrhythmias in the late hospital phase of acute myocardial infarction to sudden death after hospital discharge. Am J Med 59: 6, 1975.
17. Reeves TJ, Oberman A, Jones WB, et al.: Natural history of angina pectoris. Am J Cardiol 33: 423, 1974.
18. Burggraf GW, Parker JO: Prognosis in coronary artery disease. Circulation 51: 146, 1975.
19. Madison NP, Rutherford BD, Frye RL: Clinical course and coronary anatomy of subendocardial infarction. Am J Cardiol 35: 154, 1975.
20. Mundth ED, Austen WG: Surgical measures for coronary heart disease. N Engl J Med 293: 13, 75, 124, 1975.

Idiopathic Portal Hypertension

J. P. VILLENEUVE, M.D.
P.-M. HUET, M.D., Ph.D.
J.-G. JOLY, M.D., M.Sc.
D. MARLEAU, M.D., M.Sc.
J. CÔTÉ, M.D.
A. LÉGARÉ, M.D.
M. LAFORTUNE, M.D.
P. LAVOIE, M.D.
A. VIALLET, M.D.
Montreal, Quebec, Canada

Idiopathic portal hypertension is reported in five cases including one case of chronic arsenical intake and one case of chronic industrial vinyl chloride exposure. In all five cases the patients presented with gastrointestinal bleeding as the chief complaint. Physical examination was within normal limits except for splenomegaly in all. Results of liver function tests were normal, except for the relative clearance of sulfobromophtalein. A surgical liver biopsy specimen was obtained in all cases and showed moderate degrees of portal fibrosis, but no cirrhosis. Combined umbilicoportal, hepatic vein and superior mesenteric artery catheterization was performed in all cases. Hepatoportographies showed distortion of the intrahepatic portal venous system and cut-off of small portal venules. Portohepatic gradients ranged from 14.0 to 20.5 mm Hg. The portal hypertension was both sinusoidal and presinusoidal in nature but mainly presinusoidal. Hepatic extraction of indocyanine green and of albumin microaggregates was normal, thereby suggesting normal functional portal blood supply to the liver. The patients with arsenical or vinyl chloride exposure could not be differentiated from the other three patients with idiopathic portal hypertension. These results suggest that idiopathic portal hypertension may be related to domestic or industrial exposure to other hepatotoxins.

Idiopathic portal hypertension is a relatively uncommon disorder in America and Europe [1–14]. However, large series from India [15–21] and Japan [22,23] have revealed that in these countries, idiopathic portal hypertension is responsible for some 25 per cent of the patients with portal hypertension undergoing portal decompression. In this syndrome, portal hypertension is present, but there is no cirrhosis, extrahepatic venous obstruction or other rarer causes of portal hypertension [24]. In the majority of cases, minimal portal fibrosis is present on histology, along with some poorly defined intrahepatic vascular abnormalities on splenoportography.

Until recently, no definite etiologic factor could be identified, but recent reports suggest that prolonged exposure to inorganic arsenic [25,26] or vinyl chloride gas [27] may cause a syndrome nearly identical to the one described as "idiopathic" portal hypertension.

In the present report we describe five cases of portal hypertension, three of unknown etiology, one associated with chronic arsenical intake and one associated with chronic vinyl chloride exposure. We intend to show the similarities between these cases, and suggest that other still unidentified toxins could account for the so-called "idiopathic" portal hypertension syndrome.

From the Clinical Research Center, Hôpital Saint-Luc, and the Departments of Medicine, Pathology, Radiology and Surgery, Hôpital Saint-Luc, and University of Montreal, Montreal, Quebec, Canada. This study was supported by grants from the Medical Research Council of Canada. Requests for reprints should be addressed to Dr. André Viallet, Clinical Research Center, Hôpital Saint-Luc, 1058 St-Denis, Montreal, P.Q. Canada. Manuscript accepted January 12, 1976.

TABLE I Clinical Data

Case No.	Age (yr)	Sex	Presenting Complaint	Liver* (cm)	Spleen* (cm)
1	32	F	Hematemesis (X 3)	8	18
2	20	M	Hematemesis (X 3)	8	13
3	59	M	Melena (X 2)	12	16
4†	39	M	Melena (X 3)	17	15
5‡	60	M	Melena (X 1)	12	19

* Measured on isotopic scan.
† Chronic arsenical intake.
‡ Chronic vinyl chloride gas exposure.

TABLE II Laboratory Data

Case No.	Leukocytes (per mm³)	Platelets (per mm³)	K-BSP* (%)	K-ICG† (%)	ICG Extraction‡ (%)
1	4,920	130,000	6.6	14.4	44.8
2	7,520	40,000	6.6	18.2	47.3
3	5,300	56,000	6.0	14.4	50.2
4	3,400	29,000	11.9	24.8	60.4
5	5,140	82,000	5.3	13.6	42.8

* Normal values greater than 11 per cent.
† Normal values greater than 16 per cent.
‡ Normal values greater than 47 per cent.

MATERIAL AND METHODS

Patients. Over a three year period, a diagnosis of idiopathic portal hypertension was established in five of a total of 76 cases of portal hypertension studied before therapeutic shunt surgery in our hospital. The diagnosis of idiopathic portal hypertension was based upon the following criteria: hemodynamic evidence of "significant" portal hypertension, as defined by a portohepatic gradient of 10 mm Hg or more [26]; a surgical liver biopsy showing no cirrhosis or other lesions known to be responsible for portal hypertension, and a patent portal venous system as proved by umbilicoportography.

Radiologic and Hemodynamic Studies. Combined hepatic vein, umbilicoportal vein and superior mesenteric artery catheterization was performed in each case [29]. Retrograde splenography and portography were performed. Pressures in the hepatic vein were recorded in the wedged (WHVP) and free (FHVP) positions. Free portal venous pressure (FPVP) was recorded within 2 minutes of the hepatic vein recordings. The portohepatic gradient (PHG) was obtained by subtracting the FHVP from the FPVP value.

Using a continuous infusion method with indocyanine green, hepatic extraction of indocyanine green and estimated hepatic blood flow (EHBF) were calculated [30]. The portal fraction of the total hepatic blood flow was estimated by an indicator dilution method using ^{51}Cr labelled red blood cells [29]. Hepatic extraction of albumin microaggregates labelled with ^{125}I (^{125}I-AMA) was estimated by a double indicator dilution method using ^{51}Cr red blood cells and ^{125}I albumin microaggregates [31]. Cardiac output was measured by the indicator dilution method using either indocyanine green or ^{51}Cr red blood cells.

Other Studies. Anterior and posterior hepatosplenic scannings were obtained by a standard technic using a colloidal radioisotope. Esophagogastroduodenoscopy was performed in all cases. Fractional clearances of sulfobromophtalein (K-BSP) and indocyanine green (K-ICG) were determined as previously described [32]. Plasma volume was measured from the distribution space of indocyanine green, and total blood volume was calculated using peripheral venous hematocrit.

RESULTS

Clinical and Laboratory Data. Clinical data are shown in Table I. The patients ranged in age from 20 to 60 years. The only woman in the group was of Italian origin; the remaining four were Canadian. All five patients presented with gastrointestinal hemorrhage as the chief complaint. One (Case 4) had a history of chronic arsenical intake and has been the subject of a previous publication [26]. Another (Case 5) had been chronically exposed to industrial vinyl chloride gas. None had a history of previous jaundice or chronic alcoholism. On physical examination, splenomegaly was the only finding. None had hepatomegaly, jaundice, ascites, spider angioma or other signs of liver disease. Portosystemic encephalopathy was not observed following episodes of gastrointestinal hemorrage. Endoscopy of the upper gastrointestinal tract showed huge esophageal varices (more than 4 mm wide) in all patients with no other lesions in the upper gastrointestinal tract. In two patients (Cases 1 and 2) the endoscopy was performed during an active bleeding episode, allowing visualization of bleeding varices.

Hepatic scanning showed a homogeneous uptake of colloid by the liver and moderate extrahepatic uptake by an enlarged spleen but no vertebral bone marrow uptake. Laboratory data showed decreased white cells and platelet counts (Table II), and a hematocrit value which varied according to the bleeding status. Serum glutamic-oxaloacetic (SGOT) and glutamic-pyruvic (SGPT) transaminases, bilirubin, alkaline phosphatase, prothrombin time, total protein and protein electrophoresis were within normal limits in all patients. K-BSP was decreased in all but one patient (Case 4), whereas K-ICG was near-normal in all (Table II).

Radiologic Data. Arteriography of the celiac trunk and superior mesenteric arteriography revealed no arteriovenous fistulas in the splanchnic bed. Retrograde splenoportography demonstrated permeable splenic and portal veins, without occlusion or narrowing, and large esophageal varices originating from the coronary vein (Figure 1). In all five cases, the intrahepatic venogram revealed unexpected features: there was no occlusion of the large and medium-size portal veins (Figure 2); distortion and unusual branching of the intrahepatic portal system was observed, and cut-off of dilated small portal venules was visualized, with opacification of a capsular network (Figures 1 through 4).

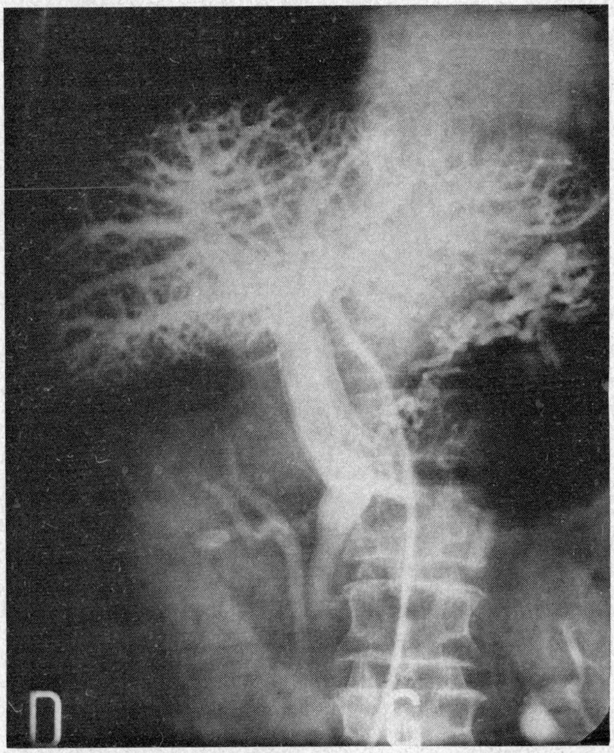

Figure 1. *The main portal trunk and the intrahepatic branches are patent. The coronary vein is dilated and shows esophageal varices (Case 5).*

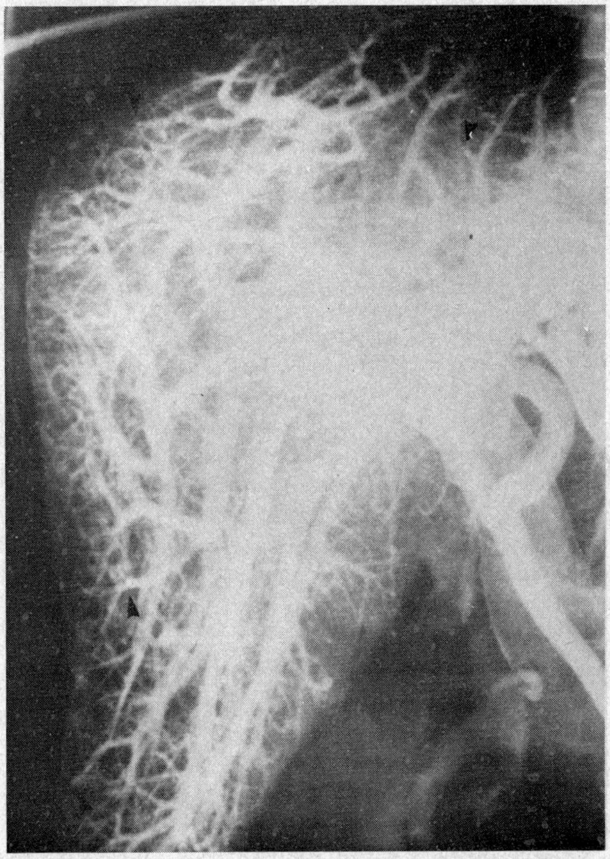

Figure 2. *The intrahepatic portal veins are patent. The distal branches of the portal venules show a cut-off appearance (**arrows**). A subcapsular network is opacified (Case 1).*

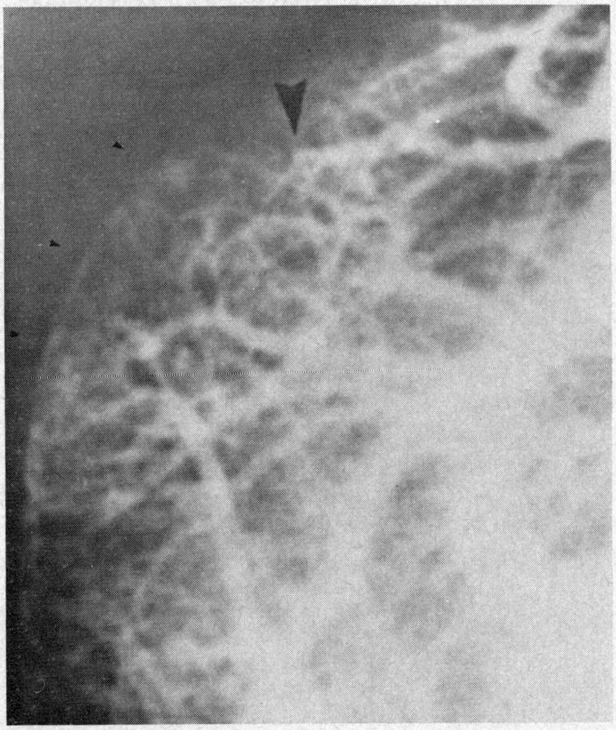

Figure 3. *Magnification of a segment of Figure 2. Cut-off of the distal branches of the portal venules (**large arrow**) and subcapsular network opacification (**small arrows**) are demonstrated (Case 1).*

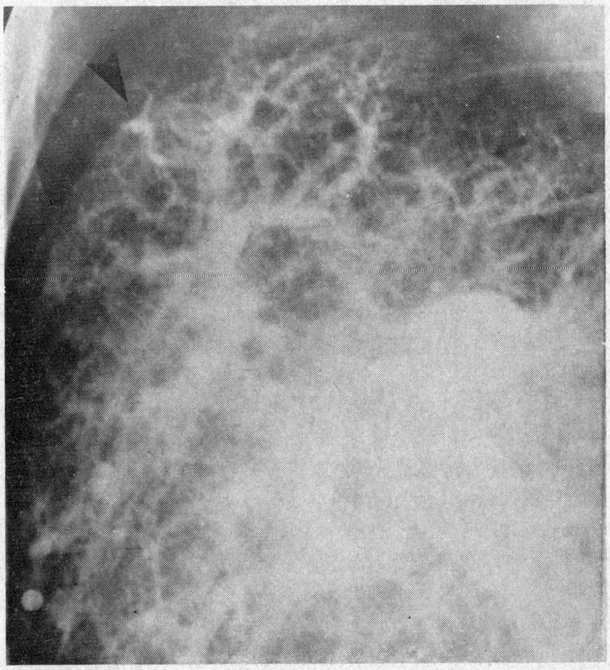

Figure 4. *Distortion of the peripheral intrahepatic portal venous system, cut-off of distal branches of the portal vein (**arrow**) and subcapsular network are revealed (Case 3).*

TABLE III Portohepatic Gradients

Case No.	FPVP (mm Hg)	WHVP (mm Hg)	FHVP (mm Hg)	PHG (mm Hg)
1	21.0	9.0	4.0	17.0
2	25.0	17.5	11.0	14.0
3	27.5	19.0	7.0	20.5
4	25.0	9.5	8.0	17.0
5	27.0	17.0	7.0	20

NOTE: FPVP = free portal vein pressure. WHVP = wedged hepatic vein pressure. FHVP = free hepatic vein pressure. PHG = portohepatic gradient (FPVP − FHVP).

Reviewed blindly by two independent radiologists, all five hepatoportograms were identified from a series of 20 cases presenting a wide variety of hepatic pathologies, also studied by umbilicoportography.

Hemodynamic Data. As shown in Table III, all patients had severe portal hypertension as evaluated by portohepatic gradients ranging from 14.0 to 20.5 mm Hg. FPVP was consistently higher than WHVP by pressure values ranging from 7.5 to 15.5 mm Hg. EHBF was within normal limits in four patients (Table IV), and was slightly increased in one (Case 4). Hepatic extraction of ^{125}I albumin microaggregates ranged from 81.5 to 100 per cent, values considered to be normal for the mammalian liver in our laboratory [31]. Cardiac index and total blood volume were increased in two patients (Cases 1 and 2), and normal in the other three (Cases 3, 4 and 5) (Table IV).

Histologic Studies. Macroscopic appearance and consistency of the liver was noted at surgery. The liver was normal in Cases 1 and 3. In Case 2, it was firmer than usual and a few small nodules, 1 cm in diameter, were observed on its inferior surface. In Case 4, the surface was slightly irregular and in Case 5, the liver was firmer than usual; there was no evidence of liver tumor. In none was there any findings suggesting partial nodular transformation of the liver [33].

Large surgical wedge biopsy specimens permitted definite exclusion of cirrhosis in all cases. On histology, large- and medium-size veins in the portal tract were normal. Portal spaces showed moderate degrees of stellate fibrosis, and some 20 to 30 per cent of the small portal veins were slightly dilated (Figure 5). The parenchyma appeared hyperplasic as evidenced by multinucleated cells and double-celled trabeculas. The hepatic capsule was thickened, and subcapsular nodularity was increased.

TABLE IV Hepatic and Cardiac Blood Flows

Case No.	EHBF (liters/min)	PF (%)	E-^{125}I AMA (%)	Cardiac Index (liters/min/m^2)	Total Blood Volume (ml/kg)
1	1.11	75.0	95.6	5.00	89.7
2	1.81	56.5	100.0	5.10	126.0
3	1.39	91.2	81.5	2.90	78.7
4	2.20	...	...	3.59	59.2
5	1.87	...	100.0	3.53	74.2

NOTE: EHBF = estimated hepatic blood flow using a continuous infusion of indocyanine green. PF = portal fraction of hepatic blood flow using ^{51}Cr red blood cell dilution curves. E-^{125}I AMA = hepatic extraction of ^{125}I albumin microaggregates.

Surgical Management and Evolution. All patients were operated on for gastrointestinal bleeding. One (Case 1) had a splenorenal shunt. Twelve days later, she had another episode of upper gastrointestinal bleeding; emergency endoscopy revealed ruptured esophageal varices and the bleeding stopped spontaneously. She died unexpectedly six weeks later. At autopsy, she had not re-bled from esophageal varices and the shunt was permeable; careful dissection of the intrahepatic portal tree showed no evidence of thrombosis. The cause of death is unknown in this case.

A terminolateral shunt with arterialization of the proximal stump of the portal vein was performed in Case 2. Except for post-transfusional HB Ag positive hepatitis, the patient is doing well 18 months after surgery.

A splenorenal shunt was performed in Case 3. The patient died 13 days after surgery because of cerebral manifestations of disseminated intravascular coagulation. At autopsy, the portal venous tree and the shunt were patent.

Case 4 has been reported elsewhere [26]. This patient responded well following a splenorenal shunt, but he died three years later after the development of a second arsenic-related cancer. An autopsy was not performed.

One patient (Case 5) is doing well nine months after splenorenal shunt.

COMMENTS

The syndrome of idiopathic portal hypertension might be responsible for some 3 per cent to 5 per cent of cases of portal hypertension in North America [34]. Our data are in agreement with these figures.

In the present study, the only clinical findings were splenomegaly and bleeding from esophageal varices without liver failure. There were no clinical or biologic signs of liver disease. After more elaborate testing, only K-BSP was abnormal in four cases, whereas K-ICG, E-ICG and E-^{131}I albumin microaggregates were normal or near-normal. Hepatic scanning showed homogeneous hepatic uptake, moderate uptake by an enlarged spleen, but no bone marrow uptake of the colloid by contrast to what is found with portal hypertension of cirrhosis [35]. The present data confirm much of what

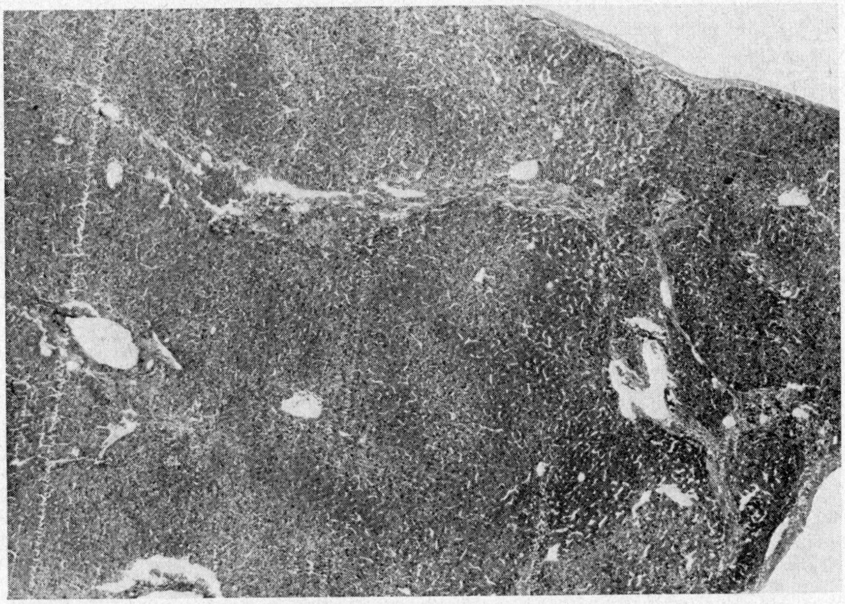

Figure 5. *Low magnification of a surgical biopsy specimen showing slight fibrosis and absence of cirrhosis (Case 3).*

has already been described in these cases [7,14,15,18,20].

Umbilicoportography permitted the study of the intrahepatic portal system, revealing some unusual features: abrupt cut-off of small portal veins along with opacification of a subcapsular network. Using splenoportography, similar findings have previously been suggested by Boyer [18], Zeegan [14] and Basu [15]. In a subsequent report [3], Boyer et al. demonstrated multiple intrahepatic portal vein thrombi using vinylite corrosion casts. It must be underlined that in that study, three of four patients previously had a portacaval shunt.

In the present cases, narrowing or occlusion of major intrahepatic portal vein branches can definitely be excluded. The radiologic "cut-off" abnormalities could not be correlated with any histologic evidence of thrombosis of small portal veins, even with serial cutting of the histologic specimens.

Pressure recordings showed that the portal hypertension was presinusoidal in Case 4, and mostly presinusoidal with an intrahepatic "sinusoidal" component in the other four cases. The normal extraction of ^{125}I AMA and indocyanine green suggest that functional portal blood supply to the liver in these patients is normal and that there is normal contact of these two substances with Kupffer cells and hepatocytes.

It would thus appear that these patients have near-normal liver functions, and that their portal hypertension is mainly presinusoidal. Thus idiopathic portal hypertension as a syndrome closely resembles portal vein thrombosis. The localization of the obstruction could be at the sinusoidal level, as already suggested by electron microscopy studies [4,20,21], or at the junction between portal vein radicles and sinusoids.

In the past few years, there have been reports [25,26] of portal hypertension without obvious cause in patients ingesting inorganic arsenic for prolonged periods. More recently, clinical manifestations of portal hypertension have been reported in patients exposed to vinyl chloride gas over long periods [27]. Both these substances are also associated with the development of hepatic angiosarcoma [35,36].

In one of the present cases (Case 5) the patient had been exposed to vinyl chloride for some time; although he had no demonstrable liver tumor, he had definite clinical as well as hemodynamic evidence of portal hypertension. Both patients with arsenical and vinyl chloride exposure could not be differentiated from the other three patients with idiopathic portal hypertension on either histologic, radiologic or hemodynamic criteria. Although the evidence presented here is only descriptive, we believe that there may be a direct relation between portal hypertension and chronic arsenical and vinyl chloride exposure in our two patients. Therefore, as has already been suggested by others [20,27], still unidentifiable chemicals may be responsible for some of the so-called "idiopathic" portal hypertension syndromes.

ACKNOWLEDGMENT

We wish to thank J. Pruneau and J. Marchi for the photographic work.

REFERENCES

1. Benhamou JP, Guillemot R, Tricot R, et al.: Hypertension portale essentielle. Presse Med 70: 2397, 1962.
2. Alvarez FB, Gil JLS, De La Marina JRA, et al.: Hipertension portal esencial: cinco casos personales. Rev Esp Enferm Apar Dig 39: 633, 1973.
3. Boyer JL, Hales MR, Klatskin G: Idiopathic portal hypertension due to occlusion of intrahepatic portal veins by organised thrombi. Medicine (Baltimore) 53: 77, 1974.
4. Kluge T, Sommerschild H, Flatmark A: Sinusoidal portal hypertension. Surgery 68: 294, 1970.
5. Leger L, Lemaigre G, Richarme J, et al.: L'hypertension portale essentielle. A propos de dix observations personnelles. Presse Med 74: 313, 1966.
6. Mendenhall CL, Sherman J, Chedid A: Intermittent idiopathic portal hypertension. A case report. Gastroenterology 67: 142, 1974.
7. Mikkelsen WP, Edmondson HA, Peters RL, et al.: Extra and intrahepatic portal hypertension without cirrhosis (hepatoportal sclerosis). Ann Surg 162: 602, 1965.
8. Miller MC, Brandt JL: Portal hypertension in the absence of both liver disease and vascular obstruction. Am J Dig Dis 7: 442, 1962.
9. Otto P, Krause PH, Jester HG, et al.: Idiopathische portale hypertension. Med Klin 67: 447, 1972.
10. Polish E, Christie J, Cohen A, et al.: Idiopathic presinusoidal portal hypertension (Banti's syndrome). Ann Intern Med 56: 624, 1962.
11. Stalder GA, Burckhardt D, Bianchi L: Idiopathic portal hypertension, manifestation of a more generalised vascular disease? Case report. Helv Med Acta 37: 281, 1973.
12. Talner LB, Boyer JL, Clemett AR: Intrahepatic portal vein occlusion. A cause of portal hypertension. Radiology 92: 1265, 1969.
13. Tisdale WA, Klatskin G, Glenn WWL: Portal hypertension and bleeding oesophageal varices. Their occurrence in the absence of both intrahepatic and extrahepatic obstruction of the portal vein. N Engl J Med 261: 209, 1959.
14. Zeegen R, Stansfeld AG, Dawson AM, et al.: Prolonged survival after portal decompression of patients with non-cirrhotic intrahepatic portal hypertension. Gut 11: 610, 1970.
15. Basu AK, Boyer J, Bhattacharya R, et al.: Non-cirrhotic portal fibrosis with portal hypertension: a new syndrome. I. Indian J Med Res 55: 336, 1967.
16. Basu Mallik KC, Sen Gupta KP, Basu AK, et al.: Non-cirrhotic portal fibrosis: a new syndrome. II. Histopathological studies. Ind J Med Res 55: 351, 1967.
17. Basu AK, Basu Mallik KC, Sen Gupta KP, et al.: Long-term follow-up studies of "non-cirrhotic portal fibrosis" after surgery. Br J Surg 56: 497, 1969.
18. Boyer JL, Sen Gupta KP, Biswas SK, et al.: Idiopathic portal hypertension. Comparison with the portal hypertension of cirrhosis and extrahepatic portal vein obstruction. Ann Intern Med 66: 41, 1967.
19. Nayak NC, Ramalingaswami V: Obliterative portal venopathy of the liver. Arch Pathol 87: 359, 1969.
20. Sama SK, Bhargava S, Gopi Nath N, et al.: Noncirrhotic portal fibrosis. Am J Med 51: 160, 1971.
21. Tandon BN, Lakshminarayanan R, Bhargava S, et al.: Ultrastructure of the liver in non-cirrhotic portal fibrosis with portal hypertension. Gut 11: 905, 1970.
22. Imanaga H, Yamamoto S, Kuroyanagi Y: Surgical treatment of portal hypertension according to state of intrahepatic circulation. Ann Surg 155: 42, 1962.
23. Nakamura S, Kera K, Sasaki K, et al.: Hepatic hemodynamics in idiopathic persinusoidal portal hypertension in Japan. Angiology 23: 7, 1972.
24. Sherlock S: Classification and functional aspects of portal hypertension. Ann Surg 127: 121, 1974.
25. Morris JS, Schmid M, Newman S, et al.: Arsenic and noncirrhotic portal hypertension. Gastroenterology 66: 86, 1974.
26. Huet PM, Guillaume E, Côté J, et al.: Non-cirrhotic presinusoidal portal hypertension associated with chronic arsenical intoxication. Gastroenterology 68: 1270, 1975.
27. Thomas LB, Popper H, Berk PD, et. al.: Vinyl-chloride-induced liver disease. From idiopathic portal hypertension (Banti's syndrome) to angiosarcomas. N Engl J Med 292: 17, 1975.
28. Viallet A, Marleau D, Huet PM, et al.: Hemodynamic evaluation of patients with intrahepatic portal hypertension. Gastroenterology 69: 1297, 1975.
29. Huet PM, Lavoie P, Légaré A, et al.: Combined hepatic vein, umbilicoportal vein, and superior mesenteric artery catheterization in portal hypertension: estimation of the portal fraction of total hepatic blood flow in cirrhotic patients. Yale J Biol Med 48: 55, 1975.
30. Leevy CM, Mendenhall CL, Lesko W, et al.: Estimation of hepatic blood flow with indocyanine green. J Clin Invest 41: 1169, 1962.
31. Huet PM, Marleau D, Lavoie P, et al.: Extraction of ^{125}I albumin microaggregates from portal blood: an index of functional portal blood supply in cirrhotics. Gastroenterology 70: 74, 1976.
32. Lefebvre M, Joubert G, Marleau D, et al.: Epuration des colorants hépatotropes dans la cirrhose. Union Med Can 98: 925, 1969.
33. Sherlock S, Feldman CA, Moran B, et al.: Partial nodular transformation of the liver with portal hypertension. Am J Med 40: 195, 1966.
34. Iber FL: Obliterative portal venopathy of the liver and "idiopathic portal hypertension." Ann Intern Med 71: 660, 1969.
35. Millette B, Chartran R, Lavoie P, et al.: The extrahepatic uptake of radioactive colloidal gold in cirrhotic patients as an index of liver function and portal hypertension. Am J Dig Dis 18: 719, 1973.
36. Block JB: Angiosarcoma of the liver following vinyl chloride exposure. JAMA 229: 53, 1974.
37. Roth F: Arsen-leber-tumoren: (Hämangioendotheliom). Z Krebsforsch 61: 468, 1957.

Ascites in Patients Undergoing Maintenance Hemodialysis

Report of Six Cases and Physiopathologic Approach

LAZARO GOTLOIB, M.D.
CIRO SERVADIO, M.D.
Afula, Israel

Six patients with chronic uremia in whom ascites developed during maintenance hemodialysis are described. Their clinical and biochemical findings are reviewed and compared with data of 10 hemodialyzed patients without ascites. Liver cirrhosis was the origin of ascites in only one case. Hypoalbuminemia, liver cirrhosis, congestive heart failure, peritonitis, peritoneal tuberculosis and carcinomatosis were uniformly absent in the other patients. Long-term and marked overhydration seems to be at the origin of ascites. Lack of peripheral edema, probably due to ascites compartmentalization, was a constant finding in every noncirrhotic patient with ascites. When long-term overhydration was stopped after successful kidney transplantation or by means of diminished water and salt ingestion, reversal of the syndrome was attained. Nevertheless, ascites because of liver cirrhosis was not influenced by means of kidney transplantation. In three patients with ascites who did not receive a transplant, a significant reduction in water and salt ingestion was reached after intensive psychotherapy which led to reversal of the ascitic syndrome. In one anephric patient ascites did not develop despite water overloading. Survival has not been influenced by the formation of ascites.

Further research is needed to determine the mechanism of sodium transfer across the peritoneal membrane. Influence of humoral factors can be considered, if an active transport mechanism could be demonstrated.

The development and technical improvement of periodic hemodialysis for the maintenance of patients with terminal uremia have created new medical, social and psychologic problems. Ascites has been recognized as an important complication [1–6]. We report our observations on six patients who presented with this complication, and we analyze the physiopathology of ascites which develops in patients treated by means of periodic hemodialysis.

MATERIAL AND METHODS

Twenty-three patients (15 men and eight women) underwent periodic hemodialysis during the observation period of four and a half years (Table I).

The patients' age at the start of hemodialysis ranged between 17 and 68 years (mean 39 years). Patients underwent maintenance hemodialysis from 1.5 to 49.75 months (mean 22.38 months/patient) (Table I). In six of the 23 patients (26 per cent), ascites developed (Table I). Ten other patients without ascites who underwent hemodialysis for more than one year (Cases 7 through 16) were included in the control group (Table I).

From the Renal Unit and Department of Urology, Central Emek Hospital, Afula, Israel. Requests for reprints should be addressed to Dr. L. Gotloib, Renal Unit, Central Emek Hospital, Afula, Israel.
Manuscript accepted January 14, 1976.

TABLE I Patients Subjected to Maintenance Hemodialysis During the Observation Period of Four and a Half Months

Case No.	Age (yr) and Sex	Original Disease	Hemodialyses No.	Hemodialyses Mo.
		Patients With Ascites		
1	40, M	Chronic glomerulonephritis	276	39.9
2	42, M	Suspected chronic glomerulonephritis	110	13.5
3	48, F	Chronic pyelonephritis	144	18
4	26, F	Familial Mediterranean fever	82	10.2
5	34, M	Chronic glomerulonephritis	346	43.1
6	50, M	Suspected chronic glomerulonephritis	207	25.8
		Selected Group of Patients Without Ascites (Control Group) Undergoing Maintenance Hemodialysis for More Than One Year		
7	17, F	Chronic glomerulonephritis; total nephrectomy	291	36.4
8	68, M	Accelerated hypertension	140	17.5
9	47, F	Familial Mediterranean fever	97	12.2
10	42, M	Chronic glomerulonephritis	186	22.8
11	31, F	Recurrent toxemia of pregnancy	273	34.6
12	44, F	Polycystic renal disease	201	25
13	43, M	Suspected chronic glomerulonephritis	121	15.3
14	41, M	Chronic glomerulonephritis	396	49.6
15	17, M	Chronic pyelonephritis	387	48.4
16	52, M	Suspected Balkanic nephropathy	398	49.8
		Patients Without Ascites Undergoing Maintenance Hemodialysis for Less Than One Year		
17	39, F	Polycystic renal disease	6	0.8
18	64, M	Left nephrectomy; right chronic pyelonephritis	55	6.8
19	33, F	Chronic pyelonephritis	30	2.7
20	46, M	Accelerated hypertension	27	3.3
21	26, M	Chronic pyelonephritis	22	2.8
22	24, M	Chronic glomerulonephritis	24	3
23	24, M	Alport syndrome	26	3.2

This study utilizes data obtained through July 31, 1973. One patient (Case 1), a transplant recipient, died of aspergillosis. Ascites and pitting edema were present until his death. Another patient (Case 3), who was free of ascites after undergoing successful renal transplantation, died because of Candida albicans septicemia. Four patients (Cases 2, 4, 5 and 6) are still undergoing hemodialysis. Only one of these (Case 6) is still affected by ascites.

Since July 1, 1973, hemodialysis has been instituted in six new patients. In none of them has ascites developed.

Hemodialysis was carried out using coil kidneys, two or three times weekly, with the standard technic [7]. Peritoneal dialyses were accomplished, using standard intraperitoneal catheters and commercially available dialysis solution, by means of the repeated peritoneal puncture technic. The administration of protein, 1 g/kg body weight, and a high caloric and low sodium diet was proposed. Aluminum hydroxide and supplemental vitamins were administered. The proposed fluid intake was established on the basis of 500 ml of fluid plus an amount equal to the 24 hour urinary output.

Results are presented as means ± standard error of the mean values. Data were analyzed and compared with control values utilizing the Student t test. P values less than 0.05 are considered significant.

RESULTS

Hepatomegaly was present in all the patients with ascites; it appeared between one and seven and a half months (mean 4.57 months) after hemodialysis was started in all but one patient in whom hepatomegaly was detected after 14.2 months of treatment. Variability of liver size was the most conspicuous feature of the hepatomegaly. Liver enlargement was related to overhydration and high central venous pressure. A reduction in liver size was frequently observed after hemodialytic ultrafiltration and weight loss. In the selected group without ascites (Cases 7 through 16), hepatomegaly was a consistent finding in one patient (Case 7) and only transiently observed in two others (Cases 9 and 13). Here again, it was related to water overloading. Liver biopsy disclosed no abnormality in three patients (Cases 3, 4 and 6). In one patient (Case 1), the histologic picture was of frank cardiac cirrhosis. Splenoportography was performed in only one patient (Case 5) with ascites and revealed a normal portal venous system. Peripheral edema was consistently found in one patient with ascites (Case 1). In the patients without ascites one (Case 7) had anasarca, despite undergoing hemodialysis three times weekly, with a 4 to 5 kg weight loss each time. Another patient (Case 8) had sporadic pitting edema of the legs (up to 2+). This sign was absent in the other patients. While undergoing dialysis, symptoms transiently appeared in two patients (Cases 2 and 6) with ascites after its development and in two others without

TABLE II Plasma Protein Values of the Two Main Groups of Patients*

	Serum Albumin (g/100 ml)		Serum Globulins (g/100 ml)	
Case No.	Mean Values	P	Mean Values	P
5 cases†	3.36 ± 0.24	>0.5	2.12 ± 0.53	>0.2
9 cases‡	3.22 ± 0.35		2.65 ± 0.25	
Case 1	3.88 ± 0.46	>0.5	3.18 ± 0.66	>0.5
5 cases‡	3.36 ± 0.24		2.12 ± 0.53	
Case 1	3.88 ± 0.46	>0.5	3.18 ± 0.66	>0.5
9 cases‡	3.22 ± 0.35		2.65 ± 0.25	
Case 7	2.88 ± 0.66	>0.5	2.86 ± 0.51	>0.5
5 cases†	3.36 ± 0.24		2.12 ± 0.53	
Case 7	2.88 ± 0.66	>0.5	2.86 ± 0.51	>0.5
9 cases‡	3.22 ± 0.35		2.65 ± 0.25	

*Values of the cirrhotic patients with ascites (Case 1) and the anephric patients without ascites (Case 7) are compared.
†Five patients with ascites (Cases 2–6).
‡Nine patients without ascites (Cases 8–16).

ascites (Cases 9 and 13). In each instance, rapid reversal was reached by means of a three times weekly hemodialysis schedule.

Serial examinations of serum total proteins (including albumin), globulins and protein electrophoresis failed to demonstrate statistically significant differences between the patients with ascites and those without ascites (Table II).

In the same way, data from two patients (Cases 1 and 7), and from the patients with and without ascites were compared. Differences were not statistically significant (Table III).

No patient presented signs of congestive heart failure. In no case was a prolonged circulation time detected. Hepatojugular reflux was constantly observed in each one of the patients with ascites, but only infrequently in those without ascites.

Four patients with ascites underwent peritoneal dialysis from one to 28 times after the development of ascites following ascites evacuation (Table III). Signs of peritonitis were not observed.

The data presented in Table IV reflect the severity of overhydration and the homogeneity of this pattern in the patients with ascites. We failed to find significant differences between these former patients and the anephric patient (Case 7), but there was a definite difference between the patients with ascites and the patients without ascites.

TABLE III Peritoneal Dialysis in Patients With and Without Ascites

	Peritoneal Dialysis	
Case No.	No. Before Ascites	Total No. Before and After Ascites
Patients With Ascites		
1	0	0
2	0	0
3	3	11
4	1	1
5	2	28
6	0	1
Patients Without Ascites (Control Group)		
7	2	2
8	1	1
9	3	3
10	0	0
11	1	1
12	0	0
13	1	1
14	2	2
15	1	1
16	1	1
$\bar{x}$ (with ascites)	1.0 ± 1.0	5.8 ± 3.2
$\bar{x}$ (without ascites)	1.3 ± 1.1	1.3 ± 1.1
p	<0.05	<0.001

Ascites appeared regularly after hepatomegaly was discovered. In five patients, ascites was detected during the first year of hemodialysis (from 2 to 11.5 months, with a mean of 7.9 months) (Table V). In one patient (Case 1) ascites developed during the 23rd month of maintenance hemodialysis.

Paracentesis had been performed for diagnostic and/or therapeutic purposes, from 1 to 33 times in each of the patients with ascites (Table V). Volume of evacuated ascitic fluid ranged between 0.010 liter and 261 liters. In three patients (Cases 1, 2 and 4) the volume of ascitic fluid was estimated by means of body weight differences ranging from 5 to 7.5 liters. In these cases, the ascitic fluid was not evacuated because of

TABLE IV Variations in Body Weight Because of Overhydration in Five Patients With Ascites (Cases 2–6) and No Cirrhosis and in Nine Patients Without Ascites* (Cases 8–16)

		Body Weight Increase Between Two Hemodialyses		Difference Between Body Weight Before Hemodialysis and Estimated Dry Weight	Percentage of Chronic Water Overloading
Patients	No.	kg	Per Cent	(kg)	
With ascites	5	2.70 ± 0.18	5.25 ± 0.24	5.82 ± 0.15	11.34 ± 2.15
Without ascites	9	1.41 ± 0.23	2.46 ± 0.53	1.71 ± 0.52	3.02 ± 1.10
P		<0.01	<0.01	<0.001	<0.001

*These nine patients did not undergo nephrectomy.

TABLE V Duration of Hemodialysis Before Formation of Ascites and Analysis of Ascitic Fluid After Paracentesis in Six Patients

Case No.	Duration of Hemodialysis Before Formation of Ascites (mo)	Ascites Functions (no.)	Total Evacuated Ascites (liters)	Tuberculosis	Total Proteins (g/100 ml)	Albumin (g/100 ml)	Globulin (g/100 ml)
1	23	1	20 ml	Neg	1.8	1.2	0.6
2	11	1	10 ml	Neg	2.1	1.1	1.0
3	11	3	11.3	Neg	2.3	1.2	1.1
4	7	1	20 ml	Neg	2.4	1.4	1.0
5	1	33	261.2	Neg	2.8	1.5	1.3
6	8	2	21.3	Neg	2.6	1.4	1.2

the absence of serious respiratory distress signs. Moreover, repeated paracentesis carried out in the three other patients (Cases 3, 5 and 6) were promptly followed by abdominal refilling.

The protein content of the ascitic fluid ranged from 1.8 g/100 ml to 2.8 g/100 ml, with a mean of 2.33 g/100 ml (Table V). After each paracentesis, samples of this transudate were examined for malignant cells and tuberculosis, without positive confirmation.

As seen in Table III, peritoneal dialysis (before the start of hemodialysis) was performed more frequently in the patients without ascites.

TREATMENT AND EVOLUTION

Different therapeutic schedules have been tried by several investigators: more frequent hemodialysis, plasma infusion, reinfusion of ascites [2–6], intravenous albumin, hyperalimentation, severe sodium restriction [2–6] and the administration of steroids [1]. None of these procedures has been successful. Wang et al. [5] reported only one successful case in which the ascites resolved completely after strict fluid restriction. Kidney transplantation has been claimed to be the treatment of choice [4,5].

In our patients, a 24-hour weekly hemodialysis schedule with a high ultrafiltration rate for three to seven months was unsuccessful. Hypovolemic shock complicated many of these hemodialyses, and patients continued to gain weight because of excessive fluid ingestion during the intervening period. One patient (Case 1), with proved liver cirrhosis, showed ascites and edema four months after undergoing kidney transplantation, with a creatinine clearance of 52 ml/min. The noncirrhotic patient (Case 3), with normal liver histology, remained ascites-free three and a half months after undergoing a successful cadaver kidney transplantation.

Attempts were made for a more comprehensive approach to the patients' problems. A psychiatrist and a social worker were routinely included in the team to help the patients with ascites. A very high degree of dependence on the team was regularly found. Patients suffered from an obsessive compulsion to drink water. Permanent and unsatisfied thirst and exaggerated fluid ingestion were followed by adamant denials of excessive water drinking. Patients claimed that they could not understand the origin of their body weight gain. One patient suggested "water formation" by his own body. Behavior of patients at home was child-like. Some of them claimed to lock the refrigerator by means of a padlock and some dreamed of enormous intakes of fluids. Patients' hostility against the team was impressive.

Intensive psychotherapy directed to diminish patients' dependence was initiated including a more permissive-like approach by the staff. Doctors' and nurses' observations about excessive weight gain stopped, and the twice weekly 8-hour hemodialysis schedule was reinstated in each case. Easily, three patients (Cases 2, 4 and 5) recovered their self control. Hostility and dependence diminished; two patients (Cases 2 and 5) started to work, and remarkable improvement of their self body image and self esteem was evident. Lower weight gain between hemodialyses was attained and ascites disappeared; nonetheless, patients continued to dream about water (Table VI). In one patient (Case 6), this therapeutic approach was unsuccessful. This is the only case in which ascites is still present and the patient remains markedly dependent on his wife and the team.

In our experience, survival is not influenced by the formation of ascites.

COMMENTS

The incidence of ascites in patients undergoing maintenance hemodialysis for less than one year was 26.1 per cent; in patients undergoing hemodialysis treatment for one year or more, it was 37.5 per cent. A much lower incidence was found in other centers: Wang et al., 4.8 per cent [5]; Singh et al., 5 per cent [4]; and Zerefos et al., 5.6 per cent [6]. Age and sex were similar in our two groups of patients.

TABLE VI Body Weight Variations Because of Overhydration During the Ascitic Period and After Reversal of the Syndrome

Patients	No.	Increase in Body Weight Between Two Hemodialyses (kg)	Increase in Body Weight Between Two Hemodialyses (%)	Difference Between Body Weight Before Hemodialysis and Estimated Dry Weight (kg)	Percentage of Chronic Water Loading
With ascites*	3	2.74 ± 0.43	5.35 ± 1.03	6.36 ± 1.26	11.90 ± 2.64
Without ascites*	3	1.24 ± 0.12	2.40 ± 0.26	1.40 ± 0.14	2.70 ± 0.23
P		<0.05	<0.01	<0.05	<0.05

*Cases 2, 4 and 5.

One of the most interesting clinical features of this syndrome is the volume of the ascites which commonly was out of proportion to that of the edema in the legs. This apparent disparity has also been noted by Wang et al. [5].

Shear and Swartz and associates [8] demonstrated that in patients without ascites, saline solution is absorbed from the peritoneal cavity at a rate ranging between 612.9 and 894.2 ml/24 hours. In cirrhosis with ascites and edema, rates of fluid mobilization from these two compartments are not related to each other. There is a ceiling for ascites mobilization, which in cirrhotic patients reaches 930 ml/24 hours, whereas the elimination rate of peripheral edema can be four or five times greater [9]; this, perhaps, could explain the lack of detectable edema in the patients with uremia and ascites. The rate of ascites mobilization is self-limited, and the interstitial edema can easily be eliminated by means of ultrafiltration. Moreover, cirrhotic patients with ascites and without edema are prone to plasma volume depletion when undergoing diuretic treatment [9]. In our patients with ascites, high ultrafiltration frequently induced hypovolemic shock.

Symptoms of heart failure were uniformly absent. Circulation time was normal in the patients with ascites. Pericardial diseases in the form of constrictive pericarditis or effusion have been excluded. Hepatomegaly was a constant finding in all the noncirrhotic patients without ascites. In addition, evidence of portal hypertension was absent.

Only one patient had histologically confirmed liver cirrhosis. This was also the only patient in whom ascites developed after the first year of maintenance hemodialysis, and the only one with constant peripheral edema.

Blood protein levels were within the low limit of normal values in the two groups of patients. Nevertheless, we failed to find statistically significant differences between the patients with ascites and the patients without ascites in serum total protein, albumin and globulin concentrations. In the published reports of patients with ascites undergoing long-term hemodialysis, hypoproteinemia was the rule [3–6]. Our experience suggests that factors other than hypoproteinemia must be considered in order to explain ascites formation.

The possibility of altered peritoneal permeability because of repeated peritoneal dialysis has been raised [5,6]. Peritoneal dialysis was performed in six of the seven patients with ascites undergoing dialysis described by Zerefos [6]. In the eight cases reported by Singh [4], the patients were receiving peritoneal dialysis from two to 20 months before they received hemodialysis. In our experience, peritoneal dialysis before hemodialysis was performed more frequently in patients without ascites. This indicates that repeated peritoneal dialysis is not etiologically related to the development of ascites.

Overhydration has been the constant feature in reported cases [2–6]. In our study, analysis of body weight variations demonstrates striking differences between the two groups of patients. An exaggerated increase in body weight in the period between dialyses, because of overhydration, not followed by a proportional weight loss by means of ultrafiltration, leads the noncirrhotic patients with ascites to a state of chronic water overloading up to 11.3 per cent of their body weight. The increase in body weight was partially attributed to ascites.

Percentage of estimated dry body weight increase between hemodialyses indicates the extent of overhydration. Nevertheless, in one chronically overhydrated anephric patient (Case 7) the ascitic syndrome did not develop.

Plasma from saline solution-loaded normal dogs and uremic patients has an inhibitory effect on para-aminohippurate (PAH) uptake by slices of renal cortex [10]. One fraction, F4, was isolated and identified as the determinant of this effect. This fraction inhibits the transepithelial transport of sodium by the isolated frog skin [11,12]. This factor, inhibiting the active transport of sodium in vivo, in systems other than the kidney, raises the possibility of its influence on the dynamics of peritoneal sodium transfer. The mechanism of transperitoneal transfer of sodium has not been defined, but there is evidence indicating that the peritoneal membrane is not an inert, unresponsive structure [13–15]. Mahony et al. [3] suggest a peritoneal membrane transport abnormality in patients with uremia and ascites. In this way, influence of humoral factors should be considered if active sodium transport mechanism across the peritoneal membrane is demonstrated.

ACKNOWLEDGMENT

We wish to thank Dr. Victor Magal and Mrs. Shula Shai for psychiatric support to our patients, and Dr. H. Basan who performed the liver biopsies.

We greatly acknowledge our nursing staff for their comprehensive and qualified care of these patients.

REFERENCES

1. Gutch CF, Mahony JF, Pinggera WJ, Holmes JH, Kolff WJ: Ascites in hemodialysis patients (abstracts). Am Soc Nephrol 5: 30, 1970.
2. Mahony JF, Gutch CF, Holmes JH: Intractable ascites in chronic dialysis patients (abstracts). Am Soc Nephrol 4: 51, 1970.
3. Mahony J, Pinggera W, Holmes J, Klein M, Gutch C, Kolff W: Ascites during maintenance hemodialysis (abstracts). Fifth International Congress on Nephrology, Mexico, 1972, p 64.
4. Singh S, Mitra S, Berman LB: Ascites in patients on maintenance hemodialysis. Nephron 12: 144, 1974.
5. Wang F, Pillay CKG, Armbruster KFW, Rosenberg JC: Ascites in patients treated with maintenance hemodialysis. Nephron 12: 105, 1974.
6. Zerefos N, Duffy B, Chrysant S, Kastagir B, Tauber J, Lavender AR: Dialysis ascites. A new syndrom? Abstracts of the Fifth International Congress on Nephrology, Mexico, 1972, p 34.
7. Hampers CL, Schupack E, Lowrie EG, Lazarus JM: Long-Term Hemodialysis, 2nd ed, New York, Grune & Stratton, 1973.
8. Shear L, Swartz Ch, Shinaberger JA, Barry KG: Kinetics of peritoneal fluid absorption in adult man. N Engl J Med 272: 123, 1965.
9. Shear L, Ching S, Gabuzda GJ: Compartmentalization of ascites and edema in patients with hepatic cirrhosis. N Engl J Med 282: 1391, 1970.
10. Klahr S, Bourgoigne JJ, Lindsey Miller C, Lubowitz M, Bricker NS: Studies on search of a natriuretic hormone in uremic patients. Proceedings of the Fourth International Congress on Nephrology, Stockholm, 1969, vol 2, Basel, Karger, 1970, p 88.
11. Bourgoigne JJ, Klahr S, Bricker N: Inhibition of transepithelial sodium transport in the frog skin by a low molecular weight fraction of uremic serum. J Clin Invest 50: 303, 1971.
12. Bourgoigne JJ, Kwang KH, Espinel C, Klahr S, Bricker N: A natriuretic factor in the serum of patients with chronic uremia. J Clin Invest 51: 1514, 1972.
13. Hare HG, Valtin M, Gosselin RE: Effect of drugs on peritoneal dialysis in the dog. J Pharmacol Exper Therap 145: 122, 1964.
14. Shear L, Barry KG: Effect of pitressin on the movement of water and solute across the peritoneum. Clin Res 12: 203, 1964.
15. Shear L, Harvey JD, Barry KG: Peritoneal sodium transport. Enhancement by pharmacologic and physical agents. J Lab Clin Med 67: 181, 1966.

Nephrotic Syndrome in Hodgkin's Disease

Evidence for Pathogenesis Alternative to Immune Complex Deposition

A. VISHNU MOORTHY, M.D.*
STEPHEN W. ZIMMERMAN, M.D.
PETER M. BURKHOLDER, M.D.
Madison, Wisconsin

The nephrotic syndrome has been reported to occur in patients with Hodgkin's disease even in the absence of amyloidosis, tumor infiltration or renal vein thrombosis. Three patients are presented with Hodgkin's disease and the nephrotic syndrome whose renal biopsy specimens studied with light, immunofluorescence and electron microscopy were compatible with "lipoid nephrosis" (minimal change disease). A review of the literature reveals 35 patients with Hodgkin's disease and the nephrotic syndrome. Renal tissue was available for examination in only 27 patients. The majority of patients apparently had glomerular alterations consistent with lipoid nephrosis. The nephrotic syndrome in most of these patients remitted with a variety of methods of therapy (including excision, irradiation, prednisone and cyclophosphamide) and tended to relapse with a recurrence of Hodgkin's disease. In three-fourths of the patients with Hodgkin's disease and the nephrotic syndrome, the Hodgkin's disease was of a mixed cellularity type. The etiology of lipoid nephrosis, although unclear, may be a consequence of altered lymphocyte function. Hodgkin's disease is a malignancy involving T lymphocytes, and the nephrotic syndrome occurring in the course of Hodgkin's disease may be a result of an adverse effect on glomeruli by products of tumor lymphocytes rather than of glomerular deposition of immune complexes.

Renal complications in the course of Hodgkin's disease due to a variety of mechanisms such as ureteral obstruction, tumor infiltration of the kidneys, amyloidosis and renal vein thrombosis have been reported. Since 1939 the occurrence of the nephrotic syndrome in patients with Hodgkin's disease in the absence of any of the symptoms listed has been reported on many occasions [1–23]. In the majority of these patients, renal tissue has usually revealed no specific abnormalities. Findings similar to those seen in lipoid nephrosis have been noted, although an occasional patient has shown more extensive glomerular changes. This is in contrast to the nephrotic syndrome associated with carcinoma of the lung and colon in which renal biopsy specimens have revealed membranous glomerulonephropathy [24], and tumor antigen has been eluted from immune complexes deposited along glomerular capillary walls [25]. We describe here three patients with the nephrotic syndrome and Hodgkin's disease in whom the findings on renal biopsy were compatible with lipoid nephrosis, and review the data on 32 other patients described in the literature.

From the Nephrology Program, Departments of Medicine and Pathology, University of Wisconsin Center for Health Sciences, Madison, Wisconsin. This study was supported in part by Research Grant AM 15159 from the National Institutes of Health, Bethesda, Maryland. Requests for reprints should be addressed to Dr. A. Vishnu Moorthy, Nephrology Section, Department of Medicine, University Hospitals, 1300 University Avenue, Madison, Wisconsin 53706. Manuscript accepted January 23, 1976.

* Recipient of a joint fellowship from the National Kidney Foundation and the Kidney Foundation of Wisconsin.

MATERIAL AND METHODS

Biochemical and hematologic analyses were made in the clinical laboratories. Surgically removed lymph nodes were examined by hematoxylin and eosin stained sections. Renal tissue obtained by percutaneous needle biopsy was processed for light microscopy by fixation in formalin. Two micron paraffin sections were stained with hematoxylin and eosin, periodic acid-Schiff and periodic acid silver methenamine Masson stain as described elsewhere [26]. A portion of renal tissue for immunofluorescence study was frozen in aqueous gelatin and 4 μ sections were stained with fluorescein-conjugated immunoglobulin fractions of antiserum to human immunoglobulins G (IgG), M (IgM), A (IgA), third component of complement (C3) and fibrinogen. A third portion of each renal biopsy specimen was processed for electron microscopy and examined as previously described [26]. Serum was assayed for macrophage migration inhibition activity against guinea pig peritoneal macrophages harvested four days after giving the guinea pigs an intraperitoneal injection of light mineral oil. A 50 per cent dilution of the patient's serum with tissue culture medium (medium 199) was used in Sykes-Moore chambers containing capillary tubes filled with guinea pig macrophages, and the areas of migration after 24 hours' incubation at 37°C in 5 per cent carbon dioxide were drawn and measured with a planimeter as described elsewhere [27]. The experiment was carried out in triplicate, using normal human serum as control. Migration inhibition was considered to be present when the area of migration decreased to less than 60 per cent of normal control migration.

CASE REPORTS

Case 1. In a 14 year old Caucasian boy, poison ivy dermatitis developed on his legs in October 1973 and responded completely to local and systemic steroid therapy. Two weeks later he was hospitalized with ankle edema and ascites. On admission to the hospital he had discrete lower cervical lymphadenopathy; three lymph nodes measured about 5 cm by 2 cm. No other lymph nodes were enlarged, and neither the spleen nor liver was palpable. His blood pressure was 100/70 mm Hg. Roentgenographic examination of the chest was within normal limits. Urinalysis revealed 4+ protein with a rare red blood cell and an occasional hyaline cast in the sediment. The daily urinary protein excretion was 5.6 g. Serum albumin was 3.0 g/dl, blood urea nitrogen 20 mg/dl and cholesterol 300 mg/dl. Antinuclear antibodies were negative and serum C3 was 108 mg/dl (normal 80 to 150 mg/dl).

A renal biopsy was performed, and therapy with prednisone, 40 mg/day, was initiated. As the cervical lymphadenopathy became more prominent, a lymph node was obtained surgically and interpreted as showing Hodgkin's disease of the mixed cellularity type. The disease was considered to be at stage I-B after abdominal lymphangiography and hepatic and splenic scan. The patient was then treated with cervical irradiation, to a total dose of 3,000 rads in three weeks; therapy was continued with prednisone, 40 mg/day, to which was added cyclophosphamide, at a dose of 1.5 mg/kg and vincristine, 1 mg daily. Proteinuria decreased and disappeared in six weeks. He has been followed for a year and has been given monthly injections of 5 mg vinblastine sulfate; during this time his urine has remained protein free.

Case 2. A 26 year old, mentally handicapped white woman presented in January 1966 with cervical lymphadenopathy. A lymph node biopsy specimen showed Hodgkin's disease of mixed cellularity type. It was staged I-A after lymphangiography and hepatic and splenic scans, and the patient was treated with upper mantle irradiation over three weeks for a total dose of 4,000 rads. Over the next five years she had three further courses of irradiation (to a total dose of 6,000 rads) for right submandibular, left cervical and iliac recurrences of Hodgkin's disease. The kidneys were shielded during irradiation. Urinalysis was negative for protein during this period.

In September 1972 she presented with pedal edema. There was no lymphadenopathy. Blood pressure was 110/70 mm Hg. Urinalysis revealed 3+ protein with Maltese crosses, hyaline casts and a few white blood cells in the sediment. The 24-hour urine protein excretion was 5 g. Urine protein was highly selective being 90 per cent albumin on electrophoresis. Serum albumin was 2.0 g/dl. The creatinine clearance was 110 ml/min. Abdominal lymphangiogram, hepatic and splenic scans, bone marrow biopsy, renal venogram and rectal biopsy for amyloid disclosed no abnormalities. Serum antinuclear antibodies were negative and serum C3 was 110 mg/dl. A renal biopsy was performed.

She was treated with vinblastine, 7 mg intravenously, twice monthly with disappearance of proteinuria in three months. Vinblastine therapy has been continued, 10 mg given intravenously monthly, and she has remained protein free.

Case 3. A 57 year old Caucasian man, a retired construction worker, presented to his local physician in May 1974 with cervical lymph node swelling of three weeks' duration. A lymph node biopsy specimen showed Hodgkin's disease of mixed cellularity type. He was transferred to the VA Hospital in Madison, Wisconsin, as he had increasing edema and a weight gain of 27 pounds over the next three weeks.

His past medical history included thrombophlebitis in the legs with recurrent pulmonary emboli necessitating inferior venacaval ligation in October 1967. He had been receiving Coumadin® for 14 months prior to this. He had a history of treated pulmonary tuberculosis 14 years earlier and an uncomplicated myocardial infarction three years earlier.

Physical examination on admission revealed a middle-aged man with gross edema of the legs, sacrum and forearms. He had multiple enlarged cervical lymph nodes on both sides. There was no hepatosplenomegaly. Blood pressure was 150/90 mm Hg. Urinalysis revealed 4+ protein with occasional red blood cells in the sediment. The 24-hour urinary protein excretion was 7.1 g. The creatinine clearance was 91 ml/min. Serum albumin was 1.8 g/dl and cholesterol 486 mg/dl. Renal venogram, abdominal lymphangiogram, hepatic and splenic scans disclosed no abnormalities. The serum was negative for antinuclear antibodies and serum C3 was 88 mg/dl. A renal biopsy was performed. The patient was treated

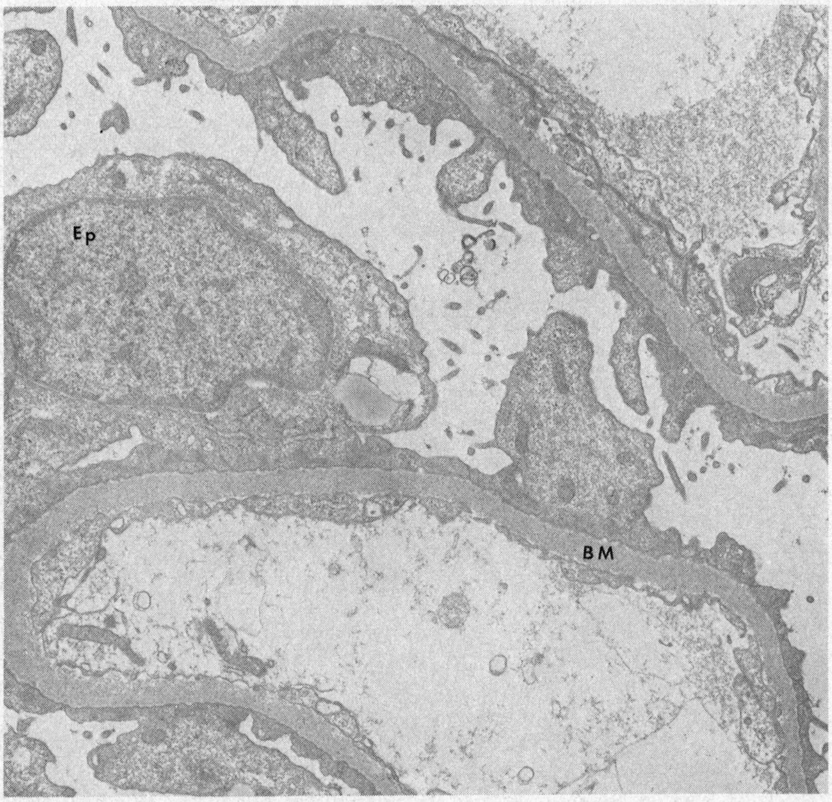

Figure 1. *Electron micrograph of a glomerulus showing normal looking basement membrane with extensive effacement of epithelial cell foot processes. Original magnification × 4,700, reduced by 45 per cent.*

with upper mantle irradiation for a total of 4,000 rads over six weeks and prednisone, 60 mg/day. The proteinuria decreased to 2.0 g/day in two weeks and disappeared in eight weeks. He has remained protein-free during follow-up for a year, without therapy.

RESULTS

Case 1. The renal biopsy specimen contained 7 glomeruli, all of which were essentially normal on light microscopy apart from showing a minimal increase in mesangial matrix material. The cells of the proximal and distal tubules were rich in lipid, and occasional tubules were filled with proteinaceous material. The blood vessels appeared normal. Immunofluorescence microscopy for immunoglobulins G, M and A, C3 and fibrin were negative. Four glomeruli were studied by electron microscopy. In all these glomeruli the basement membrane was of normal thickness without any electron-dense deposits, but there was widespread and complete effacement of the foot processes of epithelial cells (Figure 1).

Case 2. The renal biopsy specimen contained 11 glomeruli. Most glomeruli were normal on light microscopy, although in an occasional glomerulus minimal endocapillary hypercellularity was noted. Moderate hyalinization was seen in afferent arterioles. Stains for amyloid were negative. Immunofluorescence microscopy revealed IgM, C3 and fibrinogen in limited segmental streaks in a few glomeruli, but electron microscopic study of 5 glomeruli revealed uniformly thin, normal-appearing glomerular capillary basement membranes without electron-dense deposits. Epithelial cell foot processes were effaced in all the glomeruli (Figure 2).

Case 3. The renal biopsy specimen contained 8 glomeruli, one of which was sclerosed. The other glomeruli were essentially normal without any increase in cellularity and with occasional increase in mesangial matrix. Immunofluorescence microscopy was negative for immunoglobulins G, M and A, C3 and fibrin. Electron microscopic study of 3 glomeruli revealed normal basement membranes with no dense deposits. Epithelial foot processes were effaced in all glomeruli. The patient's serum showed the presence of macrophage migration inhibition activity as tested on guinea pig peritoneal macrophages. The area of macrophage migration was only 48 per cent of a normal human serum control.

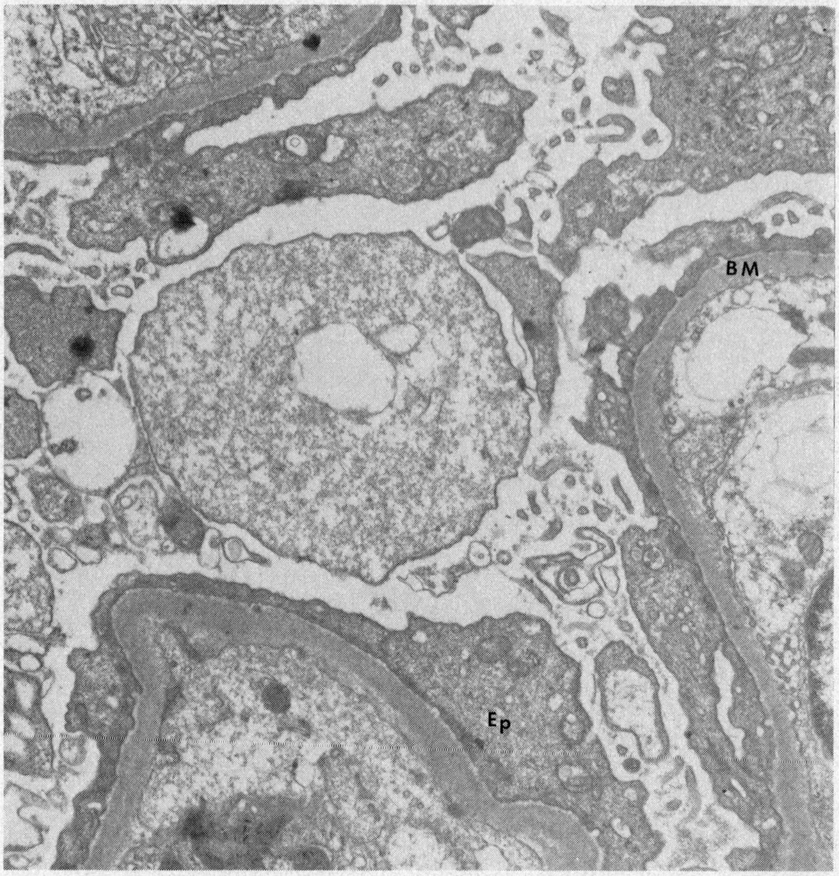

Figure 2. *Electron micrograph of a glomerulus with complete effacement of epithelial cell foot processes. The basement membrane is free of deposits. Original magnification × 6,600, reduced by 40 per cent. BM = basement membrane. EP = epithelial cells.*

COMMENTS

The relationship of the nephrotic syndrome to Hodgkin's disease is not clearly understood. Nephrotic syndrome occurring in the course of bronchogenic carcinoma, gastric carcinoma or carcinoma of the colon has been associated with membranous glomerulonephropathy [24]. However, the nephrotic syndrome associated with Hodgkin's disease has seldom been observed to be secondary to membranous glomerulonephropathy.

A review of the data on 35 patients with Hodgkin's disease and nephrotic syndrome described in the literature is presented in Table I. Eight patients did not undergo renal biopsy; of the remaining 27, only light microscopic findings in the renal biopsy specimen are available in 13 patients. Eleven of these biopsy specimens were interpreted as showing lipoid nephrosis. In Case 19, the condition was said to be "proliferative glomerulonephritis" and in Case 20, there was minimal cellular proliferation and minimal thickening of basement membranes.

In only 14 patients with Hodgkin's disease and the nephrotic syndrome was the renal biopsy specimen examined by light, electron and/or immunofluorescence microscopy. In 12 of these patients the initial renal alterations could be classified as lipoid nephrosis. In one (Case 29) the first renal biopsy specimen was initially read as membranous glomerulonephropathy on light microscopic study only, but upon subsequent review was revised to lipoid nephrosis. A repeat renal biopsy specimen showed no abnormalities by light and immunofluorescence microscopy, and electron microscopy showed, in addition to extensive loss of epithelial foot processes, only one subepithelial deposit.

In the three patients we describe here, renal biopsy specimens were interpreted as lipoid nephrosis. Immunofluorescence was negative for glomerular localization of immunoglobulins and complement except in one patient (Case 2) in whom faint, isolated streaks of IgM, C3 and fibrinogen were noted. We have noted similar streaks of IgM in the glomeruli in 17 of 31 other

TABLE I Nephrotic Syndrome in Patients with Hodgkin's Disease

Case No.	Reference	Year	Type of Hodgkin's Disease	Renal Pathology	Clinical Course
1	[1]	1939	Unknown	No renal biopsy	Remission with radiotherapy
2	[2]	1948	Unknown	No renal biopsy	Remission with radiotherapy
3	[3]	1953	Unknown	No renal biopsy	Resistant to radiotherapy
4	[4]	1957	Unknown	No renal biopsy	Remission with cervical node excision
5	[5]	1967	Unknown	LM: lipoid nephrosis	Remission with nitrogen mustard and radiotherapy
6	[6]	1967	Unknown	No renal biopsy	Remission with nitrogen mustard
7	[7]	1967	Unknown	No renal biopsy	Remission with prednisone
8	[8]	1967	Unknown	LM: lipoid nephrosis	Remission with prednisone
9	[9]	1968	Unknown	LM: lipoid nephrosis	Remission with radiotherapy
10	[10]	1968	Unknown	LM: lipoid nephrosis	Remission with radiotherapy
11	[10]	1968	Unknown	LM: lipoid nephrosis	Remission with radiotherapy
12	[11]	1969	Lymphocyte depletion	LM: membranous nephropathy EM: subepithelial deposits	No information
13	[12]	1969	Unknown	LM: lipoid nephrosis	Remission with prednisone
14	[13]	1970	Granuloma	LM, EM: lipoid nephrosis	Remission with combination chemotherapy
15	[14]	1971	Mixed cellularity	LM: lipoid nephrosis	Remission with combination chemotherapy and radiotherapy
16	[14]	1971	Mixed cellularity	LM: lipoid nephrosis	Remission with chemotherapy
17	[14]	1971	Nodular sclerosis	LM: lipoid nephrosis	Remission with chemotherapy and radiotherapy
18	[14]	1971	Lymphocyte depletion	No renal biopsy	Remission with chemotherapy
19	[15]	1971	Unknown	LM: proliferative glomerulonephritis	Remission with cyclophosphamide
20	[15]	1971	Unknown	LM: Minimal proliferation and basement membrane thickening	Remission with chemotherapy and radiotherapy
21	[16]	1972	Mixed cellularity	Biopsy 1. LM: proliferative with crescents; EM: subepithelial deposits. Biopsy 2. LM: membranous; EM: subepithelial deposits; Immuno.-positive for IgG, β_1C	Remission after two courses of radiotherapy
22	[17]	1972	Granulomatous thymoma	LM, EM: lipoid nephrosis	Remission with surgery
23	[17]	1972	Mixed cellularity	LM: lipoid nephrosis	Remission with radiotherapy
24	[17]	1972	Mixed cellularity	LM, EM: Immuno.: lipoid nephrosis	Resistant to radiotherapy
25	[18]	1972	Mixed cellularity	LM, EM: lipoid nephrosis	Remission with radiotherapy and chemotherapy
26	[18]	1972	Mixed cellularity	LM, EM: lipoid nephrosis	Resistant to prednisone; remission with radiotherapy
27	[19]	1973	Mixed cellularity	LM: focal proliferative; Immuno.: IgG and IgA-fine granular pattern; EM: subepithelial electron-dense deposits and electron-lucent areas	Remission with combination chemotherapy
28	[20]	1973	Mixed cellularity	Biopsy 1. LM, Immuno., EM: lipoid nephrosis. Biopsy 2. mesangial proliferation; Immuno.: IgG, IgM-positive	Remission with radiotherapy Remission with cyclophosphamide
29	[21]	1973	Nodular sclerosis	Biopsy 1. LM: lipoid nephrosis. Biopsy 2. LM, Immuno.: lipoid nephrosis; EM: one subepithelial deposit in 4 glomeruli	Spontaneous remission
30	[22]	1971	Unknown	LM: lipoid nephrosis	Initial response to prednisone
31	[22]	1971	Unknown	No biopsy	Remission with prednisone
32	[23]	1974	Unknown	LM: lipoid nephrosis; Immuno.: granular IgG, β_1C deposits; EM: subendothelial granular and radiolucent material	No information
33	Present report	1975	Mixed cellularity	LM, EM, Immuno.: lipoid nephrosis	Remission with chemotherapy and radiotherapy
34	Present report	1975	Mixed cellularity	LM, EM, Immuno.: lipoid nephrosis	Remission with chemotherapy
35	Present report	1975	Mixed cellularity	LM, EM, Immuno.: lipoid nephrosis	Remission with radiotherapy and prednisone

NOTE: LM = light microscopy; EM = electron microscopy; Immuno. = immunofluorescence microscopy.

TABLE II Course of Nephrotic Syndrome in 35 Patients with Hodgkin's Disease*

Therapy	No. of Cases	Remission in Nephrotic Syndrome
Surgical excision	2	Cases 4, 22
Radiotherapy only	9	Cases 1, 2, 9, 10, 11, 21, 23 (resistant in Cases 3 and 24)
Prednisone only	5	Cases 7, 8, 13, 30, 31
Chemotherapy only	7	Cases 6, 14, 16, 18, 19, 27, 34
Combination: radiotherapy, prednisone and chemotherapy	9	Cases 5, 15, 17, 20, 25, 26, 28, 33, 35
Spontaneous remission	1	Case 29

*Details unclear in Cases 12 and 32.

patients with lipoid nephrosis. Electron microscopic study of glomeruli did not reveal any electron-dense deposits. Only three patients have been described in the literature with initial renal biopsy changes other than minimal changes (Cases 12, 21 and 27). Review of reported renal alterations associated with the nephrotic syndrome seen in Hodgkin's disease reveals that the lesion noted most frequently was lipoid nephrosis. Membranous glomerulopathy in this situation seemingly occurs rarely.

Response of the nephrotic syndrome to therapy of the Hodgkin's lymphoma is reported in Tables I and II. The course of the nephrotic syndrome has usually paralleled the course of Hodgkin's disease, but occasionally the nephrotic syndrome has persisted in the absence of detectable activity of Hodgkin's disease (Cases 24 and 34). Recurrence of Hodgkin's disease seems to cause a relapse of the nephrotic syndrome, and this can happen repeatedly [14]. Disappearance of proteinuria in response to therapy has been rapid. Urine protein selectivity when studied (Cases 22 and 34) has been highly selective.

The etiology of idiopathic minimal change nephrotic syndrome itself is unclear. The response of the nephrotic syndrome to therapy with agents like prednisone and cyclophosphamide, the remission induced during measles-virus infection and the increased incidence of pneumococcal peritonitis in patients with the nephrotic syndrome all suggest an abnormality in T lymphocytes that might result in production of a "lymphokine" injurious to glomeruli [28]. Hodgkin's disease is considered a malignant tumor involving T lymphocytes. Cell-mediated immunity is often suppressed in Hodgkin's disease [29], possibly as a consequence in part of recently recognized hyperactivity of suppressor T lymphocytes [30]. It is possible that an occasional clone of T lymphocytes might produce a lymphokine injurious to glomerular basement membrane or toxic to glomerular epithelial cells. Additional evidence for a circulating lymphokine is provided by the finding of inhibition of migration of guinea pig peritoneal macrophages by serum from patients with Hodgkin's disease [31].

A review of the histologic type of Hodgkin's disease in cases in which information was available showed it to be of mixed cellularity type in 11, of nodular sclerosis in two and of the lymphocyte depletion variety in two; none was of the lymphocyte dominant type. The usual incidence of mixed cellularity type in Hodgkin's disease is about 35 per cent [29], but in 75 per cent of the patients with the nephrotic syndrome, it is of this histologic type. Whether patients with this type of Hodgkin's disease are immunologically unusual or distinctive is unknown. A possible difference is suggested in demonstrating that lymphocytes from patients with Hodgkin's disease of the mixed cellularity and lymphocyte depletion types studied in mixed lymphocyte cultures stimulated subnormal responses with normal allogeneic lymphocytes more often than lymphocytes from patients with lymphocyte predominant or nodular sclerotic tumors [30].

Very few immunologic evaluations of patients with the nephrotic syndrome and Hodgkin's disease have been performed. Sherman et al. [18] have shown diminished responsiveness of lymphocytes to phytohemagglutinin when incubated in patients' serum. The serum of one of our patients had macrophage migration inhibitor activity. Further work along these lines is needed. It is likely that the nephrotic syndrome of Hodgkin's disease is usually a variety of minimal glomerular change nephrotic syndrome related more to abnormalities of lymphocyte function, although in infrequent instances it could be related to immune complex deposition.

ACKNOWLEDGMENT

We wish to thank Ms. Kay Kirk and Mr. Kenneth Groehler for their able technical assistance. We also wish to thank Dr. Gregory Beirne of the Veterans Administration Hospital, Madison, Wisconsin, for allowing us to include one of his patients in this report.

ADDENDUM

Since preparation of this manuscript, five more cases of Hodgkin's disease have come to our attention. Larson et al. [32], Perlin et al. [33] and Yum et al. [34] each described a patient with Hodgkin's disease and lipoid nephrosis. Yum et al. [34] also described a second patient with Hodgkin's disease and nephrotic syndrome with membranous glomerulonephropathy. Row et al. [35] described one patient with Hodgkin's disease and membranous glomerulonephropathy.

REFERENCES

1. Cornig HJ: Une forme nouvelle de la maladie de Hodgkin. Lymphogranulomatose maligne à type de nephrose lipoidique. Thèse 547. Faculte de Medecine de Paris, 1939.
2. Rohmer P, Sacrez R: Un cas de nephrose lipoidique au cours d'une maladie de Hodgkin. Strasbourg Med 108: 45, 1948.
3. Solsona-Conillera J: Linfogranulomatosis maligna. Forma monoganglionary nefrosica. Med Clin (Barcelona) 20: 37, 1953.
4. Tapie J, Laporte J, Richalens J: Syndrome nephrotique au cours de la maladie de Hodgkin-Sternberg. Presse Med 65: 287, 1957.
5. Miller DG: The association of immune disease and málignant lymphoma. Ann Intern Med 66: 507, 1967.
6. Mehta SR, Kumar KK, Gupta ML: Hodgkin's disease with nephrotic syndrome and erythema multiforme. J Indian Med Assoc 48: 279, 1967.
7. Paslawska-Udolf E: Przypadek nerczycy lipoidowej w przebiegu ziarnicy zlosliwej u dziecka 2-letniego. Pediatr Pol 42: 591, 1967.
8. Kiy Y: Sindrome nefrotica associada a doenca de Hodgkin. Rev Hosp Clin Fac Med Sao Paulo 22: 186, 1967.
9. Brodovsky HS, Samuels ML, Migliore PJ, et al.: Chronic lymphocytic leukemia, Hodgkin's disease and the nephrotic syndrome. Arch Intern Med 121: 71, 1968.
10. Hamburger J, Richet G, Crosnier J, et al.: Nephrology, vol 1, Philadelphia, W. B. Saunders Co., 1968, p 226.
11. Hardin JG Jr, Coker AS, Blanton JH: Medicine grand rounds. South Med J 62: 1111, 1969.
12. Kiely JM, Wagoner RD, Holley KE: Renal complications of lymphoma. Ann Intern Med 71: 1159, 1969.
13. Ghosh (Banerji) L, Muehrcke R: The nephrotic syndrome: a prodrome to lymphoma. Ann Intern Med 72: 379, 1970.
14. Plager J, Stutzman L: Acute nephrotic syndrome as a manifestation of active Hodgkin's disease. Am J Med 50: 56, 1971.
15. Lowry WS, Munzenrider JE, Lynch GA: Nephrotic syndrome in Hodgkin's disease. Lancet 1: 1127, 1971.
16. Froom DW, Franklin WA, Hano JE, et al.: Immune deposits in Hodgkin's disease with nephrotic syndrome. Arch Pathol 94: 547, 1972.
17. Hansen HE, Skov PE, Askjaer SA, et al.: Hodgkin's disease associated with nephrotic syndrome without kidney lesion. Acta Med Scand 191: 307, 1972.
18. Sherman RL, Susin M, Weksler ME, et al.: Lipoid nephrosis in Hodgkin's disease. Am J Med 52: 699, 1972.
19. Lokich JJ, Galvenek EG, Moloney WC: Nephrosis of Hodgkin's disease. Arch Intern Med 132: 597, 1973.
20. Hyman LR, Burkholder PM, Joo PA, et al.: Malignant lymphoma and nephrotic syndrome. J Pediatr 82: 207, 1973.
21. Case Records of the Massachusetts General Hospital. Case 49, 1973. N Engl J Med 289: 1241, 1973.
22. Jackson RH, Oo M: Nephrotic syndrome with Hodgkin's disease. Lancet 2: 821, 1971.
23. Sharma HM, Hurtubise PE, Stevenson TD: The nephrotic syndrome in Hodgkin's disease. Lab Invest 30: 404, 1974.
24. Loughridge LW, Lewis MG: Nephrotic syndrome in malignant disease of non-renal origin. Lancet 1: 256, 1971.
25. Lewis MG, Loughridge LW, Phillips TM: Immunological studies in nephrotic syndrome associated with extrarenal malignant disease. Lancet 2: 134, 1971.
26. Burkholder PM: Atlas of Human Glomerular Pathology. Hagerstown, Md., Hoeber Medical Division, Harper & Row, 1974.
27. David JR, David R: In Vitro Methods in Cell Mediated Immunity. (Bloom BR, Glade PR, eds), New York, Academic Press, 1971, p 249.
28. Shalhoub RJ: Pathogenesis of lipoid nephrosis: a disorder of T-cell function. Lancet 2: 556, 1974.
29. O'Conor GT, Correa P, Christine B, et al.: International Symposium on Hodgkin's Disease, NCI Monographs, No. 36, 1973, p 7.
30. Twomey JJ, Laughter AH, Farrow S, et al.: Hodgkin's disease: an immuno-depleting and immunosuppressive disorder. J Clin Invest 56: 467, 1975.
31. Cohen S: Serum migration—inhibitory activity in patients with lymphoproliferative diseases. N Engl J Med 290: 882, 1974.
32. Larson LS, Fritz RD: Nephrotic syndrome in association with Hodgkin's disease. Wis Med J 75: S14, 1976.
33. Perlin E, Powers JM, Dickson LG, et al.: The nephrotic syndrome in Hodgkin's disease. Med Ann DC 41: 354, 1972.
34. Yum MN, Edwards JL, Kleit S: Glomerular lesions in Hodgkin's disease. Arch Pathol 99: 645, 1975.
35. Row PG, Cameron JG, Turner DR, et al.: Membranous nephropathy: long-term follow-up and association with neoplasia. Q J Med 174; 207, 1975.

Effects of Alternating Phosphorus and Calcium Infusions on Osteoporosis

MORDECAI M. POPOVTZER, M.D.*
MELVYN STJERNHOLM, M.D.
WILLIAM E. HUFFER, M.D.
Denver, Colorado

The osteoblastic effect of inorganic phosphorus and the inhibitory action of calcium on parathyroid hormone secretion formed the basis for a therapeutic trial in which both elements were given intravenously in an alternating sequence for one year to five patients with severe osteoporosis. During treatment, calcium and phosphorus balances were positive, and serum phosphorus concentrations decreased. Iliac crest bone biopsy specimens obtained one year after beginning treatment demonstrated an increase in the thickness of cortical bone. All patients experienced lasting relief of bone pain, and the rate of spontaneous fractures decreased from at least one fracture per year to none following the beginning of treatment. These findings suggest that long-term treatment with alternating phosphorus and calcium infusions may result in lasting relief of symptomatic osteoporosis. It is proposed that the observed improvement reflects an increase in bone mass resulting from enhanced bone formation.

The decrease in bone mass in relation to bone volume in osteoporosis reflects an imbalance between bone formation and resorption in which the latter prevails [1–3]. In most previous reports, treatment of osteoporosis was based on attempts to suppress bone resorption [4–9]. Both hormonal and nonhormonal agents employed in the treatment of osteoporosis demonstrated only a limited therapeutic effect [4–8]. These unsatisfactory results intensified the search for factors that primarily promote new bone formation and may lead to a net increase in bone mass [9–11].

This study was designed to evaluate the therapeutic effect of alternating phosphate and calcium infusions in patients with severe osteoporosis. This regimen conformed partly with the theoretic considerations advanced by Rasmussen and Bordier [11], and was supported by experimental findings reported by several workers, which ascribed to phosphorus a stimulating effect on new bone formation [11–15]. It has been proposed that inorganic phosphorus acts on bone by (1) increasing the conversion of osteoclasts to osteoblasts, (2) enhancing the activity of osteoblasts to synthesize new bone collagen matrix, and (3) increasing the deposition of calcium at sites of new bone formation [11]. The second therapeutic component, intravenous calcium, was added for two reasons: (1) to maintain normocalcemia and so prevent excessive secretion of parathyroid hormone and its unfavorable effects on bone metabolism [16,17] and (2) to increase the pool of active bone cells by stimulating, with calcium, the con-

From the Departments of Medicine and Pathology, University of Colorado, School of Medicine, Denver, Colorado. This study was presented at the International Workshop on Phosphate, June 5–6, 1975, Hôpital Necker, Paris, France. Requests for reprints should be addressed to Dr. M. M. Popovtzer. Manuscript accepted January 30, 1976.

* Present address: Department of Medicine, Temple University School of Medicine, Philadelphia, Pennsylvania 19140.

version of mesenchymal cells into osteoclasts which subsequently, under the influence of inorganic phosphorus, may be converted into osteoblasts [11].

MATERIAL AND METHODS

One man and four women entered the study. The pertinent clinical data are listed in Table I. All patients suffered from unremitting and intractable skeletal pains, and required increasing doses of analgesics for relief. In the selection of the patients, attempts were made to include in the study only those who had had persistent symptoms for several years and to exclude those in whom the activity of the disease was intermittent with periods of exacerbation after new fractures and periods of quiescence. The patients were admitted to the metabolic unit of the Clinical Research Center for evaluation and initiation of treatment. Four of the five patients reported a progressive decrease in height, with a loss ranging from 1 to 3 inches. The height of all patients was measured on their admission and thereafter at six month intervals for the following two years. The history of bone fractures, their frequency and the time of occurrence was obtained in great detail from the patients and their referring physicians, and was correlated with roentgenographic abnormalities seen on serial skeletal films. All patients presented evidence of recurrent spontaneous fractures; however, in one (Case 5) it was not possible to determine the exact times of their occurrence. Roentgenographic surveys of bone and soft tissues, and radiotechnetium diphosphonate scans were obtained in all patients on admission and thereafter at six month intervals for the following two years.

Open surgical biopsy specimens of the iliac crest were obtained immediately posterior to the anterior iliac spine. The bone specimens were approximately 1.5 cm long in the anteroposterior axis and included the superior cortical surface, 1 to 2 cm segments of the inner and outer cortical tables, and the enclosed cancellous bone. In order to evaluate changes in cortical thickness between biopsy specimens obtained before and after treatment, the inner and outer tables had to be distinguished from one another to ensure that the anatomic regions being compared were in fact comparable. The inner table is thinner, forming a smooth convex curve where it joins the superior surface of the crest. The outer table is thicker, concave and forms an acute angle with the superior cortical surface. To avoid errors in the interpretation of results due to variations in sampling areas [18] and structural changes induced by the trauma of the first biopsy, the second biopsy specimen was obtained after treatment from the contralateral side, in a symmetrical fashion, by the same surgical team. This was further confirmed by visualizing two symmetrical defects in the contour of the iliac bone on x-ray films taken after the second biopsy. Since in all patients the defects were symmetrical there was no need to repeat the second biopsy. Using these criteria it was possible to compare the same relative areas of superior cortex, inner and outer tables of right and left-sided biopsy specimens of iliac bone. In other unrelated studies in which symmetrical biopsy specimens were obtained at short time intervals from five patients, we found no difference between the two sides. The specimens were bissected; one half was used to prepare decalcified, paraffin-embedded sections, and the second half was used for frozen section. Frozen sections were cut at 10 to 15 μ after washing out the marrow with a strong stream of tap water, infiltrating the marrow space with frozen-section embedding media, freezing at $-30°C$ and mounting on cryostat chucks. The sections were picked up on warm albuminized slides, heated at 56°C for 2 hours and stained by the von Kossa technic, with a van Gieson counterstain. The other half of the specimen (decalcified sections) was embedded in paraffin and fixed for 24 hours in neutral buffered formalin solution, decalcified 24 hours with citric and nitric acid mixtures, sectioned at 7 μ, and stained with hematoxylin and eosin. Von Kossa stained sections were used to determine the degree of bone mineralization and to exclude the presence of osteomalacia; the hematoxylin and eosin stained sections were used to determine cortical thickness and general histologic detail. Since variations could be introduced

TABLE I Clinical Data of All Patients

Case No.	Age(yr) and Sex	Menopause (yr before admission)	Duration of Bone Pains (yr)	First Bone Fracture (yr before admission)
1	66,F	15	9	6
2	84,F	27	16	16
3	86,F	28	9	7
4	67,F	18	10	6
5	65,M	. . .	20	10

TABLE II Biochemical Data of All Patients

Case No.	Duration of treatment (days)	Total Calcium (mg/100 ml)		Ionized Calcium (mg/100 ml)		Serum Phosphorus (mg/100 ml)		Creatinine Clearance (ml/min)		Cumulative Balance		
		P	E	P	E	P	E	P	E	Duration (days)	Calcium (mg)	Phosphorus (mg)
1	365	10.1	9.5	4.6	4.2	4.5	2.7	60	80	15	+4,820	+3,450
2	400	10.0	9.4	4.5	4.5	3.7	3.0	45	52	55	+13,856	+6,489
3	445	9.1	9.2	4.2	3.8	3.5	2.2	62	60	42	+19,395	+15,388
4	410	10.2	9.9	4.7	4.2	3.9	2.3	60	72	27	+12,700	+3,250
5	405	9.5	9.0	4.3	4.1	3.7	2.0	78	85			

NOTE: P = pretreatment. E = end of treatment.

by cutting the sections at different angles, the procedure was performed with extreme care to ascertain the same angle in all sections. The volume of the cancellous bone was measured by a previously described technic [19]. The volume of the cortical bone was measured by projecting the microscopic section on graph paper, drawing the outlines of the cortical bone and estimating its volume by direct counting of the number of the squares. The change is expressed in terms of per cents of the control volume; to obtain this value the volume of biopsy specimens obtained before treatment was subtracted from the volume of biopsy specimens obtained after treatment, and the result was divided by the volume of biopsy specimens before treatment and multiplied by 100.

After admission to the hospital, daily determinations of serum and urine concentrations of creatinine and phosphorus and serum alkaline phosphatase (by Technicon Autoanalyzer®), total calcium and magnesium (by Perkin Elmer, atomic absorption spectrophotometer model 290), serum

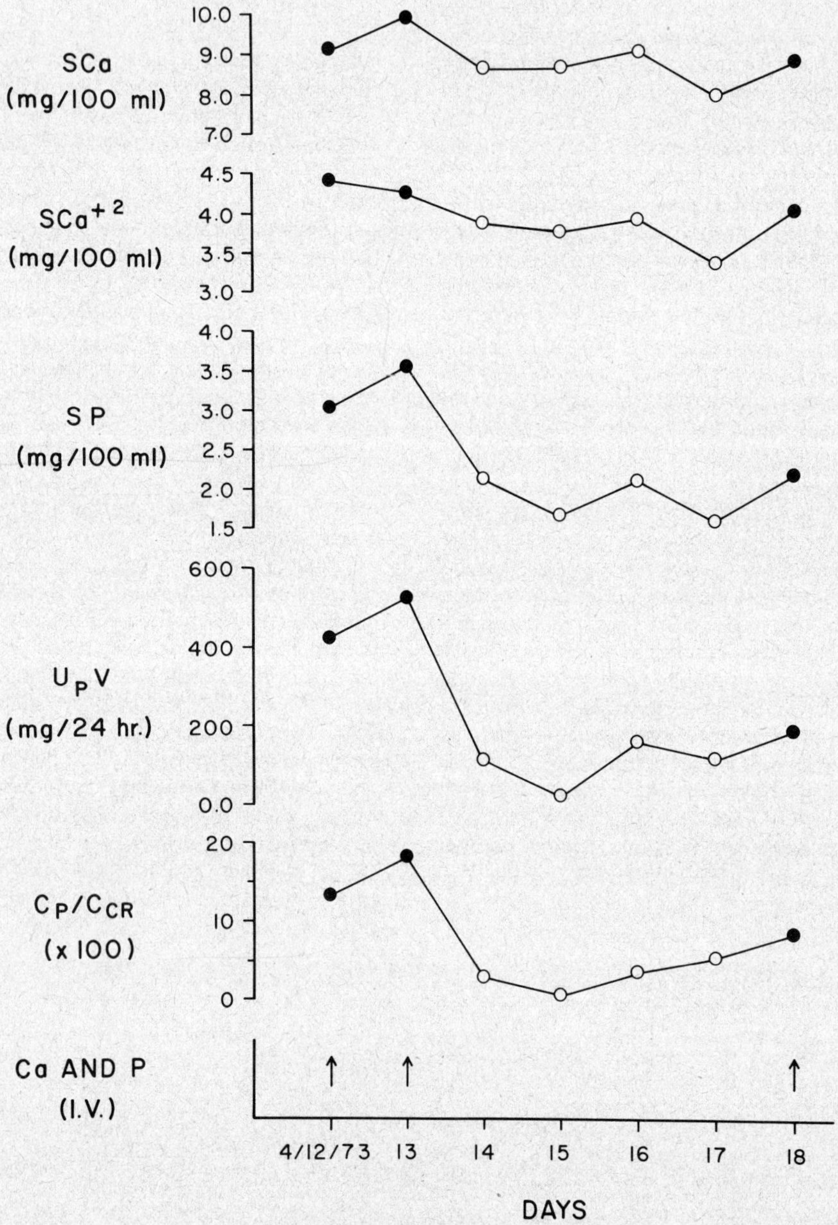

Figure 1. *Case 3. The temporal relationship between serum levels of total, ionized calcium and phosphorus and urinary excretion of phosphorus. Closed circles and arrows represent days of treatment, open circles represent days without treatment.*

ionized calcium (by Orion flow through ion exchange electrode), sodium and potassium (by flame photometer) were made. In four patients external balances of calcium and phosphorus were measured. These four patients were maintained on a constant diet containing the same amounts of minerals, electrolytes and calories as their home diets. Stool was collected in three day periods and stored frozen in stainless steel containers. A dry ashing method was used in processing the feces before chemical analysis for calcium and phosphorus [20]. The same method was applied for analysis of the diet. In two patients (Cases 1 and 2), the mineral content of the skin was measured in punch biopsy

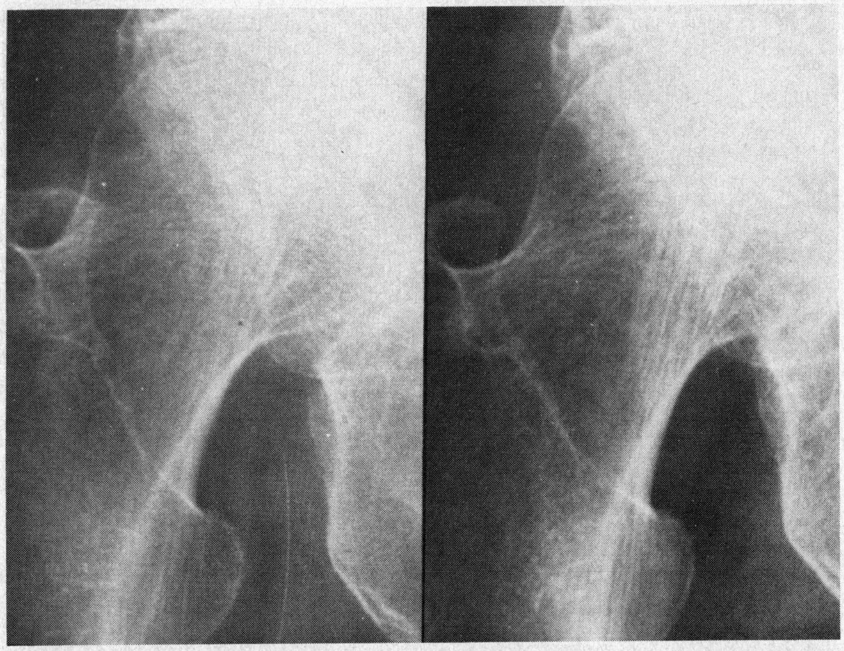

Figure 2. *Case 5. The proximal femur of patient before **(left)** and one year after beginning treatment **(right)**. Notice the increase in the trabeculation pattern of the principal compressive trabeculas which are running vertically on the medial aspect of the femoral neck from the head down to the lesser trochanter. Also notice a slight increase in the trabeculation pattern of the principal tensile trabeculas which run a horizontal course across the head of femur.*

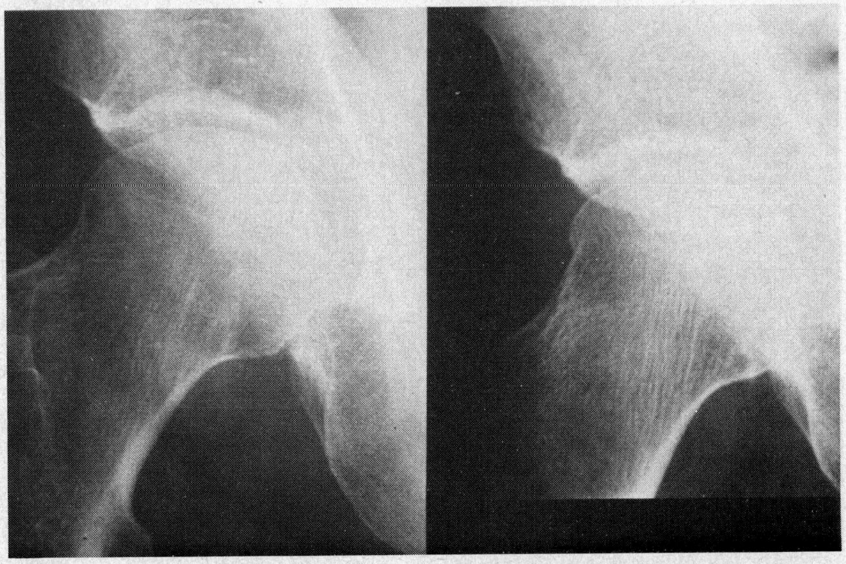

Figure 3. *Case 1. The proximal femur of patient before **(left)** and one year after beginning therapy **(right)**. Notice an increase in the trabeculation pattern of the principal compressive and the principal tensile trabeculas.*

specimens, obtained one year after the beginning of the treatment, by a micromodification of a previously described method [21].

One patient (Case 3) had been treated in another hospital with calcium infusion for about six months. This treatment failed to relieve the bone pain and was discontinued four months before her admission.

Therapeutic Regimen. Treatment consisted of alternating phosphate and calcium infusions. Phosphorus was given in the form of neutral sodium phosphate, and calcium was given in the form of calcium gluconate; both salts were dissolved in 5 per cent dextrose in water. The total daily doses of phosphorus ranged from 5 to 10 mg/kg body weight and of calcium from 8 to 15 mg/kg.

The infusions were divided evenly over 24 hours and delivered by alternating phosphorus and calcium every 4 to 6 hours. The intravenous lines were flushed with normal saline solution when switching from one salt to another to prevent precipitation of calcium phosphate. At all times serum phosphate was maintained at or below 4.5 mg/100 ml and serum calcium was maintained at or below 11.2 mg/100 ml. The calcium × phosphorus product in the serum did not exceed 45. During the first six to eight weeks the patients were in the hospital, infusions were given every day. During an additional 10 to 12 months, most infusions were given on an outpatient basis, two or three days every week, over 12 hour periods.

RESULTS

All patients experienced marked symptomatic relief two to three weeks after the institution of the therapy. They regained the ability to change positions without precipitating severe pains. Use of analgesic drugs was tapered and discontinued. As the pains subsided, the patients became more active and spent a considerable portion of the infusion time walking with portable intravenous poles. The striking subjective improvement encouraged the patients to continue to participate in the study despite the inconvenience incurred by the intravenous therapy.

All patients exhibited positive balances for calcium and phosphorus; the cumulative results are listed in Table II. Fasting serum concentrations of total and ionized calcium, and phosphorus, and clearances of creatinine, before and at the end of the treatment period are shown in Table II. Creatinine clearances did not change during the course of treatment. In all patients, creatinine clearances were also measured two years after the beginning of the study; the rates did not differ from pretreatment values. All patients exhibited a decrease in serum phosphorus concentration. When the serum levels were correlated with the urinary excretion of phosphorus, it was apparent that the decrease in serum phosphorus was associated with a parallel decline in the urinary excretion of phosphorus. A representative illustration of this phenomenon, as recorded in Case 3, is shown in Figure 1. As serum phosphorus declined, during the days when treatment was withheld (open symbols), the urinary excretion of phosphorus decreased and fractional tubular reabsorption approached 100 per cent. By measuring the urinary excretion of phosphorus, it was obvious in all patients that the decrease in serum phosphorus was not due to increased urinary losses. Serum concentrations of total and ionized calcium exhibited only minimal changes (Table II). Serum alkaline phosphatase did not change throughout the study.

The initial bone surveys demonstrated multiple vertebral compression fractures and generalized loss of bone density in all patients, these features did not change considerably throughout the study. After one year of treatment, in two patients (Cases 1 and 5) the films of the proximal femurs showed an increase in trabeculation pattern, affecting the principal compressive trabeculas and, to a lesser extent, the principal tensile trabeculas (Figures 2 and 3).

Bone biopsy specimens obtained before and after treatment showed severely reduced mass of the cortical and the cancellous bones. In two patients (Cases 1 and

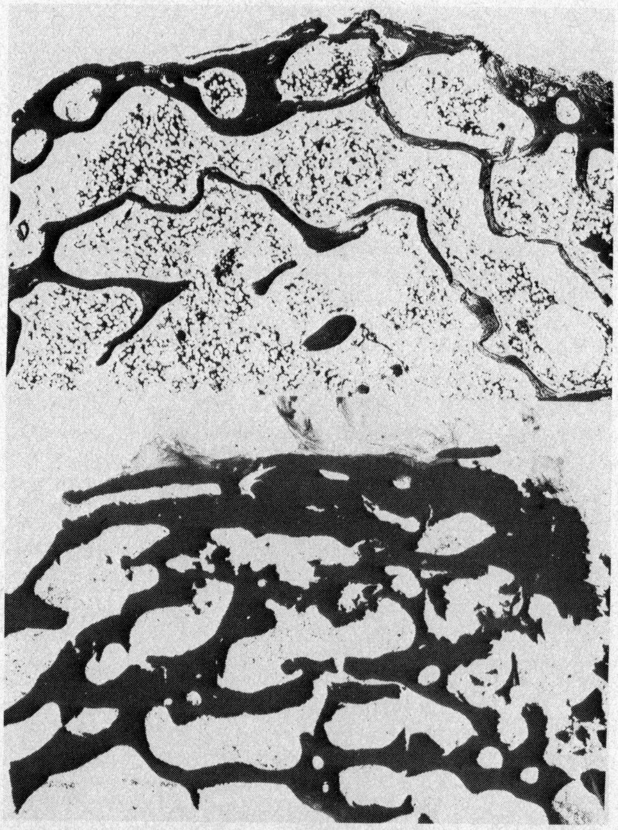

*Figure 4. Case 5. Biopsy specimens obtained before **(top)** and after **(bottom)** treatment. Both specimens are upper cortical surfaces with underlying cancellous bone. Notice that the thickness and number of trabeculas are increased in the biopsy specimen obtained after treatment. Also the cortical bone is slightly increased in thickness. Original magnification × 12, reduced by 24 per cent.*

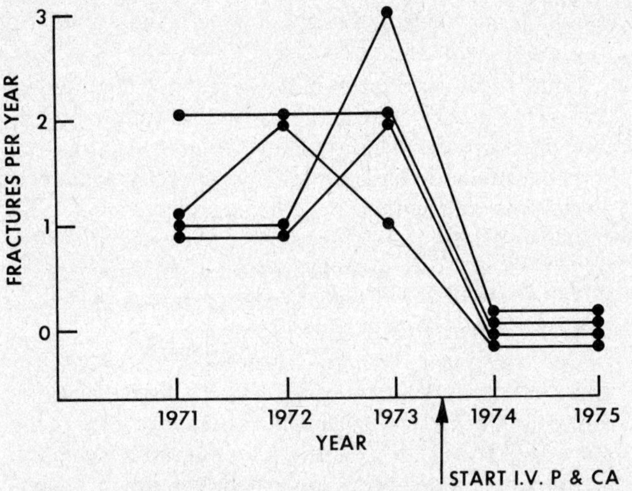

Figure 5. The annual occurrence rates of spontaneous fractures in four patients, during three years before and two years after the institution of the therapy.

3), the biopsy specimens obtained after treatment showed a considerable increase in the thickness of one of the cortical surfaces. The measured increment in the whole cortical bone volume in these two patients amounted to 163 per cent and 124 per cent of the volume before treatment. There was no substantial change in the cancellous bone. In the third patient (Case 5), there was a marked increase in the mass of cancellous bone from 7 to 11 per cent and also an increase in the thickness of the upper cortical surface. The estimated increment in total cortical bone volume amounted to 150 per cent of the pretreatment value. In the fourth patient (Case 2), there was a moderate increase in the thickness of the upper cortical surface. The measured increment in the whole cortical bone was 132 per cent of the control volume. There was no measurable substantial change in the volume of cancellous bone. In the fifth patient (Case 4), there was no difference between biopsy specimens obtained before and after treatment. Representative micrograms illustrating the changes in bone mass in Case 5 are shown in Figure 4. None of the biopsy specimens obtained before or after treatment showed any abnormalities in bone mineralization; thus, the presence of osteomalacia was excluded. No differences in the remodelling processes or cellular activities were noted.

The annual occurrence rates of spontaneous fractures during the three consecutive years before the institution of the therapy were readily available in four patients. In one patient (Case 5), it was not possible to determine that rate with certainty. In each patient, at least one fracture per year could be documented for that period of time. The follow-up extends over at least two years after the beginning of therapy. During these two years, there has been no recurrence of fractures or return of bone pains (Figure 5). Although the present study did not include a group of sham-treated control patients for comparison with the treated patients, during the same period four other patients with osteoporosis were treated symptomatically for similar disease activity. But the occurrence rate of fractures, which was 2.5 per year, did not change during the corresponding five years.

The height of all patients remained unchanged throughout the observation period, in contrast to the progressive loss noticed prior to treatment. It is noteworthy that, up to date, none of the patients exhibited clinical evidence of extraskeletal calcifications as determined by physical examinations, slit lamp inspections of the eyes, x-ray surveys and radiotechnetium scans of the soft tissues. In two patients (Cases 1 and 2), the measured calcium contents of their skin were 210 and 260 mg/kg dry weight, respectively. These values are within the normal range for this laboratory, however, the calcium contents of the skin before treatment were not available for comparison. An incidental finding in two patients (Cases 1 and 4) was a decrease in serum cholesterol concentrations from values of 320 and 410 before treatment to values of 220 and 240 mg/100 ml, respectively, after treatment.

COMMENTS

The present study demonstrated clinical improvement in five patients with severe osteoporosis following the long-term intravenous administration of phosphate and calcium. The most important finding was complete cessation of spontaneous fractures in five patients who had suffered from recurrent fractures for at least three consecutive years preceding the institution of therapy (Figure 5). Since all patients increased their physical activities following relief of bone pains; the absence of spontaneous fractures was more likely the consequence of a gain of mechanical strength than a reduced exposure to physical strain. It is well recognized that patients with osteoporosis may undergo a spontaneous phase of quiescence of their disease activity. It seems unlikely that this would have occurred in all five patients simultaneously, and then persisted for two years.

The data presented suggest that the improvement observed was the result of an increase in bone mass. The positive external balances of calcium and phosphorus recorded during the early phase of this study, and the diminishing serum concentration of phosphorus, are compatible with an increased formation of new mineralized bone, yet the exact site of deposition of the retained mineral could not be established with absolute certainty on the basis of the data available. An increase in the trabeculation pattern of various bones was noticed in two patients one year after the beginning of therapy. Although several workers considered variations in bone trabeculation as indicative of changes in bone density, the significance of these variations in our patients cannot be well defined [9,22,23]. In four patients the biopsy specimens obtained after treatment showed an increase in bone thickness, which was present in at least one of the anatomic subunits examined.

The specific nature of the therapeutic response, its reproducibility, and the cause and effect relationship to one, and/or the combination of the two agents employed, are the central questions raised by our study. Previous attempts to treat patients with osteoporosis with intravenous calcium alone have not been uniformly successful [4,7]. In one study, in which the treatment group consisted primarily of middle-aged men, clinical improvement was reported [4]. In a recent study, in which the group which was treated with intravenous calcium consisted of postmenopausal elderly women, a population comparable to ours, no improvement was observed [7]. It is also noteworthy that one of our patients (Case 3) had failed to respond to the prolonged intravenous administration of calcium prior to entering our study.

The foregoing considerations which seriously question the therapeutic action of intravenously administered calcium alone, focus the attention on intravenously administered phosphorus, and/or the combined intravenous administration of phosphorus and calcium, as possibly therapeutically effective agents in patients with osteoporosis.

It has to be emphasized, however, that the clinical use of the proposed regimen is limited because of its long duration and its complexity. Obviously, it may not be recommended as a general therapeutic modality in all patients with symptomatic osteoporosis; it has to be considered only in selected patients. Furthermore, more patients and more quantitative documentation are required before the procedure can be firmly established as uniformly effective.

Our therapeutic regimen was not associated with any apparent complications other than the inconvenience related to the intravenous route of administration of the solutions. The latter was offset by the remarkable improvement in the patients' condition. The complications related to phosphate therapy are well known [16,17]. Therefore ample caution is warranted when the clinical use of this element is contemplated. Our rule of using relatively small amounts of phosphorus and calcium, which were evenly divided over a wide range of time, and avoiding excessive increases in serum concentrations, was rigorously observed throughout our study. At present, one year after discontinuing intravenous therapy, clinical improvement continues and no side-effects are noticeable.

REFERENCES

1. Frost HM: The Bone Dynamics of Osteoporosis and Osteomalacia, Springfield, Ill., Charles C Thomas, 1966.
2. Rasmussen H, Tenenhouse A: Thyrocalcitonin, osteoporosis and osteolysis. Am J Med 43: 711, 1967.
3. Harris WH, Heaney RP: Skeletal renewal and metabolic bone disease. N Engl J Med 280: 193, 1969.
4. Pak CYC, Zisman E, Evens R, et al.: The treatment of osteoporosis with calcium infusions. Am J Med 47: 7, 1969.
5. Jowsey J, Riggs BL, Goldsmith RS, et al.: Effects of prolonged administration of porcine calcitonin in post-menopausal osteoporosis. J Clin Endocrinol Metab 33: 752, 1971.
6. Riggs BL, Jowsey J, Goldsmith RS, et al.: Short- and long-term effects of estrogen and synthetic anabolic hormone in post-menopausal osteoporosis. J Clin Invest 51: 1659, 1972.
7. Dudl RJ, Ensinck JW, Baylink D, et al.: Evaluation of intravenous calcium as therapy for osteoporosis. Am J Med 55: 631, 1973.
8. Jowsey J, Riggs BL, Kelly PJ, et al.: The treatment of osteoporosis with disodium ethane-1-hydroxy-1,1-diphosphonate. J Lab Clin Med 78: 574, 1971.
9. Jowsey J, Riggs BL: Seeking successful treatment for osteoporosis. Modern Med 41: 36, 1973.
10. Jowsey J, Riggs BL, Kelly PJ, et al.: Effects of combined therapy with sodium fluoride, vitamin D and calcium in osteoporosis. Am J Med 53: 43, 1972.
11. Rasmussen H, Bordier PH: The Physiological and Cellular Basis of Metabolic Bone Disease, Baltimore, Williams & Wilkins Co., 1974.
12. Pechet MM, Bobadilla E, Carrol EL: Regulation of bone resorption and formation. Influences of thyrocalcitonin, parathyroid hormone, neutral phosphate and vitamin D_3. Am J Med 43: 696, 1967.
13. Feinblatt J, Belanger LF, Rasmussen H: Effect of phosphate infusion on bone metabolism and parathyroid hormone action. Am J Physiol 218: 1624, 1970.
14. Raisz LG: The effect of factors implicated in osteoporosis on bone formation and resorption in tissue culture. Osteoporosis (Barzel U, ed), New York and London, Grune & Stratton, 1970.
15. Flanagan B, Nichols G Jr: Bone matrix and balance in vitro. II. The effects of aging. J Clin Invest 48: 607, 1969.
16. Laflamme GH, Jowsey J: Bone and soft-tissue reaction to an increased intake of phosphate in animals. J Clin Invest 51: 2834, 1972.
17. Jowsey J, Balasubramaniam P: Effect of phosphate supplements on soft tissue calcification and bone turnover. Clin Sci 42: 289, 1972.
18. Ellis HA, Peart KM: Quantitative observations on mineralized and nonmineralized bone in the iliac crest. J Clin Pathol 25: 277, 1972.
19. Huffer WE, Kuzela D, Popovtzer MM: Metabolic bone disease in chronic renal failure. I. Dialyzed uremics. Am J Pathol 78: 365, 1975.
20. Newell JE: Quantitative chemical assay of feces, collecting, mixing and sampling. Am J Clin Pathol 34: 189, 1960.
21. Massry SG, Coburn JW, Hartenbower DL, et al.: Mineral content of human skin in uremia; Cameron Proc EDTA, vol 7, p 146 (Pitman, London, 1970).
22. Singh M, Riggs BL, Beabout JW, et al.: Femoral trabecular pattern index for evaluation of spinal osteoporosis. Ann Intern Med 74: 63, 1972.
23. Singh M, Riggs BL, Beabout JW, et al.: Femoral trabecular pattern index for evaluation of spinal osteoporosis. A detailed methodologic description. Mayo Clin Proc 48: 184, 1973.

Steroid Myopathy in Connective Tissue Disease

ALI ASKARI, M.D.*
PAUL J. VIGNOS, Jr., M.D.
ROLAND W. MOSKOWITZ, M.D.
Cleveland, Ohio

In eight women with polymyositis (three patients), systemic lupus erythematosus (SLE) (three patients), rheumatoid arthritis (one patient) and shoulder-hand syndrome (one patient), weakness developed during high dose prednisone therapy. These women were studied using serial functional and manual muscle tests, determination of serum glutamic oxaloacetic transaminase (SGOT), creatinine phosphokinase (CPK) and serum aldolase levels, and urinary excretion of creatine. Insidious onset of weakness was characteristic. Myalgias were seen in five patients and unusual sudden weakness in two. Weakness was always most severe in the pelvic girdle muscles; there was a lesser involvement of shoulder girdle and distal muscles.

Serum muscle enzyme levels were normal in all cases, but urinary creatine excretion was invariably increased and proved to be the most sensitive laboratory indicator for clinical diagnosis and for monitoring patient improvement. Serial urinary creatine excretion and serum enzyme studies were of value in differenting steroid myopathy from a flare of myositis in patients with connective tissue disease. Diagnosis and effective management were achieved by the use of readily available laboratory and clinical procedures without resorting to muscle biopsy.

Myopathy is a well known side effect of corticosteroid therapy. Numerous clinical reports [1–25] and experimental studies [26–37] of muscle weakness during steroid therapy have appeared in the literature since the introduction of corticosteroids to clinical medicine. Clinical steroid myopathy has been reported in papers concerned principally with the effectiveness of corticosteroids in a variety of diseases in which the myopathy was observed as one of a number of undesirable side effects. A systematic study of steroid myopathy using such formal methods of evaluation as manual and functional muscle testing, serum muscle enzymes and urinary creatine excretion studies has not been reported. Such studies have been conducted on only a few patients [15,16,22]. The clinical significance of the laboratory findings, the temporal relationship between the steroid administration and the appearance of the myopathy have not received adequate attention. The management of steroid myopathy has consisted of discontinuing administration of the drug or substituting another steroid derivative without any serious attempt to determine the clinical guidelines for proper therapeutic dose adjustment (Table I).

Laboratory studies in clinical steroid myopathy have consisted mainly of muscle biopsy, electromyography and nerve conduction velocity, often with conflicting results (Table II). Noninvasive proce-

From the Division of Rheumatology, Department of Medicine, Case-Western Reserve University School of Medicine, Cleveland, Ohio. Requests for reprints should be addressed to Dr. Ali Askari.
Manuscript accepted January 28, 1976.
*Present address: St. Lukes Hospital, 11311 Shaker Boulevard, Cleveland, Ohio 44104.

TABLE I Summary of Clinical Findings Reported in Steroid Myopathy (Present Study Not Included)

Data	Findings
No. of cases	76 (1–25)
Sex	Female 33, male 15, not known 28
Incidence	7 per cent, 47 of 700 steroid-treated patients
Age (yr)	2 [16] to 75 [12]
Underlying rheumatic disease (total of 55 cases)*	SLE 8 [2,9], RA 38 [3,8,10,11,15,17,22], rheumatic fever 5 [16], temporal arteritis 1 [3], polyarteritis nodosa 1 [5], ankylosing spondylitis 2 [11,15], polymyositis not reported
Methods of evaluation	Based on subjective complaints and physicians' observation 80 per cent, serial muscle examinations 6 per cent [16], combined functional and manual muscle examinations not reported
Type of steroid causing myopathy	Triamcinolone 39 [2,3,5,8,10,11,15,18, 20], dexamethasone 11 [4,12,13,15,16,20], fludrocortisone 1 [6], prednisone 19 [5,7, 9–11,14–17,22], cortisone 4 [5,7,11], prednisolone 1 [25], methylprednisolone 1 [1]
Daily dose and duration	Triamcinolone 8–24 mg (1 to 48 weeks), dexamethasone 1.5–6 mg (3 to 12 weeks), prednisone 15–100 mg (4 to 240 weeks), cortisone 150–250 mg (3 to 48 weeks)

NOTE: SLE = systemic lupus erythematosus. RA = rheumatoid arthritis.
*In 21 reported cases the underlying disease was non-rheumatic.

dures which would assist the clinician in differentiating steroid myopathy from underlying connective tissue disease have not been attempted. Steroid myopathy occurring as a complication of therapy for polymyositis has not been reported, although this may well be an important and confusing problem in patient management.

Our purpose in reporting this study is to evaluate the clinical characteristics of steroid-induced myopathy that occurred in a group of patients with connective tissue disease, including polymyositis, in order to define more precisely the biochemical abnormalities induced with this myopathy, to correlate the clinical and the laboratory findings and, finally, to outline a practical noninvasive approach for the early detection, differential diagnosis and management of steroid-induced myopathy.

TABLE III Functional Classification of Muscle Weakness

Class	Functional Capacity
1	Has difficulty in climbing stairs
2	Cannot rise from chair
3	Cannot walk without assistance
4	Cannot elevate extremities or move in bed

MATERIALS AND METHODS

Eight patients in whom steroid myopathy developed while they were receiving prednisone therapy for their primary connective tissue disease were seen at University Hospitals of Cleveland between July 1972 and November 1973. All patients were hospitalized for evaluation which included manual and functional muscle testing, determination of serum enzyme levels and urinary excretion of creatine. These studies were made on admission and repeated every two weeks until discharge or such time as clinical improvement was obvious.

The patients were treated for their steroid myopathy by gradually reducing their prednisone dosage and monitoring both the clinical and laboratory parameters to be described.

Manual muscle testing was carried out by an experienced physical therapist using the standard technic [38]. Functional classification was made by a system of grading based on timed tests of specific activities of daily living (Table III). The method of assay for serum aldolase was essentially that of Sibley and Lehniger [39] as modified by Cook and Dounce [40]. The normal value by this method is 0.4 U (± 0.3 U).

Creatinine phosphokinase (CPK) was measured by a method similar to that of Siegel and Cohen [41]. The normal range by this method is 0 to 110 mIU/ml.

TABLE II Summary of Reported Laboratory Findings in Steroid Myopathy (Present Series Not Included)

Test	No.	Reference	Summary of Results
Muscle biopsy			
Light microscope	21	[1,5–7,13–16,18]	Fiber size variation, fiber necrosis, fiber vacuolation, increased sarcolemmal nuclei, centralization of nuclei, phagocytosis, regeneration, loss of striation, increase in fibrous or adipose tissue
Electron microscope	7	[1,15,18]	Mitochondrial structure changes (enlargement, proliferation, aggregation, vacuolation, decreased or absent), presence of lipid bodies, outpouching of sarcolemma, increased glycogen in subsarcolemmal area
Electromyography	17	[1,9,14–17,22]	Normal, myopathic, neuromyopathic, neuropathic
Urinary creatine excretion	11	[7,15,16,22]	Increased excretion in six, normal in five
CPK	1	[22]	Elevated on one occasion and normal later in the course
Aldolase	6	[1,15,22]	Elevated in two, normal in four
SGOT	4	[1,14,15]	Normal

TABLE IV Clinical Description of Patients with Steroid Myopathy

Data	Case 1	Case 2	Case 3	Case 4	Case 5	Case 6	Case 7	Case 8
Age (yr)	38	33	24	84	53	61	10	22
Sex	F	F	F	F	F	F	F	F
Chief complaint due to primary disease	Myalgia and weakness	Weakness	Arthralgia and fatigue	Arthralgia	Pain and swelling, right upper extremity	Dyspnea and weakness	Weakness	Periorbital edema and fatigue
Chief complaint due to steroid myopathy	Myalgia and weakness	Weakness	Myalgia and weakness	Weakness	Myalgia and weakness	Weakness	Myalgia and weakness	Myalgia and weakness
Onset	Insidious	Acute	Insidious	Insidious	Acute	Insidious	Insidious	Insidious

Serum glutamic oxaloacetic transaminase (SGOT) was determined by a method based on the procedure of Morgenstern et al. [42]. The normal range for SGOT by this method is 9 to 25 Henry U (HU)/ml.

Urinary creatine and creatinine were determined on aliquots of 24 hour urine samples by the methods of Clark and Thompson [43] and Anker [44]. They are reported as per cent creatinuria (per cent creatinuria = creatine/creatine + creatinine) which we have found to be relatively more reliable than the absolute creatine excretion values [45]. Creatinuria above 6 per cent after age 15 is considered abnormal by this method. Because of occasional variation in day to day creatine excretion, duplicate 24 hour collections were obtained, and the values given are averages of the two determinations [45]. Muscle biopsy specimens were taken from quadriceps and gastrocnemius muscles under local anesthesia by members of the Department of Surgery at University Hospitals of Cleveland. Pathologic description and diagnosis of these muscle specimens were made by a senior neuropathologist at the institute of Pathology, Case Western Reserve University. Electromyography was performed with concentric needle electrodes. The activity recorded was presented for interpretation, in the conventional manner, both on a cathode ray oscilloscope and through a loudspeaker.

RESULTS

The onset of steroid myopathy was insidious in six of the eight patients. Two patients (Cases 3 and 5) experienced sudden onset of weakness over a period of a few days.

Diffuse myalgia occurred in five patients at the onset of steroid myopathy but was absent in all but one patient when the primary diagnosis of connective tissue disease was made (Table IV). The diagnosis of steroid myopathy was made retrospectively in two patients (Cases 2 and 7) when muscle strength improved after the prednisone dose was reduced because of severe nonmyopathic side effects.

The correlation between weakness demonstrated by functional testing and manual muscle testing was good, but the manual muscle examination appeared to be more sensitive in uncovering mild muscle weakness (Table V).

Muscle weakness was symmetrical with initial involvement of the proximal lower extremities followed by progression to the proximal shoulder girdle and finally to the distal extremities. At the time of evaluation, the most common pattern of weakness (four of eight patients) involved mainly the proximal pelvic girdle muscles with slight proximal weakness in the upper extremity (Table VI). Weakness was never restricted to the muscles of the proximal shoulder girdle or the distal extremities. The recovery of muscle strength followed a reverse progression.

TABLE V Functional and Manual Muscle Testing in Patients with Steroid Myopathy

Data	Case 1	Case 2	Case 3	Case 4	Case 5	Case 6	Case 7	Case 8
Clinical diagnosis	SLE	Poly	SLE	RA	S-H-S	Poly	Poly	SLE
Before myopathy								
Functional class	0	2	0	0	0	1	2	0
Manual muscle grade	Normal	Fair	Normal	Normal	Normal	*	Good	Normal
During myopathy								
Functional class	3	3	4	2	3	3	3	Normal-1
Manual muscle grade	Fair	Poor	Poor	Poor—fair	Fair	Poor—fair	Fair	Fair
Following steroid reduction								
Functional class	1	1	0	0	0	1	0	0
Manual muscle grade	Good—normal	Fair—good	Good—normal	Good—normal	Normal	Good—normal		Good—normal

NOTE: Poly = polymyositis. SLE = systemic lupus erythematosus. RA = rheumatoid arthritis. S-H-S = shoulder hand syndrome.

* = No formal manual test available prior to the development of myopathy.

TABLE VI **Pattern of Muscle Weakness in Steroid Myopathy**

Muscle Weakness	No. of Cases
Predominantly proximal lower with slight proximal upper extremities	4
Generalized	2
Proximal upper and lower with slight distal extremities	1
Proximal lower extremities	1
Proximal upper or distal extremities	0

There was a wide variation in the times that symptoms of steroid myopathy appeared which correlated poorly with either the total steroid dose or the duration of therapy (Table VII). Five of the patients had been receiving maintenance steroid therapy for their connective tissue disease and had tolerated a daily dose of 15 to 60 mg of prednisone per day for 60 to 240 days without having any symptoms or signs of weakness. However, an increase in the daily dose or the initiation of 40 and 70 mg of prednisone per day was followed by the occurrence of steroid myopathy within 30 days in six patients.

There did not appear to be any correlation between the development of myopathy and the total cumulative maintenance steroid dosage (Table VII). Six of the eight patients received a total of 5,000 to 15,000 mg before myopathy developed. Two patients, however, had a low threshold for the development of myopathy as demonstrated by the onset of symptoms either after a low daily dose given for a long period of time (Case 4) or after a short period of time (10 days), with total dose of only 400 mg (Case 5). Both patients had relatively severe

TABLE VII **Relation of Prednisone Dosage to Appearance of Steroid Myopathy**

	Maintenance		Onset of Myopathy		Recovery		
Case	Dose (mg)	Duration (days)	Dose (mg)	Duration (days)	Dose (mg)	Duration (days)	Follow-up (days)
1	15	210	70*	30	15	120	360
2	25	210	60*	120	17.5	60	360
3	0	0	70*	30	17.5	30	360
4†	15	—	—	360	10	30	180
5‡	0	0	40	10	0	12	0
6	60	60	60	30	10	120	180
7	60	180	80*	30	15	60	360
8	40	240	70*	30	35	30	120

* Increased dose administered for management of flare of underlying disease.

† Steroid myopathy developed very gradually during one year when patient was receiving 15 mg prednisone/day.

‡ Patient had complete recovery within 12 days with gradual discontinuation of prednisone.

osteoporosis prior to the initiation of prednisone therapy and may have been in negative nitrogen balance. Steroid myopathy cleared when the prednisone dose was gradually reduced to a level of 10 to 35 mg/day over a period of 30 to 120 days. In Case 5 rapid resolution was noted in 12 days when prednisone therapy was withdrawn. Several patients showed complete resolution of myopathy when the steroid dosage was reduced to the level of the previous maintenance dose (Cases 1, 4 and 8). Although symptomatic improvement was observed relatively rapidly after the reduction in dose, complete resolution of the muscle weakness usually took from one to four months.

Serum muscle enzymes remained normal in all patients during the entire course of steroid myopathy (Table VIII). This was in contrast to the abnormal elevation of serum enzyme levels which occurred in the patients with polymyositis at the onset of the myopathy or during a flare of the disease. Creatine excretion, on the other hand, was consistently increased whenever symptoms of steroid myopathy appeared in a patient. At the onset of their primary disease, abnormal creatinuria developed in patients with polymyositis (Cases 2, 6 and 7); this then remained fairly constant until the appearance of steroid myopathy. The creatine excretion in these three patients did increase when steroid myopathy developed although there was no change in the serum muscle enzyme concentration. The highest creatinuria values were found in these patients (Table VIII). As the steroid myopathy diminished, creatinuria decreased toward normal levels and remained stable in all patients, including those with polymyositis. Creatinuria correlated well with the degree of weakness determined by manual muscle testing and appeared to be a very sensitive method for detecting or confirming even mild degrees of myopathy.

The patients in whom steroid myopathy developed also had at least two or more other undesirable side effects of prednisone therapy (Table IX). The presence of osteoporosis, a late manifestation of hypercortisonism, showed a particularly frequent association with the occurrence of steroid myopathy (in five of eight patients). In four patients mild mood changes developed, and three patients had steroid-induced diabetes. Hypokalemia, which may be associated with muscle weakness, was not found in any of these patients. Muscle biopsy, performed in two patients (Cases 1 and 4), showed nonspecific histologic changes including variation of fiber size, loss of striation and centralization of the nuclei with no evidence of inflammatory cells or vasculitis. Histochemical staining including NADH and phosphorylase reactions did not reveal any specific changes except that the fiber atrophy involved mainly type II fibers in one patient. Nerve conduction velocity and an electromyogram obtained in one patient

TABLE VIII **Laboratory Evaluations in Patients with Steroid Myopathy**

	Case 1	Case 2*	Case 3	Case 4	Case 5	Case 6*	Case 7*	Case 8	Normal Values
Creatinuria† (%)									
During myopathy	35	65	40	40	25	35	70	35	<10%
After improvement	14	20	5	14	—	13	25	2	
CPK									
During myopathy	40	70	65	80	20	60	25	45	<110 MIU
After improvement	—	70	30	30	—	30	40	—	
SGOT									
During myopathy	14	13	13	17	17	14	13	12	<25 HU
After improvement	12	13	12	22	—	—	—	—	

NOTE: MIU = milli-International Unit/100 ml. HU = Henry Unit (a modified Karmen Unit)/100 ml.
*Patients with polymyositis in whom creatinuria decreased during reduction of the prednisone dose but whose creatinuria remained stable due to their primary disease.
† Average values during period of clinical steroid myopathy.

(Case 1) were consistent with peripheral neuropathy.

COMMENTS

Steroid myopathy appears to exhibit threshold characteristics. The variations in tolerance to corticosteroids, reported herein and by other investigators [1,2], do not appear to be related to the age of the patient, the underlying type of connective tissue disease, the magnitude of the dose or the duration of maintenance therapy. Five patients in this study tolerated prednisone at a daily maintenance dose of 15 to 60 mg for a period of 60 to 240 days without displaying any signs or symptoms of steroid myopathy. However, increasing the maintenance dose resulted in the appearance of steroid myopathy within 30 days in four of five patients. Although the development of tolerance and the susceptibility to osteoporosis vary from one patient to another, the presence of the latter does seem to be associated with a more rapid appearance of steroid myopathy.

The appearance of myopathy associated with steroid administration is frequently insidious as shown in the cases reported herein and in the literature [1]. Caution should be exercised in interpreting progressive weakness in patients with polymyositis receiving large doses of prednisone as always due to uncontrolled polymyositis. The acute onset of weakness seen within a few days in two patients, who were not receiving maintenance prednisone therapy, is unusual and has not been reported previously. Sudden onset of muscle weakness can be confused with a flare of polymyositis but, as demonstrated in these two cases, it is not inconsistent with steroid myopathy.

Myalgia was rather common when steroid myopathy first appeared. This symptom has not previously been associated with steroid myopathy but its occurrence, during high dosage steroid therapy, should suggest the diagnosis of steroid-induced myopathy. Myalgias disappeared rapidly after the reduction of steroid dosage, although objective improvement in muscle weakness was delayed. This finding is in agreement with Byers et al. [16] who followed the time course of recovery from muscle weakness due to steroid myopathy by serial muscle examinations.

The pattern of developing muscle weakness in steroid myopathy was similar to that seen in polymyositis [45]. The progression of steroid myopathy occurred in a systematic fashion spreading from the proximal pelvic girdle to the proximal shoulder girdle muscles. When steroid therapy was continued without a reduction in dosage, the distal muscles also became involved, and eventually the weakness became generalized. Although different patterns of weakness were observed in this study, the involvement of upper extremity muscles or of distal muscles alone either in legs or arms was not observed. Such a pattern of isolated muscle weakness is not consistent with the diagnosis of steroid myopathy.

There is no satisfactory explanation for the pattern of muscle weakness found in steroid myopathy. Some insight into the pathogenesis has been gained from the

TABLE IX **Side Effects of Corticosteroids in Patients with Steroid Myopathy**

Side Effect	Total
Cushingoid facies	7
Osteoporosis	
Fracture	3
Without fracture	2
Psychiatric disorders	
Mild euphoria or depression	4
Diabetes	
Insulin	2
Diet alone	1
Hypertension	
Diastolic—blood pressure >100 mm Hg	2
Hypokalemia	
Serum potassium <3.5 meq/liter	0

study of muscle fiber types by histochemical methods. Histochemically, human skeletal muscle fibers can be divided simply into two types. Type I fibers have a low glycolytic and high oxidative activity whereas type II fibers have a high glycolytic and low oxidative activity. Histochemical technics have shown a selective atrophy of type II glycolytic fibers in Cushing's syndrome in human subjects [47]. There have also been a number of histochemical studies of corticosteroid-induced myopathy in experimental animals with a similar suggestion of preferential involvement of type II fibers [35,48]. The relative proportion of the fiber types present in different skeletal muscles might help to explain the pattern of weakness in steroid myopathy, but unfortunately only a few individual human muscles have been adequately typed due to the complex relationships of the different fiber types in various portions of a given muscle [49].

Serum enzyme levels (CPK, aldolase and SGOT) were normal at the onset of steroid myopathy in all patients and remained normal throughout the course of the disease process. This was true even in those patients with polymyositis in whom the serum muscle enzyme levels had been elevated initially in the disease before therapy with prednisone. This finding has been consistent in most of the reports of steroid myopathy although no previous systematic evaluation of serum muscle enzyme levels has been made in a series of cases involving steroid myopathy. In a few case studies of steroid myopathy in which elevated serum enzyme levels were reported, the possibility that hypokalemic myopathy caused the abnormal enzyme elevation must be considered [22].

Creatine excretion was increased in all cases of steroid myopathy at the time of diagnosis. Creatinuria returned towards normal when the daily dose of prednisone was reduced or the patient showed clinical recovery. The measurement of urinary creatine excretion appears to be a sensitive laboratory method for detecting mild degrees of muscle weakness. Abnormal creatinuria was found even in patients with early steroid myopathy and relatively well preserved functional muscle strength. The extent of creatinuria also showed a good correlation with the extent of muscle weakness as determined by manual muscle testing. Increased creatinuria in steroid myopathy has been observed previously [7], but its value in differential diagnosis has not been recognized. Serial determination of serum muscle enzyme levels and urinary creatine excretion can be very helpful in determining whether an increase in muscle weakness, occurring during steroid treatment of connective tissue disease, is due to a worsening of the disease or to steroid myopathy. Although creatinuria is increased in both situations, serum muscle enzyme levels are not elevated when the increased weakness in polymyositis is due to the onset of superimposed steroid myopathy. In contrast, serum enzyme levels frequently are elevated with a flare of polymyositis [50]. Therefore, the finding of an increase in creatinuria in the presence of normal serum enzyme levels suggests steroid myopathy rather than a flare of polymyositis.

In certain cases of polymyositis, serum enzyme levels are not elevated at the onset of a disease flare [50] or even during the entire course of the disease [45], consequently determination of serum enzyme levels is not an effective means of distinguishing steroid myopathy from the disease flare. Differentiation of disease flare from steroid myopathy in these situations can be achieved by the serial determination of creatine excretion and by the patient's clinical recovery as the steroid dose is reduced. If the increased weakness is due to steroid myopathy, a reduction in prednisone dosage results first in a decrease in urinary creatine excretion and then in clinical improvement. On the other hand, a patient with a flare of polymyositis will exhibit enhanced muscle weakness and increased creatinuria when the steroid dose is reduced.

There are few reliable clinical clues that are helpful in suggesting the diagnosis of steroid myopathy, although the appearance of accelerated osteoporosis in a patient with increasing muscle weakness should suggest that the steroid may be associated with these events. In particular, patients receiving prednisone in whom severe osteoporosis develops rapidly resulting in vertebral fracture should be suspected of having a hidden steroid myopathy. These two side effects are late manifestations of hypercortisonism and the presence of one should suggest a search for the other. When steroid myopathy appeared, all of our patients had two or more other undesirable side effects of corticosteroid therapy. The absence of nonmyopathic corticosteroid side effects in patients suspected of steroid-induced myopathy makes the diagnosis less likely. Hypokalemia, a possible cause of muscle weakness and elevated enzyme levels, was consistently absent.

Our results confirm previous reports [1,6,7,13–16,18] that the histologic study of a muscle biopsy specimen is diagnostically unhelpful in patients with steroid myopathy. To our knowledge, the histochemical study of biopsy specimens in human steroid myopathy, with predominantly type II fiber atrophy, has not been reported previously except in Cushing's syndrome [47]. Unfortunately, both histochemical and electron-microscopic studies of muscle biopsy specimens have provided little practical assistance in diagnosis [1,15,18]. Electromyographic studies have given confusing results which have been interpreted as indicating the presence of myopathy, neuropathy, neuromyopathy or even that the muscle was normal [1,9,14–17,22].

Our study suggests that the most useful laboratory approach for the diagnosis of steroid myopathy is the concomitant serial determination of the serum muscle enzymes and urinary excretion of creatine during steroid reduction. This approach has the advantage of being noninvasive.

The recovery time for steroid myopathy is variable, but most often it takes from one to four months. None of our patients showed recurrence of steroid myopathy during a follow-up period of observation of 120 to 360 days.

REFERENCES

1. Afifi AK, Bergman RA, Harvey JC: Steroid myopathy, clinical, histologic and cytologic observation. Johns Hopkins Med J 123: 158, 1968.
2. Dubois EL: Triamcinolone in the treatment of systemic lupus erythematosus. JAMA 167: 1590, 1958.
3. Fryberg RH, Bernsten CA, Helman L: Further experience with triamcinolone in treatment of patients with rheumatoid arthritis. Arthritis Rheum 1: 215, 1958.
4. Walton CHA: Clinical experience with dexamethasone. Can Med Assoc J 81: 724, 1959.
5. Williams RS: Triamcinolone myopathy. Lancet 1: 698, 1959.
6. MacLean K, Schurr PH: Reversible amyotrophy complicating treatment with fludrocortisone. Lancet 1: 701, 1959.
7. Perkoff GT, Silber R, Tyler FH, et al.: Studies in disorders of muscles. XII. Myopathy due to the administration of therapeutic amounts of 17-hydroxycorticosteroids. Am J Med 26: 891, 1959.
8. Kendal PH, Hart MF: Side effects following triamcinolone. Br Med J 1: 682, 1959.
9. Harman JB: Muscular wasting and corticosteroid therapy. Lancet 1: 887, 1959.
10. Neustadt DH: Corticosteroid therapy in rheumatoid arthritis. JAMA 170: 1253, 1959.
11. Robinson CE, Robinson HS: Triamcinolone in rheumatoid arthritis. Can Med Assoc J 80: 245, 1959.
12. Dunenci J, Chodosh S, Segal MS: Dexamethasone therapy in bronchial asthma. Ann Allerg 17: 695, 1959.
13. Syme JR: Muscle wasting complicating treatment with dexamethasone. Med J Aust 2: 240, 1960.
14. Hagstrom JWC, Roseman DM, Ellis JT: Debilitating muscular wasting and steroid therapy. Arch Neurol 5: 60, 1961.
15. Golding DN, Murray SM, Pearce GW, et al.: Corticosteroid myopathy. Ann Phys Med 5: 171, 1961.
16. Byers RK, Bergman AB, Joseph MC: Steroid myopathy: report of five cases occurring during treatment of rheumatic fever. Pediatrics 29: 26, 1962.
17. Coomes EN: The role of recovery of reversible myopathies and the effect of anabolic agents in steroid myopathy. Neurology 15: 523, 1966.
18. Engel AG: Electron microscopic observations in thyrotoxic and corticosteroid myopathies. Mayo Clinic Proc 41: 785, 1966.
19. Bauer FK, Dubois EL, Teleer N: Total exchangeable potassium in SLE with reference to triamcinolone myopathy. Proc Soc Exp Biol Med 105: 671, 1960.
20. Williams GT: A comparative evaluation of newer corticosteroids in the treatment of rheumatoid arthritis. South Med J 52: 267, 1959.
21. Boland EW: 16 α-methyl corticosteroids, a new series of anti-inflammatory compounds, clinical appraisal of anti-inflammatory compounds, clinical appraisal of antirheumatic potencies. Calif Med 88: 417, 1958.
22. Powell RJ: Steroid and hypokalemic myopathy after corticosteroids for ulcerative colitis. Am J Gastroenterol 52: 425, 1969.
23. Bunim JJ, Ziff M, McEwen C: Evaluation of prolonged cortisone therapy in rheumatoid arthritis. Am J Med 18: 27, 1955.
24. Coomes EN: Corticosteroid myopathy. Ann Rheum Dis 24: 465, 1965.
25. Stern R, Amundsen P: Diphenylhydantoin for steroid-induced muscle weakness. JAMA 223: 1287, 1973.
26. Faludi G, Gotlieb J, Meyers J: Factors influencing the development of steroid-induced myopathy. Ann NY Acad Sci 138: 61, 1966.
27. Bullock GR, Christian RA, Peters RF, et al.: Rapid mitochondrial enlargement in muscle as a response to triamcinolone acetonide and its relationship to the ribosomal defect. Biochem Pharmacol 20: 943, 1971.
28. Comez-Puyow A, Pena-Dias A, Gwzman-Garcia J, et al.: Effect of triamcinolone and other steroids on the oxidative phosphorylation reaction. Biochem Pharmacol 12: 331, 1963.
29. Kimberg DV, Loud AV, Wiener J: Cortisone-induced alterations in mitochondrial function and structure. J Cell Biol 37: 63, 1968.
30. Peter JB, Verhaag DA, Worsfold M: Studies of steroid myopathy. Examination of the possible effect of triamcinolone on mitochondria and sarcotubular vesicles of rat skeletal muscle. Biochem Pharmacol 19: 1627, 1970.
31. Tice LW, Engel AG: The effect of glucocorticoids on red and white muscles in the rat. Am J Pathol 50: 311, 1967.
32. Afifi AK, Bergman RA: Steroid myopathy. A study of evolution of the muscle lesion in rabbits. Johns Hopkins Med J 124: 66, 1969.
33. D'Agostino AN, Chiga M: Cortisone myopathy in rabbits, a light and electron microscopic study. Neurology 16: 257, 1966.
34. Ellis JT: Necrosis and regeneration of skeletal muscles in cortisone-treated rabbits. Am J Pathol 32: 993, 1956.
35. Sheahan MG, Vignos PJ: Experimental corticosteroid myopathy. Arthritis Rheum 12: 491, 1969.
36. Smith B: Histological and histochemical changes in muscles of rabbits given the corticosteroid triamcinolone. Neurology 14: 857, 1964.
37. Faludi G, Mills LD, Chayes ZW: Effects of steroids on muscle. Acta Endocrinol 45: 68, 1964.
38. Daniels L, Williams M, Worthingham C: Muscle Testing: Techniques of Manual Examination, 2nd ed, Philadelphia, W. B. Saunders Co., 1956.
39. Sibley JA, Lehninger AL: Determination of aldolase in animal tissue. J Biol Chem 177: 859, 1949.
40. Cook JL, Dounce AH: Determination of serum aldolase. Proc Soc Exp Biol Med 87: 349, 1954.
41. Siegel AL, Cohen PS: Automation in analytical chemistry. An automated determination of creatine phosphokinase. A Technicon Symposia. Medical Inc., 1966, p 474.
42. Morgenstern S, Oklander M, Auerbach J, et al.: Automated determination of serum glutamic oxaloacetic transaminase. Clin Chem 12: 95, 1966.
43. Clark LC, Thompson HL, Beck EI, et al.: Excretion of creatine and creatinine by children. Am J Dis Child 81: 774, 1951.

44. Anker RM: Determination of creatine and creatinine in the urine. J Lab Clin Med 43: 798, 1954.
45. Vignos PJ Jr, Bowling GF, Watkins MP: Polymyositis, effect of corticosteroids on final results. Arch Intern Med 114: 263, 1964.
46. Dubowitz V, Pearse AGE: A comparative histochemical study of oxidative enzyme and phosphorylase activity in skeletal muscle. Histochemie 2: 105, 1960.
47. Pleasure DE, Walsh GO, Engel WK: Atrophy of skeletal muscle in patients with Cushing's syndrome. Arch Neurol 22: 118, 1970.
48. Vignos PJ Jr, Green R: Oxidative respiration of skeletal muscle in experimental corticosteroid myopathy. J Lab Clin Med 81: 365, 1973.
49. Brooke MH, Engel WK: The histographic analysis of human muscle biopsies with regard to fiber types 1: adult male and female. Neurology 19: 221, 1969.
50. Vignos PJ Jr, Goldwyn J: Evaluation of laboratory test in diagnosis and management of polymyositis. Am J Med Sci 263: 291, 1972.

Simultaneous Antibiotic Levels in "Breakthrough" Gram-Negative Rod Bacteremia

ELIZABETH T. ANDERSON, M.D.
LOWELL S. YOUNG, M.D.
WILLIAM L. HEWITT, M.D.
Los Angeles, California

Of 237 cases of gram-negative rod bacteremia observed at the UCLA Medical Center during a 12 month period, 52 (22 per cent) occurred while the patient was receiving antibiotics which inhibited the infecting organism by disc diffusion tests. One half of the plasma samples available from 42 such patients with "breakthrough" bacteremia had subinhibitory circulating antibiotic levels when cultures were positive. Sepsis documented within 72 hours of initiation of therapy was usually due to antibiotic-sensitive Esch. coli and was associated with inadequate antibiotic levels; the patient was usually treated with a penicillin or cephalosporin. The source of bacteremia was most frequently the urinary tract or the biliary tree. In contrast, sepsis occurring more than 72 hours after the administration of antibiotics was frequently caused by multiple antibiotic-resistant Esch. coli in patients treated with gentamicin in adequate dosage and was associated with leukopenia or undrained purulent collections. Therapy ultimately failed in 20 cases (48 per cent): in early "breakthrough" bacteremia, failure was associated with subinhibitory antibiotic levels, and in late "breakthrough" bacteremias with inadequate drainage or impaired host defenses.

Septicemia caused by gram-negative bacilli continues to be associated with high morbidity and mortality. Selection of antimicrobial therapy is usually guided by in vitro tests of the antibiotic susceptibility of the infecting organism. Despite the initiation of "appropriate" therapy, however, some patients continue to be clinically ill and are found to have persistent or recurrent bacteremia [1–4]. Such failures despite appropriate therapy, here termed "breakthrough" bacteremia, may have several explanations, but little attention has been directed to the adequacy of antibiotic therapy in such cases as determined by measurements of simultaneous antibiotic blood levels at the time of "breakthrough."

The initiation of a new blood culture system at our institution in which an aliquot of heparinized plasma is obtained simultaneously with the specimen for culture permits an assessment of some of the clinical, microbiologic and pharmacologic factors associated with "breakthrough" bacteremia. During a 12 month period, 52 such instances were observed, which represented 22 per cent of the blood cultures positive for gram-negative bacilli.

From the Division of Infectious Diseases, Department of Medicine, UCLA Center for the Health Sciences, Los Angeles, California 90024. This study was supported by Research Grant No. AI-11271 and U.S. Public Health Service Training Grant No. AI-309 from the National Institute of Allergy and Infectious Diseases. It was presented at the Fourteenth Annual Interscience Conference on Antimicrobial Agents and Chemotherapy, September 12, 1974, San Francisco, California. Requests for reprints should be addressed to Dr. Lowell S. Young, Division of Infectious Diseases, Department of Medicine, UCLA Center for the Health Sciences, Los Angeles, California 90024. Manuscript accepted February 27, 1976.

MATERIALS AND METHODS

Hospital records of all patients at the UCLA Medical Center who had one or more positive blood cultures for gram-negative bacilli between July 1, 1973, and June 30, 1974, were reviewed. All patients with persistent or recurrent bacteremia, despite more than 24 hours of treatment with an antibiotic to which the infecting organism was reported as sensitive by disc-diffusion test [5], were included in this analysis. Excluded from review were patients with positive blood cultures thought to be due to contamination rather than clinical illness. Patients were considered leukopenic if less than 2,000 mature granulocytes/mm^3 were circulating in their blood at the time of sepsis. The outcome of sepsis was considered a success if the patient was cured and left the hospital, or if the febrile episode resolved and the patient survived at least a week after bacteremia. The outcome was judged a failure if the patient died febrile or if another "breakthrough" occurred 24 or more hours after the first. A control group of patients with various illnesses were selected for this study by reviewing all patients with gram-negative sepsis in whom a second blood specimen was submitted for culture (which was negative) in the week after bacteremia was documented and while the patient was receiving appropriate antibiotic therapy.

Blood for culture at the UCLA Hospital is inoculated into a thioglycollate and an enrichment broth medium. A simultaneously obtained heparinized sample from the same blood specimen (heparin 15 U/ml) must also be submitted as part of the blood culture "set." Bottles containing blood for culture and special media are incubated at 37°C for eight days. Plasma is separated from the heparinized sample and refrigerated at 4°C within 1 hour, following which it is frozen at −20°C. Serum antimicrobial assays in cases of "breakthrough" bacteremia were performed on the *same* sample from which bacteria were isolated.

An agar well diffusion technic, as previously described [6,7], was utilized for antibiotic assays using either Bacillus globigii or Klebsiella pneumoniae as the seed organism. For assaying aminoglycoside in serum also containing a penicillin or cephalosporin, the activity of the latter compounds was destroyed by use of penicillinase or cephalosporinase. Circulating levels of the latter antibiotics in the presence of an aminoglycoside were measured using the low pH agar technic of Sabath et al. [8]. Additionally, all measurements of aminoglycosides were also carried out by either radioimmunoassay for gentamicin or radioenzymatic acetylation for gentamicin, kanamycin or amikacin, using a previously described method [7]. The same set of antibiotic "standards" was consistently employed for aminoglycoside assays, and the results of gentamicin assays by the different methods showed close correlation [8]. The concentration of heparin used for anticoagulation was always below that which would interfere with the determination of aminoglycoside content.

In addition to disc sensitivity tests, which served as a screening measure, the minimum inhibitory concentration of the antibiotic used was determined for each isolate by the broth dilution technic recommended by the International Collaborative Study on Antibiotic Susceptibility Testing sponsored by the World Health Organization [9].

RESULTS

Two hundred and thirty-seven episodes of gram-negative rod bacteremia occurred during the 12 month period of this study. Fifty-two blood cultures were positive despite the patient's receiving at least 24 hours of apparently "appropriate" antibiotic therapy. Thus, "breakthrough" bacteremia occurred in 22 per cent of the patients. However, isolates from four patients that were initially reported "sensitive" by disc diffusion methods were subsequently found to be resistant by broth dilution sensitivity tests. One organism was a K. pneumoniae resistant to cephalothin; three were Esch. coli, two resistant to cephalothin, one to ampicillin. In five patients a simultaneous plasma specimen was not available for study and in one the organism was lost. After eliminating these 10 patients, a total of 42 "breakthroughs" and 29 control patients were evaluated. The 42 bacteremias occurred in 34 patients, representing one episode in 28, two in four and three in two. In one patient the two bacteremias occurred two months apart, representing two distinct episodes. The other patients were septic on two or three occasions one to four days apart. Of the 42 "breakthroughs," 13 (in 11 patients) occurred within 48 hours of admission and were considered to be community acquired; 29 (in 23 patients) occurred five or more days after hospital admission and were considered nosocomial. Twelve (in 10 patients) community-acquired infections were early "breakthroughs" and all patients survived, although two had a second "breakthrough" during the illness. In the 42 cases studied, Esch. coli was isolated in 22 cases, P. aeruginosa in eight cases, K. pneumoniae in six cases, and other gram-negative bacilli in six cases.

Antibiotic levels exceeded the minimum inhibitory concentration for the organism at the time of "breakthrough" in approximately half of both study patients with bacteremias and the control group of patients with various illnesses. Since most clinicians would observe a patient for 48 to 72 hours while receiving appropriate therapy before becoming concerned about failure of therapy, we analyzed the data separately (Table I) for "breakthrough" bacteremias that occurred between 24 and 72 hours after antibiotic therapy was started (19 episodes) and those which occurred when the patient had received 72 hours or more of "appropriate" antibiotic therapy (23 episodes). All but one episode of late "breakthrough" bacteremia was a nosocomial infection.

In the group with early "breakthrough" bacteremias, 12 of 19 (63 per cent) occurred when the antibiotic level was inadequate to inhibit in vitro the infecting organism; eight of 23 (35 per cent) late "breakthrough" bacteremias were associated with subinhibitory circulating antibiotic levels. The most common pathogen in both

TABLE I Antimicrobial Therapy, Host Factors and Outcome in 42 Cases of "Breakthrough" Bacteremia

		Early "Breakthrough" (19)		Late "Breakthrough" (23)	
		Treatment		Treatment	
	Total	Adequate (7)	Inadequate (12)	Adequate (15)	Inadequate (8)
Antibiotic therapy					
Gentamicin	27	6	3	11	7
Cephalosporin	9	2*	5	1	1†
Ampicillin	4	—	3	1	—
Other	4	—	1	2	1
Host factors					
Leukopenia	16	5	2	5	4
Urinary tract or biliary infection	13	1	8	2	2
Abscess	7	—	—	6	1
Other	6	1	2	2	1
Outcome					
Another "breakthrough"	11	2	2	5	2
Death	9	2	2	4	1
Failure	20	4	4	9	3
Success	22	3	8	6	5

NOTE: Figures in parentheses indicate the number of patients.
*The concentrations of both gentamicin and a cephalosporin were adequate in one patient given both antibiotics.
†The concentrations of both gentamicin and a cephalosporin were inadequate in one patient treated with these two agents.

groups was Esch. coli, 10 of 19 (53 per cent) and 12 of 23 (52 per cent) in early and late "breakthrough" bacteremias, respectively. Esch. coli isolates in cases of early "breakthrough" bacteremias were susceptible to a wider range of antibiotics; nine of 10 and seven of 10 strains were sensitive to kanamycin and carbenicillin and eight of 10 and seven of 10 were inhibited by cephalothin and ampicillin. The late "breakthrough" bacteremias tended to be due to more resistant organisms. As in the group with early "breakthroughs," all were sensitive to gentamicin and chloramphenicol, but only eight of 12 and seven of 12 were sensitive to kanamycin and carbenicillin, and four of 12 and three of 12 were inhibited by cephalothin and ampicillin, respectively.

Gentamicin was the most commonly used antibiotic to treat the patients with these episodes of bacteremia. Nine of 19 in the group with early "breakthroughs" and 18 of 23 in the group with late "breakthroughs" (Table I) were treated with this drug. Ten of 27 (37 per cent) of those treated with gentamicin had subinhibitory levels at the time bacteremia was proved by culture. Subinhibitory gentamicin levels were seen in three of nine with early "breakthrough" bacteremias and in seven of 18 with late "breakthrough" bacteremias. After excluding patients with renal failure, there were no systematic differences in dose selected to treat the remaining 18 patients in whom 25 cases of bacteremia occurred. Only two of the patients with early "breakthrough" bacteremias had received an initial dose of 2.0 mg/kg of gentamicin. Those with inhibitory circulating gentamicin blood levels received only an average dose of 3.3 mg/kg/day whereas those with inadequate gentamicin levels received an average dose of 5.0 mg/kg/day. Although a slightly higher proportion of patients with late "breakthrough" bacteremia received initial doses of 1.5 to 2.0 mg/kg gentamicin, by 72 hours of treatment this should have made little difference. Among the patients with late "breakthrough" bacteremia, those with adequate levels were treated with an average dose of 4.3 mg/kg/day; those with inadequate levels received an average dose of 3.5 mg/kg/day.

Thirteen "breakthrough" bacteremias occurred in patients being treated with beta-lactam antibiotics administered in usual dosage, in two patients in combination with gentamicin. Of these, most (10 of 13) were early "breakthroughs" and in nine of 13 patients circulating antibiotic levels were subinhibitory. Five "breakthrough" bacteremias occurred in patients receiving oral antibiotics, four were treated with cephalexin and one with ampicillin. All but one of these patients were found to have subinhibitory blood levels, the exception being a patient in renal failure.

Patients with "breakthrough" bacteremia all had identifiable, severe illnesses (Table I). The early "breakthrough" bacteremias occurred most frequently in patients with urinary tract infection or cholangitis for a total of nine of 19 (47 per cent). Of the remaining 10, seven early "breakthrough" bacteremias occurred in leukopenic patients, two bacteremias were from unknown sources and one occurred in a patient with septic pelvic thrombophlebitis. Eight of the nine bacteremias complicating urinary tract infection or cholangitis were associated with subinhibitory antibiotic levels.

Late "breakthrough" bacteremias occurred most frequently in patients with leukopenia (nine of 23 cases) due to leukemia [6] or aplastic anemia [3]. In the nonleukopenic population late "breakthrough" bacteremias were observed in six patients with undrained abdominal abscesses or liver abscesses. In "breakthroughs" after 72 hours of therapy, most patients (15 of 23 or 65 per cent) had adequate circulating levels of antibiotic. The bacteremias in adequately treated patients were associated with leukopenia or undrained purulent collections in 11 of 15 (73 per cent) instances.

The outcome of therapy was discouraging with 48 per cent of the bacteremias ending in a second "breakthrough" or death due to the septic episode (Table I). In general, adequate antibiotic levels did not significantly affect the outcome. Despite inadequate circulating antibiotic levels, there was a tendency for the outcome in early "breakthrough" bacteremias to be slightly more successful than in late ones, 11 of 19 (58 per cent) as opposed to 11 of 23 (48 per cent), perhaps due to less adverse host factors.

During the same year the "breakthrough" bacteremias were studied, 29 patients known to have gram-negative sepsis and in whom a second blood culture was negative while they were receiving appropriate therapy for three to seven days were similarly studied. Plasma submitted with the negative culture was assayed for antibiotic levels which were related to the minimum inhibitory concentration of the initial infecting organism. In this control group of patients with negative blood cultures, antibiotic levels were equally likely to be adequate or inadequate as judged by the minimum inhibitory concentration of the organism causing bacteremia. Specifically, levels were adequate in 13 and inadequate in 16 of this group of 29 controls. This group showed a similar predominance of Esch. coli as the cause of bacteremia (10 of 29 cases), and gentamicin was similarly the antibiotic to which the organism was sensitive (21 of 29 cases). Underlying disease was usually less severe; only 11 of 19 episodes occurred in the face of leukopenia or undrained abscesses. The outcome was more benign, as 25 of 29 cases were therapeutic successes.

COMMENTS

The significant morbidity and mortality from gram-negative rod bacteremia have led many investigators to assess factors influencing the incidence, course and outcome of this infection [10–13]. Although it has been apparent that underlying disease is the most important determinant of survival, recent reports have suggested that early, aggressive antimicrobial therapy, particularly in patients with impaired host resistance such as those with leukopenia, is associated with improved clinical results [12,14].

We have observed in our institution a surprisingly high incidence of positive blood cultures despite the patient's being treated for at least 24 hours with appropriate antibiotics—fully 22 per cent of gram-negative rod bacteremias. We wished to delineate whether therapeutic failures might be associated with inadequate antimicrobial therapy or attributed primarily to adverse host factors. Because plasma samples were available from the same blood which was culture-positive, we were able to determine circulating antibiotic levels at the time bacteremia was documented. Although previous investigators have attempted to ascertain adequacy of antibiotic therapy by examining antibiotic dose [1,2] and serum inhibitory capacity [17], little attention has been paid to simultaneous antibiotic levels in a series of patients with persistent or recurrent bacteremia despite supposedly adequate therapy.

Our data indicate that about one-half of the episodes of "breakthrough" bacteremia are associated with subinhibitory antibiotic levels. This proportion was similar to that in the "control" group of patients selected for comparison study because blood for a repeat culture (later shown to be negative) was drawn after the start of therapy. Although an equal proportion of episodes in the "breakthrough" group and the control group occurred in the face of inadequate blood levels of antibiotic, the groups were not comparable, since both sterilization of the bloodstream and the improved outcome in the "control" group could be attributed to less adverse host factors.

When our data were evaluated by dividing those with "breakthrough" bacteremia into "early" and "late" groups, we delineated two distinct groups of patients. Early "breakthrough" bacteremias originated most frequently from urinary or biliary foci, and the patients were frequently inadequately treated. In particular, inadequate levels of beta-lactam antibiotics (e.g., a penicillin or cephalosporin) could be implicated in therapeutic failures. This may reflect, in part, inadequate absorption of the antibiotic rather than inadequate dosing, as oral rather than parenteral medication was used in five of 10 cases in this group.

The clinical outcome was still poor in those with early "breakthrough" bacteremia, and it would seem that improvement in antibiotic therapy, either by use of parenteral rather than oral doses, larger loading doses or larger daily doses might have improved the outcome. Further, it was not possible to document the interval between the last antibiotic dose and the exact time that a specimen was obtained for blood culture, so we cannot evaluate whether "breakthroughs" are more likely to occur during "valleys" in intermittent antibiotic dose schedules.

Some patients with prolonged gram-negative bacteremia have been found to have serious intravascular infections [3,4], an entity we did not observe in this series. We, and other investigators, have suggested that host factors are the major cause of therapeutic failure, but we have also proposed that antibiotics with low therapeutic ratio might allow "breakthroughs" during "valleys" of therapy, particularly when using agents like gentamicin when intervals between doses may be long [1,2]. The late "breakthroughs" we observed did occur with multiple antibiotic-resistant organisms; the antibiotic most frequently used for therapy, namely, gentamicin, reflected this fact. Gentamicin has a low therapeutic ratio, and because of concern for renal toxicity in desperately ill patients with fluctuating renal perfusion, it has frequently been used in inadequate dose. However, in our hospital, rapid gentamicin assay is available and customarily used to judge adequacy of therapy. In those with late "breakthrough" bacteremias treated with gentamicin, an adequate circulating antibiotic concentration was achieved to inhibit most of the causative gram-negative bacilli in vitro. Host factors in these cases were adverse, consisting usually of marked leukopenia or undrained abscesses, and seemed to be a more important factor than antibiotic dosage.

We have four basic conclusions from this study. First, documentation of bacteremia in the face of apparently "appropriate" antimicrobial therapy should be the impetus for immediate broth or agar dilution sensitivity testing to validate the result obtained by disc diffusion tests. Four episodes of sepsis in this series were initially thought to be "breakthroughs" but instead represented erroneous determination of in vitro antibiotic susceptibility; the organism was subsequently proved to be resistant to the antibiotic used. Secondly, physicians should not assume therapeutic levels are predictably achieved with conventional drug doses. This is particularly true for drugs with low therapeutic ratios such as gentamicin. The need for a "loading dose" of gentamicin is not widely appreciated, yet in our experience the peak level following an initial dose is usually lower than that following succeeding doses of the same size. Other studies have demonstrated considerable variation in blood levels achieved with commonly used dosage regimens of this drug [2,6,15,16]. Monitoring of serum levels if readily, rapidly and reliably available may be helpful as a guide to adequacy of therapy. This may be especially true in critically ill patients in whom assurance of adequate antimicrobial levels is crucial and in patients with renal impairment in whom such levels may be less predictable [16]. Thirdly, the oral administration of antibiotics, especially oral cephalosporins, frequently does not result in blood levels sufficient to inhibit gram-negative rods in vitro and should not be used in the treatment of serious infection likely to be caused by gram-negative rods. Finally, "late" "breakthrough" bacteremias are usually associated with seriously impaired host defenses or undrained abscesses. Detection and alleviation of the latter are obviously mandatory for successful therapy, and the eventual outcome in this group is critically related to amelioration of predisposing factors and underlying disease.

ACKNOWLEDGMENT

The expert technical assistance of Nalinee Linpisal, Foek-nan Teng and Shahnza K. Raza is gratefully acknowledged.

REFERENCES

1. Young LS: Gentamicin: Clinical use with carbenicillin and in vitro studies with recent isolates of Pseudomonas aeruginosa. J Infect Dis 124 (suppl): 202, 1971.
2. Jackson G, Riff LJ: Pseudomonas bacteremia: pharmacologic and other bases for failure of treatment with gentamicin. J Infect Dis 124 (suppl): S185, 1971.
3. Harris JA, Cobbs GE: Persistent gram-negative bacteremia. Am J Surg 125: 705, 1973.
4. McHenry MC, Gavan TL, Hawk WA, et al.: Gram-negative bacteremia of long duration. Cleve Clin Q 40: 47, 1973.
5. Barry AL, Garcia F, Thrupp LD: An improved single disk method for testing the antibiotic susceptibility of rapidly growing pathogens. Am J Clin Pathol 53: 149, 1970.
6. Winters RE, Litwack KD, Hewitt WL: Relation between dose and levels of gentamicin in blood. J Infect Dis 124 (suppl): S90, 1971.
7. Stevens P, Young LS, Hewitt WL: Radioimmunoassay, acetylating radio-enzymatic assay, and microbioassay of gentamicin: a comparative study. J Lab Clin Med 86: 349, 1975.
8. Sabath LD, Casey JI, Ruch PA: Rapid microassay of gentamicin, kanamycin, neomycin, streptomycin, and vancomycin in serum or plasma. J Lab Clin Med 78: 457, 1971.
9. Ericsson HM, Sherris JC: Antibiotic sensitivity testing: report of an international collaborative study. Acta Pathol Microbiol Scand [B], No. 217, p 64, 1971.
10. McCabe WR, Jackson GG: Gram-negative bacteremia. II. Clinical, laboratory, and therapeutic observations. Arch Intern Med 110: 856, 1962.
11. Dupont HL, Spink WW: Infections due to gram-negative organisms: an analysis of 860 patients with bacteremia at the University of Minnesota Medical Center, 1958–1966. Medicine (Baltimore) 48: 307, 1969.
12. Myerowitz RL, Medeiros AA, O'Brien TF: Recent experience with bacillemia due to gram-negative organisms. J Infect Dis 124: 239, 1971.
13. McHenry MC, Gavan TL, Hawk WA, et al.: Gram-negative bacteremia; variable clinical course and useful prognostic factors. Cleve Clin Q 42: 15, 1975.
14. Schimpff S, Saterlee W, Young VM, et al.: Therapy with carbenicillin and gentamicin in febrile cancer patients. N Engl J Med 284: 1061, 1971.
15. Kaye D, Levison ME, Labovitz ED: The unpredictability of serum concentrations of gentamicin. Pharmacokinetics of gentamicin in patients with normal and abnormal renal function. J Infect Dis 130: 150, 1974.
16. Hewitt WL: Reflections on the clinical pharmacology of gentamicin. Acta Pathol Microbiol Scand [B] Suppl No. 241, p 151, 1973.
17. Klastersky J, Daneau D, Swings G, et al.: Antibacterial activity in serum and urine as a therapeutic guide in bacterial infections. J Infect Dis 129: 187, 1974.

Serious Infections in Adults Due to Group B Streptococci

Clinical and Serotypic Characterization

ARNOLD S. BAYER, M.D.
ANTHONY W. CHOW, M.D.
BASCOM F. ANTHONY, M.D.
LUCIEN B. GUZE, M.D.
Torrance, California

Serious infections in adults due to group B streptococci have been infrequently reported. We describe 24 such patients. Bacteremic pyelonephritis, pneumonitis and endometritis were the most common clinical syndromes observed. Group B streptococcal infections tended to occur in patients with underlying illnesses, particularly genitourinary disorders and diabetes mellitus. Mortality was surprisingly low (8 per cent). Type III was the serotype most commonly isolated, and there was no significant correlation of different serotypes with specific organ-system involvement. Group B streptococcal isolates from these patients were uniformly sensitive to penicillin, ampicillin, cephalothin, chloramphenicol, erythromycin and clindamycin; all were highly resistant to kanamycin. Eighty-seven per cent were resistant to tetracycline. Although consistently sensitive to penicillin, the minimal inhibitory concentrations were significantly higher for group B than group A streptococci ($p < 0.0005$).

Lancefield group B streptococci have been recently recognized as a leading cause of neonatal sepsis [1–4]. The clinical spectrum of group B streptococcal infections in adults, however, has not been fully characterized. In addition, data on the serotypic distribution of strains causing infections in adults are lacking. In the present report we describe 24 adult patients with serious group B streptococcal infections, document the prevalence of group B streptococcal bacteremia among the adult population of one general hospital and examine the distribution of serotypes and antibiotic susceptibilities of these pathogens among this patient population.

MATERIALS AND METHODS

All streptococci isolated from blood and other body fluids (e.g., synovial fluid, cerebrospinal fluid) of non-neonatal patients hospitalized at Harbor General Hospital (HGH) between September 1972 and September 1975 were studied. Presumptive identification of these isolates as groups A, B and D (both enterococcal and nonenterococcal) was carried out by screening tests including: (1) hemolysis, (2) bacitracin sensitivity, (3) hippurate hydrolysis, (4) bile-esculin hydrolysis and (5) salt tolerance, according to the criteria of Facklam et al. [5]. Such screening tests have been shown to correlate in over 90 per cent of cases with formal Lancefield serogrouping. Organisms presumptively identified as group B streptococci by positive-hippurate hydrolysis were further studied by the precipitin reaction with antiserums to Lancefield groups

From the Departments of Medicine and Pediatrics, Harbor General Hospital, Torrance, California 90509; Research and Medical Services, Wadsworth Hospital, Veterans Administration Center, Los Angeles, California 90073; and Department of Medicine, UCLA School of Medicine, Los Angeles, California 90024. This investigation was supported in part by U.S. Public Health Service Grant HD 07559. Requests for reprints should be addressed to Dr. Arnold S. Bayer, Division of Infectious Disease, Harbor General Hospital, 1000 West Carson Street, Torrance, California 90509. Manuscript accepted February 17, 1976.

A to G [6]. Confirmed Lancefield group B streptococci were serotyped as previously described [7]. Antiserums for Lancefield grouping of streptococci and serotyping of group B isolates were supplied by the Center for Disease Control, Atlanta, Georgia.

Antibiotic susceptibilities of group B isolates were determined by the Kirby-Bauer disc-diffusion technic [8] with the following disc contents: penicillin (10 U), ampicillin (10 μg), cephalothin (30 μg), kanamycin (30 μg), erythromycin (15 μg), clindamycin (2 μg), chloramphenicol (30 μg) and tetracycline (30 μg). Additionally, minimal inhibitory concentrations of penicillin, tetracycline and kanamycin for these pathogens were determined by an agar dilution technic [9].

Medical records of all patients with culture-proved group B streptococcal infections were reviewed and pertinent clinical data extracted. Multiple group B streptococcal isolates from a single patient, unless differing clearly in serotype and/or antibiotic sensitivity pattern, were regarded as a single strain.

RESULTS

During the 36-month study period, 350 streptococcal isolates were recovered from blood and other body fluids of non-neonatal patients. Of these, 28 isolates were hippurate hydrolysis-positive (8 per cent), and all 28 were subsequently confirmed as group B streptococci by Lancefield serogrouping. Of note, nine of these

TABLE I Clinical Features of 24 Adults with Serious Group B Streptococcal Infections

Case No.	Age (yr) and Sex	Predisposing Condition(s)	Type(s) of Infections	Positive Cultures: Blood	Positive Cultures: Other*	Therapy	Outcome
1	49,F	Bladder laceration	Pyelonephritis	+	Urine	Clindamycin	S†
2	33,F	Postpartum; prolonged membrane rupture	Endometritis	+	Cervix	Ampicillin	S
3	71,M	Prostatic hypertrophy	Pyelonephritis	+	Urine	Penicillin	S
4	61,M	Diabetes	Cellulitis; endocarditis; meningitis	+	Leg ulcer; cerebrospinal fluid	Penicillin	S
5	59,F	Diabetes; glioma	Pneumonia	+	Sputum	Penicillin	S
6	44,F	Diabetes; liver disease	Pneumonia	+	Sputum	Penicillin	S
7	31,M	Diabetes	Pneumonia	+	Sputum	Penicillin	S
8	29,M	Trauma	Septic arthritis	—	Synovial fluid	Penicillin	S
9	22,F	Postpartum	Endometritis; pyelonephritis	+	Urine; cervix	Ampicillin	S
10	24,M	Diabetes; renal failure	Cellulitis	+	Cutaneous abscess	Penicillin	S
11	37,M	Diabetes	Pneumonia	+	Sputum	Cephalothin	Died
12	53,F	Liver disease	Peritonitis	+	Ascitic fluid	Penicillin	S
13	20,F	Postpartum; preeclampsia	Endometritis	+	Cervix	Ampicillin	S
14	17,F	Postpartum; prolonged membrane rupture	Endometritis	+	Cervix	Ampicillin	S
15	16,F	Postpartum; preeclampsia	Endometritis	+	Cervix	Ampicillin	S
16	50,F	Diabetes	Pneumonia	+	Sputum	Penicillin	Died
17	24,M	Diabetes	Septic arthritis	—	Synovial fluid, urine	Penicillin	S
18	36,F	Diabetes; postpartum; prolonged membrane rupture	Endometritis	+	Cervix	Cephalothin; Clindamycin	S
19	89,M	Diabetes	Pyelonephritis	+	Urine	Ampicillin	Died
20	21,M	Trauma	Tracheobronchitis	+	Sputum	Erythromycin	S
21	63,M	Diabetes; chronic Foley catheter	Pyelonephritis	+	Urine	Ampicillin	S
22	61,M	Interstitial fibrosis	Pneumonia	+	Sputum	Penicillin	Died
23	70,M	Renal carcinoma; renal failure	Meningitis; pyelonephritis	+	Cerebrospinal fluid; urine	Penicillin	S
24	79,M	Prostatic hypertrophy renal failure	Meningitis; pyelonephritis	+	Cerebrospinal fluid; urine	Penicillin	Died

* Streptococci other than those from cerebrospinal fluid, ascitic fluid and synovial fluid were not specifically serogrouped or serotyped, but had hemolytic reactions, bacitracin sensitivities, bile-esculin reactions and disc antibiograms identical to concomitant blood or other body fluid isolates confirmed to be group B streptococci by Lancefield grouping. All urine cultures were pure for group B streptococcal organisms (>10^5 organisms/ml).

† S = survived.

28 isolates (32 per cent) were also bacitracin-sensitive and would have been misidentified as group A streptococci without further characterization.

These 28 group B streptococcal isolates were recovered from 24 adult patients. Twenty-two were isolated from blood, three from cerebrospinal fluid, two from synovial fluid and one from ascitic fluid. Group B streptococci, therefore, were responsible for approximately 2 per cent of all non-neonatal bacteremias (22 of 1,374), 4 per cent of non-neonatal gram-positive coccal bacteremias (22 of 528) and 8 per cent of non-neonatal streptococcal bacteremias (22 of 282) at HGH during this same period.

Clinical Features of Group B Streptococcal Infections in Adults. The salient characteristics of the 24 patients with serious group B streptococcal infections are summarized in Table I. Eleven were women and 13 men. The mean age was 44 years, with a range from 16 to 89 years.

In six cases (25 per cent), group B streptococcal infection occurred in the early (24 to 48 hours) postpartum period; prolonged rupture of membranes existed in three of these patients. Seven patients (30 per cent) had a variety of urologic disorders including prostatic hypertrophy (two patients), renal cell carcinoma (one patient), renal failure (three patients), bladder trauma (one patient) and chronic indwelling Foley catheterization (one patient). Of interest, diabetes mellitus was an underlying medical problem in 11 patients (45 per cent). Alcoholic liver disease was present in two patients and head trauma in one.

Bacteremic group B streptococcal pyelonephritis was the most common clinical syndrome, occurring in seven patients. Pneumonia (six patients) and endometritis (six patients) were also common. Other types of group B streptococcal infections included meningitis (three patients), septic arthritis (two patients), cellulitis (two patients), endocarditis (one patient), tracheobronchitis (one patient) and peritonitis (one patient). In general, the major organ system involved was also the likely source of infection. In two patients with meningitis, the primary site of group B streptococcal infection was the urinary tract. In another case, endocarditis and meningitis followed group B streptococcal cellulitis. Of the two patients with group B streptococcal septic arthritis, one had an antecedent urinary tract infection; in the other patient the primary source of infection could not be identified. There appeared to be nothing unusual about the clinical presentation or hospital course of these patients with group B streptococcal infections when compared to patients with similar infections caused by more common etiologic organisms. Of note, despite the high frequency of bacteremia associated with these infections (90 per cent), no episodes of hypotension or shock were observed.

Five patients died; however, only two deaths were directly attributable to the group B streptococcal infection. One was due to severe, purulent meningitis in an elderly man in whom death occurred within 72 hours of clinical onset. The other death, also in an elderly man, occurred within seven days of extensive group B streptococcal pneumonia. Both deaths ensued despite appropriate antimicrobial therapy.

Serotypic Distribution. Among the 28 group B streptococcal isolates, only one (4 per cent) was nontypable. Serotype III was the most prevalent (46 per cent), followed by types II (16 per cent), Ib (13 per cent), Ic (13 per cent) and Ia (8 per cent). There was no significant

TABLE II Prevalence of Group B Streptococcal Serotypes in 24 Serious Adult Infections

Type of Infection	No. of Patients	Serotype					
		Ia	Ib	Ic	II	III	NT*
Pneumonia and/or tracheobronchitis	7	...	...	2	2	3	...
Endometritis	5	...	2	...	1	2	...
Pyelonephritis	4	1	...	...	1	1	1
Pyelonephritis, meningitis	2	1	...	...	...	1	...
Pyelonephritis, endometritis	1	...	...	...	...	1	...
Septic arthritis	2	...	...	1	...	1	...
Cellulitis, meningitis, endocarditis	1	...	1	...	...	...	...
Peritonitis	1	...	...	...	...	1	...
Cellulitis	1	...	...	...	...	1	...
Totals	24	2 (8%)	3 (13%)	3 (13%)	4 (16%)	11 (46%)	1 (4%)

* Nontypable.

correlation of different serotypes with specific organ-system involvement (Table II). At least one isolate from each patient was typed.

Antibiotic Susceptibility Studies. All group B streptococcal isolates were sensitive to penicillin, ampicillin, cephalothin, erythromycin, clindamycin and chloramphenicol by the Kirby-Bauer disc-diffusion technic. In contrast, all were resistant to kanamycin, and 25 of 28 were resistant to tetracycline by this method.

Twenty-three isolates (each from a different patient) were available for sensitivity testing to penicillin, kanamycin and tetracycline by an agar dilution technic. Minimal inhibitory concentrations of penicillin ranged from 0.04 to 0.16 U/ml. Twenty-two of 23 strains were highly resistant to kanamycin with minimal inhibitory concentrations $\geq$200 μg/ml. For tetracycline, the range of minimal inhibitory concentrations was 0.8 to 100 μg/ml. However, only three strains (13 per cent) were sensitive (minimal inhibitory concentrations $\leq$3.12 μg/ml); the remaining 20 isolates were highly resistant (minimal inhibitory concentrations $\geq$25 μg/ml). Two of the three tetracycline-sensitive strains were serotype Ib and the other was type III.

The minimal inhibitory concentrations of penicillin for these 23 group B streptococcal isolates were compared with 67 group A streptococcal isolates recovered at HGH during this same period (Figure 1). Although both streptococcal groups were uniformly sensitive to penicillin, the minimal inhibitory concentrations for group B streptococci were significantly higher than those for group A streptococci ($p < 0.0005$, Student t analysis).

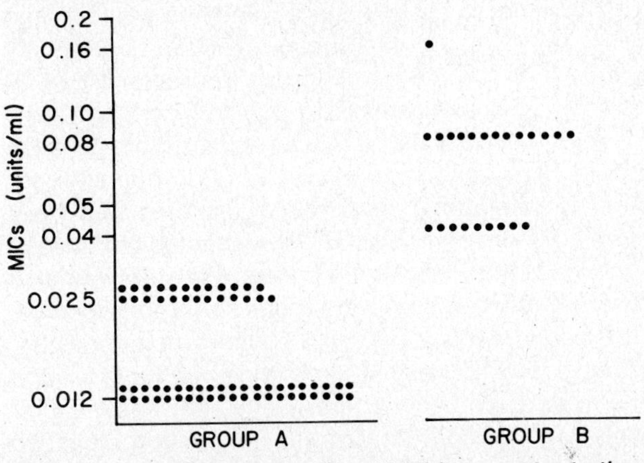

***Figure 1.** Comparison of minimal inhibitory concentrations of penicillin against 67 group A streptococcal strains and 23 group B streptococcal strains. Sensitivity data for the group A isolates were previously reported [22].*

COMMENTS

The group B streptococcus (also known as Streptococcus agalactiae), once considered a pathogen only for domestic animals, is now a well-recognized causative agent in a variety of infections in man [1–3,10,11]. Most reports of serious group B streptococcal infections have been confined to the neonatal and early infancy period (<12 weeks of age) [1,2,12–16]. Severe infections in adults caused by these organisms have been only sporadically cited. Our experience with a relatively large number of serious infections in adults (24 patients seen within a 36-month period) underscores the importance of these pathogens in the non-neonatal age group as well.

Previous reports of group B streptococcal infections in adults have alluded to a bimodal age distribution of infected patients: a young, previously healthy female population in which group B streptococcal infection occurred in association with obstetrical or gynecologic manipulations, and an older population in which this infection complicated preexisting illnesses [1,10, 11,17]. Thus, among 42 nonparturient adults with group B streptococcal infection described in the literature, the mean age was 64 years [1,10,11,17]. In the present report, a similar age distribution was seen. Eleven of the 24 patients (45 per cent) were between the ages of 16 and 36 years. Eight of the 11 had no prior medical illnesses, and group B streptococcal infection developed as a complication of parturition or trauma. Each of the other three patients had long-standing juvenile diabetes with multisystem involvement. In contrast, the mean age of the remaining 13 patients was 60 years; all but one had a chronic, underlying disease. It is intriguing that there were no pediatric cases outside of the neonatal age group in our series.

The importance of the female, both as a reservoir and a susceptible population for serious group B streptococcal infections has also been stressed in earlier reports [1,10,11,18–21]. Twenty-two of 28 previously described adults with severe group B streptococcal infections were women [1,10,11]. However, in our series, both sexes were evenly affected, suggesting that the male may be equally susceptible and may also harbor this organism in the urogenital flora.

Previous reports of group B streptococcal infections in adults have noted the common occurrence of bacteremia, meningitis and bacterial endocarditis [10,11,17]. These types of infection were also noted in our series, but the large number (seven of 24) of cases involving the respiratory tract deserves mention. Although pulmonary infections secondary to group B streptococci have rarely been commented upon in the literature, they may be more prevalent than currently recognized, since the pharynx and upper respiratory passages often harbor these organisms [10].

The frequent association of diabetes mellitus and group B streptococcal infection has been commonly noted [1,10,11]. Of the 28 group B streptococcal infections previously referred to, eight (30 per cent) were in patients with diabetes. This relationship was even more striking among our patients, 11 of whom (45 per cent) were diabetic. The type of diabetes was most often adult-onset, noninsulin dependent (eight cases), although brittle, insulin-dependent diabetes was also observed (three cases). Ketoacidosis was not observed, either as a predisposing or a complicating condition. Although Eickhoff et al. [1] emphasized the presence of severe diabetic peripheral vascular disease in their adults with group B streptococcal infection, only two of our 11 diabetic patients were so afflicted. The relationship of group B streptococcal infections to diabetes mellitus remains unexplained, but it seems that more than a casual association exists.

An impressive feature of group B streptococcal infections in both the neonate and the young infant has been the fulminant nature of infection and the high attendent mortality. Among 175 neonates and infants with group B streptococcal bacteremia and/or meningitis, recently reported on, the mortality rate was 37 per cent [13–16,22]. Earlier reports of group B streptococcal infections in adults also indicated a grave prognosis with an over-all mortality of 64 per cent [11]. This latter figure may have been related to the great proportion of cases emanating from the pre-antibiotic era. More recent publications, however, have documented a high mortality rate, despite chemotherapy, in adults with group B streptococcal infection involving the meninges and/or heart valves or in the presence of debilitating underlying diseases [10,11,17]. In contrast, a remarkably low mortality rate was observed among our patients (8 per cent) and may be partially explained by the low incidence of endocarditis and meningitis in our experience (four of 24 cases). Of interest, one of the two patients who died had a purulent meningitis, with death occurring rapidly (<72 hours) despite appropriate antibiotic therapy.

Much has been written concerning the serotypic distribution of group B streptococci in serious infections in neonates and infants. Serotype III was the most prevalent pathogen reported by some investigators [7,14], whereas others found different serotypes, notably Ia, as the predominant group B streptococcus in neonatal infections [1,17]. Thus it appears that the prevalence of specific serotypes in neonatal sepsis may differ from one population to another, and may simply reflect the predominant serotype involved in maternal-fetal and postnatal colonization, rather than the possession of unique virulence factors by specific serotypes which render them more invasive than others. In support of this, our studies indicate that the most prevalent colonizing group B streptococcal strains in healthy pregnant women and newborns and the most common etiologic strains in neonatal sepsis are identical (types III,II [22]).

Serotypic characterization in group B streptococcal infections of the adult has been inadequately described. Butter and DeMoor [17], in a description of 23 adults with group B streptococcal bacteremia and/or meningitis, noted serotype Ia to be the etiologic agent in 16 cases. However, no detailed information was provided as to the source(s) of bacteremia or other major organ systems involved. Among the 24 patients described in this report, type III was the most common serotype; however, there was no significant correlation of specific serotypes with types of infection or specific target organ involvement.

Without exception, all group B streptococcal isolates from our patients were sensitive to penicillin, ampicillin, cephalothin, erythromycin, clindamycin and chloramphenicol, and were uniformly resistant to kanamycin. Eighty-seven per cent of strains tested were resistant to tetracycline. These susceptibility data are in agreement with other recently published studies [15,22]. Of interest, although uniformly sensitive to penicillin, minimal inhibitory concentrations of this antibiotic were significantly higher for group B than for group A streptococci, and may be of clinical importance in the treatment of certain group B streptococcal infections such as meningitis or endocarditis.

ACKNOWLEDGMENT

We thank Valerie Patten and Dominick Bednorz for microbiologic identification of the streptococci, and Nelydia F. Concepcion for serogrouping and serotyping the isolates.

REFERENCES

1. Eickhoff TC, Klein JO, Daly AK, et al.: Neonatal sepsis and other infections due to group B beta-hemolytic streptococci. N Engl J Med 271: 1221, 1964.
2. Yow M: Group B streptococci—a serious threat to the newborn. JAMA 230: 1177, 1974.
3. Howard JB, McCracken GH: The spectrum of group B streptococcal infections in infancy. Am J Dis Child 128: 815, 1974.
4. Bergqvist G: Neonatal infections caused by group B streptococci. Scand J Infect Dis 6: 29, 1974.
5. Facklam RR, Padula JF, Thacker LG: Presumptive identification of Group A, B and D streptococci. Appl Microbiol 27: 107, 1974.
6. Lancefield RC: A microprecipitin-technic for classifying hemolytic streptococci, and improved methods for producing antisera. Proc Soc Exp Biol Med 38: 473, 1938.

7. Wilkinson HW, Facklam RR, Wortham EC: Distribution by serologic type of group B streptococci isolated from a variety of clinical material over a five-year period (with special reference to neonatal sepsis and meningitis). Infect Immun 8: 228, 1973.
8. Bauer AW, Kirby WMM, Sherris JC, et al.: Antibiotic susceptibility testing by a standardized single disk method. Am J Clin Pathol 45: 493, 1966.
9. Steers E, Foltz EL, Graves BS: An inocula replicating apparatus for routine testing of bacterial susceptibility to antibiotics. Antibiot Chemother 9: 307, 1959.
10. Duma RJ, Weinberg AN, Medrek TF, et al.: Streptococcal infections—a bacteriologic and clinical study of streptococcal bacteremia. Medicine (Baltimore) 48: 87, 1969.
11. Reinarz JA, Sanford JP: Human infections caused by non-group A or D streptococci. Medicine (Baltimore) 44:81, 1965.
12. Horn KA, Meyer T, Wyrick BC, et al.: Group B streptococcal neonatal infection. JAMA 230: 1165, 1974.
13. Hey DJ, Hall RT, Burry VF, et al.: Neonatal infections caused by group B streptococci. Am J Obstet Gynecol 116: 43, 1973.
14. Baker CJ, Barrett FF: Group B streptococcal infections in infants. JAMA 230: 1158, 1974.
15. Barton LL, Feigin RD, Lins R: Group B beta-hemolytic streptococcal meningitis in infants. J Pediatr 82: 719, 1973.
16. Baker CJ, Barrett FF, Gordon RC, et al.: Suppurative meningitis due to streptococci of Lancefield group B—a study of 33 infants. J Pediatr 82: 724, 1973.
17. Butter MNW, DeMoor CE: Streptococcus agalactiae as a cause of meningitis in the newborn, and of bacteremia in adults. Antonie van Leeuwenhoek 33: 439, 1967.
18. Sokol RJ, Walker RS: Beta-hemolytic streptococcus in a population of antepartum patients. Obstet Gynecol 42: 227, 1973.
19. Baker CJ, Barrett FF: Transmission of group B streptococci among parturient women and their neonates. J Pediatr 93: 919, 1973.
20. Grossman J, Tompkins RL: Group B beta-hemolytic streptococcal meningitis in mother and infant. N Engl J Med 290: 387, 1974.
21. Baker CJ, Barrett FF, Yow MD: The influence of advancing gestation on group B streptococcal colonization in pregnant women. Am J Obstet Gynecol 122: 820, 1975.
22. Anthony BF, Concepcion NF: Group B streptococcus in a general hospital. J Infect Dis 132: 561, 1975.

The Course of Pregnancy in Patients with Artificial Heart Valves

CARLOS IBARRA-PEREZ, M.D., M.Sc.
NOEL AREVALO-TOLEDO, M.D.
OCTAVIO ALVAREZ-DE LA CADENA, M.D.
LUIS NORIEGA-GUERRA, M.D.
Mexico City, Mexico

Twenty-five women with prosthetic heart valves (PHV) became pregnant 28 times. Twenty-six of the pregnancies occurred while the patients were receiving oral anticoagulants and these were continued throughout in 25 pregnancies. Dipyridamole or dipyridamole and acetylsalicylic acid were used in 22 pregnancies. Eighteen infants were delivered, one with a congenital corneal leukoma; none had hemorrhagic complications; their psychomotor development was normal. Nine women aborted 10 times, including patients with two PHV, pelvic trauma and self-induced abortion. We could not detect excess anticoagulation in eight of the nine who had spontaneous losses; excess anticoagulation occurred five weeks before an abortion. There were no maternal deaths despite numerous complications; in two women, brain embolism was related to short interruptions of anticoagulation. The details of management are mentioned. We lack enough evidence to suggest routine sterilization, routine interruption of coumarin therapy during pregnancy or routine interruption of pregnancy in women with certain types and models of PHV; however, pregnancy under such conditions, plus antithrombotic therapy, carries a high risk for the product and a potential teratogenic effect. Women with one or two PHV can have children if their management is closely supervised and if extreme care is taken with the use of oral anticoagulants.

In previous communications [1–5] we have reported the experience and concepts regarding, what we have considered to be, adequate management of pregnant women with prosthetic heart valves (PHV). This report updates our results and policy in the management of such patients, with special reference to antithrombotic drugs.

CLINICAL MATERIAL AND METHODS

Twenty-five women, aged 20 to 38 years, were managed during 28 pregnancies (Table I); 24 had Starr-Edwards PHV and one a Cooley-Bloodwell-Cutter, all of which were implanted for rheumatic heart disease; none was cloth covered. Eight women had spontaneous abortions before undergoing surgery for heart disease and one had a premature delivery. After surgery, and before coming to our care, three had had abortions (Cases 3, 7 and 21) and one a premature delivery (Case 4); five patients (Cases 3, 7, 9, 16 and 24) had had a cerebral embolism; two patients (Cases 18 and 19) had associated mild to moderate aortic lesions; and 12 women were in atrial fibrillation. One patient (Case 11) had diffuse neurofibromatosis. A prothrombin time determination (Quick) or thrombotest (Owren) was performed every two to eight weeks during the postoperative period.

From the Division of Surgery, Hospital de Enfermedades del Tórax, Centro Médico Nacional, Instituto Mexicano del Seguro Social, México City, México, and the High Risk Pregnancy Clinic, Hospital de Gineco-Obstetricia No. 2, Centro Médico Nacional, Instituto Mexicano del Seguro Social, México City, México. Request for reprints should be addressed to Dr. Carlos Ibarra-Pérez, Uxmal 689, México City 13, Mèxico. Manuscript accepted January 30, 1976.

Management During Pregnancy. Coumarinic drugs were being given at the time of conception in 26 of the 28 pregnancies. One patient (Case 11) stopped taking the medication since being lost to follow-up after a successful delivery. Another patient (Case 19) discontinued taking acenocoumarin shortly after undergoing heart surgery due to retroperitoneal bleeding and laparotomy; she was not receiving antithrombotic drugs until dipyridamole was added during the fifth month of pregnancy.

Efforts were made to hospitalize the patient as soon as pregnancy was confirmed; if this was not possible, emphasis was placed upon bed rest and avoidance of physical stress and trauma to the uterus.

The prothrombin time determination or thrombotest was performed every one to two weeks, if the subjects were outpatients, or oftener, if they were hospitalized, aiming to achieve values of one and a half to two times that of control, or from 8 to 10 per cent, respectively; anticoagulation was considered satisfactory if values fell within those ranges in more than 75 per cent of the determinations, fair if this occurred only in 60 to 74 per cent of the determinations, poor if it occurred in less than 60 per cent and excessive if it was over two and a half times that of the control or less than 6 per cent. If not already administered and tolerated, 300 to 450 mg of dipyridamole [6–8] or 100 mg of dipyridamole plus 1 g of acetylsalicylic acid [9] were given as additional protection against thrombus formation.

Electrocardiograms, chest roentgenograms, phonome-

TABLE I Data on 25 Women with Prosthetic Heart Valves Treated with Antithrombotic Drugs During 28 Pregnancies

Case No.	Pregnancy No.	Age (yr)	Heart Surgery (date) and Procedure	Rhythm	Obstetric History	Delivery
1	1	27	11/3/67, mitral SE 6100	Atrial fibrillation	Gravida 1, Para 0	2/9/70 Vaginal
2	2	28	11/24/67, mitral SE 6100	Sinus	Gravida 7, Para 4, Abortion 2	2/19/70 Vaginal
3	3	22	6/3/65, mitral SE 6100	Sinus	Gravida 2, Para 0, Abortion 1*	2/1/71 Caesarean
4	4	38	6/6/68, mitral SE 6100	Atrial fibrillation	Gravida 8, Para 7†	4/14/71 Vaginal
5	5	27	6/13/70, mitral SE 6120	Sinus	Gravida 6, Para 4, Abortion 1	7/10/71 Vaginal
6	6	31	10/30/70, mitral and aortic SE 6120, 1260	Sinus	Gravida 3, Para 1, Abortion 1	6/15/71 Abortion
7	7	28	2/24/67, mitral SE 6120	Atrial fibrillation	Gravida 4, Para 2, Abortion 1	2/22/72 Abortion*
8	8	23	5/14/71, aortic SE 1260	Sinus	Gravida 4, Para 3	3/2/72 Vaginal
9	9	33	8/29/69, mitral CBC	Atrial fibrillation	Gravida 6, Para 4, Abortion 1	8/10/72 Abortion
10	10	22	7/14/70, mitral SE 6120	Atrial fibrillation	Gravida 2, Para 2	8/30/72 Caesarean
11	11	34	6/22/67, aortic SE 1200	Sinus	Gravida 1, Para 0	9/28/72 Vaginal
7	12	29	2/24/67, mitral SE 6120	Atrial fibrillation	Gravida 5, Para 2, Abortion 2	3/10/73 Abortion
11	13	35	6/22/67, aortic SE 1200	Sinus	Gravida 2, Para 1	6/29/73 Abortion
12	14	38	4/27/72, mitral SE 6120	Atrial fibrillation	Gravida 4, Para 3	7/12/73 Vaginal
13	15	22	2/29/72, mitral SE 6120	Atrial fibrillation	Gravida 2, Para 1	8/6/73 Caesarean
14	16	32	11/17/71, mitral SE 6120 + tricuspid annuloplasty	Atrial fibrillation	Gravida 7, Para 4, Abortion 2	8/13/73 Vaginal
15	17	29	9/24/71, mitral SE 6120	Sinus	Gravida 3, Para 0, Abortion 2	12/10/73 Abortion
16	18	25	8/30/71, mitral SE 6120	Atrial fibrillation	Gravida 5, Para 3, Abortion 1	3/24/74 Vaginal
17	19	29	1/24/69, mitral SE 6120	Sinus	Gravida 1, Para 0	5/4/74 Caesarean
18	20	20	6/29/70, mitral and tricuspid SE 6120	Atrial fibrillation	Gravida 1, Para 0	12/11/74 Abortion
19	21	27	5/25/70, mitral SE 6120	Sinus	Gravida 1, Para 0	12/12/74 Caesarean
20	22	31	11/9/73, mitral SE 6120	Atrial fibrillation	Gravida 4, Para 3	12/25/74 Vaginal
21	23	25	5/20/71, mitral SE 6120	Sinus	Gravida 3, Para 0, Abortion 2	3/15/75 Abortion
22	24	32	12/5/72, mitral and tricuspid SE 6120	Sinus	Gravida 2, Para 1†	3/18/75 Vaginal
23	25	23	6/10/74, mitral SE 6120 + tricuspid annuloplasty	Sinus	Gravida 2, Para 1	4/18/75 Premature delivery
11	26	37	6/22/67, aortic SE 1200	Sinus	Gravida 3, Para 1, Abortion 1	5/22/75 Vaginal
24	27	28	12/13/72, mitral SE 6120	Sinus	Gravida 3, Para 2	6/29/75 Caesarean‡
25	28	22	12/18/73, mitral SE 6120	Sinus	Gravida 4, Para 2, Abortion 1	8/9/75 Caesarean

NOTE: SE = Starr-Edwards; the numbers following indicate the model. CBC = Cooley-Bloodwell-Cutter.

* Induced.

† Premature delivery.

‡ Transverse dead product.

chanocardiograms, hormonal determinations in blood and urine and other tests for fetal condition were performed as often as necessary [1,10].

Management During Labor and Puerperium. When spontaneous labor was permissible, the dose of coumarinics was tapered and then discontinued shortly before the expected time of delivery. When induction of labor or caesarean section was planned, administration of the anticoagulants was electively discontinued 24 to 72 hours before delivery.

Central venous pressure, blood pressure, a suitable lead of the electrocardiogram and valve sounds were constantly monitored throughout labor, delivery and at least the first 12 hours of puerperium; labor was monitored with a cardiotocograph [10].

Heparin was used during delivery and puerperium in two of the first three cases but its use has been abandoned since. Diluted dipyridamole was administered by slow intravenous drip, 30 to 60 mg every 8 hours while the mother fasted, and then orally at the usual dosage, given either alone or with acetylsalicylic acid. Antibiotics were given during the end stages of labor, delivery and the five following days. Prothrombin times were determined daily before, during and after delivery for about five to seven days. The administration of coumarinics was resumed 6 to 72 hours after delivery.

RESULTS

Complications During Pregnancy. There were numerous complications (Tables II and III), but several deserve separate description.

Two patients (Cases 2 and 12) threatened to abort around the 11th and 15th weeks, respectively; bleeding subsided after temporary interruption of acenocoumarin therapy.

One patient (Case 6) was in mild congestive failure at the time of conception; the cause of amenorrhea was not detected; the administration of acenocoumarin was continued, despite vaginal bleeding, and she had an abortion.

One patient (Case 7) had had an abortion and a brain embolism with significant neurologic sequelae after heart surgery while managed by another service; under our care, she had two more abortions with prothrombin times within the therapeutic range; at least one abortion was self-induced.

When one patient (Case 9) threatened to abort, anticoagulants were withheld for five days, maintaining an optimal dose of dipyridamole. After the danger had apparently subsided, and still without coumarinic therapy, she suffered a brain embolism; the administration of acenocoumarin was resumed to prevent further embolization. She aborted two days later with a prothrombin time short of the therapeutic range.

One patient (Case 11) aborted a macerated embryo (second pregnancy) eight weeks after she received antityphoid vaccine that produced fever, seven weeks after the cessation of fetal motility and four weeks after the resumption of anticoagulant therapy that had been stopped before a successful postoperative delivery (first pregnancy). During her third pregnancy, which occurred despite an intrauterine device in situ, she had two episodes of painless vaginal bleeding during weeks 14–16 and 36 that resolved after the dose of anticoagulants was lowered; she also had an onset of labor during weeks 27–28, but uterine contractions were inhibited with isoxsuprine hydrochloride therapy.

In another patient (Case 15) vaginal bleeding stopped after a short interruption of sodium warfarin therapy; 10 days later, the patient had a pubic contusion and aborted.

In another patient (Case 17), the onset of premature labor occurred one week before delivery; isoxsuprine hydrochloride therapy was used during 36 hours.

One patient (Case 18) aborted a macerated embryo without a detectable reason; prothrombin time was short of the therapeutic range.

One patient (Case 21) had two postoperative abortions while she was managed by another service. Under our care, she had a severe, long-lasting bacterial and trichomoniasic vaginitis with bloody discharge; there was one episode of excessive anticoagulation five weeks before increased vaginal bleeding ensued; the administration of coumarinics was not discontinued and she aborted. She was also receiving treatment for mild hypothyroidism.

One patient (Case 22) had a short interruption of warfarin sodium therapy because of a threatened abortion; 20 days later she had a stroke, with a prothrombin time just short of the therapeutic range; rupture of fetal membranes around week 34–35 led to successful induction of labor; she was given digitalis and diuretics, and sodium was restricted throughout her pregnancy because of mild congestive heart failure.

One patient (Case 23) had chest roentgenograms taken around the time of conception; petechiae, ecchymosis and bacterial vaginitis complicated her course before delivery of a 980 g macerated male. There was no detectable excess of anticoagulants or measurable defect of other coagulation factors.

Transverse position of the product appeared around week 24–25 in Case 24; fetal motility disappeared five days before caesarean section for delivery of a macerated 1,100 g female.

One patient (Case 25) had the onset of labor at week 32; contractions were inhibited until term with large doses of isoxsuprine hydrochloride.

The gestational age at the time of death was 16 weeks or less in eight cases, around 26 weeks in one and 30 to 32 weeks in another.

The rest of the complications were treated in the standard manner. In Case 11 the patient required interruption of acetyl salicylic acid therapy around week 18–20 of her third pregnancy because of the persistent formation of petechiae and ecchymosis.

Coumarinic drug therapy was interrupted 32 times during the 28 pregnancies for periods lasting from 24 hours (Case 22) to the entire length of pregnancy (Case 19, since the second postoperative month, for a total of 45 months); the causes were threatened abortion, abortion, threatened premature delivery, premature or term delivery by vaginal route or caesarean section, excessive anticoagulation, dental extraction and hematuria. Two patients (Cases 9 and 22) had cerebral embolization during pregnancy; this was related to anticoagulant interruption lasting five and three days, respectively.

Except during the periods when administration of coumarinics was withheld intentionally, anticoagulation was considered poor in four pregnancies; fair in three and supposedly satisfactory in the rest.

Hospitalization lasted from 16 days to six months. Of the 14 women hospitalized during early pregnancy five lost their products; hospital bed rest was not possible or late in 14 pregnancies of which five products were lost; at least one was self-induced.

Nine of 22 pregnancies were terminated (one self-induced) while the mother received dipyridamole, alone or with acetylsalicylic acid; in one of six pregnancies in which no one was receiving the drugs, abortion occurred.

Complications During Labor and Puerperium. Twelve women had vaginal deliveries under light general anesthesia (Case 1), epidural block (Cases 2, 8, 20, 22 and the first and third pregnancies in Case 11) or no medication (Cases 4, 5, 12, 13 and 16). Seven underwent caesarean section, two (Cases 3 and 14) under light general anesthesia, the rest with epidural block (Case 24 for delivery of a transverse dead product).

Prothrombin times at or about the time of delivery ranged from 24 to 100 per cent activity (Quick).

Prophylactic forceps were applied in Cases 1, 2, 8 and 22, and in Case 11 during the first and third pregnancies.

Results of studies of the placental tissue of several patients were no different from those of mothers who did not receive antithrombotic drugs.

In Case 1, the patient had a prothrombin time within the therapeutic range when she entered the delivery room, and she had numerous complications [1]. During the puerperium of her third pregnancy, one patient (Case 11) had anemia and was in need of fresh blood, she also had mild congestive heart failure; because of retention of placental tissue and persistent hemorrhage, she was treated by dilatation and curettage eight and 12 days after delivery, and was given more fresh blood. One patient (Case 20) had anticoagulant activity at the time of delivery; she had also been receiving other antithrombotic drugs; hemorrhage in the uterine and in the gingival and puncture sites (also that of the epidural block) during and after delivery prompted the use of vitamin K1 and fresh blood; five days later she underwent dilatation and curettage and five days later, because of puerperal infection, she was treated with large doses of antibiotics. Patients with other complications, including atrial extrasystoles and changes in central venous pressure and blood pressure, were treated in the standard manner.

Infants. Eleven males and seven females, weighing 1,660 to 3,460 g, were born and are alive. One female had a left corneal congenital leukoma (Case 14). There was Rh blood group incompatibility in the parents of product 28 (Case 25); the baby had a low prothrombin time and was markedly jaundiced at birth, but presently is doing well. The infants delivered by forceps showed no untoward effects. Premature babies were kept in the incubator until necessary. Prothrombin times from umbilical cord samples were normal in 11 of 12 infants. The psychomotor development of the 18 infants has been normal.

Follow-up. Six patients (Cases 1 through 6) are being managed by another service. One patient (Case 9) was lost to control when postembolic sequelae were mild. In Case 22, recovery was complete. In Cases 12 and 13, late postpartal brain embolism occurred when the patients were poorly anticoagulated; sequelae are moderate and mild, respectively. In Case 23, severe rheumatic fever recurred three months after delivery of a dead product. In Case 18, the patient has mild to moderate aortic stenosis and insufficiency; and in Case 19, the patient has mild to moderate aortic insufficiency. All women still under our care are considered to be in functional class I or II (New York Heart Association Classification). Six patients (Cases 10, 13, 17, 19, 24 and 25) had simultaneous caesarean and tubal section; two patients (Cases 7 and 20) had electrocoagulation of the tubouterine junctions; the rest are using temporary contraceptive methods.

COMMENTS

If able to conceive, all our female patients with PHV are routinely sent for contraceptive consultation [11], but pregnancy has occurred due to various reasons.

When the suspicion is confirmed, we have elected to proceed with the pregnancy and anticoagulation despite reports pointing out the dangers, to the mother and fetus, of anticoagulants administered during pregnancy [12,14,19], even suggesting routine sterilization of these women [16]. Several factors have influenced

TABLE II Data on 25 Women with Prosthetic Heart Valves Treated with Antithrombotic Drugs During 28 Pregnancies

Case No.	Pregnancy No.	Drug and Quality of Anticoagulation	Coumarin Therapy Before and After Delivery	% Prothrombin at Delivery	Other Antithrombotic Drugs
1	1	Acenocoumarin, satisfactory	Stopped 1 day before, resumed 2 days after	24	Heparin postpartum
2	2	Acenocoumarin, satisfactory	Stopped 1 day before, resumed 2 days after	35	None
3	3	Acenocoumarin, satisfactory	Stopped 2 days before, resumed 3 days after	90	Heparin postpartum, dipyridamole from 20th week, during caesarean, postpartum.
4	4	Acenocoumarin, satisfactory	Stopped during 13th week, resumed 3 days after	100	Dipyridamole from 13th week, labor, postpartum
5	5	Acenocoumarin, satisfactory	Stopped 1 day before, resumed 2 days after	65	None
6	6	Acenocoumarin, satisfactory	Not discontinued	...	Dipyridamole after heart surgery
7	7	Acenocoumarin, poor	Not discontinued before D & C, resumed 3 days after	35	Dipyridamole from 6th week
8	8	Acenocoumarin and warfarin, satisfactory	Stopped 4 days before, resumed 1 day after	100	Dipyridamole from 28th week, labor, postpartum.
9	9	Acenocoumarin, satisfactory	Stopped 5 days before, resumed 1 day after	70	Dipyridamole started before conception
10	10	Acenocoumarin, satisfactory	Stopped 2 days before, resumed 1 day after	100	Dipyridamole started before conception
11	11	Warfarin, satisfactory	Stopped 1 mo before, resumed 8 mo after	100	None
7	12	Warfarin, satisfactory	Not discontinued	25	Dipyridamole started before conception
11	13	Warfarin, poor	See text, resumed 3 days after	...	None
12	14	Acenocoumarin, satisfactory	Stopped 2 days before, resumed 1 day after	85	Dipyridamole started before conception, during labor, puerperium
13	15	Warfarin, satisfactory	Stopped 1 day before, resumed 1 day after	50	Dipyridamole after heart surgery, labor, puerperium
14	16	Warfarin, poor	Stopped 13 days before, resumed 7 days after	100	None
15	17	Warfarin, satisfactory	See text	70	Dipyridamole after heart surgery, abortion, puerperium
16	18	Acenocoumarin, fair	Discontinued the day of delivery	35	Dipyridamole since 8th week, labor, puerperium
17	19	Acenocoumarin, satisfactory	Stopped 2 days before, resumed 2 days after	100	Dipyridamole started before conception, labor, puerperium
18	20	Warfarin, fair	Discontinued the day of abortion	45	Dipyridamole started before conception, labor and puerperium
19	21	None	Discontinued since second postoperative month	100	Dipyridamole since 5th gestational month
20	22	Warfarin, satisfactory	Discontinued 1 day before, resumed 1 day after	50	Dipyridamole + A.S.A. since second postoperative month
21	23	Acenocoumarin, fair	Not discontinued	60	Dipyridamole before conception, abortion, puerperium
22	24	Warfarin, satisfactory	Discontinued the day of delivery	40	Dipyridamole after heart surgery, labor, puerperium
23	25	Warfarin, satisfactory	Stopped 2 days before, resumed 2 days after	...	Dipyridamole + A.S.A. since heart surgery
11	26	Warfarin, poor	Stopped 1 day before, resumed 1 day after	30	Dipyridamole + A.S.A. since 14th week
24	27	Warfarin, satisfactory	Stopped 3 days before, resumed 2 days after	45	Dipyridamole since heart surgery
25	28	Warfarin, satisfactory	Stopped 2 days before, resumed 1 day after	80	Dipyridamole since heart surgery

NOTE: D & C = dilatation and curettage. A.S.A. = acetylsalicylic acid.

TABLE III Results of 28 Pregnancies in 25 Women with Prosthetic Heart Valves

MOTHER					INFANTS		
Case No.	Pregnancy No.	Complications During Pregnancy	Delivery	Complications During Labor and Puerperium	Sex	Weight (kg)	% Prothrombin
1	1	Congestive heart failure, severe toxemia, hematuria	Vaginal	Hypotonic uterus, hemorrhage, wound hematoma, dehiscence	F	1,660	100*
2	2	Threatened abortion, mild toxemia, dental extraction, premature rupture of fetal membranes	Vaginal	None	M	2,760	100*
3	3	Pulmonary edema, angiocardiography	Caesarean	Caesarean	F	3,030	100
4	4	Congestive heart failure	Vaginal	None	F	3,000	...
5	5	None	Vaginal	None	F	2,360	...
6	6	Congestive heart failure, abortion	None	...	...	...	...
7	7	None, abortion	None	...	...	...	...
8	8	Excessive anticoagulation 1 determination (5 times the value of control)	Vaginal	None	M	3,460	100*
9	9	Congestive heart failure, cerebral embolism, abortion	None	...	...	...	...
10	10	None	Caesarean	Caesarean, paralytic ileus	F	2,500	100
11	11	None	Vaginal	None	M	2,950	...*
7	12	Abortion	None	...	...	...	...
11	13	Antityphoid vaccine, fever, abortion	None	...	...	...	...
12	14	Congestive heart failure, threatened abortion	Vaginal	Perineal laceration	F	2,500	100
13	15	None	Caesarean	Caesarean	M	2,800	100
14	16	Congestive heart failure	Vaginal	None	F	2,000	...
15	17	Pubic contusion; abortion	None	...	...	...	...
16	18	Convalescence of pre-conception cerebral embolism	Vaginal	None	M	2,080	...
17	19	Congestive heart failure, pyelonephritis, polyhydramnios, threatened premature labor	Caesarean	Caesarean	M	2,600	100
18	20	Congestive heart failure, abortion	None	...	...	...	...
19	21	Congestive heart failure, pneumoniae in lower lobe of left lung	Caesarean	Caesarean	M	2,500	100
20	22	None	Vaginal	Hemorrhage from multiple sites, D & C, puerperal infection	M	2,700	100
21	23	Mild hypothyroidism, bacterial and trichomoniasic vaginitis, excessive anticoagulation 1 determination (342″ = less than 5 per cent Owren); abortion	None	...	...	...	...
22	24	Congestive heart failure, threatened abortion, cerebral embolism, premature rupture of fetal membranes	Vaginal	None	M	2,640	75*
23	25	Exposure to radiations, petechiae, ecchymosis, premature delivery	Vaginal	None	M†	980	...
11	26	(IUD in situ); 2 episodes of painless vaginal bleeding, petechiae, ecchymosis, threatened premature labor	Vaginal	Mild congestive heart failure, anemia, D & C two times	M	2,980	...*
24	27	Transverse position of product, premature delivery	Caesarean	Caesarean	F†	1,100	...
25	28	Threatened premature labor, low and posterior insertion of placenta	Caesarean	Caesarean	M	2,520	45

NOTE: IUD = Intrauterine device. D & C = dilation and currettage.
* Product delivered by forceps.
† Macerated dead product.

our decision to go ahead with the pregnancy and the use of antithrombotic drugs, and to insist upon bed rest:

(1) Although there is a growing concern to avoid the use of oral anticoagulants during the first trimester of pregnancy because of possible teratogenic effects [14,15,17–20], our patients became pregnant without planning the date of conception. Consultation was sought because of amenorrhea, conception having occurred during the ingestion of coumarinics.

(2) Our patients are under our direct surveillance (Heart Valve Prostheses Clinic and High Risk Pregnancy Clinic) in hospitals 750 meters apart.

(3) The drugs given and their complications are familiar to the patients [11].

(4) Oral anticoagulants can be used during pregnancy, delivery and puerperium [1,2,5,21–23].

(5) There is a state of relative hypercoagulability during pregnancy [22].

(6) There is ample evidence of the increased risk of thromboembolism after the interruption of anticoagulant therapy or during poor anticoagulation in carriers of certain types and models of PHV, including pregnant and postpartal women [12,21–26].

(7) Dipyridamole and acetylsalicylic acid are efficient blockers of white thrombus formation in carriers of certain types and models of PHV when associated with coumarinic therapy [6–9], but reported results and our unreported results with their use without anticoagulants have not been uniformly good as to incite us to routinely discontinue the use of acenocoumarin or sodium warfarin in carriers of such PHV.

(8) Bed rest and other measures taken to lessen the hemodynamic burden and to avoid trauma to the product are convenient; prolonged bed rest is feasible in our socioeconomic environment.

Some USA figures of fetal mortality in the noncardiac population are 1.6 per cent, and in cardiac women from 3.2 to 10.5 per cent [27]. In our medical center [28] there have been 639 pregnancies in nonoperated women with rheumatic heart disease: 45 resulted in abortions, 13 in perinatal deaths and one in maternal death; among 20 women subjected to closed mitral valvotomy during pregnancy there were no abortions, four perinatal and one maternal death. Our figures, 10 losses in 28 pregnancies and no maternal deaths, indicate an unquestionable increased risk of death for the product, if not to the mother, in this highly selected group that includes patients with one or two PHV receiving long-term antithrombotic therapy, multiple complications during pregnancy, delivery and puerperium, including various degrees of hemodynamic derangement, and even self-induced abortion.

Although we were unable to obtain permission for necropsies of the products, none of the losses could be attributed to detectable excess of coumarinics in more than two determinations [23]; however, this does not exclude anticoagulants as potential causal factors in the spontaneous losses.

It is tempting to apply a statistical approach to several of the factors probably able to influence the outcome, live births or lost products, but we consider that this would represent the application of sound mathematical principles to a smaller number of cases of poorly chosen biologic material. Nevertheless, it has been mentioned that fetal complications are more prone to occur when oral anticoagulation is excessive and there is a previous history of miscarriages [23,29,30]; by checking anticoagulation very often and maintaining it close to the lower limits of the therapeutic range we try to avoid excessive anticoagulation in women with a pregnant uterus prone to potentially dangerous trauma; in this way we detected only two episodes of excessive anticoagulation, one without consequences and the other occurring five weeks before abortion; as to the problem of miscarriages, six products were lost in 15 pregnancies in women with a positive past history (one self-induced), and four lost in 13 pregnancies of women without such a history. There appeared to be no relationship between the quality of anticoagulation and the results, although it seemed to be important only when anticoagulant therapy was continued despite vaginal bleeding (abortions in Cases 6, 7 and 21). The use of other antithrombotic drugs seems to be important, as eight of 21 women receiving the drugs had spontaneous losses and only one of six not receiving the drugs had an abortion; this matter is under close scrutiny at the present time. Less than satisfactory myocardial function [21,32] has been mentioned as a cause of death of the product, particularly during the late months of pregnancy [12]; in our series, five of 20 pregnancies in which digoxin was required for the control of rhythm disturbances (atrial fibrillation, sinus tachycardia) or heart failure, and four of seven in which the patients were not receiving digitalis ended in spontaneous losses; regarding heart failure alone, three of 11 pregnancies were spontaneously lost to mothers under treatment for heart failure (including one with pulmonary edema).

We cannot disregard the oral anticoagulant as a causal factor of the corneal leukoma, as more reports are suggesting a relation between such therapy and congenital defects. However, the mother (Case 14) was also receiving digitalis, diuretics and diazepam, drugs which have also been used simultaneously with oral anticoagulants in other children with congenital anomalies [13–19].

We consider that no generalization can or should be made and that each case should be judged individually, weighing the consequences of policies such as continued pregnancy with coumarinic therapy which definitely increases the frequency of miscarriages and requires very close, expensive and time-consuming care without a guarantee of success, while carrying a potential risk of congenital defects in the offspring, or without such drugs and the risk of life-threatening embolism for the mother and product [12,16]. Systemic embolization occurred in four of eight pregnancies in which anticoagulant therapy was interrupted [12]; under similar conditions, we had two such episodes; the ever present danger of systemic embolism in patients with mitral and aortic Starr-Edwards PHV has been stressed in a recent review [26]. Even though we have elected to carry on with pregnancy and coumarinic therapy, we acknowledge that the subject is open to suggestions and debate with medical, ethical, economical, legal and emotional implications. There is no question that serious consideration has to be given to the use of reliable valve substitutes that do not require anticoagulation in women of child-bearing age.

CONCLUSIONS

This is largest reported series of pregnant women with PHV who were receiving antithrombotic drugs at the time of conception.

As soon as the diagnosis of pregnancy was made our management included (1) immediate bed rest, at the hospital if possible, and avoidance of pelvic trauma; (2) immediate consultation with the High Risk Pregnancy Clinic for simultaneous management; (3) prothrombin time determination or thrombotest every one to two weeks if subjects were outpatients or oftener if they were hospitalized, maintenance of prothrombin values between one and a half to two times that of control or a thrombotest between 8 and 10 per cent; (4) maintenance or addition of therapy with dipyridamole or dipyridamole and acetylsalicylic acid; (5) the performance of electrocardiograms, chest roentgenograms, phonomechanocardiograms, hormonal determinations and other tests for fetal condition, as often as necessary; (6) group decision to select the type of delivery according to cardiovascular, obstetric and fetal conditions; (7) if spontaneous delivery is possible, tapering of anticoagulant therapy and interruption from 24 to 96 hours before the expected time of delivery; (8) if induction or caesarean section is planned, the administration of oral anticoagulants is discontinued 24 to 72 hours before; (9) maintenance of other oral antithrombotic drugs; when fasting, administration of dipyridamole intravenously; (10) careful monitoring of central venous pressure, blood pressure, electrocardiogram and valve sounds during labor, delivery and first hours of puerperium; monitoring of labor by cardiotocograph; (11) the administration of prophylactic antibiotics; (12) daily determinations of prothrombin time before, during and after delivery and in samples from the infant; and (13) resumption of coumarinic therapy as soon as possible.

There were 18 live births and 10 miscarriages, one self-induced, and no perinatal mortality. A girl had a congenital corneal leukoma; warfarin sodium may have had a teratologic effect on the child; there were no maternal deaths. Review of the available information and of our own clinical material shows insufficient evidence to suggest routine sterilization, routine interruption of coumarinic therapy during pregnancy or routine interruption of pregnancy in women with certain types and models of PHV. The presence of these PHV is no contraindication, per se, for pregnancy. Due to the small number of cases we are unable to come to any conclusions about the safety of the routine use of dipyridamole and acetylsalicylic acid for the fetus as infants born to women receiving the drugs have not shown detectable defects, but more products were lost among them; on the other hand, the drugs did not appear effective in preventing embolic complications in two instances in which anticoagulant therapy was discontinued. The time necessary for the infants' coagulation factors to return to normal was not determined. The prothrombin time was normal in all but one of the infants sampled (despite therapeutic levels in a few mothers) and none had hemorrhagic complications (despite trauma of forceps in six) as a result of interrupting coumarinic therapy shortly before delivery while continuing the use of other antithrombotic drugs in some; this appears to be an indicator that under similar circumstances these drugs can be administered during pregnancy, labor and delivery. Pregnant women with certain types and models of PHV can have live births with normal psychomotor development if the use of antithrombotic drugs is closely supervised and other measures are taken. The teratogenic potential of oral anticoagulants used during the first trimester of pregnancy deserves careful consideration and should not be underestimated. The answer to the problem is related to the use of valve substitutes that do not require the use of oral anticoagulants.

ACKNOWLEDGMENT

We thank our colleagues R. Flores-Gómez, M. Cosio-Pascal, E. Ochoa, S. Portillo, R. Lezama, J. Nis, X. Palacios-Macedo, A. Lee, J. L. Lara, C. Morales Lepe, A. Ley, C. Valdez, J. Ray-Lara, G. Hagg, M. del Bosque-Ruiz and H. Zarate for their contributions to the work presented in this paper.

REFERENCES

1. Ibarra-Pérez C, Del Bosque Ruiz M: Pregnancy in 6 patients with Starr-Edwards heart valve prostheses, Am J Cardiol 30: 565, 1972.
2. Ibarra-Pérez C: El uso de anticoagulantes en la enferma embarazada portadora de prótesis valvular cardiaca. Thesis for Master of Science Degree (Cardiovascular Surgery),

University of Mexico, October 1972.

3. Del Bosque-Ruiz M, Ibarra-Pérez C, Del Bosque-Santos Jr, Monroy Izquierdo R, Zárate Sandoval H: Embarazo, parto y puerperio en pacientes con prótesis mitral de Starr-Edwards. Arch Inst Cardiol Mex 43: 149, 1973.
4. Ibarra-Pérez C, Argüero R: El manejo de anticoagulantes en enfermos con prótesis valvulares cardiacas. Prensa Med Mex 38: 17, 1973.
5. Ibarra-Pérez C: Uso de anticoagulantes en enfermas embarazadas en las que se han implantado prótesis valvulares cardiacas de Starr-Edwards. Gaceta Med Mex 106: 239, 1973.
6. Sullivan JM, Harken DE, Gorlin R: Pharmacological control of thromboembolic complications of cardiac valve replacement. N Engl J Med 279: 576, 1968.
7. Sullivan JM, Harken DE, Gorlin R: Effect of dipyridamole on the incidence of arterial emboli after cardiac valve replacement. Circulation 39 (suppl 1): 149, 1969.
8. Sullivan JM, Harken DE, Gorlin R: Pharmacological control of thromboembolic complications of cardiac valve replacement. N Engl J Med 284: 1391, 1971.
9. Harker LA, Slichter SJ: Studies of platelet and fibrinogen kinetics in patients with prosthetic heart valves. N Engl J Med 283: 1302 1970.
10. Arévalo-Toledo N, Noriega-Guerra L: Estudio de la frecuencia fetal. Bol Med IMSS 16: 159, 1974.
11. Ibarra-Pérez C, Argüero R, Cobo J: La clínica de prótesis valvulares cardiacas: filosofía método y resultados iniciales. Prensa Med Mex 38: 149, 1973.
12. Buxbaum A, Aygen MM, Shahin W, Levy MJ, Ekerling B: Pregnancy in patients with prosthetic heart valves. Chest 59: 639, 1971.
13. Villasanta U: Thromboembolic disease in pregnancy. Am J Obstet Gynecol 93: 142, 1965.
14. Di Saia PF: Pregnancy and delivery of a patient with a Starr Edwards mitral valve prosthesis. Obstet Gynecol 28: 469, 1966.
15. Kerber IJ, Warr OS, Richardson C: Pregnancy in a patient with a prosthetic mitral valve. Associated with a fetal anomaly attributed to sodium warfarin. JAMA 203: 223, 1968.
16. Bennett GG, Oakley CM: Pregnancy in a patient with a mitral valve prosthesis. Lancet 1: 616, 1968.
17. Pettifor JM, Benson R: Congenital malformations associated with the administration of oral anticoagulants during pregnancy. J Pediatr 86: 459, 1975.
18. Becker MH, Genieser NB, Finegold M, Miranda O, Spackman T: Chondrodysplasia punctata, 15: Maternal warfarin therapy a factor? Am J Dis Child 129: 356, 1975.
19. Shaul WL, Emery H, Hall JG: Chondrodysplasia punctata and maternal warfarin during pregnancy. Am Dis Child 129: 360, 1975.
20. Hirsh J, Cade JF, Gallus AS: Anticoagulants in pregnancy: a review of indications and complications. Am Heart J 83: 301, 1972.
21. Hirsh J, Cade JF, O'Sullivan EF: Clinical experience with anticoagulant therapy during pregnancy. Br Med J 1: 270, 1970.
22. Hedstrand H, Cullhed I: Pregnancy in patients with prosthetic heart valves (Starr-Edwards). Scand J Thorac Cardiovasc Surg 2: 196, 1968.
23. Fillmore SJ, McDevitt E: Effects of coumarin compounds on the fetus. Ann Intern Med 73: 731, 1970.
24. Ueland K, Tatum HJ, Metcalfe J: Pregnancy and prosthetic heart valves. Report of successful pregnancies in 2 patients with Starr-Edwards aortic valves. Obstet Gynecol 27: 257, 1966.
25. Otterson WN, McGranahan G, Freeman MVR: Successful pregnancy with Mc Govern aortic prosthesis and long term heparin therapy. Report of a case. Obstet Gynecol 31: 273, 1968.
26. Barnhorst DA, Oxman HA, Connolly DC, et al.: Long-term follow-up of isolated replacement of the aortic or mitral valve with the Starr-Edwards prosthesis. Am J Cardiol 35: 228, 1975.
27. Gilbert CS, Sullivan GJ, McLaughlin JJ: Heart disease in pregnancy; ten year report from the Lewis Memorial Maternity Hospital. Obstet Gynecol 9: 58, 1957.
28. Cobo J, Skromne KD, Cuadra J: Comisurotomía mitral en la cardiópata embarazada. Prensa Med Mex 34: 376, 1974.
29. Bloomfield DK: Fetal deaths and malformations associated with the use or coumarin derivates in pregnancy. A critical review. Am J Obstet Gynecol 107: 883, 1970.
30. Hirsh J, Cade JF, Gallus AS: Fetal effects of coumadin administered during pregnancy. Blood 36: 623, 1970.
31. McHenry MM, Smeloff EA, Savey TB, Kaufman B, Fong WY: Hemodynamic results with the full flow orifice prosthetic valves. Circulation 35 (suppl 1): 24, 1967.
32. Hultgreen H, Hubis H, Shumway N: Cardiac function following mitral valve replacement. Am Heart J 75: 302, 1968.

Splenic Abscess

Report of 10 Cases and Review of the Literature

JEFFREY D. CHULAY, M.D.*
MOHAMMAD R. LANKERANI, M.D.
Cleveland, Ohio

Ten cases of splenic abscess seen between 1964 and 1974 are reviewed. Pain referable to the abscess was the most common symptom, but was present in only five cases. Fever was present in all but one case. Tenderness in the region of the spleen was noted in six cases, in three cases the spleen was palpable and in one case a large mass in the upper left quadrant of the abdomen was palpated. Abdominal films were suggestive of the diagnosis in two cases, and the liver-spleen scan demonstrated a defect in three cases. Seven abscesses were caused by gram-negative bacilli of bowel origin; the etiologic agents in the other three were Staphylococcus aureus, Streptobacillus moniliformis and a Nocardia species. Associated conditions predisposing to splenic abscess included trauma in three cases, splenic arteritis or embolization in five cases, and foci of infection elsewhere in the body in six, including two cases of endocarditis. The mortality was 60 per cent. Half of the deaths were due to the underlying illness, but failure to diagnose splenic abscess contributed to a fatal outcome in three cases.

Splenic abscess is an uncommon entity, as evidenced by its absence from a recent review of 540 intra-abdominal abscesses [1]; when present, it is frequently diagnosed only during postmortem examination. Our experience with six cases of splenic abscess within an eight month period, three of which were diagnosed clinically, prompted this report.

MATERIAL

All medical records and pathology reports dated between 1964 and 1974 at Cleveland Metropolitan General Hospital (CMGH) were reviewed for cases coded as splenic abscess or splenitis. Only those cases in which macroscopic splenic abscess was noted were selected. In addition to the six cases seen in consultation by one of us (J.D.C.), four other cases were found, one of which has been reported elsewhere [2]. These nine previously unreported cases are presented here, and the pertinent literature is reviewed.

CASE REPORTS

Case 1. A 13 year old white girl was admitted to CMGH on August 3, 1973, with a five week history of intermittent fever, headache, chills, malaise and anorexia. Five days prior to admission she was admitted to another hospital where she had intermittent discomfort in the upper left abdominal quadrant and daily fever despite therapy with minocycline.

From the Departments of Medicine (Division of Infectious Diseases) and Pathology, Cleveland Metropolitan General Hospital and Case Western Reserve University School of Medicine, Cleveland, Ohio. Requests for reprints should be addressed to Dr. Jeffrey D. Chulay. Manuscript accepted December 10, 1975.

* Present address: Walter Reed Army Institute of Research, Washington, D.C. 20012.

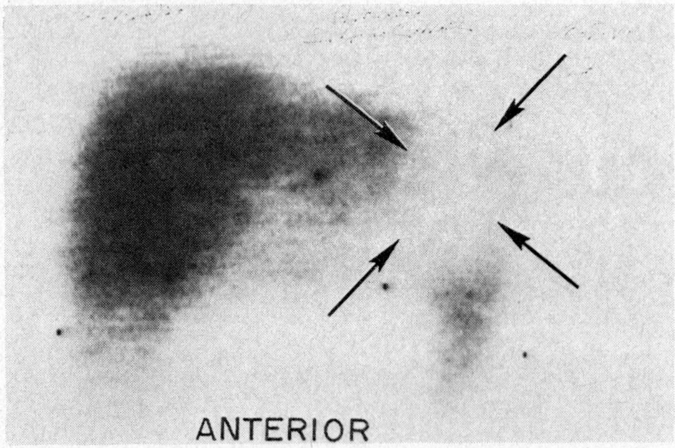

*Figure 1. Case 1. Technetium-99m-sulfur colloid liver-spleen scan. A large defect is seen in the upper pole of the spleen **(arrows).***

Temperature was 39.8°C. There was tenderness in the upper left quadrant, but the spleen was not palpable. The white blood cell count was 8,300/mm^3 with 82 per cent polymorphonuclear leukocytes and 5 per cent band forms. Urine, gastric aspirate and four blood cultures were sterile. Stool cultures grew no enteric pathogens. A chest film obtained on the seventh hospital day showed elevation of the left hemidiaphragm, and a liver-spleen scan showed a defect in the upper pole of the spleen (Figure 1). Additional history was obtained that while playing baseball three months earlier she had collided with another girl and experienced transient soreness in the upper left portion of her abdomen.

Laparotomy disclosed a splenic abscess containing 60 cc of foul-smelling pus which grew Salmonella heidelberg; anaerobic culture was negative. Microscopically, there was extensive hemorrhage with marked hemosiderosis in the wall of the abscess cavity. She was treated with ampicillin and made an uneventful recovery.

Comment: The pathologic findings suggest that this abscess developed as a complication of a hematoma, presumably caused by minor trauma three months earlier. Although repeated questioning elicited no history suggestive of previous gastroenteritis, seeding of the hematoma probably occurred as the result of a transient bacteremia arising in the gut. A similar lack of preceding gastrointestinal symptoms has been noted in some [3,4], but not all [5], previous reports of splenic abscess caused by salmonellae.

Case 2. A 73 year old white woman was admitted to CMGH on August 13, 1973, after she was found on the floor of her apartment, having slipped and fallen two days previously. Past history included a remote stroke, chronic dementia and rheumatoid arthritis. Temperature was 37.2°C. She was dehydrated and had multiple bruises. The abdomen was nontender and neither the liver nor spleen was palpable. The white blood cell count was 27,000/mm^3 with 90 per cent polymorphonuclear leukocytes. Chest roentgenogram was within normal limits.

A low grade fever persisted throughout her hospitalization. A large sacral decubitus ulcer grew Escherichia coli. A blood culture grew Klebsiella ozaenae, but she remained febrile despite therapy with gentamicin.

On the 16th hospital day a tender, tympanitic mass in the left upper quadrant developed, and porphobilinogen was found in her urine. Abdominal films were interpreted as showing massive gastric dilatation. A diagnosis of acute intermittent porphyria was made, and she was treated with chlorpromazine and intravenous glucose. She showed no improvement and died three weeks after admission.

Autopsy disclosed thrombosis of the splenic vein and a large splenic abscess containing brown fluid. Microscopically there was necrosis and pyogenic response surrounded by granulation tissue and fibroblast proliferation. Culture of the pus yielded Esch. coli. Postmortem blood culture was sterile.

When the films were reviewed it was appreciated that the large air-fluid level in the upper left portion of the abdomen was an abscess cavity and not the stomach (Figure 2).

Comment: Although this patient had clinical and roentgenographic findings typical of splenic abscess, the diagnosis was not made antemortem because of the concurrent development of acute intermittent porphyria, misinterpretation of the x-ray films and failure to consider the possibility of abscess. The antemortem Klebsiella bacteremia, taken together with the isolation of Esch. coli from splenic pus at autopsy, suggests a mixed infection. Factors which may have contributed to the development of splenic abscess include the decubitus ulcer and trauma associated with her fall.

Case 3. A 79 year old diabetic white woman was admitted to CMGH on January 3, 1974, with a four day history of anorexia, polyuria and lethargy. Temperature was 37.3°C, pulse 132/min, respirations 48/min and blood pressure 90/60 mm Hg. She was restless and disoriented. There was generalized abdominal tenderness, but no organs or masses were palpable. The white blood cell count was 16,200/mm^3, urine culture grew Esch. coli, and blood glucose was 720 mg/100 ml. She was treated with intravenous fluids and insulin. Low grade fever and abdominal tenderness, now maximal in the lower right quadrant, persisted. An abdominal paracentesis yielded turbid fluid which subsequently grew Esch. coli. Clindamycin and gentamicin therapy was begun, and on the third hospital day laparotomy disclosed seropurulent fluid within the peritoneal cavity. The small bowel, liver, stomach, kidneys, uterus and ovaries were examined and considered to be normal. The surgeon described "matting of the omentum in the area of the spleen, but no evidence that any inflammatory process was going on at this time." Postoperatively she was treated with chloramphenicol, but she remained febrile and died on the ninth hospital day.

At autopsy there was massive infarction of the spleen with thrombosis of the splenic artery and vein. A 13 by 7 by 3 cm splenic abscess contained 200 cc of chocolate brown, nonfoul-smelling pus, culture of which grew Esch. coli. There were remote and recent myocardial infarctions, with a mural

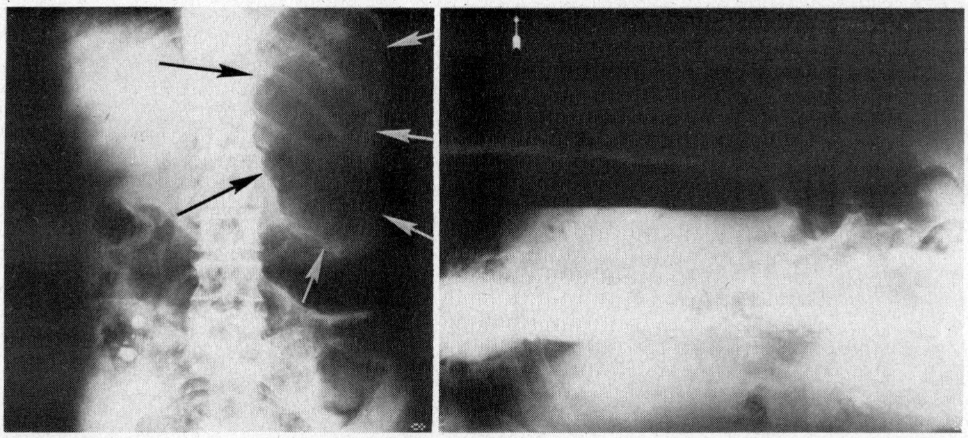

Figure 2. *Case 2. Supine anteroposterior **(left)** and lateral decubitus **(right)** abdominal films. An abscess cavity **(arrows)** occupies almost the entire left half of the abdominal cavity, with an air-fluid level apparent in the lateral decubitus view.*

thrombus partially adherent to the apex of the left ventricle. Multiple cerebral infarcts were present.

Comment: This patient had a myocardial infarction complicated by a mural thrombus. Embolization to the spleen was followed by infarction, abscess formation and peritonitis, perhaps originating from a urinary infection. Despite exploratory laparotomy, the diagnosis of splenic abscess was not made antemortem, a diagnostic difficulty reported by others [6,7].

Case 4. A 49 year old white woman was first admitted to CMGH on July 9, 1973, because of pleuritic pain in the left side of her chest for four months and fever with intermittent shaking chills for two months which did not diminish with tetracycline therapy. Past history included chemical diabetes mellitus.

Temperature was 38.6°C. She had tenderness and signs of consolidation over the lower left side of the chest. The upper left portion of the abdomen was tender, but the spleen was not palpable. The white blood cell count was 12,000/mm^3 with 67 per cent polymorphonuclear leukocytes and 3 per cent band forms. Chest film showed pleural effusion on the left. Second strength tuberculin purified protein derivative was negative. Thoracentesis yielded 40 cc of thick pus. Thoracotomy disclosed only clear fluid in the pleural space, but incision of an indurated area in the diaphragm revealed a subphrenic abscess which was drained. Smears and aerobic cultures of the wall of the cavity and pus were negative for pyogens, fungi and acid-fast bacilli. The patient was treated with cephalothin and gentamicin and discharged on July 31.

Her symptoms slowly resolved over several months, but recurrence of chest pain and wound drainage led to her readmission on January 16, 1974. She was afebrile. Purulent secretions drained from the scar and she had mild tenderness in the upper left quadrant. A liver-spleen scan (Figure 3) showed a defect in the upper half of the spleen, and a splenic abscess was removed by splenectomy. Microscopic examination disclosed a dimorphic picture consisting of both pyogenic reaction and granulomatous inflammation with caseation. Special stains showed occasional groups of acid-fast, silver-positive, branching filaments consistent with nocardia. There was evidence of preceding endarteritis with focal intimal thickening and loss of the internal elastic membrane. Aerobic and anaerobic cultures of the spleen were negative for pyogens, fungi and acid-fast bacilli, and cultures of sputum were negative for fungi and acid-fast bacilli. Sulfisoxazole therapy was started for nocardiosis, and she made an uneventful recovery.

Comment: Subphrenic abscess was diagnosed during the first admission, but recurrence of drainage led to the consideration of splenic abscess, known to be the origin of approximately 3 per cent of subphrenic abscesses [8]. Although an organism was not isolated by culture, the acid-fast filamentous forms seen in the spleen sections were probably nocardia. Antibiotic therapy prior to obtaining material for cultures may have been responsible for the inability to recover the organism. Splenic involvement is uncommon in nocardiosis, occurring in only eight of 147 cases recently reviewed [9], and is usually accompanied by multiple abscesses elsewhere [10,11]. In this case hematogenous dissemination from an occult pulmonary focus may have resulted in abscess formation limited to the spleen.

Additionally, this case demonstrates the value of the posterior view of the liver-spleen scan, since the anterior view appears normal (Figure 3).

Case 5. A six year old white girl was admitted to CMGH on January 14, 1974, because of weakness, pallor and anorexia for two weeks. Temperature was 39.5°C and cervical lymphadenopathy and hepatosplenomegaly were present. Hematocrit value was 13 per cent, reticulocyte count 0.1 per cent and white blood cell count 10,300/mm^3 with 45 per cent lymphocytes (half atypical). Heterophil antibodies were characteristic of infectious mononucleosis, a direct Coombs

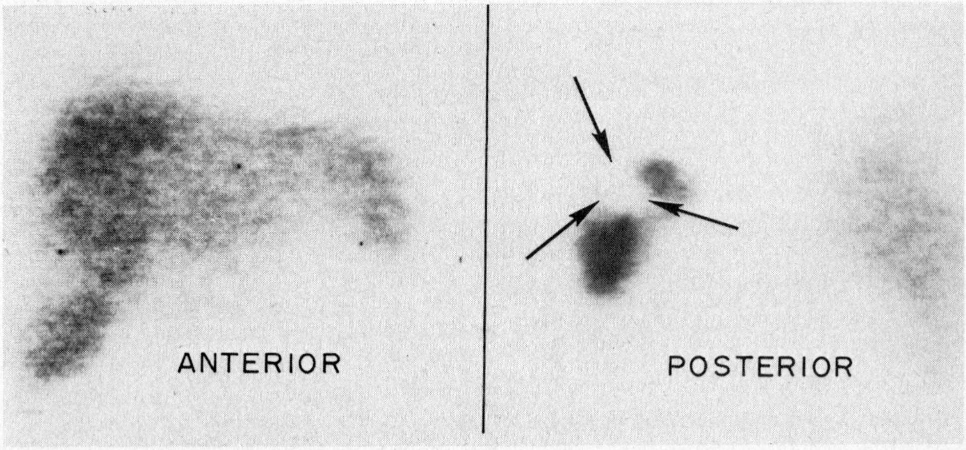

Figure 3. *Case 4. Technetium-99m-sulfur colloid liver-spleen scan. The anterior view appears normal, but a 3 by 3 cm filling defect in the upper pole of the spleen is easily seen in the posterior view* ***(arrows).***

test was positive, and anti-i and anti-I antibodies were detected in her serum.*

She was treated with large doses of prednisone and frequent blood transfusion. Her fever abated in three days but recurred during the second week of hospitalization. On the 12th hospital day signs of peritonitis developed and she was treated with gentamicin; a blood culture grew Enterobacter cloacae, sensitive to gentamicin. Despite continued therapy with gentamicin, she remained febrile and six days later a blood culture again grew E. cloacae. A liver-spleen scan showed a large defect in the upper pole of the spleen, and a diagnosis of infected subcapsular hematoma was confirmed at laparotomy. Culture of foul-smelling pus from the excised spleen grew E. cloacae plus Bacteroides fragilis, and clindamycin was added to her therapy. Recovery was uneventful.

Comment: This girl had several unusual complications of infectious mononucleosis. Hemolytic anemia is seen infrequently with this disease; it is rarely accompanied by an aplastic crisis [12]. Subcapsular splenic hematoma, often attributed to the minor trauma of physical examination, is a well known complication of infectious mononucleosis and may progress to splenic rupture. Secondary bacterial infections, however, are rarely seen in patients with infectious mononucleosis [13,14], and to our knowledge the complication of splenic abscess has not been reported previously. The mechanism of infection of the hematoma is unknown in this patient, but intravenous therapy, including multiple blood transfusions, provided an obvious portal of entry for bacteria. The role of corticosteroid therapy in the development of bacterial superinfection is only speculative. Persistent bacteremia despite appropriate antibiotic therapy led to consideration of an occult abscess, and splenic scanning pinpointed the site of infection.

* Cold agglutinins have a specificity for the I-i system of erythrocyte antigens, with virtually all having anti-I activity; the cold agglutinins seen in infectious mononucleosis are unusual in that they react with the i antigen.

Case 6. A 55 year old black woman was admitted to CMGH on January 27, 1974, with a two week history of anorexia, weakness and myalgias. Past history included multiple complications of chronic alcoholism. Temperature was 37.5°C and blood pressure 70/50 mm Hg. She was emaciated, dehydrated and disoriented. A grade 3/6 systolic ejection murmur along the left sternal border radiated to the apex. The liver was enlarged but the spleen was not palpable. The white blood cell count was 17,900/mm^3 with 76 per cent polymorphonuclear leukocytes and 20 per cent band forms. A sickling test yielded negative results.

Hypotension persisted despite intravenous fluid therapy, and a diagnosis of septic shock was entertained. Treatment with methylprednisolone, cephalothin and gentamicin was begun, but she died in shock three days after admission. Three blood cultures later grew Streptobacillus moniliformis.

Autopsy revealed acute bacterial endocarditis with vegetations on the mitral valve and perforation of both leaflets. The spleen contained a 3 by 1.5 cm area of infarction with central abscess formation. Pus from this abscess grew a few colonies of Esch. coli and an enterococcus. The brain contained multiple infarcts with a small abscess in an area of hemorrhagic infarction in the occipital lobe.

Comment: This is at least the 14th reported case of endocarditis caused by Strep. moniliformis [15,16]. Death was due to the hemodynamic effects of valve perforation, and splenic abscess can be considered an incidental finding. The significance of Esch. coli and enterococcus in cultures of splenic pus is unclear. Both organisms were present in small quantity, and cultures of postmortem blood and adjacent splenic tissue were sterile. The difficulties in interpretation of autopsy cultures are well known, and it seems likely that the splenic abscess was caused by the same organism that caused endocarditis. Antibiotic therapy, the fastidiousness of Strep. moniliformis, and the presence of other bacteria may all have contributed to the inability to culture the organism from splenic pus.

Case 7. A 62 year old white woman was admitted to CMGH on April 24, 1969, with fever, chills and hematemesis. Past history included diabetes mellitus and recurrent urinary tract infections. Temperature was 38.6°C. There was tenderness in the upper right abdominal quadrant, but liver and spleen were not palpable. The white blood cell count was 36,000/mm^3 with 48 per cent polymorphonuclear leukocytes and 46 per cent band forms.

Upper gastrointestinal tract bleeding responded to medical management, and because of pyelonephritis the patient was treated with kanamycin. Blood and urine cultures grew Esch. coli and Klebsiella. The patient remained febrile for four weeks, urine cultures persistently grew Klebsiella and/or Pseudomonas, and she was treated with varying antimicrobial agents. On the 14th hospital day a right ureterolithotomy was performed with drainage of a right perinephric abscess. On the 76th hospital day several pockets of pus were drained from the bed of the previous incision. Proteus morganii bacteremia occurred on the 94th hospital day and the patient was treated with gentamicin for two weeks. Shortly thereafter fever and renal failure developed, and she died despite therapy.

Autopsy revealed a large splenic abscess containing 1,000 cc of foul-smelling fluid. The splenic vessels were patent. Both kidneys showed evidence of acute and chronic pyelonephritis. Postmortem blood cultures grew Pseudomonas aeruginosa, and cultures of the spleen grew P. aeruginosa and Enterobacter (Serratia) liquefaciens. Anaerobic cultures were not obtained.

Comment: The origin of splenic abscess in this patient is unknown. Although hematogenous spread from a urinary tract infection was a possible source, the foul-smelling pus suggests anaerobic infection, perhaps originating from the gastrointestinal tract. Clinical diagnosis was hindered by the lack of localizing signs or symptoms referable to her spleen, and fever was attributed to urinary sepsis. There was, however, no evidence of uncontrolled renal suppuration at autopsy, and the undiagnosed splenic abscess was at least contributory to her death.

Case 8. A 64 year old black woman was admitted to CMGH on June 29, 1970, because of dyspnea and edema. She was afebrile and had periorbital edema, increased jugular venous pressure and hepatosplenomegaly. The white blood cell count was 6,100/mm^3 with a normal differential, urinalysis showed red cell casts, and urine culture was sterile. Creatinine was 7.8 mg/100 ml, antinuclear antibody was present, and renal biopsy showed membranous and proliferative glomerulonephritis.

Treatment with digitalis, diuretics and prednisone was begun, but persistent oliguria and azotemia necessitated peritoneal dialysis. On the 31st hospital day she died of ventricular fibrillation.

Autopsy disclosed atypical verrucous (Libman-Sacks) endocarditis of the tricuspid valve, pericarditis and lupus glomerulonephritis. The spleen had a subcapsular abscess cavity containing 25 cc of foul-smelling pus, culture of which grew Klebsiella. Anaerobic cultures were not obtained. The splenic vessels were free of thrombus, but microscopically there was periarterial fibrosis ("onion-skinning") of follicular arteries. Blood cultures were sterile.

Comment: This patient had systemic lupus erythematosus with renal insufficiency, and uremia may explain the lack of fever in the face of an abscess. No signs or symptoms referable to splenic abscess developed, its origin remains unknown, and it can be considered an incidental autopsy finding.

Case 9. A 45 year old white man was admitted to CMGH on December 24, 1970, because of fever and confusion. Temperature was 40°C. A grade 3/6 systolic murmur was maximal at the left sternal border, and the spleen was palpable. The white blood cell count was 11,600/mm^3 with 38 per cent polymorphonuclear leukocytes and 45 per cent band forms. Blood cultures grew Staphylococcus aureus, resistant to penicillin. Therapy for endocarditis was initiated with methicillin. Subsequent complications included aortic insufficiency, atrial fibrillation and cerebral embolism. On the 19th hospital day shock developed, and he died the next day.

Autopsy revealed acute endocarditis, with vegetations involving the aortic valve, and rupture of the left aortic cusp. Several septic infarcts and small abscesses were noted in the spleen and both kidneys. A smear of splenic pus showed clusters of gram-positive cocci, but culture was sterile.

Comment: In this patient splenic abscess developed as a complication of acute bacterial endocarditis. As in Case 6, the abscess was clinically silent and did not contribute to the patient's death.

DESCRIPTION OF SERIES

During a 10 year period, 10 cases of splenic abscess were diagnosed among the 94,460 patients admitted to CMGH. The six cases diagnosed postmortem represented 0.22 per cent of the 2,840 autopsies performed at CMGH during this period. The characteristics in these 10 cases are summarized in Table I. The patients' ages ranged from 6 to 79 years, with a mean of 46.8 years. Three patients were black and seven were white, a ratio similar to the general population at CMGH. A sickling test was negative in the one case in which it was performed. In contrast to the male predominance in other series [17–19], in nine of our 10 cases the patients were female. Although six of these cases occurred during the last year of study, no reason for an increasing incidence is apparent.

Fever was the most common finding, occurring at some time during the course of the illness in nine of 10 cases. Abdominal pain and tenderness were present in six cases, but in only three was it localized to the region of the spleen. In three cases the spleen was palpably enlarged, and in another case there was a tympanitic mass in the upper left quadrant. In eight

TABLE I Summary of Findings in Patients with Splenic Abscess at CMGH, 1964–1974

Case No.	Age (yr) and Sex	Symptoms	Fever	Physical Findings	Abnormal X-ray Films	Blood Culture	Abscess Smear or Culture	Associated Conditions	Outcome
1	13, F	Upper left quadrant pain	+	Upper left quadrant tender	Chest, spleen scan	Sterile	S. heidelberg	Trauma	Cured
2	73, F	Abdominal pain	+	Tympanitic upper left quadrant tender mass	Abdominal	K. ozaenae	Esch. coli	Decubitus ulcer, trauma	Died
3	79, F	. . .	+	Peritonitis	. . .	Sterile	Esch. coli	Urinary tract infection, myocardial infarction, diabetes mellitus	Died
4	49, F	Chest pain	+	Left side of chest and upper left quadrant tender	Chest, spleen scan	Sterile	Nocardia sp.*	Diabetes mellitus	Cured
5	6, F	Abdominal pain	+	Splenomegaly, abdomen tender	Spleen scan	E. cloacae	E. cloacae B. fragilis	Infectious mononucleosis	Cured
6	55, F	. . .	+	. . .	. . .	Strep. moniliformis	See text	Endocarditis	Died
7	62, F	. . .	+	. . .	. . .	P. aeruginosa†	P. aeruginosa E. liquefaciens	Diabetes mellitus, perinephric abscess	Died
8	64, F	. . .	0	Splenomegaly	. . .	Sterile	Klebsiella	Systemic lupus erythematosus	Died
9	45, M	. . .	+	Splenomegaly	. . .	Staph. aureus	Staphylococcus*	Endocarditis	Died
10‡	22, F	Shoulder and flank pain	+	Left costovertebral angle tender, peritonitis	Chest, abdominal	Sterile	Esch. coli "paracolon bacillus"	Septic abortion	Cured

* Culture negative. † Postmortem. ‡ Reference 2.

cases leukocytosis was present. Roentgenographic clues to the diagnosis were found in five cases, including one in which the patient had an air-fluid level in the left side of the abdomen, another in which the patient had medial displacement of the colon and extraintestinal perinephric gas, and three in which the left hemidiaphragm was elevated or pleural effusion was present, and three in which a liver-spleen scan was abnormal.

The bacteriology in our cases included Staph. aureus and Strep. moniliformis in the two cases of endocarditis, and presumed nocardiosis in one instance. In the remaining seven cases, infection was with various enteric gram-negative bacilli, including Esch. coli in three, Enterobacter in three, and Salmonella, Klebsiella, Pseudomonas, Bacteroides and "paracolon bacillus" in one each. In four cases, more than one organism was apparently involved. Although an anaerobic organism was isolated from only one abscess, three others contained foul-smelling pus, suggesting anaerobes may have been present.

The mode of infection in this series included known or presumed hematogenous spread of infection from another focus in six cases (Cases 2, 3, 6, 7, 9 and 10), in two of which bacterial endocarditis was present. Splenic trauma was possibly involved in three cases (Cases 1, 2 and 5), and embolism, thrombosis or arteritis of the splenic vessels was present in Cases 2, 3, 4, 6, 8 and 9.

There were no deaths among the four cases in which a correct diagnosis was made and treatment given, and no survivors among the six cases in which a clinical diagnosis was not made. In three cases in which no signs or symptoms were referable to the splenic abscess (Cases 6, 8 and 9) the patients died from an underlying illness, but in the other three cases failure to surgically drain the splenic abscess was at least contributory to the patients' death.

TABLE II **Causative Organisms in Splenic Abscesses from Review of Literature and Present Series***

Organism		Number of Cases†
Staphylococci		27 (21%)
Staph. aureus [Present series, 7, 17, 18, 22, 23, 37, 44, 58–62]	19	
Staph. epidermidis [5, 43, 63, 64]	5	
Not stated [7, 65, 66]	3	
Streptococci		21 (16%)
Alpha hemolytic [22, 36, 67, 68]	6	
Beta hemolytic [20, 48, 64]	4	
Nonhemolytic [17, 18, 44, 59]	5	
Enterococci [45, 69]	2	
Not stated [7, 66, 70, 71]	4	
Streptococcus pneumoniae [30, 59]		2
Nocardia species [Present series, 10, 11]		3
Salmonellae		19 (15%)
Salmonella typhi [7, 20, 72, 73]	7	
Other Salmonella species [Present series, 3–5, 18, 24, 49, 51, 68, 74]	12	
Other gram-negative bacilli		31 (24%)
Escherichia coli [Present series, 2, 5, 7, 25, 44, 53, 62, 71]	10	
Enterobacter species [Present series, 17]	4	
Brucella species [75]	4	
Proteus species [17, 26, 41]	3	
Pseudomonas aeruginosa [Present series, 17, 18]	3	
Klebsiella species [Present series, 26]	3	
"Paracolon bacillus" [2]	1	
Pseudomonas pseudomallei [76]	1	
Streptobacillus moniliformis [Present series]	1	
Yersinia enterocolitica [77]	1	
Smear only positive [78]	1	
Anaerobic organisms		7 (5%)
Streptococci [17, 22]	2	
Bacteroides species [Present series, 24]	2	
Clostridium species [22, 79]	2	
Actinomyces species [7]	1	
Mycobacterium tuberculosis [80]		1
Sterile cultures [7, 18, 26–28, 37, 44, 46, 62, 65, 81–83]		31 (24%)

* Culture results in 129 cases with adequate documentation of etiologic agent. In cases of endocarditis, the organism responsible for cardiac infection was assumed to be the cause of splenic infection, even when cultures from the abscess were negative or not reported.

† Percentages total more than 100 per cent because of multiple organisms isolated in some cases.

COMMENTS

In various autopsy series the incidence of splenic abscess has been reported to be between 0.26 per cent and 0.67 per cent [7,20,21], comparable to the incidence in our series. An antemortem diagnosis was made in only three of 66 cases among several large series [7,17,20]. More recent reports have included cases correctly diagnosed in which the patients were surgically treated [5,22–26], but few have included autopsy reviews to consider those cases which were undiagnosed during the patient's life [18,19].

The most frequent symptom occurring in patients with splenic abscess is pain, often pleuritic, located in the upper left portion of the abdomen, the left side of the chest, left flank or referred to the left shoulder. Chills, nausea, vomiting and awareness of an abdominal mass may also be present. In addition to the fever and leukocytosis usually present, objective findings may include splenomegaly, tenderness in the upper left portion of the abdomen or left side of the chest, and rarely a splenic friction rub or tympany in the region of the spleen.

Various roentgenographic signs of splenic abscess have been described, including a soft tissue mass in the upper left quadrant; extra-alimentary gas in the upper left quadrant; displacement of other organs, including the splenic flexure of the colon, the mediastinum, the left kidney or the gastric shadow; and elevation of the left hemidiaphragm with or without a pleural effusion

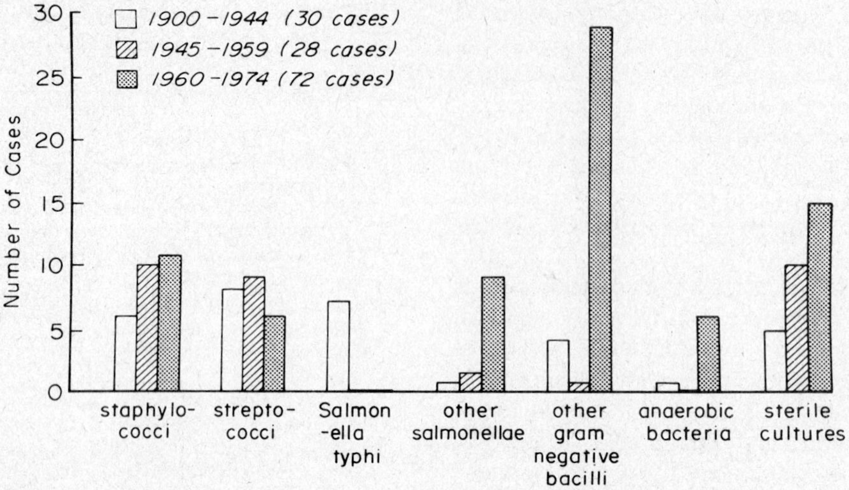

Figure 4. *Causative organisms in splenic abscesses analyzed by year of report.*

[18,27]. Perhaps the most diagnostically useful roentgenographic information is obtained from the technetium-99m-sulfur colloid liver-spleen scan. This examination was invaluable in three of our cases and in previously reported cases as well [5,22]. The importance of a posterior view when looking for splenic disease has been emphasized by others [28]. The spleen scan may not demonstrate a defect when multiple small abscesses are present, in which case selective arteriography may be helpful [19]. Total body scanning following the intravenous administration of gallium-67 may not be helpful in diagnosing splenic abscess, since uptake of this radioisotope by the abscess may not differ sufficiently from normal splenic uptake to allow visualization of even a large abscess [29].

The mechanism by which splenic abscess develops is evident in 80 per cent of cases, with infection elsewhere in the body causative in a large majority [30]. Approximately 15 per cent of cases are traumatic in origin [30,31], whereas direct extension from a neighboring process is seen occasionally [30].

Certain infections are complicated by splenic abscess with unusual frequency. A threefold increased incidence of splenic abscess has been found among patients dying with typhoid fever [7,32,33] and malaria [34], and in the pre-antibiotic era 10 per cent of the patients who died of bacterial endocarditis had suppurative lesions in their spleens [35]. In more recent years, splenic abscess has occasionally been responsible for persistent bacteremia despite appropriate antibiotic therapy of endocarditis, in which case splenectomy is often curative [36]. Splenic abscess has also been reported complicating relapsing fever [37,38] and amebic dysentery [39] as well as otitis media [17,40], mastoiditis [19,20,41], peritonsillar abscess [42], suppurative parotitis [17], cutaneous infections of various types [7,17,21,22,43], lung abscess [17,21], pneumonia [21], empyema [17,43], appendicitis [7,44–47], diverticulitis [22], cholecystitis [7], pelvic infections [2,7,48], osteomyelitis [49] and intravenous drug abuse [19].

Hemoglobinopathies also appear to predispose to the development of splenic abscess. Among reports from Nigeria, 74 per cent of patients with splenic abscess had sickle hemoglobin [18,25,26,50], an incidence three times greater than that in the general population [18]. Reports of splenic abscesses from the United States have also included patients with hemoglobin S [22,24,49,51]. The most common hemoglobinopathies reported have been sickle trait or hemoglobin SC disease, and rarely hemoglobin S-thalassemia or hemoglobin AC. The absence of patients with sickle cell anemia (hemoglobin SS disease) in reported cases of splenic abscess may reflect the functional asplenia which begins in early childhood in these patients [52].

Some insight into the pathogenesis of splenic abscess in many of the conditions cited can be gained from the work of Caldarera [53]. He was able to produce splenic abscess following intravenous injection of Staph. aureus in rabbits only when their spleens had been previously traumatized or a terminal branch of the splenic artery had been ligated prior to injection. Thus it is not surprising that the illnesses associated with splenic abscess are often those in which there is a high incidence of splenic infarction in addition to the opportunity for bacteremia.

Little attention has been paid to the bacteriology of splenic abscess. In reviewing those reports in which culture data are available, it can be seen that Staph. aureus, various streptococci and gram-negative bacilli are most frequently isolated (Table II). A variety of unusual organisms have occasionally been reported, including Brucella, Actinomyces, Pseudomonas pseudomallei, Nocardia, Strep. moniliformis and Yersinia enterocolitica. An interesting finding is the relatively frequent isolation of Salmonella species. The relationship of typhoid fever to splenic abscess has already been mentioned, but nontyphoidal salmonellae have been reported even more frequently than S. typhi. Only five of the 12 cases involving these other Salmonella species have occurred in patients known to have sickle hemoglobin [18,24,49,51]. The true incidence of splenic abscess caused by Salmonella is undoubtedly higher than indicated in Table II, since splenic abscess was present in an unknown number of the 136 abscesses caused by Salmonella reported by Saphra and Winter [54].

Although anaerobic bacteria have been isolated from only 5 per cent of splenic abscesses, these fastidious organisms probably played a role in many more cases. As shown in Table II, an additional 24 per cent of abscesses had sterile pus, many of which contained gas [18,26]. It has recently been re-emphasized that "sterile pus," especially when associated with gas, often contains anaerobic organisms recoverable by appropriate culture technics [55]. The number of sterile abscesses would be even higher if Wallace's cases [56] were included, but it is unclear in how many of his patients cultures were obtained.

When the culture data are analyzed by year of report, several trends become apparent (Figure 4). In recent years the number of cases of splenic abscess reported per year has increased. Although staphylococci and streptococci accounted for the majority of reports prior to 1960, there has been an increase during the past 15 years in the relative proportion of cases caused by gram-negative bacilli, especially Esch. coli and nontyphoidal salmonellae. A similar change in the proportion of cases due to gram-negative bacilli has been noted in many other types of infections, and may be related to a variety of factors, including the widespread use of antibiotics, improved survival of critically ill patients colonized with these bacteria, and prolonged hospitalization with its attendant risk of nosocomial infection. S. typhi have not been reported as a cause of splenic abscess since 1940, obviously related to the decreased incidence of typhoid fever in recent years. All but one of the anaerobic organisms isolated from splenic abscesses have been reported since 1960, probably reflecting improved culture technics for these organisms.

Treatment of splenic abscess consists of surgical drainage and appropriate antibiotic therapy. Although the older literature suggests a lower mortality with splenotomy than with splenectomy [7,20,57], current surgical opinion favors splenectomy when feasible [19,22,51]. The prognosis is dependent primarily on accurate diagnosis and whether infection elsewhere in the body can be controlled. Without surgical drainage, or in patients with multiple disseminated abscesses, the mortality approaches 100 per cent, but with appropriate surgical and antibiotic therapy of isolated splenic abscess, mortality during the past 25 years has been less than 10 per cent.

ACKNOWLEDGMENT

We thank Dr. Herbert Tanowitz for review of the manuscript, Dr. John Reid for help with interpretation of microscopic pathology and Dr. Emanuel Wolinsky for advice, encouragement and assistance in the preparation of the manuscript.

REFERENCES

1. Altemeier WA, Colbertson WR, Fullen WD, et al.: Intra-abdominal abscesses. Am J Surg 125: 70, 1973.
2. Knauer QF, Abrams JS: Generalized peritonitis due to a ruptured splenic abscess. Am J Surg 112: 923, 1966.
3. Sharr MM: Splenic abscess due to Salmonella agona. Br Med J 1: 546, 1972.
4. Elfving G, Parmala ME, Perttilä M: Splenic abscess caused by Salmonella paratyphi B perforating retroperitoneally. Ann Chir Gynaecol Fenn 44: 16, 1955.
5. Zook EG, Bolivar JC, Epstein LI: Value of scintiscans in the diagnosis of splenic abscess. Surg Gynecol Obstet 131: 1125, 1970.
6. Baker RE: Abscess of the spleen. US Vet Bur Med Bull 7: 264, 1931.
7. Billings AE: Abscess of the spleen. Ann Surg 88: 416, 1928.
8. Ochsner A, Graves AM: Subphrenic abscess. Ann Surg 98: 961, 1933.
9. Presant CA, Wiernik PH, Serpick AA: Factors affecting survival in nocardiosis. Am Rev Respir Dis 108: 1444, 1973.
10. Neu HC, Silva M, Hazen E, et al.: Necrotizing nocardial pneumonitis. Ann Intern Med 66: 274, 1967.
11. Murray JF, Finegold SM, Froman S, et al.: The changing spectrum of nocardiosis. Am Rev Respir Dis 83: 315, 1961.
12. Worlledge SM, Dacie JV: Haemolytic and other anaemias in infectious mononucleosis, chap 5. Infectious Mononucleosis (Carter RL, Penman HG, eds), Oxford and Edinburgh, Blackwell Scientific Publications, 1969.
13. Penman HG: Fatal infectious mononucleosis: a critical review. J Clin Pathol 23: 765, 1970.
14. Penman HG: Extreme neutropenia in glandular fever. J Clin Pathol 21: 48, 1968.
15. McCormack RC, Kaye D, Hook EW: Endocarditis due to Streptobacillus moniliformis. JAMA 200: 77, 1967.
16. Finland M, Barnes MW: Changing etiology of bacterial endocarditis in the antibacterial era. Ann Intern Med 72: 341, 1970.
17. McSherry CK, Dineen P: The significance of splenic abscess. Am J Surg 103: 618, 1962.
18. Kolawole TM, Bohrer SP: Splenic abscess and the gene for hemoglobin S. Am J Roentgenol Radium Ther Nucl Med 119: 175, 1973.
19. Gadacz T, Way LW, Dunphy JE: Changing clinical spectrum

of splenic abscess. Am J Surg 128: 182, 1974.
20. Walker IJ: Abscess of the spleen. N Engl J Med 203: 1025, 1930.
21. Krumbharr EB: Diseases of the spleen, vol 5, chap 4. Modern Medicine, 3rd ed (Osler W, ed), Philadelphia, Lea & Febiger, 1927.
22. Pickleman JR, Paloyan E, Block GE: The surgical significance of splenic abscess. Surgery 68: 287, 1970.
23. Kuiper DH, Papp JP, Thompson NW: Solitary splenic abscess. Mich Med 69: 293, 1970.
24. Frankel A, Ashikari H, Dreiling DA, et al.: Splenic abscess. J Mt Sinai Hosp NY 33: 404, 1966.
25. Anand SV, Davey WW: Surgery of the spleen in Nigeria. Br J Surg 52: 335, 1965.
26. Cockshott WP, Weaver EJM: Primary tropical splenic abscess: a misnomer. Br J Surg 49: 665, 1962.
27. Zatzkin HR, Drazan AD, Irwin GA: Roentgenographic diagnosis of splenic abscess. Am J Roentgenol Radium Ther Nucl Med 91: 896, 1964.
28. McIntyre PA: Diagnostic significance of the spleen scan. Semin Nucl Med 2: 278, 1972.
29. Silva J Jr, Harvey WC: Detection of infections with gallium-67 and scintigraphic imaging. J Infect Dis 130: 125, 1974.
30. Elting AW: Abscess of the spleen. Ann Surg 62: 182, 1915.
31. Inlow WDP: Traumatic abscess of the spleen. Ann Surg 85: 368, 1927.
32. Berg, cited in Elting AW: Abscess of the spleen. Ann Surg 62: 182, 1915.
33. Curschman, cited in Elting AW: Abscess of the spleen. Ann Surg 62: 182, 1915.
34. Anderson ARS: Splenic abscess in malarial fever. Lancet 2: 1159, 1906.
35. Blumer G: Subacute bacterial endocarditis. Medicine 2: 105, 1923.
36. Lingeman CJ, Smith EB, Battersby S, et al.: Subacute bacterial endocarditis. Splenectomy in cases refractory to antibiotic therapy. Arch Intern Med 97: 309, 1956.
37. Nasr LA: Sterile splenic abscess after relapsing fever. Lancet 1: 555, 1948.
38. Manson JK, Thornton LHD: East African relapsing fever. J Roy Army Med Corps 33: 97, 1919.
39. Frank JR: Amoebic abscess of spleen. Br Med J 1: 458, 1944.
40. Cutler EC: Abscess of the spleen. JAMA 75: 1712, 1920.
41. Davidson SG, Doig JA, Everam GJH: Acute splenic abscess. J Roy Coll Surg Edinburgh 6: 44, 1960.
42. Eliason EL: Splenic abscess. Ann Surg 97: 301, 1933.
43. Bassler A: Splenic abscess. Three cases of pyogenic infection. Am J Dig Dis 12: 223, 1945.
44. Chaffee JS, Lasher RL, Tredway JB: Splenic abscess. Report of four cases. Ann Surg 148: 979, 1958.
45. Andrus DL, Ray RC, Cottrell FW Jr, et al.: Abscess of the spleen. US Armed Forces Med J 2: 233, 1951.
46. Lang PR, James CF Jr: Abscess of the spleen with diaphragmatic perforation. Va Med Mon 72: 26, 1945.
47. Fauntleroy AM: Report of a case of splenic abscess. JAMA 56: 260, 1911.
48. Wolfson IN: Abscess of the spleen. N Engl J Med 230: 135, 1944.
49. Goldenberg IS: Sickle-cell anemia, Salmonella enteritidis osteomyelitis, and remote postoperative wound abscess. Surgery 38: 758, 1955.
50. Beet EA: Primary splenic abscess and sickle cell disease. East Afr Med J 26: 180, 1949.
51. Parrish RA Jr, Sherman HC: The surgical significance of splenic abscess. Am Surg 30: 712, 1964.
52. Pearson HA, Spencer RP, Cornelius EA: Functional asplenia in sickle-cell anemia. N Engl J Med 281: 923, 1969.
53. Caldarera E: Acute abscess of the spleen. Surg Gynecol Obstet 67: 265, 1938.
54. Saphra I, Winter JW: Clinical manifestations of salmonellosis in man. An evaluation of 7779 human infections identified at the New York Salmonella Center. N Engl J Med 256: 1128, 1957.
55. Gorbach SL, Bartlett JG: Anaerobic infections. N Engl J Med 290: 1177, 1974.
56. Wallace AF: Splenic abscess. Med J South Afr 17: 155, 1922.
57. Reid SE, Lang SJ: Abscess of the spleen. Am J Surg 88: 912, 1954.
58. Whelan TJ: Abscess of the spleen. Am J Surg 94: 945, 1957.
59. Mason LB, Crouch WL: Solitary splenic abscess associated with sickle cell anemia. NC Med J 15: 260, 1954.
60. Winterbotham J: Abscess of spleen. Indian Med Gaz 53: 340, 1918.
61. Peters UJW: Report of a case of abscess of the spleen. Ala Med J 23: 216, 1910.
62. Bell WH: Splenic abscess as a not uncommon complication of grave malarial infection. Milit Surg 21: 83, 1907.
63. Singer R: Abscess of the spleen. S Afr Med J 23: 715, 1949.
64. Pollock RW: Splenic abscess. Northwest Med 48: 853, 1949.
65. Jelliffe DB: Splenic abscess in the tropics. J Trop Med Hyg 52: 134, 1949.
66. Gelfand M: Primary splenic abscess. Trans R Soc Trop Med Hyg 40: 789, 1947.
67. Baron JM, Weinshelbaum EI, Block GE: Splenic rupture associated with bacterial endocarditis and sickle cell trait. JAMA 205: 112, 1968.
68. Schmeisser HC, Harris LC Jr: Multiple necrosis of the spleen. Am J Pathol 14: 821, 1938.
69. Shoenfeld MR, Messeloff CR, Han ST, et al.: Large abscess of the heart and spleen complicating bacterial (enterococcal) endocarditis. Am Heart J 61: 818, 1961.
70. Kerkhof A, Giere E: Rupture of splenic infarct in subacute bacterial endocarditis. Am Heart J 8: 423, 1933.
71. Pitt GN, Fagge CH: A case of splenic abscess—operation—recovery, with remarks. Practioner 86: 541, 1911.
72. Ransohoff JL, O'Rourke W: Typhoid abscess of the spleen in hemolytic jaundice. JAMA 114: 2543, 1940.
73. Morel C, Dambrin C, Tapie J: Abscess of the spleen of typhoid origin. JAMA 86: 1730, 1926.
74. Schulte WJ, Tucker KR: Surgical implications in salmonellosis. Arch Surg 96: 593, 1968.
75. Spink WW: Host-parasite relationship in human brucellosis with prolonged illness due to suppuration of the liver and spleen. Am J Med Sci 247: 129, 1964.
76. Levine S, Whelan TJ Jr: Mellioidosis of the spleen. Am J Surg 115: 849, 1968.
77. Rabsou AR, Koornhof HJ, Notman J, et al.: Hepatosplenic abscesses due to Yersinia enterocolitica. Br Med J 4: 341, 1972.
78. Podgorny G: Splenic abscess causing intestinal obstruction of the large intestine. Am Surg 37: 269, 1971.
79. Rosenblum AL, Bonner H Jr, Milder MS, et al.: Cavitating splenic infarction. Am J Med 56: 720, 1974.
80. Rumold MJ, Orr TG: Tuberculosis of the spleen. Ann Surg 98: 474, 1933.
81. Gelfand M: Primary splenic abscess. Lancet 2: 904, 1947.
82. Haskins JB: Report of two spleen cases. J Tenn Med Assoc 24: 272, 1931.
83. Brady ET: Splenic abscess. Va Med Semi-Mon 12: 538, 1908.

Metastatic Catecholamine-Secreting Paraganglioma (Extra-Adrenal Pheochromocytoma)

Stenographic reports, edited by Philip E. Cryer, M.D. and John M. Kissane, M.D., of weekly clinicopathologic conferences held in Barnes and Wohl Hospitals, are published in each issue of the Journal. These conferences are participated in jointly by members of the Departments of Internal Medicine and Pathology of Washington University School of Medicine.

A 57 year old man was admitted to Barnes Hospital on August 15, 1975, because of hypertension.

He was hospitalized elsewhere on July 14, 1975, because of pain in the upper left abdominal quadrant, constipation, weight loss and hypertension. Sigmoidoscopy, barium studies of the upper and lower gastrointestinal tract and liver-spleen scans disclosed no abnormalities. Episodes of headache and diaphoresis associated with wide fluctuations in blood pressure (diastolic pressures ranging from 100 to 150 mm Hg) were noted. The urinary excretion of catecholamines and vanillylmandelic acid (VMA) was markedly increased. Transient hypercalcemia, with a maximum value of 12.8 mg/100 ml, was noted. The patient lost 10 kg in weight over one month.

He was transferred to the Washington University Clinical Research Center on August 15, 1975. At that time he also complained of low back pain extending to the inner aspects of the thighs. There was a past history of heavy cigarette and alcohol consumption, and a family history of hypertension.

The patient appeared wasted with a body weight of 60 kg. The blood pressure was 140/100 mm Hg, the pulse rate 84/min and the temperature 36.7°C. Positive physical findings included arteriolar narrowing in the optic fundi, a multinodular goiter approximately two times normal size, tremor of the outstretched fingers, brisk reflexes in the arms, muscular weakness especially in the legs, absent ankle jerks and diminished pin perception over the distal portions of the legs. The skin was normal, there was no hepatomegaly, and no abdominal masses were felt. Although the prostate was asymmetrical, there were no hard nodules.

The administration of antihypertensive medications was discontinued for the first four hospital days. The blood pressure increased progressively to 230/130 mm Hg. Pulse rates ranged from 100 to 128/min. Postural hypotension was documented. For example, on one occasion the blood pressure with the patient supine was 180/110 mm Hg with a pulse rate of 100/min; with the patient standing the blood pressure was 90/70 mm Hg with a pulse rate of 130/min.

Initial laboratory studies included a hemoglobin level of 8.3 g/100 and a hematocrit value of 25 per cent with normal red blood cell indices. The white blood cell count was 9,200/mm^3 with 79 per cent segmented neutrophils, 4 per cent eosinophils, 13 per cent lymphocytes and 4 per cent monocytes. The reticulocyte count was 2.8 per cent. Routine serum chemistry studies were within normal limits aside from a creatinine level of 1.6 mg/100 ml, a fasting glucose level of 126 mg/100 ml and an alkaline phosphatase level of 136 mIU/ml. The serum acid phosphatase level was 2.0 King-Armstrong units. Serum calcium concentrations were 9.6, 9.5 and 9.5 mg/100 ml with corresponding phosphate values of 4.1, 4.6 and 4.0 mg/100 ml. The serum free calcium concentration (4.30 mg/100 ml) and plasma parathyroid hormone (9 μleq/ml) and calcitonin (148 pg/ml) levels were normal. Serum thyroxine concentrations were 13.6, 12.3 and 14.5 μg/100 ml (normal 5.0 to 11.0 μg/100 ml) with triiodothyronine (T_3) uptake values of 46 and 47 per cent (normal 35 to 45 per cent) on the last two samples. The thyroid uptake of radioactive iodine (^{131}I) (determined five days after an intravenous urogram) was 2 per cent at 24 hours. During an oral glucose tolerance test the plasma glucose concentrations were 125, 188, 206, 220, 204 and 142 mg/100 ml at 0, 30, 60, 90, 120 and 180 minutes.

Urinary catecholamines were 766 and 806 μg/24 hours and VMA excretion was 33.0 and 39.1 mg/24 hours. Plasma norepinephrine concentrations with the patient supine were 12,100, 9,210, 6,300 and 9,280 pg/ml (normal mean $\pm$ standard deviation [SD] = 234 $\pm$ 81 pg/ml) on four consecutive days. Corresponding plasma epinephrine levels were 587, 177, 159 and 284 pg/ml (normal mean $\pm$ SD = 35 $\pm$ 18 pg/ml).

Chest roentgenograms demonstrated a large extrapleural mass on the left with destruction of the seventh rib. Retrospectively, this lesion had been present at least since February 1975. Additional films revealed metastatic lesions in the spine, sacrum and left iliac wing. Intravenous urograms, with suprarenal laminograms, were within normal limits aside from the bone lesions.

The hypertension and tachycardia were controlled with the administration of phenoxybenzamine (30 mg twice daily) and propranolol (40 mg four times daily). Methimazole (20 mg three times daily) was administered for treatment of hyperthyroidism. Percutaneous biopsy of a bone lesion was refused and the patient was discharged.

CLINICAL DISCUSSION

Dr. Lewis Chase: The problems that we are faced with in this patient can be divided into three areas. The first is to explain the nature of the underlying process, the second is to explain the nature of the skeletal abnormalities and, the third is to consider the possibility of associated abnormalities that might be related to the primary process. These abnormalities include hypercalcemia, hyperthyroidism, hyperglycemia and the syndrome of multiple endocrine adenomas.

In terms of the major underlying pathologic process, I think there is very good evidence that this patient had a pheochromocytoma. A pheochromocytoma is a tumor that synthesizes and secretes catecholamines. Catecholamines are produced normally in the brain, the sympathic nerve endings and at sites of the body that contain chromaffin tissue. Chromaffin tissue is detectable in the adrenal medulla, in the organ of Zuckerkandl and in a variety of areas containing ectopic rests of neural crest tissue that are generally associated with sympathetic ganglia. The latter may be found from the aortic arch to the floor of the bladder. Although there are multiple sites in which pheochromocytomas occur, more than 90 per cent of them are found between the diaphragm and the bladder. Thus, thoracic pheochromocytomas are rare and usually appreciated on a chest film.

The symptoms caused by a pheochromocytoma result from excess circulating epinephrine and/or norepinephrine in the plasma. These substances are derivates of the amino acid, tyrosine. Tyrosine is converted to norepinephrine through dihydroxyphenylalanine (Dopa) and dopamine. In the presence of the enzyme phenylethanolamine N-methyltransferase, norepinephrine is converted to epinephrine. This enzyme is located primarily in the adrenal medulla and in the organ of Zuckerkandl. It has been said that if a pheochromocytoma secretes predominantly epinephrine then it is most likely located in the adrenal gland. This generalization is usually, but not always correct. The converse, however, is not true. Tumors that secrete predominantly norepinephrine can occur either along the paraganglion system or in the adrenal medulla.

The effects of these two hormones differ considerably. Norepinephrine stimulates alpha-adrenergic receptors which result in vasoconstriction and hypertension. Epinephrine stimulates both alpha- and beta-adrenergic receptors and causes a variety of physiologic effects, including vasodilation, tachycardia, supraventricular arrhythmias and relaxation of intestinal smooth muscle resulting in constipation. Beta-adrenergic agonists also increase oxygen consumption and cause a hypermetabolic syndrome which may mimic hyperthyroidism.

The secretion of catecholamines from pheochromocytomas is frequently episodic, which accounts for the classic paroxysms of hypertension, headaches, pallor, sweating and impending doom that are described in many patients with this disorder. Tumors that secrete epinephrine predominantly can also cause paroxysmal hypotension and paralytic ileus. If we postulate that this patient had a tumor that was secreting excessive catecholamines, I think we can account for most of his major symptoms and signs, namely, hypertension, postural hypotension, headache, diaphoresis, tachycardia, constipation, tremor and weight loss. In addition, he had pain in the upper left abdominal quadrant and lower back, which occurs in patients with pheochromocytoma but may also be attributable to metastatic disease in this patient. Patients with pheochromocytoma can experience paraesthesias, but peripheral neuropathy is uncommon. I would attribute the evidence of neuropathy to a complication of his skeletal disease or to his previous history of alcoholism rather than to his pheochromocytoma.

Are there laboratory data to support the diagnosis of pheochromocytoma? We know that the excretion of urinary total catecholamines and VMA was increased. Once catecholamines are secreted, their fate is threefold. Primarily, they are reaccumulated by nerve endings. A small portion is excreted as norepinephrine and epinephrine in the urine; and the remainder are metabolized by the enzyme catecholamine-O-methyl transferase to metanephrine and normetanephrine, and further by the enzyme monoamine oxidase to VMA. In the absence of the ingestion of drugs such as exogenous catecholamines (commonly found in nosedrops and bronchodilators), amphetamines, ephedrine and methyldopa, increased urinary catecholamines, metanephrines or VMA are virtually diagnostic of a pheochromocytoma. In addition to assaying catecholamines and their metabolites in the urine, it is now possible to measure catecholamines in plasma. I have asked Dr. Cryer to discuss the value of determining plasma catecholamines in patients suspected of having pheochromocytomas and to interpret the results that were obtained in this patient.

Dr. Philip Cryer: The measurement of catecholamines and their metabolites in the urine has been, and continues to be, the standard approach to the biochemical diagnosis of pheochromocytoma. Measurements of catecholamines in plasma have some conceptual advantages and some very practical limitations. Pheochromocytomas, in general, secrete excessive quantities of norepinephrine. Excessive production of epinephrine is more variable.

In contrast to epinephrine, which can be viewed as a hormone secreted largely from the adrenal medulla, norepinephrine is primarily a neurotransmitter released from sympathetic postganglionic neurons. When the sympathetic axon depolarizes, norepinephrine is released into the synaptic cleft and gains direct access to receptor sites on its effector cell and in areas in which it produces its characteristic biologic effect. As Dr. Chase indicated, the major route of biologic inactivation of released norepinephrine is reuptake into the axon terminal. In addition, some of it is metabolized locally. Thus, the portion of released norepinephrine that escapes into the circulation is a small fraction of the norepinephrine that is released. As a consequence, the concentration of norepinephrine in the cleft after the axon discharges is much higher than the normal plasma concentration, and there is a steep norepinephrine gradient from cleft to plasma. From this, it follows that if norepinephrine was introduced directly into the circulation, as it is with a pheochromocytoma, plasma concentrations would have to be very high in order to produce biologically effective concentrations in the cleft. So, one would expect a patient who has a pheochromocytoma which releases enough norepinephrine to produce a clinically recognized syndrome, such as hypertension, to have very high plasma concentrations of norepinephrine. Another point, to which Dr. Chase alluded, was that norepinephrine delivered tnto the circulation is largely metabolized. Only 1 to 3 per cent appears in the urine unaltered. Thus, one would expect increases in plasma norepinephrine to be more dramatic than those in urine norepinephrine.

Despite these conceptual advantages, there are practical limitations to measurement of plasma catecholamine concentrations in the diagnosis of pheochromocytoma. The first is methodologic. Although sensitive and highly reproducible methods for the measurement of norepinephrine and epinephrine in plasma, such as the isotope derivative method used in the patient under discussion, have been developed, they are time-consuming and expensive to perform. Second, plasma catecholamine concentrations vary widely under physiologic and pathophysiologic conditions. For example, plasma norepinephrine concentrations normally increase two- to threefold with assumption of the upright posture [1], three- to fourfold during the stress of insulin-induced hypoglycemia [2] and up to tenfold during the major stresses of acute myocardial infarction [3] or diabetic ketoacidosis [4]. Epinephrine release into the plasma is even more labile. Mean plasma epinephrine levels rose 50-fold in our studies of insulin-induced hypoglycemia [2]. Third, catecholamine release from pheochromocytomas varies considerably and a single plasma measurement reflects catecholamine release only at that point in time.

In our experience with eight patients proved to have pheochromocytomas, plasma norepinephrine concentrations ranged from 3,770 to 12,100 pg/ml, dramatically different from normal values (with the subjects supine) of approximately 100 to 400 pg/ml. The expe-

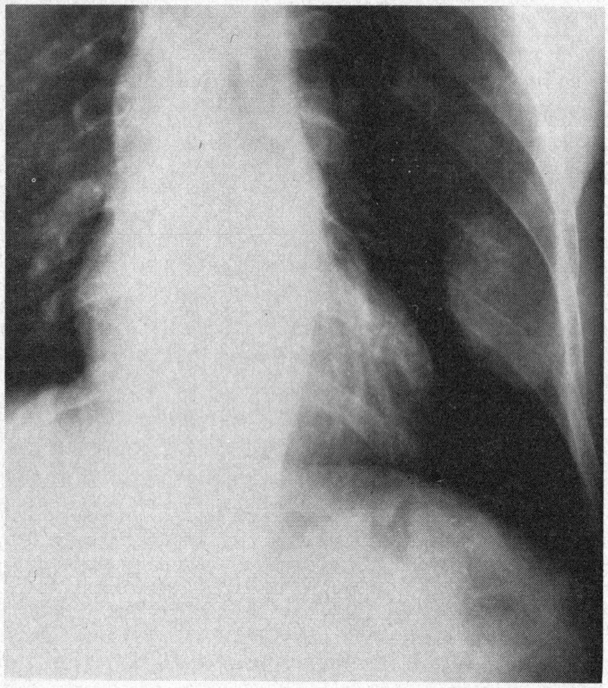

Figure 1. Lytic destruction of the left seventh rib with a surrounding intrathoracic extrapleural soft tissue mass.

rience of others is generally similar [5,6] although a few patients with values approaching 1,000 pg/ml, and a single patient with a total plasma catecholamine concentration of 540 pg/ml [5], have been described.

Dr. Chase: Thank you. Let us now turn to the skeletal lesions. Dr. Debnam, would you discuss the films?

Dr. James Debnam: The chest film obtained on admission (August 16, 1975) demonstrated metastatic destruction of the left seventh rib. The soft tissue extension of this metastasis had produced a prominent extrapleural mass (Figure 1). Metastases to the seventh and ninth thoracic vertebrae were present on the bone survey of August 20, 1975 (Figure 2). On this examination there was a 5 cm lytic metastasis in the left superior iliac wing and a 2 cm lytic metastasis in the adjacent sacral wing (Figure 3).

Laminograms of the suprarenal areas after the intravenous injection of urographic contrast material were nonrevealing. This screening examination will demonstrate at least 70 per cent of suspected adrenal tumors [7]. Catheter angiography, although not performed in this case, is the most definitive roentgenographic method for localization of a suspected pheochromocytoma [8]. Adrenal venography may be performed if all arterial studies are within normal limits. Abdominal ultrasound will image adrenal masses 3 cm or larger [9]. No significant experience localizing pheochromocytomas by total body computerized axial tomography has yet been accumulated.

Dr. Chase: At this point we can say that this patient had definite evidence of metastatic malignancy. Approximately 6 per cent of pheochromocytomas are malignant. Like many other endocrine malignancies, the diagnosis of a malignant pheochromocytoma can only be made with certainty if metastases are demonstrated. It is very difficult for the pathologist to determine whether some of these endocrine neoplasms are benign or malignant by examining only the primary tumor. The most common site of metastases from a pheochromocytoma is bone. Less common are lymph nodes, liver and then other soft tissues. In the absence of any other obvious malignancy in this patient I believe the most likely cause for the skeletal lesions is metastatic pheochromocytoma.

I would like to consider some of the other abnormalities that were noted in this case. During his initial hospitalization, the patient had a transient episode of hypercalcemia with a calcium value as high as 12.8 mg/100 ml. This returned to normal by the time he was discharged. The most likely possibilities I would consider for the hypercalcemia in this patient include

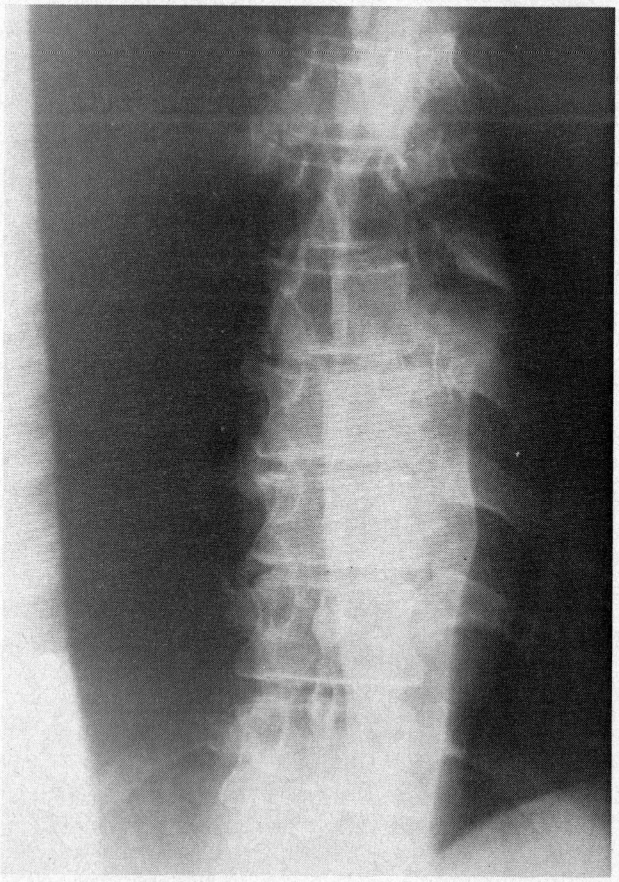

Figure 2. Metastases to the thoracic spine are demonstrated by roentgenographic absence of the left pedicle of the seventh thoracic vertebra and sclerosis of the left pedicle of the ninth thoracic vertebra.

metastatic malignancy, primary hyperparathyroidism and various secretions from the tumor. We know that the patient did have metastatic malignancy, and I think this is certainly an excellent reason for his transient hypercalcemia. Primary hyperparathyroidism is a distinct possibility, but the absence of persistent hypercalcemia and the normal concentration of parathyroid hormone in his blood make this diagnosis highly unlikely. A number of secretory products from pheochromocytomas can cause hypercalcemia. The ectopic parathyroid hormone syndrome has been reported in patients with pheochromocytomas, and parathyroid hormone has actually been detected in the tumor. Prostaglandins have been detected in pheochromocytomas and are known to cause bone resorption; however, a cause and effect relationship has not been established among pheochromocytoma, prostaglandin production and hypercalcemia. An intriguing observation is that epinephrine is known to release parathyroid hormone both in vivo and in vitro. Also of interest is that there are several case reports of patients with pheochromocytomas and hypercalcemia in which hypercalcemia reverted to normal after adrenalectomy. It has not been possible in the cases reported to exclude the ectopic parathyroid hormone syndrome as an alternate possibility. Also, in a recent prospective study [10] of 12 patients with pheochromocytomas, the serum parathyroid hormone level was normal in 10. All 10 of these patients were normocalcemic. The remaining two patients with elevated serum parathyroid hormone levels had hypercalcemia which did not revert to normal after the pheochromocytoma was removed. Both of these patients were later proved to have primary hyperparathyroidism. In examining our patient's chart it becomes apparent that at the time he was hypercalcemic, he was extremely dehydrated and that he was being treated with thiazide diuretics. When he was

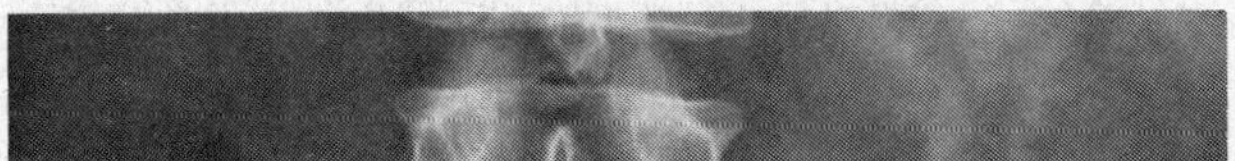

Figure 3. Lytic metastases of the left iliac wing and adjacent left sacrum. The sacral lesion has destroyed the cortical margins of neural foramina.

rehydrated and the administration of diuretics stopped, the serum calcium concentration reverted to normal. Thus, I believe that he had a tendency to increased bone resorption from his metastatic malignancy and that this resulted in hypercalcemia when he became dehydrated during thiazide therapy. The presence of hypercalcemia, however, does raise some interesting possibilities, namely, that he might have one of the multiple endocrine neoplasias syndromes. I have asked Dr. Jacobs to review the endocrine disorders associated with pheochromocytomas and also to comment on whether this patient's abnormalities in thyroid function could be attributed to our primary diagnosis.

Dr. Laurence Jacobs: Pheochromocytoma is an uncommon endocrine disorder, and patients with pheochromocytoma probably constitute 1 per cent or less of all hypertensive subjects. A great deal of interest in pheochromocytomas nonetheless persists, in part because of the frequently dramatic episodic clinical manifestations. These tumors of the adrenal medulla are usually benign and unilateral, hence curative surgery is quite feasible; this is another major reason for special interest in this disease. Most pheochromocytomas occur as sporadic, isolated instances. However, pheochromocytomas constitute an important feature in two distinct genetic syndromes of multiple endocrine neoplasia in which they occur in association with other distinctive clinical abnormalities.

In multiple endocrine neoplasia type II, initially described by Steiner, Goodman and Powers [11], pheochromocytoma, hyperparathyroidism and medullary thyroid carcinoma segregate in an autosomal dominant pattern. Roughly 15 per cent of family members demonstrate clinically apparent disease; of these, about 50 per cent have pheochromocytoma alone. The remainder of those affected also have medullary thyroid carcinoma and/or hyperparathyroidism. A single case of Cushing's syndrome was identified in Steiner's family study [11].

The recently described multiple endocrine neoplasia type III [12] has striking similarities to type II neoplasia in that medullary thyroid carcinoma and pheochromocytoma are common endocrine features. However, a sufficient number of differences between them has been delineated to suggest that they are genetically and endocrinologically distinct from each other. In patients with type III neoplasia, medullary thyroid carcinoma is a nearly universal finding and pheochromocytomas less common; in type II neoplasia, pheochromocytoma is about twice as common as medullary thyroid carcinoma. In type III neoplasia, hyperparathyroidism almost never occurs, only one such case has been reported; in type II neoplasia, hyperparathyroidism occurs in about one half of all affected family members. Most striking, however, is the unusual general physical appearance of those with multiple endocrine neoplasia type III. They tend to be slender and tall and have been described as Marfanoid; in addition, multiple mucosal neuromas, most commonly occurring in and around the eyes, mouth, lips and tongue, create such a distinctive facial appearance that subjects from different kindreds with the type III syndrome have been said to look like siblings. Especially common are thickened and "lumpy-bumpy" lips, probably caused by submucosal neuromas. These neuromas may occasionally also occur along the gastrointestinal tract and may be associated with gastrointestinal complaints.

Finally, hypertrophied, medullated corneal nerves are a very common feature of type III neoplasia, and should be specifically sought by slit-lamp examination when other clinical features point to this diagnosis.

I should mention in passing that multiple endocrine neoplasia type I, which involves adenomas or hyperplasia of the pituitary, pancreas and parathyroid glands, as well as a substantial incidence of peptic ulcer disease, has never been reported in association with pheochromocytoma.

Some of the clinical features of multiple endocrine neoplasia types II and III are worthy of special attention. First, the pheochromocytomas are frequently bilateral (50 to 70 per cent) as opposed to the uncommon (5 to 10 per cent) occurrence of bilaterality in sporadic disease. The surgical implications are clear. Second, it is quite clear that the incidence of familial syndromes increases linearly with increases in the vigor with which the family history is pursued. This makes it difficult to be certain of the epidemiology of the sporadic versus the familial occurrence of isolated endocrine components or more complete forms of the disease. However, the clinical messages seem clear: careful and detailed family histories should be taken in all patients with documented pheochromocytoma and medullary thyroid carcinoma, and patients with medullary thyroid carcinoma should have screening tests for pheochromocytoma prior to the induction of general anesthesia for surgery. Since primary hyperparathyroidism is a relatively common sporadic disease in patients coming to the attention of internists, with an incidence of about one in 800, it occurs alone far more commonly than it does in association with pituitary or pancreatic adenomas, medullary thyroid carcinoma or pheochromocytoma. It is unwise to administer ACTH to patients with the type II disorder as part of an adrenal cortical work-up since release of catecholamines with fatal paroxysms of hypertension has been reported in these circumstances. Third, the clinical course of hypertension in family members with multiple endocrine neoplasia and pheochromocytoma is most often episodic and only very rarely sustained. This is in contrast to the reported approximate 50 to 50 split in sporadic cases of pheochromocytoma. Thus, the absence of hypertension in a patient with medullary thyroid carcinoma does not minimize the need to determine urinary catecholamines, VMA or normetanephrine prior to any surgery for thyroid disease. Fourth, assay of plasma calcitonin has proved to be an extraordinarily useful biochemical marker for the presence of medullary thyroid carcinoma, and in selected familial circumstances, C cell hyperplasia has been detected when surgery was carried out after the demonstration of abnormally elevated calcitonin levels stimulated by calcium infusion [13]. Calcitonin appears to be an essentially universal product of the C cell, whether it is hyperplastic (and presumably preneoplastic) or neoplastic. However, stimulation with calcium or some other calcitonin secretagogue may be required to demonstrate abnormal values, and a normal basal calcitonin such as was found in our patient does not rule out the presence of C cell abnormalities.

In addition to the multiple endocrine syndromes, pheochromocytomas may also occur in association with von Recklinghausen's neurofibromatosis and with von Hippel-Lindau disease.

Thus, in any patient with a pheochromocytoma, one should obtain a careful and complete family history, thorough physical examination with special attention to habitus, eyes, lips and thyroid, and determinations of serum calcium and of plasma calcitonin before and after the infusion of calcium.

The patient under discussion had, in addition to evidence of excess catecholamine secretion, transient hypercalcemia (probably reflecting dehydration), a nodular goiter and clear chemical evidence of thyrotoxicosis.

Nontoxic nodular goiters are common. Thyrotoxicosis is a common disorder and its incidence in those harboring nodular goiters is increased. The parafollicular cells are the only component of the thyroid gland which have been reported to participate in the multiple endocrine neoplasia syndromes outlined.

Two questions arise regarding our patient's thyroid status. Did he have a small focus of medullary thyroid carcinoma within his goiter? Although I doubt it, calcium stimulation of calcitonin levels was not carried out, therefore, we cannot answer this question with biochemical certainty. The second question is perhaps more intriguing. Was his thyrotoxicosis an independent event, or can it be related in some way to catecholamine excess? Data in experimental animals suggest that both alpha [14] and $beta_2$ [15] adrenergic agonists can increase thyroidal secretion. The relevance of these interesting observations to human disease remains uncertain. I suspect this man had an independent garden variety toxic nodular goiter unrelated to his pheochromocytoma.

Dr. Chase: Finally, this patient had an abnormal glucose tolerance test. Dr. Pagliara, did he have diabetes mellitus?

Dr. Anthony Pagliara: Carbohydrate intolerance is very common in patients with pheochromocytoma. In a review by Gifford and co-workers [16], of clinical data on 76 patients seen at the Mayo Clinic, hyperglycemia was observed in two thirds of the patients with sustained hypertension; among patients with paroxysmal hypertension, hyperglycemia was less common. In another series [17] of 13 patients with pheochromocytoma, eight had diabetes when first seen, and in one patient who had metastatic pheochromocytoma, diabetes developed after the original tumor was removed. Therefore, it is quite clear that the incidence of abnormalities in glucose tolerance is very high in patients with pheochromocytoma.

Less well documented is the response of carbohydrate intolerance to surgical removal of the tumor. In five patients followed at the Joslin Clinic (four who required insulin therapy and one who required an oral hypoglycemic agent for control of hyperglycemia), removal of the pheochromocytoma resulted in dramatic amelioration of the hyperglycemia in four. In the one patient who continued to require insulin, the diagnosis of diabetes mellitus was made three years before hypertension developed [18].

There is ample evidence that epinephrine infusion in man results in hyperglycemia; this can be ascribed to the combined effects of this hormone on glycogenolysis, gluconeogenesis and decreased glucose utilization by peripheral tissues. In addition, and probably most important, Porte and Bagdade [19] have clearly shown that catecholamines (epinephrine and norepinephrine) are potent inhibitors of glucose-mediated insulin secretion. This results from catecholamine stimulation of alpha adrenergic receptors on the beta cell, which are inhibitors for insulin release.

In two patients with pheochromocytoma, studied before and after the tumors were removed, Spergel, Bleicher and Ertel [20] demonstrated that the glucose intolerance in both, prior to operation, was associated with a hypoinsulinemic response to oral glucose. Several days after the operation, glucose intolerance persisted in the presence of a hyperinsulinemic response to glucose challenge, implying peripheral insulin resistance. Complete normalization of glucose tolerance, with an appropriate insulin response, subsequently occurred several months after surgery. Thus, it would appear that the glucose intolerance in patients with pheochromocytoma can be ascribed to excessive circulating catecholamines, and one does not have to postulate that the patient under discussion had diabetes mellitus.

Dr. Chase: In summary, I am reasonably certain that this patient had a pheochromocytoma. I think that the skeletal lesions were due to metastases from a malignant pheochromocytoma. His hypercalcemia is best attributable to metastatic malignancy when he was dehydrated and taking thiazide diuretics. If Dr. McKeel shows me a little bit of parathyroid hyperplasia, I am prepared to argue that this was attributable to his bit of renal disease and not to a multiple endocrine neoplasia syndrome or to primary hyperparathyroidsim. His hyperthyroidism is most likely due to a toxic multinodular goiter but I cannot exclude the possibility that he had subacute thyroiditis with a transient episode of increased release of thyroid hormone which would explain his high serum T_4 and T_3 uptake test and his low ^{131}I uptake. I do not have any evidence to suggest a multiple endocrine neoplasia syndrome. His hyperglycemia has been explained nicely by Dr. Pagliara.

Dr. Cryer has some follow-up information on the patient.

Dr. Cryer: The patient did poorly, with increasingly severe pain in the sacral region, and was readmitted on October 13, 1975. While taking phenoxybenzamine and propranolol, the blood pressure was 128/80 mm Hg and the pulse rate 90/min. The weight was 58.8 kg.

Methimazole therapy was discontinued on admission. Serum thyroxine concentrations were 8.7, 9.8 and 9.2 μg/100 ml on October 14, 21 and 29, respectively. The ^{131}I thyroid uptake was 6 per cent at 24 hours on October 21. I, too, found the biochemical evidence of thyrotoxicosis convincing on his first admission. Although he had clinical findings consistent with that diagnosis, these were potentially explicable on the basis of his pheochromocytoma and metastatic tumor, as pointed out by Dr. Chase. However, after antithyroid drug treatment was withdrawn, his thyroid function remained normal. Thus, he did not appear to have an ongoing thyrotoxic state. Taking the data at face value, this patient had a transient form of thyrotoxicosis which could have been due to subacute thyroiditis without thyroid tenderness, as suggested by Dr. Chase, or to an effect of the massively elevated plasma catecholamine levels on thyroid hormone secretion which was blocked by the administration of adrenergic antagonists, as suggested by Dr. Jacobs. I know of no precedent for the latter pathogenetic mechanism.

A percutaneous biopsy specimen of the lesion in the left iliac wing was obtained The lesion was noted to be pulsatile. The histologic diagnosis was metastatic carcinoma consistent with metastatic paraganglioma.

Palliative irradiation to the iliac bones was administered (2,000 R) and the administration of phenoxybenzamine and propranolol was continued. The patient continued to do poorly after discharge and died at home on February 6, 1976.

Dr. McKeel will present the pathologic findings.

PATHOLOGIC DISCUSSION

Dr. Daniel McKeel: Postmortem examination was performed several hours after the patient was pronounced dead on arrival at the Barnes Hospital Emergency Room. The cause of death was determined to be very extensive bronchopneumonia. An acute inflammatory exudate diffusely involved the bronchi and alveoli. Gram-positive diplococci were demonstrated within abscesses. Adjacent alveoli contained organizing fibrin masses (Mallory bodies). We found some foreign bodies resembling partly digested plant material within the most intense inflammatory exudates, indicating aspiration was part of and perhaps caused the pneumonic process.

The gross examination revealed a markedly wasted person with virtually no subcutaneous or visceral adipose tissue. The serous cavities were dry. Both adrenal glands were normal in size and configuration; the right one weighed 5.0 g and the left one 6.5 g. The adrenal cortices had a fine surface nodularity which is a normal finding. Both glands were fixed in toto, sectioned at 2 mm intervals, and representative portions containing medullary tissue were examined microscopically; no adrenal pathology was found.

However, a large mass of abnormal tissue surrounded the abdominal aorta adjacent to the kidneys and adrenals, and intimately involved the origin of the celiac and both mesenteric arteries (Figure 4). On sectioning the mass, confluent lobular masses of partly necrotic tan tissue with foci of hemorrhage were evident. On microscopic examination, the mass was composed of tumor nodules intermixed with lymph nodes effaced by

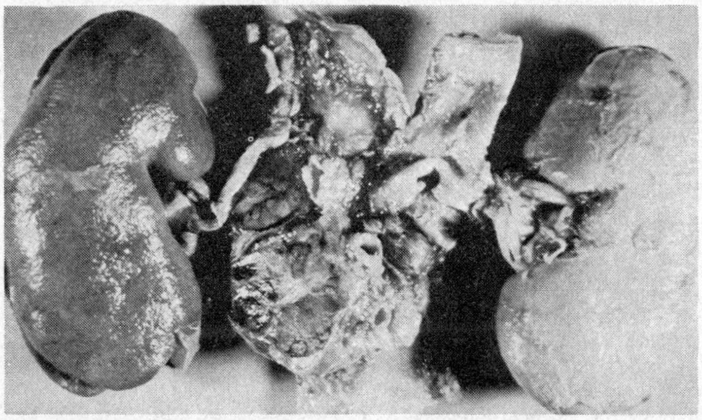

__Figure 4.__ An anterior view of the gross tumor specimen. The adrenal glands have been removed. The aorta is to the left of the inferior vena cava.

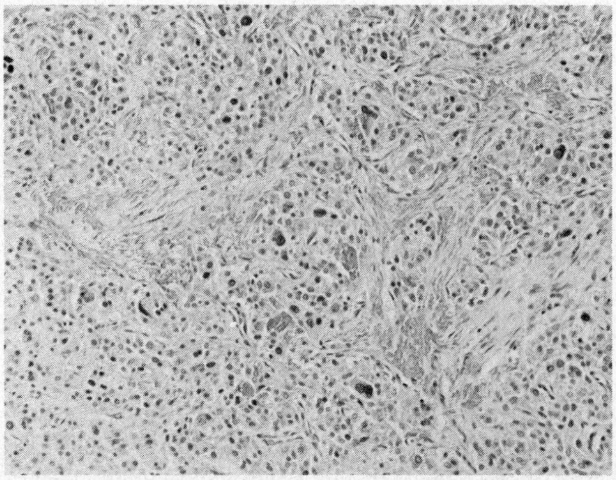

__Figure 5.__ A survey photomicrograph illustrating nests of tumor cells separated by fibrovascular stroma and sinusoids. Note the presence of scattered cells with giant and multiple nuclei. Hematoxylin and eosin stain; original magnification × 130, reduced by 12 per cent.

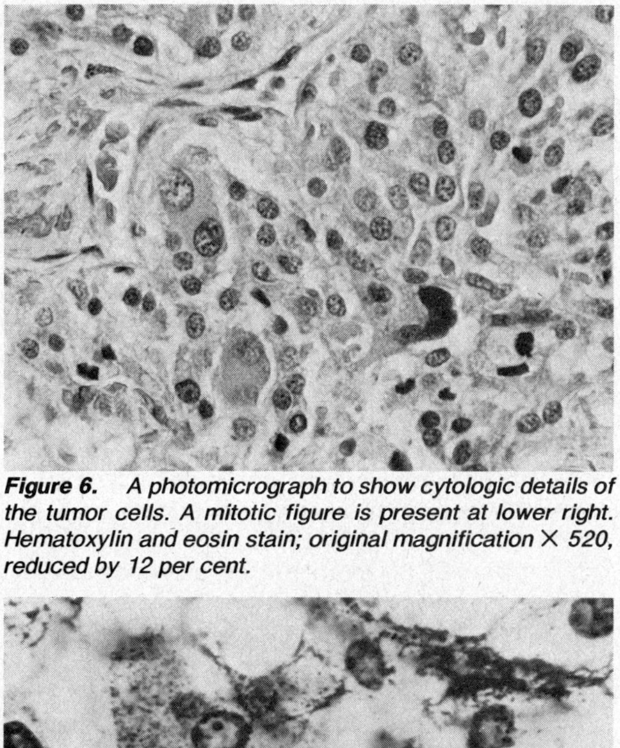

__Figure 6.__ A photomicrograph to show cytologic details of the tumor cells. A mitotic figure is present at lower right. Hematoxylin and eosin stain; original magnification × 520, reduced by 12 per cent.

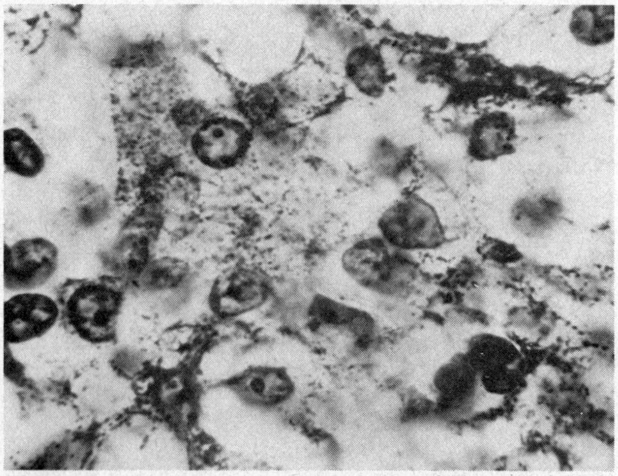

__Figure 7.__ Tumor cells contain argyrophilic cytoplasmic granules as shown in this oil immersion photomicrograph. Sevier-Munger silver stain; original magnification × 1,300, reduced by 12 per cent.

invasive tumor. Similar but more congested tumor masses destroyed portions of two ribs and the spine in the locations documented roentgenographically. The final surgical pathologic diagnosis, based on a biopsy specimen of an iliac crest lesion, was metastatic paraganglioma; this was confirmed at autopsy by excluding a pheochromocytoma of primary adrenal origin. Since clinical studies indicated that the tumor had produced large amounts of catecholamines, a gross Henle chromoreaction [21] was obtained by applying Zenker's solution to the surface of a block of unfixed tumor. A faint brown color developed after 1 minute and became maximal at 3 minutes. This weakly positive reaction was caused by brown complex formation between chromate salts in the solution and residual catechols diffusing from the tumor. Similar reactions can be elicited using adrenomedullary tissue and pheochromocytomas, strongly positive results being obtained only with freshly resected surgical specimens. The weak reaction with this tumor was probably due to postmortem autolytic diffusion of catechols from the tumor tissue. Probably for similar reasons, the expected purple chromoreaction with iodate salts and the histologic chromaffin reactions were negative. Histologically, the tumor was composed of nests of pleomorphic polygonal cells separated by thin-walled blood vessels and sinusoids (Figure 5). The pattern was indistinguishable from many examples of adrenal pheochromocytomas. Small to medium-sized polygonal cells with vesicular nuclei and granular acidophilic cytoplasm predominated. However, multinucleate, binucleate and singly nucleated giant cells were interspersed (Figure 6), as were mitotic figures, pigmented macrophages, foci of necrosis and cells with pyknotic or hyperchromatic nuclei. Argyrophilic stains disclosed silver-positive cytoplasmic granules in the cytoplasm of most of the tumor cells (Figure 7). The degree of granularity, which reflects the amount of stored catecholamines, varied greatly from cell to cell. The histologic findings were identical in the primary para-aortic tumor and in bone and lymph node metastases.

The final designation of the present tumor as a malignant para-aortic (Zuckerkandl) paraganglioma conforms to terminology suggested by Drs. Glenner and Grimley [22]. The exact site of origin of the present tumor, similar to that in most other reported cases, could not be definitely established. Histologic examination was made on tissue surrounding the origin of the inferior mesenteric artery, the usual site of the organ of Zuckerkandl. Tumor cells infiltrated nerve fascicles and abnormal ganglion cells which resembled one configuration of Zuckerkandl tissue found in infants. Whether or not this tumor actually originated in the true organ of Zuckerkandl, the clinical, laboratory, gross and microscopic findings showed that the tumor was composed of functionally active, neoplastic, sympathetic paraganglionic tissue. This entity had been reported in 27 cases by 1973; in approximately 38 per cent of the reported cases metastases were present and in 63 per cent hypersecreted catecholamines [22].

No evidence of multiple endocrine adenomatosis was found. One of four parathyroids was sectioned and showed absence of fat; chief cell hyperplasia was present.

The final anatomic diagnoses were malignant para-aortic (Zuckerkandl) paraganglioma, metastatic to regional lymph nodes, ribs, vertebra, sacrum and iliac bone; diffuse bilateral bronchopneumonia, partly due to aspiration; cachexia; hypertrophy of the left side of the heart; moderately severe generalized arteriosclerosis, with marked sclerosis of small adrenal arteries; and chief cell hyperplasia of one parathyroid gland.

Editors' note: The problem of classification of these tumors has been recently discussed [23].

REFERENCES

1. Cryer PE, Santiago JV, Shah SD: Measurement of norepinephrine and epinephrine in small volumes of human plasma by a single-isotope derivative method. J Clin Endocrinol Metab 39: 1025, 1974.
2. Garber AJ, Cryer PE, Santiago JV, et al.: The role of adrenergic mechanisms in the substrate and hormonal response to insulin induced hypoglycemia in man. J Clin Invest (in press).
3. Christensen NJ, Jorgen V: Plasma catecholamines and carbohydrate metabolism in patients with acute myocardial infarction. J Clin Invest 54: 278, 1974.
4. Christensen NJ: Plasma norepinephrine and epinephrine in untreated diabetics, during fasting and after insulin administration. Diabetes 23: 1, 1974.
5. Engelman K: Assay of plasma catecholamines. Hypertension Manual (Laragh JH, ed), New York, Yorke Medical Books, 1974, p 605.
6. Geffen LB, Rush RA, Louis WJ, et al.: Plasma catecholamine and dopamine β-hydroxylase amounts in phaeochromocytoma. Clin Sci 44: 421, 1973.
7. Pickering RS, Hartman GW, Weeks RE, et al.: Excretory urographic localization of adrenal cortical tumors and pheochromocytomas. Radiology 114: 345, 1975.
8. Zelch JV, Meaney TF, Belhobek GH: Radiologic approach to the patient with suspected pheochromocytoma. Radiology 111: 279, 1974.
9. Birnholz JC: Ultrasound imaging of adrenal mass lesions. Radiology 109: 163, 1973.
10. Miller SS, Sizemore GW, Sheps SG, et al.: Parathyroid function in patients with pheochromocytoma. Ann Intern Med 82: 372, 1975.
11. Steiner AL, Goodman AD, Powers SR: Study of a kindred with pheochromocytoma, medullary thyroid carcinoma, hyperparathyroidism and Cushing's disease: multiple endocrine neoplasia type 2. Medicine (Baltimore) 47: 371, 1968.

12. Rashid M, Khairi A, Dexter RN, et al.: Mucosal neuroma, pheochromocytoma and medullary thyroid carcinoma: multiple endocrine neoplasia type 3. Medicine (Baltimore) 54: 89, 1975.
13. Wolfe HJ, Melvin KEW, Cervi-Skinner SJ, Al Saadi AA, et al.: C-cell hyperplasia preceding medullary thyroid carcinoma. N Engl J Med 289: 437, 1973.
14. Melander A, Nilsson E, Sundler F: Sympathetic activation of thyroid hormone secretion in mice. Endocrinology 90: 194, 1972.
15. Melander A, Ranklev E, Sundler F, et al.: $Beta_2$-adrenergic stimulation of thyroid hormone secretion. Endocrinology 97: 332, 1975.
16. Gifford RW Jr, Kvale WF, Maher FT, et al.: Clinical features, diagnosis and treatment of pheochromocytoma: a review of 76 cases. Mayo Clin Proc 39: 281, 1964.
17. Evans JA: Difficulties in diagnosis of pheochromocytoma. Med Clin N Am 44: 411, 1960.
18. Kozak GP: Diabetes and other endocrinologic disorders. Joslin's Diabetes Mellitus, 11th ed (Marble A, White P, Frandley RF, Krall LP, eds), Philadelphia, Lea & Febiger, 1971, p 666.
19. Porte D Jr, Bagdade JD: Human insulin secretion: an integrated approach. Ann Rev Med 21: 219, 1970.
20. Spergel G, Bleicher SJ, Ertel NH: Carbohydrate and fat metabolism in patients with pheochromocytoma. N Engl J Med 228: 803, 1968.
21. Nichols J: Adrenal cortex. The chromoreactions. Endocrine Pathology (Bloodworth JMB, ed), Baltimore, Williams & Wilkins, 1968, p 260.
22. Glenner GG, Grimley PM: Tumors of the Extra-Adrenal Paraganglion System (Including Chemoreceptors). Armed Forces Institute of Pathology Atlas of Tumor Pathology, 2nd series, Fascicle 9, 1974.
23. Schwartz EL, Mao P, Hernried HP, et al.: Catecholamine-secreting paraganglioma. The problem of classification. Arch Intern Med 135: 978, 1975.

Acute Unilateral Adrenal Hemorrhage Following ACTH Administration in a Patient with Cushing's Syndrome

JOHN F. REDMAN, M.D.
FRED H. FAAS, M.D.
Little Rock, Arkansas

A patient with Cushing's syndrome and a concomitant unilateral adrenal hemorrhage following ACTH administration is described. Although stress is commonly associated with the onset of adrenal hemorrhage, a pathologically documented adrenal hemorrhage has not been reported previously in association with ACTH administration in Cushing's syndrome. Repeated doses of ACTH should not be given to patients with Cushing's syndrome as this has little diagnostic value and may lead to adrenal hemorrhage in such patients.

Acute adrenal hemorrhage or adrenal apoplexy has been described many times and has been attributed to or associated with numerous conditions, including pregnancy, surgical stress, endotoxic shock, anticoagulant therapy and adrenal venography [1–5]. Adrenal hemorrhage has also been noted following the administration of ACTH [6–9].

Patients with Cushing's syndrome would seem to be prone to the development of adrenal hemorrhage. There are reports of remission of Cushing's syndrome following adrenal venography [10–11]. Pratt et al. [12] observed the remission of Cushing's disease following ACTH administration. In the latter case there was no pathologic verification of the presumed adrenal hemorrhage.

Our finding of a clinically significant, pathologically verified adrenal hemorrhage following ACTH administration in a patient with Cushing's syndrome prompts this report.

CASE REPORT

A 61 year old white woman (No. 44-30-87) was admitted to the University Hospital for surgical exploration of the adrenal glands. A tentative diagnosis of Cushing's syndrome had been made eight months earlier on the occasion of a compensation examination. The patient related a two to three year history of weakness and a one year history of blackouts, staggering and falling. She reported being frequently anxious and tremulous. She volunteered that she bruised easily. For the previous five years she had been treated for hypertension and diabetes. There were no abdominal complaints.

On physical examination she presented an appearance of centripetal obesity with normal appearing extremities. Weight was 140 pounds. Blood pressure was 170/100 mm Hg. Her face was rounded and florid. A cervical hump, multiple large ecchymoses and abdominal striae were present.

From the Department of Urology, and the Department of Medicine, Division of Endocrinology and Metabolism, University of Arkansas College of Medicine, Little Rock, Arkansas. Requests for reprints should be addressed to Dr. John F. Redman, Department of Urology, University of Arkansas College of Medicine, 4301 W. Markham Street, Little Rock, Arkansas 72201. Manuscript accepted January 14, 1976.

TABLE I Steroid Data Confirming Diagnosis of Cushing's Disease*

Medication	Date (mo/yr)	24 Hour Urine 17-OHCS (mg/g creatinine)	Plasma Cortisol (μg/dl)
None	2/75	23.9	8 A.M.–21 Noon–19 4 P.M.–23 8 P.M.–16
None		17.9	
Dexamethasone (20 μg/kg/day–day 2)		4.9	13
None	3/75	19.3	
None		17.6	
2nd day of dexamethasone (20 μg/kg/day)		12.9	
2nd day of dexamethasone (8 mg/day)		4.1	
3rd day of ACTH gel (40 U twice a day IM)		222	
4th day of ACTH gel (40 U twice a day IM)		182	
None		20.9	
Day after metyrapone (3 g/day)		166	

*Urine 17-OHCS were determined by the Porter Silber method [13]. Plasma cortisol was determined fluorimetrically [14]. Normal urine 17-OHCS are 2 to 7 mg/g creatinine with normal suppression of urine 17-OHCS being to less than 1 mg/g creatinine and plasma cortisol to less than 5 μg/dl on 20 μg/kg/24 hour dexamethasone administered in four divided doses [15].

Laboratory data included a hematocrit value of 45 per cent, a fasting blood sugar of 160 mg/100 ml, a level of blood urea nitrogen 17 mg/100 ml and a serum potassium of 4.9 meq/liter. Twenty-four hour urine adrenaline was 13 μg and noradrenaline 8 μg (normal less than 25 μg adrenaline and less than 50 μg noradrenaline/24 hours). An electrocardiogram revealed left axis deviation and right bundle branch block. Endocrinologic steroid data are shown in Table I. The increased urine 17-hydroxycorticosteroids (17-OHCS), the absent diurnal variation of plasma cortisol and the inadequate suppression of urine 17-OHCS and plasma cortisol with small doses of dexamethasone confirmed the diagnosis of Cushing's syndrome. The suppression of urine 17-OHCS with large doses of dexamethasone and the excessive increase in urinary 17-OHCS following the administration of ACTH and metyrapone indicated that Cushing's syndrome was due to bilateral adrenal hyperplasia.

On the third day of an ACTH stimulation test the patient experienced severe pain in the left flank and upper abdomen which persisted for five days. The patient was never hypotensive but experienced a 10 per cent decrease in her hematocrit value. The other remarkable symptoms were her nausea and vomiting. She was treated symptomatically and did not require corticosteroids. An excretory urogram demonstrated lateral displacement of the superior pole of the left kidney. On comparison with an excretory urogram obtained three months previously, lateral displacement was also present but not as pronounced (Figure 1). B mode ultrasonography of the left adrenal area demonstrated a sonolucent area above the left kidney which measured 6 by 6 cm. Venography bilaterally was not of diagnostic quality.

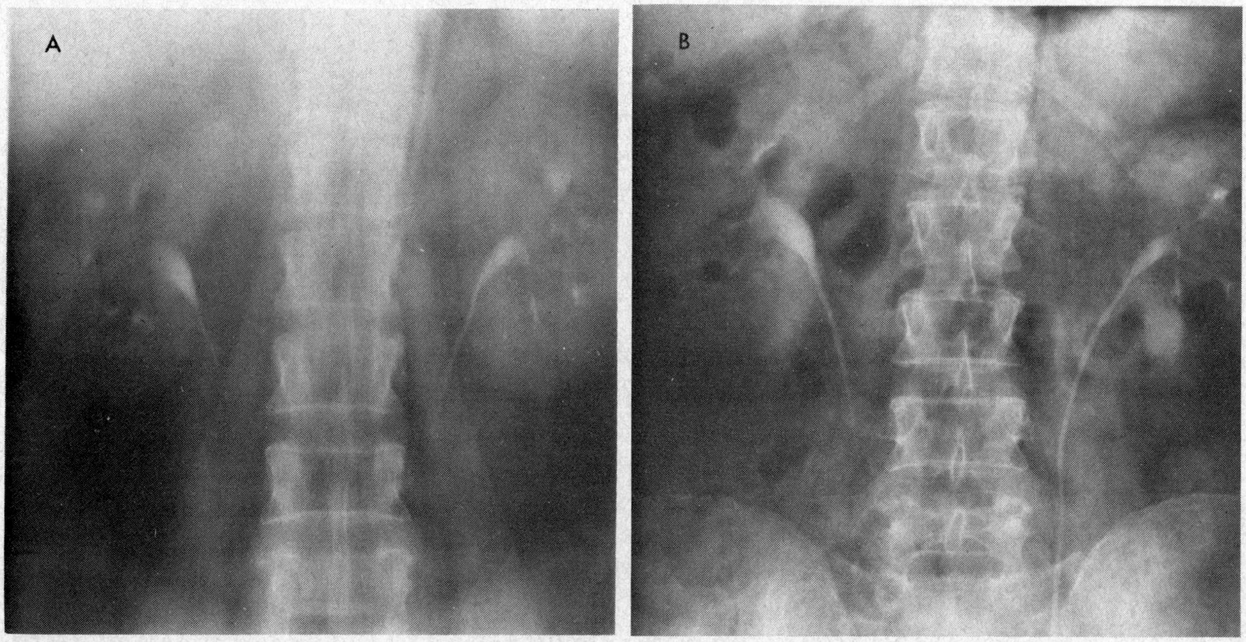

Figure 1. ***A,*** *initial excretory urogram.* ***B,*** *excretory urogram three months later demonstrating greater lateral displacement of the upper pole of the left kidney.*

Two weeks after the onset of flank pain, the adrenal glands were approached transperitoneally through a transverse upper abdominal incision. A large, firm left suprarenal mass was found. Extensive, dense fibrosis was present from the diaphragm to the renal pedicle, medially, and to the lower pole of the kidney, laterally and posteriorly. Because of the difficulty in securing a cleavage plane between the suprarenal mass and the kidney and in dissecting around the renal pedicle, the large tumor-like mass of adrenal and kidney were removed together. The right adrenal gland which was hyperplastic but otherwise normal was excised without difficulty. On cut section the left adrenal gland was identified as a thin rim surrounding a 6 by 4 cm mass of thrombus (Figure 2). No tumor was identified. The patient was discharged from the hospital feeling well on the 22nd postoperative day.

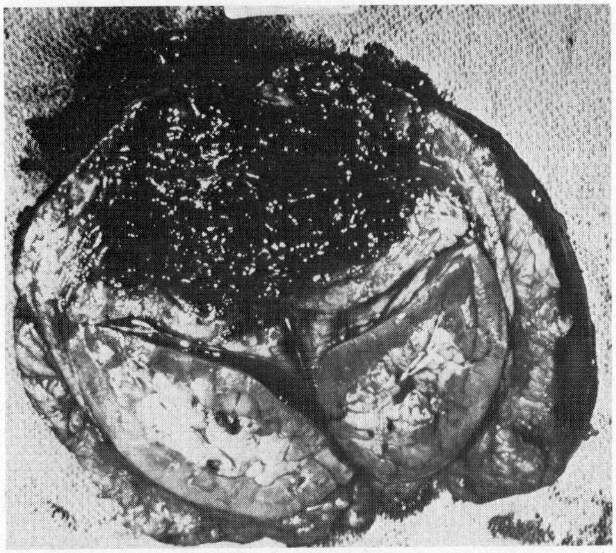

Figure 2. *Gross specimen immediately following excision. Centimeter scale is above specimen.*

COMMENTS

The pathophysiology of adrenal hemorrhage has been well reviewed [16–18]. Five etiologic groupings have been proposed: (1) hemorrhage associated with an involuting gland as found in the newborn or in postpartum women; (2) hemorrhage associated with capillary wall damage, including that occurring with convulsions, toxemia, trauma, septicemia, arteriosclerosis, hypertension and bacterial embolism; (3) hemorrhage associated with hemorrhagic diseases, such as hypothrombinemia or blood dyscrasias, and anticoagulation; (4) hemorrhage associated with adrenal vein thrombosis; and (5) adrenal hemorrhage associated with intracranial injury or lesions [16,17]. Greendyke [18] has pointed out that the majority of patients who suffered adrenal hemorrhage had been under prolonged stress. The fact that ACTH administration may induce adrenal hemorrhage has been noted experimentally and clinically [6–9,19]. It thus appears that long-term ACTH stimulation of the adrenal glands may result in adrenal hemorrhage. Adrenal hemorrhage following metyrapone administration has not been reported.

Patients with Cushing's syndrome and enlarged hypervascular adrenal glands secondary to overstimulation by endogenous ACTH would seem to be candidates for adrenal hemorrhage. The single prior report of a case of Cushing's syndrome with adrenal hemorrhage on the fourth day of ACTH administration was without pathologic verification [12]. The present case, with pathologic verification of the adrenal hemorrhage, occurred on the third day of ACTH administration. Adrenal hemorrhage associated with ACTH administration in Cushing's syndrome may be uncommon due to infrequent prolonged administration of ACTH in such patients. Evaluation of the response to adrenal glucocorticoids to ACTH in Cushing's syndrome has been advocated as an ancillary diagnostic test to separate patients with bilateral adrenal hyperplasia from patients with an adrenal tumor [20]. This is ordinarily done with ACTH administration for one or two days. ACTH administration in the present case was continued because of inadequate urine collections during the first two days of ACTH administration. In recent years it has become apparent that the ACTH stimulation test is not as good as the metyrapone stimulation and dexamethasone suppression tests in separating patients with adrenal tumor from those with bilateral adrenal hyperplasia [21]. Therefore, it would seem that in view of the risk of adrenal hemorrhage, ACTH administration should not be carried out or should be given for no more than one day in patients with Cushing's syndrome.

The diagnosis of adrenal hemorrhage is usually made postmortem [17]. Clark [17], in a report of 34 cases of adrenal hemorrhage and a review of the literature, found that the most common symptoms which might lead to a diagnosis of acute adrenal hemorrhage are pain and tenderness confined to the upper part of the abdomen, severe pain in the back and flank, emesis, profound changes in mentation with agitation, confusion or weakness [17]. The most common physical findings are fever, with a normal pulse rate, upper abdominal tenderness and hypoactive bowel sounds. Peritoneal signs are unusual unless blood has extravasated into the peritoneal cavity. The side on which the flank or abdominal pain occurs usually corresponds to the side of the adrenal hemorrhage [17].

If adrenal hemorrhage is suspected, steroids should be given to protect against possible adrenal insufficiency along with supportive measures with volume expansion if necessary. Surgical exploration may or may not be necessary depending on the amount of adrenal hemorrhage [17]. Similar to our patient, Falconer described a patient with a unilateral hemorrhage which resembled a renal tumor [22]. In regard to the simultaneous left nephrectomy we would agree with Julian that when an extensive dissection of the renal pedicle is necessary to remove an adrenal mass, nephrectomy should be considered. The procedure is not only shortened, but also iatrogenic renovascular hypertension may be prevented [23].

REFERENCES

1. Brea CA Jr, Gomes M, Connor EJ, Balch HH: Report of a case with survival. Am Surg 31: 39, 1965.
2. Fox B: Adrenal hemorrhage and necrosis resulting from abdominal operations. Lancet 1: 600, 1969.
3. Kaplan G: Endotoxin shock with massive adrenal hemorrhage. Calif Med 102: 231, 1965.
4. Markle CD, Evans EC: Adrenal hemorrhage associated with anticoagulant therapy. South Med J 63: 526, 1970.
5. Bookstein JJ, Conn J, Reuter SR: Intra-adrenal hemorrhage as a complication of adrenal venography in primary aldosteronism. Radiology 90: 778, 1968.
6. Proctor EL, Rawson AJ: Adrenal cortical failure following treatment with cortisone and ACTH. Report of a case. Am J Clin Pathol 21: 158, 1951.
7. Galin MA: Unilateral adrenal hemorrhage during ACTH therapy. N Engl J Med 258: 945, 1958.
8. Moolten SE: Symmetrical hemorrhagic necrosis of adrenal glands complicating coronary thrombosis. Case report with discussion of possible role of corticotropin and heparin. J Mt Sinai Hosp NY 24: 1042, 1957.
9. Wilson DAW, Roth D: Adrenal apoplexy occurring during corticotropin therapy of ulcerative colitis. JAMA 152: 230, 1953.
10. Fellerman H, Dalakos TG, Streeten DHP: Remission of Cushing's syndrome after unilateral adrenal phlebography. Apparent destruction of adrenal adenoma. Ann Intern Med 73: 585, 1970.
11. Melby JC: Identifying the adrenal lesion in primary aldosteronism. Ann Intern Med 76: 1039, 1972.
12. Pratt JH, Sawin CT, Melby JC: Remission of Cushing's disease after administration of adrenocorticotropin. Am J Med 57: 949, 1974.
13. Silber RH: Free and conjugated 17-hydroxycorticosteroids in urine. Stand Methods Clin Chem 4: 113, 1963.
14. Spencer-Peet J, Daly JR, Smith V: A simple method for improving the specificity of the fluorimetric determination of adrenal corticosteroids in human plasma. J Endocrinol 31: 235, 1965.
15. Streeten DHP, Stevenson CT, Dalakos TG, et al.: The diagnosis of hypercortisolism. Biochemical criteria differentiating patients from lean and obese normal subjects and from females on oral contraceptives. J Clin Endocrinol Metab 29: 1191, 1969.
16. Berte SJ: Spontaneous adrenal hemorrhage in the adult. Literature review and report of two cases. Ann Intern Med 38: 28, 1953.
17. Clark OH, Hall AD, Schambelan M: Clinical manifestations of adrenal hemorrhage. Am J Surg 128: 219, 1974.
18. Greendyke RM: Adrenal hemorrhage. Am J Clin Pathol 43: 210, 1965.
19. Wilbur OM Jr, Rich AR: A study of the role of adrenocorticotropic hormone (ACTH) in the pathogenesis of tubular degeneration of the adrenals. Bull Johns Hopkins Hosp 93: 321, 1953.
20. Soffer LJ, Geller J, Gabrilove JL: Response of the plasma 17-hydroxy-corticosteroid level to gel-ACTH in tumorous and non-tumorous Cushing's syndrome. J Clin Endocrinol Metab 17: 878, 1957.
21. Weiss ER, Rayyis SS, Nelson DH, Bethune JE: Evaluation of stimulation and suppression tests in the etiological diagnosis of Cushing's syndrome. Ann Intern Med 71: 941, 1969.
22. Falconer CD: Adrenal apoplexy. A case of unilateral hemorrhage simulating a tumor of the kidney. Br J Urol 25: 183, 1953.
23. Julian WA, Cole AT, Fried FA: Renovascular hypertension. A rare complication of excision of pheochromocytoma. J Urol 111: 722, 1974.

Unusual Electrocardiographic Finding—Bifascicular Block Due to Hyperkalemia

JAMES P. O'NEIL, M.D.
EDWARD K. CHUNG, M.D.
Philadelphia, Pennsylvania

A unique case in which the patient had bifascicular block consisting of right bundle branch block and left posterior hemiblock as a result of marked hyperkalemia is presented. To our knowledge, this is the first reported case in which such unusual electrocardiographic abnormalities due to hyperkalemia were demonstrated. The electrocardiographic abnormalities produced by hyperkalemia in this case disappeared promptly by hemodialysis, as the serum potassium level returned to normal. It has been stressed that hyperkalemia should be considered as an important etiologic factor in the differential diagnosis of bundle branch block, hemiblocks and bifascicular block, particularly when these intraventricular blocks are produced suddenly.

Various electrocardiographic abnormalities including cardiac arrhythmias have been reported in patients with hyperkalemia [1–3]. In general, hyperkalemia produces a gradual depression of excitability, conduction velocity of the specialized pacemaker cells and conducting tissues throughout the heart. High degree or complete atrioventricular block, diffuse intraventricular block and ventricular fibrillation followed by ventricular standstill have been observed in advanced hyperkalemia in experimental animals. In human studies, progression to cardiac asystole is rather unusual. In mild potassium elevation, a peaked and tent-shaped T wave is the earliest and the most common electrocardiographic abnormality [1]. As the degree of hyperkalemia progresses further, prolongation of the P-R interval is produced, and it is followed by flat or actual disappearance of P waves. In the later stage of hyperkalemia, the QRS interval will gradually widen when intraventricular block develops. The acceleration of the atrioventricular junctional pacemaker associated with conduction delays in the His Purkinje system may also occur [1–3]. In animal studies, His bundle recordings have shown that asystole is due to a block within the distal conducting system [4]. This finding is applied in man to demonstrate the prolongation of the QRS interval which is due to transient conduction defects within the fascicles of the His Purkinje system.

Our purpose here is to present a unique case in which bifascicular block developed consisting of right bundle branch block (RBBB) and left posterior hemiblock (LPHB) as a result of marked hyperkalemia which was successfully treated with hemodialysis within 5 hours. Related subjects will be briefly reviewed.

From the Jefferson Medical College of Thomas Jefferson University and the Heart Station, Thomas Jefferson University Hospital, Philadelphia, Pennsylvania 19107. Requests for reprints should be addressed to Dr. Edward Chung, Thomas Jefferson University Hospital, Philadelphia, Pennsylvania 19107. Manuscript accepted November 12, 1975.

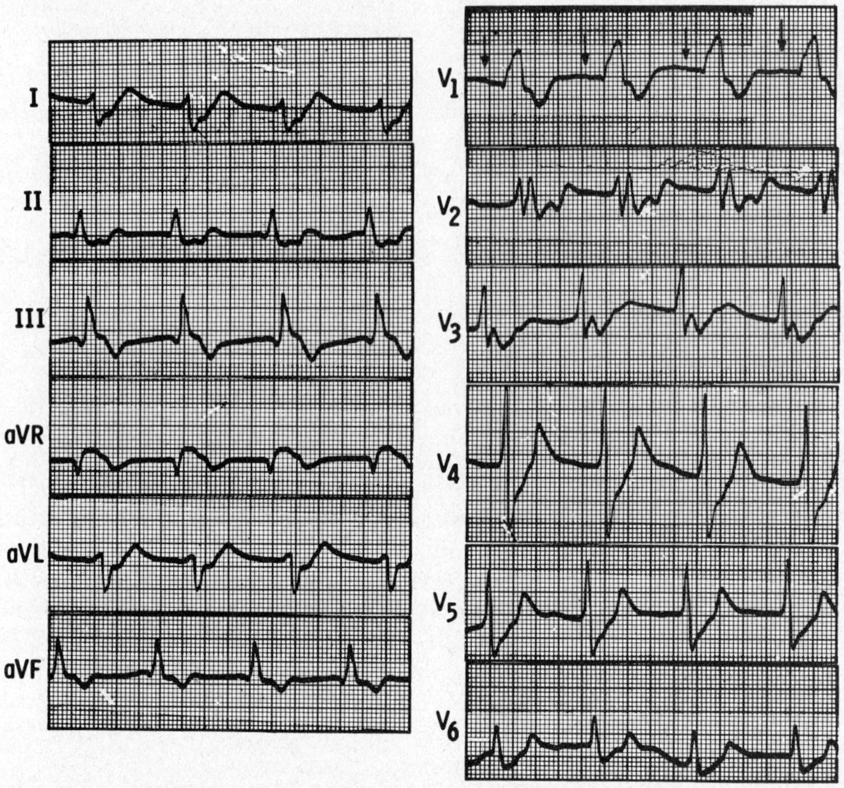

Figure 1. *This electrocardiographic tracing was taken on admission. It shows flat P waves (indicated by arrows), bifascicular block consisting of RBBB and LPHB (the QRS axis: +120 degrees) and peaked T waves due to marked hyperkalemia.*

CASE REPORT

A 58 year old man who had been followed at Thomas Jefferson University Hospital for several years because of long-term renal failure due to necrotizing glomerulonephritis proved by biopsy. He had been in the long-term hemodialysis program three times weekly for 18 months. Repetitive episodes of angina pectoris associated with congestive heart failure without documented myocardial infarction had necessitated several hospitalizations previously. For several days prior to admission, he had increased his salt and fluid intake. His shortness of breath had gradually increased and it was associated with substernal pressure-like pain, unrelieved by the ingestion of nitroglycerin. He was admitted to the cardiac care unit (CCU) because of continuous chest pain. His medications, at the time of admission, included Digoxin® 0.125 mg once, Isordil® 5 mg and Inderal® 10 mg four times each per day with nitroglycerin, aluminum hydroxide gel (Amphogel®), dihydrotachysterol (Hytakerol®) and Tabron®. His other past medical history and family history were unremarkable.

On physical examination his blood pressure was 200/100 mm Hg, with a pulse rate of 56/min and regular. The funduscopic examination disclosed grade II hypertensive retinopathy. There was no thyroid enlargement. His neck veins were distended to the mandible at 45 degrees. There were bibasilar rales to the inferior border of the scapula. The apex of his heart was felt to be at the left anterior axillary line in the sixth intercostal space. The first and second heart sounds were normal. A ventricular gallop was easily heard but there was no atrial gallop. Examinations of the abdomen and extremity disclosed no abnormalities. Neurologically, he was disoriented to time and place. Asterixis was noted. His reflexes were diffusely hypoactive.

Laboratory findings included a hemoglobin level of 7.7 mg/100 ml, blood urea nitrogen 104 mg, sodium 143 meq/liter, potassium 9.0 meq/liter, chloride 108 meq/liter, carbon dioxide 13 meq/liter, calcium 4.2 meq/liter. Chest film showed a marked cardiomegaly with bilateral pleural effusion. The electrocardiogram on admission showed flat P waves, bifascicular block consisting of RBBB and LPHB, associated with peaked and tent-shaped T waves characteristic of advanced hyperkalemia (Figure 1). Within 5 hours after hemodialysis, all of the aforementioned electrocardiographic abnormalities due to hyperkalemia disappeared (Figure 2).

Initial therapy consisted of intravenous injections of 50 cc of 50 per cent glucose, 10 units insulin, 1 ampule bicarbonate, 1 ampule calcium chloride and Kayexalate® enema. He was hemodialyzed within 2 hours of admission to the CCU with a lowering of the serum potassium level to 4.2 meq/liter from the admission value of 9.0 meq/liter, 5 hours after admission. Repeated serum enzyme determinations showed no change and the patient was discharged two days after admission fully recovered.

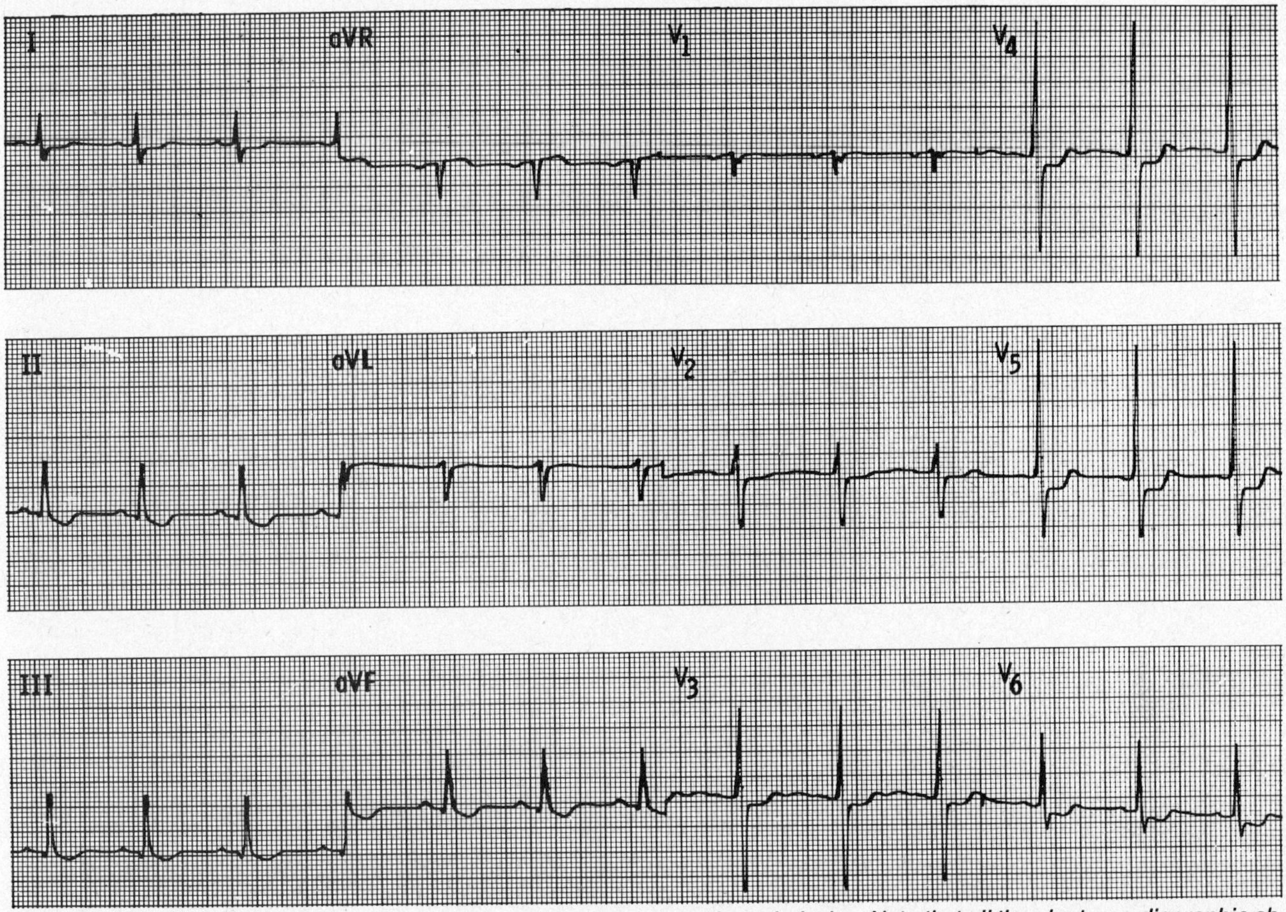

Figure 2. *This electrocardiographic tracing was obtained 5 hours after admission. Note that all the electrocardiographic abnormalities produced by hyperkalemia shown in Figure 1 have disappeared following hemodialysis. The tracing reveals left ventricular hypertrophy.*

COMMENTS

The clinical setting of hyperkalemia is not uncommon and it may occur in renal failure, diabetic keto acidosis, adrenal insufficiency, and rapid administration of potassium solution, stored blood or medications with high potassium concentration.

The increased extracellular concentration of potassium lowers the resting membrane potential and shortens the duration of action potential in all cardiac tissues. The shortening of the action potential causes a shortening of the Q-T intervals at mild hyperkalemia (6 to 7 meq/liter). At this stage of hyperkalemia, peaked T waves are often observed. Generalized conduction delay occurs as the serum potassium increases to 8 to 9 meq/liter. During this moderately severe hyperkalemia, the P wave becomes lower in amplitude with ultimate atrial arrest. In the late stage of advanced hyperkalemia, widening of the QRS complex results from diffuse intraventricular block. Numerous animal experiments have demonstrated this electrocardiographic finding but failed to clarify whether the widening was due to a localized block in the conducting tissue or diffuse conduction delay in the ventricular myocardium [4]. More recent clinical studies have demonstrated left or right QRS axis deviation in the presence of hyperkalemia, some of which reverted to normal after therapy [5]. There have been several reports of RBBB which were thought to be due to hyperkalemia [6]. In a previous report, bifascicular block consisting of RBBB and left anterior hemiblock (LAHB) considered to be due to hyperkalemia had disappeared following treatment [7]. However, to our knowledge, bifascicular block consisting of RBBB and LPHB due to hyperkalemia has not been reported previously. Clinically, LPHB is encountered much less commonly than LAHB because of the large, deeply situated fascicle and its dual blood supply in comparison to the left anterior fascicle [1]. The bifascicular block in the present case was corrected promptly by restoring the potassium level to normal by hemodialysis. Our case study clearly demonstrates that the widening of the QRS complex due to hyperkalemia may actually be due to a localized block in the His-Purkinje system. This case report stresses further that hyperkalemia must be considered as an important etiologic factor in the differential diagnosis of a true bundle branch block, hemiblocks and bifascicular block, particularly when these intraventricular blocks are acute in onset.

REFERENCES

1. Chung EK: Electrocardiography. Practical Application with Vectorial Principles. Hagerstown, Md., Harper & Row, 1974.
2. Ettinger PO, Regan TJ, Oldewurtel HA: Hyperkalemia, cardiac conduction and the electrocardiogram. A review. Am Heart J 88: 360, 1974.
3. Fisch C: Relation of electrolyte disturbances to cardiac arrhythmias. Circulation 47; 408, 1973.
4. Lanari A, Chait L, Capurro C: Electrocardiographic effects of potassium. Perfusion through the coronary bed. Am Heart J 67: 357, 1964.
5. Ewy GA, Karliner J, Bedyner J: Electrocardiographic QRS axis as a manifestation of hyperkalemia. JAMA 215: 429, 1971.
6. Fisch C, Knoebel S, Feigenbaum H, Greenspan K: Potassium and monophasic action potentials, electrocardiogram, conduction and arrhythmias. Prog Cardiovasc Dis 8: 387, 1966.
7. Punja M, Schneebaum R, Cohen J: Bifascicular block induced by hyperkalemia. J Electrocardiol 6: 71, 1973.

Bilateral Scalp Necrosis in Temporal Arteritis

A Rare Complication of Horton's Disease

CARL W. SODERSTROM, M.D.
JAMES R. SEEHAFER, M.D.
Peoria, Illinois

In an elderly man bilateral temporal scalp necrosis complicating temporal (systemic giant cell) arteritis developed. The patient also demonstrated other features characteristic of this entity: (1) exquisite scalp tenderness and headache, (2) onset late in life, (3) visual disturbances, (4) general debility, (5) diagnostic temporal artery biopsy, and (6) gradual healing with glucocorticosteroid therapy. A computer assisted review revealed 13 similar cases of scalp necrosis associated with temporal arteritis published in the English literature.

Hutchinson [1] first reported the clinical picture of temporal arteritis in 1890, and Horton [2] and his colleagues, in 1932, clarified the clinical and histologic features of the disease. In 1941 Gilmour [3] noted systemic vascular involvement by giant cells in temporal arteritis. The first case of scalp necrosis in temporal arteritis was reported by Cooke [4] in 1946, 56 years after the original description of the disease. Wilske and Healey [5], in 1967, proposed the phrase "systemic giant cell arteritis," thus describing a disease now recognized as an illness of the elderly, affecting any of the major arteries or the aorta in a segmental manner, but having an unusual predilection for the vessels of the carotid system.

The clinical manifestations of systemic giant cell arteritis are protean, and the various syndromes observed have been subclassified according to the region of the vascular system involved. The symptoms which most frequently bring a patient to the physician are unilateral or bilateral intermittent temporal or retrobulbar aching, or excrutiating, throbbing headaches with a clinical finding of exquisite scalp tenderness over the temporal arteries [6]. Additional symptoms of systemic giant cell arteritis as reported by Fairbairn et al. [6] include low grade fever, anorexia, malaise, the polymyalgia rheumatica syndrome, facial pain, pain in the temporomandibular joint, intermittant claudication of the jaw, mononeuritis multiplex, symmetrical peripheral neuropathy, depression, delirium, confusion, photophobia and visual disturbances, including blurred vision, diplopia, amaurosis fugax and, frequently, complete ophthalmic artery occlusion and blindness. Other symptoms include sweats, weakness and weight loss.

Objective clinical findings, as reviewed by Hitch [7], include decreased or absent temporal pulses, a thickened, nodular, tender temporal artery, urticaria, edema, erythema, ecchymosis, vesicles, hemorrhagic bullae, crusting, necrosis, ulceration, purpura, alopecia and hyperpigmentation in the area of distribution of the temporal arteries. Other clinical manifestations occur in relationship to the arteries involved.

From the Department of Dermatology, Peoria School of Medicine, University of Illinois College of Medicine, and St. Francis Hospital Medical Center, Peoria, Illinois 61606. Requests for reprints should be addressed to Dr. Carl W. Soderstrom, 81 Queenwood, Morton, Illinois 61550.
Manuscript accepted December 31, 1975.

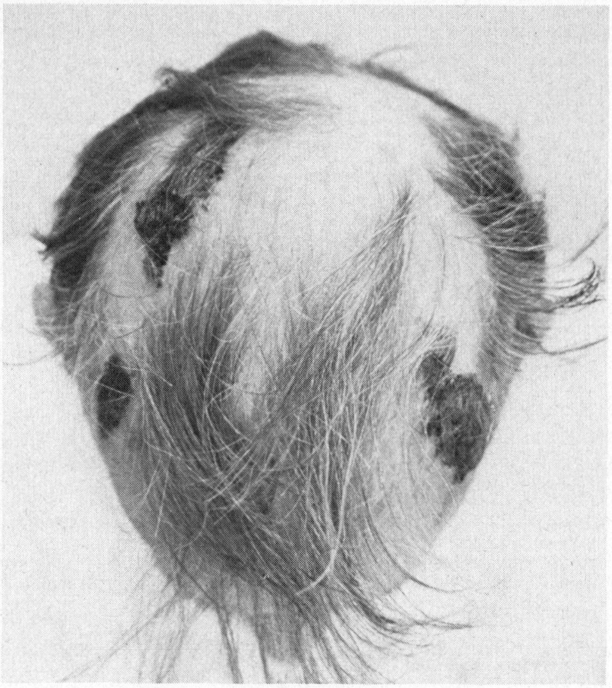

Figure 1. Bilateral ulcerations with eschar formation and scarring alopecia extending over temporoparietal scalp areas prior to therapy.

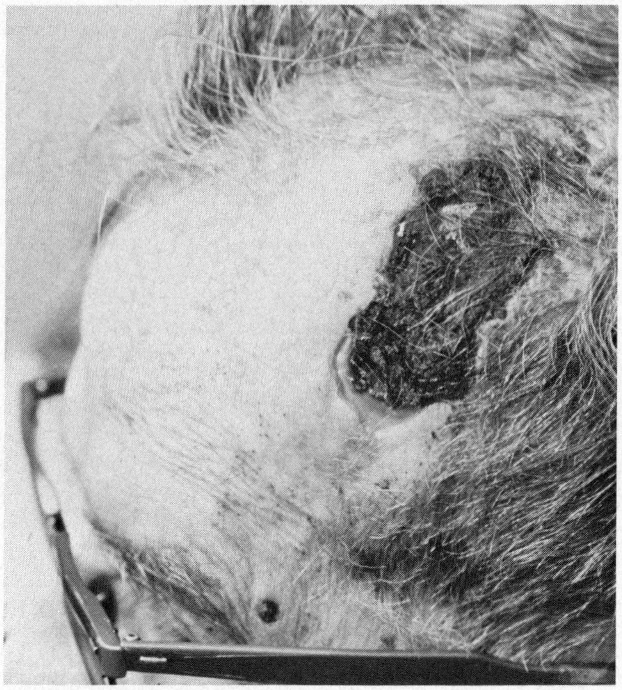

Figure 2. Large 7 by 3.5 cm crusted, necrotic ulceration showing calvarium at its inferior border and a basal cell carcinoma lateral to the left eye.

Laboratory findings supporting a diagnosis of temporal arteritis include a mild leukocytosis with a shift to the left, anemia, low serum iron, an increased erythrocyte sedimentation rate and, frequently, an increased alpha$_2$-globulin.

Total or partial obliteration of the lumen of the involved arteries is a feature frequently noted on biopsy of vessels in patients with systemic giant cell arteritis; however, necrosis or gangrene of the scalp secondary to this is a rare observation. A computer assisted review of the English literature revealed 13 previously reported cases of scalp necrosis in temporal arteritis. Because of the rarity and the diagnostic and therapeutic importance of this finding, we wish to report an additional case.

CASE REPORT

An 81 year old man was admitted to St. Francis Hospital, Peoria, Illinois, on September 14, 1973, with the chief complaint of bilateral, painful, crusted scalp lesions.

In April 1973, he noted the onset of rather severe, throbbing and recurrent headaches followed on July 2, 1973, by an initial ulceration of the left anterior scalp. This was followed two weeks later by multifocal ulcerations of the right side of the scalp that enlarged progressively over the next two and a half months until his admission. No history of vesicles, bullae or the polymyalgia rheumatica syndrome was elicited. During the time prior to hospitalization, a working diagnosis was bilateral Herpes zoster, but the ulcerations developed into necrotic lesions, the pain became more intense and persistent, and hospitalization was required.

Also during this interval, the patient's visual acuity was affected and he saw his optometrist for refitting of his corrective lenses for the first time in 10 years. In 1963, his visual acuity was 20/40 in the right eye and 20/50 in the left eye. In August 1973, his visual acuity was 20/100 in the right eye and 20/200 in the left eye.

Angina pectoris developed in 1959 and the patient suffered a probable myocardial infarction in 1961. In 1971, he experienced intermittent claudication with absent posterior tibial and dorsalis pedis pulses, and he was treated with a vasodilator.

The patient was slightly cachectic, depressed and remorseful, and resting quietly in a darkened room; any breeze, slight touch or positional change initiated severe and lasting paroxysms of bilateral temporal pain. He also suffered from photophobia. He was afebrile with a blood pressure of 140/74 mm Hg.

Evaluation of the scalp revealed scarring alopecia bilaterally over the temporoparietal areas (refer to Figure 1). The left temporal region had a 7 by 3.5 cm eschar covering an erythematous bordered area of necrotic gangrenous scalp tissue whose depth reached to the calvarium (refer to Figure 2). The right temporoparietal scalp showed two similar necrotic gangrenous crusted ulcerations, one anteriorly measuring 2.5 by 3.5 cm and the more posterior lesion measuring 8.5 by 3 cm.

Ophthalmologic examination disclosed normal muscle movements, corneas and lenses. Vision was 20/30 bilaterally with corrective lenses; tension was normal; macula, arteries,

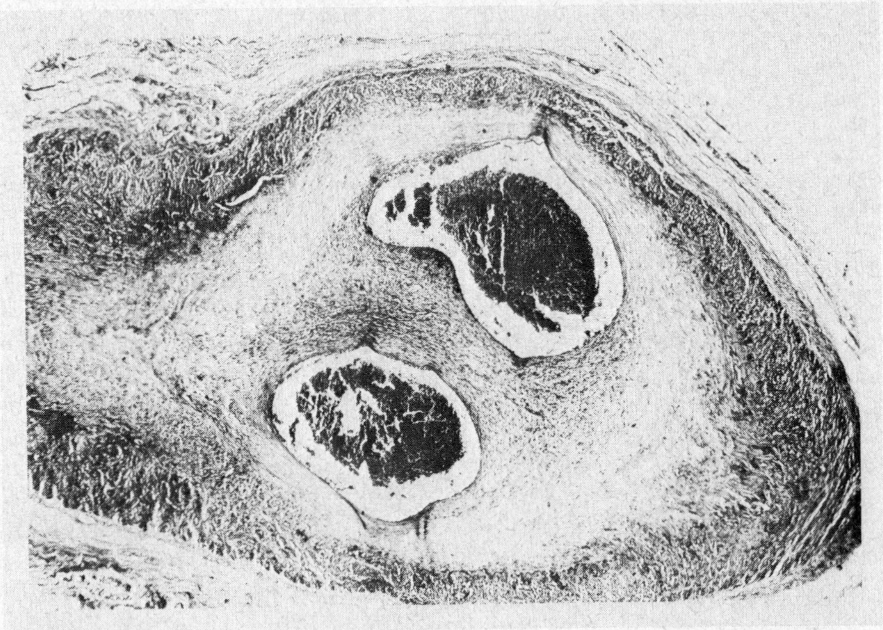

Figure 3. *Section of temporal artery prior to treatment showing chronic inflammation, marked intimal proliferation, narrowed vessel lumen and involvement with giant cells.*

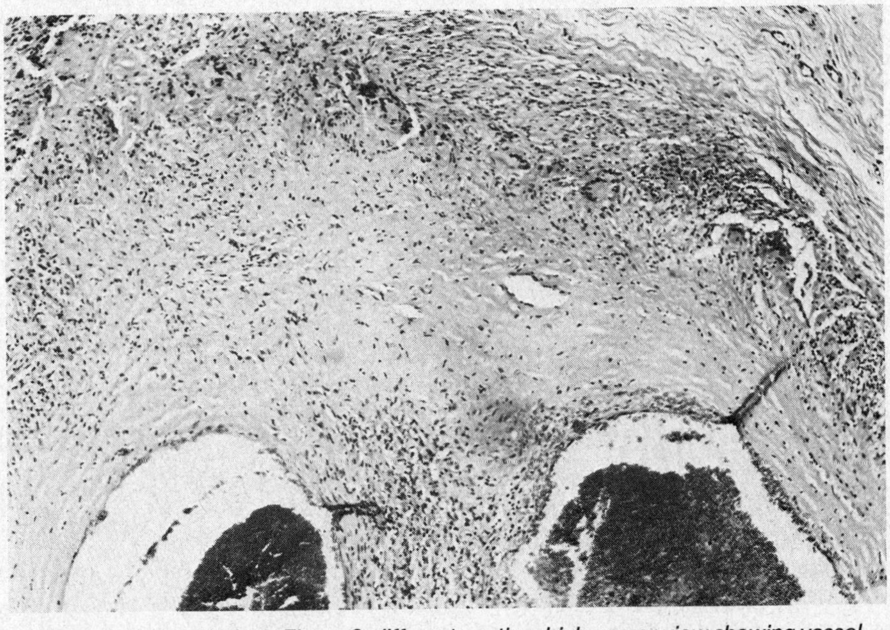

Figure 4. *Same artery as Figure 3, different section, high-power view showing vessel lumen and giant cell in area of chronic inflammation and intimal proliferation.*

venules and discs were normal. Several soft exudates were present in the temporal field of the right eye; no other retinopathy or evidence of ischemic optic neuritis was present.

Other positive physical findings included a 1 cm basal cell carcinoma lateral to the left eye (refer to Figure 2) and mild stasis dermatitis.

The hemoglobin level was 14.1 g/100 ml, and the white cell count was 7,900/mm^3 with a normal differential. Fasting blood sugar was 114 mg/100 ml, a lupus erythematosus preparation was negative, and the erythrocyte sedimentation rate was 30 mm/hour (Wintrobe). Total serum protein was 6.3 g/100 ml, albumin 3.5 g/100 ml and globulins were 2.8

g/100 ml. Serum electrolytes were all within normal limits. A chest film showed mild cardiomegaly with no active pulmonary or pleural pathologic processes.

Left temporal artery biopsy was performed; it showed a thickened, firm vessel on gross inspection.

Histologic examination (refer to Figures 3 and 4) revealed a markedly narrowed lumen with collections of chronic inflammatory cells and areas infiltrated with multinucleated giant cells. The internal elastic lamina was fragmented, and there was marked intimal proliferation and evidence of recannalization of the vessel lumen. Very little bleeding occurred when the biopsy was performed.

The administration of prednisone, 30 mg twice a day, was begun immediately, and within 72 hours the headaches were much less severe and less frequent. The necrotic scalp areas were covered with wet dressings which were held in place with a stockinette. He was instructed to adhere to a 90 meq sodium diet, Maalox® four times a day, and to use Jobst leg stockings. On the sixth day of prednisone therapy, the erythrocyte sedimentation rate was 15 mm/hour and by the 10th day of therapy, he estimated a 70 per cent over-all improvement in his condition. Scalp tenderness abated, and active healing began to take place about the edges of the necrotic areas. Photophobia had diminished. He was discharged to weekly follow-up visits after a 17 day hospitalization.

On the 19th day of therapy his prednisone was decreased to 20 mg twice a day. Slow but steady healing of the necrotic areas continued, and on the 56th day of therapy, the dose of prednisone was altered to 30 mg once a day. The basal cell carcinoma was removed by electrodesiccation and curettage on November 1, 1973.

On the 69th day of therapy, the crusts on the right side of the scalp had fallen off, and scalp tissue had healed over the ulcerated areas. The left side continued to improve, but much more slowly. By this time the patient was relatively asymptomatic and in much brighter spirits. On the 82nd day of therapy, the dose of prednisone was decreased to 20 mg once a day.

On the 91st day of therapy he was readmitted to the hospital with a chief complaint of epigastric distress which was relieved by the intake of Maalox. On this admission, the left temporal ulcer measured 3 by 4 cm with an exposed area of clean, dry calvarium at the base of the ulceration. Plastic surgical consultation recommended continued local care, which was done with wet dressings.

Peripheral blood studies at this time were essentially unchanged from his first hospitalization except that the erythrocyte sedimentation rate was 15 mm/hour. X-ray studies of the skull, gallbladder, colon and upper gastrointestinal tract were all within normal limits.

Outpatient care was then continued with wet dressings and stockinette, prednisone 15 mg once daily and Maalox every 2 hours. By the 116th day of therapy, the left temporal ulcer had healed to 1.9 by 2.7 cm.

On April 27, 1974, he presented to the emergency room and was admitted with the chief complaint of acute substernal chest pain. An electrocardiogram obtained at that time was consistent with posterior-lateral ischemia. The patient died on April 30, 1974. Permission for a postmortem examination was not obtained.

COMMENT

The majority of reported cases of temporal arteritis are in patients greater than 55 years old with no predilection for either sex. Of those patients with scalp necrosis noted in Table I, the ages range from 66 to 85 years, with a mean age of 76 years. The male to female ratio is 1:2. Of those patients in whom a clear description of the area of ulceration or necrosis was made, six had bitemporal involvement, two had right parietal ulceration and one had a midline ulceration sparing the parietal and temporal regions; the case we report represents another of bitemporal involvement.

In addition to scalp necrosis, several reports of tongue necrosis in patients with temporal arteritis have been made [13,17,18]. Ulcerations and gangrene of the lower extremities [19] and a syndrome characterized by an acutely painful hand [20] have also been reported which may have represented peripheral vascular involvement in systemic giant cell arteritis.

Confirming a diagnosis of temporal arteritis early in the course of the disease is an urgent matter as evidenced by the frequent occurrence of variable degrees of visual loss or blindness, complications which may be prevented but not usually reversed by early initiation of proper therapy. Of 175 patients described by Hollenhorst et al. [21] who had temporal arteritis not associated with scalp necrosis, approximately 40 per cent suffered partial or complete visual loss. In those described in this review, eight of 12 patients suffered irreversible visual loss and one exhibited tongue necrosis, emphasing the aggressive nature of temporal arteritis when associated with scalp necrosis.

An increased erythrocyte sedimentation rate is often considered the most useful laboratory test associated with temporal arteritis, where values greater than 100 mm/hour are not unusual. When the erythrocyte sedimentation rate is normal or only slightly increased, a diagnosis of temporal arteritis is often not considered [22]. We believe that this could be misleading in patients with associated scalp necrosis. Boyd and Hoffbrand [23] have suggested an upper normal limit of 40 mm/hour for hospital inpatients greater than 65 years of age, but the erythrocyte sedimentation rates in those patients with scalp necrosis, when reported, ranged from 24 mm/hour to 65 mm/hour with a mean of 43 mm/hour and four patients had an erythrocyte sedimentation rate less than 40 mm/hour. Our patient's highest erythrocyte sedimentation rate was 30 mm/hour.

If the clinical picture of temporal arteritis is present, we believe that a temporal artery biopsy should be performed on an emergency basis with immediate institution of therapy. Adrenocorticosteroids are the agents of choice and Sandok [24] has clearly stressed

TABLE I 13 Documented Cases of Scalp Necrosis Associated with Temporal (Systemic Giant Cell) Arteritis

Investigator	Date Reported	Age (yr) and Sex	Description of Scalp	Erythrocyte Sedimentation Rate	Associated Findings	Treatment	Outcome
Cooke et al. [4]	1946	73, F	Ulceration	—	Complete visual loss	None	Patient died 14 mo after onset
	1946	66, F	Vesicles with crusts	—	Right eye visual loss	Compress and sulfonamides	
Whitfield et al. [8]	1953	66, F	Large area necrosis	—	Restricted visual fields	Cortisone	Scalp healed in 4 mo
Kendall [9]	1953	78, F	Necrosis right parietal scalp	—	Necrosis of nasal septum, complete visual loss	None	Scalp healed in 4 mo
Russell [10]	1959	...	Case not described in detail		...	...	...
Clark [11]	1960	75, M	Bitemporal necrosis	65	Left eye visual loss	Prednisone	Scalp unchanged over 9 wk; died of myocardial infarction secondary to arteriosclerotic heart disease
Fleischl, Oldham [12]	1960	85, M	Bitemporal necrosis	48	Right eye visual loss	Prednisone	Scalp healed in a few mo
Brearley, MacDonald [13]	1961	82, F	Right parietal necrosis	34	Necrosis anterior two-thirds of tongue	Prednisone	Not healed 30 days after treatment began
Kinmont, McCallum [14]	1964	79, F	Bitemporal necrosis	53	None	Prednisone	Scalp healed in 3 mo
	1964	75, F	Central scalp necrosis	33	Complete visual loss	Prednisone	Not healed in 8 mo; patient died of pulmonary causes
Barefoot, Lund [15]	1966	80, M	Necrosis anterior two-thirds of scalp	24	Marked visual loss	Prednisone	Scalp healed in 2 mo
Folan [16]	1969	78, F	Extensive (80%) scalp necrosis	45	None	Topical antibodies and pinch grafts	Lost to follow-up
Hitch [7]	1970	76, M	Bitemporal necrosis	54	None	Prednisone	Cardiorespiratory death on 83rd treatment day

the importance and urgency of adequate dosages suggesting an initial amount of 60 to 80 mg of prednisone/day with slow tapering of the dosage relative to the healing process. If biopsy for diagnosis must be delayed, treatment nevertheless should begin if the diagnosis is highly suspected.

Of those patients in whom clear reports were given, seven of 12 were alive, none of whom had yet completed treatment courses. Five died, three of cardiopulmonary causes, during their treatment courses. The autopsy reports described atheromatous vessel disease in the three cardiopulmonary deaths, but interestingly, none showed coronary vessel arteritis at postmortem examination. Despite diagnosis and treatment, scalp necrosis in temporal arteritis carries a grave prognosis.

SUMMARY

An 81 year old man is described with bilateral scalp necrosis, an infrequent but important diagnostic clue, following the onset of temporal (systemic giant cell) arteritis. Diagnosis was confirmed by biopsy, and the necrotic areas responded nicely to prednisone therapy. Ulceration, necrosis and blindness may be prevented in such cases, with early diagnosis and treatment; however, the over-all prognosis is guarded due to the multivessel involvement, patient's age, long-term steroid therapy and aggressive nature of this disease.

REFERENCES

1. Hutchinson J: Diseases of the arteries. Arch Surg 1: 323, 1890.
2. Horton BT, Magath TB, Brown GE: An undescribed form of arteritis of the temporal vessels. Proc Staff Meet Mayo Clinic 7: 700, 1932.
3. Gilmour JR: Giant cell chronic arteritis. J Pathol 53: 263, 1941.
4. Cooke WT, Cloake PCP, Govan ADT, Colbeck JC: Temporal arteritis. Q J Med 15: 47, 1946.
5. Wilske KR, Healey LA: Polymyalgia rheumatica: a manifestation of systemic giant-cell arteritis. Ann Intern Med 66: 77, 1967.
6. Fairbairn JF, Juergens JL, Spittell JA: Peripheral Vascular Diseases, Philadelphia, W.B. Saunders Co., 1972, p 362.
7. Hitch JM: Dermatologic manifestations of giant-cell (temporal, cranial) arteritis. Arch Dermatol 101: 409, 1970.
8. Whitfield AWG, Cooke WT, Jameson-Evans P, Rudd C: Temporal arteritis and its treatment with cortisone and ACTH. Lancet 1: 408, 1953.
9. Kendall D: Some complications of temporal arteritis. Br Med J 2: 418, 1953.
10. Russell RWR: Giant cell arteritis: a review of 35 cases. Q J Med 28: 471, 1959.
11. Clark J: Gangrene of the scalp. Br Med J 2: 1160, 1960.
12. Fleischl P, Oldham BE: Temporal (giant-cell) arteritis associated with gangrene of the scalp. Br Med J 2: 439, 1960.
13. Brearley BF, MacDonald JG: Temporal arteritis resulting in infected gangrene of tongue. Br Med J 1: 1151, 1961.
14. Kinmont PDC, McCallum DI: Skin manifestations of giant-cell arteritis. Br J Dermatol 76: 299, 1964.
15. Barefoot SW, Lund HZ: Temporal (giant-cell) arteritis associated with ulcerations of scalp. Arch Dermatol 93: 79, 1966.
16. Folan DW: Polymyalgia rheumatica with purpura necrotica of the entire scalp. Cutis 5: 278, 1969.
17. Howard S, Cremin MD: Acute parenchymatous glossitis with gangrene of the tongue. Lancet 2: 410, 1959.
18. Reed C, Inglis MJ: Acute massive gangrene of tongue. Br Med J 2: 575, 1965.
19. Finlayson R, Robinson JO: Giant-cell arteritis of the legs. Br Med J 2: 1595, 1955.
20. Bugg EI, Coonrad RW, Grim KB: Giant-cell arteritis. An acute hand syndrome. J Bone Joint Surg 45: 1269, 1963.
21. Hollenhorst RW, Brown JR, Wagener HP, Schick RM: Neurologic aspects of temporal arteritis. Neurology 10: 490, 1960.
22. Kinmont PDC, McCallum DI: Hemorrhagic and necrotic leg ulcers in the elderly. Aust J Dermatol 9: 95, 1967.
23. Boyd RV, Hoffbrand BI: Erythrocyte sedimentation rate in elderly hospital in-patients. Br Med J 1: 901, 1966.
24. Sandok BA: Part 3: Temporal arteritis. JAMA 222: 1405, 1972.

Chronic Intravascular Coagulation Associated with Chronic Myelocytic Leukemia

Use of Heparin in Connection with a Surgical Procedure

HAROLD J. GERMAN, M.D.
JEANNE A. SMITH, M.D.
JOHN LINDENBAUM, M.D.
New York, New York

A woman with Philadelphia chromosome-positive chronic myelocytic leukemia lived nearly 12 years from the time of diagnosis. During most of this period she received no therapy, and marked cyclic oscillations in the white blood cell count were documented. The last two years of her illness were marked by a hemorrhagic disorder associated with hypofibrinogenemia, thrombocytopenia, increased plasma fibrinopeptide A concentration and markedly elevated serum levels of fibrin degradation products. The coagulation disorder was rapidly reversible on several occasions with heparin therapy. After treatment with heparin and platelet transfusions, the patient underwent successful resection of a large ovarian cyst with excellent hemostasis during the procedure. Postoperatively, the administration of heparin and platelets was discontinued and a large wound hematoma developed. After resumption of therapy with heparin and platelets, the remainder of her postoperative course was uneventful. The literature on the subject is reviewed and tentative guidelines are offered concerning the management of patients with intravascular coagulation who require diagnostic or therapeutic surgical procedures.

In recent years increasing numbers of patients have been described to have a chronic state of intravascular coagulation associated with underlying malignancies, hemangiomas, aortic aneurysms, vasculitides and liver disease [1–4]. Such patients may require diagnostic or therapeutic surgical procedures, which may be complicated by disastrous operative or postoperative hemorrhage [5–10].

The defibrination syndrome has frequently been encountered in the acute leukemias [11], but it is not a recognized complication of chronic myelocytic leukemia (CML). We describe a patient with CML in whom a coagulation disorder developed consistent with intravascular coagulation and who also required surgical excision of an enlarging pelvic mass. Based on our experience with this patient and that of others described in the literature, we have attempted to develop guidelines which may be useful in the management of other patients with chronic intravascular coagulation who may require surgery or invasive diagnostic procedures.

From the Medical Service, Harlem Hospital Center; and the Department of Medicine, Columbia University, College of Physicians and Surgeons, New York, New York. Requests for reprints should be addressed to Dr. John Lindenbaum, Medical Service, Harlem Hospital Center, Lenox Avenue and 135th Street, New York, New York 10037.
Manuscript accepted December 31, 1975.

CASE REPORT

In September 1962, at age 35, a previously healthy Puerto Rican housewife was found to have CML when she presented to another hospital with painful splenomegaly. The white blood cell count was 364,000/μl, with 43 per cent neutrophils, 15 per cent band forms, 17 per cent metamyelocytes, 14 per cent myelocytes, 3 per cent promyelocytes, 1 per cent myeloblasts, 3 per cent basophils, 3 per cent eosinophils and 1 per cent monocytes. The hemoglobin value was 6.4 g/dl and the platelet count 490,000/μl. A bone marrow aspirate was hypercellular with increased myelopoiesis. She was treated with busulfan. By March 1963 she felt well, the spleen was no longer palpable, the white blood cell count was 8,900/μl, and the hemoglobin value and platelet count were normal.

The patient did well without further therapy until July 1967, when she was admitted to Bellevue Hospital with acute tuberculous pericarditis. At that time the spleen was not palpable. The white blood cell count was 13,800/μl with a normal differential, the hematocrit value was 35 per cent, and the platelet count 360,000/μl. She had an uneventful recovery on antituberculous therapy and was subsequently followed at 1 to 2 month intervals in the hematology clinics of Bellevue and Harlem Hospitals from October 1967 to April 1972; during this period she remained asymptomatic and received no antileukemic therapy. Her peripheral blood values fluctuated markedly during this period.

In April 1972 she noted the onset of multiple ecchymoses on both legs, and evaluation at that time showed an increase in the size of the spleen to 5 cm below the left costal margin, a more marked leukocytosis, thrombocytopenia and evidence of a disorder in blood coagulation. Results of liver function tests were within normal limits. Over the next several months she was treated with prednisone and busulfan, with lowering of the white blood cell count to 31,000/μl but no change in her coagulation abnormalities and a slight diminution in the purpuric tendency. In December 1972, she noted the onset of menorrhagia, and a 10 by 15 cm nontender lower abdominal mass was noted on pelvic examination. She was admitted to Harlem Hospital and after further evaluation and heparin therapy, underwent resection of a benign mucous cyst of the left ovary weighing 1,200 g. Her postoperative course was complicated by the development of a wound hematoma which caused a superficial dehiscence, requiring operative incision and drainage, and by pulmonary infection. She was discharged in May 1973.

During the last year of her life she had multiple admissions to Harlem Hospital Center for recurrent episodes of gout, massive splenomegaly with splenic infarction, generalized lymphadenopathy due to infiltration with immature leukocytes, and a severe peripheral neuropathy. The peripheral blood showed a worsening anemia, and advancing leukocytosis with increasing numbers of promyelocytes and blast cells. Transient responses to therapy with vincristine, prednisone, splenic irradiation and hydroxyurea were documented. In May 1974, the patient had convulsive seizures, congestive heart failure, ascites and worsening liver function test results associated with the presence of hepatitis B antigen in her serum. She died 11 2/3 years after her initial presentation. Permission for postmortem examination was denied.

HEMATOLOGIC FINDINGS

White Cells. The patient had a complete blood count with platelet and reticulocyte counts and 200 to 500 cell differentials on 171 occasions during the period 1967–1974. Review of these findings revealed certain trends. Between 1967 and 1972 the white blood cells fluctuated in a cyclic fashion, with a periodicity of approximately two to three months, between 9,000 and 98,000/μl. At the time of the cyclic white blood cell peaks, there were higher percentages of immature myeloid cells in the peripheral blood, with 2 to 4 per cent promyelocytes and 0 to 1 per cent blast forms. At the nadirs of the white blood cell cycles, when counts were below 25,000, no blast forms and 0 to 1 per cent promyelocytes were seen. The spleen was palpable at 1 to 2 cm below the left costal margin at the time of peak leukocytosis, but it could not be felt during the white blood cell nadirs. The percentage of basophils remained at 1 per cent or less.

In April 1972, at the time of development of her coagulation disorder, the white blood cell count had risen to 88,000/μl with 6 per cent promyelocytes and 1 per cent myeloblasts. A bone marrow aspirate was hypercellular with 15 per cent promyelocytes and 5 per cent myeloblasts. The promyelocyte granules showed no unusual morphologic features. Over the next month (before therapy), the white blood cell count rose to 194,000/μl with 10 to 11 per cent promyelocytes and 1 to 4 per cent myeloblasts. A bone marrow aspirate was hypercellular with 15 per cent myeloblasts. A basophilia of 2 to 7 per cent was noted from April 1972 until her death two years later. The cycling of the white blood cells was interrupted by multiple courses of chemotherapy and irradiation during her last two years, but during a 10 month period without any therapy in 1973, the white blood cells cycled between 17,000 and 374,000/μl. The percentage of blast cells in the peripheral blood was approximately 16 per cent in late 1973 (at which time the bone marrow showed more than 90 per cent myeloblasts) and increased to 44 per cent during the month before her death in 1974.

The Philadelphia chromosome was present in bone marrow cultures obtained in 1969 and 1970. Leukocyte alkaline phosphatase determinations were low in 1967 and 1969, but rose to well within the normal range in late 1970 and were again normal in 1972 and 1973, at times of marked leukocytosis.

Erythrocytes. Rare nucleated red blood cells and mild anisocytosis and poikilocytosis with occasional ovalocytes and tear drop shaped red blood cells were noted in the peripheral blood in 1968 and 1969. The morphologic abnormalities gradually became more severe until April 1972, after which time marked anisopoikilocytosis was present, with 3 to 10 nucleated red blood cells/100 white blood cells. The hematocrit value remained in the 30 to 35 per cent range until April 1972 when it declined to 15 to 20 per cent, where it remained (except after transfusions) during the last two years of her life, associated with a 6 to 20 per cent reticulocytosis. On several occasions, the serum bilirubin and haptoglobin levels, plasma hemoglobin and urinary hemosiderin were within normal limits. No myelofibrosis could be demonstrated on connective tissue stains of bone marrow biopsy specimens obtained in 1972 and 1973.

Platelets. During 1967 to 1971, the platelet count varied between 134,000 and 480,000/μl; cyclic oscillations appeared to be present which were out of phase with the fluctuations in white blood cells. Significant thrombocytopenia was noted for the first time in April 1972, when the platelet count fell to 34,000/μl in association with her coagulation disorder. During the previous two years the platelet count had been in the range of 150,000 to 480,000/μl. Increased numbers of megathrombocytes were noted in the peripheral blood as early as 1969. Bone marrow biopsy specimens in 1972 and 1973 showed decreased numbers of megakaryocytes. The platelet count remained at 25,000 to 75,000/μl, except after platelet transfusions, during the last two years of her life.

Coagulation Studies. When the onset of ecchymoses and severe thrombocytopenia occurred in April 1972, a coagulation profile (Table I) showed marked hypofibrinogenemia, with minimal prolongations of the prothrombin time, activated partial thromboplastin time and thrombin time. The staphylococcal clumping titer was markedly elevated, and the euglobulin lysis time (performed on a 1:1 mixture of the patient's plasma and normal plasma) was 3 hours (normal 2 to 4 hours). A cryofibrinogen could not be demonstrated. The coagulation profile was essentially unchanged when repeated on 18 occasions when she was not receiving heparin during the last two years of her life, except for a marked prolongation of the thrombin time, that was not corrected by the addition of normal plasma, on one occasion in May 1973. The fibrinogen concentration fluctuated between 34 and 175 mg/dl except on two occasions when it rose to 234 to 262 mg/dl in association with acute gouty arthritis and splenic infarction in October 1973 and in the week before her death in May 1974. The fluctuations in the fibrinogen concentration could not be correlated with variations in the platelet or white counts. The fibrinogen remained low following various courses of therapy with busulfan, vincristine and prednisone, which resulted in temporary depressions of the white blood count to normal or near normal levels and regression of splenomegaly.

Effects of Heparin Therapy. Since the only clinical manifestations of the patient's coagulation disorder were occasional recurrent ecchymoses over the lower extremities, it was initially elected to withhold any therapy directed specifically at the hypofibrinogenemia. In February 1973, when exploratory abdominal surgery for diagnosis and treatment of the pelvic mass was under consideration, a trial of heparin therapy was undertaken. Following two intravenous injections of heparin, 5,000 U (75 U/kg), separated by a 6 hour interval, the plasma fibrinogen concentration rose to normal (Table II). An initially elevated plasma fibrinopeptide A level fell to within normal limits within an hour of the first heparin injection (Table II).

Two weeks later, the patient was prepared for surgery by being given intravenous injections of 5,000 U of heparin, 12 and 6 hours preoperatively. The fibrinogen concentration rose from 91 mg/dl before the administration of heparin to 147 mg/dl at the time of surgery. Twenty units of platelet concentrates were infused during the operation. The surgeons noted no excessive bleeding during resection of the large ovarian cyst. Immediately after the operation, the platelet count was 198,000/μl, and the fibrinogen concentration 139 mg/dl. Heparin and platelet transfusions were not given during the first six postoperative days. On day 7, a large wound hematoma was noted. The fibrinogen concentration was 131 mg/dl, thrombin time 18 seconds (control, 12 seconds), platelet count 59,000/μl, and staphylococcal clumping titer 1:1024. Heparin therapy was resumed, the patient was given platelet transfusions, and the wound was opened and drained in the operating room. Twelve hours after heparin therapy was resumed, the fibrinogen level rose to 223 mg/dl. Intravenous heparin, 5,000 U every 8 hours, was given over the remaining seven weeks in the hospital, which were uncomplicated except for an episode of pneumonia. The fibrinogen level measured on nine occasions while the patient was receiving heparin was between 208 and 352 mg/dl except for one value of 156 mg/dl. No definite effect of heparin therapy on the platelet count or the staphylococcal clumping titer was apparent. Heparin therapy was discontinued at the time of discharge in April 1973, and one month later in the clinic the fibrinogen concentration was 87 mg/dl.

During the two years between the discovery of the coagulation disorder and the patient's death, the fibrinogen level was measured on 19 occasions when she was not receiving heparin (mean ± 1 SE, 126 ± 14 mg/dl) and 10 times when she was receiving heparin (mean, 257 ± 20 mg/dl, $p < 0.001$).

TABLE I Coagulation Studies

Test	Normal Range	Patient 4/17/72	Range* 1972–1974
Prothrombin time (sec)	11–13	13.8	12.7–16.3
Partial thromboplastin time (sec)	37–41	46.9	31.0–47.0
Thrombin time (sec)	11–13	15.1	11.6–>120
Fibrinogen [36] (mg/dl)	200–400	52	34–262
Staphylococcal clumping titer [37]	<1:8	1:1024	1:64–1:1024

* Range of 18 determinations when patient was not receiving heparin, between April 1972 and May 1974.

COMMENTS

Intravascular coagulation appears to have been the cause of the disorder of hemostasis that was manifested two years before the death of this patient with Philadelphia chromosome-positive CML. This is strongly supported by a number of findings, including the decreased fibrinogen level and platelet count, markedly elevated staphylococcal clumping titer, elevated fibri-

TABLE II Effects of Heparin Therapy

Time After First Heparin Injection (hour)	Plasma Fibrinogen (mg/dl)	Plasma Fibrinopeptide A [38] (ng/ml)	Platelet Count (cells/μl)
0*	87	11.4	46,000
0.5	...	3.8	...
1	...	1.7	...
6*	154	...	...
12	306	...	...
28	138	...	60,000

* Heparin, 5,000 U given intravenously at 0 and 6 hours.

nopeptide A level, and prompt response of the abnormalities in fibrinogen and fibrinopeptide A concentrations to heparin therapy. At the time of discovery of the hypofibrinogenemia, there were no abnormalities in liver function; surgical removal of the ovarian cyst had no effect on the coagulation abnormalities. In the absence of other underlying causes associated with chronic intravascular coagulation, such as an aortic aneurysm, hemangioma, carcinoma, vasculitis or severe liver disease [1–4], we suspect that the defibrination syndrome in this patient was in some way related to the presence of CML.

Defibrination has been reported to be a common complication of the various *acute* leukemias, and it is especially common in the acute promyelocytic variety [11]. Hypofibrinogenemia appears to be an unusual complication of CML. Normal fibrinogen concentrations were found in all of 26 patients studied with CML [12]. Fibrinogen and platelet survival times were reported to be normal or increased in six patients with CML who also had normal fibrinogen levels and platelet counts [13]. Low fibrinogen concentrations have been recorded in four previously described patients with CML [14–17]. In two, hypofibrinogenemia was clearly associated with blastic transformation [14,15], and in a third it was first noted at a time of busulfan resistance in the sixth year of illness, two weeks before the death of the patient [17]. In the fourth patient, an eight year old child with CML, the disease was still responsive to busulfan therapy, and the patient was reported well after 14 months of follow-up, although no subsequent coagulation data were presented [16]. In none of the reported cases was therapy with heparin attempted; in one of the patients, fibrin degradation products were measured and found to be slightly increased [17].

Our patient survived more than two years after the appearance of the defibrination syndrome, but even at that time evidence of impending blastic transformation [18,19] was present, including increased percentages of myeloblasts and promyelocytes in the peripheral blood and bone marrow, basophilia, worsening anemia, decreased marrow megakaryocyte numbers, and an increase to within the normal range of a previously depressed leukocyte alkaline phosphatase level. Subsequently unequivocal evidence of myeloblastic transformation developed. Intravascular coagulation may therefore have been a harbinger of the accelerated phase of her disease, and may have been related to the increased numbers of promyelocytes in the blood, bone marrow and spleen. Increased procoagulant or "tissue factor" activity has been reported in the promyelocytes of patients with promyelocytic leukemia, and it has been postulated that tissue factor present on the promyelocyte cell membranes or released from these cells is responsible for initiating intravascular coagulation [11].

Subsequent to the development of the coagulation disorder, an enlarging pelvic mass was noted in our patient. Since the underlying cause for the intravascular coagulation was not established, and defibrination has been reported in association with ovarian carcinoma [20], pelvic surgery was deemed to be of both diagnostic and potentially curative value. There are no guidelines in the literature regarding the surgical management of patients with underlying intravascular coagulation. Several cases have been published in which the coagulation disorder was due to disease in the spleen (such as the presence of splenic hemangiomas), and splenectomy in the absence of heparin therapy resulted in cure of the coagulation disorder, followed by an uneventful postoperative course [21–24]. In other patients with inoperable hemangiomas who were not prepared for surgery by heparinization, severe, even fatal, operative or postoperative bleeding occurred, or massive wound hematomas developed [5–10,25,26], as in our patient.

Two patients have been described who received heparin in preparation for surgery [27,28]. In one an above-elbow amputation of an arm bearing a large hemangioma was successfully performed during a continuous intravenous infusion of heparin; administration of the anticoagulant was gradually discontinued postoperatively after the wound had healed [28]. In a patient with metastatic colonic carcinoma associated with defibrination, heparin was given preoperatively, omitted on the day of surgery, and resumed 24 hours later [27]. Fibrinogen levels remained normal until anticoagulation was discontinued on the fifth postoperative day. Hypofibrinogenemia recurred within 24 hours of heparin withdrawal and promptly responded to reinstitution of therapy [27]. In two other patients with multiple hemangiomas that were not resected, heparin treatment was instituted on the fifth [26] and ninth [25] postoperative days in order to control profuse bleeding from the operative site. In our patient, heparin was administered immediately prior to surgery and platelet infusions were given during the operation. A large ovarian cyst was removed without excessive operative hemorrhage. The administration of heparin was discontinued postoperatively, and platelets were withheld to determine whether resection of the ovarian tumor would cure the defibrination. A massive wound hematoma developed and therapy with these measures was resumed, enabling an uneventful second operative procedure and postoperative course.

From our experience and that reported in the literature, we would suggest that patients with intravascular coagulation who require surgical procedures be managed in the following fashion: (1) Heparin therapy should be given preoperatively using a dosage shown in that patient to be adequate to reverse hypofibrinogenemia. (2) Platelet concentrates can be infused immediately before and during the procedure, if heparinization has not resulted in a normal platelet count. (The platelet count is slow to respond to heparin therapy in patients with defibrination [2]. In our patient, decreased platelet production was an additional cause of the thrombocytopenia). (3) On the basis of the limited experience in our patient and that of Merskey and colleagues [27], heparin does not need to be given during the operative procedure, unless hemostasis proves to be unsatisfactory. (4) The administration of heparin should be resumed 24 hours after the operation and continued (for at least one week) until excellent wound healing has occurred. Platelet transfusions should be given for thrombocytopenia noted during this period. (5) Daily monitoring of fibrinogen and platelet levels during the postoperative period is advisable.

Two other features of our patient's course are worthy of comment: the cyclic leukocytosis and prolonged survival. Cyclic oscillations of the white blood cell count have been well documented in certain patients with treated or untreated CML [29–32]. Periodic increases in the numbers of immature cells in the peripheral blood and in the size of the spleen at the time of the peaks of the white blood cell cycles were noted in our patient and have been reported by others [32]. The relationship of these phenomena to elevations in urinary white cell colony stimulating factor levels is presently uncertain [31,32].

Our patient survived for nearly 12 years after her first presentation with marked leukocytosis. After an initial remission following busulfan administration, she did well for more than nine years without any antileukemic therapy. The average survival time in CML is in the order of three to four years [33]; however, approximately 2 per cent of patients live more than 10 years after the onset of symptoms [34], and several well documented cases have been reported in which survival lasted from 16 to 19 years [35]. There is too little information in the literature published to date to determine whether long survival is more likely to occur in those patients with marked cyclic fluctuations in the circulating white blood cell count.

ACKNOWLEDGMENT

We thank Drs. Hymie L. Nossel and Harold S. Ballard for their assistance and advice. Dr. Nossel and Dr. Ian Yudelman performed the fibrinopeptide A assays.

REFERENCES

1. Owen CA Jr, Oels HC, Bowie EJW, Didisheim P, Thompson JH: Chronic intravascular coagulation syndrome. Thromb Diath Haemorrh 36 (suppl): 197, 1969.
2. Minna JD, Robboy JS, Colman RW: Disseminated Intravascular Coagulation in Man, Springfield, Ill., Charles C Thomas, 1974.
3. Bieger R, Vreeken J, Stibbe J, Loeliger EA: Arterial aneurysm as a cause of consumption coagulopathy. N Engl J Med 285: 152, 1971.
4. Verstraete M, Vermylen J, Collen D: Intravascular coagulation in liver disease. Ann Rev Med 25: 447, 1974.
5. Gilon E, Ramot B, Sheba C: Multiple hemangiomata associated with thrombocytopenia: remarks on the pathogenesis of thrombocytopenia in this syndrome. Blood 14: 74, 1959.
6. Dargeon HW, Adiao AC, Pact GT: Hemangioma with thrombocytopenia. J Pediatr 54: 285, 1959.
7. Blix S, Aas K: Giant haemangioma, thrombocytopenia, fibrinogenopenia and fibrinolytic activity. Acta Med Scand 169: 63, 1961.
8. Blix S, Jacobsen CD: The defibrination syndrome in a patient with haemangioendotheliosarcoma. Acta Med Scand 173: 377, 1963.
9. Behar A, Moran E, Izak G: Acquired hypofibrinogenemia associated with a giant cavernous hemangioma of the liver. Am J Clin Pathol 40: 78, 1963.
10. Thompson LR, Umlauf HJ: Hemangioma associated with thrombocytopenia: report of two cases and review of the literature with emphasis on methods of therapy. Milit Med 129: 652, 1964.
11. Gralnick HR, Sultan C: Acute promyelocytic leukaemia: haemorrhagic manifestation and morphologic criteria. Br J Haematol 29: 373, 1975.
12. Didisheim P, Trombold JS, Vandervoort RLE, Mibashan RS: Acute promyelocytic leukemia with fibrinogen and factor V deficiencies. Blood 23: 717, 1974.
13. Brodsky I, Kahn SB, Ross EM, Petkov G: Platelet and fibrinogen kinetics in the chronic myeloproliferative disorders. Cancer 30: 1444, 1972.
14. Ben-Zeev D, Schwartz SO, Friedman IAL: Promyelocytic-myelocytic leukemia as a terminal manifestation of chronic granulocytic leukemia. Report of a case. Blood 27: 863, 1966.
15. Hirsh J, Buchanan JG, de Gruchy GC, Baikie AG: Hypofibrinogenemia without fibrinolysis in leukemia. Lancet 1: 418, 1967.
16. Pochedly C: Unusual manifestations of chronic granulocytic leukemia in a child. Cancer 24: 1017, 1969.
17. Seligman BR, Rosner F, Solomon RB: Chronic myelogenous leukemia. Disseminated intravascular coagulation and chloromas containing sea-blue histiocytes. NY State J Med 65: 1271, 1975.
18. Karanas A, Silver RT: Characteristics of the terminal phase of chronic granulocytic leukemia. Blood 32: 445, 1968.
19. Canellos GP, DeVita VT, Whang-Peng J, Carbone PP: Hematologic and cytogenetic remission of blastic transformation in chronic granulocytic leukemia. Blood 38: 671, 1971.
20. Mosesson MW, Colman RW, Sherry S: Chronic intravascular coagulation syndrome. Report of a case with special studies of an associated plasma cryoprecipitate ("cryofibrinogen"). N Engl J Med 278: 815, 1968.
21. Fisher S: Cryptogenetic congestive severe coagulopathy in splenomegaly. JAMA 205: 101, 1968.
22. Zervos N, Vlachos J, Karpathios T, Mantas J: Giant hemangioma of the spleen with thrombocytopenia and fibrinogen deficiency. Acta Pediatr Scand 172: 206, 1967.
23. Thatcher LG, Clatanoff DV, Stiehm ER: Splenic hemangioma with thrombocytopenia and afibrinogenemia. J Pediatr 73: 345, 1968.
24. Stathakis NE, Papayannis AG, Dervenoulas J, et al.: Multiple coagulation abnormalities in a case of cryptogenic splenomegaly. Br Med J 4: 142, 1974.
25. Kelly, GL: Heparin therapy for bleeding associated with hemangioma. Surgery 65: 894, 1969.

26. (a) Lang PG, Dubin HV: Hemangioma-thrombocytopenia syndrome. A disseminated intravascular coagulopathy. Arch Dermatol 111: 105, 1975.
(b) Hillman, RS, Phillips LL: Clotting-fibrinolysis in a cavernous hemangioma. Am J Dis Child 113: 649, 1967.
27. Merskey C, Johnson AJ, Pert JH, Wohl H: Pathogenesis of fibrinolysis in defibrination syndrome: effect of heparin administration. Blood 24: 701, 1974.
28. Rodriquez-Erdmann F, Murray JE, Moloney WC: Consumption coagulopathy in Kasabach-Merritt syndrome. Trans Assoc Am Physicians 83: 168, 1970.
29. Morley AA, Baikie AG, Galton DAG: Cyclic leukocytosis as evidence for retention of normal homeostatic control in chronic granulocytic leukemia. Lancet 2: 1320, 1967.
30. Kennedy BJ: Cyclic leukocyte oscillations in CML during hydroxyurea therapy. Blood 35: 751, 1970.
31. Vodopick H, Rupp EM, Edwards CL, et al.: Spontaneous cyclic leukocytosis and thrombocytosis in chronic granulocytic leukemia. N Engl J Med 286: 284, 1972.
32. Gatti RA, Robinson WA, Deinard AS, et al.: Cyclic leukocytosis in chronic myelogenous leukemia: new perspectives in pathogenesis and therapy. Blood 41: 771, 1973.
33. Stryckmans PA: Current concepts in chronic myelogenous leukemia. Semin Hematol 11: 101, 1974.
34. Shimkin MB, Mettier SR, Bierman HR: Myelocytic leukemia—an analysis of incidence, distribution, and fatality, 1910–1948. Ann Intern Med 35: 194, 1951.
35. Rak C, Macher T: Chronic granulocytic leukemia with unusually long duration. Folia Hematol N.F. 9: 131, 1964.
36. Ellis BC, Stransky AA: A quick and accurate method for the determination of fibrinogen in plasma. J Lab Clin Med 58: 477, 1961.
37. Hawiger J, Niewiarowski S, Gurewich V, Thomas DP: Measurement of fibrinogen and fibrin degradation products in serum by staphylococcal clumping test. J Lab Clin Med 75: 93, 1970.
38. Nossel HL, Yudelman I, Canfield RE, et al.: Measurement of fibrinopeptide A in human blood. J Clin Invest 54: 43, 1974.

Immunoblastic Lymphadenopathy

Evolution into a Malignant Lymphoma with Plasmacytoid Features

RICHARD I. FISHER, M.D.
ELAINE S. JAFFE, M.D.
RAUL C. BRAYLAN, M.D.
JUDITH C. ANDERSEN, M.D.
HENRY K. TAN, M.D.
Bethesda, Maryland

In the patient described progressive lymphadenopathy, splenomegaly and interstitial pulmonary disease developed two months after the development of immunoblastic lymphadenopathy. Light microscopic examination of a lymph node biopsy specimen suggested a diagnosis of immunoblastic sarcoma. Evolution of this malignant lymphoma into a leukemic phase allowed detailed studies of the malignant cells by electron microscopy, cytochemical staining and immunologic technics. Evidence is presented that this is a case of malignant lymphoma with plasmacytoid and not lymphoid features. Review of the literature on immunoblastic sarcoma suggests that light microscopy and clinical setting are not sufficient to define a homogeneous clinicopathologic disease.

Immunoblastic lymphadenopathy has been defined morphologically by the obliteration of normal lymph node architecture by prominent immunoblasts, arborizing small vessels and amorphous acidophilic interstitial material [1]. However, the histologic characteristics of a malignant process have not been seen in biopsy sections. Clinically, the patients have often presented with marked constitutional symptoms, generalized lymphadenopathy, hepatosplenomegaly and, occasionally, rash. Most patients have had polyclonal hypergammaglobulinemia and some have Coombs' positive hemolytic anemia. Although the disorder has been regarded as a benign process microscopically, the median survival of the patients in Lukes' 18 fatal cases was only 15 months. Three patients later died from a malignant lymphoma, termed immunoblastic sarcoma.

Dameshek [2] originally used the term immunoblast to describe a lymphocyte that had been transformed by a mitogen in vitro into a hyperbasophilic, pyrinophilic blast cell. Lukes and Collins [3] subsequently described immunoblastic sarcoma as a malignant lymphoma composed of cells microscopically similar to immunoblasts. The development of this pathologic entity has been reported in patients with connective tissue disorders and presumed chronic immune stimulation, as well as in patients with immunoblastic lymphadenopathy [1]. Mathe et al. [4] recently described an immunoblastic variant of acute lymphocytic leukemia.

Thus, immunoblastic sarcoma has been reported in many diverse clinical settings. Since light microscopy may not be capable of defining a homogeneous clinicopathologic entity, we have studied (by electron microscopy, cytochemical staining and immunologic technics) the neoplastic cells from a patient in whom a malignant lymphoma de-

From the Medicine Branch and Laboratory of Pathology, National Cancer Institute, and the Hematology Service, Clinical Pathology Department, Clinical Center, National Institutes of Health, Bethesda, Maryland 20014. Requests for reprints should be addressed to Dr. Richard I. Fisher, Medicine Branch, Bldg. 10, Rm. 12N226, National Institutes of Health, Bethesda, Maryland 20014.
Manuscript accepted January 9, 1976.

veloped after immunoblastic lymphadenopathy. Evidence is presented that this is a case of malignant lymphoma with plasmacytoid and not lymphoid features.

CASE REPORT

A 28 year old white man was admitted to the NIH on August 21, 1974, for evaluation of fever and lymphadenopathy of three weeks' duration. Previously in excellent health, he was not taking any medication, had no allergies and had no family history of malignant disease. Right inguinal lymphadenopathy and a temperature of 39.5°C had developed three weeks prior to his admission. His fever had abated temporarily with oral tetracycline therapy, but adenopathy persisted and then became more prominent. Low grade fever recurred one week before his admission. Physical examination on admission was entirely within normal limits except for a temperature of 39.2°C and marked tender femoral and inguinal adenopathy. Laboratory studies on admission including a complete blood count, routine chemistry studies, chest and abdominal films, cultures of blood, urine and stool were within normal limits. Direct and indirect Coombs' tests were negative. Serum protein electrophoresis and immunoelectrophoresis disclosed no abnormalities. Concentrated urine did not contain Bence Jones protein.

Pain developed in the lower right quadrant soon after his admission, associated with guarding, rebound tenderness and a positive psoas sign. Exploratory laparotomy revealed striking adenopathy of para-aortic and iliac nodes; the liver and spleen were of normal size. Microscopic examination revealed a reactive process histologically consistent with immunoblastic lymphadenopathy. Liver-spleen scan, liver biopsy and gallium scan were all within normal limits. Bone marrow aspirate and biopsy specimens revealed a hypercellular marrow with mild lymphocytosis and eosinophilia, and a moderate degree of erythro- and thrombophagocytosis. Repeat culture of urine, sputum, blood and bone marrow grew no organisms. Bacterial and fungal agglutinins were negative; an elevated anti-Toxoplasma gondii titer was noted but had been similarly elevated one year prior to admission. The patient's fever was unresponsive to an empiric trial of combination antibiotic therapy.

One month after admission, the patient became acutely dyspneic, hypoxic and tachycardic. Chest film revealed perihilar interstitial infiltrates. Splenomegaly was noted for the first time. Bilateral inguinal adenopathy had become more prominent and a left inguinal lymph node biopsy was performed. The specimen was interpreted as showing "malignant lymphoma with plasmacytoid features." Therapy with cyclophosphamide, vincristine and prednisone was initiated [5]. A dramatic decrease in respiratory distress was noted within 12 hours. Over the ensuing two days, the patient's temperature returned to normal, his pulmonary infiltrate resolved, and adenopathy and splenomegaly regressed. His course was complicated only by drug-induced leukopenia. He was discharged to the outpatient clinic. Treatment with cyclophosphamide, vincristine, procarbazine and prednisone was empirically chosen to attempt to consolidate his clinical remission [5].

The patient remained well for the next three weeks until November 7, 1974, when he experienced fever, myalgias and diarrhea. Physical examination revealed him to be weak and apprehensive with a temperature of 39.7°C, pulse rate of 124 beats/min and respirations of 40/min. The chest was clear, the liver was of normal size, and the spleen was minimally enlarged and tender. There was fullness in the left supraclavicular area, but groin adenopathy was much diminished.

The hemoglobin level was 12.0 g/100 ml, the platelet count 37,000/mm^3 and the white blood cell count 17,000/mm^3 with an abnormal leukocyte differential. Peripheral blood smears revealed 15 to 20 per cent abnormal leukocytes; a few were plasmacytic cells of intermediate maturity, but most were poorly differentiated blast forms. Bone marrow aspirate and biopsy confirmed the presence of abnormal immature plasmacytic cells. Because of the appearance of a leukemic picture, therapy was re-instituted with cytoxan, vincristine, cytosine arabinoside and prednisone with a decrease in the number of circulating abnormal cells [6]. The patient was transferred to a hospital near his home on November 17. Adenopathy, splenomegaly and bone marrow involvement with a leukemic peripheral blood picture proved resistant to the administration of imidazole carboxamide, bleomycin and splenic irradiation in sequence. His condition continued to deteriorate with progressive leukopenia and thrombocytopenia unresponsive to supportive therapy. On December 4, an acute right hemiplegia developed and he died shortly thereafter. Postmortem examination revealed malignant lymphoma, plasmacytic type, involving lymph nodes, spleen, liver, bone marrow, heart, lungs, esophagus, kidneys and dura mater; nonbacterial thrombotic mitral valvulitis with left parietal, frontal and occipital lobe embolism; focal and confluent hemorrhage in skin and myocardium.

MATERIALS AND METHODS

Light and Electron Microscopic Studies. Para-aortic lymph node biopsy specimens were obtained during exploratory laparotomy. Superficial inguinal lymph node biopsies were performed under local anesthesia. Lymph node material and bone marrow biopsy material (after decalcification) were processed routinely by formalin fixation, paraffin embedding and hematoxylin and eosin staining. Methyl green pyronin, Masson trichrome (for collagen) and periodic acid-Schiff stains were obtained on lymph node material. Bone marrow aspirate material was processed for smear morphology, by using a modified Romanovsky stain on an Ames automatic stainer, and for aspirate clot section morphology, by routine methods already described. Material for electron microscopy was fixed in sucrose-buffered 3 per cent glutaraldehyde at 4°C for 1 1/2 hours, washed overnight in buffer solution and post-fixed for 1 hour in 2 per cent osmium tetroxide. The specimens were dehydrated in increasing concentrations of ethanol and infiltrated with 50 per cent Epon® and 50 per cent propylene oxide. Subsequently, the specimen was embedded in Epon and cut to silver-gold thickness sections on an LBK Ultratome.

Surface Markers. Cells were obtained for study from peripheral blood. Heparinized peripheral blood was purified through a Ficoll-Hypaque gradient, and the mononuclear cell-rich fraction was obtained [7]. The cells were washed

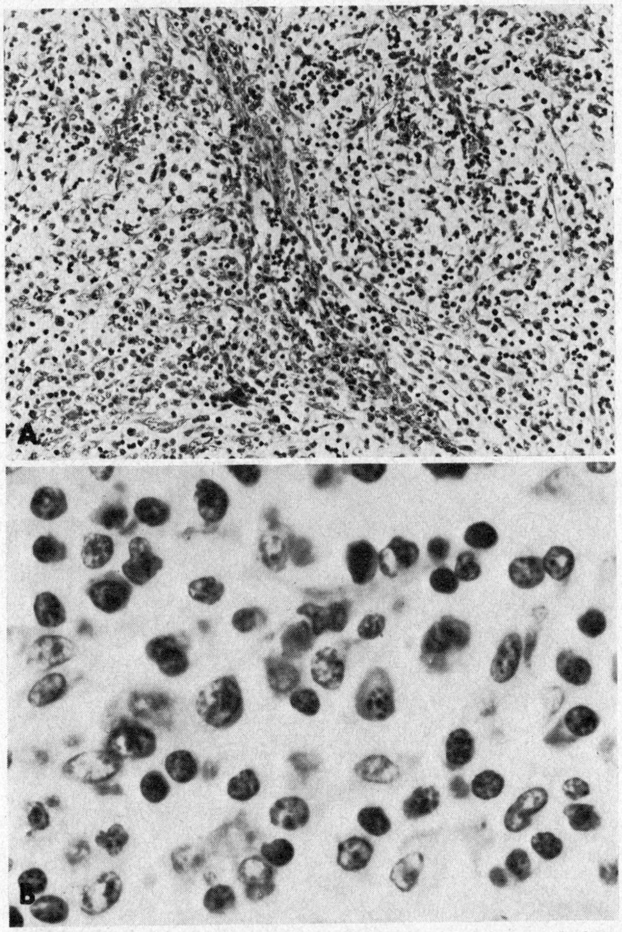

Figure 1. *Para-aortic lymph node biopsy specimen.* ***A,*** *low power view showing obliteration of normal architecture with arborizing vessels, interstitial edema and a diffuse cellular infiltrate. Hematoxylin and eosin stain; original magnification × 160, reduced by 28 per cent.* ***B,*** *high power view showing a polymorphous infiltrate. Lymphocytes, plasma cells and immunoblasts are seen. Hematoxylin and eosin stain; original magnification × 1,000, reduced by 28 per cent.*

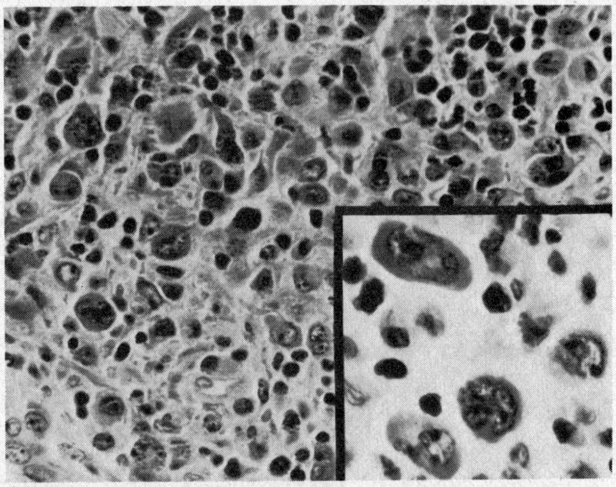

Figure 2. *Inguinal lymph node biopsy specimen showing histologic features of malignant lymphoma. Numerous pleomorphic plasmacytoid cells are present. Hematoxylin and eosin stain; original magnification × 400, reduced by 30 per cent. Insert shows large bizarre cells in greater detail. Hematoxylin and eosin stain; original magnification × 800, reduced by 30 per cent.*

three times in RPMI-1640 (Grand Island Biological Co., Grand Island, N.Y.) and brought to the appropriate concentration for subsequent studies.

The rosette assays for cells bearing complement receptors (EAC) or receptors for cytophilic antibody (IgGEA) were performed as previously described with slight modification [8]. Normal mouse serum was used as the source of complement (C). Equal volumes of the white cell suspensions (2.5 × 10^6/ml) and the IgGEA, EAC or IgMEA suspensions (1 × 10^8/ml) were mixed in plastic tubes, centrifuged at 200 g at room temperature for 10 minutes and then incubated at 37°C for 30 minutes. The pellet was resuspended, the aliquot was mixed with trypan blue, and the percentage of rosetted cells was determined. Only viable cells were counted. Conditions producing E rosette formation, i.e., 37°C to 4°C, were never used, and IgMEA rosette formation was never observed.

Determination of E rosette-forming cells, a T cell characteristic, was made as previously described [9]. Equal volumes of white cells (2.5 × 10^6/ml and sheep red blood cells (E) (1 × 10^8/ml) previously treated with neuraminidase were mixed and incubated under appropriate conditions.

For cytologic identification of rosetted cells, Shandon cytocentrifuge (Shandon Scientific Co., Inc., Sewickley, Pa.) preparations were stained with Wright's stain. For identification of monocytes, the cytocentrifuge preparations were stained for nonspecific esterase using alpha-naphthyl butyrate as substrate [10].

Immunofluorescent staining was performed as follows: One million white cells in 0.05 ml of medium were incubated in ice with 0.05 ml of a fluoresceinated polyvalent goat antiserum against human gamma, alpha, mu, kappa and lambda chains. After three washings the cells were resuspended in phosphate-buffered glycerine and examined with an American Optical microscope equipped with a vertical illuminator and phase contrast. At least 200 cells were counted. For the detection of cytoplasmic immunoglobulins, washed cells in suspension were centrifuged onto glass slides by cytocentrifugation and incubated in a moist chamber with fluorescein-conjugated antiserums against human immunoglobulins. Monospecific antiserums against human gamma, alpha, mu, delta, kappa and lambda chains were used separately. After 30 minutes at room temperature, the slides were thoroughly washed in phosphate buffer saline solution, mounted in glycerine and examined by fluorescent light. All antiserums were obtained from Meloy Laboratories, Springfield, Va. The activity and specificity of these antiserums were tested by immunoelectrophoresis and double diffusion, using the appropriate purified human antigens.

RESULTS

Lymph Nodes. Sections of para-aortic lymph nodes revealed marked young fibroblastic proliferation and some stromal edema. A polymorphous infiltrate was

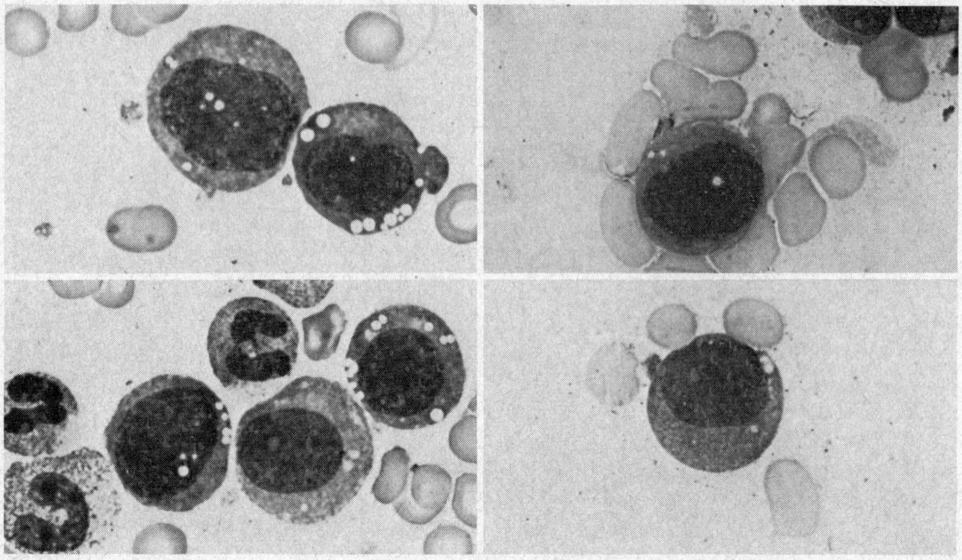

*Figure 3. **Upper left,** abnormal cells in peripheral smear demonstrating blastic appearance, cytoplasmic and nuclear vacuoles and finely dispersed nuclear chromatin. **Upper right,** abnormal cell in bone marrow smear. Note similarity to cells in periphery. **Lower left,** abnormal cells in peripheral smear. Note lack of any similarity with mature plasma cells. **Lower right,** abnormal cell in bone marrow. Note lack of perinuclear Golgi zone in this cell, finely stippled cytoplasm and nuclear and cytoplasmic vacuoles. Original magnification × 950, reduced by 19 per cent.*

present throughout the node and was composed of lymphocytes, occasional immunoblasts, numerous plasma cells and occasional eosinophils. Frequent capillary buds were seen and some vessels were surrounded by eosinophilic material. Although numerous binucleate plasma cells were present, no atypical plasma cells were observed (Figure 1).

Inguinal lymph nodes biopsied one month later demonstrated extensive infiltration with pleomorphic plasmacytoid cells (Figure 2). Marked variations in size and shape were evident in different areas of the same node. Sheets of mature plasma cells were noted focally. Very large anaplastic cells 30 to 40 μ in diameter were frequently seen. Fibroblastic proliferation and endothelial hyperplasia were conspicuous features, but amorphous acidophilic interstitial material was not present. Methyl green pyronin stains demonstrated intense pyrinophilia not only in mature plasma cells but also in the more anaplastic cytologic types.

Bone Marrow and Peripheral Smear. Initial bone marrow examination did not disclose lymphomatous involvement. Subsequent examination six weeks later showed increasing numbers of large blast-like cells with a moderately high nuclear-cytoplasmic ratio, basophilic cytoplasm, nuclear and cytoplasmic vacuoles, and moderately dispersed nuclear chromatin without clumping. Peroxidase, periodic acid-Schiff and oil red O stains were negative. Following relapse from the first cycle of chemotherapy, peripheral blood buffy coat concentrates contained 15 to 20 per cent abnormal cells with features similar to the abnormal marrow blast-like cells (Figure 3). Mature plasma cells were not seen. Occasional cells in the buffy coat smear were suggestive of plasmacytic cells possessing a slightly eccentric nucleus with prominent perinuclear clear zone. Nucleoli were not prominent in Romanovsky-stained material from bone marrow and peripheral smear.

Electron microscopy of the abnormal bone marrow cells showed prominent cytoplasmic rough endoplasmic reticulum that was irregularly lined with ribosomal particles and could be traced over long distances in the cytoplasm. A true Golgi apparatus was not evident in most cells. Occasional spherical vacuoles filled with granular electron-dense material were present. The nuclei of all abnormal cells contained two or more prominent well-developed nucleoli, with smaller electron-dense clusters of chromatin clustered circumferentially along the inner nuclear membrane. Mitochondria were remarkably infrequent (Figure 4).

Cell Surface Membrane Markers. Twelve per cent of the mononuclear cells isolated from the patient's peripheral blood formed rosettes with EAC. These cells were all identified as monocytes on the cytocentrifuge preparations, both by morphology and the presence of nonspecific esterase. Twenty-two per cent of the cells formed rosettes with IgGEA, and again, all were monocytes. Ten per cent of the cells bore surface immu-

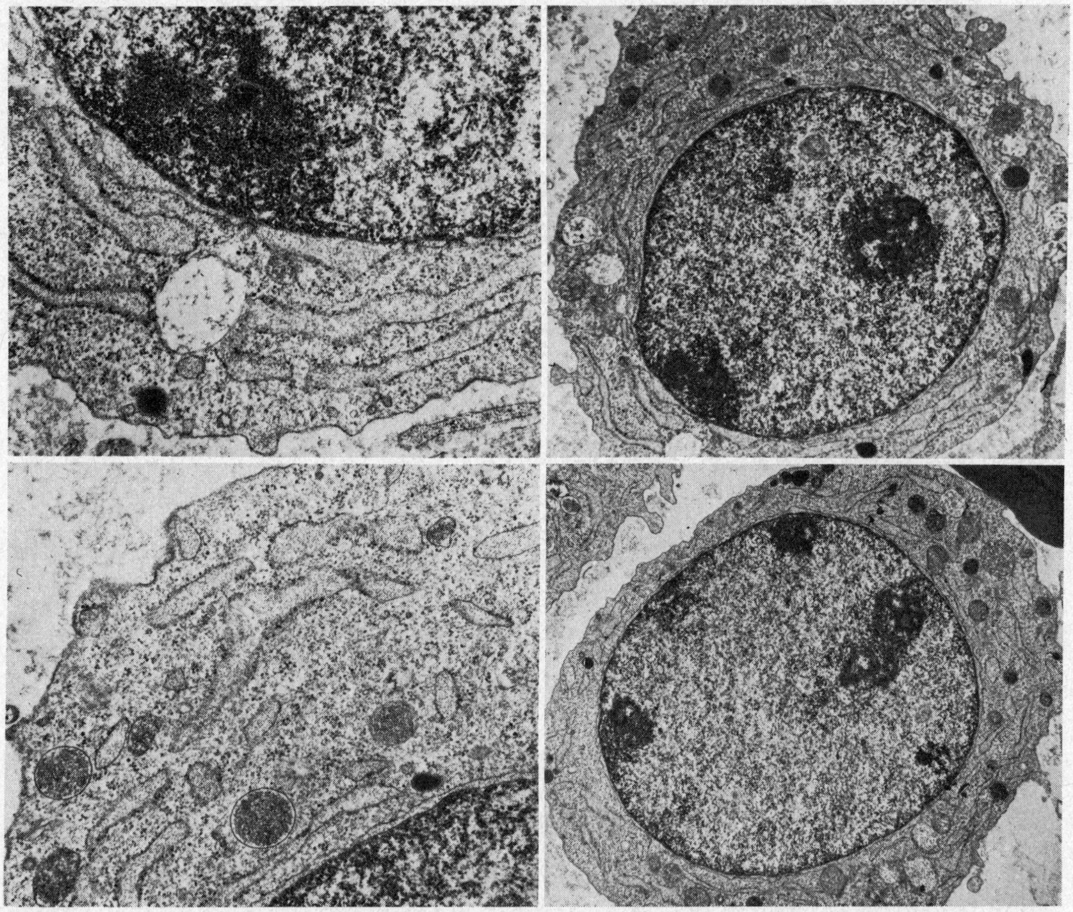

Figure 4. ***Left,*** *electron micrographic views of abnormal cells in bone marrow demonstrating well developed nucleoli, high nuclear:cytoplasmic ratio, partially dilated endoplasmic reticulum, multiple cytoplasmic vesicles and lack of evidence for a developed Golgi apparatus. Original magnification × 8,000, reduced by 15 per cent.* ***Right,*** *detailed view of cytoplasm of abnormal cells in bone marrow showing clear vesicle (probable counterpart of light microscopic cytoplasmic vacuoles), fairly abundant endoplasmic reticulum-lined by ribosomal particles and spherical single membrane-lined vesicles filled with amorphous granular material.*

noglobulin, but all appeared to be monocytes when examined by phase contrast illumination. Thirteen per cent of the cells formed E rosettes, and all were cytologically small lymphocytes. These results indicate no B lymphocytes could be identified with certainty among the peripheral blood mononuclear cells. No surface markers could be demonstrated on the neoplastic cells which, at times, represented as much as 70 per cent of the mononuclear cells in peripheral blood.

Previous studies in our laboratory and elsewhere have demonstrated that EAC is bound to both B lymphocytes [11] and monocytes [12]. IgGEA is bound preferentially to monocytes [13], but under certain conditions, as used in this study (i.e., incubation after centrifugation), it is bound to some lymphocytes, mainly B lymphocytes [14]. Easily detectable surface immunoglobulin is a B cell characteristic [15], although monocytes may bear nonspecifically bound surface immunoglobulins via Fc receptors. T cells are characterized by E rosette formation [9]. Mature plasma cells lack complement receptors [11] and Fc receptors [16,17], and may lack surface immunoglobulin [18].

Cytoplasmic Immunoglobulins. No cytoplasmic staining was demonstrated by the use of specific fluorescein-conjugated antihuman immunoglobulins on the cytocentrifuged preparations of washed cells.

COMMENTS

Immunoblastic lymphadenopathy is a recently described clinicopathologic syndrome. Lukes and Tindle [1] described 32 patients with constitutional symptoms, generalized lymphadenopathy, hepatosplenomegaly and, occasionally, rash. Microscopically, the lymph nodes were replaced by prominent immunoblasts, arborizing small vessels and amorphous acidophilic interstitial material. The process was considered a nonneoplastic hyperimmune proliferation of B cells. However, the median survival of the patients in 18 fatal cases was only 15 months. In three patients a malignant lymphoma, termed immunoblastic sarcoma, developed. Frizzera et al. [19] described 15 patients with a very similar clinical and pathologic syndrome [19]. They named the syndrome "angio-immunoblastic lymphadenopathy with dysproteinemia." In none of their patients did a malignant lymphoma develop [20].

Immunoblastic sarcoma has been defined as a pathologic entity based on the light microscopic resemblance of the malignant cell to a transformed lymphocyte or immunoblast [3]. The cells are large (20 to 30 μ) with oval nuclei, finely distributed chromatin, prominent nucleoli and a moderate amount of deeply staining cytoplasm. Few cases have been described, yet the clinical syndrome has varied greatly. Lukes and Collins observed the development of immunoblastic sarcoma in patients with systemic lupus erythematosus, rheumatoid arthritis, Sjögren's syndrome, alpha chain disease and during immunosuppression for graft rejection. They regarded the disorder as a disease of B cells on the basis of "the type of abnormal immune disorder, the frequency of plasmacytoid features and the evidence usually of monoclonal gammapathy." The development of three cases was reported following immunoblastic lymphadenopathy [1]. The change from immunoblastic lymphadenopathy to immunoblastic sarcoma was apparently heralded by a rapid deterioration of the patients' clinical status and a more malignant appearing nodal histopathology.

Mathe et al. [4] described eight patients with what they termed "immunoblastic acute lymphoid leukemia." Several patients presented with a leukemic picture whereas in others the condition began as a lymphoma and quickly evolved into a leukemic phase. Circulating abnormal cells were described as large blast forms with basophilic cytoplasm resembling immunoblasts. Hypogammaglobulinemia was common. Responses to chemotherapy occurred but were of short duration. Electron microscopy of "immunoblasts" demonstrated abundant polyribosomes and large cytoplasmic vacuoles without evident endoplasmic reticulum. The cells carried "T" or "B" or, in one case, no surface membrane immunologic markers.

In our case the patient presented with fever and lymphadenopathy. A para-aortic lymph node biopsy specimen showed a reactive process histologically consistent with immunoblastic lymphadenopathy. Progressive lymphadenopathy, splenomegaly and interstitial pulmonary disease led to a second lymph node biopsy one month later. At that time the lymph node histopathologically was definitely malignant with obliteration of normal nodal architecture by pleomorphic cells with plasmacytic features. Very large anaplastic cells 30 to 40 μ in diameter were seen. There was considerable debate among pathologists whether this biopsy specimen represented immunoblastic sarcoma (a disorder of transformed lymphocytes) since Lukes [1] had extended the pathologic features to occasionally include prominent abnormal plasma cells. The pathologic findings also suggested a plasmacytic reticulum cell sarcoma but such cases have been associated with classic multiple myeloma [21]. The patient was initially responsive to combination cytotoxic chemotherapy but the tumor rapidly recurred between cycles of chemotherapy and evolved a leukemic phase allowing detailed study of the malignant cells by cytochemical staining, electron microscopy and immunologic technics. Light microscopy revealed immature blast-like cells with eccentric nuclei, a high nuclear: cytoplasmic ratio, a prominent perinuclear clear zone and basophilic cytoplasm. Electron microscopy of the blast-like cells showed prominent rough endoplasmic reticulum irregularly lined with ribosomal particles. This is in marked contrast to electron micrographs of the immunoblasts of Mathe et al. in which a relatively low nuclear:cytoplasmic ratio, prominent cytoplasmic vacuoles and a paucity of endoplasmic reticulum were evident. This is consistent with a plasmacytic origin for the blast forms in our case in contrast to a lymphoid origin in Mathe's cases. In this case, cell surface markers of the neoplastic cells including surface immunoglobulin, Fc receptors, complement receptors and E rosettes were all absent. These membrane markers were compatible with a plasma cell origin of the tumor [11,16–18], but the absence of cytoplasmic immunoglobulin was unexpected. However, plasma cells lacking cytoplasmic immunoglobulin have been reported in nonsecretory multiple myeloma [22] in which it has been postulated that immunoglobulin was not produced, could not be detected by available technics or was rapidly metabolized.

The preceding reports suggest that the term immunoblastic sarcoma has not been applied to a homogeneous clinicopathologic entity. In previous cases, the characteristic cell appeared similar to a transformed lymphocyte thereby leading to the diagnosis of immunoblastic sarcoma. However, some cases in which the patients had marked plasmacytoid features have been included in the same syndrome. The associated disorders have varied from connective tissue disorders to immunoblastic lymphadenopathy to acute lymphocytic leukemia. In all patients the course was rapidly progressive, with death occurring in several months. Finally, the malignant cell has been reported to have "B" or "T" or no surface membrane markers. In our patient with immunoblastic lymphadenopathy a malignant lymphoma developed with plasmacytoid and not lymphoid features.

In conclusion, we suggest that the light microscopic appearance of immunoblasts and clinical setting are not sufficient to define a precise clinicopathologic disease. Future cases should be studied by immunologic and electron microscopic means in an attempt to further define this entity.

REFERENCES

1. Lukes RJ, Tindle BH: Immunoblastic lymphadenopathy. N Engl J Med 292: 1, 1975.
2. Dameshek W: Immunoblasts and immunocytes, an attempt at a functional nomenclature. Blood 21: 243, 1963.
3. Lukes RJ, Collins RD: Immunologic characterization of human malignant lymphomas. Cancer 34: 1488, 1974.
4. Mathe G, Belpomme D, Dantchev D, et al.: Immunoblastic acute lymphoid leukemia. Biomedicine 20: 333, 1974.
5. Schein PS, Chabner BA, Canellos GP, et al.: Potential for prolonged disease free survival following combination chemotherapy of non-Hodgkin's lymphoma. Blood 43: 181, 1974.
6. Whitecar JP, Bodey GP, Freireich EJ, et al.: Cyclophosphamide, vincristine, cytosine arabinoside, and prednisone (COAP) combination chemotherapy for acute leukemia in adults. Cancer Chemother Rep 56: 543, 1972.
7. Boyum A: Separation of leukocytes from blood and bone marrow: with special reference to factors which influence and modify sedimentation properties of hematopoietic cells. Scand J Clin Lab Invest 21 (suppl 97): 1, 1968.
8. Jaffe ES, Shevach EM, Frank MM: Nodular lymphoma—evidence for origin from follicular B lymphocytes. N Engl J Med 290: 813, 1974.
9. Jondal M, Holm G, Wigzell H: Surface markers on human T and B lymphocytes. I. A large population of lymphocytes forming nonimmune rosettes with sheep red blood cells. J Exp Med 136: 207, 1972.
10. Li CY, Yam LT, Crosby WH: Histochemical characterization of cellular and structural elements of human spleen. J Histochem Cytochem 20: 1049, 1972.
11. Bianco CR, Patrick R, Nussenzweig V: A population of lymphocytes bearing a membrane receptor for antigen-antibody complement complexes. I. Separation and characterization. J Exp Med 132: 702, 1970.
12. Huber H, Polley JM, Linscott WD, et al.: Human monocytes: distinct receptor sites for the third component of complement and for immunoglobulin G. Science 162: 1281, 1968.
13. Huber H, Douglas SD, Fudenberg HH: The IgG receptor: an immunological marker for the characterization of mononuclear cells. Immunology 17: 7, 1969.
14. Kedar E, Ortiz de Landazure M, Fahey J: Comparative studies of immunoglobulin receptors and antibody-dependent cell cytotoxicity (ADCC) in rat lymphoid organs. J Immunol 112: 37, 1974.
15. Raff MC: Two distinct populations of peripheral lymphocytes in mice distinguishable by immunofluorescence. Immunology 19: 637, 1970.
16. Ramasamy R, Munro A, Milstein C: Possible role for the Fc receptor on B lymphocytes. Nature (Lond) 249: 573, 1974.
17. Brown G, Greaves MF, Lister TA, et al.: Expression of human T and B lymphocyte cell-surface markers on leukaemic cells. Lancet 2: 753, 1974.
18. Fu SM, Winchester RJ, Feizi T, et al.: Idiotypic specificity of surface immunoglobulin and the maturation of leukemic bone marrow derived lymphocytes. Proc Natl Acad Sci USA 71: 4487, 1974.
19. Frizzera G, Morna EM, Rappaport H: Angio-immunoblastic lymphadenopathy with dysproteinemia. Lancet 1: 1070, 1974.
20. Rappaport H, Moran EM: Angio-immunoblastic (immunoblastic) lymphadenopathy. N Engl J Med 292: 42, 1975.
21. Okano H, Azar HA, Osserman EF: Plasmacytic reticulum cell sarcoma. Am J Clin Pathol 46: 546, 1966.
22. River GL, Tewksbury DA, Fudenberg HH: "Nonsecretory" multiple myeloma. Blood 40: 204, 1972.

INFORMATION FOR AUTHORS

PREPARATION OF MANUSCRIPTS

Manuscripts should be typed on one side of the sheet, doublespaced, on white bond paper, 8½ by 11 inches, with margins of 1 inch. Two copies of the manuscript and illustrations should be sent to the Editor at 666 Fifth Avenue, New York, New York 10019. Title page should include full name, degrees and affiliation of all authors, the source from which the article emanates, and the name and address of the person to whom requests for reprints should be addressed.

All manuscript pages including tables and legends should be numbered consecutively in the upper right hand corner.

The number of manuscript pages, the number of illustrations and the number of tables should be indicated at the bottom of the covering letter.

Every article must be preceded by an abstract (not to exceed 350 words). This obviates the need for a summary. In addition, for the convenience of our readers, we require a brief abstract (not exceeding 100 to 125 words) and key words for indexing purposes. These brief abstracts appear in the back of the *Journal* in the same issue in which the paper appears.

Since all manuscripts submitted for publication in the *Journal* are sent out for review before a final decision is made, there is generally a lapse of three to six weeks before contributors are notified. If you have received an acknowledgment of receipt, there is no need to call the *Journal* office; your manuscript has not gone astray. The decision will be forthcoming shortly.

PREPARATION OF ILLUSTRATIONS AND TABLES

Illustrations must be black and white glossy prints or professional drawings in india ink; they should be unmounted. The name of the lead author and the title of the article should be typed on a label and affixed to the back of each illustration; the top should be indicated.

Reference to all illustrations should be inserted in the text in consecutive order. Legends for the illustrations should be typed, double spaced, on a separate sheet with numbers corresponding to those on the photographs or drawings. They should not be attached to the pictures.

Tables should be typed on separate sheets and should be set up in accordance with the style of the Journal. Units of measure should be confined to column headings. Abbreviations should be kept to a minimum and should conform with those used by the *Journal* or listed as acceptable in the Council of Biology Editors Style Manual. Any variations should be explained. All vertical rules should be omitted.

The publisher allows a fixed amount towards the reproduction of illustrations and tables. Charges in excess of this amount must be assumed by the authors. The Editor reserves the right to limit the number of illustrations and/or tables.

PREPARATION OF BIBLIOGRAPHY

Bibliographic references should be listed chronologically on a separate sheet (not in footnotes) as referred to in the text and should be typed (double-spaced) in accordance with the style and abbreviations (open punctuation) used by Index Medicus; only the first page of the journal citation is necessary. Examples follow:

For periodical references:

22. Theologides A, Kennedy BJ: Toxoplasmic myocarditis and pericarditis. Am J Med 47: 169, 1969.

For book references (with chapter):

18. Schiebler GL, Van Mieron LHS, Krovetz LJ: Diseases of the tricuspid valve, chap 2. Heart Disease in Infants, Children and Adolescents (Moss AJ, Adams F, eds), Baltimore, Williams & Wilkins, 1968.

For book references (without chapter):

13. Berne E: Principles of Group Treatment, New York, Oxford University Press, 1966, p 26.

Authors are responsible for the accuracy of all references.

REPRINTS

Price schedules and order cards for reprints are mailed to the person so listed in the footnote on the title page.

The American Journal of Medicine, 666 Fifth Avenue, New York, New York 10019

Abstracts of papers in this issue

Osteoporosis **Phosphorus and calcium infusions**
Parathyroid hormone secretion **Bone pain**

Popovtzer MM, Stjernholm M, Huffer WE: Effects of alternating phosphorus and calcium infusions on osteoporosis. Am J Med 61: 478–484, 1976.

The osteoblastic effect of inorganic phosphorus and the inhibitory action of calcium on parathyroid hormone secretion formed the basis for a therapeutic trial in which both elements were given intravenously in an alternating sequence for one year to five patients with severe osteoporosis. During treatment, calcium and phosphorus balances were positive, and serum phosphorus concentrations decreased. Iliac crest bone biopsy specimens obtained one year after treatment demonstrated an increase in the thickness of cortical bone. All patients experienced lasting relief of bone pain, and the rate of spontaneous fractures decreased from at least one fracture per year to none. Long-term treatment with alternating phosphorus and calcium infusions may result in lasting relief of symptomatic osteoporosis.

Steroid myopathy **Connective tissue disease** **Urinary creatine**
Prednisone therapy **Myalgias** **Sudden weakness**

Askari A, Vignos PJ Jr, Moskowitz RW: Steroid myopathy in connective tissue disease. Am J Med 61: 485–492, 1976.

In eight women with polymyositis, weakness developed during high dose prednisone therapy. These women were studied using serial functional and manual muscle tests, serum glutamic oxaloacetic transaminase, creatinine phosphokinase and serum aldolase determinations and urinary creatine excretion. Insidious onset of weakness was characteristic. Weakness was most severe in the pelvic girdle muscles with lesser involvement of shoulder girdle and distal muscles. Serum muscle enzyme levels were normal in all cases but urinary creatine excretion was invariably increased and proved to be the most sensitive laboratory indicator for clinical diagnosis and monitoring of patient improvement. Serial urinary creatine excretion and serum enzyme studies proved of value in differentiating steroid myopathy from myositis in patients with connective tissue disease. Diagnosis and effective management were achieved by the use of readily available laboratory and clinical procedures without resorting to muscle biopsy.

Gram-negative rod bacteremia **Urinary tract** **Esch. coli sepsis**
Biliary tree **Gentamicin** **Cephalosporin**

Anderson ET, Young LS, Hewitt WL: Simultaneous antibiotic levels in "breakthrough" gram-negative rod bacteremia. Am J Med 61: 493–497, 1976.

Of 237 cases of gram-negative rod bacteremia observed during a 12 month period, 52 (22 per cent) occurred while the patient was receiving antibiotics which inhibited the infecting organism by disc diffusion tests. Sepsis documented within 72 hours of therapy was usually due to antibiotic sensitive Esch. coli, was associated with inadequate antibiotic levels, and was usually treated with a penicillin or cephalosporin. Source of bacteremia was most frequently the urinary tract or biliary tree. In contrast, sepsis occurring more than 72 hours after therapy was frequently caused by multiple antibiotic-resistant Esch. coli, treated with gentamicin in adequate dosage, and was associated with leukopenia or undrained purulent collections. Therapy ultimately failed in 20 cases and was associated with subinhibitory antibiotic levels (early "breakthrough") or with inadequate drainage or impaired host defenses (late "breakthrough").

Group B streptococci infections **Bacteremic pyelonephritis**
Pneumonitis **Endometritis** **Genitourinary disorders**

Bayer AS, Chow AW, Anthony BF, Guze LB: Serious infections in adults due to group B streptococci. Clinical and serotypic characterization. Am J Med 61: 498–503, 1976.

Serious infections in adults due to group B streptococci have been infrequently reported. We describe 24 such patients. Bacteremic pyelonephritis, pneumonitis and endometritis were the most common clinical syndromes observed. Group B streptococcal infections tended to occur in patients with underlying illnesses, particularly genitourinary disorders and diabetes mellitus. Mortality was surprisingly low (8 per cent). Type III was the serotype most commonly isolated. Group B streptococcal isolates from these patients were uniformly sensitive to penicillin, ampicillin, cephalothin, chloramphenicol, erythromycin and clindamycin, and highly resistant to kanamycin. Eighty-seven per cent were resistant to tetracycline. Minimal inhibitory concentrations were significantly higher for group B than group A streptococci ($p < 0.0005$).

C1q Deficiency Associated with Urticarial-Like Lesions and Cutaneous Vasculitis

R. J. MARDER, B.S.*
ROSEMARIE RENT, M.S.
E. Y. C. CHOI, M.D.
H. GEWURZ, M.D.†
Chicago, Illinois

We describe a 46 year old woman with a seven year history of urticarial-like symptoms and cutaneous vasculitis with marked deficiency of C1q in the presence of normal levels of C1r and C1s and high titers of low molecular weight (7S) C1q precipitins. Hemolytic C1 activity, which was greatly reduced, was restored upon the addition of purified C1q. The other complement components were present in moderately reduced or normal levels. This patient bears resemblance to several other persons previously described with urticarial-like lesions in association with selective deficiency of C1q. The similarity of the clinical features, pathologic diagnosis, C1q levels disproportionately deficient in relation to other complement components and low molecular weight C1q precipitins support the conclusion that these are causally related in a symptom complex. The underlying basis is yet to be defined.

We recently observed a patient who presented with episodic urticarial-like lesions, angioedema, markedly reduced serum concentrations of the complement component C1q and low molecular weight C1q precipitins. As such, she was similar to patients previously described by Agnello et al. [1,2] with erythema multiforma and a lupus-like syndrome with depressed C1q, a group of patients described by McDuffie et al. [3] who had urticarial-like lesions associated with depletion of C1q and two persons described by Sissons et al. [4] with cutaneous lesions, angioedema, renal disease (one patient) and hypocomplementemia. The other proteins with which C1q is found in the functional C1 macromolecule were present in normal amounts. We describe this patient to further call attention to the association of urticarial-like symptoms and cutaneous vasculitis with deficiency of C1q.

MATERIALS AND METHODS

Blood samples, including aliquots drawn into citrate as an anticoagulant, were collected and centrifuged at 37°C; serum and plasma samples were stored at −70°C and thawed at 37°C immediately before use. Hemolytic complement (C) and C component activities and C protein concentrations were measured by standard procedures as previously described [5,6]. C1q also was measured by agglutination of gamma globulin-coated latex particles by the method of Ewald and Schubart [7] as previously described [8]. C1-esterase inhibitor ($\bar{C1}$-INH) activity was measured according to Donaldson [9]. C1q was purified according to the method of Yonemasu and Stroud [10]. Serums initially were tested for complexes which precipitated with C1q and monoclonal rheumatoid factor by Dr. Robert J. Winchester [1,11]; assays for C1q precipitins were also subsequently performed in these laboratories. Cryoprecipitates were obtained from plasma and centrifuged at 4°C after incubation for two days at 4°C; the cryoprecipitate was collected by cen-

From the Department of Immunology, Rush Medical College, and the Department of Microbiology, University of Illinois at the Medical Center, Chicago, Illinois. Requests for reprints should be addressed to Dr. Henry Gewurz, Department of Immunology, Rush Medical College, 1753 West Congress Parkway, Chicago, Illinois 60612.
Manuscript accepted January 9, 1976.

* Recipient of a Boothroyd Foundation Medical Student Fellowship.

† Holder of the Thomas J. Coogan, Sr. Chair in Immunology established by Majorie Lindheimer Everett.

TABLE I C Component Profile

	CH_{50}	C1	C4	C2	C3	C5	C6	C7	C8	C9
Hemolytic C activity (% normal)	70	8	43	100	31	95	102	87	119	225

	C1q	C1r	C1s	C4	C3	C5	Properdin	Factor B
C Protein (μg/ml)								
Patient	10	105	38	130	630	110	9	167
Normal range	110–210	77–107	23–38	200–800	800–1,800	70–170	10–20	175–275

trifugation, resuspended in half its original volume and redissolved at 37°C for 1 hour prior to assay. C1q precipitins were characterized by ultracentrifugation (55,000 rpm, 4°C, 5 1/2 hours) of a 10 to 20 per cent isokinetic sucrose gradient [12] using a Beckman Model L265B ultracentrifuge and a SW56Ti rotor; fractions were assayed by the method of Agnello et al. [11], using a 0.01 M sodium phosphate buffer (pH 7.0, relative salt concentration (RSC) 0.09 M).

CASE REPORT

A 46 year old Caucasian woman presented because of repeated episodes over the past five years of "burning" urticarial-like lesions which had appeared abruptly on her head and neck, arms, legs and back. These lesions were 1 to 5 cm in diameter, raised, erythematous and well-circumscribed; periodically, they persisted for one to five days. The patient also had suffered cluster-headaches, arthralgias, bouts of asthma, conjunctivitis, periorbital edema, nonpitting edema of the wrists and oral mucosa, and pitting edema of the legs for three years, with which the skin lesions were frequently associated; because of these episodes she had required multiple hospitalizations. The frequency of her symptoms had increased to the point where she was rarely free of them. Treatment had included intravenous histamine desensitization, antihistamines, steroids, diuretics and analgesics; only high dose steroids was effective, and lowering the steroid dosage was associated with a recurrence of symptoms. She also had experienced psychiatric depressions for which she was hospitalized.

Allergen testing had revealed insignificant reactions, and triggering events for the eruptions were not defined. She had no apparent sensitivity to sunlight, cold or heat, no increased propensity to infection, no joint effusion and no renal, hepatic, intestinal or central nervous system dysfunction. There was no ancestral history of urticaria, allergy, asthma or propensity to infection. One daughter recently had a single transient episode of urticaria with a reported concomitant decrease in C3. Her husband and two of the three children tested had cryofibrinogen levels of 45, 30 and 20 mg/100 ml, respectively (normal, < 5 mg/100 ml); each had a normal complement profile.

Reduced levels of C3 and hemolytic C, which ultimately brought this patient to our attention, had been present for at least three years. This was the basis for a plasma transfusion she was given prior to referral which was said to have resulted in a diminution of both the cutaneous and conjunctival symptoms for one week. At the time of the present admission, C3 and hemolytic C were partially reduced, whereas C1q was almost completely depleted; yet C1r, C1s and $C\bar{1}$-INH levels were normal. Complement and complement component activities are discussed extensively herein. The erythrocyte sedimentation rate was 54 mm/hour (Westergren), and the C-reactive protein level was 17 μg/ml. The immunoglobulin M (IgM) level was elevated (6.5 mg/ml), whereas the immunoglobulin G (IgG) (14.6 mg/ml), immunoglobulin A (IgA) (1.4 mg/ml), immunoglobulin D (IgD) (0.08 mg/ml) and immunoglobulin E (IgE) (245 ng/ml) concentrations were within normal limits. Serum protein electrophoresis revealed no abnormalities. No antinuclear, antimitochondrial or antismooth muscle antibodies, rheumatoid factors, cryoglobulins or cold agglutinins were detectable, but cryofibrinogens (40 mg/100 ml) were present. The plasma prekallikrein level was within normal limits. Phytohemagglutinin (PHA), mixed leukocyte culture and E rosette reactions were normal. The hemogram (except for mild anemia), coagulation profile, urinalysis and basic biochemistry studies were within normal limits.

A biopsy specimen of an involved cutaneous area showed leukocytoclastic angiitis, atypical for urticaria; adjacent asymptomatic tissue showed mild vasculitis. Granular IgG deposits were seen on the basement membrane in both involved and asymptomatic tissue; this was associated with deposition of C3 in the active lesion. IgM, IgA, C4, C1q and properdin were not detected, and perivascular fluorescence was not seen.

RESULTS

The patient's complement component protein levels and total C and C component hemolytic activities are presented in Table I. Most notable was a dramatic reduction of C1q protein (10 μg/ml), whereas the C1r and C1s protein levels were normal. C1 hemolytic activity and C1q agglutination titers were both reduced 5 to 10 per cent of normal. The C1 hemolytic activity was similar when antibody-sensitized cells were reacted with the patient's serum and washed in buffer (0.075 M RSC) prior to reactivity with C4 and later-acting C components [13], indicating that the intact C1 macromolecule was present and that the activity was not resulting from free $C\bar{1}s$. C1-esterase inhibitor activity was normal, whereas C4 protein (130 μg/ml) and hemolytic activity (43 per cent normal), and C3 protein

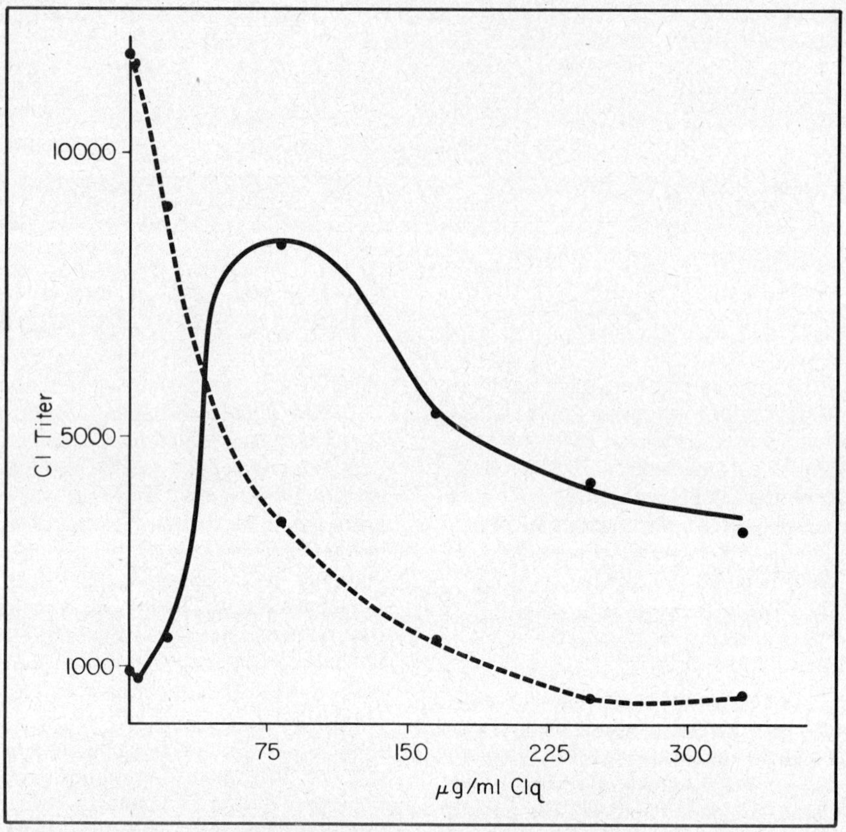

Figure 1. Effect of highly purified human C1q upon C1 hemolytic activity in patient's serum (●——●) and in normal serum (●- - - -●). C1q restored C1 hemolytic activity to normal levels in patient's serum, while inhibiting hemolytic C1 activity in normal serum, presumably on a competitive basis; this suggested that free C1r and C1s were present selectively in the patient's serum.

(630 μg/ml) and hemolytic activity (31 per cent normal) were partially reduced; C2, C5, C6, C7, C8, and C9 hemolytic activities, and C5, factor B and properdin protein concentrations each were within normal or near normal limits. The total complement hemolytic activity was 70 per cent normal, showing the insensitivity of this parameter to fluctuations of C1 and its subcomponents.

The deficiency of C1q relative to the other subcomponents of the C1 macromolecule was emphasized when a highly purified preparation of this subcomponent was added to patient and normal serum, respectively, and the effect on C1 hemolytic activity was assayed. Strikingly different patterns were observed (Figure 1). Although C1q inhibited C1 activity in normal serum, it elevated the level of C1 activity in the patient's serum; when sufficient amounts were added, normal C1 function was restored. This suggested that free C1r and C1s were available to combine with C1q selectively in the patient's serum, and furter, in amounts sufficient for complete restoration of C1 activity. As the concentration of C1q was further increased, hemolytic activity was inhibited. This most likely indicates that saturation of the available C1r and/or C1s had occurred and that the excess C1q was "anticomplementary," as it was in normal serum.

C1q protein and C1 hemolytic activity were deficient in the patient's plasma and serum collected and assayed at both 37°C and 4°C immediately after venipuncture. Precipitation occurred as her plasma, but not serum, was brought from 37°C to 4°C; the cryoprecipitate (40 mg/100 ml) contained C1q as well as fibrinogen, IgG, IgM, C3 and C4. However, only 12 μg of C1q was found to precipitate from 1 ml of patient serum, an amount insufficient to account for the depletion of C1q. The patient's serum contained complexes which precipitated with C1q to a serum dilution of 1:8 [1,11]; it was not reactive with monoclonal rheumatoid factor, and no anti-C1 activity was detected. Preparative sucrose ultracentrifugation showed that the precipitins sedimented with 7S characteristics (Figure 2).

Interestingly, although there was no ancestral history of similar disease, the episode of "urticaria" in one daughter with a transiently low C3, and the presence of cryofibrinogens in the patient's husband and two of their children, raises the possibility of a common agent or process. Their C profiles now are normal. Although we do not know the basis for the cryofibrinogenemia, the normal C1q levels in family members with cryofibrinogens and the absence of symptoms similar to those of the patient suggest that the cryofibrinogens alone were not responsible for the underlying immunopathology.

COMMENTS

In this patient, episodic urticarial-like symptoms and cutaneous vasculitis were associated with a selective deficiency of C1q; C1r and C1s levels were normal and hemolytic C1 activity was reconstituted upon the addition of C1q. Thus, there was a clear dissociation of the levels of the subcomponents which comprise C1. Of interest was that C1q reconstituted C1 activity in the patient's serum whereas it inhibited C1 activity in normal serum, presumably on a competitive basis [19].

C1q, the thermolabile combining portion of the C1 macromolecule [14,15], is known to react with IgG and IgM [16], C-reactive protein [17] and certain polyanions [11,18]. C1q has been found to be depressed in certain diseases including agammaglobulinemia [8,9,20–22], systemic lupus erythematosus [23–25], serum sickness nephritis [26] and nephrotic syndrome [27]. Dissociation of serum levels of the proteins which comprise the C1 macromolecule now has been seen in multiple conditions. A selective deficiency of C1q has been seen in multiple patients with agammaglobulinemia [28], single patients with systemic lupus erythematosus, juvenile rheumatoid arthritis or viral hemorrhagic fever, respectively [29], and in a child with mixed connective tissue disease syndrome [30]. C1s levels have been found to rise in excess of levels of C1q in the postsurgical state as well as in the "acute phase" of certain infectious and inflammatory diseases [5]. Persons with selective, apparently inborn, deficiency of C1r with normal levels of C1q have been described [31,32], as has a person with systemic lupus erythematosus in whom C1s was depressed whereas C1q was normal [33].

Our patient seems to have the greatest similarity to those previously described by Agnello et al. [1,2], McDuffie and his colleagues [3] and Sissons et al. [4]. Agnello et al. [1] observed a patient with erythema multiforma with C1q levels of 2 μg/ml, who had circulating factors which bound and precipitated C1q; Agnello and his colleagues [2] later observed three similar patients. McDuffie et al. [3] observed four patients with C1q levels between 20 and 50 μg/ml in association with urticarial-like skin lesions, and the two with the lowest C1q levels had demonstrable C1q precipitins. Sissons et al. [4] observed two similar patients except C1q precipitins were not detected and one had renal disease. Our patient is strikingly similar to these groups of patients in the appearance, distribution, size and abruptness of onset of the skin lesions, their association with arthralgia and transitory low grade fevers, skin biopsy histopathology (leukocytoclastic angiitis rather than urticarial pathology), complement profile, C1q precipitins and relative lack of detectable antinuclear antibodies, rheumatoid factors and renal disease. Our patient did not manifest intestinal complaints as did certain of the patients cited and her symptoms of periorbital edema, cluster-headaches, asthma and conjunctivitis were unique. Like our patient, those previously studied had only partially lowered levels of C4 and C3 [2–4], whereas C5 and later-acting components were normal [2,4]. Levels of C1s were elevated in the three patients of Agnello et al. [2], whereas levels of C1r and of C1s in the other patients were not reported.

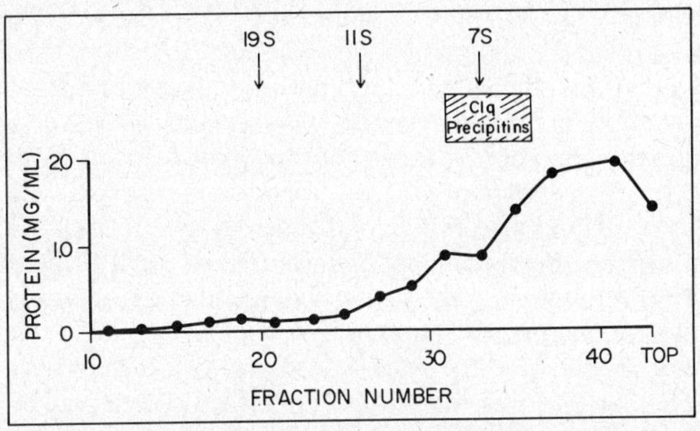

Figure 2. *Sucrose density gradient ultracentrifugation of patient's serum, with 19S (IgM), 11S (C1q) and 7S (IgG) markers; the C1q precipitins were associated with the 7S proteins.*

Sorter et al. [34] described eight patients with cutaneous vasculitis presenting as urticaria. These patients had increased sedimentation rates (except one), negative antinuclear antibodies (except one) and absent rheumatoid factors (except one); skin biopsy specimens showed leukocytoclastic angiitis. C1q levels were greatly reduced in two patients. C1q precipitins, however, were not reported. It is possible these patients may have the same syndrome as our patient and those discussed previously.

Oishi et al. [35] reported recently a case of lupus-like disease with low molecular weight C1q precipitins, antibodies to RNA and DNA, and elevated antibody titers to multiple viruses. C1r and C1s levels were not measured.

C1q precipitins were readily demonstrable in our patient although her serum was not "anticomplementary." The nature of these precipitins, which seem similar to those observed in the study of Agnello et al. [2], is not yet clear. The determination of a 7S sedimentation coefficient for the precipitins raised the possibility of an anti-C1q antibody, a complex involving a single 7S immunoglobulin molecule and a low molecular weight antigen such as the univalent hapten-antibody complexes recently described [36], or a nonimmunoglobulin factor or complex reactive with C1q. The amount of C1q in 1 ml of patient serum was equivalent to the amount of C1q in the cryoprecipitate formed from this amount of serum; thus, most or all of the C1q present may have been bound in complexes, clearance of which in turn may have contributed to the low levels of C1q. However, we do not yet know whether C1q was more rapidly depleted or less rapidly synthesized than the other C1 subcomponents, or whether our patient has an intrinsic abnormality of the C system [4]; these factors have been discussed by others [1,2,4,22].

It does seem that the constellation of urticarial-like lesions, cutaneous vasculitis, arthralgias, low molecular weight C1q precipitins with depletion of C1q, and the relative lack of antinuclear antibodies and of significant renal disease comprise a syndrome as described by Agnello et al. [1,2], McDuffie et al. [3] and Sams [37]. Patients with this syndrome clearly present with numerous manifestations generally associated with immune complex disease; whether it can be so categorized and involves a predominant antigen different from those seen in systemic lupus erythematosus, or indeed, whether an immune or "nonimmune" complex is involved at all, remains to be determined. Since the dominant serologic feature is the extreme and selective depletion of C1q among the C1 subcomponents along with the presence of 7S C1q precipitins, it seems critical to define the source and chemical nature of these precipitins, the characteristics of their interaction with C1q and the C1 macromolecule, and the relationship of these interactions to the cutaneous and systemic manifestations of the disease.

ACKNOWLEDGMENT

We thank Dr. Robert J. Winchester of the Rockefeller University for performing assays for complexes precipitating with C1q and monoclonal rheumatoid factor, and Drs. Winchester and Vincent Agnello of the New England Medical Center for valuable suggestions at critical phases in these studies. We also wish to thank Dr. Robert H. Painter of the University of Toronto for performing the assays for C1r. This work was supported by a grant from the Fay-Hunter Trust.

REFERENCES

1. Agnello V, Koffler D, Eisenberg JW, et al.: C1q precipitins in the sera of patients with systemic lupus erythematosus and other hypocomplementemic states: characterization of high and low molecular weight types. J Exp Med 134: 228s, 1971.
2. Agnello V, Ruddy S, Winchester RJ, et al.: Hereditary C2 deficiency in systemic lupus erythematosus and acquired complement abnormalities in an unusual SLE-related syndrome. Birth Defects 11: 312, 1975.
3. McDuffie FC, Sams WM Jr, Maldonado JE, et al.: Hypocomplementemia with cutaneous vasculitis and arthritis. Possible immune complex syndrome. Mayo Clin Proc 48: 340, 1973.
4. Sissons JGP, Williams DG, Peters DK, et al.: Skin lesions, angio-oedema, and hypocomplementemia. Lancet 2: 1350, 1974.
5. Gewurz H, Page AR, Pickering RJ, et al.: Complement activity and inflammatory neutrophil exudation in man. Studies in patients with glomerulonephritis, essential hypocomplementemia and agammaglobulinemia. Int Arch Allergy Appl Immunol 32: 64, 1967.
6. Schutte M, DiCamelli R, Murphy P, et al.: Effects of anesthesia, surgery, and inflammation upon host defense mechanisms. I. Effects upon the complement system. Int Arch Allergy Appl Immunol 48: 706, 1975.
7. Ewald RW, Schubart AF: Agglutinating activity of the complement component C1q in the F-II latex fixation test. J Immunol 97: 100, 1966.
8. Gewurz H, Pickering RJ, Christian CL, et al.: Decreased C1q protein concentration and agglutinating activity in agammaglobulinemia syndromes: an inborn error reflected in the complement system. Clin Exp Immunol 3: 437, 1968.
9. Donaldson VH: Mechanisms of activation of C1 esterase in hereditary angioneurotic edema plasma in vitro. The role of Hageman factor, a clot-promoting agent. J Exp Med 127: 411, 1968.
10. Yonemasu K, Stroud RM: C1q: rapid purification method for preparation of monospecific antisera and for biochemical studies. J Immunol 106: 304, 1971.
11. Agnello V, Winchester RJ, Kunkel HG: Precipitation reactions of the C1q component of complement with aggregated γ-globulin and immune complexes in gel diffusion. Immunology 19: 909, 1970.
12. McCarty KS Jr, Vollmer RT, McCarty KS: Improved computer program data for the resolution and fractionation of macromolecules by isokinetic sucrose density gradient sedimentation. Anal Biochem 61: 165, 1974.
13. Nagaki K, Stroud RM: The relationship of the hemolytic activity of active C1s to its TAMe esterase action: a new method of purification and assay. J Immunol 102: 421, 1969.
14. Müller-Eberhard HJ, Kunkel HG: Isolation of a thermolabile serum protein which precipitates γ-globulin aggregates and participates in immune hemolysis. Proc Soc Exp Biol 106: 291, 1961.
15. Lepow IH, Naff GB, Todd WD, et al.: Chromatographic resolution of the first component of human complement into three activities. J Exp Med 117: 983, 1963.
16. Müller-Eberhard HJ: Complement. Ann Rev Biochem 44: 899, 1975.
17. Volanakis JE, Kaplan MH: Interaction of C-reactive protein complexes with the complement system. II. Consumption of guinea pig complement by CRP complexes: requirement for C1q. J Immunol 113: 9, 1974.
18. Rent R, Ertel N, Eisenstein R, et al.: Complement activation by interaction of polyanions and polycations. I. Heparin-protamine induced consumption of complement. J Immunol 114: 120, 1975.
19. Messner RP, Jelinik JG: Inhibition of γG-mediated in vitro phagocytosis by the C1q component of complement. Clin Immunol Immunopathol 1: 203, 1973.
20. O'Connell RM, Enriquez P, Linman JW, et al.: Absence of

activity of the first component of complement in man: association with thymic alymphoplasia and defective inflammatory response. J Lab Clin Med 70: 715, 1967.

21. Kohler PF, Müller-Eberhard HJ: Complement-immunoglobulin relation: deficiency of C1q associated with impaired immunoglobulin G synthesis. Science 163: 474, 1969.
22. Kohler PF, Müller-Eberhard HJ: Metabolism of C1q. Studies in hypogammaglobulinemia, myeloma and systemic lupus erythematosus. J Clin Invest 51: 868, 1972.
23. Hanauer LB, Christian CL: Clinical studies of hemolytic complement and the 11S component. Am J Med 42: 882, 1967.
24. Gewurz H, Pickering RJ, Mergenhagen SE, et al.: The complement profile in acute glomerulonephritis, systemic lupus erythematosus and hypocomplementemic chronic glomerulonephritis. Int Arch Allergy Appl Immunol 34: 556, 1968.
25. Kohler PF, Ten Bensel R: Serial complement component alterations in acute glomerulonephritis and systemic lupus erythematosus. Clin Exp Immunol 4: 191, 1969.
26. Gewurz H, Pickering RJ, Moberg A, et al.: Reactivities to horse anti-lymphocyte globulin. II. Serum sickness nephritis with complement alterations in man. Int Arch Allergy Appl Immunol 39: 210, 1970.
27. Lewis EJ, Carpenter CB, Schur PM: Serum complement levels in human glomerulonephritis. Ann Intern Med 75: 555, 1971.
28. Stroud RM, Nagaki K, Pickering RJ, et al.: Subunits of the first component in immunologic deficiency syndromes. Independence of C1s and C1q. Clin Exp Immunol 7: 133, 1970.
29. DeBracco MM, Manni JA: Serum levels of C1q, C1r, and C1s in normal and pathologic sera. Arthritis Rheum 17: 121, 1974.
30. Wara DW, Reiter EO, Doyle NE, et al.: Persistent C1q deficiency in a patient with systemic lupus erythematosus-like syndrome. J Pediatr 86: 743, 1975.
31. Pickering RJ, Naff GB, Stroud RM, et al.: Deficiency of C1r in human serum. Effects on the structure and function of macromolecular C1. J Exp Med 131: 803, 1970.
32. Day NK, Geiger H, Stroud RM, et al.: C1r deficiency: an inborn error associated with cutaneous and renal disease. J Clin Invest 51: 102, 1972.
33. Pondman KW, Stoop KW, Stoop JW, et al.: Abnormal C1 in a patient with systemic lupus erythematosus. J Immunol 101: 811, 1968.
34. Sorter NA, Austen KF, Gigli I: Urticaria and arthralgias as manifestations of necrotizing angiitis (vasculitis). J Invest Dermatol 63: 485, 1974.
35. Oishi M, Takano M, Miyachi K, et al.: A case of unusual SLE related syndrome characterized by erythema multiforma, angioneurotic edema, marked hypocomplementemia, and C1q precipitins of low molecular weight type. Int Arch Allergy Appl Immunol 50: 463, 1976.
36. Goers J, Ziccardi B, Glovsky M, et al.: Studies on the activation of C1 by a univalent hapten-antibody complex. J Immunol 116: 1734, 1976.
37. Sams WM: Hypocomplementemia with cutaneous vasculitis and arthritis. A new syndrome. Arch Dermatol 110: 290, 1974.

Purpura Fulminans

THOMAS E. SPICER, M.D.*
JEROLD M. RAU, M.D.
Kansas City, Kansas

Purpura fulminans is a rare disease characterized by cutaneous ecchymosis, hypotension and fever associated with disseminated intravascular coagulation. It usually follows a preparatory infectious illness. A case in a 55 year old woman challenges the concept that this disease is limited to childhood. A review of 100 case reports is presented in which the often quoted high mortality of 90 per cent is found to be no longer tenable.

Purpura fulminans is generally reported to be a rare disease of childhood with a mortality rate approaching 90 per cent. The three primary clinical features of this syndrome, which follows a nonspecific preparatory, usually infectious, illness, are: (1) large purpuric ecchymotic areas of the skin, (2) fever and (3) hypotension. Characteristically, the hematologic picture is one of consumption coagulopathy; the pathologic picture is one of venule and capillary thrombosis, involving primarily the skin, but occasionally other organs. The pathogenesis of the disease, although never fully elucidated, closely parallels the generalized Shwartzman reaction of laboratory animals.

It is our purpose here to report an unusual case of purpura fulminans in a 55 year old white woman and to review the literature to more clearly define the confines of the syndrome.

CASE REPORT

This patient was referred to the University of Kansas Medical Center for admission because of a sudden onset of shock and associated purpura. Ten days prior to admission, she had the onset of a febrile upper respiratory tract illness for which she was hospitalized at another facility. Symptomatically improved on conservative therapy, including oral erythromycin estolate, the patient was discharged after three days. Five days later, she began to experience persistent abdominal pain, followed in two days by diarrhea, for which she was given an opiate for symptomatic relief. Ten days after discharge, a rapidly spreading petechial rash appeared, first on the dorsum of the feet and then spreading to become ecchymotic involving the legs to the mid-thigh, the arms, abdomen and face. On the morning of admission, she presented to her personal physician in shock. Her past medical history revealed multiple drug hypersensitivities including opiates. A variety of cutaneous eruptions had previously occurred with the use of multiple antibiotics, but the patient denied any previous reaction to erythromycin. Physical examination revealed a white woman who was confused but oriented. Her blood pressure was 60/40 mm Hg, pulse rate 140 beats/min, respirations 24/min, and temperature 38°C rectally. Examination of her skin disclosed violaceous ecchymoses, which were nonraised and nontender over the areas previously noted. Examinations of the head and neck disclosed no abnormalities. There were no conjunctival, retinal or oral hemorrhages. Examination of the chest and heart showed no abnormalities other than hypotension with tachycardia as already noted. Bowel sounds were hypoactive, but present. Rectal ex-

From the Department of Medicine, Section of Dermatology, University of Kansas Medical Center, 29th and Rainbow Boulevard, Kansas City, Kansas 66103. Requests for reprints should be addressed to Dr. Jerold M. Rau. Manuscript accepted January 9, 1976.

*Present address: 3480 East 3020 South, Salt Lake City, Utah 84109.

amination produced a small amount of bloody mucous. There were no focal neurologic signs.

Laboratory data disclosed a hemoglobin level of 14.2 g/dl, falling to 6.8 g/dl despite a 12 unit transfusion. The white cell count was 23,900/mm^3 with 50 per cent segmented forms, 29 per cent band forms, 5 per cent lymphocytes and 4 per cent metamyelocytes. Platelet count was 51,000/mm^3. Examination of the peripheral blood smear demonstrated an occasional schistocyte. Fibrinogen level on admission was 139 mg/dl (normal 200 to 400 mg/dl). Prothrombin time was 16.3 sec with a control of 11.1 sec, and activated partial thromboplastin time was 66.3 sec (normal 30 to 40 sec) which corrected to normal with a 1:1 mix with normal plasma. Thrombo Wellco was positive for fibrin degradation products greater than 40 μg/ml. Urinalysis revealed 4+ protein, 25 to 50 white blood cells per high power field (hpf), 10 to 20 red blood cells/hpf, 1+ bilirubin and 1+ hemoglobin. Examination of sternal marrow aspirate disclosed myeloid hyperplasia with an increased number of megakaryocytes.

The patient's intial course was complicated by shock responsive to volume expansion with electrolyte and protein solutions. Two units of whole blood and 10 units of packed red cells were required to maintain the hemoglobin level. Abdominal pain was evaluated by a surgical consultant who, on proctosigmoidoscopy, observed ecchymotic mucosal changes and performed a rectal biopsy with some subsequent bleeding in the lower gastrointestinal tract. A hematologic picture of disseminated intravascular coagulation was apparent but bleeding in the gastrointestinal tract precluded early heaprinization. Bleeding was controlled by the seventh hospital day, and heparinization at that point produced a remarkable rebound in platelet count, and fibrinogen levels approached normal (see Figure 1). The administration of heparin was discontinued on the 13th hospital day and those

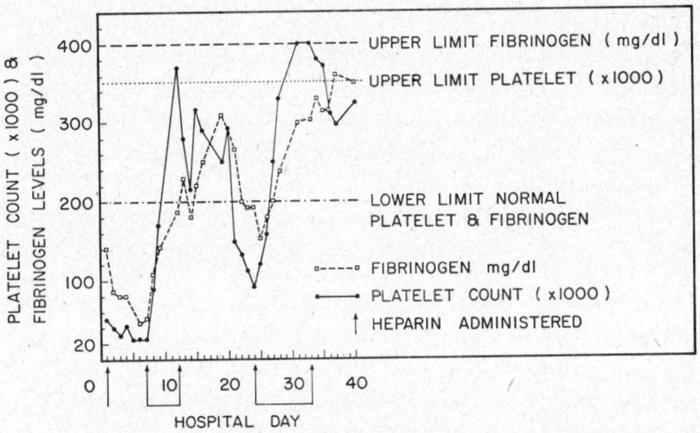

Figure 1. *Platelet and fibrinogen data of patient.*

parameters remained stable for the following week, but the patient suffered a relapse on the 20th hospital day with a shaking chill and subsequent development of falling platelet and fibrinogen levels. Heparin therapy was reinstituted on the 24th hospital day and maintained for a further eight days after which it was discontinued without a deterioration in the hematologic status during the week before discharge.

During the patient's hospital stay, the areas of the skin most severely involved became necrotic with associated bullae formation (Figure 2). Following debridement, the underlying areas were treated successfully as secondary degree burns with reverse isolation and strict asepsis. Thick eschar subsequently developed which gradually separated resulting in only minimal scar formation.

Skin biopsy specimens both from involved and uninvolved areas demonstrated the presence of fibrin thrombi compatible with disseminated intravascular coagulation [3,38]. In addition, from clinically involved skin, focal necrosis of small

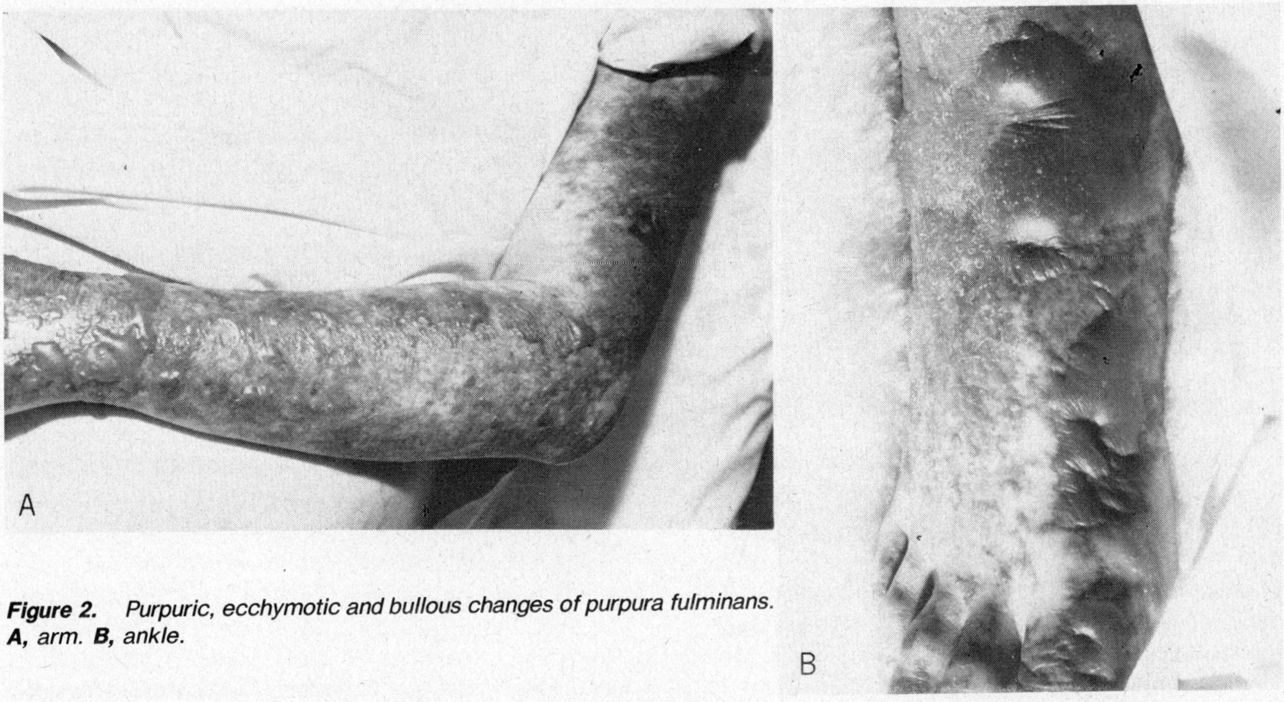

Figure 2. *Purpuric, ecchymotic and bullous changes of purpura fulminans.* ***A,*** *arm.* ***B,*** *ankle.*

vessel walls was noted. In the same sections, fibrin thrombi were often present with a mild perivascular inflammatory reaction. No evidence of a primary vasculitis was observed in any of the sections. Direct immunofluorescent staining for immunoglobulins G (IgG), A (IgA), M (IgM), third component of complement (C_3) and fibrinogen was negative. Biopsy specimens of the rectal mucosa also revealed intravascular fibrin thrombi without evidence of a primary vasculitis. In in vitro cultures, the patient's lymphocytes failed to undergo blastic transformation on exposure to the medications which she had taken in the immediate premorbid period (Ilosone®, Parepectolin® and isoniazid). Using the serotonin-release method [44], antiplatelet antibodies were not demonstrated in the patient's serum.

COMMENTS

The syndrome of purpura fulminans was first described by Guelliot [1] in 1884; the name was first applied by Henoch in 1887 [2]. Since the original description of the disease, many case studies of a fulminating disease associated with purpura have been published usually as single case reports. Such reports included many cases of other similar syndromes, including meningococcemia and Henoch-Schoenlein purpura, and the reporting of these cases with the title of purpura fulminans has caused much confusion. It was not until the report of Hjort et al. [3] that an attempt was made to extract from those reports a homogeneous group of patients in whom a single syndrome could be defined. In that previous literature review, the following criteria were proposed: (1) Purpura fulminans is a disease of children which (2) is preceded by a benign disorder, usually an infection (3) after which, with a variable but definite latent period, bleeding into the skin begins and spreads rapidly, often in waves resulting in severe anemia. With survival beyond the initial acute episode, (4) the most extensively involved skin undergoes necrosis with bullae formation and occasionally with necrosis of an entire extremity. (5) In the cases described since adequate methods have been available, coagulation abnormalities compatible with disseminated intravascular coagulation have been demonstrated. The pathologic findings described include (6) widespread thrombosis of venules and capillaries with a perivascular inflammatory infiltrate. Using the first four of these criteria, Hjort et al. extracted a total of 50 cases from the literature prior to 1964 and provided a unifying description of the syndrome. During the past 10 years, a further 50 cases meeting those criteria [4–33] have been combined with the cases reviewed by Hjort et al. [3] to give an updated overview of the syndrome.

Age. In the past, the disease was defined as a disease of children. Of the 100 cases reported, only four have occurred in subjects over the age of 12. The age range in the 100 cases was 0 (at birth) to 74 years, with a median age at 46 months.

Sex. The sex incidence is almost equal: 53 males and 47 females.

Familial. No reports of the familial incidence of purpura fulminans were discovered to complement the two cases cited by Hjort et al. [3].

Season. There are slight seasonal variations; cases are more likely to appear in the winter and spring, possibly reflecting an increased incidence of upper respiratory tract illness during those months. Of the 71 cases in which information is available, 31 or 44 per cent occurred during the first quarter of the calendar year, 22 or 31 per cent during the second quarter, 6 or 8 per cent during the third quarter and 12 or 17 per cent during the fourth quarter.

Preparatory Disease. Twenty-seven per cent of the patients had a history of scarlet fever immediately preceding the development of purpura fulminans [3,6,30]. Even so, purpura fulminans is a rare complication of scarlet fever occurring in only 1 of 20,000 cases [42,43].

The second most common, 23 per cent is "post-infectious" following an unverified upper respiratory tract infection [3,4,11,13,14,15,20,22,25,26,28,30]. Presumably, most such infections are viral in origin; however, there are no viral cultures or other data to substantiate a viral etiology. Varicella was the third most common preceding illness, occurring in 20 per cent of the patients [3,5,7,8,9,10,12,15,17,19,23,29].

Other streptococcal infections accounted for an additional 11 cases: four in which pneumonia was secondary to S. pneumoniae [3,21,33], four in which pharyngitis was secondary to a beta hemolytic streptococcus [3,13,15,16], two with skin infections [10,30] and one with empyema [3].

The remaining preparatory disorders included rubella [13], roseola [3], a second injection of diphtheria antiserum [3] and smallpox vaccination [3]. These disorders were followed by a latent period, varying between 0 and 90 days [3]. In 44 of 48 cases in which the information is available, the onset occurred within four weeks of the "preparatory illness." In five cases, no preparatory disorder could be elucidated [3,18,27, 32].

With the exception of these previous disorders, no other significant unifying event could be identified. In eight cases, however [6,13,14,33], there was a history of intramuscular injections of penicillin for the treatment of the preparatory disease.

Presentation. The sites of cutaneous hemorrhage at the time of presentation tended to be symmetrical, with a strong predilection for the lower extremities. In virtually every one of the latter 50 cases presently reviewed, there was some involvement of the lower extremities, most often the lateral buttocks, lateral thighs or ankle areas. Other commonly involved areas included the upper extremities and the abdomen. Rarely involved were the chest, face, scalp or neck.

Skin bleeding tended to occur in large confluent patches of ecchymoses which, if seen in the active phase, advanced behind a small erythematous, well-defined border to produce nonpalpable purpura. As the lesions matured, those areas most extensively involved became necrotic with bullae formation as in the patient we describe herein. Those bullae contained a serous fluid which, if uncontaminated, was sterile. With further progression, obvious necrosis was followed by a thick hard eschar which separated from the underlying tissue as new skin was formed. Initially, peripheral pulses were intact. Later in the disease, however, these pulses may disappear, either because of subsequent large vessel thrombosis [6,22], or because of the development of concentric rings of eschar which further compromise the vasculature of an already edematous extremity. Both events may lead to the development of ischemic necrosis of an entire extremity often requiring amputation, a complication which occurred in the 19 per cent of the 100 cases [3,8,11,12,13,15,19,26]. Large areas of skin grafting are frequently required [7,11,12,19,24,30]. Bleeding into mucous membranes is unusual, but it has been reported [27]. In the present 100 cases, conjunctival bleeding was noted in four cases [3], epistaxis in five [3], hematemesis in five and hematochezia in nine [4,7,8,20,26]. Hematuria was noted in 17 cases [3,13,20,21,26].

Hematologic Findings. On initial examination, the hemoglobin level often is normal. With hydration and treatment of shock, levels fall dramatically, and hemoglobin levels below 9 mg/dl are not unusual. In 25 of the latter 50 cases, the initial hemoglobin determination was below 12 g/dl, and in 11 it was below 9 g/dl. Examination of the peripheral smear in those few cases reported, is remarkable for schistocytes with burr and helmet cells characteristic of a microangiopathic hemolytic process [40].

White blood cell counts are rarely below 10,000/mm^3 and are often dramatically increased. Of the 90 patients for whom the data are available, only eight had levels less than 10,000/mm^3 and 50 had levels greater than 20,000/mm^3. Also notable is a strong tendency for a shift to the left with a large proportion of early "band" forms present. The platelet count was included in 68 reports: in 31 per cent it was below 50,000/mm^3, also in 31 per cent the count was greater than 150,000/mm^3. The Rumple Leede tourniquet test was reported in 23 cases and was positive in three [3,9] (in these three, platelet counts were 54,000, 154,000 and 164,000/mm^3). A bone marrow examination was performed in 12 patients and yielded consistent findings of a hypercellular marrow often with an increase in megakaryocytes [3,8,10,14].

Bacteriology. Cultures of the skin lesions were all negative initially although in several colonization and infection developed later in the courses with Pseudomonas and Streptococcus. Blood cultures were consistently negative with the exception of streptococci cultured in two cases [3], and both streptococci and staphylococci in an additional case [30]. These organisms were recovered late in the courses of the disease and were probably related to concomitant skin infection. In two cases of infected ventriculoatrial shunts, blood cultures for Staphylococcus albus [28] were positive.

Hemostasis. Bleeding time was abnormal in 41 per cent of 34 patients in whom it was reported, and clotting time was markedly abnormal in 50 per cent of 49. Prothrombin time was moderately to markedly prolonged in 83 per cent of 55 patients, and partial thromboplastin time was prolonged in 79 per cent of nine for whom it was reported. Fibrinogen levels were reported in 38 patients. In 66 per cent, it was below 100 mg/dl and in only 18 per cent was it greater than 150 mg/dl. Specific assays for clotting factors were performed in only 18 patients; the most remarkable abnormality was a marked depression of factor V activity in 73 per cent of the 11 patients for whom values were given. Factor VII was low in 50 per cent of six patients, and factor VIII was mildly depressed in 73 per cent of 11 patients for whom values were available.

Duration of the Active Phase. The active phase is the time period from the onset of skin lesions until their progression has stabilized. In 66 patients, the active phase lasted less than three days.

Mortality. The total mortality for the 100 cases was 35 per cent. There is a large disparity in comparing the mortality in the 50 cases reported prior to 1964 (52 per cent) with the mortality in the 50 cases reported since that date (18 per cent). The difference presumably reflects not only new approaches to the treatment of this disease, but also particularly improved methods of managing critically ill patients.

Pathology. Pathologic material is available in 27 autopsy reports and in 18 biopsy reports most of which are skin biopsy specimens. The most remarkable finding is that of diffuse and extensive hemorrhage into skin with subsequent development of necrosis [3,10,13,27]. A similar pathologic picture is occasionally found in larger vessels and in organs other than skin [3,22], particularly bowel, bladder, brain and serosal surfaces. Other pathologic findings which are occasionally described include a particular "perivascular cuffing" of small vessels by polymorphonuclear leukocytes [11], and focal fibrinoid necrosis of the walls of small arteries [21,26]. Of some interest in the consideration of the pathogenesis of this disorder is the fact that similar findings are often found in skin involved with the

Shwartzman phenomenon [34,37]. A more extensive review of the similarity of this disorder with the generalized Shwartzman phenomenon is available [3,41].

Treatment. The treatment of purpura fulminans can logically be divided into the acute phase and the rehabilitative phase. The acute phase is characterized by rapidly spreading skin lesions with severe constitutional signs of shock and fever, and a laboratory picture consistent with disseminated intravascular coagulation. Treatment during this phase is largely supportive. The shock component results from intravascular volume depletion and responds to replacement of that deficit. Some have warned against the use of vasopressors in fear of exacerbating dermal ischemia [3]. The most controversial element is the treatment of the coagulopathy. Because of the relative rarity of the disease, no comparison of therapeutic regimens is available and the choice of treatment can only be guided by anecdotal experiences with single patients. Heparin therapy has been advocated by many with favorable experiences in its use in this disease [3–6,10,12,13,17,22, 23,25,27,28,30]. Its mode of action involves inhibition of the coagulation cascade inhibiting the development of intravascular thrombosis [39]. In the case presented herein, the patient initially responded to heparin therapy with a remarkable rebound in platelet and fibrinogen levels. Seven days after discontinuation of heparin therapy, the patient suffered a hematologic relapse which responded abruptly to reinitiation of heparin therapy. Those reports with unfavorable experiences result largely from the use of this agent as a final effort in a moribund patient [10,20]. Various dose levels have been advocated although there is general agreement that large doses are required initially (100 U/kg/4 hours) based upon the evidence of massive intravascular coagulation which is found in these patients and the fact that the generalized Shwartzman reaction has been shown to be inhibited by heparin, but only when given in large doses [35–37]. In any event, the dose levels must be adjusted to provide evidence that the ongoing process of disseminated intravascular coagulation has been interrupted. The length of therapy is equally confusing. On the basis that the active phase of the disease may last from one to two weeks, plus the experience of others that the early discontinuation of heparin therapy may result in relapse [6,13,17,22,28], many have recommended that heparin therapy be continued at least two to three weeks; some recommend that oral anticoagulation be continued for an extended period following heparin therapy [17]. Control of the coagulopathy has not been shown to affect the progression of cutaneous ecchymoses early in the disease, nor has it been shown to affect the incidence of gangrene.

Other therapeutic maneuvers are frequently used. The presenting picture is very similar to that of septic shock and until adequate bacteriologic information is available, antibiotic therapy has been started in most patients. In addition, most patients have empirically been given large doses of parenteral steroids. Of some interest is the fact that the generalized Shwartzman reaction is potentiated by steroids [34], therefore, they may be contraindicated. Other modalities used in occasional cases with good results include dextran [11,13,29,30], hyperbaric oxygen [13,20,30,33], epsilon amino caproic acid [24] and replacement of the hemostatic components as they are consumed [10,15,16,18,22,23,29,31,32].

The treatment of the rehabilitative phase of the disease involves meticulous skin care to prevent secondary infections. Skin grafting is usual and amputations are occasionally necessary.

SUMMARY

Purpura fulminans is primarily, but not solely, a disease of childhood which follows a benign, usually infectious, illness. It is characterized by the rapid progression of ecchymotic areas of skin associated with the development of hypovolemic shock and disseminated intravascular coagulation. Although most evidence is circumstantial, it is currently thought to represent a human equivalent of the generalized Shwartzman reaction of laboratory animals. Because of the paucity of cases, no absolute treatment regimens can be recommended to the exclusion of others; however, the most consistently good reports include the use of heparin and steroids. The once quoted 90 per cent mortality is no longer tenable; the mortality rate in the 50 cases reported since 1964 is 18 per cent.

REFERENCES

1. Guelliot O: Note sur trois cas de purpura infectieux foudroyant. Un Med Sci Norde-Est 8: 25, 1884.
2. Henoch E: Ueber Purpura Fulminans. Prag Med Wochnschr 11: 494, 1886.
3. Hjort PF, Rapaport SI, Jorgensen I: Purpura fulminans—report of a case successfully treated with heparin and hydrocortisone. Review of 50 cases from the literature. Scand J Haematol 1: 169, 1964.
4. Ainer MM, Kauff RE, Sherman JD: Purpura fulminans in a child with pneumococcal septicemia two years after splenectomy. JAMA 213: 1681, 1970.
5. Allen DM: Heparin therapy of purpura fulminans. Pediatrics 38: 211, 1966.
6. Antley RM, McMillan CW: Sequential coagulation studies in purpura fulminans. N Engl J Med 276: 1287, 1967.
7. Becker FT, Buckley RP: Purpura fulminans associated with varicella. Arch Dermatol 94: 613, 1966.
8. Bogunull GP: Bilateral above the knee amputations. A complication of chickenpox. J Bone Joint Surg 47: 371, 1965.

9. Bouhasin JP: Purpura fulminans. Pediatrics 34: 265, 1964.
10. Castleman B, McNeely BU: Case records of the Massachusetts General Hospital. N Engl J Med 281: 153, 1969.
11. Cram PL, Soley RL: Purpura fulminans. Br J Dermatol 80: 323, 1968.
12. Crocker AM, Middlekamp JN: Varicella gangrenosa. J Pediatr 54: 104, 1959.
13. Dudgeon DL, Gilchrist GS, Woolley MW: Purpura fulminans. Arch Surg 103: 351, 1971.
14. Geigin RD, San Joagquin V, Middlekamp JN: Purpura fulminans associated with Neisseria catarrhalis septicemia and meningitis. Pediatrics 44: 120, 1969.
15. Fishbein RH: Purpura fulminans: an analysis of the lesion and its treatment. J Pediatr Surg 4: 320, 1969.
16. Fredricks E, Huffstadt AJC: Two cases of purpura fulminans. Br J Plast Surg 23: 90, 1970.
17. Hattersley PG: Purpura fulminans, complete recovery with IV administered heparin. Am J Dis Child 120: 467, 1970.
18. Hollingsworth JH, Mohler DN: Microangiopathic hemolytic anemia caused by purpura fulminans. Ann Intern Med 68: 1310, 1968.
19. Horder M: Purpura fulminans following varicella. Dan Med Bull 15: 221, 1968.
20. Kuzemko JA, Loder RE: Purpura fulminans treated with hyperbaric oxygen. Br Med J 4: 157, 1970.
21. Leavell UW: Cutaneous changes in a case of purpura fulminans following pneumococcal pneumonia. J Ky Med Assoc 70: 853, 1972.
22. Little JR: Purpura fulminans treated successfully with anticoagulation. JAMA 169: 36, 1959.
23. McGovern JP, Dawson JP: Purpura fulminans: report of a case coincident with varicella. Clin Proc Child Hosp 10: 114, 1954.
24. Morse TS, Rowe MI, Hartigan M: Purpura fulminans. Arch Surg 93: 268, 1968.
25. Nagi NA, Al-Hasso ARA: Purpura fulminans with hemolytic anemia. Postgrad Med J 50: 750, 1974.
26. Dodge WF, Travis LB, Daeschner CW: Anaphylactoid purpura, polyarteritis nodosa and purpura fulminans. Pediatr Clin North Am 10: 879, 1963.
27. Rainier-Pope CRC: Purpura fulminans and disseminated intravascular coagulation. A report of five cases in childhood. S Afr Med J 47: 1420, 1973.
28. Shennan AT: Purpura necrotica as a complication of ventriculoatrial shunts in hydrocephalus. Arch Dis Child 47: 821, 1972.
29. Smith H: Purpura fulminans complicating varicella. Recovery with low molecular weight dextran and steroids. Med J Aust 2: 685, 1967.
30. Urbaniak JR, O'Neil MT, Meyer LC: Purpura fulminans. J Bone Joint Surg 55: 69, 1973.
31. Van Creveld S, van der Kolk WFJ, Mochtaic JA: Purpura fulminans; a case of recovery. Clin Pediatr 4: 23, 1965.
32. Van der Horst RL: Purpura fulminans in a newborn baby. Arch Dis Child 37: 436, 1962.
33. Waddell WB, Saltzman HA, Fuson RL, Harris J: Purpura gangrenosa treated with hyperbaric oxygenation. JAMA 191: 971, 1965.
34. Thomas L, Good RA: The effect of cortisone on the Shwartzman reaction. J Exp Med 95: 409, 1952.
35. Thomas L, Smith RT, VonKorff R: Studies of the generalized Shwartzman reaction. J Exp Med 102: 263, 1955.
36. Good RA, Thomas L: Studies on the generalized Shwartzman reaction. J Exp Med 97: 871, 1953.
37. Cluff LE, Berthrong M: The inhibition of the loca Shwartzman reaction by heparin. Johns Hopkins Med J 92: 353, 1953.
38. Robboy SJ, Mihm MC, Colman RW, et al.: The skin in disseminated intravascular coagulation. Prospective analysis of 36 cases. Br J Dermatol 88: 221, 1973.
39. Rodriguez-Erdman F: Bleeding due to increased intravascular blood coagulation. N Engl J Med 273: 1370, 1965.
40. Rodriguez-Erdman F: Experimental in vivo production of helmet cells. Fed Proc 27: 500, 1968.
41. Hjort PF, Rapaport ST: The Shwartzman reaction. Pathogenic mechanisms and clinical manifestations. Ann Rev Med 16: 135, 1965.
42. Frodin M: Purpura fulminans and its relation to scarlatina. Acta Paediatr 34: 217, 1946.
43. Hoyne AL, Smoller L: Gangrene as a complication of scarlet fever. J Pediatr 18: 242, 1941.
44. Hirschman RJ, Shulman NR: The use of platelet serotonin release as a sensitive method for detecting anti-platelet antibodies and a plasma anti-platelet factor in patients with idiopathic thrombocytopenic purpura. Br J Haematol 24: 793, 1973.

A Complement Independent Erythropoietic Inhibitor Acting on the Progenitor Cell in Refractory Anemia

G. P. BROWMAN, M.D.
M. H. FREEDMAN, M.D.
Toronto, Ontario, Canada
M. A. BLAJCHMAN, M.D.
J. A. McBRIDE, M.B.
Hamilton, Ontario, Canada

An erythropoietic inhibitor was detected in the serum of a patient with refractory anemia. Using an in vitro heme synthesis method, the patient's serum produced tenfold inhibition of erythropoietin-stimulated radioactive iron (Fe^{59}) incorporation into heme of normal human marrow at 72 hours, as compared with AB serum. In a separate experiment the patient's serum produced threefold inhibition, whereas immunoglobulin G (IgG) prepared from the same serum sample produced 12-fold inhibition. To identify the site of action of the inhibitor, serum was tested in a cell culture system whereby human marrow cells, grown in a plasma clot, respond to exogenous erythropoietin with the appearance of nucleated erythroid colonies. Each colony arises from a committed erythroid progenitor. The patient's serum produced a two- to tenfold reduction in the number of colonies from normal human marrow. The effect was also demonstrated on autologous marrow obtained when the patient was in "partial clinical remission." Serum samples obtained at various times during the course of the patient's illness all demonstrated a suppressive effect on colony growth. All serums were heat-inactivated, and total hemolytic complement could not be detected in either culture system. It is concluded that the anemia is due to an inhibitor, probably of IgG class, that acts on the erythroid progenitor cell. The absence of heat-labile complement components in the culture systems suggests that the mechanism is not due to immune cytolysis.

It is now well documented in vitro [1] and in vivo [2] that an erythropoietic inhibitor is present in some adult patients with acquired pure red cell aplasia and refractory anemia. The mechanism of inhibition is not entirely understood, but the inhibitor in many cases has been found in the serum immunoglobulin G (IgG) fraction [3,4]. The demonstration of an IgG erythropoietic inhibitor, the association of red cell aplasia with thymoma and autoimmune phenomena [5,6] and the hematologic response to immunosuppressive therapy [7] have stimulated many investigators to a search for antibody-like activity to explain the pathogenesis of the anemia.

Jepson and Lowenstein [2] suggested that the inhibitor may be an antibody directed against erythropoietin; this idea has recently received some experimental support [8]. On the other hand, Krantz et al. [7] hypothesized that the action of the inhibitor may be in the form of cytotoxicity, and they convincingly demonstrated a cytolytic effect of an inhibitor on erythroblasts. This cytolytic effect was complement-

From the Departments of Medicine and Laboratory Medicine, Henderson General Hospital, McMaster University, Hamilton, Ontario and the Division of Hematology, Hospital for Sick Children, University of Toronto, Toronto, Ontario, Canada. This study was supported in part by Medical Research Council of Canada Grant MA-4982. Requests for reprints should be addressed to Dr. J. A. McBride, Department of Laboratory Medicine, Henderson General Hospital, 711 Concession Street, Hamilton, Ontario, Canada L8V 1C3. Manuscript accepted January 12, 1976.

dependent [9]. The demonstration of erythroblast cytolysis measured by the release of heme-incorporated Fe^{59} suggested that inhibition of erythropoiesis in red cell aplasia is due to damage of previously formed cells.

In this study, the nature of an erythropoietic inhibitor in an adult patient with refractory erythroblastopenic anemia was examined. The inhibitor was demonstrated in the serum and in the IgG fraction of serum, and a site of action at the committed erythroid progenitor cell level was demonstrated in vitro. The inhibitory effect was not dependent on the presence of complement. It is suggested that this inhibitor acts by suppressing new erythroblast development rather than through immune cytolysis.

CASE REPORT

A 49 year old woman presented in April 1974 with chronic fatigue and anemia, and a recent need for transfusions. She had a 20 year history of anemia associated with intermittent rectal bleeding. Two years previously, a diagnosis of iron deficiency was made on the basis of a low serum iron level and a high total iron-binding capacity associated with the absence of stainable marrow iron. The patient had only a partial response to oral iron therapy. She had no history of exposure to chemical toxins, and the only medication she took was thyroid extract which she had been taking for eight years following thyroidectomy for Hashimoto's thyroiditis. She had no other illnesses. Examination revealed a pale but healthy-looking woman with no abnormal physical findings.

Hematologic investigations were as follows: hemoglobin 6.0 g/dl, white blood cells 5.1×10^9/liter (66 per cent neutrophils, 30 per cent lymphocytes, 2 per cent monocytes, 2 per cent eosinophils), platelets 210×10^9/liter, reticulocytes less than 0.1 per cent. The red blood cells appeared normochromic and normocytic. Bone marrow revealed markedly depressed erythropoiesis (myeloid:erythroid ratio 30:1) with normal iron stores. Plasma cells were morphologically normal and not increased in number. Granulopoiesis and megakaryocytes were normal. Serum iron was 48 μmol/liter, total iron-binding capacity 54 μmol/liter. The half-clearance time ($T_{1/2}$) of intravenously injected transferrin-bound Fe^{59} was 180 minutes (normal: 80 to 120 minutes) and red cell utilization at 10 days was 3 per cent (normal: 70 to 90 per cent). Serum vitamin B_{12} and folate and red cell folate levels were normal. Results of Ham's test for acid hemolysis and the sucrose-lysis test were negative. The erythropoietin level was 15 mU/ml in serum obtained on April 19, 1974 (normal: 37 $\pm$ 22 mU/ml).* The serum protein electrophoretic pattern showed a monoclonal peak of 1.17 g/dl which on immunoelectrophoresis was shown to be an IgG kappa paraprotein; in addition, free light chains were demonstrated in the urine. There was no other evidence of myeloma, plasmacytoma or amyloid disease. The serum total protein was 7.2 g/dl, serum albumen 4.15 g/dl, immunoglobulin A (IgA) 650 mg/dl, IgG 1,800 mg/dl, immunoglobulin M (IgM) 90 mg/dl. Renal and hepatic function were normal. Antithyroid antibody by complement fixation was positive to a titer 1:8. Antismooth muscle, antimitochondrial, antiparietal cell, anti-intrinsic factor and antiskeletal muscle antibodies were negative. Antinuclear factor, demonstrated by indirect immunofluorescence on rat liver, was positive to a titer 1:4 with a speckled pattern. Rheumatoid factor and lupus erythematosus cells were negative. Chest roentgenogram, skeletal survey and tomograms of the mediastinum disclosed no abnormalities.

* In vitro hemagglutination inhibition kindly performed by JCL Laboratories, Knoxville, Tennessee.

A summary of the hematologic course is presented in Figure 1. From 1972 on, the patient had had chronic, moderate anemia; for an episode of red cell aplasia in March 1974 she was treated with 10 units of blood within one month. From mid-April to November 1974 there was a spontaneous "partial remission" during which the hemoglobin remained stable at 10 g/dl without transfusion. At the start of this "remission," the reticulocyte count was 5.2 per cent; throughout this period, the reticulocyte count varied from 0.4 per cent to 4.8 per cent. Repeat ferrokinetic studies in mid-August revealed an improvement of red cell utilization at 10 days to 40 per cent, and a repeat bone marrow performed at that time revealed active normal erythropoiesis. There was no change in the quantity of serum paraprotein.

During 1974, serum was obtained for study of the erythropoietic inhibitor on April 5, April 19 and August 16.

METHODS

Isolation of IgG. Immunoglobulins were extracted from serum and purified by the standard technics of ammonium sulfate precipitation and DE52 column chromatography. The purity of the gamma G globulin fraction was verified by immunoelectrophoresis. The gamma G globulin was concentrated by ultracentrifugation and the protein content measured by absorbance of ultraviolet light at 280 nm. It was then lyophlized, pooled and adjusted to a concentration equal to the concentration in the patient's serum for use in the heme synthesis assay system.

All serum specimens and culture materials used in the heme synthesis and erythroid colony assay that could serve as a complement source were heat-inactivated. To determine the completeness of inactivation, total hemolytic complement was measured by a micromethod [10] in which 1 per cent sensitized sheep red cells are mixed with serial dilutions of test serum in normal saline solution, incubated 30 minutes at 37°C, agitated and then read for lysis. No complement was detected in any of the samples tested.

Heme Synthesis. Marrow specimens were cultured by the method of Krantz [11]. Buffy coat from 4 ml of heparinized marrow was washed three times in NCTC-109 medium containing penicillin, 100 units/ml, and streptomycin, 50 μg/ml, and resuspended in a medium of 60 per cent NCTC-109 and 40 per cent human AB serum obtained from a hematologically normal adult volunteer.

One milliter of marrow suspension containing 5×10^6 nucleated cells was plated in 35 by 10 mm plastic tissue culture dishes and incubated for 72 hours with and without 0.2 units/ml erythropoietin* in 5 per cent carbon dioxide in

* Erythropoietin (sheep plasma, step III) obtained from Connaught Laboratories, Toronto, Ontario.

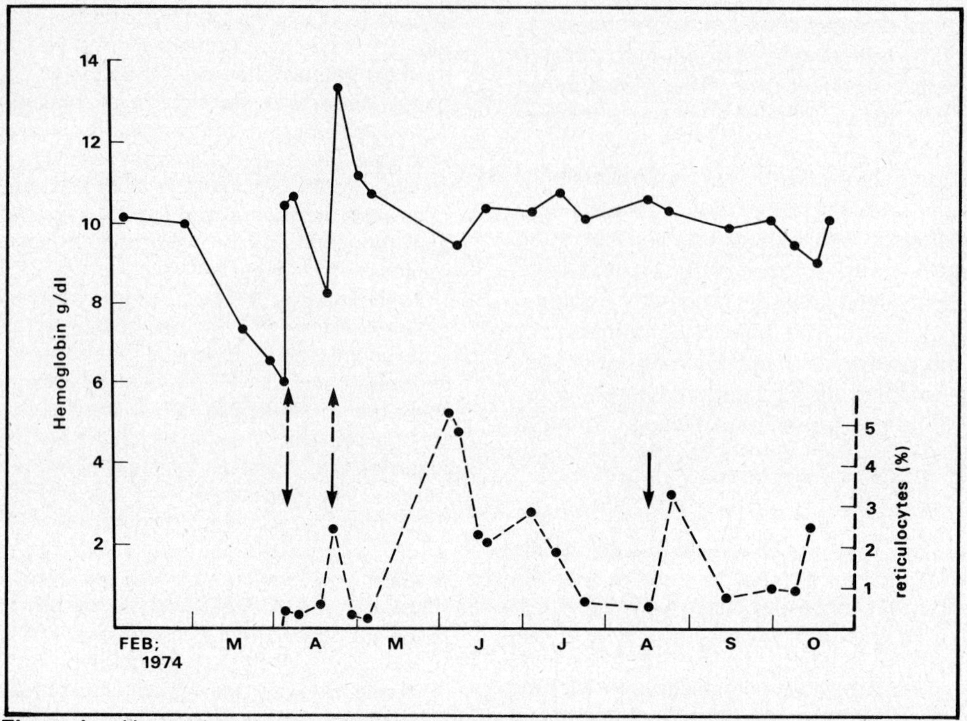

Figure 1. *Hematologic course. Dotted arrows indicate times of transfusion and solid arrows indicate times when test serums were obtained. Throughout this period white blood cells and platelets remained normal.*

air at 37°C. Erythropoietin had a potency of 2.8 to 4.7 units/mg dry weight and was dissolved in NCTC-109 and frozen until use.

Six hours prior to harvesting, 1 μc of ferric chloride ($^{59}FeCl_3$), pre-incubated for 1 hour with AB serum as a source of transferrin, was added to each culture.

At the end of incubation, the dishes were chilled at 4°C for 10 minutes. The contents were transferred to plastic centrifuge tubes, washed three times with cold phosphate-buffered saline solution, and the heme fraction was extracted with methylethylketone [12]. An aliquot of the heme was removed from each specimen and the radioactivity counted.

Each culture was made in duplicate, and the results were averaged. Heme synthesis was expressed in disintegrations per minute and results were compared to those in cultures without erythropoietin.

To detect serum inhibitors of erythropoiesis, the patient's serum obtained on April 5 and April 19, 1974 (Figure 2) was substituted for AB serum in the culture medium; IgG prepared from serum obtained on April 19 (Figure 3) was added to heat-inactivated AB serum in other studies.

Erythroid Colonies. Colonies were grown as originally described [13] with some modification. Three milliliters of bone marrow were aspirated in a dry syringe and transferred to 5 ml supplemented Eagle's minimum essential medium (GIBCO), 2 per cent fetal calf serum and 10 units/ml of preservative-free heparin. After centrifugation the supernatant was discarded; the cells were resuspended in the same solution without heparin and recentrifuged. Buffy coat was removed and suspended in Eagle's medium in a final concentration of 1×10^7 nucleated cells/ml.

A mixture was made from 0.7 ml bovine serum albumen (Miles Laboratories), 0.7 ml beef embryo extract (GIBCO), 0.7 ml L-asparagine (1 mg/ml) (Sigma Chemical), 1.4 ml NCTC-109 (Microbiological Assoclates) and 2.1 ml fetal calf serum. From this combination, 0.8 ml was placed into each of five separate tubes; into each tube, 0.1 ml of bovine plasma was added, mixed with the contents and plated rapidly before clotting into the wells of plastic titration plates (Linbro). Cultures were incubated at 37°C in air with 5 per cent carbon dioxide in high humidity for seven days with 2.0 U of erythropoietin/ml.

At the end of the incubation, the plasma clots were removed from the wells, placed on microscope slides, flattened and then fixed in 5 per cent glutaraldehyde in 0.01 M phosphate buffer for 10 minutes. After washing in distilled water and drying, the slides were stained in 1 per cent 3-dimethoxybenzidine (Eastman Kodak Co.) in methanol for 3.5 minutes, then in 3 per cent hydrogen peroxide in 70 per cent ethanol for 1 minute. After rinsing in distilled water, they were counterstained with Harris' hematoxylin for 2 minutes, air-dried and mounted with coverslips.

The clots were scanned at 10X magnification, and the total number of colonies per clot was counted. A colony is defined as a clump of 8 or more nucleated cells showing a positive benzidine reaction. All determinations were made in quadruplicate and the results averaged. The counts were expressed as number of colonies per 1×10^5 nucleated cells plated.

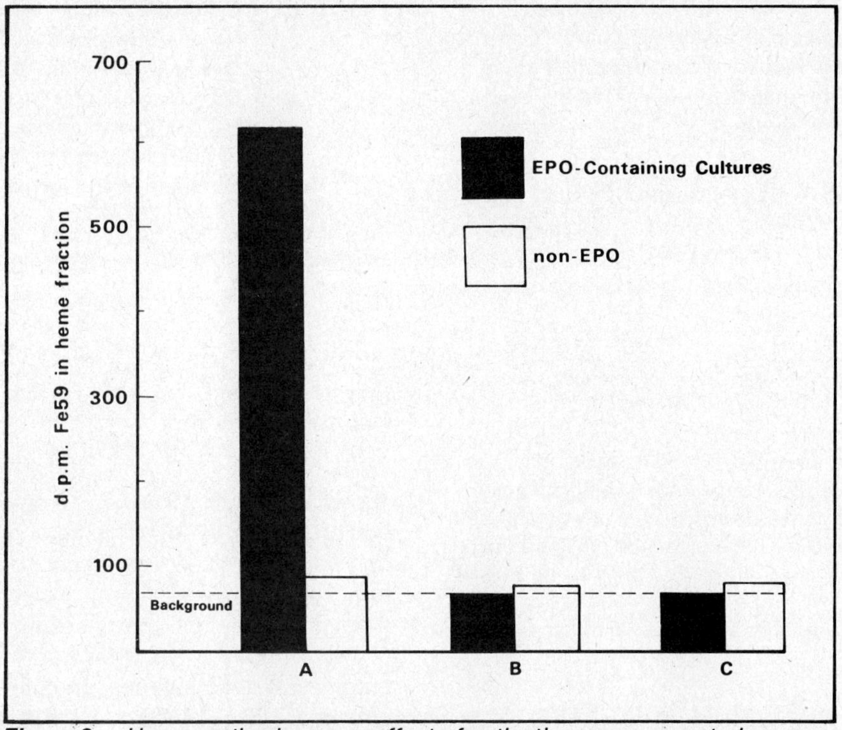

Figure 2. *Heme synthesis assay: effect of patient's serum on control marrow. EPO = erythropoietin 0.2 U/ml. The stimulated cultures to which the patient's serum had been added differed significantly from the AB serum (p <0.01).* ***A,*** *cultures with AB serum.* ***B,*** *cultures with patient's serum (April 5).* ***C,*** *cultures with patient's IgG (April 19).*

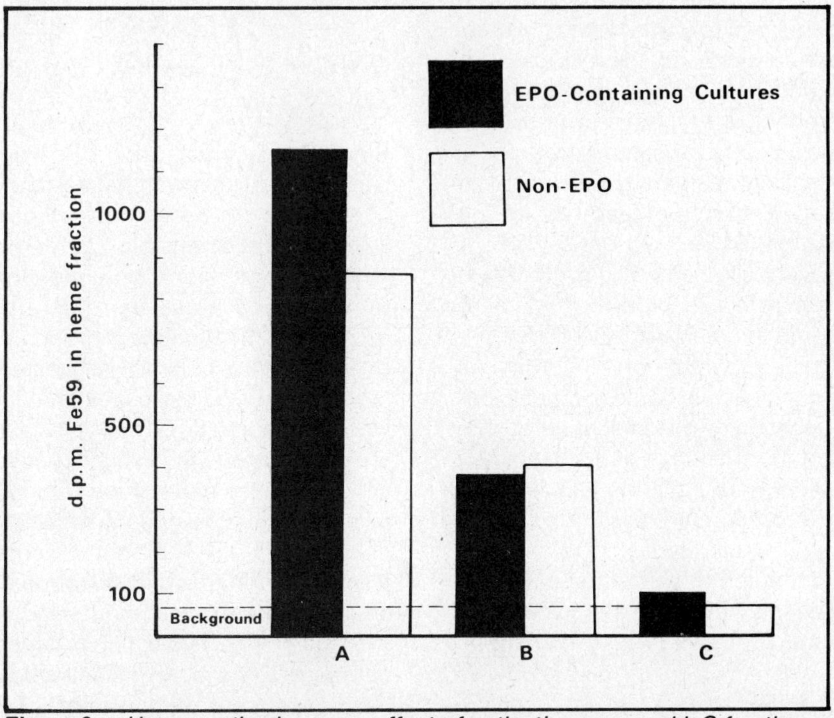

Figure 3. *Heme synthesis assay: effect of patient's serum and IgG fraction on control marrow. EPO = erythropoietin 0.2 U/ml. Addition of patient's serum and IgG fraction prepared from that serum significantly reduced heme synthesis (p <0.05).* ***A,*** *cultures with AB serum.* ***B,*** *cultures with patient's serum (April 19).* ***C,*** *cultures with patient's IgG (April 19).*

TABLE I Results of an Experiment Made in Quadruplicate in Erythroid Colony Growth in Control Marrow Comparing the Patient's Serum Obtained at Various Times to Control Serum

Source of Serum	Date Obtained	No. of Colonies/10^5 Cells				Mean
Normal AB		158	196	210	214	195
Patient	4/5/74	41	34	32	40	37
Patient	4/19/74	9	15	31	25	20
Patient	8/16/74	0	0	0	0	0

NOTE: The results obtained from the three samples of the patient's serum do not differ significantly from each other but differ substantially from the normal AB serum ($p < 0.001$).

TABLE II Erythroid Colony Growth of Patient's Marrow; Results of Experiments Carried Out in Quadruplicate When the Patient's Own Marrow Was Incubated in the Patient's Serum Obtained at Various Times Compared with the Number of Colonies Obtained with Normal Serum

Source of Serum	Date Obtained	No. of Colonies/10^5 Cells				Mean
Normal AB		129	80	98	77	96
Patient	4/9/74	46	30	38	40	39
Patient	8/16/74	0	0	0	0	0

NOTE: The results obtained from the samples to which patient's serum had been added differ significantly from those obtained when normal AB serum was added (p 0.005).

Mixing experiments were performed to detect the presence of an inhibitor. Marrow from control subjects with normal erythropoiesis or marrow from the patient was cultured with 2.0 U erythropoietin/ml in the presence of AB serum or the patient's serum obtained on April 5, April 19, and August 16, 1974.

Standard statistical methods were used in the analysis of the data [14].

RESULTS

Heme Synthesis. The results of culturing normal marrow in AB serum and in serum obtained from the patient on two separate days are shown in Figure 2. In the cultures with AB serum there was a greater than sevenfold increase of heme synthesis in the presence of erythropoietin as compared to unstimulated cultures. When the patient's serum was used, there was no difference between erythropoietin-containing cultures and those without erythropoietin. If heme synthesis in erythropoietin-containing cultures is compared, there was at least tenfold inhibition when the patient's serums were used in place of AB serum. These results are significantly different $p < 0.01$.

The effect of the patient's IgG on heme synthesis of normal marrow is shown in Figure 3. Once again, there was stimulation of heme synthesis in erythropoietin-containing cultures in the presence of AB serum. As before, there was no difference in heme synthesis between erythropoietin-containing and unstimulated cultures in the presence of the patient's serum. This effect was also demonstrated by the patient's IgG. If heme synthesis in erythropoietin-containing cultures is compared, there was at least threefold inhibition in the presence of the patient's serum and at least 12-fold inhibition when the patient's IgG was used in place of AB serum. Since heme synthesis of this marrow in unstimulated cultures was active, inhibition of cultures without erythropoietin by the patient's serum and IgG, was also demonstrated.

Erythroid Colonies. The effect of the patient's serums obtained at various times during the clinical course is shown in Table I. All serum samples resulted in reduction of the number of colonies of normal marrow when compared to AB serum. An unexpected result was the total suppression of colony growth by serum obtained during the patient's "partial remission."

Table II shows the effect of the patient's serums, obtained at various times, on colony growth of autologous marrow obtained during the patient's "partial remission." Serum obtained just prior to her "partial remission" (April 19) continued to demonstrate a suppressive effect. The total suppressive effect of serum obtained during her "partial remission" (August 16) was confirmed on autologous marrow.

The size of the colonies which developed was uninfluenced by the serum used.

COMMENTS

Since the demonstration of serum erythropoietic inhibitors in patients with red cell aplasia, the mechanism of their action has provoked considerable interest. Jepson and Lowenstein [2] originally proposed that inhibition was due to an antierythropoietin, but more recently Jepson and Vas [15] concluded that it was most probably mediated through a cytolytic effect on erythroblasts as originally suggested by Krantz et al. [7]. More recent studies suggest that there are at least two types of inhibitor in red cell aplasia, an antierythropoietin and an inhibitor which acts directly on cells [8]. Krantz [7] recognized that reduced heme synthesis produced by an inhibitor could be the result of suppression of new erythroblast development or destruction of already formed erythroblasts. Subsequently he provided evidence for the existence of an IgG molecule in patients with red cell aplasia which produced cytolysis specifically directed at erythroblasts and which was complement-dependent [9]. It was concluded that at least part of the inhibitory effect was due to an immune-cytolytic action mediated through an antibody or an immune-complex.

The in vitro heme synthesis method is useful for demonstrating the inhibitory effect of plasma, serum and of the IgG fraction on erythropoiesis of human marrow [1,3]. Since the heme synthesis system and the in vivo polycythemic mouse assay system measure only an end product of erythropoiesis, namely, incorporation of radioactive iron, the actual mechanism of inhibition cannot be deduced from these methods.

Field et al. [16] tested the hypothesis that the inhibitor suppresses new erythroblast development with an effect on stem cells; however, the results did not clarify whether or not cytolysis was involved.

With the development of the culture method for detecting erythroid colony growth [13], a technic became available to study the behavior of erythroid precursor cells (CFU-E). CFU-E are erythropoietin-responsive committed cells [17,18] which are progenitors of recognizable erythroblasts [19,20]. Each colony in the erythroid colony system is derived from a single CFU-E. Any effect demonstrated on the number of colonies is therefore a reflection of an effect on erythroid precursors.

In the present study, the heme synthesis system was used to demonstrate the presence of an IgG erythropoietic inhibitor in the serum of a patient with refractory anemia. The inhibitor in this patient is unlikely to represent an antierythropoietin since erythropoietin could be measured in her blood. The erythroid colony system was used to test the effect of the inhibitor on progenitor cells, and an action at this level was demonstrated. However, since erythropoietin acts on differentiated cells as well, inhibition in vivo may not be restricted to the precursor cell [21].

All serum specimens and test materials that could provide complement in the cultures were heat-inactivated. Heat destroys C1 and C2 of the classic complement pathway, as well as factor B of the alternate pathway. The completeness of the heat-treatment was reflected by the lack of detectable total hemolytic complement in the specimens and culture ingredients. However, it is always possible that activated components beyond C3 were present in the treated specimens, but that their presence was not detected. Nevertheless, the action of the IgG inhibitor in our patient seems to differ from that described by Zaentz and Krantz [9], since heat-treatment abolished the inhibitor mechanism in their studies, suggesting complement mediation. Heat had no obvious effect in our experiments, so complement-dependent immune cytolysis is probably not the mechanism of inhibition. Possibly, the action is by direct suppression of new erythroblast development. This hypothesis fits with the observations made by Marmont et al. [8] in exhypoxic polycythemic mice. However, until the patient's serum and/or IgG is tested in the appropriate system, cytolysis of erythroblasts cannot be excluded. Bone marrow lymphocytes may be present in the cultures, and IgG-dependent lymphocyte-mediated cytotoxicity cannot be ruled out.

Two observations argue against a cytolytic mechanism as an explanation of the anemia and in vitro erythropoietic inhibition. Firstly, although the number of colonies was reduced, the size of the colonies that developed was not influenced by the patient's serum. If the inhibitor represented an antierythroblast antibody one would have expected a reduction in the number of cells per colony. Secondly, the inhibitory effect was demonstrated by serum obtained when the patient was in "partial remission" and able to produce a compensatory reticulocytosis, albeit suboptimal, to a fall in hemoglobin level (Figure 1). Such a demonstrable increase in erythropoiesis would be unexpected in the presence of a cytotoxic anitbody; however, it is consistent with a mechanism whereby the marrow may overcome a suppressing influence.

The anemia in this patient has been documented for over two years and its exact etiology is uncertain. Although iron deficiency was suggested in 1972, the red cells were normochromic and normocytic, and the response to iron therapy was incomplete. The studies here were inspired by an episode of severe anemia during which the marrow demonstrated erythroblastopenia when other cellular elements appeared normal. A diagnosis of pure red cell aplasia was considered, and the patient's subsequent recovery was thought to represent an example of the transient spontaneous remissions which patients with this diagnosis may experience. However, the prolonged maintenance of spontaneous remission, with erythroid hyperplasia, and the similarity of this clinical picture to that seen for two years suggest the more likely diagnosis of refractory anemia interrupted by an episode of red cell aplasia. In fact, despite her present anemia, the patient exhibits a compensatory reticulocytosis when her hemoglobin level falls below the usual level of about 10 g/dl (Figure 1).

The most surprising finding in this study is the total inhibitory effect demonstrated by serum obtained during "partial remission." This was a consistent effect which persisted in the serum even after storage at $-20°C$ for three months. The culture plates exposed to this serum have no resemblance to culture plates contaminated with yeast or bacteria, and the inhibition seems to be a true one. This finding casts doubt on the usefulness of the erythroid colony system to predict the clinical course of patients who have inhibitors with the properties observed in our patient. However, there is little doubt that the ability to study the behavior of erythroid precursors and the effects of inhibitors on autologous and isologous marrow can greatly contribute to the understanding of anemias characterized by decreased or abnormal erythropoiesis.

The results reported here confirm and expand other data reported elsewhere [22] and suggest that a similar erythropoietic inhibitor may be present in other patients with idiopathic refractory anemia. Confirmation of this hypothesis would have important implications regarding the true nature of these disorders and would offer hope for new therapeutic approaches.

ACKNOWLEDGMENT

We wish to express our thanks to W. Hiddleston for technical assistance and to L. Leeming and K. MacMillan for their help in preparing the manuscript.

REFERENCES

1. Krantz SB, Kao V: Studies on red cell aplasia. I. Demonstration of a plasma inhibitor to heme synthesis and autoantibody to erythroblast nuclei. Proc Natl Acad Sci USA 58: 493, 1967.
2. Jepson JH, Lowenstein L: Inhibition of erythropoiesis by a factor present in the plasma of patients with erythroblastopenia. Blood 27: 425, 1966.
3. Krantz SB, Kao V: Studies on red cell aplasia. II. Report of a second patient with an antibody to erythroblast nuclei and a remission after immunosuppressive therapy. Blood 34: 1, 1969.
4. Jepson JH, Gardner FH, Degnan T, et al.: A gammaglobulin inhibitor of erythropoiesis in erythroblastopenic plasma from patients with thymoma. Clin Res 16: 536, 1968.
5. Hirst E, Robertson TI: The syndrome of thymoma and erythroblastopenic anemia. Medicine 46: 225, 1967.
6. Krantz SB: Pure red cell aplasia. Br J Haematol 25: 1, 1973.
7. Krantz SB, Moore WH, Zaentz SD: Studies on red cell aplasia. V. Presence of erythroblast cytotoxicity in G-globulin fraction of plasma. J Clin Invest 52: 324, 1973.
8. Marmont A, Peschle C, Sanguineti M, et al.: Pure red cell aplasia (PRCA): response of three patients to cyclophosphamide and/or antilymphocyte globulin (ALG) and demonstration of two types of serum IgG inhibitors to erythropoiesis. Blood 45: 247, 1975.
9. Zaentz SD, Krantz SB: Studies on pure red cell aplasia. VI. Development of two-stage erythroblast cytotoxicity method and role of complement. J Lab Clin Med 82: 31, 1973.
10. Bradstreet CMP, Taylor CED: Technique of complement fixation testing applicable to diagnosis of virus diseases. Mon Bull Min Hlth Publ Hlth Lab Serve 21: 96, 1972.
11. Krantz SB: The effect of erythropoietin on human bone marrow cells in vitro. Life Sci 4: 2393, 1965.
12. Teale FWJ: Cleavage of the heme-protein link by acid methylethylketone. Biochim Biophys Acta 35: 543, 1959.
13. Stephenson JR, Axelrad AA, McLeod DC, et al.: Induction of colonies of hemoglobin-synthesizing cells by erythropoietin in vitro. Proc Natl Acad Sci USA 68: 1542, 1971.
14. Sokal RR, Rolf FJ: Biometry, San Francisco, W.H. Freeman & Co., 1969.
15. Jepson JH, Vas M: Decreased in vivo and in vitro erythropoiesis induced by plasma of ten patients with thymoma, lymphosarcoma, or idiopathic erythroblastopenia. Cancer Res 34: 1325, 1974.
16. Field EO, Caughi MN, Blackett NM, et al.: Marrow-suppressing factors in the blood in pure red-cell aplasia, thymoma and Hodgkin's disease. Br J Haematol 15: 101, 1968.
17. Iscove NN, Sieber F, Winterhalter KH: Erythroid colony formation in cultures of mouse and human bone marrow: analysis of the requirement for erythropoietin by gel filtration and affinity chromatography on agarose—concanavalin A. J Cell Physiol 83: 309, 1974.
18. Cooper MC, Levy J, Cantor LN, et al.: The effect of erythropoietin on colonial growth of erythroid precursor cells in vitro. Proc Natl Acad Sci USA 71: 1677, 1974.
19. Gregory CJ, McCulloch EA, Till JE: Erythropoietic progenitors capable of colony formation in culture: state of differentiation. J Cell Physiol 81: 411, 1973.
20. Tepperman AD, Curtis JE, McCulloch EA: Erythropoietic colonies in cultures of human marrow. Blood 44: 659, 1974.
21. Necheles TF, Sheehan RG, Meyer HJ: Studies on the control of hemoglobin synthesis: nucleic acid synthesis and normoblast proliferation in the presence of erythropoietin. Ann NY Acad Sci 149: 449, 1968.
22. Browman GP, Freedman MH, Blajchman MA, et al.: An erythropoietic inhibitor acting at the "Stem Cell" level in refractory anaemia. Clin Res p 742 A, 1974.

Hypertension, Hyperreninemia and a Solitary Renal Cyst in an Adolescent

H. JOSEPHINE ROSE, M.D.
ALBERT W. PRUITT, M.D.
Atlanta, Georgia

Solitary renal cysts associated with hypertension and documented hyperreninemia are relatively uncommon. A 13 year old boy with these findings is described (pressure 160/120 mm Hg). Contrast studies of the urinary tract and arteriography with selective renal vein sampling demonstrated a solitary cyst in the right kidney. The ratio of plasma renin activity in the right renal vein to left renal vein (RRV:LRV) was 2.35:1. After drainage of the cyst, there was a marked reduction in both systolic and diastolic pressures (126/84 mm Hg). Hypertension has not recurred during 14 months' follow-up.

Hypertension in children and adolescents is often secondary to an underlying condition and has been associated with renal, adrenal, cardiac and other causes [1].

We recently treated a patient in whom increased blood pressure was associated with the relatively uncommon disorder of a solitary renal cyst and documented hyperreninemia. Upon drainage of the cyst and partial removal of the sac, the patient's hypertension and increased plasma renin activity decreased immediately.

CASE REPORT

A 13 year old black boy was admitted to the Grady Memorial Hospital for evaluation of hypertension discovered during a routine physical examination for school. Repeated measurements prior to admission revealed a blood pressure of 160/120 mm Hg in the arm. The patient was asymptomatic.

There was no known past history or family history of hypertension, renal disease or heart disease.

Physical examination on admission revealed a slightly overweight adolescent who appeared in excellent health. His weight was 61 kg (greater than the 84th percentile) and his height was 136 cm (slightly less than the 84 per cent percentile using the growth charts from the State University of Iowa). Blood pressure measurements in the arm were 150/110 mm Hg with the patient supine, 164/108 mm Hg with the patient standing and 150/100 mm Hg in the leg. All measurements were made using the appropriate size cuff. The cardiovascular examination was otherwise within normal limits. The optic fundi were normal. There were no bruits over the flank or abdomen, and femoral pulses were present bilaterally.

A complete blood count was within normal limits. Other blood studies disclosed the following: sodium 144 meq/liter, potassium 4.2 meq/liter, chloride 107 meq/liter, carbon dioxide 23 meq/liter, fasting blood sugar 105 mg/100 ml, blood urea nitrogen 14 mg/100 ml and creatinine 1.0 mg/100

From the Departments of Pediatrics and Pharmacology, Emory University School of Medicine, Atlanta, Georgia. This study was supported by U.S. Public Health Grants D-001031 and HD 01275 (H.J.R.). Requests for reprints should be addressed to Dr. H. Josephine Rose, Emory University School of Medicine, Woodruff Memorial Building, Atlanta, Georgia 30322. Manuscript accepted February 25, 1976.

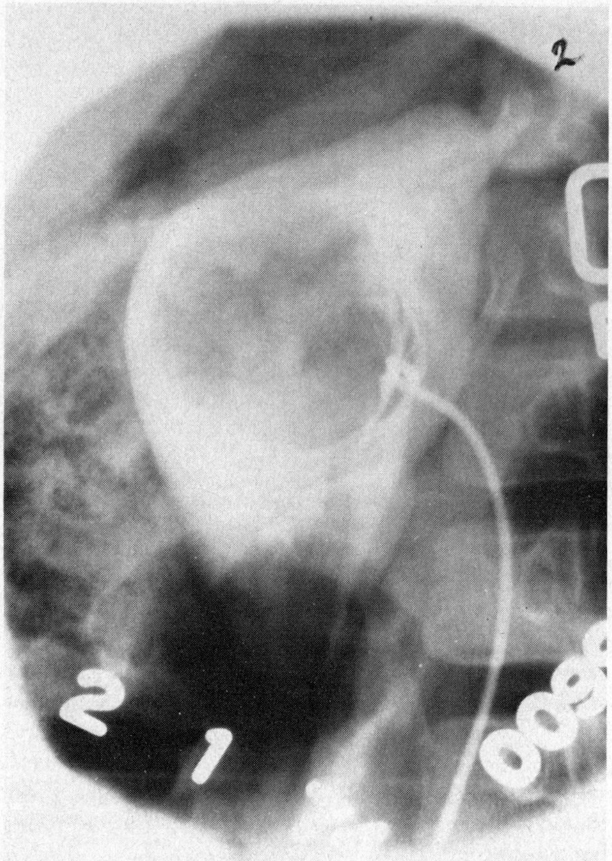

Figure 1. *Pyelogram. A constrast study of the urinary tract showing a mass in the upper pole of the right kidney.*

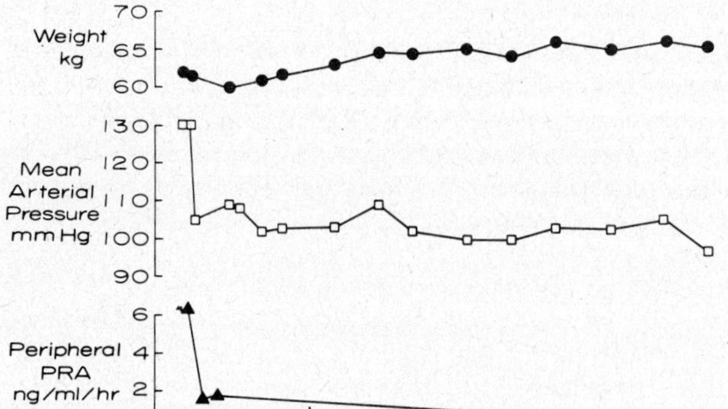

Figure 3. *Changes in mean arterial pressure, peripheral plasma renin activity (PRA) and weight with time. Drainage of the cyst coincides with the marked decrease in mean arterial pressure and PRA. (Mean arterial pressure calculated as diastolic + one-third pulse pressure.)*

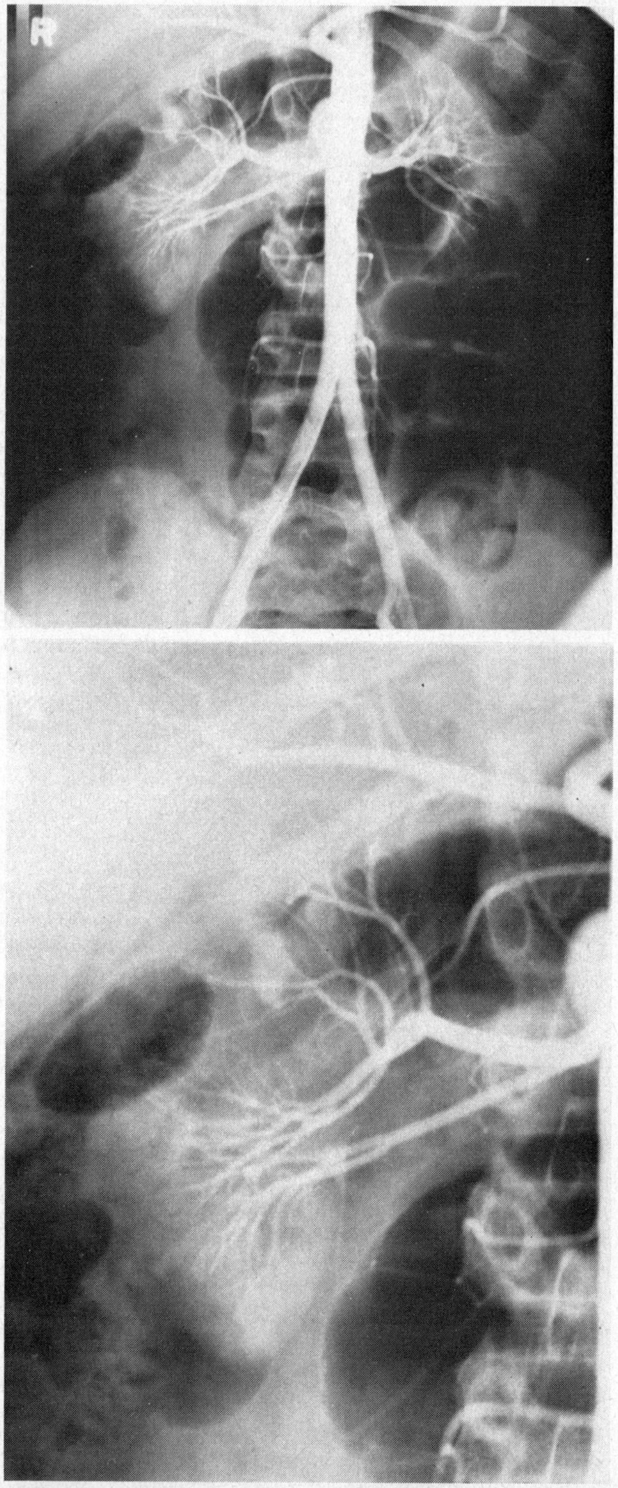

Figure 2. *Arteriogram demonstrating both renal arteries and intrarenal vessels and the avascular cystic mass in the mid-portion of the right kidney **(top),** and more detail of the avascular mass in the mid-portion **(bottom).***

TABLE I Plasma Renin Activity Before Surgery

Site	ng/ml/hour*
Right renal vein	18.13
Left renal vein	7.71
Inferior vena cava	6.31

* Normal values = with preparation <4.5 ng/ml/hour, without preparation <3.0 ng/ml/hour.

ml. Creatinine clearance was 92 ml/min/1.73 m^2 body surface area. Results of urine studies, including a urinalysis, 24-hour excretion of vanillylmandelic acid, urinary 17-hydroxycorticosteroids and 17-ketosteroids, were within normal limits. Chest film and electrocardiogram were also within normal limits. Contrast studies of the urinary tract disclosed splaying of the right renal pelvis with a mass in the upper pole of the kidney (Figure 1). No ureteral obstruction of the kidney was noted. The left kidney appeared normal.

Selective renal arteriography with injection into the right renal artery demonstrated an avascular cystic mass in the mid-portion of the right kidney with stretching of several superior and middle intrarenal vessels. The left renal artery and intrarenal vessels appeared normal (Figure 2). Plasma samples for measurement of plasma renin activity were obtained from the renal veins and inferior vena cava (Table I). The patient was treated with a low sodium diet and furosemide the day before the study so that 2 per cent of the body weight was lost. Samples were obtained with the patient in a supine position. Plasma renin activity was measured by the radioimmunoassay of angiotensin I using a technic similar to that described by Haber et al. [2]. Plasma was collected in chilled Vacutainer tubes (Becton, Dickinson & Co., Rutherford, N.J.) containing EDTA, centrifuged in the cold and stored at −20°C until the time of assay. After the addition of neomycin, dimercaprol and 8-hydroxyquinoline, and adjustment of pH to 7.4 ± 0.05 with 1.5 N hydrochloric acid, incubation for generation of angiotensin I was carried out at 37°C for 3 hours. Each sample was assayed in duplicate. Results are expressed in nanograms per milliliter per hour.

After completion of these studies the patient underwent surgery and a solitary cyst was located in the upper pole of the right kidney. The pressure within the cyst was 11 to 12 cm H_2O. The cyst was drained and most of the wall was removed. Immediately after surgery blood pressure in the arm was 126/84 mm Hg (supine); five days later it was 134/70 (supine) and 128/82 mm Hg (standing). Plasma renin activity measured in a peripheral vein with the patient ambulatory, eight days after surgery and after the patient had been pretreated with furosemide, was 1.57 ng/ml/hour (normal). The patient was discharged; no medication was prescribed. On microscopic examination, the cyst was benign.

Subsequently, the patient continued asymptomatic. Three weeks after surgery, the plasma renin activity in a peripheral vein was 1.78 ng/ml/hour (normal). All values in peripheral veins were obtained without pretreating the patient and while he was ambulatory. His blood pressure during this time was 130/90 mm Hg and, because a slight increase persisted, he was treated with trichlormethiazide (4 mg daily). After three months administration of the drug was discontinued, and during the next six months the patient's blood pressure was not greater than 134/92 mm Hg (Figure 3). Plasma renin activity in a peripheral vein 11 1/2 months after surgery was 0.4 ng/ml/hour. The patient's blood pressure 14 months after drainage of the cyst was 128/80 mm Hg.

COMMENTS

Goldblatt et al. [3] in 1934 demonstrated reproducible hypertension by renal artery constriction in the dog. Since then, unilateral renal disease has been considered a significant cause of hypertension. Subsequently, many conditions relating hypertension to disease of the renal vasculature and parenchyma have been discussed. These have included renal artery stenosis, Wilms' tumor and solitary renal cysts [1]. More recently, increased plasma renin activity has been associated with many causes of hypertension associated with kidney disease.

In 1942, the first case of a solitary renal cyst and hypertension was reported [4] in an 18 year old person in whom the renal cyst was secondary to blunt abdominal trauma. Since then, several other cases have been reported and the coexisting hypertension in all these cases was corrected by nephrectomy [5,6]. Also, Smith in 1956 [7] reported on the surgical treatment of hypertension in 149 cases, in two of which a solitary renal cyst was present. In a review of 500 cases of hypertension and renal disease [8], 100 patients with single or multiple renal cysts were matched with an equal number of patients with glomerulonephritis, pyelonephritis and renal tumor or primary hypertension with renal disease. Nine patients in the first group had solitary cysts, but none became normotensive after nephrectomy. Plasma renin activity was not determined in these earlier studies.

Solitary renal cysts in patients with documented increases in plasma renin activity have only recently been reported in the literature. There are two other reports of the association between a solitary renal cyst and hyperreninemia [9,10]. In a 14 year old boy, whose blood pressure was 130/90 mm Hg, the ratio of angiotensin I generated in the right renal vein to left renal vein (RRV:LRV) was 2.67:0.77 ng/ml/hour [9]. One and a half years after drainage of the cyst, his blood pressure was 120/80 mm Hg. The other case with documented hyperreninemia was in a 60 year old man whose blood pressure ranged from 140 to 210/110 mm Hg with RRV:LRV ratio 570:98 ng angiotensin II/100 ml plasma [10]. After surgery his blood pressure remained at 130/80 mm Hg for nine months.

Thus it appears that renal cysts can produce localized areas of renal ischemia, and associated renovascular hypertension and hyperreninemia. The RRV:LRV ratio of 2.35:1 in our patient and the increased plasma renin activity in a peripheral vein initially indicated that excess renin production could be responsible for the hypertension. Postoperatively both peripheral plasma renin activity and the blood pressure decreased and have remained so for one year. It has been reported that plasma renin activity between the affected and unaffected kidney of greater than 1.5:1 in renal artery stenosis [11] predicts a favorable result from surgery. Our patient responded well to surgery and one year later has had no recurrence of his hypertension.

REFERENCES

1. Loggie JMH: Hypertension in children and adolescents. I. Causes and diagnostic studies. J Pediatr 74: 331, 1969.
2. Haber E, Koerner T, Page LB, et al.: Application of a radioimmunoassay for angiotensin I to the physiologic activity in normal subjects. J Clin Endocrinol Metab 29: 1349, 1969.
3. Goldblatt H, Lynch J, Hanzal RF, et al.: Studies on experimental hypertension. I. The production of persistent elevation of systolic blood pressure by means of renal ischemia. J Exp Med 59: 347, 1934.
4. Farrell JI, Young RH: Hypertension caused by unilateral renal compression. JAMA 118: 711, 1942.
5. Pearce AE, Bower JO, Burns JC: Uncomplicated, solitary, serous renal cyst with hypertension relieved by nephrocystectomy. Ann Intern Med 29: 994, 1944.
6. Kreutzmann HAR: Hypertension associated with solitary renal cyst: report of two cases. J Urol 57: 467, 1947.
7. Smith HW: Unilateral nephrectomy in hypertensive disease. J Urol 76: 685, 1956.
8. Hunt JC, Strong CG, Harrison EG, et al.: Management of hypertension of renal origin. Am J Cardiol 26: 280, 1970.
9. Babka JC, Cohen MS, Sode J: Solitary intrarenal cyst causing hypertension. N Engl J Med 291: 343, 1974.
10. Rockson SG, Stone RA, Gunnells JC: Solitary renal cyst with segmental ischemia and hypertension. J Urol 112: 550, 1974.
11. Michelakis AM, Foster JH, Liddle GW, et al.: Measurement of renin in both renal veins: its use in diagnosis of renovascular hypertension. Arch Intern Med 120: 444, 1967.

Letters to the Editor will be published, if suitable, and as space permits. They should not exceed 500 words in length, typed double space, and may be subject to editing or abridgment. If bibliographic references are necessary, they should not exceed five and should conform to the standards of the Journal. When a single table, graph, diagram or photograph will amplify or clarify the thoughts, it will be printed if space and expense permit. Letters should be addressed, To the Editor, and mailed to The American Journal of Medicine, 666 Fifth Avenue, New York, New York 10019.

LEAD NEPHROPATHY

To the Editor:

In the paper "Occupational Lead Nephropathy" by Wedeen and associates (Am J Med 59: 630, 1975), the authors conclude that "The finding of three cases of lead nephropathy in workers whose blood lead levels would be considered acceptable (<80 μg/100 ml) suggests that a reevaluation of these criteria (NIOSH-blood lead under 80 μg/100 ml is safe) may be warranted." The first patient had heavy exposure to lead for five years, anemia four years before admission, repeated hospitalization for epigastric pain and frequent vomiting lasting five days each month. Blood lead levels during this period are not reported. From the history of heavy exposure to lead and the chronic symptoms, it is quite likely that the blood lead levels in the past were periodically unacceptably high (over 80 μg/100 ml). In the other two cases classified as preclinical renal dysfunction, the patients showed slightly reduced glomerular filtration rate. Without some indication of the variability of glomerular filtration rate values obtained in an adequate control population, the significance of a slightly reduced glomerular filtration rate is open to question. No changes in tubular function were noted. Blood lead levels in the past are not reported. In one other case of preclinical renal dysfunction with least impairment, the patient's blood lead levels in the past were unacceptably elevated at 182 μg/100 ml (current level 98 μg/100 ml) with a history of lead colic within one week of the study. The renal pathologic changes are not pathognomonic for lead nephropathy as presently recognized. The authors state, "In the absence of a specific reversible renal tubular lesion, the diagnosis of lead nephropathy is more difficult to prove in the three other patients we describe here." Renal damage from exposure to lead after persistent elevations of blood lead levels *over* 80 μg/100 ml has been documented. The National Institute for Safety and Health requires that blood lead level be *maintained* under 80 μg/100 ml to protect the worker from lead toxicity. The data in the present study do not show that renal damage occurs when blood leads have been *maintained* below this level. The data do warrant another look at nephropathy in lead workers. In the future, to draw firm conclusions about the relationship of blood lead levels to lead nephropathy, more data on blood lead concentration in the past will be needed than was apparently available to Dr. Wedeen and his associates. Perhaps a more appropriate title for the paper would have been "Nephropathy in Lead Workers."

Sidney Lerner, M.D.
Assistant Professor of Environmental Health
Paul B. Hammond, D.V.M., Ph.D.
Professor of Environmental Health

The Author's Reply:

Drs. Lerner and Hammond point out that our patients with lead nephropathy may have had elevated blood lead levels before examination by us and imply that maintenance of the blood lead level under 80 μg/100 ml affords satisfactory protection. Unfortunately, although the blood lead level may be used to estimate current lead exposure, our data indicate that it fails to provide a reliable assessment of the cumulative hazard of lead. At any given time after exposure, blood lead levels may be in the "acceptable" range despite lead-induced organ damage. With one exception at the time of our study, the blood lead level did not indicate the possibility of lead toxicity. The potential hazard to workers who are removed from lead exposure for any reason may therefore easily be overlooked.

Monitoring of blood lead levels is inadequate to protect workers from lead nephropathy and may lead to inappropriate and ill-advised treatment. As long as the blood lead level standard is solely relied upon, elevated blood lead levels may be lowered simply to comply with Federal regulations. There is good reason to doubt that treatment of the patient's "blood lead" will protect against lead nephropathy. Removal of persons with excessive body lead burdens from heavy exposure to lead may lead to "acceptable" blood lead levels despite progression of renal disease from lead. Dr. Lerner is not unaware of this problem, as indicated in the following quotation from a recent AFL-CIO health bulletin [1]:

> "The use of chelating agents in pill form in the National Lead plant had been limited by an agreement between the company's medical consultant, Dr. Sidney Lerner, and George Becker, the Steelworkers' safety representative. At a meeting on lead last year, sponsored by the Society for Occupational and Environmental Health, Becker accused the company of

> improperly using chelating drugs for prophylactic purposes. Under pressure from members of the ethics committee of the American Occupational Medical Association, Lerner agreed to stop the illegal practice."

Our recent data suggest that blood lead values greater than 25 μg Pb/100 ml may be associated with occupational lead nephropathy in workers who have been removed from continuous exposure. Even the 60 μg Pb/100 ml standard recently proposed by OSHA [2] would fail to arouse suspicion of lead toxicity in 12 of the 17 patients we have identified with occupational lead nephropathy. The diagnosis of "renal disease" in our paper is based mainly on the glomerular filtration rate, although in each case the effective renal plasma flow (C_{PAH}) was comparably reduced. Histologic changes confirmed the physiologic abnormalities in all nine cases in which renal biopsy specimens have been obtained. Glomerular filtration rate is particularly valuable for assessing renal dysfunction because of the plethora of normal data in the literature. We referred to the data of Homer Smith for the normal range because of its universal acceptance. The term "renal dysfunction" was reserved for lead workers whose glomerular filtration rates were more than 2 SD below the "normal" mean value. In the same issue of *The American Journal of Medicine* as our report, Berger and Yü presented extensive data on the glomerular filtration rate in patients with gout. These subjects may well represent more appropriate "controls" than normal subjects for our lead workers. Our corrected standards for age and body surface area remain valid when compared with their data.

I nevertheless agree that obtaining appropriate controls remains important and dfficult. Although there are many approaches, my view is that the most reliable method is to use the patient as his own control. This ideal has been met in two cases in which chelation therapy resulted in an increase in glomerular filtration rate. Although reversal of renal dysfunction by chelation therapy provides both the best "control" data and the strongest evidence of a causal relationship, such compelling information will be difficult to accumulate. Less conclusive, but suggestive evidence is appropriate during the interim. Diagnosis by "exclusion" is an essential step in making rational decisions. When no other cause of renal disease can be identified, it seems appropriate to offer chelation therapy to workers with renal dysfunction and excessive body lead burdens. I therefore believe the term "occupational lead nephropathy" is both appropriate and essential even at this stage of investigation. We have now examined renal function in 41 lead workers including the eight described in our report. Of these, 17 have had glomerular filtration rates less than 90 ml/min/1.73 m^2. In each case, C_{PAH} and renal biopsy specimens showed concordant renal abnormalities. It is difficult for me to imagine that we are seeing coincidence or trivial renal findings. With these additional data, to doubt that occupational lead nephropathy occurs with normal blood lead levels strains credulity.

RICHARD P. WEDEEN, M.D.
Director, Department of Medicine
Jersey City Medical Center
Jersey City, New Jersey 07304

References

1. IUD Spotlight on Health and Safety, Industrial Union Department, American Federation of Labor—Congress of Industrial Organizations, vol 5 (No. 1), First Quarter, 1976.
2. Federal Register, vol 40, No. 193, October 3, 1975.

LUNG BIOPSY IN IMMUNOCOMPROMISED HOSTS

To the Editor:

In "Lung Biopsy in Immunocompromised Hosts" (Am J Med 59: 488, 1975), Table X states that our specific diagnoses totalled only 31 per cent. Since no such figure appeared in our report [1], the authors may have interpreted our classification of "interstitial pneumonitis and fibrosis" as nonspecific. Quite the reverse is true [2]. Our patients had microscopic examination of transbronchial biopsy specimens of the lung. The common clinical features were dry rales, digital clubbing, altered immune activity and a characteristic pattern on chest films. With many biopsy findings now correlated with the clinical picture, we believe that in most patients with classic interstitial pneumonitis with fibrosis, lung biopsy is not needed to prove the illness. Therefore, the separation of these patients with diffuse interstitial pneumonitis from those with a specific diagnosis seems unjustified.

HOWARD A. ANDERSEN, M.D.
Mayo Clinic
Rochester, Minnesota 55901

References

1. Andersen HA, Fontana RS: Transbronchoscopic lung biopsy for diffuse pulmonary diseases: technique and results in 450 cases. Chest 62: 125, 1972.
2. DeRemee RA, Harrison EG Jr, Andersen HA: The concept of classic interstitial pneumonitis-fibrosis (CIP-F) as a clinicopathologic syndrome. Chest 61: 213, 1972.

The Authors' Reply:

The source of the data in Table X is exactly as Doctor Andersen described. We took similar license with other reports to obtain comparable data for the same table. We do not argue with the entity of classic interstitial pneumonitis with fibrosis. The thrust of our paper was to define the frequency with which a specifically treatable lesion was encountered in progressive pulmonary lesions in compromised hosts. Accordingly we defined our terms as "specific" (treatable) and "nonspecific" (untreatable) under "Diagnostic Yield" in our results. For internal consistency, we kept this division when reviewing the literature, and we intended no slight upon classic interstitial pneumonitis with fibrosis as a clinicopathologic syndrome. We commented that our experience with transbronchial biopsy was limited.

RICHARD L. GREENMAN, M.D.
PATRICK T. GOODALL, M.D.
DONALD KING, A.B.
Division of Infectious Diseases
Department of Medicine
School of Medicine
University of Miami
Miami, Florida 33152

NOVEMBER 1976

The American Journal of Medicine

VOLUME 61

NUMBER 5

EDITORIAL

Intravascular Coagulation Associated with the Adult Respiratory Distress Syndrome

ROGER C. BONE, M.D.*
P. BAILEY FRANCIS, M.D.†
ALAN K. PIERCE, M.D.
Dallas, Texas

In seven of 30 consecutive patients with the adult respiratory distress syndrome, disseminated intravascular coagulation (DIC) developed. Increasing respiratory dysfunction characterized by decreased effective static compliance and increased hypoxemia coincided with the development of DIC. Patients in whom DIC developed were characterized by a high incidence of bleeding, gangrene of the extremities, renal dysfunction, mortality and autopsy evidence of fibrin microthrombi in the lungs, kidney and skin.

In 12 of 23 patients who did not meet the criteria for DIC, the platelet count decreased by at least 50 per cent of the initial values at some time during their illness. Fibrin microthrombi were found in the lungs in the majority of the patients subjected to autopsy. These data support the concept that deposition of platelets on damaged pulmonary capillary endothelium may be more common in the adult respiratory distress syndrome than the DIC syndrome.

The adult respiratory distress syndrome is characterized by diffuse pulmonary capillary endothelial injury [1] leading to predictable clinical, physiologic and pathologic manifestations [2]. A relationship between pulmonary capillary endothelial damage and thrombocyte function has been demonstrated in experimental animal models [3–6]. Such injury in dogs and rabbits has resulted in a prolonged platelet transit time through the lung and decreased platelet recovery from the lung compared to animals with normal pulmonary vasculature. Moreover, decreased platelet recovery was correlated with a decrease in pulmonary compliance and an increase in physiologic shunting. Histologically, platelet thrombi were observed in small blood vessels.

From the Pauline and Adolph Weinberger Laboratory for Cardiopulmonary Research, Department of Internal Medicine, University of Texas Southwestern Medical School at Dallas, Dallas, Texas. Requests for reprints should be addressed to Dr. Roger C. Bone. Manuscript accepted April 5, 1976.

* Present address: Department of Medicine, University of Kansas Medical Center, Rainbow Boulevard at 39th Street, Kansas City, Kansas 66103.

† Trainee, U.S. Public Health Service Training Grant HE 05812. Present address: Department of Medicine, Atlanta Veterans Administration Hospital, Atlanta, Georgia 30033.

TABLE I Features of Patients with Disseminated Intravascular Coagulation (DIC)

Etiology of ARDS	Platelets Within 72 hr of ARDS (mm^3)	Hypo-tension*	Abnormal Hemorrhage†	Ischemic Necrosis	Autopsy Evidence of DIC‡
Viral pneumonia	56,000§	+	VS	Right forearm and hand (arterial catheter)	No autopsy
Gastric acid aspiration	19,500	+	VS	None	No autopsy
Gastric acid aspiration	119,000	+	VS, GI, P	Right thumb and index finger (arterial catheter)	Lungs, kidneys, skin
Gastric acid aspiration	38,000§	–	VS, GI	All extremities	Lungs, kidneys, skin
Viral pneumonia	10,000§	–	VS, GI	All extremities	Lungs, kidneys, skin
Pseudomonas aeruginosa septicemia	69,000	+	VS, GI, P	Acrocyanosis	Lungs, kidneys
Noxious gas inhalation	93,000	+	VS	Right thumb and index finger (arterial catheter)	Lungs

NOTE: ARDS = adult respiratory distress syndrome. + = present. – = absent.
* Hypotension was defined by a systolic blood pressure less than 90 mm Hg for 1 hour or longer within 72 hours of beginning PEEP.
† VS = venipuncture sites, GI = gastrointestinal, P = petechiae and/or purpura.
‡ Fibrin microthrombi of small blood vessels was taken as evidence of DIC.
§ Schistocytes seen on microscopic examination of peripheral blood.

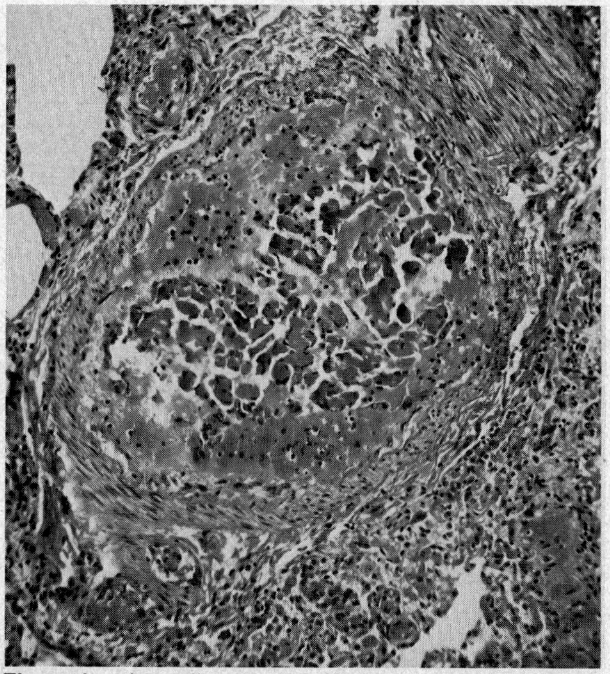

Figure 1. *A small muscular pulmonary artery from one of our patients with DIC. Hematoxylin and eosin stain; original magnification × 100, reduced by 12 per cent. Multiple small vessels were largely occluded by fibrin microthrombi. Beginning fibroblastic proliferation and endothelialization can be seen.*

A possible association between the adult respiratory distress syndrome and the clinical manifestations of intravascular platelet deposition, disseminated intravascular coagulation (DIC), has been suggested by an occasional case report [7,8]. However, a relationship between the adult respiratory distress syndrome and DIC has not been established. This study was undertaken to determine if such exists.

METHODS

The records of 30 consecutive patients with the adult respiratory distress syndrome admitted to the Parkland Memorial Hospital medical intensive care unit from July 1, 1972, to June 1, 1974, were reviewed. All patients were treated by one of us. In order to compare patients with an illness of similar severity, only patients with arterial oxygen tensions (PaO_2) of 70 mm Hg or less, despite inspired oxygen concentrations (F_IO_2) of 50 per cent or greater during assisted ventilation with positive end-expiratory pressure (PEEP), were included. Patients whose adult respiratory distress syndrome was associated with trauma or surgery, or who received blood transfusions or antifibrinolytic agents before the onset of bleeding secondary to intravascular coagulation, were excluded from analysis.

Patients were diagnosed as having DIC only when all the following abnormalities of blood coagulation existed: the platelet count was less than 125,000/mm^3, the Quick prothrombin time was 3 seconds greater than control [9], the activated partial thromboplastin time [10] was greater than

47 seconds, the thrombin time [11] was greater than 25 seconds and fibrin split products, analyzed by the staphylococcal clumping technic [12], were greater than 40 μg/ml.

Two measurements of lung function were analyzed. First, the effective static compliance of the lungs and thorax was determined by dividing the exhaled tidal volume by inflation hold pressure minus the PEEP as measured by the ventilator manometer. Second, the ratio of arterial:alveolar oxygen tension was computed [13]. A value less than 0.75 represents abnormal oxygen transfer by the lung. This ratio was used because it is more reliable than other parameters as an index of gas exchange when comparing patients receiving different concentrations of inspired oxygen [13].

Statistical analysis was performed by Student's t test or Chi square analysis. The probability of an observation occurring by chance alone less than 5 per cent of the time ($P < 0.05$) was considered significant.

RESULTS

In seven of 30 (23 per cent) consecutive patients with adult respiratory distress syndrome, DIC developed. Clinical and pathologic data for these seven patients are recorded in Table I. All patients had clinical as well as laboratory evidence of abnormal blood coagulation. All these patients died. Five of the seven patients who died were examined at autopsy and fibrin microthrombi were present in their lungs (Figure 1); four of five had thrombi in additional tissues (Table I).

Data in patients with DIC are compared with those in patients without intravascular coagulation in Table II. We were unable to distinguish the two groups on the basis of the presumed etiology of the adult respiratory distress syndrome, age, sex, the presence of bacteremia, hypotension, adrenal cortical steroid treatment, renal function, survival or survival time. There was a marked difference in sequential platelet counts in patients in whom DIC developed compared to patients in whom it did not develop (Figure 2).

Respiratory function in the two groups of patients is compared in Figures 3 and 4. In those patients in whom DIC developed oxygen exchange and compliance were significantly worse after the onset of DIC than in those in whom this syndrome did not develop, although the two groups had similarly deranged functions at the outset. In patients with DIC, lung function was also significantly worse after the syndrome developed than it was previously.

In 23 of the patients who did not meet our laboratory criteria for DIC, clinical symptoms of this syndrome did not develop. However, 12 of these patients had a decrease in circulating platelets of at least 50 per cent of their intial values at some time during their illness. Five of these patients who died were subjected to autopsy; two had megakaryocytic hyperplasia of the bone marrow and four had fibrin microthrombi in the lungs but not in other tissues.

TABLE II **Comparison of Seven Patients With and 23 Patients Without Disseminated Intravascular Coagulation (DIC)**

	Patients With DIC	Patients Without DIC	P
Age (yr, $\overline{M} \pm SD$)	42 ± 14	38 ± 16	NS*
Men	5	14	NS
Positive blood cultures (%)	57	30	NS
Hypotension (%)†	71	61	NS
Adrenal cortical steroids (%)‡	57	30	NS
Blood urea nitrogen (mg/100 ml, $\overline{M} \pm SD$)	46 ± 37	19 ± 11	NS
Mortality (%)	100	71	NS
Survival time (days, M ± SD)	8 ± 1	10 ± 3	NS

* NS = not significant ($p > 0.05$).
† Hypotension was defined by a systolic blood pressure less than 90 mm Hg for 1 hour or longer within 72 hours of beginning PEEP.
‡ Each patient received the equivalent of 5 mg/kg body weight of hydrocortisone or more each 24 hours.

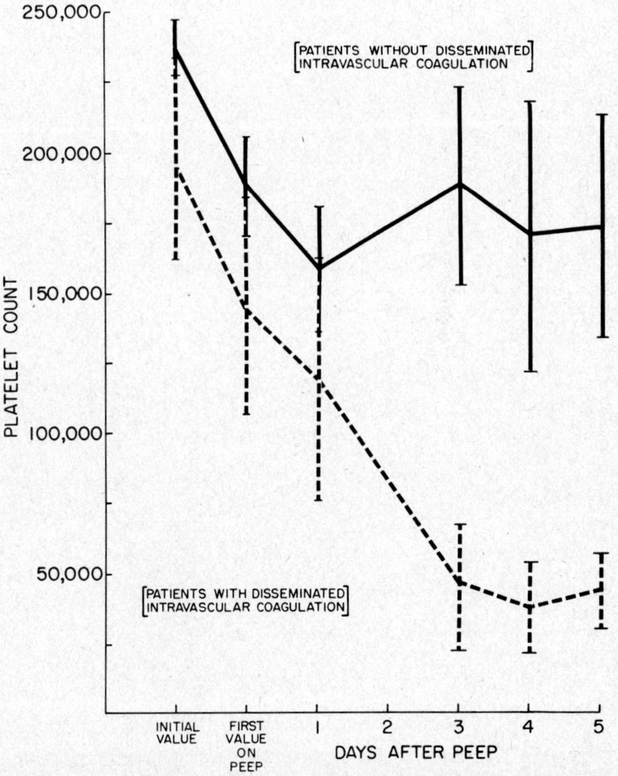

Figure 2. Platelet count of patients with DIC (continuous line) compared to patients without DIC (dashed line). The brackets indicate 1 standard deviation around the mean value. There are no significant differences between the values initially obtained, when PEEP was begun, or during the first day of PEEP. From the third through the fifth days, the platelet counts are significantly different ($P < 0.05$).

COMMENTS

Our data indicate that DIC is a frequent complication in patients with severe adult respiratory distress syndrome. The original etiology of the adult respiratory distress syndrome does not apparently alter the likelihood of DIC developing in patients observed in a medical intensive care unit. Our data do not assess the incidence among patients with surgery or blood transfusions; such patients were excluded from this study, since blood transfusions may independently be associated with thrombocytopenia and selective factor deficiencies. Further, only patients with severe hypoxemia necessitating high concentrations of inspired oxygen and the use of PEEP were studied. The role of any of these factors in the genesis or incidence of DIC in the adult respiratory distress syndrome cannot be determined from this report.

Patients in whom DIC developed had the expected clinical manifestations of excessive hemorrhage and ischemic necrosis of extremities. In addition, the onset of DIC was associated with deterioration of pulmonary function indicated by a progressive fall in compliance and worsening of oxygen transfer by the lung. Since these events were coincidental, it is not clear which are cause and which effect.

Many of the patients in whom DIC did not develop had a decrease in circulating platelets during the course of the adult respiratory distress syndrome. At autopsy, four of five of these patients had fibrin microthrombi in the lungs, and two of five had megakaryocytic hyperplasia of the bone marrow. Pulmonary-capillary endothelial-platelet interaction may be the first step in establishing DIC. In our patients without other clinical evidence of DIC, the presence of thrombocytopenia suggests that platelet aggregation may occur frequently in patients with the adult respiratory distress syndrome. Platelet sequestration may be important in altering vascular permeability. Compensatory increase in platelets and coagulation factors may mask the clinical syndrome of DIC in many patients with the adult respiratory distress syndrome. Pathologic evidence of microthrombi in our patients suggest that intravascular coagulation may be a more frequent event in the adult respiratory distress syndrome than the clinical syndrome of DIC.

Our data in conjunction with the experimental models of others [3–6] suggest a causal relationship between

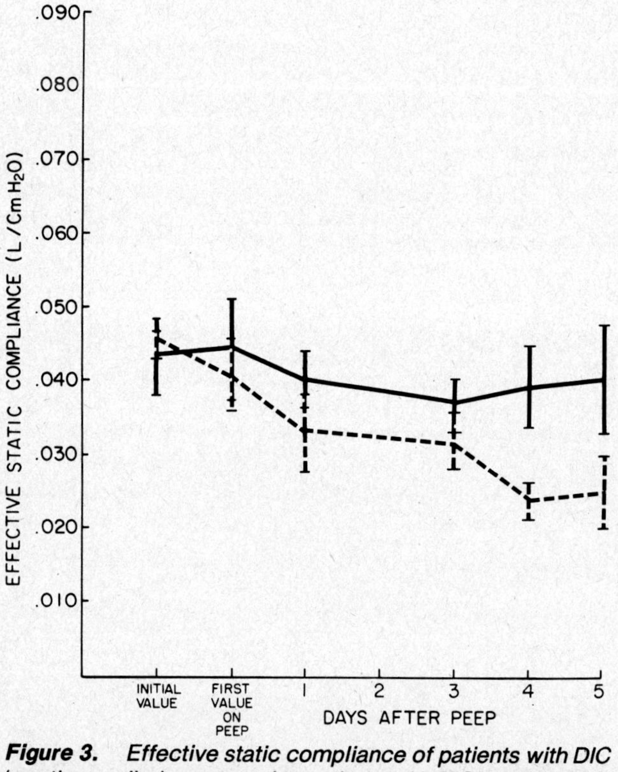

Figure 3. *Effective static compliance of patients with DIC (continuous line) compared to patients with DIC (dashed line). The brackets indicate 1 standard deviation around the mean values. Although this measurement of lung stiffness was similar at the onset of disease and of PEEP therapy, those patients in whom DIC developed had significantly lower effective static compliance than patients without DIC ($P < 0.05$).*

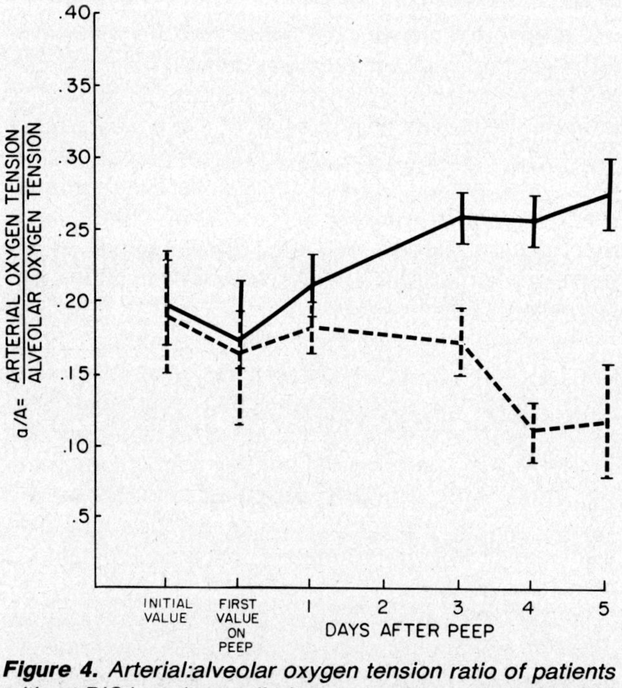

Figure 4. *Arterial:alveolar oxygen tension ratio of patients without DIC (continuous line) compared to patients with DIC (dashed line). The brackets represent 1 standard deviation around the mean values. There are no significant differences between the values initially obtained, when PEEP was begun or during the first day of PEEP. From the third through the fifth days, the ratios in two groups are significantly different ($P < 0.05$).*

limited intravascular coagulation initiated by damage to pulmonary capillary endothelial cells and a perpetuation of the adult respiratory distress syndrome. The platelet release reaction associated with the adherance of platelets to collagen liberates a variety of vasoactive mediators [14]. It is possible that local changes in pulmonary capillary permeability mediated by these substances compound the existing pulmonary edema. Further clinical and experimental studies are needed utilizing labelled fibrinogen and platelets to delineate the importance of fibrin deposition and intravascular coagulation to acute respiratory insufficiency.

REFERENCES

1. Robin ED, Cross CE, Zelis R: Pulmonary edema. N Engl J Med 288: 239, 1973.
2. Pontoppidan H, Geffin B, Lowenstein E: Acute respiratory failure in the adult. N Engl J Med 287: 690, 1972.
3. White MK, Shapiro D, Hechtman HB: Pulmonary function and platelet lung interaction. J Appl Physiol 34: 697, 1973.
4. Moritz E, Border JR, Schueller EF, Schenk WG: Experimental pulmonary fat embolism: effects on pulmonary function by reserpine pretreatment. Arch Surg 105: 275, 1972.
5. Evans G, Mustard JF: Inhibition of the platelet-surface reaction in endotoxin shock and the generalized Schwartzmann reaction. J Clin Invest 47: 31a, 1968.
6. Stein M, Thomas DP: Role of platelets in the acute pulmonary responses to endotoxin. J Appl Physiol 23: 47, 1967.
7. Pleet AB: "Shock lung." Syndrome following diabetic ketoacidosis: treatment with heparin. Chest 63: 434, 1973.
8. Greipp PR, Brown JA, Gralnick NR: Defibrination in acute pancreatitis. Ann Intern Med 76: 73, 1972.
9. Quick AK: Hemorrhagic Diseases and Thrombosis, Philadelphia. Lea & Febiger, 1966, p 395.
10. Proctor RR, Rapoport SI: The partial thromboplastin time with kaolin. Am J Clin Pathol 36: 212, 1961.
11. Verrmylen C, Verstraete M: Antithrombi V: critical evaluation of its assessment and properties. Thromb Diath Haemorrh 5: 267, 1961.
12. Satterwhite TK, Hawiger J, Burklow SL, et al.: Degradation products of fibrinogen and fibrin in bacteremia due to gram-negative rods. J Infect Dis 127: 437, 1973.
13. Gilbert R, Keighley JF: The arterial/alveolar oxygen tension ratio: an index of gas exchange applicable to varying inspired oxygen concentrations. Am Rev Respir Dis 109: 142, 1974.
14. Deykin D: Emerging concepts of platelet function. N Engl J Med 290: 144, 1974.

Diagnosis and Evaluation of Patients with an Enlarged Sella Turcica

LEON A. WEISBERG, M.D.*
EARL A. ZIMMERMAN, M.D.†
ANDREW G. FRANTZ, M.D.
New York, New York

A prospective analysis of the roentgenographic and laboratory parameters in 100 patients with an enlarged sella turcica was made. Seventy-five patients had no visual symptoms: 27 had primary intrasellar tumor; 25 had the empty sella syndrome; 13 had an extrasellar process; and in 10, no final diagnosis was made because air study was omitted. However, these patients remained asymptomatic for up to three years. Eighteen of the patients with a primary intrasellar tumor had symptomatic pituitary dysfunction; nine were asymptomatic. Five of 14 patients studied had elevated plasma prolactin levels. Of the 25 patients with the empty sella syndrome and the 10 patients in whom no final diagnosis was made, none had any clinical endocrine or visual abnormalities, although in 10 of these 35 patients, results of laboratory studies were compatible with pituitary dysfunction. In these cases, air study was necessary to differentiate a clinically silent pituitary tumor from the empty sella syndrome. This emphasizes the high incidence of the empty sella syndrome in patients with enlarged sella, and also confirms the high incidence of hyperprolactinemia in patients with pituitary tumors.

Roentgenographic evidence of an enlarged sella turcica is frequently found in patients suspected of harboring an expanding intracranial tumor.* Sellar enlargement may be seen in patients with increased intracranial pressure, the empty sella syndrome, internal carotid artery aneurysm, primary hypothyroidism and juxtasellar tumors, but it is most frequently seen in patients with a primary intrasellar pituitary tumor. Ninety per cent of patients with any clinical signs of a pituitary adenoma have an enlarged sella; if laminograms are included, more subtle abnormalities in sella configuration can be detected [1,2]. Patients with pituitary tumors may present with symptoms of pituitary dysfunction and visual abnormalities. Sometimes patients with an enlarged sella are asymptomatic or present with only headaches. The correct diagnosis and management of these patients may be difficult, because the enlarged sella may be empty and contain no tumor, or it may contain a pituitary tumor which is clinically silent and "burned out." This study is a prospective analysis of patients who were evaluated for an enlarged sella turcica.

From the Department of Neurology of the Neurological Institute and the Department of Medicine, Columbia Presbyterian Medical Center, New York, New York 10032. This study was supported by U.S. Public Health Service Grants CA-11704 and CA-13696. Requests for reprints should be addressed to Dr. Leon A. Weisberg. Manuscript accepted March 3, 1976.

* Present address: Department of Neurology and Psychiatry, Tulane Medical School, 1430 Tulane Avenue, New Orleans, Louisiana 70112.

† Recipient of the NIH Teacher-Investigator Award NS 02005.

*The diagnosis of sella enlargement was made according to the criteria of Taveras and Wood [1].

MATERIALS AND METHODS

Patients. One hundred consecutive patients who were admitted to the adult neurology service of the Neurological Institute, Columbia Presbyterian Medical Center, for evaluation of an enlarged sella turcica were studied. Skull roentgenograms were taken because of headache, endocrine symptoms, syncope, dizziness, sinusitis, seizures, arterial hypertension or rhinorrhea. Twenty-two patients were excluded because their primary complaint was related to visual impairment; these patients either had visual symptoms, decreased corrected visual acuity or a visual field defect detected by confrontation examination. Also excluded were three patients with clinical signs and symptoms of acromegaly. Evaluation of the other 75 patients included isotope brain scan, electroencephalogram (EEG), tomograms of the sella, cerebrospinal fluid examination, tangent screen visual field examination, endocrine studies, arteriogram and pneumoencephalogram. Final diagnosis was made by pneumoencephalogram, arteriogram or craniotomy. These patients were classified into three groups: primary intrasellar tumor, extrasellar process and empty sella syndrome. The pneumographic diagnosis of primary intrasellar tumor was made if there was upward bulging of the diaphragma sellae above the interclinoid line, and there was no intrasellar extension of air seen in the brow-up position with the head fully extended. The roentgenographic diagnosis of the empty sella syndrome was made if subarachnoid air was seen to extend below the level of the diaphragma sella to fill the anterior and superior portion of the sella; the presence of air within the sella was confirmed by tomography. The pituitary tissue usually appeared compressed in the posterior-inferior region of the sella. In addition, none of the patients with a diagnosis of the "empty sella" had had prior surgery or radiation therapy of the pituitary region. Ten patients in this series did not have a pneumoencephalogram. No final diagnosis was made in these patients. Observation of these 10 patients has extended for up to three years.

Endocrine Studies. Some or all of the following tests of endocrine function were carried out on all patients: serum thyroxine, 24-hour urinary 17-ketogenic steroids, plasma follicle-stimulating hormone (FSH) and luteinizing hormone (LH) by radioimmunoassay or 24-hour urinary gonadotropins by bioassay, A.M. and P.M. plasma cortisol and serum thyroid-stimulating hormone (TSH). More specialized tests included plasma prolactin [3], plasma growth hormone response to insulin hypoglycemia [4] and plasma cortisol response to the intravenous administration of ACTH [5].

RESULTS

Final Diagnosis. Twenty-seven patients had a primary intrasellar tumor and these were classified as pituitary adenomas (Table I). Twenty-five patients had the empty sella syndrome. Thirteen patients had an extrasellar process and the specific diagnoses are listed in Table II. Follow-up observation of the 10 undiagnosed patients for up to three years demonstrated a benign course with no endocrine, visual or neurologic signs or symptoms, and no change in sella size or contour was demonstrated on skull films.

Clinical Variables. The 27 patients with primary intrasellar tumor studied were 20 to 69 years old; 67 per cent were women. Twenty-four of the 25 patients with the empty sella syndrome and all 10 undiagnosed patients were women. They ranged in age from 35 to 60 years; the majority were in their forties. The age and sex distributions of patients with the primary intrasellar tumor or extrasellar process were more variable (Tables III and IV).

TABLE I Final Diagnosis in 75 Patients With an Enlarged Sella Without Visual Symptoms

Final Diagnosis	No. of Patients
Primary intrasellar tumor	27
Empty sella syndrome	25
Extrasellar processes	13
No diagnosis	10

TABLE II Diagnosis in 13 Patients With Extrasellar Conditions

Etiology	No. of Patients
Craniopharyngioma	2
Chordoma	2
Sarcoidosis	2
Obstructive hydrocephalus	2
Metastasis to sella	1
Eosinophilic granuloma	1
Atypical pinealoma	1
Parasellar meningioma	1
Pseudotumor cerebri	1

TABLE III Age Distribution in 75 Patients With an Enlarged Sella Without Visual Symptoms

Age (yr)	Primary Intrasellar Tumor (no.)	Extra-sellar Process (no.)	Empty Sella Syndrome (no.)	No Diagnosis (no.)
20–29	1	10	0	0
30–39	2	2	4	1
40–49	16	0	17	7
50–59	7	1	4	2
60–69	1	0	0	0

TABLE IV Sex Incidence in 75 Patients With an Enlarged Sella Without Visual Symptoms

Diagnosis	Male (no.)	Female (no.)
Primary intrasellar tumor	9	18
Extrasellar processes	6	7
Empty sella syndrome	1	24
No final diagnosis	0	10
Total	16	59

TABLE V Clinical Symptoms in 75 Patients With Enlarged Sella

	Primary Intrasellar Tumor (no.)	Extrasellar Process (no.)	Empty Sella Syndrome (no.)	No Diagnosis (no.)
Clinical symptom				
Headache	23	13	11	8
Rhinorrhea	0	0	2	0
Endocrine	18	7	0	0
Visual	0	4	0	0
Asymptomatic	4	0	12	2
Presenting symptom				
Headache	5	13	6	4
Rhinorrhea	0	0	2	0
Endocrine	18	4	0	0
Visual	0	0	0	0
Asymptomatic	4	0	17	2

Symptoms of pituitary dysfunction were present in 18 of 27 patients with primary intrasellar tumor and in seven of 13 patients with extrasellar process (Table V). In 15 women with primary intrasellar tumor, the earliest symptom was a change in frequency or regularity of the menstrual pattern which later progressed to amenorrhea. This was the most frequent presenting symptom. Other endocrine symptoms of pituitary dysfunction included infertility, decreased libido, recent weight gain, cold intolerance, galactorrhea and change in skin texture or pigmentation (Table VI). No patient in this series had diabetes insipidus. Only one of the eight men with primary intrasellar tumor presented with endocrine symptoms. No patient with the empty sella syndrome or in the undiagnosed group noted any similar endocrine symptoms suggestive of pituitary dysfunction. Twenty-four of 25 patients with the empty sella syndrome and eight of the 10 undiagnosed patients were obese, but none reported recent weight gain or amenorrhea. Two patients with the empty sella syndrome presented with cerebrospinal fluid rhinorrhea, a symptom not described by patients in the other groups. Six patients with extrasellar process had diplopia which was associated with lateral rectus paresis, papilledema and increased intracranial pressure. No other patients had any visual symptoms which were suggestive of optic pathway involvement.

Fifty-five of the 75 patients studied complained of headache. The pattern of headache differed in the four groups. All 13 patients with extrasellar process presented with headache. The headache was recent in onset, awakened the patient from sleep, was most severe in the morning, increased with change in position, and was associated with nausea and vomiting; this pattern was suggestive of increased intracranial pressure. Of the 42 patients with primary intrasellar tumor, and the empty sella syndrome or of the 10 in the undiagnosed group, headache was frequent but less characteristic in pattern than in patients with extrasellar process. In these 42 patients the headache was usually frontal or temporal in location, dull or aching in quality, not altered by change in position, not associated with nausea or visual symptoms, and present for months to years; it did not awaken the patient. In these three groups, headache was not a frequent presenting symptom (Table V). Four patients with primary intrasellar tumor were asymptomatic and five had only headache. Eleven of the 25 patients with the empty sella syndrome were asymptomatic and 12 complained of only headache. Of the 10 undiagnosed patients, two were asymptomatic and eight presented with only headache (Table V).

In 25 of 27 patients with primary intrasellar tumor, skull films demonstrated sellar enlargement in addition to evidence of demineralization of the sella, erosive changes in the clinoid processes or the presence of a double sella floor (Table VII). The other two patients with primary intrasellar tumor had a symmetrically enlarged sella with no changes in its configuration, but tomo-

TABLE VI Endocrine Symptoms in Patients With an Enlarged Sella Without Visual Symptoms

Symptom	Primary Intrasellar Tumor (no.)	Empty Sella Syndrome (no.)	Extrasellar Process (no.)	No Diagnosis (no.)
Amenorrhea	15	0	7	0
Infertility	3	0	0	0
Decreased libido	1	0	0	0
Galactorrhea	3	0	2	0
Recent weight gain	6	0	2	0
Recent weight loss	0	0	0	0
Cold intolerance	1	0	0	0
Change in skin texture	1	0	0	0
Change in skin pigmentation	1	0	0	0

TABLE VII Roentgenographic Finding in 75 Patients With an Enlarged Sella Without Visual Symptoms

	Primary Intrasellar Tumor (no.)	Empty Sella Syndrome (no.)	Extrasellar Process (no.)	No Diagnosis (no.)
Enlarged sella with normal shape	2	18	5	6
Enlarged sella with abnormal shape	25	7	8	4
Abnormality of shape				
Demineralization of dorsum	25	7	8	4
Erosion of clinoids	19	5	8	3
Undercutting of clinoids	12	2	5	2
Asymmetrical of double floor	16	5	3	2
Abnormal calcification	0	0	2	0

grams were not obtained. Of the 35 patients with the empty sella syndrome or in the undiagnosed group, 24 were found to have a symmetrically enlarged sella with normal shape. In the other 11 patients the sella was enlarged, and an abnormality was detected in mineralization, symmetry of the sella floor, dorsum or clinoid processes. In these 11 patients and in the two patients with primary intrasellar tumors whose whole sella was symmetrically enlarged, air study was necessary to make the correct diagnosis. In the 13 patients with extrasellar process, the roentgenographic changes in the sella were indistinguishable from those produced by primary intrasellar tumor, but the results of neurologic and tangent screen visual field examination, isotope brain scan, electroencephalogram, cerebrospinal fluid examination, arteriogram and pneumoencephalogram were diagnostic (Table VIII).

Despite the absence of visual symptoms suggestive of optic pathway involvement and a negative confrontation visual field examination, all patients with an enlarged sella were thoroughly investigated with a tangent screen visual field study. Four patients in whom no field defect was detected on confrontation examination were found to have a partial or total superior bitemporal quadrant defect on careful tangent screen study. This was most readily demonstrated using a small (1 or 2 mm) test object which was colored (red). Subsequent air study in these patients demonstrated a primary intrasellar tumor with suprasellar extension. No visual field abnormality was detected in patients with the empty sella syndrome or in the undiagnosed group.

Endocrine studies showed various abnormalities. Of the 27 patients with primary intrasellar tumor, 20 were found to have an abnormality in at least one parameter. The most frequent changes detected were inadequate

TABLE VIII Laboratory Studies in 75 Patients With an Enlarged Sella Without Visual Symptoms

Study	Primary Intra-sellar Tumor (no.)	Extra-sellar Process (no.)	Empty Sella Syn-drome (no.)	No Diag-nosis (no.)
Positive brain scan	2/27	5/13	0/13	0/10
Abnormal EEG	0/27	6/13	0/13	0/10
Cerebrospinal fluid examination				
Increased pressure (>200 mm H_2O)	0/27	8/13	0/13	0/10
Pleocytosis (>3/hpf)	0/27	2/13	0/13	0/10
Increased protein content (>45 mg/100 ml)	10/27	9/13	0/13	0/10
Decreased sugar content	0/27	2/13	0/13	0/10
Abnormal arteriogram	6/17	6/10	0/2	0/0

NOTE: Positive/number of studies.

TABLE IX Endocrine Studies in Patients With an Enlarged Sella Without Visual Symptoms

Studies	Primary Intra-sellar Tumor (no.)	Empty Sella Syn-drome (no.)	Extra-sellar Process (no.)	No Diag-nosis (no.)
1. Inadequate GH response to insulin hypoglycemia (0.1 unit/kg)*	12/14	7/16	6/9	3/6
2. Inadequate cortisol response to IV ACTH†	10/24	0/18	6/11	0/7
3. Low urinary or plasma gonadotropins	10/27	0/22	4/11	0/6
4. Loss of diurnal rhythm of plasma cortisol	6/16	0/16	8/10	0/6
5. Low urinary ketogenic steroids	8/25	0/22	4/11	0/6
6. Elevated plasma prolactin‡	5/14	1/12	2/11	0/6
7. Low serum thyroxine	1/20	0/20	0/11	0/8

NOTE: Number abnormal/number studied. GH = growth hormone. IV = intravenous.
* Normal response: rise of plasma GH level to at least 10 ng/ml provided blood glucose level falls to <50 per cent of initial fasting level.
† Normal response: rise of plasma cortisol level to at least 30 μg/100 ml 4 hours after start of infusion containing 25 units ACTH.
‡ Normal A.M. values: men, <1 to 20 ng/ml; women, 1 to 25 ng/ml.

response of growth hormone to insulin-induced hypoglycemia, low or borderline gonadotropin values in patients with amenorrhea, inadequate response of plasma cortisol to the administration of ACTH and an elevated serum prolactin level (Table IX). Seven patients with the empty sella syndrome and three undiagnosed patients had an inadequate growth hormone response to insulin-induced hypoglycemia, but all had a normal cortisol response to the intravenous administration of ACTH, normal gonadotropins, prolactin, thyroid and adrenal function values on the studies carried out. None of the patients with the empty sella syndrome or undiagnosed patients who had an abnormal growth hormone response had any symptoms suggestive of pituitary dysfunction.

COMMENTS

Analysis of these 75 patients demonstrates several clinical points. First, the cause of the sellar enlargement was extrasellar in 13 patients; in these conditions neurologic examination and additional studies including cerebrospinal fluid examination, brain scan, arteriogram or pneumoencephalogram were necessary to make the correct diagnosis. In these patients the sellar enlargement and erosive changes were probably related to increased pulsatile pressure in the third ventricle transmitted to the sellar region. Second, 32 patients in whom an enlarged sella was demonstrated on skull films were asymptomatic or presented with headache only.

Of these 32 patients, nine were subsequently found to have a primary intrasellar tumor and 23 were found to have the empty sella syndrome; the diagnosis was confirmed by pneumoencephalogram. In the absence of visual or endocrine disturbance in these patients, findings on films of the skull and endocrine laboratory studies were not sufficient to differentiate these two conditions. Third, 10 asymptomatic patients with an enlarged sella did not have a pneumoencephalogram, but in follow-up observation no visual, endocrine or neurologic abnormality was subsequently detected. It is probable that these patients have the empty sella syndrome, but it is also possible that they harbor a clinically silent intrasellar pituitary tumor.

Several studies derived from necropsy material have demonstrated that pituitary microadenomas and macroadenomas occur relatively frequently: an incidence of up to 25 per cent in unselected cases. These adenomas may be the cause of asymptomatic sellar enlargement [6,7]. In a study of patients with pituitary tumors, Younghusband et al. [8] described 164 patients who presented with endocrine, visual or neurologic symptoms. In addition, they identified 44 patients who were found to have an enlarged sella but, because of lack of clinical symptoms, were not studied further. These investigators suggested that the sella enlargement was not caused by a pituitary tumor or, possibly, that not all pituitary tumors produce clinical symptoms.

Other investigators have suggested that not all enlarged sellas are filled with tumor but may be "empty." Dobben and Caplan [9] studied 17 patients with an enlarged sella; an "empty sella" was demonstrated by pneumoencephalogram in six. Faglia et al. [10] diagnosed the "empty sella" syndrome in seven of 45 patients evaluated for sella enlargement who had no symptoms of pituitary dysfunction.

The roentgenographic appearance of an enlarged sella with a smoothly curving regular cavity with the clinoid processes in normal position, no evidence of erosion of cortical bone, symmetrical sella floor and normal appearing dorsum is believed to be characteristic of the "empty sella" [11]. This is in contrast to the roentgenographic findings in patients with primary intrasellar tumor in whom there usually is marked cortical bone erosion, separation and erosion of both anterior and posterior clinoid processes, distortion of the dorsum and asymmetry of the sella floor. In this present series, the findings on plain skull films were not specific enough to permit differentiation between primary intrasellar tumor and the empty sella syndrome without an air study. In seven of 25 patients with the empty sella syndrome and in four of 10 undiagnosed patients, roentgenographic abnormalities were compatible with primary intrasellar tumor, and two patients with primary intrasellar tumor had a symmetrically enlarged ballooned sella. Standard tomograms add to diagnostic accuracy, but the only definitive diagnostic technic is air study or, possibly, the recently developed technic of computerized axial tomography (CAT).

In asymptomatic patients with an enlarged sella, pneumographic analysis or CAT is necessary. Pneumographic analysis can present difficulties in technic and interpretation. Air must be maneuvered into the sella from the suprasellar cisterns by fully extending the head to the brow-up position, with tomograms taken in the coronal and sagittal sections. If this is accomplished, failure of air to enter the enlarged sella, usually also accompanied by upward bulging of the diaphragma sellae, confirms the presence of an intrasellar mass. If this is not accomplished, one cannot be certain that the enlarged sella is indeed filled with tumor and not with subarachnoid space. An incomplete study can give the roentgenographic impression of an intrasellar mass when, in fact, no tumor is present. An additional problem arises if the optic chiasm or other forebrain structures are depressed into the pituitary fossa; this may prevent air from penetrating below the clinoid processes and thus simulate the appearance of an intrasellar mass [12]. In the future, improvements in CAT technic may obviate the need for pneumoencephalography in many patients.

If patients with an enlarged sella have visual symptoms suggestive of optic pathway impairment, a pituitary tumor is usually found. Typical visual symptoms include dimming or haziness of vision, difficulty in focusing, diminished visual acuity, faulty peripheral vision, polyopia or nonparetic diplopia. Visual involvement is a not uncommon symptom in patients with pituitary tumors; it has been reported in 58 to 88 per cent of patients, and objective visual acuity or field defect abnormality is detected in 80 to 97 per cent of patients [13–22]. High figures for the incidence of visual disturbances tend to be reported in those series in which an initial patient selection was derived by referral from ophthalmologists or in which the patients were treated primarily by surgery. The present series, including the 22 patients who had definite visual impairment and who were not considered in detail in this report, suggests that in an unselected series which includes cases of small pituitary tumors or of primarily intrasellar tumors, only 50 per cent or less of the patients with pituitary tumors will have any kind of visual defect.

Occasionally patients with an enlarged sella will have no visual symptoms, and no field defect will be detected on confrontation examinations. Tangent screen examination is necessary to detect early evidence of chiasmal involvement due to a primary intrasellar tumor. The earliest visual field abnormality caused by primary intrasellar tumor, which compresses the chiasm from below, is a superior bitemporal quadrantopsia. This early defect is usually symmetrical, but it may be unilateral and may not be associated with any loss of visual acuity. As already stated, it is important to perform tangent screen visual field examination with a small red colored test object and to test perception of color vision with the pseudoisochromatic color charts to detect a field defect in any patient suspected of having a possible pituitary tumor [21,22]. This method of testing will detect abnormalities in the temporal field early in the course of the disease and also scotomatous hemianopic defects which may be missed when only the peripheral fields are tested by confrontation examination. In this present series, four patients without visual symptoms in whom no defect was detected on confrontation examination were found to have a bitemporal superior quadrantopsia by tangent screen examination; a pneumoencephalogram demonstrated an intrasellar tumor with suprasellar extension in these patients. In no patient with an enlarged sella, in whom a subsequent diagnosis of the empty sella syndrome was made, was a visual field impairment detected by these careful methods of visual field testing.

The presence of clinical symptoms suggestive of pituitary dysfunction is helpful in differentiating primary intrasellar tumor from the empty sella syndrome. In this present series no patient with the empty sella syndrome or in the undiagnosed group had any endocrine symptoms. This is in agreement with the lack of well documented cases of symptomatic pituitary dysfunction in patients with the empty sella syndrome, although some endocrine laboratory disorders have been reported [10,24]. Eighteen of 27 patients with primary intrasellar tumor had clinical symptoms of pituitary dysfunction. The earliest symptom was amenorrhea in women; in this series no change in libido was reported by any man or was detected in the course of an evaluation for infertility. Galactorrhea occurred in three patients, all of whom had elevated prolactin levels. Six patients reported recent weight gain; the endocrine basis for this has not been defined. Only one patient had symptoms of thyroid dysfunction, consisting of cold intolerance.

In the absence of endocrine symptoms in patients with an enlarged sella, laboratory endocrine data were not sufficient to differentiate primary intrasellar tumor from the empty sella syndrome. In patients with pituitary tumors, Rabkin and Frantz [23] reported a high incidence of inadequate response of growth hormone to insulin-induced hypoglycemia, accompanied by a nearly equal incidence of decreased urinary gonadotropins; decreased thyroid and adrenal function was less common but could be demonstrated by special tests in approximately half the patients. Nieman, Landon and Wynn [19] also described the frequent inadequate response of growth hormone and low gonadotropins in patients with primary intrasellar tumor. In this present series, 20 of 27 patients with primary intrasellar tumor had abnormalities of at least one of the following parameters of endocrine function: gonadotropins, growth hormone response to insulin-induced hypoglycemia, cortisol response to intravenously administered ACTH, cortisol diurnal rhythm, urinary ketogenic steroids or serum prolactin. Two patients had elevated prolactin levels without galactorrhea. The present study confirms our earlier findings [3,24] that prolactin hypersecretion is found in approximately one third of all chromophobe adenomas, with or without accompanying galactorrhea, making it the most commonly hypersecreted of all anterior pituitary hormones. Its measurement is, therefore, of considerable diagnostic importance.

Endocrine abnormalities similar to those documented in primary intrasellar tumor have been observed in some patients with the empty sella syndrome [10,11,25]. The most frequent abnormality has been an inadequate response of growth hormone to insulin-induced hypoglycemia associated with normal gonadotropins and normal corticosteroid response. Faglia et al. [10] reported an impaired corticotropin and growth hormone response to lysine-vasopressin, pyrogen-induced stress and insulin-induced hypoglycemia in the empty sella syndrome. In the present series, seven patients with the empty sella syndrome and three in the undiagnosed group had a blunted response of growth hormone to hypoglycemia but normal results for other endocrine tests.

In the empty sella syndrome, it has been postulated that the sellar remodeling leads to pituitary atrophy with flattening of the gland in the posterior-inferior part of the pituitary fossa [26]. Paucity of clinical evidence of endocrine dysfunction with only mild abnormalities in laboratory studies indicates the vast reserve capacity of the hypothalamic-pituitary system [27]. In addition, these findings demonstrate that the differential diagnosis between primary intrasellar tumor and the empty sella syndrome cannot be made on endocrine laboratory data alone; the presence of clinical symptoms of pituitary dysfunction, however, suggests that the enlarged sella is caused by an intrasellar pituitary tumor.

This prospective analysis of the roentgenographic and laboratory parameters involved in evaluating patients with an enlarged sella indicates the surprisingly high incidence of the empty sella syndrome, and points out the difficulty in differentiating primary intrasellar tumor from the empty sella syndrome. Air study or, in the future, computerized axial tomography is necessary to make the correct diagnosis. This series also confirms a high incidence of hyperprolactinemia, often unaccompanied by galactorrhea, in patients with pituitary tumors.

REFERENCES

1. Taveras JM, Wood EH: Diagnostic Neuroradiology, 1st ed, Baltimore, Williams & Wilkins Co., 1964, p 109.
2. Vexina JL, Sutton TJ: Prolactin-secreting pituitary microadenomas. Am J Roentgenol 120: 46, 1974.
3. Frantz AG: The regulation of prolactin secretion in humans. Frontiers in Neuroendocrinology 1973 (Ganong WF, Martini L, eds), New York, Oxford University Press, 1973, p 337.
4. Frantz AG, Rabkin MT: Human growth hormone: clinical measurement, response to hypoglycemia and suppression by corticosteroids. N Engl J Med 271: 1375, 1964.
5. Christy NP, Wallace EZ, Jailer JW: The effect of intravenously-administered ACTH on plasma 17, 21-dihydroxy-20-ketosteroids in normal individuals and in patients with disorders of the adrenal cortex. J Clin Invest 34: 899, 1955.
6. Costello RT: Subclinical adenoma of the pituitary gland. Am J Pathol 12: 205, 1936.
7. Kraus JE: Neoplastic diseases of the human hypophysis. Arch Pathol 39: 343, 1945.
8. Younghusband OZ, Horrax G, Hurxthal LM, et al.: Chromophobe pituitary tumors. J Clin Endocrinol Metab 12: 611, 1952.
9. Caplan RH, Dobben GD: Endocrine studies in patients with the "empty sella syndrome." Arch Intern Med 123: 611, 1969.
10. Faglia G, Ambrosi B, Beck-Peccoz P, et al.: Disorders of growth hormone and corticotropin regulation in patients with empty sella. J Neurosurg 38: 59, 1973.
11. Neelon FA, Goree JA, Lebovitz HE: The primary empty sella. Clinical and radiographic characteristics and endocrine function. Medicine (Baltimore) 52: 73, 1973.
12. Hodgson SF, Randall RV, Holman CB, et al.: Empty sella syndrome. Med Clin North Am 56: 897, 1972.
13. Hollenhorst RW, Younge BR: Ocular manifestations produced by adenomas of the pituitary gland: analysis of 1000 cases. Diagnosis and Treatment of Pituitary Tumors (Kohler PO, Ross GT, eds), Amsterdam, Excerpta Medica, 1973, p 53.
14. Poppen JL: Changing concepts in the treatment of pituitary adenomas. Bull NY Acad Med 39: 21, 1963.
15. Lyle TK, Clover P: Ocular symptoms and signs in pituitary tumours. Proc Roy Soc Med 54: 611, 1961.
16. Davidoff LM, Feiring EH: Surgical treatment of tumors of the pituitary body. Am J Surg 75: 99, 1948.
17. Bakay L: The results of 300 pituitary adenoma operations (Prof. Herbert Olivecrona's series). J Neurosurg 7: 240, 1950.
18. Henderson WR: The pituitary adenomata. A follow-up of the surgical results in 338 cases (Dr. Harvey Cushing's series). Br J Surg 26: 811, 1939.
19. Nieman EA, Landon J, Wynn V: Endocrine function in patients with untreated chromophobe adenomas. Q J Med 36: 357, 1967.
20. Sheline GE: Treatment of chromophobe adenomas of the pituitary gland and acromegaly. Diagnosis and Treatment of Pituitary Tumors (Kohler PO, Ross GT, eds), Amsterdam, Excerpta Medica, 1973, p 201.
21. Wilson P, Falconer MA: Patterns of visual failure with pituitary tumours. Br J Ophthal 52: 94, 1968.
22. Knight CL, Hoyt WF, Wilson CB: Syndrome of incipient prechiasmal optic nerve compression. Arch Ophthal 87: 1, 1972.
23. Rabkin MT, Frantz AG: Hypopituitarism. A study of growth hormone and other endocrine functions. Ann Intern Med 64: 1197, 1966.
24. Zimmerman EA, Defendini R, Frantz AG: Prolactin and growth hormone in patients with pituitary adenomas. A correlative study of hormone in tumor and plasma by immunoperoxidase technique and radioimmunoassay. J Clin Endocrinol Metab 38: 577, 1974.
25. Brisman R, Hughes JEO, Holub DA: Endocrine function in nineteen patients with empty sella syndrome. J Clin Endocrinol Metab 34: 570, 1972.
26. Bergland RM, Ray BS, Torack RM: Anatomical variations in the pituitary gland and adjacent structures in 225 human autopsy cases. J Neurosurg 28: 93, 1968.
27. Ganong WF, Hume DM: The effect of graded hypophysectomy on thyroid, gonadal, and adrenocortical function in the dog. Endocrinology 59: 293, 1956.

The Effect of Anti-Inflammatory Agents and Inflammation on Granulocyte Adherence

Evidence for Regulation by Plasma Factors

ROB ROY MACGREGOR, M.D.
Philadelphia, Pennsylvania

Significant inhibition of granulocyte adherence to nylon fiber columns followed the administration of alcohol, aspirin, sodium salicylate, acetaminophen, indomethacin, phenylbutazone, colchicine or prednisone to normal subjects. The addition of salicylates and glucocorticoids to blood in vitro had no effect on adherence, but plasma from volunteer subjects treated with either drug contained a factor which inhibited the adherence of normal granulocytes. The factor is heat stable, nondialyzable and not present in serum; it produces a linear dose response in normal cells. When mixed with the adherence-increasing factor found in inflammatory diseases, it neutralizes the augmenting effect and normal granulocyte adherence results.

The effect of anti-inflammatory therapy on inflammatory disease was studied in aspirin-treated patients with rheumatoid arthritis. Their granulocyte adherence fell into two categories based on the clinical control of their disease: patients in good control had only slightly increased granulocyte adherence, but those in poor control had an average adherence more than twice normal. Mean blood aspirin levels were equivalent for the two groups (11.0 mg/100 ml for the well controlled and 13.4 mg/100 ml for those poorly controlled). Thus, clinical response to anti-inflammatory therapy correlates well with granulocyte adherence, not with aspirin levels. The potential pathogenetic role of adherence-modifying factors in inflammatory diseases remains to be determined.

The adherence of metazoan cells to surfaces requires glycolytic metabolism [1] and is achieved without morphologic change in cell membrane [2]. The granulocyte, primary effector cell in acute inflammation, utilizes this ability to adhere to capillary endothelium before diapedesis through the vessel wall into the tissue. Thus, granulocyte adherence is an important step in the development of the inflammatory reaction. Previously, we reported a new simple assay system for measuring granulocyte adherence to surfaces in vitro [3] and used it to show that in vivo administration of ethanol, prednisone and aspirin inhibited adherence. All three drugs are potent anti-inflammatory agents, and their inhibition of granulocyte adherence suggested a possible mechanism for this action. To see if impaired granulocyte adherence was an effect common to the anti-inflammatory drugs, granulocyte adherence before and after administration of the

From the Infectious Disease Section, Department of Medicine, University of Pennsylvania, Philadelphia, Pennsylvania 19174. This study was supported in part by U.S. Public Health Grant AA00332. Requests for reprints should be addressed to Dr. R. R. MacGregor, 552 Johnson Pavilion, University of Pennsylvania School of Medicine, Philadelphia, Pennsylvania 19174. Manuscript accepted February 17, 1976.

TABLE I Effect of Anti-Inflammatory Drugs on Granulocyte Adherence (GA)

Drug	Subjects* (no.)	Average Maximum Change from Control GA (%)	Time Maximum Inhibition (hr)	Time of Return to Normal (hr)
Ethanol†	4 (rabbits)	↓ 50.3‡	1	3
Aspirin†	4	↓ 33.4‡	2–4§	4
Sodium salicylate	5	↓ 37‡	1	2–3
Indomethacin	5	↓ 34.8‡	1–2§	4
Acetaminophen	6	↓ 31.9‖	1	4
Phenylbutazone	4 (rabbits)	↓ 28.8‖	1–2§	2–4
Colchicine	5	↓ 29.2¶	2–4§	6
Prednisone†	5	↓ 38.4**	4–8§	24
Chloroquine	4	↓ 7.3††	1–2§	2–4
Dipyridamole	4	↑ 10.6††	None	1–4

*All subjects were normal human beings except as indicated.
†Reported previously, MacGregor et al. [3].
‡p <0.01, Student's t test for each subject.
§ Different subjects had maximum inhibition at different times.
‖p <0.02, Student's t test for each subject.
¶p <0.05, Student's t test for each subject.
**p <0.01, paired sample t test for the group.
††No significant change from pretreatment values.

drug was compared in normal volunteer subjects receiving these agents. Finding that inhibition was a general phenomenon, we questioned whether it was mediated by a plasma factor or whether it was a direct effect of the drug on granulocytes. Finally, because previous studies had shown that acute inflammatory illnesses are associated with augmented granulocyte adherence [4], the combined effect of inflammation and anti-inflammatory agents on adherence was investigated. This paper presents our findings.

MATERIALS AND METHODS

The adherence assay uses 1 ml of heparinized whole blood (15 units/ml) filtered through 15 mm columns of nylon fiber packed into Pasteur pipettes [3]. Three columns are set up for each specimen and the number of granulocytes adhering in each column is determined; the per cent granulocyte adherence for each specimen is the mean of results from the triplicate columns and is calculated as follows: No. of granulocytes adhering/No. of granulocytes precolumn = per cent of granulocyte adherence. Results are quite reproducible when care is given to precise measurement of fiber weight, column length and pipette tip diameter.

The degree of granulocyte adherence is dependent upon both the weight of fiber in the column and the sex of the blood donor: columns which trap the majority of granulocytes ("high-adherence" columns) are packed with 80 mg of fiber for males and 70 mg for females, leading to an average granulocyte adherence in the normal population of 76 ± 12 per cent and 70.8 ± 4.3 per cent, respectively [3]. Because it was anticipated that anti-inflammatory agents might decrease granulocyte adherence, "high-adherence" columns were used in all experiments except the one that evaluated the effect of aspirin treatment on rheumatoid arthritis. For all experiments other than the arthritis study, the actual per cent of granulocyte adherence was not important because the study design compared adherence values before treatment with those after treatment in the same cell donor. Thus, the changes in per cent adherence were of concern and were submitted to statistical analysis.

All medications were obtained from the hospital pharmacy and given orally between 8 and 9 A.M. to fasting 21 to 40 year old normal volunteer subjects not receiving any other medication. Whole blood samples were drawn into heparinized evacuated tubes (Vacutainer Co., Becton-Dickenson, Rutherford, N.J.) before and generally 1, 2 and 4 hours after medication. The following drugs and doses were used: aspirin 1.2 g, sodium salicylate 1.2 g, acetaminophen 1.3 g, prednisone 40 mg, indomethacin 50 mg, colchicine 1.8 mg and chloroquine 500 mg. Because of potential toxicity, the effects of phenylbutazone and ethanol were studied only in 2.5 to 3.0 kg New Zealand white rabbits following the intravenous administration of 20 mg/kg. Dipyridamole, an agent which inhibits platelet aggregation, was also tested in a dose of 100 mg. As control, several drugs not known to have an anti-inflammatory effect were tested: diphenylhydantoin 100 mg orally, furosemide 40 mg orally, chlorpromazine 50 mg orally and diazepam 5 to 10 mg intravenously.

The effect of long-term administration was evaluated for two drugs: seven patients with brain tumors had received glucocorticoid doses, equivalent to 100 mg or more of prednisone, for from 14 days to six months prior to study. They had no evidence of infection or inflammation and were not taking other medications. Aspirin, 900 mg, was given every 6 hours for seven to 10 days to four normal volunteer subjects and their granulocyte adherence was measured before, and on the last day of medication.

Blood was separated into cellular and plasma fractions by centrifugation at 250 G for 10 minutes. Plasma was decanted and kept on wet ice if used the same day, or frozen at −70°C if used later. The cell pellet was washed three times with

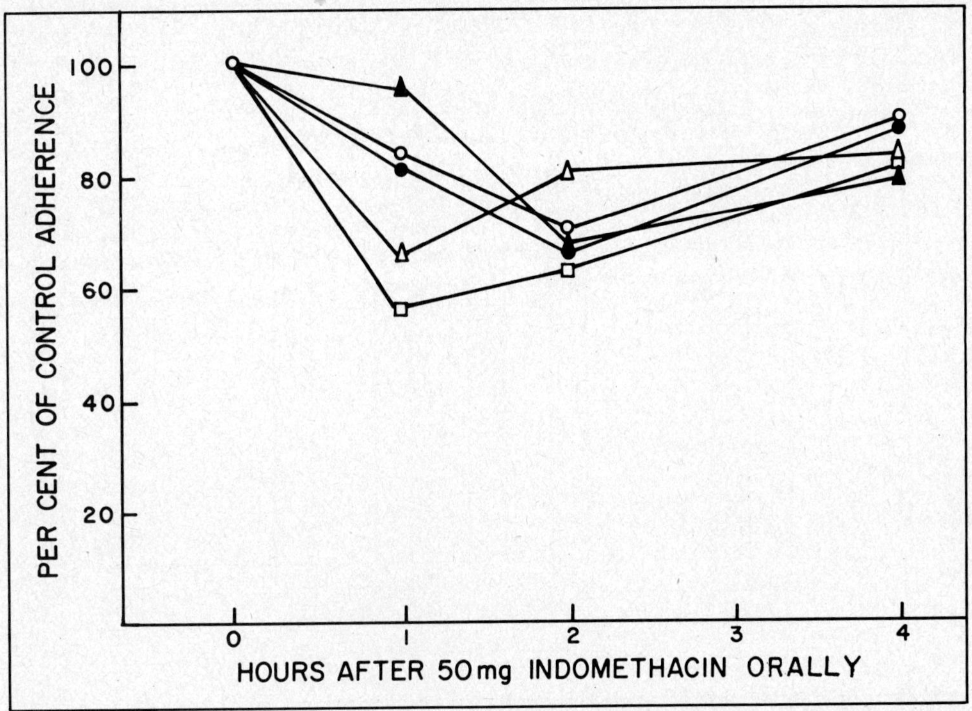

Figure 1. *The difference between adherence before treatment and that at time of maximum inhibition is statistically significant for each normal volunteer subject ($p < 0.01$, Student's t test).*

modified Hank's solution and resuspended in an equal volume of the supernatant to be tested (plasma, serum, modified Hank's solution, normal saline solution, etc.). The mixture then was incubated at 37°C for 30 minutes before determining granulocyte adherence. In all studies involving the mixture of supernatants and cells from different donors, ABO-compatible subjects of the same sex were used. Heat stability of plasma factors was assessed by incubating the samples at 56°C for 30 minutes, followed by centrifugation at 2,000 G for 10 minutes to remove precipitate. To look for dialyzable factors that might alter adherence, 5 ml of plasma was dialyzed for 24 hours at 4°C in cellulose dialysis tubing (No. 3787-D20, Arthur H. Thomas, Philadelphia, Pa.) against 400 ml of modified Hank's solution.

To evaluate the sequential effect of acute inflammation and anti-inflammatory therapy on granulocyte adherence, sterile peritonitis was induced in 2 to 3 kg male New Zealand white rabbits by the intraperitoneal injection of 120 cc of sterile normal saline solution. Granulocyte adherence was measured 4 hours later, at which time the animals had marked abdominal tenderness, and a peritoneal exudate containing 1,000 to 5,000 granulocytes. The animals then received 8 to 10 mg/kg of sodium salicylate intravenously over 5 minutes, and adherence was measured 15 minutes later.

RESULTS

The change in granulocyte adherence produced in normal subjects by single doses of the various anti-inflammatory drugs is presented in Table I. For each drug, except prednisone, the timing and degree of maximum inhibition varied from volunteer subject to volunteer subject. Therefore, to assess the statistical significance of the changes, the maximum inhibition for each volunteer was compared with his own premedication value, using the Student's t test. The significance of the changes varied among the subjects, and Table I lists the least significant p value for each group (e.g., for phenylbutazone, the inhibition in the least affected rabbit had a p value of <0.02, the two others were <0.01). Maximum inhibition was significantly different from control in all subjects, and the minimum p value was <0.02 with the Student's t test. For prednisone, the changes were similar in time and degree in the five subjects, and so their data were grouped for analysis by the paired sample t test ($p < 0.01$). Figure 1 demonstrates the variability in time course and intensity of indomethacin's effect on granulocyte adherence in five subjects; the variation is similar to that seen with all drugs except prednisone. Maximum inhibition occurred 1 to 2 hours after administration of the dose, and adherence had returned to normal by 4 hours with all agents other than colchicine and prednisone, which had a more prolonged effect. Significant inhibition lasted for 6 hours in most subjects given colchicine; in those given prednisone, maximum inhibition was between 4 and 8 hours, and was still significant at 16 hours; adherence was not back to normal until 24 hours after

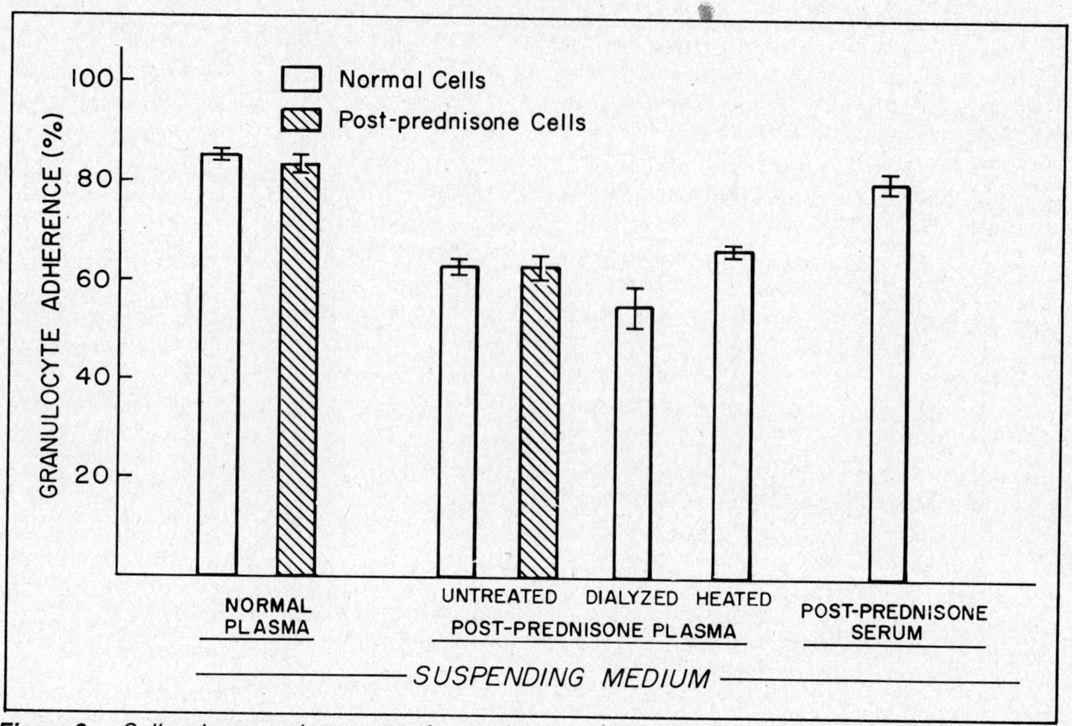

Figure 2. *Cells, plasma and serum are from a donor treated with 40 mg of prednisone orally 4 hours before. Plasma from a donor treated with prednisone inhibits the adherence of normal granulocytes when compared to plasma from a normal subject ($p < 0.01$, Student's t test). Dialysis and heating do not significantly affect adherence found with plasma from a prednisone-treated donor. Adherence of normal granulocytes in serum from such a donor is not significantly different from that found with normal plasma.*

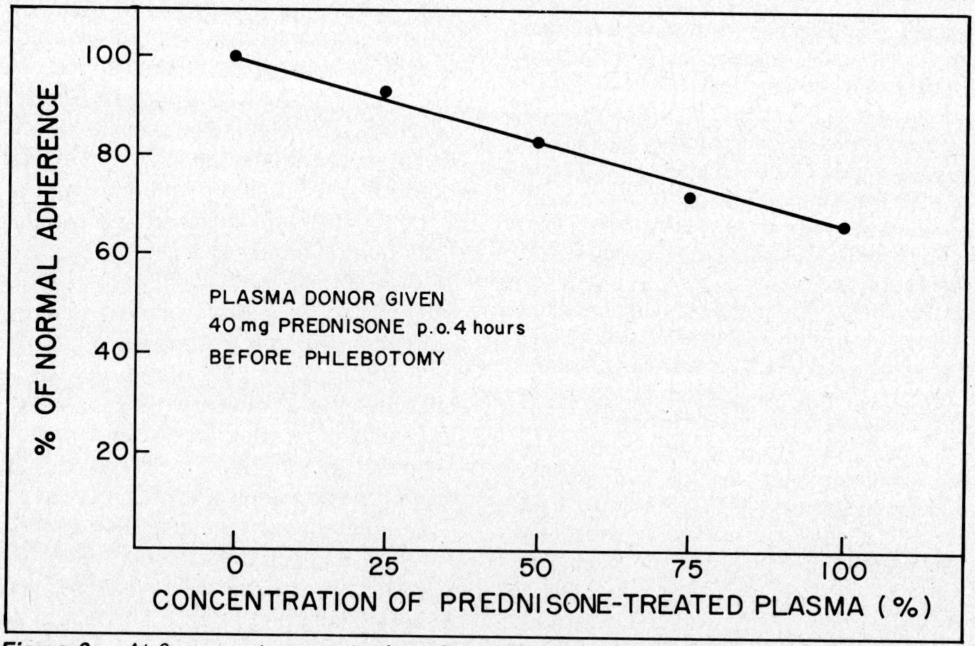

Figure 3. *At 0 per cent concentration of prednisone-treated plasma, the normal cells are suspended only in their own normal plasma, and the adherence is thus 100 per cent of normal. With 25 per cent plasma from a prednisone-treated donor, the other 75 per cent of the volume is normal plasma; and so forth.*

administration of the dose. In contrast, there was no significant change in granulocyte adherence following the administration of chloroquine or dipyridamole.

Inhibition continued with prolonged administration of glucocorticoids and aspirin. The seven patients receiving glucocorticoids daily for prolonged periods all showed impaired granulocyte adherence; using "high-adherence" columns, women had a mean granulocyte adherence of 41.9 per cent (normal for women = 70.8 ± 4.3 per cent) and the mean for men was 50.9 per cent (normal for men = 76.0 ± 12 per cent). Following the intake of aspirin, 900 mg every 6 hours for seven days, volunteer subjects showed a mean reduction in granulocyte adherence (from pretreatment levels) of 38.2 per cent (range 31.2 to 44 per cent); the average level of aspirin in the blood at the same time (2 hours after last dose) was 18.7 mg/100 ml.

Figure 2 shows that plasma from a donor given 40 mg prednisone 4 hours before, impaired adherence of normal cells (clear bars) to the same degree found when the donor's cells (cross-hatched bars) were suspended in his own plasma. Conversely, after washing and resuspension in normal plasma, granulocytes from the donor given prednisone had the same level of adherence shown by normal cells in normal plasma. Thus, the degree of granulocyte adherence was dependent on the plasma, not the cell source. The factor inhibiting granulocyte adherence (impaired granulocyte adherence factor) was not affected by heating at 56°C for 30 minutes, nor was it removed from plasma by dialysis. It was present in the prednisone-treated donor's plasma, but not in the serum. This experiment was performed three separate times, using three different pairs of prednisone-treated and normal control blood donors. In all cases, the degree of granulocyte adherence found when cells were suspended in plasma from the donor given prednisone was significantly less than when suspended in normal plasma ($p < 0.01$, Student's t test). For this experiment, male donors were tested with "high-adherence" columns. However, it is the differences in adherence which the same cells show in different plasmas that is to be noted rather than their absolute degrees of adherence. Incubation of normal cells in increasing concentrations of the prednisone-inhibited granulocyte adherence plasma caused a linear inhibition of granulocyte adherence on the three occasions the experiment was performed using plasma from different donors. Figure 3 displays the data from a representative experiment. Aspirin induced a similar factor in vivo as shown in Figure 4: cells from the aspirin-treated volunteer subject demonstrated normal adherence when suspended in normal plasma; the aspirin-inhibited granulocyte adherence factor was present only in plasma, was heat-stable but not dialyzable, and produced a linear dose-response inhibition of normal granulocyte adherence. This experiment also was

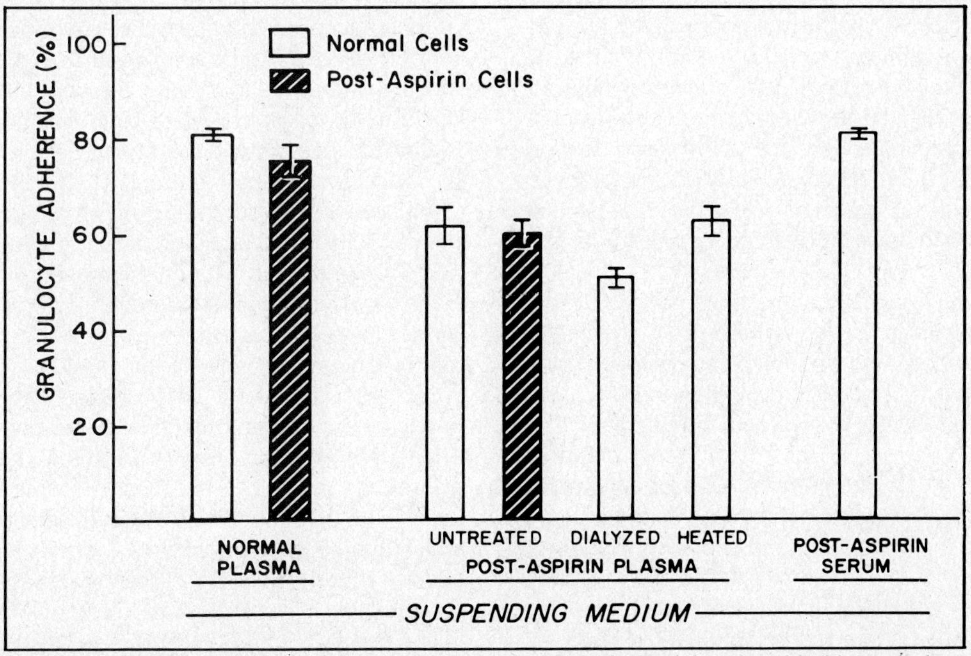

Figure 4. Cells, plasma and serum are from a donor treated with 1.2 g of aspirin 2 hours before. The difference in adherence between cells in plasma from a normal or aspirin-treated donor is significant at the 0.01 level (Student's t test). The effect of plasma from an aspirin-treated donor is not altered significantly by dialysis or heating. Adherence in serum from such a donor is the same as in normal plasma.

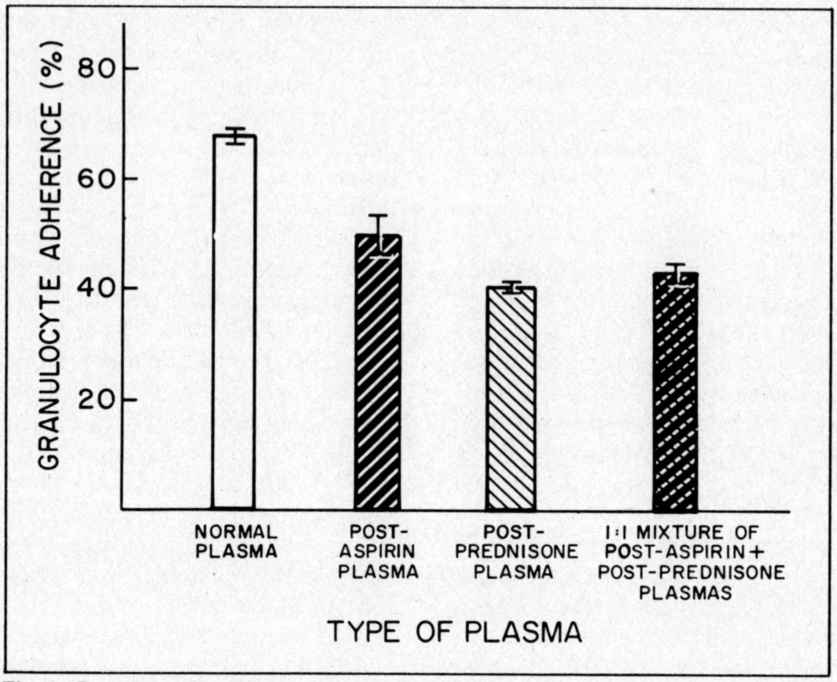

Figure 5. *Normal volunteer subjects were given 1.2 g of aspirin 2 hours before obtaining their plasma, and 40 mg of prednisone 4 hours before obtaining their plasma. Granulocyte adherence in both of these specimens, and in the mixture, is significantly less than in normal plasma ($p < 0.01$, Student's t test).*

performed three times, with different pairs of aspirin-treated and normal donors. The difference demonstrated by either subject's cells when suspended in normal plasma versus the plasma from a donor given aspirin was statistically significant ($p < 0.01$, Student's t test). Moreover, an equal-volume mixture of aspirin-induced and prednisone-induced impaired granulocyte adherence plasmas inhibited adherence to the same degree as a full concentration of either inhibited granulocyte adherence plasma alone (Figure 5). This experiment was performed with three different donor pairs, with the same results.

The change in granulocyte adherence caused by the competing influences of an inflammatory disease (rheumatoid arthritis) and an anti-inflammatory agent (aspirin) is shown in Figure 6. "Low-adherence" columns were used in this experiment because of the known enhancing effect which inflammatory disease exerts on granulocyte adherence. (Use of "high-adherence" columns would have blunted this effect, because they trap most granulocytes under **normal** conditions.) For blood from both normal males and females, "low-adherence" columns (packed with 50 mg of fiber) lead to an average adherence of only 27.7 ± 3.6 per cent. The normal volunteer data were described previously in reference to the effect of long-term aspirin administration on granulocyte adherence. Patients with untreated rheumatoid arthritis are difficult to find; however, with the help of our hospital Arthritis Group, four patients were studied who had either not yet begun therapy [2] or who had discontinued treatment because of toxicity, depression, and the like (Figure 6, last bar). Fifteen other patients with rheumatoid arthritis were studied only while receiving therapy; all had attended our arthritis clinic for more than two years and were judged to have classic rheumatoid arthritis, confirmed by rheumatoid factor titers >1:320; their symptoms were sufficient to require frequent clinic visits and the intake of 3.6 to 6.0 g aspirin daily for at least six months prior to study. None was taking other medications known to inhibit aspirin absorption. After discussion with their clinic physicians, review of their charts and examination by me before their granulocyte adherence was measured, they were divided into two groups, based on the degree of clinical control of their disease. Those described as "well controlled" had only minor arthralgias, no joint effusions, morning stiffness that lasted less than 1 hour, erythrocyte sedimentation rates which averaged 43.3 mm/hour (normal: <20 mm/hour) and felt much improved with aspirin therapy. They had a mean level of aspirin in their blood of 11.0 mg/100 ml, with a range from 3.5 to 29.3 mg/100 ml. Their granulocyte adherence was above normal but not strikingly so (40.6 per cent versus 29.2 per cent). Note that their granulocyte adherence was more than twice the level seen in the normal volunteer subjects taking the same

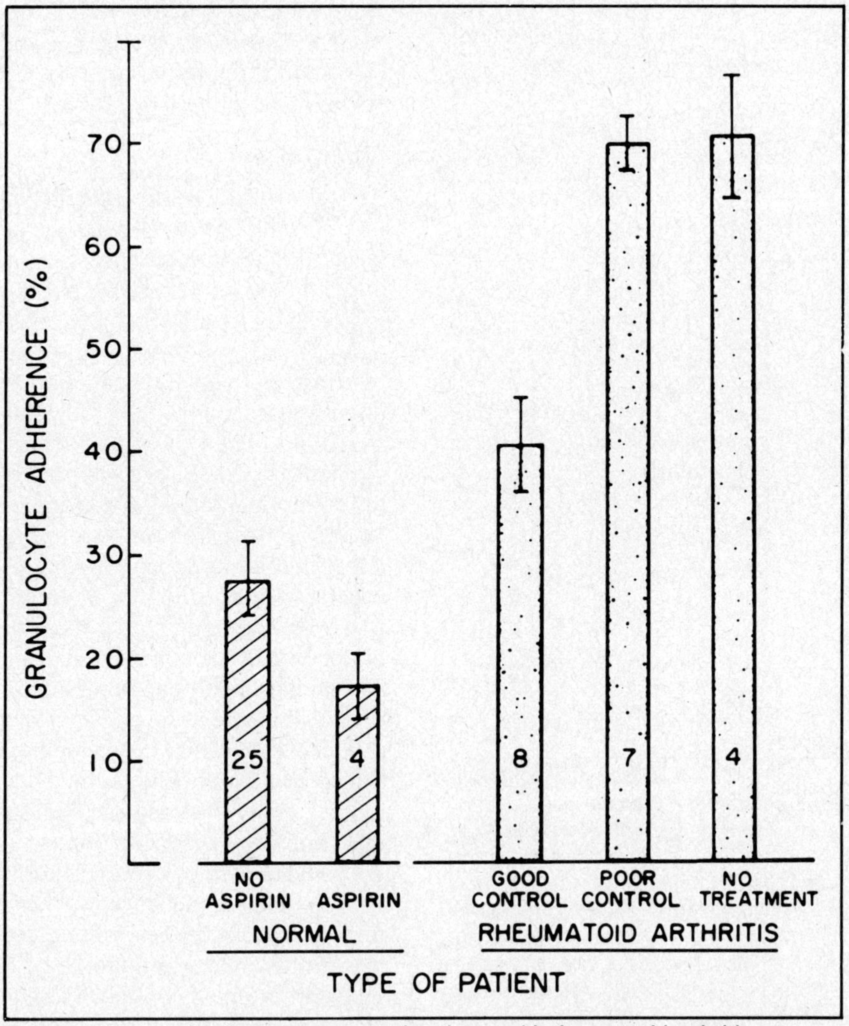

Figure 6. *Only the first two groups of patients with rheumatoid arthritis were receiving aspirin (3.6 to 6.0 g/day); the third group was untreated. Numbers in bars signify ± standard error of the mean. The difference between the means of the two normal groups was statistically significant ($p < 0.05$, Student's t test), as was the difference between the well-controlled group with arthritis and the other two. The difference between the well-controlled group with arthritis and the normal subjects not receiving aspirin was significant at the 0.05 level (Student's t test).*

amount of aspirin but without inflammatory disease ($p < 0.01$ Student's t test). The patients with rheumatoid arthritis described as "poorly controlled" had persistent, debilitating arthritis, often with effusions and pain limiting joint motion. Some required repeated arthrocenteses, with injection of glucocorticoid locally, and most were being considered for gold, indomethacin or other forms of therapy. Their average level of aspirin in blood was 13.4 mg/100 ml (range 1.5 to 22.0 mg/100 ml). Their erythrocyte sedimentation rates averaged 87.7 mm/hour and their granulocyte adherence averaged more than twice normal, equivalent to that of the *untreated* patients with rheumatoid arthritis. The difference between the mean granulocyte adherence for the two groups of treated patients with rheumatoid arthritis was significant at the 0.01 level (Student's t test), but their mean blood levels of aspirin were not significantly different.

The sequential effects of inflammation and anti-inflammatory therapy are demonstrated in Figure 7: 4 hours after the induction of sterile peritonitis, the animals had a mean increase in granulocyte adherence of 193.7 ± 10.8 per cent from values before the induction of peritonitis ($p < 0.01$, paired sample t test). Fifteen minutes after the intravenous administration of sodium salicylate, adherence had returned to normal (112.0 ± 18.2 per cent of values before the induction of peritonitis). The mean granulocyte adherence after the ad-

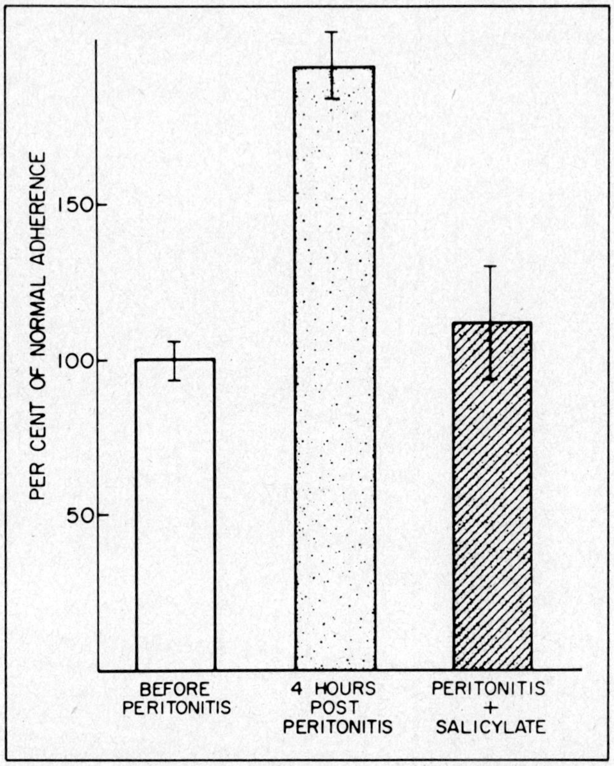

Figure 7. *Three New Zealand white rabbits were studied sequentially. Normal adherence is that found in each animal just before the induction of peritonitis with sterile normal saline solution. The second bar represents mean adherence 4 hours after the induction of peritonitis. The peritonitis and salicylate bar represents the mean adherence for the same animals 15 minutes later, following the intravenous administration of 8 to 10 mg/kg of sodium salicylate. The difference in adherence for the animals with peritonitis before versus after salicylate therapy is significant at the 0.02 level (paired sample t test).*

ministration of salicylate was significantly lower than the value for the animals before they were treated for inflammation ($p < 0.02$, paired sample t test).

To evaluate the interaction of granulocyte adherence-inhibiting and granulocyte adherence-augmenting factors in vitro, plasma samples were obtained from a patient with vasculitis, and a normal donor with a compatible blood-type who had been given 40 mg of prednisone 4 hours before. Cells from a second blood type-compatible normal donor were suspended in the two plasmas, and granulocyte adherence was measured (Figure 8). The patient's plasma augmented adherence by 36.5 per cent above that seen with normal plasma, and the plasma from the prednisone-treated volunteer inhibited adherence by 28.9 per cent (both of these deviations from normal were statistically significant, $p < 0.01$, Student's t test). Adherence in the 1:1 mixture of the two plasmas was not significantly different from that in normal plasma. Similar results were obtained when the experiment was repeated using a patient with untreated rheumatoid arthritis as the "inflammatory" donor.

COMMENTS

A recent review of anti-inflammatory agents began with the following quote: "There has been no truly dramatic breakthrough in our understanding of inflammation or anti-inflammatory drugs in recent years" [5]. Attempts to define the mechanism of action of anti-inflammatory agents have referred to their effects on lysosomal membranes [6,7], prostaglandin production [8,9], chemotaxis [10,11], phagocytosis [12] or microtubule formation [13]. However, each of these proposals has significant counter-arguments, relating predominantly to the fact that attainable blood levels of the drugs fail to affect these various functions. At present, there is no generally accepted theory proposing a common mechanism of action for the anti-inflammatory agents [14,15]. The agents may have different mechanisms of action, but it is striking that all produced a prompt and statistically significant inhibition of granulocyte adherence when given to normal volunteer subjects. This reduced adherence could inhibit the inflammatory reaction by blocking diapedesis and exudation of granulocytes out of the vascular compartment. In contrast to this general inhibition, no change in adherence occurred with single-dose chloroquine administration, consistent with the clinical observation that an anti-inflammatory effect can be noted only after prolonged use of the drug. Nor did granulocyte adherence change following the administration of diphenylhydantoin, furosemide, diazepam or chlorpromazine, all potent agents but without known anti-inflammatory action. Thus, inhibition of granulocyte adherence appears to be an effect both unique to the anti-inflammatory agents and common to them.

The inhibition seen with acetaminophen can be viewed as an exception to this principle. Generally, it is not thought to have much if any anti-inflammatory effect, but it has been reported to suppress some experimental inflammatory lesions, for example, adjuvant-induced arthritis [16].

The adherence of platelets and granulocytes appears to be a separate phenomenon: dipyridamole inhibits platelet aggregation [17] but has no effect on granulocyte adherence, whereas sodium salicylate and prednisone do not affect platelet adherence but do block granulocyte adherence. Other investigators also have found the adherence of these two blood elements to be independent [18,19].

The inhibition of granulocyte adherence produced by prednisone and aspirin is mediated by a heat-stable, nondialyzable plasma factor. Although they have im-

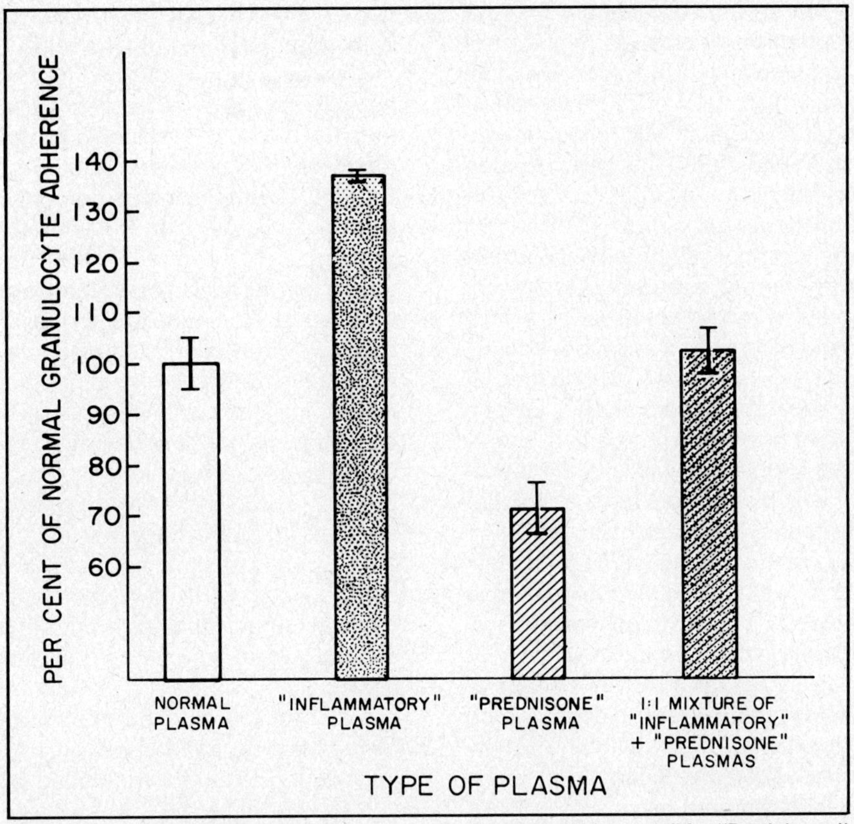

Figure 8. *"Inflammatory" plasma was from a patient with vasculitis. "Prednisone" plasma was from a normal volunteer subject given 40 mg of prednisone 4 hours before. The degree to which each modified the adherence of normal granulocytes was statistically significant ($p < 0.01$, Student's t test).*

paired granulocyte adherence in their own plasma, the adherence of cells from aspirin- or prednisone-treated donors returns to normal when they are resuspended in normal plasma, demonstrating that the effect of the inhibiting factor is reversible. Each drug may induce its own unique factor, but evidence suggests that they are the same: both are heat-stable, nondialyzable, not found in serum, strictly additive in their effect on cells when mixed in equal volume and linear in their dose-response curve. That the factors are nondialyzable and present only in plasma suggest that they are not the anti-inflammatory agents themselves. Moreover, we have shown previously [3] that the direct addition of hydrocortisone (500, 1,500 and 3,000 μg/100 ml) or sodium salicylate (5, 10, 20 and 50 mg/100 ml) to whole blood does not affect granulocyte adherence. Bryant and Sutcliffe [20] have shown that cyclic adenosine monophosphate (AMP) and its inducers can inhibit granulocyte adherence in vitro; anti-inflammatory agents may stimulate the production of such an AMP inducer in vivo, which may be the adherence-inhibiting factor we have described.

Previous work from our laboratory has shown that inflammatory states induce augmented granulocyte adherence, also mediated by a plasma factor [4]. The fact that plasma from patients with different clinical situations can both increase and decrease granulocyte adherence suggests that all adherence might be governed by a single plasma mediator whose relative concentration determines the degree of adherence; thus anti-inflammatory therapy would lower the mediator's concentration and result in poor granulocyte adherence, whereas high concentrations would be induced by inflammation and lead to the augmented adherence found with inflammatory diseases. However, two facts argue against this theory: first, the factor found in inflammatory states is heat-labile, whereas the inhibited granulocyte adherence factor is stable at 56°C for 30 minutes. Second, the same normal degree of adherence is seen when cells are suspended in normal plasma, serum or various physiologic salt solutions not containing proteins; thus, normal adherence does not require any plasma factor.

The relationship between in vitro adherence of granulocytes to nylon fiber and the in vivo events of endothelial adherence and diapedesis remains unproved. Nonetheless, our data are consistent with the hypothesis that anti-inflammatory agents might exert their clinical effect by stimulating the production of an anti-adherence factor which counteracts the adherence-augmenting factor associated with inflammation. Thus granulocyte adherence of patients being treated with anti-inflammatory agents for inflammatory disease might be determined by the interplay in vivo of these two opposing factors. Data from in vitro studies support this view: normal cells have normal adherence when suspended in an equal-volume mixture of plasmas from a patient with inflammation and from a volunteer subject treated with aspirin. When used alone, the former increases granulocyte adherence and the latter inhibits it. The in vivo data from patients with rheumatoid arthritis also support the hypothesis: untreated patients have a plasma factor which augments granulocyte adherence; normal volunteer subjects taking aspirin have a factor which inhibits granulocyte adherence. Patients with rheumatoid arthritis with a good clinical response to aspirin therapy showed granulocyte adherence only slightly higher than normal; in contrast, those with a poor response had markedly increased adherence (equivalent to untreated patients) despite aspirin doses which caused a 50 per cent inhibition of granulocyte adherence in normal volunteer subjects. Since blood levels of aspirin were equivalent in both groups of arthritis patients, their degree of granulocyte adherence correlated much better with their clinical response than did their aspirin levels. Additional evidence for the interplay in vivo between the adherence-modifying factors is found in the sequential data from animals with peritonitis. The augmented adherence associated with untreated inflammation was rapidly reversed by treatment with an anti-inflammatory agent.

The variations in granulocyte adherence described herein may have wider implications for granulocyte kinetics because they could provide a simple mechanism for regulating movement of granulocytes from marrow to intravascular compartment to tissue. For example, immature myeloid cells have poor adherence to glass, a high degree of cellular rigidity and difficulty squeezing through small apertures [21]; these characteristics may regulate the cells' egress from the marrow. Furthermore, leukemic cells show poor adherence [22–24], which could account for their prolonged intravascular lifespan [25,26]. Similarly, glucocorticoid treatment has been shown to prolong the granulocytes' intravascular lifespan [27], and the present study shows that such treatment markedly impairs granulocyte adherence. The findings with marrow and leukemic cells suggests that their reduced adherence is intrinsic to the cell, and improves with maturation; our findings with mature cells shows that their degree of adherence can be modified rapidly and reversibly by different plasma factors. Thus, the body has at least two mechanisms for affecting the intensity of granulocyte adherence which, in turn, may be an important method for regulating granulocyte kinetics.

ACKNOWLEDGMENT

I am grateful to Mrs. Elvira Ventura for her expert technical assistance, to Drs. Elias Abrutyn and Richard Root for helpful editorial comments, and to the many laboratory personnel who volunteered for the normal control studies.

REFERENCES

1. Garvin JE: Factors affecting the adhesiveness of human leukocytes and platelets in vitro. J Exp Med 114: 51, 1961.
2. Marchesi VT, Florey HV: Electron micrographic observations on the emigration of leukocytes. Q J Exp Physiol 45: 343, 1960.
3. MacGregor RR, Spagnuolo PJ, Lentnek AL: Inhibition of granulocyte adherence by ethanol, prednisone, and aspirin, measured with a new assay system. N Engl J Med 291: 642, 1974.
4. Lentnek AL, Schreiber AD, MacGregor RR: The induction of augmented granulocyte adherence by inflammation. J Clin Invest 57: 1098, 1976.
5. Weiner M, Piliero SJ: Nonsteroid anti-inflammatory agents. Ann Rev Pharmacol 10: 171, 1970.
6. Allison A: The role of lysosomes in the action of drugs and hormones. Adv Chemother 3: 253, 1968.
7. Weissman G: Interaction of Drugs and Subcellular Components in Animal Cells (Campbell PN, ed), London, Churchill, 1968, p 203.
8. Vane JR: Prostaglandins and the aspirin-like drugs. Hosp Practice 7: 61, 1972.
9. Willis AL, Davidson P, Smith JB, et al.: Prostaglandins in Cellular Biology and the Inflammatory Process (Pharriss BB, Ramwell PW, eds), New York, Plenum, 1972, p 227.
10. Ward PA: Chemotaxis of polymorphonuclear leukocytes. Biochem Pharmacol 17 (suppl): 99, 1968.
11. Caner JEZ: Colchicine inhibition of chemotaxis. Arthritis Rheum 8: 757, 1965.
12. Lehrer RI: Effects of colchicine and chloramphenicol on the oxidative metabolism and phagocytic activity of human neutrophils. J Infect Dis 127: 40, 1973.
13. Malawista SE, Bensch KG: Human polymorphonuclear leukocytes: demonstration of microtubules and effect of colchicine. Science 156: 521, 1967.
14. Paulus HE, Whitehouse MW: Nonsteroid anti-inflammatory agents. Ann Rev Pharmacol 13: 107, 1973.
15. Mills JA: Nonsteroidal anti-inflammatory drugs. N Engl J Med 290: 781, 1002, 1974.
16. Van Arman CG, Nuss GW: Interactions of aspirin, indomethacin, and other drugs in adjuvant-induced arthritis in the rat. J Pharmacol Exp Ther 187: 400, 1973.
17. Hampton JR, Harrison MJG, Honour AJ, et al.: Platelet behavior and drugs used in cardiovascular disease. Cardiovasc Res 1: 101, 1967.
18. Penny R, Galton DAG, Scott JT, et al.: Studies on neutrophil function. I. Physiological and pharmacological aspects. Br J Haematol 12: 623, 1966.

19. Banks DC, Mitchell JR: Leukocytes and thrombosis. II. Relationship between leukocyte behaviour and divalent cations, sulphydryl groups, red cells and adenosine diphosphate. Thromb Diath Haemorrh 30: 47, 1973.
20. Bryant RE, Sutcliffe MC: The effect of 3′,5′-adenosine monophosphate on granulocyte adhesion. J Clin Invest 54: 1241, 1974.
21. Lichtman MA, Weed RI: Alteration of the cell periphery during granulocyte maturation: relationship to cell function. Blood 39: 301, 1972.
22. Lichtman MA, Weed RI: Peripheral cytoplasmic characteristics of leukocytes in monocytic leukemia: relationship to clinical manifestations. Blood 40: 52, 1973.
23. Lichtman MA: Rheology of leukocytes, leukocyte suspensions, and blood in leukemia. J Clin Invest 52: 350, 1973.
24. Brandt L: Adhesiveness to glass and phagocytic activity of neutrophilic leukocytes in myeloproliferative diseases. Scand J Haematol 2: 126, 1965.
25. Athens JW, Raab SO, Haab OP, et al.: Blood granulocyte kinetics in chronic myelocytic leukemia. J Clin Invest 44: 765, 1965.
26. Duvall CP, Perry S: The use of 51-chromium in the study of leukocyte kinetics in chronic myelocytic leukemia. J Lab Clin Med 71: 614, 1968.
27. Bishop CR, Athens JW, Boggs DR, et al.: Leukokinetic studies. XIII. A non-steady-state kinetic evaluation of the mechanism of cortisone-induced granulocytosis. J Clin Invest 47: 249, 1968.

Effect of Sodium Depletion on Plasma Renin Concentration Before and During Adrenergic β-Receptor Blockade with Propranolol in Normotensive Man

PER OMVIK, M.D.*
ERIK ENGER, M.D.
IVAR EIDE, M.D.
Oslo, Norway

Plasma renin levels have been used to discriminate between different forms of hypertension, but how to define the normal range of plasma renin levels has not been agreed upon. Sodium depletion stimulates renin release. Evaluation of plasma renin would, therefore, seem possible only in relation to sodium balance.

Plasma renin concentration and concurrent daily sodium excretion were determined in 33 healthy normotensive subjects (control group) ingesting high, normal and low sodium diets. A well-defined hyperbolic relationship was found between the two variables indicating that the physiologic level of plasma renin concentration depends on the state of sodium balance. An increase in plasma potassium concentration may reduce plasma renin concentration, but this appeared to be overruled by the stimulating effect of sodium depletion.

To examine whether β-adrenergic stimulation contributes to the increase in plasma renin concentration during sodium depletion, the relationship between plasma renin concentration and concurrent sodium excretion was studied during β-receptor blockade with propranolol. In 20 healthy normotensive subjects in whom β-receptor blockade was verified by a significant reduction in pulse rate, the same hyperbolic relationship was found between plasma renin concentration and sodium excretion as in the control group showing that sodium depletion stimulates renin release independent of sympathetic nervous activity.

Plasma renin activity increases during sodium depletion both in experimental animals [1,2] and in man [3–5], but the mechanisms involved have not been fully elucidated. In man, the relationship between sodium balance and plasma renin has been most extensively studied by Laragh and associates [4,6]. They have repeatedly claimed a hyperbolic correlation between urinary sodium excretion and plasma renin activity. The significance of this correlation has been challenged [7], and other measures of sodium balance have been used to define the normal range of plasma renin [3,5,8]. The first aim of this study was, therefore, to re-examine the changes in plasma renin in normotensive man in response to changes in sodium excretion.

Various stimuli, including a decrease in sodium excretion [6], activation of the sympathetic nervous system [9,10] and autoregulated

From the Medical Department VII, Ullevaal Hospital, Oslo, and Institute for Experimental Medical Research, University of Oslo, Ullevaal Hospital, Oslo, Norway. Requests for reprints should be addressed to Dr. Ivar Eide, Medical Department VII, Ullevaal Hospital, Oslo, Norway. Manuscript accepted March 3, 1976.

* Present address: Medical Department A, Haukeland Hospital, 5000 Bergen, Norway.

renal vasodilatation by reducing blood pressure [11–13], increase plasma renin concentration by increasing the release of renin from the kidney. A negative sodium balance reduces tubular sodium delivery at the macula densa. This might stimulate the release of renin from juxtaglomerular cells [14], but since a negative sodium balance also leads to a reduction in plasma volume and thereby to increased sympathetic activity, the inverse relationship between plasma renin concentration and sodium excretion might be caused by stimulation of the sympathetic nervous system [15,16]. These possibilities were examined by comparing the effect of sodium depletion on plasma renin concentration in normotensive man before and during adrenergic β-receptor blockade with propranolol.

METHODS

Plasma renin concentration was determined in 53 healthy normotensive medical students and members of the medical staff ingesting high, normal and low sodium diets. In 33 subjects adrenergic β-receptor blockade was not given (control group) whereas 20 subjects received β-receptor blockade with propranolol (Inderal®, Imperial Chemical Industries). The drug was administered orally at 40 mg/day, divided into two daily doses for two days and then gradually increased to 160 mg/day. This dosage was reached within two days prior to the study and was maintained for one week.

The volunteers were of both sexes (nine female and 44 male), ranging in age between 20 and 36 years with an average of 25 ± 3 years (mean ± SD). Only volunteers with blood pressure levels less than 140/90 mm Hg were accepted. Blood pressure levels and pulse rate were measured after the subject had had 5 minutes of rest in a chair. Systolic and diastolic (fifth phase) blood pressure levels were determined with a conventional mercury sphygmomanometer.

The relationship between plasma renin activity and daily sodium excretion has previously been shown to be similar in outpatients and in subjects examined in metabolic wards [6]. Therefore, in this study, the subjects were treated as outpatients, but the meals were prepared at the hospital by the dietitian. Three different diets were used, calculated to contain approximately 15, 150 and 250 meq sodium/day, respectively. Potassium intake was approximately 80 meq/day under all three dietary regimens. The control group was studied during the ingestion of all three diets, whereas the subjects blocked with propranolol were examined during the ingestion of low and normal sodium diets only. Each diet was administered for five days except to four students who, during the last two days of the low salt diet period, received an almost sodium-free rice and fruit diet.

Plasma concentrations of renin, electrolytes and creatinine were determined in venous blood samples drawn at 12 noon on the fifth day (experimental day) of the respective sodium diet. The students were ambulatory from 7 A.M. and were seated during blood samplings. They received their meals as usual. A 24 hour urine sample was collected from 7 A.M. to determine creatinine clearance and daily excretion rates of sodium and potassium. Concentrations of electrolytes and creatinine in plasma and urine were measured with a Technicon® autoanalyzer (Ardsley, New York). Peripheral venous plasma renin concentrations were determined by radioimmunoassay according to the method of Haber et al. [17] following incubation of the buffered plasma samples with an excess of exogenous renin substrate. Angiotensinases were inhibited by ethylenediaminetetraacetic acid (EDTA), dimercaprol (BAL), and 8-hydroxyquinoline as previously described [11]. Internal standards of human renin (Dr. Erwin Haas, Mt. Sinai Hospital, Cleveland, Ohio) were used according to Haas and co-workers [18]. Analysis of urinary sodium concentrations and plasma renin concentration were performed at different laboratories. Data are presented as means ± 1 standard error (SE) of the mean. The statistical probability (P) of differences was calculated with Wilcoxon's tests for two samples and for paired comparison [19]. The differences were regarded as significant at $P < 0.05$. Correlation coefficients were calculated by the method of least squares.

RESULTS

Effect of Sodium Depletion on Plasma Renin Concentration. Figure 1 depicts the inverse relationship between plasma renin concentration and sodium excretion in 33 normotensive, healthy subjects, each given three different sodium diets. Sodium depletion led to a marked decrease in urinary sodium excretion and an increase in plasma renin concentration. Despite a fixed sodium content of the diet for five days, the sodium excretion on the experimental day varied widely due to

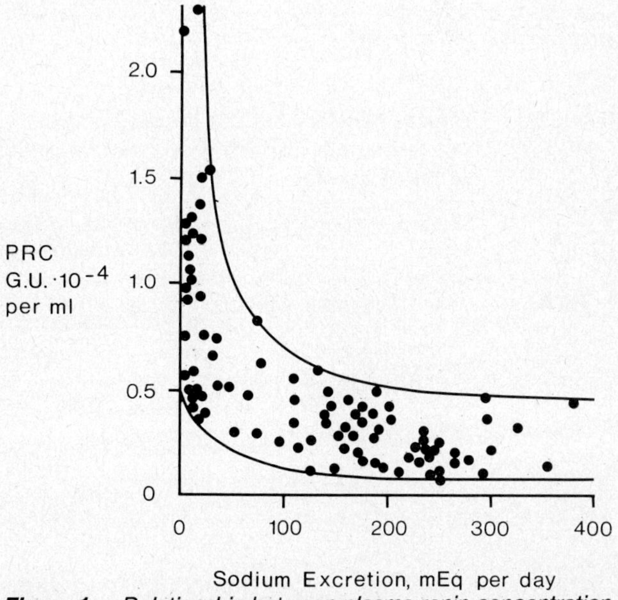

Figure 1. *Relationship between plasma renin concentration (PRC) expressed in Goldblatt Units (GU) and daily sodium excretion in 33 healthy normotensive subjects of both sexes (control group). The dots indicate single observations during high, normal and low sodium diets. Curves are drawn as the visual best fit of the range of observations.*

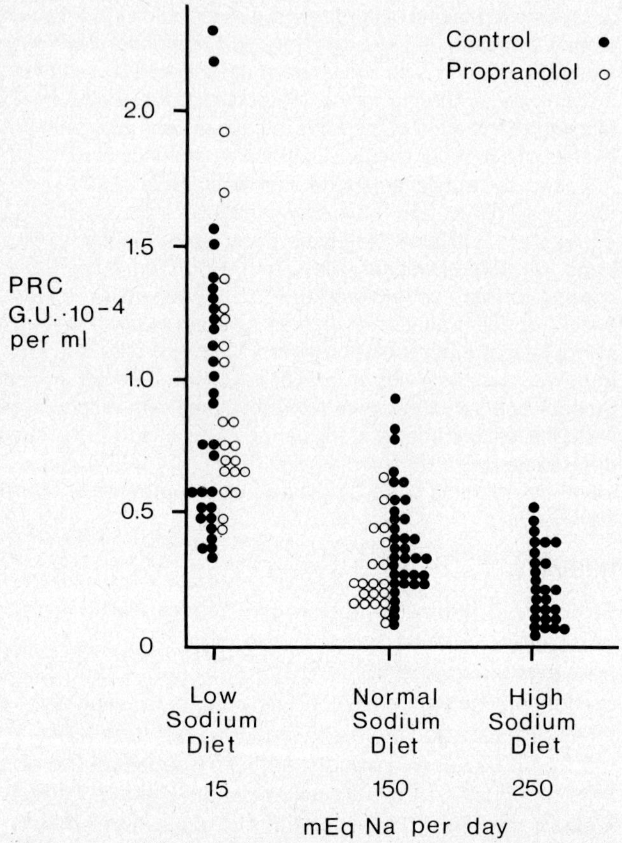

Figure 2. *Filled circles represent rearrangement of the plasma renin concentrations of Figure 1 according to sodium intake during high (250 meq/day), normal (150 meq/day) and low sodium (15 meq/day) diets, respectively. Open circles represent observations during β-receptor blockade with propranolol (160 mg/day).*

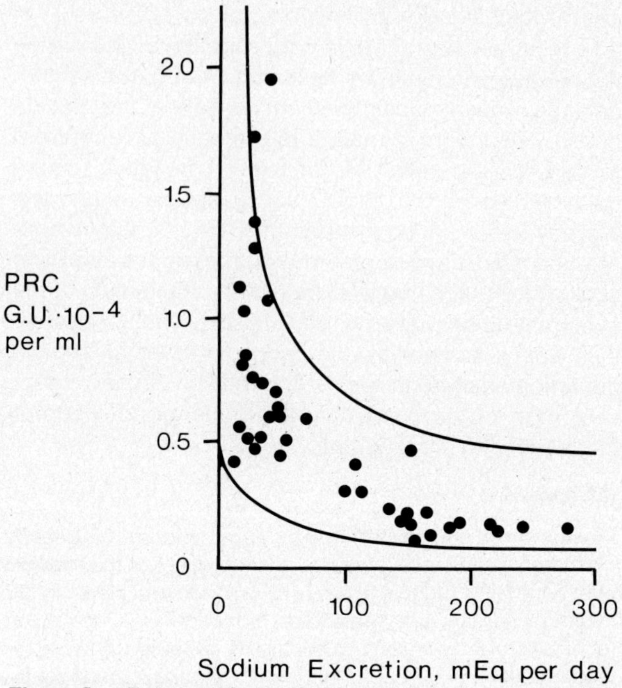

Figure 3. *Relationship between plasma renin concentration and daily sodium excretion in 20 healthy normotensive subjects of both sexes during adrenergic β-receptor blockade with propranolol. The dots indicate single observations during normal or low sodium diets. Curves show the range of observations in the control group.*

TABLE I **Effect of Dietary Sodium Intake on Urinary Electrolyte Excretion, and on Plasma Renin and Electrolyte Concentrations in Healthy Normotensive Subjects Before and During Adrenergic β-Receptor Blockade with Propranolol**

Period	Pulse Rate (beats/min)	Blood Pressure (mm Hg) Systolic	Diastolic	Plasma Renin Concentration (GU · 10⁻⁴/per ml)	$U_{Na}V$ (meq/24 hr)	U_KV (meq/24 hr)	Plasma Na^+ (meq/liter)	K^+ (meq/liter)	Cr (mg/100 ml)	C_{Cr} (ml/min)
Low Sodium Diet										
Control	72 ± 2	119 ± 3	83 ± 2	0.96 ± 0.10	12 ± 2	73 ± 4	139 ± 0.4	4.3 ± 0.1	1.0 ± 0.03	112 ± 4
Propranolol	52 ± 2	117 ± 2	79 ± 1	0.90 ± 0.09	29 ± 3	89 ± 4	139 ± 0.1	4.4 ± 0.1	1.2 ± 0.1	107 ± 6
P	<0.05	NS	NS	NS	<0.05	<0.05	NS	NS	<0.05	<0.05
Normal Sodium Diet										
Control	71 ± 3	122 ± 2	80 ± 1	0.41 ± 0.03	150 ± 10	82 ± 4	140 ± 0.4	4.1 ± 0.1	0.9 ± 0.04	119 ± 4
Propranolol	53 ± 2	118 ± 2	77 ± 2	0.28 ± 0.03	148 ± 13	92 ± 4	144 ± 0.1	4.1 ± 0.04	1.0 ± 0.03	125 ± 4
P	<0.05	NS	NS	<0.05	NS	<0.05	<0.05	NS	NS	NS
High Sodium Diet										
Control	72 ± 4	115 ± 5	81 ± 1	0.23 ± 0.02	255 ± 13	84 ± 5	139 ± 0.6	4.1 ± 0.1	1.1 ± 0.03	114 ± 5

NOTE: Each diet was used for five days. Control = 33 subjects without β-adrenergic blockade. Propranolol = 20 subjects blocked with propranolol at 160 mg/day. Data represent mean values ± 1 SE. $U_{Na}V$ = urinary sodium excretion and U_KV = urinary potassium excretion. Na^+, K^+ and Cr = plasma concentrations of sodium, potassium and creatinine, respectively. C_{Cr} = endogenous creatinine clearance according to $C_{Cr} = Plasma_{Cr} \cdot V/Urine_{Cr}$ where V = urine flow. NS = not significant. GU = Goldblatt units.

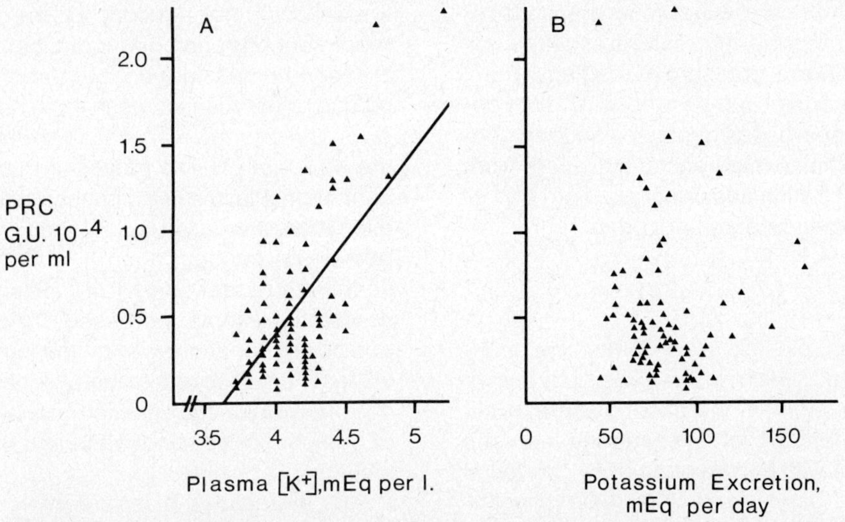

Figure 4. ***A,*** *relationship between plasma renin concentration and plasma potassium concentration (K^+) in 33 normotensive healthy subjects during high, normal and low sodium diets. Curve indicates the regression line of the data ($y = 1.12x - 4.07$, $r = 0.63$, $P < 0.001$).* ***B,*** *relationship between plasma renin concentration and daily potassium excretion during high, normal and low sodium diets.*

a different intake of food: during the period of low sodium intake, sodium excretion ranged between 0 and 43 meq/24 hours and during the period of high sodium intake, sodium excretion ranged between 109 and 376 meq/24 hours. Thus, a less consistent relationship was found when plasma renin concentration was plotted against calculated daily sodium intake (Figure 2) than against daily sodium excretion. At a sodium excretion below 100 meq/24 hours plasma renin concentration increased significantly in all subjects studied: with a sodium excretion between 0 and 49 meq/24 hours, plasma renin concentration averaged 0.95 ± 0.09 Goldblatt Units (GU)·10^{-4}/ml; between 50 and 99 meq/24 hours, plasma renin concentration averaged 0.53 ± 0.12 GU·10^{-4}/ml; and above 100 meq/24 hours, plasma renin concentration averaged 0.29 ± 0.02 GU·10^{-4}/ml. Although plasma renin concentration decreased when daily sodium intake increased, the concentration of renin, measured in the plasma of all subjects, was significant.

Effect of Propranolol on the Relationship Between Sodium Excretion and Plasma Renin Concentration. Twenty healthy normotensive subjects were studied during the intake of normal and low sodium diets after β-receptor blockade with propranolol. During a normal sodium intake, with a sodium excretion rate exceeding 100 meq/24 hours, plasma renin concentration was lower ($P < 0.05$) in subjects receiving propranolol than in the control group (Table I, Figure 2). However, when sodium intake was reduced, plasma renin concentration increased and, as shown in Figure 3, the same hyperbolic relationship between urinary sodium excretion and plasma renin concentration was found in patients during β-blockade with propranolol as in those who did not receive β-blockade. During low sodium intake there was no significant difference between the plasma renin concentration in the two groups (Table I). In all subjects, β-adrenergic blockade was indicated by a decrease in pulse rate during propranolol administration: from the control conditions with the resting pulse rate averaging 72 ± 2 beats/min, the pulse rate decreased during β-blockade by an average of 28 per cent to 52 ± 2 and 53 ± 2 beats/min during the intake of low and normal sodium diets, respectively. After the administration of propranolol had been discontinued for 10 days, the resting pulse rate returned to an average of 69 ± 2 beats/min. β-receptor blockade did not reduce blood pressure, which averaged 121/79 mm Hg before and 117/79 mm Hg during the administration of propranolol, respectively.

Table I summarizes blood pressures and laboratory data of the two groups during the intake of the different sodium diets. Urinary potassium excretion was not significantly altered during sodium depletion whereas plasma potassium concentration increased slightly. Consequently, a low but significant correlation was found between plasma renin concentration and plasma potassium concentration both without ($r = 0.63$, $P < 0.001$) (Figure 4A) and with ($r = 0.43$, $P < 0.01$) β-adrenergic blockade. However, correlations were low and might depend on extreme points. No correlation was found between plasma renin concentration and potassium excretion (Figure 4B). Blood pressure remained constant during the decrease in sodium excretion, with mean arterial pressure averaging 91 ± 2 mm Hg. During propranolol administration, sodium depletion led to slight decreases in plasma sodium concentration and creatinine clearance, but apart from plasma renin concentration and urinary sodium excretion, the other parameters summarized in Table I remained unchanged.

COMMENTS

In normotensive man, plasma renin concentration increases during reduced sodium intake. This study shows that sodium depletion may increase plasma renin concentration independent of sympathetic nervous activity. In agreement with Laragh et al. [4,6], we found that the relationship between plasma renin concentration and urinary sodium excretion is curvilinear and that the normal range of plasma renin concentration is determined by the rate of sodium excretion. The same hyperbolic relationship between plasma renin concentration and sodium excretion applies after β-adrenergic blockade. Finally, it might appear that the stimulating effect of reduced sodium excretion on plasma renin concentration is stronger than the inhibitory effect exerted by the accompanying increase in plasma potassium concentration during sodium depletion.

During antinatriuresis due to sodium depletion, the concentration of renin in plasma may be more than ten times the concentration during natriuretic conditions (Figure 1). Thus, to evaluate plasma renin concentration as high, normal or low, it is essential to relate plasma renin concentration to sodium balance. This has also been achieved by relating plasma renin to dietary sodium [3,5]. As shown in Figure 2, plasma renin concentration is inversely correlated to sodium intake (Figure 2), but a more consistent relationship is found when plasma renin concentration is related to sodium excretion (Figure 1). At a sodium intake of about 150 meq/day, 20 per cent of the observations of plasma renin concentration exceeded the upper range of normal when compared to the relationship between plasma renin concentration and sodium excretion. This indicates that the exact intake of sodium is difficult to assess despite a fixed sodium content of the diet for five days, and that sodium excretion is a better index of sodium balance.

Sodium depletion led to an increase in plasma potassium concentration [20,21], and positive correlations between plasma potassium and plasma renin concentration were observed. However, these correlations were low and might depend on extreme single observations (Figure 4A). The correlation between potassium concentration and plasma renin concentration could not account for the increase in plasma renin concentration during antinatriuresis since an increase in potassium concentration has been found to reduce rather than increase renal renin release [22,23]. Thus, the decrease in sodium excretion might overrule the effect of plasma potassium on plasma renin concentration. Plasma renin concentration might have been even more increased by low sodium excretion if plasma potassium concentration had remained constant. Indeed, in a recent study [24], plasma renin in sodium-depleted subjects increased during the reduction of potassium concentration by the intravenous infusion of glucose, suggesting that the plasma renin concentration observed when sodium excretion is low is the net result of sodium-linked stimulation and potassium-linked inhibition.

The increase in plasma renin concentration during sodium depletion is probably due to increased renin secretion from the kidney [2,25], although an effect of reduced inactivation by the liver cannot be ruled out [26]. In addition to sympathetic stimulation [9,10], two intrarenal mechanisms might account for an increase in renin release: the renal autoregulation mechanism [11–13] and reduction of tubular sodium delivery at the macula densa [14]. Renin release increases as the blood pressure level falls towards the lower limit of renal blood flow autoregulation, but this mechanism was obviously not activated in the present study since blood pressure remained unchanged during sodium depletion both before and during β-adrenergic blockade.

During sodium depletion and decrease in plasma volume, sympathetic nervous activity increases and might thereby contribute to the increase in plasma renin concentration [9,10]. Previously, attempts have therefore been made to block the possible stimulating effect of sodium depletion on plasma renin by the administration of propranolol to different groups of patients, but the results are conflicting. In hypertensive subjects given low sodium diets combined with diuretic treatment [27] or in patients with hypoparathyroidism [28], propranolol was found to reduce peripheral plasma renin activity, whereas in hypertensive patients receiving long-term propranolol therapy no such reduction was observed [29]. Thiazides and loop diuretics [30,31] might increase renin release considerably by stimulating β-adrenergic receptors. A reduction of plasma renin by β-receptor blockade might, therefore, be anticipated during combined dietary sodium depletion and administration of diuretics.

In the present study of 20 normotensive subjects, propranolol reduced plasma renin concentration by about 30 per cent (Table I) during normal, unrestricted sodium intake. Statistically, this might not be significantly different from the reduction observed in three normotensive subjects by Michelakis and McAllister

[32]. However, by relating plasma renin concentration to the urinary excretion of sodium we found that sodium depletion had the same stimulating effect on plasma renin concentration whether propranolol was used or not. In the three normotensive subjects of Michelakis and McAllister [32], sodium depletion increased plasma renin during β-receptor blockade approximately three times. This increase might well fall within the range limits in Figure 1. Thus, the increase in plasma renin concentration during sodium depletion seems to be virtually unaffected by the β-adrenergic nervous system. Adequate β-receptor blockade of propranolol was indicated by a significant decrease in pulse rate since lower plasma concentrations of propranolol are needed to produce maximum suppression of adrenergically-mediated increases in plasma renin than to reduce the heart rate [33].

Arterial blood pressure remained normal during propranolol administration. Thus, the finding of a small reduction in plasma renin concentration following β-receptor blockade when sodium excretion is normal is in agreement with the previous observations that the inhibitory effect of β-adrenergic blockade with propranolol [34,35] and the stimulating effect of β-adrenergic activation with isoproterenol [35] on renin release is small at normal blood pressure levels compared to the respective effects at low arterial blood pressure levels. In normotensive subjects, therefore, a decrease in sodium excretion seems to be a more potent stimulus to increase plasma renin concentration than activation of the β-adrenergic nervous system.

Propranolol may be a potent antihypertensive agent. Bühler et al. [36] found roughly proportional reductions in blood pressure and plasma renin activity suggesting a better effect of β-receptor blockade in patients with high renin hypertension than in patients with other subgroups of hypertension. In other studies, however, such a positive correlation between changes in plasma renin and blood pressure were not observed [27,32,33]. As different estimates of sodium balance were used, part of the discrepancies might be due to dissimilar criteria in evaluating plasma renin. Since in the present investigation propranolol had no significant effect on plasma renin concentration during low sodium excretion, different mechanisms seem to be responsible for the increase in plasma renin concentration during high renin hypertension and during sodium depletion in normotensive subjects.

ACKNOWLEDGMENT

We thank The Central Laboratory, Ullevaal Hospital for analysis of electrolytes and creatinine. The skilled assistance of Mrs. Ellen Dahl, Mrs. Irene Eggen, Mrs. Mildred Lewis and Mrs. Ellen Schinnes is gratefully acknowledged. This work was supported by the Norwegian Council for the Promotion of Science.

REFERENCES

1. Peart WS: The renin-angiotensin system. Pharmacol Rev 17: 143, 1965.
2. Brubacher ES, Vander AJ: Sodium deprivation and renin secretion in unanesthetized dogs. Am J Physiol 214: 15, 1968.
3. Brown JJ, Davies DL, Lever AF, et al.: Influence of sodium loading and sodium depletion on plasma-renin in man. Lancet 2: 278, 1963.
4. Laragh JH, Sealey JE, Sommers SC: Patterns of adrenal secretion and urinary excretion of aldosterone and plasma renin activity in normal and hypertensive subjects. Circ Res 18–19 (suppl 1): 158, 1966.
5. Gunnells JC, Grim CE, Robinson RR, et al.: Plasma renin activity in healthy subjects and patients with hypertension. Arch Intern Med 119: 232, 1967.
6. Laragh JH, Baer L, Brunner HR, et al.: Renin, angiotensin and aldosterone system in pathogenesis and management of hypertensive vascular disease. Am J Med 52: 633, 1972.
7. Doyle AE, Chua KG, Duffy S, et al.: Plasma renin, urinary sodium excretion and vascular disease. Clin Sci Molec Med 48: 127s, 1975.
8. Davies DL, Schalekamp MA, Beevers DG, et al.: Abnormal relations between exchangeable sodium and the renin-angiotensin system in malignant hypertension and in hypertension with chronic renal failure. Lancet 1: 683, 1973.
9. Vander AJ: Effect of catecholamines and the renal nerves on renin secretion in anesthetized dogs. Am J Physiol 209: 659, 1965.
10. Davis JO: The control of renin release. Am J Med 55: 333, 1973.
11. Eide I, Løyning E, Kiil F: Evidence for hemodynamic autoregulation of renin release. Circ Res 32: 237, 1973.
12. Ayers CR, Harris RH, Lefer LG: Control of renin release in experimental hypertension. Circ Res 24 (suppl): 103, 1969.
13. Gottschall RW, Davis JO, Blaine EH, et al.: Increased renin release during renal arteriolar dilatation in dogs. Am J Physiol 227: 251, 1974.
14. Vander AJ, Miller R: Control of renin secretion in the anesthetized dog. Am J Physiol 207: 537, 1964.
15. Vander AJ, Luciano JR: Neural and humoral control of renin release in salt depletion. Circ Res 20–21 (suppl 2): 69, 1967.
16. Mogil RA, Itskovitz HD, Russell JH, et al.: Renal innervation and renin activity in salt metabolism and hypertension. Am J Physiol 216: 693, 1969.
17. Haber E, Koerner T, Page LB, et al.: Application of a radioimmunoassay for angiotensin I to the physiologic measurements of plasma renin activity in normal human subjects. J Clin Endocrinol Metab 29: 1349, 1969.
18. Haas E, Gould AB, Goldblatt H: Estimation of endogenous renin in human blood. Lancet 1: 657, 1968.
19. Snedecor GW, Cochran WG: Statistical Methods, 6th ed, Iowa State University Press, 1967.
20. Howell DS, Davis JO: Relationship of sodium retention to potassium excretion by the kidney during administration of desoxycorticosterone acetate to dogs. Am J Physiol 179: 359, 1954.

21. Anderson HM, Laragh JH: Renal excretion of potassium in normal and sodium depleted dogs. J Clin Invest 37: 323, 1958.
22. Brunner HR, Baer L, Sealey JE, et al.: The influence of potassium loading and potassium deprivation on plasma renin in normal and hypertensive subjects. J Clin Invest 49: 2128, 1970.
23. Vander AJ: Direct effects of potassium on renin secretion and renal function. Am J Physiol 219: 455, 1970.
24. Himathongkam T, Dluhy RG, Williams GH: Potassium-aldosterone-renin interrelationships. J Clin Endocrinol Metab 41: 153, 1975.
25. Vander AJ: Control of renin release. Physiol Rev 47: 359, 1967.
26. Johnson JA, Davis JO, Baumber JS, et al.: Effects of hemorrhage and chronic sodium depletion on hepatic clearance of renin. Am J Physiol 220: 1677, 1971.
27. Geyskes GG, Boer P, Leenen FHH, et al.: Effect of volume depletion and subsequent propranolol treatment on blood pressure and plasma renin activity in patients with essential and with renovascular hypertension. Clin Sci Molec Med 48: 69s, 1975.
28. Weber MA, Kleerekoper M, Thornell IR, et al.: Effects of sodium depletion on plasma renin activity and on the urinary excretion of cyclic AMP and aldosterone in hypoparathyroid patients. J Clin Endocrinol Metab 40: 982, 1975.
29. Bravo EL, Tarazi RC, Dustan HP: On the mechanism of suppressed plasma-renin activity during β-adrenergic blockade with propranolol. J Lab Clin Med 83: 119, 1974.
30. Attman PO, Aurell M, Johnsson G: Effects of metoprolol and propranolol on furosemide-stimulated renin release in healthy subjects. Europ J Clin Pharmacol 8: 201, 1975.
31. Eide I, Løyning E, Langaard Ø, et al.: Influence of ethacrynic acid on intrarenal renin release mechanisms. Kidney Int 8: 158, 1975.
32. Michelakis AM, McAllister RG: The effect of chronic adrenergic receptor blockade on plasma renin activity in man. J Clin Endocrinol 34: 386, 1972.
33. Bravo EL, Tarazi RC, Dustan HP, et al.: Dissociation between renin and arterial pressure responses to β-adrenergic blockade in human essential hypertension. Circ Res 36–37 (suppl 1): 241, 1975.
34. La Grange RG, Sloop CH, Schmid HE: Selective stimulation of renal nerves in the anesthetized dog. Effect on renin release during controlled changes in renal hemodynamics. Circ Res 33: 704, 1973.
35. Eide I, Løyning E, Kiil F: Potentiation of renin release by combining renal arterial constriction and β-adrenergic stimulation. Scand J Clin Lab Invest 34: 301, 1974.
36. Bühler FR, Laragh JH, Vaughan ED Jr, et al.: Antihypertensive action of propranolol. Specific antirenin responses in high and normal renin forms of essential, renin, renovascular and malignant hypertension. Am J Cardiol 32: 511, 1973.

A Nationwide Outbreak of Reye's Syndrome

Its Epidemiologic Relationship to Influenza B

LAWRENCE COREY, M.D.*
ROBERT J. RUBIN, M.D.†
MICHAEL A. W. HATTWICK, M.D.
GARY R. NOBLE, M.D.
EDWARD CASSIDY, B.A.‡
Atlanta, Georgia

Between December 15 and June 30, 1974, 379 cases of confirmed Reye's syndrome were reported to the Center for Disease Control. Of these, 316 occurred during February and March 1974. A simultaneous surveillance system for influenza B indicated that this clustering of cases of Reye's syndrome correlated both temporally and geographically with influenza B outbreaks. The incidence of Reye's syndrome was higher in rural than in urban centers. Epidemiologically, two groups of cases of Reye's syndrome emerge: those which occur in older children (median age 11 years), cluster in time and geographic region, and are associated with antecedent influenza B infection; and those which occur sporadically throughout the year, are isolated in occurrence, occur in younger children (median age 6 years), and are associated with a wide variety of antecedent viral illnesses.

Although encephalopathy with fatty degeneration of the viscera was described as early as 1929 [1,2], this clinicopathologic entity did not receive widespread attention until it was described by Reye in 1963 [3]. Over 500 cases have since been reported in the medical literature, but the etiology of Reye's syndrome remains unknown. In most patients an antecedent viral-like illness has been noted prior to the onset of vomiting and encephalopathy [4,5]. Many viruses, including adenovirus type 3 [6], Coxsackie A [7], A9, B1 [8], B4 [9], Epstein-Barr virus [10], ECHO 8 [9], 11 [11], polio type 1 [12], parainfluenza [13], reovirus [14], rubella virus [15], measles [16], varicella [17–19], herpes simplex [4], influenza A [20] and influenza B [21], have been associated with this antecedent illness. However, most of these viruses have been isolated in single cases widely separated in time and geographic area, and have not been associated with the temporal and geographic clustering of cases of Reye's syndrome that have been reported [22,23]. Although a few cases of varicella-associated Reye's syndrome in siblings have been reported [24], the virus which has been associated most frequently in clusters of cases is the influenza B virus. Since 1967, eight clusters of cases of Reye's syndrome have been investigated by the Center for Disease Control (CDC); seven were associated temporally with the presence of influenza B infection in the community [22,25–28] (Table I). Typically, however, influenza B occurs sporadically in focal outbreaks within states and regions; thus, in previous studies linking Reye's syndrome and influenza B, (1) surveillance for both entities has been retrospective and confined to small areas within states, (2) regional and nationwide influenza activity has

From the Bureau of Epidemiology, Center for Disease Control, Public Health Service, U.S. Department of Health, Education and Welfare, Atlanta, Georgia 30333. Requests for reprints should be addressed to Dr. Lawrence Corey. Manuscript accepted March 5, 1976.

* Fellow in Medicine. Present address: Division of Infectious Diseases, University of Washington, Seattle, Washington 98115.

† Fellow in Medicine. Present address: New England Medical Center, Boston, Massachusetts 02111.

‡ Present address: U.S. Food and Drug Administration, Room 460, 220 Milvia Street, Berkeley, California 94704.

TABLE I Cases of Reye's Syndrome Reported to CDC, January 1967–June 1974

Year	Cases Reported (no.)	Cases Clustered in Time and Region (no.)	Viral Agent Implicated in Antecedent Illnesses	Reference
1967	11	6 Tampa	Influenza B/Mass/1/66	[22]
1968	17			
1969	41	6 Oklahoma	Influenza B/Mass/1/66	[25]
		6 Atlanta	Influenza B/Mass/1/66	[22]
1970	13			
1971	83	14 Chicago	Influenza B/Mass/1/71	[26]
		36 New England	Influenza B/Mass/1/71	[27]
		10 North Carolina	3/10 parainfluenza	[28]
		6 Guam	Influenza B	
1972	30	0	...	
1973	32	0	...	
1974 (Jan-June)	379	326	Influenza B/Hong Kong/5/72	

not been evaluated and (3) observations have been limited to small numbers of cases. In this paper we describe data gathered prospectively through a nationwide surveillance system for Reye's syndrome initiated by CDC in 1973; we also describe a nationwide outbreak of Reye's syndrome that occurred between February and March 1974, and that was epidemiologically associated with a widespread outbreak of influenza B.

METHODS

In the summer and early fall of 1973, a new variant of the influenza B virus—influenza B/Hong Kong/5/72—caused outbreaks of influenza in Japan, Australia and Great Britain. Anticipating substantial influenza B activity in this country, we designed a prospective study to monitor the association between influenza B and Reye's syndrome, with the cooperation of state and territorial epidemiologists. Although active surveillance of the occurrence of Reye's syndrome had already been undertaken in many areas of the United States, in December 1973 all state health departments were asked to report any confirmed or suspected cases to CDC on standardized case report forms. The form had been modified in the fall of 1973 to elicit information on demographic characteristics, signs and symptoms experienced during the prodromal and acute neurologic phase of the illness, treatment modalities, virologic studies and outcome. In addition, private physicians were urged by the American Academy of Pediatrics and through bulletins in the Morbidity and Mortality Weekly Report (MMWR) to report cases.

Thus, information on cases was gathered by a review of case report forms and hospital records submitted by attending physicians (51 per cent), by direct investigation of suspected cases by CDC or state health department epidemiologists (33 per cent), or through telephone interviews with health personnel reporting suspected cases (16 per cent).

Data on influenza activity was derived from CDC's influenza surveillance system, which received reports each week by telephone, telegraph and postcard from state epidemiologists. These reports included data on absenteeism in sentinel schools and industries, hospital emergency room visits and physician reporting of influenza-like disease; they also supplied data on the extent and duration of influenza activity in the area. Forty-seven states participated in this system. In addition, influenza activity was monitored through reports from World Health Organization (WHO) Cooperating Laboratories located throughout the United States. Of 56 such laboratories, 33 supplied information weekly from January 1 through April 30, 1974, on the total number of specimens taken from the respiratory tract submitted for viral isolation, and the number and type of influenza viruses isolated from these specimens. This system provided the most specific data available on the initial occurrence and disappearance of influenza virus activity in the communities surveyed.

In February 1974, we requested that state laboratories send serum specimens from any patients with confirmed Reye's syndrome to CDC. Serum samples were analyzed for hemagglutination inhibition antibody to influenza B by standard microtiter technics, and nonspecific agglutinins were removed with receptor destroying enzyme [29]. As evidence of recent infection with influenza B we accepted either a fourfold increase in the hemagglutination inhibition titer in paired serum specimens or a titer of $>$1:80 to B/Hong Kong/5/72 in a specimen obtained during the convalescent phase and within 30 days after the onset of influenza. Antigenic analyses of influenza B isolates were performed by the Respiratory Virology Laboratory at CDC.

CASE DEFINITION

A case of Reye's syndrome was defined as an acute noninflammatory encephalopathy demonstrated by either the presence of less than 8 white blood cells/mm^3 in the cerebrospinal fluid or cerebral edema without perivascular or meningeal inflammation on histologic sections of brain associated with (1) fatty metamorphosis of the liver, diagnosed either by biopsy or autopsy, or (2) a serum glutamic oxaloacetic transaminase (SGOT) greater than three times normal and a high blood ammonia level* [1,2].

* The ammonia level was one and a half times greater than normal (48 μg/ml) in all but eight cases.

RESULTS

The Outbreak. Of the 450 suspected cases of Reye's syndrome reported to CDC between December 15, 1973, and June 30, 1974, 379 fit our case definition. Of the reported suspected cases that did not fit our case definition, 56 (79 per cent) were excluded because the necessary laboratory data were not available: no cerebrospinal fluid data (30 cases), no blood ammonia determinations (18 cases), no SGOT levels (eight cases). In 15 other suspected cases, another diagnosis was subsequently made: encephalitis (six cases), meningitis (three cases), salicylate toxicity (four cases) and sudden infant death syndrome (two cases).

The first reported case occurred in the third week of December in New York; the last reported case occurred in the last week of June in South Carolina. There was a marked increase in cases during the first week of February 1974, and in 316 (83 per cent) of 379 cases reported the patients were hospitalized in February and March 1974 (Figure 1).

Of the 379 cases reported, 179 (47 per cent) were in males and 200 (53 per cent) in females. The median age for all patients with Reye's syndrome was 11 years, with 139 (37 per cent) patients in the 11 to 14 year age range and 4 per cent over 16 years (Figure 2). The patients' ages ranged from three months to 28 years. The 28 year old, the only patient over 18 years of age, was a woman in whom the diagnosis at autopsy was noninflammatory encephalopathy and microvesicular fatty metamorphosis of the liver.

The nationwide case fatality ratio was 41 per cent (157 of 379 patients) (Table II). Age-specific case fatality ratios ranged from a low of 30 per cent in 8 year olds to 60 per cent in 17 year olds; however, these differences in mortality were not statistically significant. Data on ethnic (race) affiliation were available in 224 cases (59 per cent); 211 patients (94 per cent) were white, nine (4 per cent) were black, two (1 per cent) were (American) Indian and two (1 per cent) were Asian.

Of the 379 cases, there was either biopsy or autopsy evidence of fatty regeneration of the liver in 156 (41 per cent), whereas 223 (59 per cent) of these cases fit our clinical and laboratory criteria. No differences between biopsy-confirmed or autopsy-confirmed cases and clinically diagnosed cases were noted with respect to antecedent illness, age, sex and temporal or geographic distribution.

Antecedent Illness. Three types of antecedent illness in patients with Reye's syndrome were identified: upper respiratory illness, varicella infection and gastrointes-

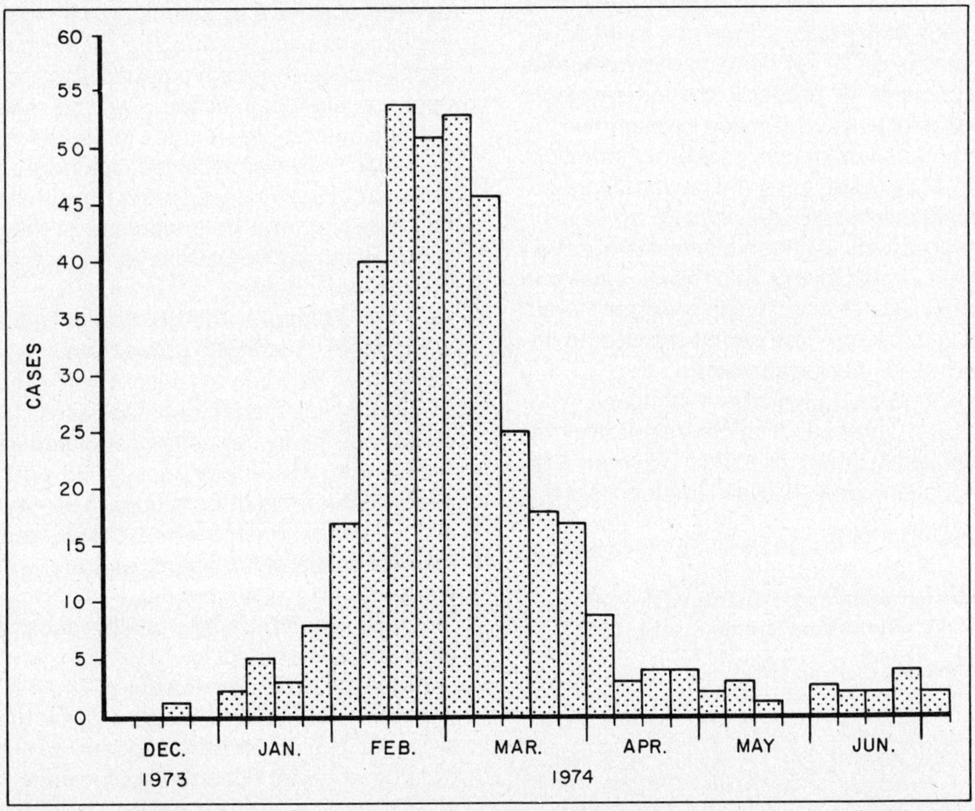

Figure 1. Cases of Reye's syndrome reported in the United States, December 15, 1973 to June 30, 1974.

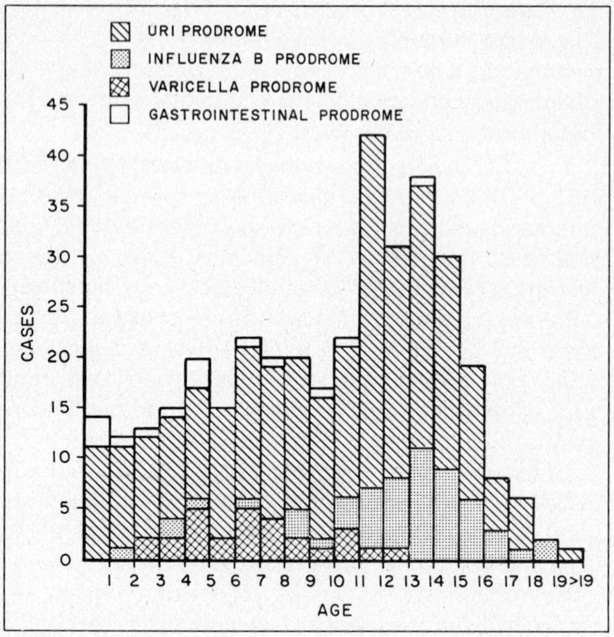

Figure 2. *Cases of Reye's syndrome (367) arranged according to patient's age, United States, December 15, 1973 to June 30, 1974.*

tinal illness. In 340 (90 per cent) cases, the patient had an antecedent upper respiratory infection with a mean duration between onset of upper respiratory symptoms and hospitalization of 5.7 days (range one to 17 days). In most reported cases (79 per cent) no early attempts to obtain viral isolates or properly spaced serologic studies for respiratory virus were made to determine the etiology of the antecedent upper respiratory infection. However, in 58 (17 per cent) cases there was laboratory evidence of recent influenza B infection, 26 by isolation and 32 by serologic tests. Antigenic analysis of seven influenza B isolates from patients with Reye's syndrome and 24 influenza B isolates from patients without Reye's syndrome during the same time period showed no detectable differences in hemagglutinins.

In addition to influenza B, five other viral agents were associated with an antecedent upper respiratory infection. In two patients, influenza A/Port Chalmers was isolated; in one, adenovirus 14 was isolated from the cerebrospinal fluid, and in one there was serologic evidence of parainfluenza virus infection. Three patients with Reye's syndrome had double viral infections; one had influenza A (titer rise) and herpes simplex (isolated from brain), one had clinical varicella and cytomegalovirus (isolated from lung), and one had adenovirus 17 (isolated from throat washings) and influenza B (titer rise). In five other patients with an antecedent upper respiratory infection in whom specimens were cultured for viral agents or who underwent properly spaced serologic studies for respiratory viruses, no viral agent was identified.

TABLE II Mortality Data on Patients with Reye's Syndrome United States, 1974

	Survived		Died		Total	
	No.	%	No.	%	No.	%
Male	107	60	72	40	179	47
Female	115	58	85	42	200	53
Total	222	59	157	41	379	

Twenty-eight patients had antecedent varicella infections before the onset of Reye's syndrome. All 28 had the characteristic exanthem, and one also had a high complement-fixation titer to varicella virus. The mean duration between onset of the rash in patients with varicella-associated cases and their hospitalization was 5.8 days, range three to 20 days; all but one case occurred within 10 days after the rash appeared.

The third clinical prodrome was reported in 15 patients and consisted of primarily gastrointestinal symptoms and signs, such as diarrhea and abdominal cramping followed by nausea, vomiting and a change in mental status. The mean duration between the onset of these prodromal symptoms and hospitalization was 4.8 days (range one to 14 days).

Recent vaccinations were not related to the development of Reye's syndrome. In only five patients were vaccinations reported in the month before hospitalization, and all these patients had also had an antecedent upper respiratory infection. Two had received measles, mumps and rubella vaccine in the week before hospitalization, one had received diphtheria, pertussia, tetanus vaccine two days before hospitalization, and two had received oral polio vaccine in the month before hospitalization. No patient had a history of recent influenza vaccination.

Age and Temporal Distribution in Cases Associated with Upper Respiratory Infection. Age differences were noted between the patients without and with upper respiratory infection-associated cases. The median age of patients with varicella-associated cases was six years, with 26 (93 per cent) of 28 patients under 11 years. Patients with both upper respiratory infection- and influenza B-associated cases were older; their median age was 11 years, and the greatest number were 11 to 14 years old (Figure 2). No significant differences in death-to-case fatality ratios and antecedent illnesses were noted.

Figure 3 shows the cases of Reye's syndrome by date of the patient's admission to the hospital and antecedent illness. Both the varicella and gastrointestinal prodromal cases occurred sporadically throughout the surveillance period, and no distinct temporal clustering was noted. The 28 varicella-associated cases were

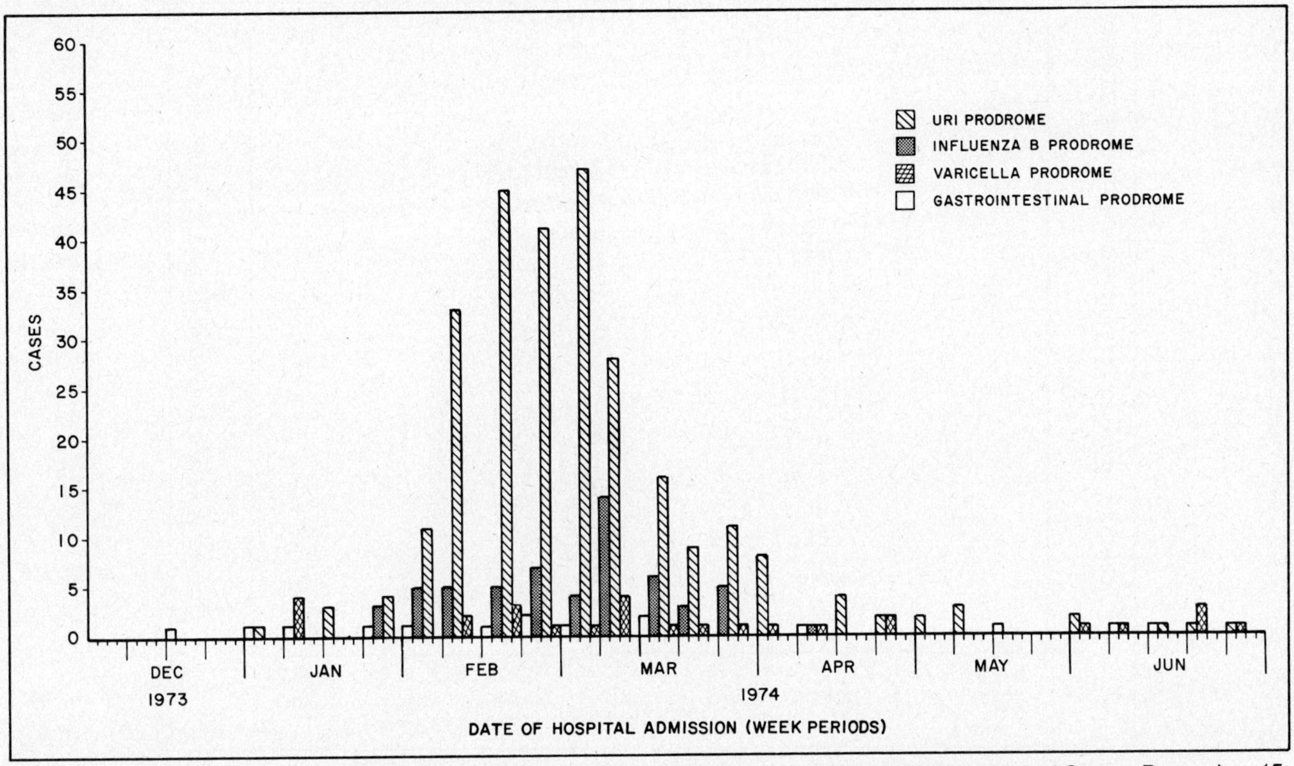

Figure 3. Reported cases (374) of Reye's syndrome, by date of patient's hospital admission, United States, December 15, 1973 to June 30, 1974.

spread nearly evenly over the six-month surveillance period, with four to seven cases occurring per month. In addition, none of the patients with an antecedent upper respiratory infection in which either double viral infections or influenza A, adenovirus or parainfluenza virus infection was documented were clustered temporally or geographically. In contrast the majority of cases associated with upper respiratory infection were clustered markedly between the second week of February and the third week of March, the period in which the cases of Reye's syndrome associated with influenza B were also at a peak.

Temporal Relationship Between Influenza B and Reye's Syndrome. Influenza surveillance data for the 1973–1974 influenza season indicated that the incidence of Reye's syndrome was associated temporally with the occurrence of widespread outbreaks of influenza B. Weekly data collected from the WHO Cooperating Laboratories on the per cent of respiratory isolates which were influenza showed that influenza B activity began in the second week of January 1974 and that nationwide influenza activity peaked in the second week of February, one week before the peak of cases of Reye's syndrome (Figure 4). Both the incidence of Reye's syndrome and influenza B activity decreased markedly by the first week of April 1974. A subsequent outbreak of influenza A/Port Chalmers occurred along the eastern seaboard in April, but it was not associated with an increase in reported cases of Reye's syndrome.

This temporal association between influenza B and Reye's syndrome was also noted on a regional, state and county level. Influenza B activity started initially in the Midwest and peaked in the second week of February in that region. In contrast, widespread community outbreaks of influenza were not recorded in the northeastern United States until early March 1974. Admission dates of patients with Reye's syndrome followed a similar pattern, with hospitalizations in the Midwest occurring in early to mid-February and markedly decreasing when influenza B activity was no longer present (Figure 5). This same association was also seen in the Northeast where an increase in the cases of Reye's syndrome was not seen until community-wide outbreaks of influenza B began in early and mid-March, and where cases continued to occur in large numbers as long as influenza B activity was widespread in the region. Although there was an increase in influenza B activity as indicated by influenza B isolates from patients in the Northeast early in February, these isolates came from college students in two localized campus outbreaks, a population in which Reye's syndrome is not often seen. Again, a widespread influenza A outbreak in the Northeast in April was not associated with any

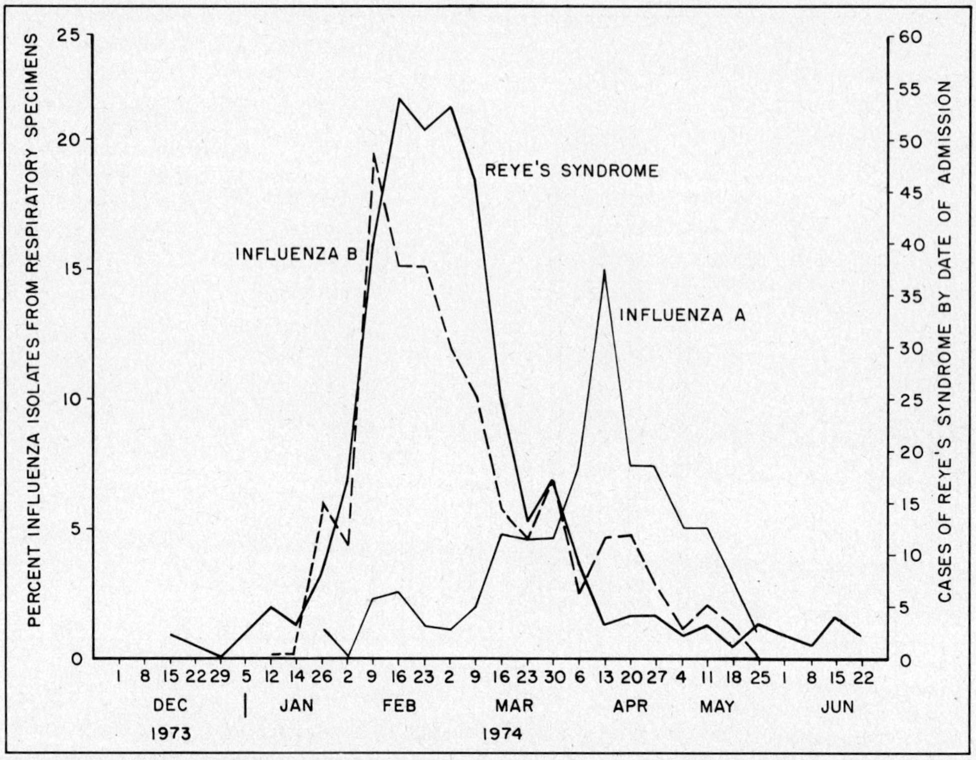

Figure 4. *Reported cases of Reye's syndrome and influenza isolates (33 regularly reporting, WHO Cooperating Laboratories) by week of isolation, United States, January through May 1974.*

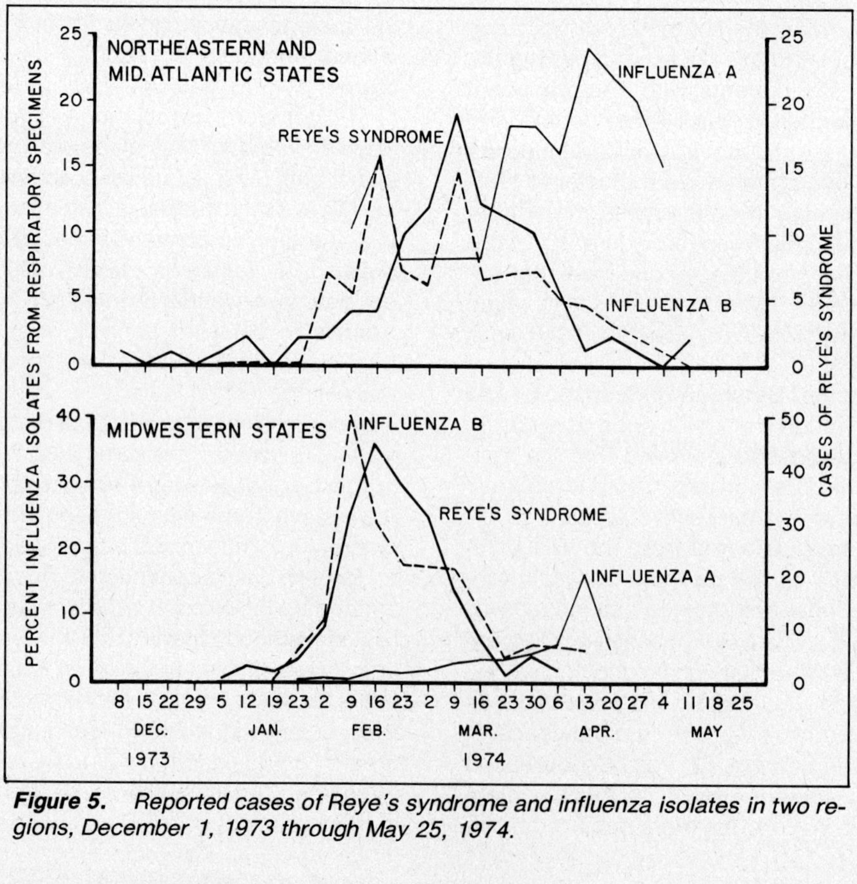

Figure 5. *Reported cases of Reye's syndrome and influenza isolates in two regions, December 1, 1973 through May 25, 1974.*

substantial increase in the number of reported cases of Reye's syndrome.

Other parameters of influenza activity, such as school absenteeism and physician reporting of influenza-like disease, also demonstrated this temporal association between influenza B and Reye's syndrome. Figure 6 illustrates the association between influenza activity monitored in the Cook County, Illinois, area with dates of admission of patients with Reye's syndrome seen in Cook, Lake and DuPaige counties. The simultaneous occurrence of Reye's syndrome and influenza B activity as monitored by both school absenteeism and reported cases of influenza is again evident.

Geographic Distribution. Geographical clustering of cases also occurred. Although 40 of the 50 states reported cases of Reye's syndrome, 188 cases (nearly 50 per cent) were reported by Michigan, Indiana, Ohio, Wisconsin, Minnesota and Illinois. The over-all nationwide incidence for the population less than 18 years of age was estimated to be 0.58/100,000. An analysis of incidence data by state showed that almost every state that reported an incidence of Reye's syndrome of >0.5/100,000 also reported influenza B outbreaks (Figures 7 and 8).

Rural Clustering. The home addresses of all patients with Reye's syndrome reported from Michigan (46

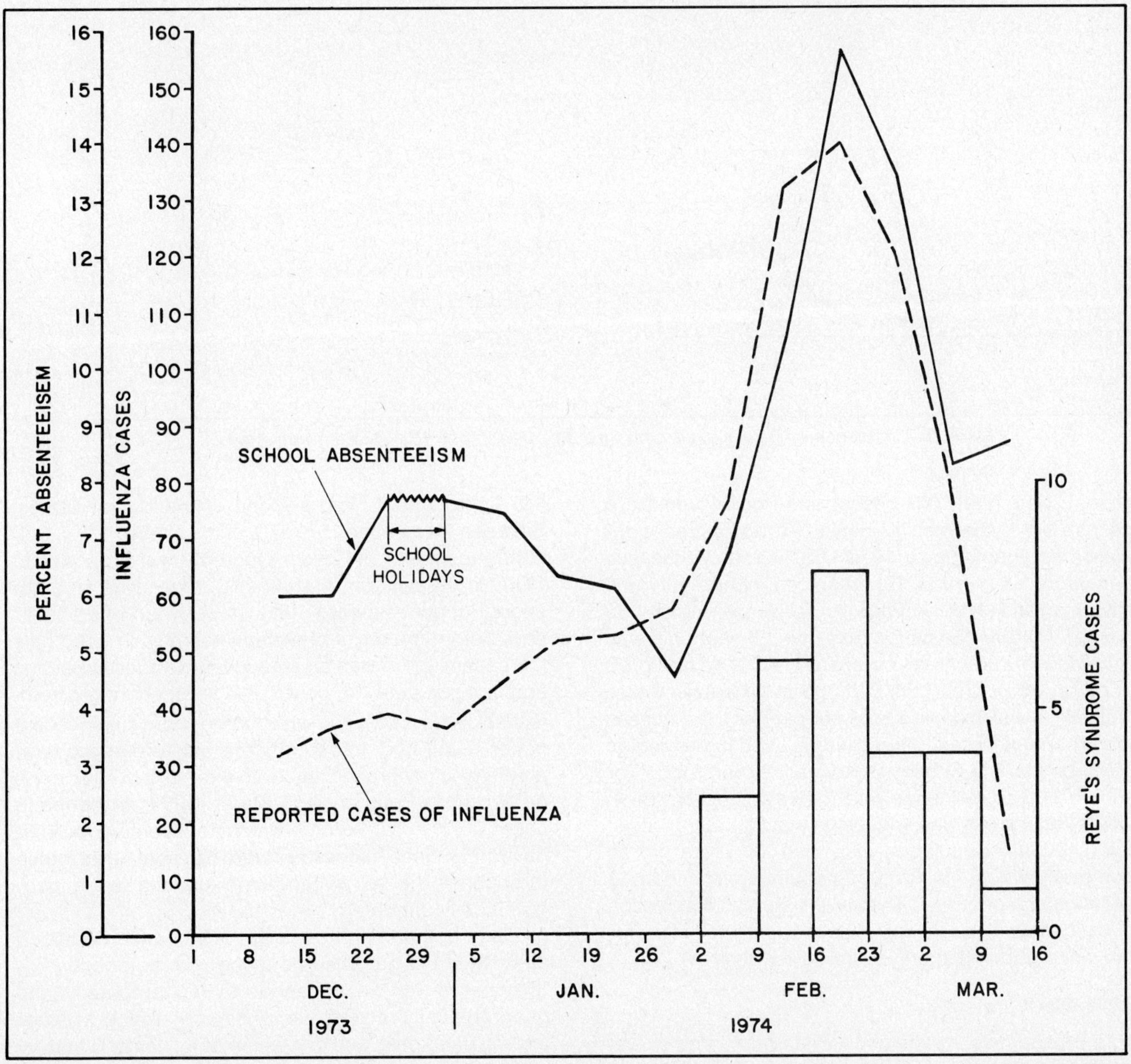

Figure 6. Relationship between influenza surveillance and incidence of Reye's syndrome, Cook County, Illinois, December 1, 1973 through March 16, 1974.

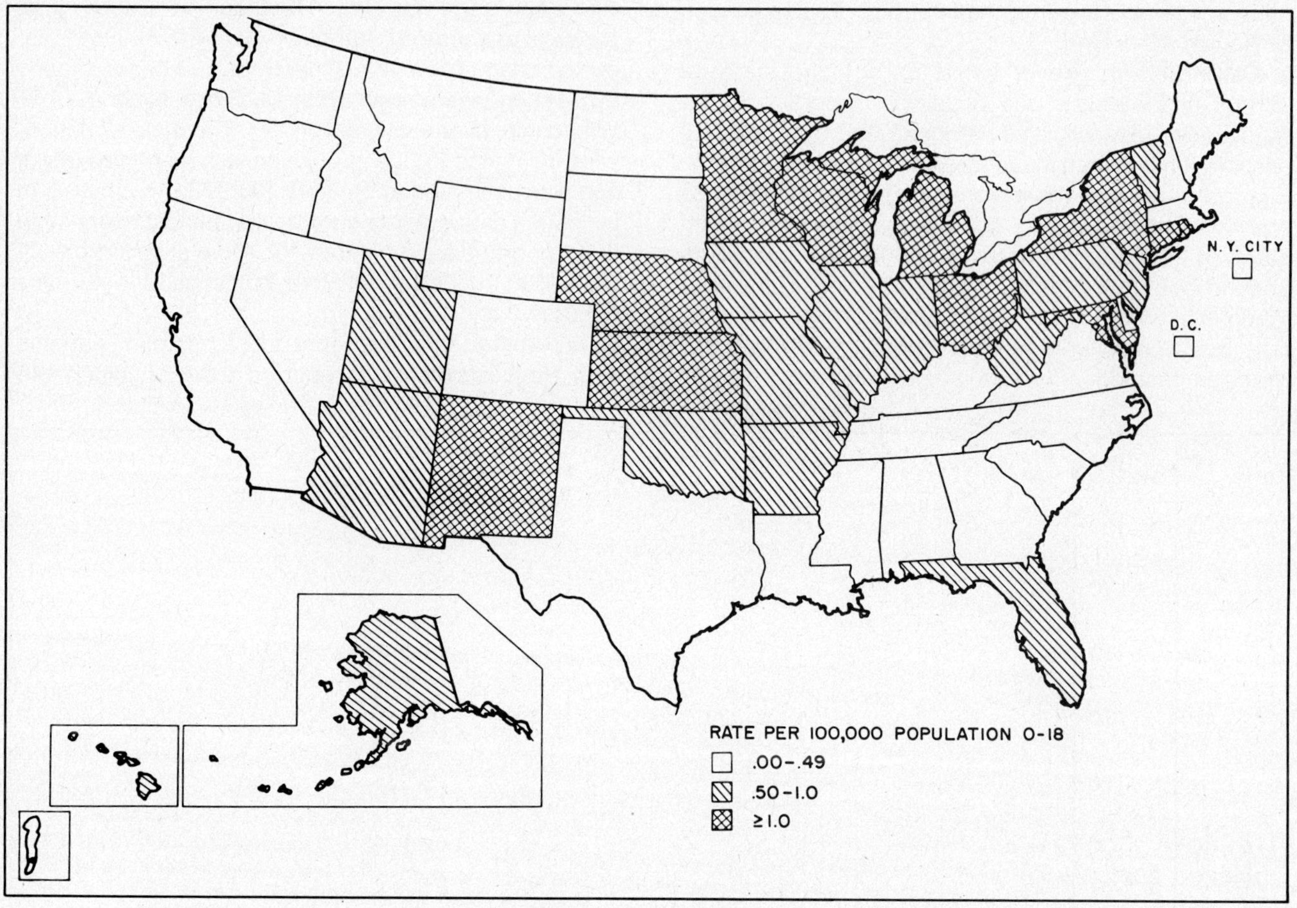

Figure 7. *Incidence of Reye's syndrome by state, December 15, 1973 through June 30, 1974.*

cases), New York (40 cases) and Pennsylvania (26 cases) were analyzed in detail. All addresses were classified according to 1970 U.S. Bureau of Census definitions as (1) rural, (2) urbanized (central city and suburban) and (3) other urban. An incidence rate of 1.80 cases/100,000 population less than 18 years old was recorded for rural areas compared with 0.42/100,000 in other urban and 0.58/100,000 in urbanized areas (Table III). In addition, in 31 (61 per cent) of the 51 cases in "urbanized areas," the patients lived in the region described by the Census Bureau as "urban fringe" or suburban. The incidence rate for Reye's syndrome in urban fringe areas was 1.65 times that for central cities, 0.81/100,000 population less than 18 years old as compared with 0.49/100,000 population less than 18 years old, respectively. This rural-suburban distribution of cases was also present when the incidence rates for the white population only were calculated.

COMMENTS

This prospective surveillance system initiated in December 1973 indicated that an outbreak of Reye's syndrome occurred during February, March and April 1974 throughout most regions of the United States. Between December 15, 1973, and June 30, 1974, 379 confirmed cases of Reye's syndrome were reported to CDC. In 88 per cent (340 cases), there was an antecedent upper respiratory illness between one and 17 days before the onset of encephalopathy. In 7 per cent (28 cases), there was an antecedent varicella infection and in 4 per cent (15 cases), an antecedent gastrointestinal illness. Cases in which there was an antecedent upper respiratory infection were clustered both temporally and geographically, with over 295 (87 per cent) occurring in February and March 1974. In contrast, cases of Reye's syndrome with antecedent varicella or gastrointestinal illnesses were evenly distributed throughout the surveillance period and were geographically unrelated.

Since both the proved cases of influenza B-associated Reye's syndrome and those with antecedent influenza-like illness appeared to be temporally and geographically related, we tried to determine whether the initiation, peak and diminution of influenza B activity within communities was related to the occurrence of Reye's syndrome. The isolation of influenza virus is the

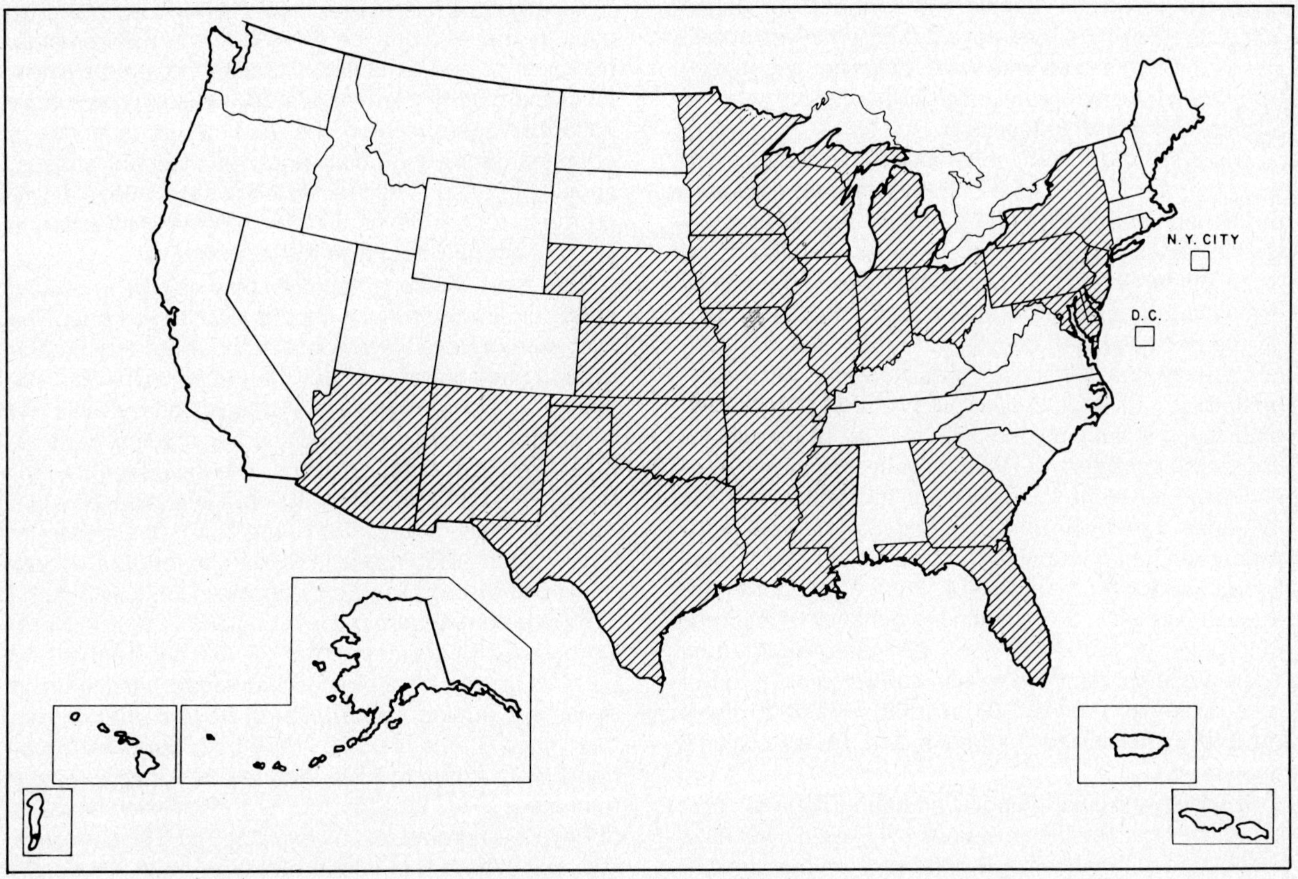

Figure 8. *States reporting influenza B outbreaks from December 1, 1973 to March 1, 1974.*

most objective measure of determining the beginning and duration of influenza activity in a community. Data collected weekly from 33 WHO Cooperating Laboratories indicated that influenza activity first occurred in the midwestern United States in mid-January 1974 and spread over a six week period to the northeastern and southern sections of the country. The peak activity for influenza B in the Midwest occurred in the second week of February, whereas that in the Northeast occurred in the second week of March. This same three week separation was noted in the occurrence of Reye's syndrome in these areas. Other parameters of influenza surveillance, such as school absenteeism and private physician reporting, also reflected this association between community outbreaks of influenza B and outbreaks of Reye's syndrome. The markedly increased incidence of cases of Reye's syndrome following the increase in influenza B activity in the community, the short separation between peak influenza B activity and the peak in admissions of patients with Reye's syndrome, and the simultaneous diminution of cases of Reye's syndrome and influenza B in the area, all indicated that influenza B was the predominant cause of the antecedent upper respiratory infection in the cases of Reye's syndrome that occurred in February–March 1974. Although in three cases the antecedent upper respiratory infection was shown to be influenza A infection, these cases were widely spaced geographically and no epidemiologic association between a widespread outbreak of influenza A/Port Chalmers, which

TABLE III **Distribution of Cases of Reye's Syndrome by Home Address, Michigan, New York, Pennsylvania, December 1973–June 1974**

	Rural	Other Urban	Urbanized
Total population <18 years old	3,096,854	1,175,378	8,659,498
Total white population <18 years old	3,047,349	1,119,483	7,008,489
No. of cases of Reye's syndrome	56	5	50 (31 suburban)
Cases/100,000 population <18 years old	1.80	0.42	0.58
Cases/100,000 white population <18 years old	1.83	0.44	0.71

occurred in the mid-Atlantic and northeastern United States in April 1974, and Reye's syndrome was noted. Cases of Reye's syndrome were, however, associated temporally and geographically in this region with an earlier outbreak of influenza B.

The first cases of encephalopathy and fatty degeneration of the viscera in the United States were reported by Johnson et al. in 1962 [9], before Reye characterized this entity. This cluster of 16 cases was also noted to be epidemiologically associated with influenza B. Previous increases in reported cases of Reye's syndrome occurred in 1969 and 1971. Fifty-five per cent of cases reported in these years were due to "microepidemics" of Reye's syndrome related to localized outbreaks of influenza B [22,26–28]. Although increased awareness of Reye's syndrome may be responsible for some increase in its incidence, in 1974 influenza B activity in the United States was more widespread than in any of the years 1967–1973. Between January and April 1974, 38 states reported influenza B activity, 20 recording regional or widespread outbreaks. In 1970–1971 only 23 states reported influenza B; eight recorded widespread outbreaks and two recorded regional ones [30]. In 1969, eight of 20 states reported widespread outbreaks and seven regional activity [31].

In addition to this temporal and geographical clustering, the age distribution in cases of Reye's syndrome associated with influenza B differed from that in varicella-associated and probable enterovirus (gastrointestinal)-associated cases. Patients with influenza B-associated Reye's syndrome were older (median age 11 years) than those without upper respiratory infection prodromes. This observation probably reflects the age-specific attack rates of influenza B and varicella [32].

Epidemiologically, two distinct groups of cases of Reye's syndrome have emerged from our analyses:

(1) Cases which cluster both temporally and geographically. These children tend to be older (median age of 11 years), to have preceding upper respiratory infections and, as shown in outbreaks in 1962, 1967, 1969 and 1974, to be epidemiologically associated with influenza B. These cases comprise 400 (66 per cent) of the 606 cases reported to CDC since 1967.

(2) Cases which occur sporadically throughout the year and are usually isolated in time and geographic area. These cases tend to occur in younger children (median age 6 years) and are associated with a number of viral agents, the most common being the varicella virus.

What unique role viruses, especially influenza B virus, play in the etiology of Reye's syndrome remains, however, to be elucidated. Detailed virologic studies, including cultures for respiratory viruses grown from nasopharyngeal specimens and serum specimens obtained during the acute and convalescent phases, should be made in all suspected cases of Reye's syndrome to further delineate the role of viral infection in the pathogenesis of Reye's syndrome.

However, additional factor(s) may also be important contributory agents in the etiology of this syndrome. The incidence of Reye's syndrome in our series was greater in rural and suburban areas than in central cities. Although all 121 patients from Michigan, Pennsylvania and New York were hospitalized in urban medical centers, most lived in nonurban locales. The incidence rate for Reye's syndrome for white children less than 18 years of age in these states was nearly 2.7 times greater in rural than in urban areas (1.83 versus 0.68). A review of the outbreaks of Reye's syndrome in 1971 in Chicago [26] (western suburbs), New England [29] and North Carolina [28], indicated that 50 (83 per cent) of 60 patients lived in rural or suburban areas. In addition, in Johnson's original description of Reye's syndrome in the United States in 1962, 13 (81 per cent) of 16 patients were noted to have "come from predominately rural areas" [9]. Whether this rural distribution of cases of Reye's syndrome can be explained by a higher attack rate of influenza B in rural areas is unknown. However, preliminary analysis of a serologic survey within the county of Kalamazoo, Michigan, indicated that influenza B attack rates for urban and rural locales did not differ [32]. Thus, another factor, in addition to an antecedent influenza B infection, a factor that is most likely environmental, may be important in the pathogenesis of this syndrome. Although many exogenous and endogenous substances such as organophosphate exposure [34], aflatoxin [35], 4-pentenoic acid ingestion [36] and acquired or inherited hepatic ornithene transcarbamylase deficiency [37,38] have been suggested as contributory factors in either isolated cases or animal models of Reye's syndrome, none of these substances has been subjected to detailed epidemiologic surveys as to whether the prevalence and distribution of these agents in the United States follow the epidemiologic pattern of cases of Reye's syndrome.

Detailed studies into the dietary, chemical, environmental and genetic "mileau" of patients with Reye's syndrome are needed in order to delineate further possible viral-environmental interactions in the pathogenesis of this syndrome.

REFERENCES

1. Brain WR, Hunter D, Turnbull HM: Acute meningo-encephalomyelitis of childhood. Lancet 1: 221, 1929.
2. Brain WR, Hunter D: Encephalopathy and fatty degeneration of the viscera. Lancet 1: 881, 1963.
3. Reye RDK, Morgan G: Encephalopathy and fatty degeneration of the viscera. A disease entity in childhood. Lancet 2: 749, 1963.
4. Becroft DMO: Syndrome of encephalopathy and fatty degeneration of the viscera in New Zealand children. Br Med J 2: 135, 1966.
5. Riley HD Jr: Reye's syndrome. J Infect Dis 125: 77, 1972.
6. Dvorackova I, Vortel V, Hroch M: Encephalitic syndrome with fatty degeneration of viscera. Arch Pathol 81: 240, 1966.
7. Utian HL, Wagner HM: White liver disease. Lancet 2: 1043, 1964.
8. Barr R, Glass IHJ, Chawla G: Reye's syndrome: massive fatty metamorphosis of the liver with acute encephalopathy. Can Med Assoc J 98: 1038, 1968.
9. Johnson GM, Scurletis TD, Carroll NB: A study of 16 fatal cases of encephalitis-like disease in North Carolina children. NC Med J 24: 464, 1963.
10. Rahal JJ, Henle G: Infectious mononucleosis and Reye's syndrome. A fatal case with studies for Epstein-Barr virus. Pediatrics 46: 776, 1970.
11. Golden GS, Duffell D: Encephalopathy and fatty change in the liver and kidney. Pediatrics 36: 67, 1965.
12. Bell WE: Reys syndrome: an association with type I vaccine-like poliovirus. Arch Neurol 30: 304, 1974.
13. Powell HC, Rosenberg RN, McKellar B: Reye's syndrome: isolation of parainfluenza virus. Arch Neurol 29: 135, 1973.
14. Joske RA, Keall DD, Leak PJ, et al.: Hepatitis-encephalitis in humans with reovirus infection. Arch Intern Med 113: 811, 1964.
15. Sherman FE, Michaels RH, Kenny FM: Acute encephalopathy (encephalitis) complicating rubella. JAMA 192: 675, 1965.
16. Ferraro A, Scheffer IH: Toxic encephalopathy in measles. Arch Neurol 27: 1209, 1932
17. Blair AW, Jamieson WM, Smith GH: Complications and death in chickenpox. Br Med J 2: 981, 1965.
18. Breen GE, Emond RTD: Chickenpox associated with fulminating hepatitis. The Medical Press 232: 251, 1954.
19. Mortimer EA, Lepow ML: Varicella with hypoglycemia possibly due to salicylates. Am J Dis Child 103: 583, 1962.
20. Hall BD: Reye's syndrome: an association with influenza A infection. J Ky Med Assoc 67: 269, 1969.
21. Norman MG, Lowden JA, Hill DE, et al.: Encephalopathy and fatty degeneration of the viscera in childhood. II. Report of a case with isolation of influenza B virus. Can Med Assoc J 99: 549, 1968.
22. Glick TH, Likosky WH, Levitt LP, et al: Reye's syndrome: an epidemiologic approach. Pediatrics 46: 371, 1970.
23. Bourgeois CH, Keschamras N, Comer DS, et al.: Udorn encephalopathy. Fatal cerebral edema and fatty degeneration of the viscera in Thai children. J Med Assoc Thai 52: 552, 1969.
24. Glick TH, Ditchek NT, Salitsky S, et al.: Acute encephalopathy and hepatic dysfunction associated with chickenpox in siblings. Am J Dis Child 119: 68, 1970.
25. Reynolds DW, Riley HD Jr, LaFont DS, et al.: An outbreak of Reye's syndrome associated with influenza B. J Pediatr 80: 429, 1972.
26. Hochberg FH, Nelson K, Janzen W: Influenza type B-related encephalopathy. JAMA 231: 817, 1975.
27. Center for Disease Control: Morbidity and Mortality Weekly Report 20: 99, 1971.
28. Roe CR, Schonberger LB, Gelbach SH: Enzymatic alterations in Reye's syndrome. Pediatrics 55: 119, 1975.
29. Hierholzer JC, Suggs MT, Hall EC: Standardized viral hemagglutination and hemagglutination inhibition tests. II. Description and statistical application. Appl Microbiol 18: 824, 1969.
30. Center for Disease Control: Influenza and Respiratory Disease Surveillance Report No. 85, June 1969.
31. Center for Disease Control: Influenza and Respiratory Disease Surveillance Report No. 87, December 1971.
32. Corey L, Rubin RJ, Thompson TR, et al.: Incidence and potential for prevention of influenza-B associated Reye's syndrome. J Infect Dis (in press).
33. Ross AH: Modification of chickenpox in family contacts by administration of gamma globulin. N Engl J Med 267: 369, 1962.
34. Crocker JFS, Ozere RL, Rozee KR: Insecticide and viral interaction as a cause of fatty visceral changes and encephalopathy in the mouse. Lancet 2: 22, 1974.
35. Shank RC, Bougoeis CH, Keschamras N, et al.: Aflatoxins in autopsy specimens from Thai children with an acute disease of unknown aetiology. Food Cosmet Toxicol 9: 501, 1971.
36. Glasgow AM, Chase HP: Reye's syndrome, Jamaican vomiting sickness and 4-pentenoic acid. Reye's Syndrome (Pollack JD, ed), New York, Grune & Stratton, p 273, 1975.
37. Thaler MM, Hoogenraad NJ, Boswell M: Reyes syndrome due to novel protein tolerant variant of ornithine transcarbamylase deficiency. Lancet 2: 438, 1974.
38. Tang TT, Siegesmund KA, Sedmak GV, et al.: Reye's syndrome. JAMA 232: 1339, 1975.

Pulmonary Aspergilloma

A Rational Approach to Treatment

BASIL VARKEY, M.D.
HAROLD D. ROSE, M.D.
Milwaukee, Wisconsin

A prospective study of 15 patients with pulmonary aspergilloma was undertaken over an 11 year period. Serious underlying diseases, particularly chronic obstructive pulmonary disease and alcoholic cirrhosis, were present in 12 of them. Eight of 15 patients whose clinical and roentgenographic course was followed for an average of 50 months, received no specific therapy. There were four deaths in this group, none attributable to aspergilloma. The aspergilloma had lysed spontaneously in two, decreased in size in one and was unchanged in one. In the four surviving patients who had no treatment, the aspergilloma lysed spontaneously in one, remained unchanged in two and increased in size in one. Of the seven patients who were treated medically or surgically, three died. Among the seven deaths (untreated and treated patients combined), six were clearly related to underlying disease. The prognosis of aspergilloma is related primarily to the nature and severity of the underlying disease(s). Contrary to the conclusions of previous reports, the experience in our series of patients suggests that routine surgical excision of aspergilloma is not indicated.

The intracavitary aspergilloma results from saphrophytic colonization of areas of lung tissue that have been destroyed by tuberculosis [1,2], sarcoidosis [2], pulmonary infarcts [3], bronchiectasis [4], lung abscesses [4], neoplasms [5] and various pulmonary mycoses [1,6,7]. Proliferation of the fungus in an air-containing cavity is eventually recognized by the distinctive roentgenographic appearance of a crescent of air separating the mycetoma from the well of the cavity [8].

The natural history of this infection is not well documented, and the mode of treatment therefore remains controversial. Medical treatment with intravenous amphotericin B has been shown to be ineffective [6,9,10] and the number of patients treated with endobronchial instillation of amphotericin and sodium iodide has been too small to draw conclusions [11]. Surgical excision of all aspergillomas has been recommended by numerous investigators [3,4,12,13]. Others have recommended surgery for patients with hemoptysis [2,14]. A conservative approach with careful observation has also been proposed [7].

This report is an analysis of 15 cases of aspergilloma seen during an 11 year period and focuses on the outcome of patients who received no treatment for the infection.

From the Pulmonary and Infectious Disease Sections, Medical Service, Veterans Administration Center, Wood (Milwaukee), Wisconsin, and the Department of Medicine, Medical College of Wisconsin, Milwaukee, Wisconsin. Requests for reprints should be addressed to Dr. Basil Varkey, Pulmonary Disease Section, Veterans Administration Center, Wood, Wisconsin 53193. Manuscript accepted March 16, 1976.

MATERIALS AND METHODS

To select patients with aspergilloma, a prospective study was undertaken at the Veterans Administration Center, Wood, Wisconsin, to include (1) those specimens submitted to the Mycology Laboratory for fungus culture that yielded Aspergillus species; (2) chest roentgenograms showing an intracavitary density, and (3) surgical and autopsy specimens showing aspergilli in tissue sections. The study period included the 11 years from January 1964 through December 1974. Aspergilloma was identified in 15 patients who fulfilled one of the following criteria: (1) chest roentgenograms showed an intracavitary mass with a "crescent sign" and either Aspergillus was demonstrated in sputum or there was a positive Aspergillus serum precipitin test, and (2) there was gross and histologic evidence of aspergilloma in resected lung tissue.

RESULTS

The incidence of aspergilloma in the general population is unknown. MacPherson [15] found an incidence of 0.01 per cent in reviewing 60,000 chest films. The 15 cases presented here represent an incidence of one case per 6,000 admissions (0.017 per cent) to this Center.

All patients were male and ranged in age from 40 to 76 years, with an average of 54.3 years. There were 12 Caucasians, two Blacks and one American Indian. All patients smoked tobacco and had averaged approximately 20 cigarettes a day for over 20 years.

The clinical data of these 15 patients are shown in Table I. Tuberculosis or atypical mycobacterial disease was the predisposing disease in seven patients. Two of these patients had undergone previous resective surgery, and one had roentgenographic evidence of a postoperative residual space. The mycobacterial disease was inactive in these seven patients. Primary lung abscess was the predisposing disease in two patients, one of whom had active tuberculosis when the aspergilloma was discovered. Two patients had ankylosing spondylitis. Other probable predisposing conditions included pulmonary infarct, silicosis and chronic tracheocutaneous fistula.

Twelve patients had other serious underlying conditions. Six patients had chronic obstructive pulmonary disease; pulmonary function studies revealed significant ventilatory impairment (1 second forced expired volume of 22 to 56 per cent of predicted). Four patients had

TABLE I Clinical Data on 15 Patients with Aspergilloma

Age (yr)	Predisposing Disease; Associated Conditions	Presenting Manifestations	Intracavitary Mass with "Crescent"	Sputum Culture	Serum Precipitins
51	Ankylosing spondylitis; cirrhosis	Abnormal chest film	+	+	0
40	Tuberculosis—lung, spine; paraplegia	Abnormal chest film	+	+	0
71	Silicosis; chronic obstructive pulmonary disease	Abnormal chest film	+	—	+
43	Ankylosing spondylitis	Productive cough, abnormal chest film	+	+	0
40	Tracheocutaneous fistula; seizures, hemiplegia	Abnormal chest film	+	—	+
55	Atypical mycobacterial disease; status postoperative lobectomy, thoracoplasty, chronic obstructive pulmonary disease, cirrhosis	Cough with hemoptysis (streaks)	+	+	0
47	Atypical mycobacterial disease; chronic obstructive pulmonary disease	Cough with hemoptysis (streaks), weakness, weight loss	+	+	+
49	Lung abscess	Abnormal chest film	+	+	+
50	Tuberculosis; status postoperative segmentectomy	Productive cough	+	—	+
74	Pulmonary infarct; heart failure, thrombophlebitis	Abnormal chest film, cough	+	+	+
56	Lung abscess; tuberculosis, cirrhosis, chronic obstructive pulmonary disease	Hemoptysis (gross)	+	+	+
51	Tuberculosis; cirrhosis	Hemoptysis (gross)	+	+	+
76	Esophageal carcinoma*	Vomiting, weight loss	—	0	0
54	Tuberculosis; chronic obstructive pulmonary disease	Hemoptysis (gross)	+	+	+
58	Tuberculosis; chronic obstructive pulmonary disease	Hemoptysis (gross)	+	+	+

Note: + = present. — = absent. 0 = not performed.
*Diagnosis of aspergilloma not made preoperatively.

TABLE II Course and Outcome in Seven Treated Patients with Aspergilloma

Age (yr)	Treatment	Follow-Up (mo) Total	Follow-Up (mo) After Rx	Course: Clinical	Course: Roentgenologic	Outcome	Cause of Death
51	Amphotericin (intracavitary) 70 mg	75	70	No respiratory symptoms, hepatic decompensation	Aspergilloma disappeared in 6 mo	Died	Autopsy—aspiration pneumonia, hepatic failure
47	Amphotericin (intravenously 2 g), 5-flurocytosin (oral) (100 mg/kg/day for 2 weeks)	22	20	Mild exertional dyspnea, occasional blood-streaked sputum	Aspergilloma increased in size in 20 mo	Alive	. . .
43	Lobectomy (elective)	24	23	Stable	No recurrence of aspergilloma	Alive	. . .
50	Lobectomy (for hemoptysis)	103	7	Repeat surgery for bleeding, heart failure	No recurrence	Died	Autopsy—pneumonia, hepatic failure
51	Lobectomy (for hemoptysis)	30	27	Chronic chest wall sinus, fistulotomy	No recurrence	Died	Autopsy—pneumonia, hepatic failure
76	Segmentectomy (diagnostic)	48	1/2	Cerebrovascular accident	. . .	Died	No autopsy, had esophageal surgery for carcinoma
54	Lobectomy (for hemoptysis)	3	1	Lost for follow-up	. . .	. . .	. . .

TABLE III Course and Outcome in Eight Untreated Patients with Aspergilloma

Age (yr)	Follow-Up (mo)	Course: Clinical	Course: Roentgenologic	Outcome	Cause of Death
40	13	Paraplegia due to tuberculosis of spine, no cough or hemoptysis	Aspergilloma unchanged in 13 mo	Died	Died 5 mo after discharge, cause of death unknown
71	40	Progressive silicosis, dyspnea, cough (chronic obstructive pulmonary disease and corpulmonale)	Aspergilloma disappeared in 14 mo	Died	No autopsy, respiratory failure, chronic obstructive lung disease
40	48	Hemiplegia, tracheocutaneous fistula corrected, no cough or hemoptysis	Aspergilloma unchanged in 48 mo	Alive	. . .
55	39	Progressive dyspnea, cough (chronic obstructive pulmonary disease and corpulmonale)	Aspergilloma disappeared in 9 mo	Died	No autopsy, respiratory failure, chronic obstructive lung disease
49	64	Asymptomatic	Aspergilloma increased in size in 64 mo	Alive	. . .
74	96	Cardiac failure, cough with recurrent blood-streaked sputum	Aspergilloma unchanged in 92 mo	Lost for further follow-up	. . .
56	7	Progressive dyspnea (chronic obstructive pulmonary disease), upper gastrointestinal bleeding (peptic ulcer)	Aspergilloma decreased in size in 3 mo	Died	Autopsy—aspiration pneumonia, respiratory failure, chronic obstructive pulmonary disease, hepatic failure, cirrhosis, no aspergilloma seen in lung
58	92	Exertional dyspnea (chronic obstructive pulmonary disease)	Aspergilloma disappeared in 16 mo	Alive	. . .

alcoholic cirrhosis, and four had either paraplegia, hemiplegia, congestive heart failure or carcinoma of the esophagus.

In 13 of 15 patients, the major presenting manifestation was either hemoptysis or the discovery of an abnormal chest film. Hemoptysis varied from blood-streaked sputum to several hundred milliliters of gross blood and was the presenting complaint in six patients. A single abnormal chest film or a change noted in a previously abnormal but stable film accounted for the referral of seven patients for evaluation. Fourteen patients had the distinctive roentgenographic finding of an intracavitary mass with a "crescent sign" on chest films or laminagrams. The aspergilloma was present in the upper lobes of all patients; the upper lobe of the left lung was involved in 10.

The diagnosis was established in one patient after surgical resection and histologic examination of the resected lung segment. Sputum cultures were positive for aspergilli in 11 patients; Aspergillus fumigatus was isolated in eight and Aspergillus niger in three. A strongly positive serum precipitin test by immunodiffusion was obtained in all 10 patients tested. However, the precipitin test in one patient with aspergilloma caused by A. niger was negative to A. fumigatus antigen, but it was strongly positive when retested with A. niger antigen.

After the diagnosis of aspergilloma was established, patients were seen at intervals of four to 16 weeks in the Chest Clinic, and their roentgenographic and clinical course followed. Although no attempt was made to group them for different modalities of treatment, episodes of hemoptysis were recorded, and surgical consultation was obtained. During the 11 year study period two patients were treated medically, five underwent surgical resection and eight received no specific treatment. The course and outcome in the 15 patients are summarized in Tables II and III.

Treated Cases (Table II). Two patients were treated with amphotericin B. One patient received a small dose of intracavitary amphotericin B (complicated by chemical pneumonitis) and the aspergilloma lysed six months later. A combination of an intravenous course of 2.0 g of amphotericin B and oral 5-fluorocytosine for two weeks had no appreciable effect in the other patient.

Surgical resection was performed in five patients: indications for surgery were hemoptysis (blood streaking to 50 ml/day) in three patients, diagnostic evaluation in one, and one patient had surgery as an elective treatment. Lobectomy was the surgical procedure in four patients and segmentectomy in one. A postoperative death due to a cerebrovascular accident occurred in a patient who underwent resective surgery for esophageal carcinoma combined with a diagnostic segmentectomy. Postoperative complications occurred in two patients; in one a chest wall fistula developed and in another repeat surgery was required for control of wound bleeding. One patient was lost for follow-up. During a follow-up period of seven to 27 months, one patient had heart failure, one died of hepatic failure and pneumonia, and one's condition remained stable. In none of the patients did aspergilloma recur.

Untreated Cases (Table III). The follow-up period of the eight patients who received no treatment ranged from seven to 96 months (average 50 months). Four patients experienced hemoptysis, three as a presenting manifestation and one during the course of the infection. The amount of hemoptysis varied; two had blood streaking of sputum only, and in the other two hemoptysis was estimated at a total of 200 and 500 ml, respectively. Surgery was not performed in either patient because of severe underlying chronic obstructive lung disease. Blood transfusions and supportive therapy were instituted, and hemoptysis ceased in five to seven days. Neither patient had recurrent hemoptysis during a follow-up period of seven and 92 months.

There were four deaths among the eight patients who received no treatment which occurred from seven to 40 months after the diagnosis was established. Respiratory failure due to chronic obstructive pulmonary disease was the cause of death in three patients, and the cause was unknown in one. Aspergilloma could not be implicated as a causative factor in any of the deaths. Roentgenographically, the aspergilloma disappeared or decreased in size in three patients and was unchanged prior to death in one. Of the four surviving patients followed from 48 to 96 months, the aspergilloma increased in size in one patient, was stable in two and spontaneously disappeared in one.

COMMENTS

The natural history of the intracavitary aspergilloma is not well documented. This is due to the scarcity of reports of long-term follow-up, the difficulty in separating the course of the underlying diseases from that of the aspergilloma, and the fact that elective surgical resection is performed in many cases. The eight untreated patients in this study were closely followed for an average of 50 months. The aspergilloma disappeared spontaneously in four patients, remained unchanged in size in three and enlarged in one. Disappearance ("lysis") of the aspergilloma over a four year period is shown in Figure 1; enlargement of an aspergilloma over a five year period is shown in Figure 2.

Although roentgenographic evidence of spontaneous lysis has been observed by many groups [2,3,9,16,17], the frequency of this phenomenon is difficult to ascertain. In two cooperative studies, spontaneous lysis was found in 7 and 10 per cent of the patients [16,17]. As

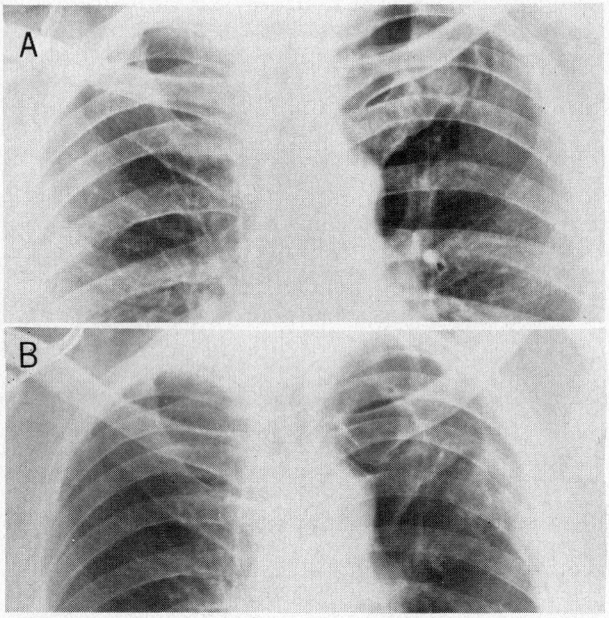

Figure 1. ***A,*** *aspergilloma of the upper lobe of the left lung.* ***B,*** *roentgenogram taken four years later shows no intracavitary density.*

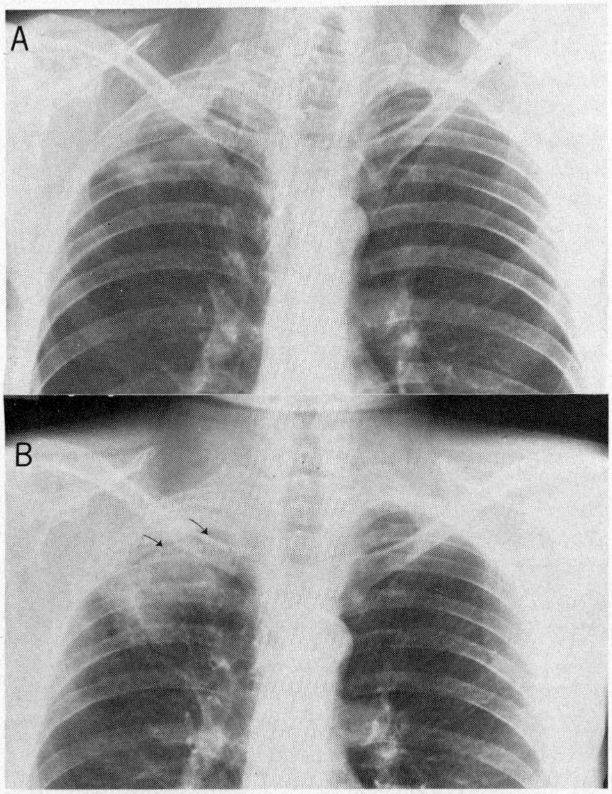

Figure 2. ***A,*** *aspergilloma of the upper lobe of the right lung.* ***B,*** *roentgenogram taken five years later shows increased size of the aspergilloma.* ***Arrows*** *indicate the "crescent."*

in this study, lysis occurred within 36 months after the diagnosis was established. Hammerman et al. [17], however, described one patient in whom lysis occurred after 69 months of follow-up. In the absence of a history of expectorating a "fungus ball," devitalization of the fungus and gradual elimination in the sputum, as suggested by Pimental [18], may be the explanation for the spontaneous lysis. It has been suggested that growth and death of the fungus go on continuously within the cavity, and death of the fungus can be hastened by a supervening bronchopulmonary infection [19,20]. The dead fungus, if not expectorated in sputum, may calcify. In one series of 30 aspergillomas, the fungus was reported dead in nine and calcified in four [21].

The risk of an aspergilloma progressing to invasive pulmonary disease or causing hematogenous dissemination of the organism is negligible. Israel and Ostrow [2] made the interesting observation that seven of their patients with sarcoidosis were undergoing treatment with adrenal corticosteroids prior to the appearance of an aspergilloma. Corticosteroid therapy was continued in three of the patients without evidence of dissemination of the infection. Furthermore, in another report, two patients with aspergilloma appeared to actually benefit from treatment with corticosteroids [22]. In our patients, there was no evidence of invasive or disseminated Aspergillus infection. Specimens obtained from patients who underwent surgical resection of the lesion revealed that the mycelial mass was confined to the intracavitary space, and microscopic sections did not show invasion through the wall of the cavity (Figure 3).

The prognosis in a patient with aspergilloma appears related more to the nature and severity of the underlying diseases than to the aspergilloma itself. All of our patients had a long history of cigarette smoking. Chronic

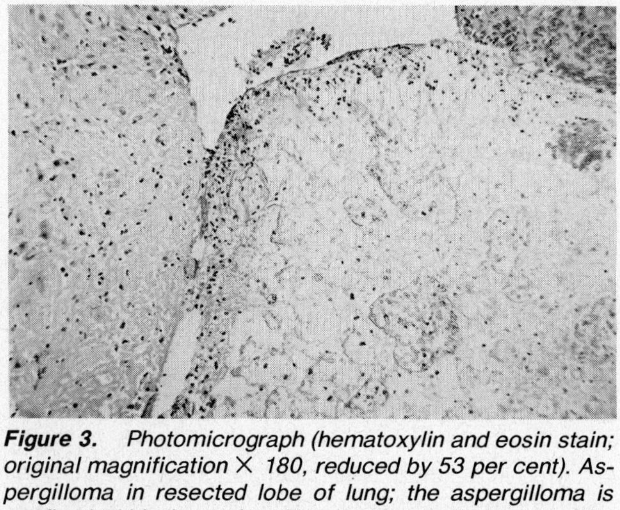

Figure 3. *Photomicrograph (hematoxylin and eosin stain; original magnification × 180, reduced by 53 per cent). Aspergilloma in resected lobe of lung; the aspergilloma is confined within the cavity with no evidence of invasion of the surrounding lung.*

obstructive lung diseases, alcoholic cirrhosis and other serious diseases were common. Among the seven deaths that occurred during the follow-up period, six were clearly related to underlying disease. The cause of death in one patient is unknown.

Our experience seriously questions many previous reports that favor surgical excision of all aspergillomas. We reviewed the data on 140 pulmonary resections for aspergilloma reported in the literature [1,3,4,12, 13,23–25]. Although the over-all mortality rate was less than 7 per cent, major postoperative complications occurred in 22 per cent of the patients. Bronchopleural fistulas, persistent air space problems, hemorrhage and empyema were most common. The nature and severity of underlying disease or diseases, particularly chronic lung disease, was a major determinant of morbidity and mortality.

Although hemoptysis occurs in from 55 to 85 per cent of the patients with aspergilloma [4,12,13], the precise pathogenetic mechanism of the bleeding is unknown. Intracavitary growth of the fungus and friction caused by its movements have been implicated as a likely cause [18,25]. Trypsin-like proteolytic enzymes, an endotoxin with hemolytic property and an anticoagulant produced by the fungus may be causative factors in the bleeding [2,27]. Patients with massive hemoptysis, measuring 600 ml or more in 24 hours, are candidates for emergency surgery if their underlying pulmonary disease permits resective surgery and bronchoscopic identification of the bleeding site has been achieved [28]. The indications for surgery in patients with lesser degrees of hemoptysis are not clearly defined. Solit and associates [4] noted that 19 of their patients (12 presented with hemoptysis) either refused surgery or had severe lung disease that precluded surgery. Five of these patients subsequently died of massive hemoptysis. They recommended pulmonary resection whenever the diagnosis of aspergilloma is made and the patient is a suitable operative candidate.

The experience in our series of patients suggests that the routine surgical excision of aspergilloma in acceptable risk patients is not indicated. Consequent to our study, we have adopted a conservative approach: careful follow-up in patients with aspergilloma who have mild to moderate hemoptysis, and surgical intervention in those with massive hemoptysis. A well controlled cooperative study of patients with aspergilloma who present with mild to moderate hemoptysis seems warranted.

REFERENCES

1. Reddy PA, Christianson CS, Brasher CA, et al.: Comparison of treated and untreated pulmonary aspergilloma; an analysis of 16 cases. Am Rev Respir Dis 101: 928, 1970.
2. Israel HL, Ostrow A: Sarcoidosis and aspergilloma. Am J Med 47: 243, 1969.
3. Aslam PA, Eastridge CE, Hughes FA: Aspergillosis of the lung—an 18 year experience. Chest 59: 28, 1971.
4. Solit RW, McKeown JJ Jr, Smullens S, et al.: The surgical implications of intracavitary mycetomas (fungus balls). J Thorac Cardiovasc Surg 62: 411, 1971.
5. Mays EE, Hawkins JA: Cavitary bronchiolar carcinoma with an intracavitary aspergilloma. Am Rev Respir Dis 95: 1056, 1967.
6. Schwartz J, Baum GL, Straub M: Cavitary histoplasmosis complicated by fungus ball. Am J Med 31: 692, 1961.
7. Sarosi GA, Silberfarb PM, Saliba NA, et al.: Aspergillomas occurring in blastomycotic cavities. Am Rev Respir Dis 104: 581, 1971.
8. Twining EW, Kerley P: A Textbook of X-ray Diagnosis (Shanks SC, Kerley P, eds), London, H. K. Lewis, 1951, p 441.
9. Parker JD, Sarosi GA, Doto IL, et al.: Pulmonary aspergillosis in sanatoriums in the South Central United States. A National Communicable Disease Center Cooperative mycoses study. Am Rev Respir Dis 101: 551, 1970.
10. Hammerman KJ, Sarosi GA, Tosh FE: Amphotericin B in the treatment of saprophytic forms of pulmonary aspergillosis. Am Rev Respir Dis 109: 57, 1974.
11. Ramirez RJ: Pulmonary aspergilloma—endobronchial treatment. N Engl J Med 271: 1281, 1964.
12. Pecora DV, Toll MW: Pulmonary resection for localized aspergillosis. N Engl J Med 263: 785, 1960.
13. Kilman JW, Ahn C, Andrews NC, et al.: Surgery for pulmonary aspergillosis. J Thorac Cardiovasc Surg 57: 642, 1969.
14. Riley EA, Tennebaum J: Pulmonary aspergilloma or intracavitary fungus ball. Report of five cases. Ann Intern Med 56: 896, 1962.
15. MacPherson P: Pulmonary aspergillosis in Argyll. Br J Dis Chest 59: 148, 1965.
16. Davis D (ed): Aspergilloma and residual tuberculous cavities—the results of a resurvey. A report from the Research Committee of the British Thoracic and Tuberculosis Association. Tubercle 51: 227, 1970.
17. Hammerman KJ, Christianson CS, Huntington I, et al.: Spontaneous lysis of aspergillomata. Chest 64: 697, 1973.
18. Pimental JC: Pulmonary calcification in the tumor-like form of aspergilloma. Am Rev Respir Dis 94: 208, 1966.
19. Pimental JC: Aspergilose polmonar tumoriforme ("aspergilloma pulmonar"). Estuda anatamo-pathologico de quatro casos e discussao da sua patogenia. Gac Med Port 11: 455, 1958.
20. Monod O, Pesle G, Meyer A: L'aspergillome bronchectasiant. Sem Hop Paris 33: 3588, 1957.
21. Villar TG, Pimental JC, Avila R: Some aspects of pulmonary aspergilloma in Portugal. Dis Chest 51: 402, 1967.
22. Davies D, Somner AR: Pulmonary aspergillomas treated with corticosteroids. Thorax 27: 156, 1972.
23. Belcher JR, Plummer NS: Surgery in bronchopulmonary aspergillosis. Br J Dis Chest 54: 335, 1960.
24. Saliba A, Pacini L, Beatty DA: Intracavitary fungus balls in pulmonary aspergillosis. Br J Dis Chest 55: 65, 1961.
25. Robinson CLN, McPherson AR: Bronchopulmonary aspergilloma. Can J Surg 5: 411, 1962.
26. Villar TG, Pimental JC, Costa MF: The tumor-like forms of aspergillosis of the lung (pulmonary aspergilloma). Report of five new cases and review of the Portuguese literature. Thorax 17: 22, 1962.
27. Campbell MJ, Clayton YM: Bronchopulmonary aspergillosis. A correlation of the clinical and laboratory findings in 272 patients investigated for bronchopulmonary aspergillosis. Am Rev Respir Dis 89: 186, 1964.
28. Mattox KL, Guinn GA: Emergency resection for massive hemoptysis. Ann Thorac Surg 17: 377, 1974.

Visceral Fungal Infections Due to Petriellidium boydii (Allescheria boydii)

In Vitro Drug Sensitivity Studies

LARRY I. LUTWICK, M.D.*
JOHN N. GALGIANI, M.D.†
RUDOLPH H. JOHNSON, M.D.‡
DAVID A. STEVENS, M.D.
Stanford, California

Four patients with visceral infections due to the fungus Petriellidium boydii, who were recently hospitalized in our institutions, are described. Three of the patients were compromised hosts; in the fourth patient, infection occurred after trauma. All had received prior steroid and antibiotic therapy. Studies of patients with mycetoma or secondary infection of a pulmonary cavity due to this organism and of patients with visceral infections are reviewed. Because of histologic similarities to Aspergillus species, infections due to P. boydii may have been misdiagnosed in the past if the infecting fungus was not isolated in culture. The fungus has been shown to be resistant in vitro to currently available antifungal agents. Resistance to amphotericin and 5-fluorocytosine is demonstrated in our studies. There are few reports of successful chemotherapy of any manifestation of this infection, and no such reports of visceral disease. We demonstrate in vitro sensitivity of isolates in our cases and in others to miconazole, a new antimicrobial agent; this drug may be indicated for treatment of disease due to P. boydii.

From the Stanford University Medical Center, Stanford, California and the Santa Clara Valley Medical Center, San Jose, California. This study was supported by National Research Service Award 5F22-CA01680-02 (L.I.L.), National Research Service Award 1F32-A105170-01 (J.N.G.) and an Advanced Research Fellowship (R.H.J.) from the Bay Area Heart Research Committee. This study was presented in part in abstract form at the Western Section, American Federation for Clinical Research, Carmel, California, February 1976. Requests for reprints should be addressed to Dr. D. A. Stevens, Santa Clara Valley Medical Center, 751 South Bascom Avenue, San Jose, California 95128. Manuscript accepted March 24, 1976.

* Present address: Naval Regional Medical Clinic, Treasure Island, San Francisco, California 94130.

† Present address: Department of Medicine, Pacific-Presbyterian Hospital, Clay and Webster Streets, San Francisco, California 94115

‡ Present address: Section of Infectious Diseases, Medical Service, Veterans Administration Hospital, Memphis, Tennessee 38104.

Allescheria boydii and Monosporium apiospermum have been isolated from human subjects with mycetomas. Not until 1944 did Emmons [1] demonstrate that A. boydii was the perfect (ascocarpic) form of M. apiospermum, that is, that it was a different growth form of the same fungus. Twenty case reports of nonmycetoma infections have appeared, and one report of three saprophytic pulmonary infections [2]. Based on more recent concepts, Malloch [3] has proposed the new genus Petriellidium for the organism (this nomenclature will be used here). In this review, the first reported series of systemic infections, we discuss four recent cases in our institutions, report the results of antifungal drug susceptibility studies and summarize the literature.

MATERIALS AND METHODS

Sensitivity studies were performed on fungal isolates from three patients (Case 1, 2 and 4). Five other clinical isolates of P. boydii were tested in their imperfect morphologic form (kindly supplied by Dr. Libero Ajello, Center for Disease Control, Atlanta).

Isolates were grown for three days in liquid Synthetic Amino Acid Media for Fungi (SAAMF). This completely defined medium [4] was modified by substituting L-cysteine (0.24 g/liter) for L-cystene. A fraction of this growth was homogenized with a pasteur pipette and adjusted to 10^4 conidia/ml with a hemocytometer.

Miconazole, 5-fluorocytosine and amphotericin B were obtained from Janssen R & D, Hoffman-LaRoche and Squibb, respectively. The drugs were reconstituted at the time of study, or aliquots frozen at −20°C were thawed. The drugs were serially diluted in SAAMF. Equal volumes (0.5 ml) of drug and inocula solutions were mixed in tubes and incubated at 37°C. Tube dilutions with amphotericin B were wrapped in aluminum foil during incubation. Minimal inhibitory concentrations were read at 48 hours as the lowest drug concentration that showed no growth.

Miconazole tissue concentrations were determined by an agar well method [5] with a sensitive Candida albicans isolate as the indicator organism. This assay detects miconazole concentrations $\geqslant$0.3 μg/ml.

CASE REPORTS

Case 1. A 32 year old Mexican-American woman was admitted to Stanford University Hospital for the first time on January 24, 1975, because of an exacerbation of her lupus erythematosus.

Her disease was diagnosed in December 1972. She had been followed in the Stanford Clinic since April 1973, without evidence of active renal disease, receiving prednisone (10 mg/day), hydroxychloroquine (200 mg/day) and azathioprine (50 mg/day). In December 1974, she departed on a one month trip to Mexico, where she discontinued taking all medication. Subsequently, she had the gradual onset of fever, sweats, cough, right-sided pleuritic chest pain, shortness of breath, and facial and lower extremity swelling. She was hospitalized on her return to the Stanford area.

On admission she had a cushingoid appearance. The fundi were normal, except for minimal arteriolar narrowing. Her chest examination revealed dullness to percussion in the lower half of the posterior right chest, with absent breath sounds. There was a grade 3/6 systolic ejection murmur at the lower left sternal border without radiation and 3+ pitting edema of the lower extremities.

Laboratory data revealed a leukocyte count of 4,300/mm^3 (50 per cent polymorphonuclear leukocytes, 29 per cent band forms, 21 per cent lymphocytes) and a hematocrit value of 30 per cent. The creatinine was 3.7 mg/dl, albumin 1.8 g/dl, calcium 6.4 mg/dl and phosphate 5.7 mg/dl. Urinalysis revealed a specific gravity of 1.020 with 3+ protein, 30 to 40 erythrocytes, 20 to 30 leukocytes/hpf and granular casts. The urine culture was sterile. A chest film obtained on admission revealed bilateral pleural effusions, greater on the right side than the left, and left ventricular enlargement.

Pleural fluid examination revealed 640 leukocytes/mm^3 (92 per cent mononuclear cells), glucose 140 mg/dl, total protein 1.4 g/dl, negative fluorescent antinuclear antibody and negative cultures for bacteria, mycobacteria and fungi. An echocardiogram was interpreted as showing a small to moderate pericardial effusion. The administration of prednisone (30 mg/day) was started on the day of admission.

The patient's urine output ranged between 200 and 300 ml/24 hours, and her serum creatinine and uric acid levels rose. On January 27, the dose of prednisone was doubled to 60 mg/day, and azathioprine (100 mg/day) and allopurinol were added. On January 30, a percutaneous biopsy of the right kidney was performed. Histologic examination of the specimen showed a generalized diffuse necrotizing glomerulonephritis with extensive crescent formation, consistent with active grade 3 lupus nephritis. Immunofluorescence and electron microscopic evaluation of the biopsy specimen confirmed the diffuse immune complex nephritis. Renal function deteriorated further, and on February 13 an arteriovenous fistula was inserted and hemodialysis was initiated.

About February 12, intermittent epistaxis occurred, for which the patient required nasal packing. Evaluation revealed that her platelet count had decreased to 16,000/mm^3, with 900 white blood cells/mm^3 (18 per cent polymorphonuclear leukocytes, 41 per cent band forms, 6 per cent metamyelocytes, 35 per cent lymphocytes). Bone marrow aspirate showed hypoplasia. The administration of both azathioprine and allopurinol was discontinued on February 15, and blood counts returned gradually to normal (by March 1).

On February 17, temperatures of 38.3° to 38.5°C occurred daily. A chest film revealed an infiltrate in the lower lobe of the left lung. Sputum culture for bacteria and fungi, urine culture and several blood cultures were unrevealing. On February 24, empirical treatment with cefazolin and gentamicin was initiated. Administration of the antibiotics was continued for five days, and her temperature returned to normal.

The patient began to complain of a throbbing pain in her right eye on February 28. Prednisone eye drops were prescribed. The pain continued for two days, and she began to complain of diminished vision. Examination of the eye on March 2 revealed marked conjunctival irritation and edema, 4 mm proptosis and visual acuity limited to discrimination between light and dark. The anterior chamber was filled with cells, and the ocular fundus contained what appeared to be several retinal-vitreal abscesses. A vitreous aspiration removed 0.5 ml of fluid. Gram stain of this revealed many polymorphonuclear leukocytes without organisms. Six blood cultures were also obtained, and chloramphenicol, gentamicin and amphotericin B therapy was started. Amphotericin B, 150 μg was also administered once to the subconjunctiva.

Cultures of blood and pleural fluid were sterile, but the vitreous culture showed heavy growth of a filamentous fungus, identified as P. boydii, on several plates. A partial vitrectomy was performed on March 4, and 5 μg of amphotericin B was instilled in the vitreous cavity. Skull films at this time showed normal sinuses, and the cerebrospinal fluid was normal. There was no vision in the affected eye just prior to the vitrectomy, and none subsequently.

On March 7, because of data in the literature indicating resistance of this organism to amphotericin therapy, this was discontinued and miconazole therapy was initiated (200 mg three times a day intravenously). This was increased by 600 mg/day every other day to 1,000 mg three times a day. Examination of the eye showed no change during treatment. Evisceration of the right eye on March 15 was performed; no evidence of extraocular orbital disease was noted.

P. boydii grew from the excised vitreous. Histologic examination revealed chronic inflammation with numerous

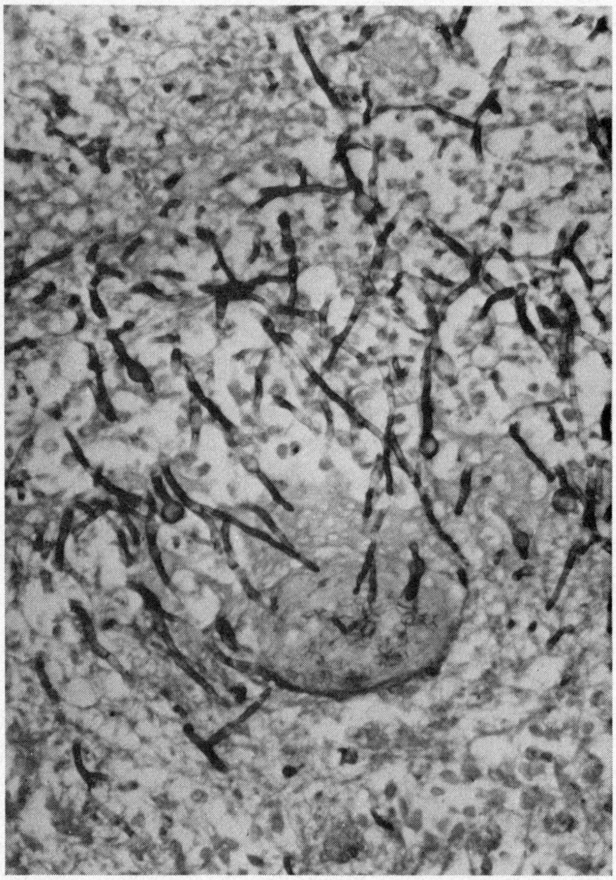

Figure 1. Vitreous removed from patient showing clearly the branching septate hyphae with terminal conidia. Gomori-methenamine-silver stain.

branching hyphae (Figure 1) in the vitreal cavity. No fungi were noted in the retinal or uveal tissue. Miconazole therapy was continued until March 22. Side effects were limited to nausea and phlebitis. The right eye healed without incident, and she was discharged on April 3, 1975.

At nine months follow-up, no evidence of orbital infection was present, and an ocular prosthesis was used. Chronic hemodialysis is being continued.

Comment: This is the first reported case of endogenous endophthalmitis caused by this fungus. There was no clear portal of entry. It is postulated that the primary infection was pulmonary (with spontaneous resolution following correction of granulocytopenia) with hematogenous spread to the eye.

Case 2. A 66 year old white housewife was in good health until December 1972 when she noted a mass in the right side of her neck. An excisional biopsy in January 1973 revealed nodular histiocytic-lymphocytic lymphoma. In March 1973, at staging laparotomy, her condition was staged IVA on the basis of nodular lymphoma in the spleen, para-aortic and jejunomesenteric nodes, and marrow. Chemotherapy with cytoxan, vincristine and prednisone was given in conjunction with total nodal irradiation. She responded to therapy with a decrease in the size of the lymph nodes as seen on a roentgenogram.

In July 1974, she was admitted with severe thrombocytopenia, epistaxis, intermittent fever and cough of two weeks' duration. Gingival bleeding, ecchymoses and petechiae were noted. A chest film disclosed the presence of a left pleural effusion. She was given multiple platelet and red blood cell transfusions. Temperatures as high as 38.8°C occurred after each transfusion. Because of the possibility of pneumonitis, she was given six days of intravenous cefazolin followed by seven days of oral cephalexin. An abdominal film revealed an increase in the size of the left para-aortic and iliac lymph nodes, and a bone marrow biopsy revealed lymphomatous infiltration. Because of the increased activity of the lymphoma she was treated with a five day course of oral prednisone, 100 mg/day. Lingual and oral herpes simplex infection developed, but the patient became afebrile. The left pleural effusion resolved.

She was admitted for evaluation of pancytopenia in October 1974. She denied recent constitutional symptoms but had a dry, hacking cough. The chest film was clear. Pancytopenia was thought to be secondary to chemotherapy and radiotherapy, and lymphoma was believed to be persistent in bone marrow and abdominal lymph nodes. The administration of oral prednisone, 60 mg/day, was started, and she was subsequently followed as an outpatient for transfusions of platelets and red blood cells.

In November 1974, she was admitted for evaluation of an infiltrate in the right lung with a history of a hacking, nonproductive cough and right pleuritic chest pain of several days' duration. She specifically denied having fever, sweats, chills, weight loss, hemoptysis and dyspnea. Examination of the chest showed bilateral diffuse rhonchi and right posterior chest wall tenderness. Laboratory studies revealed a hematocrit value of 28 per cent, a white cell count of 5,300/mm^3 (32 per cent polymorphonuclear leukocytes, 19 per cent band forms, 3 per cent metamyelocytes, 28 per cent lymphocytes, 16 per cent monocytes, 2 per cent myelocytes) and platelets 9,000/mm^3. The erythrocyte sedimentation rate was 28 mm/hour. A chest film revealed a 5 cm round infiltrate in the superior segment of the lower lobe of the right lung adjacent to the posterior pleural surface. Skin tests with intermediate purified protein derivative, histoplasmin and coccidioidin were negative, and the Candida precipitin test and the test for complement-fixing antibody to Coccidioides immitis were nonreactive. Her prednisone dose was decreased. Platelet and red blood cell transfusions were given. Sputum cultures showed a heavy growth of Staphylococcus, coagulase-positive. Examination of acid-fast stained and potassium hydroxide-prepared sputums were negative. Cultures of the sputum for fungi grew P. boydii and an Aspergillus species. Acid-fast bacilli cultures grew small numbers of Runyan group III organisms. Fiberoptic bronchoscopy disclosed no abnormalities, but cultures of bronchial washings and brushings grew Aspergillus, Penicillium and Pseudomonas species. Needle aspiration of the lesion in the lower lobe of the right lung revealed many fungi on silver-stained smears and in cytologic preparations. P. boydii and Aspergillus subsequently grew from cultures of this specimen. Gram stain of the aspirate showed rare gram-negative bacilli, and Pseudomonas was also grown from it. No acid-fast bacilli were seen on smear of the needle aspirate and acid-fast bacilli cultures were negative. Two sputums examined after the bronchoscopy and aspiration showed many acid-fast bacilli on smear; from these Runyan group III organisms were cultured.

On the fifth hospital day the patient had a spike in temperature to 39°C. The lesion in the lower lobe of the right lung progressively increased. On the seventh hospital day, she became lethargic and multiple, widespread, pustular, cutaneous lesions, some with erythematous margins, were noted. Stained smears of these lesions showed structures resembling septate hyphae, but no bacteria or acid-fast bacilli. Bacterial and acid-fast bacilli cultures of these pustules were negative, fungal cultures were not obtained. Lumbar punctures on two occasions on the same day were presumed traumatic (spinal fluid red blood cells 25 and 1,022/mm^3, glucose normal, protein 72 and 98 mg/dl and white blood cells 5 and 12/mm^3, all mononuclear). Smears for acid-fast bacilli and cultures, potassium hydroxide and India ink preparations, and fungal cultures of spinal fluid were negative. Despite antimicrobial therapy with cefazolin, gentamicin, carbenicillin, amphotericin B, isoniazid and ethambutol, she died on the ninth hospital day.

Postmortem examination failed to demonstrate evidence of lymphoma. Disseminated fungal infection was manifested by multiple cardiac abscesses containing large numbers of filamentous septate hyphae with true septums, involving the aortic valve and the coronary sinus. Multiple bilateral pulmonary and renal abscesses containing similar hyphae were noted. Multiple fungal abscesses of the brain (involving the left frontal cortex, corpus callosum, left temporal lobe, right occipital lobe and cerebellum) and cervical spinal cord were also seen; all contained septate hyphae with true septums. Cultures of antemortem and postmortem blood and postmortem lung tissue and spinal fluid were negative for bacteria, acid-fast bacilli and fungi. Acid-fast smears, and India ink and potassium hydroxide preparations were also negative.

Comment: In this woman pulmonary infection developed with Pseudomonas, atypical mycobacteria, Aspergillus and Petriellidium while she was under treatment for lymphoma. Differentiation between the two fungi could not be made histologically, but the organisms in the cardiac, cerebral and renal lesions more closely resembled Aspergillus species than Petriellidium. Postmortem cultures, after amphotericin therapy, were negative.

Case 3. A 50 year old Mexican-American man was admitted on August 9, 1973, following an auto accident in which he sustained severe head trauma and lacerations of the face, elbows and knees.

On admission he responded only to painful stimuli. Pertinent physical findings were lacerations of the forehead and chin, nasal bone fracture, a fixed midposition left pupil without papilledema, separation of the costal cartilages of the right sixth, seventh and eighth ribs with paradoxic chest wall motion, absent bowel sounds and deep lacerations of both knees with exposure of the patellas. On peritoneal aspiration, blood-tinged fluid was withdrawn. Roentgenograms did not show pneumothorax, or fractures of the skull or extremities.

The patient was admitted to the intensive care unit where his multiple lacerations were sutured, and his nasal fracture reduced. Cephalothin and dexamethasone therapy was started. A cerebral arteriogram did not indicate focal lesions. The steroid dose was decreased over two weeks, and discontinued. Over the next three weeks, his major problem was pulmonary (fever, hypoxia and pulmonary infiltrates). Sputum cultures grew Escherichia coli and Pseudomonas aeruginosa. He was treated with carbenicillin and gentamicin, with gradual resolution. His neurologic status improved slightly.

On August 27, the patient's right knee was aspirated because of increasing swelling and redness. Fifteen milliliters of blood-tinged fluid were removed. The initial fluid and several subsequent arthrocenteses all grew a fungus identified as P. boydii. Discharge from the knee grew the fungus and several gram-negative rods including P. aeruginosa, Esch. coli and Klebsiella pneumoniae. On August 31, the knee was opened, irrigation tubes were inserted, and specimens of joint capsule and synovium obtained. Gomori-silver stain of both specimens showed septate hyphae. The knee was irrigated with amphotericin B solutions throughout September, while cultures from the joint continued to grow P. boydii.

On October 2, synovectomy and meniscectomy were performed. Sections of the synovium again showed the fungus, but culture was sterile as were subsequent cultures of material from the knee. The patient was transferred to a chronic care facility for custodial care, without evidence of active knee infection.

Comment: P. boydii joint infection developed after open trauma and corticosteroid administration. The gram-negative rods isolated from the discharge alone with the fungus most likely represented colonization as they were never isolated from arthrocentesis fluid. This is the first reported case of joint infection due to P. boydii, and demonstrates the effect of local surgery in contrast to amphotericin as a therapeutic maneuver.

Case 4. A 56 year old man was admitted to the Palo Alto Veterans Hospital in May 1969 because of advancing systemic lupus erythematosus. During treatment with prednisone for advancing renal disease, intermittent pulmonary infiltrates developed, and he was treated with penicillin. Sputum cultures grew P. boydii, but by the time of the report the pneumonia cleared, and fever and cough subsided. Subsequent cultures did not grow the fungus.

One month later the patient had an acute neurologic decompensation. Brain scan revealed a brain abscess, which was drained through a burr hole. Stains and subsequent cultures of the material were negative. The patient died within 27 hours.

At postmortem examination two brain abscesses were found which contained septate branching fungi. A smaller abscess was found in the thyroid, and fungi were seen on section. Cultures of material from one of the brain abscesses grew P. boydii. No fungi were noted in the lung. Other aspects of this case have been reported in detail elsewhere [6].

COMMENTS

Several aspects of the biology of this fungus, and of the infections it causes, are briefly reviewed.

Mycology and Diagnosis. The fungus belongs to the ascomycete family. It grows as septate, branched hyphae on which ovoid light brown spores called conidia, measuring 3 μ by 5 μ, are found. The conidia may occur at the ends of the hyphae or on short side branches, usually singly, but sometimes in groups of two to five. In cultures, bundles of parallel hyphae termed coremia may be found bearing conidia on their free ends. The perfect or ascocarpic stage is formed when the usual slender hyphal elements swell into large thick cells [7]. These twist upon one another forming ball-like structures which develop into the mature perithecia or fruiting bodies containing ascospores. The perithecia, 50 to 200 μ in diameter, are cleistogamous, that is, without an opening, and have a thin easily-ruptured wall. The fragility of the structure, and the fact that the formation of perithecia is dependent on the type of media used [8], may explain why the imperfect form (formerly M. apiospermum) is often the one initially isolated from clinical specimens.

In pathologic section, it may be difficult to distinguish the hyphal forms of Petriellidium from those of Aspergillus species. Rosen et al. [9] found it impossible to distinguish the two in a case of mixed pulmonary infection except in sections in which the conidiophores and echinulated conidia of Aspergillus were present. Other investigators [2,10,11] state that culture is needed for differentiation. In one case [11] the presumed diagnosis was aspergilloma based on histologic criteria until cultures grew P. boydii. These workers believed that other cases of petriellidosis may be missed unless appropriate cultures are obtained. The growth characteristics of P. boydii can also be helpful if it is found in tissues as a fungal granule typical of mycetoma, in contrast to the diffuse growth of Aspergillus hyphae (B. Fetter, personal communication). Skin test antigens and serologic tests may be of some value in diagnosis [11–16], but currently these are not generally available.

Ecology and Epidemiology. This fungus is ubiquitous in the environment and has been isolated both from soil [17–19] and polluted water and sewage [20]. The most common manifestation of disease is the mycetoma ("Madura foot"), a chronic mycotic infection usually involving the lower extremity. This is characterized by disfiguring swelling, multiple draining sinuses, prolonged disability and, ultimately, amputation in many cases. It has been presumed that the organism is introduced into the tissues at sites of major or minor trauma. The disease is uncommon and sporadic in the United States; most of the cases are reported in the warm climates of the South and Southwest. In a series from Texas of 19 cases of Madura foot [21], 11 were due to this organism.

Pulmonary Petriellidosis. The most commonly described extracutaneous site of human petriellidosis is the lung. Creitz and Harris [22] in 1955 first described this entity in a patient with a long history of cavitary lung disease, presumably due to a pyogenic abscess. The same patient was described in follow-up in a later publication [23] and subsequently other patients with pulmonary petriellidosis have been reported [2,9–13,24–28]. Of the 14 patients, all but one had definite evidence of previous cavitation of various etiologies (in one the possible presence of prior cavitation was unclear). In these patients with cavities, P. boydii presumably acted as a secondary infectious agent. In none of the 11 specimens examined pathologically was there evidence of tissue invasion outside the cavity wall. Thus, it seems that one form of pulmonary petriellidosis is similar to intracavitary saprophytic infections with Aspergillus, that is, as a secondary infection without tissue invasion in patients who have structural lung disease but are otherwise immunocompetent. Such secondary infection by P. boydii has also been observed in two cases of chronic otitis externa [29,30] and one case of chronic bacterial prostatitis [31]. Our Case 2 is, therefore, of greater interest, since it demonstrates a type of lung infection rarely encountered, i.e., in the absence of cavitary disease. Petriellidium pneumonia may have been present in our Case 4 and cleared spontaneously, or this patient may have been colonized by the organism in his respiratory tract while receiving corticosteroid therapy. A similar sequence is suggested by the patient's course in Case 1.

It appears necessary to separate secondary pulmonary petriellidosis, as described in the literature, from mycetomas and deep visceral infections, as patients with the former disease may not need specific antifungal therapy. This is analogous to saprophytic aspergillosis. A recent retrospective study in the latter disease suggested that the intravenous administration of amphotericin B with pulmonary drainage is no more effective than drainage alone [32]. The effectiveness of surgical treatment of saprophytic aspergillosis, however, has been well demonstrated [33], and the situation with petriellidosis seems analogous [11].

P. boydii As Primary Pathogen. In contrast to pulmonary petriellidosis, P. boydii has been isolated as a primary pathogen, in addition to mycetoma. Benham and Georg [7] describe a woman in whom an indolent, progressive meningoencephalitis developed which began one month after spinal anesthesia. Ten of 13 cultures of spinal fluid grew P. boydii, which was thought to have been introduced during anesthesia. The small ovoid bodies seen repeatedly on stained cerebrospinal fluid smears may have been individual fungal conidia. Selby [34] describes a patient in whom an extradural

TABLE I Classic Antifungal Agents and P. boydii

Agent	Minimal Inhibitory Concentration (μg/ml)	Reference	Maximum Achievable Serum Level (μg/ml)	Reference
2-Hydroxystilbamidine	10	[24]	Insufficient data	
	"Moderate inhibition" at 10	[23]		
Nystatin	125	[24]	20–40*	[39]
	200	[37]		
Potassium iodide	>1,000	[24]	Insufficient data	
Amphotericin B	Most >2 at 48 hours incubation	[24,34,37,38,40,41]	2	[42]
5-Fluorocytosine	>128	[43]	40	[44]

*Deemed too toxic for systemic use.

abscess of the thoracic spine developed with P. boydii identified only histologically (no material for cultures were obtained). In contrast to the preceding patient, no penetrating injury or procedure preceded the infection. Zaffiro [35] described a military physician in whom multiple subcutaneous abscesses and spiking fevers developed following a prolonged nonhealing puncture wound of a hand. The case was presented as one of disseminated petriellidosis because P. boydii was isolated from several abscesses. However, incomplete culture data were presented. Rosen et al. [36] present a young woman with proliferative glomerulonephritis treated with corticosteroids and azathioprine who died in renal failure. At postmortem examination, abscesses caused by P. boydii were found in the brain and thyroid gland (compare with our Case 4). Endophthalmitis with P. boydii following cataract extraction has also been recently reported [37]. One of the P. boydii isolates tested by Nielsen [38] reportedly came from a knee infection, but no clinical details are given.

Thus, it appears that P. boydii may cause significant disease in an immunoincompetent host or when it is inadvertently introduced into certain sites. Benham and Georg [7] were, however, unable to induce a meningitis by the intrathecal instillation of spores in rabbits. This suggests relatively low pathogenicity in this animal model. Travis et al. [24], however, have been able to induce hepatic and splenic fungal abscesses by intraperitoneal injection of P. boydii in mice. Of note is that of our four patients, three were clearly immunocompromised hosts, all four had received prior corticosteroid therapy, and two had renal insufficiency. All had also received antibiotic therapy before the development of the P. boydii infection.

In vitro Sensitivity Studies. There is fragmentary data in the literature on the in vitro sensitivity of P. boydii to different compounds. The summary of these results is shown in Tables I and II. The minimal inhibitory concentration is presented next to the maximum serum levels that can be obtained with systemic therapy, as reported in the literature. The methods and conditions of sensitivity testing are not described in some papers.

Nielsen [38] assayed amphotericin B against 15 isolates of P. boydii. He found seven (47 per cent) sensitive to ≤2 μg/ml (maximum achievable blood level) at 24 hours incubation but only three (20 per cent) sensitive to that minimal inhibitory concentration at 48 hours. Hoeprich and Huston [49] indicate that 48 hour incubation with amphotericin for determinations of minimal inhibitory concentration correlates best with clinical response in coccidioidomycosis. Reddy et al.

TABLE II Uncommonly Used and Generally Unavailable Agents in P. boydii Therapy

Agent	Minimal Inhibitory Concentration (μg/ml)	Reference	Maximum Achievable Serum Level (μg/ml)	Reference
Chloramphenicol	"75% inhibition" at 20	[23]	20–40	[45]
	"100% inhibition" at 100	[23]		
	>50	[24]		
Polymyxin B	125	[24]	1–8	[46]
Amphotericin A	2.4 at 48 hours' incubation	[40]	Insufficient data	
Diamidinodiphenylamine	5–10	[47]	Insufficient data	
2,2'dichloro,5,5'-diphenylsulfide	20–50	[47]	Insufficient data	
4,4'diaminodiphenyl-sulphone (Dapsone, DDS)	200	[47]	Insufficient data	
2,2'hydroxy,5,5'dichloro-phenylsulfide (Fentachlor)	1.56 at 56 hours' incubation	[48]	25–65	[48]
2,2'thiobis,4,4'dichloro-phenol (Win 4227, dithidol)	5	[24]	Insufficient data	

[2] claim that one culture of P. boydii was highly sensitive in vitro to 5-fluorocytosine (no minimal inhibitory concentration given). However, the minimal inhibitory concentration to 5-fluorocytosine of only one isolate has been reported [43], and this was resistant to the drug. In Table III we present our results with the two most commonly used antifungal agents, amphotericin and 5-fluorocytosine, assayed against isolates from our patients as well as from other patients. These studies, and the in vitro studies reviewed, generally indicate resistance of this fungus to currently available antifungal agents.

Chemotherapy. There are few in vivo drug studies of P. boydii. Buckley et al. [48] treated a patient with mycetoma intralesionally with amphotericin B, with transient improvement, followed by local fenticlor, apparently resulting in control of the disease. However, the extremity was amputated because of bacterial infection. No fungi could be cultured from the specimen. Seeliger and Reifferschied [50] reported good results in a similar case with the oral and intralesional administration of 2,2′dihydroxy, 5,5′-dichlorodiphenyl sulfide, another aromatic compound (two year follow-up). There have been no encouraging reports of systemic treatment of P. boydii mycetoma with amphotericin. Adelson and Malcolm [27] describe direct endocavitary instillation of sodium iodide for pulmonary mycetomas. It produced a transient absence of P. boydii from sputum cultures, possibly secondary to bronchorrhea due to the irritative nature of the sodium iodide. Tong et al. [23] treated a patient with pulmonary petriellidosis with chloramphenicol (which initially partially inhibited the isolate in in vitro testing), with transient clearing of P. boydii from the sputum. Retreatment with chloramphenicol and 2-hydroxystilbamidine had no effect on the disease. The remarkable cyclic nature of one P. boydii mycetoma, with complete quiescence during three successive pregnancies, led Mohr and Muchmore [51] to suppress menstruation with oral contraceptives. This resulted in diminution of the mycetoma, but the follow-up was brief.

Miconazole. Miconazole is a substituted 1-phenylimidazole which inhibits the growth of many pathogenic fungi and gram-positive bacteria. In vitro it is inhibitory at concentrations of ≤10 μg/ml against such fungi as Cryptococcus neoformans, Candida species, Saccharomyces cerevisiae, Blastomyces dermatiditis, Histoplasma capsulatum, Sporotrichum schenckii and Trichophyton species [52]. It is being used as an alternative to amphotericin B in coccidioidomycosis [53]. There has been no demonstration of development of resistance in vitro or in vivo. The mechanism of action at low dosages appears to be on the cell wall and plasma membrane, inducing permeability changes, and at higher dosage, inducing structural changes in the endoplasmic reticulum leading to decreased bud formation and cell wall synthesis. Stevens, Levine and Deresinski [53] showed that peak serum levels >1.0 μg/ml can be most consistently obtained with intravenous doses ≥9 mg/kg. Table IV presents the body fluid drug levels determined in Case 1. The minimal inhibitory concentration of eight P. boydii isolates, including those from the patients in Cases 1, 2 and 4, were <0.25 μg/ml (Table III), a level easily obtained in the blood (and obtained in the eye in Case 1) and spinal fluid [54] with systemic therapy with miconazole. These data suggest that miconazole may be a useful drug for the chemotherapy of P. boydii infection.

Fungal Endophthalmitis Therapy. Green et al. [55] have shown in a rabbit keratitis model that amphotericin does not penetrate the vitreous after subconjunctival or intravenous therapy. Both routes produced detectable and similar drug levels in the aqueous. Possibly because of the low minimal inhibitory concentrations of Candida and some other fungi, systemic or subconjunctival treatment with amphotericin can be effective in this disease [55–57]. Spontaneous resolution of endogenous Candida endophthalmitis complicating hyperali-

TABLE III Minimal Inhibitory Concentration (μg/ml) of Miconazole and Other Antifungal Drugs in P. boydii Isolates

	Drug		
	5-Fluorocytosine	Amphotericin B	Miconazole
Isolate			
Case 1			
Before therapy	>250	>12.5	0.125
After therapy	NT*	NT	0.063
Case 2	>250	6.25	0.16
Case 4	>250	6.25	0.08
CDC strain			
1581	>250	NT	<0.016
1437	>250	NT	<0.016
1535	>250	NT	0.125
1396	>250	NT	0.032
1505	>250	NT	0.032

* Not tested.

TABLE IV Fungal Endophthalmitis: Drug Concentration in Body Fluids (Case 1)*

Specimen	Time After End of Infusion (hr)	Miconazole Concentration (μg/ml)
Blood	0.25	0.8
	7.5	0.3
Vitreous	2.25	0.6

* Patient receiving 1,000 mg three times a day at time of study.

mentation has been reported, with retention of vision [58].

A patient with P. boydii endophthalmitis [37] following cataract extraction recovered after treatment with topical amphotericin, 4 mg/ml every 2 hours, for three months. The good results may have been due to the anterior location of the infection or easier penetration of the drug following surgery.

Intravitreal injection of amphotericin B has been studied in rabbits. Five to 10 μg of the drug can be tolerated without toxic changes [59], and that dose is effective in reversing the course of Candida endophthalmitis as compared to the course in untreated controls [60].

In our case, even though miconazole was detected in the vitreous, the fungus could still be grown from that site. Perhaps longer systemic treatment, initiated earlier, would have given better results. Direct inoculation of miconazole into the eye, as another therapeutic approach, needs study. Intracutaneous injection of the drug, and injection into the central nervous system by intracisternal, intraventricular and lumbar intrathecal routes, have been studied and do not appear to produce adverse effects [54].

REFERENCES

1. Emmons CW: Allescheria boydii and Monosporium apiospermum. Mycologia 36: 188, 1944.
2. Reddy PC, Christianson CS, Gorelick DF, et al.: Pulmonary Monosporosis: an uncommon pulmonary mycotic infection. Thorax 24: 722, 1969.
3. Malloch D: New concepts in the microascaceae illustrated by two new species. Mycologia 62: 727, 1970.
4. Hoeprich PD, Finn PD: Obfuscation of the activity of antifungal antimicrobics by culture media. J Infect Dis 126: 353, 1972.
5. Bennett JV, Brodie JL, Benner EJ, et al.: Simplified accurate method for antibiotic assay of clinical specimens. Appl Microbiol 14: 170, 1966.
6. Forno LS, Billingham ME: Allescheria boydii infection of the brain. J Pathol 106: 195, 1972.
7. Benham RW, Georg LK: Allescheria boydii, causative agent in a case of meningitis. J Invest Dermatol 10: 99, 1948.
8. Gordon MA: Nutrition and sporulation of Allescheria boydii. J Bacteriol 73: 199, 1957.
9. Rosen P, Adelson HT, Burleigh E: Bronchiectasis complicated by the presence of Monosporium apiospermum and Aspergillus fumigatus. Am J Clin Pathol 52: 182, 1969.
10. Louria DB, Lieberman PH, Collins HS, et al.: Pulmonary mycetoma due to Allescheria boydii. Arch Intern Med 117: 748, 1966.
11. Arnett JC, Hatch HB: Pulmonary Allescheriasis. Arch Intern Med 135: 1250, 1975.
12. McCarthy DS, Longbottom JL, Riddell RW, et al.: Pulmonary mycetoma due to Allescheria boydii. Am Rev Respir Dis 100: 213, 1969.
13. Hainer JW, Ostrow JH, MacKenzie DWR: Pulmonary monosporosis. Chest 66: 601, 1974.
14. May LK, Knight RA, Harris HW: Allescheria boydii and Aspergillus fumigatus skin test antigens. J Bacteriol 91: 2155, 1966.
15. Murray IG, Mahgoub EL: Discussion. Systemic Mycoses (CIBA Foundation Symposium) (Wolstenholme GEW, Porter R, eds), Boston, Massachusetts, 1972, p 72.
16. Seeliger HPR: Recent applications of immunological techniques in the diagnosis of the deep mycoses. Systemic Mycoses, ibid, p 54.
17. Ajello L, Zeidberg LD: Isolation of Histoplasma capsulatum and Allescheria boydii from soil. Science 113: 662, 1951.
18. Ajello L: The isolation of Allescheria boydii Shear, an etiologic agent of mycetomas, from soil. Am J Trop Med Hyg 1: 227, 1952.
19. Dabrowa N, Landau JW, Newcomer VD, et al.: A survey of tide-washed coastal areas of Southern California for fungi potentially pathogenic to man. Mycopathologia 24: 137, 1964.
20. Cooke WB, Kabler P: Isolation of potentially pathogenic fungi from polluted water and sewage. Pub Health Rep 70: 689, 1955.
21. Green WO, Adams TE: Mycetoma in the United States. Am J Clin Pathol 42: 75, 1964.
22. Creitz J, Harris HW: Isolation of Allescheria boydii from sputum. Am Rev Tuberc 71: 126, 1955.
23. Tong JL, Valentine EH, Durrance JR, et al.: Pulmonary infection with Allescheria boydii. Am Rev Tuberc 78: 604, 1958.
24. Travis RE, Ulrich EW, Phillips S: Pulmonary Allescheriasis. Ann Intern Med 54: 141, 1961.
25. Scharyj M, Levene N, Gordon H: Primary pulmonary infection with Monosporium apiospermum. J Infect Dis 106: 141, 1960.
26. Stoeckel H, Ermer C: Ein fall von Monosporium-mycetom der lunge. Beitr Klin Tuberk 122: 30, 1960.
27. Adelson HT, Malcolm JA: Endocavitary treatment of pulmonary mycetomas. Am Rev Respir Dis 98: 87, 1968.
28. Belitsos NJ, Merz WG, Bowersox DW, et al.: Allescheria boydii mycetoma complicating pulmonary sarcoid. J Hopkins Med J 135: 259, 1974.
29. Belding DL, Umanzio CB: A new species of the genus Monosporium associated with chronic otomycosis (abstract). Am J Pathol 11: 856, 1935.
30. Blank F, Stuart EA: Monosporium apiospermum Sacc., 1911, associated with otomycosis. Can Med Assoc J 72: 601, 1955.
31. Meyer E, Herrold RD: Allescheria boydii isolated from a patient with chronic prostatitis. Am J Clin Pathol 35: 155, 1961.
32. Hammerman KJ, Sarosi GA, Tosh FE: Amphotericin B in the treatment of saprophytic forms of pulmonary aspergillosis. Am Rev Respir Dis 109: 57, 1974.
33. Kilman JW, Ahn C, Andrews NC, et al.: Surgery for pulmonary aspergillosis. J Thorac Cardiovasc Surg 57: 642, 1969.
34. Selby R: Pachymeningitis secondary to Allescheria boydii. J Neurosurg 36: 225, 1972.
35. Zaffiro A: Forma singolare di mycosi cutanea do Monosporium apiospermum a sviluppo clinicamente setticemico. Giorn Med Milit 86: 636, 1938.
36. Rosen F, Deck JHN, Rewcastle NB: Allescheria boydii—unique systemic dissemination to thyroid and brain. Can Med Assoc J 93: 1125, 1965.
37. Glassman M, Henkind P, Alture-Werber E: Monosporium apiospermum endophthalmitis. Am J Ophthal 76: 821, 1973.
38. Nielsen HS: Effects of amphotericin B in vitro on perfect and imperfect strains of Allescheria boydii. Appl Microbiol 15:

86, 1967.
39. Weinstein L: Miscellaneous antimicrobial agents. The Pharmacological Basis of Therapeutics (Goodman LS, Gilman A, eds), New York, Macmillan, 1970, p 1293.
40. Gold W, Stout HA, Pagano JF, et al.: Amphotericins A and B, antifungal antibiotics produced by a Streptomycete. Antibiotic Annal 1955–56, New York, Medical Encyclopedia, Inc., 1956, p 579.
41. MacKinnon JE, Garcia-Zorron N: Amphotericin B and causal organisms of Maduromycosis (letter). Trans Roy Soc Trop Med Hyg 53: 362, 1959.
42. Bindschadler DD, Bennett JE: A pharmacologic guide to the clinical use of amphotericin B. J Infect Dis 120: 427, 1969.
43. Wagner G, Shadomy S, Paxton LD, et al.: New method for susceptibility testing with antifungal agents. Antimicrob Agents Chemother 8: 107, 1975.
44. Schonebeck J, Polak A, Fernex M, et al.: Pharmokinetic studies on the oral antimycotic agent 5-fluorocytosine in individuals with normal and impaired kidney function. Chemotherapy 18: 321, 1973.
45. Weinstein L: Reference 39, page 1261, 1970.
46. Weinstein L: Reference 39, page 1279, 1970.
47. MacKinnon JE, Artagaveytia-Allende RC, Garcia-Zorron N: The inhibitory effect of chemotherapeutic agents on the causal organisms of exogenous mycetomas and nocardiosis. Trans Roy Soc Trop Med Hyg 52: 78, 1958.
48. Buckley CE, Mathews RS, Grant JA, et al.: Local chemotherapy of Maduromycosis caused by Monosporium apiospermum. Arch Intern Med 124: 748, 1967.
49. Hoeprich PD, Huston AC: Susceptibility of Coccidioides immitis, Candida albicans and Cryptococcus neoformans to amphotericin B, Flucytosine and Clotrimazole. J Infect Dis 132: 133, 1975.
50. Seeliger H, Reifferscheid M: Successful treatment of mycetoma caused by Monosporium apiospermum. Therapy of Fungus Diseases (Sternberg TH, Newcomer VD, eds), Boston, Little, Brown & Co., 1955, p 328.
51. Mohr JA, Muchmore HG: Maduromycosis due to Allescheria boydii. JAMA 204: 125, 1968.
52. Van Cutsem JM, Thienpont D: Miconazole, a broad spectrum antimycotic agent with antibacterial activity. Chemotherapy 17: 392, 1972.
53. Stevens DA, Levine HB, Deresinski SC: Miconazole in coccidioidomycosis. II. Am J Med 60: 191, 1976.
54. Deresinski SC, Lilly RB, Levine HB, et al.: Treatment of fungal meningitis with miconazole. Am Rev Respir Dis (in press).
55. Green WR, Bennett JE, Goos RD: Ocular penetration of amphotericin B. Arch Ophthal 73: 769, 1965.
56. Fishman LS, Griffin JR, Sapico FL, et al.: Hematogenous candida endophthalmitis—a complication of candidemia. N Engl J Med 286: 675, 1972.
57. Meyers BR, Lieberman TW, Ferry AP: Candida endophthalmitis complicating candidemia. Ann Intern Med 79: 647, 1973.
58. Dellon AL, Stark WJ, Chrehen PB: Spontaneous resolution of endogenous Candida endophthalmitis complicating intravenous hyperalimentation. Am J Ophthal 79: 648, 1975.
59. Axelrod AJ, Peyman GA, Apple DJ: Toxicity of intravitreal injection of amphotericin B. Am J Ophthal 76: 578, 1973.
60. Axelrod AJ, Peyman GA: Intravitreal amphotericin B treatment of experimental fungus endophthalmitis. Am J Ophthal 76: 584, 1973.

Atrial Pacing in Patients with Sinus Node Dysfunction

MELVIN M. SCHEINMAN, M.D.*
FREDERICK W. KUNKEL, M.D.
ROBERT W. PETERS, M.D.
DAVID S. HIRSCHFELD, M.D.
PHILIPPE L. SCHOENFELD, M.D.
JOSEPH A. ABBOTT, M.D.
GUNNARD MODIN, B.S.
San Francisco, California

Sinus node recovery time (SNRT) at paced atrial rates of 100 ($SNRT_{100}$) and 120 ($SNRT_{120}$) beats/min, atrial effective refractory periods at spontaneous heart rates (AERP) and at paced rates of 100 ($AERP_{100}$) and 120 ($AERP_{120}$) beats/min, and premature atrial stimulation were among the studies used in evaluating 33 patients with symptomatic sinus node disease and 42 normal subjects. Although mean $SNRT_{100}$ and $SNRT_{120}$ were statistically significantly greater in patients than in control subjects, there was a significant overlap between patient and control groups, and $SNRT_{100}$ or $SNRT_{120}$ was associated with a 30.3 per cent false-negative and 5 per cent false-positive incidence. Correction for heart rate (SNRT–spontaneous cycle length) failed to improve the sensitivity or specificity of this test. There was no significant difference in mean AERP, $AERP_{100}$ or $AERP_{120}$, or in sinoatrial conduction time in patients compared with control subjects.

Analyses of curves derived from plots of test and return cycles showed abnormal curves in only five of the 24 patients studied by progressively premature atrial stimulation. Two of these five patients showed normal zones I and II phenomena followed by a progressive linear increase in the return cycle that was thought to be due to abnormal refractoriness of the perinodal fibers.

In several reports [1–6], the clinical spectrum and management of patients with sinus node dysfunction have been reviewed. More recent work also focused on the value of atrial pacing in the diagnosis of sinus node dysfunction. Mandel et al. [7,8] and Narula et al. [9] emphasized the importance of abnormal depression of sinus node automaticity after pacing in patients with sinus node dysfunction. Langendorf et al. [10] described a method for assessing sinoatrial conduction in patients with atrial parasystole, and Strauss et al. [11] extended this approach by using progressively premature atrial stimulation in patients with sinus node dysfunction, and they first defined 1st degree sinoatrial entrance block by this technic. The objective of our study was to define the sensitivity and specificity of these methods in distinguishing patients with or without sinus node dysfunction. In addition, because previous postmortem studies of patients with sinus node dysfunction [12,13] showed that the disease process also involves the atria, we studied the effects of atrial pacing on atrial effective refractory periods (AERP) in subjects with and without sinus node dysfunction.

From the Medical Service, San Francisco General Hospital, and the Department of Medicine and the Cardiovascular Research Institute, University of California, San Francisco, California. This study was presented in part at the World Congress of Electrocardiology, Bombay, India, 1975. It was supported in part by Grant GM 16496 from the National Institutes of Health, Bethesda, Maryland. Requests for reprints should be addressed to Dr. Melvin M. Scheinman, San Francisco General Hospital, 1001 Potrero Avenue, San Francisco, California 94110. Manuscript accepted February 23, 1976.

* This study was performed during tenure of the American Heart Association Teaching Scholar in Cardiology.

METHODS AND MATERIALS

Thirty-three patients with symptomatic sinus node dysfunction were studied. Detailed clinical and electrocardiographic findings as well as results of exercise stress and autonomic nervous function tests in these patients were reported previously [14–16]. In brief, all patients had symptoms of either dizziness or syncope along with electrocardiographic evidence of sinus node dysfunction. In addition, results of exercise and/or autonomic tests were qualitatively normal except for a blunted heart rate response. Patients with metabolic, neurogenic, orthostatic or other cardiac causes of these symptoms were excluded. Sixteen patients showed predominately chronic sinus bradycardia (group I). These patients all had either frank syncope or dizzy spells and documented episodic severe sinus bradycardia (<45

TABLE I Electrophysiologic Data for Patient Groups*

Case No.	SCL Mean (msec)	SCL Range (msec)	$SNRT_{100}$ (msec)	$SNRT_{120}$ (msec)	AERP (msec)	$AERP_{100}$ (msec)	$AERP_{120}$ (msec)	SACT (msec)
Group I: Sinus Bradycardia								
1	1,162	1,135–1,270	1,050	900	...	...	...	...
2	1,053	1,000–1,120	1,370	1,230	...	...	...	...
3	1,207	1,180–1,256	1,500	1,690	...	...	...	...
4	1,305	1,290–1,520	1,560	>1,580	420	320	330	64
5	1,090	980–1,080	1,280	1,420	<310	220	220	37
6	1,094	1,034–1,198	1,490	1,470	420	240	<220	119
7	1,040	1,033–1,174	1,480	1,580	220	250	180	77
8	985	945–1,069	>1,060	950	...	...	...	...
9	1,083	1,035–1,175	1,205	1,470	240	145	175	1st degree sinoatrial entrance block
10	1,204	1,130–1,297	900	1,020	<270	205	220	†
11	1,133	1,045–1,259	1,640	1,560	...	...	...	...
12	1,104	1,051–1,246	1,100	1,620	305	255	170	1st degree sinoatrial entrance block
13	1,550	1,470–1,620	>1,090	1,550	325	270	260	Zone II only
14	1,152	1,109–1,210	1,550	2,550	310	<260	230	‡
15	991	805–1,015	1,000	1,000	240	200	220	‡
16	1,109	920–1,140	1,450	1,250	230	<180	170	111
Mean ± SD	1,141 ± 144	...	1,295 ± 237	1,428 ± 398	299 ± 70	231 ± 48	218 ± 47	87 ± 29
CSRT	...	...	211 ± 245	306 ± 381	...	...	...	...
Group II: Bradycardia-Tachycardia								
17	890	875–910	2,000	...	...	...	...	...
18	1,080	1,030–1,095	>1,440	1,400	...	...	...	...
19	788	720–840	1,170	1,180	225	185	180	85
20	1,159	940–1,280	1,330	1,065	<285	265	260	28
21	969	840–1,060	1,270	1,140	375	155	<285	59
22	1,026	1,000–1,045	1,380	1,060	360	270	230	100
23	1,190	1,130–1,245	800	1,050	...	...	...	...
24	880	860–990	1,460	1,380	...	...	...	...
25	946	910–1,040	5,600	4,500	280	240	230	161
26	1,124	1,020–1,245	>1,480	1,400	390	280	260	56
27	1,200	1,175–1,295	1,570	1,590	285	<240	230	74
28	1,078	930–1,215	1,745	1,800	270	310	280	57
29	1,066	885–1,290	930	1,050	240	260	<210	80
Mean ± SD	1,044 ± 43	...	1,706 ± 1,211	1,601 ± 936	312 ± 62	245 ± 48	241 ± 34	76 ± 38
CSRT	...	...	662 ± 1,207	557 ± 930	...	...	...	...
Group III: Sinus Arrest								
30	810	750–850	650	840	230	180	200	57
31	1,080	970–1,145	870	1,060	185	160	170	82
32	1,620	1,480–1,720	1,020	1,420	330	285	220	90
33	615	600–740	1,190	1,245	270	230	200	59
Mean ± SD	981 ± 479	...	932 ± 229	1,141 ± 249	254 ± 62	214 ± 56	198 ± 21	72 ± 17
CSRT	...	...	49 ± 492	160 ± 360	...	...	...	...

*SCL = spontaneous cycle length, $SNRT_{100}$ = sinus node recovery time after atrial pacing at a rate of 100 beats/min, $SNRT_{120}$ = sinus node recovery time after atrial pacing at a rate of 120 beats/min, $CSRT_{100}$ + $CSRT_{120}$ = $SNRT_{100}$ or $SNRT_{120}$ − mean spontaneous cycle length, AERP = atrial effective refractory periods determined during spontaneous cycle length, $AERP_{100}$ = AERP determined at a paced rate of 100 beats/min, $AERP_{120}$ = AERP at a paced rate of 120 beats/min, SACT = sinoatrial conduction time.
† See text and Figure 6.
‡ See text and Figure 5.

beats/min). Five of these 16 showed episodic sinoatrial exit block, 13 of the 33 patients studied showed alternating sinus bradycardia and supraventricular tachycardia (group II), and four of the 33 showed episodic sinus arrest (group III). Control subjects were patients with chest pain referred for atrial pacing to evaluate the possible presence of ischemic heart disease. Forty-two control subjects who had no clinical or electrocardiographic evidence of sinus node dysfunction or ischemic heart disease (judged by history and exercise stress or atrial pacing studies or coronary arteriography, which was performed in seven) were included in this study. There was no significant difference in mean age between patients (62 ± 12 years) or control subjects (58 ± 18), and the administration of all medications was discontinued at least 48 hours prior to study.

A quadripolar electrode catheter was inserted in a vein and advanced against the high lateral wall of the right atrium for pacing. The atrium was paced by means of a Medtronics research stimulator (Model No. 1348) or by a programmed stimulator (Blum Associates, Philadelphia, Pa.) with a rectangular pulse of 1 msec in duration at four to five times diastolic threshold. The high stimulus current was used to maintain consistent atrial capture during these studies. Each subject underwent atrial pacing at rates of 100 and 120 beats/min for 2 minutes, and sinus node recovery time was taken as the interval from the last paced atrial beat to the next spontaneous atrial depolarization using the high right atrial electrogram. The corrected sinus node recovery time was determined as the difference between the sinus node recovery time and the mean spontaneous cycle length. In five

TABLE II Electrophysiologic Data for Control Group*

Case No.	SCL Mean (msec)	SCL Range (msec)	$SNRT_{100}$ (msec)	$SNRT_{120}$ (msec)	AERP (msec)	$AERP_{100}$ (msec)	$AERP_{120}$ (msec)	SACT (msec)
				Control Group				
34	676	645–708	950	870	285	200	180	88
35	636	600–734	800	830	280	<170	175	66
36	738	652–793	950	1,050	190	170	180	47
37	650	652–680	770	700	225	...	...	64
38	760	709–820	790	900	...	...	...	...
39	1,014	978–1,055	1,230	1,220	<245	110	180	71
40	798	750–803	1,060	1,080	210	200	170	44
41	720	685–876	880	890	...	...	...	...
42	720	672–755	730	810	190	175	185	75
43	807	792–897	1,020	1,000	215	180	150	47
44	656	617–694	900	920	...	...	...	...
45	636	622–670	810	990	<300	280	250	101
46	742	664–855	900	985	275	230	220	70
47	755	730–824	1,020	1,065	320	250	200	71
48	694	631–713	800	865	...	...	...	...
49	849	810–890	990	1,050	285	220	200	58
50	926	805–1,000	1,070	980	250	<230	220	86
51	738	708–799	810	1,030	330	190	200	78
52	803	782–895	1,050	1,100	360	320	330	69
53	825	743–872	865	860	350	<300	270	70
54	735	660–800	950	950	285	210	140	82
55	768	735–805	980	1,010	315	308	270	87
56	750	712–790	945	930				
57	710	680–760	850	875				
58	655	590–685	780	820				
59	678	612–750	794	770				
60	612	598–692	815	800				
61	640	540–690	870	840				
62	810	770–884	925	930				
63	875	684–937	970	960				
64	830	782–959	995	1,000				
65	725	689–820	900	930				
66	650	610–698	920	970				
67	820	790–868	1,070	1,050				
68	870	775–920	870	890				
69	730	637–820	875	880				
70	900	840–950	1,040	950				
71	550	510–584	740	700				
72	850	745–892	950	840				
73	820	739–889	1,100	980				
74	680	589–757	830	1,020				
75	760	698–795	950	920				
Mean ± SD	755 ± 99	...	917 ± 110	934 ± 107	273 ± 52	220 ± 57	207 ± 49	71 ± 16
CSRT	...	...	160 ± 73	177 ± 80	...	...	...	...

*See Table I for definitions of abbreviations.

patients, the sinus node recovery time was actually greater than the designated value because the postpacing pause was terminated by an ectopic atrial or junctional depolarization.

The atrial effective refractory periods (AERPs) were determined by extrastimulus methods [17] in 24 of the 33 patients and in 18 of the 42 control subjects. Successively coupled premature atrial stimulation at 10 to 20 msec decrements were introduced every 7 to 10 beats during spontaneous rhythm and at paced atrial rates of 100 and 120 beats/min. The longest interval between spontaneous atrial depolarization (A_1) and stimulated beat (S_2) that failed to depolarize the atrium during spontaneous rhythm was denoted as the AERPs and the longest interval between the last driven beat and the induced premature beat (S_1S_2) in which atrial capture failed at paced rates of 100 and 120 beats/min as $AERP_{100}$ and $AERP_{120}$, respectively. The atrial functional refractory period was defined as the shortest interval between spontaneous and premature depolarization (A_1A_2) for any given A_1S_2 or S_1S_2 during either spontaneous rhythm or at paced rates of 100 or 120 beats/min. Because of the known variation of atrial refractoriness with rate, patients with marked sinus arrhythmia were excluded from study, and the mean and range of the spontaneous cycle length for each patient were recorded (Tables I and II). When the coupling interval of the test stimulus was longer than the AERP, the AERP was designated as being less than the shortest induced A_1S_2 or S_1S_2. In most instances, the given cycle length was repeatedly scanned to obtain the AERP.

The sinoatrial conduction time was determined from analyses of test (A_1A_2) and return cycles (A_2A_3) during spontaneous rhythm in 24 patients and 18 control subjects. To allow comparison of data despite wide variations in heart rate, both test (A_1A_2) and return cycles (A_2A_3) were normalized by dividing each by the preceding spontaneous cycle length (A_1A_1). In each of the 24 patients and 18 control subjects who underwent premature atrial stimulation, A_2A_3:A_1A_1 was plotted as a function of A_1A_2:A_1A_1. Both zones I and II were determined by analyses of point aggregates, and lines drawn through these points represent the best curve fit derived from a computer program using the least squares method. The sinoatrial conduction time was computed by

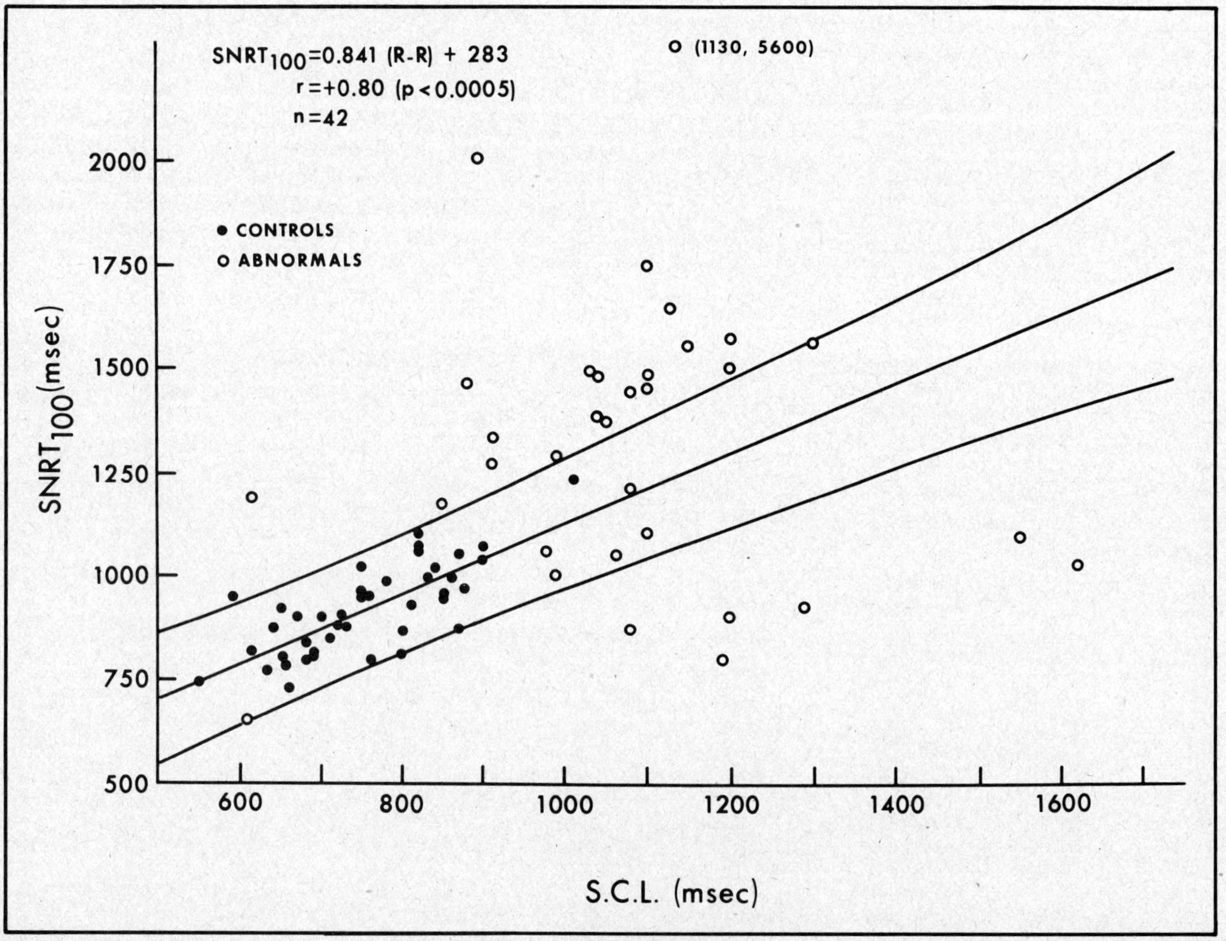

Figure 1. *Plot of sinus node recovery times (SNRT) at a paced rate of 100 beats/min and spontaneous cycle lengths (SCL) (R-R) for control subjects (●) and patients (○). Denoted are the regression line and 95 per cent confidence band of $SNRT_{100}$ and spontaneous cycle length for control subjects. Twenty patients with sinus node disease were outside the 95 per cent confidence band. Control cycle length in one subject (Case 71) was 550 msec (point farthest to the left on figure) but spontaneous cycle length increased allowing for atrial capture at a cycle length of 600 msec.*

taking one half of the difference between mean plateau return cycles and mean spontaneous cycle lengths. Very early atrial premature depolarizations that resulted in abrupt shortening of the return cycle were noted but excluded from analyses.

All recordings were obtained using an Electronics for Medicine DR-12 oscilloscope recorder at a paper speed of 100 mm/sec. All subjects gave written, informed consent prior to the study according to a protocol approved by the University of California, San Francisco, Committee on Human Experimentation.

RESULTS

Sinus Node Recovery Time and Spontaneous Cycle Length. The pertinent electrophysiologic data are summarized in Tables I and II. Both the mean maximal sinus node recovery time (SNRT) at paced rates of 100 and 120 beats/min ($SNRT_{100}$ and $SNRT_{120}$) as well as mean spontaneous cycle length were significantly longer for patients in groups I and II compared with those in control subjects, but there was no significant difference between either mean sinus node recovery time at 100 or 120 beats/min or spontaneous cycle length for the four patients in group III when compared with those in the control subjects. There was no significant difference and good correlation between mean $SNRT_{100}$ and $SNRT_{120}$ for both patients and control subjects ($r = +0.77$, $p < 0.0005$). In addition, spontaneous cycle length and $SNRT_{100}$ or $SNRT_{120}$ correlated closely ($r = +0.80$ and 0.70, respectively) ($p < 0.0005$) (Figure 1) for control subjects. Thus, in normal subjects roughly 50 to 64 per cent of the variance observed in $SNRT_{100}$ or $SNRT_{120}$ was related to the spontaneous cycle length. Extrapolation of this linear relationship found among normal subjects (Figure 1) to spontaneous cycle lengths > 1,000 msec showed that the $SNRT_{100}$ (in 20 of the 33 patients) fell above the 95 per cent confidence band predicted from the control data. Similar extrapolation of the linear regression equation for $SNRT_{120}$ and spontaneous cycle length showed that in only 18 of the 33 patients did these fall above the corresponding 95 per cent confidence level (not shown). There was no significant difference in mean corrected sinus node recovery time (CSRT) at paced rates of 100 or 120 beats/min for all subjects, but mean $CSRT_{100}$ and $CSRT_{120}$ values were significantly greater for patients in group II than in control subjects ($p < 0.05$).

The sensitivity and specificity of mean spontaneous cycle length, $SNRT_{100}$, $SNRT_{120}$, $CSRT_{100}$, and $CSRT_{120}$ in distinguishing subjects with or without abnormal sinus node function were determined by the most significant p value found by means of serial 2 by 2 chi square analyses at 50 msec increments for these variables with at least one entry into each of four cells (Table III). The atrial pacing tests showed a low order of sensitivity (with the incidence of false-negatives ranging from 30.3 to 48.5 per cent), but a high order of specificity (with the incidence of false-positives ranging from 2.4 to 9.6 per cent). Also of note is the finding that analyses of spontaneous cycle length, using a cutoff of 950 msec, proved to be more sensitive (21.2 per cent false-negative) and equally as specific (2.4 per cent false-positive) as any of the atrial pacing procedures. Linear discriminant analysis [18] of $SNRT_{100}$ or $SNRT_{120}$ and spontaneous cycle length yielded the highest order of sensitivity (5 per cent false-positive) and a high order of specificity (9 per cent false-negative). It must be appreciated, however, that this analysis is strongly weighted by the spontaneous cycle length.

Atrial Effective Refractory Period. Progressively premature atrial depolarizations were induced in 24 of the 33 patients and in 18 of the 45 control subjects to determine AERP and sinoatrial conduction time. Because there was no significant difference between mean atrial functional refractory period and AERP either at spontaneous cycle length or during atrial pacing in control or patient groups, only analyses of AERP are discussed. No significant differences in mean AERP, $AERP_{100}$ or $AERP_{120}$ were found between control and patient groups. There was, however, a statistically significant decrease in mean $AERP_{100}$ compared with AERP in all groups (group I $p < 0.01$, group II $p < 0.02$, group III $p < 0.01$ and control subjects $p < 0.01$). Although mean $AERP_{120}$ was less than $AERP_{100}$ for each group, the differences were not statistically significant. There was a statistically significant correlation between mean AERP and spontaneous cycle length ($r = +0.48$), but no significant difference in the mean slope of AERP and spontaneous cycle length between the control and patient groups. Of interest were two patients in group I (Cases 4 and 5) who had AERPs of 420 msec (which exceeded the highest AERP, 360 msec, found among control subjects). However, all AERP values for patients with sinus node dysfunction fell within the 95 per cent confidence band generated from the regression equation of cycle length and AERP in control subjects (not shown). Thus, AERP, $AERP_{100}$ and $AERP_{120}$ were not useful in separating subjects with normal sinus function from patients with sinus node dysfunction.

Sinoatrial Conduction Time. There was no statistically significant difference in mean sinoatrial conduction time

TABLE III Sensitivity and Specificity of Atrial Pacing Studies

Parameter	Cutoff (msec)	False-Negative		False-Positive	
		Incidence	Per Cent	Incidence	Per Cent
SCL	950	7/33	21.2	1/42	2.4
$SNRT_{100}$	1,100	10/33	30.3	2/42	5
$SNRT_{120}$	1,100	10/33	30.3	2/42	5
$CSRT_{100}$	300	13/33	39.4	1/42	2.4
$CSRT_{120}$	300	16/33	48.5	4/42	9.6

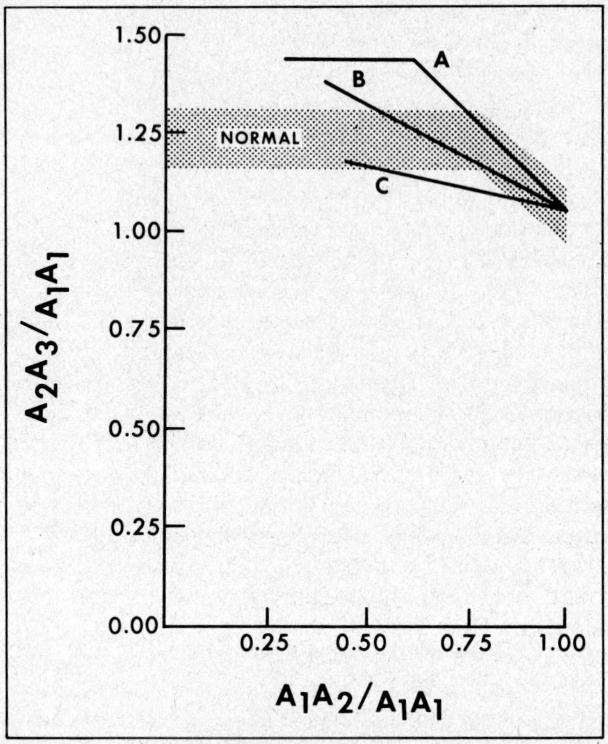

Figure 2. *Relationship between test (A_1A_2) and return cycles (A_2A_3). The ordinate and abscissa represent test and return cycles normalized for spontaneous length for each person tested. Points along the abscissa represent fractions of A_1A_1 at which premature atrial beats were induced. For each A_1A_2 interval, the recovery cycle (A_2A_3) was also recorded and expressed as a fraction of A_1A_1. Thus, recording the corrected recovery time (A_2A_3:A_1A_1) for every corrected test cycle (A_1A_2:A_1A_1) allows for direct comparison of patients with different cycle lengths. Cumulative points of test (A_1A_2) and return cycles (A_2A_3) for all subjects are shown. A, B and C are three abnormal curves and the stippled area is the composite of "normal" curve points. The stippled area is diagrammatically extended to zero on the abscissa while the actual earliest induced atrial premature depolarization (APD) was approximately 25 per cent of spontaneous cycle lengths (SCL).*

between the control and each of the patient groups (Tables I and II). In each of the 24 patients and 18 control subjects, normalized test (A_1A_2:A_1A_1) and return cycles (A_2A_3:A_1A_1) were plotted and analyzed. Sinus node entrance block ($A_1A_1 = A_1A_3$) [19] was responsible for abrupt shortening of A_2A_3 in three patients and two control subjects, whereas sinus node or atrial reentry resulted in shortening of the return cycle in three patients and two control subjects [20].

For the 18 normal subjects, late atrial premature depolarizations resulted in reciprocal lengthening of the return cycle (zone I) until plateau levels were achieved (zone II). The composite curve for normalized test and return cycles in control subjects is shown in Figure 2. Plots of normalized test and return cycles for 18 of the 24 patients fell within the range of control determinations.

Clearly abnormal curves were found in five patients: one patient (Case 25, group II) reached zone II (reset) at atrial premature depolarizations equal or less than 61 per cent of the spontaneous cycle length, and sinoatrial conduction time was markedly prolonged, whereas two patients (Cases 9 and 12, group I) showed the pattern of 1st degree sinoatrial entrance block in that a zone of reset was never reached (Figure 2). Plots of test and return cycles in two (Cases 14 and 15) of four patients showing spontaneous antegrade sinoatrial node exit block were of particular interest in that normal zones I and II were observed after relatively late atrial premature depolarizations. Atrial premature depolarizations occurring earlier than 70 per cent of spontaneous cycle length in one and 60 per cent in the other resulted in further progressive prolongation of the return cycle. The point aggregates for these patients could not be fitted by a single diagonal line and appeared to be best represented by two diagonal lines as seen in Figure 3. The secondary progressive increase in return cycles occurred well outside the atrial relative refractory period and could not be explained by increasing latency between stimulus and atrial response or by slowed interatrial conduction. Finally, in one additional patient (Case 10, group I) all return cycles were either equal to or only slightly different from the spontaneous cycle length (Figure 4). The calculated sinoatrial conduction time for this patient was close to zero.

COMMENTS

Methods of assessing the postpacing pause vary among different laboratories. Some prefer to use a fixed value as the upper limits of normal [8,21] whereas others apply a correction factor based upon the spontaneous cycle length [9,22]. Our study shows a clear relationship between spontaneous cycle length and $SNRT_{100,120}$ for normal subjects and therefore sinus node recovery time should be corrected for spontaneous cycle length. Correction by subtraction of spontaneous cycle length from sinus node recovery time ($CSRT_{100,120}$), as suggested by Narula et al. [9], however, was less sensitive than $SNRT_{100}$ or $SNRT_{120}$ alone in distinguishing patients from control subjects (Table III). We, therefore, suggest an alternative approach; namely, extrapolation of the regression equation derived from our normal subjects to spontaneous cycle length $>$1,000 msec (into the spontaneous cycle length range generally found in patients with sinus node dysfunction), and consider sinus node recovery times falling above 2 standard deviations from this regression line (95 per cent confidence limits) as abnormal. Using this formulation, the "normal" sinus node recovery time is neither

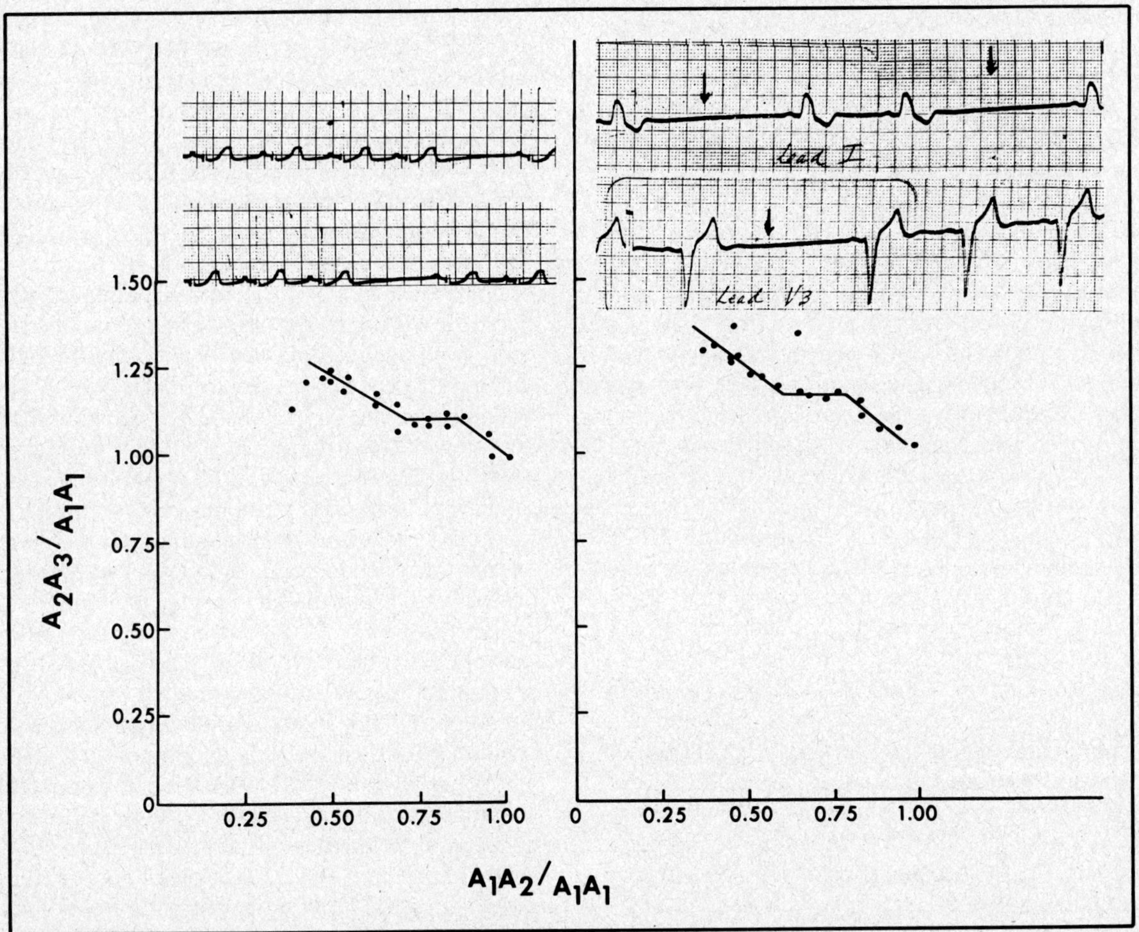

Figure 3. *Ordinate and abscissa as in Figure 2. Electrocardiographic rhythm strips from two patients showing sinoatrial exit block (Wenckebach conduction on the left side and 3:2 exit block on the right side) along with respective plots of test and return cycles. Both patients show normal zones I and II, but earlier atrial premature depolarizations (APD) result in progressive lengthening of the return cycle.*

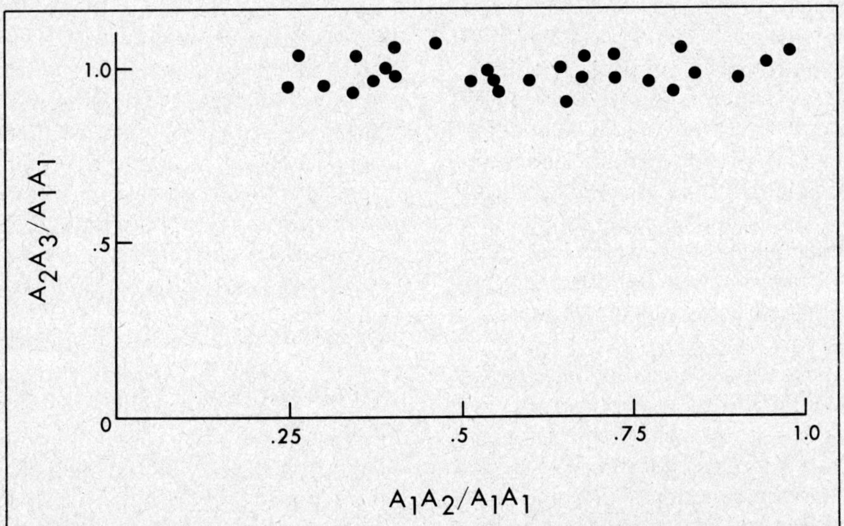

Figure 4. *Ordinate and abscissa as in Figure 2. Plot of normalized test and return cycles for one patient (Case 10, group I) shows that normalized return cycles were almost identical to the test cycles and the calculated sinoatrial conduction time was −5 msec.*

a fixed value nor is it determined by merely subtracting spontaneous cycle length, but it is related to spontaneous cycle length in the following manner: $SNRT_{100} = 0.841$ (spontaneous cycle length) + 117 or $SNRT_{120} = 0.76$ (spontaneous cycle length) + 367. Thus, for a patient with a heart rate of 60 beats/min (spontaneous cycle length = 1,000 msec), an abnormal $SNRT_{100}$ would be expected to be >1,275 msec; for a heart rate of 50 beats/min (1,200 msec), abnormal $SNRT_{100}$ would be expected to be >1,470 msec; and for a heart rate of 40 beats/min (1,500 msec), an abnormal $SNRT_{100}$ would be expected to be >1,770 msec. The 95 per cent confidence band relating sinus node recovery time and spontaneous cycle length must, however, be interpreted as a very rough approximation at spontaneous cycle length >1,000 msec because only one of our control subjects had a spontaneous cycle length in this range. Similarly, caution must be used in interpreting relative sensitivity and specificity of these tests since a truly appropriate control group (namely, subjects with sinus bradycardia without sinus node dysfunction) is not currently available.

Sinoatrial Conduction Time. The mean sinoatrial conduction time was greater while mean spontaneous cycle length was significantly longer ($p < 0.0005$) in patients versus control subjects. Since in a given patient sinoatrial conduction time varies inversely with spontaneous cycle length [23], the converse would have been expected; namely, patients with long spontaneous cycle length would be expected to show shorter sinoatrial conduction time. Thus, sinoatrial conduction time might, in fact, be abnormally prolonged in many of the patients when corrected for heart rate. We were, however, unable to correct sinoatrial conduction time for variations in heart rate since there was no significant correlation between sinoatrial conduction time and spontaneous cycle length among the control subjects, and there are no data on sinoatrial conduction time in "normal" subjects with sinus bradycardia. In addition, particularly troublesome was one patient whose return cycles were always either equal to or only slightly different from the mean spontaneous cycle length, thus yielding a sinoatrial conduction time which was close to zero (Figure 4). Similar findings were reported by Reiffel et al. [23] in patients with sinus bradycardia and marked sinus arrhythmia, and their findings may be related to the extreme variations observed in sinoatrial cycle length; our patient (Case 10, group I) did not have a sinus arrhythmia. Conceivably, this finding was related to pacemaker shift to a very peripheral position in the sinus node explaining the marked foreshortening of the sinoatrial conduction time.

On the other hand, analyses of plots of tests and return cycles occasionally produced evidence of marked abnormalities in sinoatrial conduction. For example, two patients (of four studied) with spontaneous antegrade sinoatrial exit block showed a heretofore undescribed relationship between test and return cycles in that late atrial premature depolarizations produced relatively normal zones I and II, whereas atrial premature depolarizations initiated during the middle of the atrial cycle resulted in further linear prolongation of the return cycle. These phenomena were not related to increases in either latency between stimulus and atrial depolarization or changes in sinus rate, interatrial conduction time or paper recording speed. We believe that this phenomenon can best be explained by abnormal refractoriness of the perinodal fibers. Strauss and Bigger [24] clearly defined a zone of perinodal fibers using a rabbit preparation with electrophysiologic properties intermediate between sinus node and atrial fibers. Klein et al. [25] found that very early atrial premature depolarizations (coupling intervals <150 msec) resulted in increased atrial to sinus node conduction times that clearly could not be ascribed solely to increasing latency. Ticzon et al. [26] reported abrupt increases in the return cycle (as much as 10 per cent of plateau A_2A_3) for atrial premature depolarizations induced in early zone II in seven of 25 dogs and attributed these findings to atrial premature depolarizations encountering the sinoatrial junctional relative refractory period. In our patients, the observed secondary increase in return cycle length that began after relatively late atrial premature depolarizations (60 per cent and 70 per cent of spontaneous cycle length) suggests that atrial premature depolarizations falling in this zone encountered perinodal fibers with abnormally prolonged refractoriness resulting in progressive prolongation of sinoatrial conduction. Klein et al. [25] further showed that atrial premature depolarizations initiated during the middle of the atrial cycle usually resulted in return atrial cycles slightly longer than corresponding sinoatrial nodal cycles and the difference reflected antegrade and retrograde sinoatrial conduction time. On occasion, such atrial premature depolarizations resulted in marked prolongation of sinoatrial conduction with corresponding increases in the atrial return cycle. The chance occurrence of induced progressively premature atrial premature depolarizations in succeeding cycles resulting in almost linear prolongation of the return cycle would appear to be most unlikely.

CONCLUSION

It is apparent that present laboratory procedures lack sufficient sensitivity in distinguishing normal subjects from patients with sinus node dysfunction. For the present, we suggest that only sinus node recovery times clearly falling outside the 95 per cent confidence band predicted by the regression equation of sinus node recovery time and spontaneous cycle length be considered abnormal. Likewise, measurements of sinoatrial conduction time lacked sufficient specificity to be of value in distinguishing patients from control subjects. Of special interest were the atrial test-response curves in two of four subjects with spontaneous sinoatrial node exit block which is best explained on the basis of abnormal refractoriness of perinodal fibers and suggests that conduction failure from the sinoatrial node to the atrium might be related to abnormalities in perinodal refractoriness.

REFERENCES

1. Rubenstein JJ, Schulman CL, Yurchak PM, et al.: Clinical spectrum of the sick sinus syndrome. Circulation 46: 5, 1972.
2. Easley RM Jr, Goldstein S: Sino-atrial syncope. Am J Med 50: 166, 1971.
3. Chokshi DS, Mascarenhas E, Samet P, et al.: Treatment of sinoatrial rhythm disturbances with permanent cardiac pacing. Am J Cardiol 32: 215, 1973.
4. Conde CA, Leppo J, Lipski J, et al.: Effectiveness of pacemaker treatment in the bradycardia-tachycardia syndrome. Am J Cardiol 32: 209, 1973.
5. Ferrer MI: The sick sinus syndrome. Circulation 47: 635, 1973.
6. Moss AJ, Davis RJ: Brady-tachy syndrome. Prog Cardiovasc Dis 16: 439, 1974.
7. Mandel W, Hayakawa H, Danzig R, et al.: Evaluation of sinoatrial node function in man by overdrive suppression. Circulation 44: 59, 1971.
8. Mandel WJ, Hayakawa H, Allen HN, et al.: Assessment of sinus node function in patients with the sick sinus syndrome. Circulation 46: 761, 1972.
9. Narula OS, Samet P, Javier RP: Significance of the sinus-node recovery time. Circulation 45: 140, 1972.
10. Langendorf R, Lesser ME, Plotkin P, et al.: Atrial parasystole with interpolation. Observations on prolonged sinoatrial conduction. Am Heart J 63: 649, 1962.
11. Strauss HC, Saroff AL, Bigger JT Jr, et al.: Premature atrial stimulation as a key to the understanding of sinoatrial conduction in man. Circulation 47: 86, 1973.
12. Kaplan BM, Langendorf R, Lev M, et al.: Tachycardia-bradycardia syndrome (so-called "sick sinus syndrome"). Am J Cardiol 31: 497, 1973.
13. Rosen KM, Rahimtoola SH, Gunnar RM, et al.: Transient and persistent atrial standstill with His bundle lesions. Circulation 44: 220, 1971.
14. Scheinman MM, Peters R, Hirschfeld DS, et al.: The sick sinus and ailing atrium. West J Med 121: 473, 1974.
15. Abbott JA, Kunkel F, Hirschfeld DS, et al.: Effects of cardiac pacing and heart rate acceleration on exercise-induced symptoms in patients with sick sinus syndrome. Circulation 50 (suppl III): III-9, 1974.
16. Scheinman MM: Sinus node dysfunction. Proceedings of the World Congress of Electrocardiology, Bombay, India, 1975 (in press).
17. Wit AL, Weiss MB, Berkowitz WD, et al.: Patterns of atrioventricular conduction in the human heart. Circ Res 27: 345, 1970.
18. Truett J, Cornfield J, Kannel W: A multivariate analysis of the risk of coronary heart disease in Framingham. J Chronic Dis 20: 511, 1967.
19. Goldreyer BN, Damato AN: Sinoatrial-node entrance block. Circulation 44: 789, 1971.
20. Paulay KL, Varghese PJ, Damato AN: Atrial rhythms in response to an early atrial premature depolarization in man. Am Heart J 85: 323, 1973.
21. Dhingra RC, Rosen KM, Rahimtoola SH: Normal conduction intervals and responses in GI patients using His bundle recordings and atrial pacing. Chest 64: 55, 1973.
22. Gupta PK, Lichstein E, Chedda KD, et al.: Appraisal of sinus node recovery time in patients with sick sinus syndrome. Am J Cardiol 34: 265, 1974.
23. Reiffel JA, Bigger JT, Konstam MA: The relationship between sinoatrial conduction time and sinus cycle length during spontaneous sinus arrhythmia in adults. Circulation 50: 924, 1974.
24. Strauss HC, Bigger JT Jr: Electrophysiological properties of the rabbit sinoatrial perinodal fibers. Circ Res 31: 490, 1972.
25. Klein HO, Singer DH, Hoffman BF: Effects of atrial premature systoles on sinus rhythm in the rabbit. Circ Res 32: 480, 1973.
26. Ticzon AR, Strauss HC, Gallagher JJ, et al.: Sinus nodal function in the intact dog heart evaluated by premature atrial stimulation and atrial pacing. Am J Cardiol 35: 492, 1975.

Local Characteristics of the Normal and Asynergic Left Ventricle in Man

MONTY M. BODENHEIMER, M.D.
VIDYA S. BANKA, M.D.
ROBERT G. TROUT, M.D.
GEORGE A. HERMANN, M.D.
HOMAYOON PASDAR, M.D.
RICHARD H. HELFANT, M.D.
Philadelphia, Pennsylvania

The significance of ventricular asynergy in determining medical prognosis and surgical risk in patients with coronary artery disease and its delineation by ventriculography have been of increasing interest. To determine the underlying histopathologic and electrographic features of left ventricular asynergy, 39 patients undergoing open heart surgery were studied. Thirty-six histopathologic specimens were obtained in 31 patients (26 as transmural needle biopsies and 10 as aneurysm resections). In four normally contracting areas and 12 hypokinetic areas, neither fibrosis nor early changes of myocardial damage was evident. In contrast, of eight akinetic areas there was more than 50 per cent muscle loss in four and from 30 to 35 per cent muscle loss in three, in only one area was there less than 10 per cent muscle loss. Of 12 dyskinetic zones there was more than 75 per cent muscle loss in 10 zones, 35 per cent in one and no pathologic abnormalities in one.

Epicardial electrograms were obtained from 35 areas in 29 patients. Of 10 normally contracting ventricles, in one, pathologic Q waves were demonstrated only over the inferior area. Progressive increases in the severity of asynergy were associated with a progressive increase in frequency of initial abnormal Q waves. In only one of nine hypokinetic areas were epicardial Q waves exhibited, but they were present in six of 10 akinetic and five of six dyskinetic areas.

Both histopathologic and electrographic data were available from 20 asynergic areas in 16 patients. Initial epicardial R waves were associated with normal biopsy specimens in seven of eight hypokinetic areas. Of seven akinetic areas, initial R waves were associated with 30 to 35 per cent muscle loss in three; of four areas with initial Q waves, there was a 35 per cent muscle loss in one and more than 50 per cent muscle loss in three. Similarly, of five dyskinetic segments, a QS pattern was associated with more than 75 per cent fibrosis in four. In one dyskinetic area there was an initial R wave in association with a normal appearing biopsy specimen.

In summary, a good correlation exists between the severity of asynergy by ventriculography, the degree of muscle loss and the presence of epicardial Q waves. However, a significant amount of histologically and electrographically normal myocardium may be present even in severely asynergic areas.

Ventricular asynergy (abnormal contraction) is a major factor in defining the medical prognosis [1,2] and surgical risk [3–5] of patients

From the Departments of Cardiology, Cardiovascular Surgery and Pathology, Presbyterian-University of Pennsylvania Medical Center, Philadelphia, Pennsylvania. This study was presented in part at the American Heart Association National Meeting, Anaheim, California in November 1975. It was supported in part by a grant from the American Heart Association—Southeastern Pennsylvania Chapter. Requests for reprints should be addressed to Dr. Richard H. Helfant, Division of Cardiology, Presbyterian-University of Pennsylvania Medical Center, 51 North 39th Street, Philadelphia, Pennsylvania 19104. Manuscript accepted March 31, 1976.

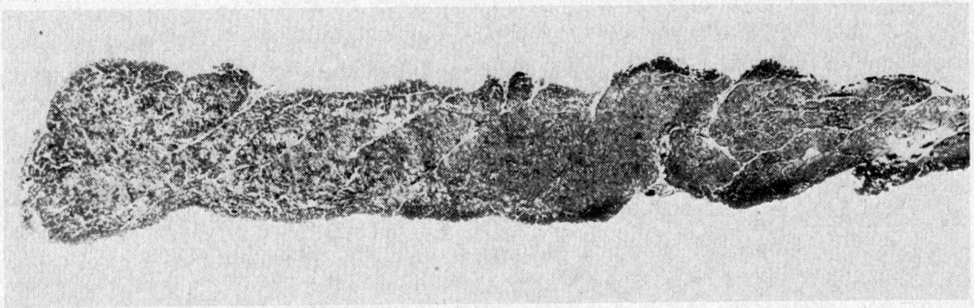

Figure 1. *Biopsy specimen from a hypokinetic apical area (hemiaxis shortening 15 per cent). Muscle fibers appear normal without evidence of fibrosis or inflammatory cells. Hematoxylin and eosin stain; original magnification X 15, reduced by 35 per cent.*

with coronary artery disease. At present, ventriculography provides the best method for assessing the presence and severity of asynergy in living man [6]. However, little is known about the underlying histopathology or electrographic status of asynergic zones of the left ventricle.

This study was undertaken, therefore, to better understand the histopathologic and electrographic features of left ventricular asynergy depicted by ventriculography in 39 patients at the time of open heart surgery for coronary heart disease.

METHODS

Thirty-nine patients undergoing cardiac surgery form the basis of this study. Twenty-nine patients underwent aortocoronary bypass surgery because of angina associated with significant (>75 per cent) obstruction of at least one major coronary artery (right coronary, left anterior descending or left circumflex coronary artery); six patients underwent combined resection of the aneurysm and aortocoronary bypass, and four had resection of the aneurysm alone. None of the patients included in the study sustained an acute myocardial infarction within four weeks prior to surgery.

Cardiac catheterization was performed in the postabsorptive state after premedication with 50 mg of Nembutal®, 50 mg of Demerol® and 0.4 mg of atropine. Right heart catheterization was performed via an antecubital vein cutdown, and left heart catheterization either percutaneously through a femoral artery or via a right brachial arteriotomy. Following recordings of left ventricular pressure (using Statham P23Db transducers) and cardiac output (indicator dilution method using indocyanine green), left ventriculography was performed in the 30 degree right anterior oblique projection using 30 to 40 cc of meglumine diatrizoate (Renografin-76) injected into the left ventricle. In no case was this performed during or immediately after the onset of anginal symptoms. Selective cinecoronary arteriography was then performed using either the Sones' or Judkins' technic. Cines were taken on a 10 by 6 inch dual field image intensifier (Siemens) at 64 frames/sec using Kodak Shellburst film. Hemodynamics were monitored and recorded on an Electronics for Medicine oscillographic recorder.

Epicardial electrograms were obtained before or immediately after the institution of cardiopulmonary bypass and before elective ventricular fibrillation [7,8]. Unipolar electrograms were obtained using three silver electrodes mounted in acrylic plastic in the shape of a triangle and recorded between 0.1 to 100 Hz on a Grass model 7B polygraph at 25, 50 and 100 mm/sec paper speeds. A flat probe on a flexible handle was utilized to facilitate recordings from the posterior surface of the left ventricle.

With the patient on cardiopulmonary bypass for less than 5 minutes and before elective ventricular fibrillation, a full thickness punch biopsy specimen was obtained using a punch sucker technic [9,10]. A 14-gauge needle with a square, keenly sharpened tip was connected to an aspiration suction line with a Likens' tube interposed and a sponge covering the outflow arm of the collecting tube. This technic avoided undue compression, trauma or distortion (Figure 1). The biopsy specimen was processed routinely, serially sectioned longitudinally and stained with both hematoxylin and eosin and a connective tissue stain for semiquantitative estimate of the amount of fibrosis.

To facilitate the correlation of ventriculographically determined asynergic sites with the corresponding anatomic location at the time of surgery, the antero-apical and inferior zones were specifically examined. These areas were chosen for their ease of demarcation by right anterior oblique ventriculography. In addition, their low vascularity rendered biopsy a safe procedure. During surgery, epicardial electrograms were recorded from multiple sites beginning over the right ventricle and then sequentially from the region next to the septum, antero-apical area, lateral wall and the inferior aspect of the left ventricle. The antero-apical area was taken as the zone between the anterior interventricular groove and a line 4 to 5 cm parallel and lateral to it extending towards the apex. The inferior area was taken as the epicardial surface bounded by the atrioventricular groove, the posterior interventricular groove and a line 3 to 4 cm parallel and lateral to it. Recordings were obtained in an average of six sites from each area. All recordings were obtained during sinus rhythm.

The electrogram pattern from the proposed biopsy site (antero-apical and/or inferior) was then specifically noted. Following institution of cardiopulmonary bypass, a biopsy specimen was taken from this site, permitting correlation of electrogram and biopsy data.

Severity of asynergy during ventriculography was evaluated both qualitatively and quantitatively [11,12]. A quantitative analysis was performed by superimposing tracings of

TABLE I Correlation of Severity of Asynergy and Muscle Loss

Ventricular Contraction	Muscle Loss (% by volume)			
Severity of asynergy (hemiaxis shortening mean ± SEM)	0–9	10–49	50–74	75–100
Normal (35.0 ± 5.6%)	4	—	—	—
Hypokinetic (13.8 ± 1.2%)	12	—	—	—
Akinetic (3.6 ± 1.2%)	1	3	2	2
Dyskinetic (−4.4 ± 0.7%)	1	1	—	10

NOTE: Values in table represent number of ventricular areas biopsied.

end-diastolic and end-systolic frames using the apex and mid-aortic valve as fixed points. Hemiaxes were drawn which quadrisected the long axis at right angles to it. Each hemiaxis was recorded as a percentage change from end-diastole. Segmental contraction was thus classified as normal (≥25 per cent hemiaxis shortening), hypokinetic (decreased contraction; <25 per cent hemiaxis shortening), akinetic (absence of contraction; 0 to 5 per cent hemiaxis shortening) and dyskinetic (paradoxical systolic expansion; hemiaxis lengthening) [11,12].

Epicardial electrograms were analyzed for the presence and duration of Q waves. Previous studies have indicated that Q waves are normally absent over the left ventricle immediately lateral to the septum with Q waves of ≤0.01 sec in duration occasionally seen over the anterior free wall and initial Q waves of ≤0.03 sec inferiorly [13–15]. Thus, anterior Q waves ≥0.03 sec and inferior Q waves of ≥0.04 sec were considered abnormal. In addition, electrogram sites over each area were analyzed for the relative distribution and frequency of initial R and Q waves providing an index of homogeneity of a specific zone.

Each biopsy specimen was examined independently and blindly by at least two observers and classified according to the per cent muscle loss present in the biopsy material. This included both fibrosis and evidence of myocardial necrosis (healing infarct) which may not have progressed to complete fibrosis; namely, the presence of leukocytic infiltration, removal of muscle fibers, appearance of macrophages and fibroblasts and early signs of collagen formation [16]. The percentage muscle loss and fibrosis was assessed, graded as 0 to 9 per cent, 10 to 49 per cent, 50 to 74 per cent and 75 to 100 per cent of the biopsy specimen by volume and then correlated with the severity of asynergy.

Statistical analysis was performed using the Student's t test, and all values are given as mean ± standard error of the mean (SEM).

TABLE II Correlation of Severity of Asynergy and Epicardial Electrogram

	Epicardial Electrogram	
	Initial R Wave	Initial Q Wave*
Severity of Asynergy (hemiaxis shortening)		
Normal (36.1 ± 3.9)	9	1
Hypokinetic (15.5 ± 1.2)	8	1
Akinetic (2.7 ± 1.6)	4	6
Dyskinetic (−4.6 ± 1.2)	1	5

* Anterior Q ⩾ 0.03 sec, inferior Q ⩾ 0.04 sec.

RESULTS

Normal Segmental Contraction. There were 10 patients with an average of 2.3 major coronary arteries involved and a normal ventricular contraction pattern.

Biopsy specimens obtained from four areas all demonstrated normal myocardial structure (Table I). Epicardial electrograms were normal in nine of 10 patients (Table II). In one patient with obstructive lesions involving both the right coronary and left circumflex arteries, pathologic epicardial Q waves were localized to the inferior area.

Segmental Asynergy. There were 29 patients with an average of 2.4 major coronary arteries demonstrating obstructive lesions.

Ventriculographic-histopathologic correlation: Histopathologic specimens were obtained from 32 areas in 27 patients, via aneurysmal resection in 10 and biopsy in 22.

None of the 12 hypokinetic zones demonstrated fibrosis or classic early changes indicating myocardial damage (Table I and Figure 1). In contrast, four of the eight akinetic areas exhibited more than 50 per cent (Table I and Figure 2), whereas the specimens from three additional areas showed a 30 to 35 per cent muscle loss. One akinetic area showed minimal evidence of muscle loss (Figure 3).

Ten of the 12 dyskinetic segments demonstrated more than 75 per cent fibrosis (Figure 4). One patient had 35 per cent muscle loss and another (with a three week history of unstable angina and normal enzymes) demonstrated antero-apical dyskinesis without evidence of significant muscle loss.

Ventriculographic-electrographic correlation: Of the 25 asynergic areas (in 19 patients) from which local multiple site electrograms were recorded, nine were hypokinetic, 10 akinetic and six dyskinetic (Table II). In 24 of the 25 zones there was a consistent pattern of either R or Q waves over the entire area. One showed significant local Q waves in two thirds of the recorded sites.

In eight of the nine hypokinetic segments initial R waves were recorded from all epicardial sites (Figure 5), whereas in one inferior zone there was an initial wide Q wave in two thirds of the sites. Of the 10 akinetic segments, there were associated initial R waves in four

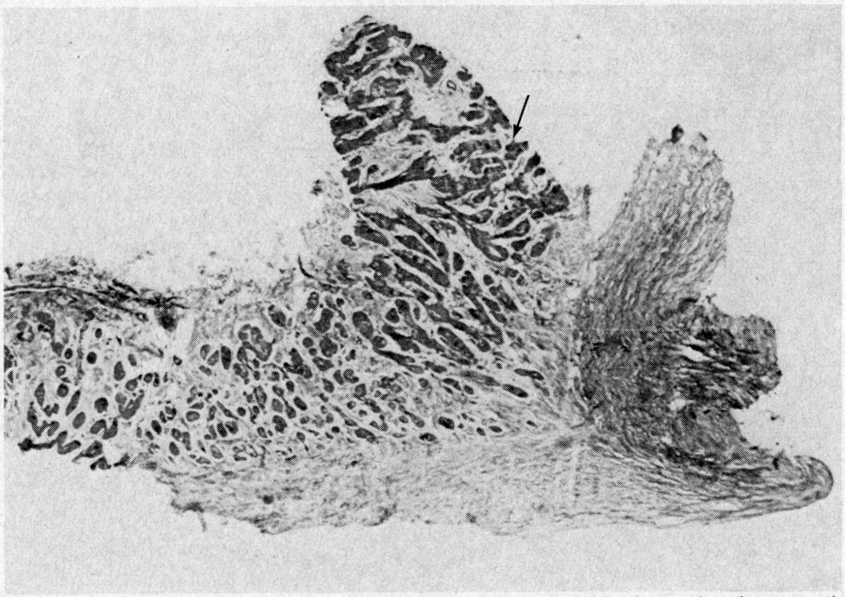

Figure 2. *Biopsy specimen from an akinetic area (hemiaxis shortening 4 per cent). More than 50 per cent of the specimen is replaced by fibrous tissue with areas of normal residual muscle fibers (arrow). Hematoxylin and eosin stain; original magnification ×75, reduced by 33 per cent.*

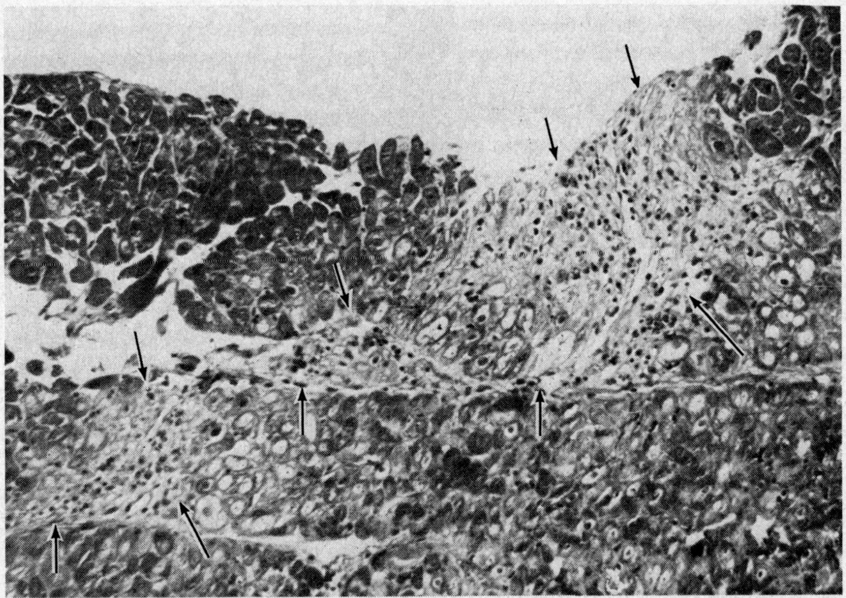

Figure 3. *Biopsy specimen from an akinetic area (hemiaxis shortening 3 per cent). Arrows outline a small area of muscle loss comprising less than 10 per cent of the total volume with replacement by a micro-infarct with moderately early organization. Hematoxylin and eosin stain; original magnification ×125, reduced by 33 per cent.*

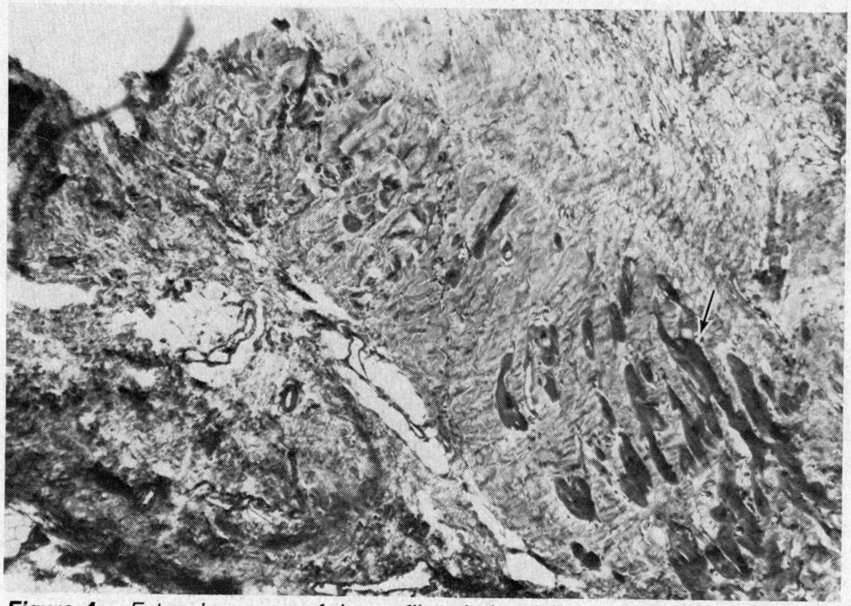

Figure 4. *Extensive areas of dense fibrosis involving over 75 per cent of the specimen (apical aneurysmectomy) with only widely scattered areas of muscle still present (arrow). No inflammatory cells are seen. Masson-trichrome stain; original magnification × 125, reduced by 33 per cent.*

and local Q waves in six. In contrast, in five of six dyskinetic segments, there were either local Q waves or no electrical activity over the sites recorded (Figure 6).

A transitional zone consisting of abnormal but smaller Q waves could be demonstrated adjacent to a fibrotic aneurysm (Figure 7). However, no such intermediate area could be demonstrated in the absence of frank fibrotic tissue.

Ventriculographic-electrographic-histopathologic correlation. Histopathologic specimens were available from 20 electrographic sites (recorded prior to biopsy) in 16 patients.

Initial R waves were associated with normal biopsy specimens in seven of eight hypokinetic areas. In one area with electrographic evidence of a Q wave in two thirds of the leads, only small foci of structural damage were found which resulted in less than 10 per cent muscle loss.

In three of the seven akinetic zones, initial R waves were present in all recordings with 30 to 35 per cent muscle loss in the corresponding biopsy specimens. In contrast, in four segments with an initial Q wave, there was more than a 75 per cent muscle loss in one, more than a 50 per cent loss in two and a 35 per cent muscle loss in one.

In four of the five dyskinetic zones, there was a QS pattern and more than 75 per cent fibrosis. In one dyskinetic area, there was an initial R wave in association with no significant degree of muscle loss.

COMMENTS

The present study indicates that there is a good over-all correlation between ventriculographically depicted segmental contraction and the amount of muscle loss as determined histopathologically. The histopathologic appearance of both normally contracting and hypokinetic segments is normal. In contrast, as shown in Table I, in the more severe forms of asynergy (akinesis and dyskinesis) muscle destruction and replacement by fibrotic tissue are increased. However, it is of considerable interest that significant asynergy, including akinetic or even frankly dyskinetic segments, is also quite compatible with the presence of structurally intact myocardium (Table I). This suggests that the asynergy in such areas depicted ventriculographically is secondary to ischemia and not frank muscle destruction [17]. Thus, potentially, if this ischemia were alleviated, the structurally intact myocardium might show improved contraction.

Local electrograms have been of considerable value in demarcating areas of transmural infarction [7,8,14,15,18], and data obtained in man have confirmed that a QS complex is recorded over fibrotic aneurysmal areas [7,8]. However, it has been shown in experimental studies that a pathologic Q wave can also be seen over areas containing structurally intact myocardium [7,18]. This is consistent with our observations in man that electrograms demonstrating Q waves may be associated with only partially fibrotic myocardium (Table II). In addition, the electrogram recordings from

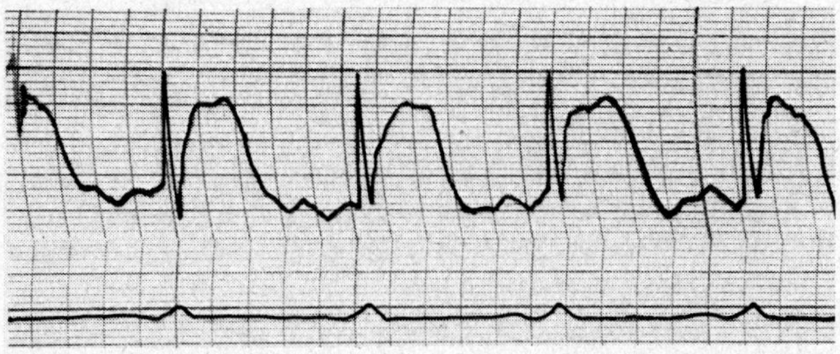

Figure 5. *Epicardial unipolar recording (upper trace) demonstrates initial R wave over a hypokinetic area (hemiaxis shortening 15 per cent). Bottom trace is lead II of the electrocardiogram. Recording speed 25 mm/sec.*

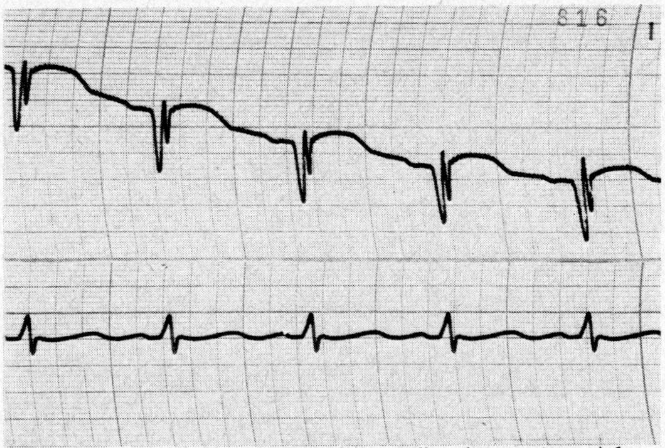

Figure 6. *Unipolar epicardial recording (upper trace) from a dyskinetic area (hemiaxis shortening 4 per cent). An initial wide Q wave (0.05 sec) is seen. Recording speed 50 mm/sec.*

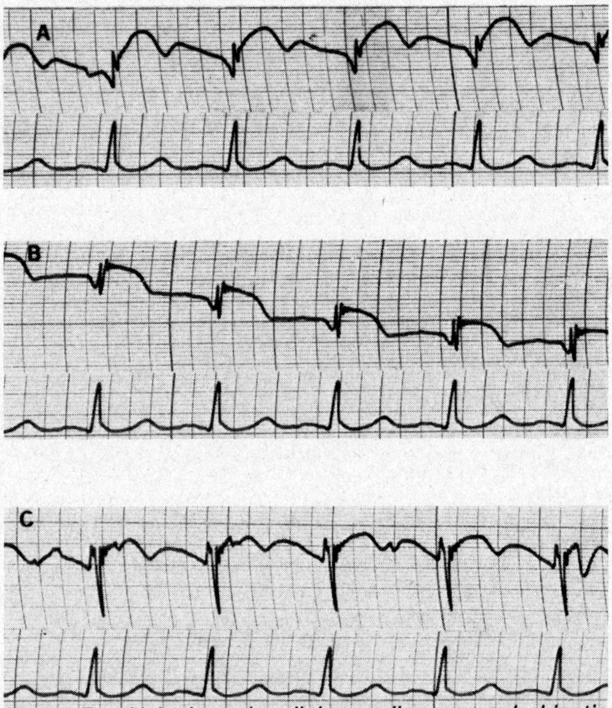

Figure 7. *Unipolar epicardial recording over a dyskinetic fibrotic area at the apex (A) reveals an initial Q wave of 0.05 sec. As the electrode is moved laterally, the Q wave is seen to decrease to 0.03 sec (B) (transitional zone) and to disappear entirely with an initial R wave 1 cm lateral to the scar (C). Recording speed 50 mm/sec. In each panel, upper trace is the epicardial electrogram, and the lower trace is lead II of the standard electrocardiogram.*

such a site appear homogeneous without evidence of a transitional area. Thus, local electrograms appear to detect the presence of fibrotic tissue but are unable to provide consistent quantification.

A biopsy technic provides a relatively small amount of tissue, raising the possibility of sampling error. For this reason, discrete, easily demarcated ventriculographic zones of the left ventricle were chosen for analysis. Therefore, the lateral wall of the left ventricle, which is difficult to visualize in the right anterior oblique view, and the proximal areas of the anterior wall, with its high vascularity interfering with the biopsy technic, were excluded. Moreover, care was taken to obtain the biopsy specimen from a site from which electrograms had been previously recorded. This should have minimized, to the extent possible, the potential error of sampling site and should have permitted a relatively accurate correlation of ventriculographic, electrographic and histopathologic data in living patients to be made.

In conclusion, the severity of asynergy as depicted by ventriculography correlates well with the degree of myocardial loss and, to a lesser extent, with the presence or absence of a Q wave on the local electrogram. However, even in the presence of more severe forms of asynergy (akinesis and dyskinesis), a significant amount of histologically normal myocardium remains. Thus, significant asynergy depicted ventriculographically may occasionally be associated with histologically and electrographically normal myocardium.

ACKNOWLEDGMENT

We wish to thank Ms. Marlene Fauerbach, Ms. Sandy Hicks, Ms. Janice Phillips and Mr. Joseph Lewandowski for their technical assistance.

REFERENCES

1. Bruschke AVG, Proudfit WL, Sones FM: Progress study of 590 consecutive nonsurgical cases of coronary disease followed 5–9 years. II. Ventriculographic and other correlations. Circulation 47: 1154, 1973.
2. Burgraff GW, Parker JO: Prognosis in coronary artery disease. Angiographic, hemodynamic and clinical factors. Circulation 51: 146, 1975.
3. Spencer FC, Green GE, Tice DA, et al.: Coronary artery bypass grafts for congestive heart failure. J Thorac Cardiovasc Surg 62:529, 1971.

4. Manley JC, Johnson WD: Effects of surgery on angina (pre- and post-infarction) and myocardial function (failure). Circulation 46: 1208, 1972.
5. Kouchoukos NT, Kirklin JW, Oberman A: An appraisal of coronary bypass grafting. Circulation 50: 11, 1974.
6. Herman MV, Heinle RA, Klein MD, et al.: Localized disorders in myocardial contraction. Asynergy and its role in congestive heart failure. N Engl J Med 277: 222, 1967.
7. Kaiser GA, Waldo AL, Harris PD, et al.: New method to delineate myocardial damage at surgery. Circulation 39 (suppl): I, 1969.
8. Kaiser GA, Waldo AL, Bowman FO, et al.: The use of ventricular electrograms in operation for coronary artery disease and its complications. Ann Thorac Surg 10: 153, 1970.
9. Sutton GC, Driscoll JF, Gunnar RM, et al.: Exploratory mediastinotomy in primary myocardial disease. Progr Cardiovasc Dis 7: 83, 1964.
10. Bjork VO, Hultquist G: Left ventricular biopsy for evaluation of the myocardium before and after perfusion. Ann Surg 163: 179, 1966.
11. Helfant RH, Pine R, Meister SG, et al.: Nitroglycerin to unmask reversible asynergy. Correlation with post-coronary bypass ventriculography. Circulation 50: 108, 1974.
12. Banka VS, Bodenheimer MM, Helfant RH: Determinations of reversible asynergy. Effect of pathologic Q waves, coronary collaterals, and anatomic location. Circulation 50: 714, 1974.
13. Roos JP, Van Dam R, Durrer D: Epicardial and intramural excitation of normal heart in six patients 50 years of age and over. Br Heart J 30: 630, 1968.
14. Daniel TM, Boineau JP, Sabiston DC: Comparison of human ventricular activation with a canine model in chronic myocardial infarction. Circulation 44: 74, 1971.
15. Daniel TM, Boineau JP, Cox JL, et al.: Mapping of epicardial and intramural activation of the heart. J Thorac Cardiovasc Surg 60: 704, 1970.
16. Mallory GK, White PD, Salcedo-Salgar J: The speed of healing of myocardial infarction. A study of the pathologic anatomy in seventy-two cases. Am Heart J 18: 647, 1939.
17. Sonnenblick EH, Gorlin R: Reversible and irreversible depression of ischemic myocardium. N Engl J Med 286: 1154, 1972.
18. Durrer D, Van Lier AAW, Buller J: Epicardial and intramural excitation in chronic myocardial infarction. Am Heart J 68: 765, 1964.

Pulmonary Hypertension and Foreign Body Granulomas in Intravenous Drug Abusers

Documentation by Cardiac Catheterization and Lung Biopsy

CHARLES H. ROBERTSON, Jr., M.D.*
ROLLAND C. REYNOLDS, M.D.
JAMES E. WILSON, III, M.D.
Dallas, Texas

In this report we confirm the presence of pulmonary hypertension by cardiac catheterization in four intravenous drug abusers with biopsy-documented foreign body granulomas in the pulmonary vessels and interstitium. Each patient had a history of intravenous injections of alpha-sympathomimetic agents obtained from nasal inhalers. These agents may have contributed to the disease by constricting small vessels when simultaneously injected foreign bodies were passing through the vasculature of the lung. The severity of the pulmonary hypertension correlated well with the decrease in single breath diffusing capacity in each case. Pulmonary hypertension may contribute significantly to the increased morbidity and mortality observed in intravenous drug users.

A recently recognized pulmonary complication of intravenous drug abusers is a vascular and interstitial granulomatous response to the foreign bodies injected with psychotropic agents: talc [1–19] and starch [3–5,14,17] from diluents of heroin and from pulverized tablets, cotton used for filtering illicit solutions [8,20,21] or unknown substances [22–26]. Pulmonary hypertension has been suspected on pathologic [6,9,10,12,15,16,23], roentgenographic [2,14,22] or physical findings [2,11,22,23] in such patients. However, in no report has pulmonary hypertension, documented by cardiac catheterization, been correlated with these clinical and pathologic features. In this communication we describe four intravenous drug abusers in whom catheterization data and lung biopsy studies allowed such correlation.

METHODS

A rolling-seal waterless spirometer was utilized for measuring forced expiratory volumes and flows. Normal prediction values for spirometry are those of Morris et al. [27] with values reduced by 15 per cent for black males [28].

Total lung capacity was obtained by adding inspiratory capacity to functional residual capacity determined in a volume displacement body plethysmograph [29]. Normal values were obtained by multiplying predicted forced vital capacity by a factor related to age [30]. Airway resistance was obtained in the plethysmograph utilizing the protractor developed by Comroe et al. [31].

Diffusing capacity was determined by the single breath carbon monoxide method [32]. Prediction values are pooled data from five sources [33–37].

From the Pauline and Adolph Weinberger Laboratory for Cardiopulmonary Research, Departments of Internal Medicine and Pathology, University of Texas Health Science Center at Dallas, Dallas, Texas 75235. This study was supported in part by a grant (HL14187) from the National Heart and Lung Institute, National Institutes of Health. Request for reprints should be addressed to Dr. Charles H. Robertson, Jr., Pulmonary Division, University of Texas Health Science Center, 5323 Harry Hines Blvd., Dallas, Texas 75235. Manuscript accepted March 19, 1976.

$$D_{L_{CO}} = 1.068\ Ht - 0.249\ age - 35.5$$

where Ht = height in inches

$$\frac{D_{L_{CO}}\ (STPD)}{V_A\ (BTPS)} = 6.63 - 0.05\ age$$

Pulmonary angiograms were performed with pressure injection of Renografin® 76, 1 ml/kg up to a maximum of 70 ml through a No. 7 or 8 NIH or Eppendorf catheter with the tip in the main pulmonary artery. A Shonander rapid film changer was used, taking 3 frames per second for 3 seconds during the expected arterial filling phase.

Pathologic specimens were fixed in 4 per cent buffered formalin, dehydrated and embedded in parafin. Sectioned tissues were stained with hematoxalin and eosin, and reviewed by transmission and polarized light microscopy.

CASE REPORTS

Case 1. A 33 year old woman was admitted to the hospital because of progressively increasing dyspnea on exertion, edema and orthopnea of one year's duration. She related a four year habit of injecting, intravenously, the liquid squeezed from the cotton pledget of mephenteramine nasal inhalers. There were numerous injection marks on both arms, an increased right ventricular pulsation with a loud pulmonic sound, a grade 3/6 holosystolic murmur heard best at the lower left sternal border, tender hepatomegaly 2 cm below the right costal margin and moderate peripheral edema. The lungs were clear to auscultation. Electrocardiographic interpretation was right atrial overload with right ventricular hypertrophy and strain. A chest film was compatible with pulmonary hypertension and right ventricular failure, but there was no interstitial infiltrate. Macroaggregated albumin lung scan showed patchy defects more severe in the superior segment of the lower lobe of the left lung. Serologic tests were not suggestive of connective tissue disease. Bed rest and thiazide diuretic administration resulted in a 22 pound weight loss prior to the time of right heart catheterization which documented the severe pulmonary hypertension and persistent right ventricular failure without shunts. Angiography revealed large central pulmonary arteries with poor fine branching and, in the lower lobe of the left lung, two filling defects in arteries too small ($<$1.5 mm diameter) to allow definitive interpretation. Pulmonary function tests showed well preserved vital capacity and flows, a markedly decreased diffusing capacity and hypoxemia at rest out of proportion to a small increase in the right to left shunting. Open lung biopsy disclosed class III pulmonary hypertension [38] and interstitial fibrosis greatest around arterioles, some of which were completely obliterated (Figure 1). Focal collections of hemosiderin-laden macrophages were present in the alveolar spaces. No granulomas or foreign bodies were seen.

This patient was lost to follow-up shortly after discharge from the hospital. She returned approximately three years later and died within 1 hour of staphylococcal sepsis from multiple cutaneous abscesses. At autopsy the lungs demonstrated class II pulmonary hypertension and less interstitial fibrosis than was evident on the previous biopsy specimen. There were birefringent foreign bodies with granuloma formation in moderate amounts in the interstitial space.

Case 2. This 30 year old woman presented with a one year history of progressive breathlessness, orthopnea, edema and syncopal episodes with exercise or Valsalva maneuvers. She was essentially bedridden prior to seeking medical assistance. She related intermittent intravenous use over two years of the liquid squeezed from the cotton pledget of mephenteramine nasal inhalers. She denied the use of other intravenous drugs. Examination showed a prominent right ventricular heave, an increased pulmonic sound, a pulmonary ejection click and a grade 5/6 murmur of tricuspid insufficiency (confirmed by intracardiac phonocardiography). There was neck vein distention 4 cm above the suprasternal notch, and peripheral edema was present. There were multiple injection sites. The lungs were clear to auscultation. Chest roentgenograms showed pulmonary hypertension, right ventricular enlargement and no interstitial infiltrate. The electrocardiogram was consistent with right ventricular strain and biatrial overload. An echocardiogram was not consistent with mitral stenosis or myxoma. Serologic tests were not suggestive of connective tissue disease. A macroaggregated albumin lung scan was normal. The patient underwent diuresis and digitalization with resolution of clinical right ventricular decompensation. Results of pulmonary function tests were compatible with a restrictive ventilatory defect with normal flow rates and airways resistance (predicted 1.2 to 4.3 cm H_2O/liter/sec). Diffusing capacity was significantly decreased out of proportion to the decrease in lung volumes, and slight hypoxemia was present at rest. Right heart catheterization disclosed moderate pulmonary hypertension without failure and no shunts. An angiogram confirmed large central arteries, but the fine branching was intact. Open lung biopsy demonstrated class II pulmonary hypertension with very little interstitial fibrosis and many pericapillary interstitial granulomas containing birefringent foreign bodies and giant cells. There were a moderate number of alveolar macrophages, some with hemosiderin, in these areas of granulomas. In approximately six months of outpatient follow-up she has abstained from further injections, but there have been no changes in pulmonary function.

Case 3. This 26 year old man was admitted to the hospital with a three month history of dyspnea on exertion. He related a four to five year habit of giving himself intravenous injections of ground amphetamine capsules and the liquid squeezed from the cotton pledget of propylhexedrine nasal inhalers. No history of occupational or environmental exposure to noxious materials was uncovered. One week before his admission he had a syncopal episode. Physical examination disclosed a right ventricular heave, palpable pulmonic closure, a grade 2/6 brief systolic murmur at the lower sternal border, which increased on inspiration, and a loud pulmonic sound. Needle tracks were present. There was no edema or hepatomegaly, and the lungs were clear to auscultation. The electrocardiographic interpretation was right ventricular strain. A chest film was compatible with pulmonary hypertension and right ventricular enlargement without failure (Figure 2). There was no interstitial infiltrate. Serologic tests were not suggestive of connective tissue disease. Pulmonary function tests revealed normal vital capacity and flow rates with a significantly decreased diffusing capacity. Moderate hypoxemia was present at rest out of proportion to a mild

1

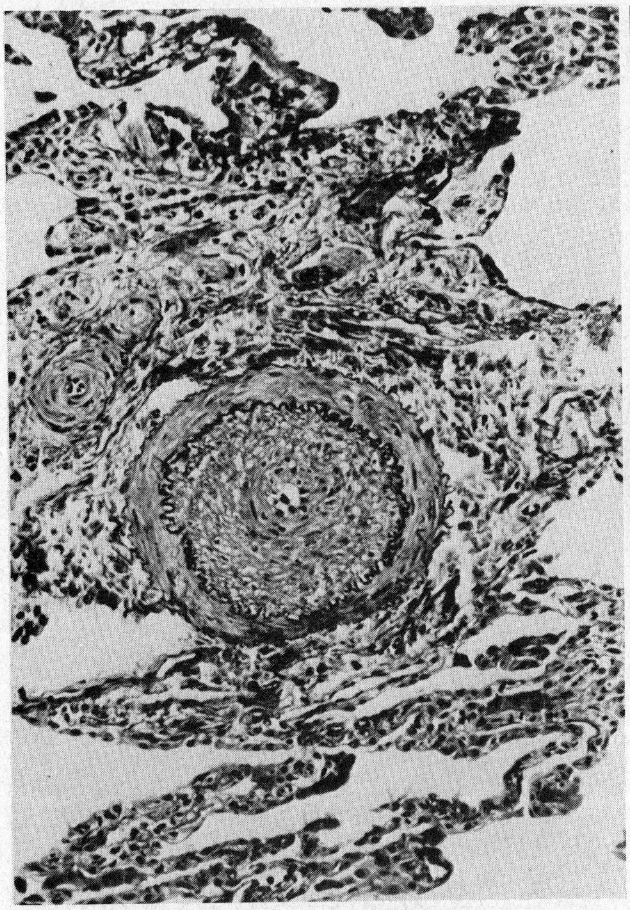

2

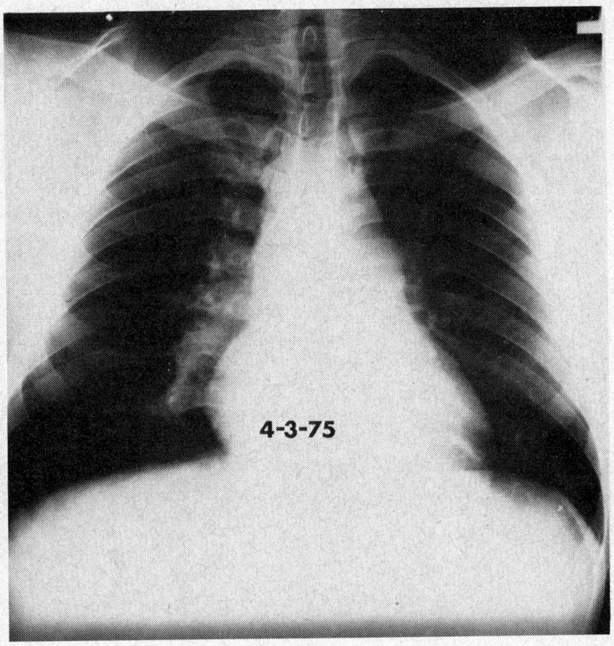

Figure 1. *Histologic section from a patient (Case 1) showing class III pulmonary hypertension with muscular hypertrophy and fibrous intimal proliferation. Just above and left of the larger pulmonary artery are several arterioles in various stages of obliteration.*

Figure 2. *Chest film from a patient (Case 3) illustrating enlarged main pulmonary artery and hilar arteries but normal peripheral vessels and no fibrosis.*

A

B

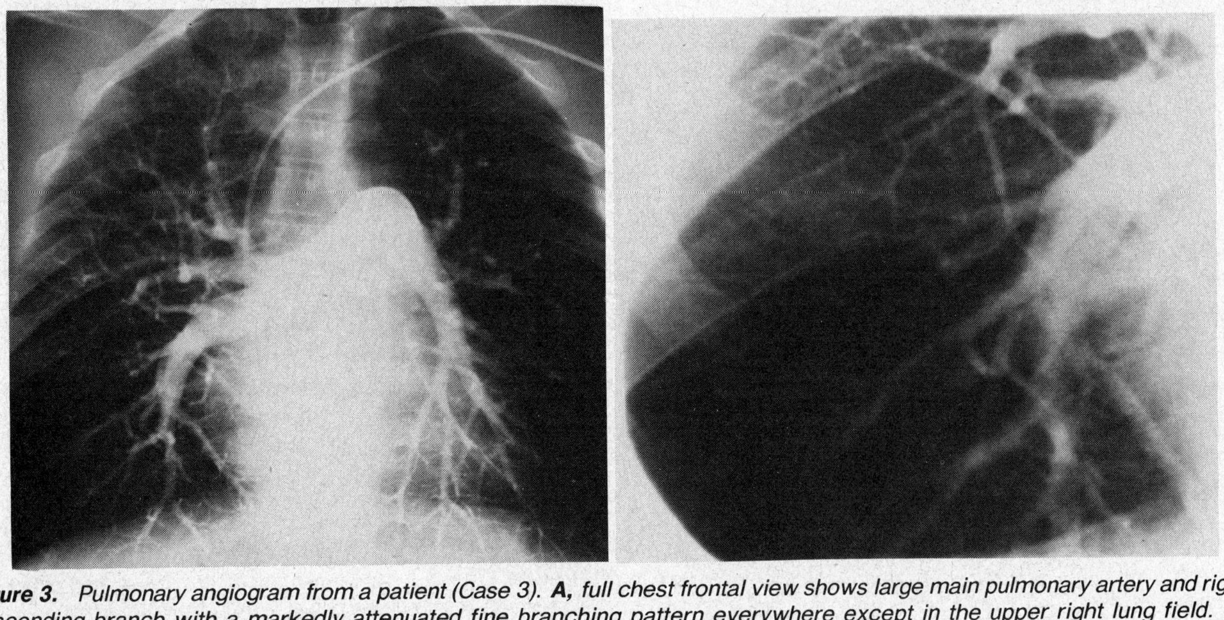

Figure 3. *Pulmonary angiogram from a patient (Case 3).* ***A,*** *full chest frontal view shows large main pulmonary artery and right descending branch with a markedly attenuated fine branching pattern everywhere except in the upper right lung field.* ***B,*** *cone-down view of the lower right lung field to emphasize the loss of fine branching compared to the upper zone just at top edge of the view.*

A

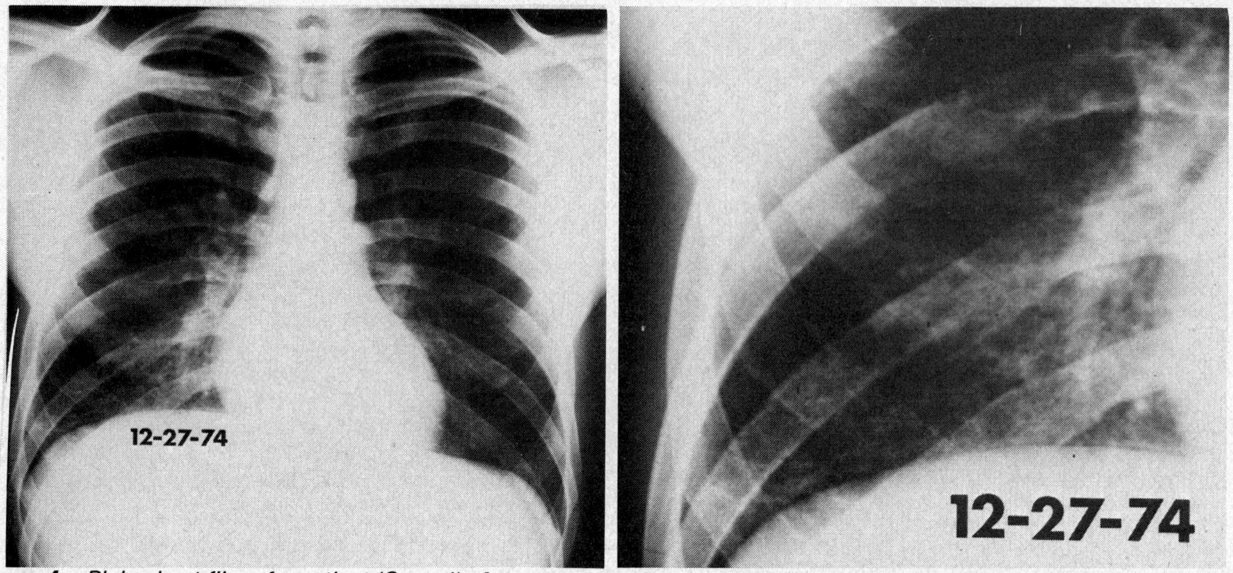

B

Figure 4. *Plain chest film of a patient (Case 4).* ***A,*** *posteroanterior view discloses normal pulmonary arteries with bibasilar interstitial pattern.* ***B,*** *close-up view of lower right lung field displays diffuse fine reticular pattern more clearly.*

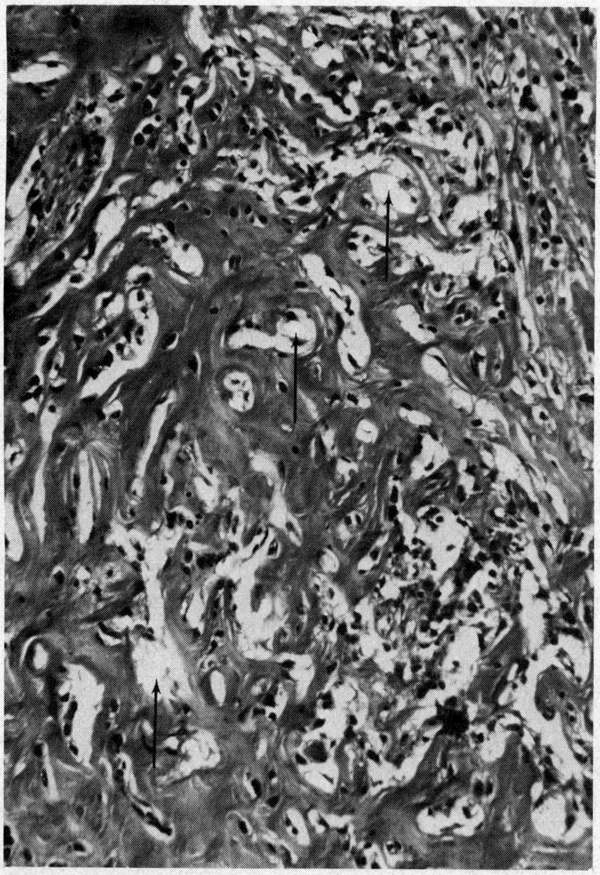

Figure 5. *Histologic section from open lung biopsy specimen obtained from lower lobe of right lung of a patient (Case 4). There is a dense fibrosis with many birefringent foreign bodies which show as white clefts on this reproduction (see* ***arrows****).*

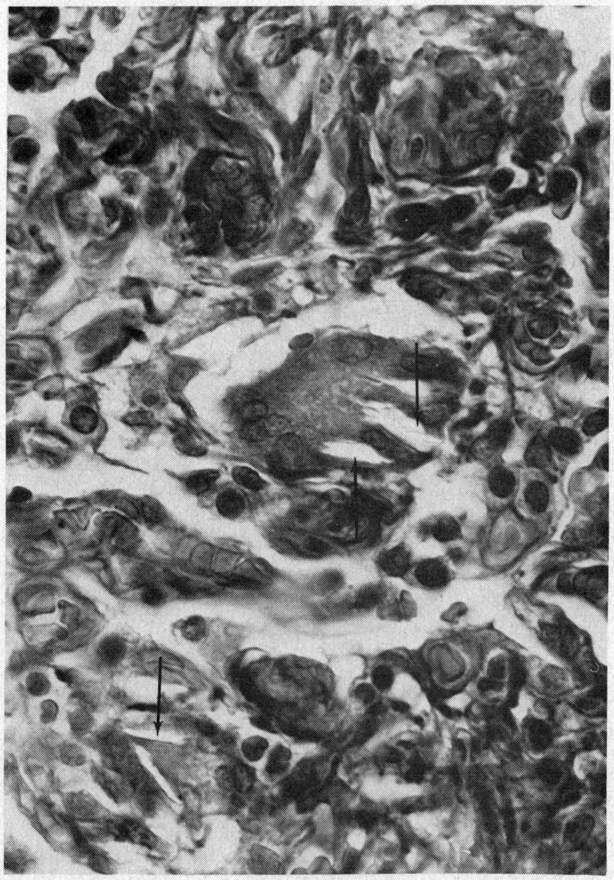

Figure 6. *Another area from the biopsy specimen (Case 4) shows one of the granulomas with giant cell formation surrounding birefringent foreign bodies* ***(arrows).***

increase in right to left shunt. Cardiac catheterization demonstrated modest pulmonary hypertension without shunts. An angiogram showed pulmonary artery enlargement with a dramatic diminution of fine branching except in the upper lobe of the right lung (Figure 3). A transbronchial lung biopsy specimen showed an arteriole with obliterated lumen containing birefringent particles and a modest generalized interstitial fibrosis. The small biopsy specimen did not include enough vessels to assess changes of pulmonary hypertension. There was a moderate number of hemosiderin-laden macrophages.

Case 4. This 28 year old man had been seen intermittently for cellulitis of his arms due to injections and for an overdose of intravenous barbiturate. He was admitted again with a one year history of progressive dyspnea on exertion, nonproductive cough and occasional hemoptysis. He related intravenous injection of barbiturate capsule contents, pulverized amphetamine tablets, heroin and liquid squeezed from the cotton pledget of mephenteramine nasal inhalers. There was no occupational or environmental exposure to dusts or organic materials. Examination disclosed diffuse dry end-inspiratory rales. The pulmonic component was louder than the aortic component of the second heart sound. There were no murmurs, edema or hepatomegaly. An electrocardiogram was interpreted as normal. Serologic test results were not suggestive of connective tissue disease. A chest film showed a bibasilar interstitial infiltrate without hypertensive changes in pulmonary vasculature, and the heart size was within normal limits (Figure 4). Pulmonary function tests disclosed a moderate restrictive ventilatory defect, with diffusing capacity decreased only slightly more than would be expected from the decrease in lung volumes. Minimal arterial hypoxemia was present at rest. A limited right heart catheterization disclosed a slightly increased mean pulmonary artery pressure and no shunts. Angiography was normal. An open lung biopsy specimen from the lower lobe of the right lung showed class I pulmonary hypertension with dramatic interstitial fibrosis (Figure 5) and an equally impressive amount of birefringent foreign material in the fibrosis with surrounding granulomas with giant cell formation (Figure 6).

This patient has been followed for six months as an outpatient, with progressive symptoms while continuing his intravenous drug use. His diffusing capacity has remained unchanged at 12.09 ml/min/mm Hg, after an initial decrease associated with the lung biopsy and a complicating empyema. After obtaining informed consent, a two month experimental trial of high dose oral prednisolone (60 mg/day) was undertaken; there was no improvement in diffusing capacity, vital capacity or symptoms.

COMMENTS

Three other cases have been reported in which cardiac catheterizations were performed on similar patients. In one, pulmonary artery pressures were normal [11].

TABLE I Summary of Physiologic Data

	Case 1	Case 2	Case 3	Case 4
Pulmonary Function Tests				
TLC (liters)	4.00 (96)	3.38 (79)	...	4.24 (76)
FVC (liters)	3.32 (100)	2.25 (65)	4.56 (99)	2.65 (59)
$FEV_{1.0}$ (liters/sec)	2.73 (98)	2.00 (73)	3.54 (90)	2.26 (63)
R_{aw} (cm H_2O/liter/sec)	0.7	2.3	...	...
$D_{L_{CO}}$ (SB) (ml/min/mm Hg)	4.24 (18)	9.02 (41)	12.85 (40)	16.00 (51)
$D_{L_{CO}}$: Va (ml/min/mm Hg/liter)	1.09 (22)	2.85 (56)	2.60 (49)	4.17 (80)
Qs:Qt (%)	6.1	5.2	7.9	...
pH_a	7.43	7.45	7.42	7.45
$PaCO_2$ (mm Hg)	32	38	39	38
PaO_2 (mm Hg)	62	70	70	78
SaO_2 (%)	93	94	94	97
Cardiac Catheterization				
Pressures (mm Hg)				
RA (mean)	7.5	2.5	3	...
RV (systolic/diastolic)	90/13	65/5	40/3	...
PA (systolic/diastolic/mean)	95/35/55	65/30/45	40/22/30	22 (mean)
Wedge (mean)	8.0	1	5	...
BA (systolic/diastolic/mean)	150/70/100	160/90/100	110/84/93	130/90/103
Cardiac output (liters/min)	4.1	3.9	5.2	...
Cardiac index (liters/min/m²)	2.4	2.4	2.4	...
PVR (dyne sec cm^{-5})	920	882	386	...
$C_aO_2 - C_{\bar{v}}O_2$ (ml O_2/100 ml)	5.0	5.0	...	4.3
Oxygen content step-up	No	No	No	...
SVC dye curve	No shunt	No shunt	No shunt	No shunt

NOTE: TLC = total lung capacity; FVC = forced vital capacity; $FEV_{1.0}$ = 1 second forced expiratory volume; R_{aw} = airway resistance; $D_{L_{CO}}$ (SB) = diffusing capacity for carbon monoxide by the single breath method; $D_{L_{CO}}$:Va = ratio of diffusing capacity to alveolar volume; Qs:Qt = per cent of total cardiac output that is shunted right to left, bypassing the lungs; pH_a = arterial pH; PaO_2 = arterial oxygen tension; $PaCO_2$ = arterial carbon dioxide tension; SaO_2 = per cent of arterial hemoglobin that is saturated with oxygen; RA = right atrium; RV = right ventricle; PA = pulmonary artery; BA = brachial artery; PVR = pulmonary vascular resistance; $C_aO_2 - C\bar{v}O_2$ = difference in oxygen content between arterial blood and mixed venous blood; SVC = superior vena cava. Numbers in parentheses indicate per cent of predicted.

TABLE II Summary of Pathologic Data

	Case 1		Case 2	Case 3	Case 4
	Open Biopsy	Autopsy	Open Biopsy	Transbronchial Biopsy	Open Biopsy
Pulmonary hypertension class	III	II	II		I
Interstitial fibrosis	2+	1+	1+	2+	4+
Foreign bodies	0	2+	3+	1+	4+
Granulomas	0	1+	3+	0	2+
Macrophages with hemosiderin	2+	2+	2+	2+	3+

In two patients, pulmonary hypertension was present; but in one, coexisting chronic obstructive lung disease may have contributed to this finding [19], and in the other, pressure measurements were not reported [2]. Our patients with this syndrome had pulmonary hypertension at cardiac catheterization without any other recognizable etiology (Table I). In two, it was severe enough to induce cor pulmonale.

All of our patients had foreign bodies consistent with talc in their lungs (Table II) and a history of injection of alpha sympathomimetic agents obtained from nasal inhalers, which may have induced pulmonary arteriolar constriction at times when simultaneously injected foreign bodies were in the pulmonary vessels [39]. Venous injections of talc [5], cotton fibers [20,40,41] and starch [5,17], which might be present in the materials injected by drug abusers, induce pulmonary granulomas in animals; starch causes a mild, transient reaction [5,17] whereas the other materials are poorly degraded and produce a permanent lesion. Injection of totally inert materials, such as plastic spherules, induces a pulmonary hypertension which resolves quickly [42], whereas carborundum particles that induce a granulomatous response cause an increase in pulmonary arterial pressure which resolves slowly over months [43]. These animal studies support growing evidence that intravenous injection of foreign bodies by drug abusers may induce the pathologic [6,9,10,12,15,16,23], roentgenographic [2,14,22], clinical [2,11,22,23] and hemodynamic (this report) changes of pulmonary hypertension.

Two patients (Case 1 and 3) also showed a marked paucity of fine branching on angiograms (Figure 3 and Table III). This probably relates to the major site of granulomatous reaction, since the two patients with this finding had a significant number of arterioles with obliterated lumens on biopsy (Figure 1 and Table II) whereas the other two had more of a reaction at the alveolar capillary level. In one patient (Case 1) involvement of small vessels (<1.5 mm) was visible on angiogram as vascular cutoffs and avascular areas. This patient also had an abnormal lung scan. Another patient (Case 2) had a normal perfusion lung scan despite a low diffusing capacity, which is unusual in the experience of Soin [26].

Roentgenographic changes suggesting pulmonary hypertension or cardiomegaly were present in three of our patients, but they were not present in the patient with the smallest increase in pulmonary artery pressure (Table III). Only the patient with very marked histologic interstitial fibrosis (Figure 5) had an interstitial infiltrate on chest films (Figure 4). The lung scan was abnormal in only one of the two patients in whom it was performed. A restrictive ventilatory defect was present in only two patients. Conversely, all patients had decreases in the diffusing capacity as measured by the single breath carbon monoxide method. Moreover, the

TABLE III Summary of Roentgenographic Data

	Case 1	Case 2	Case 3	Case 4
Plain Chest Film (posteroanterior + lateral)				
Pulmonary hyptertension				
Main pulmonary artery enlarged	+	+	+	−
Hilar size increased	−	±	+	−
Peripheral vasculature decreased	−	−	−	−
Interstitial pattern	−	−	−	+
Cardiomegaly	+	+	+	−
Cardiothoracic ratio	17:30	13.6:25.0	16.8:33.8	13.2:30.0
Anterior space obliterated	±	+	+	−
Azygous vein enlarged	+	−	−	−
Pulmonary Angiography				
Main pulmonary artery size	Large	Slightly large	Large	Normal
Right descending branch (mm)	17	14	18	11
Fine branching	Poor	Good	Poor	Good
Cutoffs and filling defects	Left lower lobe (<1.5 mm artery)	None	None	None
Avascular areas	Few	None	None	None
Delayed venous phase	None	None	None	None

degree of decrease in diffusing capacity correlated well ($R = 0.99$, $P < 0.003$) with the mean pulmonary artery pressure (Figure 7) and apparently with the pulmonary vascular resistance in these few cases. Similar correlations between pulmonary vascular resistance and diffusing capacity have been reported for two other diseases in which pulmonary hypertension occurs: sarcoidosis [44] and recurrent pulmonary thromboembolism [45]. The poor correlation between vital capacity and diffusing capacity, and between interstitial fibrosis and pulmonary hypertension argue that the interstitial fibrosis and vascular obstruction are independent responses in these patients and that the pulmonary hypertension and reduction in diffusing capacity are mainly due to pulmonary vascular obstruction rather than pulmonary fibrosis. Thus, diffusing capacity might be the best screening test for pulmonary hypertension in intravenous drug abusers. Two previous studies [13,25] have noted a decrease in diffusing capacity in these patients, although it was not correlated with the degree of pulmonary hypertension.

Finally, many of the drugs injected by addicts have significant vasodilatory properties which could reduce right ventricular filling pressure enough to be catastrophic to cardiac output in the setting of a high pulmonary vascular resistance. Shock and sudden death would ensue. Indeed, granulomas were seen in 15 per cent of a series of autopsies performed on patients in whom sudden death occurred [16]. Thus, pulmonary hypertension may explain a significant incidence of sudden death in drug addicts.

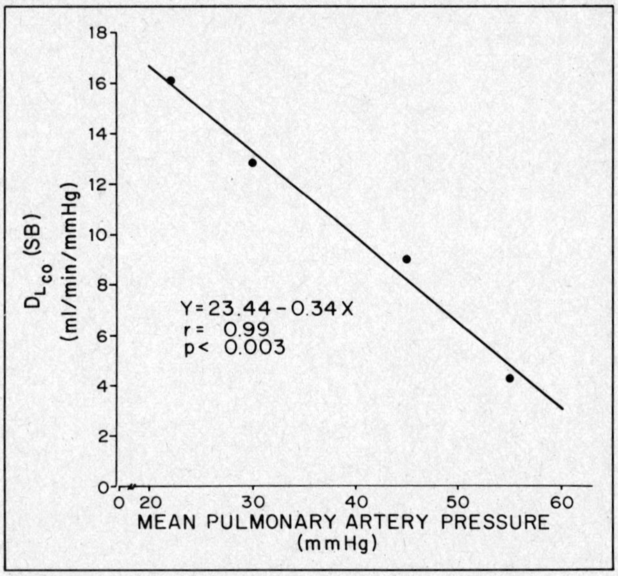

Figure 7. *Relationship between single breath diffusing capacity of carbon monoxide [$D_{L_{CO}}$ (SB)] and mean pulmonary artery pressure at rest.*

REFERENCES

1. Krainer L, Berman E, Wishnick SD: Parenteral talcum granulomatosis: complication of narcotic addiction (abstract). Lab Invest 11: 671, 1962.
2. Wendt VE, Puro HE, Shapiro J, et al.: Angiothrombotic pulmonary hypertension in addicts: "blue velvet" addition. JAMA 188: 755, 1964.
3. Burton JF, Zawadzki ES, Wetherell HR, et al.: Mainliners and blue velvet. J. Forensic Sci 10: 466, 1965.
4. Lerner AM, Oerther FJ: Characteristics and sequellae of paregoric abuse. Ann Intern Med 65: 1019, 1966.
5. Puro HE, Wolf PL, Skirgaudas J, et al.: Experimental production of human "blue velvet" and "red devil" lesions. JAMA 197: 1100, 1966.
6. Butz WC: Pulmonary arteriole foreign body granulomata associated with angiomatoids resulting from the intravenous injection of oral medications. J Forensic Sci 14: 317, 1969.
7. Hahn HH, Schweid AI, Beaty HN: Complications of injecting dissolved methylphenidate tablets. Arch Intern Med 123: 656, 1969.
8. Johnston EH, Goldbaum LR, Whelton RL: Investigation of sudden death in addicts. Med Ann DC 38: 375, 1969.
9. Bainborough AR, Jericho KWF: Cor pulmonale secondary to talc granulomata in the lungs of a drug addict. Can Med Assoc J 103: 1297, 1970.
10. Hopkins GB, Taylor DG: Pulmonary talc granulomatosis. Am Rev Respir Dis 101: 101, 1970.
11. Szwed JJ: Pulmonary angiothrombosis caused by "blue velvet" addiction. Ann Intern Med 73: 771, 1970.
12. Zientara M, Moore S: Fatal talc embolism in a drug addict. Human Pathol 1: 324, 1970.
13. Douglas FG, Kafilmont KJ, Patt NL: Foreign particle embolism in drug addicts: respiratory pathophysiology. Ann Intern Med 75: 865, 1971.
14. Atlee WE: Talc and cornstarch emboli in eyes of drug abusers. JAMA 219: 49, 1972.
15. Groth DH, Mackay GR, Crable JV, et al.: Intravenous injection of talc in a narcotics addict. Arch Pathol 94: 171, 1972.
16. Hopkins GB: Pulmonary angiothrombotic granulomatosis in drug offenders. JAMA 221: 909, 1972.
17. Lamb D, Roberts G: Starch and talc emboli in drug addicts' lungs. J Clin Pathol 25: 876, 1962.
18. Gross EM: Talc embolism: sudden death following intravenous injection of phenyltoloxamine. Forensic Sci 2: 475, 1973.
19. Vevaina JR, Civantos F, Viamonte M, et al.: Emphysema associated with talcum granulomatosis in a drug addict. South Med J 67: 113, 1974.
20. Von Glahn WC, Hall JW: The reaction produced in the pulmonary arteries by emboli of cotton fibers. Am J Pathol 25: 573, 1949.
21. Ortuno G, Vazquez JJ: Intraarterial granulomas due to lung embolization of cotton fibers. Zentralbl Chir 41: 2671, 1967.
22. Jaffe RB, Koschmann EG: Intravenous drug abuse. Am J Roentgenol Radium Ther Nucl Med 109: 107, 1970.
23. Spain DM: Patterns of pulmonary fibrosis as related to pulmonary function. Ann Intern Med 33: 1150, 1950.
24. Soin JS, McKusick KA, Wagner HN: Regional lung-function abnormalities in narcotic addicts. JAMA 244: 1717, 1973.
25. Camargo G, Culp C: Pulmonary function studies in ex-heroin users. Chest 67: 331, 1975.
26. Soin JS, Wagner HN, Thomashaw D, et al.: Increased sensi-

tivity of regional measurements in early detection of narcotic lung disease. Chest 67: 325, 1975.
27. Morris JF, Koshi A, Johnson LC: Spirometric standards for healthy nonsmoking adults. Am Rev Respir Dis 103: 57, 1971.
28. Oscherwitz M, Eldavich SA, Baker TR, et al.: Differences in pulmonary functions in various racial groups. J Epidemiol 96: 319, 1972.
29. Mead J: Volume displacement body plethysmograph for respiratory measurements in human subjects. J Appl Physiol 19: 813, 1964.
30. Fowler WS: Specific tests of lung function: lung volumes. Methods in Medical Research (Comroe J, ed), Chicago, Yearbook Publishers, 1960, p 197.
31. Comroe JH Jr, Botelho SY, Dubois AB: Design of a body plethysmograph for studying cardiopulmonary physiology. J Appl Physiol 14: 439, 1959.
32. Ogilvie CM, Forster RE, Blakemore WS, et al.: A standardized breath holding technique for clinical measurement of the diffusing capacity of the lung for carbon monoxide. J Clin Invest 36: 1, 1957.
33. Hamer NAJ: Variations in the components of the diffusing capacity as the lung expands. Clin Sci 24: 275, 1963.
34. Johnson RL Jr: Unpublished data.
35. Miller JM, Johnson RL Jr: Effect of lung inflation on pulmonary diffusing capacity at rest and exercise. J Clin Invest 45: 493, 1966.
36. Johnson RL Jr, Spicer WS, Bishop JM, et al.: Pulmonary capillary blood volume, flow and diffusing capacity during exercise. J Appl Physiol 15: 893, 1960.
37. McGrath MW, Thompson ML: The effect of age, body size and lung volume change on alveolar-capillary permeability and diffusing capacity in man. J Physiol (London) 146: 572, 1959.
38. Heath D, Edwards JE: The pathology of hypertensive pulmonary vascular disease. Circulation 18: 533, 1958.
39. Innes IR, Nickerson M: Norepinephrine, epinephrine and the sympathomimetic amines, chap 24. The Pharmacological Basis of Therapeutics (Goodman LS, Gilman A, eds), New York, Macmillan Publishing Co., 1975, p 503.
40. Wartmann WB, Hudson B, Jennings RB: Experimental arterial disease. II. The reaction of the pulmonary artery to emboli of filter paper fibers. Circulation 4: 756, 1951.
41. Von Glahn WC, Hall JW, Sun S: Arteritis in guinea-pigs produced by emboli of cotton. Am J Pathol 30: 1129, 1954.
42. Weidman WH, Marshall RJ, Wagenvoort CA, et al.: Relation in dogs of pulmonary vascular obstruction to pulmonary vascular "resistance." Lab Invest 12: 821, 1963.
43. Kittle CF, Bianchini L, Hostetler T, et al.: The development of chronic pulmonary hypertension. Surg Forum 9: 360, 1958.
44. Svanborg N: Studies on the cardiopulmonary function in sarcoidosis. Acta Med Scand 366 (suppl): 125, 1961.
45. Daum S: Oxygen transferring factor (diffusing capacity) of the lungs in pulmonary embolism. Bull Physiopathol Respir (Nancy) 6: 135, 1970.

The Cardiovascular Effects of Lithium in Man

A Review of the Literature

ARA G. TILKIAN, M.D.
JOHN S. SCHROEDER, M.D.
JOHN JUE KAO, M.D.
HERBERT N. HULTGREN, M.D.
Palo Alto, California

The medical literature since 1900 has been reviewed to determine the nature of lithium's cardiovascular effects. In therapeutic doses, lithium produces reversible T wave flattening and inversion in the electrocardiogram; rarely, it may cause sinus node dysfunction or ventricular arrhythmias. Patients with lithium toxicity almost always present with neurologic signs and symptoms. "Hypotension and cardiovascular collapse," alleged cardiotoxic manifestations of lithium, invariably follow days of coma. Given the possible cardiotoxic effect of other psychopharmacologic agents and the hazards of withholding effective therapy in mania, it is concluded that lithium may be used safely in patients with cardiac disease if the dose is adjusted to the rate of lithium excretion and if serum levels of lithium are followed carefully. When used in patients with cardiac arrhythmias, frequent electrocardiographic monitoring is advised.

The use of lithium salts is now well established in psychiatric pharmacotherapy. Presently, lithium carbonate is the treatment of choice for the long-term control of mania, and it is also used effectively to prevent relapse in bipolar manic-depressive illness [1–4]. It has been used in a variety of other psychiatric disorders, including psychoses, neuroses and personality disorders, although its therapeutic value in these conditions remains to be established [5]. The increasingly widespread administration of lithium in such cases has exposed to its use many psychiatric patients who have cardiac disease or arrhythmias. Although in most reviews of lithium's adverse effects and toxicity the presence of cardiovascular disease and arrhythmias is a contraindication to its use [5,6], a search of the literature reveals contradictory and inconclusive reports [7–17]. In this article we summarize the available knowledge of the effect of lithium chloride on the heart.

The use of lithium in medicine dates back to 1841 when it was proposed as an effective therapy for gout, but it was soon declared ineffective for this purpose. In the late 1940's, with the appreciation of the value of salt restriction in patients with hypertension and congestive heart failure, it was again introduced in medicine, in the form of lithium chloride, as a salt substitute, "West Sal"®. Following its indiscriminate use in patients whose salt intake was restricted, several cases of lithium toxicity, some fatal, were reported, precipitating its withdrawal from the market under the blanket indictment that lithium was specifically toxic and, therefore, contraindicated in patients with cardiovascular disease [5,6]. After the serendipitous discovery of the

From The Cardiology and Psychiatry Divisions, Stanford University School of Medicine; and the Veterans Administration Hospital, Palo Alto, California 94305. This work was supported in part by the Palo Alto Veterans Administration Hospital, NIH Grant No. HL-5866 and Program Project Grant No. 1-PO1-HL-15833. Requests for reprints should be addressed to Dr. John S. Schroeder, Cardiology Division, Stanford University School of Medicine, Stanford, California 94305. Manuscript accepted January 14, 1976.

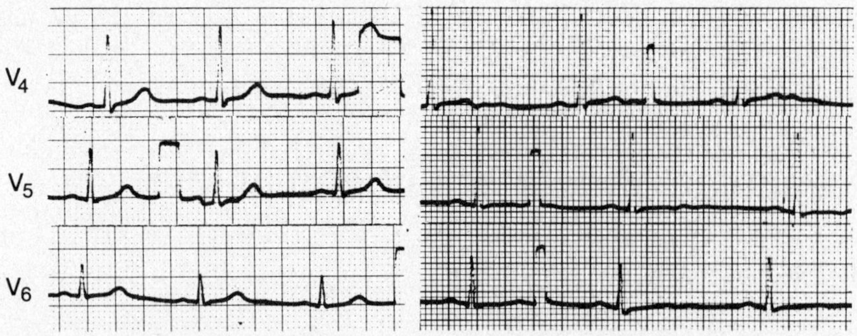

Figure 1. *Leads V_4 through V_6 of the electrocardiogram before **(left)** and during lithium therapy **(right)**. T wave changes include flattening and minor degree of inversion. Small U waves have appeared. Serum potassium was normal.*

beneficial effect of lithium in mania by Cade [1] in 1949 and confirmation of this by numerous studies, it was released by the Federal Drug Administration in April 1970 for use in the treatment of manic episodes of manic-depressive psychosis. A Federal Drug Administration statement accompanying the release declared this agent to be contraindicated in patients with significant cardiovascular or renal disease [18].

The Effect of Lithium on the Heart in Animals. In 1875 Hess [19] reported that lithium chloride, injected intravenously into frogs, rabbits and doves, caused "diastolic stopping of the heart." Krumhoff [20] in 1885 reported on the effect of large doses of lithium salts, given intravenously, in animals. He concluded that "lithium salts depressed the heart's action and caused a fall of blood pressure, and if the dose was large enough, stopped the heart in diastole." He also mentioned occasional small hemorrhages into the heart muscle. In 1903, Good [21] induced lethal gastroenteritis in animals by the subcutaneous administration of lithium chloride for four to 17 days. None of the animals died of cardiac causes, five of six had no cardiac abnormality at postmortem examination, whereas the sixth had "a few small hemorrhages under the endocardium." In none of these experiments were serum levels of lithium or other electrolytes measured. Roberts and Magida [22] in 1952 infused lithium chloride into dogs at the rate of 0.95 meq/min, and after a total dose of 114 to 190 meq, they noted characteristic changes of progressive hyperkalemia, although the serum potassium concentration ranged from 4.8 to 6.3 meq/liter only. In 1954, McKusick [23] infused lithium chloride into dogs, cats, rabbits and guinea pigs at a rate of 3.5 to 20 meq/min, and he noted characteristic changes of hyperkalemia in all animals which progressed to ventricular standstill or fibrillation. He observed that (1) the serum concentration of potassium increased in all animals reaching a level of 10 meq/liter at the time of cardiac arrest; (2) the serum potassium level continued to rise after the lithium infusion was discontinued, and changes noted on the electrocardiogram continued to progress; (3) the serum potassium levels at the point of cardiac arrest were lower than those produced by direct infusion of potassium chloride. McKusick concluded that lithium displaced intracellular potassium ion, producing hyperkalemia, and caused a proportionately larger drop in the K_{IC}:K_{EC} ratio, accounting for the appearance of cardiac arrest at relatively lower serum potassium levels. Ricciutti et al. [24] reported decreased cardiac output and left ventricular pressure, and delayed atrioventricular and intraventricular conduction within 2 hours of an intravenous infusion of lithium chloride (300 mg/kg) in dogs. At this infusion level, ventricular fibrillation developed in 17 of 22 dogs whereas asystole developed in five of 22.

Three recent studies have demonstrated an **antiarrhythmic** effect of lithium in animals [13–15]. Polumbo et al. [13] infused lithium chloride into dogs at 0.5 meq/min and noted a marked shortening of the duration of ouabain-induced arrhythmias. No consistent changes in serum potassium were noted, although increased T voltage was reported. Serum magnesium was not measured. Horgan et al. [14] reported that the administration of lithium chloride at 5 mg/kg/min for 60 minutes in dogs reverted digitalis-induced ventricular tachycardia to normal sinus rhythm in approximately 22.4 minutes or less. Serum potassium was not reported, but intra-atrial atrioventricular conduction, QRS duration and QTc intervals were unchanged. Extending these studies, these investigators also reported that the intraperitoneal administration of lithium chloride prevented the development of ventricular tachyarrhythmias during chloroform-induced apnea in mice and in dogs, significantly increased the ventricular fibrillation threshold [15] and increased left ventricular dp/dt and cardiac output [17].

The relevance of these animal studies to man is questionable. In all these studies, lithium was used in large doses (five to 15 times that used in human subjects) and was administered intravenously. Given the present knowledge of the mechanism of action of lithium [25,26], we suspect that the reported antiarrhythmic or arrhythmogenic effect was probably secondary to lithium-induced hyperkalemia and hypermagnesemia [27]. Such electrolyte changes are not seen with the long-term oral administration of lithium in man.

The Effect of Trace Amounts of Lithium on the Heart in Man. A protective action of hard water has been shown repeatedly in epidemiologic studies on the development of atherosclerotic cardiovascular disease [28] and the incidence of sudden death [29]. Lithium has been proposed as the element responsible for this presumed antiarrhythmic effect [28]. The amount of lithium under discussion in these studies is minute in proportion to the amount used in the therapeutic application of this agent [30]; thus, findings from these epidemiologic reports can hardly be applied to patients receiving lithium therapy.

The Effect of Therapeutic Doses of Lithium on the Heart in Man. The effect of lithium therapy observed on the resting electrocardiogram has been reported in a total of 79 patients [7,9,10,16,31]. Abnormalities were limited to reversible T wave changes (T wave depression, rarely inversion, not unlike that seen in hypokalemia) (Figure 1). These changes were all reversed when the administration of lithium was discontinued, and no QT prolongation was seen. It was postulated that these reversible T wave abnormalities reflected intracellular myocardial potassium depletion by displacement with lithium. Only two cases have been reported in which arrhythmias appeared during controlled lithium therapy and these disappeared after cessation of therapy; in neither case was the patient known to have heart disease. In the first case, premature ventricular contractions were noted during lithium therapy; these resolved when administration of the drug was discontinued and reappeared when lithium therapy was resumed [12]. In the second case, symptomatic sinus node dysfunction occurred during lithium therapy, subsided after its withdrawal, and was reproduced and documented by intracardiac electrography five days after lithium therapy was resumed [32]. In both cases, serum lithium levels were in the therapeutic range.

The occurrence of acute myocardial infarction during lithium therapy has been reported in a 42 year old man [11]. Serum lithium levels were in the therapeutic range, the course was not complicated, and the investigators concluded that a causal relationship could not be inferred. In two patients receiving long-term lithium therapy, fatal idiopathic myocarditis developed [33,34]. The first patient [33] was also taking other medications and had hypothyroidism, late latent syphilis and an undiagnosed generalized skin lesion. In the second patient [34], careful review of his history strongly suggests the presence of unexplained heart failure prior to the initiation of lithium therapy. Despite the serious shortcomings in these two cases, and the implicit likelihood of encountering unrelated primary myocardial disease in the large number of patients receiving lithium therapy, these two cases cannot be easily dismissed, considering the present understanding of the distribution of lithium in the body [25]. Lithium partially replaces intracellular potassium in the heart. Myocardial degeneration and "cardiomyopathy" have been documented in animals with severe potassium depletion [35], and hypokalemia has been proposed as the cause of myocarditis in man [36,37]. Thus, it will require careful reporting of further suspected cases of myocarditis, serial endomyocardial biopsies in such cases after the discontinuation of lithium therapy and autopsy studies in psychiatric hospitals before a causative relationship between lithium and idiopathic myocarditis can be established. The fact that these two patients also had hypothyroidism (before lithium therapy in one patient) warrants a search of this association in possible future cases.

Nonfatal Lithium Intoxication in Man. All cases of nonfatal lithium toxicity in which information concerning the cardiovascular system was available were reviewed. A cluster of toxicity reports occurred in 1949 and 1950 during the uncontrolled use of lithium salts as a salt substitute in patients with hypertension and/or congestive heart failure [38–42]. Of the 12 patients who recovered, none was described as having manifested signs of cardiac toxicity, either in the form of arrhythmias or worsening congestive heart failure. With the present increasing use of lithium, the number of reported cases of serious toxicity remains small. In a total of 25 cases reported in 11 studies [8,43–53] in which the cardiovascular system is mentioned, transient T wave abnormalities on the electrocardiogram and borderline hypotension in the setting of dehydration and coma were described. In nearly all these cases, the manifestations of toxicity were central nervous system disorders, including coma and seizures.

During an episode of coronary insufficiency in a 57 year old patient who was receiving lithium therapy, atrioventricular dissociation, with atrioventricular block and junctional rhythm, was observed [54]. A year and a half later, while still receiving lithium therapy, this patient presented with Adams-Stokes attacks secondary to sinoatrial block, and a slow idionodal rhythm, with hypokalemia (K = 2.5 meq/liter) and lithium intoxication (lithium = 2.15 meq/liter). The bradyarrhythmia persisted after correction of the hypokalemia

TABLE I Fatal Cases of Lithium Intoxication in Which Information About the Heart is Mentioned

Patient	Age (yr) and Sex	Preexisting Heart Disease	Mode of Presentation	ECG	Course	Autopsy	Reference
1	70, F	ASCVD, CHF	Tremor, confusion	Not known	Coma and death	Not done	[40]
2	66, F	ASCVD	Tremor, confusion	Not known	Coma for 7 days → hypotension, death	Not done	[40]
3	58, M	ASCVD, COPD, premature beats	Lethargy	Transient I-ventricular conduction delay	Coma for 2 days → hypotension and death	Not done	[42]
4	57, F	None	Vomiting, confusion, ataxia	Not known	Satus epilepticus and coma for 5 days → irregular pulse 150/min → hypotension, fever (105.5°F), death	No cardiovascular disease, nonrevealing	[57]
5	71, F	ASCVD	Confusion	Atrial flutter: 1 day before death	Coma for 4 days, fever, death	Pneumonia, pulmonary edema	[8]
6	59, M	None	Confusion	T wave abnormality	Coma for 2 days, fever, death	Pneumonia, pulmonary edema	[8]
7	57, F	None	Confusion	T wave abnormality	Atelectasis, fever, death	Pneumonia, pulmonary edema	[8]
8	45, M	None	Ataxia, seizures	Not known	Confusion, muscle incoordination, 8–12 days → death	Myocardial fiber segmentation and interstitial fibrosis	[58]

NOTE: ASCVD = arteriosclerotic cardiovascular disease. CHF = congestive heart failure. COPD = chronic obstructive pulmonary disease.

and a permanent pacemaker was inserted. A myocardial toxic effect of lithium was postulated as the cause.

Regular bradycardia at 40 beats/min, with no atrial activity, was described in a 61 year old patient with severe lithium intoxication who presented with mental confusion and neurologic signs [55]. During the course of her therapy, she lapsed into coma, hyperkalemia developed (8.1 meq/liter) and progressed to ventricular fibrillation, from which she was successfully resuscitated. The electrocardiogram taken after recovery was normal.

Lithium-induced sinoatrial block was considered as a possible cause of syncope recorded on an electrocardiogram of a 49 year old patient with toxic serum levels of lithium (2.5 meq/liter) [56]. The sinoatrial block disappeared as lithium levels decreased and reappeared when administration of the drug was resumed. The patient did not manifest other signs of lithium intoxication.

Thus, it appears that arrhythmias in the course of controlled lithium therapy are rare. Their occurrence should prompt a search for lithium intoxication or associated electrolyte abnormalities.

We reviewed reports of eight cases of fatal lithium intoxication in which the cardiovascular system was mentioned [40,42,57,58] and have summarized these in Table I. It is apparent that the mode of presentation and the course in these patients was dominated by central nervous system toxicity. Cardiovascular collapse and death occurred after two to 12 days of stupor, and coma with bronchopneumonia in three of the five cases in which autopsy was performed. Myocardial pathology findings were reported in one patient (Case 8), and although these findings were somewhat different from those reported in the two cases of myocarditis associated with lithium therapy [33,34], no other cause for such changes was noted.

In almost all cases, the "pulse irregularities, fall in blood pressure levels, peripheral circulatory failure and circulatory collapse," generally listed as the cardiac toxicity of lithium [59], occurred terminally in patients who died after prolonged coma.

Mechanism of Action of Lithium. The mechanism of action of lithium remains unknown, although its biologic effects are widely recognized [60]. Present concepts of lithium's mechanism of action have been summarized recently [25]. It has been proposed that lithium participates in ionic transfer and distribution as an imperfect substitute for other cations, as well as affecting multiple hormonal systems through its effect on the cellular microenvironment. Since our present knowledge about its mechanism of action is limited, few conclusions can be drawn about its effect on cardiac conduction or contractile tissue. It is known that lithium partially replaces intracellular potassium and in a single large dose oral administration produces hyperkalemia [23]. This action can explain the effect noted on the cardiac conduction system in animal and tissue experiments, i.e., decreased resting membrane potential of Purkinje fibers, prolonged depolarization and decreased velocity of conduction [61]. These changes may have been responsible for the antiarrhythmic effect of lithium which has been reported in animals. As noted earlier, these effects have questionable relevance to the use of lithium in man, except perhaps in cases of acute, massive overdose.

The slow, partial intramyocardial depletion of potassium and its replacement with lithium may explain the commonly observed T wave flattening on the electrocardiogram. There have been no electrophysiologic studies in this setting in man or animal models. It appears to be well established that chronic potassium depletion can cause myocardial degeneration in animals [35], but it is entirely unknown whether a similar situation exists in hearts with intracellular potassium depletion secondary to lithium.

There have been no reported investigations of the effects of *long-term* lithium administration on myocardial contractility. Singer et al. [25] mention dog studies showing decreased cardiac output and intraventricular pressure, but we have been unable to locate the source of this information. Since lithium may interfere with the action of catecholamines and indoleamines, this action may affect myocardial contractility as well as excitability.

Thus, until there is a clearer understanding of lithium's mode of action, no conclusive statements can be made about its expected effects on cardiac arrhythmias or contraction.

Use of Lithium in Patients with Heart Disease. There is a general reluctance to use lithium in cardiac patients, although one study reports its use in the presence of major cardiac disease [49]. This reluctance is based on three reasons: (1) the unfortunate experience in 1949 and 1950, when its *uncontrolled* use as a salt substitute led to several fatalities [40,42]; (2) the unquestioning acceptance that "cardiac arrhythmia, hypotension and peripheral circulatory collapse" [18] were manifestations of lithium toxicity on the heart; and (3) the increased susceptibility of patients with congestive heart failure, or those on salt restriction, to lithium intoxication [62]. The third reason remains valid; a decreased glomerular filtration rate, presence of heart failure, dietary salt restriction or the *prolonged* use of loop-acting diuretics [63], singly or in combination, will interfere with the renal clearance of lithium and ultimately result in its toxic accumulation. Acute administration of commonly used diuretics do not significantly affect lithium clearance [64], but prolonged thiazide treatment decreases its clearance by 24 per cent [63].

Based on our review of the literature, it appears that inadequate data are available to contraindicate the administration of lithium chloride to patients with heart disease when there are clear psychiatric indications for its use, since the cardiotoxicity of other psychotherapeutic agents which would be required probably exceed that of lithium [65,66]. If lithium is used, factors interfering with the renal clearance of lithium (heart failure, salt restriction, long-term use of diuretics) must be identified and appropriate adjustments in dosage made. If this agent is used in patients with cardiac arrhythmias, electrocardiographic monitoring is essential in order to detect any possible, although unlikely, aggravation of the arrhythmia. Studies in *long-term* animal models and further investigation in human subjects are necessary for better understanding of the cardiac effects of long-term lithium administration.

REFERENCES

1. Cade JF: Lithium salts in the treatment of psychotic excitement. Med J Aust 2: 349, 1949.
2. Prien RF, Caffey EM Jr, Klett CJ: A comparison of lithium carbonate and chlorpromazine in the treatment of mania. Arch Gen Psychiatry 26: 146, 1972.
3. Stallone F, Shelley E, Mendlewicz J, et al.: The use of lithium in affective disorders. III. A double-blind study of prophylaxis in bipolar illness. Am J Psychiatry 130: 1006, 1973.
4. Baldessarini RJ, Lipinski JF: Lithium salts: 1970–1975. Ann Intern Med 83: 527, 1975.
5. Prien RF, Caffey, EM, Klett JC: Lithium carbonate. A survey of the history and current status of lithium in treating mood disorders. Dis Ner Syst 31: 521, 1971.
6. Brown WT: The use of lithium carbonate in the treatment of mood disorders. Can Med Assoc 108: 742, 1973.
7. Schou M: Electrocardiographic changes during treatment with lithium and with drugs of imipramine-type. Acta Psychiat Scand 38: 331, 1962.
8. Schou M, Amdisen A, Trap-Jensen J: Lithium poisoning. Am J Psychiatry 125: 520, 1968.
9. Demers RG, Heninger GR: Electrocardiographic changes during lithium treatment. Dis Nerv Syst 31: 674, 1970.
10. Idem: Electrocardiographic T wave changes during lithium carbonate treatment. JAMA 218: 381, 1971.
11. Baldessarini RJ, Stephens JH: Lithium carbonate for affective disorders: clinical pharmacology and toxicology. Arch Gen Psychiatry 22: 72, 1970.
12. Tangedahl TN, Gau G: Myocardial irritability associated with lithium carbonate therapy. N Engl J Med 287: 867, 1972.
13. Polumbo RA, Branzi A, Schroeder JS, et al.: The antiarrhythmic effect of lithium chloride for experimental ouabain induced arrhythmias. Proc Soc Exp Biol Med 142: 1200, 1973.
14. Horgan JH, Proctor JD, Velandia J, et al.: Antiarrhythmic effect of lithium. Arch Int Pharmacodyn 206: 105, 1973.
15. Horgan JH, Ford GD, Proctor JD, et al: The effect of prophylactic and therapeutic administration of lithium on ventricular tachycardia. Arch Int Pharmacodyn 207: 77, 1974.
16. Andreani G: Electrocardiographic findings during treatment with lithium salts. G Clin Med 38: 1759, 1957.
17. Horgan JH, Proctor JD, Ford GD, et al.: The acute effects of lithium chloride infusion on some hemodynamic parameters. Arch Int Pharmacodyn Ther 210: 5, 1974.
18. Federal Drug Administration Statement. Ann Intern Med 73: 291, 1970.

19. Hess A: Lithion. Inaugural Dissertation, 1876. (Quoted by Good [21].)
20. Krumhoff E: Experimentalle Beitrage zur wirkung des lithium. Inaugural Dissertation, 1884. (Quoted by Good [21].)
21. Good CA: An experimental study of lithium. Am J Med Sci 125: 273, 1903.
22. Roberts KE, Magida MG: Electrocardiographic alterations produced by a decrease in plasma pH, bicarbonate and sodium as compared with those produced by an increase in potassium. Circ Res 1: 206, 1953.
23. McKusick VA: The effect of lithium on the electrocardiogram of animals and relation of these effects to the ratio of the intracellular and extracellular concentrations of potassium. J Clin Invest 33: 598, 1954.
24. Ricciutti MA, Lisi KR, Damato AN: A metabolic basis for the electrophysiological effects of lithium. Circulation 44 (suppl II): 217, 1971.
25. Singer I, Rotenberg D: Mechanism of lithium action. N Engl J Med 289: 254, 1973.
26. Birch NJ, Jenner FA: The distribution of lithium and its effect on the distribution and excretion of other ions in the rat. Br J Pharmacol 47: 586, 1973.
27. Ghani MF, Smith JR: The effectiveness of magnesium chloride in the treatment of ventricular tachyarrhythmias due to digitalis intoxication. Am Heart J 88: 621, 1974.
28. Voors AW: Lithium in drinking water and atherosclerotic heart disease. Am J Epidemiol 92: 164, 1970.
29. Anderson TW, Riche WH, MacKay JS: Sudden death and ischemic heart disease. Correlation with hardness of local water supply. N Engl J Med 280: 805, 1969.
30. Livingston HD: Lithium depletion and atherosclerotic heart disease. Lancet 2: 99, 1970.
31. Kochar MS, Wang RH, D'Cunha GF: Electrocardiographic changes simulating hypokalemia during treatment with lithium carbonate. J Electrocardiol 4: 371, 1971.
32. Wellens HJ, Cats VM, Duren DR: Symptomatic sinus node abnormalities following lithium carbonate therapy. Am J Med 59: 285, 1975.
33. Tseng HL: Interstitial myocarditis probably related to lithium carbonate intoxication. Arch Pathol 92: 444, 1971.
34. Swedberg K, Winblad B: Heart failure as complication of lithium treatment. Acta Med Scand 196: 279, 1974.
35. Harrison CD, Cooper G, Zujko KJ, et al.: Myocardial and mitochondrial function in potassium depletion cardiomyopathy. J Mol Cell Cardiol 4: 633, 1972.
36. Rodriguez CE, Wolfe AL, Bergstrom VW: Hypokalemic myocarditis. Am J Clin Pathol 20: 1050, 1950.
37. McAllen PM: Myocardial changes occurring in potassium deficiency. Br Heart J 17: 5, 1955.
38. Stern RL: Severe lithium chloride poisoning with complete recovery. JAMA 139: 710, 1949.
39. Waldron AM: Lithium intoxication. JAMA 139: 733, 1949.
40. Corcoran AC, Taylor RD, Page IH: Lithium poisoning from the use of salt substitutes. JAMA 139: 685, 1949.
41. Talbott JH: Use of lithium salts as a substitute for sodium chloride. Arch Intern Med 85: 1, 1950.
42. Hanlon LW, Romaine M, Gilroy FJ, et al.: Lithium chloride as a substitute for sodium chloride in the diet. JAMA 139: 688, 1949.
43. Noack CH, Trautner EM: The lithium treatment of maniacal psychosis. Med J Aust 11: 219, 1951.
44. Daumézon G, Guibert M, Chanoit P: Un cas d'intoxication grave par le lithium. Ann Med Psychol 113: 673, 1955.
45. Coats DA, Trautner EM, Gershon S: The treatment of lithium poisoning. Aust Ann Med 6: 11, 1957.
46. Allgén LG: Laboratory experience in lithium toxicity in man. Acta Psychiatr Scand Suppl 207, p 98, 1969.
47. Verbov JL, Phillips JD, Fife DG: A case of lithium intoxication. Postgrad Med J 41: 190, 1965.
48. Horowitz CL, Fisher GU: Acute lithium toxicity. N Engl J Med 281: 1369, 1970.
49. McKnelly WV, Tupin JP, Dunn M: Lithium in hazardous circumstances with one case of lithium toxicity. Compr Psychiatry 11: 279, 1970.
50. Aoki FY, Ruedy J: Severe lithium intoxication. Management without dialysis and report of a possible teratogenic effect of lithium. Can Med Assoc J 105: 847, 1971.
51. Herrero FA: Lithium carbonate toxicity. JAMA 226: 1109, 1973.
52. Hurtig HI, Dyson WL: Lithium toxicity enhanced by diuresis. N Engl J Med 290: 748, 1974.
53. Bouletreau P, Petit P, Ducluzeau R, et al.: Intoxication accidentelle au lithium. Bull Med Leg Toxicol 17: 385, 1974.
54. Kleinert M: Myokardiopathie unter lithiumtherapie. Med Klin 69: 494, 1974.
55. Humbert G, Fillastre JP, Leroy J, et al.: Intoxication par le lithium. Sem Hop Paris 50: 509, 1974.
56. Tobin RJ, Nemickas R, Scanlon JP, et al.: EKG of the month. Ill Med J 146: 45, 1974.
57. Roberts EL: A case of chronic mania treated with lithium citrate and terminating fatally. Med J Aust 2: 261, 1950.
58. Glesinger B: Evaluation of lithium in treatment of psychotic excitement. Med J Aust 1: 277, 1954.
59. Gershon S, Shopsin B: Lithium: Its Role in Psychiatric Research and Treatment, New York, Plenum Press, 1973, p 108.
60. Ibid: p 51.
61. Ettinger PO, Regan TJ, Oldewurtel HA: Hyperkalemia, cardiac conduction and the electrocardiogram. A review. Am Heart J 88: 360, 1974.
62. Gershon S, Shopsin B: Lithium: Its Role in Psychiatric Research and Treatment, New York, Plenum Press, 1973, p 171.
63. Peterson V, Hvidt S, Thomsen K, et al.: Effect of prolonged thiazide treatment on renal lithium clearance. Br Med J 3: 143, 1974.
64. Thomsen K, Schou M: Renal lithium excretion in man. Am J Physiol 215: 823, 1968.
65. Raisfeld IH: Cardiovascular complications of antidepressant therapy. Am Heart J 83: 129, 1972.
66. Muller V, Burckhardt D: Effect of tricyclic and tetracyclic antidepressant drugs on heart and circulation. Schweiz Med Wochenschr 104: 1911, 1974.

Systemic Mastocytosis

Stenographic reports, edited by Philip E. Cryer, M.D. and John M. Kissane, M.D., of weekly clinicopathologic conferences held in Barnes and Wohl Hospitals, are published in each issue of the Journal. These conferences are participated in jointly by members of the Departments of Internal Medicine and Pathology of Washington University School of Medicine.

A 58 year old Caucasian woman was admitted to Barnes Hospital on February 27, 1976, for evaluation because of multiple skeletal fractures.

The patient was well until 1967 when she sustained a fracture of the left femoral neck after minimal trauma. Attempts to pin the hip were unsuccessful, but in 1975 total hip replacement was performed with a good functional result. During this time she took analgesics in substantial quantities for chronic pain in that hip. Among these was indomethacin which was continued until 1974 when symptomatic peptic ulcer disease developed. Subsequently, antacids (including aluminum hydroxide) were taken occasionally to relieve epigastric pain. Between 1967 and 1976 there were several episodes of acute back pain, and compression fractures of the vertebrae were documented roentgenographically. Approximately one month before admission the right seventh rib was fractured with no recognized trauma. These fractures occurred despite the administration of calcium supplements and estrogens. The patient had noticed a progressive skin rash for approximately two to three years. She denied having gastrointestinal symptoms and weight loss.

Physical findings included marked kyphosis, bilateral cataracts, a palpable 1 by 1.5 cm left axillary lymph node and a profusion of brownish red, small, maculopapular skin lesions, particularly over the trunk. There was no bone tenderness. The vital signs were normal.

Routine serum chemistry values were normal including a serum calcium of 9.8 mg/100 ml, a serum phosphate of 4.1 mg/100 ml, a serum alkaline phosphatase of 61 mIU/ml and a serum cholesterol of 173 mg/100 ml. The urine calcium was 90 mg/24 hours, the urine phosphate 270 mg/24 hours and the serum parathyroid hormone concentration was 3 μl eq/ml (normal $<$10 μl eq/ml). The white blood cell count was 5,400/mm^3 with 5 per cent eosinophils, the erythrocyte sedimentation rate 8 mm/hour and the prothrombin time normal. Serum immunoglobulin electrophoresis revealed an immunoglobulin G (IgG) paraprotein; the total serum IgG level was 1,800 mg/100 ml. Immunoglobulin electrophoresis of the urine disclosed no abnormalities. The urine pH was 6.0; 10 white blood cells per high power field were noted in the urine sediment, and Escherichia coli were cultured from the urine.

Roentgenograms of the chest showed a large calcified lesion, believed to be a granuloma, in the right mid-lung field. Multiple bone films demonstrated widespread osteopenia, particularly marked in the axial skeleton; there were several compressed vertebrae. Pseudofractures were not seen. Bone density, by photon absorption osteodensitometry, was normal at the radial mid-shaft. A duodenal deformity, consistent with chronic peptic ulcer disease, was noted on an x-ray series of the upper gastrointestinal tract.

Biopsies of skin and bone were performed.

CLINICAL DISCUSSION

Dr. Charles Parker: In summary, this 58 year old woman had symptoms of bone disease for nine years, and of peptic ulcer disease and skin rash for two years. We will begin the discussion with the roentgenograms.

Dr. R. Gilbert Jost: The roentgenogram of the chest demonstrated cardiomegaly and an ill defined infiltrate in the right mid-lung field. Laminograms, however, showed definite calcification within the infiltrate, indicating that it most likely represented the residual effects of some old inflammatory disease. A lateral view of the chest indicated severe demineralization of the skeleton with multiple compression deformities in the thoracic spine; the compression deformities were even more pronounced in the lumbar area. Severe generalized demineralization of this kind has a variety of causes. Osteoporosis, of course, needs to be considered with its many underlying etiologies such as osteogenesis imperfecta tarda, exogenous steroid therapy, endogenous Cushing's syndrome or poor diet. Osteomalacia could also present this roentgenographic picture. In fact, it is often difficult to distinguish between osteomalacia and osteoporosis simply on the basis of the roentgenograms. Looser's zones, or pseudofractures, when they are present, offer a means of differentiating between osteomalacia and osteoporosis; Looser's zones are characteristic of osteomalacia, but none was present in this patient.

Hyperparathyroidism is another condition which can present with severe demineralization, although this patient's films showed none of the accessory findings to support that diagnosis. In the hand films there was periarticular demineralization, but there was certainly no evidence of subperiosteal resorption. A good place to look for the characteristic lace-like appearance of subperiosteal resorption is on the radial surface of the middle phalanx of either the third or fourth finger. However, the cortices in the patient's hands were sturdy and thick. There was certainly no evidence of cortical resorption of the kind that we associate with hyperparathyroidism. Incidentally, the mineralization of the radius was nearly normal. In this patient, demineralization was much less severe in the appendicular skeleton than it was in the axial skeleton. This would account for the rather high bone densitometry reading which was obtained.

A final consideration in an older patient with demineralization would be multiple myeloma. Multiple myeloma certainly can present with diffuse demineralization, although more characteristically it presents with discrete punched out lesions. There was no roentgenographic evidence of the characteristic lesions of multiple myeloma in this patient.

In summary, we have a patient with generalized demineralization of the skeleton with no specific roentgenographic findings to support any one diagnosis. This is not an unusual situation. On the basis of films alone, it is frequently very difficult to explain the underlying cause of generalized demineralization. Bone biopsy is often necessary.

Dr. Parker: Thank you. When I read through the protocol the first time, I found myself wondering why an immunologist had been selected to discuss a case in which the most prominent manifestations were in the skin and bone. The only thing I could think of was that the Residents had decided that I needed to learn more about those areas, which is no doubt true. But, after a second reading, it occurred to me that this whole story might be put together as mastocytosis involving both the skin and bone. At the risk of spending a considerable amount of time describing a disease that the patient may conceivably not have, I have decided to orient my discussion almost exclusively from that point of view.

The term mastocytosis is used to describe a disease in which focal collections of mast cells involve one or a combination of organs. As a rule, these mast cells have a normal morphologic appearance with no suggestion of malignant change. Only approximately 1,000 cases of mastocytosis have been reported, but the true incidence is undoubtedly higher with an estimated frequency of one in every 1,000 to 2,500 new patient visits in dermatologic practice [1]. Since mast cells are secretory cells, the clinical manifestations of mastocytosis fall into two general categories: (1) Infiltrative manifestations. In organs infiltrated by mast cells, discrete lesions can often be seen, particularly in the skin. In addition, marked degrees of infiltration can occur in a wide variety of other tissues, including bone, liver, spleen, lymph nodes, gastrointestinal tract, heart and lung, leading to localized collections of mast cells, organomegaly or functional impairment. (2) Pharmacologic manifestations. The mast cells that accumulate in this condition appear to be perfectly normal from a biosynthetic point of view and, therefore, contain histamine and other mediators of immediate hypersensitivity. Under a variety of circumstances, these substances are released and produce acute pharmacologic changes either locally or systemically.

The organ involvement in mastocytosis varies, and five distinct clinical syndromes [2] are possible. (1) Involvement of the skin (urticaria pigmentosa) without obvious systemic involvement. This is the most common form of mastocytosis accounting for about 90 per cent of all the cases in affected persons [1]. (2) Skin lesions in association with bone changes. This appears to be the second most common mode of presentation of mastocytosis and may well be the form of the disease in our patient, assuming mastocytosis is indeed her problem. (3) Systemic mastocytosis and skin involvement. In perhaps as many as 10 per cent of the patients with involvement of the skin, there are clinical manifestations referable to involvement of systemic organs. Of the ones I have just mentioned, the most common are bone, liver, spleen and lymph nodes. (4) Mastocytosis in association with leukemia. In up to 4 or 5 per cent of the patients with mastocytosis some form of leukemia ultimately develops. Although this can be a mast cell leukemia it usually is not, and all forms of leukemia are represented. (5) Systemic mastocytosis without urticaria pigmentosa. This is a rare presentation, although it may be a challenging one from the diagnostic point of view.

Let us now consider the individual organ manifestations of mastocytosis in greater detail. Since Dr. Bauer will also discuss the skin manifestations, I will limit my remarks to a consideration of whether or not the changes shown by our patient fit with the diagnosis of cutaneous mastocytosis. To begin with, her age is not a problem. To be sure, skin involvement in this condition most commonly begins in infancy or early childhood, but in some 25 per cent of all cases of recognized mastocytosis, the onset is in adults. In addition, the occurrence of initial symptoms in above the age of 70 years has been described. Secondly, the lesions described in our patient conform, at least superficially, to what is usually found in mastocytosis in that they were macular, round or oval, and especially marked on the trunk. Moreover, although the color of urticaria pigmentosa lesions varies widely, among the colors listed is red-brown which was the color of the lesions in our patient. There is one other very common clinical feature of urticaria pigmentosa that I would prefer to have had before making this diagnosis—urtication, that is, the occurrence of a local urticarial exacerbation when involved areas of skin are stroked.

The bone lesions also appear to fit with a diagnosis of mastocytosis in that bone lesions, when they occur in this condition, are very likely to appear in cases of adult onset, especially in those beginning in people over the age of 50. As will be discussed in more detail by Dr. Haddad, both osteosclerosis and osteoporosis are seen, either together or separately [1]. The lesions may be static or slowly or rapidly progressive; therefore, the course of our patient's illness, dating back over a period of nine years, is perfectly consistent with this diagnosis. The only reservation I have in ascribing the bone involvement to mastocytosis is the presence of paraprotein in her serum which, of course, raises the possibility of multiple myeloma. It is well recognized that diffuse myelomatous involvement of bone can cause the roentgenologic changes of osteopenia without the typical punched out lesions of myeloma being demonstrable. But, I find it hard to believe that this patient had multiple myeloma with diffuse bone involvement back in 1967 and that she still does not have any punched out bone lesions or, for that matter, is still alive. How then can the presence of paraprotein be explained? Although the association of bone disease and paraproteinemia in this patient may be coincidental (e.g., she may have a benign monoclonal gammapathy and also happen to have bone involvement), there are now a handful of cases in the literature in which both severe idiopathic or postmenopausal osteoporosis and a paraprotein were present [3]. Several of these patients have been followed for six years or longer with no change being noted in the level of paraprotein in their serum and with no clinical evidence of myeloma, either initially or later. In addition, at least one case in which the patient had both amyloidosis and mastocytosis has been reported, and it is now recognized that many persons with amyloidosis have paraproteins [4]. In any event, I am unable to make a diagnosis of myeloma and, although the bone lesions in this patient might be explained by osteoporosis per se without mast cell infiltration, I strongly suspect that mastocytosis is, indeed, present and that it does involve her bones.

Systemic symptoms of mastocytosis include weight loss, fever and flushing. The flushing varies in intensity, sometimes to the point that the malignant carcinoid syndrome is simulated. Originally, episodic flushing was thought to be rare in mastocytosis but Dr. Joseph Demis, who was Professor of Dermatology here in the early 1960's, pointed out that as many as 35 per cent of the patients with mastocytosis have this symptom [5]. The flush is typically bright red and involves primarily the face and upper thorax. It may be provoked by a variety of stimuli including emotional stress, exposure to cold and drugs, such as aspirin, which also produce exacerbations of chronic idiopathic urticaria. Several subjects have been described in whom symptoms of an upper respiratory tract infection developed followed by marked exacerbations of symptoms of flushing which continued until the infection was brought under control. It seems likely that these subjects had large numbers of mast cells in their respiratory tract and that, in response to a local immunologic or nonspecific irritant reaction, these cells were releasing their intracellular content of mediators. Other symptoms of systemic release include pounding headaches, bronchospasm, hypotension, diarrhea, rhinorrhea, urticaria, palpitation and dyspnea; many of these are probably due largely to histamine. Mastocytosis is similar to epinephrine-secreting pheochromocytoma in that hypotension and other systemic symptoms may be precipitated by trauma or surgery, although this is unusual. Occasionally fever is a prominent clinical finding with episodes lasting from a few hours to several days or, rarely, for many weeks, leading to diagnostic difficulties as a fever of unknown origin. Facial or peripheral edema or ascites occasionally occurs, presumably as a manifestation of mediator effects on vascular permeability.

Differentiation of the episodes of flushing seen in mastocytosis from those seen in the carcinoid syndrome should not present serious difficulties. In mastocytosis, the flush is bright red and usually lasts for 10 to 30 minutes. The skin is warm and permanent telangiectatic changes in the skin are unusual, even in those with repeated flushing [1]. In the carcinoid syndrome, the flush tends to be cyanotic near its periphery, it usually lasts 10 minutes or less, the skin may be cool and, not infrequently, permanent skin changes eventually occur. Moreover, urticaria pigmentosa is not a feature of the carcinoid syndrome. As further verification, measurements of histamine and 5-hydroxyindoleacetic acid in the urine will ordinarily clearly differentiate between these two conditions.

Physical findings associated with systemic mastocytosis include hepatomegaly (70 per cent), splenomegaly (50 per cent) and lymphoadenopathy (30 per cent) [6]. Often, the enlarged organs contain markedly increased numbers of mast cells. However, this is not always true even when the tissue appears to have been properly fixed. In the liver, it has been suggested that mast cell products, particularly histamine, may be capable of stimulating hepatic cell proliferation and fibrosis. As far as our patient is concerned, she did not have splenic or hepatic enlargement, but she did have axillary lymphadenopathy which may be a manifestation of systemic mastocytosis.

Gastrointestinal manifestations also are common in systemic mastocytosis. Bleeding occurs in up to 10 per cent of the patients either on the basis of peptic ulcer disease or, less commonly, some other factor. The incidence of peptic ulcer in this condition is listed as 5 to 10 per cent which is no higher than in the general population. Nonetheless, the occurrence of ulcer symptoms has been observed for the first time in association with other symptoms of systemic mastocytosis and, certainly, histamine is a potent stimulator of acid secretion. In addition to peptic ulcer disease and gastrointestinal bleeding, giant rugae have been described in the stomach. Diarrhea, with or without associated steatorrhea, may occur and can be quite severe. One case has been reported in which the diarrhea was quite well controlled by disodium cromoglycate [7], a drug currently being used to control mediator release in bronchial asthma. The patient under discussion does have a peptic ulcer which was first described in 1974 and, although she has also received drugs which promote ulcer formation, it seems quite possible that mastocytosis is an important contributing factor.

A variety of hematologic manifestations are seen in association with systemic mastocytosis including anemia, leukocytosis, leukopenia, eosinophilia, basophilia, peripheral blood mastocytosis and, more rarely, one of a variety of different types of leukemias [1]. The anemia seen in association with this condition is not completely understood, but possible contributing factors include bone marrow infiltration by mast cells, splenomegaly and the enhancing effects of heparin on erythrophagocytosis. Mast cells contain sizeable quantities of heparin but, aside from occasional episodes of gastrointestinal bleeding or local ecchymosis in the skin, in which heparin may or may not be a contributing factor, bleeding manifestations are not a problem. The one hematologic manifestation that our patient may have is eosinophilia. Eosinophilia is seen in about 15 per cent of the subjects with systemic mastocytosis and is presumably due to release of eosinophil chemotactic factors from mast cells. Our patient also has a serum cholesterol value which is near the lower limits of normal for her age and sex. Hypocholesterolemia is seen in about 10 to 20 per cent of the patients with mastocytosis and is probably secondary to the effects of heparin on cholesterol metabolism. Results of urine or serum measurements of histamine or other mast cell products are not available to us and presumably were not obtained prior to biopsy.

In summary, taking the skin, bone and peptic ulcer manifestations together, including their apparent onset after the age of 50 years within seven years of one another, and perhaps the eosinophilia and suggestion of hypocholesterolemia, I believe this patient does, indeed, have systemic mastocytosis. We will now hear from Dr. Bauer and Dr. Haddad, both of whom have seen the patient, for a more detailed discussion of her skin and bone manifestations.

Dr. Eugene Bauer: The skin lesions in this patient consist of numerous erythematous to tan macules and papules localized primarily on the trunk. Lesions are less prominent on the extremities and on the face. The lesions on the skin are clinically quite typical of urticaria pigmentosa and are urticated upon gentle stroking.

The dermatologic differential diagnoses here should include several erythematous or pigmented lesions.

Benign pigmented nevi are somewhat more sharply circumscribed and usually palpable, although they need not be. To find them so profusely, as in this patient, would be unusual. Perhaps a more realistic consideration in the differential diagnosis is multiple lentigines, but these lesions would not urticate when stroked. Furthermore, in addition to the lentigines, several other features of the lentiginosis profusa syndrome may be present, such as ocular hypertelorism, prognathism, deafness, electrocardiographic abnormalities and pulmonary stenosis [8,9]. A third possibility would be neurofibromatosis. The typical café au lait spots, which are somewhat more well defined than we see in our patient with urticaria pigmentosa, axillary freckling and a family history of the disease would help to confirm the diagnosis. Older lesions of eruptive xanthomas might superficially resemble lesions of urticaria pigmentosa. However, early in the course of the eruption there should be little confusion, since they began as pink papules, often with a slight yellow color. They later tend to form rosettes and become slightly tan. In addition, the dermal character of these lesions is easily appreciated.

In briefly discussing the types of urticaria pigmentosa, we should consider at least two important parameters: the number of lesions and the age of onset. The solitary mastocytoma is usually present at birth or in infancy and resolves spontaneously within the first few years. The prognosis is very good in the absence of systemic involvement, including both bone and other organ involvement [10]. Not only solitary mastocytomas, but also multiple pigmented papules and nodules occurring early in childhood are associated with a good prognosis. The lesions often resolve spontaneously, and the chances of extracutaneous involvement are slim. It is important to note, however, that cases of systemic mast cell disease have been reported even in young children. [6]. There may be such a vigorous response to stroking the skin that a blistered lesion will actually develop. An important aside with respect to obtaining a skin biopsy specimen in these patients is that the mast cell degranulation involved in urtication may make it difficult for the pathologist to visualize the mast cells with a metachromatic stain [11]. Thus, if one wishes to induce urtication (Darier's sign), the biopsy specimen should be taken from a different lesion. With the onset of lesions later in childhood, adolescence or adult life, the prognosis becomes more guarded [12,13]. In these patients, the skin lesions often persist throughout life and, just as we have seen in this patient, the possibility of extracutaneous involvement is greater. Finally, there is the telangiectatic variety of urticaria pigmentosa called telangiectasia macularis eruptiva perstans. This disease occurs primarily in middle-aged patients and clinically there are few, if any, palpable lesions. The most prominent feature is mottled pigmentation and telangiectasia of the skin of the trunk. Rarely is there extracutaneous involvement, and the prognosis is very good.

Dr. Parker: Dr. Bauer, when you saw this patient, what was your clinical impression?

Dr. Bauer: Our clinical impression was urticaria pigmentosa. Her lesions did urticate.

Dr. Parker: Dr. Haddad will discuss the patient's bone problem.

Dr. John Haddad: This patient's skeletal difficulties seem to be more appropriate for a woman 10 to 20 years older, and yet they mimic idiopathic osteoporosis best of all. Normal serum and urine values undermine the likelihood of intestinal malabsorption, renal tubular osteomalacia, myelomatosis, thyroid and parathyroid disorders. There is no important history of excessive aluminum hydroxide, heparin or corticosteroid therapy. In brief, then, she appears to have experienced an earlier onset of severe osteopenia than would be reasonably explained by idiopathic osteoporosis, and a more protracted course than would be likely for osteolysis secondary to common neoplasias. Despite her impressive history of vertebral, femoral and rib fractures, the radius bone density was not subnormal. This resembles a recently reported case of urticaria pigmentosa with vertebral osteoporosis and a roentgenographically normal appendicular skeleton [14]. As many as 40 per cent of patients with urticaria pigmentosa have roentgenographically detectable bone lesions [15] which often include a focal or generalized sclerotic process in addition to a cystic or stippled demineralization or apparent trabecular loss and thinning [16]. It is of interest that sclerotic lesions can dominate [17], and argues for a complex, imperfectly understood effect of mast cells on the skeleton.

The link between one of the mast cell products, heparin, and bone has derived from "cofactor" promotion of bone resorption in vitro [18], and its association with clinical osteoporosis in subjects receiving 15,000 to 30,000 units/day [19]. Further, an increase in bone mast cells has been observed in animals receiving low calcium diets [20], as well as in the bone marrow of human subjects with osteoporosis [21]. However, the bone lesions in mast cell disorders often show sclerotic foci which are not observed in heparin-induced osteopenia. Therefore, it is likely that other products of the mast cell do contribute directly or indirectly to the disordered skeletal formation and resorption seen in these conditions.

PATHOLOGIC DISCUSSION

Dr. Raul Garza: The skin biopsy specimen did show urticaria pigmentosa. A low power view of the specimen showed clusters of cells around blood vessels in the superficial dermis (Figure 1) beneath a normal epidermis. Under high power view, these cells were oval to

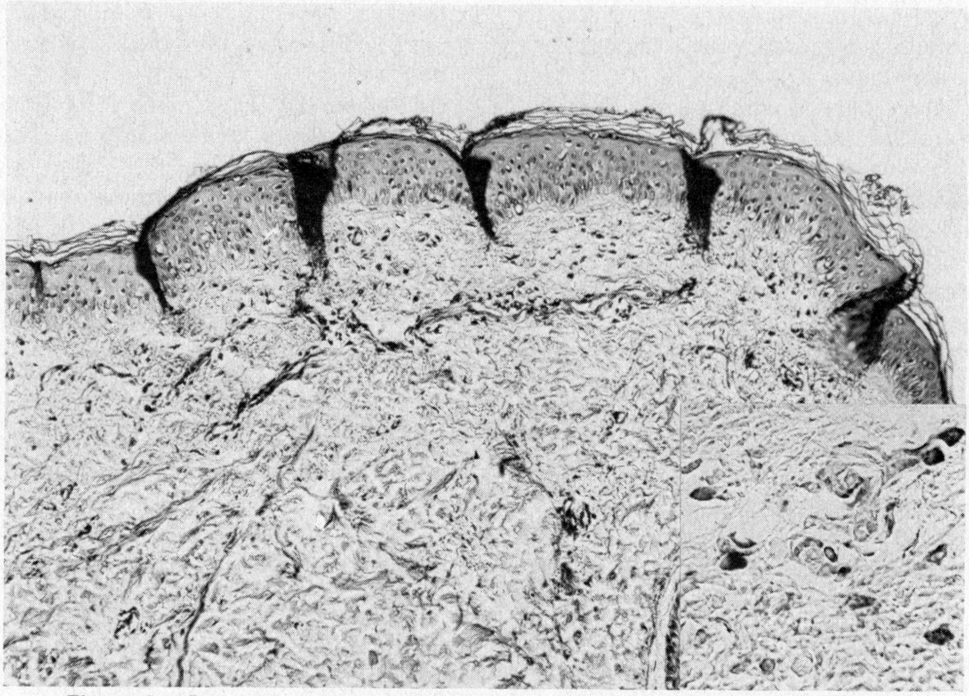

Figure 1. *Punch biopsy specimen of the skin showing an increase in cellularity in the upper dermis mainly around blood vessels. Hematoxylin and eosin stain; original magnification × 150, reduced by 28 per cent.* ***Inset,*** *5 mast cells are seen with a dark cytoplasm (granules). Toluidine blue stain; original magnification × 350, reduced by 28 per cent.*

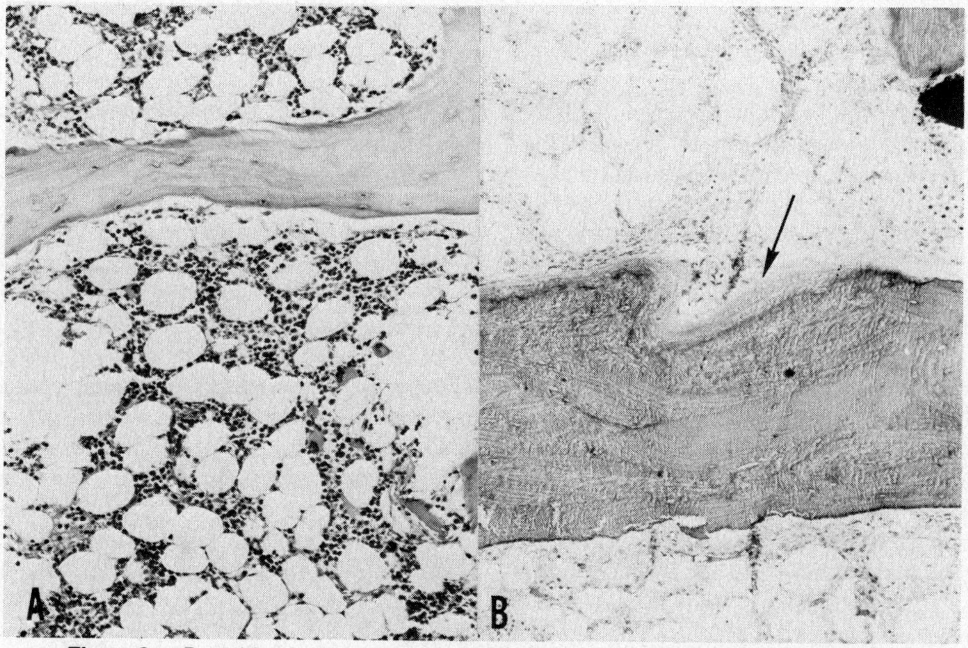

Figure 2. *Bone biopsy specimen showing thinning of the bone spicules and normal looking bone marrow* **(*A*)** *and undecalcified bone section with a rim of osteod* **(*arrow*)** *in the periphery of a bone trabeculum* **(*B*).** *Hematoxylin and eosin stain (A) and Phloxine-Taitrazine stain (B); original magnification × 150, reduced by 28 per cent.*

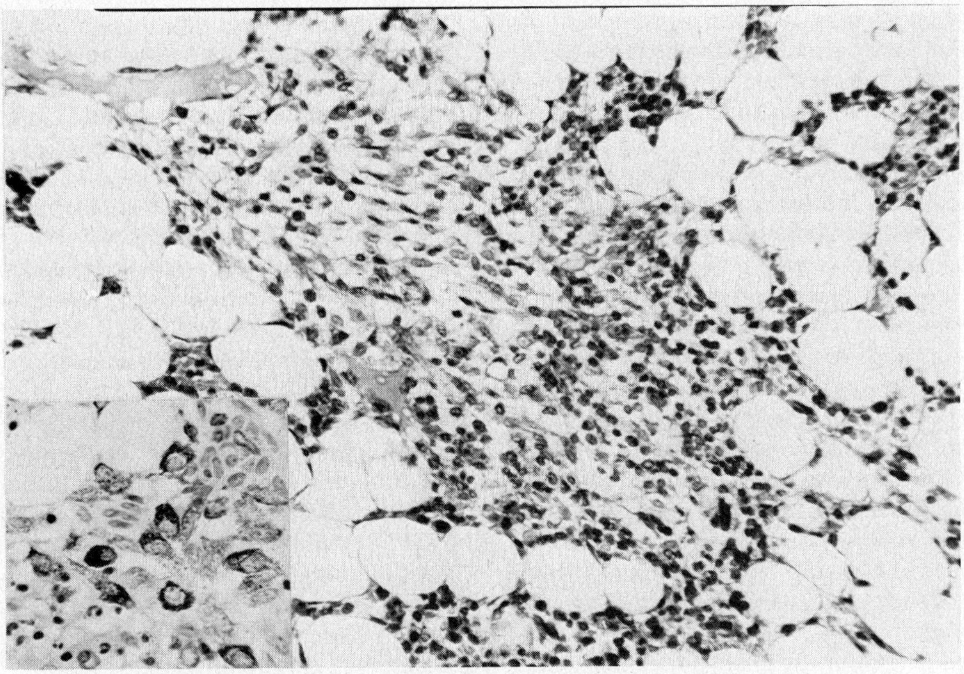

Figure 3. *Bone biopsy specimen under high power showing a granuloma-like formation with mononuclear cells.* ***Inset,*** *mast cells in perivascular arrangement. Hematoxylin and eosin stain; original magnification × 350, reduced by 28 per cent.*

spindle-shaped with a round hyperchromatic nucleus and a slightly basophilic granular cytoplasm. Special stains demonstrated the granules of mast cells; these granules are metachromatic, and with toluidine blue they stain red (Figure 1, inset). The von Leder (nonspecific esterase) stain colors the granules bright orange to red. There were not too many mast cells in the punch biopsy specimen of the skin, but there were enough to make an adequate diagnosis.

The bone biopsy was an open surgical biopsy from the iliac crest. Under low power view, there was thinning of the bone spicules with areas of total or partial loss of the bone trabeculation (Figure 2A). The bone marrow cellularity was about normal in relation to erythroid, myeloid and megakaryocytic series. Scattered throughout the marrow, however, were small granuloma-like foci composed of a slight increase in fibrous tissue and inflammatory cells (Figure 3). With metachromatic staining, these foci showed scattered cells with red granules in their cytoplasm. I must say that this bone biopsy specimen was slightly overdecalcified; this procedure causes granules in mast cells to lose their staining properties but, even with that consideration, there were a good number of mast cells scattered in a perivascular arrangement and they were easily seen in the granuloma-like areas in which they tended to cluster. The Giemsa stain is also useful in showing the mast cells, staining them purple-blue in color.

Fortunately, the surgeon at the time of biopsy sent a piece of bone to Dr. Teitelbaum for uncalcified sections. These sections showed a marked increase in mast cells in the bone marrow with striking perivascular arrangement (Figure 3, inset). The bone itself showed an increase in osteoblastic and osteoclastic activity with prominent deposition of osteoid at the periphery of the trabeculae (Figure 2B) and an over-all decrease in bone mass. In summary, this patient has urticaria pigmentosa with bone lesions consistent with systemic mastocytosis.

Dr. Parker: Thank you. Several of the sources I used in preparing my presentation commented on the danger of missing the diagnosis in decalcified bone samples, due to mast cell degranulation, so I think your suggestion that the decalcification process is responsible for the failure to find large numbers of mast cells in all the bone specimens is correct.

Fortified by a tissue diagnosis of mastocytosis, I would like now to continue my discussion. To begin with, what is known about the etiology of mastocytosis? Since mast cells are critically involved in immediate hypersensitivity reactions, one might wonder about the relationship of mastocytosis to chronic allergic stimulation. In point of fact, there is no evidence whatever that allergies or parasitic infections, in which increased levels of immunoglobulin E (IgE) are incurred over sustained periods of time, in any way predispose to mastocytosis. Nonetheless, it does appear that if mastocytosis is already present and a systemic allergic reaction then occurs the reaction is more likely to be severe; this is not terribly surprising considering the large reservoir of mast cell mediators available in subjects who have this condition. There is one very interesting case report of a patient with carcinoma of the colon associated with mastocytosis in whom the tumor was resected and in whom the mastocytic involvement of the skin disappeared entirely only to reappear when the tumor recurred [22]. Thus, it would appear that mastocytosis may rarely occur as a reaction to a systemic disease. Even though only one such case has been described, further efforts to identify systemic factors which might be chemotactic for mast cells or basophils or which otherwise might promote mast cell infiltration into tissues appear to be well worth pursuing. On the other hand, mastocytosis has been observed to occur with increased frequency in certain families and often begins in infancy, suggesting that it may often be congenital in origin.

Let us now consider how mast cells function under ordinary circumstances. Mast cells contain or rapidly generate a number of substances with potent physiologic activities including histamine, heparin, various mucopolysaccharides, eosinophil chemotactic factor A, slow reacting substance of anaphylaxis (SRS-A), serotonin, one or more kinin generating enzymes and prostaglandins. All these substances appear to be present either in a preformed or a precursor state in granules and are released into the extracellular medium at the time of the releasing stimulus. Histamine is the best known mast cell mediator. It is present in large quantities in mast cells and no doubt contributes importantly to the changes in vascular permeability and smooth muscle tone seen in acute allergic responses. Serotonin, another vasoactive substance, is present in variable amounts in animal mast cells, and probably in human mast cells as well, although this has not been conclusively established. On one or two occasions, increased amounts of 5-hydroxyindoleacetic acid have been demonstrated in the urine of patients with mastocytosis, but as a rule no alterations are found. Enzymes released from stimulated mast cells, and presumably derived from the granules, are capable of activating kinins, which also are vasoactive. SRS-A is another substance of considerable interest in immediate hypersensitivity reactions which Dr. Barbara Jakschik in our Division has recently shown to be definitely present in rat mast cells. It is an acidic lipid of unknown structure with potent bronchoconstrictor activity and less marked effects on vascular reactivity. SRS-A is generated de novo in mast cells at the time of the releasing stimulus and may be the most important pharmacologic mediator in human bronchial asthma. Moreover, mast cells presumably have the synthetic capacity to produce prostaglandins, which also act on smooth muscle and blood vessels. Thus, at least four vasoactive or smooth muscle reactive agents, in addition to histamine, are released when mast cells are stimulated. Heparin, which is also preformed, is well known for its anticoagulant activity, but why it is present in mast cells and what role, if any, it plays in the early or late stages of immediate hypersensitivity responses are not presently clear. Several substances present in mast cells stimulate the directional migration of eosinophils and may be involved in the eosinophilia of bronchial asthma and acute allergic reactions. These include histamine itself as well as two acidic tetrapeptides recently characterized and synthesized in Austen's laboratory [23]. In addition, studies in progress by Dr. Seth Eisen in our group indicate that there is at least one other potent eosinophil chemotactic factor in rat basophilic leukemia cells, presumably in normal basophils and mast cells as well, which has not yet been structurally characterized.

Mast cells are prominently represented in the lung and skin in close association with blood vessels whereas a functionally and morphologically analogous cell, the basophil, is present in peripheral blood. The possibility has been raised that acute hypersensitivity reactions in the lung and skin involve mast cells whereas systemic anaphylactic responses involve circulating basophils, but this is difficult to establish conclusively. Both cell types contain high affinity glycoprotein receptors for IgE on their surfaces. The bond formed between IgE and the receptor is reversible, but it is sufficiently stable that skin sites passively sensitized with IgE antibody sometimes remain reactive for at least several weeks. The cell is unaffected by bound IgE unless antigen is present. Antigen appears to act by cross-linking IgE molecules on the cell surface; when this occurs, there is a very rapid release of granule contents into the extracellular fluid. Exactly how this is achieved is not altogether clear, but studies by Dr. Sullivan in our laboratory as well as those of others suggest that an initial plasma membrane event is followed both by increased uptake of calcium into the cell and alterations in intracellular cyclic adenosine monophosphate [24].

A number of nonimmunologic stimuli, including drugs, polycations, ionophores and extremes of temperature or pH, also result in histamine release. During release, some granules are physically extracted from the cell. Others remain within the cell but, nonetheless, release their mediator content through channels, formed at the time of the allergic stimulus, which communicate directly with the cell exterior. The over-all result of the release reaction is to increase local vascular permeability and fluid accumulation, produce contraction of smooth muscle and stimulate an influx of eosinophils and other leukocytes into the area. Although the utility of this reaction is not altogether clear, IgE-mediated reactions may be of help in resisting parasitic and other infections. In addition to their well recognized role in immediate hypersensitivity, mast cells are important in cellular immune reactions as evidenced by the frequent presence of marked basophilic infiltration in delayed cutaneous reactions to foreign protein antigens.

As far as the syndrome of systemic mastocytosis is concerned, it seems logical to assume that histamine is important in the urticaria, flushing, hypotension, peptic ulceration, facial edema, rhinorrhea and bronchospasm. It is more questionably involved in the eosinophilia, fever and intestinal hypermotility. Since SRS-A, kinins, prostaglandins and serotonin overlap in their pharmacologic effects with histamine, quite possibly they contribute to some of the symptoms. The reason symptoms of flushing tend to be episodic may relate to partial depletion of mast cell mediators after an acute release reaction. In addition, as in pheochromocytoma, sustained low grade mediator release may result in reduced end-organ responsiveness. At a more speculative level, a marked atrophy of lymph node follicles has been noted in mastocytosis on occasion [1]. Moreover, at least one person with this condition has been described as having an impairment of cell-mediated immunity. This is of interest in regard to the observation that lymphocytes appear to have receptors for histamine and that, under appropriate circumstances, histamine inhibits both lymphocyte transformation and lymphocyte-mediated cytotoxicity. It is, therefore, possible that, in at least a few people with mastocytosis, exposure to continuing high levels of histamine might be associated with partial impairment of lymphocyte reactivity. Histamine may also be involved in the liver fibrosis sometimes seen in this condition although this also is speculative. As far as what heparin may be doing, Dr. Haddad mentioned the work that suggests that heparin may be directly involved in the pathogenesis of the osteoporosis. I find that evidence very provocative, although certainly more work is needed. Since prostaglandins are known to have potent effects on bone resorption, they may also be involved. Clinically significant coagulation defects appear to be rare in these patients but, as noted, occasionally there are bleeding manifestations in the skin or gastrointestinal tract in which heparin may be a contributory factor. Heparin stimulates lipoprotein lipase and has been used on occasion as a cholesterol lowering agent helping to explain the moderate degree of hypocholesterolemia seen not infrequently in people with mastocytosis. Finally, it may be worth noting that only about 10 to 15 per cent of the patients with systemic mastocytosis have eosinophilia, which is somewhat surprising if histamine and the acidic tetrapeptides are as potent as chemotactic factors for eosinophils in vivo as they appear to be in vitro. This may be a clue that sensitized lymphocytes are at least as important as mast cells in chronic eosinophilic states.

REFERENCES

1. Sagher F, Even-Paz Z: Mastocytosis and the Mast Cell, Chicago, Year Book Medical Publishers, Inc., 1967.
2. Szweda JA, Abraham JP, Fine G, et al.: Systemic mast cell disease. Am J Med 32: 227, 1962.
3. Maldonado JE, Riggs BL, Bayrd ED: Pseudomyeloma. Arch Intern Med 135: 267, 1975.
4. Rukavina JG, Dickison G, Curtis AC: The simultaneous occurrence of urticaria pigmentosa and primary systemic amyloidosis. Report of a case with autopsy findings. J Invest Dermatol 28: 243, 1975.
5. Demis DJ: The mastocytosis syndrome. Clinical and biological studies. Ann Intern Med 59: 194, 1963.
6. Mutter RD, Tannenbaum M, Ultmann JE: Systemic mast cell disease. Ann Intern Med 59: 887, 1963.
7. Dolovich J, Punthakee ND, MacMillan AB, et al.: Systemic mastocytosis: control of lifelong diarrhea by ingested disodium cromoglycate. Can Med Assoc J 111: 684, 1974.
8. Capute AJ, Rimoin DL, Konigsmark BW, et al.: Congenital deafness and multiple lentigenes. Arch Dermatol 100: 207, 1969.
9. Smith RF, Pulicicchio LU, Holmes AV: Generalized lentigo. Electrocardiographic abnormalities, conduction disorders and arrhythmias in three cases. Am J Cardiol 25: 501, 1970.
10. Klaus SN, Winkelmann RK: Course of urticaria pigmentosa in children. Arch Dermatol 86: 68, 1962.
11. Parker F, Odland GF: The mastocytosis syndrome. Dermatology in General Medicine (Fitzpatrick TB, Arndt KA, Clark WH Jr, Eisen AZ, Van Scott EJ, Vaughn JH, eds), New York, McGraw-Hill Book Co., 1971.
12. Caplan RM: Urticaria pigmentosa and systemic mastocytosis. JAMA 194: 1077, 1965.
13. Caplan RM: The natural course of urticaria pigmentosa. Arch Dermatol 87: 146, 1963.
14. Ives DR: Urticaria pigmentosa with spinal osteoporosis. Proc Roy Soc Med 66: 175, 1973.
15. Poppel MH, Gruber WF, Sibber R, et al.: Roentgen manifestations of urticaria pigmentosa (mastocytosis). Am J Roentgenol Radium Ther Nucl Med 82: 239, 1959.
16. Sagher F, Schorr S: Bone lesions in urticaria pigmentosa. Report of central registry on skeletal x-ray survey. J Invest Dermatol 26: 431, 1956.
17. Bendel WL Jr, Race GJ: Urticaria pigmentosa with bone in-

volvement. J Bone Joint Surg 45: 1043, 1963.
18. Goldhaber P: Heparin enhancement of factors stimulating bone resorption in tissue culture. Science 147: 407, 1964.
19. Griffith GC, Nichols G Jr, Asher JD, et al.: Heparin osteoporosis. JAMA 193: 85, 1965.
20. Urist MR, McLean FC: Accumulation of mast cells in endosteum of bones of calcium-deficient rats. Arch Pathol 63: 239, 1957.
21. Frame B, Nixon RK: Bone marrow mast cells in osteoporosis of aging. N Engl J Med 279: 626, 1968.
22. Cohen HJ, Raisbeck MJ, Baer RL: Acquired (adult) urticaria pigmentosa. Disappearance after removal of intestinal carcinoma. Dermatologica 121: 386, 1960.
23. Goetzl EJ, Austen FK: Purification and synthesis of eosinophilotactic tetrapeptides of human lung tissue. Identification as eosinophil chemotactic factor of anaphylaxis. Proc Natl Acad Sci 72: 4123, 1975.
24. Sullivan TJ, Parker CW: Pharmacological modulation of the inflammatory mediator release by rat mast cells. Am J Pathol (in press).

Selected and edited by Richard T. Silver, M.D. and Alexander G. Bearn, M.D.
Department of Medicine, The New York Hospital-Cornell Medical Center, New York, New York

Prostaglandins and Blood Pressure Control

Moderator:
HENRY O. HEINEMANN, M.D.
New York, New York

Lecturer:
JAMES B. LEE, M.D.*
Buffalo, New York

From the Department of Medicine, The New York Hospital-Cornell Medical Center, New York, New York; and the Section of Hypertension, Department of Medicine, State University of New York at Buffalo, School of Medicine, Buffalo General Hospital, Buffalo, New York. Requests for reprints should be addressed to Dr. James B. Lee, Department of Medicine, Buffalo General Hospital, 100 High Street, Buffalo, New York 14203. The lecturer is grateful to Dr. Bas Mookerjee, Veterans Administration Hospital, Buffalo, New York for critically reviewing this manuscript. Manuscript accepted February 27, 1976.

* Research supported by grants-in-aid from Hoechst AG, Frankfurt, Germany and Hoechst-Roussel, Somerville, New Jersey, U.S.A.

The prostaglandins are a group of ubiquitous, hormone-like substances that participate in numerous processes in the human body. The immense accumulation of information about these compounds, first described more than 40 years ago [1–3], leave the noninitiated reader bewildered and uncertain about their physiologic role.

Prostaglandins are a family of 20 carbon unsaturated lipids which differ in their side chains. They are formed by an enzyme system present in many tissues from several precursors, of which the most common is arachidonic acid. Prostaglandins are not stored in tissues but appear in response to stimuli originating locally or reaching the site of formation via humoral or neurogenic pathways. The newly synthesized prostaglandins may enter the circulation via effluent blood and, depending on their structural characteristics, are effectively inactivated in either the pulmonary vascular bed or the liver.

In this Combined Clinical and Basic Science Seminar the discussion will be limited to the potential involvement of prostaglandins in blood pressure control. This subject cannot be reviewed without mentioning the role of these compounds in modulating renal blood flow. The kidneys, as an integral part of the circulatory system, are intimately concerned with the control of the composition and volume of extracellular fluid. It is not surprising, therefore, that the kidneys, which have a unique capacity to modulate the flow and distribution of blood reaching this organ, are also involved in the control of systemic blood pressure which has such immediate effects upon renal blood flow and glomerular filtration.

To what extent the kidneys depend upon prostaglandins for autoregulation of the total renal blood flow, that is, maintenance of flow despite wide variations in blood pressure, remains a controversial subject. The role of prostaglandins in the intrarenal distribution of total blood flow between cortical and medullary components of the organ is also uncertain at this time.

The control mechanisms regulating renal blood flow rely on the negative feedback principle. One of these feedback loops which becomes operative in situations characterized by reduced renal blood flow has been well defined and involves the renin-angiotensin system as the messenger and the kidneys, and the adrenal glands as the target organs. Angiotensin II, generated from its precursor angiotensin I by a converting enzyme mainly localized within the lung, contributes via its pressor effect to blood pressure control and via the formation of aldosterone in the adrenal gland and subsequent sodium retention to extracellular fluid volume regulation. In disease, in which the signals for this feedback principle are distorted, angiotensin II may contribute to inappropriate increases in blood pressure and to body fluid retention.

A question frequently raised is whether there is a second feedback loop which serves to lower blood pressure and promote sodium and water excretion; if, in fact, such a control system does exist, does it originate in the kidneys and do prostaglandins play a role in it? It is easy to ask these questions, but it is difficult to examine the available evidence in a meaningful way. We are fortunate to have as our guest today Dr. James B. Lee, Professor of Medicine at the State University of New York in Buffalo, one of the pioneers in this field of rapidly expanding research, who will review for us the role of prostaglandins in blood pressure control.

HISTORICAL ASPECTS

James B. Lee: Biologic activity of a class of compounds now known as prostaglandins was discovered independently in the early 1930's by von Euler [1], Goldblatt [2] and Kurzrok and Lieb [3]. They independently observed that extracts of sheep seminal vesicles or human semen given to animals lowered blood pressure and produced contraction of nonvascular smooth muscle. Von Euler further characterized the responsible compounds as fatty acids and named them prostaglandins. For the next 25 years the field remained relatively quiescent. Then, in 1960, Bergström and Sjövall [4,5] reported the isolation of two classes of prostaglandins, prostaglandin E (PGE) and prostaglandin F (PGF) from sheep seminal vesicles. Bergström and his co-workers [6] subsequently elucidated the chemical structure of these two classes of prostaglandins. Figure 1 shows that the prostaglandins are 20 carbon fatty acids with a five membered cyclopentane ring. The PGE class differs from the PGF class by virtue of a ketone group at position 9 in the five membered ring. The PGF class has a hydroxyl in this position. Otherwise, the two compounds are identical. The prostaglandins are called PG_1, PG_2 or PG_3 depending on whether there are one, two or three double bonds in the aliphatic side chains, respectively. It was observed that these compounds not only have an effect on blood pressure but that they also have other biologic actions affecting virtually every tissue or organ system in the body. For instance, depending on the species and the type of prostaglandin, prostaglandins are important in central nervous system neurotransmission; they mediate light adapted myosis in the eye, stimulate thyroidal and steroidal hormonogenesis, dilate or constrict bronchiolar smooth muscle, inhibit gastric hydrochloric acid secretion and experimental peptic ulcer production, produce or inhibit platelet aggregation, induce labor and act as abortifacients at all stages of pregnancy, produce bone reabsorption, and are important mediators of inflammatory and immune responses. These examples are not the only actions of this ubiquitous class of compounds but they illustrate their diverse biologic activity.

Unaware of these early developments, we observed in 1961 that extracts of rabbit renal medulla, when injected into rats treated with pentolinium and pentobarbital [7,8], lowered blood pressure. The rationale for these early experiments was that hypertension may not solely be due to mechanisms which increase blood pressure but that it may be the consequence of a deficiency of compounds which lower blood pressure. Thus "normal" vascular tone and normotension might be the net result of vasoconstrictor influences being equally offset by vasodilating influences. An acquired or hereditary deficiency of vasodilators might allow vasoconstrictors to act unopposed producing arteriolar vasoconstriction and hypertension even when levels of these pressor factors are normal. Space does not permit a detailed analysis of the evidence for this so-called "deprivation theory" or renal antihypertensive endocrine function. The interested reader is referred to reviews dealing with this controversial subject [9,10].

The material in the rabbit renal medulla responsible for its blood pressure lowering effects was found to be a dialyzable, ethanol-soluble fatty acid of low molecular weight [8]. Three compounds were subsequently isolated, two of which were capable of lowering blood pressure [11]. These were compound 1, compound 2 and medullin (Figure 2). Now aware of the earlier observations on prostaglandins, we believed compound 1 to be prostaglandin F since it had no vasodepressor activities but possessed marked nonvascular smooth muscle stimulating activity. Compound 2 was believed to be a prostaglandin E since it had both vasodepressor and nonvascular smooth muscle stimulating activities. However, the third isolate, originally called medullin, was devoid of nonvascular stimulating smooth muscle activity, but had potent vasodepressor activity. This compound was subsequently identified as 15-hydroxy-9-oxoprosta 5, 10, 13 trienoic acid [12,13] and was the first of the prostaglandin A (PGA) compounds to be isolated (Figure 3). PGA_1 as well as PGA_2 were also independently identified in human semen by Hamberg and Samuelsson [14]. Compound 1 was identified as $PGF_{2\alpha}$ and compound 2 as PGE_2 (Figure 3).

BIOSYNTHESIS AND METABOLISM

Synthesis. Prostaglandins are biosynthesized from essential fatty acids. PGE_1, PGE_2 and PGE_3 are formed when the precursor fatty acids di-homo-γ-linolenic acid, arachidonic and cis-eicosapentanoic acid are, respectively, incubated with sheep vesicular gland homogenates [15,16]. $PGF_{2\alpha}$ can also be formed using arachidonic acid as substrate [17]. In Figure 4 the pathway for the formation of the PG_2 class from di-homo-γ-linolenic acid is shown. The conversion requires molecular oxygen and is accomplished by an enzyme conglomerate, prostaglandin synthetase. An intermediate cyclic endoperoxide is in turn converted to PGE_2 and $PGF_{2\alpha}$. Although most of the studies of biosynthesis of prostaglandins have been carried out with sheep seminal vesicles, the same general reaction appears to be true in most tissues in which prostaglandins are formed. Although these biosynthetic pathways are well known for PGE and PGF compounds, little is known about the synthesis of PGA or PGE by the renal medulla, and convincing evidence for enzymatic conversion of arachidonic acid or PGE_2 to PGA_2 in renal medulla is lacking [18]. Studies in other tissues suggest that there is an enzymatic mechanism for the conversion of arachidonic acid to PGA_2 [19]. It is possible that the correct conditions of incubation with renal medulla have yet to be defined, particularly with regard to the presence of glutathione and variations in oxygen tension and sodium chloride concentration in the medium [20,21]. The oxygen tension of the renal medulla is normally low. Changes in renal medullary blood flow would alter the oxygen tension and also modify the sodium chloride concentration in this tissue. Thus the many variables which can affect PGA biosynthesis will have to be studied before it can be concluded that this compound is not synthesized by this tissue.

The distribution of prostaglandin synthetase was studied in detail by Larsson and Änggård [22] who showed that the formation of PGE_2 was highest in the papilla and that it decreased toward the outer medulla. The cortex, which contains only trace amounts of PGE_2, nevertheless, has a significant capacity to synthesize PGE_2. Prostaglandin synthetase activity is located mainly in the microsomal fraction [23] and over-all synthesis is markedly inhibited by nonsteroidal anti-flammatory agents such as aspirin, indomethacin and phenylbutazone [24]. Formed prostaglandins are predominantly recovered in the cytosol fractions suggesting that on completion of prostaglandin synthesis by the endoplasmic reticulum, the prostaglandins are released into the extracellular space almost immediately.

Utilizing histochemical technics, Nissen and Andersen [25] found high prostaglandin biosynthetic activity in the inner medulla of rabbits, particularly in the collecting ducts and in the renal medullary interstitial cells. The latter cells are believed to be in large part responsible for renal prostaglandin synthesis. They are fibroblastic-like cells containing numerous lipid droplets composed of triglycerides and phospholipids presumably containing prostaglandin precursors such as arachidonic acid in esterified form (Figure 5). Tissue cultures of these cells from renomedullary transplants convert arachidonic acid to PGA_2, PGE_2 and $PGF_{2\alpha}$ [26]. The composition and number of the lipid droplets can be altered by manipulations such as induction of experimental hypertension, administration of the prostaglandin synthetase inhibitor, indomethacin and sodium chloride loading. In man, the interstitial cells are not only located at random throughout the renal papilla, but also appear as clusters in the outer medulla [27,28]. These prostaglandin-rich cell clusters are visible as discrete, yellow, nonencapsulated nodules [27]. The exact role of the cluster of renal medullary interstitial cells remains unclear, but it has been suggested that they may represent an evolutionary modification of the renal medullary interstitial cell system which may have a function in either sodium homeostasis or blood pressure regulation [27].

Metabolism. The PGE and PGF compounds are largely inactivated by the lung [29,30]. This would preclude that these substances have a role as circulating hormones. By contrast, the PGA compounds are not metabolized during a single passage through the lungs [31,32]. These circulating compounds may, therefore, have a role in the regulation of systemic blood pressure. Both PGA_1 and PGA_2 are transformed by the liver [32], and PGA_2 is converted to less polar metabolites by homogenates of the renal cortex but not the outer medulla [33,34]. In vivo, PGA_2 is converted in almost a single passage through the kidney to less polar metabolites. The enzymes responsible for degradation of prostaglandins are located primarily in the renal cortex with little activity in the renal medulla [22]; they appear to be specific PGA dehydrogenases which are competitively inhibited by ethacrynic acid and do not require NAD^+ [35].

Transport. The prostaglandins are transported in plasma primarily bound to albumin [36,37]. The affinity of PGE compounds to plasma proteins decreases as the number of polar groups in the cyclopentane ring increases. PGA, the least polar of the prostaglandins, is bound more tightly than PGE which, in turn, is more firmly bound than the PGF class. The metabolism of PGA to less polar metabolites is albumin-dependent [38]. In the absence of albumin, almost 65 per cent of PGA is metabolized, whereas in the presence of 4.5 g/100 ml of human serum albumin only 35 per cent PGA_1 is metabolized. The lack of PGA transformation by the lung may be a consequence of the binding to albumin, and the ability of the kidney cortex to metabolize PGA may result from the presence of specific binding sites [39] which are, in fact, PGA metabolizing enzymes [35].

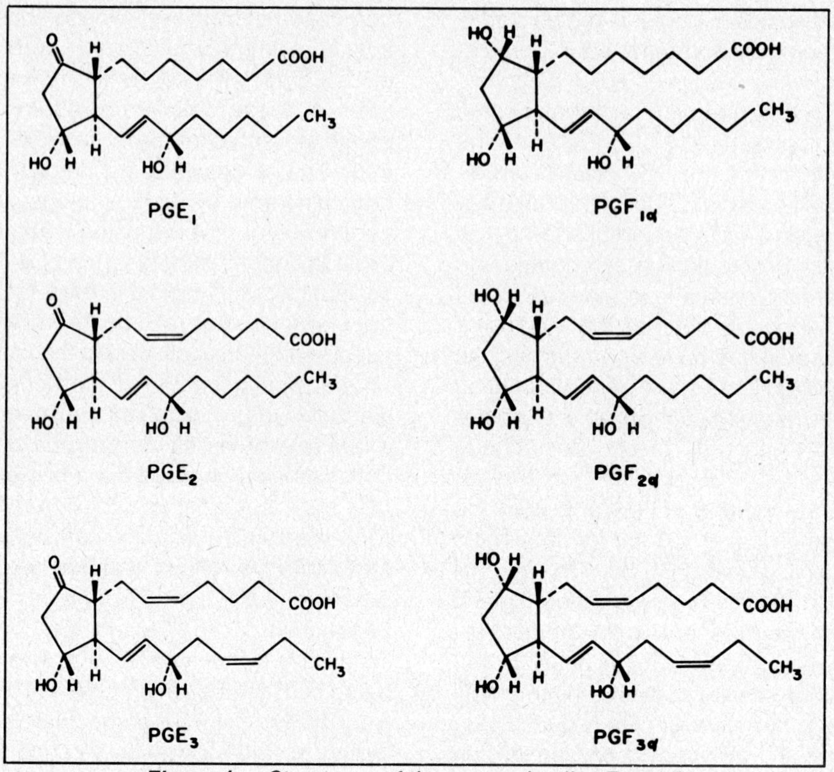

Figure 1. *Structures of the prostaglandins E and F.*

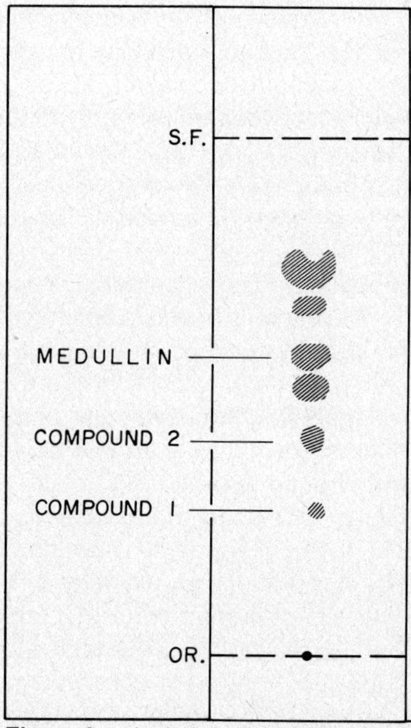

SPOT	R_f	DEPRESSOR ACTIVITY	JEJUNAL STIM.
6	.68–.80	–	–
5	.66–.67	–	–
4	.57–.60	++++	+
3	.50–.55	–	–
2	.40–.45	++++	+++
1	.27–.30	+	+++
0	0	–	–

Figure 2. *Isolation of medullin, compound 1 and compound 2 from rabbit medulla by thin layer chromatography. Unlike compound 1 and 2, medullin was devoid of nonvascular smooth muscle stimulating activity. OR = origin; SF = solvent front. From Lee et al. [11] with permission of the publisher.*

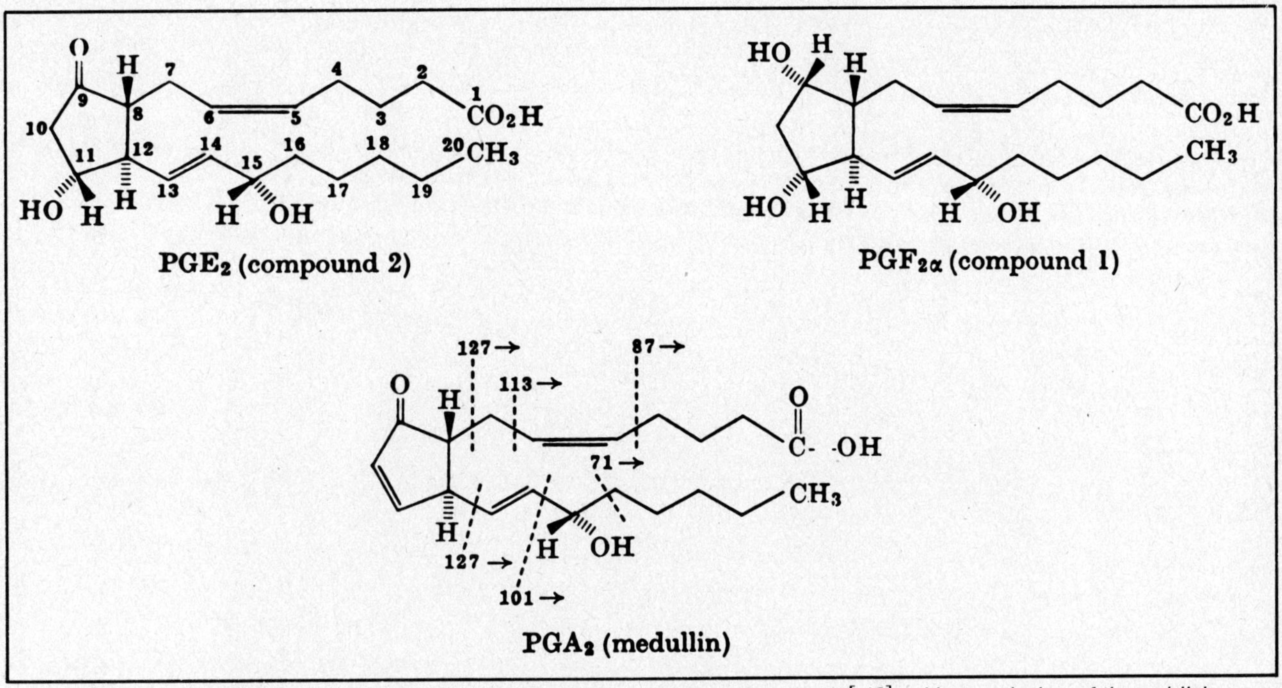

Figure 3. *Identification of the renomedullary prostaglandins. From Lee et al. [13] with permission of the publisher.*

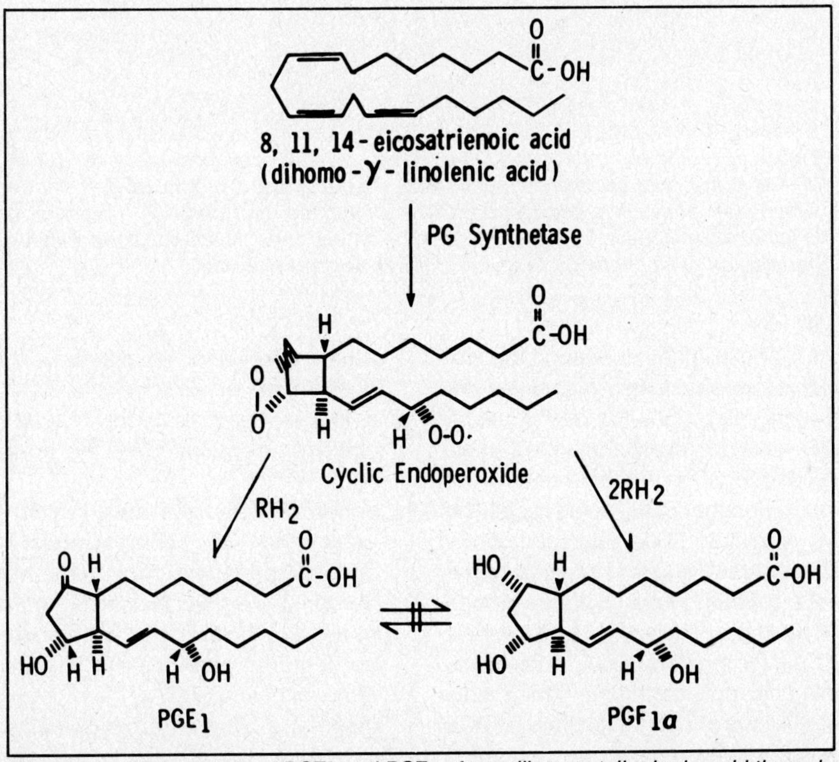

Figure 4. *Biosynthesis of PGE_1 and $PGF_{1\alpha}$ from dihomo-γ-linolenic acid through the intermediate cyclic endoperoxide.*

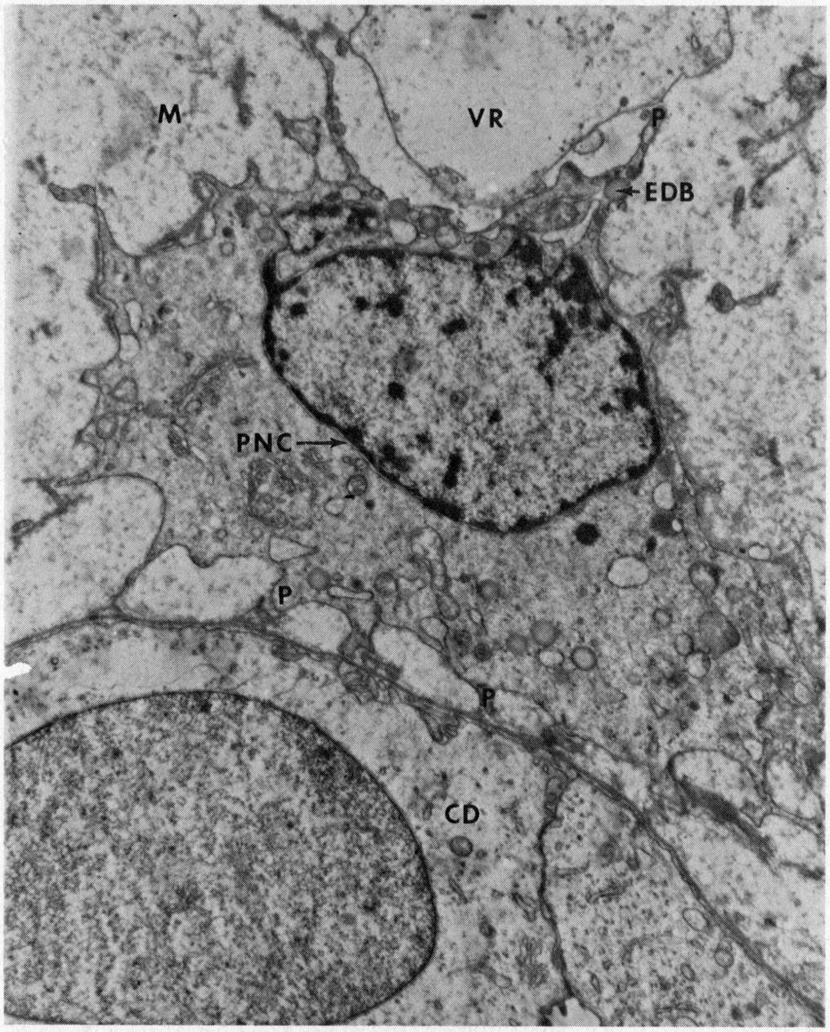

Figure 5. Electron microscopy of a rabbit interstitial cell from the renal papilla. M = acid mucopolysaccharide matrix; PNC = perinuclear cycterna; EDB = electron dense (fat) body; P = pseudopod; CD = collecting duct cell; VR = vasarecta. Original magnification × 8,130, reduced by 44 per cent. Illustration used with kind permission of Dr. Anthony Prezyna, Buffalo General Hospital.

PGA Fact or Artifact. The original studies on the isolation and identification of renomedullary prostaglandins suggested that they were fatty acids for they could be extracted from acid but not from alkaline aqueous media [11]. During the final identification procedures of these compounds, it was observed that PGE_2 could readily be dehydrated nonenzymatically to PGA_2 upon addition of acid to the media. This led us to suggest that part of the PGA identified from the renal medulla could have been formed by the acidification procedures [13]. Crowshaw [18] failed to detect biosynthesis of PGA in homogenates of renal medulla utilizing glutathione in the media and concluded that PGA is probably an artifact of PGE dehydration. Others [40,41] more recently also failed to detect PGA_2 in either fresh preparations of rabbit renal medulla or in plasma. This has led many to question the existence of the PGA compounds. Although it now appears that freshly removed rabbit renal medulla does not contain PGA_2, the conclusion that all PGA_2 observed under any condition is an artifact of PGE_2 dehydration appears unwarranted. As mentioned before, enzymatic PGA_2 synthesis from PGE_2 in other tissues, under appropriate conditions, has been convincingly demonstrated. Furthermore, in the studies of Frohlich et al. [41] the technics were such that only PGA_2 could be detected and thus the possibility could not be excluded that (1) PGA_1 might be circulating in human plasma, or (2) that a biologically active metabolite of PGA might be present. In summary, certain classes of PGA arise as an artifact of PGE dehydration, but this does not warrant the conclusion that all PGA is an artifact. Rather, it points out the need for carefully designed experiments to exclude artifactual dehydration of PGE to PGA.

HEMODYNAMIC MECHANISMS

Normotensive Animals and Man. Extrarenal effects: Investigations of the mechanism of the blood pressure lowering action of the prostaglandins have shown that both PGE and PGF compounds lower blood pressure by direct peripheral arteriolar dilation. Figure 6 shows the results of early experiments with PGA_2 (medullin). This compound caused a greater decrease in diastolic than systolic blood pressure, leading to an increase in pulse pressure. The cardiac output increased significantly at the time of maximal vasodepression, and the calculated total peripheral resistance decreased. The increase in cardiac output was almost entirely due to a reflex (baroreceptor-mediated) increase in heart rate. In vitro preparations have shown that PGA has little, if any, effect on cardiac contractility or cardiac rate in the isolated perfused Langendorf rabbit heart preparation [11].

The precise biochemical mechanism by which prostaglandins dilate peripheral arterioles is unknown. Studies on the microcirculation have shown that prostaglandins appear to dilate almost all segments of this system including arterioles, metarterioles, precapillary sphincters and venules [42]. There is also an increase in the capillary filtration coefficient suggesting enhanced capillary permeability [43]. In contrast to the action of PGA and PGE in producing peripheral arteriolar dilation, PGF tends to increase blood pressure primarily by increasing venous constriction [44].

In animals, the intravenous administration of PGE and PGA induces a decrease in blood pressure which is not sustained. The blood pressure returns to control levels despite continuing infusion of PGE or PGA. In normotensive man, the intravenous infusion of PGE or PGA has little effect upon systemic hemodynamics [45,46].

The infusion of PGE or PGA into regional vascular beds of both animals and man uniformly increased blood flow [47–49]. The increase in regional blood flow observed with PGA and PGE is not associated with any significant changes in blood pressure, with one notable exception. The infusion of PGA or PGE into the splanchnic artery results in a concomitant decrease in blood pressure, suggesting that the splanchnic vascular bed is a major resistance bed whose dilation by prostaglandins results in decreasing systemic blood pressure [48]. In man, as in animals, it is likely that prostaglandin-induced splanchnic vasodilation is the major cause for blood pressure reduction.

Although PGA and PGE both produce peripheral arteriolar dilation and a decrease in blood pressure, there

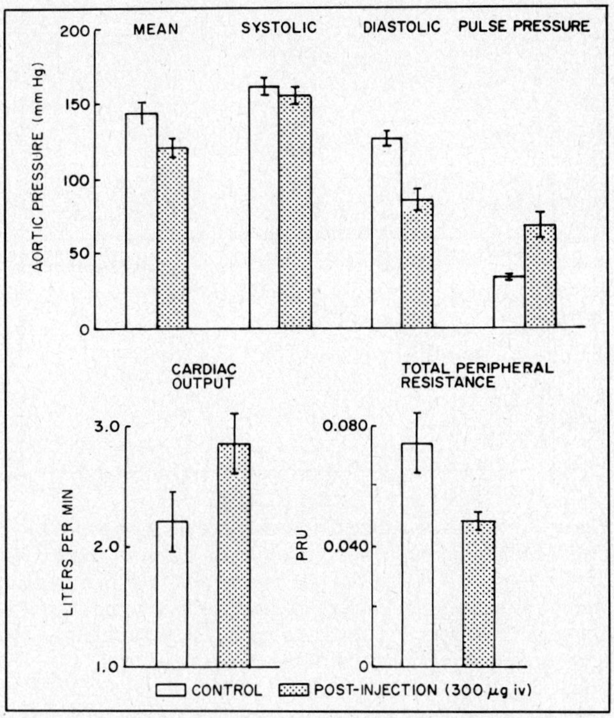

Figure 6. *Hemodynamic effects of medullin (PGA_2) in the pentobarbital anesthetized dog. Decrease in blood pressure is associated with the increase in cardiac output secondary to a decrease in total peripheral resistance. PRU = peripheral resistant unit. From Lee et al. [11] with permission of the publisher.*

are notable differences between these two compounds. First, as already mentioned, PGA, but not PGE, escapes degradation by the lung [31]. Second, PGA does not have the nonvascular smooth muscle stimulating activity of PGE. Third, the onset and duration of the action of PGA and PGE is quite different. Injection of PGE into the aorta of the anesthetized cat results in an immediate reduction in blood pressure [50]. This reflects events taking place between the aorta and the lung since PGE is ineffective upon intravenous administration. The action of PGA is much slower in onset, the decrease in blood pressure not becoming maximal for a period of some 80 seconds (Figure 7). Since PGA is not metabolized by the lung, it is possible that it recirculates producing a secondary series of events (conversion to an active metabolite? release of vasoactive peptides such as bradykinin?) leading to peripheral arteriolar dilation.

The fourth major difference is that in vitro, unlike PGE, PGA markedly inhibits oxygen consumption and sodium, potassium ATPase activity in cortical and outer medullary renal tissue. This has raised the possibility that the natriuretic effects of PGA might be mediated through inhibition of energy-releasing reaction sequences necessary for sodium reabsorption. These differences between PGA and PGE may underlie their potential

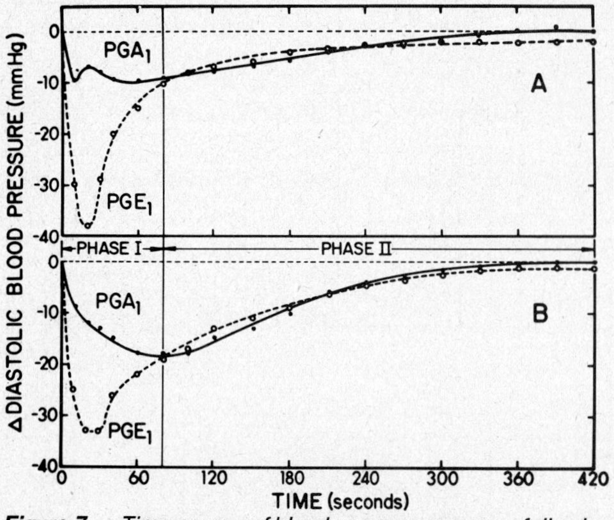

Figure 7. *Time course of blood pressure response following prostaglandin administration high in the aorta of the anesthetized cat. A = nonpentolium treated animals. B = pentolium treated animals. Each point represents the mean of six animals. Prostaglandin dose: 80 ng ia. From Kennegiesser et al. [50] with permission of the publisher.*

physiologic role in regulating systemic blood pressure, renal blood flow and sodium balance which will be discussed.

Renal effects: The actions of PGA and PGE compounds on the kidney are extremely complex. As with other regional vascular systems, the infusion of PGE or PGA into the renal artery uniformly leads to an increase in renal blood flow (Figure 8) [12]. This increase in renal blood flow is accompanied by an increased formation of urine from the infused but not the control kidney. The increase in urine formation is the result of an osmotic diuresis owing to large increments in sodium and potassium excretion. The increase in renal blood flow [51,52] may be caused by redistribution of blood flow to the inner cortex and medulla [53–55] by PGA or PGE, or by prostaglandin vasodilator action on the arterioles of the inner cortex.

The redistribution of renal blood flow and natriuresis by prostaglandins are not unique for these compounds, since similar response patterns have been observed after the administration of furosemide, acetylcholine, ethacrynic acid and saline solution. Thus, the natriuretic effects of these and other agents might be mediated by intrarenal release of prostaglandin. In fact, Williamson et al. [56] recently observed that the increase in renal blood flow induced by ethacrynic acid was practically eliminated by the prior administration of indomethacin, a prostaglandin synthetase inhibitor.

The conflicting data on the physiologic role for PGAs and PGEs synthesized in the renal medulla will have to await additional information before any definite conclusions can be drawn. Nonetheless, currently available information suggests that PGE_2 or PGA_2 are synthesized in the renal medulla, circulate to inner cortex to produce inner cortical efferent arteriolar vasodilation in response to many stimuli. For example, prostaglandins released concomitantly with vasoconstrictor stimuli would, because of their antagonistic action, promote normalization of cortical blood flow. Vasodilator stimuli which would primarily increase inner cortical blood flow, such as diuretics or saline infusion, may stimulate prostaglandin synthesis in the medulla leading to a prostaglandin-mediated increase in inner cortical blood flow with associated natriuresis.

The mechanism of action whereby PGE and PGA compounds promote sodium excretion is unknown. It appears that the PGE_2 is much more potent than PGA_2 in its action on renal blood flow, sodium and water excretion. Both compounds, in common with infusion of saline solution, markedly increase sodium, potassium and water excretion with an increase in free water and total solute clearance, there is an increase in inner

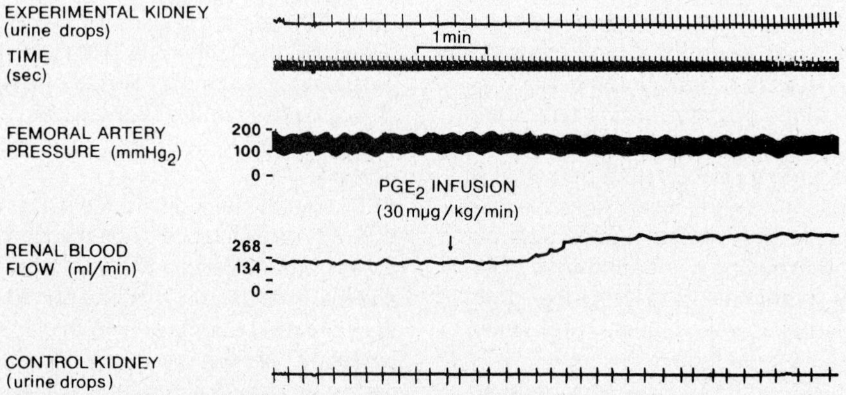

Figure 8. *Effect of PGE_2 on renal blood flow and urine formation in the pentobarbitalized anesthetized dog. From Lee et al. [12] with permission of the publisher.*

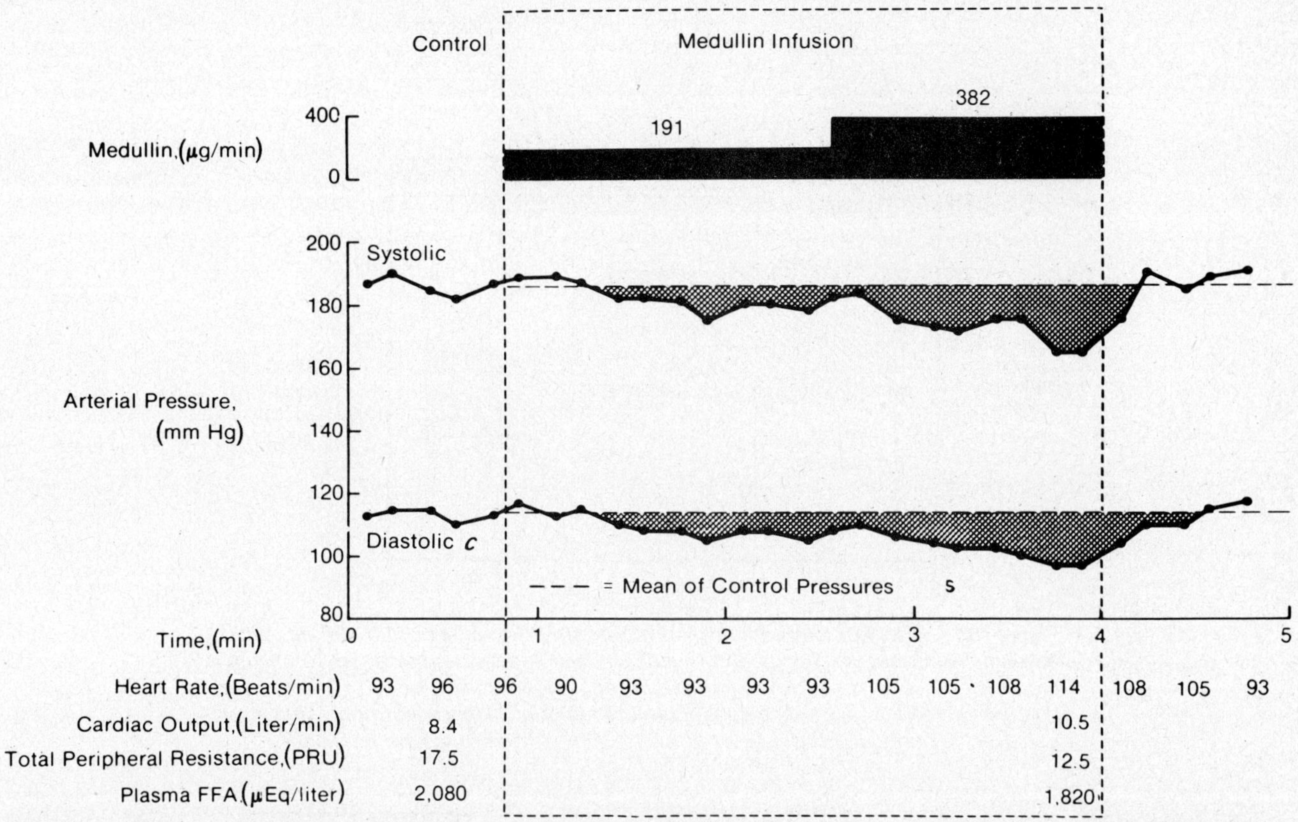

Figure 9. *Effect of intravenous administration of medullin (PGA_2) in a patient with fixed diastolic hypertension. Decrease in blood pressure is associated with an increase in cardiac output (heart rate) secondary to a decrease in total peripheral resistance. FFA = free fatty acids. From Lee et al.* [12] *with permission of the publisher.*

cortical blood flow with an unchanged or slightly increased glomerular filtration rate. The similarities between the infusion of prostaglandin and of saline solution have led to the suggestion that the prostaglandins which are normally present in the renal medulla may be responsible, at least in part, for the activity attributed to the so-called renal natriuretic "hormone" [57].

The increase in free water clearance is quite small since the increase in osmolal clearance accounts for over 90 per cent of the increase in urinary flow. Nevertheless, it is possible that the prostaglandins may have a direct action on water reabsorption conceivably by an inhibitory effect on renal medullary adenyl cyclase activity [58].

Hypertensive Animals and Man. Animals: Prostaglandins of the A and E series, given in large doses, have been shown to reduce blood pressure in animals with renoprival hypertension, renovascular hypertension and in those with spontaneous hypertension when given as intravenous infusions [59,60]. The mechanism of action is similar to that observed in normotensive animals, for the reduction in blood pressure is primarily the result of a decrease in peripheral resistance. On the other hand, Muirhead and his co-workers have presented data which suggest that PGAs may also alter the arterial blood pressure in the spontaneously hypertensive rat by indirect mechanisms including a central action mediated by the vagus nerve [60]. In the spontaneously hypertensive rat the administration of arachidonic acid, PGE_1 and PGE_2 results in a decrease in arterial blood pressure accompanied by an increase in heart rate [61]. After the administration of prostaglandin synthetase inhibitors, the cardiovascular responses to arachidonic acid are inhibited whereas those to PGEs are not. These results were interpreted to mean that the blood pressure lowering effects in hypertensive animals induced by arachidonic acid are mediated by its conversion to PGE_2. Thus, prostaglandins are capable of lowering blood pressure not only in normotensive animals but also in animals with various forms of experimental hypertension.

Patients with Essential Hypertension. The first prostaglandin to be infused into a patient with essential hypertension was PGA_2 isolated from the kidney as medullin [12]. The patient was a 25 year old woman with fixed diastolic essential hypertension. Her blood pressure, which averaged 190/120 mm Hg, was resistant to diuretic therapy, guanethidine and hydralazine. Figure 9 shows that at an infusion rate of 191 μg/minute of medullin (PGA_2) the blood pressure level fell from

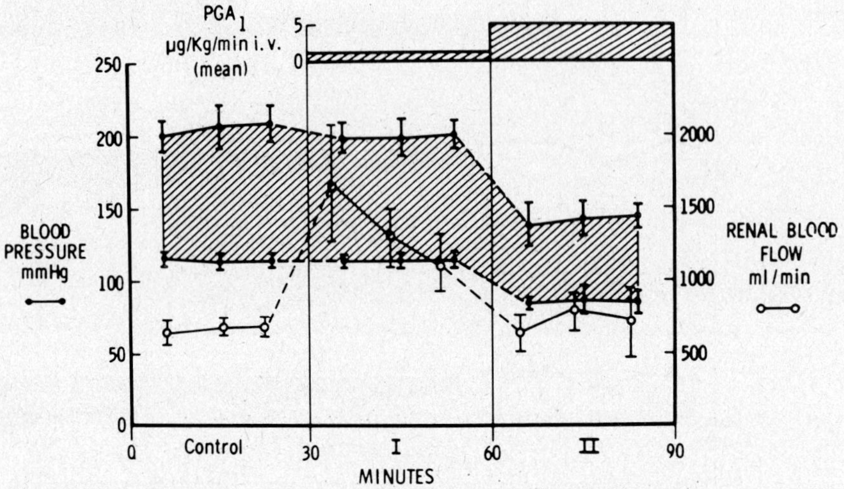

Figure 10. *Effect of intravenously administered PGA_1 in six of 20 patients with essential hypertension. Each period (control, I and II) consisted of three 10 minute clearance observations. Note increase in renal blood flow in period I before any change in blood pressure and subsequent fall to control when normotension was achieved in period II. From Lee et al. [63] with permission of the publisher.*

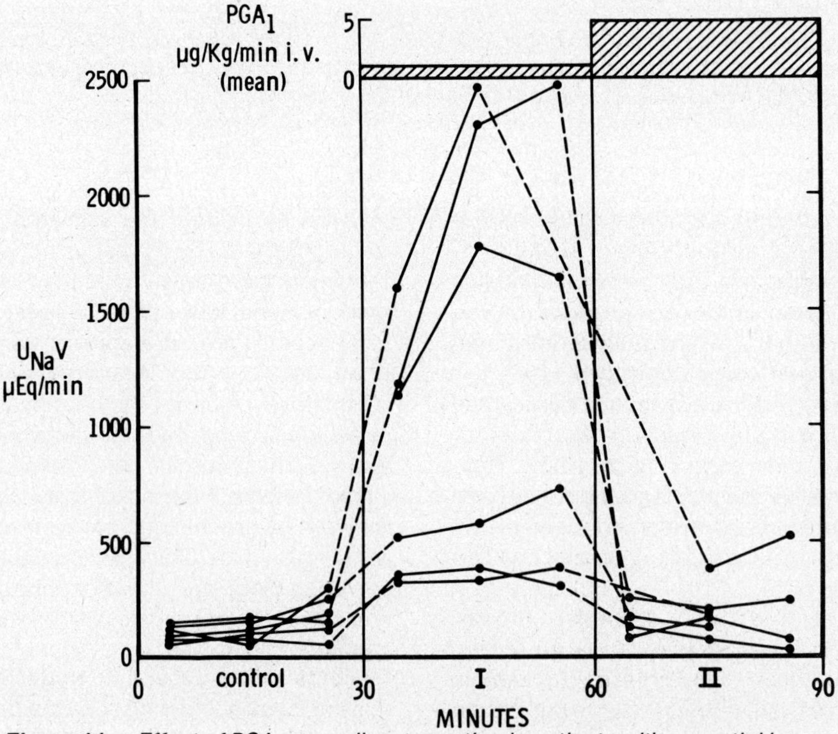

Figure 11. *Effect of PGA_1 on sodium excretion in patients with essential hypertension. Same conditions as Figure 10. From Lee et al. [63] with permission of the publisher.*

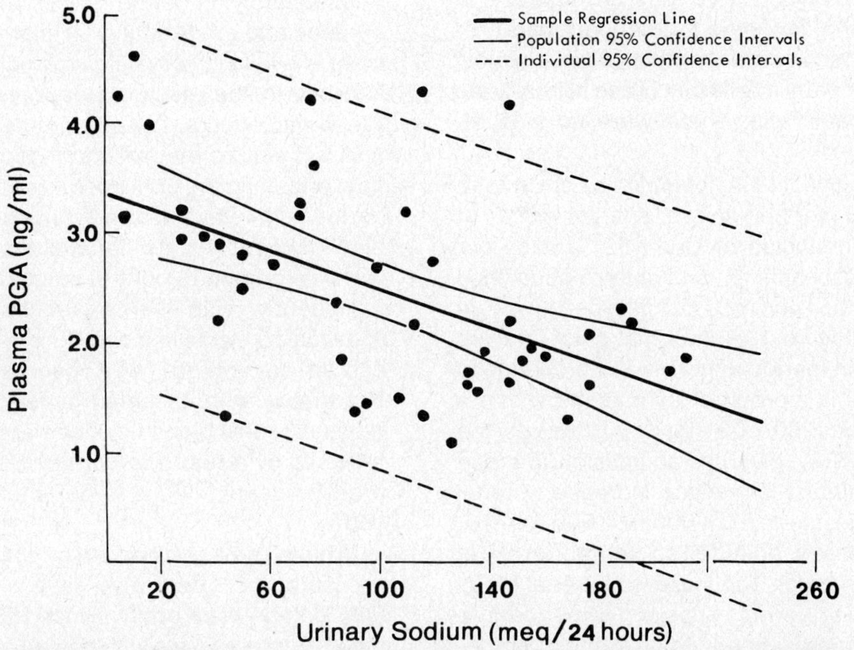

Figure 12. *Effect of sodium intake on plasma PGA in normotensive man. Each value represents the mean ± SEM. n = 65, y = 3.37-0.0089x. From Payakkapan et al. [73] with permission of the publisher.*

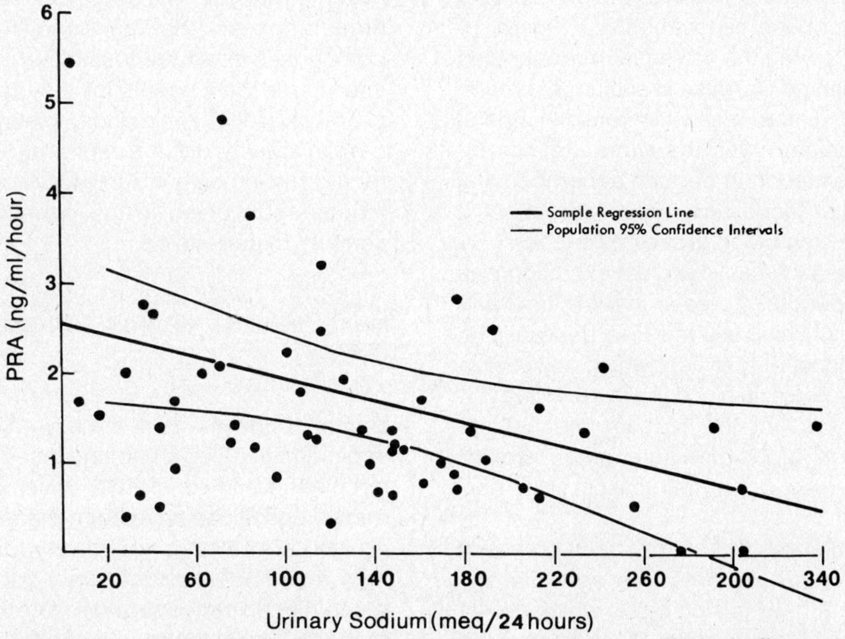

Figure 13. *Confidence intervals of plasma renin activity on urinary sodium excretion. y = 2.51-0.0059x. From Payakkapan et al. [73] with permission of the publisher.*

control values of 186/115 to 180/106 mm Hg. When the infusion rate was increased to 382 μg/minute, there was a further decline in blood pressure to 165/95 mm Hg. As in animal studies, there was an increase in cardiac output and a decrease in total peripheral resistance. The increase in cardiac output could be almost entirely accounted for by a reflex increase in heart rate from 96 to 114 beats/min. There were no side effects.

With the availability of PGA_1 obtained by enzymatic dehydration of PGE_1 for human use, a larger series of patients have been studied by Carr [62] and by our group [63,64]. Mechanisms and interrelationships between renal function and reduction in blood pressure were determined. Figure 10 shows that at an infusion rate of 1 μg/kg/min (period I) there was no change in the blood pressure in a group of 20 patients with essential hypertension (200/100 mm Hg). However, the earliest action of PGA_1, given as an infusion to these patients, was an almost immediate increase in renal blood flow, in this instance from 600 to 1,600 ml/min. Blood pressure subsequently fell to normal levels in period II (140/85 mm Hg). The increase in renal blood flow observed during period I subsided in period II to control values of approximately 600 ml/min. The decrease in blood pressure in period II, when the PGA infusion had been increased to 5 μg/min, was again the result of a decrease in total peripheral resistance accompanied by an increase in cardiac rate and cardiac output similar to that observed with PGA_2. Figure 11 shows that accompanying the increase in renal blood flow, there was a marked increase in sodium excretion in some patients and a more modest increase in others. Nevertheless, the pattern was the same, i.e., an increase in sodium excretion in period I accompanying the increase in renal blood flow and a decrease to control in period II when blood pressure reached normotensive levels. The increase in sodium excretion was accompanied by a parallel increase in urine flow and potassium excretion. This resulted in a decrease in plasma volume by about 10 per cent which could have contributed to the decrease in blood pressure. However, volume depletion was not the primary mechanism causing reduction in blood pressure since similar changes were observed when fluid losses were corrected.

In brief, the following mechanism has been proposed for the action of PGA_1 in patients with essential hypertension: initially, at low infusion rates, which do not alter extrarenal resistance vessels, PGA_1 dilates the extremely sensitive renal vessels. This renal vasodilation results in an increase in renal blood flow associated with a high renal artery perfusion pressure secondary to the hypertensive state [65]. This is accompanied by increased excretion of sodium and water presumably in large part because of alterations in the physical factors affecting the reabsorption process such as peritubular hydrostatic and oncotic pressures. Subsequently, in period II when the infusion rate is increased and extrarenal arteriolar dilation takes place, there is a fall in the systemic blood pressure level which is primarily the result of peripheral arteriolar dilation. When this occurs, the ensuing decrease in renal perfusion pressure may lead to a decrease in renal blood flow offsetting the continued vasodilating effect of PGA on the renal vasculature. This normalization of renal blood flow results in a parallel decrease in sodium and water excretion to control values.

Recently, with the availability of synthetic PGA_2 (identical to medullin isolated from the kidney), Hornych and his co-workers [66] observed similar responses in patients with essential hypertension: an initial increase in renal blood flow, natriuresis and diuresis was followed by a return to control values when the blood pressure level fell due to peripheral arteriolar dilation [66].

Whatever the mechanism by which PGA lowers blood pressure, the effect may have clinical importance if PGA can be used orally. Since PGA results in a fall in blood pressure levels with normal blood flow and normal sodium and water excretion, its clinical use may have certain advantages over other current therapeutic regimens which compromise renal blood flow, particularly in patients with borderline renal function. At this time, it appears that intravenously administered PGA compounds in intravenous experiments act as "ideal" antihypertensive agents for they favorably affect blood pressure, renal resistance, plasma volume, baroreceptor activity, total peripheral resistance and, indirectly, cardiac output. All these factors are known to be intimately involved in the genesis of so-called "essential" hypertension.

MEASUREMENT OF PGA IN HUMAN KIDNEYS AND PLASMA

Human Kidneys. With the advent of relatively specific and sensitive radioimmunoassay for PGA [67,68], circulating and renal PGA under a variety of experimental conditions have been measured. Vance and his co-workers [69] observed very low concentrations of PGA and PGE in human renal cortex (15 pg/ml), and much higher concentrations (1,500 and 2,000 pg/ml, respectively) in the renal papilla. Thus, prostaglandins are present in the medulla and, to a much lesser degree, in the cortex of the human kidney. This is similar to observations in animals and may allow greater extrapolation of animal data to man. It is also likely that in man as in the animal the site of prostaglandin synthesis is in the renal papilla and that its action and degradation takes place in the renal cortex.

Plasma PGA in Normotensive Man. Since infusion of PGA into hypertensive man was associated with a marked, albeit transient, natriuresis, it was proposed that an increase in either intrarenal PGA or PGE or circulating PGA might, in part, mediate saline-induced natriuresis and might, in part, be responsible for the activity of the so-called "natriuretic hormone" [57]. In fact, an increase in intrarenal PGA in renal cortex and outer medulla was observed in chronically salt-loaded rabbits [68]. This increase was inhibited by the administration of indomethacin and was associated with a decrease in sodium excretion. To investigate the possibility that circulating PGA might be a natriuretic factor, plasma PGA, renin and urine aldosterone were measured in normotensive subjects on an ad libitum sodium chloride diet [70–73]. Surprisingly, the highest plasma PGA concentration (3.06 ng/ml) was observed in those receiving sodium intakes below 50 meq/liter (Figure 12). As the intake of sodium increased, there was a highly significant decrease in plasma PGA, reaching 1.76 ng/ml in subjects ingesting more than 200 meq of sodium. This decrease in plasma PGA with a high sodium intake was not the result of individual variations.

Figure 13 shows that under conditions of low sodium intake there is an increase in plasma renin activity. This increase is significant only when extremes of sodium intake are compared. It is notable, therefore, that the increase in PRA is much less in magnitude that that of plasma PGA under conditions of low sodium intake. There is a significant linear correlation between plasma PGA and urinary aldosterone and although there is a similar correlation between plasma PGA and PRA, it is much less striking. These findings raise the possibility that under conditions of low sodium intake, the increase in PGA might participate in either the synthesis or release of aldosterone. In fact, evidence in support of this has been presented by Fichman et al. [74] who showed that infusions of PGA for 1 hour into normotensive subjects significantly increased plasma aldosterone but not PRA. It is noteworthy in this regard that the increase in plasma aldosterone is not secondary to any effect of volume depletion by PGA-induced natriuresis, since a significant increase in plasma aldosterone was observed upon infusion of PGA into four anephric subjects. Figure 14 illustrates a schema by which PGA, rather than mediating volume-induced natriuresis, might act in precisely the reverse fashion, that is, by acting as an antinatriuretic factor in normotensive, but not necessarily hypertensive, subjects. Current evidence suggests that volume depletion gives rise to both an increased plasma PGA and PRA which together might stimulate aldosterone release leading to sodium retention. A

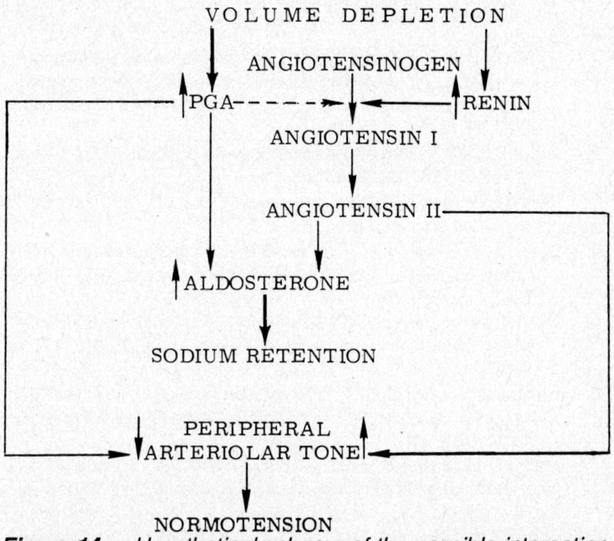

__Figure 14.__ Hypothetical scheme of the possible interaction of increased plasma PGA in the biosynthesis of angiotensin I, aldosterone production and maintenance of normotension in normotensive subjects. Stimulation solid arrow, inhibition "hatched" arrow. From Payakkapan et al. [73] with permission of the publisher.

second action of the increase in PGA might be its inhibition of conversion of angiotensinogen to angiotensin I. Kotchen and Miller [75] have shown that low concentrations of PGA (10^{-6M}) inhibit this conversion in vitro. An interesting third effect might be on blood pressure. During volume depletion, such as that caused by sodium restriction, blood pressure in normotensive as well as hypertensive subjects remains unchanged or tends to decrease. On the other hand, there is reason to believe that during volume depletion there might be an increase in blood pressure since there is an increase in the prohypertensive factors of the renin-angiotensin-aldosterone axis. It is possible, therefore, that the increase in circulating peripheral vasodilating PGA offsets the vasoconstrictor effects of the associated increase in angiotensin, leading to a preservation of normotension or even lowering of blood pressure. It seems clear from these studies, however, that circulating PGA most likely does not participate in mediating natriuresis induced by administration of saline solution. If prostaglandins are natriuretic factors in normotensive subjects, their most plausible role would be local, affecting the regulation of intrarenal blood flow and sodium excretion. Thus, current preliminary evidence is in support of the fact that (1) PGA may have a circulatory role acting as an antihypertensive agent by interaction with the renin-angiotensin, norepinephrine pro-hypertensive system and that (2) PGA or PGE may participate in the regulation of renal blood flow and sodium balance by functioning as so-called "local" intrarenal vasodilator compounds.

REFERENCES

1. Euler US von: Zür Kenntnis der pharmakologischen Wirkungen von Nativsekreten and Extrakten männlicher accessorischer Geschlechtsdrüsen. Arch Expt Pathol Pharmakol 175: 78, 1934.
2. Goldblatt MW: Depressor substance in seminal fluid. Chem Ind 52: 1056, 1933.
3. Kurzrok R, Lieb CC: Biochemical studies of human semen II. Proc Soc Exp Biol Med 26: 268, 1930.
4. Bergström S, Sjövall J: The isolation of prostaglandin F from sheep prostate gland. Acta Chem Scand 14: 1693, 1960.
5. Bergström S, Sjövall J: The isolation of prostaglandin E from sheep prostate gland. Acta Chem Scand 14: 1701, 1960.
6. Bergström S, Ryhage R, Samuelsson B, Sjövall J: The structure of prostaglandin E, F_1, and F_2. Acta Chem Scand 16: 501, 1962.
7. Lee JB, Hickler RB, Saravis CA, Thorn GW: Sustained depressor effects of renomedullary extracts. Circulation 26: 747, 1962.
8. Lee JB, Hickler RB, Saravis CA, Thorn GW: Sustained depressor effect of renal medullary extract in the normotensive rat. Circ Res 13: 359, 1963.
9. Muirhead EE, Jones F, Stirman JA: Antihypertensive property in renoprival hypertension of extract from renal medulla. J Lab Clin Med 56: 167, 1960.
10. Lee JB: Prostaglandins and the renal antihypertensive and natriuretic endocrine function. Recent Prog Hormone Res 30: 481, 1974.
11. Lee JB, Covino BG, Takman BH, Smith ER: Renomedullary vasodepressor substance, medullin: Isolation, chemical characterization and physiological properties. Circ Res 17: 57, 1965.
12. Lee JB: Chemical and physiological properties of renal prostaglandins: The antihypertensive effects of medullin in essential human hypertension. Prostaglandins, Proceedings of the 2nd Nobel Symposium, 1966, p 197.
13. Lee JB, Crowshaw K, Takman BH, et al.: The identification of prostaglandin E_2, $F_{2\alpha}$ and A_2 from rabbit kidney medulla. Biochem J 105: 1251, 1967.
14. Hamberg M, Samuelsson B: Prostaglandins in human seminal plasma. J Biol Chem 241: 257, 1966.
15. Bergström S, Danielsson H, Samuelsson B: The enzymatic formation of prostaglandin E_2 from arachidonic acid. Biochim Biophy Acta 90: 207, 1964.
16. Van Dorp DA, Beerthuis RK, Nugteren DH, et al.: The biosynthesis of prostaglandins. Biochim Biophy Acta 90: 204, 1964.
17. Änggård E, Samuelsson B: Biosynthesis of prostaglandins from arachidonic acid in guinea pig lung. J Biol Chem 240: 3518, 1965.
18. Crowshaw K: The incorporation of I-^{14}C arachidonic acid into the lipids of rabbit renal slices and conversion to prostaglandins E_2 and $F_{2\alpha}$. Prostaglandins 3: 607, 1973.
19. Schlegel W: Prostaglandin biosynthesis in human placenta (abstract). Fed Proc 33: 590, 1974.
20. Ham EA, Oien HG, Ulm EH, Kuehl Jr FA: The reaction of PGA_1 with sulfhydryl groups; A component in the binding of A-type prostaglandins to protein. Prostaglandins 10: 217, 1975.
21. Corey EJ, Washburn WN, Chen JC: Studies on the prostaglandin A_2 synthetase complex from plexaura homomalla. J Am Chem Soc 95: 2054, 1973.
22. Larsson C, Änggård E: Regional differences in the formation and metabolism of prostaglandins in rabbit kidney. Eur J Pharmacol 21: 30, 1973.
23. Änggård E, Bohman SO, Griffin III JE, et al.: Subcellular localization of the prostaglandin system in the rabbit renal papilla. Acta Physiol Scand 84: 231, 1972.
24. Vane JB: Inhibition of prostaglandin synthesis as a mechanism of action for aspirin-like drugs. Nature (New Biol) 231: 232, 1971.
25. Nissen HM, Andersen H: On the localization of a prostaglandin-dehydrogenase activity in the kidney. Histochemie 14: 189, 1968.
26. Muirhead EE, Germain GS, Leach BE, et al.: Production of renomedullary prostaglandins by renomedullary interstitial cells grown in tissue culture. Circ Res (suppl II) 30: II-161, 1972.
27. Prezyna A, Attallah A, Vance K, et al.: The renomedullary body. A newly recognized structure of renomedullary interstitial cell origin associated with high prostaglandin content. Prostaglandins 3: 669, 1973.
28. Lerman RJ, Pitcock JA, Stephenson P, et al.: Renomedullary interstitial cell tumor (formerly fibroma of renal medulla). Human Pathol 3: 559, 1972.
29. Änggård E, Samuelsson B: Metabolism of prostaglandin E_1 in guinea pig lung: The structure of two metabolites. J Biol Chem 239: 4097, 1964.
30. Hamberg M, Samuelsson B: Metabolism of prostaglandin E_2 in guinea pig liver. J Biol Chem 246: 1073, 1971.
31. McGiff JC, Terragno NA, Strand JC, et al.: Selective passage of prostaglandins across the lung. Nature (Lond) 223: 742, 1969.
32. Horton EW, Jones RL: Prostaglandins A_1, A_2 and 19-hydroxy A_1: Their action on smooth muscle and their inactivation on passage through the pulmonary hepatic portal vascular beds. Br J Pharmacol 37: 705, 1969.
33. Attallah AA, Payakkapan W, Lee JB: Metabolism of prostaglandin A: The kidney cortex as a major site of PGA_2 degradation. Life Sci 14: 1521, 1974.
34. Attallah AA, Duchesne MJ, Lee JB: Metabolism of prostaglandin A. II. Isolation, characterization, and synthesis of PGA_1 renal metabolites. Life Sci 16: 1743, 1975.
35. Oien HG, Ham EA, Zanetti MA, et al.: A 15-OH prostaglandin dehydrogenase specific for A prostaglandins in rabbit kidney. Proc Natl Acad Sci (in press).
36. Attallah AA, Schussler GC: Prostaglandin binding in human serum follows the polarity rule. Prostaglandins 4: 479, 1973.
37. Raz A: Interaction of prostaglandins with blood plasma proteins. Comparative binding of prostaglandins A_2, $F_{2\alpha}$ and E_2 to human plasma proteins. Biochem J 130: 631, 1972.
38. Duchesne MJ, Attallah AA, Lee JB: Human serum albumin (HSA) decreases prostaglandin A_1 (PGA_1) metabolism: Biochem Biophy Res Comm 64: 196, 1975.
39. Attallah AA, Lee JB: Specific binding sites in the rabbit kidney for prostaglandin A. Prostaglandins 4: 703, 1973.
40. Larsson C, Änggård E: Mass spectrometric determination of prostaglandins in regions of the rabbit kidney. Proceedings of the International Conference on Prostaglandins, Florence, Italy, May 26–30, 1975, p 179.
41. Frohlich JC, Sweetman BJ, Carr K, et al.: Assessment of the levels of PGA_2 in human plasma by gas chromatography-mass spectrometry. Prostaglandins 10: 185, 1975.
42. Weiner R, Kaley G: Influence of prostaglandin E_1 on the terminal vascular bed. Am J Physiol 217: 563, 1969.
43. Horton EW: Action of prostaglandin E_1 on tissues which respond to bradykinin. Nature (London) 200: 892, 1963.
44. DuCharme WM, Weeks JR, Mortgomery RG: Studies on the mechanism of the hypertensive effect of prostaglandin $F_{2\alpha}$. J Pharmacol Exp Therap 160: 1, 1967.
45. Bergström S, Carlson LA, Ekelund LG, et al.: Cardiovascular and metabolic response to infusions of prostaglandin E_1 in man. Acta Physiol Scand 64: 332, 1965.
46. Montgomery RG, Patel NC, Lee JG: A comparison of the di-

uretic effects of prostaglandin A_1, sodium ethacrynate and placebo. Prostaglandins 4: 381, 1973.
47. Nakano J, McCurdy JR: Hemodynamic effects of prostaglandins E_1, A_1 and $F_{2\alpha}$ in dogs. Proc Soc Exp Biol Med 128: 39, 1968.
48. Covino BG, Lee JB, McMorrow JV: Circulatory effects of prostaglandins. Circulation 38 (suppl 6): 60A, 1968.
49. Barner HB, Kaiser GC, Jellinek M, et al.: Effect of prostaglandin A on several vascular beds in man. Am Heart J 85: 584, 1973.
50. Kannegiesser H, Lee JB: Difference in haemodynamic response to prostaglandin A and E. Nature (London) 229: 498, 1971.
51. Johnston HH, Herzog JP, Lauler DP: Effect of prostaglandin E_1 on renal hemodynamics, sodium and water excretion. Am J Physiol 213: 939, 1967.
52. Vander AJ: Direct Effects of prostaglandin on renal function and renin release in anesthetized dog. Am J Physiol 214: 218, 1968.
53. Barger AC, Herd JA: Study of renal circulation the unanesthetized dog with inert gases: external counting, "Proceedings of the Third International Congress of Nephrology, Basel, S. Karger, 1966, p 174.
54. Kirschenbaum MA, White N, Stein H, et al.: Redistribution of renal cortical blood flow during inhibition of prostaglandin synthesis. Am J Physiol 227: 801, 1974.
55. Solez K, Fox JA, Miller M, et al.: Effects of indomethacin on renal inner medullary plasma flow. Prostaglandins 7: 91, 1974.
56. Williamson HE, Bourland WA, Marchand GR: Inhibition of ethacrynic acid induced increase in renal blood flow by indomethacin. Prostaglandins 8: 297, 1974.
57. Lee JB: Hypertension, natriuresis, and the renal prostaglandins. Ann Intern Med 70: 1033, 1969.
58. Orloff J, Grantham J: The effect of prostaglandin (PGE_1) on the permeability response of rabbit collecting tubules to vasopressin. Nobel Symp 2, Prostaglandins (Bergstrom S, Samuelsson B, eds), Stockholm, Almquist and Wiksell, 1967, p 143.
59. Murihead EE, Leach B, Brooks B, et al.: Antihypertensive action of prostaglandin E_2. Prostaglandin Symposium of Worchester Foundation for Experimental Biology Ramwell PW, Shaw JE, eds), New York, Interscience 1968.
60. Muirhead EE, Leach BE, Armstrong FR Jr, et al.: Vasodepressor action of renomedullary prostaglandins (PGE_2 and PGA_2) in the spontaneously hypertensive rat (SH Ray). Evidence for a central action mediated by the vagus. Adv Biosci 9 (suppl): 60, 1972.
61. Cohen M, Sztokalo J, Hinsch E: The antihypertensive action of arachidonic acid in the spontaneous hypertensive rat and its antagonism by antiinflammatory agents. Life Sci 13: 317, 1973.
62. Carr AA: Effect of PGA_1 on renin and aldosterone in man. Prostaglandins 3: 621, 1973.
63. Lee JB, McGiff JC, Kannegiesser H, et al.: Prostaglandin A_1. Antihypertensive and renal effects. Ann Intern Med 74: 703, 1971.
64. Westura EE, Kannegiesser H, O'Toole JD, et al.: Antihypertensive effects of prostaglandin A_1 in essential hypertension. Circ Res 27 (suppl 1): 131, 1970.
65. Lee SJ, Johnson JG, Smith CJ, et al.: Renal effects of prostaglandin A_1 in patients with essential hypertension. Kidney Int 1: 254, 1972.
66. Hornych A, Safar M, Papanicolaou N, et al.: Renal and cardiovascular effects of prostaglandin A_2 in essential hypertension. Eur J Clin Inv 2: 289, 1972.
67. Zusman RM, Caldwell BV, Speroff L: Radioimmunoassay of the A prostaglandins. Prostaglandins 2: 41, 1972.
68. Attallah AA, Lee JB: Radioimmunoassay of prostaglandin A. Intrarenal PGA_2 as a factor mediating saline-induced natriuresis. Circ Res 33: 696, 1973.
69. Vance VK, Attallah AA, Prezyna A, et al.: Human renal prostaglandins. Prostaglandins 3: 647, 1973.
70. Lee JB: Hypertension, natriuresis and the renomedullary prostaglandins. Prostaglandins 3: 551, 1973.
71. Zusman RM, Caldwell BV, Mulrow PJ, et al.: The role of prostaglandin A in control of sodium homeostasis and blood pressure. Prostaglandins 3: 679, 1973.
72. Zusman RM, Spector D, Caldwell BV, et al.: The effect of chronic sodium loading and sodium restriction on plasma prostaglandin A, E and F concentrations in normal humans. J Clin Invest 52: 1093, 1973.
73. Payakkapan W, Attallah AA, Lee JB, et al.: Effect of sodium intake on prostaglandin A, renin and aldosterone in normotensive humans. Kidney Int 8: S-283, 1975.
74. Fichman M, Littenburg G, Brooker G, et al.: Effect of Prostaglandin A_1 on renal and adrenal function in man. Circ Res 31 (suppl): 19, 1972.
75. Kotchen TA, Miller MC: Effect of prostaglandins on renin activity. Am J Physiol 226: 314, 1974.

INFORMATION FOR AUTHORS

PREPARATION OF MANUSCRIPTS

Manuscripts should be typed on one side of the sheet, doublespaced, on white bond paper, 8½ by 11 inches, with margins of 1 inch. Two copies of the manuscript and illustrations should be sent to the Editor at 666 Fifth Avenue, New York, New York 10019. Title page should include full name, degrees and affiliation of all authors, the source from which the article emanates, and the name and address of the person to whom requests for reprints should be addressed.

All manuscript pages including tables and legends should be numbered consecutively in the upper right hand corner.

The number of manuscript pages, the number of illustrations and the number of tables should be indicated at the bottom of the covering letter.

Every article must be preceded by an abstract (not to exceed 350 words). This obviates the need for a summary. In addition, for the convenience of our readers, we require a brief abstract (not exceeding 100 to 125 words) and key words for indexing purposes. These brief abstracts appear in the back of the *Journal* in the same issue in which the paper appears.

Since all manuscripts submitted for publication in the *Journal* are sent out for review before a final decision is made, there is generally a lapse of three to six weeks before contributors are notified. If you have received an acknowledgment of receipt, there is no need to call the *Journal* office; your manuscript has not gone astray. The decision will be forthcoming shortly.

PREPARATION OF ILLUSTRATIONS AND TABLES

Illustrations must be black and white glossy prints or professional drawings in india ink; they should be unmounted. The name of the lead author and the title of the article should be typed on a label and affixed to the back of each illustration; the top should be indicated.

Reference to all illustrations should be inserted in the text in consecutive order. Legends for the illustrations should be typed, double spaced, on a separate sheet with numbers corresponding to those on the photographs or drawings. They should not be attached to the pictures.

Tables should be typed on separate sheets and should be set up in accordance with the style of the Journal. Units of measure should be confined to column headings. Abbreviations should be kept to a minimum and should conform with those used by the *Journal* or listed as acceptable in the Council of Biology Editors Style Manual. Any variations should be explained. All vertical rules should be omitted.

The publisher allows a fixed amount towards the reproduction of illustrations and tables. Charges in excess of this amount must be assumed by the authors. The Editor reserves the right to limit the number of illustrations and/or tables.

PREPARATION OF BIBLIOGRAPHY

Bibliographic references should be listed chronologically on a separate sheet (not in footnotes) as referred to in the text and should be typed (double-spaced) in accordance with the style and abbreviations (open punctuation) used by Index Medicus; only the first page of the journal citation is necessary. Examples follow:

For periodical references:

22. Theologides A, Kennedy BJ: Toxoplasmic myocarditis and pericarditis. Am J Med 47: 169, 1969.

For book references (with chapter):

18. Schiebler GL, Van Mieron LHS, Krovetz LJ: Diseases of the tricuspid valve, chap 2. Heart Disease in Infants, Children and Adolescents (Moss AJ, Adams F, eds), Baltimore, Williams & Wilkins, 1968.

For book references (without chapter):

13. Berne E: Principles of Group Treatment, New York, Oxford University Press, 1966, p 26.

Authors are responsible for the accuracy of all references.

REPRINTS

Price schedules and order cards for reprints are mailed to the person so listed in the footnote on the title page.

The American Journal of Medicine, **666 Fifth Avenue, New York, New York 10019**

Influenza A Viral Infection Associated with Acute Renal Failure

ADEL SHENOUDA, M.D.*
FRED E. HATCH, M.D.
Memphis, Tennessee

The clinical and laboratory findings in four cases of acute renal failure following the onset of influenza A viral infection (Port Chalmers/1/73) are presented.

Although the pathophysiologic mechanisms affecting the kidney in these cases varied, the ensuing renal failure in each patient was severe. Findings suggestive of acute myoglobinuria developed in one patient, and disseminated intravascular coagulation (DIC) occurred in another.

The role of viruses in the pathogenesis of renal disease is reviewed. Despite inconclusive evidence that the influenza virus can cause human renal disease, the secondary pathways that can be triggered by viral infections may be even more significant in producing various degrees of renal dysfunction. The occurrence of renal failure during an episode of influenza represents a serious complication which may influence significantly the morbidity and mortality of patients with this viral infection.

The development of acute renal failure subsequent to the onset of influenza viral infection has been the subject of sporadic reports in various areas of the world in recent years [1–6]. When viral or serologic identification has been possible, influenza A infections (London/72, Hong Kong/68, England/42/72) have provided the closest association with renal disease [1–6]. Inherent difficulties in viral isolation in renal tissue have hampered attempts to demonstrate a direct etiologic role. Other well defined pathogenetic mechanisms, however, appear to have been responsible for the renal failure in many of these cases. Acute myoglobinuria has developed in several patients [5,6], and disseminated intravascular coagulation (DIC) has occurred in others [2–4]. Myking and Schreiner [1] reported a case of severe renal failure following an influenza virus A infection in which a possible immunologic mechanism was suggested. Until the definitive role of viruses in the pathogenesis of renal disease has been fully established, additional observations on the course of viral-associated renal failure continue to be of clinical interest.

In this study we report four cases of acute renal failure following influenza A/Port Chalmers/1/73 viral infection during a recent midwinter epidemic. Although the pathophysiologic mechanisms affecting the kidney in these cases varied, the ensuing renal failure in each patient was severe. This report serves to emphasize that the occurrence of renal failure during an episode of influenza represents a serious complication which may influence significantly the morbidity and mortality of the patient with this viral infection.

From the Division of Nephrology, Department of Medicine, University of Tennessee Center for the Health Sciences, Memphis, Tennessee. Requests for reprints should be addressed to Dr. Fred E. Hatch, 353 D, 951 Court Avenue, Memphis, Tennessee 38163. Manuscript accepted March 5, 1976.

* Present address: Department of Nephrology, Baroness Erlanger Hospital, Chattanooga, Tennessee 37403.

TABLE I Clinical Data in Patients with Acute Renal Failure Following Influenza

Case No.	Age (yr) and Sex	Clinical Presentation	Renal Status on Admission	Arterial Blood Gasses: pH	pO$_2$ (mm Hg)	pCO$_2$ (mm Hg)	O$_2$ Saturation (%)	Serum Enzymes: SGOT (mU/ml)	LDH (mU/ml)	CPK (mU/ml)	Outcome
1	26,F	Dyspnea, cyanosis	Anuria	7.38	35	34	66	5,084	5,310	>50,000	Recovery
2	33,F	Dyspnea, cyanosis, confusion	Normal	7.42	55	25	88	140	1,200	200	Death
3	47,F	Dyspnea, peripheral edema	Oliguria	7.36	62	21	90	135	940	690	Death
4	28,M	Cough, peripheral edema	Oliguria	7.47	75	24	94	70	480	300	Chronic renal failure

NOTE: pO$_2$ = oxygen tension; pCO$_2$ = carbon dioxide tension; O$_2$ = oxygen.

CASE REPORTS

Case 1. An upper respiratory tract infection, characterized by low grade fever, nonproductive cough and myalgia, developed in a 26 year old white woman. During the second week of her illness, she began to have moderate respiratory distress that resulted in mild cyanosis of all extremities. Profound generalized muscle weakness occurred, and she became unable to walk. Two days before admission, her urine became dark brown and decreased in amount. She was known to have had normal renal function previously and had no history of kidney disease. Because of increasing respiratory distress and progressive cyanosis, she was admitted to a local hospital.

Physical examination revealed an acutely ill woman without palpable blood pressure. Her fingers and toes, lips and face were cyanotic (Table I). The lungs were clear, and a chest film was within normal limits. A white blood cell count was 26,900/mm^3, hematocrit value 44 per cent and blood urea nitrogen 40 mg/100 ml. She was treated with intravenous saline solutions, intermittent intravenous hydrocortisone and antibiotics. Her vital signs returned to normal, and the cyanosis showed marked diminution. The urinary output was low and did not respond to the intravenous administration of mannitol or furosemide. The urine was dark brown in color, with a specific gravity of 1.023, pH 6.5, albumin 4+ and orthotolidin (Hematest®) 4+; microscopic examination showed an occasional white blood cell and red blood cell/hpf. Serum enzyme levels were markedly elevated (Table I). Because of the renal failure, the patient was transferred to the City of Memphis Hospital.

Physical examination on admission revealed a critically ill but alert young woman in moderate respiratory distress. The vital signs were stable, but the extremities were cold and mildly cyanotic. Examination of the chest showed diffuse rales and rhonchi throughout both lung fields. The cardiac size was normal; the heart rate was 150 beats/min with a gallop rhythm. Laboratory values included a blood urea nitrogen of 72 mg/100 ml, creatinine 7.5 mg/100 ml, calcium 5.3 mg/100 ml, phosphorus 7.6 mg/100 ml, and sputum and blood cultures that were negative.

Treatment was started with 6 liters of nasal oxygen. The arterial blood gases showed persistent hypoxia, however (Table I), and a volume-controlled ventilator and positive end-expiratory pressure were employed for ventilatory assistance. A Swan-Ganz catheter was inserted into the pulmonary artery for monitoring pressure. The intravenous administration of hydrocortisone was continued (400 mg/day), and the administration of aqueous penicillin G (8 million units/day) was begun. Because of continued renal failure, hemodialysis was performed regularly over a two week period.

The patient showed marked clinical improvement with these measures, and all mechanical assistance was discontinued by the third week. She underwent a spontaneous diuresis during the recovery phase of acute renal failure, and renal function slowly returned to normal. Attempts to identify myoglobinuria during the diuretic phase by 80 per cent saturation with ammonium sulfate were unsuccessful. Serum was obtained during the acute and convalescent phases for influenza virus antibody determinations. The serologic response to A/Hong Kong/68 and Port Chalmers/1/73 influenza viruses was measured by hemagglutination inhibition as described by Fazekas and Webster [7]. An increase in hemagglutination inhibiting antibody titers to 1:10,000 dilution was detected (Table II). Extreme soreness and weakness persisted in the quadriceps muscles and prevented ambulation without assistance. Intensive physiotherapy produced gradual improvement in muscle strength. The patient was discharged on the 38th hospital day.

Case 2. A 33 year old white woman was admitted to the City of Memphis Hospital in acute respiratory distress (Table I). Three days earlier, she had been treated for symptoms of an upper respiratory tract infection. One day prior to admission, she became disoriented and progressive dyspnea developed.

Physical examination revealed a well developed, slender woman who was confused and agitated. She had a temperature of 100.4° F, blood pressure 118/70 mm Hg, pulse rate 120 beats/min and respiratory rate 48/min. Pertinent physical findings included cyanotic lips, coarse rales heard in bases of both lungs, a normal-sized heart without murmurs or gallop, and a neurologic examination within normal limits except for the altered mentation.

Laboratory studies showed a hematocrit value of 43 per cent and a white blood cell count of 26,900/mm^3; blood urea nitrogen was 16 mg/100 ml and creatinine 0.8 mg/100 ml. Arterial blood gases indicated severe hypoxia (Table I). The urine was yellow in color, with a specific gravity of 1.019, pH 6 and albumin negative; microscopic examination showed 0 to 4 white blood cells/hpf. Other pertinent laboratory values included a direct platelet count of 417,000/mm^3, negative protamine sulfate test and fibrinogen 460 mg/100 ml. Serum enzyme levels were moderately elevated (Table I). Gram-stain of the tracheal aspirate revealed rare gram-positive diplococci. Blood and sputum cultures were negative. A chest film showed bilateral diffuse infiltrates consistent with pulmonary edema.

The impression on admission was influenza viral pneumonitis with severe respiratory failure. The hypoxia did not diminish with oxygen administration, and positive end-expiratory pressure was begun. In addition, penicillin (8 million units/day) and gentamicin (120 mg/day) were administered. The patient's condition improved clinically over the next 48 hours, but subsequently a persistent fever developed with a temperature of 103°F. A lumbar puncture was performed which was within normal limits. Acute renal failure developed as manifested by a decreased urine output and progressive azotemia.

Repeat laboratory studies revealed a white blood cell count of 54,000/mm^3; the red blood cell morphology showed many fragmented cells, burr cells and target cells; the platelet count was 152,000/mm^3, fibrinogen 365 mg/100 ml; protamine sulfate test was positive.

The patient received intravenous heparin therapy for DIC, and hemodialysis was started. The platelet count fell subsequently to 44,200/mm^3 and the fibrinogen was 265 mg/100 ml. Bleeding developed subcutaneously and in the gastrointestinal tract. The patient had a cardiac arrest, but cardiac resuscitation was unsuccessful. Permission for an autopsy was not obtained. Blood was obtained for assays of influenza antibodies shortly before the patient's death (Table II). Values determined during convalescence could not be obtained for comparison.

Case 3. A 47 year old white woman had been in good health until two weeks prior to admission when fever, cough, malaise and a sinus infection developed. Four days later, she noticed progressive dyspnea, weight gain, and edema of her feet and ankles (Table I). She was admitted to a local hospital where she was found to be in moderate respiratory distress. A 20 pound weight gain was documented, and her urinary output was diminished.

Laboratory data included a hematocrit value of 20.5 per cent and a white blood cell count of 11,700/mm^3; the blood urea nitrogen was 114 mg/100 ml, serum creatinine 7.5 mg/100 ml and creatinine clearance 7.7 ml/min. The patient had no prior history of renal disease and had been seen by her physician at regular intervals for routine physical examinations including urinalyses.

TABLE II Serologic Response to A/Hong Kong/68 and A/Port Chalmers/1/73 Influenza Viruses as Measured by Hemagglutination Inhibition

Case No.	No. of Days After Admission	Antibody Titers to Viral Antigens*	
		Hong Kong/68	Port Chalmers/73
1	9	1:9,300	1:7,100
	22	>1:10,000	1:10,000
2†	8	<1:20	<1:20
3	7	<1:20	<1:20
	19	1:160	1:46
4	15	1:160	1:200
	32	1:260	1:2,000
	53	1:260	1:4,000

*The figures represent the lowest dilution of serum that inhibited hemagglutination.
† Convalescent viral titers could not be obtained for comparison.

She was transferred to the City of Memphis Hospital because of acute renal failure. On admission she had a temperature of 100.8°F, blood pressure 200/100 mm Hg, pulse rate 100 beats/min and respiration 36/min. Diffuse, moist rales were present in the bases of both lungs and over the left anterior portion of the chest. The heart was enlarged moderately and showed a sinus tachycardia with a ventricular gallop. She had 2+ edema over the legs and sacral area.

Pertinent laboratory studies included a hematocrit value of 25.3 per cent, a white blood cell count of 29,300/mm^3, and a platelet count of 343,000/mm^3; the urine was amber in color, with a specific gravity of 1.013, pH 6 and albumin 3+; microscopic examination showed 30 to 40 red blood cells/hpf. Multiple sputum and blood cultures were negative. Initial arterial blood gases were determined while the patient was receiving 6 liters of nasal oxygen (Table I). Blood urea nitrogen was 138 mg/100 ml and creatinine 14 mg/100 ml. Serum enzyme levels were moderately elevated. A chest film showed extensive pulmonary vascular congestion compatible with pulmonary edema. The heart was moderately enlarged with left ventricular preponderance. Results of laboratory studies for myoglobinuria and DIC were negative.

The patient was treated with oxygen, antibiotics and hemodialysis. Approximately 30 pounds of edema fluid were removed. Two weeks after admission, she had a sudden massive gastrointestinal hemorrhage followed by shock and cardiorespiratory arrest. Resuscitation was successful, but aspiration pneumonia developed and ventilatory assistance was required. Over the next week, the patient became more alert, but she remained anuric and required continued use of the respirator. Serum was obtained during the acute and convalescent phases for influenza virus studies and showed a fourfold increase in antibody titer to A/Hong Kong/68 influenza (Table II). On the 19th hospital day, gastrointestinal bleeding recurred. Coagulation studies disclosed no abnormalities. The platelet count was 132,000/mm^3; protamine sulfate was negative. A cardiac arrest developed, and the

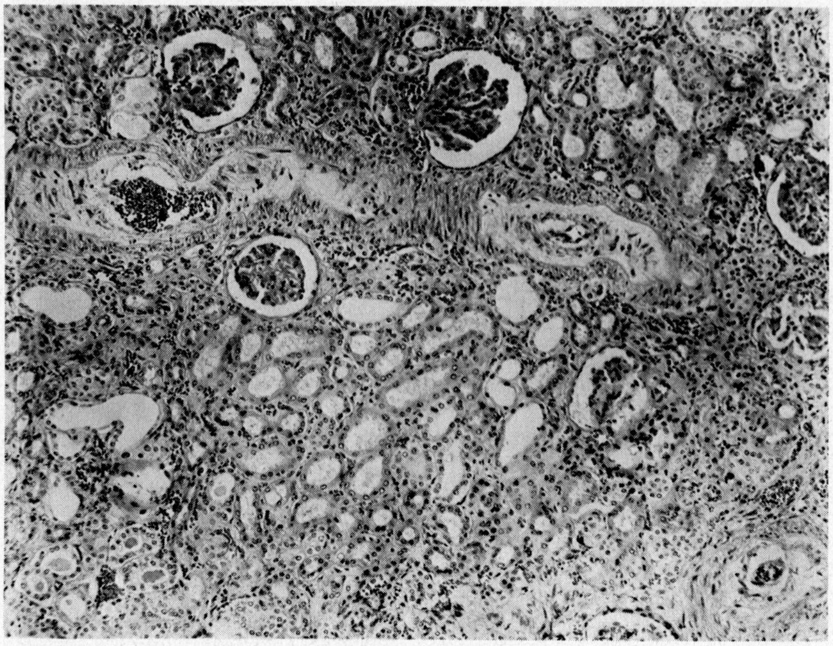

Figure 1. *Case 3. Section of the kidney at autopsy in a patient with acute renal failure following influenza viral infection. There is moderate thickening of the arterioles with deposition of mucoid ground substance characteristic of arteriolonephrosclerosis. The glomeruli and tubules are unremarkable. Hematoxylin and eosin stain; original magnification × 100, reduced by 4 per cent.*

patient died. At postmortem examination a perforated duodenal ulcer was found with massive bleeding into the gastrointestinal tract. Atelectasis was present in the lower portion of the left lung and in the lower portion of the right lung. There were patchy areas of bronchopneumonia. The kidneys showed moderate arteriolonephrosclerosis (Figure 1). Viral studies of renal tissue were not obtained.

Case 4. An upper respiratory tract infection, manifested by coryza, pharyngitis, nonproductive cough and fever, developed in a 28 year old black man two weeks before his admission. He was known to have sickle cell anemia and was treated by his local physician for a mild sickle cell crisis. The fever and cough persisted and were followed by pedal edema, vomiting and a marked decrease in urinary output during the second week of his illness (Table I). The patient had been in relatively good health except for occasional sickle cell crises. He denied a previous history of renal disease and had had a normal urinalysis on a routine clinic visit shortly before the respiratory tract infection began. The patient was referred to the City of Memphis Hospital.

Physical examination on admission revealed a well developed thin man who appeared acutely ill. His temperature was 101°F, blood pressure 140/90 mm Hg, pulse rate 100 beats/min and respiratory rate 22/min. Pertinent physical findings included mild periorbital edema, moist rales at the base of the left lung posteriorly, a grade 2/6 early systolic ejection murmur heard best along the left sternal border, and moderate edema of his feet and hands.

Initial laboratory values included a hematocrit value of 19 per cent, a white blood cell count of 16,400/mm^3 and a reticulocyte count of 20.1 per cent. The urine was cloudy and yellow in color, with pH 5 and albumin 4+; there were 15 to 25 red blood cells/hpf, 30 to 40 white blood cells/hpf, oval fat bodies, and moderate numbers of hyaline and granular casts. Initial arterial blood gases, determined while the patient was receiving 4 liters of nasal oxygen, showed moderate hypoxia (Table I). Blood urea nitrogen was 83 mg/100 ml and creatinine 9.7 mg/100 ml. Serum enzyme levels were moderately elevated. Cultures of the sputum, blood and urine were negative. A chest film revealed an infiltrate in the lower lobe of the left lung. The cardiac size was normal. A film of the abdomen showed the kidneys to be normal in size.

The patient was treated with antibiotics, oxygen and intermittent positive pressure breathing. He remained oliguric, and hemodialysis was begun for acute renal failure. Progressive respiratory distress and somnolence developed. Arterial blood gases failed to improve, and assisted ventilation was begun. Shortly thereafter, he had a cardiorespiratory arrest as a result of hypoxia, but he was resuscitated successfully.

The patient was maintained with dialysis and assisted ventilation over the next three week period. Repeat laboratory examination included a urine which was negative for myoglobin. Cultures of the tracheal aspirate and blood continued to be negative. During the fourth hospital week, he entered the diuretic phase of acute renal failure. His renal function improved progressively, but his urinary protein excretion was 11.5 g/24 hours. Because of a persistant prolonged bleeding time, a renal biopsy could not be performed. Films of his chest showed marked clearing of the pulmonary infiltrates. Serum obtained during the acute and convalescent phases for influenza viral antibody determination showed a significant increase in titer for influenza A/Port Chalmers/1/73 (Table II). The patient continued to show improvement and was discharged on the 47th hospital day. Subsequent follow-up has revealed the development of chronic renal disease that has persisted six months after his initial illness.

COMMENTS

Influenza in Tennessee reached epidemic proportions during the winter months of 1974–1975. The peak incidence occurred in January 1975 when 32,244 cases were reported to the Tennessee Department of Public Health. The mean age of the patients in the present study was 33.5 years (range 26 to 47 years) (Table I). Despite their relatively young age, all the patients became critically ill after the onset of their respiratory tract infection. Severe respiratory failure developed and ventilatory assistance was required for control of hypoxia. None of the patients had a prior history of renal disease, yet renal failure developed in all of them shortly after their illness began. Three of the patients were oliguric and uremic on admission. One patient (Case 1) passed dark brown urine after the onset of profound generalized muscle weakness, and had clinical and laboratory findings suggestive of myoglobinuria. One patient (Case 2) had normal renal function on admission, but acute renal failure developed after the onset of DIC. Bacteriologic studies were negative in all the patients on admission. Three of the patients had a significant increase in influenza viral antibody titer during the course of their illness. The fourth patient had the clinical picture of influenza during the epidemic period but died before serum could be obtained during the convalescent phase.

Attempts to establish a direct causative relationship between viral infections and renal disease in man have proved disappointing in most instances. Despite a growing body of evidence which suggests that at least certain viruses can induce acute renal disease, the mechanisms involved remain unknown. Isolated reports of glomerulonephritis associated with mumps [8], Coxsackie B [9], vaccinia [10], ECHO [11], varicella [12], hepatitis [13] and adenovirus [14] infections have been recorded. In addition, transient alterations of the urinary sediment, proteinuria and an occasional mild decrease in renal function have been observed during acute viral infections [15–17], but they usually subside without renal sequelae. Viruses have been isolated from the urine during the clinical course of mumps [15], enterovirus [18], vaccinia [19], cytomegalovirus [20], measles [21] and many others. The presence of viruria, however, does not necessarily indicate virus infection in the kidney since seeding of the urine by viruses from infected cells of the genitourinary tract has been observed during the course of disseminated infection [22].

The demonstration of viral antigens in the urinary sediment [23] and within the glomeruli and interstitium of the kidney [9] by immunofluorescent technics has suggested a possible immunologic basis for viral-renal damage. More recently, the finding of glomerulonephritis, immune complex deposits and intracellular cytoplasmic inclusion bodies in kidney biopsy specimens of patients with viral hepatitis and their possible association with hepatitis B antigen [24,25] have strengthened this concept. Experimental animal models of virus-induced renal disease also have shown immune pathogenetic mechanisms. Chronic viral infections with lymphocyte choriomeningitis virus [26], Maloney sarcoma virus [27], Aleutian disease of mink [28] and others [29,30] have been associated with immune complex deposition along the glomerular capillary wall and in the mesangia that bear striking similarities to glomerulonephritis in man.

Despite the paucity of direct evidence that the influenza virus can cause human renal disease, the secondary pathways that may be triggered by viral infection may be even more significant in producing various degrees of renal dysfunction. At least two of these pathways, rhabdomyolysis and DIC, were present in our series and most likely contributed largely towards the development of acute renal failure in two patients (Cases 1 and 2).

The occurrence of rhabdomyolysis has been reported after influenza [5,6] and other viral [31] infections. In addition to the leakage of myoglobin through the damaged muscle-cell membrane, other muscle components including creatine, serum glutamic oxaloacetic transaminase (SGOT), lactic dehydrogenase (LDH), creatine phosphokinase (CPK), potassium and many others are released into the circulation. Grossman et al. [32] observed 15 patients with acute renal failure after nontraumatic myoglobinuria. These investigators found that a presumptive diagnosis of myoglobinuria can be made easily when the triad of orthotolidin-positive urine (Hematest), pigmented granular casts in the urinary sediment and a marked increase in CPK was present. The patient in Case 1 of our series fulfilled these criteria in addition to having profound muscle weakness extending into the convalescent period. The pathophysiologic mechanism by which myoglobinuria produces acute renal failure remains poorly understood, but the prognosis for recovery of the nontraumatic type appears to be excellent when an early diagnosis is made and adequate facilities for management of the renal failure are available [5,6,32].

Acute renal failure may also develop in patients with influenza viral infections as a result of DIC [2–4]. Previous studies have shown that certain viral infections can induce intravascular coagulation [33]. Possible mechanisms by which viruses can trigger the blood coagulation system include agglutination and lysis of platelets [34] with release of coagulation factors into the circulation, the formation of procoagulant immune complexes from the combination of virus with circulating antibody [33], and intravascular destruction of red blood cells producing hemolysis and a hemolytic uremic-like syndrome [2,35]. Additional factors commonly present in critically ill patients that have been shown to cause intravascular coagulation include anoxia, acidosis, tissue trauma and hypotension. Many of these factors were present at various times in all of our patients, yet in only one patient (Case 2) did intravascular coagulation develop as the probable cause of her acute renal failure. This complication of influenza viral infections may be more common than was realized formerly. It was demonstrated in all six of the patients referred to the Renal Unit of the Princess Alexandra Hospital because of acute renal failure that occurred after an influenza infection during the 1970 influenza epidemic in Australia [2]. The favorable environment for the development of this syndrome in influenza viral infections warrants careful scrutiny of the coagulation system in these patients when acute renal failure ensues.

ACKNOWLEDGMENT

We gratefully acknowledge Dr. R. G. Webster of the St. Jude Childrens Research Hospital who performed the influenza viral studies. Dr. Webster's work was supported by NIH Grant AI08831. We also thank Dr. Mark Weisburst for assistance in the case preparations.

REFERENCES

1. Myking O, Schreiner A: Influenza virus infection complicated by severe renal failure. Scand J Infect Dis 6: 205, 1974.
2. Whitaker AN, Bunce I, Graeme ER: Disseminated intravascular coagulation and acute renal failure in influenza A2 infection. Med J Aust 2: 196, 1974.
3. Davison AM, Thomson D, Robson JS: Intravascular coagulation complicating influenza A virus infection. Br Med J 1: 654, 1973.
4. Talley NA, Assumpcao CAR: Disseminated intravascular clotting complicating viral pneumonia due to influenza. Med J Aust 2: 763, 1971.
5. Morgensen JL: Myoglobinuria and renal failure associated with influenza. Ann Intern Med 80: 362, 1974.
6. Simon NM, Rovner RN, Berlin BS: Acute myoglobinuria associated with type A2 (Hong Kong) influenza. JAMA 212: 1704, 1970.
7. Fazekas de St. Groth S, Webster RG: Disquisitions on original antigenic sin. I. Evidence in man. J Exp Med 124: 331, 1966.
8. Hughes WT, Steigman AJ, Delong HF: Some implications of fatal nephritis associated with mumps. Am J Dis Child 111: 297, 1966.
9. Burch GE, Colcolough HL: Progressive coxsackie viral pancarditis and nephritis. Ann Intern Med 71: 963, 1969.
10. Herbut PA: Diffuse glomerulonephritis following revaccination for smallpox. Am J Pathol 20: 1011, 1944.
11. Yuceoglu AM, Berkovich S, Minkowitz S: Acute glomerulonephritis associated with ECHO virus type 9 infection. J Pediatr 69: 603, 1966.
12. Yuceoglu AM, Berkovich S, Minkowitz S: Acute glomerulonephritis as a complication of varicella. JAMA 202: 879, 1967.
13. Conrad ME, Schwartz FD, Young AA: Infectious hepatitis—a generalized disease. Am J Med 37: 789, 1964.
14. Chany C, Lepine P, Lelong M, et al.: Severe and fatal pneumonia in infants and young children associated with adenovirus infections. Am J Hyg 67: 367, 1958.
15. Utz JP, Houk VN, Alling DW: Clinical and laboratory studies of mumps. N Engl J Med 270: 1283, 1964.
16. Mary AS, Swallow JH: An epidemic of ECHO 6 virus infection. Postgrad Med J 46: 265, 1970.
17. Van Der Veen J, Van Der Ploeg G: An outbreak of pharyngoconjunctival fever caused by types 3 and 4 adenovirus at Waalwijk, the Netherlands. Am J Hyg 68: 95, 1958.
18. Utz JP, Shelokov AI: Coxsackie B virus infection. JAMA 168: 264, 1958.
19. Gresser I, Kibrick S: Isolation of vaccinia virus and type 1 adenovirus from urine. N Engl J Med 265: 743, 1961.
20. Weller TH, Hanshaw JB: Virologic and clinical observations on cytomegalic inclusion disease. N Engl J Med 266: 1233, 1962.
21. Gresser I, Katz SL: Isolation of measles virus from urine. N Engl J Med 263: 452, 1960.
22. Schultz I, Nev FA: Relationship between blood clearance and viruria after intravenous injection of mice and rats with bacteriophage and polioviruses. J Immunol 94: 833, 1965.
23. Hinuma Y, Miyamoto T, Murai Y, et al.: Detection of coxsackie virus antigen in urinary cells by immunofluorescence. Lancet 2: 179, 1962.
24. Eknoyan G, Gyorkey F, Dichoso C, et al.: Renal morphological and immunological changes associated with acute viral hepatitis. Kidney Int 1: 413, 1972.
25. Knieser MR, Jenis EH, Lowenthal DT, et al.: Pathogenesis of renal disease associated with viral hepatitis. Arch Pathol 97: 193, 1974.
26. Oldstone M, Dixon F: Lymphocytic choriomeningitis: production of antibody by "tolerant" infected mice. Science 158: 1193, 1967.
27. Hirsch M, Allison A, Harvey J: Immune complex in mice infected neonatally with Moloney leukaemogenic and murine sarcoma viruses. Nature (Lond) 223: 739, 1969.
28. Porter D, Larsen A, Porter H: The pathogenesis of Aleutian disease of mink. I. In vivo viral replication and the host antibody to viral antigen. J Exp Med 130: 575, 1969.
29. Banks K, Henson J: Glomerular deposition of gamma globulin and complement (C'3) in equine infectious anemia. Fed Proc 28: 752, 1969.
30. Cheville N, Mengeling W: The pathogenesis of chronic hog cholera. Lab Invest 20: 261, 1969.
31. Favara BE, Vawter GF, Wagner R, et al.: Familial paroxysmal rhabdomyolysis in children. A myoglobinuric syndrome. Am J Med 42: 196, 1967.
32. Grossman RA, Hamilton RW, Morse BM, et al.: Nontraumatic rhabdomyolysis and acute renal failure. N Engl J Med 291: 807, 1974.
33. McKay DG, Margaretten W: Disseminated intravascular coagulation in virus diseases. Arch Intern Med 120: 129, 1967.
34. Terada H, Baldini M, Ebbe S, et al.: Interaction of influenza virus with blood platelets. Blood 28: 213, 1966.
35. Ray CG, Tucker VL, Harris DJ, et al.: Enteroviruses associated with the hemolytic-uremic syndrome. Pediatrics 46: 378, 1970.

Herpesvirus Hominis Type 2 Meningoencephalitis Following Renal Transplantation

CALVIN C. LINNEMANN, Jr., M.D.
M. ROY FIRST, M.D.
MARIANO M. ALVIRA, M.D.
J. WESLEY ALEXANDER, M.D.
GILBERT M. SCHIFF, M.D.
Cincinnati, Ohio

Herpesvirus hominis (HVH) type 2 meningoencephalitis, confirmed by isolation of the virus from cerebrospinal fluid and brain biopsy specimens, is described in a 44 year old man following renal transplantation. An HVH type 2 genital infection developed two weeks after renal transplantation, which was followed by meningoencephalitis 10 days later. Subsequently an intracerebral hemorrhage developed with evidence of diffuse vasculitis on arteriography. In a second transplant patient a similar clinical syndrome also developed after an HVH type 2 genital infection, but viral studies were not made to confirm the etiology of the meningoencephalitis. HVH has been recognized as a cause of mucocutaneous diseases in recipients of renal transplants, but involvement of the central nervous system has not been reported.

Herpesvirus hominis (HVH) infections are a recognized complication of renal transplantation, but the virus usually produces only mucocutaneous disease [1–4]. However, both HVH type 1 and 2 can produce central nervous system disease [5]. HVH type 1, which causes herpes labialis, produces encephalitis in the adult patient, whereas HVH type 2, which causes herpes genitalis, produces encephalitis in the neonate or aseptic meningitis in the adult [6]. In this report we describe the occurrence of HVH type 2 meningoencephalitis after renal transplantation. Although HVH type 2 has been isolated from cerebrospinal fluid in the past, this represents the first report of HVH type 2 recovered from brain biopsy specimens. Intracerebral hemorrhage and a unique arteriographic finding, compatible with a diffuse vasculitis, were observed in this patient. A second patient is also described who was seen with a similar clinical syndrome following renal transplantation, including an HVH type 2 genital infection, meningoencephalitis, intracerebral hemorrhage and an abnormal cerebral arteriogram. Since viral infection of the central nervous system was not considered in the second patient, brain specimens and cerebrospinal fluid for viral culture were not taken. These two patients suggest that HVH infection should be considered in patients in whom central nervous system disease develops after renal transplantation.

From the Departments of Medicine, Pathology and Surgery, University of Cincinnati College of Medicine, Cincinnati, Ohio. This study was supported in part by U.S. Public Health Service Research Grant 1 R01 AI 12309. Requests for reprints to Dr. Calvin C. Linnemann, Jr., Infectious Disease Division, 7064 Medical Science Building, 231 Bethesda Ave., Cincinnati, Ohio 45267. Manuscript accepted January 14, 1976.

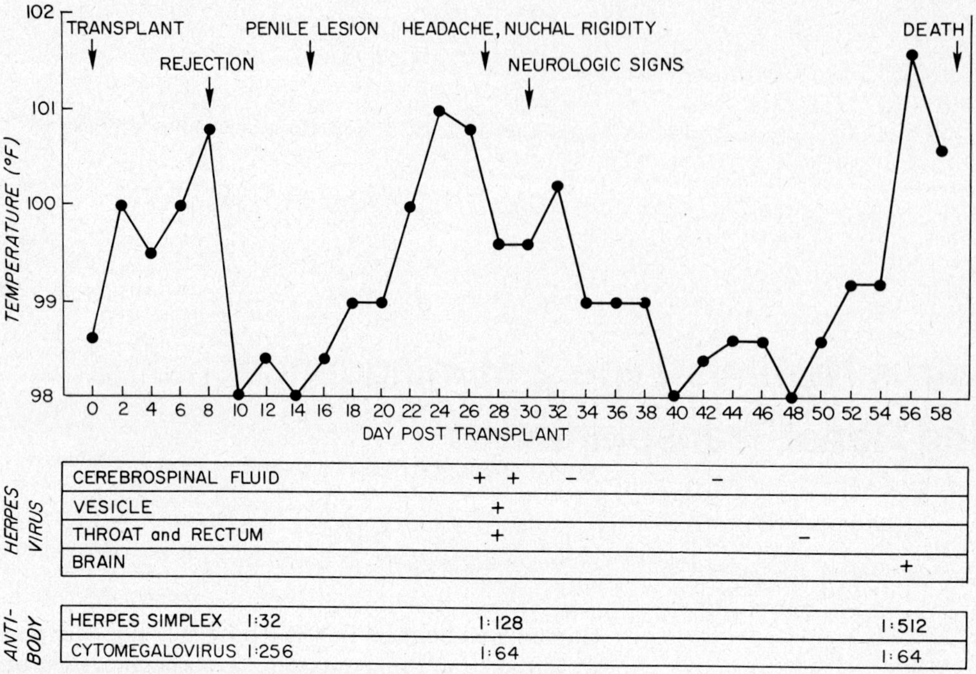

Figure 1. *Clinical and virologic findings in type 2 herpesvirus hominis meningoencephalitis.*

CASE REPORTS

Case 1. A 44 year old white man was admitted to the Cincinnati General Hospital on June 27, 1974, for a cadaveric renal allograft. He had been found to have proteinuria at age 30, and renal function had declined progressively in subsequent years. In November 1973 he required peritoneal dialysis for the first time, and in December he received a living donor kidney transplant at another hospital. He rejected the transplant and was transferred to Cincinnati General Hospital where he underwent an allograft nephrectomy on February 21, 1974. In March 1974, he underwent a bilateral nephrectomy, splenectomy and fulguration of rectal condylomas. Renal tissue showed chronic end-stage renal disease. He was maintained on hemodialysis until the present admission.

The transplant was completed without incident on the night of admission and good renal function was established with the creatinine level falling from 9.1 to 1.8 mg/100 ml. He received 150 mg of azathioprine/day and 150 to 300 mg of prednisone/day. A low grade fever, with temperatures of 100°F, developed on post-transplant day 2 and persisted for seven days; no etiology was discovered (Figure 1). On day 8, the allograft was noted to be enlarged, firm and tender, and the patient was treated for acute rejection with 150 R of external radiation to the kidney on three occasions, and 500 mg of methylprednisolone/day for five days. He became afebrile, but the serum creatinine did not begin to decrease until day 16. At that time, he was receiving 150 mg of azathioprine and 90 mg of prednisone/day.

On day 15, a small ulcer was noted on the dorsum of the penis for the first time. Fever developed again on day 21 (Figure 1). Physical examination did not reveal the source of the fever, and both blood and urine cultures were negative. Renal function remained good and the administration of azathioprine was continued with decreasing doses of prednisone. On day 25, a small vesicular lesion was noted under the right nostril. Because of persistent fever with temperatures to 101°F and leukopenia of 4,200 white blood cells/mm^3, the administration of azathioprine was discontinued. The patient felt extremely weak and began to complain of diffuse fronto-occipital headaches. On physical examination, he had minimal nuchal rigidity, and multiple superficial ulcers were present around the anus. A lumbar puncture was performed on day 27 and the cerebrospinal fluid contained 41 white blood cells/mm^3, 86 per cent polymorphonuclear leukocytes, 8 red blood cells/mm^3, a protein level of 178 mg/100 ml and a sugar level of 42 mg/100 ml with a blood sugar level of 160 mg/100 ml. Bacterial cultures were negative and viral culture grew HVH (Figure 1). The headache persisted with photophobia, and in addition to generalized weakness, coarse tremors of both upper extremities were noted. On neurologic examination, there was a question of some impairment of finger-to-nose coordination of the left hand. The lumbar puncture was repeated on day 29 and showed a decrease in the number of cells but an increase in protein to 252 mg/100 ml. The cerebrospinal fluid glucose content was 34 mg/100 ml, but a blood glucose level was not obtained. An electroencephalogram and brain scan were within normal limits. On day 30, a right supranuclear facial nerve paresis and ptosis developed, and two days later, a dilated right pupil and a left Babinski reflex. A right retrograde brachial arteriogram was performed, which was within normal limits. The following day, a third lumbar puncture was performed which showed 190 red blood cells/mm^3, 200 white blood cells/mm^3 and 86 per cent lymphocytes.

By day 34, his fever disappeared and his neurologic signs

slowly diminished, with the disappearance of pyramidal tract signs and cranial nerve involvement, but the dilated right pupil was persistent. During this time his renal function remained good, and azathioprine therapy was reinstituted on day 36. At that time he was receiving 50 mg of prednisone/day. On day 40, he complained of a mild right-sided headache; this was followed by blurring of the vision in the right eye two days later. Examination of the right eye revealed blurring of the disk and clouding of the vitreous. A repeat lumbar puncture showed 38 red blood cells/mm^3, 176 white blood cells/mm^3 and 80 per cent polymorphonuclear leukocytes, with a protein level of 218 mg/100 ml and a glucose level of 64 mg/100 ml. The patient's condition continued to improve except for occasional right-sided headaches and the visual impairment. On day 47, the skin lesions were noted to be healing. A repeat electroencephalogram and brain scan were within normal limits.

By day 55, discharge from the hospital was being contemplated. His blood pressure was 150/90 mm Hg and his creatinine 1.2 mg/100 ml. At 8:00 P.M. that night, the patient complained of a severe headache, and at 9:30 P.M. he was found in bed unresponsive. The blood pressure level was elevated to 220/120 mm Hg, Doll's eye movements were present, the right pupil was dilated and unreactive as before, and a right Babinski reflex was present. By morning, both pupils were dilated and bilateral plantar reflexes were present. Bilateral carotid arteriograms were performed, which demonstrated numerous focal dilatations of branches of both the anterior and middle cerebral arteries on the right and left, and a mass effect indicating a large avascular mass in the right temporal fossa and in the right frontal area (Figure 2). These were interpreted to be mycotic aneurysms with intracerebral hemorrhage. A right temporal craniotomy was performed with evacuation of a hematoma, and biopsy of the brain. There was no neurologic improvement after surgery, the pupils remained fixed and dilated; there were no spontaneous respirations and there was no response to pain. The patient was pronounced dead on August 25, 1974, 59 days after receiving the renal transplant.

An autopsy was not performed, but the brain biopsy specimen was available for pathologic examination. Tissue from the temporal lobe showed focal necrotizing lesions accompanied by a severe vasculitis (Figure 3). There were focal infiltrations of lymphocytes, mononuclear cells and a few polymorphonuclear leukocytes. Neuronal and glial cells showed severe pyknotic degeneration, and the neuropil was very edematous. Early basophilic intranuclear inclusion bodies were seen in necrotic neurones, glial cells and endothelial cells. These inclusion bodies were large and single. Some had a peripheral halo, and the nuclei exhibited margination of the nuclear chromatin. There were no cytoplasmic inclusion bodies. Blood vessels were focally necrotic and infiltrated by numerous inflammatory cells. Mononuclear cell infiltration predominated. Numerous perivascular "ring" hemorrhages were also present.

Between the 26th and 28th days after the transplant, viral cultures of material from the cerebrospinal fluid, throat, rectum, urine and skin lesions were taken. These were inoculated into human fibroblastic lung (WI-38), HeLa, primary monkey kidney and Vero monkey kidney cell cultures, and HVH was isolated from all specimens except the urine (Figure 1). HVH was cultured again from the cerebrospinal fluid obtained at the time of the second lumbar puncture. Cerebrospinal fluid from the 33rd and 43rd days after transplant and throat and rectal cultures on the 49th day were negative. The urine culture was negative for cytomegalovirus. Tissue obtained from the brain biopsy specimen on the 56th day grew HVH. Three of the isolates (brain, cerebrospinal fluid and rectal) were typed by the immunofluorescent technic by Dr. Andre J. Nahmias and identified as HVH type 2.

Serum specimens obtained prior to renal transplantation and on post-transplant days 12, 29 and 56 were tested for complement-fixing antibody to HVH, cytomegalovirus, Epstein-Barr (EB) and varicella zoster virus. HVH antibody was present prior to transplantation and remained at the same level on the 12th day after the transplant. Subsequently there was a 16-fold rise in antibody titer. Cytomegalovirus antibody

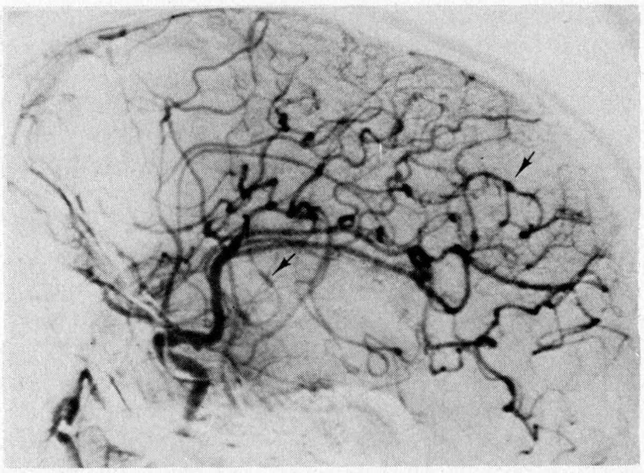

Figure 2. *Cerebral arteriogram taken on post-transplant day 55, prior to brain biopsy. Arrows indicate representative areas of dilatation in cerebral vessels, some associated with localized constriction.*

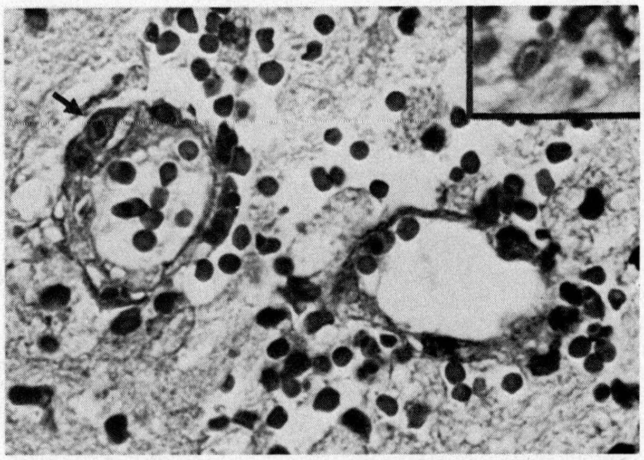

Figure 3. *Brain biopsy specimen from temporal lobe showing necrotic blood vessels with abundant mononuclear inflammatory cell infiltration. Arrow points to an intranuclear inclusion body in an endothelial cell. A typical intranuclear inclusion body is shown in the inset. Original magnification 4,400, reduced by 50 per cent.*

was also present prior to the transplant and this showed a fourfold rise in antibody titer by day 12. Subsequently, there was a fourfold fall in antibody titer. EB and varicella zoster virus antibody remained low or undetectable after renal transplantation. Cerebrospinal fluid obtained at the time of the third lumbar puncture did not contain measurable complement fixation antibody to HVH.

Case 2. A 24 year old white woman was admitted to CGH on October 7, 1973, for a cadaveric renal allograft. She had a history of chronic renal failure secondary to chronic pyelonephritis and had been undergoing regular hemodialysis for eight months. Following the kidney transplantation she had a fever for three days; she then showed improvement until post-transplant day 7, when acute rejection developed. For this, she was treated with external radiation and methylprednisolone, in addition to her azathioprine and prednisone.

On day 9, a vesicular lesion was noted on the left buttock, from which HVH type 2 was isolated. On day 18 a fever developed, followed by a headache. Because of persistent fever and headache, a lumbar puncture was performed. The cerebrospinal fluid had an initial pressure of 260 mm water and contained 26 red blood cells/mm^3, 25 white blood cells/mm^3, a glucose level of 21 mg/100 ml with a blood glucose level of 108 mg/100 ml. Bacterial cultures were sterile. Therapy with intravenous ampicillin was started and her azathioprine therapy was discontinued. Nuchal rigidity and photophobia developed on day 25, and a repeat lumbar puncture showed 2,617 red blood cells/mm^3 and 50 white blood cells/mm^3, 62 per cent lymphocytes. A brain scan was within normal limits. She became afebrile on day 30 and the administration of azathioprine was restarted.

On day 39, a right facial nerve paresis, right homonymous hemianopsia, and right hemiplegia suddenly developed. A brain scan showed increased uptake in the left parietal, occipital and temporal areas, and an arteriogram showed a mass effect on the left side with a questionable small aneurysm in a vessel over the central Sylvian area. It was believed that she might have a mycotic aneurysm with intracranial hemorrhage. A burr hole was made and the hematoma aspirated. Bacterial cultures were sterile and viral cultures were not performed.

Subsequently, her condition improved, but on day 55 a fever developed with temperatures of 100.5°F. A repeat lumbar puncture two days later showed an initial pressure of 270 mm water and contained 1,211 red blood cells/mm^3, 16 white blood cells/mm^3, predominantly lymphocytes, a glucose level of 39 mg/100 ml and a protein level of 131 mg/100 ml. On day 61, a left hemiparesis developed. The brain scan was within normal limits. Six days later, the cerebrospinal fluid showed no significant change, but an arteriogram showed numerous small dilations of the cerebral arteries bilaterally. All cultures were sterile, but she was treated for bacterial endocarditis because of the possibility that she had mycotic aneurysms in the brain.

The remainder of her hospital course was complicated by hypercalcemia, for which she required parathyroidectomy, recurrent renal rejection and hypertensive encephalopathy followed by death on post-transplant day 123. At autopsy, neuropathologic examination revealed multiple infarcts and hemorrhages, attributed to her hypertensive encephalopathy. There were small areas of perivascular lymphocytic infiltration and rare multinucleated giant cells, but intranuclear inclusion bodies were not seen. Serum specimens obtained during the acute and convalescent phases showed a fourfold rise in complement fixation antibodies to HVH.

COMMENTS

Herpesvirus infections, including cytomegalovirus, herpes zoster and HVH, are common in renal transplant recipients [2]. HVH infections are usually asymptomatic, although Lopez et al. [7] suggested, on the basis of a temporal relationship, that these infections may be associated with renal allograft rejection. In the present two cases, rejection preceded the HVH infection. When HVH produces clinical disease in the transplant patient, it is usually limited to mucocutaneous disease [1–3,8,9]. Most of these are perioral or intraoral lesions, which may take weeks to months to heal; occasionally they may involve the esophagus. These HVH isolates are presumably type 1. Arora et al. [4] described a generalized cutaneous infection in a transplant recipient in whom HVH type 2 was isolated. The only fatal HVH infection in a renal transplant recipient was reported by Montgomerie et al. [8]. Interestingly, that patient also had chronic genital herpetic lesions which would suggest that this was also HVH type 2. These genital lesions persisted for months and oral lesions subsequently developed. At autopsy, HVH was grown in cultures of specimens from the mouth, vulva, lung and ileum. Examination of the brain, spinal cord and cerebrospinal fluid was not reported. Our report represents the first central nervous system infection with HVH in a renal transplant recipient. A possible explanation for the failure to see fatal HVH infections in transplant recipients despite the frequency of such infections in this population is due to the type of HVH involved. Most infections in transplant recipients are probably due to HVH type 1; it may be that HVH type 2 has a greater pathogenic potential in the immunosuppressed patient. To resolve this question, HVH isolates from renal transplant recipients in the future will need to be typed and related to the clinical illness.

HVH types 1 and 2 are associated with different patterns of neurologic involvement: HVH type 1, with encephalitis in the adult; and HVH type 2, with neonatal encephalitis and with aseptic meningitis in the adult [6]. Craig and Nahmias [2] postulated that HVH reached the central nervous system by neural spread in the case of HVH type 1 and by hematogenous dissemination for HVH type 2. They emphasized the importance of differentiating the bad prognosis of HVH type 1 encephalitis in adults and HVH type 2 in neonates from the good prognosis of HVH type 2 infection of the central nervous system in adults. These differences in neurologic involvement may be true for the normal host, but it would now appear that the immunosuppressed host, such as the renal transplant recipient, may be the exception to these generalizations. Disseminated HVH type 2 infection similar to that seen in neonates has been reported in an adult with thymic dysplasia [10]. However, HVH type 2 has not been isolated from a brain biopsy specimen in an adult patient prior to the present report. Disseminated infections have also been documented in six other adult patients, but the viral isolates were not typed [10]. All these patients had predisposing factors, including steroid treatment, burns, Hodgkin's disease and malnutrition. Unusual HVH type 1 infections of the central nervous system have also been reported in compromised hosts, including aseptic meningitis in a patient with leukemia, and a slowly progressive encephalitis with atypical pathologic findings in a patient with Hodgkin's disease [11,12].

The present case presented as typical HVH type 2 aseptic meningitis occurring nine to 10 days after the appearance of genital herpetic lesions. Hypoglycorrhachia was present, which has been reported in HVH meningoencephalitis [13]. Neurologic signs subsequently developed, including involvement of the cranial nerves, pyramidal tract and the eyes. In this case, HVH type 2 was present in the cerebrospinal fluid and disappeared with the clinical improvement of the patient. Antiviral chemotherapy was considered at this point, but was not used because of the disappearance of the virus in cerebrospinal fluid. Subsequently, the patient experienced an intracerebral hemorrhage, and a cerebral arteriogram indicated the presence of a diffuse vasculitis with multiple aneurysmal dilatations. This patient and the second patient had the only arteriograms with this pattern which have been seen at the University of Cincinnati over the past five years (Dr. R. Lukin, Department of Radiology, personal communication). In both cases, it was thought that these represented rupture of a mycotic aneurysm with intracerebral hemorrhage. However, bacterial cultures were sterile. A cerebral vasculitis has been demonstrated in herpes zoster virus infection, which can be demonstrated on angiography, but it has not been demonstrated previously on arteriograms in HVH encephalitis [14,15]. The absence of complete autopsy studies at the time of the acute illness prevents absolute proof that the findings on the arteriogram were the direct result of HVH type 2 infection. However, the isolation of HVH type 2 from the brain four weeks after the onset of HVH type 2 meningoencephalitis and the finding of a vasculitis in the brain biopsy specimen support this possibility. Intranuclear inclusion bodies were found in both endothelial cells and neural tissue. These were very suggestive of HVH, although only basophilic inclusion bodies were seen. The basophilic intranuclear inclusion bodies in HVH infections represent actual viral particles and are seen at an early stage of infection, whereas the eosinophilic inclusion bodies occur later, after the release of viral particles from the nucleus [16]. Larger tissue specimens than those available from the brain biopsy specimen may have demonstrated eosinophilic inclusions.

The present cases suggest that HVH infection should be considered in renal transplant recipients in whom central nervous system disease develops. When HVH infection of the central nervous system occurs, antiviral chemotherapy with adenine arabinoside may be considered, since uncontrolled observations in neonates with HVH type 2 encephalitis have suggested that it may be of some benefit [17]. However, the value of this drug is unproved and it should be used only in controlled studies.

ACKNOWLEDGMENT

The HVH isolates were typed by Dr. Andre J. Nahmias, Atlanta, Georgia.

REFERENCES

1. Spencer ES, Andersen HK: Clinically evident, non-terminal infections with herpesviruses and the wart virus in immunosuppressed renal allograft recipients. Br Med J 3: 251, 1970.
2. Pien FD, Smith TF, Anderson CF, et al.: Herpesviruses in renal transplant patients. Transplantation 16: 489, 1973.
3. Koranda FC, Dehmel EM, Kahn G, et al.: Cutaneous complications in immunosuppressed renal homograft recipients. JAMA 229: 419, 1974.
4. Arora KK, Karalakulasingam R, Raff MJ, et al.: Cutaneous herpesvirus hominis (type 2) infection after renal transplantation. JAMA 230: 1174, 1974.
5. Nahmias AJ, Roizman B: Infection with herpes-simplex viruses 1 and 2 (in three parts). N Engl J Med 289: 667, 719, 781, 1973.
6. Craig CP, Nahmias AJ: Different patterns of neurologic involvement with herpes simplex virus types 1 and 2. Isolation of herpes simplex virus type 2 from the buffy coat of two adults with meningitis. J Infect Dis 127: 365, 1973.
7. Lopez C, Simmons RL, Mauer SM, et al.: Association of renal allograft rejection with virus infections. Am J Med 56: 280, 1974.
8. Montgomerie JZ, Becroft DMO, Croxson MC, et al.: Herpes-simplex-virus infection after renal transplantation. Lancet 2: 867, 1969.
9. Logan WS, Tindall JP, Elson ML: Chronic cutaneous herpes simplex. Arch Dermatol 103: 606, 1971.
10. Sutton AL, Smithwick EM, Seligman SJ, et al.: Fatal disseminated herpesvirus hominis type 2 infection in an adult with associated thymic dysplasia. Am J Med 56: 545, 1974.

11. Cappel R, Klastersky J: Herpetic meningitis (type 1) in a case of acute leukemia. Arch Neurol 28: 415, 1973.
12. Price R, Chernik NL, Horta-Barbosa L, et al.: Herpes simplex encephalitis in an anergic patient. Am J Med 54: 222, 1973.
13. Morrison RE, Miller MH, Lyon LW, et al.: Adult meningoencephalitis caused by herpesvirus hominis type 2. Am J Med 56: 540, 1974.
14. Walker RJ, EL Gammal T, Allen MB Jr: Cranial arteritis associated with herpes zoster. Radiology 107: 109, 1973.
15. Radcliffe WB, Guinto FC Jr, Adcock DF, et al.: Herpes simplex encephalitis; a radiologic-pathologic study of 4 cases. Am J Roentgenol Radium Ther Nucl Med 112: 263, 1971.
16. Rhodes AJ, Van Rooyen CE: Textbook of Virology, 5th ed. Baltimore, Williams & Wilkins, 1968.
17. Ch'ien LT, Whitley RJ, Nahmias AJ, et al.: Antiviral chemotherapy and neonatal herpes simplex virus infection. A pilot study—experience with Adenine Arabinoside (ARA-A). Pediatrics 55: 678, 1975.

Diurnal Pattern of Water and Electrolyte Excretion and Body Weight in Idiopathic Orthostatic Hypotension

The Effect of Three Treatments

C. DAVIDSON, M.B., M.R.C.P.
D. SMITH, M.B., Ph.D.
D. B. MORGAN, M.D., M.R.C.Path.
Leeds, England

The diurnal pattern of water and solute excretion and body weight were examined in five control subjects and in a patient with idiopathic orthostatic hypotension before and during treatment. The patient had a reversed diurnal pattern of excretion of sodium, urea and water but not of potassium and creatinine, and there was an excessive diurnal variation in body weight. The effects of three treatments, high salt diet alone and then with the addition of head-up tilt, and later fludrocortisone, were studied. Fludrocortisone caused marked clinical improvement and retention of sodium and water. Once a steady state was achieved none of the treatments had any significant effect either on the diurnal variation in weight or on the water and solute excretion pattern except for a small reduction in sodium excretion at night when the patient slept with a head-up tilt. It is concluded that these treatments cause symptomatic improvement in idiopathic orthostatic hypotension through an increase in extracellular fluid volume rather than through any change in the abnormal diurnal pattern of water and salt excretion.

An abnormal diurnal pattern of water and electrolyte excretion may occur in a number of common diseases such as heart failure, cirrhosis [1] or idiopathic steatorrhea [2], and during steroid treatment [3]. The abnormality is a "reversal" of the normal pattern with the urinary excretion of water and sodium being greater at night than in the day, and this may cause nocturia. Idiopathic orthostatic hypotension is a rare disorder of the autonomic nervous system in which nocturia may be prominent due to a reversed diurnal pattern of water excretion [4]. Studies suggest that there is also a reversed pattern of sodium excretion [5,6] and, therefore, an excessive loss of extracellular fluid during the night. This may explain why the hypotension and fainting in these patients is often worse in the morning [7].

There is other evidence that sodium and water balance influences the severity of symptoms in this condition. Firstly, the most effective treatment is with sodium-retaining steroids and not, as might be expected, with sympathomimetic agents [8]. Secondly, sodium-retaining steroids, such as desoxycorticosterone or fludrocortisone, are only effective when adequate salt intake is ensured, and successful treatment is usually associated with sodium retention and expansion

From the Departments of Medicine and Chemical Pathology, Leeds General Infirmary, Leeds, England. Requests for reprints should be addressed to Dr. D. B. Morgan, Department of Chemical Pathology, Leeds General Infirmary, Leeds LS1 3EX, England. Manuscript accepted January 14, 1976.

of the extracellular fluid. Thirdly, MacLean and Allen [9] reported that sleeping with a head-up tilt of 25 degrees lessened the severity of the symptoms, and it was later shown that this sleeping posture increased extracellular fluid and blood volume [10,11].

Studies of the diurnal pattern of solute excretion in idiopathic orthostatic hypotension are, however, surprisingly limited and have involved urine collections over single 24 hour periods [5,6]. The effect of treatment on the diurnal pattern has not, to our knowledge, been studied in detail. We recently saw a patient with the classic features of idiopathic orthostatic hypotension whose symptoms were more severe in the mornings. In her, we studied the diurnal pattern of solute and water excretion, and the diurnal changes in body weight during a control period and during treatment with a high salt intake, at first alone and later in combination with "head-up tilt" at night and then fludrocortisone. We have compared the findings in this patient during the control period with those in five women without orthostatic hypotension who were studied under the same conditions.

CASE REPORT

The patient was a 65 year old woman who had had orthostatic hypotension for four years at the time of the study, and who had become completely housebound. Autonomic dysfunction was shown by the characteristic anhidrosis, absent reflex vasodilation and a fixed pulse rate. The general examination, including full neurologic examination, was otherwise within normal limits.

The patient had normal values for full blood count, erythrocyte sedimentation rate, serum vitamin B_{12}, plasma proteins, Wasserman reaction, glucose tolerance test and synacthen test.

A rectal biopsy specimen showed no evidence of amyloid, and nerve conduction studies disclosed no abnormalities. Thus there was no evidence for any of the known causes of orthostatic hypotension, and the patient was, therefore, considered to have idiopathic orthostatic hypotension.

The patient will be described in detail elsewhere together with a review of the literature (Davidson and Morgan; in preparation).

DESIGN OF STUDY

The patient was studied in a metabolic ward for six weeks. She was ambulant during the daytime and was in bed from about 10 P.M. each evening until after the 8 A.M. observations next day. She adhered to a constant low salt diet (20 mmol a day) throughout the study. During the control period, this diet was supplemented with salt capsules to give a total sodium chloride intake of 70 mmol a day. This intake was chosen as it was the amount of sodium she excreted daily in the urine during a preliminary study made when she was at home. The salt intake was subsequently increased with extra salt capsules. Three therapeutic regimens were tested so that the total study was in four periods.

Period I. Control period: salt intake 70 mmol a day (10 days).

Period II. High salt period: salt intake 150 mmol a day (10 days).

Period III. Tilting: Salt intake as in period II, but the patient slept with her bed tilted to 25 degrees (10 days).

Period IV. Salt intake as in period III but with fludrocortisone, 0.5 mg twice a day (12 days). During the last six days of this period she was given 90 mmol of potassium (as potassium chloride) a day to correct hypokalemia.

Table I shows the details of the five women who served as controls. Each woman had osteoporosis and was in a metabolic ward for calcium balance measurements. The women were ambulant and adhered to a constant diet throughout the study.

Clinical Measurements. Each 24 hour period started at 8 A.M. Observations and measurements were made throughout the study at four-hourly intervals and included the number of faints, the pulse rate, blood pressure and body weight. The blood pressure was measured with the patient lying down and after she had been standing for 2 minutes. On many occasions, particularly in the early part of the study, the patient fainted before the 2 minutes had passed, and the standing blood pressure was then recorded as zero. Body weight was measured on Baxendale chair scales; the patient always wore night clothes and emptied her bladder before she was weighed. Urine was collected in 4 hour periods throughout the study. In preliminary investigations, venesection produced a severe but transient deterioration in symptoms, and further blood tests were, therefore, kept to a minimum.

Each control subject was studied over a six day period. Body weight was measured as described at four hourly intervals (except 4 A.M.), and urine was collected over 4 hour periods with the exception of one 8 hour period (12 midnight to 8 A.M.).

Laboratory Measurements and Methods. Creatinine, urea and electrolyte levels were measured in urine and plasma by standard autoanalyzer methods (Technicon®). Exchangeable sodium was measured with sodium (Na^{24}) and plasma volume with ^{131}I-labeled albumin [12]. On one occasion when plasma volume was measured twice in a day, ^{125}I-labeled albumin was used for the second measurement.

RESULTS

Clinical Response to Treatment. Figure 1 and Table II show the effect of therapy on the number of faints, standing blood pressure, body weight and sodium excretion. In period I (the control period), there was no trend in any of these variables. An increased salt intake (period II) resulted in a decrease in the frequency of faints and retention of sodium, and an increase in body weight ($p < 0.01$). When the patient slept tilted at 25 degrees (period III) there was a further small gain in body weight (not statistically significant) and a higher average standing blood pressure, but no further decrease in the frequency of faints.

TABLE I Details of the Patient and the Five Control Subjects*

Data	Patient	Control Subjects 1	2	3	4	5
Age (yr)	65	55	64	67	63	53
Weight (kg) 8 A.M.	63.38 ± 0.09	49.54 ± 0.04	57.60 ± 0.04	58.91 ± 0.09	71.85 ± 0.10	51.29 ± 0.08
Height (cm)	157	159	156	147	167	149
Plasma						
Sodium (mmol/liter)	142	140	141	141	142	140
Potassium (mmol/liter)	3.95	4.1	4.1	3.9	4.2	4.4
Urea (mmol/liter)	8.2	3.8	6.3	6.5	5.7	5.7
Creatinine (μmol/liter)	101.7	77.4	84	84	84	97.2
Urine						
Volume (ml/day)	2,211 ± 72	1,650 ± 150	2,022 ± 85	1,725 ± 99	1,544 ± 72	1,815 ± 67
Sodium (mmol/day)	59.3 ± 6.0	123 ± 5.8	76.8 ± 4.6	109 ± 5.4	106 ± 4.6	65.5 ± 7.1
Potassium (mmol/day)	62.4 ± 2.0	39.2 ± 1.6	44.0 ± 1.7	40.6 ± 1.5	45 ± 1.1	37.5 ± 1.7
Urea (mmol/day)	341.3 ± 13.3	311.4 ± 3.3	259.7 ± 6.7	378 ± 10	383 ± 10	289.7 ± 13.3
Creatinine (mmol/day)	11 ± 0.43	10.4 ± 0.24	9.66 ± 0.13	10.6 ± 0.40	12.4 ± 0.27	9.93 ± 0.36

* Values shown are mean (± SEM) for the six day periods.

The administration of fludrocortisone (period IV) had a striking effect on each of the four variables. Initially, there was sodium retention and weight gain, followed by a period of escape when the weight remained steady but sodium excretion returned to its previous value. This retention of sodium and water was associated with a cessation of fainting, a higher blood pressure when standing and an increase in plasma volume. Two further measurements of plasma volume were made after the patient had returned home and showed that this increase in plasma volume following the administration of fludrocortisone was sustained, although the increase was less than at the beginning of treatment. At two months, the value was 2.40 liters; at six months, the value was 2.57 liters in the morning and 2.71 liters in the evening, when measured on the same day.

Diurnal Variation: Control Periods. Figure 2 compares the variation in the patient's body weight during period I with that of the five control subjects. The variation in weight is expressed as the difference of each measurement from the weight at 8 A.M. on the same day. In the patient and the control subjects there was a weight gain during the daytime (8 A.M. to 12 midnight) and a weight loss during the nighttime (12 midnight to 8 A.M.). These gains and losses were greater in the patient than in any of the controls, and much greater in the patient than in four of the five control subjects.

In order to compare the diurnal pattern of each variable, both between persons and between treatment periods, we calculated hourly excretion rates for the daytime (8 A.M. to 12 midnight) and for the nighttime (12 midnight to 8 A.M.). Figure 3 shows that in the patient excretion rates for sodium, water and urea were greater in the nighttime than in the daytime, but this was not so for potassium or creatinine. In contrast, in the control subjects, with one exception, the excretion rate for water, sodium, potassium, urea and creatinine was greater during the daytime than the nighttime. In one control subject the nighttime excretion rate for sodium was just greater than the daytime excretion rate; this woman also had a greater diurnal variation in body weight than any of the other control subjects.

Diurnal Variations: Effect of Treatment. At the beginning of each treatment there was a transient period of change in the variables followed by a new steady state. In order to examine the effect of treatments on the diurnal pattern of each variable, only the results obtained during the steady state were used, that is the last six days of each treatment period.

Figure 2 shows that none of the treatments changed the diurnal variation in body weight. Figure 3 shows that the treatments had no effect on the diurnal excretion of potassium, urea or creatinine but that there were some changes in the excretion patterns of water and sodium. The intake of extra salt (period II) increased the daytime and nighttime excretion rates of sodium, but it did not change the relation between them. The intake of extra salt did, however, increase the ratio of nighttime to daytime urine flow rate. Tilting (period III) caused the excretion patterns of water and sodium to change

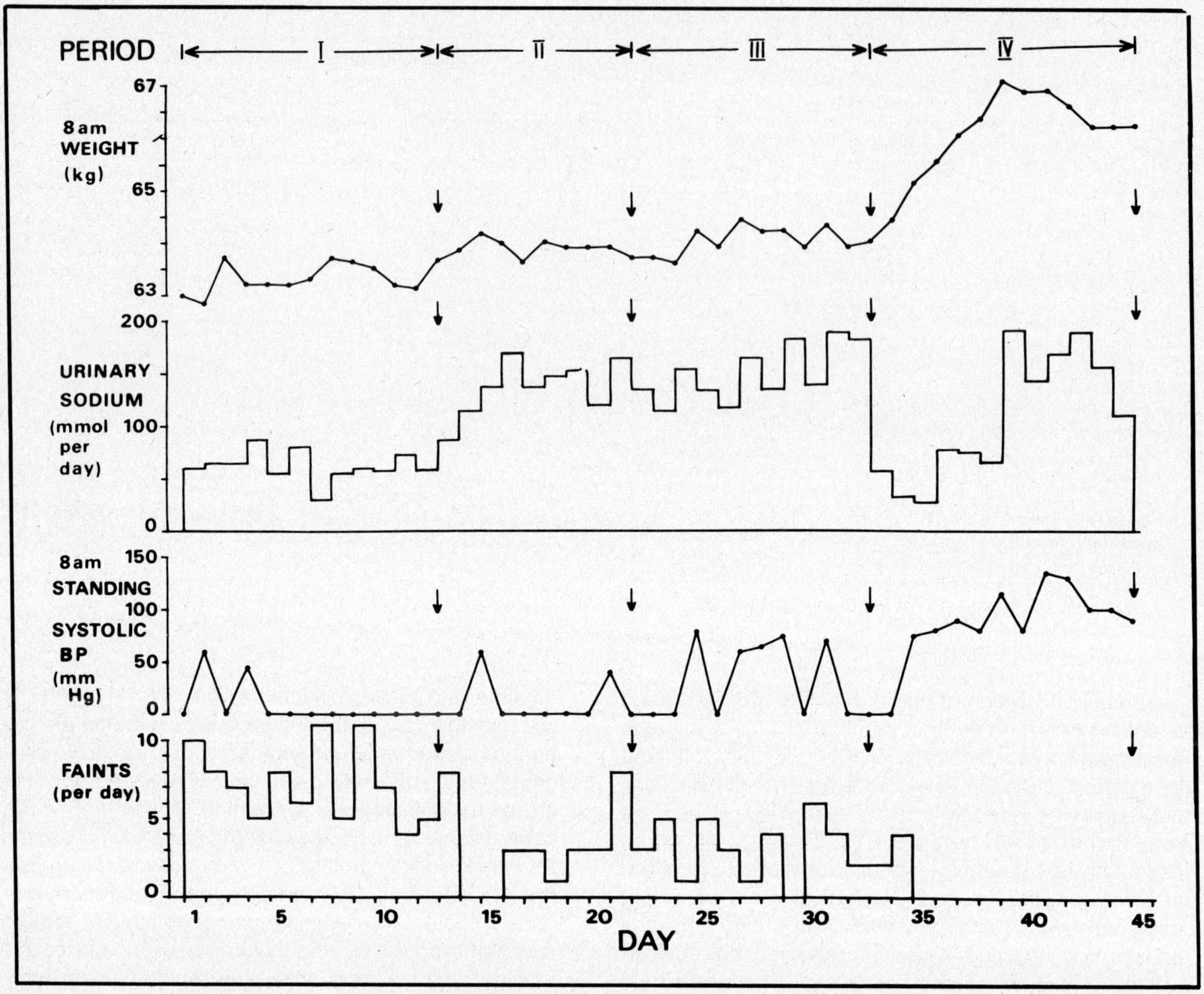

Figure 1. *Body weight, sodium excretion, standing blood pressure and frequency of faints in the patient before (I) and during treatment with high salt diet alone (II), and together with tilting (III) and fludrocortisone (IV).*

TABLE II **Details of the Patient During the Control (I) and Three Treatment Periods (II–IV)***

Data	Control Period I	Treatment Period II	Treatment Period III	Treatment Period IV
Weight (kg)	63.38 ± 0.09	63.92 ± 0.06	64.11 ± 0.08	66.55 ± 0.16
Plasma				
Sodium (mmol/liter)	142.3 ± 0.61	137.1 ± 0.87	138.5 ± 1.03	146.4 ± 0.30
Potassium (mmol/liter)	3.88 ± 0.06	3.97 ± 0.04	4.03 ± 0.06	3.11 ± 0.09
Urea (mmol/liter)	7.95 ± 0.08	6.97 ± 0.16	7.18 ± 0.16	4.19 ± 0.08
Creatinine (μmol/liter)	105.2 ± 0.02	102.54 ± 0.02	101.66 ± 0.01	81.33 ± 0.01
Urine				
Volume (ml/day)	2,211 ± 72	2,398 ± 108	1,905 ± 144	2,197 ± 76
Sodium (mmol/day)	59.3 ± 6.0	147 ± 6.6	159 ± 10	159 ± 12
Potassium (mmol/day)	62.4 ± 2.0	65.4 ± 1.4	49 ± 3.5	166 ± 12
Urea (mmol/day)	341.2 ± 13.3	363.1 ± 9.5	317 ± 13	280.4 ± 10.5
Creatinine (mmol/day)	11 ± 0.43	10.9 ± 0.58	9.58 ± 0.32	9.19 ± 0.31
Aldosterone (nmol/day)	18.7	17.2	9.6	0.7
Plasma volume (liters)	1.89	...	...	2.75
Exchangeable sodium (mmol)	2,395	2,564	2,589	3,019

* Values shown are the mean ± SEM for the last six days of each period.

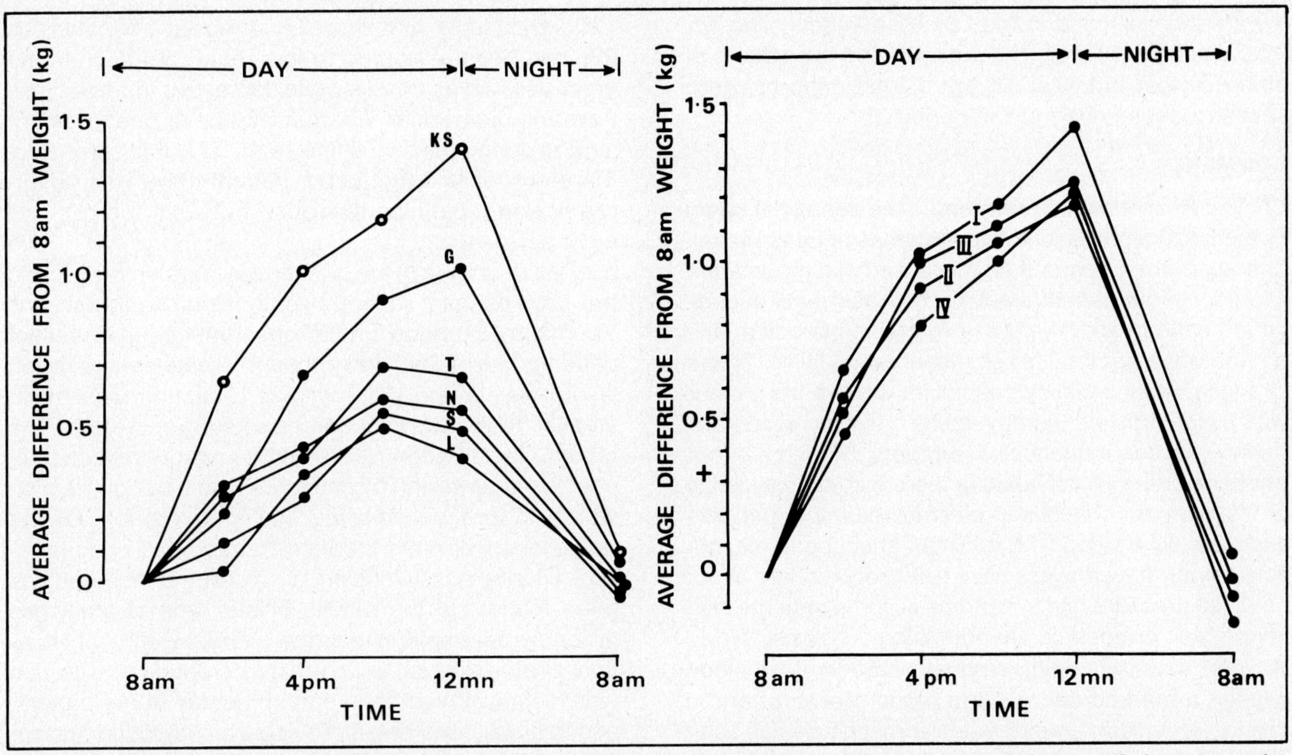

Figure 2. *Diurnal variation in body weight in patient and in the control subjects. Each point is the mean of six consecutive days. mn = midnight.* ***Left,*** *comparison of patient data in the control period (open circles) with data of the control subjects (closed symbols).* ***Right,*** *comparison of data in the four study periods in patient (details are given in the text).*

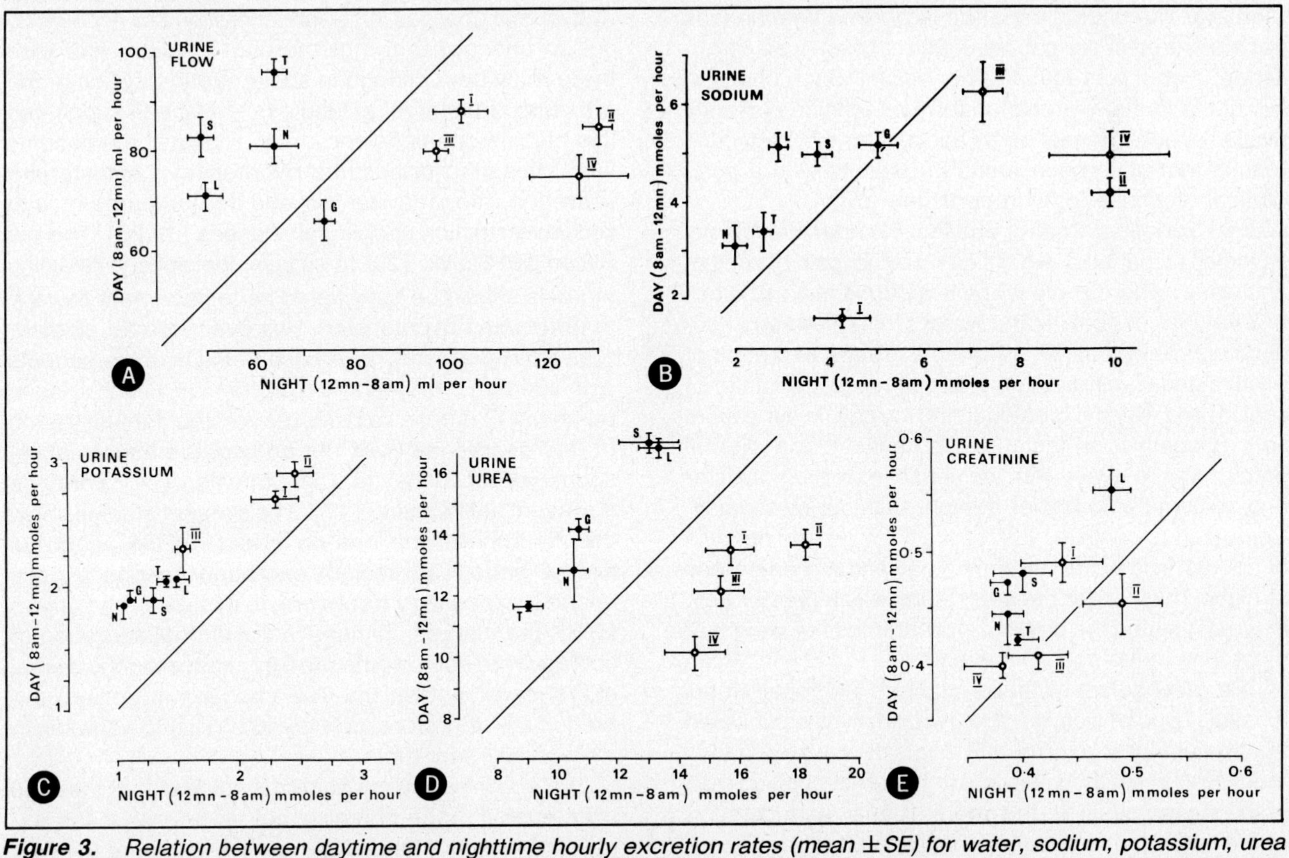

Figure 3. *Relation between daytime and nighttime hourly excretion rates (mean ± SE) for water, sodium, potassium, urea and creatinine in five control subjects (closed symbols) and in patient during the last six days of each of the four study periods (open symbols). The diagonal indicates an equal daytime and nighttime excretion rate. Potassium results are not given for period IV as the patient was taking potassium supplements, and the excretion rates were much higher.*

towards those found in the control subjects. The administration of fludrocortisone reversed the effects of tilting so that in period IV the diurnal patterns were similar to those observed in period II.

COMMENTS

Clinical Response to Treatment. The beneficial effect of the treatments used in this study has been attributed to sodium retention and an increased plasma volume [10,13]. In our patient, each of the treatments caused an increase in body weight, a retention of sodium and an increase in total exchangeable sodium. These changes, like the clinical response, were much greater with fludrocortisone therapy. It has been suggested that fludrocortisone influences symptoms through a direct effect on arteriolar tone, since there may be only small or insignificant changes in plasma volume in patients successfully treated with it. Small changes in plasma volume may nevertheless have a disproportionate effect on blood pressure and symptoms in some patients with idiopathic orthostatic hypotension. Wagner [14] showed that the rapid removal of 500 ml of blood caused a marked decrease in blood pressure, and a change in blood volume of a similar magnitude has been noted as part of the diurnal variation in blood volume in one patient with idiopathic orthostatic hypotension [7] in whom it was sufficient to worsen symptoms in the morning. The diurnal variation in plasma volume was not measured in our patient until treatment was established; then it was found to be 140 ml. Such changes are at the limits of precision for the technics currently available, and this may partly account for the conflicting results that have been found in patients with a good clinical response to fludrocortisone [13].

Diurnal Variation: Control Studies. In normal subjects, daytime is a period of weight gain and net gain of sodium and water, whereas nighttime is a period of weight loss and net loss of sodium and water. This retention of sodium and water happens despite a greater excretion of sodium and water during the day because the intake of sodium and water is greater during the day. In our patient with idiopathic orthostatic hypotension, the diurnal pattern was reversed with the urinary excretion of water and sodium being higher at night than during the day. Compared to controls, this resulted in a greater net gain of sodium and water during the day and a greater loss at night. Thus, in our patients, there was a greater gain in weight during the day and a greater loss of weight at night than in the control subjects.

The mechanism of these changes in idiopathic orthostatic hypotension is not known. It is well established that the ability to excrete either a salt or water load is much less when the subject is in the erect position than in the supine position; this represents an exaggeration of the response to postural changes in healthy people [15]. In patients with idiopathic orthostatic hypotension this has been attributed to low renal perfusion in the erect position as considerable decreases in renal blood flow and glomerular filtration rate have been demonstrated during passive tilting [6,16,17]. It is surprising, therefore, to find that in our patient there was no difference in creatinine excretion between the day and night periods, and this suggests that there was a little over-all decrease in the glomerular filtration rate during the day, despite severe hypotension. Bachman and Youmans [5] made similar observations in ambulant patients; they found that although creatinine excretion was lower during the day, this reduction was much smaller than the reduction in sodium excretion. The glomerular filtration rate could be maintained despite poor renal perfusion by an increase in filtration fraction which, in turn, would lower sodium excretion. On the occasions when the filtration fraction has been measured during passive tilting [6,17,18], no increase has been found, but the results of this type of study are probably not applicable to the everyday clinical situation. Urea excretion in contrast to creatinine excretion was higher at night than during the day in our patient, and this has been noted previously in idiopathic orthostatic hypotension [5]. There has been no satisfactory explanation for the abnormal urea handling, but it may be related to the higher urine flow rates at night.

If diurnal changes in sodium excretion are not directly due to changes in the glomerular filtration rate, then there must be a change in sodium reabsorption in the proximal or distal renal tubules. It has been suggested that aldosterone deficiency may exist in some patients with idiopathic orthostatic hypotension; aldosterone secretion rates may be low and do not increase with sodium restriction or postural changes [19,20]. This led Slaton and Biglieri [20] to suggest that sodium-retaining steroids should be considered as replacement therapy in orthostatic hypotension. However, normal aldosterone excretion rates have been found in some patients with idiopathic orthostatic hypotension [21,22], as in our own (19 nmol a day). Moreover, the administration of fludrocortisone does not correct the abnormal response of the kidney to saline infusion [14], nor does it prevent salt wasting [17]. The present studies show that fludrocortisone had no effect on the abnormal diurnal pattern of sodium excretion despite a good clinical response to treatment; in this study and others [5,6], the marked changes in the diurnal excretion of sodium were not accompanied by changes in the diurnal excretion of potassium. The changes in sodium excretion are, therefore, unlikely to be due to variation in aldosterone secretion.

The abnormal diurnal pattern in idiopathic orthostatic hypotension could primarily be due to either the excessive retention of sodium and water during the day, or to excessive loss at night, but this loss might merely represent the excretion of excessive amounts of sodium and water retained during the day. Studies with salt loading in patients with idiopathic orthostatic hypotension have shown that sodium and water retention in the erect position is abnormal [5] and that sodium loss in the supine position is excessive [14]; this suggests that the responses are abnormal in both positions. The data from this study do not clarify the problem further, but it is interesting that both the day and night excretion of sodium could change in response to salt loading or tilting, indicating that in neither period was sodium excretion fixed. The same difficulty in interpreting changes in diurnal rhythm has been encountered in relation to the effect of steroid treatment [3].

Diurnal Variation: Effect of Treatment. The results of this study suggest that the beneficial effect of treatment is due to sodium retention, and there are at least two mechanisms through which this might occur. Firstly, there might be a direct effect of the treatment on the abnormal excretion patterns so that diurnal fluctuations in extracellular fluid and plasma volume would become less marked and approach those in the control subjects. Secondly, treatment might cause sufficient sodium retention and expansion of the extracellular fluid so that despite continuing diurnal fluctuations the volume would never fall below a critical level associated with fainting. We found that none of the treatments had any significant effect on the diurnal weight pattern and that none caused the diurnal pattern of water and solute excretion to return to normal. Tilting caused a reduction in sodium and water loss at night, but the change in water excretion was comparatively small and there was no change in the night weight loss. However, each treatment was associated with an increase in body weight, expansion of extracellular fluid and probably of plasma volume. The findings taken together suggest that treatments were effective through an expansion of extracellular fluid volume rather than through any effect on the diurnal variation in weight and extracellular fluid volume.

ACKNOWLEDGMENT

We would like to thank Dr. O. Maxwell Telling and Professor B. E. C. Nordin for permission to study patients under their care, Sister Walker and Sister Dyer and staff of the Metabolic Ward, Leeds General Infirmary, Miss P. Jolliff and Mr. D. Brown of the Department of Chemical Pathology who made the chemical analyses, Dr. C. Hayter of the Department of Nuclear Medicine for isotopic measurements and Dr. M. Levell for the aldosterone measurements.

REFERENCES

1. Goldman R: Studies in diurnal variation of water and electrolyte excretion; nocturnal diuresis of water and sodium in congestive cardiac failure and cirrhosis of the liver. J Clin Invest 30: 1191, 1951.
2. Flear CTG, Cooke WT, Quinton A: Water diuresis and steatorrhoea. Clin Sci 18: 137, 1959.
3. Thomas JP, Coles GA, El-Shaboury AH: Nocturia in patients on long term steroid therapy. Clin Sci 38: 415, 1970.
4. Bradbury S, Eggleston C: Postural hypotension: a report of three cases. Am Heart J 1: 73, 1925.
5. Bachman DM, Youmans WB: Effects of posture on renal excretion of sodium and chloride in orthostatic hypotension. Circulation 7: 413, 1953.
6. Scherba EJ: Orthostatic hypotension and orthostatic tachycardia. Am J Med 17: 880, 1954.
7. Bannister R, Ardull L, Fentem P: An assessment of various methods of treatment of idiopathic orthostatic hypotension. Q J Med 38: 377, 1969.
8. Shear L: Pathophysiology and treatment of orthostatic hypotension. Am Heart J 77: 715, 1969.
9. MacLean AR, Allen EV: Orthostatic hypotension and orthostatic tachycardia; treatment with "head-up" bed. JAMA 115: 2162, 1940.
10. MacLean AR, Magrath TB: Orthostatic hypotension and orthostatic tachycardia; defects in return of venous blood to heart. Am Heart J 27: 145, 1944.
11. Veirsma HJ, Ven Holt SP: The three types of "natural" diuresis quoted by Boorst JGG, De Vries LA. Lancet 2: 1, 1950.
12. Belcher EH, Vetter H: Radioisotopes in Medical Diagnosis, London, Butterworths, 1971.
13. Shear L: Orthostatic hypotension: treatment with sodium chloride and sodium retaining hormones. Arch Intern Med 122: 467, 1968.
14. Wagner HN: Influence of autonomic vasoregulatory reflexes on rate of sodium and water excretion in man. J Clin Invest 36: 1319, 1957.
15. Epstein FH, Kleeman CR, Lamdin E, et al.: Studies of the antidiuresis of quiet standing: observations upon electrolyte and acid base excretion during sulphate diuresis. J Clin Invest 35: 308, 1956.
16. Corcoran AC, Browning JS, Page IH: Renal haemodynamics in orthostatic hypotension. JAMA 119: 793, 1942.
17. Shear L: Renal function and sodium metabolism in idiopathic orthostatic hypotension. N Engl J Med 268: 347, 1963.
18. Brodwell EK: Study of renal function in orthostatic hypotension. Circulation 21: 38, 1960.
19. Wagner HN: Orthostatic hypotension. Bull Johns Hopkins Hosp 105: 322, 1959.
20. Slaton PE, Biglieri EG: Reduced aldosterone excretion in patients with autonomic insufficiency. J Clin Endocrinol Metab 27: 37, 1967.
21. Schirger A, Hines EA, Molnar GD, et al.: Idiopathic orthostatic hypotension. JAMA 181: 822, 1962.
22. Hedeland H, Dymling JF, Hohfelt B: Catecholamines, renin and aldosterone in postural hypotension. Acta Endocrinol (Kbh) 62: 399, 1969.

Post-Transplant Malignant Lymphoma

Distinctive Morphologic Features Related to Its Pathogenesis

ARTHUR J. MATAS, M.D.
BRUCE F. HERTEL, M.D.
JUAN ROSAI, M.D.
RICHARD L. SIMMONS, M.D.
JOHN S. NAJARIAN, M.D.
Minneapolis, Minnesota

Malignant lymphoma developed in two patients after renal transplantation. In both, the central nervous system was involved. Histologic study of the tumors showed that they were composed of a monomorphous proliferation of cells characterized by a large vesicular nucleus, prominent basophilic nucleolus and strongly pyroninophilic cytoplasm. The tumors thus would be classified as "diffuse large lymphoid lymphomas with pyroninophilia" or "immunoblastic sarcomas" as described in the literature. Tumor cells resembled cells observed in the paracortex of antigenically stimulated lymph nodes, cells from malignant lymphomas in mice that were antigenically stimulated and from malignant lymphomas in patients with immunodeficiency diseases or autoimmune disorders. The distinctive morphologic features of the tumors in the transplant recipients described provide further evidence that long-term antigenic stimulation may be important in their pathogenesis.

The incidence of malignancy is increased in allograft recipients [1], and epidemiologic data show that the incidence of lymphoproliferative tumors has the greatest increase [2]. These lesions have an unusual anatomic distribution; brain and spinal cord involvement occurred in 46 per cent of affected patients, and in 33 per cent the lesion was confined to these areas. This is in contrast to a 0.4 to 1.5 per cent involvement of the central nervous system in patients with malignant lymphoma who have not received transplants. Why malignant lymphomas in organ transplant recipients behave in such a bizarre fashion is unclear, although several hypotheses have been put forth [3–5].

From January 1, 1968, to October 1, 1974, 523 renal transplants were performed in 452 patients at the University of Minnesota Hospitals. Patient selection, operative technic and postoperative management have been described previously [6,7]. In brief, following acceptance into the program, bilateral nephrectomy and splenectomy are performed prior to renal transplantation. Post-transplant immunosuppression therapy consists of the administration of antilymphocyte globulin, azathioprine and prednisone. Following renal transplantation, de novo lymphoreticular tumors have developed in two patients. We describe the pathologic findings in these two patients in order to further define the difference between these lesions and malignant lymphomas in patients who do not receive organ transplants.

CASE REPORTS

Case 1. A 50 year old woman with renal failure secondary to chronic glomerulonephritis received a cadaver renal transplant. Histocompatibility typing

From the Departments of Surgery and Pathology, University of Minnesota, Minneapolis, Minnesota 55455. This study was supported by Grant AM 13083 from the U.S. Public Health Service. Requests for reprints should be addressed to Dr. Richard L. Simmons, Box 185—Mayo Memorial Building, University of Minnesota Hospitals, Minneapolis, Minnesota 55455. Manuscript accepted January 14, 1976.

revealed two HL-A antigens in common between donor and recipient. Initial immunosuppression therapy consisted of the administration of antilymphoblast globulin [8], azathioprine and prednisone [7]. The postoperative course was uneventful and she was discharged three weeks after receiving the transplant, with normal renal function. Within six months of the transplantation, she was receiving 2.5 mg/kg azathioprine and 0.3 mg/kg prednisone. One year after the transplantation she experienced occipital headaches and expressive aphasia. Brain scan and cerebral angiography revealed a mass in the left mediofrontal region. Craniotomy was performed and a biopsy specimen was obtained. Postoperatively she received 4,000 rads to the left cerebral hemisphere and 5,500 rads to the left frontal lobe. She was discharged without weakness or aphasia.

Ten months later behavioral changes developed; she had difficulty with mentation, emotional lability and a progressively deteriorating course until death 25 months after renal transplantation. No autopsy was performed.

Case 2. A 10 year old girl with renal failure secondary to hypocomplementemic glomerulonephritis received a renal transplant from her mother. She did well the first year after the transplant with the exception of two rejection episodes which responded well to therapy. One year after the transplant, she was receiving 1.5 mg/kg azathioprine and 0.27 mg/kg prednisone. Thirteen months after the transplant she was admitted to the hospital with weakness, lethargy, fever and leukopenia. A chest roentgenogram showed bilateral nodular infiltrates. Bronchoscopy revealed a creamy exudate, but no bacteria, fungi or protozoa were seen. Open lung biopsy was performed to define a presumptive opportunistic infection. Histologic sections, at that time, were interpreted as showing only chronic pneumonitis and pleuritis. Antibiotic treatment was begun and immunosuppression therapy discontinued. Three weeks after admission, cytomegalovirus (CMV) was reported in cultures of urine, sputum, bronchial washings and lung biopsy specimens. The patient had a progressive downhill course which was attributed to the systemic viral infection. Seven weeks after admission a Jacksonian seizure developed which started on the right side and became generalized. The seizure was associated with cardiopulmonary arrest, for which intubation and resuscitation were required. A postictal right hemiparesis persisted. An electroencephalogram was markedly abnormal with continuous spike and wave activity over the left hemisphere and independent foci in the left central and left occipital areas that suggested multiple lesions. She could not be weaned from the respirator and her condition continued to deteriorate. She had a second cardiopulmonary arrest on the 59th hospital day (15 months after the transplant) from which she could not be resuscitated.

MORPHOLOGY

Case 1. Histologic evaluation of the brain biopsy specimen showed a highly cellular, widely infiltrating neoplasm with large areas of necrosis (Figure 1). Distention of Virchow-Robin spaces by tumor cells was a prominent feature. The tumor was composed of a monomorphous proliferation of cells characterized by large [10–12] oval nuclei containing one or several prominent basophilic nucleoli and finely distributed chromatin (Figure 2). The nuclear membranes were regular without significant wrinkling or cleaving. There was a moderate amount of amphophilic cytoplasm which was strongly pyroninophilic. Occasional plasmacytoid cells and mature plasma cells were present. No phagocytic activity was observed in the tumor cells.

Case 2. At autopsy, malignant lymphoma was identified in the brain, liver and transplanted kidney, in the lung, heart and lymph nodes, but not in the bone marrow. The tumor was composed of a monomorphous proliferation of cells with large oval nuclei, prominent basophilic nucleoli and strongly pyroninophilic cytoplasm (Figure 3). The pattern was similar in all involved organs and the cytologic features were similar to those seen in Case 1. In the central nervous system, the tumor was present as multiple masses and diffusely in a perivascular distribution, frequently distending Virchow-Robin spaces. The liver grossly contained numerous tumor nodules up to 5 cm in diameter; microscopically, it also showed diffuse portal infiltration without significant sinusoidal involvement. The transplanted kidney showed widespread diffuse interstitial infiltration by tumor. Small aggregates of neoplastic cells were present in the myocardium. Lymph nodes were diffusely replaced by tumor. Retrospective review of the open lung biopsy specimen showed that the malignant lymphoma was present in the lung at the time of biopsy.

COMMENTS

Penn et al. [9] and McKhann [10] independently reported an increased incidence of cancer in the transplant recipient in 1969; since that time 241 de novo malignancies in transplant recipients have been reported to Penn's informal registry [1]. This represents a significant increase over the number that would be expected to develop in the age-matched general population.

Epidemiologic data compiled by Hoover and Fraumeni [2] disclosed that the incidence of lymphoreticular tumors showed the greatest increase. We have previously described our over-all experience with malignancy in patients before and after organ transplantation [11], and the two patients we describe in this report are the only ones in whom lymphoproliferative disorders developed.

Most cases of malignant lymphoma reported in immunosuppressed patients have been classified under the broad term "reticulum cell sarcoma" or "histiocytic lymphoma," the latter according to the Rappaport classification [12]. Based on our material, we believe that many of these tumors represent a distinctive histologic entity. The classic histiocytic lymphoma is

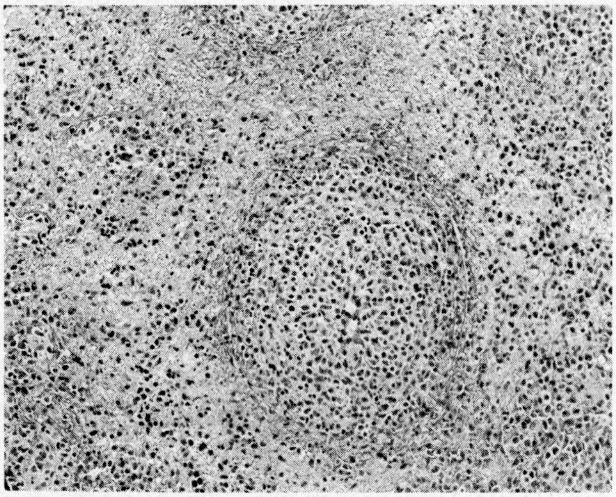

Figure 1. *Case 1. Brain biopsy specimen of the tumor mass demonstrating perivascular infiltration typical of central nervous system lymphomas. Hematoxylin and eosin stain; original magnification × 120, reduced by 34 per cent.*

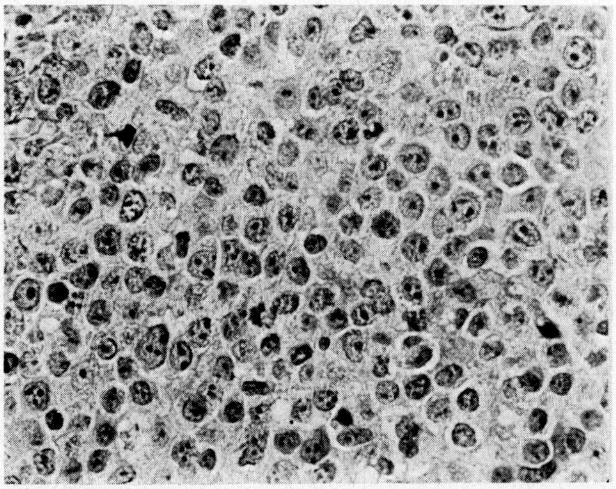

Figure 2. *Case 1. Higher magnification of the brain biopsy specimen demonstrating the monotonous population of uniform large cells with round to oval nuclei, multiple basophilic nucleoli and abundant cytoplasm. Hematoxylin and eosin stain; original magnification × 600, reduced by 32 per cent.*

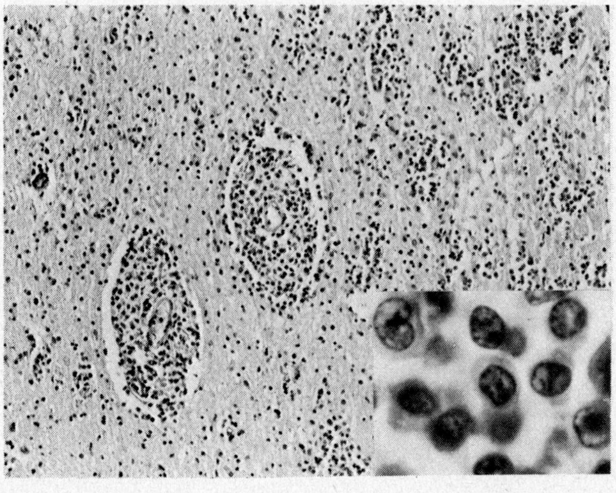

Figure 3. *Case 2. Specimen of autopsy tissue from the cerebrum illustrating the perivascular as well as diffuse pattern of central nervous system involvement. Hematoxylin and eosin stain; original magnification × 120, reduced by 34 per cent.* ***Inset,*** *higher magnification shows cells similar to those seen in Case 1 with more prominent plasmacytoid appearance. Hematoxylin and eosin stain; original magnification × 1,000, reduced by 34 per cent.*

characterized by a large, irregular, vesicular nucleus with a prominent eosinophilic nucleolus and abundant eosinophilic cytoplasm which is not pyroninophilic. By contrast, the lymphomas in our transplant recipients are composed of a monotonous proliferation of cells with large regular nuclei, diffusely distributed chromatin, several basophilic nucleoli and strongly pyroninophilic cytoplasm (Figures 1, 2 and 3). Similar cells are observed in the paracortex of antigenically-stimulated lymph nodes [13,14] and can be produced by stimulating peripheral lymphocytes with phytohemagglutinin in cultures [15]. Dameshek [13] proposed the term "immunoblast" for such cells, and experimental evidence strongly supports their lymphocytic origin [15–18]. In their functional classification of lymphomas, Lukes and Collins [16,17] propose the term "immunoblastic sarcoma" for lymphomas composed of these cells. They state that they have observed only B cell variants of such tumors, although it is not clear what studies were performed in determining cell types. Dorfman [19] uses the term "diffuse large lymphoid lymphomas with pyroninophilia" for such neoplasms in his working classification of non-Hodgkin's lymphomas. At present, Dorfman's terminology is appealing because it indicates the accepted cell of origin while describing the distinctive features whose significance is unclear. Regardless of the nomenclature used, these neoplasms should be recognized as a distinctive morphologic entity with a peculiar association with immunoglobulin abnormalities, congenital immune defects, Dilantin® ingestion and chronic immune disorders such as severe rheumatoid arthritis, Sjögren's syndrome and systemic lupus erythematosus [16,17,20]. The two malignant lymphomas we have observed in transplant recipients should be included in this subgroup of lymphomas. Review of photomicrographs published with case reports of post-transplant lymphoma reveals a similar histologic picture in some cases [21]. Lukes and Collins [16,17] state that the lymphomas in transplant recipients that they reviewed have been immunoblastic sarcomas. A complete morphologic review of the lymphomas recorded in the transplant tumor registry may be of value in substantiating these observations.

The pathogenesis of the increased incidence of de novo cancer in the transplant recipient is unknown. It was at first thought that the immunosuppressive treatment used in these patients to prevent allograft rejection resulted in decreased immunosurveillance allowing neoplastic clones to develop and multiply. However, a number of observations suggest that this is not the entire explanation. First, all tumors are not increased in proportion to their occurrence in the general population as would be expected if decreased immunosurveillance were the sole pathogenic factor. Second, in other groups of patients who did not receive transplants but who did receive the same medications, the risk of cancer is not the same. Third, cure of disseminated tumor in a transplant recipient during maintenance of immunosuppressive therapy has been reported [22]. Fourth, the anatomic location of these lymphoproliferative tumors is unusual—in transplant recipients 46 per cent involve the central nervous system compared to 0.5 to 1.5 per cent in those who do not receive transplants. Finally, the histopathology of the lymphoreticular tumors differs from those occurring in the general population.

Both long-term and repeated intermittent antigenic stimulation have previously been associated with an increased incidence of lymphoreticular neoplasms. Repeated injection of bovine serum albumin [23] or cells differing at weak histocompatibility loci [24] in mice results in a significantly increased incidence of lymphomas. A long-term graft versus host reaction results in a similar increase [25]. These tumors differ histologically from spontaneous lymphomas in mice and are similar to lymphoproliferative tumors in the transplant recipient in their monomorphous appearance [26,27]. In man, long-term antigenic stimulation of repeated malarial infection has been associated with the development of Burkitt's lymphoma [28]. This tumor predominates in areas in which malaria is endemic, and children in these areas are probably exposed repeatedly. Areas in which malaria is eradicated show a corresponding drop in the incidence of Burkitt's lymphoma [29]. Interestingly, Burkitt's lymphoma is also a monomorphous pyroninophilic tumor.

Each of the tumor systems mentioned has been associated with virus infection. Long-term antigenic stimulation due to the graft versus host reaction or due to allogenic stimulation has been shown to result in oncogenic virus activation in the mouse [30,31], and Burkitt's lymphoma has been linked to the Epstein-Barr virus (EBV) [32], a herpesvirus in man. Herpesviruses (cytomegalovirus [CMV], herpes simplex virus type 1 [HSV-1], herpes simplex virus type 2 [HSV-2] and Epstein-Barr virus [EBV]) infections are a common problem in transplant recipients [33]. The oncogenicity of these viruses has previously been demonstrated in both animals and man. These viruses have been associated with lymphoproliferative tumors, as well as carcinoma of the skin, lip, nasopharynx and cervix [34,35].

If long-term antigenic stimulation and viral activation play a role in the pathogenesis of the increased incidence of cancer in the transplant recipient, a possible explanation may be found for the unusual pattern of central nervous system involvement by these tumors. Herpesviruses have previously been shown to be neurotropic, EBV has been implicated in the pathogenesis of Bell's palsy and the Guillain-Barré syndrome [36],

HSV-1 and HSV-2 have been shown to reside in dorsal root ganglia between overt infections [37,38], primary HSV-1 infection can result in encephalitis, and congenital CMV infection often affects the brain [36]. This neurotropism of the herpesviruses may thus explain the frequent central nervous system involvement by lymphoproliferative tumors in the transplant recipient.

In summary, the morphologic features of these lymphoproliferative disorders occurring after organ transplantation are consistent with the theory that long-term antigenic stimulation may play an important role in their pathogenesis. Whether potentially oncogenic herpesviruses also play an important role is still speculative. The distinctive morphologic features described here offer additional support to the idea that long-term antigenic stimulation rather than lost immunosurveillance is important in the pathogenesis of this disease.

REFERENCES

1. Penn I: The incidence of malignancies in transplant recipients. Transplant Proc 7: 323, 1975.
2. Hoover R, Fraumeni JF: Risk of cancer in renal transplant recipients. Lancet 2: 55, 1973.
3. Penn I: Malignant Tumors in Organ Transplant Recipients, New York, Springer-Verlag, 1970.
4. Schwartz RS: A new concept of immunoregulation and its application to leukemia and lymphoma. Tumori 59: 383, 1973.
5. Matas AJ, Simmons RL, Najarian JS: Chronic antigenic stimulation, herpesvirus infection and cancer in transplant recipients. Lancet 1: 1277, 1975.
6. Kjellstrand CM, Simmons RL, Buselmeier TJ, Najarian JS: Recipient selection, medical management, and dialysis. Transplantation (Najarian JS, Simmons RL, eds), Philadelphia, Lea & Febiger, 1972, p 415.
7. Simmons RL, Kjellstrand CM, Najarian JS: Kidney: Technique, complications, and results. Transplantation (Najarian JS, Simmons RL, eds), Philadelphia, Lea & Febiger, 1972, p 445.
8. Najarian JS, Simmons RL: The clinical use of antilymphocyte globulin. N Engl J Med 285: 158, 1971.
9. Penn I, Hammond A, Brett Scheider L, Starzl TE: Malignant lymphomas in transplantation patients. Transplant Proc 1: 106, 1969.
10. McKhann CF: Primary malignancy in patients undergoing immunosuppression for renal transplantation: a request for information. Transplantation 8: 209, 1969.
11. Matas AJ, Simmons RL, Kjellstrand CM, Buselmeier TJ, Najarian JS: Increased incidence of malignancy during chronic renal failure. Lancet 1: 883, 1975.
12. Rappaport H: Malignant lymphomas, Atlas of Pathology, section III, fascicle 8, Tumors of the Hematopoietic System, Washington, D.C., Armed Forces Institute of Pathology, 1966, p 91.
13. Dameshek W: "Immunoblasts" and "Immunocytes"—an attempt at a functional nomenclature. Blood 21: 243, 1963.
14. Dorfman RF, Warnke R: Lymphadenopathy simulating the malignant lymphomas. Human Pathol 5: 519, 1974.
15. Biberfeld P, Morphogenesis in blood lymphocytes stimulated with phytohemagglutinin (PHA). A light and electron microscopic study. Acta Pathol Microbiol Scand [A], suppl 223, p 1, 1971.
16. Lukes RJ, Collins RD: A functional classification of malignant lymphomas. The Reticuloendothelial System (Rebuck JW, Berard CW, Abell MR, eds), Baltimore, Williams & Wilkins, 1975, p 213.
17. Lukes RJ, Collins RO: Immunologic characterization of human malignant lymphomas. Cancer 34: 1488, 1974.
18. Nowell PC: Phytohemagglutinin: an initiator of mitosis in cultures of normal human lymphocytes. Cancer Res 20: 462, 1960.
19. Dorfman RF: The Non-Hodgkin's lymphomas. The Reticuloendothelial System (Rebuck JW, Berard CW, Abell MR, eds), Baltimore, Williams & Wilkins, 1975, p 262.
20. Brand MM, Marinkovich VA: Primary malignant reticulosis of the brain in Wiskott-Aldrich syndrome. Report of a case. Dis Child 44: 536, 1969.
21. Cho ES, Connolly E, Porro RS: Primary reticulum cell sarcoma of the brain in a renal transplantation recipient. J Neurosurg 41: 235, 1974.
22. Simmons RL, Kelly WD, Tallent MB, Najarian JS: Cure of dysgerminoma with widespread metastases appearing after renal transplantation. N Engl J Med 283: 190, 1970.
23. Metcalf D: Reticular tumors in mice subjected to prolonged antigenic stimulation. Br J Cancer 15: 769, 1961.
24. Walford RC: Increased incidence of lymphoma after injection of mice with cells differing at weak histocompatability loci. Science 152: 78, 1966.
25. Schwartz RS, Beldotti L: Malignant lymphomas following allogenic disease: transitor from an immunological to a neoplastic disorder. Science 149: 1511, 1965.
26. Kersey JH: Personal communication, 1975.
27. Gleichmann E, Gleichmann H, Schwartz R: Immunologic induction of malignant lymphoma: genetic factors in the graft-versus-host model. J Natl Cancer Inst 49: 793, 1972.
28. O'Connor G: Persistent immunologic stimulation as a factor in oncogenesis with special reference to Burkitt's lymphoma. Am J Med 48: 279, 1970.
29. Burkitt DP, Wright DH: Burkitt Lymphoma, Edinburg, Livingstone, 1970.
30. Hirsch MS, Phillips SM, Solnik C, et al.: Activation of leukemia viruses by graft versus host and mixed lymphocyte reactions in vitro. Proc Natl Acad Sci USA 69: 1069, 1972.
31. Armstrong MY, Black FL, Richards FL: Tumor induction by cell-free extracts derived from mice with graft versus host disease. Nature (New Biol) 235: 153, 1972.
32. Epstein MA, Achong BG, Barr YM: Virus particles in cultured lymphoblasts from Burkitt lymphomas. Lancet 1: 702, 1964.
33. Simmons RL, Lopez C, Balfour H, et al.: Cytomegaloviruses: clinical virological correlations in renal transplant recipients. Ann Surg 180: 623, 1974.
34. Klein G: Herpesviruses and oncogenesis. Proc Natl Acad Sci 69: 1056, 1972.
35. Rapp F: Question: Do herpesviruses cause cancer? Answer: Of course they do. J Natl Cancer Inst 50: 825, 1973.
36. Grose C, Henle W, Henle G, Feorino PN: Primary Epstein-Barr-virus infections in acute neurologic diseases. N Engl J Med 292: 392, 1975.
37. Baringer JR, Swoseland P: Recovery of herpes-simplex virus from human trigeminal ganglions. N Engl J Med 288: 648, 1973.
38. Baringer JR: Recovery of herpes simplex virus from human sacral ganglions. N Engl J Med 291: 828, 1974.

Introduction to Part II of the Hypertension Symposium

Prorenin, Renal Hypertension
Diuretics and Hyperlipidemia
Angiotensin Receptors and Blocking Drugs
A New Treatment System

JOHN H. LARAGH, M.D.
New York, New York

This second section of the Symposium on Hypertension concludes the up-dating of this timely and provocative subject. Part I appeared in the May 31st issue [1] of *The American Journal of Medicine,* and other parts have been published in three recent issues of *The American Journal of Cardiology* [2–4]. Altogether, the format employed allows in depth treatment of the subject. Experimental, clinical and animal data have been blended together with the goal of formulating modern viewpoints for diagnosis and management.

This issue of the Symposium begins with a thoughtful reconsideration of a problem of interest to clinicians and investigators alike. The very active group from Hôpital Louis Mourier in Paris, headed by Joel Menard and Pierre Corvol, presents a critical analysis of some methodologic problems encountered in performing plasma renin measurements. Since these measurements promise to have increasing application both experimentally and clinically, it may be helpful for those interested in the subject to be aware of methodologic pitfalls which perhaps explain some of the conflicting results of various clinical studies. In particular, it has become apparent that exploration of the subnormal range is increasingly important for a useful clinical method. This is because low renin states are quite common in hypertension and suggest either the presence of adrenocortical hypertension, or alternatively, of low renin essential hypertension with the latter often being responsive to diuretic treatment alone. Accordingly, plasma renin activity measurements should have sensitivity adequate to discriminate accurately between subnormal values. This is most effectively accomplished by the use of the acid pH optimum for renin during the incubation procedure, by using a method in which the incubation period can be prolonged for up to 18 hours, and by the use of inhibitors of angiotensinase which are fully effective. In our hands, BAL and 8-hydroxy quinoline at acid pH have proved ineffective and appear to add nothing to the procedure [5].

The second paper by Jean Sealey and associates extends her original description of an inactive cryoactivatable form of renin which she has called prorenin. The new study defines more precisely the conditions for cryoactivation to active renin. In so doing, it makes the clinical pathologist and the clinician aware of the disquieting fact that prolonged cooling of plasma samples without freezing could activate prorenin and lead to artificially higher plasma renin activity measurements. The practical implication of these results is that plasma should remain at room temperature during collection and transfer, and then be rapidly frozen, until the time of analysis. The study indicates that there is potentially a large reservoir of prorenin in plasma so that activation could have a considerable effect on the plasma renin activity measurement. From a theoretic standpoint, the role of this renin reservoir remains to be clarified.

The next paper by Dr. Beretta-Piccoli and his associates from Berne, Switzerland, provides a critical analysis of the role of sodium and volume retention, and of renin suppression in the pathogenesis of hypertension associated with early stage kidney disease. Their data suggest that a subtle failure of suppression of the renin feedback mechanism and hypervolemia may participate in pathogenesis.

The next paper by Drs. Ames and Hill of New York City demonstrates that long-term diuretic therapy can produce small but significant increases in the serum concentration of cholesterol and triglycerides. Even if this is simply due to dehydration and hemoconcentration, the questions raised by these observations seem pertinent. Could it be that the hyperlipidemia induced by the administration of diuretics increases the risk of atherosclerosis, and, if so, could it be that this increased risk, consequent to diuretic therapy, cancels out the benefit obtained from lowering blood pressure? It seems that this will be a difficult question to answer, but if the concentration of lipid is a factor in the causation of coronary disease and atherosclerosis, then one must now view with circumspection the classic long-term use of diuretic therapy to control blood pressure. Certainly this paper will provoke reexamination of a number of long held beliefs.

The paper by Drs. Devynck and Meyer from Hôpital Necker in Paris reviews the current state of knowledge of the biology of angiotensin II receptors located in vascular tissue. The characterization of the biochemical and physiologic properties of these vascular receptors could be a critical step forward in analyzing the ultimate role of angiotensin II in blood pressure control and in the pathogenesis of hypertensive vascular diseases. In the immediately following paper by Dr. Herbert Thurston from Leicester, England, the in vivo, physiologic behavior of angiotensin receptors is reviewed. In particular, Dr. Thurston critically analyzes our current knowledge of the role of sodium balance and of changes in plasma volume in determining the reactivity of receptors to angiotensin II. His experiments suggest that the major determinant of angiotensin II receptor activity is the preexisting level of the hormone itself. Thus, the blunted response to exogenous angiotensin following sodium deprivation seems to be due to prior occupancy of receptor sites by endogenous hormone, either resulting from increased plasma levels or from local tissue generation. If this impression is correct, there is no need to postulate any change in the number or affinity of angiotensin II receptors to explain the changes produced by sodium or volume depletion. Whatever the case, the change in receptor behavior associated with sodium and volume depletion seems to be an important component of the control system in which blood pressure is regulated by the renin axis.

In the next paper, Dr. Joseph Levy reviews his interesting animal studies dealing with the effects of a group of well-known beta-blocking drugs in spontaneous hypertension occurring in the rat. This animal study is included since it deals with a most timely subject, the mechanism of antihypertensive action of beta-adrenergic drugs. Propranolol, whose antihypertensive action was first recognized in clinical studies, has now also been shown to be pressor in certain hypertensive patients, usually those with low renin hypertension [6]. Accordingly, Levy's study is of special interest because he has been able to show that a group of beta-blockers may be either pressor or depressor in the spontaneously hypertensive rat. However, the conditions which predetermine whether a beta-adrenergic blocking drug will raise or lower the blood pressure remain to be fully defined. Nonetheless, the results are provocative since these drugs as a group will probably be widely used in man, and clinicians should be alerted to their amphibaric potential.

The following paper by Dr. David B. Case and his associates of the Cardiovascular Center at the New York Hospital-Cornell Medical Center complements two previous reports in Part I of this Symposium describing the clinical effects of two exciting new angiotensin blocking drugs. The first of these, the octapeptide saralasin, was characterized in depth in the reports by Case et al. [7] and by Streeten and his group [8]. In the present paper, Case and his associates provide a critical comparison between the effects of saralasin and another blocker, the nonapeptide converting enzyme inhibitor. The octapeptide, saralasin, is clearly a partial agonist so that it underestimates the true renin component involved in hypertension. In fact, saralasin is overtly pressor in both patients with low renin activity and in anephric subjects. In contrast, the nonapeptide converting enzyme inhibitor is never pressor; also, unlike saralasin, it induces depressor responses not only in patients with high renin activity but also in nearly all patients with "normal" renin [9]. This new experience suggests that in most patients with "normal renin," a significant renin factor is involved in the maintenance of their blood pressure.

Since patients with normal renin and high renin activity, together, comprise perhaps 70 per cent of all hypertensive patients, one can make the reasonable extrapolation, albeit from a very small sample, that a significant renin factor is involved in the maintenance of blood pressure in the majority of patients with essential and other common forms of hypertensive vascular disease. This new impression seems to parallel the earlier view about the role of renin in essential hypertension derived from studies using the beta-adrenergic drug, propranolol [9]. Thus, because of its intrinsic agonism, saralasin testing underestimates renin participation in a hypertensive state. Prior sodium depletion with induced hyperreninemia will increase the frequency of positive saralasin tests, but then one is exposing reactive reninemia rather than any native involvement of renin in the hypertension. On the other hand, future studies may show that the agonistic property of saralasin can actually be exploited to identify and characterize the volume component which seems important in patients with low renin activity. It thus seems possible that in the near future routine base-line testing with these blocking drugs will provide the clinician with a powerful tool for planning more specific treatment. Certainly, we are only beginning to explore the exciting research and diagnostic potentials of these new angiotensin blocking drugs.

In the final paper of the Symposium, I have proposed and presented a new system for the treatment of hypertensive patients based on experience using our *vasoconstriction-volume* hypothesis to sort out mechanisms and to plan treatment for the whole spectrum of patients with hypertension. In testing this hypothesis we first used renin profiling with the renin-sodium index to identify the degree to which renin-induced vasoconstriction participates in the maintenance of the blood pressure [10]. Our subsequent serial studies in human subjects, using three different pharmacologic probes to block either renin secretion, angiotensin action or its formation (propranolol, saralasin and converting enzyme inhibitor), have validated this use of renin profiling while, at the same time, indicating that a physiologically significant renin factor participates in maintaining part or all of the high blood pressure in the majority of patients with so-called essential hypertension (i.e., all patients with high renin and most patients with "normal" renin activity). Moreover, at the same time, these studies collectively support the view [11] that the antirenin action of propranolol is after all a major element in its antihypertensive action.

Our cumulative experience in applying the new reference framework points to the operation of both a renin factor and a volume factor in the majority of hypertensive patients (i.e., the group with normal renin activity), with patients with high renin activity (about 20 per cent) being largely renin-dependent and the subgroup with low renin activity (about 30 per cent of the whole) being almost entirely volume-dependent.

In this context one can consider anew the possibility of rearranging priorities in the treatment strategy. Traditionally, diuretic therapy has been the first step in initiating therapy. However, our new treatment system proposes instead a first-line role for beta-adrenergic blocking drugs, such as propranolol. It is our view that, in the majority of patients, administration of this type of drug may be a better first step than the classic approach of administering a diuretic first. Diuretic therapy, of course, has the credibility of a long-standing experience. On the other hand, it is reasonable to suspect that long-term dehydration may not be as desirable as the use of an agent which effectively reduces peripheral resistance without producing hypovolemia and, therefore, promises to enable better peripheral tissue perfusion for the long-term. Beyond this cogent theoretic consideration is the fact that probably a significant fraction of the total hypertensive population will respond effectively to therapy with propranolol or a similar type of antirenin drug alone. This opportunity for complete long-term correction with a single palatable agent of greater specificity should not be missed. Moreover, the response is apt to be achieved with even fewer side effects than with diuretics and, certainly, without dehydration and its possibly adverse accompaniments (hypovolemia, hemoconcentration, hyperuricemia and hyperlipidemia).

When renin profiling becomes more generally available, the capacity to select that minor subgroup of patients who should receive diuretics first (the group with low renin activity) as opposed to those who can best be treated with antirenin drugs as a first step (patients with normal and high renin activity) will make the new approach more efficient and more certain. Meanwhile, in the absence of renin profiling, a system can be devised in which the clinician can explore and exploit this new concept using first a trial of beta-blockers alone and then of diuretics alone. The residual group of partial responders to the use of either alone, who probably have both a renin and volume factor, can be treated with the two drugs together. Then only a small group will remain in which the ad seriatum addition of more potent agents will be required in the traditional trial and error fashion.

This new treatment system may be viewed as a second generation offspring, in which the empiric therapy, which gave us the initial validation for antihypertensive drug therapy, will be superseded by more specific and rational treatments that are based on our new knowledge of the workings of the renin system as either a causal or a predictably reactive factor in all hypertensive diseases.

More studies in the near future promise to shed further light on the numerous questions of current interest that have been reviewed in this Symposium. The ultimate goal of exposing and understanding the primary causes of hypertension seems within our grasp if we persevere. Meanwhile, useful information of considerable practical value has already emerged from the new framework of analysis provided in particular by our new understanding of blood pressure control by the renin axis.

REFERENCES

1. Laragh JH (ed): Symposium on Hypertension. Am J Med 60: 733, 1976.
2. Laragh JH (ed): Symposium on Hypertension. Am J Cardiol 36: 651, 1975.
3. Laragh JH (ed): Symposium on Hypertension. Am J Cardiol 37: 635, 1976.
4. Laragh JH (ed): Symposium on Hypertension. Am J Cardiol 38: 766, 1976.
5. Sealey JE, Laragh JH: Searching out low renin patients. Limitations of some commonly used methods. Am J Med 55: 303, 1973.
6. Drayer JIM, Keim HJ, Weber MA, et al.: Unexpected pressor responses to propranolol in essential hypertension. An interaction between renin, aldosterone and sympathetic activity. Am J Med 60: 879, 1976.
7. Case DB, Wallace JM, Keim HJ, et al.: Usefulness and limitations of saralasin, a partial competitive agonist of angiotensin II, for evaluating the renin and sodium factors in hypertensive patients. Am J Med 60: 825, 1976.
8. Streeten DHP, Anderson GH Jr, Dalakos TG: Angiotensin blockade. Its clinical significance. Am J Med 60: 817, 1976.
9. Case DB, Wallace JM, Keim HJ, et al.: Identifying angiotensin-dependent hypertension. A comparison of two different angiotensin inhibitors and renin profiling (abstract). Clin Res 24: 418A, 1976.
10. Laragh JH: Vasoconstrictor-volume analysis for understanding and treating hypertension. The use of renin and aldosterone profiles. Am J Med 55: 261, 1973.
11. Bühler FR, Laragh JH, Vaughan ED Jr, et al.: Antihypertensive action of propranolol. Specific antirenin responses in high and normal renin forms of essential, renal, renovascular and malignant hypertension. Am J Cardiol 32: 511, 1973.

Methodologic Problems in Plasma Renin Activity Measurements

ANNE DELORME, M.D.
PHAN TAM GUYENE, M.D.
PIERRE CORVOL, M.D.
JOEL MENARD, M.D.
Paris, France

The influence of pH and angiotensinase inhibitors on the in vitro generation of angiotensin I during PRA measurements has been investigated. PRA values obtained at pH 5.7 are higher than those obtained at pH 7.4. At pH 5.7, values obtained using diisopropylfluorophosphate (DFP 9 mM) as an angiotensinase inhibitor are higher than values obtained with a mixture of dimercaprol (BAL, 1.6 mM) and hydroxyquinoline (8-OHQ, 3 to 4 mM). Since the two methods for inhibiting angiotensinase are completely and equally efficient, it is suggested that these inhibitors might interfere with the renin angiotensinogen reaction.

Significant correlations are observed between the PRA values obtained by the different methods which have been studied. Using an incubation pH of 5.7, and BAL and 8-OH quinoline as angiotensinase inhibitors, the distribution of PRA values in a population of 124 hospitalized hypertensive patients ingesting a normal sodium diet has been studied, and it has been demonstrated that the sensitivity of this method of measurement can detect small changes in PRA in patients with low renin activity.

A great dispersion is being observed in the values of plasma renin activity (PRA) obtained by different methods of measurement [1]. Many factors can explain this dispersion, some are physiologic, others biochemical. Because it was proposed that PRA could have a prognostic meaning in hypertension [2] and that it could direct the choice of treatment with diuretic [3] or beta-blocking [4] agents, it is becoming important to assert that it is actually the same parameter that is being measured by the different methods. Otherwise, normal values in different laboratories are determined under various physiologic circumstances: upright or supine position, during normal sodium intake or during sodium restriction, intravenous or oral diuretic treatment [5]. This variability becomes an obstacle when the classifications of patients must be compared and may make this comparison illusive.

Apart from the sampling circumstances, the in vitro-incubation conditions of plasma for the determination of PRA must be rigorously controlled. PRA means that no homologous or heterologous substrate has been added, and no inhibitor or activator of the angiotensinogen-renin reaction has been eliminated by a previous extraction of the renin. Contradictory results dealing with the influence of various factors in this method of measurement have already been related [6,7]. The effects of pH and of two inhibitors of angiotensinases and converting enzyme on the in vitro generation of angiotensin I are now examined.

From the Hôpital Louis Mourier and the Unité de Recherches INSERM U_{36}, Paris, France. This work was supported by grants from DGRST and INSERM. Requests for reprints should be addressed to Dr. Joel Menard, Unité de Recherches INSERM U_{36}, 17 rue du Fer-à-Moulin, 75005 Paris, France.

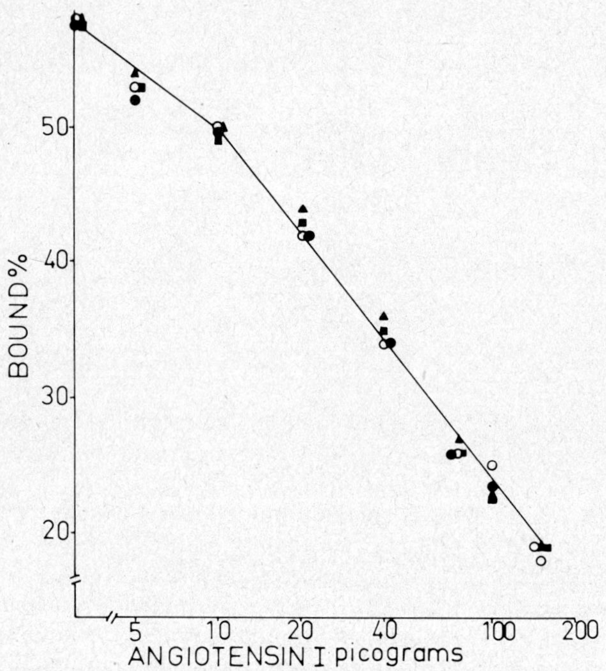

Figure 1. Binding of antiangiotensin I antiserum with angiotensin I. The standard curve was determined by adding increasing amounts of angiotensin (○). Three binding curves were determined after the addition to the standard curves of 25 μl aliquots of the nonincubated mixture which contained all reagents for PRA measurements: (●) mixture without inhibitors; (■) mixture with BAL and 8-OHQ; (▲) mixture with DFP.

MATERIAL AND METHODS

Determination of Plasma Renin Activity. Endogenous angiotensin I was removed from plasma samples by passage through a column of moist resin Dowex WX_2 (ammonium ion). When PRA was measured at pH 5.7, 250 μl of stripped plasma were added to 200 μl of 0.2 M citrate-phosphate buffer, pH 5.7, containing 1.5 per cent EDTA (ammonium ion) (2.10^{-2} M final concentration), 25 μl of 0.6 N hydrochloride, and 25 μl of angiotensinase inhibitor. When PRA was measured at pH 7.4, the incubation mixture contained 200 μl of 0.2 M citrate-phosphate buffer, pH 7.4 with 1.5 per cent EDTA (ammonium ion), 25 μl of 0.2 M citrate-phosphate buffer, pH 7.4 and 25 μl of angiotensinase inhibitor. The incubation lasted 3 hours at 37°C. The reaction was stopped by cold. Ten and 25 μl of the incubation mixture were put into tubes for immediate angiotensin I radioimmunoassay. The results were expressed as nanograms of angiotensin I produced per milliliter of plasma per hour. Two inhibitors of angiotensinases and converting enzyme were used. One was the mixture of dimercaprol (BAL) (1.6 mmol final concentration) and 8-hydroxyquinoline (8-OHQ) (3.4 mmol final concentration) in water-ethanol; the other was diisopropyl fluorophosphate (DFP) (9 mmol final concentration) in isopropyl alcohol.

Determination of Plasma Renin Substrate. Ten microliters of 1:50 plasma renin samples were incubated at pH 5.7 in the same mixture as the one used for the measurement of PRA in the presence of an excess of human renin (0.05 Goldblatt Units (GU) of a renin purified until step 5 of the Haas et al. method [8]). The incubation lasted 2 hours. The angiotensin concentrations were expressed as nanograms of angiotensin I which could be liberated per milliliter of plasma by an excess of renin.

Radioimmunoassay of Angiotensin I. A ^{125}I-monoiodinated angiotensin I, purified by polyacrylamide gel electrophoresis [9], was used. Its specific activity was 1,750 μCi/μg. The angiotensin I antiserum was obtained by rabbit immunization against angiotensin I coupled to bovine gamma globulin by carbodiimide condensation; it does not recognize angiotensin II [10]. When utilized for the purification of hog renin, this antiserum permitted the realization of successive steps resulting in a highly purified and stable preparation which contained 240 GU/mg protein [11,12]. Assay of this purified renin in the laboratory of Haas and Goldblatt verified that the results obtained with this bioassay in dogs were the same as those obtained with radioimmunoassay of angiotensin I produced in vitro [12].

Radioimmunoassays were performed with standards of synthetic ileu-5 angiotensin I (Schwartz-Mann). One milliliter aliquots of diluted antiangiotensin I serum (diluted: 1:110,000 in 0.1 M Tris hydrochloride buffer pH 8.5 containing bovine albumin 0.5 mg/ml) was added to tubes containing angiotensin I standards (5 to 150 pg) or samples to be assayed. After mixing, 1 ml aliquots of tracer solution containing 20,000 dpm of ^{125}I-angiotensin I were added, followed by incubation at 4°C for 48 hours. Bound and free tracer were then separated by the addition of 0.3 ml of a suspension containing 2.5 per cent Norit A (Fisher) and 0.5 per cent Dextran 70 (Pharmacia) in 0.1 M Tris hydrochloride buffer pH 8.5. After 10 minutes the tubes were centrifuged at 1,200 g for 15 minutes at 4°C; the supernatant solutions were aspirated, and the charcoal counted in a Packard automatic-gamma spectrometer with ^{125}I counting efficiency of 55 per cent.

The complete absence of nonspecific interference in the radioimmunoassay was a characteristic of the standard curve using this tracer and this antiserum. The addition of a 25 μl aliquot of the nonincubated mixture which was used for PRA measurement did not change the standard curve (Figure 1).

Destruction of Endogenous Angiotensinogen. Two plasma samples were treated according to Skinner's method of substrate denaturation [13]. In these conditions, more than 97 per cent of the endogenous substrate was destroyed, and the angiotensinases were inactivated.

RESULTS

Influence of the Incubation pH on the Angiotensin I Generation. Whatever the angiotensinase inhibitor used is, the amount of angiotensin I generated is greater at pH 5.7 than at pH 7.4 (Figure 2). The correlation coefficient between incubations performed at pH 5.7 and pH 7.4 is $r = 0.97$ in the presence of DFP and $r = 0.93$ in the presence of BAL and 8-OHQ.

Influence of the Angiotensinase Inhibitors on Angiotensin I Generation. At pH 5.7, the amount of angio-

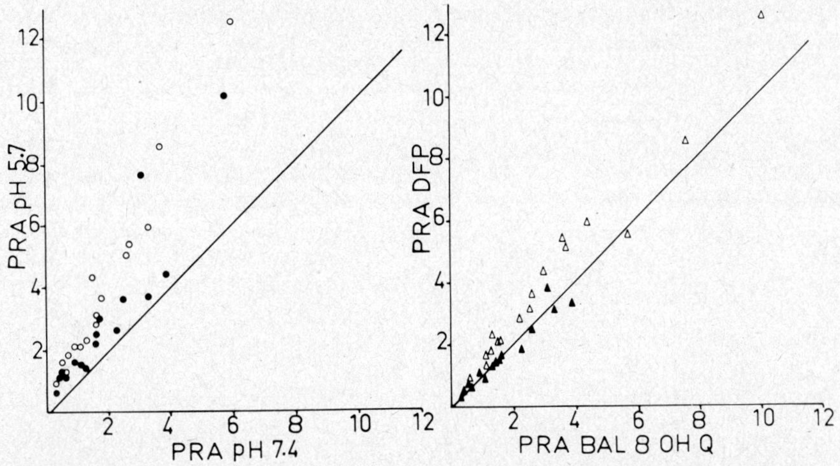

Figure 2. *Influence of the incubation pH and the angiotensinase inhibitors on angiotensin I generation. Sixteen plasma samples were incubated in standard conditions. Correlations between pH 5.7 and pH 7.4 in the presence of BAL and 8-OHQ (○) or of DFP (●) are shown at the left side of the graph. Correlations between BAL and 8-OHQ, and DFP at pH 5.7 (△) or at pH 7.4 (▲) are shown at the right side.*

tensin I generated is greater in the presence of DFP than of BAL and 8-OHQ. On the contrary, at pH 7.4, the amount of angiotensin I produced does not depend on the inhibitor (Figure 2). This correlation coefficient between BAL and 8-OHQ, and DPF is r = 0.99 at pH 5.7 and r = 0.98 at pH 7.4.

The correlation is highly significant among 70 plasma samples from hypertensive patients with low, normal or high renin activity levels: $r = 0.99$, $Y_{DFP} = 1.55 X_{BAL\text{-}8\ OHQ}$.

Influence of the Incubation Time on Angiotensin I Generation. At pH 5.7, in the presence of BAL and 8-OHQ as well as DFP, the amount of angiotensin I increases with the incubation time in a linear manner. More angiotensin I is produced in the presence of DFP (Table I).

Influence of the Angiotensinase Inhibitors on the Recovery of Angiotensin I at Various pH. The production of angiotensin I at pH 5.7, which differs according to the inhibitor used, is not due to an unequal inhibition of angiotensinases and converting enzyme. Two aliquots of a renin-free plasma, obtained from a binephrectomized male patient were incubated at pH 5.7 after having added 0.25 ng and 5 ng of angiotensin I, respectively. A pool of plasma was incubated under standard conditions, with or without 2.5 ng of angiotensin I. In the two experiments, the amounts of angiotensin I added were completely recovered after 3 hours of incubation, at pH 5.7 and pH 7.4, in the presence of BAL and 8-OHQ as well as DFP (Table II).

Influence of the Incubation pH and Angiotensinase Inhibitors on the Reaction of Acidified Plasma Renin with Human Angiotensinogen. PRA and plasma renin substrate (PRS) of two plasma samples were measured at pH 5.7, in the presence of BAL and 8-OHQ, and of DFP. Afterwards, the substrate of these plasmas was denatured according to Skinner's method [13]. In a 500 μl volume, 50 μl of these acidified samples were added to 100 μl of binephrectomized human plasma which contained 2,800 ng of angiotensin I liberable/ml. The angiotensin I production was measured after 2 hours of incubation. The angiotensin I produced by the substrate-free plasma incubated with similar amounts of binephrectomized plasma substrate, is two to four times greater than that produced by the incubation of the plasma by itself, before any acidification. However, the effects of pH and inhibitors remain the same: at pH 5.7, but not at pH 7.4, more angiotensin I is generated in the presence of DFP than of BAL and 8-OHQ (Table III).

TABLE I Kinetics of Angiotensin Generation (ng angiotensin I/ml) of Three Different Plasmas at pH 5.7

		Incubation Time			
Plasma	Inhibitor	0 hr	1 hr	2 hr	4 hr
1	BAL + 8-OHQ	0	15.3	28.9	54.5
	DFP	0	26.0	49.3	104
2	BAL + 8-OHQ	0	2.4	4.1	8.6
	DFP	0	3.8	7.5	13.8
3	BAL + 8-OHQ	0	...	0.5	0.9
	DFP	0	...	0.7	1.3

NOTE: BAL = British antilewisite; 8-OHQ = 8-hydroxyquinoline; DFP = diisopropyl (dimercaprol)fluorophosphate.

TABLE II Influence of Angiotensinase Inhibitors on the Recovery of Angiotensin I (ng angiotensin I/500 μl incubation) at Two Different pH's

		Incubation Time			
		0 hr		3 hr	
Plasma	pH	BAL + 8-OHQ	DFP	BAL + 8-OHQ	DFP
Plasma*	5.7	0	0	2.77 ± 0.14	3.77 ± 0.10
	7.4	0	0	2.47 ± 0.18	2.28 ± 0.15
Plasma + 2.5 ng angiotensin I	5.7	2.51 ± 0.13	2.60 ± 0.08	4.96 ± 0.19	6.44 ± 0.36
	7.4	2.40 ± 0.18	2.40 ± 0.18	4.37 ± 0.24	4.35 ± 0.34
Renin-free plasma + 0.25 ng angiotensin I	5.7	0.22	0.21	0.29	0.24
Renin-free plasma + 5 ng angiotensin I	5.7	5.0	5.0	4.75	4.79

NOTE: Abbreviations as in Table I.
*Five determinations (mean ± standard deviation) were made on each plasma containing endogenous renin and one determination on the renin-free plasma.

Influence of the Angiotensinase Inhibitors on the Renin Substrate. The amount of angiotensin I liberated by exhaustion of plasma by an excess of renal renin is not altered by the presence of the angiotensinase inhibitors, whether the plasma is preincubated in their presence (at 37°C 2 or 4 hours before the addition of renal renin) or not preincubated. Kinetics of plasma angiotensinogen exhaustion do not depend on the inhibitors (Figure 3).

Searching out Patients with Low Renin Activity. From 1972 to 1974, among 180 patients who were investigated, a solitary adenoma of the adrenal glands overproducing aldosterone was found in 16 patients. PRA was measured at pH 5.7, with BAL and 8-OHQ as inhibitors, after a 3 hour incubation time. It has been observed that PRA was always detectable in patients adhering to a diet containing under 110 meq of sodium, and that the PRA could be increased by having them assume the upright posture. The same observation was made in four cases of licorice-induced hypertension (Table IV). In these two syndromes, PRA is sharply decreased by comparison with a mean PRA (measured with the patient upright) of 1.59 ± 0.7 ng of angiotensin I/ml of plasma/hour in 20 normotensive subjects, aged 25 to 55 years, with a mean urinary sodium excretion of 107 ± 27 meq/day. During the same period of time, among 124 essential hypertensive patients aged 25 to 55 years and investigated under the same conditions, PRA was lower in 35 and higher in 25 than in control normotensive subjects.

COMMENTS

The investigation of the renin-angiotensin system in hypertensive diseases supplies three types of information. It is very useful in making the diagnosis of surgically curable hypertension due to renal artery disease or to overproduction of mineralocorticoids [1]. It helps in the choice of treatment with diuretics or beta-blocking agents [3,4]. It is a part of the cardiovascular prognosis of the disease [2]. The PRA measurement is now very often carried out using the easy assay of angiotensin I by radioimmunoassay. Although it is a very incomplete method by which to explore the renin-angiotensin system, it is a sufficient routine index to appreciate the basal or stimulated state of this system. The comparison of the PRA results obtained in several laboratories shows a big dispersion [1]. A critical study of the different parameters in assay methods is thus necessary, especially as opposite conclusions concerning PRA

TABLE III Influence of the Incubation pH and Angiotensinase Inhibitors on the Reaction Between Two Substrate-Free Plasmas with Renin-Free Renin-Substrate

		Before Acidification		After Acidification		
					PRA	
Plasma	Inhibitors	PRA pH 5.7	Renin Substrate	Added Renin Substrate	pH 5.7	pH 7.4
1	BAL + 8-OHQ	3.0	1,120	1,120	14.6	9.6
	DFP	5.1	1.120	1,120	19.0	10.1
2	BAL + 8-OHQ	7.7	1,380	1,120	18.6	14.2
	DFP	11.3	1,380	1,120	22.0	13.2

NOTE: Abbreviations as in Table I. PRA values are given in ng/angiotensin I/ml/hr. Renin substrate values are given in ng/angiotensin I/ml.

meanings for the choice of treatments [14,15] as well as for the prognosis [2,16–18] were reported. As for any radioimmunoassay, a great sensitivity and a high specificity of the antibody for its hapten are absolutely required. Another difficulty appears as some antibodies cross react with nonspecific substances in plasma. This "blank" leads, if it is not subtracted, to falsely high values, or, if it is substracted from low renin plasma, to negative values [7]. In the present assay, the minimum detectable dose defined as a dose 2 standard deviations away from mean for zero-dose tubes is 5 pg, and the presence of 25 μl of incubated stripped plasma does not interfere. Consequently, the sensitivity of this PRA measurement is 0.08 ng of angiotensin I/ml of plasma/hour, and it makes it easy to detect patients with low renin activity with 3 hours' incubation time.

In order to measure PRA, it is important to protect the angiotensin I produced in vitro from the action of converting enzyme and angiotensinases. BAL and 8-OHQ mixture and DFP are the generally used inhibitors [20,21]. Oparil et al. [6] recently reported that the efficiency of these inhibitors was incomplete and that it varied with pH at incubation. At pH 7.4, the BAL and 8-OHQ mixture would permit a ^{125}I-angiotensin recovery of 90 per cent, DFP of only 10 per cent. At pH 5.5, the BAL and 8-OHQ mixture is less efficient, and DFP would result in a 90 per cent recovery. Using nonradioactive angiotensin I amounts which are detectable by radioimmunoassay, the present study shows that the two inhibitors are completely and equally efficient, at pH 5.7 as well as pH 7.4.

An incomplete inhibition of converting enzyme and angiotensinases does not explain the different PRA values observed in the presence of these two different inhibitors at two different pH's. More angiotensin I is always detected at pH 5.7 than at pH 7.4, regardless of the angiotensinase inhibitors used. At pH 5.7, angiotensin I generation is always greater in the presence of DFP than of BAL and 8-OHQ, during incubation times from 1 to 4 hours. This difference persists when plasma, free of endogenous substrate and angiotensinases through acidification [13], is then incubated in the presence of the same amount of a renin-free substrate obtained in plasma from a binephrectomized male patient. In these conditions, the angiotensin I production becomes more important. This may be due to the use of binephrectomized plasma as substrate, or to the activation of the plasma renin by the acidification at pH 3.3 [22]. Whatever the cause of this increased angiotensin I production, the incubation in the presence of DFP at pH 5.7 leads once more to greater values than in the presence of BAL and 8-OHQ. At pH 7.4, production of the angiotensin I is smaller than at pH 5.7 and similar in the presence of one or another of the inhibitors. It was proved that the use of these inhibitors does

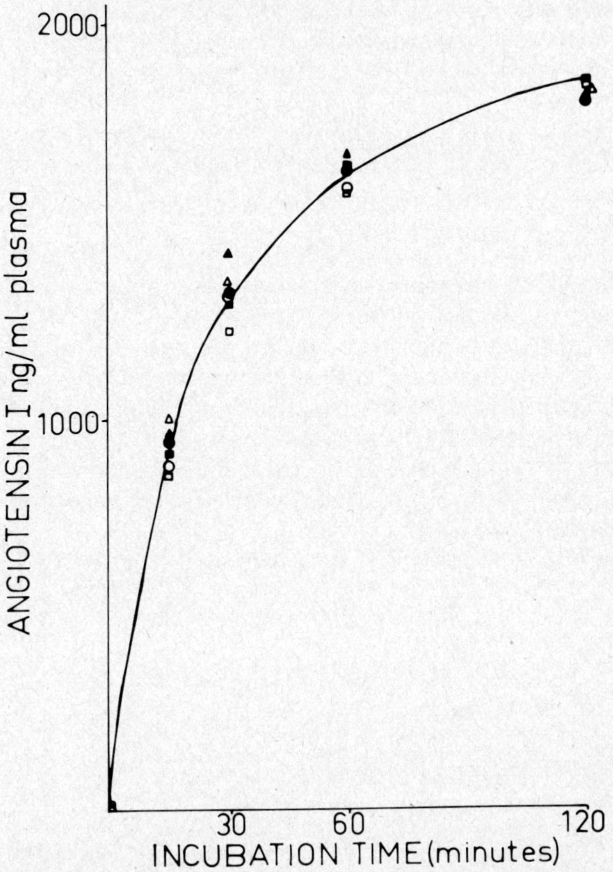

Figure 3. *Influence of angiotensinase inhibitors on plasma renin substrate measurements. No preincubation (○); 2 hours preincubations (△); 4 hours preincubations (□). In the presence of BAL and 8-OHQ, white; of DFP, black.*

not change endogenous substrate, thus it is concluded that the addition of DFP to plasma at pH 5.7 might modify, directly or not, the renin-substrate reaction and increase the rate of the enzymatic reaction.

The correlations between the PRA values obtained at two pH's, and with two inhibitors are highly significant. Within the same laboratory, the high or low PRA values determined in hypertensive patients are compared to the values obtained in normal subjects. The correlations

TABLE IV **Influence of Upright Posture on PRA in 16 Cases of Surgically Confirmed Adrenal Adenomas (p 0.01) and in Four Cases of Licorice-Induced Hypertension**

Condition	No. of Cases	Recumbent	Upright
Primary aldosteronism	16	0.15 ± 0.09	0.20 ± 0.21*
Licorice-induced hypertension	4	0.23 ± 0.09	0.37 ± 0.09

*$p < 0.01$.

just described might suggest that different methods should lead to similar clinical conclusions. Thus in our laboratory, when PRA is measured at pH 5.7 in the presence of BAL and 8-OHQ, in 124 subjects with essential hypertension receiving 110 meq of sodium a day, PRA was lower in 28 per cent and higher in 23 per cent than the PRA of control normotensive subjects of the same age; this distribution approaches the one reported by Bühler et al. [4] using a different method. Moreover, among 20 low renin hypertensive cases secondary to primary aldosteronism or licorice intoxication, it is possible to demonstrate that even in this low range, renin secretion in such patients is regulated in the same way as in normal subjects. Using a sensitive method of measurement for plasma renin concentration, Stockigt et al. [22] have already reported postural responses in patients with aldosterone-producing adenomas and hyperplastic aldosteronism.

In conclusion, the results show that absolute PRA values can be modified either by changing the incubation pH or by utilizing various angiotensinase inhibitors. However, the fact that PRA values correlate significantly within different methods suggest that differences in methodology cannot explain differences in clinical conclusions. Indeed, using its own method, in reference to its own normal range, each laboratory should obtain a similar classification of patients.

This is illustrated by the identity of PRA distribution as measured by two different methods in two different hospitalized groups of hypertensive patients. Moreover, when the method is sufficiently sensitive, PRA can be equally valuable as plasma renin concentration changes for detecting small variations in renin secretion of patients with low renin activity.

ACKNOWLEDGMENT

We wish to thank Mrs. M. F. Gonzales for her skillful technical help.

REFERENCES

1. Oparil S, Haber MD: The renin angiotensin system. N Engl J Med 292: 389, 1974.
2. Brunner HR, Laragh JH, Baer L, et al.: Essential hypertension: renin and aldosterone, heart attack and stroke. N Engl J Med 286: 441, 1972.
3. Dunn MJ, Tanner RL: Low renin hypertension. Kidney Int 5: 317, 1974.
4. Bühler FR, Laragh JH, Baer L, et al.: Propranolol inhibition of renin secretion. A specific approach to diagnosis and treatment of renin-dependent hypertensive diseases. N Engl J Med 287: 1209, 1972.
5. Drayer J, Kloppenborg PWC, Benraad TJ: Detection of low-renin hypertension. Evaluation of out-patient renin-stimulation methods. Clin Sci Mol Med 48: 91, 1975.
6. Oparil S, Koerner JT, Haber E: Effects of pH and enzymes inhibitors on apparent generation of angiotensin I in human plasma. J Clin Endocrinol Metab 39: 965, 1974.
7. Sealey JE, Laragh JH: Searching out low renin patients: limitations of some commonly used methods. Hypertension Manual (Laragh JH, ed), New York, Yorke Medical Books, 1974, p 87.
8. Haas E, Goldblatt H, Gipson EC, et al.: Extraction, purification, and assay of human renin free of angiotensinase. Circ Res 19: 739, 1966.
9. Corvol P, Rodbard D, Drouet J, et al.: Monoiodinated angiotensins: preparation and characterization by polyacrylamide gel electrophoresis and isoelectric focusing. Biochim Biophys Acta 322: 392, 1973.
10. Menard J, Catt KJ: Measurement of renin activity, concentration and substrate in rat plasma by radioimmunoassay of angiotensin I. Endocrinology 90: 422, 1972.
11. Corvol P, Devaux C, Menard J: Pepstatin, an inhibitor for renin purification by affinity chromatography. FEBS Lett 34: 189, 1973.
12. Devaux C, Menard J, Sicard A, et al.: Partial characterization of hog-renin purified by affinity chromatography. Eur J Biochem 64: 621, 1976.
13. Skinner SL: Improved assay methods for renin concentration and activity in human plasma: methods using selective denaturation of renin substrate. Circ Res 20: 391, 1967.
14. Stokes GS, Weber MA, Thornel IR: Beta-blockers and plasma renin activity in hypertension. Br Med J 1: 60, 1974.
15. Hansson L: Beta-adrenergic blockade in essential hypertension. Effects of propranolol on hemodynamic parameters and plasma renin activity. Acta Med Scand 194 (suppl): 550, 1973.
16. Doyle AE, Jerums G, Johnston CI: Plasma renin levels and vascular complications in hypertension. Br Med J 2: 206, 1973.
17. Genest J, Boucher R, Kuchel O: Renin in hypertension. How important as a risk factor? Br Med J 2: 206, 1973.
18. Mroczek WJ, Finnerty FA, Catt KJ: Lack of association between plasma-renin and history of heart-attack or stroke in patients with essential hypertension. Lancet 2: 464, 1973.
19. Stockigt JR, Collins RD, Biglieri EG: Determination of plasma renin concentration by angiotensin I immunoassay; diagnostic importance of precise measurements of subnormal renin hyperaldosteronism. Circ Res 28 (suppl II): 175, 1970.
20. Haber E, Koerner T, Page LB: Application of a radioimmunoassay for angiotensin I to the physiologic measurements of plasma renin activity in normal human subjects. J Clin Endocrinol Metab 29: 1349, 1969.
21. Sealey JE, Gerten-Banes J, Laragh JH: The renin-system: variations in man measured by radioimmunoassay or bioassay. Kidney Int 1: 240, 1972.
22. Day RP, Luetscher JA: Biochemical properties of big renin extracted from human plasma. J Clin Endocrinol Metab 40: 1085, 1975.

Plasma Prorenin: Cryoactivation and Relationship to Renin Substrate in Normal Subjects

JEAN E. SEALEY, D.Sc.
CAROL MOON, B.A.
JOHN H. LARAGH, M.D.
MICHAEL ALDERMAN, M.D.
New York, New York

We previously demonstrated an inactive form of renin, termed prorenin, in the plasma of normal, hypertensive and anephric patients. Prorenin activity can be determined in plasma from the total renin activity after activation, minus the prior endogenous plasma renin activity.

In the present study, conditions for cryoactivation of prorenin have been defined. Plasma prorenin is slowly converted to active renin-like material at −5°C at pH 7.4. Activation takes four days and does not occur at pH 5.0. The degree of activation increases above pH 5 and is greatest between pH 7 and pH 9. Thus, almost no cryoactivation of prorenin occurs at the pH optimum for renin (5.7) in contrast to maximum activation at pH 7.4. No activation has been observed in the frozen state, but it does occur with decreasing rapidity at temperatures from −5° to +4°C. Since blood samples obtained for the determination of plasma renin activity are routinely chilled upon collection by most laboratories, some activation of prorenin most likely occurs in all routine renin assays.

The pH optimum of the enzymatic reaction of the activated prorenin in plasma is 5.8, the same as for renal renin, and the shape of the pH optimum curve is similar to that of renal renin added to human plasma.

In a group of 23 normal subjects with plasma renin activity of 3.5 ± 2.9 (SD), the activated prorenin increment was found to be significantly higher, 6.3 ± 5.0 (SD) ng/ml/hour. Unlike plasma renin activity, prorenin activity in these normal subjects was directly related to the concentration of renin substrate ($p < 0.001$). When the actual "concentration" of prorenin was calculated using renal renin as the reference standard, a direct relationship was also found between the concentration of prorenin and renin substrate ($p < 0.01$). The observed relationship between prorenin and renin substrate concentrations might be a consequence of their regulation by common factors.

Several different forms of renin have been reported. Evidence has come from the demonstration of variable pressor characteristics of crude renal extracts [1], and different separation characteristics of renin in chromatographic and electrophoretic systems [2–10]. Differences in molecular weight for some of these various forms have been described. Most of these forms of renin were observed in studies of renal renin of various species. The physiologic significance of thee different renins is still unknown.

More recently, inactive forms of renin have been described in human plasma. One form, which has been described, exhibits increased

From the New York Hospital-Cornell Medical Center, New York, New York 10021. Requests for reprints should be addressed to Dr. Jean E. Sealey, New York Hospital-Cornell Medical Center, 525 East 68th Street, New York, New York 10021. This study was supported by U.S. Public Health Service Grant HL18323-SCR.

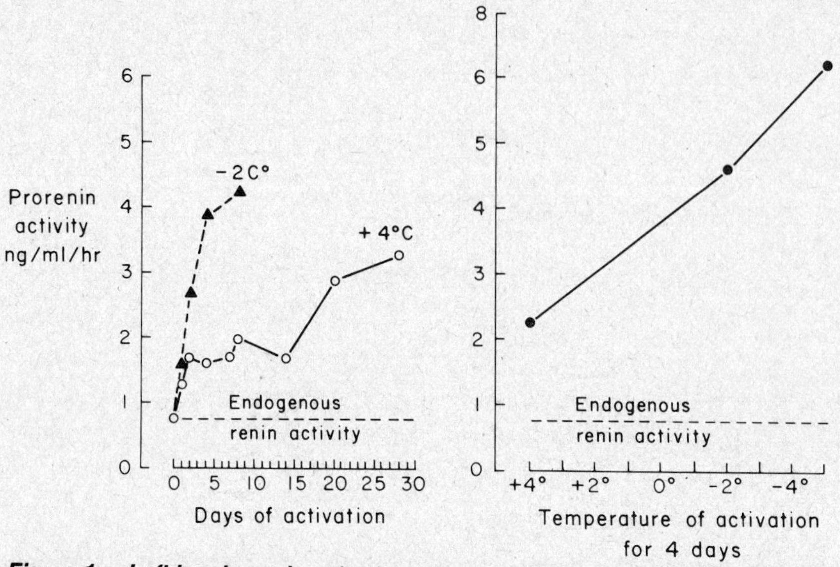

Figure 1. ***Left hand panel,*** *activation of prorenin is more rapid at −2° C than at +4° C and reaches close to equilibrium by four days. At +4° C the conversion of prorenin to renin-like activity is erratic and has not reached equilibrium by four weeks.* ***Right hand panel,*** *relationship between the amount of prorenin converted to renin-like activity and the temperature of storage of the plasma. All samples were at pH 7.4 and remained at the designated temperature for four days. Activation of prorenin was most rapid at −5° C. Below this temperature plasmas often froze and activation ceased.*

enzymatic activity after acidification of plasma to pH 3.3 [6,9,11]. Another inactive form of renin in human plasma can be activated by cold [12–14]. We have tentatively called this cold-activated substance "prorenin." Our recent studies show that it is, at least in part, of extrarenal origin since it is present in plasma of anephric patients [14].

We report here further characterization of this cold-sensitive prorenin in studies of normal subjects.

METHODS

Human plasma collected in dipotassium-ethylenediamine tetraacetate (K_2 EDTA) vacutainers was used as the source of prorenin. One pool, which was used for most of the studies, was from hypertensive patients with low plasma renin activity, some of whom were taking antihypertensive medications. Renin activity of the pool was 0.75 ng/ml/hour, and renin substrate concentration was 1,800 ng/ml. The pool was divided into 1 ml aliquots and stored frozen at −40°C. This pool is also used as a reference standard in all activation studies and is routinely included with every set.

For studies of prorenin in normal subjects, plasma was collected from 23 normal subjects who ranged in age from 25 to 64 years. Ten were male and 13 female, 12 were black and 11 white. The subjects were on random sodium intakes. They were ambulatory and the blood was drawn at their work site between 9 AM and 11 AM. In the previous 24 hours, they had saved a complete 24-hour urine collection which was analyzed for sodium and creatinine content.

Endogenous plasma renin activity was measured by radioimmunoassay of the angiotensin generated by the reaction of plasma renin with renin substrate during 3- or 18-hour incubations at 37°C in the presence of neomycin, EDTA and phenylmethylsulfonyl fluoride (5 μl of 5 per cent alcoholic phenylmethylsulfonyl fluoride per ml plasma) [15,16]. **Total renin activity** was measured in plasmas which were first activated (described herein) and then incubated for 3 and 18 hours at pH 5.7 and 37°C using the same inhibitors. The angiotensin I measured in unincubated plasma was subtracted from the total renin measurement. **Prorenin activity** was calculated from the difference between total and endogenous renin activity. Renin substrate concentration and renin reactivity were measured as previously described [15]. Renin reactivity is the hourly rate of angiotensin I generated in plasma in response to the addition of a fixed amount of renin. Renal renin used for these measurements was prepared according to the method of Haas et al. [17]. The concentrations used were 6.6×10^{-2} Goldblatt units (GU)/ml for measurement of renin substrate and 3.3×10^{-4} GU/ml for measurement of renin reactivity. The concentration of renin was based on its activity relative to the British Medical Research Council renin standard No. 68/356.

Cold Activation Studies. To determine the effects of repeated freezing and thawing, 1 ml aliquots of the pool were thawed rapidly by placing them in a 37°C water bath for 90 seconds and then plunging them into a propylene glycol bath at −40°C. These steps were repeated 30 times. In another study, three aliquots of the pool were allowed to thaw slowly at +4°C for 18 hours and then plunged into the propylene glycol bath at −40°C. These steps were repeated three times.

To determine the effect of reduced temperature without

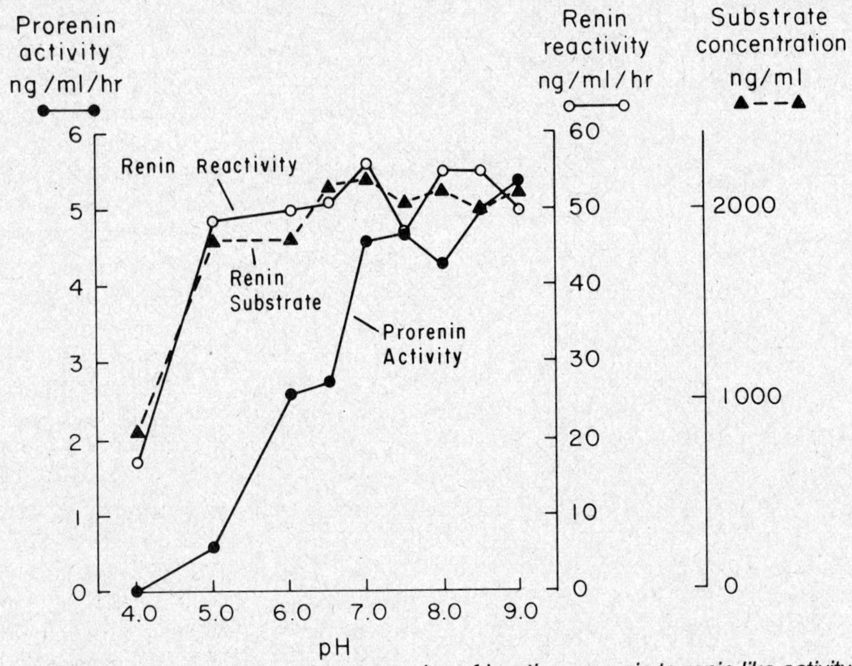

Figure 2. *Effect on pH on the conversion of inactive prorenin to renin-like activity. All aliquots of plasma were placed at −5° C for four days. Activation was most rapid at pH 7 or higher and declined between pH 7 and 5. Below pH 5 destruction of renin substrate masked any conversion of prorenin to renin that may have occurred.*

freezing on activation, 1 ml aliquots of the pool were placed in a cold room at +4°C for one, two, three and four weeks and then reassayed. Other aliquots were placed in a shaker water bath at +4°, −2° or −5°C for four days. To achieve temperatures below 0°C, crushed ice and sodium chloride were mixed together in a water bath which was placed in a cold room at +4°C.

The pH optimum for activation of prorenin was determined by adjusting aliquots of the pool to pH's ranging from 4 to 9. The aliquots were placed in a shaker water bath at −5°C for four days. The pH of each aliquot was then adjusted to 5.7 prior to incubation at 37°C for 0 and 3 and 18 hours as described.

For all other activation studies the routine procedure was to place the samples in a shaker water bath at −5°C and pH 7.4 for four days.

RESULTS

Effect of Freezing and Thawing on Prorenin Activation. Neither rapid freezing to −40°C followed by rapid thawing to 37°C nor rapid freezing to −40°C followed by slow thawing to 4°C over 18 hours resulted in any activation of prorenin. Also, samples stored frozen at −40°C for over a year have exhibited no activation of prorenin.

Effect of Temperature and Time on Prorenin Activation (Figure 1). When samples were stored at +4°C a slow, somewhat erratic, activation of prorenin was observed over four weeks (Figure 1, left). However, when the temperature was reduced to −2°C, activation was more rapid. During the first 24 hours at −2°C, renin activity increased by 110 per cent and by the fourth day it had increased by 420 per cent. Only an additional 50 per cent activation occurred when the samples were kept at −2°C for an additional four days.

As illustrated in Figure 1, right panel, there was an inverse relationship between the temperature of activation, down to −5°C, and the degree of activation that occurred during four days. It remains possible that, if the temperature of plasma could be lowered further without freezing, a greater degree of activation might occur. On the basis of these studies, four days at −5°C was chosen as the most suitable condition for future activation studies.

The Effect of pH on the Activation Process (Figure 2). As illustrated in Figure 2, activation at −5°C for four days was most effective when the pH was 7 or higher. However, increasing the pH above 7.0 did not result in a further increase in activation of prorenin. Between pH 7 and 5 there was a gradual and consistent decline in activation which was not related to differences in substrate concentration or in the response of plasma to the addition of a fixed amount of exogenous renal renin (renin reactivity). At pH 4.0 destruction of renin substrate occurred and no activation was apparent.

Reproducibility of Activation. The same plasma pool was activated six times at −5°C and pH 7.4 for four days. These samples were assayed in six different radioimmunoassay sets. Mean prorenin activity was 5.2

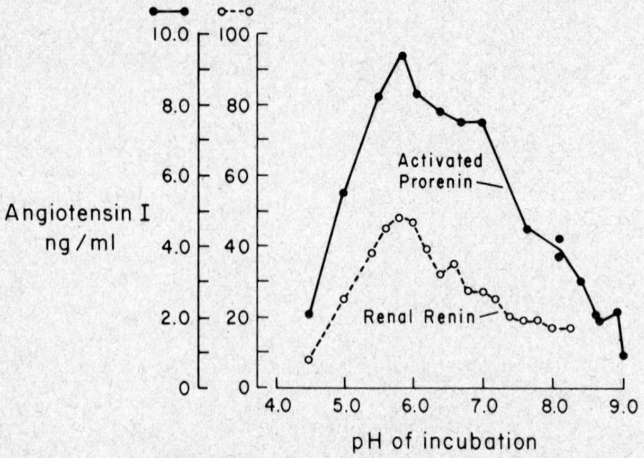

Figure 3. *The pH optima of activated prorenin and endogenous renin are quite similar, suggesting that the two enzymes may be identical.*

ng/ml/hour with a coefficient of variation of 12 per cent. This pool was used as a standard reference pool in all activation sets.

pH Optimum of Activated Prorenin (Figure 3). In Figure 3 is presented the influence of pH on prorenin activity for a pool of activated plasmas. The endogenous renin activity of this pool was 1.8 ng/ml/hour and the total renin activity, after activation, was 9.4 ng/ml/hour. Therefore only 19 per cent of the total activity was due to endogenous renin activity whereas 81 per cent could be attributed to activated prorenin. The pH optimum for this activated plasma was 5.8, a value identical to that already described for human renal renin added to plasma [18,19]. Moreover, the shape of the two curves was quite similar. Both exhibited a steep decline below pH 5.5 and a more gradual fall above pH 6.

Relationship of Activated Prorenin to Plasma Renin and Renin Substrate in Normal Subjects. Plasma prorenin activity in 23 normal subjects ranged from 0 to 20 ng/ml/hour, mean = 6.3 ± 5.0 (SD). There was no relationship between the prorenin measurement and the age, sex or race of these normal subjects. Endogenous plasma renin activity in these same subjects was much lower than the prorenin values, 3.5 ± 2.8 ng/ml/hour, and there was a weak, but direct, correlation between the two measurements ($r = 0.45$). In one subject, in whom the prorenin measurement was 20 ng/ml/hour, the measurement fell outside 2 SD of the normal range and his data were omitted from further analyses. For the remaining 22 normal subjects, there was a highly significant correlation between prorenin activity and renin substrate concentration (Figure 4) $r = 0.68$, $p < 0.001$.

Relationship Between Prorenin Activity and Renin Reactivity in Normal Human Plasma (Figure 5). In the same 22 normal subjects there was also a highly significant direct relationship between prorenin activity and renin reactivity, i.e., the rate of angiotensin I generation in plasma in response to the addition of 3.3×10^{-4} GU/ml of exogenous human renal renin, $p < 0.001$, $r = 0.77$. This relationship suggests that activated prorenin reacts with plasma renin substrate to generate angiotension I and that substrate concentration is rate-limiting for prorenin, just as has previously been shown for renin. Therefore, since the measurement of

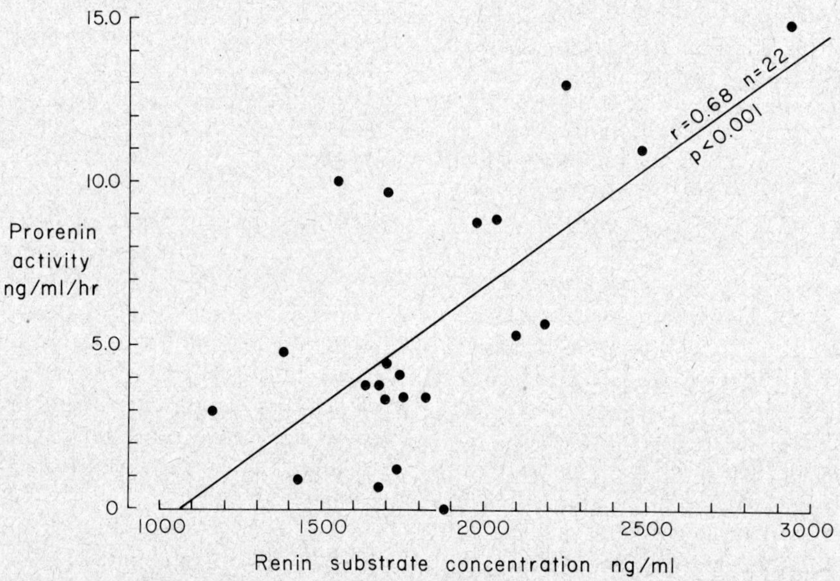

Figure 4. *The normal range of plasma prorenin activity was 6.3 ± 5.0 (SD). There was a direct relationship between prorenin activity and renin substrate concentration in 22 normal subjects.*

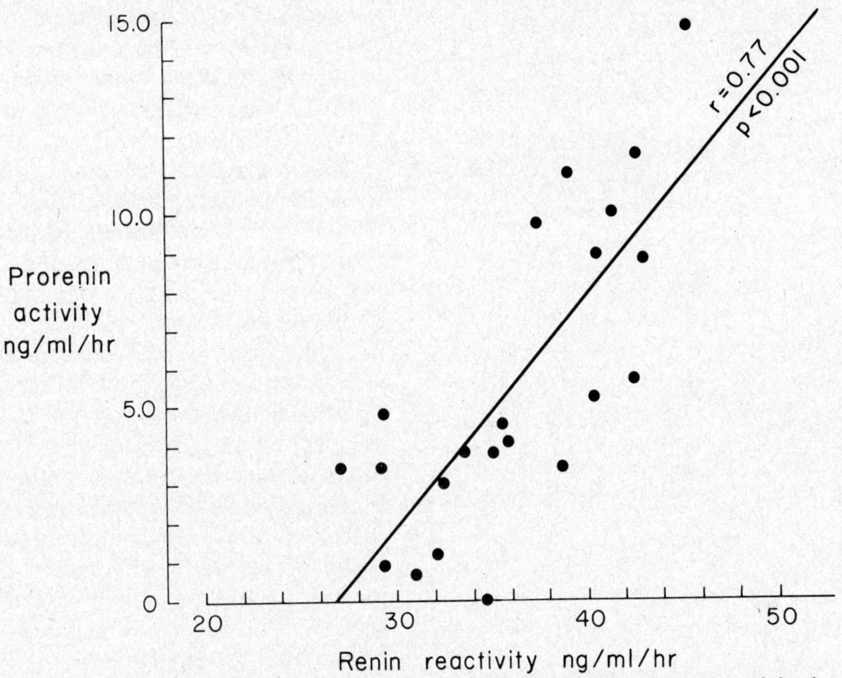

Figure 5. *A highly significant direct relationship between prorenin activity in normal subjects and the angiotensin I generated in each plasma sample in response to addition of 3.3 × 10^{-4} GU/ml of renal renin (renin activity). This suggests that the enzymatic activity of activated prorenin is determined by the same factors that affect renal renin.*

prorenin in plasma as determined herein is a function of both prorenin concentration and renin substrate concentration, the results are termed prorenin *activity*.

Estimation of Prorenin Concentration. Prorenin concentration was calculated using renal renin as a reference standard. The relationship between renin reactivity and renin substrate concentrations was first determined for 29 normal subjects (including three receiving estrogen therapy) using a Lineweaver-Burke plot (Figure 6). Prorenin concentration was derived from prorenin activity using the following formula:

Prorenin concentration

$$= \frac{\text{prorenin activity} \times 3.3 \times 10^{-4}}{\text{renin reactivity}} \text{GU/ml}$$

The value used for renin reactivity was derived from the relationship between renin substrate and renin reactivity presented in Figure 6.

Prorenin concentration was calculated in each normal subject and its relationship to the substrate concentration was evaluated (Figure 7). A direct relationship between the concentration of substrate and prorenin was found, $r = 0.61$, $p < 0.01$. Mean prorenin concentration for the 22 normal subjects was 5.4 (± 4.1) × 10^{-4} GU/ml.

COMMENTS

In this communication we have further characterized an inactive form of renin in the plasma of normal subjects. We have tentatively called this material prorenin [13]. Prorenin can be converted to active renin-like activity by treatment at −5°C for four days at pH 7.4. The activation process is both pH and temperature dependent. Activation is most effective at pH 7 and above and declines at mildly acid pH. No activation occurs during four days at pH 5 and −5°C. Thus, cryoactivation is minimal at the pH optimum for renin, pH 5.7, and maximal at physiological pH, 7.4. The lower the temperature without freezing the greater the speed of activation. Although activation does occur at +4°C, after four weeks at this temperature the total renin activity was not as great as was found after four days at −5°C. Freezing totally prevents activation. It now seems that our previous observation that activation occurs during storage at −20°C was a misinterpretation most likely due to the failure of freezer equipment to maintain samples constantly frozen.

The amounts of prorenin in the plasma of normal subjects varied quite a lot, ranging from 0 to 20 ng/ml/hour. Differences within this range could not be explained on the basis of age, race or sex of the

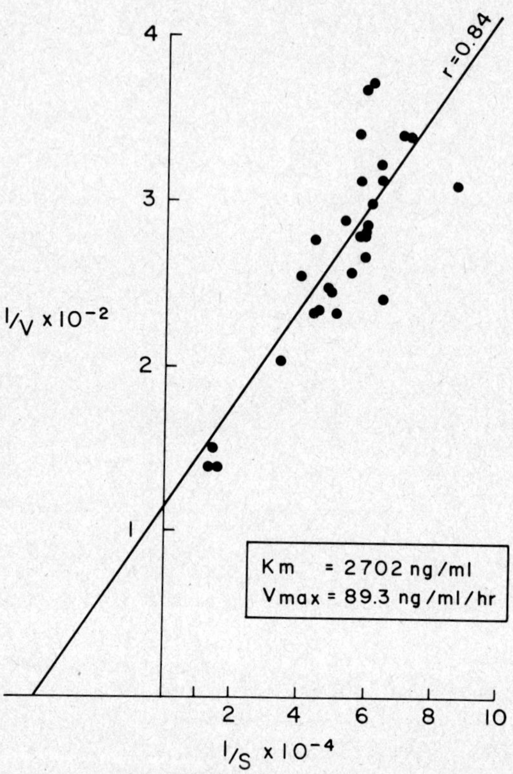

Figure 6. *Lineweaver-Burke plot of the relationship between substrate concentration and reaction velocity (renin reactivity; 3.3 $\times$ 10^{-4} GU/ml) in normal subjects who exhibit a wide natural range of renin substrate concentrations or who have very high substrate concentrations due to oral contraceptive therapy (n = 3). This relationship was then used to calculate prorenin* ***concentration*** *in the 22 normal subjects (see Figure 7).*

subjects. In general, prorenin activity was higher than renin activity. This difference was proportionally greater when plasma renin activity was low. Thus, in three normal subjects whose plasma renin activity was under 2 ng/ml/hour, prorenin activity was fivefold higher.

These observations have application in routine measurements of plasma renin activity. It has become common practice to collect the blood into chilled tubes, place them in an ice bucket and then centrifuge them in the cold. Accordingly, activation might well occur during processing of the blood. Moreover, in many instances plasma is shipped elsewhere for analysis during which time temperatures which might be optimal for prorenin activation may be maintained for considerable periods oftime. Studies in nephrectomized human subjects suggest that an average of 8 per cent of the prorenin can be activated during routine processing of the blood [14]. Since the prorenin level is normally twice as high as the renin level, this could have considerable impact on renin measurements, especially in those plasmas in which the prorenin level is much higher than the renin level.

The similarity between the enzymatic pH optimum of activated prorenin and renal or plasma renin suggests that the two enzymes may be identical [18,19]. The strong direct relationship between the response of plasma to the addition of renal renin (renin reactivity) and prorenin activity in plasma also supports this possibility since it suggests that activated prorenin reacts with the renin substrate and that renin substrate is rate-limiting for both plasma renin [20] and activated prorenin. Another interesting finding was the strong relationship between "concentration" of prorenin and

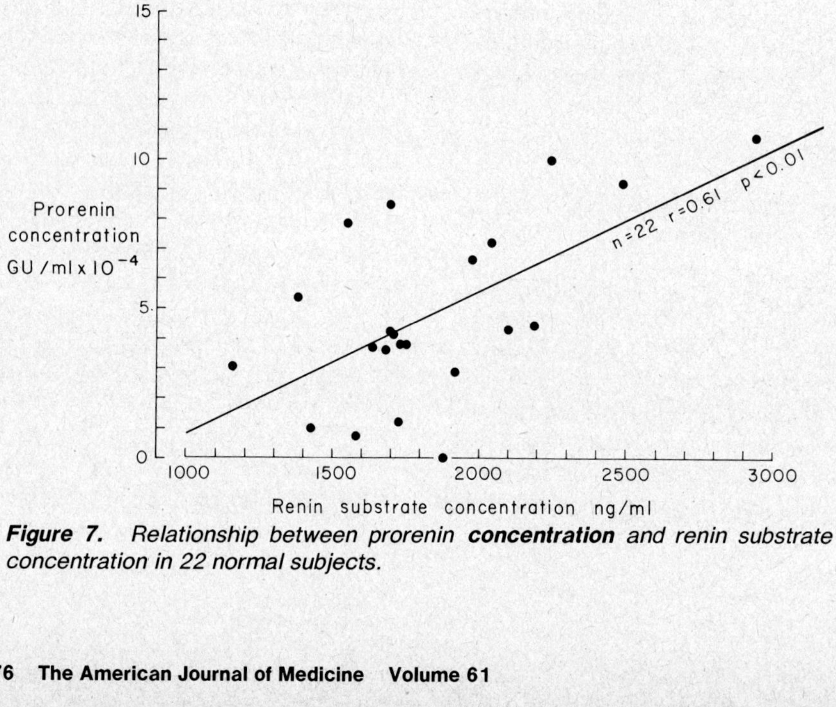

Figure 7. *Relationship between prorenin* ***concentration*** *and renin substrate concentration in 22 normal subjects.*

renin substrate. It is possible that a calculation error could perhaps partially explain this relationship since the concentration of prorenin was calculated using renal renin as a reference standard. If the Michaelis constant (K_m) for activated prorenin were higher than for renal renin the estimation of prorenin concentration would be incorrect and might result in an apparent relationship between the renin substrate and activated prorenin "concentration" when, in fact, none existed. More work, using purified components of the system, will be required to determine whether or not the relationship between the concentration of renin substrate and prorenin is real and whether plasma renin is identical to activated prorenin.

Notwithstanding, the strong relationship between prorenin activity and renin substrate concentration suggests that the prorenin secretion rate is regulated in part by different stimuli than those which regulate renin secretion. Thus, in contrast to prorenin, there is no relationship between endogenous plasma renin activity and renin substrate concentration [15], and renal renin secretion appears to autoregulate in response to changes in renin substrate concentration to maintain the same net ability to generate the angiotensin required by physiologic demands [20]. However, prorenin plasma levels do not appear to autoregulate to fluctuations in plasma renin substrate concentration. In fact the opposite occurs.

One explanation for the lack of a feedback relationship between prorenin and renin substrate concentration is that prorenin may not normally react with plasma renin substrate. If prorenin has a biologic action, it may react with a particular pool of substrate. If this were the case, it would be expected to autoregulate in response to changes in this particular pool. If such is the case, the relationship between substrate and prorenin is intriguing. It might be the appropriate response of a second renin system in which both prorenin and substrate change together physiologically. The fact that women in whom plasma renin substrate concentration is very high during estrogen therapy have normal prorenin activity and low prorenin concentration perhaps supports this viewpoint since, when substrate is stimulated by this apparently different mechanism, prorenin concentration is not also stimulated.

Altogether, these data suggest that both prorenin concentration and its activity should be determined in plasma until the relationships of the enzyme to its substrate and/or the renin substrate are resolved.

Changes in biochemical characteristics induced by reduction in temperature are not unique to prorenin. However, prorenin is unusual in that its activity is in fact enhanced by prolonged cooling. Pyruvate carboxylase from chicken liver mitochondria is rapidly inactivated by exposure to 0°C [21]. Exposure of purified 17β-hydroxysteroid dehydrogenase to temperatures below 10°C also results in loss of enzymatic activity [22]. It has been proposed that the mechanism of these changes could be related to differences in aggregation, changes in the configuration of the active site or disruption of hydrophobic bonds which are known to become significantly weaker as the temperature is lowered.

The physiologic role of prorenin, if any, remains to be defined. We previously demonstrated increases in prorenin activity in patients with low renin levels in response to sodium depletion [13] and, more recently, have shown that prorenin does not necessarily originate in the kidneys since it is present in close to normal amounts in the plasma of anephric patients [14]. Our demonstration that these same anephric patients have very low, almost unmeasurable, plasma aldosterone levels suggests that prorenin is not involved in the regulation of aldosterone biosynthesis. The lack of an apparent negative feedback link between prorenin and the circulating renin substrate concentration suggests either that prorenin does not normally react with plasma renin substrate or that factors affecting prorenin secretion simultaneously affect plasma renin substrate levels. Since the potential activity of prorenin is usually greater than that of plasma renin activity itself, the impact of this system could be highly significant if physiologic or pathologic conditions exist in which prorenin is converted to renin.

REFERENCES

1. Goldblatt H, Haas E: Renal mechanism in hypertension. Proceedings of the 6th Annual Conference on Nephrotic Syndrome (Metcott J, ed), New York, National Nephrosis Foundation, Inc., 1955, p 117.
2. Haas E, Lamfrom H, Goldblatt H: Ultraviolet spectroscopy of renin. Arch Biochem Biophys 44: 79, 1953.
3. Skeggs LT, Lentz KE, Kahn JR, et al.: Multiple forms of human kidney renin. Hypertension 1972 (Genest J, Koiw E, eds), Berlin-Heidelberg-New York, Springer-Verlag, 1972, p 149.
4. Newsome HH: Purification of bovine renin. Biochim Biophys Acta 185: 247, 1959.
5. Rubin L: Purification of hog renin. Properties of purified hog renin. Scand J Lab Invest 29: 51, 1972.
6. Lumbers ER: Activation of renin in human amniotic fluid by low pH. Enzymologia 40: 329, 1971.
7. Boyd W: A protein-bound form of porcine renal renin. Circ Res 35: 426, 1974.
8. Leckie B: Activation of a possible zymogen of renin in rabbit kidney. Clin Sci 44: 301, 1973.
9. Day RP, Luetscher JA, Zager PG: Big renin: identification, chemical properties and clinical implications. Am J Cardiol 37: 667, 1976.
10. Inagami T, Murakami K: Purification of renin precursor from

hog kidney (abstract). Circulation 51, 52 (suppl II): 14, 1975.

11. Skinner SL, Cran EJ, Gibson R, et al.: Angiotensins I and II, active and inactive renin, renin substrate, renin activity and angiotensinase in human liquor amnii and plasma. Am J Obstet Gynecol 121: 626, 1975.
12. Osmond DH, Ross LJ, Sciaff KD: Increased renin activity after cold storage of human plasma. Can J Physiol Pharmacol 51: 705, 1973.
13. Sealey JE, Laragh JH: "Prorenin" in human plasma. Circ Res 36, 37 (suppl I): 10, 1975.
14. Sealey JE, White RW, Laragh JH, et al.: Plasma prorenin in anephric patients. Circ Res (suppl) (in press) 1976.
15. Sealey JE, Gerten-Banes J, Laragh JH: The renin system: variations in man measured by radioimmunoassay or bioassay. Kidney Int 1: 240, 1972.
16. Sealey JE, Laragh JH: Radioimmunoassay of plasma renin activity. Semin Nucl Med 5: 189, 1975.
17. Haas E, Goldblatt H, Gipson EC: Extraction, purification and acetylation of human renin and the production of antirenin to human renin. Arch Biochem Biophys 110: 534, 1965.
18. Pickens PT, Bumpus F, Merlin F, et al.: Measurement of renin activity in human plasma. Circ Res 17: 438, 1965.
19. Sealey JE, Laragh JH: Searching out low renin patients. Limitations of some commonly used methods. Am J Med 55: 303, 1973.
20. Newton MA, Sealey JE, Ledingham JGG, et al.: High blood pressure and oral contraceptives. Am J Obstet Gynecol 101: 1037, 1968.
21. Irias JJ, Olmstead MR, Utter MF: Pyruvate carboxylase. Reversible inactivation by cold. Biochemistry 8: 5136, 1969.
22. Jarabak J, Seeds AE Jr, Talalay P: Reversible cold inactivation of a 17β-hydroxysteroid dehydrogenase of human placenta; protective effect of glycerol. Biochemistry 5: 1269, 1966.

Hypertension Associated with Early Stage Kidney Disease

Complementary Roles of Circulating Renin, the Body Sodium/Volume State and Duration of Hypertension

CARLO BERETTA-PICCOLI, M.D.*
PETER WEIDMANN, M.D.†
RUDOLF DE CHÂTEL, M.D.‡
FRANÇOIS REUBI, M.D.§
Berne, Switzerland

Interrelations among blood pressure, exchangeable sodium, blood volume and plasma renin activity were studied in 40 normal subjects and in 40 patients with early stage kidney disease (mean plasma creatinine, 2 mg/100 ml). Findings in eight normotensive patients did not differ significantly from those in normal subjects. However, 32 hypertensive patients showed increases ($p < 0.05$) in mean exchangeable sodium and in the products of the logarithm of plasma renin activity and exchangeable sodium or blood volume. In normal subjects, blood pressure did not correlate with any of the parameters measured. In the patients, it correlated significantly ($p < 0.05$) with duration of hypertension ($r = 0.70$), exchangeable sodium ($r = 0.34$) and with sodium-renin ($r = 0.38$) or volume-renin ($r = 0.30$) products, but not with blood volume or circulating renin individually. Multiple regression analysis with blood pressure as a dependent variable, and duration of hypertension and the sodium-renin or volume-renin products as independent variables, revealed correlation coefficients of 0.77 and 0.76, respectively. These findings suggest that hypertension accompanying early stage kidney disease may depend at least partly on subtle abnormalities in the sodium/volume-renin feedback mechanism as well as on a factor related to the duration of preexisting hypertension.

Previous studies have indicated that certain forms of hypertension may be at least partly related to abnormalities in the physiologic body sodium-volume-renin feedback mechanism [1]. Thus, a deranged relationship between the body sodium-volume state and circulating renin has been described in malignant hypertension and in hypertension associated with end-stage kidney disease [1–4]; in the latter category of patients, blood pressure was found to correlate significantly with the combined values of plasma renin and exchangeable sodium [3,5,6] or blood volume [3,6]. In contrast, in patients with essential hypertension and without impairment of excretory kidney function plasma renin levels were usually normal or even low in relation to their extracellular sodium and fluid contents [7,8], and blood pressure did not correlate with the calculated product of blood volume and plasma renin activity [9].

The quantitative aspects between impairment of renal function and derangements of body sodium-volume-renin homeostasis are presently unclear. Although these factors have been studied extensively in patients undergoing hemodialysis little is known about the interrelations between sodium-water metabolism and the renal pressor system in nonoliguric patients with lesser degrees of renal insufficiency. Therefore, this study was undertaken to evaluate the interrelations

From the Medical Policlinic, University of Berne, Switzerland. This work was supported by the Swiss National Foundation for Scientific Research. Requests for reprints should be addressed to Dr. Peter Weidmann.

* Present address: Department der Inneren Medizin, Kantonspital, 8006 Zurich, Switzerland.
† Present address: Division of Nephrology, LAC-USC Medical Center, 2025 Zonal Ave, Los Angeles, California 90033.
‡ Present address: 1st Department of Medicine, Koranyi—u. 2/a, H-1083 Budapest, Hungary.
§ Present address: Medizinische Polikklinik, Inselspital, Freiburgstrasse 3, 3010 Bern, Switzerland.

between blood pressure, exchangeable body sodium, blood volume and plasma renin activity in a population of patients who had a slight to moderate reduction in renal function.

SUBJECTS AND METHODS

Studies were carried out in 40 normal volunteer subjects and in 40 patients with renal disease. The normal subjects included 17 women and 23 men, ranging in age from 19 to 66 years. The patients included 18 women and 22 men ranging in age from 20 to 65 years. The diagnosis of the renal disease, based on clinical signs, laboratory tests and, in 11 patients, renal biopsy findings, was chronic glomerulonephritis in nine patients, chronic pyelonephritis in 13, interstitial nephritis of various etiology in five, renal tuberculosis in two, unilateral hydronephrosis in three, nephroangiosclerosis in five, and polycystic kidney disease, medullary sponge kidney and bilateral renal arterial narrowing, in one patient each. All patients were clinically stable and showed no signs of congestive heart failure or edema.

Normal subjects and patients were instructed to maintain their usual dietary habits but to avoid salt in their food during at least five days prior to the study. The administration of antihypertensive drugs was withdrawn at least two weeks before the test. Twenty-four hour total exchangeable sodium was measured by the radioisotope dilution technic using radioactive sodium (^{24}Na) [10]; the standardized method in this laboratory has been described previously [11]. During the last hour of this 24 hour period, the subjects remained in the supine position, and blood pressure, plasma sodium, potassium and creatinine concentrations, plasma volume and plasma renin activity were determined. Blood pressure measurements were obtained with standard pressure cuff and sphygmomanometer. The pressure at the disappearance of the Korotkoff sounds was taken as diastolic blood pressure. Each blood pressure recording was the mean of three readings. Mean blood pressure was calculated as the sum of the diastolic pressure andone third of the pulse pressure.

Plasma and urinary sodium and potassium concentrations were determined using the Instrumentation Laboratory flame photometer. Plasma creatinine was determined with the Greiner-Analyzer II. Plasma volume was determined by the isotope dilution technic using radioiodinated (^{131}I) human serum albumin [10,12]; ^{131}I plasma concentration at time zero was obtained by extrapolation of the values measured 10, 20 and 30 minutes after its injection. The radioactivity of peripheral venous blood was used to calculate blood volume assuming:

$$\text{whole blood volume} = \text{measured volume} \times \frac{100 - \text{hematocrit}}{100 - 0.91 \times \text{hematocrit}}$$

Exchangeable sodium, and plasma and blood volume were expressed as meq/kg lean body mass and ml/kg lean body mass, respectively. Lean body mass was estimated by using the leanness index of Nicholson and Zilva [13]; this index is the ratio of body height^3:weight. For comparison with other published data, plasma volume was also calculated as ml/cm body height, and results were expressed in per cent of normal, taking the sex of patient into consideration [14]. Plasma renin activity was measured in duplicate samples utilizing the radioimmunoassay method of Sealey et al. [15]; within assay variation in 214 duplicate samples averaged 4.1 per cent and between assay variation in 36 samples was 6.4 per cent.

In 33 of the 40 patients, glomerular filtration rate and effective renal plasma flow were also measured by constant infusion clearance methods using ^{51}Chromium-ethylenediamine tetraacetate and paraamino hippuric acid, respectively, as previously reported from this laboratory [16,17]; the filtration fraction was calculated as the ^{51}Cr-EDTA:PAH clearance ratio. The interval between the clearance studies and the determinations specified was two weeks or less.

For statistical analysis of plasma renin activity, the natural logarithm transformation of the respective values was used.

RESULTS

Various Clinical, Biochemical and Functional Parameters (Table I). In six of the patients included in this study the blood pressure level never rose, whereas 34 had either transient or persistent hypertension during the course of their illness. The known duration of the elevated blood pressure levels in these 34 patients ranged from 0.5 to 23 years, with a mean of 7.3 years. At the time of this study, eight of 40 patients had a mean blood pressure of $<$110 mm Hg and were considered normotensive. Thirty-two patients had a mean blood pressure $>$110 mm Hg and were considered hypertensive. No patient showed grade 3 or 4 (Keith-Wagener) hypertensive retinopathy.

Blood pressure averaged 119/78 mm Hg in the normal subjects, 132/82 mm Hg in the patients with normal blood pressure and 177/117 mm Hg in the hypertensive patients (Table I). The normotensive patients had a significantly higher systolic blood pressure level than the normal subjects ($p < 0.025$). Mean pulse rate was 68 $\pm$ 10 ($\pm$ standard deviation [SD]) beats/min in the normal subjects, 78 $\pm$ 14 beats/min in the patients with normal blood pressure and 77 $\pm$ 15 beats/min in the hypertensive patients; the values in the two patient groups were significantly higher than the mean pulse rate in the normal subjects ($p < 0.01$) (Table I). Mean hematocrit, plasma sodium and potassium concentrations, and 24 hour urinary sodium excretion were comparable in the normal subjects and in the patients with normal or elevated blood pressure levels.

A slight to moderate increase in plasma creatinine concentration or a comparable decrease in glomerular filtration rate and/or effective renal plasma flow was noted in all patients. Twenty-eight of the 33 patients in whom constant infusion clearance measurements were performed showed a decrease in both glomerular filtration rate (normal range, 93 to 159 ml/min/1.73 m^2) and effective renal plasma flow (normal range, 478 to 814 ml/min/1.73 m^2); in the remaining five patients, only one of the two clearance parameters was reduced below normal. Normal control subjects showed a mean

TABLE I Various Clinical, Biochemical and Functional Parameters in Normal Subjects and in Patients with Renal Disease (Mean ± SD)

Parameter	Normal Subjects	Patients: All	Patients: $\overline{BP}$ <110 mm Hg	Patients: $\overline{BP}$ >110 mm Hg
Blood pressure (mm Hg)	119/78 ± 9/8	168/110* ± 33/20	132/82 ± 14/7	177/117* ± 30/16
Pulse rate (beats/min)	68 ± 10	78* ± 13	78* ± 14	77* ± 15
Hematocrit value (%)	44.7 ± 3.8	44.1 ± 4.4	44.0 ± 4.3	44.2 ± 4.5
Plasma				
Sodium (meq/liter)	141.0 ± 2.0	140.9 ± 1.6	140.6 ± 1.9	141.0 ± 1.5
Potassium (meq/liter)	4.0 ± 0.3	4.06 ± 0.44	4.0 ± 0.36	4.08 ± 0.46
Creatinine (mg/100 ml)	1.21 ± 0.15	2.00* ± 1.12	1.89* ± 0.86	2.02* ± 1.18
Urinary sodium (meq/24 hr)	127 ± 64	125 ± 51	132 ± 81	121 ± 40
Glomerular filtration rate† (ml/min/1.73 m^2)	126 ± 17	59 ± 29	79‡ ± 31	53 ± 27
Effective renal plasma flow† (ml/min/1.73 m^2)	646 ± 84	285 ± 121	384‡ ± 133	245 ± 104
Filtration fraction†	0.195 ± 0.019	0.214 ± 0.043	0.208 ± 0.042	0.223 ± 0.044

NOTE: $\overline{BP}$ = mean blood pressure
*Significant difference versus normal subjects ($p < 0.0125$).
†Values shown for normal subjects are those established previously in a different study population of 203 normal volunteer subjects.
‡Significant difference versus hypertensive patients ($p < 0.01$)

plasma creatinine concentration of 1.21 ± 0.15 mg/100 ml, a glomerular filtration rate of 126 ± 17 ml/min/1.73 m^2 and an effective renal plasma flow of 646 ± 84 ml/min/1.73 m^2. The patients with renal disease had a mean plasma creatinine of 2.00 ± 1.12 mg/100 ml, a glomerular filtration rate of 59 ± 29 ml/min/1.73 m^2 and an effective renal plasma flow of 285 ± 121 ml/min/1.73 m^2. Furthermore, the hypertensive patients had a significantly lower mean glomerular filtration rate and renal plasma flow than the patients with normal blood pressure ($p < 0.01$) (Table I).

Exchangeable Body Sodium and Blood Volume (Table II). Mean exchangeable body sodium was 51.9 ± 0.8 (± standard error [SE]) meq/kg lean body mass in the normal subjects, 53.9 ± 1.7 meq/kg lean body mass in the patients with normal blood pressure and 58.0 ± 1.3 meq/kg lean body mass in the hypertensive patients; the latter value is significantly higher ($p < 0.001$) than that found in normal controls, without a significant difference between the patient groups with normal or elevated blood pressure levels. Mean blood volume was 83.1 ± 2.1 ml/kg lean body mass in the normal subjects, 84.5 ± 5.3 ml/kg lean body mass in the normotensive patients and 88.6 ± 2.9 ml/kg lean body mass in the hypertensive patients; these values do not differ significantly. When calculated as ml/cm body height and expressed in per cent of normal, taking the sex of the patient into consideration [14], mean plasma volume was 100.5 per cent of normal in the patients with normal blood pressure and 100.6 per cent of normal in the hypertensive patients.

Exchangeable sodium correlated significantly with blood volume when the patients were analyzed separately ($r = 0.68$, $p < 0.001$) or together with the normal subjects ($r = 0.63$; $p < 0.001$).

Plasma Renin Activity (Table II). Although patients with either normal or elevated blood pressure levels tended to have slightly higher plasma renin levels than the normal subjects, mean values did not differ significantly between any of these groups. More specifically, mean plasma renin activity was 2.04 ± 0.19 ng/ml/hour in the normal subjects, 3.16 ± 1.10 ng/ml/hour in the patients with normal blood pressure and 3.05 ± 0.52 ng/ml/hour in the hypertensive patients.

TABLE II Exchangeable Body Sodium, Blood Volume and Plasma Renin Activity in Normal Subjects and in Patients with Renal Disease (Mean ± SE)

	No.	Exchangeable Sodium (meq/kg LBM)	Blood Volume* (ml/kg LBM)	Plasma Renin Activity (ng/ml/hour)
Normal Subjects	40	51.9 ± 0.8	83.1 ± 2.1	2.04 ± 0.19
Patients				
$\overline{BP}$ < 110 mm Hg	8	53.9 ± 1.7	84.5 ± 5.3	3.16 ± 1.10
$\overline{BP}$ > 110 mm Hg	32	58.0 ± 1.3†	88.6 ± 2.9	3.05 ± 0.52

NOTE: $\overline{BP}$ = mean blood pressure. LBM = lean body mass.
*Blood volume was measured in 37 normal subjects and in 38 patients.
†Significant difference versus normal subjects ($p < 0.01$).

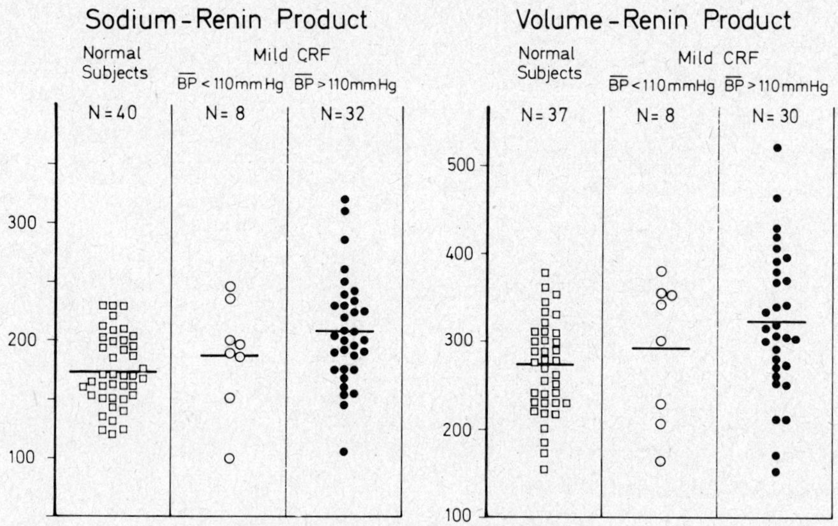

Figure 1. *The sodium-renin and the volume-renin products in normal subjects and patients with mild to moderate chronic renal failure (CRF) and normal or elevated blood pressure levels.*

In the normal subjects, plasma renin activity correlated inversely with blood volume ($r = -0.39$; $p < 0.02$) but not with exchangeable sodium ($r = -0.24$) or blood pressure ($r = -0.20$). In the patients with normal blood pressure, plasma renin correlated inversely with exchangeable sodium ($r = -0.71$; $p < 0.025$), but due to the small number of cases, the relationship with blood volume ($r = -0.47$) did not achieve the level of statistical significance. In the hypertensive patients, circulating renin correlated significantly with exchangeable sodium ($r = -0.39$; $p < 0.05$) but not with blood volume ($r = -0.17$). Analyzing the patients with renal disease as one group, no significant correlations were noted among plasma renin and blood pressure, glomerular filtration rate, renal plasma flow or filtration fraction.

Sodium/Volume-Renin Products (Figure 1). The sodium-renin product [5] was obtained by multiplying exchangeable sodium (expressed as meq/kg lean body mass) by the natural logarithm of plasma renin activity (expressed as ng/liter/min); the blood volume-renin product was derived accordingly. Mean sodium-renin or volume-renin products were significantly higher in hypertensive patients ($p < 0.0025$) than in normal subjects, and there were no significant differences between normotensive patients and normal subjects.

Relationship Between Blood Pressure and Various Parameters. In patients with renal disease, blood pressure did not correlate significantly with filtration fraction, blood volume or plasma renin activity; however, it correlated inversely ($p < 0.05$) with glomerular

TABLE III Correlations Between Mean Blood Pressure and Various Parameters

	Patients			Normal Subjects		
	No.	r	p	No.	r	p
Mean blood pressure versus						
GFR	33	–0.33	<0.05			
ERPF	33	–0.41	<0.01			
FF	33	–0.04	NS			
Na_e	40	0.34	<0.025	40	0.10	NS
PV	38	0.08	NS	37	–0.12	NS
BV	38	0.17	NS	37	–0.07	NS
ln PRA	40	0.20	NS	40	0.15	NS
lnt BP ↑	40	0.70	<0.001			
Na_e, ln PRA	40	0.38	<0.01	40	0.23	NS
BV, ln PRA	38	0.30	<0.05	37	0.16	NS
Na_e, ln PRA, lnt BP ↑	40	0.77	<0.001			
BV, ln PRA, lnt BP ↑	38	0.76	<0.001			

NOTE: GFR = glomerular filtration rate; ERPF = effective renal plasma flow; FF = filtration fraction; Na_e = exchangeable sodium; PV = plasma volume; BV = blood volume; ln PRA = natural logarithm of plasma renin activity; lnt BP ↑ = natural logarithm of known duration of hypertension. NS = not significant.

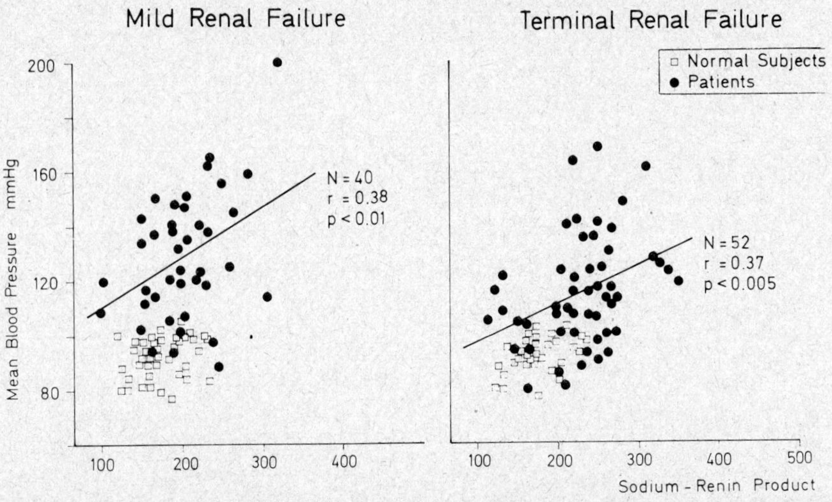

Figure 2. *Relationship between blood pressure and the product of exchangeable sodium and renin in mild and terminal renal failure. The regression lines and the r and p values refer to findings in patients with renal failure. The data from patients with terminal renal failure have been reported previously [6] and they are reproduced by permission of the International Society of Nephrology.*

filtration rate (r = −0.33) and the effective renal plasma flow (r = −0.41), and positively with the duration of previous hypertension (r = 0.70), exchangeable body sodium (r = 0.34), and with the products of renin and exchangeable sodium (r = 0.38) or blood volume (r = 0.30) (Table III). In the normal subjects, no significant correlations were found between blood pressure and any of the measured parameters (Table III).

Figure 2 illustrates the relationship between blood pressure and the sodium-renin product and compares the present results in patients with mild renal failure with our previous findings in patients with terminal renal failure undergoing maintenance hemodialysis [6]. The quantitative relationship between blood pressure and the sodium-renin or blood volume-renin products appeared to be quite comparable in early and terminal renal failure.

Multiple regression analysis, including the logarithm of the known duration of previous hypertension as a second independent variable, further improved these correlations (Table III). With blood pressure as a dependent variable, and the sodium-renin product and duration of hypertension as independent variables, the correlation coefficient for patients with renal lesions was increased to 0.77 ($p < 0.001$); with the volume-renin product and duration of previous hypertension as independent variables, it was 0.76 ($p < 0.001$).

To demonstrate these relationships in a two-dimensional graph, the product of exchangeable sodium and the logarithms of plasma renin activity and duration of hypertension were calculated and found to correlate equally well with blood pressure. Figure 3 shows these data and compares the present findings in patients with mild to moderately impaired kidney function with those obtained previously from patients with terminal renal failure [6]. Again, quantitative interrelations between the measured parameters were quite comparable in these two groups of patients.

Furthermore, there was also a highly significant correlation between blood pressure and the product of blood volume, and the logarithms of plasma renin and duration of hypertension (Figure 4).

COMMENTS

Renal lesions may affect blood pressure regulation by a variety of mechanisms, ranging from disturbances in the body sodium water homeostasis to the inappropriate release of pressor and depressor substances. In recent years, emphasis has been laid especially on two of these mechanisms. These are the impaired capacity of the diseased kidneys to fulfill their important role in adapting body sodium and fluid balance and circulatory volume with sodium intake and systemic blood pressure [18–20], and alterations in the function of the renin-angiotensin-aldosterone system [1,2,4]. In this study, mean exchangeable body sodium, plasma volume and plasma renin activity in eight normotensive patients with a mean serum creatinine concentration of 1.9 mg/100 ml did not differ significantly from the values found in 40 normal subjects. However, 32 hypertensive patients with a mean serum creatinine level of 2 mg/100 ml showed a slight but significant ($p < 0.05$) increase in mean exchangeable sodium, whereas plasma renin activity and blood volumes did not differ significantly from those in normal subjects. Furthermore, in these patients in whom glomerular filtration rates ranged from

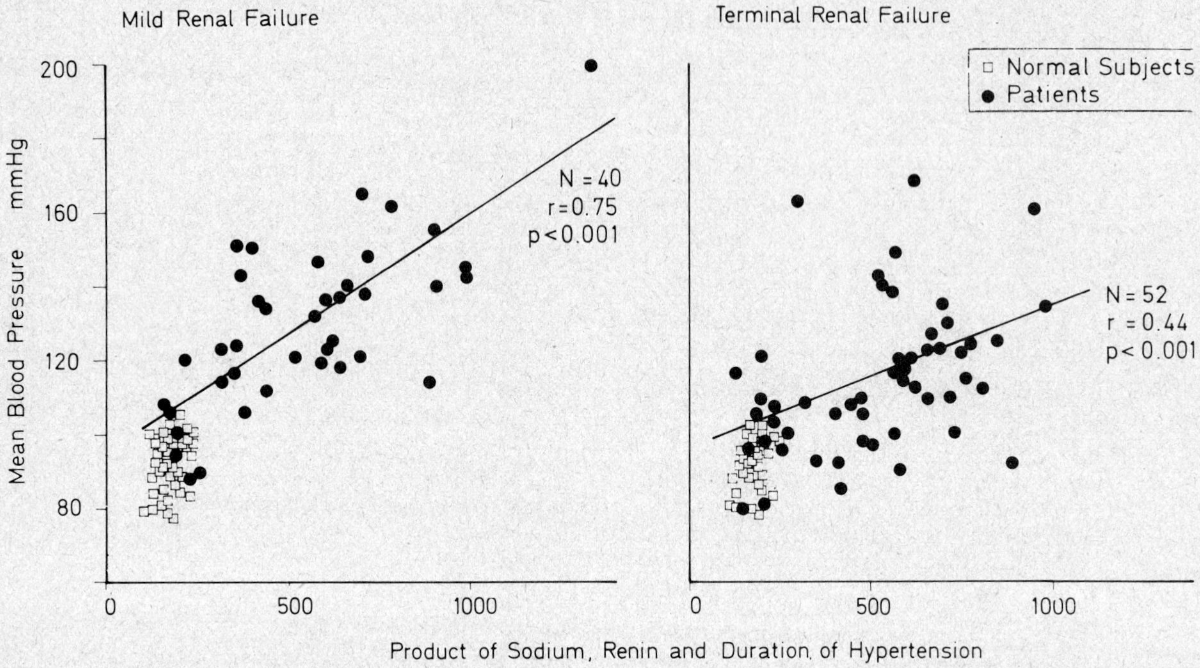

Figure 3. *Relationship between blood pressure and the product of exchangeable sodium, renin and duration of preexisting hypertension in mild and terminal renal failure. The regression lines and the r and p values refer to the findings in patients with renal failure. The data from patients with terminal renal failure have been reported previously [6] and they are reproduced by permission of the International Society of Nephrology.*

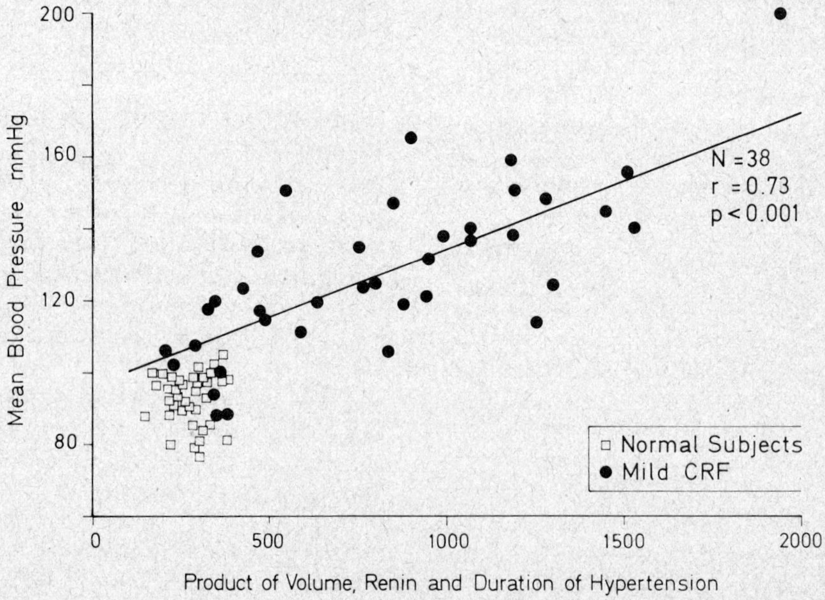

Figure 4. *Relationship between blood pressure and the product of volume, renin and duration of hypertension in normal subjects and patients with mild to moderate chronic renal failure. The regression line and the r and p values refer to the findings in patients with renal failure.*

10 to 126 ml/min/1.73 m^2 and effective renal plasma flows from 70 to 514 ml/min/1.73 m^2, blood pressure was found to correlate significantly with exchangeable sodium ($r = 0.34$; $p < 0.025$), but not with plasma, blood volumes or plasma renin activity.

The finding of normal plasma volumes in hypertensive patients with slight to moderate renal failure is consistent with previous data [14,21]. However, Nickel et al. [21], who studied six patients with inulin clearances ranging from 7 to 50 ml/min, noted consistent increases in extracellular fluid volumes. In addition, in a study of 16 hypertensive patients with primary renal parenchymal diseases and creatinine clearances ranging from 15 to 105 ml/min, Tarazi et al. [14] described a highly significant positive relationship between systemic pressure and plasma volume. It was considered whether the absence of a significant blood pressure-volume relationship in our patients could be related to the inclusion of six patients with primary vascular lesions of the kidneys, five of whom had nephrosclerosis and one of whom had bilateral renal arterial lesions. However, separate analysis of the remaining 34 patients with primary parenchymal kidney disease failed to improve the correlation between systemic pressure and plasma volume to the level of significance ($r = 0.18$).

In patients with more advanced stages of nonoliguric renal failure in whom blood pressure has been normalized, the capacity of the kidneys to excrete sodium is frequently impaired [22]. While on a liberal salt intake, such patients are prone to the development of sodium retention and hypertension. By enhancing renal sodium excretion, the increased systemic pressure may in turn help to reestablish a balance between sodium intake and output [20,22]. The present data suggest that even in the early stages of renal disease causing only a slight reduction in glomerular filtration, mild accumulation of body sodium may occur and contribute to the development of high blood pressure levels.

The impact of slight to moderate renal failure on the function of the renin-angiotensin-aldosterone system has not been studied systematically. However, patients with normal blood pressure and without gross abnormalities in plasma electrolyte composition were usually found to have normal or slightly elevated plasma renin [23–25], angiotensin II [26] and aldosterone [25] levels. In patients with slight to moderate renal failure and benign hypertension, circulating renin was found to range from low to markedly elevated values [23,24,27,28]. Whereas several investigators described significant correlations between blood pressure and circulating renin or angiotensin II levels in this category of patients [24,26], other investigators, like ourselves, were unable to demonstrate such a relationship [23,27].

Linked by a complex feedback mechanism, the body sodium-volume state and circulating renin-angiotensin activity are normally in equilibrium, and in subjects with normal renal excretory function plasma renin levels can be judged in relation to dietary sodium intake or sodium excretion [1,12,29]. However, in patients with renal lesions, who may not be in normal fluid or sodium balance, interpretation of plasma renin levels without a direct measurement of body sodium and fluid compartments may be unreliable [2,4]. Based on (1) the known reciprocal relationship between the pressor effect of exogenous angiotensin II and body sodium balance [30,31] and (2) the well established finding that increases in blood pressure during angiotensin II infusion correlate with the logarithm of the dose [32], Rosen and Robinson [5] suggested to estimate "effective" circulating renin in an individual patient by calculating the product of exchangeable body sodium and the logarithm of plasma renin concentration. Using this type of approach, blood pressure was found to correlate with the "sodium-renin" and "blood volume-renin" products in end-stage kidney disease [5,6]; whereas in patients with benign essential hypertension no significant correlation was apparent between blood pressure and the "blood volume-renin" product [9]. These data are in support of a complementary role of the body sodium/volume state and circulating renin in hypertension of end-stage kidney disease and they militate against an important part of these factors in the maintenance of benign essential hypertension.

In our patients with slight to moderate renal failure, blood pressure correlated significantly with the "blood volume-renin" product ($r = 0.30$; $p < 0.05$), but not with blood volume or plasma renin activity individually. Furthermore, systemic pressure in these patients showed a closer relationship with the "sodium-renin" product ($r = 0.38$) than with exchangeable sodium alone ($r = 0.34$). Finally, quantitative interrelations between the sodium-renin or volume-renin products and blood pressure in the patients with slight to moderate renal failure were almost similar to those observed previously in patients with terminal renal failure treated with hemodialysis (Figure 2). These data suggest that subtle abnormalities in the body sodium-volume renin feedback mechanism may be already operative in hypertension associated with early stage renal disease.

Nevertheless, despite the existence of statistically significant correlations between blood pressure and the sodium-renin or blood volume-renin products in both the early and the terminal stages of renal failure [6], the considerable splay of the data indicates that other factors are also operative in renal hypertension.

It is a well established clinical observation that with increasing duration of the disease, hypertension in any given patient tends to become more severe. Indeed, in a previous study from this laboratory, blood pressure in patients undergoing hemodialysis was found to be partly related to the total duration of hypertension [6]. In the present series, this trend is even more conspicuous. Blood pressure in our patients with slight renal failure correlated significantly with the duration of preexisting hypertension ($r = 0.70$; $p < 0.001$); furthermore, introduction of this factor as a second independent variable increased the coefficients for the relationships between blood pressure and the sodium-renin or volume-renin products from 0.38 and 0.30 to 0.77 and 0.76, respectively (Table III).

The pathophysiologic basis for the observed relationship between blood pressure and duration of preexisting hypertension is presently unclear. There is no doubt that, in chronic parenchymatous nephropathies, the severity of the kidney lesions increases with the duration of the illness, thus resulting in progressive functional impairment and in inappropriate release of renin and, possibly, some other vasoactive substances. In this view, the blood pressure should correlate inversely with the glomerular filtration rate and with PAH clearance. In the present series, this was found to be the case. However, the correlation coefficients ($r = -0.33$ and -0.41, respectively) were definitely lower than those for the relationship between blood pressure and duration of hypertension ($r = 0.76$). This indicates that the parameter "duration of hypertension" includes other variables than the renal functions.

One of them could be the development of peripheral arteriolar lesions. Persistent increases in blood pressure lead to hypertrophic structural changes of the resistance vessels with a raised wall to lumen ratio, and it has been suggested that the hemodynamic consequences of these alterations, namely, increased vascular resistance, may participate in both the development and the maintenance of hypertension [33,34]. The time course for the occurrence of such adaptive blood vessel changes in human hypertension has not been clearly delineated, but it would appear probable that their magnitude is at least partly related to the duration of hypertension [6].

ACKNOWLEDGMENT

We are indebted to Miss Irene Bollinger, Mrs. Josefina Bürki and Miss Irene Stuber for their skilled technical assistance. We would also like to thank Dr. and Mrs. John H. Laragh, New York, U.S.A., for their generous supply of angiotensin I antibody, and Dr. A. Blumberg for his help in the evaluation of a patient under his care.

REFERENCES

1. Laragh JH: Vasoconstrictor—volume analysis for understanding and treating hypertension. The use of renin and aldosterone profiles. Am J Med 55:261, 1973.
2. Davies DL, Schalekamp MA, Beevers DG, et al.: Abnormal relation between exchangeable sodium and the renin-angiotensin system in malignant hypertension and in hypertension with chronic renal failure. Lancet 1: 683, 1973.
3. Goodwin FJ, Dathan JRE, Greenwood RH, et al.: Influence of renin and volume on the blood pressure in renal failure. Proceedings of the 5th International Congress of Nephrology (Villareal H, ed), Basel, S. Karger, 1974, p 81.
4. Weidmann P, Maxwell MH: The renin-angiotensin-aldosterone system in terminal renal failure. Kidney Int 7 (suppl 5): S-219, 1975.
5. Rosen SM, Robinson PJA: Interdependence of exchangeable sodium and plasma renin concentration in determining blood pressure in patients treated by maintenance dialysis. Br Med J 4: 139, 1973.
6. Weidmann P, Beretta-Piccoli C, Steffen F, et al.: Hypertension in terminal renal failure. Kidney Int 9: 294, 1976.
7. Lebel M, Schalekamp MA, Beevers DG, et al.: Sodium and the renin-angiotensin system in essential hypertension and mineralocorticoid excess. Lancet 2: 308, 1974.
8. Distler A, Keim HJ, Philipp T, et al.: Exchangeable sodium, total body potassium, plasma volume, and hypotensive effect of various diuretics in patients with essential hypertension and low plasma renin levels. Dtsch Med Wochenschr 99: 864, 1974.
9. Weidmann P, Hirsch D, Beretta-Piccoli C, et al.: Interrelations between blood pressure, blood volume, plasma renin activity and urinary catecholamines in benign essential hypertension. Am J Med (to be published).
10. Veall N, Vetter H: Radioisotope Techniques in Clinical Research and Diagnosis, London, Butterworth Co., 1958, p 189.
11. Vorburger C: Flüssigkeits- und Elektrolyträume bei der chronischen Niereninsuffizienz. Beziehungen zum Blutdruck und zur Kohlenhydrattoleranz. Helv Med Acta suppl 51, p 1, 1971.
12. Weidmann P, DeMyttenaere-Bursztein S, Maxwell MH, et al.: Effect of aging on plasma renin and aldosterone levels in normal man. Kidney Int 7: 325, 1975.
13. Nicholson JP, Zilva JF: Body constituents and functions in relation to height and weight. Clin Sci 27: 97, 1964.
14. Tarazi RC, Dustan HP, Frohlich ED, et al.: Plasma volume in chronic hypertension. Arch Intern Med 125: 835, 1970.
15. Sealey JE, Gerten-Banes J, Laragh JH: The renin system. Variations in man measured by radioimmunoassay or bioassay. Kidney Int 1: 240, 1972.
16. Reubi F: Nierenkrankheiten, Berne, Hans Huber Verlag, 1960, p 91.
17. Vorburger C, Riedwyl H, Reubi F: Vergleichende Studien zwischen den renalen Clearances von Na-Cr_2Cr^{51}-äthylendiamintetraacetat, Inulin und Natriumthiosulfat beim Menschen. Klin Wochenschr 47: 415, 1969.
18. De Wardener HE: Control of sodium reabsorption. Br Med J 3: 611, 676, 1969.
19. Selkurt EE: Effect of pulse pressure and mean arterial pressure modification on renal hemodynamics and electrolyte and water excretion. Circulation 4: 541, 1951.
20. Guyton AC, Coleman TG, Cowley AW Jr, et al.: Arterial pressure regulation. Am J Med 52: 584, 1972.
21. Nickel JF, Lowrance PB, Leifer E, et al.: Renal function, electrolyte excretion and body fluids in patients with chronic

renal insufficiency before and after sodium deprivation. J Clin Invest 32: 68, 1953.
22. Ulvila JM, Kennedy JA, Lamberg JD, et al.: Blood pressure in chronic renal failure. Effect of sodium intake and furosemide. JAMA 220: 233, 1972.
23. Reubi F, Hodler J: L'activité rénine au cours des nephropathies parenchymateuses avec et sans hypertension. Actualités Néphrologiques de l'Hôpital Necker, Paris, Editions Médicales Flammarion, 1968, p 221.
24. Kleinknecht D, Maxwell MH: Étude statistique des variations de l'activité rénine plasmatique dans les nephropathies bilatérales, résultats préliminaires. Actualités Néphrologiques de l'Hôpital Necker, Paris, Editions Médicales Flammarion, 1970, p 63.
25. Weidmann P, Maxwell MH, Rowe P, et al.: Role of the renin-angiotensin-aldosterone system in the regulation of plasma potassium in chronic renal disease. Nephron 15: 35, 1975.
26. Catt KJ, Cain MD, Coghlan JP, et al.: Metabolism and blood levels of angiotensin II in normal subjects, renal disease and essential hypertension. Circ Res 26 & 27 (suppl II): 177, 1970.
27. Brown JJ, Davies DL, Lever AF, et al.: Plasma renin concentration in human hypertension II: renin in relation to etiology. Br Med J 2: 1215, 1965.
28. Del Greco F, Simon NM, Goodman S, et al.: Plasma renin activity in primary and secondary hypertension. Medicine (Baltimore) 46: 475, 1967.
29. Brown JJ, Davies DL, Lever AF, et al.: Influence of sodium loading and sodium depletion on plasma-renin in man. Lancet 2: 278, 1963.
30. Ames RP, Borkowski AJ, Sicinski AM, et al.: Prolonged infusions of angiotensin II and norepinephrine and blood pressure, electrolyte balance, and aldosterone and cortisol secretion in normal man and in cirrhosis with ascites. J Clin Invest 44: 1171, 1965.
31. Reid WD, Laragh JH: Sodium and potassium intake, blood pressure, and pressor response to angiotensin. Proc Soc Exp Biol Med 120: 26, 1965.
32. Chinn RH, Düsterdieck G: The response of blood pressure to infusion of angiotensin II. Relation to plasma concentrations of renin and angiotensin II. Clin Sci 42: 489, 1972.
33. Sivertsson R: The hemodynamic importance of structural vascular changes in essential hypertension. Acta Physiol Scand suppl 343, p 1, 1970.
34. Folkow B: The hemodynamic importance of structural vascular changes in the resistance vessels in hypertension. Clin Sci 41: 1, 1971.

Elevation of Serum Lipid Levels During Diuretic Therapy of Hypertension

RICHARD P. AMES, M.D.
PETER HILL, Ph.D.
New York, New York

In a study attempting to improve coronary risk status, serum cholesterol and triglyceride levels were measured before and during treatment of 74 patients with mild primary hypertension. In 35 patients there was a satisfactory reduction in elevated blood pressure levels with diet therapy alone. In the remaining 39 patients a diuretic drug was required in addition to the diet. Diet therapy alone was followed by a decrease of 11 mg/100 ml in mean serum cholesterol ($p < 0.01$ versus pretreatment value) and no change in serum triglyceride. The use of diuretics was accompanied by an average increase of 11 mg/100 ml in serum cholesterol and of 34 mg/100 ml in serum triglyceride ($p < 0.01$ versus pretreatment level for both). In a subgroup of 21 patients with greatest elevations in lipid levels during the administration of diuretics, little improvement in coronary risk status occurred because the increase in serum cholesterol balanced the decrease in systolic blood pressure, according to Framingham risk tables. If the level of serum lipids is a factor in the pathogenesis of coronary atherosclerosis, then the observed effect of diuretic drugs to elevate serum cholesterol and triglyceride levels may explain, in part, the continuing high rate of occurrence of myocardial infarction during the treatment of hypertension.

Treatment of increased arterial pressure sharply reduces the incidence of the major complications of hypertension except for myocardial infarction [1,2]. Coronary atherosclerosis has become the leading cause of death in treated patients with hypertension [3]. The reason for the lack of substantial benefit of treatment on coronary disease remains unexplained. It has been suggested that earlier treatment may be required to avert the initiation of coronary atherosclerosis [4]. It is not certain how earlier treatment can be accomplished. If this involves treating patients with slight elevations in blood pressure with antihypertensive drugs, then the evidence to date does not suggest that the standard therapeutic approach will produce dramatic results. In one study of the drug treatment of large numbers of patients with diastolic blood pressures under 105 mm Hg for periods up to five years, there was no significant reduction in the incidence of cardiac infarction [1].

The proposal for earlier treatment of patients with hypertension (i.e., before the initiation of atherosclerosis) is based, in part, on the assumption that atherosclerotic plaques, once initiated in coronary vessels, progress inexorably despite adequate antihypertensive therapy. This hypothesis is not yet certain because at least one study

From the American Health Foundation, 1370 Avenue of the Americas; the Department of Medicine, the Roosevelt Hospital, 428 West 59th Street; and The College of Physicians and Surgeons, Columbia University, New York, New York. This study was supported in part by U.S. Public Health Service Grant CA12376 from the National Cancer Institute. An abstract of this work has appeared in J Clin Pharmacol 15: 552, 1975. Requests for reprints should be addressed to Dr. Richard P. Ames, American Health Foundation, 1370 Avenue of the Americas, New York, New York 10019.

TABLE I Effect of Diuretics on Serum Lipids: Treatment Prescribed and Grouping for Analysis

			Diet Prescribed (no.)			
Subgroup	No. of Patients	Blood Pressure (mm Hg)	Low Sodium	Caloric Restriction	Lipid Lowering	Drug Prescribed
			Status at Intake			
I	35	90–104*	35	29	27	None
II	12	90–104*	12	11	11	None
III	27	104*	27	22	20	Diuretic
			Status at Four Months			
I	35	<140/90		Continue same		None
II	12	>140/90		Continue same		Add diuretic
III	27	Receiving drug		Continue same		Continue diuretic
			Status During Subsequent Months			
I	35			Continue follow up		
II	12			Continue follow up		
III	27			Continue follow up		

NOTE: Subgroup I—treated with diet alone. Subgroup II—treated with diet initially, diuretic added later. Subgroup III—treated with diet and diuretics from start of study. Subgroup II and III combined for presentation in Tables II and III.
* Diastolic.

has shown that atherosclerosis in coronary and other vessels, when associated with hyperlipidemia, may be slowed by diet therapy given to lower serum lipid levels [5]. Thus, atherosclerosis associated with other presumed pathogenetic mechanisms does not seem to be necessarily a relentless process.

An alternative explanation for the high incidence of myocardial infarction in patients treated for hypertension is that coronary atherosclerosis is a multifactorial condition and other causative processes have been neglected or aggravated in the treatment of the high blood pressure. We have evaluated an aspect of this latter possibility by measuring serum cholesterol and triglyceride levels serially in patients before and during the treatment of hypertension in a study attempting to control both blood pressure and serum lipids.

MATERIAL AND METHODS

Patients. Seventy-four patients with hypertension were studied in an outpatient setting. These patients were referred from a multiphasic screening center engaged in annual and biennial examinations of urban office and union workers and their spouses. Most patients had newly discovered hypertension and elected to be treated in our clinic because they had no personal physician. Seven patients were receiving drug treatment for hypertension when screened and elected to continue treatment in our clinic for a variety of reasons. They were included in this report because lipid determinations were obtained after they had been without drug therapy for three or more weeks. All patients in our clinic who were treated with diet alone or with diet plus diuretic drugs are included in this report. Patients treated with antiadrenergic drugs or combinations of diuretics and antiadrenergic drugs were omitted from this analysis.

Blood pressure was taken by the auscultatory method using mercury manometer and arm cuff. Blood pressures were recorded after the patient had been sitting for 5 minutes. An average of right and left arm measurements was used as the arterial pressure level. A patient was considered to be hypertensive if the blood pressure recordings at three clinic visits, usually at intervals of one week, were consistently greater than 140 mm Hg systolic or 90 mm Hg diastolic. Patients with known diabetes mellitus or fasting blood sugar levels above 130 mg/100 ml were excluded from this analysis. In all patients a complete medical history, physical examination, urinalysis, chest film and electrocardiogram were obtained. When symptoms were suggestive of pheochromocytoma, vanillylmandelic acid (VMA) excretion was measured. In one of seven patients so studied, VMA excretion was increased. This patient refused further diagnostic evaluation. In four patients with clinical evidence suggestive of renal or renovascular disease, rapid sequence intravenous pyelography was performed. Results were normal in all four. Eight patients had normal thyroid function by plasma thyroxine measurement.

Design of the Study. During the three clinic visits to establish the diagnosis of hypertension, blood samples were obtained from all patients after a 12-hour fast for determinations of cholesterol and triglyceride levels. In addition, blood was also taken for measurement of serum sodium, potassium, creatinine and uric acid. In 60 patients, a second blood sample was obtained for determining cholesterol and triglyceride levels before starting therapy. After the third blood pressure recording, therapy was started. Twenty-seven patients whose diastolic blood pressure was 105 mm Hg or more were placed on a regimen of diet and drugs after obtaining the base line data. Forty-seven patients whose diastolic blood pressure was 104 mm Hg or less were given a four-month trial of diet alone. This cut-off level for drug therapy was chosen because present information does not indicate a clear-cut benefit of drug therapy on the incidence of complications when pretreatment blood pressure is below 105 mm Hg [1]. After the four-month trial of diet, if blood pressure readings remained above 140 mm Hg systolic or 90 mm Hg diastolic, drug therapy was added. Twelve of the 47 patients required drug therapy; the remaining 35 did not (Table I).

TABLE II Characteristics of Patients with Hypertension Entering Two Different Therapeutic Regimens

	Diet	Diuretics
Number	35	39
Male/Female	21/14	18/21
Age (yr)	50 ± 13*	49 ± 10
Black/White/Yellow	5/30/0	13/25/1
Obese† (% of group)	26	36
Systolic blood pressure (mm Hg)	155 ± 15*	159 ± 20
Diastolic blood pressure (mm Hg)	97 ± 10*	102 ± 11
Serum cholesterol (mg/dl)	231 ± 35*	227 ± 39
Serum triglyceride (mg/dl)	120 ± 61*	142 ± 110

* Mean ± SD.
† > 19 per cent above ideal weight.

TABLE III Changes in Serum Lipids, Weight and Blood Pressure During Two Different Therapeutic Regimens in Hypertension

Parameter	Diet	Diet + Diuretics
Cholesterol (mg/100 ml)	−11 ± 3*	+11 ± 3*†
Triglyceride (mg/100 ml)	−3 ± 7	+34 ± 11*†
Weight (lb)	−3 ± 1*	−5 ± 1*
Systolic blood pressure (mm Hg)	−11 ± 2*	−22 ± 1*†
Diastolic blood pressure (mm Hg)	−8 ± 2*	−12 ± 2*

NOTE: All values represent the mean ± standard error of the mean.
* $p < 0.01$ versus pretreatment value.
† $p < 0.005$ versus diet group.

Diet therapy had three components: (1) All patients were instructed in mild sodium restriction. This consisted principally in the elimination of sodium in cooking and at the table. In addition, foods high in sodium content were restricted. Specially prepared foods low in sodium content, such as low sodium milk and bread, were not advocated. (2) Patients who were overweight were urged to attain ideal weight by caloric restriction. In 29 of the 35 patients treated with diet alone, and in 33 of the 39 treated with diuretics, caloric intake was restricted. (3) A lipid-lowering diet was given to patients with a serum cholesterol level above 220 mg/100 ml or a serum triglyceride level above 150 mg/100 ml.* Twenty-seven of the 35 patients treated with diet alone were instructed in lipid-lowering diets as were 31 of the 39 patients treated with diuretics.

For patients with a serum cholesterol level above 220 mg/100 ml, a low saturated fat, low cholesterol diet was prescribed. Foods containing polyunsaturated fats were also recommended, but liquid supplements of unsaturated oils were not given. When the serum triglyceride level was above 150 mg/100 ml, a reduction in carbohydrate intake, especially those foods containing refined sugar, was advocated. Patients were urged to reduce ethanol consumption as well. For patients with both serum cholesterol and triglyceride levels above the stated limits, a balanced reduction in dietary cholesterol, saturated fats and high carbohydrate foods was urged. Weight reduction was emphasized, when appropriate, in this latter group.

Of the 39 patients who were treated with a diuretic agent, 25 received chlorthalidone. The dose ranged from 50 mg twice weekly to 100 mg daily depending on the level of blood pressure before treatment and the response to therapy. Eleven patients were treated with hydrochlorothiazide, 25 to 50 mg daily, and three with spironolactone, 25 to 50 mg daily.

* These limits of serum lipids were arbitrarily chosen for intervention for two reasons. First, the Framingham data indicate a relatively low incidence of coronary artery disease in groups with serum cholesterol below 220 mg/100 ml [6]. Second, with respect to serum triglyceride, the upper limit of normal is generally considered to be 150 mg/100 ml. Serum triglyceride correlates with coronary artery disease in a number of studies [7–11].

During therapy, blood was sampled for serum lipid levels at each clinic visit (intervals of 1 to 3 months).

The characteristics of the patients in the two therapeutic groups are tabulated in Table II. The concentration of serum lipids before treatment was based on 57 measurements in the group treated with diet alone and on 81 measurements in the group treated with diuretics. In all patients receiving drug therapy, all serum lipid measurements obtained before the start of drug therapy were averaged for each subject and used as the pretreatment concentration for statistical analyses.

Laboratory Methods. Serum cholesterol and triglyceride levels were determined by the method of Kessler and Lederer [12] as modified by the Technicon AA II methodology. Serum was extracted with isopropanol and further treated with zeolite. This extract was subsequently processed using the Lieberman-Burchard reagent for cholesterol and the acetylacetone reagent of Fletcher [13] following saponification for triglycerides. The precision of serum cholesterol determinations was ±4 per cent (coefficient of variation) for specimens having a range of values from 120 to 350 mg/100 ml. The precision of the triglyceride measurement was ±6 per cent for specimens having a range of values from 50 to 300 mg/100 ml. The accuracy of both methods was within 4 per cent of the stated value.

Serum sodium and potassium were analyzed by flame photometry using lithium as internal standard. Creatinine was determined by the method of Chasson, Grady and Stanley [14]. Uric acid was measured by the method of Wheat [15]. Plasma renin activity was estimated by the radioimmunoassay of angiotensin I [16,17].

RESULTS

The effect of the two therapeutic regimens on serum lipids is listed in Table III. The treatment values of serum lipids are based on 56 measurements in the group treated with diet alone and 84 measurements in the group treated with diuretics. Patients maintained on the dietary regimen without drugs showed a small but significant decrease in serum cholesterol during an average observation period of seven months. The slight

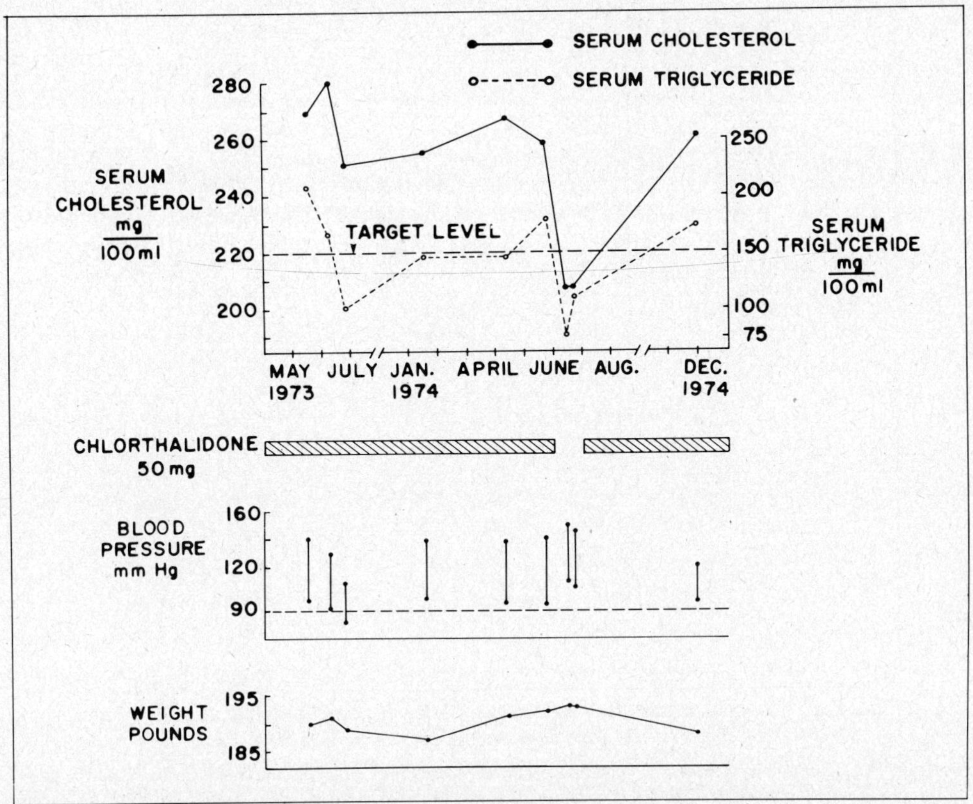

Figure 1. *Decrease in serum lipids during cessation of diuretic antihypertensive therapy. While this patient was receiving diuretic drugs, adherence to a low saturated fat, low cholesterol diet did not reduce serum cholesterol. During the third and fourth weeks after discontinuing the intake of chlorthalidone, serum cholesterol and triglyceride levels were sharply lower and below target levels; the diastolic blood pressure level was higher. Reinstitution of the diuretic drug was followed by a rise in serum lipid levels and a reduction in blood pressure.*

decrease in serum triglyceride was not significant. This group lost an average of 3 pounds in weight. Mean diastolic blood pressure levels fell 8 mm Hg.

Patients given diuretic drugs in addition to the diet showed a significant rise in both cholesterol and triglyceride levels. The serum cholesterol level rose from a mean value of 227 to 238 mg/100 ml and the triglyceride level from 142 to 176 mg/100 ml ($p < 0.01$ versus pretreatment for both). There was no correlation in individual patients between the rise in cholesterol and the rise in triglyceride above pretreatment levels. The change in serum cholesterol from control levels in the group treated with both diet and diuretics was significantly different from that observed in the group treated with diet alone ($p < 0.005$). Patients treated with diuretics had an average weight loss of 5 pounds. They showed a greater reduction in systolic blood pressure than those treated with diet alone. Figure 1 illustrates a well-marked change in serum cholesterol observed in one patient during the temporary interruption of diuretic therapy.

Further analysis of the diuretic-treated group was undertaken in an attempt to obtain information on the cause of the elevation in lipid levels and to identify indexes which might predict its occurrence.

The influence of the dose of diuretic on the elevation of lipid levels was studied. For this analysis, 11 patients treated with 100 mg of chlorthalidone daily were compared to 24 patients receiving 50 mg or less of chlorthalidone daily, or equivalent low doses of other diuretics. The patients receiving 100 mg of chlorthalidone showed a mean increase in serum cholesterol of 20 mg/100 ml whereas patients receiving smaller doses showed an increase of only 6 mg/100 ml ($0.1 > p > 0.05$). The increase in serum cholesterol observed in the group receiving a low dosage of diuretics, although small, was significantly different from the change seen in patients treated with diet alone ($p < 0.05$). There was no difference in the response of triglycerides between patients receiving a large dose and a smaller dose of diuretic drugs.

The response in serum lipids during diuretic therapy

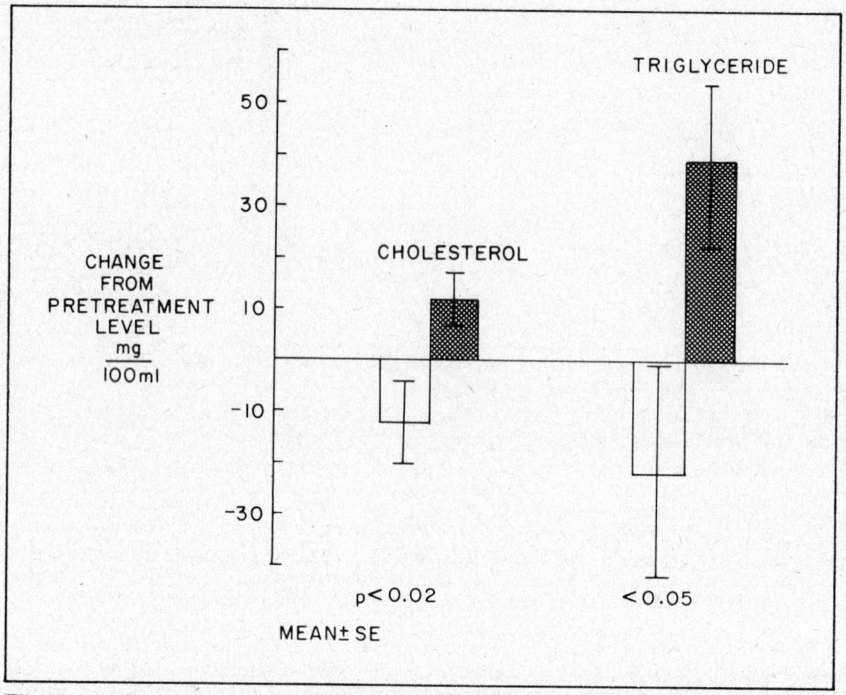

Figure 2. *Changes in serum cholesterol and triglyceride during weight loss induced by two different therapeutic regimens in hypertensive patients. Serum lipids decreased during caloric restriction in eight patients shown by open bars (mean ± SE). Serum lipids increased in 13 patients treated with caloric restriction and diuretic drugs as represented by stippled bars. Mean weight loss was 11 pounds per patient in each group. The response of serum lipids to the two regimens was significantly different for both cholesterol (p <0.02) and triglyceride (p <0.05). □ = diet. ▩ = diet plus diuretics.*

was compared between obese and nonobese patients. Obesity was defined as a weight 20 per cent or more above ideal weight (in relation to height). The 15 obese patients showed a mean increase in serum cholesterol of 20 mg/100 ml whereas the 24 nonobese patients had a mean increase of 5 mg/100 ml ($p < 0.025$). Here again the slight increase in serum cholesterol of 5 mg/100 ml in the nonobese subgroup was significantly different from the decrease of 11 mg/100 ml seen in the 35 patients following the dietary regimen without drug therapy ($p < 0.025$). There was no difference in the response of serum triglyceride to diuretic therapy between the obese and nonobese patients. The obese patients were receiving a larger average daily dose of diuretic drugs (equivalent of 73 versus 45 mg of chlorthalidone, $p < 0.025$).

To assess the effect of successful caloric restriction on the serum lipid changes during diuretic therapy, 13 patients who lost more than 5 pounds were compared to 24 patients who lost 5 pounds or less during treatment. Thirteen patients lost an average of 11 pounds during diuretic therapy. These 13 showed a mean increase in serum cholesterol of 12 mg/100 ml whereas those losing less weight showed a mean increase of 10 mg/100 ml (p, not significant). Similarly, there was no difference in serum triglyceride changes between those two groups during diuretic treatment. As a point of comparison, eight patients losing more than 5 pounds during diet therapy without diuretic drugs (mean weight loss, 11 pounds) showed a decrease in serum cholesterol of 12 mg/100 ml and in triglyceride of 22 mg/100 ml. The differences in the serum cholesterol and triglyceride response during weight loss of more than 5 pounds between the group treated with diuretics and the group treated with diet were significant at the $p < 0.02$ and $p < 0.05$ level, respectively (Figure 2).

The elevation of serum lipid levels appeared to develop quickly during diuretic therapy. The rise was observed in one patient within one week of starting treatment, within two weeks in two others, and within one month in an additional three patients. The increases in serum lipids listed in Table III represent the mean values of all determinations for the 39 patients during the course of diuretic therapy. The average follow-up period of patients receiving diuretic drugs was six months.

To determine whether the increase in serum lipids persisted during therapy of even longer duration, the

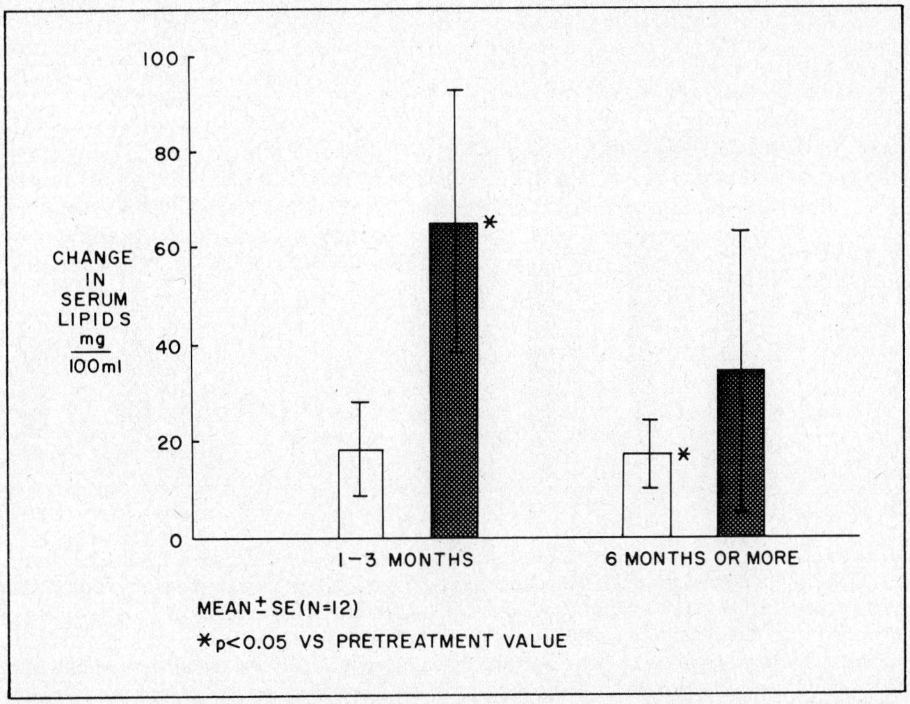

Figure 3. *Sustained elevation of serum lipid levels in 12 patients with hypertension observed for more than six months during diuretic therapy. In the early phase shown by the bars at left the increment in serum triglyceride above pretreatment levels was significant ($p < 0.05$). Serum cholesterol was significantly increased ($p < 0.05$) during the later phase. Weight loss averaging 6 pounds and drug dose were similar in both periods.* □ = *cholesterol.* ▩ = *triglyceride.*

data in the 12 patients observed for more than six months were analyzed separately. The increase in serum lipids above control levels during an early and a later period of therapy were compared. The elevations of serum cholesterol and triglyceride levels were not significantly different when measurements made during the first three months were compared to measurements obtained six months or more after the start of therapy. The median duration of treatment in these patients was 12 months (Figure 3).

There was no significant difference in serum lipid alterations during diuretic therapy between blacks and whites, men and women, or those older than 50 years compared to those 50 years old or less.

The patients receiving diuretic drugs were retrospectively divided into two subgroups on the basis of their serum lipid response to drug therapy. One subgroup was formed of patients who had an increase in cholesterol of more than 20 mg/100 ml or in triglyceride of more than 50 mg/100 ml or both (hereafter termed lipid reactors). The other subgroup was composed of patients showing lesser alterations during diuretic treatment (hereafter termed lipid nonreactors). The mean change in serum lipids in these two subgroups is depicted in Figure 4. Of the 21 patients having a substantial increase in serum lipids during treatment, 14 had an increase in cholesterol of this magnitude, 12 in triglyceride, and five in both. In this group the mean serum cholesterol level rose from 220 to 243 mg/100 ml and the mean triglyceride level from 146 to 216 mg/100 ml. Only five of 35 patients in the group treated with diet showed increases in serum lipids of this magnitude ($p < 0.02$ versus the group treated with diuretics). Numerous clinical and laboratory features in the two subgroups of diuretic-treated patients were compared in a further attempt to identify significant correlates of the increases in lipids. The following characteristics were compared: age, race, drug dose, duration of drug treatment, pretreatment weight and per cent of ideal weight, weight loss during therapy, pretreatment serum cholesterol and triglyceride levels, pretreatment fasting glucose levels, plasma renin activity before therapy (18 patients studied), serum potassium and uric acid before and during treatment, serum glutamic oxaloacetic transaminase (SGOT) before the administration of drugs, creatinine clearance before treatment and the decline in systolic and diastolic blood pressure from pretreatment levels (ΔSBP and ΔDBP). Only two features showed a significant difference between the subgroups: The level of SGOT and the decrease in systolic blood pressure.

Concerning the SGOT level, 13 lipid reactors had a

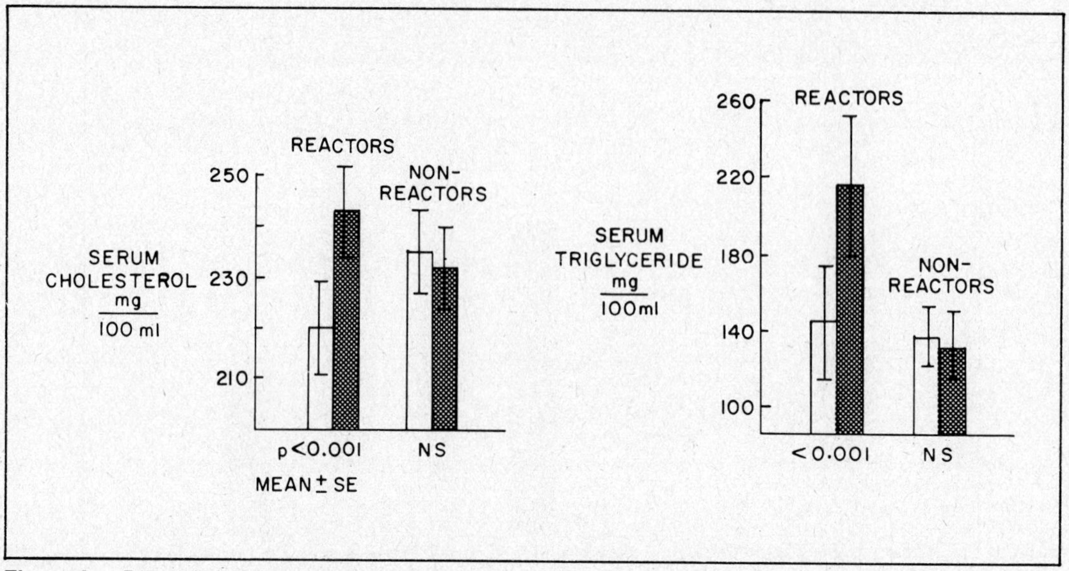

Figure 4. *Different patterns of serum lipid response to the administration of diuretic drugs. Patients with hypertension could be divided retrospectively into two subgroups on the basis of the response of serum lipids to diuretic drugs. One subgroup of 21 patients (here termed reactors) showed substantial increases in serum cholesterol or triglyceride or both. Serum lipids changed little in the remaining 18 patients (termed nonreactors). Reactors had a greater prevalence of elevated SGOT levels (38 per cent versus 0 per cent, $p < 0.05$) but none of 16 other variables was significantly different. Bars represent mean ± SE. □ = before diuretic therapy. ▩ = during diuretic therapy.*

SGOT measurement; in five of these, the level was above 45 units (range 59 to 180 units). In 14 lipid nonreactors, the SGOT determination was not elevated ($x^2 = 4.6$, $p < 0.05$). There was no other evidence of liver disease or of other organ damage in the five patients with elevated SGOT levels. Three of the five admitted to moderate ethanol intake. Two denied ethanol ingestion; one of these gave a history of hepatitis in the remote past.

The average decrease in systolic blood pressure during diuretic therapy was of similar magnitude in lipid reactors and nonreactors. However, in the reactors there was a linear correlation between the decrease in systolic blood pressure and the increase in serum triglyceride (Figure 5). In the lipid nonreactors, this correlation did not obtain. Diastolic blood pressure did not correlate with the serum triglyceride elevations. Increments in serum cholesterol did not correlate with the declines in either systolic or diastolic blood pressure during diuretic therapy.

COMMENTS

In this study, simultaneous control of serum lipids and elevated blood pressure levels was attempted by diet and, when required, by diuretic therapy in patients with mild hypertension. In 35 patients treated with diet alone, there was a small but significant decrease in serum cholesterol. In contrast, when diuretic drugs were used in addition to diet in the treatment of 39 patients with hypertension, serum cholesterol and triglyceride levels rose significantly. The elevation in serum lipid levels during diuretic therapy occurred, therefore, despite dietary instructions which ordinarily result in a lowering of serum cholesterol levels and little change in serum triglyceride.

The relatively small decrease in serum cholesterol in our diet-treated group may be explained by two facts: (1) Average control levels were not very high and thus the dietary contribution to serum levels might not be large for most patients. (2) Only patients with serum cholesterol levels above 220 mg/100 ml were instructed in low saturated fat, low cholesterol diets, and these patients comprised 60 per cent of the diet group. The remaining 40 per cent of the diet group was not placed on a cholesterol-lowering diet at all, and thus would not be expected to show a change in serum cholesterol.

Serum lipid levels increased during diuretic therapy, but the responses varied considerably from patient to patient. In an attempt to identify indexes which might predict an increase in serum lipids, a number of clinical and laboratory measurements was evaluated. For the group of 39 patients as a whole, only two indexes were found to be important: obesity and drug dosage. Both obesity and larger drug dosage were associated with greater elevations in serum cholesterol levels during

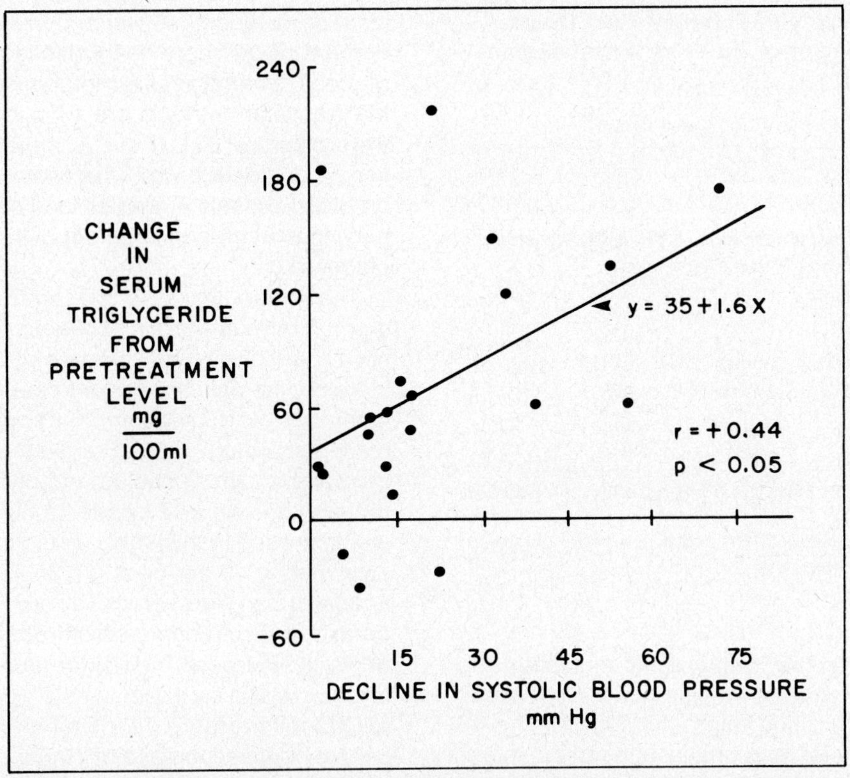

Figure 5. *Relation of the change in serum triglyceride to the decline in systolic blood pressure during diuretic therapy for hypertension. In the 21 lipid reactors a linear correlation was observed between these two variables during therapy. No such relationship existed among the 18 lipid nonreactors.*

therapy. This trend attained statistical significance only for obesity. However, the obese patients were also receiving larger doses of diuretic drugs; therefore, the relative influence of the two factors on the elevation of serum cholesterol levels could not be resolved.

It should be noted that successful caloric restriction, as judged by a weight loss of more than 5 pounds during diuretic therapy, did not affect the increases in serum cholesterol observed during diuretic therapy. The 13 patients who lost more than 5 pounds during diuretic therapy showed increases in serum lipids that were, on average, of similar magnitude to those seen in patients with little weight change. Thus, dietary control alone did not appear to offset fully the diuretic-induced rises in serum lipid levels.

In a further attempt to identify possible causes of the elevations in serum lipid levels during treatment, the 39 patients receiving diuretic drugs were divided into two subgroups depending on the response of their serum lipids to treatment. Twenty-one patients, in whom the increase in serum cholesterol was more than 20 mg/100 ml or in serum triglyceride more than 50 mg/100 ml, formed one subgroup, here termed lipid reactors. Eighteen patients who showed lesser changes in serum lipids during diuretic therapy formed the other subgroup, termed lipid nonreactors. Of 16 variables compared between the two subgroups, only two were significantly different. The pretreatment level of serum glutamic-oxaloacetic transaminase was above 45 units in five of 13 reactors who were so studied. None of 14 nonreactors so studied showed an increase in SGOT. The meaning of this association, if any, is unclear.

The other significant difference between the lipid reactors and nonreactors concerned the relation of the increase in serum triglyceride to the decrease in systolic arterial pressure during diuretic therapy. In the lipid reactors, the change in serum triglyceride correlated in a roughly linear fashion with the decrease in systolic blood pressure (Figure 5). This association raises the possibility that triglyceride metabolism is affected by the level of arterial pressure in some patients with hypertension. Alternatively, compensatory mechanisms may be activated proportionally to the fall in blood pressure levels in certain hypertensive patients, and these processes may influence triglyceride metabolism. Whether synthesis is enhanced or removal is impaired remains for further study. We did not carry out lipoprotein electrophoresis and thus did not characterize the type(s) of lipoprotein disturbance associated with these rises in serum lipid levels.

TABLE IV Probability of Coronary Heart Disease Developing in Six Years (Framingham Study)*

Cholesterol (mg/100 ml)	Systolic Blood Pressure 120 mm Hg	135 mm Hg	150 mm Hg	165 mm Hg
A. 35 Year Old Man, Nonsmoker, LVH–ECG Negative, Normal Glucose Tolerance				
210	0.5†	0.7	0.8	1.0
235	0.8	0.9	1.1	1.4
B. 60 Year Old Man, Smoker, LVH–ECG Positive, Glucose Intolerance Present				
210	22.2	25.5	29.2	33.3
235	23.8	27.3	31.2	35.3

NOTE: LVH–ECG = left ventricular hypertrophy by electrocardiography.
*Table modified from Kannel [21] with permission from the American Heart Association, Inc.
†Per hundred.

Further study will be required to elucidate the mechanism of the increases in lipids induced by diuretic drugs. Hemoconcentration might account for the increase in serum cholesterol because the mean increment was small, approximating 5 per cent of the pretreatment value. Contraction of plasma volume during diuretic treatment averages 1 to 10 per cent [18], but in occasional patients it has been recorded at 20 per cent [19]. In this study, four patients had a sustained increase in serum cholesterol of 20 to 26 per cent above pretreatment levels. Thus, the magnitude of the increase in cholesterol raises doubt that hemoconcentration can fully explain it.

Elevations in serum triglycerides during diuretic treatment could not be readily ascribed to hemoconcentration. In 10 patients, serum triglyceride levels rose 50 per cent or more above pretreatment levels. Furthermore, in three patients with serum cholesterol increments of 20 mg/100 ml or more (possibly explained by hemoconcentration), serum triglyceride actually decreased during diuretic therapy. In addition, there was no correlation between the changes in cholesterol and triglyceride levels from pretreatment levels in individual patients. Thus, it seemed unlikely that the alterations in triglyceride levels during diuretic therapy were related to hemoconcentration. However, no other explanation for the change was identified in this study.

With respect to the development of coronary heart disease, the significance of an increase in serum cholesterol, if caused by hemoconcentration or other mechanisms, is unclear. The cholesterol and lipoprotein synthetic rate may not be affected. Nevertheless, the Framingham data indicate that it is the concentration of cholesterol in the blood, irrespective of the mechanism of its induction, which correlates with the development of coronary heart disease. Furthermore, with respect to blood vessel metabolism, one theory holds that vascular nutrients are supplied by direct diffusion from plasma [20]. If this is the case, an increase in serum cholesterol, by whatever means, may impose on blood vessels a greater load of this substance and may thus accelerate the deposition of cholesterol in plaques.

The mean increase in serum cholesterol of 11 mg/100 ml in this group of diuretic-treated patients was not large. However, an increase of this magnitude would increase the risk of coronary heart disease developing within six years by about 20 per cent in a 35 year old man, according to the Framingham data. The mean increase in serum cholesterol of 23 mg/100 ml seen in the subgroup of 21 patients (lipid reactors) treated with diuretics in this study would increase the risk approximately 40 per cent in a 35 year old man. For example, it can be seen in Table IV (part A) that an increase in serum cholesterol from 210 to 235 mg/100 ml would increase the risk of having a myocardial infarction within six years in a 35 year old man with systolic blood pressure of 165 mm Hg from 1.0 to 1.4 per cent, a relative increase of 40 per cent. The magnitude of the cholesterol change and the serum concentration as well as the level of systolic blood pressure in this example approximate the average levels in our subgroup of lipid-reactors. To offset this increased risk, a decrease in systolic blood pressure of 15 to 30 mm Hg would be required. It can be noted in Table III that diuretics produced an average decrease in systolic pressure of 22 mm Hg. On the basis of these data, the two changes just balanced each other and no diminution in coronary risk occurred. In older persons and in women of any age, increases in serum cholesterol of this magnitude do not entail so great an increase in coronary risk. Consequently, the increased risk of higher cholesterol levels in these patients during diuretic therapy can be offset by lesser reductions in blood pressure (see Table IV, part B). For these patients, diuretics might be expected to yield a net beneficial effect with respect to the development of coronary heart disease. On the other hand, an enhanced risk contributed by an increase in serum triglycerides would have to be considered [7–11]. However, the magnitude of such risk has neither been established nor quantitated to the same extent as for cholesterol. Thus, the net benefit to be expected of diuretic drugs in reducing the coronary risk status of any patient with hypertension remains unclear. Coronary risk status may not be appreciably improved during treatment of large populations with hypertension when diuretic drugs represent the primary therapeutic modality. Especially in populations with milder degrees of hypertension (diastolic blood pressure under 105 mm Hg) in which atherosclerotic complications would be expected to be more prevalent than pressure-mediated complications [22], this effect of diuretics requires consideration.

The findings of this study should not be construed as proof that diuretic drugs are disadvantageous in the treatment of mild hypertension. For it is not clear that serum cholesterol or triglyceride, or for that matter hypertension itself, causes coronary atherosclerosis. These three variables are known to correlate with the incidence of coronary disease, but a causative relationship cannot be proved by this type of evidence. However, when studies are designed to test the possible causal relationship of these conditions, an appreciation of this subtle effect of diuretics to elevate serum lipid levels may be useful in planning therapeutic regimens for treating hypertensive patients.

ADDENDUM

Since submission of this manuscript we have published a preliminary communication on this topic using different data [23].

REFERENCES

1. Veterans Administration Cooperative Study Group on Antihypertensive Agents. II. Results in patients with diastolic blood pressure averaging 90 through 114 mm Hg. JAMA 213: 1143, 1970.
2. Beevers DG, Hamilton M, Fairman MJ, et al.: Antihypertensive treatment and the course of established cerebral vascular disease. Lancet 1: 1407, 1973.
3. Hodge JV, Smirk FH: The effect of drug treatment of hypertension on the distribution of deaths from various causes. Am Heart J 73: 441, 1967.
4. Freis ED: The chemotherapy of hypertension. JAMA 218: 1009, 1971.
5. Miettinen M, Turpeinen O, Karvonen MJ, et al.: Effect of cholesterol lowering diet on mortality from coronary heart disease and other causes. Lancet 2: 835, 1972.
6. Kannel WB, Castelli WP, Gordon T, et al.: Serum cholesterol, lipoproteins, and the risk of coronary heart disease. The Framingham study. Ann Intern Med 74: 1, 1971.
7. Carlson LA, Bottinger LE: Ischemic heart disease in relation to fasting values of plasma triglycerides and cholesterol. Lancet 1: 865, 1972.
8. Albrink MJ: Triglycerides, lipoproteins, and coronary artery disease. Arch Intern Med 109: 345, 1962.
9. Brown DF: Blood lipids and lipoproteins in atherogenesis. Am J Med 46: 691, 1969.
10. Heinle RA, Levy RI, Fredrickson DS, et al.: Lipid and carbohydrate abnormalities in patients with angiographically documented coronary artery disease. Am J Cardiol 24: 178, 1969.
11. Falsetti HL, Schnatz JD, Green DG, et al.: Serum lipids and glucose tolerance in angiographically proved coronary artery disease. Chest 58: 111, 1970.
12. Kessler G, Lederer H: Fluorometric measurement of triglyceride. Automation in Analytical Chemistry (Technicon Symposium), vol 1, New York, Mediad Inc., 1965, p 341.
13. Fletcher MJ: Colorimetric method for estimating serum triglyceride. Clin Chim Acta 22: 393, 1968.
14. Chasson AL, Grady HJ, Stanley MA: Determination of creatinine by means of automatic chemical analysis. Am J Clin Pathol 35: 83, 1961.
15. Wheat JL: Determination of uric acid. An automated phosphotungstate method utilizing NaOH as alkali. Clin Chem 14: 630, 1968.
16. Goodfriend TL, Ball DL, Farley DB: Radioimmunoassay of angiotensin. J Lab Clin Med 72: 648, 1968.
17. Haber E, Koerner T, Page LB, et al.: Application of a radioimmunoassay for angiotensin I to the physiologic measurements of plasma renin activity in normal human subjects. J Clin Endocrinol Metab 29: 1349, 1969.
18. Leth A: Changes in plasma and extracellular fluid volumes in patients with essential hypertension during long-term treatment with hydrochlorothiazide. Circulation 42: 479, 1970.
19. Tarazi RC, Dustan HP, Frohlich ED: Long-term thiazide therapy in essential hypertension. Circulation 41: 709, 1970.
20. Walton KW: Pathogenetic mechanisms in atherosclerosis. Am J Cardiol 35: 542, 1975.
21. Kannel WB: Handbook of Coronary Risk Probability. New York, American Heart Association, 1972.
22. Paul O: Risks of mild hypertension. A ten-year report. Br Heart J 33 (suppl): 116, 1971.
23. Ames RP, Hill P: Increase in serum lipids during the treatment of hypertension with chlorthalidone. Lancet 1: 721, 1976.

Angiotensin Receptors in Vascular Tissue

MARIE-A. DEVYNCK, Ph.D.
PHILIPPE MEYER, M.D.
Paris, France

The biologic effect of angiotensin II is triggered by its interaction with components of target organs, which specifically recognize the hormone. These receptors have been studied with the use of radioactive angiotensin and, as for other peptidic hormones, have been localized in the plasma membrane of target cells. Such angiotensin receptors have been characterized in three target organs: vascular tissue, uterus and adrenal cortex. The binding characteristics differ in contractile tissue and in adrenal glands, the N and C terminal ends of angiotensin being involved in the former, whereas the N terminus does not appear to have the same importance in the latter. Numerous factors, including ionic composition, seem to be able to modify angiotensin-receptor interaction in vascular smooth muscle. However, the molecular mechanisms responsible for angiotensin binding and for the transmission of the signal determined by receptor-angiotensin interaction are not yet understood. As observed with other peptidic hormones, the number of angiotensin receptors seems to be susceptible to variation under certain conditions. In uterine smooth muscle, it was shown that the number of receptors increased after nephrectomy, a phenomenon which was prevented by the prolonged infusion of angiotensin. The significance of such a variation remains unknown, but it may be partially responsible for the inverse relationship that exists between the endogenous angiotensin level and the pressor effect of exogenous angiotensin. In the near future, investigation of the angiotensin-receptor mechanism will probably answer whether the variation in angiotensin receptors is similar in all target tissues and whether an angiotensin-receptor mechanism is involved in the pathogenesis of certain varieties of hypertension. In addition, a precise understanding of the angiotensin-receptor interaction will help the development of new angiotensin antagonists.

A hormone receptor is a particular cellular component possessing the dual function of recognition and stimulation. Recognition is specific for certain structural elements of a given hormone which interact with complementary structures on the binding site of the receptor. Stimulation results from the interaction between active groups in the hormone and the receptor, and initiates the series of cellular events leading to the biologic response. The mechanism of receptor activation is not well understood, but it may be related to variations in receptor conformation or charge distribution.

Before the interaction of a radioactive hormone with a cellular binding site can be considered to correspond to a receptor interaction, it should fulfil the criteria of a hormonal response, exhibiting specificity, high affinity, reversibility and saturability. In addition, the kinetic characteristics of the binding should correlate with those of the hor-

From the Vascular and Renal Pharmacology and Physiology Unit (INSERM U7), Hôpital Necker, 75015 Paris, France. Requests for reprints should be addressed to Dr. Marie-A. Devynck, Vascular and Renal Pharmacology and Physiology Unit (INSERM U7), Hôpital Necker, 161 rue de Sèvres, 75015 Paris, France.

monal effect or, ideally, with those of the first biochemical event in the series culminating in the biologic response. Employing these precise characteristics, it is possible to distinguish between the binding of a hormone to "receptor" sites and to "acceptor" sites [1,2]. The function of these latter binding sites remains uncertain. Since they usually exhibit some specificity for the hormone, they may represent enzymes involved in its metabolism, or receptors responsible for as yet unidentified biologic effects, or they may correspond to immature receptors not yet coupled to the biologic response. For numerous technical reasons, it is difficult to prove that the binding sites in subcellular fractions are the actual receptors. It is possible that the target tissue is altered during its preparation or that the hormone is inactivated by degradative enzymes released from damaged subcellular material. Many of these difficulties have been overcome, and numerous hormone receptors have been characterized [3]. The study of the interaction of angiotensin with its receptors is associated with such problems that their detailed analysis seems justified. In this review we will summarize the present state of the studies on the binding of angiotensin II to vascular smooth muscle and compare them with the binding of angiotensin II to receptors in other target organs.

SPECIFIC PROBLEMS ENCOUNTERED IN THE CHARACTERIZATION OF ANGIOTENSIN II RECEPTORS

The physiologic concentration of angiotensin II in the plasma of the many species studied is in the order of 10^{-11} M. In order to study the binding of the hormone at these low concentrations, it is necessary to use a radioactive hormone of high specific activity. This is usually achieved by introducing atoms of radioactive iodine into the hormone molecule. However, the major drawback resulting from the iodination of small peptide hormones is a loss of biologic activity. This has been established for oxytocin [4] as well as for angiotensin II, at least as far as the contractile response is concerned [5–7] (Table I). In the case of angiotensin II, the halogenation is mainly made on the tyrosine (the fourth amino acid) in the α position of the hydroxyl group. This results both in a lowering of the pK of the hydroxyl group, which is necessary for biologic activity [8–11], and a steric hindrance, which is appreciable by a comparison of the dimensions of iodine and the benzene ring of tyrosine (about 2.1 and 2.7 Å, respectively). This modification is particularly important since the integrity of the tyrosine is necessary for the initiation of contraction [12,13]. In addition, halogenation may be performed on the histidine (the sixth amino acid).

The substitution of hydrogen by tritium or carbon by ^{14}C does not provoke major structural changes and

TABLE I **Biologic Activities of Iodinated Angiotensin (expressed as per cent of the activity of angiotensin II considered as 100 per cent)**

Effect	Mono-Iodinated Angiotensin II	Di-Iodinated Angiotensin II	References
Pressor response	33	13	[5]
Contractile effect on			
Rat uterus	—	2	[5]
	—	23	[6]
Rat colon	25	24	[5]
	—	24	[6]
	70	21	[7]
Rabbit aorta	—	10	[6]

does not perturb the biologic activity of the hormone [14]. However, the specific activities obtained are much lower than those of the iodinated hormone. Since ^3H bears 29 Ci/mAtom the maximum specific activity of an angiotensin II possessing 2 to 3 atoms of tritium per molecule is 58 to 87 Ci/mmol, whereas that for a monoiodinated (^{125}I or ^{131}I) angiotensin II can reach 2,000 Ci/mmol. It is clear that one must either work with physiologic concentrations of an iodinated hormone, which interacts badly with its receptor, or with higher pharmacologic concentrations of a tritiated hormone, which interact normally with the receptor. We preferred this latter solution in our own studies and chose the rabbit aorta as a model. This target organ has the advantage of being a vascular segment whose contractile responses to angiotensin have been extensively studied [11,15–18]. In addition, the rabbit aorta has a sympathetic innervation which is so weak [19] that the eventuality that tritiated (^3H) angiotensin II could bind to nervous receptors (reasonable in view of the effects of the hormone on sympathetic nerve terminals) is unlikely. There are obvious problems in generalizing the results obtained on the rabbit aorta to all vascular tissue, and in particular to those which respond physiologically to angiotensin II [20]. Nonetheless, the angiotensin II receptors in the rabbit aorta exhibit the major characteristics of angiotensin receptors in other arteries inasmuch as can be judged from their contractile responses. The second difficulty in the study of the angiotensin II receptor arises from a lack of knowledge concerning the first intracellular biochemical event provoked by the hormone-receptor interaction. The action of angiotensin II on smooth muscle adenylcyclase is uncertain [21,22], and its effect on the binding of membrane calcium has not been explained satisfactorily [23,24]. Thus, in the case of this hormone, one is reduced to correlating its specific binding with a global biologic effect, contraction measured in vitro, without being absolutely certain of the existence of a linear relationship between the occupation of receptors and the contraction, given the large number of intermediate steps. In this respect, the choice of the rabbit aorta has a great advantage in that pharmacologic studies have demonstrated a direct proportionality between the number of angiotensin II receptors and the contractile response [10]. This proportionality implies firstly, that all the receptors are coupled to the response, i.e., that a contractile response is obligatorily provoked by the occupation of receptors and that there are no spare receptors; secondly, that the receptors are comprised of homogeneous molecular entities which function independently (noncooperatively); and thirdly, that the mean effective dose (ED_{50}) corresponds to the affinity constant of the hormone (apparent dissociation constant, K_d) [25].

LOCALIZATION OF ANGIOTENSIN II RECEPTORS

It seemed very likely that the angiotensin II receptors would be localized on the plasma membrane since the receptors for most other polypeptide hormones are situated at this level. Furthermore, the contractile response of angiotensin II is extremely rapid in onset, in contrast to the slow onset of action of hormones which act inside the cell, such as steroids [26].

The contractile response of angiotensin II is closely associated with measurable membrane phenomena. During the first seconds after exposure to the hormone, there is a depolarization due to changes in the membrane permeability to various ions [27,28]. An essentially membranous effect of the hormone is suggested more directly by the fact that the contractile effect of polymerized angiotensin II (N-poly-O-acetyl-1-angiotensin II) and angiotensin II bound covalently by its N terminal to a macromolecule (gamma globulin, cytochrome C or horseradish peroxidase [29,30]) is quantitatively reduced but not delayed. These results are not conclusive since the angiotensin II molecules could eventually, under the influence of tissue hydrolases, be dissociated from their macromolecular support and have free access to smooth muscle cells. The problem was complicated by the demonstration of a possible direct action of angiotensin II on isolated mitochondria [31] and by autoradiographic results showing a nuclear localization in myocardial and arterial cells short time intervals after the intravenous injection of tritiated angiotensin II [32].

In reality, the autoradiographic results cannot be considered conclusive because the specificity of the nuclear localization was not demonstrated and could be due to radioactive fragments of the hormone. Other investigators have been unable to confirm these autoradiographic findings in myocardial cells [33] and kidney [34]. Furthermore, the stimulation of nucleic acid synthesis apparently induced by angiotensin II in myocardial cells does not appear to correlate with the much more rapid induction of contraction.

Localization of the angiotensin II receptors on the plasma membrane is directly demonstrable biochemically. By ultracentrifugation of a tissue homogenate in a density gradient, it is possible to obtain membranous fractions enriched in plasma membranes which are recognized by their high concentration of marker enzymes, such as adenylate cyclase and 5′nucleotidase. The enrichment of this membrane fraction in angiotensin receptors has been shown to be as great as that of the marker enzymes in vascular smooth muscle (rabbit aorta) [35], nonvascular smooth muscle (rat uterus) [36] and in bovine adrenal cortex [37]. This result is a strong argument supporting localization of angiotensin II receptors at the level of the plasma membrane.

CHARACTERIZATION OF AORTIC RECEPTORS

Tritiated angiotensin II binding sites exhibiting characteristics expected for receptors were demonstrated initially in the intact rabbit aorta [38] and subsequently in membrane fractions [35]. Table II shows the association and dissociation constants measured on microsomes and establishes the reversibility of the binding reaction. Study of the binding as a function of angiotensin II concentration demonstrated two classes of sites. The first high affinity sites are saturable at a ligand concentration of 2 to 3×10^{-8} M, whereas the second class of sites exhibits low affinity and is not saturable under our experimental conditions (up to 5×10^{-7} M). Identification of the first class of sites as angiotensin II receptors is strongly supported by the similarity between the apparent dissociation constant and the ED_{50} (Table II). Nevertheless, positive identification of these sites as the angiotensin II receptors was hampered in our initial studies by the absence of a correlation between the biologic activity and the binding of some analogues and fragments of angiotensin [35,39]. In these experiments, the affinity of these components for the angiotensin II receptor was studied by measuring the decrease in ^{3}H angiotensin II binding (2.5-5 $\times 10^{-8}$ M) in the presence of a twentyfold excess of the nonradioactive angiotensin II derivative. Recently, we realized that in using such high concentrations we would, in fact, principally be measuring the affinity of these structural analogues for the second, low affinity class of angiotensin II binding sites. The competition experiments, repeated subsequently employing lower concentrations of both ^{3}H angiotensin II and the nonradioactive derivatives, showed that their affinity for the first class of sites correlated well with their biologic activity (Figure 1). This observation is interesting for a number of reasons. Firstly, it permits definite identification of the first class of angiotensin II binding sites as

TABLE II **Binding Parameters for Angiotensin II Receptors**

Parameter	Rabbit Aorta: Membranes (29°C)	Rabbit Aorta: DOC-Solubilized Material (29°C)	Rat Uterus: Membranes (29°C)
Association rate constant k_1 ($10^5\ M^{-1} \times sec^{-1}$)	1.3	2.5	1.6
Dissociation rate constant k_{-1} ($10^{-4} \times sec^{-1}$)	8	41	13
Equilibrium constant K_d			
From $\frac{k_{-1}}{k_1}$	6.0	16	8.3
From Scatchard plots (10^{-9} M)	6.2	20	20
Contractile response ED_{50} (10^{-9} M)	7.8 [13] 8.5 [53]		10 [6]

NOTE: DOC = deoxycholate.

the angiotensin II receptors. Secondly, it poses the problem of the significance of the second class of low affinity sites. According to the competition experiments, these sites have a marked specificity for the C terminal of angiotensin II, whereas both the N and the C terminal are necessary for the correct interaction with the first class of sites. The existence of a membranous class of sites, with a lower affinity than that of the hormone receptor, has been demonstrated for numerous other polypeptide hormones, but their significance remains obscure [1]. One of the more commonly advanced hypotheses is that these sites, which are hormonal acceptors, could correspond to the enzymes implicated in the inactivation of the hormone. This, however, is unlikely since we have been unable to detect significant degradation of angiotensin II in contact with aortic microsomal membranes under our experimental conditions.

As has been achieved with membrane receptors for many other polypeptide hormones, it has been possible to separate the angiotensin II receptors from their membranous environment by treating them with detergents [38] (sodium deoxycholate in the case of angiotensin).

Biochemical studies performed so far cannot explain the phenomena of desensitization or tachyphylaxis. Desensitization could perhaps be related to dissociation of the hormone-receptor complex, or to a conformational change which shifts the receptor from an active to an inactive form. Similarly, tachyphylaxis has been interpreted in many different ways [20,40]. It may result from events occurring at the receptor level, such as an occupation of all the receptors by the added hormone, or from a slowly reversible conformational change in the receptor which makes it incapable of conveying the hormonal response.

Since many factors are able to modify the contractile

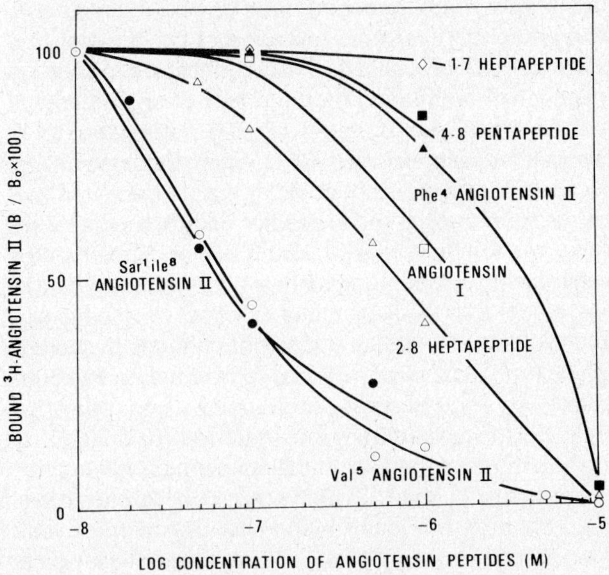

Figure 1. Specificity of angiotensin binding on rabbit aorta microsomal membranes. Displacement of ^3H angiotensin II by unlabelled angiotensin derivatives. The ordinate shows the percentage of specific binding after competition with unlabelled analogues added simultaneously. In these experiments ^3H angiotensin II concentration was 10^{-8} M, corresponding to the high affinity binding sites. The incubation was performed at 29°C for 8 minutes. The relative affinity of these compounds, determined from their contractile effects on rabbit aorta strips are: 100 for Val^5-angiotensin II, 5.6 for the heptapeptide 2–8 and 5.1 for Asp^1-angiotensin I, < 0.1 for the pentapeptide 4–8 and 0 for the heptapeptide 1–7 [13]. The Phe^4-angiotensin II analog was reported to have 10 to 20 per cent of the angiotensin II pressor response on the nephrectomized rat [11] and a relative affinity of 0.54 on rabbit aorta strip [10]. Sar^1,Ile^8-angiotensin II is a competitive antagonist with a pA$_2$ of 9.33 on rabbit aorta [12].

TABLE III Effect of Various Compounds on ^{3}H-Angiotensin II Specific Binding (% of control)*

	Concentration	Specific Binding
Ions		
Sodium	$200 - 10^{-3}$ M	100
Potassium	$80 - 10^{-3}$ M	63
Magnesium	$90 - 10^{-3}$ M	39
Calcium	$6 - 10^{-3}$ M	50
EDTA	$1 - 10^{-3}$ M	109
—SH and —S—S—Reagents		
N-ethylmaleimide	10^{-4} M	61
Dimercaprol	10^{-3} M	20
Glutathione	10^{-3} M	100
"High energy" compounds		
Adenosine triphosphate	10^{-3} M	55
Guanosine triphosphate	10^{-3} M	22
{Phosphoenol pyruvate / Pyruvate kinase	5.10^{-3} M	100
Enzymatic treatment		
Trypsine (E.C.3.4.4.4)	5 μg ml^{-1} — 20 min 37°C	200
	5 μg ml^{-1} — 40 min 37°C	70
Pepsine (E.C.3.4.4.1)	20 μg ml^{-1} — 30 min 37°C	180
Phospholipase A (E.C.3.1.1.4)	10 μg ml^{-1} — 30 min 37°C	121
Phospholipase C (E.C.3.1.4.3)	50 μg ml^{-1} — 30 min 37°C	109
Phospholipase C + 5.10^{-4} M Ca^{++}	50 μg ml^{-1} — 30 min 37°C	105
Neuraminidase (E.C.3.2.1.18)	120 μg ml^{-1} — 15 min 37°C	60

NOTE: —SH = sulfhydryl; —S═S— = disulfide.
* Each value is the mean of four to six determinations.

effect of angiotensin II, it seems reasonable that certain of them may act by modifying the binding of angiotensin to its vascular receptors. Although the available evidence is still fragmentary and derives principally from our own laboratory, we have summarized it in Table III. (1) Increasing the concentration of divalent cations (calcium and magnesium) strongly inhibits the specific binding of angiotensin II. Transmembrane movements of calcium occur during variations in mechanical activity of vascular smooth muscle and could thus be able to subtly modulate the hormone-receptor interaction at the same time. Such a phenomenon has been described with adrenocorticotropic hormone at the level of the adrenal cortical cell [41]. The inhibitory effect of magnesium on the contractile effect of angiotensin II [42] is often interpreted as being secondary to a competition with extracellular calcium. Binding studies suggest that magnesium could also act directly on the formation of the hormone-receptor complex. Potassium has a weak inhibitory effect on the specific binding of angiotensin II, and sodium has no effect. This is in agreement with the absence of an effect on angiotensin contractile response as a result of changes in sodium concentration in vitro [43]. The lack of a direct sodium effect on angiotensin-elicited contraction must be clearly distinguished from the variations resulting from modifications of the sodium balance which will be discussed subsequently. (2) Sulfhydryl (—SH) groups have been implicated in contraction and relaxation of vascular smooth muscle [44,45]. N-ethylmaleimide, which binds covalently to sulfhydryl groups, nonspecifically decreases the reactivity of the rabbit aorta, whereas dithiothreitol, which reduces disulfide bridges, specifically abolishes the response to angiotensin II [45]. During recent experiments (unpublished), we showed that 10^{-4} M N-ethylmaleimide decreased the specific binding of 5×10^{-8} M angiotensin II by 40 per cent and that 10^{-3} M dimercaprol decreased it by 80 per cent. These results do not, however, provide conclusive proof that —SH groups are part of the receptor structure; it is possible that modification of sulfhydryl groups in close proximity to the receptor on the membrane could indirectly modify the hormone-receptor interaction. (3) The same problems are associated with the analysis of the studies on the alteration of the membranes provoked by different enzymatic treatments, the results of which are presented in Table III. The increase in the binding capacity of the membranes following hydrolysis of phospholipids or proteins does not suggest that the receptor does not contain either phospholipid or protein, but rather that a disorganization of the membrane structure increases the accessibility of the receptor. However, prolonged treatment with either trypsin or phospholipase C reduced the binding of ^{3}H-angiotensin II. The physiologic significance of the angiotensin II binding sites exposed by hydrolysis is unknown. An analogous phenomenon was observed with insulin receptors [46]. The results obtained after treatment with neuraminidase are more easy to interpret since the decrease in ^{3}H angiotensin II specific binding was found both in the membrane preparations as well as on the solubilized material. The resistance of angiotensin binding sites to moderate proteolysis suggests that receptors are integral proteins in the sense proposed by Singer and Nicolson [47]. The effects of neuraminidase suggest that the receptor is a glycoprotein, the sialic acid of which is directly implicated in the formation of the angiotensin II-receptor complex. (4) Nucleotides appear to be able to modify the binding of diverse polypeptide hormones [48,49]. The results obtained with angiotensin II on vascular smooth muscle cell membranes (Table III) show that at high concentrations, adenosine triphosphate and to a lesser extent guanosine triphosphate, inhibit the specific binding of angiotensin II to aortic microsomal membranes. This decrease in binding is correlated with phosphorylation since the presence of the energy generating system, phosphoenol pyruvate-pyruvate kinase, prevents specific binding to these membranes. It is conceivable that changes in phosphorylation could be implicated in the receptor activation-inactivation process. (5) The specific binding of angiotensin II is not modified by l-noradrenaline [35], but it is increased by the prostaglandins of the E series. The interpretation of this phenomenon is more difficult in view of the variability of the experimental results of studies aimed at demonstrating an interference by endogenous prostaglandins in the angiotensin II contractile response [10,50,51] and merits further investigation.

COMPARISON OF THE VASCULAR RECEPTORS WITH RECEPTORS IN OTHER ANGIOTENSIN II TARGET ORGANS

The angiotensin receptors of contractile tissues have been studied essentially with the use of classic pharmacologic methods. According to Schild [52], it is possible to demonstrate a difference in a hormone receptor in various target organs if the pharmacologic studies take into account the following parameters: (1) apparent affinity and intrinsic activity of the agonists. In the case of a linear coupling, the apparent affinity corresponds to the apparent dissociation constant and is indicated by the ED_{50} value. (2) Apparent affinity of competitive antagonists or pA_2* values. (3) Measurement of contractile effects of analogues in organs rendered tachyphylactic with angiotensin II. In the case of smooth muscle, pharmacologic results suggest that differences may exist among angiotensin receptors in the rabbit aorta, the rat uterus and the rat colon [53]. However, other studies did not demonstrate any difference between vascular and intestinal smooth muscles of two different species [53]. These investigations should be completed by direct studies on the binding of angiotensin II, which offer obvious advantages in comparison to pharmacologic studies. Results obtained so far in our laboratory have not demonstrated any difference between vascular smooth muscle receptors (rabbit aorta) and nonvascular smooth muscle receptors (rat uterus) [36].

However, great differences exist between the receptors of vascular smooth muscle and those of the adrenal gland. These differences are particularly marked in the adrenal cortex. (1) Although the N terminal of the hormone is indispensable for full contractile activity, it is not necessary for the steroidogenic action: the 2–8 heptapeptide, sometimes referred to as angiotensin III, stimulates the secretion of aldosterone as well as [55–57] or better [58] than angiotensin II even though it only has 10 to 50 per cent of its contractile activity. It is worth noting here that the competitive antagonists Sar^1,Ala^8-angiotensin II and Sar^1,Ile^8-angiotensin II, which are relatively resistant to aminopeptidase degradation, inhibit the myotropic response more than the steroidogenic response [58,59]. These pharmacologic observations suggest that receptor occupancy in the adrenal cortex is maximally insured by a seven amino acid hormone. However, binding experiments on the adrenal cortex produced conflicting results: on the one hand, they have confirmed that the 2–8 heptapeptide angiotensin II binds nearly as well as the intact angiotensin II [37,60], and yet, on the other hand, these studies have shown that Sar^1-angiotensin derivatives are also capable of binding as efficiently to receptor sites. Further studies are obviously needed to determine whether angiotensin II receptors are identical to those of angiotensin III. (2) In contrast to vascular smooth muscle the binding of angiotensin II to the adrenal cortex is unaffected by calcium [37], variably affected by sodium [61,62] and greatly inhibited by guanosine triphosphate [49]. As discussed previously, these differences may stem from variations occurring at the level of the receptor or from changes occurring in the environment of the membrane receptor.

In the adrenal medulla, the possible differences in the receptor can only be discussed in terms of pharmacologic studies. Interestingly, the C terminal of angiotensin II can be modified without greatly affecting its activity in the adrenal medulla [63]: for example, the decapeptide angiotensin II, without apparently being converted to the octapeptide, and the Ala^8-angiotensin derivative stimulate catecholamine release. Binding studies would seem to be indispensable to better characterize this phenomenon and to demonstrate eventually that the angiotensin-receptor interaction in the adrenal medulla does not involve the C terminal of angiotensin, contrary to other target tissues.

HYPOTHESES CONCERNING THE REGULATION OF THE VASCULAR RESPONSE TO ANGIOTENSIN II MEDIATED BY CHANGES AT THE LEVEL OF THE ANGIOTENSIN II RECEPTORS

The pressor effect of angiotensin II is modified by numerous factors. Two of them, the plasma concentration

* pA_2 = negative logarithm of the concentration of antagonist that reduces the effect of a double dose of agonist to that of a single dose.

of endogenous angiotensin II and the sodium balance (acting perhaps via endogenous angiotensin II), are specific for this hormone in the sense that they do not affect (or very little) the pressor action of other vasoconstrictor agents [64–70]. The specificity of these factors implies that their action cannot be attributed to a modification of the intracellular machinery responsible for the mechanical activity of vascular smooth muscle. Their action is probably related either to the events occurring at the level of the angiotensin II receptor and concerning the formation of angiotensin II receptor complexes, or to modifications affecting the coupling of the receptors to intracellular events ultimately responsible for contraction.

The results of variations in sodium balance on the pressor effect of angiotensin II are well established. Vascular reactivity to exogenous angiotensin II increases in positive sodium balance and decreases in negative sodium balance. It is interesting to note that these effects of variations in sodium balance are the opposite in the adrenal cortex in which the steroidogenic effect of angiotensin II is potentiated by a negative sodium balance. The variations in sodium balance, via their influence on renin secretion, modify the plasma concentration of angiotensin II which increases and decreases with a deficiency or an excess of sodium, respectively. The fluctuations in endogenous angiotensin II are obviously involved in the development of specific hypersensitivity to angiotensin which occurs after bilateral nephrectomy. When plasma angiotensin II has been lowered by nephrectomy, the pressor effect of an injection of exogenous angiotensin is markedly enhanced. Several hypotheses may be proposed to explain the inverse relationship between the contractile effect and the endogenous hormone level. (1) A first hypothesis could be that the variations in pressor activity of exogenous angiotensin II are inversely proportional to the occupation of these vascular receptors by the endogenous angiotensin II. During negative sodium balance, circulating angiotensin II is increased and the proportion of free receptors accessible to the exogenous hormone is decreased, resulting in a reduction in the pressor response. During positive sodium balance and after nephrectomy, the inverse results are obtained and are related to an increase in the proportion of free vascular receptors. This reasoning has often been proposed to explain the variations in the pressor response to angiotensin II as an inverse function of the circulating level of angiotensin II as in the test of Kaplan and Silah [67]. This interpretation has been applied to the variations in angiotensin II liberated in the vascular wall under the action of iso-renin [71]. (2) A second hypothesis could be that the changes in endogenous angiotensin II, produced by variations in sodium balance or by nephrectomy, modify the "avidity" of vascular receptors for the hormone [72]. The nature of the events involved in this phenomenon is not clear. (3) The third hypothesis is that the variation in the pressor effect of exogenous angiotensin II is explained by a variation in the number of total angiotensin receptors in vascular tissues. Assuming an unmodified coupling between receptor occupancy and contraction and the law of mass action, an increase in the total number of receptors would, of course, if the hormone concentration is able to saturate binding sites, increase the angiotensin response. The difficulties of conducting studies of receptors in arterial wall due to scarcity of material led us to study this question on receptors in the uterine membrane. Our results [73,74] have established that the total number of uterine angiotensin II receptors increases by 20 per cent and 80 per cent, respectively, 19 hours and 22 hours after nephrectomy. This increase in the number of sites is not associated with a significant variation in their affinity for the hormone. The increase in uterine receptors after nephrectomy is real and does not correspond to freeing of sites secondary to the disappearance of endogenous angiotensin II following nephrectomy. In fact, the appearance of the increased number of receptors following nephrectomy is not apparent until after 18 hours and is much slower than the disappearance of renin and endogenous angiotensin II [71,75,76], and also much slower than the dissociation of angiotensin II from its membrane receptors. In addition, the increased number of receptors is not suppressed by the injection of a dose of hormone capable of occupying all the receptors immediately before sacrifice. The mechanism of the increase in the total number of receptors after suppression of the endogenous hormone is not yet understood. However, it provides a satisfactory explanation for the supersensitivity observed in vitro in the uterus of a rat previously nephrectomized. Under normal experimental conditions, this supersensitivity can no longer be explained by a freeing of receptors [77]. Although direct binding studies have not yet been conducted with vascular receptors, one may conceive that the same variation occurs at this level and causes the supersensitivity observed in vivo when endogenous angiotensin is low (in case of positive sodium balance and after nephrectomy).

Comparable observations have been made with other polypeptide hormones and transmitters, such as prostaglandins and catecholamines [78–84]. In most of these studies the effect provoked by a given hormone is specifically reduced by the prior exposure of a target tissue to this same hormone; conversely, there appears to be a specific supersensitivity after suppression of the endogenous hormone. This effect has been attributed to a variation in the total number of receptors without modification of their affinity with many substances such as insulin [85–90] and the catecholamines [91]. This effect could also concern steroid hormones: the number of estrogen-induced cytosolic receptors of progesterone in the uterus progressively decreases when plasma progesterone increases in the dioestrus phase [92]. In the case of insulin it has been clearly shown that the variation of receptor number develops directly as an inverse function of the concentration of endogenous hormone. This inverse relation between the number of receptors and the concentration of circulating hormone has been verified in the case of angiotensin and its uterine receptors, when long-term infusions of suppressor doses of angiotensin II were capable of inhibiting the increase in the maximum binding capacity.

Gavin et al. [86] have suggested that the inverse relationship between the total number of receptors (and hence the hormonal effect) and the level of circulating hormone is a regulatory phenomenon occurring in target tissues and counteracting the variations in secretion of the hormone. It is conceivable that an abnormality in this regulatory phenomenon could be the origin of certain pathologic conditions.

Before admitting such a modulatory process at the receptor level as a general phenomenon, one must demonstrate that it occurs in all target tissues of a given hormone. In the case of insulin the phenomenon seems still to be controversial in some tissues [93]. As previously emphasized, in the case of angiotensin II the vascular receptor has not been investigated. In addition, since the effects of changes in sodium balance on the steroidogenic effect of angiotensin are opposite to those of its myotropic action, one should expect a different receptor mechanism in the adrenal cortex.

Only after completion of these physiologic studies may the angiotensin receptor mechanism in hypertension be understood. The search for an abnormality at the receptor level in pathologic states is legitimized by the discovery of a decreased number of receptors in various pathologic conditions such as genetic and experimental diabetes [85,87–90] and myasthenia gravis [94].

ACKNOWLEDGMENT

We wish to acknowledge the help of V. Koreve and M. G. Pernollet for their contribution in the unpublished experiments presented in this paper, and to K. O'Dea and S. Hamon for their help with the manuscript.

ADDENDUM

Since completion of this article, Le Morvan and Palaic [95] have reported results concerning binding of ^{14}C-angiotensin II on guinea pig aorta, confirming previous results on rabbit aorta from our laboratory [35].

REFERENCES

1. Birnbaumer L, Pohl SL, Kaumann AJ: Receptors and acceptors: a necessary distinction in hormone binding studies. Advances in Cyclic Nucleotide Research. IV (Greengard P, Robison GA, eds), New York, Raven Press, 1974, p 239.
2. Cuatrecasas P, Hollenberg MD: Binding of insulin and other hormones to non-receptor material. Saturability, specificity and apparent negative cooperativity. Biochem Biophys Res Commun 62: 31, 1975.
3. Cuatrecasas P: Membrane receptors. Ann Rev Biochem 43:169, 1974.
4. Thomson EE, Freychet P, Roth J: Monoiodoocytocin: demonstration of its biological activity and specific binding to isolated fat cells. Endocrinology 91: 1199, 1972.
5. Lin SY, Ellis H, Weisblum B, Goodfriend TL: Preparation and properties of iodinated angiotensins. Biochem Pharmacol 19: 651, 1970.
6. Papadimitriou A, Worcel M: Dose-response curves for angiotensin II and synthetic analogues in three types of smooth muscle: existence of different forms of receptor sites for angiotensin II. Br J Pharmacol 50: 291, 1974.
7. Kurcbart H, Coli A, Vancheri L, et al.: Chemical and biological effects associated with the iodination of angiotensin II. Biochim Biophys Acta 230: 160, 1971.
8. Schröder E: Synthese von Lys^6Val^5, von Tyr^3Val^4, von $Tyr(Me)^4Val^5$ und von Tyr^8Val^5 angiotensin II-Asp^1-β-amid. Justus Liebigs Ann Chem 684: 243, 1965.
9. Park WK, Choi C, Rioux F, et al.: Synthesis of peptides with the solid-phase method. II. Octapeptide analogues of angiotensin II. Can J Biochem 52: 113, 1974.
10. Rioux F, Park WK, Regoli D: Application of drug-receptor theories to angiotensin. Can J Physiol Pharmacol 51: 665, 1973.
11. Schwyzer R: Synthetische Analogue des Hypertensin. I Eileitung. Helv Chim Acta 44: 667, 1961.
12. Khosla MC, Smeby RR, Bumpus FM: Structure-activity relationship in angiotensin analogues. Angiotensin (Page IH, Bumpus FM, eds), Heidelberg, Springer-Verlag, 1974, p 126.
13. Regoli D, Park WK, Rioux F: Pharmacology of angiotensin. Pharmacol Rev 26: 69, 1974.
14. Morgat JL, Hung LT, Fromageot P: Preparation of highly labelled ^3H-angiotensin II. Biochim Biophys Acta 207, 374, 1970.
15. Helmer OM: Action of natural angiotensin II and synthetic analogues on strips of rabbit aorta. Am J Physiol 207: 368, 1964.
16. Pals DT, Masucci FD, Sipos F, et al.: A specific competitive antagonist of the vascular action of angiotensin II. Circ Res 29: 664, 1971.
17. Türker RK, Yamamoto M, Khairallah PA, et al.: Competitive antagonism of 8-Ala-angiotensin II to angiotensin I and II on isolated rabbit aorta and rat ascending colon. Eur J Pharmacol 15: 285, 1971.
18. Saltman S, Baukal A, Waters S; et al.: Competitive binding activity of angiotensin II analogues in an adrenal cortex radioligand-receptor assay. Endocrinology 97: 275, 1975.
19. Burnstock G: Innervation of vascular smooth muscle: histochemistry and electron microscopy. Clin Exp Pharmacol Physiol suppl 2, p 7, 1975.
20. Bohr DF: Angiotensin on vascular smooth muscle. Angiotensin (Page IH, Bumpus FM, eds), Heidelberg, Springer-Verlag, 1974, p 424.
21. Volicer L, Hynie S: Effect of catecholamines and angiotensin

on cyclic AMP in rat aorta and tail artery. Eur J Pharmacol 15: 214, 1971.
22. Anglès d'Auriac G, Meyer P: Variation of cyclic AMP production induced by adrenaline and angiotensin in rat uterus. Advances in Cyclic Nucleotide Research. 1 (Greengard P, Robison GA, eds), New York, Raven Press, 1972, p 505
23. Baudouin M, Meyer P, Fermandjian S, et al.: Calcium release induced by interaction of angiotensin with its receptors in smooth muscle cell microsomes. Nature (Lond) 235: 336, 1972.
24. Limas CJ, Cohn JN: Alkaline phosphatase in vascular smooth muscle. Nature New Biol 245: 53, 1973.
25. Ariens EJ: Receptor theory and structure-action relationships. Adv Drug Res 3: 235, 1966.
26. Feldman D, Funder JW, Edelman IS: Subcellular mechanisms in the action of adrenal steroids. Am J Med 53: 545, 1972.
27. Somlyo AV, Somlyo AP: Electromechanical and pharmacomechanical coupling in vascular smooth muscle. J Pharmacol Exp Ther 159: 129, 1968.
28. Cuthbert AW, Sutter MC: The effects of drugs on the relation between the action potential discharge and tension in a mammalian vein. Br J Pharmacol 25: 592, 1965.
29. Smeby RR: Angiotensin, hormone of the kidney. Angiotensin Systems and Experimental Renal Diseases (Metcoff J, ed), Boston, Little, Brown & Co., 1963, p 29.
30. Richardson JB, Beaulnes A: The cellular site of action of angiotensin. J Cell Biol 51: 419, 1971.
31. Goodfriend TL, Fyhrquist F, Gutmann F, et al.: Clinical and conceptual use of angiotensin receptors, Hypertension '72. International Symposium on the Renin-Angiotensin-Aldosterone-Sodium System in Hypertension (Genest J, Koix E, eds), Heidelberg, Springer-Verlag, 1972, p 549.
32. Robertson AL, Khairallah PA: Angiotensin II: rapid localization in nuclei of smooth and cardiac muscles. Science 172: 1138, 1971.
33. Osborne-Pellegrin MJ, Meyer P: Unpublished data.
34. Osborne MJ, Droz B, Meyer P, et al.: Angiotensin II: renal localization in glomerular mesangial cells by autoradiography. Kidney Int 8: 245, 1975.
35. Devynck MA, Pernollet MG, Meyer P, et al.: Angiotensin receptors in smooth muscle cells membranes. Nature New Biol 245: 55, 1973.
36. Rouzaire-Dubois B, Devynck MA, Chevillotte E, et al.: Angiotensin receptors in rat uterine membranes. FEBS Letters 55: 168, 1975.
37. Glossmann H, Baukal AJ, Catt KJ: Properties of angiotensin II receptors in the bovine and rat adrenal cortex. J Biol Chem 249: 825, 1974.
38. Baudouin M, Meyer P, Worcel M: Specific binding of ^{3}H-angiotensin II in rabbit aorta. Biochem Biophys Res Commun 42: 434, 1971.
39. Devynck MA, Pernollet MG, Meyer P, et al.: Solubilization of angiotensin II receptors in rabbit aorta membranes. Nature New Biol 249: 67, 1974.
40. Stewart JM: Tachyphylaxis to angiotensin. Angiotensin (Page IH, Bumpus FM, eds), Heidelberg, Springer 1974, p 170.
41. Lefkowitz RJ, Roth J, Pricer W, et al.: ACTH receptors in the adrenal: specific binding of ACTH ^{125}I and its relation to adenyl cyclase. Proc Natl Acad Sci USA 65: 745, 1970.
42. Altura BM, Altura BT: Influence of magnesium on drug-induced contractions and ion content in rabbit aorta. Am J Physiol 220: 938, 1971.
43. Napodano RJ, Caliva FS, Lyons C, et al.: The reactivity to angiotensin of rabbit aorta strips after either alterations of external sodium environment or direct addition of benzydroflumethiazide. Am Heart J 64: 498, 1962.
44. Needleman P, Jakschik B, Johnson EM: Sylfhydryl requirement for relaxation of vascular smooth muscle. J Pharmacol Exp Ther 187: 324, 1973.
45. Fleisch JH, Krzan MC, Titus E: Pharmacologic receptor activity of rabbit aorta: effect of dithiothreitol and N-ethylmaleimide. Circ Res 33: 284, 1971.
46. Cuatrecasas P: Unmasking of insulin receptors in fat cells and fat cell membranes: perturbation of membrane lipids. J Biol Chem 246: 6532, 1973.
47. Singer SJ, Nicolson GL: The fluid mosaic model of the structure of cell membranes. Science 175: 720, 1972.
48. Rodbell M, Lin MC, Salomon Y: Evidence for interdependent action of glucagon and nucleotides on the hepatic adenylate cyclase system. J Biol Chem 249: 59, 1974.
49. Glossmann H, Baukal A, Catt KJ: Angiotensin II receptors in bovine adrenal cortex. Modifications of angiotensin binding by guanyl nucleotides. J Biol Chem 249: 664, 1974.
50. Eckenfels A, Vane JR: Prostaglandins, oxygen tension and smooth muscle tone. Br J Pharmacol 45: 451, 1972.
51. Chong EKS, Downing OA: Selective inhibition of angiotensin-induced contractions of smooth muscle by indomethacin. J Pharm Pharmacol 25: 170, 1973.
52. Schild HO: Receptor classification with special reference to beta adrenergic receptors. Drug Receptors (Rang HP, ed), Baltimore, University Park Press, 1973, p 29.
53. Meyer P, Papadimitriou A, Worcel M: Possible existence of different types of angiotensin II receptors. Br J Pharmacol 40: 541P, 1970.
54. Park WK, Regoli D, Rioux F: Characterization of angiotensin receptors in vascular and intestinal smooth muscles. Br J Pharmacol 48: 288, 1973.
55. Blair-West JR, Coghlan JP, Denton DA, et al.: Effect of the heptapeptide (2–8) and hexapeptide (3–8) fragments of angiotensin II on aldosterone secretion. J Clin Endocrinol 32: 575, 1971.
56. Campbell WB, Brooks SN, Pettinger WA: Angiotensin II- and angiotensin III-induced aldosterone release in vivo in the rat. Science 184: 994, 1974.
57. Lohmeier TA, Davis JO, Freeman RH: Des-Asp^1-angiotensin II: possible role in mediating responses of the renin-angiotensin system. Proc Soc Exp Biol Med 149: 515, 1975.
58. Peach MJ, Chiu AT: Stimulation and inhibition of aldosterone synthesis in vitro by angiotensin II and analogues. Clin Res 34–35 (suppl I): 1, 1974.
59. Steele JM, Lowenstein J: Differential effects of an angiotensin II analog on pressor and adrenal receptors in the rabbit. Circ Res 35: 592, 1974.
60. Brecher P, Tabacchi M, Pyun HY, et al.: Angiotensin binding to rat adrenal capsular cell suspensions. Biochem Biophys Res Commun 54: 1511, 1973.
61. Glossmann H, Baukal A, Catt KJ: Cation dependence of high-affinity angiotensin II binding to adrenal cortex receptors. Science 185: 281, 1974.
62. Gurchinoff S, Khairallah PA, Devynck MA, et al.: Angiotensin II binding to zona glomerular cells from rabbit adrenal glands. Biochem Pharmacol 25: 1031, 1976.
63. Peach MJ: Adrenal medulla. Angiotensin (Page IH, Bumpus FM, eds), Heidelberg, Springer-Verlag, 1974, p 400.
64. Laragh JH: Dependence of the vasoactivity of angiotensin on the state of sodium balance, l'Hypertension Artérielle (Milliez P, Tcherdakoff P, eds), Paris, l'Expansion Scientifique, 1966, p 92.
65. Samwer KF, Schreiber M, Molzahn M, et al.: Pressor effect of angiotensin II in sodium replete and deplete rats. Pfluegers Arch 346: 307, 1974.
66. Reid WD, Laragh JH: Sodium and potassium uptake, blood pressure and pressor response to angiotensin. Proc Soc Exp Biol 120: 26, 1965.
67. Kaplan NM, Silah JG: Effect of angiotensin II on the blood pressure in patients with hypertensive disease. J Clin Invest 43: 659, 1964.
68. Hollenberg NK, Solomon hs, Adams DF, et al.: Renal vascular

responses to angiotensin and norepinephrine in normal man: effect of sodium intake. Circ Res 31: 750, 1972.
69. Stewler GJ, Hinrichs K, Guidd LR, et al.: Sodium intake and vascular smooth muscle responsiveness to norepinephrine and angiotensin in the rabbit. Circ Res 31: 758, 1972.
70. Stouder DA, Wathen RL: Augmented vascular response of the nephrectomized rat to angiotensin. Proc Soc Exp Biol Med 141: 548, 1972.
71. Swales JD, Tange JD, Thurston H: Vascular angiotensin II receptors and sodium balance in rats. Role of kidneys and vascular renin activity. Circ Res 37: 96, 1975.
72. Brunner HR, Chang P, Wallach R, et al.: Angiotensin vascular receptors: their avidity in relationship to sodium balance, the autonomic nervous system and hypertension. J Clin Invest 51: 58, 1972.
73. Chevillotte E, Devynck MA, Fyhrquist F, et al.: Angiotensin-induced variations of receptors in rat uterine membranes. Clin Sci Mol Med 48: 235, 1975.
74. Rouzaire-Dubois B, Devynck MA, Chevillotte E, et al.: Variations in the number of uterine angiotensin receptors following changes in plasma angiotensin levels. Eur J Pharmacol (in press).
75. Osborne MJ, Pooters N, Anglès d'Auriac G, et al.: Metabolism of tritiated angiotensin II in anaesthetized rats. Pfluegers Arch 326: 101, 1971.
76. Ryan JW: The fate of angiotensin II. Angiotensin (Page IH, Bumpus FM, eds), Heidelberg, Springer-Verlag, 1974, p 81.
77. Meyer P, Papadimitriou A, Worcel M: Specific supersensitivity of smooth muscle to angiotensin II after nephrectomy. Br J Pharmacol 51: 435, 1974.
78. Franklin TJ, Foster SJ: Hormone-induced desensitization of hormonal control of cyclic AMP levels in human diploid fibroblasts. Nature New Biol 246: 146, 1973.
79. Remold-O'Donnel E: Stimulation and desensitization of macrophage adenylate cyclase by prostaglandins and catecholamines. J Biol Chem 249: 3615, 1974.
80. Deguchi T, Axelrod J: Supersensitivity and subsensitivity of the β-adrenergic receptor in pineal gland regulated by catecholamine transmitter. Proc Natl Acad Sci USA 70: 2411, 1973.
81. Sayers G, Beall R: Isolated adrenal cortex cells: hypersensitivity to adrenocorticotropic hormone after hypophysectomy. Science 179: 1330, 1973.
82. Ciosek CP, Ortel RW, Thanassi NM, et al.: Indomethacin potentiates PGE_1 stimulated cyclic AMP accumulation in human synoviocytes. Nature (Lond) 251: 148, 1974.
83. Zor U, Lamprecht SA, Kaneko T, et al.: Functional relations between cyclic AMP, prostaglandins and luteinizing hormone in rat pituitary and ovary. Advances in Cyclic Nucleotide Research I (Greengard P, Paoletti R, Robison GA, eds), New York, Raven Press, 1972, p 503.
84. Birnbaumer L, Bockaert J, Dunn M, et al.: On the modes of regulation of intracellular cyclic AMP: desensitization of adenylcyclases to hormonal stimulation and compartmentalization of cyclic AMP. Regulation of Function and Growth of Eukaryotic Cells by Intracellular Cyclic Nucleotides (Dumont JE, Butcher RW, Brown B, eds), New York, London, Plenum Press, 1975.
85. Soll AH, Kahn CR, Neville DM, et al.: Insulin receptor deficiency in genetic and acquired obesity. J Clin Invest 56: 769, 1975.
86. Gavin JR, Roth J, Neville DM, et al.: Insulin-dependent regulation of insulin receptor concentration: a direct demonstration in cell culture. Proc Natl Acad Sci USA 71: 84, 1974.
87. Forgue ME, Freychet P: Insulin receptors in the heart muscle. Demonstration of specific binding sites and impairment of insulin binding in the plasma membrane of the obese hyperglycemic mouse. Diabetes 24: 715, 1975.
88. Freychet P, Laudat MH, Laudat P, et al.: Impairment of insulin binding to the fat cell plasma membrane in the obese hyperglycemic mouse. FEBS Letters 25: 339, 1972.
89. Hepp DK, Langley J, Von Funcke HJ, et al.: Increased insulin binding capacity of liver membranes from diabetic Chinese hamsters. Nature 258: 154, 1975.
90. Hollenberg MD, Cuatrecasas P: Insulin: interaction with membrane receptors and relationship to cyclic purine nucleotides and cell growth. Fed Proc 34: 1556, 1975.
91. Kebabian JW, Zatz M, Romero JA, et al.: Rapid changes in rat pineal β-adrenergic receptor: alterations in 1-[^{3}H]-alprenolol binding and adenylate cyclase. Proc Natl Acad Sci USA 72: 3735, 1975.
92. Milgrom E, Luu Thi, Atger M, et al.: Mechanisms regulating the concentration and conformation of progesterone receptor(s) in the uterus. J Biol Chem 248: 6366, 1973.
93. Lockwood DH, Livingston JN, Amatruda JM: Relation of insulin receptors to insulin resistance. Fed Proc 34: 1564, 1975.
94. Satyamurti S, Drachman DB, Slone F: Blockade of acetylcholine receptors: a model of myasthenia gravis. Science 187: 955, 1975.
95. Le Morvan P, Palaic D: Characterization of the angiotensin receptor in guinea pig aorta. J Pharmacol Exp Ther 195: 167, 1975.

Vascular Angiotensin Receptors and Their Role in Blood Pressure Control

H. THURSTON, B.Sc., M.B., Ch.B., M.R.C.P.*
Leicester, England

The renin angiotensin system has an important role in regulating arterial blood pressure in homeostasis and disease. A reciprocal relationship exists between sodium balance and the circulating levels of renin and angiotensin II. The vascular responsiveness to angiotensin II, the major vasoconstrictor component of the renal pressor system, can be impaired by numerous factors including sodium depletion or a reduction in effective plasma volume. In situations in which the renin-angiotensin system is activated, a negative relationship between the angiotensin II pressor response and the circulating angiotensin II level is observed.

This effect seems to involve a change of the angiotensin II receptor interaction in the vascular smooth muscle. The prevention of angiotensin II generation by the inhibition of converting enzyme causes an immediate increase in the pressor response to angiotensin; after bilateral nephrectomy, it takes much longer to develop. In addition, the depressor response to angiotensin antagonists and converting enzyme inhibitor is preserved after bilateral nephrectomy for much longer periods than can be accounted for by the disappearance of circulating renin. These observations support the view that the decrease in vascular response to angiotensin II during sodium deprivation or when body fluid volumes are reduced is the result of prior occupancy of the receptor sites by endogenous hormone generated both in the plasma and locally within blood vessel walls. Therefore, a change in the number or affinity of receptors consequent to a change in sodium balance or as a modulating function of the renin-angiotensin system need not be postulated to explain changes in angiotensin vascular responsiveness.

The regulation of arterial blood pressure is a complex process, but in simplistic terms it can be resolved into two main components, the cardiac output and the resistance to flow offered by peripheral vessels. Hypertension could, therefore, arise by an increase in either of these variables, but a sustained elevation in blood pressure levels is usually associated with an increase in peripheral resistance [1,2].

Peripheral arteriolar vasoconstriction can be modified by the renin-angiotensin system, but it is also under the influence of the central and autonomic nervous system and other hormonal systems such as catecholamines, kallikrein-bradykinin and prostaglandin systems. In addition, structural modifications of the vascular tree play a major part in determining basal sensitivity, when other constrictor influences have been eliminated, and may also bring about a nonspecific increase in the vascular reponse to vasopressor agents [3].

Over the past decade a mass of data has accumulated supporting a major role for the renin-angiotensin system in regulating arterial blood

From the Department of Medicine, The General Hospital, Leicester, England. This research was supported in part by the National Kidney Fund and the Peel Medical Trust. Requests for reprints should be addressed to Dr. H. Thurston, Department of Medicine, The General Hospital, Gwendolen Road, Leicester, LE 5 4 PW England.

*Recipient of a Medical Research Council (Sir Henry Wellcome) Travelling Fellowship (1973–1974).

pressure and controlling aldosterone secretion in normal homeostasis and disease [4,5]. It is now clear that the octapeptide, angiotensin II, is the major active vasoconstrictor of the renin-angiotensin system, acting upon arterial smooth muscle [6] and the adrenal glomerulosa [7]. In this review I will deal with the peripheral vascular receptor for angiotensin II and factors which modulate its action, since it is the receptor which is best identified and which probably plays the major role in blood pressure control. Other receptors in the brain stem may also be of importance, but they are less well defined. In addition, zona glomerulosa angiotensin II receptors are important in regulating aldosterone secretion, and therefore they also play an indirect role in blood pressure homeostasis.

THE ANGIOTENSIN II RECEPTOR

There is substantial evidence from experiments with radioactively labelled angiotensin II for a direct relationship between specific binding of the hormone in the arterial wall and adrenal cortex, and its biologic effect [8–11]. Thus, in rabbit aorta the specific binding site is completely saturated at an angiotensin II concentration of 10^{-7} M [8]. This concentration also produces a maximum contractile response. In addition, the rate of binding or release of labelled angiotensin II from isolated aorta parallels the rate at which contraction or relaxation develops [8]. More recently, studies using an angiotensin II antagonist have shown a proportional reduction in both tissue binding (recently reviewed by Devynck and Meyer [11]) and contractile response [12].

These specific binding sites or receptors appear to be modified by various factors; therefore, changes in their affinity for angiotensin II or the response evoked by receptor-angiotensin complexes may modulate the effect of the renin-angiotensin system on arterial blood pressure.

ANGIOTENSIN-RECEPTOR REACTION

The action of angiotensin II upon the biologic system may be explained in terms of an interaction between the peptide and specific molecular binding sites within the target tissues [13]. The latter have been described as specific receptors but this and other terms, such as active site, biologic reactive site, should not imply that we understand the mode of action. However, the receptor hypothesis is a useful approach for evaluating drugs in molecular terms [14].

To understand the vascular action of angiotensin II, it is necessary to summarize the basic points of the receptor theory. Pharmacologists interested in drug reactions have developed mathematical models to describe the relationship between the concentration and the effector response. The most widely held theory suggests that the interaction follows the law of mass action [14]. Thus the relationship can be expressed by the following equation:

$$\frac{[RAII]}{[Rt]} = \frac{[AII]}{Ka + [AII]}$$

Where [RAII] is the angiotensin receptor complex concentration, [Rt] is the total number of receptors and [AII] is the angiotensin II concentration. Ka is then the association constant for the reaction [15].

However, the relationship between receptor occupancy and biologic response is more complicated [14]. Furchgott [16] suggested that the biologic effect can be described as a series of steps from binding to mechanical response as shown in Figure 1. This analysis involves a series of steps, each governed by its own equation. Thus, formation of an angiotensin II receptor complex induces a "stimulus" of varying magnitude depending upon an intrinsic efficacy factor (E) for the receptor, i.e., "Stimulus" = E × concentration of angiotensin-receptor complex.

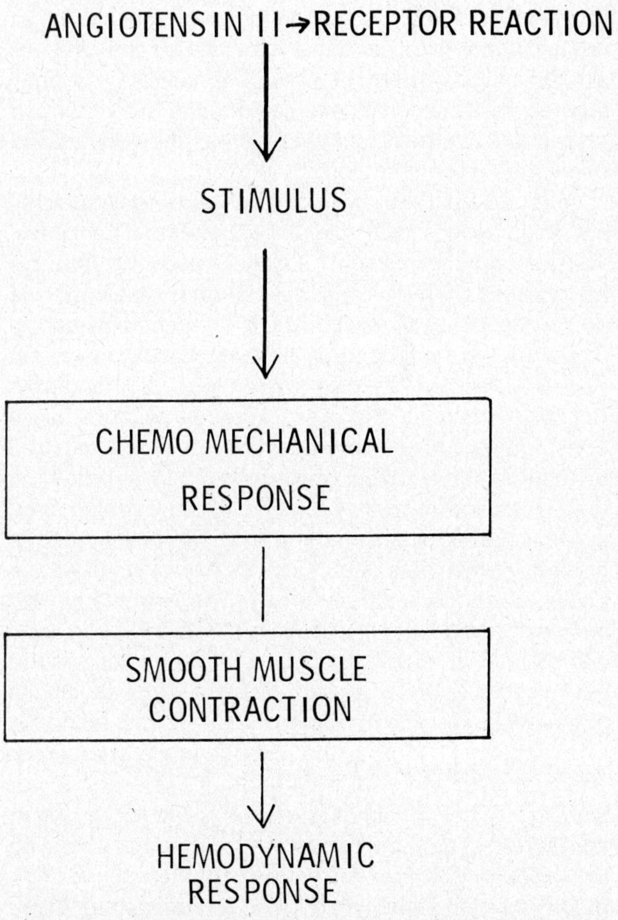

Figure 1. *Shown here is the postulated sequence of events from angiotensin II receptor binding to smooth muscle contraction.*

Potent vasoconstrictor peptides, such as angiotensin, may be considered to have a high efficacy factor whereas in certain analogues, for example sarcosine[1] alanine[8] angiotensin II (a competitive antagonist [17]), the efficacy factor is very small.

Smooth muscle contraction depends finally upon the chemomechanical response evoked by the "stimulus." This latter step may not necessarily correspond proportionally to the "stimulus" so that a 50 per cent receptor occupancy may not give rise to a half maximal response.

Angiotensin II receptor complex concentration and total receptor concentration cannot be readily determined experimentally. In addition, binding alone does not imply a given effect, since receptor sites may be inactive (so-called "silent receptors") [18].

Many observations, therefore, have been made using drug concentration and measurements of effector response. Consequently, studies involving the pressor response to angiotensin II or the contractility of isolated smooth muscle need to be interpreted with caution.

ANGIOTENSIN II VASCULAR RESPONSE

In 1940 it was first recognized that angiotensin and not renin is the active vasoconstrictor of the renal pressor system [19,20]. Early observations, utilizing partially purified natural angiotensin, demonstrated constriction of arterioles in the rabbit ear whereas the venules and capillaries were unaffected [21].

Angiotensin II is by weight the most potent naturally occurring agonist [22] with a direct effect on peripheral arteriolar smooth muscle [23]. Its pressor effects can be modified by numerous factors. Thus, the systemic pressor response to angiotensin II is impaired by sodium depletion but enhanced by sodium loading in the rat [24–26], rabbit [27], dog [28], sheep [29] and man [30,31]. However, the pressor action of other vasoconstrictors, such as norepinephrine, is hardly affected by manipulating sodium balance [25,31]. A reduction in the vascular response to angiotensin II is also seen in the isolated, perfused, hind limb preparation and in fresh in vitro studies of aortic strips from rabbits whose intake of salt is restricted [32]. The explanation for sodium-conditioned changes in pressor response to angiotensin II cannot, therefore, lie in a reduction in plasma volume or cardiac output. Equally, the specificity of the effect of sodium balance on the pressor response to angiotensin II implies that change in the chemomechanical machinery of the smooth muscle cell is not involved. The modulating action of sodium must, therefore, occur at the receptor level by either changing the receptor complex formation of angiotensin II or by modifying the "stimulus" (Figure 1) produced by these complexes.

In body fluid volume depletion, such as in hemorrhage, diarrhea and renal salt-wasting (Bartter's syndrome), angiotensin pressor reactivity is similarly reduced [33–35] whereas in salt-loaded states [24,36], especially if a mineralocorticoid is also administered, or in patients with primary aldosteronism [30] the pressor reactivity is enhanced. On the other hand, pressor response is reduced in normal pregnancy [37] and in the pathologic conditions of liver cirrhosis [38] and the nephrotic syndrome [39] in which the effective plasma volume may be reduced despite the formation of edema. Adrenal insufficiency is also associated with hyporesponsiveness [40].

In normal man [41] and in patients in whom the renin-angiotensin system is activated by disease [42], a negative relationship between the pressor response to angiotensin II and the circulating plasma renin and angiotensin II levels is observed. Similarly, pressor reactivity to both renin [43] and angiotensin II [44] is enhanced following bilateral nephrectomy.

Thus, it appears probable that either changes in sodium balance or fluctuations in circulating angiotensin II are directly involved in the specific modification of angiotensin II pressor action.

The Nature of the Sodium Balance, Pressor Reactivity Relationships. Several theories have been advanced to explain this relationship in terms of angiotensin-receptor interaction. The hypotheses fall info four main subheadings (1) Changes in absolute numbers of receptor sites with different physiological states. (2) Change in angiotensin II receptor affinity as a direct or indirect action of the sodium ion per se. (3) Receptor saturation by the high levels of endogenous angiotensin II. (4) Local renin-generating angiotensin II within the vascular wall saturating the receptor sites.

Variation in the Numbers of Receptors in the Vascular Tissue. Here it is postulated that nephrectomy or salt-loading produces a change in the total number of binding sites. Devynck and Meyer [11] summarized evidence in support of such receptor variation in their recent review. It is suggested that changes in the total number of receptor sites may exert a regulatory effect on the renin-angiotensin system. Indeed, it has been further suggested that a decrease in receptors could explain the low normal blood pressure levels observed in patients with Bartter's syndrome. Meyer and his co-workers [45] showed an increase in the total mass of binding sites in rabbit uterus from the 19th to 22nd hours after bilateral nephrectomy. This occurrence could not possibly correlate with the disappearance of renin and angiotensin II, although it should be noted that renin-like activity can be detected in vascular tissues for more than 6 hours after nephrectomy [46]. The findings in uterine receptor studies may not necessarily be representative of the findings in other vascular tissues, especially in view of the evidence for renin synthesis

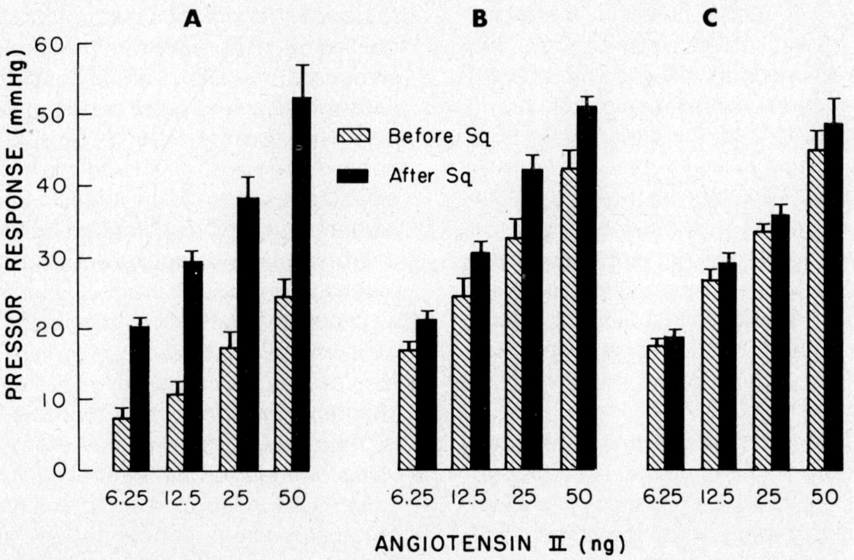

Figure 2. *Angiotensin II pressor responses (means ± SEM) in animals receiving low salt (**A**) and high salt (**B**) diets, and in nephrectomized (**C**) rats before and during converting enzyme blockade with SQ20881 (from Thurston and Laragh [48], by permission of the American Heart Association).*

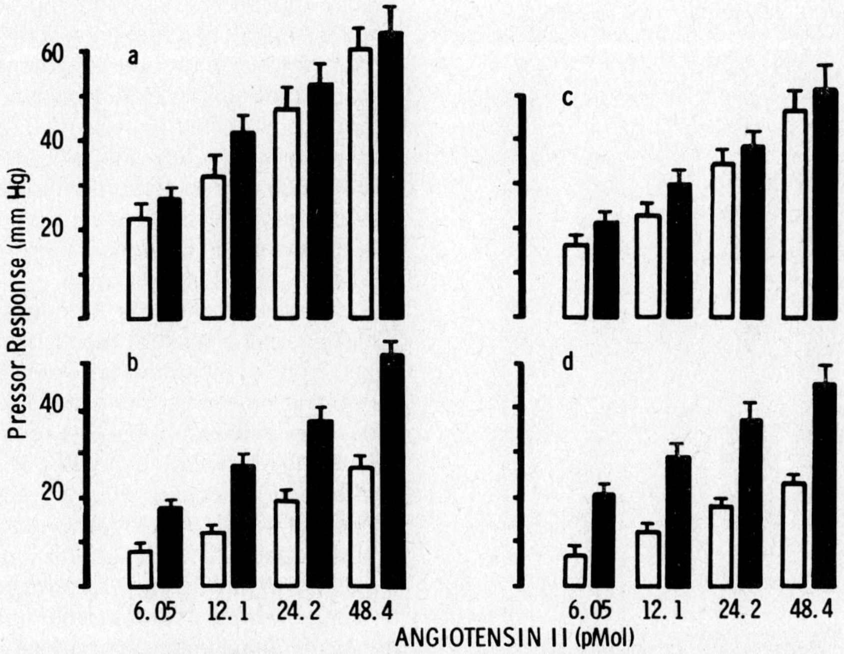

Figure 3. *Angiotensin II pressor responses (means ± SEM) in DOCA (desoxycorticosterone acetate)-treated rats receiving a normal diet (**a**) and a low salt diet (**b**), and in DOCA-treated adrenalectomized rats receiving 1 per cent saline solution (**c**) and adrenalectomized rats receiving 1 per cent saline solution (**d**) before and after converting enzyme blockade. These results indicate that the reduction in the pressor responsiveness of angiotensin II following adrenalectomy is due to activation of the renin-angiotensin system secondary to sodium depletion and that it is not a direct mineralocorticoid effect.*

within the uterus [47]. It seems possible, therefore, even at this stage after bilateral nephrectomy, that local renin may have an important influence on receptor occupancy. Moreover, the administration of converting enzyme inhibitor (SQ20881) to salt-depleted and adrenalectomized rats results in an *immediate* increase in the pressor reactivity of angiotensin II [48] to levels observed in nephrectomized rats (Figures 2 and 3). Thus, the absence of a delay in onset of this effect would argue against a major contribution by new receptor synthesis to changes in vascular reactivity: similarly, the immediacy of the change in pressor sensitivity after the infusion of renin would militate against this hypothesis [49].

Variation in Angiotensin II Receptor Affinity Produced by Sodium. According to this hypothesis "receptor affinity" for angiotensin II varies with changes in sodium balance or as a result of nephrectomy [50]. Thus, salt

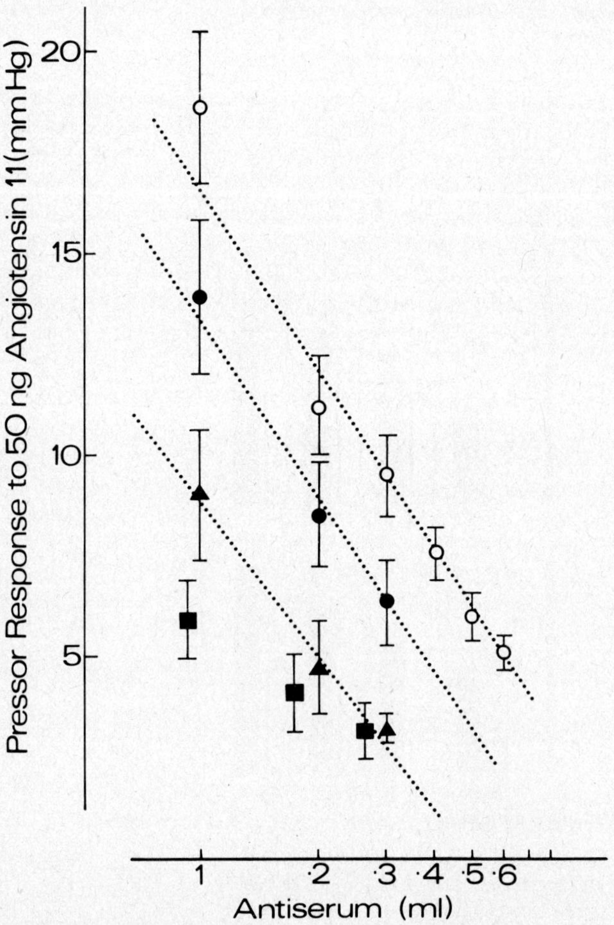

Figure 4. *Pressor responses to the administration of a 50 ng bolus of angiotensin II after the administration of 0.1 ml doses of angiotensin II antiserum. Open circles = high salt, pretreated rats; closed circles = normal rats; triangles = salt-restricted rats; squares = high salt, pretreated renin-infused rats (from Swales and Thurston [49]).*

restriction decreases receptor sensitivity and salt loading or nephrectomy increases receptor responsiveness. Vascular "affinity" for angiotensin II was determined by the pressor response to a fixed dose of hormone and the volume of specific angiotensin II antibody required to block this response. The blood pressure response to angiotensin II was impaired by salt depletion and readily blocked by the administration of small amounts of antiserum. It is not clear how this mechanism would operate. It is unlikely to be mediated by changes in the sodium concentration of the perfusing medium, i.e., plasma, since sodium depletion primarily results in a decrease in extracellular volume without a change in the sodium concentration of plasma [51]. It is, therefore, difficult to see the relevance of studies using isolated bovine adrenal cells which have shown a decrease in labelled angiotensin II binding when the external sodium concentration was lowered [52]. Brunner et al. [50] found that bilateral nephrectomy did not increase the receptor "affinity" of salt-restricted rats. However, subsequent studies have demonstrated an enhanced pressor response after nephrectomy in salt-depleted rats which was associated with an increase in the antibody blocking requirement [49]. In addition, the increase in blood pressure with angiotensin II in salt-loaded and nephrectomized rats could be readily impaired by administering a small dose of renin (Figure 4) [49], and removing sodium by peritoneal dialysis did not alter the angiotensin II reactivity in nephrectomized rats [53]. However, peritoneal dialysis in animals with intact kidneys markedly reduced pressor sensitivity with a low antibody blocking requirement [53]. Thus, a direct action of the sodium ion upon the receptor angiotensin II reaction would seem less likely than a change in responsiveness conditioned by the presence or absence of renin.

Receptor Saturation by Circulating Angiotensin II. Variations in the vascular reactivity of angiotensin might result from competition between endogenous angiotensin and infused hormone at the receptor level. In the presence of elevated plasma renin levels in salt-depleted subjects, large quantities of angiotensin will be formed and will occupy many receptor sites. Thus, few receptors will be free to respond to infused hormone, and the resultant increase in blood pressure will be small. When renin release is suppressed by salt loading or after bilateral nephrectomy, little angiotensin II is generated leaving the majority of receptors available to react with exogenous hormone. This hypothesis formed the basis of the Kaplan and Silah [30] angiotensin infusion test. It is suggested that the increase in blood pressure following the infusion of angiotensin is inversely proportional to the circulating renin and angiotensin levels [42].

However, this explanation, although attractive, cannot satisfy all the known facts. Of particular importance is the persistence of this effect in isolated preparations of rabbit aorta [32]. In addition, the well established exaggerated responsiveness to renin and angiotensin II following bilateral nephrectomy needs 6 hours to become maximal [53]. However, the circulating renin and angiotensin II levels fall to low values in less than an hour after bilateral nephrectomy [54]. Therefore, receptor saturation by high circulating concentrations of angiotensin is only a partial answer to the problem.

Local Generation of Angiotensin II by Vascular Wall Renin. It is suggested that renin accumulates within peripheral arterioles leading to the intramural formation of angiotensin II [33,49,53,56]. Renin-like activity has been demonstrated in the isolated hog arterial wall [57] with the greatest activity in the adventitia and the outer media. Vascular renin has also been detected in other species and in other arteries [58], and the amount present has changed in parallel to the plasma renin level after water deprivation or adrenalectomy [46]. Moreover, the other components needed for angiotensin generation have been demonstrated in isolated tissues. Thus, converting enzyme activity is present in the vascular bed of the hind limb of the dog [59] and sheep [60] and in the mesenteric circulation [61]. Recently, using fluorescein antibody technic, Cadwell et al. [62] showed that converting enzyme activity localized entirely to the vascular endothelium in the rabbit.

Observations that the increase in blood pressure in response to the injection of renin in nephrectomized rats persists well beyond the point at which such renin can be detected in the circulation [63,64] lend further support to this thesis. Gabelman and Rondell [44] were able to reproduce the protracted renin pressor curve by a short burst of angiotensin II injections in the nephrectomized rat. They suggested that the prolonged action of renin results from a persistent vascular smooth muscle response and that this explained the failure to detect pressor material in the circulation. However, the administration of converting enzyme inhibitor to nephrectomized rats with renin-induced hypertension, causes a rapid fall in blood pressure to basal levels (Figure 5). Thus the renin pressor response is maintained by continued generation of angiotensin II.

First experiments in which specific physiologic changes were attributed to vascular renin were those of Daum et al. [55]. They found that the infusion of aminopeptidase depressed the angiotensin II pressor response in rats but had a much less conspicuous effect on renin response. It was concluded that locally formed angiotensin within the blood vessel wall was less liable to destruction by aminopeptidase. The peculiar in vivo properties of angiotensin II antiserums are also explicable by generation of vasoconstrictor quantities of angiotensin II at a site inaccessible to the antibody. Thus in salt-depleted rats, in which the plasma renin activity

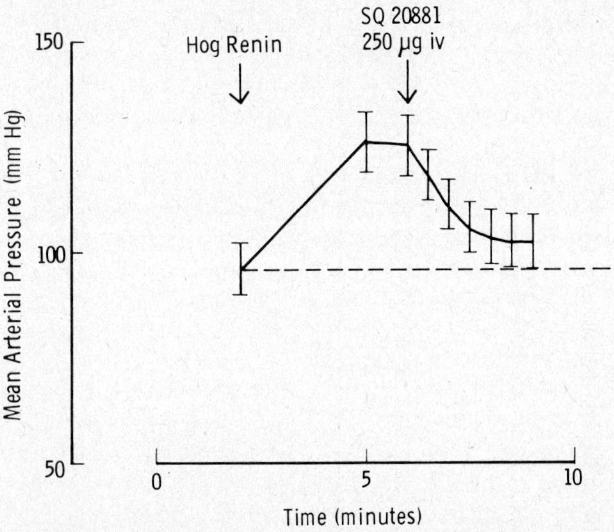

Figure 5. *Effect of converting enzyme blockade on the blood pressure of renin-infused nephrectomized rats (N = 6, values mean ± SEM).*

is high, administration of a small amount of antiserum was required to block the exogenous angiotensin II pressor response. Conversely a large dose of antiserum was needed in salt-loaded animals [50]. Swales and Thurston [49] confirmed these results using antibody dose-response curves but, in addition, they showed that the infusion of small amounts of renin changed the dose-response curve of salt-loaded animals so that it approximated to that of salt-depleted rats (Figure 4). There was also a positive correlation between angiotensin II pressor response and the volume of antiserum needed to block the response to a standard dose [53]. Clearly, saturation of the antibody-binding sites is not the answer because the blocking volume of antiserum is lowest when circulating renin levels are high. However, these contradictions are easily reconciled by postulating angiotensin II generation at a site inaccessible to antibody.

Since the vascular receptor site is obviously accessible to angiotensin II itself, it should be easily reached by substances of the same molecular size and configuration, particularly angiotensin II antagonists. Hence, infusion of the angiotensin II antagonist sarcosine^1 alanine^8 angiotensin II lowers the blood pressure in renin-induced hypertension whereas blocking doses of antibody are relatively ineffective [65] (Figure 6). Similar observations have been made in acute Goldblatt two-kidney hypertensive rats in which, in many studies, active [66,67] or passive immunization [68,69] neither prevents nor ameliorates the hypertension. Even when a fall in the blood pressure level occurred in this model, the animals did not become normotensive [70,71]. However, infusion of an angiotensin II antagonist has a marked depressor effect of a similar degree

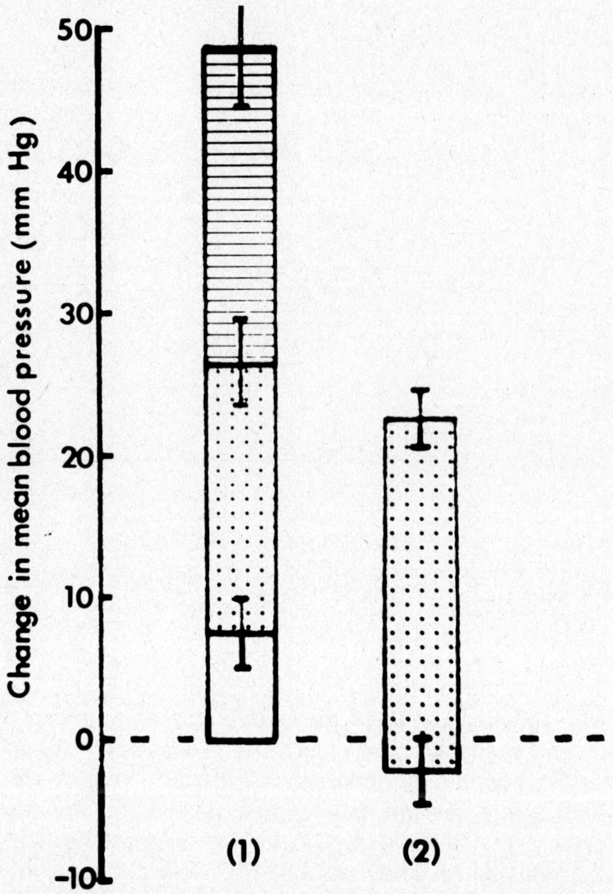

Figure 6. Response to angiotensin II antibody and antagonist infusion on renin-induced hypertension. Height of the columns shows the rise in blood pressure levels in response to the administration of renin, cross hatched part of the column represents the antibody-induced decrease in pressure, and the dotted portion of the column represents the decrease in blood pressure in response to the antagonist infusion. In group 1 (1) renin was infused before antibody and in group 2 (2) afterwards. In each group, administration of the antagonist caused a further decrease in blood pressure.

to the decrease in blood pressure that occurs after the ischemic kidney is removed (Table I) [69]. Oster et al. [72] have offered an alternative explanation for the comparative impotence of antiserums with the suggestion that high levels of circulating angiotensin II exist even in the presence of antibody. The main evidence quoted in support of this view is that plasma renin levels are normal in both actively [72,73] and passively immunized animals. It is argued, therefore, that sufficient free angiotensin II must be present to maintain feedback inhibition of renin release. But, these observations are equally consistent with feedback inhibition by locally generated angiotensin II inaccessible to antibody within the juxtaglomerular apparatus. In addition, our antibody was fully effective in blocking bolus or constant angiotensin II infusions [49,56]. Further, the similarity between our results using angiotensin antibodies and those of Daum et al. using an irreversible inhibitor of angiotensin II suggests that the explanation of Oster et al. is not the correct one.

The decrease in blood pressure caused by sarcosine[1] alanine[8] angiotensin II in Goldblatt two-kidney hypertensive rats occurs within a few minutes of the peptide reaching the circulation. Therefore, if the angiotensin-dependent mechanism is inhibited by removal of renin by bilateral nephrectomy, the blood pressure level should fall in parallel with the plasma renin activity. However, although the plasma renin activity level falls to a low level in the first hour (Figure 7) only a minute fall in the blood pressure level occurs (Figure 8). In order to confirm that the blood pressure level in this situation is maintained by the renin which persists outside the circulation, we infused converting enzyme inhibitor (SQ20881) into Goldblatt two-kidney hypertensive rats at intervals after bilateral nephrectomy. A marked depressor response was observed at 1 and 2 hours with only a small decrease at the sixth hour (Figure 9). Prior infusion of 1 μg/min of sarcosine[1] alanine[8] angiotensin blocked the depressor response confirming that the effect was the result of converting enzyme inhibition rather than bradykinin potentiation. The angiotensin II antagonist itself produced a decrease in blood pressure in this situation, but this was less marked presumably because of intrinsic agonist activity. Converting enzyme inhibitor, which has no agonist activity, gave a better and more consistent depressor response.

RECEPTOR MODULATION OF THE RENIN ANGIOTENSIN SYSTEM

Most studies of the renin-angiotensin system have depended upon assaying the circulating levels of renin and angiotensin II, but it is obvious from the foregoing discussion that such measurements may not reflect happenings at the receptor site. Normally, however, it seems likely that circulating renin levels reflect renin activity at the vascular site. This view is supported by the parallelism between angiotensin II responsiveness and circulating renin levels in a wide variety of physio-

TABLE I Effect of Antiserums, Antagonist and Removal of the Ischemic Kidney on the Mean Arterial Blood Pressure (mean ± SEM mm Hg) of Goldblatt Two-Kidney Hypertensive Rats (N = 8)

Study	Results	
Initial	144.8 ± 4.5	
After antiserum	143.7 ± 5.1	($p > 0.05$)
After antagonist	119.3 ± 3.6	($p < 0.005$)
After nephrectomy	110.9 ± 6.5	($p < 0.005$)

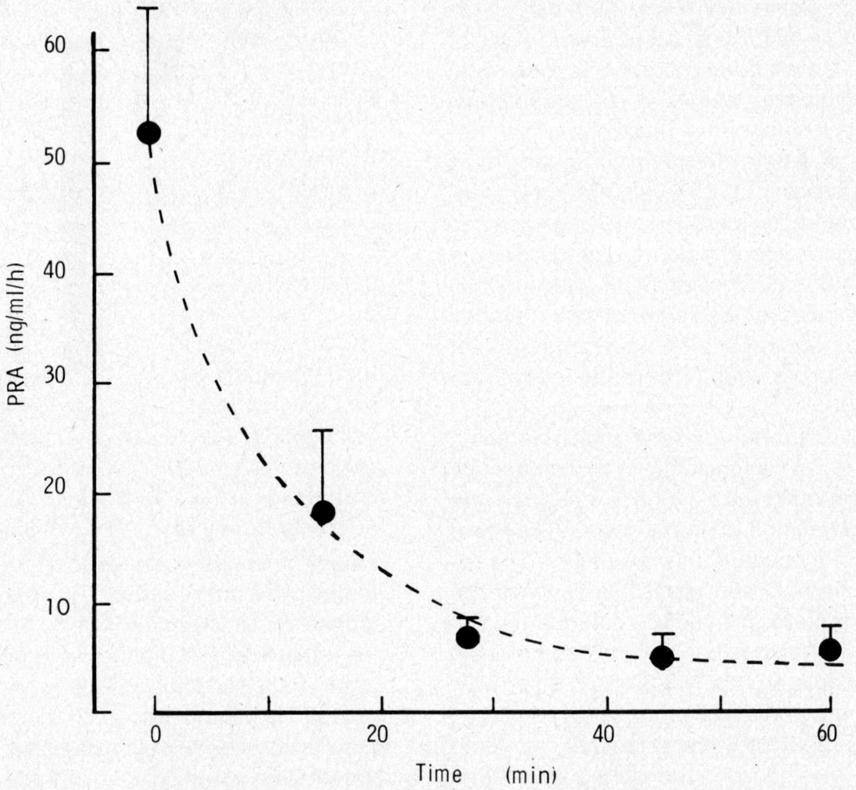

Figure 7. *Decrease in plasma renin activity (mean ± SEM) in Goldblatt two-kidney hypertensive rats after bilateral nephrectomy.*

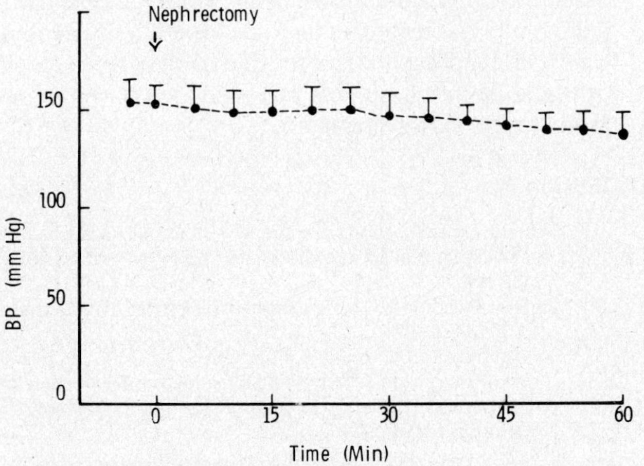

Figure 8. *Decrease in blood pressure of rats with Goldblatt two-kidney hypertensive rats for the first hour after bilateral nephrectomy.*

Figure 9. *Decrease in arterial blood pressure in rats with Goldblatt two-kidney hypertension which were bilaterally nephrectomized at 1 hour, 2 hours and 6 hours before receiving the converting enzyme inhibitor.*

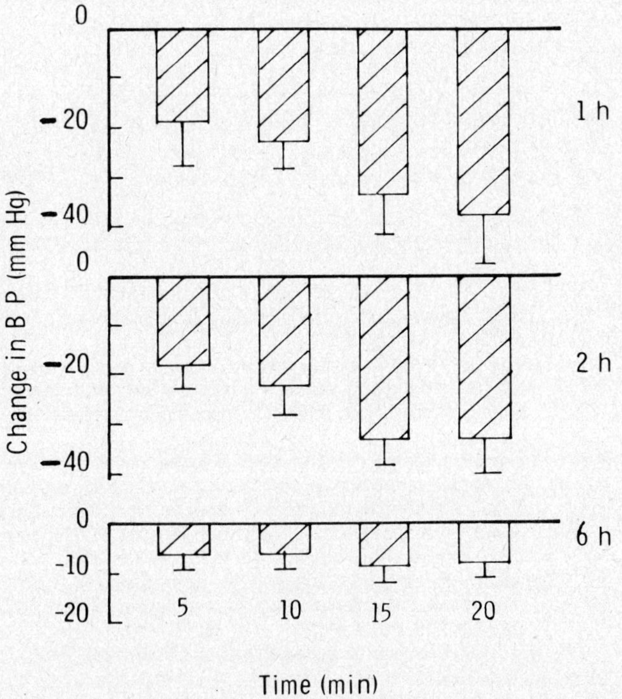

logic and pathologic states in which sodium balance is altered [24–26,30,31,42]. Thus, a prodigious body of data has been collected demonstrating a reciprocal relationship among plasma renin [74–76], angiotensin [77–79] and sodium balance. In situations of salt deprivation [74,76] or when effective circulating fluid volumes are decreased [33–35], plasma renin concentrations are markedly increased. Conversely, in sodium loading, mineralocorticoids suppress plasma renin release [74,80]. However, it is theoretically possible that modulation of the receptor site changes responsiveness of angiotensin II independently of changes in receptor occupancy by endogenous angiotensin II.

The recent development of new pharmacologic agents which interrupt renin angiotensin by competitive inhibition at the receptor site [17,81] or block the conversion of angiotensin I to angiotensin II [82] provides one means of evaluating the possibility. The reciprocal relationship between pressor activity of the renin angiotensin system and sodium balance is confirmed by studies with sarcosine[1] alanine[8] angiotensin II infusions in salt-depleted rats [83,84] and dogs [85] and in dogs with thoracic caval ligation [86]. Similarly, in the Goldblatt single-kidney hypertensive rat, renin dependency can be exposed or abolished by sodium loading [83]. Moreover, infusion of the nonapeptide converting enzyme inhibitor decreases the blood pressure of salt-depleted rats [48] (Figure 10), rabbits [87] and dogs, and of adrenalectomized dogs with an initially low blood pressure [88]. Thus, these agents uncover a major role for angiotensin II in the maintenance of arterial blood pressure in low output states (for more details see Davis et al. [5]). However, since in all these studies there was a close relationship between the decrease in blood pressure and endogenous renin activity, there is no evidence for receptor modulation as distinct from receptor occupancy. The reduced responsiveness to angiotensin II in salt depletion or when the effective circulating volume is reduced, as in hemorrhage, Addison's disease and Bartter's syndrome, can readily be understood on the basis of prior receptor occupancy. The excellent pressor responses following conversion of enzyme blockade in salt-depleted or adrenalectomized animals confirm this view [48].

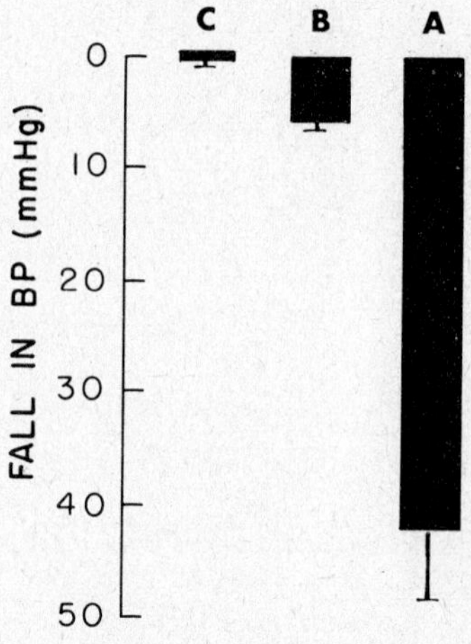

*Figure 10. Decrease in blood pressure (means ± SEM) of nephrectomized (**C**), salt-loaded (**B**) and salt-restricted (**A**) rats.*

In conclusion, there is little physiologic evidence in support of the hypothesis that variations in either receptor "affinity" or total receptor numbers exercise a modulatory role in the operation of the renin-angiotensin system. It would seem more likely that changes in angiotensin II reactivity in situations in which the system is activated represent receptor saturation by angiotensin formed in both the plasma and also locally within peripheral blood vessel walls.

REFERENCES

1. Frohlich ED, Tarazi RC, Dustan HP: Reexamination of the haemodynamics of hypertension. Am J Med Sci 257: 9, 1969.
2. Frohlich ED, Tarazi RC, Dustan HP: Haemodynamics in two renal hypertensions: arterial and pyelonephritis. Am J Med Sci 261: 189, 1971.
3. Folkow B, Hallback M, Lundgren Y, et al.: Importance of adaptive changes in vascular design for establishment of primary hypertension studied in man and in spontaneously hypertensive rats. Circ Res 32 (suppl 1): 2, 1973.
4. Laragh JH, Sealey JE: The renin angiotensin-aldosterone hormonal system and regulation of sodium, potassium and blood pressure homeostasis. Handbook of Physiology: Renal Physiology (Orloff J, Berliner RW, eds), Washington DC, American Physiological Society, 1973, p 831.
5. Davis JO, Freeman RH, Johnson JA, Spielman WS: Agents which block the action of the renin-angiotensin system. Circ Res 34: 279, 1974.
6. Peart WS: The renin-angiotensin system. Pharmacol Rev 17: 143, 1965.
7. Davis JO: The renin-angiotensin system in the control of aldosterone secretion. Angiotensin: (Page IH, Bumpus FM, eds), Berlin, Heidelberg, New York, Springer-Verlag, 1974, p 323.
8. Lin S-Y, Goodfriend TL: Angiotensin receptors. Am J Physiol 218: 1319, 1970.
9. Goodfriend TL, Fyhrquist F, Futmann F, et al.: Clinical and conceptual uses of angiotensin receptors. Hypertension '72 (Genest J, Koiw E, eds), Berlin, Heidelberg, New York, Springer-Verlag, 1972, p 549.
10. Meyer P, Baudouin M, Fermandjian S, et al.: Angiotensin receptors in smooth muscle cells. Hypertension '72 (Genest J, Koiw E, eds), Berlin, Heidelberg, New York, Springer-Verlag, 1972.
11. Devynck M-A, Meyer P: Angiotensin receptors in vascular tissue. Am J Med 61: 758, 1976.
12. Khairallah PA, Toth A, Bumpus FM: Analogs of angiotensin II. II. Mechanisms of receptor interaction. J Med Chem 13: 181, 1970.
13. Regoli D, Park WK, Rioux F: Pharmacology of angiotensin. Pharmacol Rev 26: 69, 1974.
14. Ariens EJ: Receptor theory and structure action relationships.

Advances in Drug Research, vol 3 (Harper NJ, Simmonds AB, eds), London, New York, Academic Press, 1966, p 235.

15. Johansson B: Determinants of vascular reactivity. Fed Proc 33: 121, 1974.
16. Furchgott RF: Importance of Fundamental Principles in Drug Evaluation, New York, Raven, 1968, p 277.
17. Pals DT, Masucci FD, Sipos F, Denning GS: A specific competitive antagonist of the vascular action of angiotensin II. Circ Res 29: 664, 1971.
18. Collier HOJ: Tolerance, physical dependence and receptors. Advances in Drug Research, vol 3 (Harper NJ, Simmonds AB, eds), London, New York, Academic Press, 1966, p 171.
19. Braun-Menendez E, Fascicolo JC, Leloir LF, Munoz JM: The substance causing renal hypertension. J Physiol 98: 283, 1940.
20. Page IH, Helmer OM: A crystalline pressor substance (angiotonin) resulting from the reaction between renin and renin activator. J Exp Med 71: 29, 1940.
21. Abell RG, Page IH: The reaction of peripheral blood vessels to angiotensin, renin and other pressor agents. J Exp Med 75: 305, 1942.
22. De Bono E, Lee G De J, Mottram FR, Pickering GW: The action of angiotensin in man. Clin Sci 25: 123, 1963.
23. Bohr DF: Angiotensin on vascular smooth muscle. Angiotensin (Page IH, Bumpus FM, eds), Berlin, Heidelberg, New York, Springer-Verlag, 1974, p 424.
24. Reid WD, Laragh JH: Sodium and potassium intake, blood pressure and pressor response to angiotensin. Proc Soc Exp Biol 120: 26, 1965.
25. Samwer KF, Schreiber M, Molzahn M, Oelkers W: Pressor effect of angiotensin II in sodium replete and deplete rats. Pfluegers Arch 346: 307, 1974.
26. Slack BL, Ledingham JM: The influence of sodium intake on the pressor response to angiotensin II in the unanaesthetized rat. Clin Sci Mol Med 50: 285, 1976.
27. Barraclough MA, Jones NF, Marsden CD, Bradford BC: Renal and pressor effects of angiotensin in salt loaded and depleted rabbits. Experientia (Basel) 23: 553, 1967.
28. Davis JO, Hartroft PM, Titus EO, et al.: The role of the renin-angiotensin system in the control of aldosterone secretion. J Clin Invest 41: 378, 1962.
29. Blair-West JR, Coghlan JP, Denton DA, et al.: Humoral stimulation of adrenal cortex secretion. J Clin Invest 41: 1606, 1962.
30. Kaplan NM, Silah JG: Effect of angiotensin II on the blood pressure in humans with hypertensive disease. J Clin Invest 43: 659, 1964.
31. Hollenberg NK, Solomon HS, Adams DF, et al.: Renal vascular responses to angiotensin and norepinephrine in normal man: effect of sodium intake. Circ Res 31: 750, 1972.
32. Strewler GJ, Hinrichs KJ, Guiod LR, Hollenberg NK: Sodium intake and vascular smooth muscle responsiveness to norepinephrine and angiotensin in the rabbit. Circ Res 31: 758, 1972.
33. Laragh JH: Hormones and pathogenesis of congestive heart failure: vasopressin, aldosterone and angiotensin II. Further evidence for renal-adrenal interaction from studies in hypertension and cirrhosis. Circulation 25: 1015, 1962.
34. Laragh JH: Interrelationships between angiotensin, norepinephrine, epinephrine, aldosterone secretion, and electrolyte metabolism in man. Circulation 25: 203, 1962.
35. Bartter FC, Pronove P, Gill JR Jr, MacCardle RC: Hyperplasia of the juxtaglomerular complex with hyperaldosteronism and hypokalemic alkalosis. A new syndrome. Am J Med 33: 811, 1962.
36. Healey JK, Suszkiw JB, Dennis VW: Effect of aldosterone and salt intake on renal and pressor actions of angiotensin. Nephron 3: 329, 1966.
37. Chesley LC, Talledo E, Bohler CS, Zuspan FP: Vascular reactivity to angiotensin II and norepinephrine in pregnant and non-pregnant women. Am J Obstet Gynecol 91: 837, 1965.
38. Laragh JH, Cannon PJ, Bentzel CJ, et al.: Angiotensin II, norepinephrine and renal transport of electrolytes and water in normal man and in cirrhosis with ascites. J Clin Invest 42: 1179, 1963.
39. Johnson CJ, Dose AD: Reduced vascular response to angiotensin II in secondary hyperaldosteronism. J Clin Invest 42: 1411, 1963.
40. Kuchel O, Horky K, Pazourek M, Gregorova I: Pressor hyporeactivity to angiotensin in Addison's disease. Lancet 2: 1316, 1964.
41. Chinn RH, Dusterdieck G: The response of blood pressure to infusion of angiotensin II: relation to plasma concentrations of renin and angiotensin II. Clin Sci 42: 489, 1972.
42. Silah JG, Strong CG, Nowaczynski W, Genest J: The angiotensin infusion test and peripheral venous renin activity. Can Med Assoc J 96: 1397, 1967.
43. Blaquier P, Hoobler SW, Schroeder J, et al.: Effect of bilateral nephrectomy on pressor response to renin. Am J Physiol 203: 339, 1962.
44. Gabelman EH, Rondell PA: Protracted pressor response to angiotensin after bilateral nephrectomy in rats. Circ Res 18: 705, 1965.
45. Chevillotte E, Devynck MA, Fyhrquist F, et al.: Angiotensin-induced variations of receptors in rat uterine membranes. Clin Sci Mol Med 48: 235, 1975.
46. Rosenthal J, Boucher R, Rojo-Ortega JM, Genest J: Renin activity in aortic tissue of rats. Can J Physiol Pharamacol 47: 53, 1969.
47. Gordon P, Ferris TF, Mulrow JP: Rabbit uterus as a possible site of renin synthesis. Am J Physiol 212: 703, 1967.
48. Thurston H, Laragh JH: Prior receptor occupancy as a determinant of the pressor activity of infused angiotensin II in the rat. Circ Res 36: 113, 1975.
49. Swales JD, Thurston H: Generation of angiotensin II at peripheral vascular level: studies using angiotensin II antisera. Clin Sci Mol Med 45: 691, 1973.
50. Brunner HR, Chang P, Wallach R, et al.: Angiotensin II vascular receptors: their avidity in relationship to sodium balance, the autonomic nervous system and hypertension. J Clin Invest 51: 58, 1972.
51. McCance RA: Medical problems in mineral metabolism. Lancet 1: 823, 1936.
52. Glossman H, Baukal A, Catt KJ: Cation dependence of high-affinity angiotensin II binding to adrenal cortex receptors. Science 185: 281, 1974.
53. Swales JD, Tange JD, Thurston H: Vascular angiotensin II receptors and sodium balance in rats: role of kidneys and vascular renin activity. Circ Res 37: 96, 1975.
54. Oates HF, Fretton JA, Stokes GS: Disappearance rate of circulating renin after bilateral nephrectomy in the rat. Clin Exp Pharmacol Physiol 1: 547, 1974.
55. Daum A, Uehleke H, Lkaus D: Unterschiedliche Beeinflussung der Blutdruckwirkung von Renin und Angiotensin durch Aminopeptidase. Naunyn Schmiedebergs Arch Pharmacol 254: 327, 1966.
56. Swales JD: Antagonists, inhibitors and antisera in the evaluation of vascular renin activity: the role of local generation of angiotensin II. Prog Biochem Pharmacol (in press).
57. Gould AB, Skeggs LT, Kahn JR: The presence of renin activity in blood vessel wall. J Exp Med 119: 389, 1964.
58. Haduk K, Ganten D, Boucher R, Genest J: Arterial and urinary renin activity. Hypertension '72 (Genest J, Koiw E, eds), Berlin, Springer-Verlag, 1972, p 435.
59. Aiken JW, Vane JR: Inhibition of converting enzyme of the renin-angiotensin system in kidney and hind limbs of dogs. Circ Res 30: 263, 1972.

60. Osborn EC, Tildesley G, O'Gorman LP, Mahler RF: The effect of angiotensin I and II on hind-limb blood flow in sheep. J Pharm Pharmacol 23: 466, 1971.
61. Disalvo J, Montefusco CB: Conversion of angiotensin I to II in the canine mesenteric circulation. Am J Physiol 221: 1576, 1971.
62. Cadwell RB, Seegal BC, Hsu KC: Angiotensin-converting enzyme: vascular endothelial localization. Science 191: 1050, 1976.
63. Schaechtelin G, Regoli D, Gross F: Quantitative assay and disappearance rate of circulating renin. Am J Physiol 206: 1361, 1964.
64. Bing J, Nielson K: Cause of the prolonged pressor action of renin in nephrectomized rats. Acta Pathol Microbiol Scand [A] 81: 247, 1973.
65. Thurston H, Swales JD: Action of angiotensin antagonists and antiserum upon the pressor response to renin: further evidence for the local generation of angiotensin II. Clin Sci Mol Med 46: 273, 1974.
66. Eide I: Renovascular hypertension in rats immunized with angiotensin II. Circ Res 30: 149, 1972.
67. Oates HF, Stokes GS, Storey BG, et al.: Renal hypertension in rats immunized against angiotensin I and angiotensin II. J Exp Med 139: 239, 1974.
68. MacDonald GJ, Pessina A, Boyd GW, Peart WS: Angiotensin antibodies in two kidney hypertension in the rat. Second Meeting of the International Society of Hypertension, Milan, September 1972.
69. Thurston H, Swales JD: Comparison of angiotensin II antagonist and antiserum infusion with nephrectomy in the rat with two kidney Goldblatt hypertension. Circ Res 35: 325, 1974.
70. Brunner HR, Kirshman JD, Sealey JE, Laragh JH: Hypertension of renal origin: evidence for two different mechanisms. Science 174: 1344, 1971.
71. Carretero OA, Kuk P, Piwonska S, et al.: Role of the renin-angiotensin system in the pathogenesis of severe hypertension in rats. Circ Res 29: 654, 1971.
72. Oster P, Bauknecht H, Hackenthal E: Active and passive immunization against angiotensin II in the rat and rabbit: evidence for normal regulation of the renin-angiotensin system. Circ Res 37: 607, 1975.
73. Oates HF, Stokes GS: Plasma renin activity of rats and rabbits immunized against angiotensin II. Clin Exp Pharmacol Physiol 1: 161, 1974.
74. Brown JJ, Davies DL, Lever AF, Robertson JIS: Influence of sodium deprivation and loading on plasma renin in man. J Physiol (Lond) 173: 408, 1964.
75. Gross F, Brunner H, Ziegler M: Renin angiotensin system, aldosterone and sodium balance. Recent Prog Horm Res 21: 119, 1965.
76. Laragh JH, Sealey JE, Sommers SC: Patterns of adrenal secretion and urinary excretion of aldosterone secretion and plasma renin activity in normal and hypertensive subjects. Circ Res 18 (suppl 1): 158, 1966.
77. Gocke DJ, Gertan J, Sherwood LM, Laragh JH: Physiological and pathological variations of plasma angiotensin II in man. Circ Res 34, 35 (suppl 1): 131, 1969.
78. Brown JJ, Frazer R, Lever AF, et al.: Raised plasma angiotensin II and aldosterone during dietary sodium restriction in man. Lancet 2: 1106, 1972.
79. Boyd GW, Adamson AR, Arnold M, et al.: The role of angiotensin II in the control of aldosterone in man. Clin Sci 42: 91, 1972.
80. Brown JJ, Chin RH, Davies DL, et al.: Plasma electrolytes, renin and aldosterone in the diagnosis of primary aldosteronism. Lancet 2: 55, 1968.
81. Needleman P, Johnson EM Jr, Vine W, et al.: Pharmacology of antagonists of angiotensin I and II. Circ Res 31: 862, 1972.
82. Engel SL, Schaeffer TR, Gold BI, Rubin B: Inhibition of pressor effects of angiotensin I and augmentation of depressor effects of bradykinin by synthetic peptides. Proc Soc Exp Biol Med 140: 240, 1972.
83. Gavras H, Brunner HR, Vaughan ED, Laragh JH: Angiotensin-sodium interaction in blood pressure maintenance of renal hypertensive and normotensive rats. Science 180: 1369, 1973.
84. Spielman WS, Davis JO: The renin-angiotensin system and aldosterone secretion during sodium depletion in the rat. Circ Res 35: 615, 1974.
85. Johnson JA, Davis JO: Effects of a specific competitive antagonist of angiotensin II on arterial blood pressure and adrenal steroid secretion in dogs. Circ Res 32 (suppl 1): 159, 1973.
86. Johnson JA, Davis JO: Angiotensin II. Important role in the maintenance of arterial blood pressure. Science 179: 906, 1973.
87. Mimran A, Guiod L, Hollenberg NK: The role of angiotensin in the cardiovascular and renal response to salt restriction. Kidney Int 5: 348, 1974.
88. Samuels AI, Miller ED, Fray CS, et al.: Regulation of pressure by the renin-angiotensin system (abstract). Fed Proc 32: 320, 1973.

Beta-Adrenergic Receptor Blocking Drugs in Spontaneous Hypertension

JOSEPH V. LEVY, Ph.D.
San Francisco, California

Eleven beta-adrenergic receptor blocking agents and derivatives were evaluated for their ability to affect systolic arterial blood pressure and pulse rate in unanesthetized, male spontaneously hypertensive rats (SHRs) and normotensive Wistar Kyoto (WKY) controls. Animals ranged from 7 to 76 weeks of age. The subcutaneous injection of 5 and 45 mg/kg metoprolol in 52 to 64 week old SHRs and 45 mg/kg twice a day to 26 to 29 week old SHRs produced a significant decrease in blood pressure. The subcutaneous injection of pindolol (0.1 and 1.0 mg/kg) produced a greater and more consistent depressor effect in mature SHRs. The subcutaneous administration of sotalol (100 mg/kg) and alprenolol (20 mg/kg) resulted in a depressor action which was significant 120 minutes after injection of the drug. In the doses used, propranolol, oxprenolol, 4-hydroxypropranolol and KO-1366 produced pressor effect in SHRs. Propranolol did not cause this pressor effect in prehypertensive (seven week old) SHRs. Practolol, *dextro*-propranolol and KO-1313 had no effect on blood pressure in the doses used. Propranolol, pindolol, metoprolol, *dextro*-propranolol, 4-hydroxypropranolol, practolol, oxprenolol, KO-1366 and KO-1313 produced no significant effects on blood pressure in normotensive WKY controls in the doses tested. Placing oral doses of 160 mg/kg/day of metoprolol in the drinking water for seven days significantly lowered blood pressure in 14 week old SHRs previously exposed to ineffective doses of 77 mg/kg/day for 24 days. The administration of oral doses of oxprenolol (40 mg/kg/day) in drinking water for three weeks had a slight but insignificant pressor effect. Smaller doses of metoprolol (15 and 39 mg/kg/day for three to four weeks) and practolol (70 to 85 mg/kg/day for two weeks) had no effect on 52 week old SHRs. Oral doses of pindolol, metoprolol, practolol and oxprenolol had no significant effect on blood pressure in WKY controls. There was no clear relationship between the effects of the drugs on blood pressure and their ability to affect the pulse rate. Similarly, there did not appear to be any consistent relationship between the potency of the beta-blocking drug and the blood pressure lowering action. In addition, neither cardioselective beta-blockade nor sympathomimetic properties allowed the prediction of blood pressure responses to the administration of those agents possessing these features. Although SHRs provide a valuable model of human essential hypertension, the variable effects reported here and elsewhere in the literature require caution as to the applicability and usefulness of testing and evaluating beta-adrenergic blocking drugs for their potential antihypertensive effects in this particular form of experimental hypertension.

From the Laboratory of Pharmacology and Experimental Therapeutics, The Institute of Medical Sciences; and the School of Medical Sciences, University of The Pacific, San Francisco, California. This study was presented in part at the Sixth International Pharmacology Congress, Helsinki, Finland, July 20–25, 1975. It was supported in part by a grant from the National Heart and Lung Institute, N.I.H. Requests for reprints should be addressed to Dr. Joseph V. Levy, The Institutes of Medical Sciences, P.O. Box 7999, San Francisco, California 94120.

One of the major factors which has hampered a better understanding of the mechanism of the antihypertensive effect of beta-adrenergic receptor blocking drugs has been the lack of a consistent and predictable response to these drugs in a convenient animal model of human essential hypertension. The advent and availability of the spontaneously hypertensive rat (SHR) of the Okamoto-Aoki strain [1,2] appeared to offer great potential, since many of its characteristics were likened to those seen in human disease [2,3]. Yet, despite this potential, an array of conflicting reports has appeared dealing with the effects of this group of drugs on the arterial blood pressure of the SHR. Thus, some investigators reported that these drugs have no effect on the blood pressure of SHRs [4–7,13,22]; others showed that the agents caused a further increase in arterial pressure [8–10], whereas in some studies varying degrees of a depressor effect were shown depending on the age and sex of the animal, the drug and dosage used, the route of administration and the duration of treatment [8,10–12,14–16,22]. In contrast, the SHR shows consistent depressor responses to a variety of other known antihypertensive agents [8,13,16–21,23]. Clearly, the diverse and conflicting reports of the effects of the beta-blockers on the SHR make it difficult to study and evaluate potential new antihypertensive beta-blockers, let alone understand the mechanism and mode of action of those which are already demonstrably effective in man.

One approach to this enigma is to study the effects of beta-blockers possessing diverse pharmacologic properties using SHRs of various ages. Hopefully, such an investigation might reveal the experimental condition (i.e., age, dose, route of administration) or drug characteristic that consistently would relate to the desired pharmacologic effect, i.e., an antihypertensive action. This report describes my studies with 11 beta-blocking agents and derivatives using SHRs and normotensive controls which ranged from seven to 76 weeks of age.

MATERIALS AND METHODS

Animals. Studies were performed on SHRs of the Okamoto-Aoki strain derived from breeder stock provided by Dr. Carl Hansen of the Animal Resources Branch of the National Institutes of Health. All animals were bred and raised in our own animal facility. Sister-brother mating was used to assure a uniformly consistent pattern of development of the spontaneous hypertensive state. Animals were weaned at three weeks of age; each litter being housed in its own multiple rat holding cage. The colony was checked daily for new births to assure accurate birth dating. The intake of water and Purina Rat Chow was allowed ad libitum. Animals were exposed to a 12 hour light, 12 hour dark cycle. The animal quarters were air conditioned; ambient temperature ranged from 22° to 24°C. A normotensive colony of Wistar rats of the Kyoto strain (WKY) was developed simultaneously with the SHRs, using WKY breeder stock provided by the National Institutes of Health. These WKY controls were derived from the Wistar strain from which the SHR line was originally developed [1,2]. These normotensive WKY controls are thought to be pertinent and reliable control animals for comparison with the SHRs [2,24]. Only male SHRs and WKY controls were used.

Blood Pressure Measurements. All systolic blood pressure measurements were made on unanesthetized rats using a Narco Bio-Systems model PE-300 automatic sphygmomanometer for indirect measurement of blood pressure in the tail artery. Animals were transferred from their holding cages to a warming cage with an ambient temperature of 38° to 39°C. They were held at this temperature for approximately 10 to 15 minutes before being placed into the restraining device (Narco) for the measurement of blood pressure. After being placed in the holder, the occluding cuff and pressure sensor were attached and the animal was allowed to acclimate for approximately 2 to 5 minutes before blood pressure measurements were undertaken. Arterial pulse was displayed on an oscilloscope which was calibrated to allow readings to within ± 2 mm Hg. Pulse rate was also determined from a faster sweep tracing on a memory oscilloscope. Following the short period of acclimation, three or four systolic blood pressure and pulse rate readings were made.

Subcutaneous Injections. In those experiments in which the drug was to be administered subcutaneously, the injection was made while the animal was still in the holder. Injection volumes did not exceed 0.5 ml. Appropriate saline solution or solvent controls also were tested. The animals were left in the holder for 5 minutes after the injection. In some experiments, blood pressure and pulse rate reading were taken at that time. The animals were then returned to their holding cages and maintained at temperatures of approximately 30° to 32°C. Additional blood pressure and pulse rate measurements were made usually 15, 30, 60 and 120 minutes after the injection. The animals were returned to their cages between measurements. SHRs and WKY controls were handled identically. During the total experimental period, the animals had free access to food and water when their blood pressure was not being taken.

Chronic Oral Doses. Several agents were tested for their effects on blood pressure by exposing the animals to the drug via their drinking water. In these experiments, animals were singly housed, and calibrated drinking bottles were used. All test and control animals were allowed to acclimate to their environment for one week. Their blood pressure levels and pulse rates were then determined as described. These were recorded as their control values. They were then returned to their cages and either given drinking water that contained an active drug in a known concentration, or an inactive placebo. Water consumption was measured daily. From the volume of water consumed, the daily consumption of drug was estimated and expressed as milligram of drug per kilogram of body weight. Blood pressure levels and pulse rates were determined at either daily or weekly intervals, depending on the protocol and duration of the experiment.

Drugs. The following substances were tested: Racemic propranolol hydrochloride, (+)-propranolol; 4-hydroxypropranolol; sotalol (MJ-1999); metoprolol (H 93/26); practolol (ICI 50172); pindolol (LB-46); alprenolol (H 56/28); KO-1366 (o-2-hydroxy-3-(tert butylamino)-propoxybenzonitrile); and KO-1313, a congener of KO-1366; oxprenolol. Solutions were made fresh daily. In the case of 4-hydroxypropranolol, solutions to be used for injection were made up just prior to use since this substance undergoes rapid degradation in vitro.

Statistical Evaluation. In those experiments in which each animal served as its own predrug control, subsequent changes in pulse rate and systolic blood pressure for any series of experiments were tested for statistical significance using Student's t test for paired data. A P value of 0.05 or less was regarded as significant.

RESULTS

Propranolol. The subcutaneous injection of propranolol in a dose of 0.1 mg/kg produced a significant increase in systolic blood pressure in mature (52 to 55 week old) SHRs. This pressor effect was accompanied by a slight but insignificant decrease in pulse rate (Table I). Age-matched WKY controls showed no significant response to this dose. A dose of 1.0 mg/kg produced an 11 ± 8 to 18 ± 3 per cent increase in systolic blood pressure in mature SHRs, the maximum effect being noted 15 minutes after the injection. Four of the five SHRs died from 60 to 120 minutes after receiving the injection.* In contrast to this effect, a 1.0 mg/kg subcutaneous injection of the drug into younger SHRs (25 to 28 weeks old) caused a transient significant pressor effect at 5 minutes, but no significant change in systolic blood pressure 30, 60 and 120 minutes after the injection. However, there was a significant decrease in pulse rate at these times (Table II). Five young (seven week old) SHRs with a control mean systolic blood pressure of 144 ± 8 mm Hg showed no significant change in blood pressure to a subcutaneous dose of 1.0 mg/kg over a period of 120 minutes after administration of the drug, even though the pulse rate was immediately and significantly decreased.

* In another experiment, six mature (52 to 56 week old) SHRs were given injections of 1.0 mg/kg, subcutaneous propranolol following control blood pressure and pulse rate measurements. Measurements were repeated only at 2 hours after the injection, thus obviating the repeated heating procedures required with the usual 5, 15, 30, 60 minute readings. One of the six animals died before 120 minutes. The other five showed no significant change in systolic blood pressure from the value before administration of the drug, although pulse rate was significantly lowered in all animals. It thus appears that the apparent toxicity to this dose of propranolol in mature SHRs may be, in part, due to the enhancement of a stress response to repeated environmental heating procedures required with frequent blood pressure measurements. This explanation also may apply to the lethality noted with subcutaneous injections of 0.1 mg/kg KO-1366. It should be emphasized, however, that neither a pressor response nor deaths were seen with saline solution or solvent injections in age-matched SHRs undergoing repeated heatings identical to the drug-treated groups. Similarly, no pressor response nor deaths occurred in any of WKY controls receiving the drug or saline injection and undergoing the same repeated heating procedures as used in the SHR experiments.

TABLE I Effect of Propranolol (0.1 mg/kg, subcutaneously) on Systolic Blood Pressure and Pulse Rate of Four Mature SHRs

		Minutes After Administration of Drug			
Parameter	Control	15′	30′	45′	60′
Blood pressure (mm Hg)	202 ± 6.7	240* ± 10	236* ± 2	219* ± 7	219* ± 6
Pulse rate (beats/min)	416 ± 15	404 ± 16	383 ± 8	383 ± 8	370 ± 36

* $p < 0.05$.

Pindolol. Pindolol is 2.5 to 40 times more potent than propranolol as a beta-blocker [25–29]. In addition, in small doses, it possesses intrinsic sympathomimetic effects [25,27], including the ability to increase plasma renin activity (PRA) [29–31].

Pindolol, given in doses of 0.1 and 1.0 mg/kg subcutaneously, caused a significant decrease in systolic blood pressure in mature (52 to 60 week old) SHRs (Table III). In five age-matched normotensive WKY controls with control mean systolic blood pressure of 115 ± 5 mm Hg, the subcutaneous administration of 1.0 mg/kg of pindolol caused a slight (3.4 ± 2 to 9 ± 3 per cent) but insignificant decrease in blood pressure over a period of 15 to 120 minutes after the drug was given. No deaths occurred with the 0.1 or 1.0 mg/kg doses of the drug either in mature SHRs or WKY controls. Pulse rate was increased, but not significantly, in animals receiving 1.0 mg/kg subcutaneously.

The administration of pindolol in the drinking water (estimated daily dose 5 mg/kg) failed to lower the systolic blood pressure level in mature SHRs over a period of 10 days. In fact, at the end of the 10th day, the systolic blood pressure level was higher than the control level (226 ± 12 versus 209 ± 15 mm Hg). There was

TABLE II Effect of Propranolol (1.0 mg/kg, subcutaneously) on Systolic Blood Pressure and Pulse Rate of Five 25 to 28 Week Old SHRs

		Minutes After Administration of Drug			
Parameter	Control	5′	30′	60′	120′
Blood pressure (mm Hg)	189 ± 7	203* ± 7	194 ± 7	190 ± 5	188 ± 6
Pulse rate (beats/min)	343 ± 23	300 ± 6	275† ± 8	278‡ ± 9	290‡ ± 7

* $p < 0.01$.
† $p < 0.02$.
‡ $p < 0.05$.

TABLE III Changes in Systolic Arterial Blood Pressure Produced by Pindolol (0.1 and 1.0 mg/kg, given subcutaneously) in Five Mature SHRs

Control Blood Pressure (mm Hg)	Dose (mg/kg)	% Change in Blood Pressure* — Minutes After Administration of the Drug: 15′	30′	45′	60′	90′	120′
188 ± 7	0.1	−2.5 ± 2.7	−8.1† ± 2.8	−6.2 ± 2.8	−12.5† ± 3.2	−14.9† ± 4.3	−8.1 ± 3.4
203 ± 15	1.0	−14.5 ± 6.8	−16.1† ± 5.1	−23.2† ± 5.6	−26.8† ± 6.8	−27.5† ± 4.5	−25.1† ± 5.4

* Mean ± standard error of the mean.
† $p \leqq 0.05$.

a variable but significant decrease in pulse rate during the observation period of 10 days. A dose of 45 mg/kg/day administered in drinking water to five 16 week old SHRs caused no significant decrease in blood pressure (control 204 ± 7 mm Hg) over a period of four weeks. The pulse rate was not significantly affected during the same period of observation (control, 338 ± 8 beats/min versus 342 ± 8 beats/min at the fourth week). Similarly, age-matched WKY controls showed no significant changes in blood pressure or pulse rate over a four week period at this dose.

Metoprolol. Metoprolol (H 93/26) is a cardioselective beta-blocker with demonstrated antihypertensive action in man [15]. It is essentially devoid of intrinsic sympathomimetic or local anesthetic actions.

A dose of 45 mg/kg subcutaneously produced a highly significant decrease in pulse rate when tested in mature (52 to 64 week old) SHRs. Systolic blood pressure in these animals was significantly reduced at the 60 and 120 minute period of observation (Table IV). In 28 to 36 week old SHRs, the subcutaneous administration of 0.5 mg/kg of the drug, while producing a significant negative chronotropic effect, failed to significantly change systolic blood pressure observed over a period of 5 to 60 minutes. Thus, in six animals the mean systolic blood pressure before injection of the drug was 206 ± 12 mm Hg, whereas 60 minutes after the drug was given, the value was 205 ± 15 mm Hg.

TABLE IV Effect of Metoprolol (45 mg/kg, subcutaneously) on Systolic Blood Pressure and Pulse Rate of Six Mature SHRs

Parameter	Control	Minutes After Administration of Drug: 5′	30′	60′	120′
Blood pressure (mm Hg)	217 ± 6	212 ± 6	206 ± 5	194* ± 2	185* ± 2
Pulse rate (beats/min)	356 ± 8	310† ± 9	288† ± 5	287† ± 6	290† ± 5

* $p < 0.01$.
† $p < 0.001$.

Five one year old SHRs, with a mean systolic blood pressure of 220 ± 12 mm Hg before administration of the drug, showed a decrease in blood pressure with a subcutaneous dose of 5 mg/kg metoprolol, although this effect was statistically significant only for the 120 minute period after the drug was given. Pulse rate was decreased during the entire 120 minute period of observation, but it was only statistically significant at the first 5 minute measurement period. Interestingly, a subcutaneous dose of 15 mg/kg given to five 52 to 64 week old SHRs resulted in a significant increase in systolic blood pressure 5 and 30 minutes after the injection. There was no significant difference between control blood pressures (219 ± 6 mm Hg) and those measured at 60 and 120 minutes, however. Pulse rate was significantly decreased in these animals throughout the 2 hour period of observation. Metoprolol, in a dose of 0.5 mg/kg given subcutaneously, failed to cause any significant change in systolic blood pressure or pulse rate in five 20 week old WKY controls with control systolic blood pressure levels of 107 ± 4 mm Hg and pulse rates of 323 ± 17 beats/min.

Metoprolol was administered to five mature (50 to 52 week old) SHRs at a dose of 15 mg/kg/day via drinking water. At this dose, the drug failed to significantly change systolic blood pressure from control values (220 ± 19 mm Hg) or pulse rate (412 ± 38 beats/min) over a four week exposure to the drug. A dose of 39 mg/kg/day administered in the drinking water of three mature (48 to 62 week old) SHRs also failed to significantly affect blood pressure or pulse rate from control values over an observation period of three weeks.

In view of the report that very large doses of metoprolol (0.1 per cent in drinking water) may retard the development of hypertension in young SHRs [32], experiments were carried out to test the effects of the drug at a dose level of 77 mg/kg/day in three 10 week old SHRs (systolic blood pressure before administration of the drug = 165 ± 4 mm Hg; pulse rate 355 ± 9 beats/min). At the end of 24 days of treatment, the blood pressure level was not significantly different from the control levels. Pulse rate was significantly decreased by this treatment. Increasing the daily dose to 160 mg/kg/day in these animals caused a 10 mm Hg decrease in blood pressure which was observed one week after the institution of the larger dosage. However, pulse rate was not decreased any further than the value noted at the end of therapy with the smaller dose.

In another group of experiments, five 26 to 29 week old SHRs were given metoprolol subcutaneously in a total daily dose of 90 mg/kg (half at 9 AM and half at 5 PM) over a period of seven days. This treatment caused a significant reduction in the systolic blood pressure level of 184 ± 2 mm Hg before administration of the drug. Pulse rate at the end of the seven day treatment was not significantly different from control, however.

Mature (48 to 60 week old) WKY controls receiving metoprolol in a daily dose of 12 mg/kg in their drinking water showed no significant changes in blood pressure or pulse rate over a two week period of treatment.

Sotalol. This beta-adrenergic blocking agent is less potent than propranolol, is devoid of intrinsic sympathomimetic and local anesthetic action, and has a high degree of hydrophilicity that minimizes its penetration into the central nervous system [33–35]. The drug was tested in 25 to 28 week old SHRs at a dose of 100 mg/kg subcutaneously. There was an immediate and highly significant decrease in pulse rate. However, there was no significant change in systolic blood pressure except at 120 minutes after the injection, when the pressure was significantly reduced from the value obtained before the drug was administered (Table V).

Alprenolol. This agent is characterized by its significant intrinsic sympathomimetic action in addition to its moderate nonselective beta-blocking effects [36]. When administered in a dose of 10 mg/kg subcutaneously to five 19 week old SHRs, it caused a significant and immediate (5 minute reading) decrease in pulse rate that was observed for the 2 hour period of study. There was neither a significant increase or decrease in systolic blood pressure from the mean control value of 171 ± 4 mm Hg during this observation period. A dose of 20 mg/kg subcutaneously resulted in a significant decrease in blood pressure and pulse rate 120 minutes after the injection to five 16 to 21 week old SHRs. No significant changes were seen during the prior 5, 30 and 60 minute periods.

Dextro-Propranolol. In order to investigate whether or not the observed effects of racemic propranolol might be partially explained by the activity of the (+)-isomer, experiments were performed with this substance which has been reported to have from 2 to 10 per cent of the beta-blocking activity of the racemic mixture or (−)-isomer of the drug [37–39]. The (+)-isomer possesses the same local anesthetic-like activity of the racemic compound, however [38].

A dose of 5 mg/kg, subcutaneously, of (+)-propranolol caused no significant change in systolic blood pressure in six mature SHRs with a mean systolic pressure of 230 ± 11 mm Hg. In contrast to the effects of racemic propranolol, no exacerbation of the hypertensive state was seen with the (+)-isomer. A significant decrease in pulse rate was observed, however, over the 60 minute period of observation (Table VI). In age-matched normotensive WKY controls, a 5 mg/kg subcutaneous dose of the (+)-isomer failed to significantly alter the systolic blood pressure at those times when pulse rate was significantly lowered (Table VI).

4-Hydroxypropranolol. This substance is the main metabolite of propranolol in both animals and man [40]. It has been postulated to have an important role in the antihypertensive effect of propranolol, since the metabolite possesses similar beta-adrenergic blocking potency compared to the parent compound [41]. The metabolite has been found to have some intrinsic sympathomimetic action, as well as membrane stabilizing action [41,42].

A dose of 5 mg/kg, subcutaneously, produced a

TABLE V Effect of Sotalol (100 mg/kg, subcutaneously) on Systolic Blood Pressure and Pulse Rate of Five 25 to 28 Week Old SHRs

		Minutes After Administration of Drug			
Parameter	Control	5′	30′	60′	120′
Blood pressure (mm Hg)	177 ± 3	182 ± 4	177 ± 2	174 ± 2	165* ± 2
Pulse rate (beats/min)	361 ± 6	309† ± 4	283† ± 7	271† ± 6	267† ± 3

* $p < 0.01$.
† $p < 0.001$.

TABLE VI Effect of (+)-Propranolol (5 mg/kg, subcutaneously) on Systolic Blood Pressure and Pulse Rate of Six Mature SHRs and WKY Controls

			Minutes After Administration of Drug		
Parameter	Control		5′	30′	60′
Blood pressure (mm Hg)	230 ± 11	SHR	232 ± 7	231 ± 5	231 ± 6
	118 ± 3	WKY	118 ± 5	120 ± 4	119 ± 3
Pulse rate (beats/min)	382 ± 20	SHR	343* ± 18	325† ± 12	329* ± 10
	329 ± 19	WKY	291‡ ± 15	291‡ ± 14	300§ ± 21

* $p < 0.02$.
† $p < 0.05$.
‡ $p < 0.01$.
§ $p < 0.05$.

significant pressor response in mature (28 to 32 week old) SHRs. Thus, at 5 and 30 minutes after the injection, there was a 20 and 14 mm Hg increase in systolic blood pressure, respectively, above the control value (193 ± 5 mm Hg). In nine animals, this pressor response was associated with a significant decrease in pulse rate from the values that existed before the drug was given (mean = 362 ± 9 beats/min). The same dose administered to six age-matched WKY controls produced a similar significant reduction in pulse rate at 30 to 60 minutes. There was no significant change in systolic blood pressure in these animals, however, over the 60 minute period of observation.

Practolol. This agent was the first reported cardioselective beta-adrenergic blocker [43]. It also possesses significant antihypertensive action in man [44–46]. It is less potent than propranolol as a beta-blocker, having some degree of sympathomimetic action with little or no local anesthetic or membrane stabilizing effects [43].

Tested in six 32 to 44 week old SHRs, at a dose of 5 mg/kg subcutaneously, this drug did not cause a statistically significant change in systolic blood pressure over a 60 minute period of measurement compared to control values. Pulse rate tended to be lower at all periods of measurement but was only barely (P = 0.05) significant at 30 minutes after administration of the drug.

When administered in drinking water to five 52 week old SHRs and five age-matched WKY controls, daily consumption of 70 to 85 mg/kg failed to significantly affect the systolic blood pressures in either group over a 14 day period. Pulse rates in both groups also were not affected significantly with the dose and treatment schedule used.

Oxprenolol. This substance is nearly equipotent with propranolol; it does not have cardioselectivity, yet it has some intrinsic sympathomimetic effects [47,48]. Given in a dose of 10 mg/kg subcutaneously to five 32 to 44 week old SHRs, the drug produced an immediate and sustained decrease in pulse rate that was significant 5, 30 and 60 minutes after injection. For the same time intervals, systolic blood pressure levels in these animals were significantly elevated above the control values obtained before the drug was given (mean systolic = 196 ± 9 mm Hg). The peak increase in pressure was 23 mm Hg above the control value.

Nine mature (56 to 76 week old) SHRs were treated with a daily dose of 4 mg/kg administered in drinking water. At the end of three weeks, there was a slight but insignificant increase in systolic blood pressure above the control values. Pulse rate was significantly lower during the second and third week of the observation period. Age-matched WKY controls that received the same dosage over the same period showed no significant change in systolic blood pressure, whereas their pulse rate was reduced.

Increasing the estimated daily drug consumption to 40 mg/kg for a two week period produced a further increase in systolic blood pressure in the SHRs, whereas in WKY controls the blood pressure levels were essentially unchanged from those seen with the end of the treatment with the smaller dose. Pulse rate changes in both SHRs and WKY controls following two weeks of treatment with the 40 mg/kg/day dose were insignificant compared to the values measured at the end of treatment with the small dose.

KO-1366 and KO-1313. The benzonitrile compound KO-1313 has been described as being equipotent with propranolol as a beta-blocker [49,50]. In contrast, the congener KO-1366 is approximately 10 times more potent than propranolol as a beta-blocker [50–52].

Administered subcutaneously at a dose of 0.05 mg/kg to 24 to 40 week old SHRs, KO-1366 produced a marked and significant pressor effect. This effect was associated with a significant reduction in pulse rate. When a dose of 0.1 mg/kg subcutaneously was tried in another group of 20 to 32 week old SHRs, the drug caused death in four of the seven animals tested. Death occurred from 30 to 120 minutes after injection of the drug. No significant changes in the pulse rate or blood pressure were observed in any of the seven animals 5 minutes after the injection, or in the surviving animals when measured 30 and 60 minutes after the injection (Table VII).

In a dose of 0.1 mg/kg, given subcutaneously, KO-1313 produced no significant effects on systolic blood pressure in six mature SHRs even though the pulse rate was significantly decreased during the 5 to 60 minute period of observation (Table VIII).

Seven age-matched WKY controls showed no significant changes in either systolic blood pressure or pulse rate when given subcutaneous injections of 0.1 mg/kg KO-1366. No deaths were observed in this group. Similarly, KO-1313, administered subcutaneously in a dose of 0.1 mg/kg, produced no significant changes in blood pressure or pulse rate in six WKY controls (mean age = 30 weeks).

Saline Solution Treated and Untreated Controls. Four mature (52 week old) SHRs with a mean control systolic blood pressure of 225 ± 8 mm Hg showed no significant changes in pulse rate or blood pressure over an observation period of 2 hours when given saline solution or drug solvent subcutaneously in volumes used in active drug experiments. Changes in blood pressure ranged from −4 per cent to +5 per cent from the values obtained before they received any injections. No deaths occurred.

Five 12 week old SHRs allowed tap water over a period of time comparable to the two week metoprolol oral treatment trial showed a progressive increase in systolic blood pressure as expected. Thus, at the end of two weeks, the mean systolic blood pressure in these animals was 13 per cent higher than at the start of the observation period. This increase was statistically significant. Pulse rate, although slightly higher than at the start of the observation period, was not significantly different. For the older, mature (48 to 62 week old) SHRs, neither systolic blood pressure nor pulse rate changed significantly during an observation period of three weeks during which they had free access to normal tap water used to dissolve drugs used in oral treatment experiments. This indicates the stability of these measurements in the mature animal under the conditions of the experiments.

COMMENTS

Of the 11 substances tested under the conditions of the present experiments, pindolol, metoprolol and, to a lesser degree, alprenolol and sotalol decreased systolic blood pressure in SHRs. With the doses used, subcutaneous and/or oral administration of the other agents either had no effect or increased arterial pressure. The blood pressure lowering effect of pindolol and metoprolol was not seen in age-matched normotensive WKY controls. This suggests a basic difference between SHRs and WKY controls in regards to beta-adrenergic mechanisms that participate in regulating arterial blood pressure. However, there does not appear to be any significant difference in the beta-adrenergic receptor responses of cardiac muscle from SHRs and normotensive rats [53].

The pressor effects of beta-blockers seen in our series have been described by other investigators using not only SHRs [8–10] but other models of hypertension [54]. Yet, under certain circumstances, these drugs have been shown to reduce blood pressure in both SHRs and rats with other forms of experimentally-induced hypertension [54–56]. Often, the doses of propranolol required to produce an antihypertensive effect in these animals is extraordinarily large (e.g., 60 or 75 mg/kg/day, orally) [11,14] compared with the doses that lower blood pressure in man (2 to 6 mg/kg orally).

In the present study, the doses selected are capable of producing the expected decrease in pulse rate. Propranolol's antihypertensive action in the SHR and man has been reported to be independent of changes in the heart rate [12,14,57]. The present data indicate that agents such as alprenolol, sotalol, metoprolol, (+)-propranolol, 4-hydroxypropranolol, oxprenolol, KO-1313 and KO-1366 may cause an immediate, significant and persistent reduction in the pulse rate of SHRs; yet no parallel or consistent lowering of systolic blood pressure was observed. This suggests and confirms that the negative chronotropic effects of these drugs are separable from their ability (or predictability) to produce an antihypertensive action [4,5,7,9,12–14].

The *dextro*-isomer of propranolol did not produce either a pressor or depressor response in SHRs or WKY controls. In both groups, however, a significant decrease in pulse rate was observed. This emphasizes that the *dextro*-isomer of propranolol is not totally devoid of beta-blocking activity [37–38]. The *dextro*-isomer is also capable of suppressing renin release from the dog kidney [58].

The presence of cardioselective beta-blocking properties does not appear to be a prerequisite for antihypertensive action. Metoprolol may be effective in lowering blood pressure in SHRs under certain conditions of dose, route of administration and treatment schedule. The doses required for this action are many

TABLE VII Effect of KO-1366 on Systolic Blood Pressure and Pulse Rate of Seven SHRs

Dose (mg/kg, subcutaneously)	Control	Minutes After Administration of Drug 5′	30′	60′
		Blood Pressure (mm Hg)		
0.05	206 ± 8	226* ± 18	235† ± 10	240† ± 9
0.10§	203 ± 7	207‡ ± 10	218‡ ± 16	191‡ ± 29
		Pulse Rate (beats/min)		
0.05	419 ± 18	376* ± 15	348* ± 9	329‖ ± 9
0.10§	378 ± 23	346‡ ± 9	356‡ ± 8	327‡ ± 23

* $p < 0.02$.
† $p < 0.01$.
‡ $p > 0.05$.
§ Four deaths at 30 to 120 minutes after administration of the drug.
‖ $p < 0.05$.

TABLE VIII Effect of KO-1313 (0.1 mg/kg, subcutaneously) on Systolic Blood Pressure (mm Hg) and Pulse Rate (beats/min) of Six Mature SHRs

Parameter	Control	Minutes After Administration of the Drug 5′	30′	60′
Blood pressure (mm Hg)	202 ± 12	203* ± 14	210* ± 14	198* ± 16
Pulse rate (beats/min)	361 ± 19	328† ± 11	329† ± 9	315† ± 6

* $p > 0.05$.
† $p < 0.05$.

times higher than those reported to be effective in man [15,59]. This discrepancy may be due to the unique metabolism of the drug in rats [60]. Other explanations are not excluded.

Practolol, on the other hand, was ineffective in lowering blood pressure in the SHR with the doses and treatment schedule used. This cardioselective beta-blocker has been shown to be an effective antihypertensive drug in man [44–46]. The doses used to produce this clinical effect are difficult to reconcile with the drug's action as a selective cardiac beta$_1$-adrenergic receptor blocking agent [61].

Absolute beta-blocking potency also provides no important clue as to the critical feature underlying the ability to lower blood pressure in SHRs. For example, agents such as pindolol and KO-1366, which are more potent than propranolol, differ in their effects on the SHR. Pindolol was capable of lowering blood pressure levels significantly when administered subcutaneously, whereas propranolol and KO-1366 exacerbated the hypertension in the animals tested. Others have reported a similar discrepancy between their beta-blocking potency and ability to lower arterial blood pressure in rodent hypertension models [62–64].

Several of the agents (e.g., pindolol, practolol, alprenolol, KO-1313 and KO-1366) chosen for study have significant intrinsic sympathomimetic actions. Pindolol and alprenolol lowered blood pressure levels when given in small doses, whereas practolol, KO-1313 and KO-1366 either had no effect or increased arterial blood pressure. It appears that sympathomimetic properties of these agents do not predict antihypertensive effects in SHRs.

The influence of the age of the animals used on the responses obtained are best exemplified by the differences seen with propranolol and metoprolol. Although the doses of propranolol used were pressor in mature SHRs, administration of the drug failed to significantly affect blood pressure in 25 to 28 week old SHRs or in young prehypertensive SHRs. In both of these latter groups, the drug produced its expected negative chronotropic effect. The pressor effect of propranolol has been reported by others using SHRs and normal rats of varying ages, and different doses and route of administration [9,65,66]. The long-term administration of sotalol to young SHRs did not prevent the development of the hyptertensive state [7]. Mature SHRs appear invulnerable to the antihypertensive effects of propranolol and metoprolol even when given in doses of 100 mg/kg/24 hours [5]. Younger (2.5 months) SHRs given propranolol or metoprolol treatment until eight months of age showed blood pressure levels in the prehypertensive range, indicating a significant attenuation of the expected increase in arterial pressure.

One may also consider the importance of the sex of the animals used. In this investigation, only males were studied. The failure (or ability) of the drugs to affect blood pressure in SHRs might be sex-dependent. In one instance, female SHRs were shown to be responsive to the administration of metoprolol for seven months [67]. No comparative data for age-matched males were available for comparison, however. At the present time, there is no theoretical reason for suspecting that differences in blood pressure response to various beta-blockers (or other antihypertensive drugs?) are sex-linked. Practically, however, it is well documented that the male SHR shows a much more severe hypertensive state than a comparably aged female SHR [2]. Other important physiologic differences between developing male and female SHRs have been described [2,68–70]. There is no compelling evidence to suggest that the efficiency of beta-blockers as antihypertensive drugs in human subjects is dependent on the sex of the patient.

Is the success or failure of the beta-blocking agents used in SHRs related to their ability to affect plasma renin activity (PRA)? SHRs show a complex pattern of PRA changes with age [9,71–74]. Propranolol's antihypertensive effect in many patients has been related to its ability to suppress PRA [75,76]. Other beta-blockers that are antihypertensive in man have been reported to do the same [31,77]. However, pindolol, which was effective in the present series of experiments, actually causes an increase in PRA in animals and hypertensive patients [29–31]. This effect is not blocked by propranolol and is apparently related to the intrinsic sympathomimetic action of the drug. Other agents, such as alprenolol or practolol, have inconsistent effects on PRA [30,45]. It may be prudent not to select a beta-blocker for its potential as an antihypertensive agent in man solely on the basis of its ability to lower PRA [78].

Finally, one may speculate on the value of the SHR as a model for screening potential antihypertensive beta-blockers. Based on the results of the present series, and the conflicting reports from other laboratories, it seems that prediction of antihypertensive action of beta-blockers in man from studies of SHRs may be difficult. This is not to completely negate the value of the SHR in pharmacologic screening, since certain beta-blockers and many other classes of antihypertensive drugs are consistently effective in this model. What is at issue is the relationship between beta-blocking properties and the ability to lower blood pressure in SHRs, under any given experimental condition. The fact that the doses required, or treatment schedule, or route of administration are often difficult to relate to the clinical situation, prompts the observation that the SHR be used with some reservation in screening and evaluating potential antihypertensive beta-blockers.

The results presented here and elsewhere [8] certainly emphasize the probability of false-negative results being obtained in this model. Perhaps, it might be wiser to accept the view that once a drug has been characterized as possessing beta-adrenergic blocking properties, it might be evaluated for its antihypertensive action in man, and thus minimize the chances of missing an active agent. Other rodent models besides the SHR do not seem to offer much better performance characteristics insofar as predicting or evaluating antihypertensive potential.

Sir George Pickering probably did not have the beta-blockers in mind when he made the statement that ". . . whereas the experimental production of hypertension in animals has yielded results of the greatest interest, its relevance to human disease is, in many instances, still not established" [79]. Nonetheless, his observations may be particularly well suited to the current complexities of the effects of the beta-blockers in the SHR.

ACKNOWLEDGMENT

The following people kindly supplied the drugs used in this investigation: Dr. R. Davies (Ayerst Laboratories, Montreal); Dr. A. Engelhardt (Boehringer and Sohn, Ingelheim); Dr. B. Ablad (AB Hassle, Sweden); Dr. J. Trapold (Sandoz Laboratories, New Jersey); Dr. W. Darrow (Ciba, Summit, New Jersey); Dr. Carl Hansen of the National Institutes of Health provided the breeder animals from which the SHR and WKY colonies were developed.

REFERENCES

1. Okamoto K, Aoki K: Development of a strain of spontaneously hypertensive rats. Jap Circ J 27: 282, 1963.
2. Okamoto K (ed): Spontaneous Hypertension. Tokyo, Igaku Shoin Ltd., Berlin, Heidelberg, New York, Springer-Verlag, 1972.
3. Tobian LJ Jr: Experimental models for the study of hypertension. Hosp Practice 9: 99, 1974.
4. Numao Y, Iriuchijima J: Effects of alpha and beta blockers on hemodynamics of SHR. Jap Heart J 15: 166, 1974.
5. Weiss L, Lundgren Y, Folkow B: Effects of prolonged treatment with adrenergic β-receptor antagonists on blood pressure, cardiovascular design and reactivity in spontaneously hypertensive rats (SHR). Acta Physiol Scand 91: 447, 1974.
6. Weiss L: Aspects of the relation between functional and structural cardiovascular factors in primary hypertension. Acta Physiol Scand 92 (suppl 409): 1, 1974.
7. Pfeffer MA, Frohlich ED, Pfeffer JM, et al.: Pathophysiological implications of the increased cardiac output of young spontaneously hypertensive rats. Circ Res 34-35 (suppl): I-235, 1974.
8. Tabei R, Spector S, Louis WJ, et al.: Effects of antihypertensive drugs in the spontaneously hypertensive rat. Clin Pharmacol Ther 11: 269, 1970.
9. Forman BH, Mulrow PJ: Effect of propranolol on blood pressure and plasma renin activity in the spontaneously hypertensive rat. Circ Res 35: 215, 1974.
10. Levy JV: Blood pressure changes in mature spontaneously hypertensive rats (SHR) following orally and subcutaneously administered beta-adrenergic receptor blocking drugs. Proceedings of the Sixth International Congress of Pharmacology, Helsinki, July 1975, p 569.
11. Lee DR, Simpson FO: Effect of propranolol on blood pressure, heart rate and exchangeable sodium in genetically hypertensive and normotensive rats. Proceedings of the University of Otago Medical School 51: 51, 1973.
12. Vavra I, Tom H, Greselin E: Chronic propranolol treatment in young spontaneously hypertensive and normotensive rats. Can J Physiol Pharmacol 51: 727, 1973.
13. Scriabine A, Ludden CT, Bohidar NR: Potentiation of the antihypertensive action of hydralazine by timolol in spontaneously hypertensive rats. Proc Soc Exp Biol Med 146: 509, 1974.
14. Roba J, Lambelin G, De Schaepdryver AF: Antihypertensive activity of four β blocking agents in spontaneously hypertensive rats. Arch Int Pharmacodyn Ther 200: 182, 1972.
15. Ablad B, Borg KO, Carlsson E, et al.: Animal and human pharmacological studies on metoprolol—a new selective adrenergic β_1 receptor antagonist. Acta Pharmacol Toxicol (Kbh) 36 (suppl 5): 1, 1975.
16. Wellens D, Snoeckx L, De Reese R, et al.: Antihypertensive activity of erythro1-{1-[2-(1,4-Benzodioxan-2-yl)-2-OH-ET]-4-Piperidyl}-2-Benzimidazolinone (R 28935). Arch Int Pharmacodyn Ther 215: 119, 1975.
17. Ebihara A, Martz BL: Comparative effects of currently available antihypertensive agents on spontaneously and renal hypertensive rats. Am J Med Sci 259: 257, 1970.
18. Freis ED, Ragan D, Pillsbury H, et al.: Alteration of the course of hypertension in the spontaneously hypertensive rat. Circ Res 31: 1, 1972.
19. Leach BE, Armstrong FB Jr, Germain GS, et al.: Vasodepressor action of prostaglandins A_2 and E_2 in the spontaneously hypertensive rat (SH rat): evidence for an action mediated by the vagus. J Pharmacol Exp Ther 185: 479, 1973.
20. Sen S, Tarazi RC, Khairallah PA, et al.: Cardiac hypertrophy in spontaneously hypertensive rats. Circ Res 35, 775, 1974.
21. Kohler C, Berkowitz BA, Spector S: Antihypertensive drugs and catecholamine metabolism: effects of reserpine and hydralazine on tyrosine hydroxylase activity and norepinephrine concentrations in the spontaneously hypertensive rat. J Pharmacol Exp Ther 193: 443, 1975.
22. Garvey HL, Ram N: Comparative antihypertensive effects and tissue distribution of beta adrenergic blocking drugs. J Pharmacol Exp Ther 194: 220, 1975.
23. Akashi A, Chiba T, Kasahara A: Antihypertensive activity of 1-[2-(1,3-Dimethyl-2-Butenylidene)- Hydrazino]-Phthalazine (DJ-1461), a new phthalazine derivative. Eur J Pharmacol 29: 161, 1974.
24. Hansen CT: Personal communication.
25. Levy JV: Cardiovascular effects of LB-46 (Prindolol), a potent beta-adrenergic receptor antagonist. J Clin Pharmacol 11: 249, 1971.
26. Lubawski I, Wale J: Studies with LB 46, a new β-receptor blocking drug. Eur J Pharmacol 6: 345, 1969.
27. Moore GE, O'Donnell SR: A potent β-adrenoreceptor blocking drug: 4-(2-hydroxy-3-isopropylaminopropoxy) indole. J Pharm Pharmacol 22: 180, 1970.
28. Giudicelli JF, Schmitt H, Boissler JR: Studies on dl-4-(2-hydroxy-3-isopropylaminopropoxy) indole (LB 46), a new potent beta adrenergic blocking drug. J Pharmacol Exp Ther 168: 116, 1969.
29. Anavekar SN, Louis WJ, Morgan TO, et al.: The relationship

of plasma levels of pindolol in hypertensive patients to effects on blood pressure, plasma renin and plasma noradrenaline levels. Clin Exp Pharmacol Physiol 2: 203, 1975.
30. Weber MA, Stokes GS, Gain JM: Comparison of the effects on renin release of beta adrenergic antagonists with differing properties. J Clin Invest 54: 1413, 1974.
31. Weber MA, Thornell IR, Stokes GS: Effects of beta adrenergic blocking agents on plasma renin activity in the conscious rabbit. J Pharmacol Exp Ther 188: 234, 1974.
32. Ablad B, Borg KF, Carlsson E, et al.: A survey of the pharmacological properties of metoprolol in animals and man. Acta Pharmacol Toxicol 36 (suppl 5): 7, 1975.
33. Levy JV, Richards V: Inotropic and metabolic effects of three beta-adrenergic receptor blocking drugs on isolated rabbit left atria. J Pharmacol Exp Ther 150: 361, 1965.
34. Stanton HC, Kirchgessner T, Parmenter K: Cardiovascular pharmacology of two new β-adrenergic receptor antagonists. J Pharmacol Exp Ther 149: 174, 1965.
35. Lish PM, Shelanski MV, LaBudde JA, et al.: Inhibition of cardiac chronotropic action of isoproterenol by sotalol (MJ 1999) in rat, dog and man. Curr Ther Res 9: 311, 1967.
36. Ablad B: Pharmacological studies on H 56/28 (1-(o-allylphenoxy)-3-isopropylamino-2-propanol)—A new β-adrenergic receptor antagonist. Acta Pharmacol Toxicol 25 (suppl 2): 5, 1967.
37. Levy JV, Richards V: Inotropic and chronotropic effects of a series of β-adrenergic blocking drugs. Some structure-activity relationships. Proc Soc Exp Biol Med 122: 373, 1966.
38. Levy JV: Myocardial and local anesthetic actions of β-adrenergic receptor blocking drugs. Relationship to physicochemical properties. Eur J Pharmacol 2: 250, 1968.
39. Howe R, Shanks R: Optical isomers of propranolol. Nature (Lond) 210: 1336, 1966.
40. Patterson JW, Conolly ME, Dollerg CT, et al.: The pharmacodynamics and metabolism of propranolol in man. Pharmacol Clin 2: 127, 1970.
41. Fitzgerald JD, O'Donnell SR: Pharmacology of 4-hydroxypropranolol, a metabolite of propranolol. Br J Pharmacol 43: 222, 1971.
42. Fitzgerald JD, O'Donnell SR: A comparison of the haemodynamic effects of propranolol, 4-hydroxypropranolol and practolol in anaesthetized dogs. Br J Pharmacol 45: 207, 1972.
43. Dunlop D, Shanks RG: Selective blockade of adrenoceptive beta receptors in the heart. Br J Pharmacol 32: 201, 1968.
44. Prichard BN, Boakes AJ, Day G: Practolol in the treatment of hypertension. Postgrad Med J 47 (suppl 1): 84, 1971.
45. Esler MD: Effect of practolol on blood presssure and renin release in man. Clin Pharmacol Ther 15: 484, 1974.
46. Sundquist H, Anttila M, Arstila M: Antihypertensive effects of practolol and sotalol. Clin Pharmacol Ther 16: 465, 1974.
47. Brunner H, Hedwall PR, Maier R, et al.: Pharmacological aspects of oxprenolol. Postgrad Med J 46 (suppl): 5, 1970.
48. Barrett AM, Carter J: Comparative chronotropic activity of β-adrenoceptive antagonists. Br J Pharmacol 40: 373, 1970.
49. Engelhardt A, Traunecker W: Pharmacology of some phenoxypropranolamine derivatives with beta-adrenergic blocking action. Paper presented at 31st Meeting of German Pharmacological Society, Dusseldorf, September 26, 1968.
50. Mylecharane EJ, Raper C: Nitrilophenoxypropranolamines. Influence of ring substitution on β-receptor blockade. Eur J Pharmacol 29: 93, 1974.
51. Nayler WG, Tay J: Effect of o-2-hydroxy-3-(tert.-butylamino) propoxybenzonitrile HCL (KO 1366) on beta adrenergic receptors in the cardiovascular system. J Pharmacol Exp Ther 180: 302, 1972.
52. Miyahara M, Fujise Y, Osanai S, et al.: Influence of the β-adrenergic blocking drug Ko-1366 on haemodynamics in healthy volunteers and patients with ischaemic heart disease. Jap Heart J 15: 455, 1974.
53. Antonaccio MJ, Cavaliere T: A comparison of the effects of some inotropic and chronotropic agents on isolated atria from normotensive (NTR) and spontaneously hypertensive (SHR) rats. Arch Int Pharmacodyn Ther 209: 273, 1974.
54. Dusting GJ, Rand MJ: An antihypertensive action of propranolol in DOCA/salt-treated rats. Clin Exp Pharm Physiol 1: 87, 1974.
55. Brunner H, Hedwall PR, Meier M: Influence of an adrenergic β-receptor blocking agent on the effect of various hypotensive agents in the hypertensive rat. Experientia 21: 1, 1965.
56. Karppanen H: Effect of propranolol on the blood pressure of normotensive and pinealectomized hypertensive rats. Arch Pharmacol 281: 1, 1974.
57. Wall HJ: Hypotensive action of propranolol. Clin Pharmacol Ther 7: 588, 1966.
58. Kopp U, Aurell M, Fellenius E, et al.: The effect of β-receptor blockers on renin release induced by sympathetic nerve stimulation in the anaesthetized dog. Proceedings of the VIth International Congress of Pharmacology, Helsinki, July 1975, p 111.
59. Bengtsson C, Johnsson G, Regardh CG: Plasma levels and effects of metoprolol on blood pressure and heart rate in hypertensive patients after an acute dose and between doses during long-term treatment. Clin Pharmacol Ther 17: 400, 1975.
60. Bodin NO, Borg KO, Johansson R, et al.: Tissue distribution of metoprolol-(^{3}H) in the mouse and the rat. Acta Pharmacol Toxicol 36 (suppl 5): 116, 1975.
61. Lertora JJ, Mark AL, Johannsen UJ, et al.: Effects of oral practolol on vascular beta receptors in man. Clin Res 22: 598A, 1974.
62. Menard J, Alexandre JM, Giudicelli JF, et al.: Lack of antihypertensive effects of chronic administration of dl-propranolol in Grollman rats. Arch Int Pharmacol Ther 202: 298, 1973.
63. Douglas JR, Johnson EM, Marshall GR, et al.: Development and maintenance of renal hypertension in normal and guanethidine sympathectomized rats. Circ Res 36-37 (suppl 1): 1-171, 1975.
64. Lundgren Y: Blood pressure and vascular design in renal hypertension in rats after prolonged propranolol treatment. Acta Physiol Scand 91: 409, 1974.
65. Yamamoto J, Sekiya A: Further studies on the pressor action of propranolol in the rat. Arch int Pharmacol Ther 198: 347, 1972.
66. Yamamoto J, Sekiya A: Differences in the cardiac and pressor responses to propranolol of rats and guinea pigs. Jap J Pharmacol 24: 253, 1974.
67. Ablad B, Dahlof C, Henning M, et al.: Is the antihypertensive effect of beta blockade related to an impaired vasoconstrictor nerve function? Proceedings of the VIth International Congress of Pharmacology, Helsinki, July 1975, p 110.
68. Albrecht I: The hemodynamics of early stages of spontaneous hypertension in rats. I. Male study. Jap Circ J 38: 985, 1974.
69. Tobia AJ, Walsh GM, Lee JY: Hemodynamic alterations in the young spontaneously hypertensive rat. Elevated total systemic and hindquarter vascular resistance. Proc Soc Exp Biol Med 146: 670, 1974.
70. Albrecht I: Critical period for the development of spontaneous hypertension in rats. Mechanisms of Aging and Development, vol 3, 1974, p 75.

71. Jong W, Lovenberg W, Sjoerdsma A: Increased plasma renin activity in the spontaneously hypertensive rat. Proc Soc Exp Biol Med 139: 1213, 1972.
72. Sen S, Smeby RR, Bumpus FM: Renin in rats with spontaneous hypertension. Circ Res 31: 876, 1972.
73. Campbell WB: Renin in the spontaneously hypertensive rat. Circ Res 35: 961, 1974.
74. Sinaiko A, Mirkin BL: Ontogenesis of the renin-angiotensin system in spontaneously hypertensive and normal Wistar rats. Circ Res 34: 693, 1974.
75. Bühler FR, Laragh JH, Vaughan ED, et al.: Antihypertensive action of propranolol. Am J Cardiol 32: 511, 1973.
76. Hansson L: Beta-adrenergic blockade in essential hypertension. Acta Med Scand 194 (suppl 550): 5, 1973.
77. Kuramoto K, Kurihara H, Murata K, et al.: Hemodynamic effects and variations in plasma renin activity after single oral administration of oxprenolol. Cardiology (Basel) 59: 41, 1974.
78. Hansson L, Zweifler AJ, Julius S, et al.: Propranolol therapy in essential hypertension. Observations on predictability of therapeutic response. Int J Clin Pharmacol 10: 79, 1974.
79. Pickering GW: High Blood Pressure, New York, Grune & Stratton, 1955, p 85.

Estimating Renin Participation in Hypertension: Superiority of Converting Enzyme Inhibitor Over Saralasin

DAVID B. CASE, M.D.
JOHN M. WALLACE, M.D.*
HANS J. KEIM, M.D.†
MICHAEL A. WEBER, M.D.
JAN I. M. DRAYER, M.D.
ROBERT P. WHITE, M.D.
JEAN E. SEALEY, D.Sc.
JOHN H. LARAGH, M.D.
New York, New York

This study was designed to examine more closely the differences in blood pressure responses in hypertensive patients to two agents which block the renin-angiotensin system. Accordingly, 39 seated patients received under the same conditions both saralasin, an octapeptide competitive antagonist of angiotensin II, and the nonapeptide converting enzyme inhibitor, SQ20881, which blocks the generation of angiotensin II from angiotensin I. A second component of the study involved administration of these agents in 10 additional studies in anephric subjects.

Although both agents produced maximal responses in blood pressure that correlated well with each other ($p < 0.001$) and with the pretreatment plasma renin levels ($p < 0.001$), analysis of the results by renin subgroups revealed significant differences. Thus, both drugs lowered the diastolic pressures of patients with high renin levels, but converting enzyme inhibitor produced changes of greater amplitude ($p < 0.05$). In contrast, saralasin was consistently pressor in both patients with low renin levels and anephric patients in whom converting enzyme blockade produced no significant changes in blood pressure. Another impressive disparity in the responses to the two agents occurred in the group with normal renin levels in whom saralasin produced either neutral or pressor responses (mean change was $+2.0 \pm 1.5$ standard error of the mean (SEM) per cent control diastolic pressure) whereas the converting enzyme inhibitor consistently induced depressor responses (mean change was -10.2 ± 1.2 per cent, $p < 0.001$).

Altogether, the results suggest that converting enzyme inhibitor tests for angiotensin II-dependent blood pressure with more sensitivity than the partial agonist saralasin. Moreover, it is unlikely that the differences between the responses to the two agents were due to bradykinin accumulation, since depressor responses to converting enzyme inhibitor were not observed in the patients with low renin levels and the anephric patients.

The development of agents which specifically block angiotensin II has provided the opportunity to document involvement of the renin-angiotensin system in hypertension that was originally indicated by measurements of plasma renin activity [1,2] and by therapeutic re-

From the Cardiovascular Center, The New York Hospital-Cornell Medical Center, New York, New York. This study was supported by Grant HL-18323 from the National Institutes of Health. SQ20881 was supplied by E. R. Squibb & Sons, Inc., Princeton, New Jersey. Saralasin was supplied by Eaton Laboratories, Norwich, New York. Requests for reprints should be addressed to Dr. David B. Case, Cardiovascular Center, 525 East 68th Street, New York, New York 10021.

* Present address: University of Texas Medical Branch, Galveston, Texas 77550.

† Present address: Klinikum der Johannes Gutenberg Universität, 65 Mainz, Langenbeckstr. 1, West Germany.

sponses to drugs which activate or suppress this system [2,3]. Two different blocking agents have emerged for clinical use: one, an octapeptide competitive analogue of angiotensin II, 1-Sar, 8-Ala angiotensin II (saralasin) and the other, an inhibitor of kininase II, the enzyme which converts the decapeptide angiotensin I to angiotensin II (converting enzyme inhibitor).

In earlier studies, the infusion of saralasin blocked the pressor action of infused angiotensin II [4] and lowered the blood pressure in patients with high plasma renin activity, i.e., with renovascular [5–7], essential [5,7] or malignant hypertension [5,7]. However, the drug produced pressor effects in 50 per cent of the patients with normal plasma renin activity and in all the patients with low plasma renin activity [7], thereby characterizing in man the agonistic properties of the drug which were first observed in animal studies [8,9]. Thus, as a partial agonist of angiotensin II, it appeared likely that saralasin would underestimate true renin dependency.

On the other hand, recent studies with the nonapeptide converting enzyme inhibitor, SQ20881, did not reveal pressor activity, and depressor responses correlated well with pretreatment levels of plasma renin activity [10]. In the present study, 39 patients with different forms of hypertension were selected and given both saralasin and converting enzyme inhibitor under the same conditions. The results provide evidence that converting enzyme inhibitor testing is more sensitive in detecting angiotensin II dependency in hypertension than saralasin testing.

METHODS

Patients. After complete clinical examination, 39 hypertensive patients were selected to receive both saralasin acetate (1-Sar, 8-Ala angiotensin II, P113) and the nonapeptide converting enzyme inhibitor, SQ20881. They ranged in age from 16 to 57 years, and 25 were male. All patients had been previously profiled by the renin-sodium index [3] and had not received antihypertensive medication for three weeks prior to study. Of the six patients with low renin activity, two had primary aldosteronism, one bilateral renal artery stenosis and three essential hypertension. Of the 23 patients with normal renin activity, all had essential hypertension except one who had unilateral renal artery stenosis with collateral blood flow and symmetrical renal vein renin values. Four of the 10 patients with high renin activity had renal artery stenosis (one bilateral), two had malignant hypertension, and four had essential hypertension. In addition to these patients, six patients receiving long-term dialysis who had undergone bilateral nephrectomy were also studied with either one or both agents. All patients consented to be studied according to the procedures specified by the Human Rights in Research Committee of Cornell University Medical College-The New York Hospital.

Study Procedure. The studies were carried out with the patients seated in a comfortable lounge chair where a quiet, nondistracting atmosphere was maintained. Blood pressure was measured continuously either by Arteriosonde® (16 patients) set at 2 minute intervals or by direct arterial recordings (23 patients). All patients adhered to their normal sodium intake and collected a 24-hour urine sample which started on the day before study. Values for 24-hour sodium excretion were similar in each renin subgroup (Table I). After a stable period of 30 minutes, blood samples for the determination of plasma renin activity were drawn through a previously positioned indwelling venous catheter. Saralasin was then infused at the rate of 10 μg/kg/min for 30 minutes. Afterwards, following a period of at least 1 hour but less than 24 hours during which blood pressure returned to control levels, a second blood sample was drawn, and SQ20881 was administered as a slow intravenous bolus in the dose of 1 mg/kg. Plasma renin activity was measured according to the method of Sealey and Laragh [11]. Pretreatment plasma renin activity levels did not differ before the administration of either saralasin or SQ20881 (Table I) in any renin subgroup.

Analytical Methods. The control blood pressure for each patient was the average blood pressure over 20 minutes prior to blood sampling. Unless otherwise stated, the maximal change in diastolic pressure, expressed as a per cent of the control pressure, was used for analysis. These maximal deflections were obtained as averages over 4 to 6 minute periods only at 10, 20 or 30 minute intervals after administration of the drug. By analyzing the data in this manner, the initial pressor effect of saralasin reported previously [4,7] was excluded from analysis.

As appropriate in small samples, often without a normal distribution, nonparametric statistical methods were used to detect differences between two groups (Wilcoxon's two-sample test) and to calculate correlation coefficients between variables (Spearman's correlations coefficient). All results are expressed as the means ± SEM.

RESULTS

Responses of Renin Subgroups. When the patients were divided into groups according to their renin-sodium profiles, the blood pressure responses to each drug were significantly different in each subgroup (Figure 1). Whereas the administration of saralasin produced an 8.5 ± 2.9 per cent increase in blood pressure in patients with low renin activity, the response to the converting enzyme inhibitor was neutral, −1.2 ± 2.4 per cent ($p < 0.05$). In the group of patients with normal renin activity, saralasin infusion produced a minimal response in diastolic pressure (+2.0 ± 1.5 per cent), whereas after injection of the converting enzyme inhibitor, a 10.2 ± 1.2 per cent decline was observed ($p < 0.001$). Even in patients with high renin activity in whom depressor responses occurred after the administration of both drugs, the converting enzyme inhibitor produced slightly greater depressor responses than saralasin (−18.7 ± 1.9 per cent versus −13.6 ± 2.0 per cent, $p < 0.01$). Pretreatment plasma renin levels did not differ in each subgroup before the administration of the blocking agents (Figure 1 and Table I).

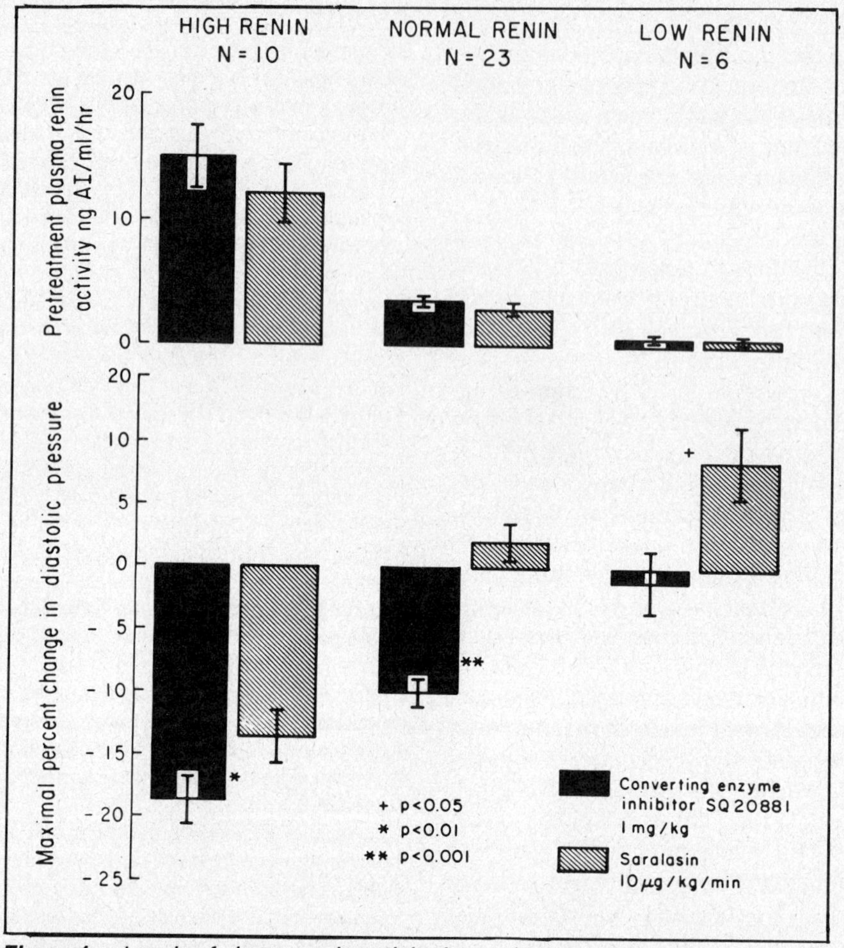

Figure 1. *Levels of plasma renin activity for each renin subgroup prior to angiotensin blockade (upper panel) and the maximal induced per cent change in diastolic pressure for each treatment group directly below (lower panel). Mean values ± standard error are shown for renin and blood pressure measurements.*

Relationship of Renin Levels to Blood Pressure Responses. When the maximal blood pressure deflections following the administration of each drug were compared relative to the pretreatment level of plasma renin activity, the decrements for any level of plasma renin activity were greater following the administration of the converting enzyme inhibitor than those following the administration of saralasin. However, the blood pressure depressor responses correlated well ($p < 0.001$ for both) with the pretreatment renin level. The differences in responses to the administration of these blocking drugs under matched conditions is represented in Figure 2. In this diagram, the consistent depressor responses to the administration of the converting enzyme inhibitor are aligned in descending magnitude (lower panel). The changes induced by the administration of saralasin in the same sequence of patients (upper panel) show a similar trend, but increasing numbers of pressor responses to saralasin occurred whereas depressor responses to converting enzyme inhibitor diminished.

TABLE I Pretreatment Renin Levels and Urinary Sodium Excretion

	No.	$U_{Na}V$ (meq/24 hr)	Control Plasma Renin Activity (ng AI/ml/hr): Before Saralasin		Before SQ20881
Low renin	6	115 ± 17	0.7 ± 0.2	NS	0.8 ± 0.3
Normal renin	23	124 ± 10	3.0 ± 0.5	NS	3.6 ± 0.4
High renin	10	103 ± 19	12.4 ± 2.3	NS	15.0 ± 2.5

NOTE: Plasma renin activity was measured in samples obtained immediately before drug was given. Values are means ± standard error. $U_{Na}V$ = 24-hour urinary sodium excretion; NS = not significant.

Effects of Saralasin and Converting Enzyme Inhibitor in Anephric Patients. In order to determine the effects of these drugs in patients in whom there is no circulating renin, the converting enzyme inhibitor and saralasin

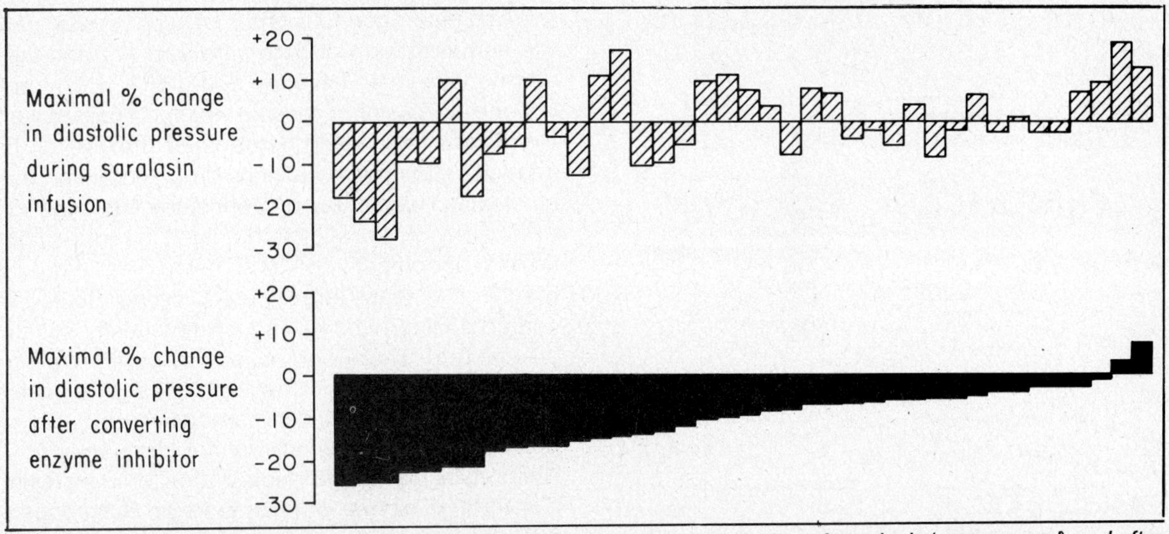

Figure 2. Maximal per cent change in diastolic pressure during the infusion of saralasin (upper panel) and after the administration of converting enzyme inhibitor (lower panel). Patients are aligned in the same sequence in both upper and lower panels according to the magnitude of their depressor responses to converting enzyme inhibitor.

were given to eight anephric patients, two of whom received both drugs. Saralasin in doses of 1 or 10 μg/kg/min was uniformly pressor in four studies (11.5 ± 1.5 per cent increase in diastolic pressure) (Table II). In contrast, SQ20881 produced no discernible trend in diastolic pressures, the mean change after 10 minutes being +2.3 ± 2.0 per cent, and after 20 minutes +1.3 ± 2.3 per cent. Blood pressures in these studies, measured by Arteriosonde, tended to be unstable.

Comparative Responses in Renovascular Patients. Since a major thrust of the diagnostic use of these drugs will be in screening procedures for renovascular hypertension, four matched studies using both agents are shown in detail in Figure 3. Arteriography in each of these patients subsequently revealed single or bilateral stenosis with high peripheral renin levels and lateralizing renal vein renin secretion. In each case, administration of the converting enzyme inhibitor produced slightly greater depressor responses, although both drugs consistently lowered blood pressure. None of these patients were sodium-restricted nor had they received diuretic pretreatment.

Data obtained in one patient presented in Table III is shown in greater detail in Figure 3. Of interest in this patient is that comparable depressor responses were obtained to the administration of both agents during the intake of very high and low salt diets.

COMMENTS

The diagnostic importance of renin levels in hypertensive disease is now well-established. The ability to separate hypertensive patients according to their native levels of plasma renin activity has provided physicians with a rationale for further diagnostic measures as well as for initial therapeutic measures [2]. Moreover, a refined classification system, relating renin levels to the state of sodium balance, i.e., the renin-sodium index, has evolved, establishing a range for normal subjects for renin values indexed against the daily urinary sodium excretion rate [3]. Implicit in this relationship is the fact that high levels of renin are normal and appropriate during sodium deprivation, but they become increasingly abnormal when the rate of sodium excretion is increased. The present study was conducted without

TABLE II Effect of Angiotensin Blockade in Anephric Patients

		Control Diastolic Pressure (mm Hg)	Change in Diastolic Pressure (mm Hg after) 10 min	20 min
I. Converting enzyme inhibitor SQ20881 (1 mg/kg)	A	72	−2	−6
	B	77	+11	+7
	C	82	−1	+3
	D	87	−1	−4
	E	91	+4	+8
	F	100	+3	0
Mean ± SE			+2.3 ± 2.0	+1.3 ± 2.3*
			15 min	
II. Saralasin (1 or 10 μg/kg/min)	G	62	+16	
	H	72	+10	
	F	89	+10	
	E	93	+10	
Mean ± SE			+11.5 ± 1.5	

*p <0.05 when compared to diastolic pressure change in patients receiving saralasin.

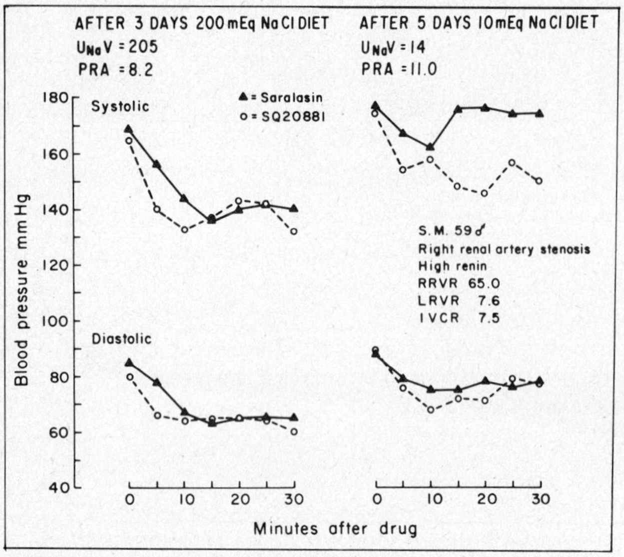

Figure 3. *The left panel shows comparable depressor responses in a patient with renovascular hypertension to both the administration of saralasin and converting enzyme inhibitor during high salt intake ($U_{Na}V$ = 205 meq/day). After five days of a 10 meq sodium chloride isocaloric diet, the control blood pressure (direct arterial recording) was slightly higher. Depressor responses of similar magnitude were observed.*

sodium depletion, so that responses would reflect renin involvement under normal dietary conditions.

Critical for the clinical application of angiotensin blocking agents is the understanding of how responses to these blockers correspond to this standard reference framework of the renin-angiotensin system, i.e., the renin-sodium index. In previous reports, we have shown that in a heterogeneous group of hypertensive patients, the administration of both saralasin [7] and the converting enzyme inhibitor SQ20881 [10] induced changes in diastolic pressure which correlated well with the plasma renin levels determined immediately before administration of the blocking drug. Moreover, in those studies and also in the present study, the experimental design closely paralleled that used in renin-sodium indexing, specifically, patients being free of drug treatment for at least three weeks, being studied in the seated position and having a known daily sodium excretion rate. Therefore, studies by other investigators in which patients were studied in the supine position or after furosemide-induced stimulation [5,6,12] of the renin-angiotensin system are not comparable.

Responses to the Administration of Saralasin and Converting Enzyme Inhibitor in Renin Subgroups. The findings in the 39 patients of the present study are congruent with our observations in larger groups of hypertensive subjects [7,10]. Saralasin was uniformly depressor only in subjects with high renin activity when administered during normal sodium intake. In contrast, the drug was pressor in patients with low renin activity and in nephrectomized patients who had no circulating renal renin. In patients with normal renin activity neutral or pressor responses occurred.

However, paired observations of saralasin and converting enzyme inhibitor-induced maximal responses were consistently different in the three renin subgroups. Indeed, the magnitude of depressor responses in the subjects with high renin activity was consistently greater with the administration of converting enzyme inhibitor. Moreover, whereas saralasin was agonistic in patients with low renin activity and in nephrectomized patients,

TABLE III Angiotensin Blockade in Patients with Renovascular Hypertension with High Plasma Renin Activity

					Lowest Blood Pressure After: (mm Hg)	
Case	Lesion	$U_{Na}V$ (meq/day)	Control PRA (ng/ml/hr)	Blood Pressure (mm Hg)	Saralasin (10 μg/kg/min)	Converting Enzyme Inhibitor (1 mg/kg)
1	Bilateral atherosclerotic renal artery stenosis, atrophic right kidney LRV = 7.1 RRV = 17 IVC = 6.1	148	7.1	230/118	205/107	191/89
2	Unilateral atherosclerotic renal artery stenosis LRV = 7.6 RRV = 65 IVC = 7.5	205	8.2	169/85	140/65	132/60
3	Unilateral fibromuscular hyperplasia of left renal artery and atrophy of left kidney LRV = 35 RRV = 11	103	13	172/119	151/97	139/84
4	Unilateral fibromuscular hyperplasia of right renal artery LRV = 7.6 RRV = 13.0 IVC = 7.2	63	26	184/113	154/100	158/96

NOTE: $U_{Na}V$ = 24-hour urinary sodium excretion; PRA = plasma renin activity; LRV = left renal vein renin; RRV = right renal vein renin; IVC = inferior vena cava renin.

the converting enzyme inhibitor induced no consistent response trends in these groups.

However, the most strikingly different responses to these two agents occurred in subjects with normal renin activity. In contrast to the neutral or pressor responses to saralasin, the administration of converting enzyme inhibitor consistently produced a 10 per cent decrease in diastolic pressure. Saralasin, apparently due to its properties as a partial agonist of angiotensin II, underestimates renin involvement, most critically in patients with normal renin activity. In fact, saralasin fails to identify a renin factor in this large group of patients, whereas under identical conditions, renin involvement is exposed by converting enzyme inhibitor.

Unlike converting enzyme inhibitor [10], our previous studies have shown that saralasin-induced responses can also be correlated with the state of sodium balance estimated by the rate of urinary sodium excretion [7]. Moreover, in a group of 13 patients in whom renin levels were similar and low, the induced pressor responses to the administration of saralasin also correlated with the rate of daily sodium excretion [7]. Altogether, these findings suggest that the state of sodium balance of a patient, perhaps even independent of its effect on the renin level, plays a determining role in the response to saralasin. The potential value of the response to saralasin as a determinant of the sodium or volume factor in hypertension remains to be fully explored.

Screening with Saralasin and Converting Enzyme Inhibitor for High Renin Hypertension. It is apparent from these results revealing good correspondence between responses to the administration of drugs and renin levels, and, consequently, separation of renin subgroups, that both of these agents have diagnostic value in screening hypertensive patients. When studied during normal sodium intake and in the upright position, only subjects with high renin activity exhibited depressor responses to saralasin. Therefore, in this context, saralasin infusion should reliably screen out the subgroup in which the majority of surgically remediable renovascular hypertension exists. Thus, as exemplified by the patient in Figure 4, a depressor response to the administration of saralasin may be achieved even when the study is conducted in the setting of a large sodium intake.

All patients with high renin activity had even greater depressor responses to the administration of the converting enzyme inhibitor than to saralasin (Figure 1). Administration of the converting enzyme inhibitor produced an 18.7 per cent decrease in diastolic pressure during normal sodium intake whereas saralasin induced only a 13.6 per cent decline. Moreover, converting enzyme inhibitor also identified angiotensin II involvement in normal-renin hypertensive patients by inducing depressor responses in 91 per cent of them as opposed to only 10 per cent with saralasin. Furthermore, the response to the converting enzyme inhibitor appears to assess angiotensin II participation in the level of blood pressure which is independent of the state of sodium balance, since in other studies involving larger numbers of patients, also unlike saralasin, there was no correlation between the blood pressure response to it and the rate of sodium excretion [10].

Is Renin Primarily Involved in the Hypertensive Process? The data from this study suggests a major role for renin in sustaining all or some part of the elevated blood pressure levels found in most normal and high-renin patients. Equally important, renin does not seem to be involved to any great extent in low-renin forms of hypertension under normal dietary conditions.

However, it should be clearly understood that, in the absence of parallel data in normotensive subjects, it may be premature to impugn renin as a primary causative factor in the hypertension of patients with normal-renin profiles. Thus, it is possible that renin participates to the same or to a greater or a lesser extent in supporting normotension. However, whatever the ultimate solution to this pathogenetic question, it is now clear that deletion of renin activity has diagnostic and therapeutic value in normal and high-renin patients.

Subtracting renin participation by using converting enzyme inhibitor did not always fully correct the hypertension in normal and high-renin subgroups. Although this latter observation may have resulted from incomplete blockade by this agent, it is also possible or likely that other factors may coparticipate in sustaining the hypertension.

Other investigators have raised the possibility that bradykinin accumulation may be involved in mediating the hypotensive response to converting enzyme inhibitor [13,14]. This matter cannot be settled by our present data. However, there are three cogent lines of evidence which argue against this possibility. The first is the good correlation between the depressor responses to the drug and the pretreatment renin levels. The second is the impressive parallelism between the results using converting enzyme inhibitor and saralasin, a drug not known to exert any effect on the kinin system. Thirdly, converting enzyme inhibition did not reduce blood pressure in either low-renin or anephric patients in whom renin levels are either low or absent.

Clinical Application of the Two Different Angiotensin Blockers. In view of the close correspondence between responses to angiotensin blocking agents and renin-sodium indices, it is pertinent to examine whether these technics are interchangeable. Angiotensin blockade may have some advantages over measurements of plasma renin activity. These are (1) the response is known in 10 to 20 minutes, as opposed to the delay involved in the radioimmunoassay, (2) it circumvents the problems involved in the methods of measuring plasma renin activity, and (3) it can be done in the office setting as easily as common endocrinologic stimulation/suppression tests. On the other hand, renin-sodium indexing takes into account the concurrent state of sodium balance which, in turn, provides a valid classification for the renin measurement. Moreover, indexing has the practical advantage of wider application since it is less time-consuming. Nonetheless, as larger numbers of patients are studied, it should be possible to establish nomograms relating response to angiotensin blocking agents to the rate of urinary sodium excretion. This latter technic should provide a physiologic renin-indexing that does not require measurement of plasma renin activity yet is interchangeable.

Of the two angiotensin blocking drugs available, converting enzyme inhibitor appears to have two advantages: (1) unlike saralasin it is not a partial agonist, a property which may obscure assessment of renin dependency and which may lead to potentially harmful pressor responses [15,16], and (2) converting enzyme inhibitor may be given as a single intravenous bolus, whereas saralasin probably should not be given in this way since an unexpected pressor response might be difficult to reverse.

Both agents may produce untoward hypotension, but this event seems limited to patients already receiving other antihypertensive and diuretic agents at the time of study [17,18] and in normal subjects on a tilt table after sodium depletion [13]. The treatment for this occurrence involves restoration of central blood volume by the infusion of saline solution, elevation of the legs and cessation of other antihypertensive agents. This complication underscores the recommendation that patients not be receiving other antihypertensive drugs (particularly vasodilators and diuretics), since these reactions have not been described otherwise.

In summary, direct comparison of a converting enzyme inhibitor and a partial agonist competitive inhibitor of angiotensin II reveals that both drugs may be used to assess renin dependency in hypertensive patients. However, the converting enzyme inhibitor appears more sensitive in exposing renin involvement in blood pressure maintenance at any level of plasma renin activity. Studies in anephric patients suggest that the converting enzyme inhibitor does not exert a nonspecific hypotensive action related to bradykinin accumulation.

REFERENCES

1. Kohlstaedt KG, Page IH: The liberation of renin by perfusion of kidneys following reduction of pulse pressure. J Exp Med 72: 201, 1940.
2. Laragh JH: Vasoconstriction-volume analysis for understanding and treating hypertension: the use of renin and aldosterone profiles. Am J Med 55: 261, 1973.
3. Laragh JH, Baer L, Brunner HR, et al.: Renin, angiotensin and aldosterone system in pathogenesis and management of hypertensive vascular disease. Am J Med 52: 633, 1972.
4. Pals DT, Masucci FD, Denning GS Jr, et al.: Role of the pressor action of angiotensin II in experimental hypertension. Circ Res 29: 673, 1971.
5. Brunner HR, Gavras H, Laragh JH: et al.: Hypertension in man: Exposure of the renin and sodium components using angiotensin II blockade. Circ Res 34 (suppl 1): I-35, 1974.
6. Streeten DHP, Anderson GH, et al.: Use of an angiotensin II antagonist (saralasin) in the recognition of "angiotensinogenic" hypertension. N Engl J Med 292: 657, 1975.
7. Case DB, Wallace JM, Keim HJ, et al.: Limitations and usefulness of saralasin, a partial competitive agonist of angiotensin II for evaluating the renin and sodium factors in hypertensive patients. Am J Med 60: 825, 1976.
8. Bing J, Nielson K: Role of the renin system in normo- and hypertension. Acta Pathol Microbiol Scand (A) 81: 254, 1973.
9. Gavras H, Brunner HR, Laragh JH, et al.: Malignant hypertension resulting from deoxycorticosterone acetate and salt excess. Circ Res 36: 300, 1975.
10. Case DB, Wallace JM, Keim HJ, et al.: Identifying angiotensin-dependent hypertension: a comparison of two different angiotensin inhibitors and renin profiling (abstract). Clin Res 24: 418A, 1976.
11. Sealey JE, Laragh JH: Radioimmunoassay of plasma renin activity. Semin Nuc Med 5: 189, 1975.
12. Gavras H, Brunner HR, Laragh JH, et al.: Use of angiotensin-converting enzyme inhibitor in diagnosis and treatment of hypertension. Clin Sci Molec Med 48: 575, 1975.
13. Saucho J, Re R, Burton J, et al.: The role of the renin-angiotensin-aldosterone system in cardiovascular homeostasis in normal human subjects. Circulation 53: 400, 1976.
14. Miller ED, Samuels AI, Haber E, et al.: Inhibition of angiotensin conversion and prevention of renal hypertension. Am J Physiol 228: 448, 1975.
15. Wallace JM, Case DB, Keim HJ, et al.: The immediate pressor responses to saralasin (in preparation).
16. Keim HJ, Drayer JI, Case DB, et al.: A role for renin in rebound hypertension and encephalopathy after infusion of Sar^1-Ala^8-Angiotensin II. N Engl J Med (in press).
17. Pettinger WA, Mitchell HC: Renin release, saralasin and vasodilator-beta-blocker interaction. N Engl J Med 292: 1214, 1975.
18. Duhme DW, Sancho J, Athanasoulis C, et al.: Hypotension during administration of angiotensin converting enzyme inhibitor SQ20881. Lancet 1: 408, 1974.

Modern System for Treating High Blood Pressure Based on Renin Profiling and Vasoconstriction-Volume Analysis: A Primary Role for Beta Blocking Drugs Such as Propranolol

JOHN H. LARAGH, M.D.
New York, New York

A new system is proposed for treating the spectrum of patients with high blood pressure. It is based on studies of the renin axis using renin profiling, pharmacologic probes and our bipolar vasoconstriction-volume hypothesis. The new system does not require renin profiling, pharmacologic testing or a vasoconstriction-volume analysis for widespread application. But these procedures, whenever available, will make treatment more efficient and more certain, and at the same time provide better base line definition.

In the new system, all patients, except the elderly and those with congestive heart failure, bradycardia or a history of asthma, are treated first with propranolol alone, a procedure which will diminish or normalize blood pressure in many patients with high and normal renin levels. For nonresponders, diuretic therapy is then superimposed. Subsequently, a propranolol subtraction trial picks out the low-renin patients who will usually respond to a diuretic alone. This program is likely to be fully effective in possibly up to 85 per cent of patients. For the residual smaller fraction, drugs such as hydralazine, methyl DOPA, clonidine, reserpine or guanethidine are then added in traditional trial and error fashion.

The proposed system has the theoretic attraction for long-term commitment, implicit in antihypertensive therapy, of achieving blood pressure control in large fractions with one drug instead of two or with two drugs instead of three or more. Moreover, the large groups who respond to therapy with propranolol alone (most high-renin and normal-renin patients) or to diuretics alone (most low-renin patients) gain the advantage of simpler, more specific, long-term (i.e., antirenin or antivolume) therapy.

The use of propranolol alone has practical and theoretic advantages over diuretics. Control may be achieved with even fewer side effects and without hypokalemia and chronic dehydration with its possibly adverse consequences (hyperuricemia, azotemia, hyperlipidemia, hyperreninemia, increased blood viscosity). Also, propranolol provides more direct control of the increased peripheral resistance and of neurogenically-induced swings in blood pressure. At the same time, the new system efficiently exploits the long-term use of diuretic therapy alone in low-renin patients in whom volume excess seems a causal factor. And it tends to avoid the use of diuretics in high-renin patients and of beta-blockers in low-renin patients in whom these drug types may be contraindicated.

From the Cardiovascular Center, The New York Hospital-Cornell Medical Center, New York, New York 10021. Requests for reprints should be addressed to Dr. John H. Laragh, Hypertension and Cardiovascular Center, New York Hospital–Cornell Medical Center, 525 East 68th Street, New York, New York 10021.

NOTE: As used herein, "low-renin," "normal-renin" and "high-renin" patients refer specifically to a subgroup of patients (as classified by the standard sodium-renin index) whose plasma renin levels may rise and fall in a way that is characteristic of others within that subgroup.

The art and the science of antihypertensive drug therapy, like many other valid pursuits in medicine, have evolved largely on an empiric basis with doctors administering one drug after another or on top of another until a successful therapeutic response is achieved. In this pursuit, probably because of an inability to identify causes, there has been little understanding of why different patients may respond or fail to respond to a particular drug and, consequently, no way that a physician or a pharmacologist could predict which type drug was likely to be effective in which hypertensive patient. This lack of predictive power is well illustrated by the fact that major types of antihypertensive drugs, the diuretics, methyl DOPA and propranolol as well as reserpine and clonidine, were not recognized at all as antihypertensive agents in animals and were only identified during subsequent clinical use. Accordingly, implicit to this therapeutic approach has been the assumption that the important issue is to lower the blood pressure, and much less consideration has been given to the relevance of the means by which it may be accomplished.

Presently, considering the various analogs, there are about 50 antihypertensive drugs available for general use in the United States and about 100 or more in most European countries. Accordingly a whole variety of more or less effective treatment systems, using various combinations of these drugs, has been developed and applied. In most systems diuretic therapy is recommended as the first step in treatment, and then when the response is incomplete various other agents are superimposed by trial and error, and by physician preference and experience.

Diuretic administration has become the first step and the cornerstone of almost all treatment systems because these agents are usually palatable and safe, and the side effects, such as hypokalemia or hyperuricemia and excess dehydration, are not usually clinical problems. Moreover, diuretic therapy alone is thought to be effective to some extent in most patients, and it enhances the effectiveness of most other drugs especially when their antihypertensive action becomes limited by reactive salt and water retention. Theoretically, too, there is support for this primary role for diuretic therapy since abnormal sodium intake or renal retention has long been suspected as a key pathogenetic factor in essential hypertension. Indeed one investigator has recently suggested again that hypertension could be controlled as a public health problem by large scale reduction in dietary sodium intake [1].

On the other hand, despite the established effectiveness and possible virtues of long-term diuretic therapy, it is perhaps appropriate to continue to question and examine its broad scale indiscriminate long-term application in hypertensive patients. Indeed a reexamination of this blanket usage may be especially appropriate in view of the new level of understanding of hypertensive mechanisms which has emerged from recent research.

This recent research has characterized and defined the biochemical heterogeneity of so-called essential hypertension, [9], a condition long thought to be genetically and biochemically uniform. Moreover, it has revealed that this biochemical heterogeneity can be correlated with the responsiveness to antihypertensive drug therapy so that, for the first time, it has become possible to predict for many patients which among them will respond to a particular type of antihypertensive drug.

This new level of understanding has emerged in particular from research in human subjects which exposed the renin-angiotensin-aldosterone system (the renin axis) as a blood pressure control system [2] and from the development of renin profiling [6,7] as a technic for monitoring the system which thereby provided a biochemical basis for reclassifying all hypertensive patients. Moreover, this renin profiling technic using a renin-sodium index can also be used to identify vasoconstrictor and volume elements [8] and to predict which patients will respond to which type of drug [2–5]. This method for predicting drug responsiveness has been validated by physiologic testing using pharmacologic probes which block the renin axis at various sites [9–14]. This new reference framework promises to lead to more predictable specific and selective therapies for increasing numbers and to open the door to separating those patients for further study who do not respond in the predicted manner.

It is known that specific derangements of the renin axis can cause special forms of hypertension, such as malignant and renovascular hypertensions associated with renin excess, and primary and pseudoprimary aldosteronism associated with excess adrenal mineralocorticoid secretion. However, our analysis of all states of hypertension in terms of the renin axis does not assume that abnormalities in the axis are necessarily causing the high blood pressure. We simply reason that if the renin axis is a blood pressure control system, measurements of its components will always have meaning since, even if the derangement is not the primary cause, it will express a predictable reaction to the hypertension which can be used to dissect mechanisms involved.

Based on these developments, in this paper a new system is proposed for treatment of the entire spectrum of patients with high blood pressure. The new treatment system (as shown in Figure 4) assigns a major and first-line role to beta-adrenergic blocking drugs such as propranolol. In the system most patients are treated first with propranolol alone—a procedure which can normalize pressure in most high renin patients (15 per cent of the whole) and many normal-renin (55 per cent of the whole) patients. For those who do not show a full response, a diuretic is then added. This combination will probably control up to 85 per cent of all patients. Patients with low renin levels, who comprise about 30 per cent of the whole and who usually respond to the administration of a diuretic alone, are identified by a subsequent propranolol subtraction trial. This new system can be applied even when renin profiling or the capacity to evaluate the renin axis with blocking drugs is not available.

The basis for this new treatment system can best be appreciated in the context of a brief review of what is known and speculated about the renin system and the physiologic and pharmacologic controls used to study it.

The Renin Axis. The workings of the renin-angiotensin-aldosterone system for regulating arterial blood pressure and sodium balance are depicted in Figure 1. When renin, an enzyme secreted by the juxtaglomerular cells of the kidneys, reacts with a circulating alpha$_2$-globulin substrate, angiotensin I is generated. The decapeptide angiotensin I is biologically inactive, but in passage through the lungs it encounters pulmonary converting enzymes that hydrolyze it into the octapeptide angiotensin II. This product, by weight the most potent pressor known, is believed by many investigators to be a central effector hormone in the day to day, hour to hour regulation of blood pressure.

Angiotensin II's effects are immediate in constricting the arteriovasculature, thus increasing blood pressure by influencing one side of the blood pressure equation—that of vasoconstriction (Figure 1). At the same time, but in a slower and more prolonged timetable, angiotensin influences the other side of the equation—volume—by signalling adrenocortical release of aldosterone, a hormone that stimulates renal sodium and fluid retention. The reduced caliber of the arterial tree on the one hand and the increase of its fluid content on the other together raise the blood pressure level, and this phenomenon, in cybernetic turn, acts on the juxtaglomerular cells by way of baroreceptor mechanisms and on the macula densa cells by increasing distal tubule sodium delivery, and both work to shut off the renin secretion that started the cycle.

It should be noted that the sodium retention induced by aldosterone is slight and gradual in comparison with the bulk of sodium-retaining transport mechanisms operating along the tubules and other hemodynamic factors acting on the kidneys. However, a slight increase in sodium retaining action, of the order of 1 to 2 per cent, will in time produce major changes in sodium balance. Most probably, in the steady state the pressor effect of aldosterone-induced fluid retention is buffered to some extent by a consequent pressure natriuresis. This is the so-called "escape" phenomenon. Thus, for all intents, although the principal renin-angiotensin effect must be considered to be vasoconstrictive, its physiologic appropriateness and the degree of its action must always be weighed on the scale of concurrent volume effects induced by aldosterone and by other factors influencing renal sodium and fluid retention, and by determining the effective volume filling the arterial tree.

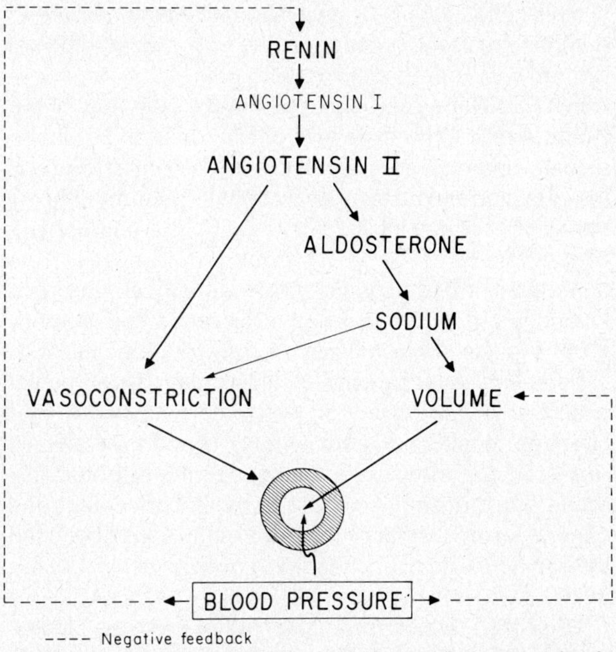

Figure 1. *The renin-angiotensin-aldosterone hormonal axis and the vasoconstriction volume hypothesis for blood pressure regulation. This hypothesis proposes that, although many imputs may be involved, the two ultimate determinants of blood pressure are the degree of* ***vasoconstriction*** *of the arterial bed between the aortic valves and the capillaries and the* ***volume*** *of fluid filling this bed. Our studies indicate that the activity of the renin axis exerts major long-term governance over those two factors via angiotensin-induced* ***vasoconstriction*** *and aldosterone-induced sodium and volume retention. Accordingly, measurement of changes in the renin axis reflecting either a primary derangement or a reactive change in the axis can be used to identify mechanisms involved in the hypertension.*

The renin axis operates to determine the pressor capacity of the blood pool container and by interacting with the physiologic changes induced by the sodium ion supplied in the diet it also determines the second component of the pressor force, the volume of the blood pool itself. The renin axis governs this second component, too, by eliciting the secretion of aldosterone. The long-term power of this sodium factor is well illustrated by many clinical and experimental observations. Thus, Ames and associates [15] showed that the pressor responsiveness to angiotensin II in human subjects is directly related to the state of sodium balance and that this relationship constitutes a secondary gain in the control system (Figure 1). And in animal studies Guyton and his colleagues [16] have shown that the natriuretic response to blood pressure is the only pressor control system with a potentially infinite gain.

Renin Profiling as a Technic to Monitor Behavior of the Renin Axis. With exposure of the renin-angiotensin-aldosterone axis as a blood pressure control system, the question next arose as to how to best monitor its behavior in states in which it might have a pathophysiologic role such as in hypertensive diseases. This question seemed especially relevant since numerous investigators in the past had often failed to relate abnormal levels of plasma renin to any form of clinical or experimental hypertension, including even experimental Goldblatt hypertension. It was clear, however, that changes in plasma renin activity practically always reflected commensurate changes in the effector hormone angiotensin II so that the more convenient and sensitive renin activity measurement could be used instead as an index of changes in over-all activity of the axis.

Recognizing the inconsistencies of previous studies and also taking into account the known feedback controls of the renin axis, we reasoned that for renin measurements to have any meaning the measurements must be evaluated in terms of their *appropriateness* to the concurrent physiologic setting. Appropriate to what? In our view it is primarily to salt balance. As already indicated, the unopposed candidate for the chief counterbalancing factor in the renin system and also in the blood pressure equation is the sodium ion, the major osmotic determinant of extracellular and intravascular volumes. This interaction between renin secretion and volume takes place always in relation to pressure circumstances arising from the volume determinants: salt intake and salt output. Conversely, too, the consequences of changes in salt balance are at the same time modulated by vasoconstrictive adaptations from the renin angiotensin limb of the bipolar concept (Figure 1).

Early investigators studying renin often failed to take into account the fact that body fluid volume varies widely among people corresponding to a wide variation in dietary sodium. Sometimes they accounted for it by relating renin measurements to bracketed ranges of normal renin activity for controlled levels of sodium balance. But such bracketed ranges, too, often overlap, and therefore fail to discern subtle deviations from normal.

The Renin Profiling Technic. Because we were aware that changes in plasma renin activity are normally finely tuned to and continuously related to changes in sodium intake and balance, we decided at the outset to reference all our renin measurements against the concurrent 24 hour rate of sodium excretion and to determine their normalcy by spotting the test value against a nomogram curve (the renin-sodium index) derived from studies of normal control subjects studied over the full range of variation in sodium intake [6,7]. We also established that the 24 hour urine collection method, except in patients who cannot maintain salt balance, reliably reflects the state of sodium balance, being about as sensitive as the balance method to changes in sodium intake, and it is applicable to large scale evaluation of outpatients on random diets [8]. Moreover, there was a hidden bonus in this approach since the sodium measurement gave us rapidly a more reliable insight into each patients salt appetite than did prolonged interrogation.

Ideally a base line renin sodium profile is best obtained in a hypertensive patient who has not received any antihypertensive drugs for about three weeks, since most of these drugs have predictable effects on the renin axis [2–5]. The blood for renin assay is collected with the patients in the seated position after they have been ambulatory so that this neurogenic component as well as the sodium volume component to renin secretion are both routinely included in the assessment. In addition, whenever possible we now utilize a preliminary five to seven day period of mild sodium deprivation. This mild stimulation of renin secretion increases the capacity to separate patients into subgroups with low, normal or high renin levels.

Methodologic Problems in Measuring Plasma Renin Activity. In addition to these physiologic considerations, the full diagnostic exploitation of renin profiling requires the use of a renin method which is sufficiently reliable and sensitive to explore and discriminate renin values below the normal range. This requires the use of a laboratory method that provides for complete inhibition of plasma angiotensinases for prolonged periods of time so that with low activity samples plasma can be incubated up to 18 hours. The prolonged incubation obviates the need for blank subtraction and therefore greatly increases the accuracy as well as the sensitivity and simplicity of the measurements. To date, such complete angiotensinase inhibition can only be achieved by the use of EDTA and a bacteriostatic agent plus either DFP or PMSF at the acid pH optimum for renin [17–19]. Another confusion, and error that should be avoided, which produces artificially high values for renin concentration occurs in those methods which acidify plasma to below pH 4 to destroy substrate and angiotensinases [20]. It is now clear that this step produces falsely high values by activating an inactive form of renin which may be prorenin [21]. Our very recent studies indicate that chilling should also be avoided in the collection period because of cryoactivation of prorenin [22]. These problems can all be avoided by the use of methods and procedures which we have described [17–19]. Failure to take the aforementioned crucial physiologic and methodologic considerations into account undoubtedly explains many of the discrepant findings of clinical reports in the current literature.

Renin Profiling in Hypertensive Diseases. Renin profiling using the prescribed renin sodium reference index combined with a reliable and sensitive method for measuring plasma renin has enabled a greatly increased range of clinical investigative and diagnostic utility, and has allowed the detection of subtle renin abnormalities obscured by previous methods. In particular, it has become apparent that plasma renin values in many hypertensive patients considered by former methods to be normal might in fact be either high or low and those heretofore considered low could in fact be normal. Accordingly our classifications of hypertensive patients into low-, normal- and high-renin groups is based entirely on this renin-sodium profiling technic.

Using renin profiling the high values characteristic of malignant hypertension and the low values characteristic of adrenal cortical hypertensions (primary and pseudoprimary aldosteronism) can be precisely characterized [2]. And renin profiling was used in exposing oral contraceptive hypertension to define inappropriateness of the renin levels and to relate them to abnormal substrate levels [2,23]. Moreover, using renin profiling we showed that the peripheral circulating renin level is after all usually abnormal in relation to sodium excretion in patients suspected of having surgically curable renovascular hypertension so that this technic could become a powerful tool indeed for screening for such patients [24]. This view is contrary to a long held belief [25,26] which has maintained that peripheral plasma renin levels are often normal in Goldblatt hypertension and so of little diagnostic value.

Beyond these diagnostic uses of renin profiling, we have used the technic to recharacterize the more subtle abnormalities associated with essential hypertension on a physiologic basis and thus to demonstrate that what was long thought to be a genetically and biochemically uniform condition is in fact heterogeneous so that essential hypertensive patients can be subdivided into subgroups with low renin levels (about 30 per cent of the whole), normal renin levels (55 per cent) and high renin levels (about 15 per cent of the whole). Our associated clinical studies suggest that these subgroups have significant differences in clinical course with the patients with low renin levels being relatively protected from the major cardiovascular complications of stroke or heart attack [7].

Antihypertensive Drug Responses Related to Renin Profiling. However, from the point of view of the present discussion, having demonstrated biochemical heterogeneity within essential hypertension we were faced with the challenge of investigating the physiologic utility and the pharmacologic relevance of our renin profile data. The questions were whether renin profiles could be used to identify and quantify mechanisms operating in various patients? And could such an analysis be diagnostic so that a corresponding therapy would be more predictable and specific?

To answer these questions, in serial studies we have (1) evaluated the effects of treatment with selected antihypertensive drugs on blood pressure and on the renin system, and then (2) compared these results with the effects on blood pressure produced by administering pharmacologic probes known to block the renin system at different points.

Propranolol, the First Antirenin Drug. For our first test of the question, we chose propranolol. This beta adrenergic drug had long been used for treatment of angina pectoris and cardiac arrhythmias. It was first used for the treatment of hypertension by Prichard in 1964 [32c]. But it had an undistinguished record as an antihypertensive agent with many investigators, especially in the United States, reporting no unique benefits and a high percentage of treatment failures. Most theories attributed its apparently spotty beneficial effects to its depressant action on cardiac performance.

However we knew that propranolol could reduce renin secretion, and from our earlier work we knew that malignant hypertension usually was caused by excessive renin and aldosterone secretion [2]. Accordingly, we decided to administer oral propranolol alone to a group of patients with malignant hypertension. We showed that in half or more of them complete correction could be achieved, and in most others the improvement was impressive [3,4] even though they required other drugs, diuretics in the main, to bring their pressure to normal. Moreover, associated with a striking clinical benefit was a dramatic correction of the characteristic biochemical abnormalities in the renin axis. The increased renin secretion and aldosterone secretion, and the attendant hypertension and hypokalemia, uniformly and dramatically returned to normal within a few days. This clinical and pharmacologic bull's-eye effect reaffirmed our view of the causation of malignant hypertension while demonstrating that a major factor in the antihypertensive action of propranolol is closely related to its antirenin effect.

We then quickly demonstrated similar unique and striking benefits of propranolol in renovascular hypertension [4]. Thus, in both of these high renin states we found its antihypertensive benefit closely related to the control renin profile and also to the degree to which the drug lowered the renin level. The results suggested that the response to propranolol might even be used diagnostically to quantify the renin factor and as an aid for identifying renin dependency and surgical curability.

Propranolol in the Subgroups of "Essential" Hypertension. Excited by these results we examined the effectiveness of propranolol in 74 patients with untreated essential hypertension, but only after obtaining base line renin profiles using our renin-sodium index to preclassify patients into the subgroups with low, normal or high renin levels [4]. We found that with an average dose of 40 mg of propranolol four times daily, there was a dramatic decrease in the hypertension of most patients with high renin levels, often all the way to normal. A majority of patients with "normal" renin levels also exhibited impressive benefit. But what confirmed our reasoning very elegantly was the fact that the patients with low renin levels and essential hypertension exhibited no significant blood pressure responses. Again, therefore, in the whole spectrum of patients, the antihypertensive benefit was closely related to the control renin level and to the degree to which the renin level was reduced suggesting that the antirenin action of propranolol is a major factor in its antihypertensive action.

Accordingly, these data provided the first real evidence that an absolute or relative excess of renin plays a major and at least a participatory role in the blood pressure level of major segments of patients with so-called essential hypertension (those with high and normal renin levels) and a minor role in patients with low renin levels, that renin-profiling is a means of identifying such patients and that propranolol confirms the identification, quantifies the involvement and provides the first specific treatment for the renin factor. We tend to the probability that propranolol's antirenin action involves a beta-adrenergic blockade preferential for the renal receptor sites associated with renin production.

Low Renin Essential Hypertension: A Volume-Sensitive Subgroup. Now what then are the mechanisms involved in those patients with low renin levels and essential hypertension who we found uniquely *unresponsive* to the administration of propranolol? What does the low renin state imply? Other investigators had studied this aspect of the problem before us [27–31]. Most had developed the view that this state was uniquely sensitive to antimineralocorticoid therapy, and therefore their hypertension was claimed to be due to oversecretion of either aldosterone or another mineralocorticoid.

Our own studies do not support this opinion [5]. In fact, we found this subgroup to be normokalemic with little evidence for mineralocorticoid excess. Moreover, we found that spironolactone therapy was in no way uniquely beneficial since volume depletion using sulfonamide diuretics instead induced an equally good decrease in blood pressure which could be normalized in about two-thirds of this subgroup by treatment with either chlorthalidone alone or spironolactone alone using a maximum of 100 mg daily of either drug. These results suggested to us the presence of abnormal renal sodium retention correctable by diuretic therapy irrespective of type.

Therefore, in our view, in this subgroup it is not necessary to postulate any unique adrenal cortical participation in causation. Volume depletion is the common basis for antihypertensive effect. Therefore, conceptually, a subtle volume excess in the arterial bed is a major basis for this type of essential hypertension and this volume excess may induce the low renin secretion.

According to our results this volume factor is not altogether unique for patients with low renin levels. It also appears operative in some hypertensive patients with normal renin levels since the blood pressure level in a third of these patients, too, could be normalized by the administration of a single volume-depleting drug [5].

It should be appreciated that most but not all patients with low renin levels do respond to diuretic therapy. Up to a third may exhibit either a partial or no response. Similarly not all patients with high renin or normal renin levels respond to propranolol alone. In the case of diuretics one reason for these failures may be a vigorous reactive increase in renin secretion which sustains the blood pressure at control levels [5]. Accordingly, these resistant patients can be rendered normotensive by superimposing antirenin therapy [11].

The Vasoconstriction-Volume Hypothesis to Analyze and Treat All Hypertension. The results of these two sets of clinical studies suggested to us [8] that two major mechanisms are operative in all hypertension so that either excessive *vasoconstriction* related to excessive renin secretion or alternatively excessive *volume* as a consequence of sodium retention are two prime and ultimate mechanisms operating to sustain all chronic hypertension. Thus chronic hypertension is viewed as an inappropriate excess of volume relative to capacity of the arterial tree or vice versa.

These deductions and the implications of them form a basis for our vasoconstriction-volume hypothesis [8] which we use to analyze, understand and treat all patients with hypertension. The hypothesis (Figure 1) simply proposes that, in the final analysis, the level of blood pressure can always be explained in terms of an excessive arterial vasoconstriction, an excessive volume of fluid filling the arterial bed (between the aortic valve and the capillaries) or an inappropriate excess of one relative to the other.

This analytical model in no way excludes the operation of a myriad of other factors such as catecholamines, neural activity, local tissue autoregulation and so on. It simply states that in the final analysis, whatever these other inputs may be, they must influence the blood pressure by affecting these two ultimate determinants, i.e., the level of arterial *vasoconstriction* or the *volume* available to fill the arterial bed. Moreover, our extensive experience in examining the renin axis in patients with high blood pressure leads us to believe that, in the chronic situation, most of the time, the degree of participation of the vasoconstriction and volume factors can be evaluated from renin-sodium profiling, indicating in turn to us that the renin axis is playing a major, primary or reactive role in the long-term governance of these final determinants.

Our vasoconstriction-volume hypothesis, which is pictured in Figure 1, is not only based on our clinical studies of antirenin and antivolume drugs. It was also built from our parallel animal and human studies of the problem of renovascular hypertension. In this research, not discussed here, we have similarly identified two different mechanisms at work in renovascular hypertensions, vasoconstriction (renin excess) and/or sodium-volume excess. In animals we showed, using angiotensin blocking drugs and angiotensin antibodies, that the two mechanisms can explain two different types of experimental renovascular hypertension. The one kidney clip model with the opposite kidney left untouched is explained by *excess renin-angiotensin* [24]. In contrast, the model in which one kidney is clipped and the opposite removed is explained by *volume* excess. In the course of time the models can switch from a vasoconstrictor to a volume-dependent type or vice versa.

Parallel studies in human subjects have defined surgically curable renovascular hypertension as resembling the two-kidney model in being renin-dependent [24]. In contrast, the hypertension of chronic renal insufficiency resembles the one-kidney model. It is usually volume-dependent and exhibits low circulating renin levels. These observations defining the role of renin and volume, have allowed us to develop a mathematical approach using first the peripheral renin level to identify renin hypersecretion and then renal vein renin levels to lateralize the renin dependency and quantify the renal ischemia. And with all three indicators, one can predict with precision the potential surgical curability.

Accordingly, the vasoconstriction-volume hypothetical model derives strong support from both the clinical pharmacologic studies of antirenin or antivolume drug effectiveness in renin subgroups, and from experimental and clinical studies of the role of vasoconstriction and volume in different forms of renal hypertensions. But over and above this, the vasoconstriction-volume hypothesis passes the test of being able to explain the whole spectrum of clinical phenomena. Thus, in the hypothesis, malignant hypertension and renovascular hypertension (renin excess) and primary aldosteronism or anephric man (volume excess) become clinical examples of the polar extremes of the spectrum. Moreover, our renin-sodium profiling technic can be used to identify which mechanisms are at work in individual patients. In fact, as I will discuss, pharmacologic probes which block the renin axis can now be used to quantify both the vasoconstriction and the volume factors in each and every patient, an approach which at the same time provides the ultimate validation of the hypothesis.

The Use of Angiotensin Blocking Drugs to Quantify the Renin Factor in Hypertension and to Verify the Use of Renin Profiling and the Vasoconstriction-Volume Hypothesis. We now come to what television drama detectives call "the clincher." Two investigative drugs, recently made available, specifically block the renin-angiotensin-aldosterone system (Figure 2). One of them, saralasin, is a structural analog of angiotensin II with terminal sarcosine and alanine replacements. Its effects stems from its competition for angiotensin II receptor sites. Thus, although it does not bar the production of angiotensin II, it does block the hormone's effect. The other agent is a nonapeptide, SQ20881 by current investigative name, which interferes with the action of pulmonary and plasma enzymes that convert angiotensin I to angiotensin II. Both agents have short-term effects and can be administered only by injection or infusion, which limits their clinical applicability largely to inhospital circumstances. We have studied both drugs extensively and have reported our findings [9–14]. Let me summarize them briefly after pointing out what may be obvious, that a specific wipe-out of angiotensin activity is indeed an indicator of the renin component, considering the renin-angiotensin relationship.

In patients with high renin levels, saralasin infusions reduced blood pressure levels either to normal or near normal. In those cases in which the response was not total, normalization was achieved by the infusion of the diuretic furosemide, demonstrating again and quantifying our postulated two-component maintenance of the hypertension in those cases (i.e., vasoconstriction [renin] and volume [sodium]) [9,10]. Indeed, when normalization was achieved with saralasin, the additional administration of sodium chloride could again raise the blood pressure level, converting the condition in these patients from renin-vasoconstrictive hypertension to sodium-volume hypertension, and verifying the usefulness of the vasoconstriction-volume hypothesis.

Comparison Studies of Three Different Anti-Renin Drugs: Propranolol, Saralasin, Converting Enzyme Inhibitor. Importantly, too, among patients with high renin levels the response to saralasin consistently paralleled the response to oral propranolol treatment. The consistency was similar among patients with low renin levels in whom, expectedly, neither saralasin nor propranolol administration lowered blood pressure. What puzzled us at first was an inconsistency in the patients with normal renin levels; in some of them sa-

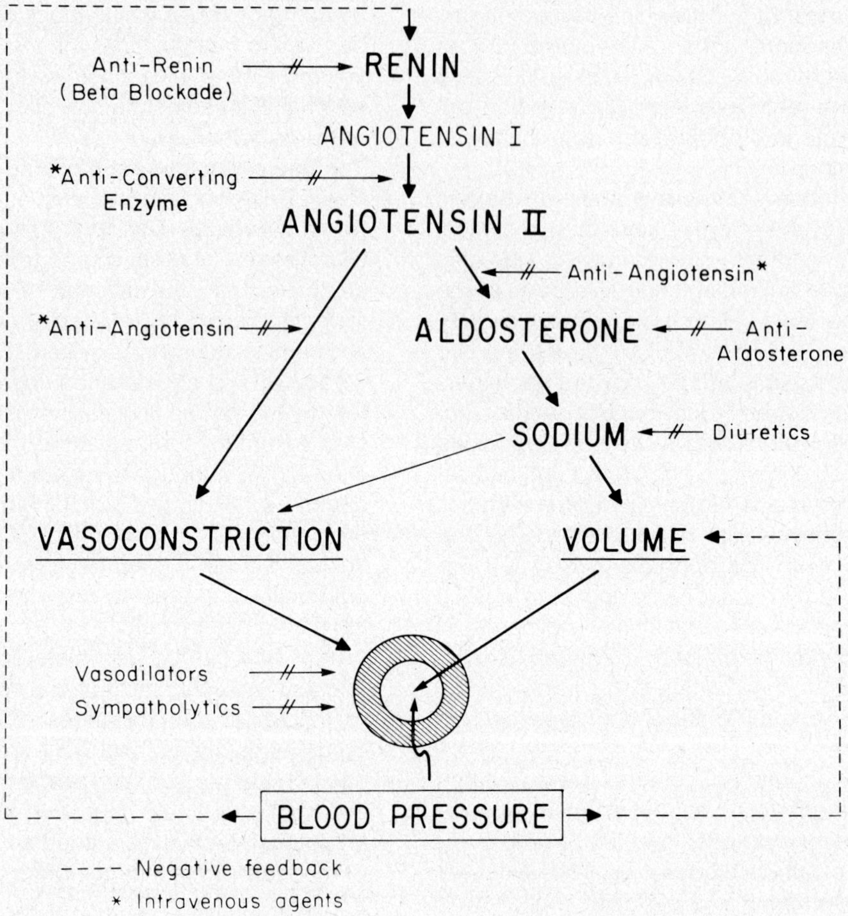

Figure 2. *Sites of intervention of various orally active antihypertensive drugs and of the two peptide inhibitors of angiotensin II formation or action.*

ralasin was either ineffective or actually slightly *pressor* even though many of these patients responded favorably to propranolol. Then we realized that this angiotensin analogue was not a true competitive antagonist [12]. It was, rather, a competitive partial agonist with pressor properties—diminished, it is true—of its own. This idea was most easily verified by more studies of patients with an absence of endogenous renin. Thus we found that saralasin was overtly *pressor* in hypertensive patients with low renin levels and also in anephric man [13] and that propranolol, too, could be pressor in low-renin patients [33].

On the other hand, no intrinsic agonism could be attributed to SQ20881, the converting-enzyme inhibitor. In repeating all studies with this newer agent [11,14], all the previous inconsistencies were eliminated. The converting enzyme blocker either reduced blood pressure or did not affect it; but it never increased it. When compared with saralasin the drug achieved greater depressor responses in all patients with high renin levels. Moreover, it identified a renin factor of one degree or another in 91 per cent of patients with normal renin levels, a result which could be achieved in only 10 per cent of them with saralasin because of its own agonism. Actually, converting enzyme blockade paralleled more closely our earlier description of the antihypertensive responses to propranolol, thereby giving strength to our antirenin theory of propranolol action.

The new studies [14] further strengthened a concept that has increasingly entered our discussions. A "normal" level of renin activity in a hypertensive patient might indeed represent an *inappropriate* renin response to the specific physiologic challenge posed to that patient's regulatory mechanisms. A "normal" renin profile therefore should not rule out the feasibility of targeting treatment against renin. Very likely these patients who now appear to have inappropriate renin levels for their hypertension should be considered to have "medium renin" levels.

For us the evidence was persuasive that an inappropriate renin activity participates in all or part of the hypertension in a wide spectrum of patients with either normal or high renin values and with very high to slightly high blood pressure levels. Indeed, a renin factor may even participate in the hypertension of a few patients with low renin levels.

Altogether, our studies now suggest that a significant renin factor is at work in maintaining the hypertension of some 50 to 70 per cent of all patients with hypertension [14]. The residual 30 per cent who have completely turned off their renin appear to have instead "volume" hypertension amenable to antivolume therapy with diuretics as the first step. These results do not necessarily mean that excessive renin secretion is the primary or initiating event in 70 per cent of all hypertensive patients. But we now know that renin is participating in the high blood pressure. Now that we know renin participates, it remains for future studies to determine whether or not the renin axis is primarily involved and, if not, to determine why it does not shut itself off.

Meanwhile, it is clear that renin profiling provides a valid means of identifying those who will most probably respond to specific treatment with either antirenin type drugs, whose number is growing daily, or alternatively with antivolume agents. The increasing availability of angiotensin blocking agents just discussed provides a further means for pharmacologic identification and for quantification of the vasoconstriction or volume factors in each and every patient, and it also provides a basis for more effective and specific diagnosis and treatment of hypertensive emergencies.

How to Make a Quantitative Vasoconstriction-Volume Analysis of the Individual Patient Using Angiotensin Blockade with Diuretic Response. The matter of physiologic identification has real and practical implications for base line diagnosis and for planning treatment even when facilities for renin profiling are not available or are overburdened. A programmed diagnostic approach employing monitored trials of renin blockers and diuretics can locate and quantify the hypertensive lesion. This is explained in Figure 3. The amount by which angiotensin blockade reduces blood pressure reflects the renin involvement of vasoconstriction, and the portion of blood pressure reduction achieved by subsequent diuretic administration will reflect the participation of the volume factor. By retesting with the angio blocker during diuretic therapy, the pressure component due to *reactive* renin can also be quantitated. By subtraction, the native volume component can then be quantitated too. Ideally, converting enzyme inhibitor should be used to test for the angiotensin II factor, but it is possible that oral propranolol could be used in this way instead. The treatment plan follows accordingly. Future research involving periodic re-evaluations of the changing hormonal scene using this type of testing during various treatments promises to tell us a lot more about changes in long-term mechanisms too, and how to cope with them.

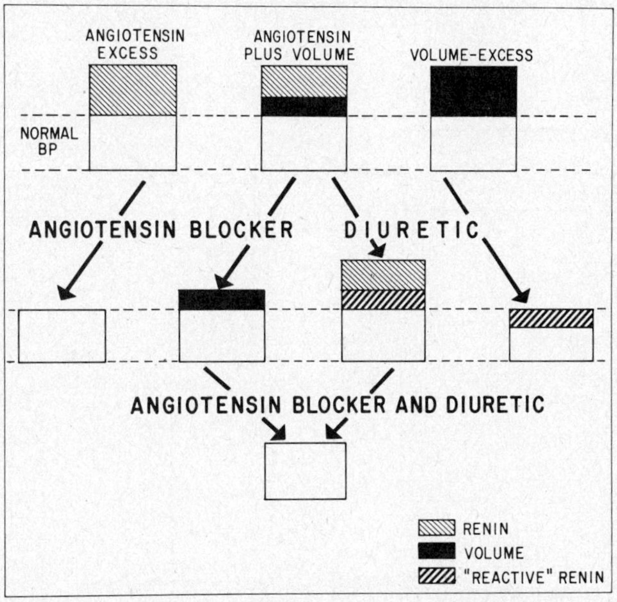

Figure 3. *Technic for quantifying the vasoconstriction and volume factors in individual patients. The vasoconstriction-volume hypothesis proposes that all hypertension can be explained in terms of appropriately excessive arterial* ***volume*** *relative to the arterial capacity (i.e.,* ***vasoconstriction****) or vice versa. At the top from left to right are shown three model expressions of the hypothesis. First, a largely vasoconstrictor hypertensive patient (i.e., high renin levels), a mixed type with an inappropriate excess of volume relative to capacity (i.e., normal renin levels) and a largely volume-dependent hypertensive (low renin levels). The vasoconstrictor component of hypertension can be quantitated in mm Hg in each individual patient by determining the blood pressure response to angiotensin blockade using converting enzyme inhibitor. The volume and vasoconstrictor components together can be quantitated by repeating the angiotensin blockade during diuretic therapy. Then by subtraction, the volume element can also be quantitated. See text.*

How to Use the Vasoconstriction-Volume Hypothesis to Plan Treatment Even When Renin Profiling is not Available. When one takes into account the lifetime commitment to maintain drug treatment that hypertension therapy usually requires, it is obvious that the most complete base line definition possible is highly desirable before commencing any therapeutic regimen. Ideally renin profiling should be made on all patients before the treatment program is begun. Whatever the expense of this procedure, and it promises to be relatively small, it cannot be compared with staggering costs of long-term therapy especially if the therapy uses unneeded drugs or drugs not designed to deal with the biochemical and the physiologic problem. Accordingly, we are convinced that in the best of all possible worlds,

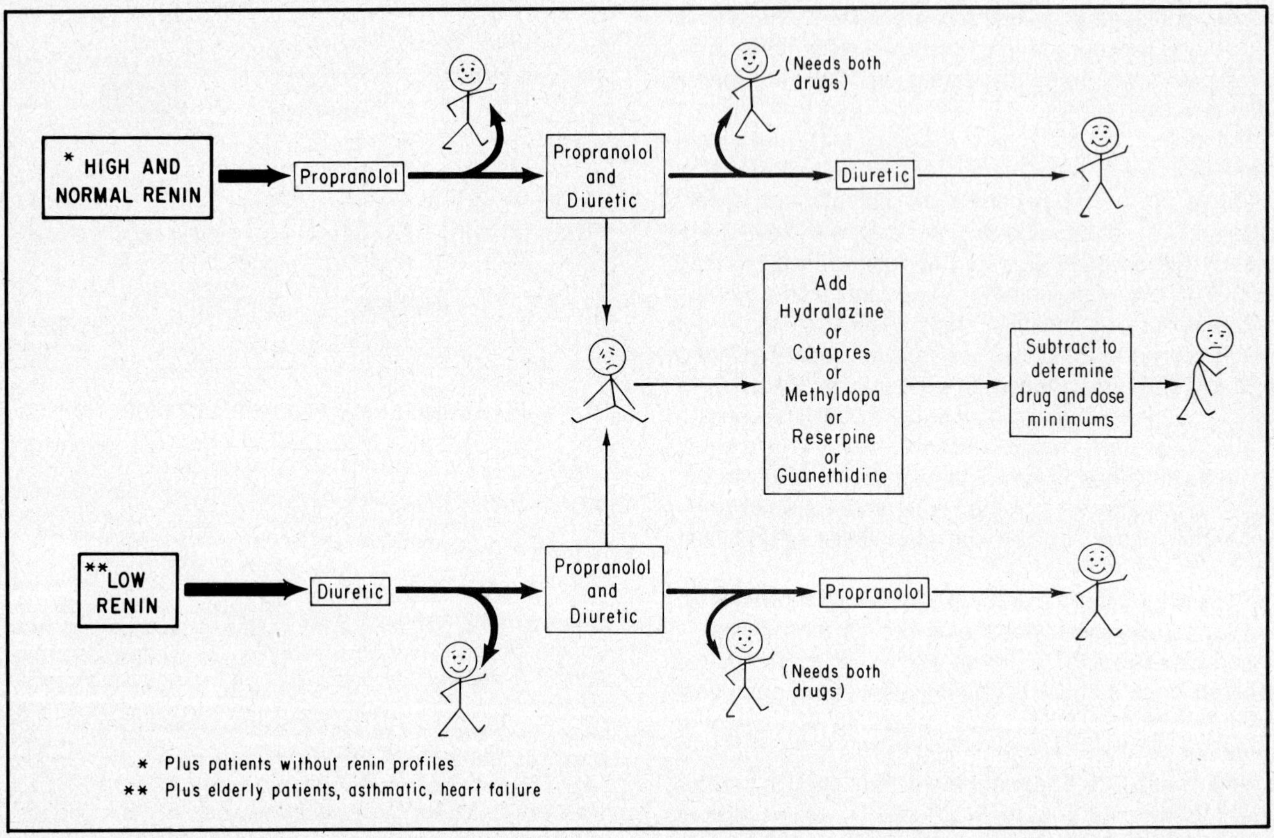

Figure 4. *Flow diagram depicting the proposed new treatment system and its application whether or not renin profiling is available as part of the base line evaluation. See text for additional discussion of relative and absolute contraindications and the use of alternative back-up regimens.*

renin profiling should be done on all patients prior to starting treatment. But, in the present state of our technologic development, renin profiling is, unfortunately, not yet available to the large majority of patients; in fact, we are not yet able to provide it for all of our own patients. But it should soon become widely available as commercial laboratories and other medical centers adopt and apply what now seems to be a relatively simple technology.

Meanwhile, how can the clinician use the information that I have just discussed to provide a more rational basis for treatment? If he becomes familiar with and accepts at least part of the information contained herein, he can use the vasoconstriction-volume hypothesis and other information that we have derived from renin profiling to work out a therapeutic system, without having renin testing available, which in most patients will produce, on a systematic trial and error basis, the same end result.

The New System. The protocol suggested by our research is disarmingly simple and can be carried out in the physicians office (Figure 4). In the large majority of patients with essential hypertension a vasoconstriction-volume analysis can be applied in the office by using a trial of propranolol therapy to test for the existence of the renin factor. If there is no response or a partial response, a diuretic agent can then be added to test for a volume factor. The combined regimen is likely to be fully effective in up to 85 per cent of all patients with a minimum of unpleasant side-effects. Subsequently a propranolol subtraction trial is tested to pick out those patients with low renin levels who will respond to therapy with a diuretic alone. Patients whose blood pressure is controlled with propranolol alone will enjoy, among other advantages, the fact that this agent produces no effect on mentation, no postural or postexercise hypotension and no interference with sexual potency.

When propranolol and a diuretic are combined, the beta blocker tends to dampen the hyperreninemic response to the diuretic. But this real bonus in practice may look smaller than expected. Thus, propranolol dramatically lowers renin levels in patients not receiving diuretics but has less apparent effect against the renin rise of sodium depletion. Our current view is that the drug acts primarily to block only that major component of renin secretion which is under neurogenic governance.

We have found that a propranolol dosage of 40 mg orally four times a day is usually sufficient. And it may prove possible to administer this instead at 80 mg twice daily. We have not usually pushed the dosage above 120 mg four times daily although some European physicians have claimed additional successes with the long-term use of up to several grams daily. Indeed, some of our patients exhibit complete correction with as little as 20 mg twice daily. Unfortunately, despite the great clinical importance of this type of drug, no alternatives to propranolol are available in the United States. In Europe, at least eight different beta receptor blockers are now commercially available, some with greater selectivity and potency than propranolol.

The diuretic one employs is dealers choice. We use chlorthalidone because it is long-acting and need only be given once daily. We start with 50 mg and then double the dose. A number of other sulfonamides such as hydrochlorthiazide (25 mg twice a day increasing to 50 mg twice a day) as well as spironolactone 50 to 100 mg a day are examples of acceptable alternatives.

Using this approach, the linician can identify those patients with a large renin factor because they will be completely responsive to the administration of propranolol and those with a large volume factor because they will instead be completely responsive to a diuretic. For the residual patients, most of whom will probably have normal renin levels, combined therapy with propranolol and a diuretic should control most of them. There will, in fact, be a residual group of perhaps 10 to 15 per cent who are not controlled with either specific antivolume or antirenin therapy or the combination. For them, the clinician will have to revert to the classic empiric approach and add serially less palatable drugs, such as hydralazine, methyldopa, clonidine, reserpine or guanethadine, until complete control is achieved.

For every step along the way, we recommend that after control has been achieved, serial subtraction be again applied to be sure that the minimum effective regimen is given for the longer term. The final regimen will then be one in which the smallest amount of each drug and the fewest number of drugs will be maintained.

In using this new system, it is difficult to be absolutely precise about the absolute percentages of patients who might be treatable for the long-term with monotherapy. This is because of the variations in proportions of patients with low normal and high renin levels which might occur in different medical populations. This variation is partly age, sex and race related since hypertension with low renin levels is more frequent in older patients, in blacks and in women. Notwithstanding these varying influences, our experience [3,4] and that of others [32,42] suggests that up to 40 to 50 per cent of patients with essential hypertension may respond to beta blockade alone whereas perhaps in some 25 to 30 per cent blood pressure levels may be fully corrected by diuretic therapy alone [5].

This new treatment system has the charm of offering, for major fractions of all patients, treatment with one drug instead of two and, for other major fractions, two drugs instead of three, with the particular attraction of the system being the likelihood that in most patients the right drug will have been given to correct the particular biochemical lesion involved in pathogenesis. Conversely too, the new system tends to avoid the use of diuretics in vasoconstricted patients with high renin levels when they may, in fact, be contraindicated [8], and it also tends to avoid the use of beta adrenoreceptor blocking drugs in patients with low renin levels in whom they are not only ineffective but in whom they can, in fact, produce paradoxical pressor responses [33]. Moreover, the over-all approach offers, for the patient, a lesser likelihood of untoward effects or unpleasant side effects and toxicity, and a lower total cost.

Some Relative Contraindications, Exclusions and Back-up Treatment Alternatives in Using the New System. Although the new treatment system should be applicable in the large majority of patients, certain contraindications and exclusions along with the back-up treatment alternatives are inevitably required. Thus, although beta-adrenergic blocking drugs, such as propranolol, are in general unusually well tolerated and without side effects, there are certain well known situations in which their use should be avoided. First of all, beta-adrenergic blocking drugs are progressively less likely to be effective in lowering blood pressure levels in the elderly in whom autonomic activity is often already reduced and in whom the low renin level-volume type hypertension is increasingly more likely. Accordingly, as suggested by Bühler [32a], therapy with propranolol and related drugs may become a second choice to diuretics in patients over the age of 60. In this group, too, underlying bradycardia may pose another relative contraindication. In this regard, although there have been very few clinical problems from propranolol-induced bradycardia, we tend to prefer other agents whenever the resting pulse rate during treatment is maintained below 50 beats/min. Whenever there is a history of bronchial asthma, use of the drug should be avoided or it should be given cautiously since asthmatic attacks can be exacerbated. In actual practice with cautious trial, often a history of asthma does not necessarily mean that the drug cannot be used.

Another situation limiting the use of beta-adrenergic blocking drugs is the presence or likelihood of congestive heart failure. This is because the negative inotropic action of beta blockade weakens cardiac contractility. In fact, this contraindication too may be relative rather than absolute since, whenever the blood pressure level is lowered, the major factor involved in causing heart failure is thereby removed. Accordingly, this possibility, too, can be cautiously tested with close follow-up of the patient. Still another contraindication to the use of beta-adrenergic blocking drugs is the presence of peripheral vascular disease or of Raynaud's-like phenomena. This is because beta-blockade often leaves unopposed alpha-tone operating to amplify peripheral vasoconstriction. In addition, in certain patients fluid accumulation and peripheral edema may occur with the use of beta-blocking drugs. This can often be controlled by superimposition of a diuretic rather than by discontinuing administration of the drug itself. However, because of its antirenin antialdosterone action, fluid accumulation is clearly much less of a problem with propranolol than with the other antiadrenergic or vasodilator agents. In certain patients with diabetes mellitus maintained on insulin, propranolol may be contraindicated because it can mask the protective symptoms of insulin-induced hypoglycemia. Finally, idiosyncrasy or rash, of course, are contraindications too. In areas outside the United States some of these problems can be effectively dealt with by using one of the many other beta-adrenergic blocking drugs now commercially available.

Diuretic therapy, too, although usually extremely well tolerated, may pose a problem in particular patients. Thus, in certain patients receiving the sulfonamide agents undue hypokalemia may develop, or hyperuricemia with or without gout, and in others overt diabetes mellitus can develop. When any of these three situations develop, they may often be dealt with effectively by changing to spironolactone. In areas outside the United States, amiloride is also a most effective alternative [34] and within the United States, triamterene, although a weaker diuretic agent, can often be substituted or added.

Beyond these particular contraindications and exclusions, alternative back-up treatment schedules are necessary since, although there is a high degree of effectiveness and specificity associated with the new program, the predictability and certainty of the regimen is still far short of 100 per cent. Thus, some patients will fail to respond to the administration of either propranolol or a diuretic alone or in combination. For these patients, who either do not tolerate or do not respond to the program, serial administration of the back-up drugs in traditional fashion is indicated. Accordingly, there will still be a large back-up role for these other effective agents in the new system.

A Conceptual Perspective. It is perhaps appropriate to close by placing the proposed new treatment system in perspective with previous more established approaches. To me, the new approach signals the transition into a second generation of research in antihypertensive therapy in which we have passed from empiricism into a more rational era. This new reference framework need not be perfect in order to reveal still more new information. In fact, it is quite clear that not all patients respond to antivolume and antirenin therapy even when fully applied together to our current limit of capability. Thus, it is possible that there may be other volume or vasoconstrictor mechanisms which are unidentified or, alternatively, that the same mechanisms already postulated are operative but that a portion of them remain beyond the reach of currently available antirenin and antivolume drugs. Some of these problems seem amenable to near term solution.

Beyond the already proved practical values of the new analytical model and the new treatment system suggested by it, it is perhaps worth considering the major conceptual change from traditional therapy that is implicit in the new system. In our new system, beta-adrenergic therapy with propranolol becomes the cornerstone of treatment and the major drug, with diuretic therapy moving into a secondary, albeit still very important position. The major physiologic issue raised by this change in modus operandi is the question of whether chronic volume depletion and dehydration is preferable to or inferior to a method of antihypertensive therapy which instead invokes long-term beta blockade of the autonomic nervous system to accomplish the reduction in peripheral resistance.

Diuretic therapy has going for it the credibility and the validation of a longer and larger experience. There is no question that this type of therapy is well tolerated and seems without dangerous side effects. On the other hand, in addition to prolonged hypokalemia, one can at least speculate about the possible hazards of long-term dehydration. These include sustained hyperuricemia, azotemia, hemoconcentration, increased blood viscosity and hypercoagulability, increased renin and aldosterone levels in the blood as well as hypercholesterolemia [35]. Moreover, the quality of life under these conditions may not be ideal. Thus, whether or not this state of dehydration leads to subtle weakness and impaired exercise tolerance remains to be tested. It is clear, however, that for whatever reason certain populations existing without dietary salt and exhibiting chronic hemoconcentration and high renin levels also have a much shortened life expectancy [36].

One cannot be entirely certain, therefore, that diuretic therapy is always the best way to maintain normotension. That the coronary circulation may not be favored by dehydration and hypokalemia may hinder cardiac rhythm and function. Thus, in studies using diuretics that established the protective benefits of antihypertensive therapy, it has been difficult to demonstrate protection from myocardial infarction in particular [37]. This may be contrasted with reports suggesting the long-term protective value of beta blockade against ischemic heart disease [38,39] so often an accompaniment or sequel of hypertension. And these impressive benefits of beta-blockade therapy in ischemic heart disease are backed up by animal experiments suggesting propranolol protection from cholesterol-induced atherosclerosis [40].

The conceptual alternative offered by the new treatment system seems, on paper at least, to have attractive features. Thus, when the blood pressure is controlled with beta-adrenergic blockade there is no attendant dehydration, renin and aldosterone levels are instead lowered, cholesterol and uric acid levels are not raised, and blood viscosity and platelet aggregation [43] are reduced [41] rather than increased. These factors have been suspected as possibly being critical to the production of vascular complications and impaired microcirculatory flow. Beyond this, the beta-adrenergic blocking drugs act more directly to reduce peripheral resistance via reduction in neurogenic and angiotensin governance rather than indirectly as appears to be the case with diuretics. Moreover, beta-adrenergic blocking drugs may also take the flings out of blood pressure associated with sudden neural and emotional discharge [42] while at the same time, being free of the unpleasant autonomic postural and central depressant effects of other antiadrenergic drugs. One can even speculate that as civilizations developed, people outgrew the need for the vigorous autonomic nervous system required for primitive life. If so, hypertension may sometimes be related causally to persisting excessive neural discharges for which we now have more effective and pinpointed treatment. Altogether then, the control of blood pressure by this route promises to be more physiologic and promises, therefore, to improve the quality and expentancy of life to an even greater extent than previous modes of therapy. But, of course, these projections will require careful prospective examination.

The new thesis requires further corroboration to be sure, and more research into the mechanisms of hypertension and of the action of antihypertensive drugs. I have not had time to explore with you all the unanswered questions, and you may be sure there are many of them, but hopefully this presentation will stimulate further communication and research, and provide even better therapy.

REFERENCES

1. Freis ED: Salt, volume and prevention of hypertension. Special article. Circulation 53: 589, 1976.
2. Laragh JH, Baer L, Brunner HR, et al.: Renin, angiotensin and aldosterone system in pathogenesis and management of hypertensive vascular disease. Am J Med 52: 633, 1972.
3. Bühler FR, Laragh JH, Baer L, et al.: Propranolol inhibition of renin secretion. A specific approach to diagnosis and treatment of renin-dependent hypertensive diseases. N Engl J Med 287: 1209, 1972.
4. Bühler FR, Laragh JH, Vaughan ED Jr, et al.: The antihypertensive action of propranolol: specific anti-renin responses in high and normal renin forms of essential, renal, renovascular and malignant hypertension. Am J Cardiol 32: 511, 1973.
5. Vaughan ED Jr, Laragh JH, Gavras I, et al.: The volume factor in low and normal renin essential hypertension: Its treatment with either spironolactone or chlorthalidone. Am J Cardiol 32: 523, 1973.
6. Laragh JH, Sealey JE, Sommers SC: Patterns of adrenal secretion and urinary excretion of aldosterone and plasma renin activity in normal and hypertensive subjects. Circ Res 18 (suppl 1): 158, 1966.
7. Brunner HR, Laragh JH, Baer L, et al.: Essential hypertension: Renin and aldosterone, heart attack and stroke. N Engl J Med 286: 441, 1972.
8. Laragh JH: Vasoconstriction-volume analysis for understanding and treating hypertension. The use of renin and aldosterone profiles. Am J Med 55: 261, 1973.
9. Brunner HR, Gavras H, Laragh JH: Angiotensin II blockade in man by Sar^1-ala^8-angiotensin II for understanding and treatment of high blood pressure. The Lancet 2: 1045, 1973.
10. Brunner HR, Gavras H, Laragh JH, et al.: Hypertension in man. Exposure of the renin and sodium components using angiotensin II blockade. Circ Res (suppl I): 35, 1974.
11. Gavras H, Brunner HR, Laragh JH, et al.: An angiotensin converting enzyme inhibitor to identify and treat vasoconstrictor and volume factors in hypertensive patients. N Engl J Med 291: 817, 1974.
12. Case DB, Wallace JM, Keim HJ, et al.: Limitations and usefulness of saralasin, a partial competitive agonist of angiotensin II for evaluating the renin and sodium factors in hypertensive patients. Am J Med 60: 825, 1976.
13. Case DB, Wallace JM, Keim HJ, et al.: Estimating renin participation in hypertension: superiority of converting enzyme inhibitor over saralasin. Am J Med 61: 790, 1976.
14. Case DB, Wallace JM, Keim HJ, et al.: Exposure of angiotensin II as a pressor factor in normal renin hypertension (abstract). Proceedings of the Endocrine Society, 58th Annual Meeting, 1976.
15. Ames RP, Borkowski AJ, Sicinski AM, et al.: Prolonged infusions of angiotensin II and norepinephrine and blood pressure, electrolyte balance, aldosterone and cortisol secretion in normal man and in cirrhosis with ascites. J Clin Invest 44: 1171, 1965.
16. Guyton AC, Coleman TG, Cowley AW Jr, et al.: Arterial pressure regulation. Overriding dominance of the kidneys in long-term regulation and in hypertension. Am J Med 52: 584, 1972.
17. Sealey JE, Gerten-Banes J, Laragh JH: The renin system: variations in man measured by radioimmunoassay or bioassay. Kidney Int 1: 240, 1972.
18. Sealey JE, Laragh JH: Searching out low renin patients: limitations of some commonly used methods. Am J Med 55: 303, 1973.
19. Sealey JE, Laragh JH: Radioimmunoassay of plasma renin activity. Sem Nucl Med 5: 189, 1975.
20. Derkx FHM, GvGool JM, Wenting GJ, et al.: Inactive renin in human plasma. Lancet 2: 496, 1976.

21. Sealey JE, Laragh JH: "Prorenin" in human plasma? Circ Res 36: 11, 1975.
22. Sealey JE, Moon C, Laragh JH, et al.: Plasma prorenin: cryoactivation and relationship to renin substrate in normal subjects. Am J Med 61: 731, 1976.
23. Laragh JH, Sealey JE, Ledingham JGG, et al.: Oral contraceptives. Renin, aldosterone and high blood pressure. JAMA 201: 918, 1967.
24. Laragh JH, Sealey JE, Bühler FR: The renin axis and vasoconstriction volume analysis for understanding and treating renovascular and renal hypertension. J Med 58: 4, 1975.
25. Williams GH: Editorial: Management of renin activity—when is it useful? N Engl J Med 294: 1176, 1976.
26. Simon NM: Letter to the editor. Measurement of renin activity. N Engl J Med 295: 622, 1976.
27. Crane MG, Harris JJ: Effect of spironolactone in hypertensive patients. J Med Sci 260: 311, 1970.
28. Spark RF, Melby JH: Hypertension and low plasma renin activity: presumptive evidence for mineralocorticoid excess. Ann Intern Med 75: 831, 1971.
29. Crane MG, Harris JJ, Johns VJ: Hyporeninemic hypertension. Am J Med 52: 457, 1972.
30. Carey RM, Douglas JG, Schweikert JR, et al.: The syndrome of essential hypertension and suppressed plasma renin activity. Normalization of blood pressure with spironolactone. Arch Intern Med 130: 849, 1972.
31. Woods JW, Liddle GW, Stant EG, et al.: Effect of an adrenal inhibitor in hypertensive patients with suppressed renin. Arch Intern Med 123: 366, 1969.
32. (a) Bühler FR, Burkart F, Lütold BE, et al.: Antihypertensive beta blocking action as related to renin and age: a pharmacologic tool to identify pathogenetic mechanisms in essential hypertension. Am J Cardiol 36: 653, 1975.
(b) Hansson, L: The use of propranolol in hypertension. A review. Postgrad Med J 52 (suppl 4): 77, 1976.
(c) Gillam PMS, Prichard BNC: Discovery of the hypotensive effect of propranolol. Postgrad Med J 52 (suppl): 70, 1976.
(d) Zacharias FJ: Patient acceptability of propranolol and the occurrence of side effects. Postgrad Med J 52 (suppl 4): 87, 1976.
33. Drayer JIM, Keim HJ, Weber MA, et al.: Unexpected pressor responses to propranolol in essential hypertension. An interaction between renin, aldosterone and sympathetic activity. Am J Med 60: 897, 1976.
34. Laragh JH: The proper use of newer diuretics. Ann Intern Med 67: 606, 1967.
35. Ames RP, Hill P: Elevation of serum lipid levels during diuretic therapy of hypertension. Am J Med 62: 1976.
36. Nell JV, Weiss KM: The genetic structure of a tribal population, the Yanomama indians. Am J Phys Anthropol 42: 25, 1976.
37. Veterans Administration Cooperative Study Group on Antihypertensive Agents. Effect of treatment on morbidity and mortality: results in patients with diastolic blood pressure averaging 115 through 129 mmHg. JAMA 202: 1028, 1967.
38. Chamberlain DS, Multi-centre International Study. Improvement in prognosis of myocardial infarction by long-term beta-adrenoceptor blockade using practolol. Br Med J 3: 735, 1975.
39. Mueller H, Ayres SM: Propranolol in acute myocardial infarction in man. Effect on haemodynamics and myocardial oxygenation. Postgraduate Medical Journal 53: 141, 1976.
40. Whittington-Coleman PJ, Carrier O Jr, Douglas BH: The effects of propranolol on cholesterol-induced atheromatous lesions. Atherosclerosis 18: 337, 1972.
41. Dintenfass L, Lake B: Beta blockers and blood viscosity. Letter to the Editor. The Lancet, 1: 1026, 1976.
42. Lorimer AR, Dunn FG, Jones JV, et al.: Beta-adrenoreceptor blockade in hypertension. Am J Med 60: 877, 1976.
43. Frishman WH, Weksler B, Christodoulou JP, et al.: Reversal of abnormal platelet aggregability and change in exercise tolerance in patients with angina pectoris following oral propranolol. Circulation 50: 887, 1974.

DECEMBER 1976

The American Journal of Medicine

VOLUME 61

NUMBER 6

EDITORIAL

Labile Hypertension

Precursor of Sustained Essential Hypertension?

ROBERT M. CAREY, M.D.*
CARLOS R. AYERS, M.D.†
Charlottesville, Virginia

Arterial blood pressure sometimes below and sometimes above 140/90 mm Hg is "labile hypertension" (stage I WHO classification) [1]. This fluctuation of blood pressure implies no hypertensive damage to organs. Identifying people as having labile hypertension is not easy because so little is known about the spontaneous variation of blood pressure in the labile hypertensive state in contrast to that in normal persons or in those with sustained hypertension [2,3]. The small number of patients evaluated and the lack of uniform assessment of blood pressure within each investigation have precluded isolation of these three groups. Despite the use of an intermittent increase in blood pressure above 140/90 mm Hg as the bottom marker for establishing hypertensive hemodynamic and hormonal characteristics [4–7], a very wide fluctuation in blood pressure has not been proved unequivocally in the labile hypertensive state. It is often called "borderline hypertension," "transient hypertension" or "prehypertension" [8,9]. The prevalence of labile hypertension exceeds 10 per cent and the estimated new case rate is 1 per cent per year [8]. The blood pressure survey of 12,371 persons aged 15 years or older in Charlottesville, Virginia (Figure 1) showed an 11 per cent prevalence of the labile hypertensive state after correlation with subsequent blood pressure measurements [10]. This high frequency of labile hypertension cannot be dismissed by statistical regression toward the mean. Since sequential blood pressure measurement in these people disclosed an increasing frequency of diastolic blood pressure above 90 mm Hg, justification appears to classify them as having labile hypertension.

The Charlottesville blood pressure survey, which showed a high prevalence of labile hypertension in the young which decreased with advancing age (Figure 2), contrasts with the belief that the prevalence of labile hypertension increases with age [8].

From the Department of Internal Medicine, University of Virginia School of Medicine, Charlottesville, Virginia. Requests for reprints should be addressed to Dr. Robert M. Carey, Box 146, University of Virginia Hospital, Charlottesville, Virginia 22901. Manuscript accepted June 16, 1976.

* Established Investigator of the American Heart Association.
† Virginia Heart Association Professor of Cardiovascular Research.

The most complete examination of the relation between blood pressure and age which showed "transient hypertension" with increasing age is limited to a retrospective analysis of male U.S. Army officers [11]. The Charlottesville study showed a high prevalence of labile hypertension in white men which conforms to the greater prevalence of labile hypertension in men [8].

Retrospective analyses indicate that in 10 to 25 per cent of these patients the labile hypertension may progress to sustained hypertension [8]. Other investigations which suggest a much higher percentage are not limited to labile hypertension and include patients with mild sustained hypertension with subsequent progressive increases in blood pressure [12,13]. In 12 per cent of young airmen with labile hypertension, sustained hypertension developed over the subsequent 20 years whereas in only 2 per cent of those who were initially normotensive did sustained hypertension develop [14]. During the past year in the Charlottesville survey, 169 patients with labile hypertension, aged 15 to 55 years, were reassessed at six month intervals

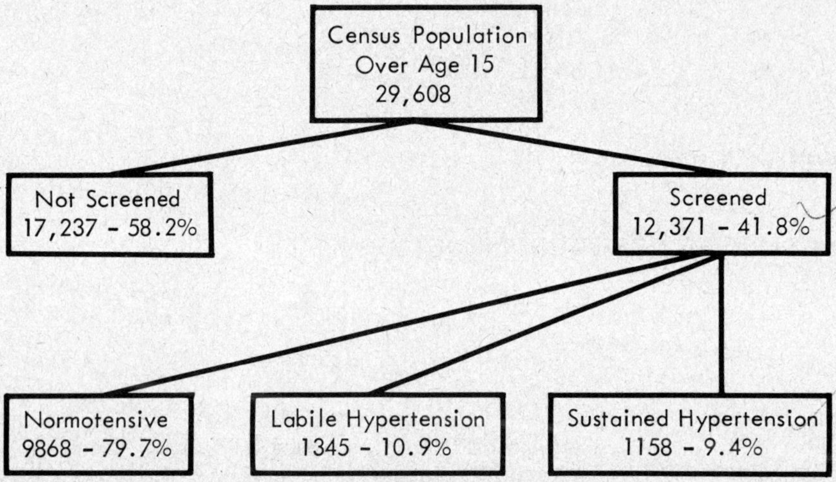

Figure 1. *Prevalence of labile and sustained hypertension in the population of Charlottesville, Virginia, after initial home screening, repeat blood pressure measurements of persons initially hypertensive and confirmation of hypertension in treated patients by chart review. (Criteria for hypertension: diastolic blood pressure ≥ 90 mm Hg < age 55; ≥ 100 mm Hg ≥ age 55.)*

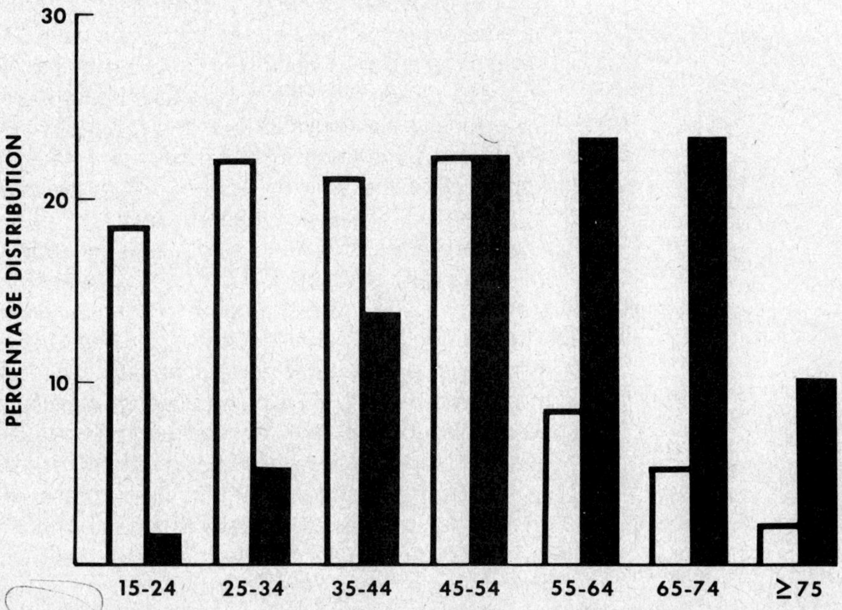

Figure 2. *Distribution of labile hypertension (open bars) and sustained hypertension (closed bars) in Charlottesville, Virginia, by age.*

[15]. During the first six months, sustained essential hypertension developed in nine patients (5.3 per cent), and 20 patients (12 per cent) became hypertensive within the year.

Most longitudinal studies of labile hypertensive patients suggest that they have increased risk of subsequent cardiovascular morbidity and mortality when compared to control subjects [9,16,17], and the risk in all age groups appears twice that of the normotensive population [18]. Retrospective assessment suggests that the risk of cardiovascular mortality and morbidity is probably increased only when labile hypertension progresses to sustained essential hypertension. The natural history of labile hypertension has not been prospectively examined, and the number of people with labile hypertension who acquire sustained hypertension remains unknown.

Many investigators have hypothesized that a number of patients with essential hypertension once had labile hypertension before their elevated diastolic blood pressure level became fixed [2,3,19]. In the hyperkinetic circulatory state of increased cardiac output, heart rate, systolic pressure, left ventricular ejection rate and ejection fraction, the peripheral vascular resistance is normal, but it may be inappropriately high relative to the cardiac output. This state resembles the "hyperdynamic beta-adrenergic circulatory state" with its increased sensitivity of the cardiovascular system to catecholamines during upright tilting, exercise or infusion of isoproterenol [20,21]. The hyperkinetic state mimics cardiovascular changes of emotional stress and of the defense response of animals during vagal inhibition [22,23]; it may be associated with decreased parasympathetic and increased sympathetic tone [6].

Half of the patients in the first report of the hyperkinetic heart syndrome had labile hypertension [24]; later workers suggested that the hyperkinetic circulatory state and labile hypertension represented an early stage in the development of fixed hypertension [5]. In these patients with labile hypertension the resting cardiac outputs and ventricular ejection rates are high when compared to those in normal subjects and in patients with fixed essential hypertension [4]. Total peripheral resistance appeared normal in labile hypertension, but increased progressively in mild, moderate and severe essential hypertension. Plasma renin activity was increased in labile hypertension. The decrease in blood pressure during treatment with the beta-adrenergic antagonist, propranolol, was directly related to the decrease in cardiac output. Although the hemodynamic abnormalities of labile hypertension are known, the relationship of the catecholamine and renin-angiotensin hormonal systems to the development and maintenance of the hyperkinetic circulatory state is unknown. Since most studies of labile hypertension are retrospective, its natural history and the evolution of hemodynamic and hormonal influences are not clearly defined.

Now, well-performed prospective study of a large population of patients can be accomplished by employing noninvasive technics, including echocardiography and vectorcardiography, for quantification of cardiovascular structure and function. Blood pressure, cardiac output, peripheral vascular resistance, left ventricular wall thickness, systolic time intervals, left ventricular circumferential fiber shortening rate and mean normalized posterior ventricular wall velocity can be measured at periodic intervals. Thus, a dynamic profile of cardiovascular physiology during the generation of the hypertensive process is now feasible.

Since we now have precise methods for measuring basal hormone levels in outpatients, the contribution of vasoactive compounds to the evolution of labile to fixed hypertension can be accessed concomitantly.

The hypothesis that labile hypertension progresses in severity with concomitant hormonal and hemodynamic changes to fixed essential hypertension needs testing urgently. Elucidation of the pathophysiology and natural history of labile hypertension will provide the basis for rational, specific therapeutic and preventive interventions in the future.

REFERENCES

1. Brod J, Hilleboc HE, Kimura N, et al.: Arterial hypertension and ischemic heart disease: preventative aspects: report of an expert committee. WHO Technical Report Service 231: 3, 1961.
2. Thacker EA: A comparative study of normal and abnormal blood pressures among university students. Am Heart J 20: 89, 1940.
3. Robinson SC, Brucer M: Range of normal blood pressure: a statistical and clinical study of 11,383 persons. Arch Intern Med 64: 409, 1939.
4. Frolich ED, Kozul VJ, Tarazi RC, et al.: Physiological comparison of labile and essential hypertension. Circ Res 26 and 27 (suppl I): I-55, 1970.
5. Eich RH, Peters RJ, Cuddy RP, et al.: The hemodynamics of labile hypertension. Am Heart J 63: 188, 1972.
6. Julius S, Pascual AV, London R: Role of parasympathetic inhibition in the hyperkinetic type of borderline hypertension. Circulation 44: 413, 1971.
7. Hamet P, Kuchel O, Genest J: Effect of upright posture and isoproterenol infusion on cyclic adenosive monophosphate excretion in control subjects and patients with labile hypertension. J Clin Endo Met 36: 218, 1973.
8. Julius S, Schork MA: Borderline hypertension—a critical review. J Chronic Dis 23: 723, 1971.
9. Safar ME, Weiss YA, Levenson JA, et al.: Hemodynamic study of 85 patients with borderline hypertension. Am J Cardiol 31: 315, 1973.
10. Carey RM, Reid RA, Ayers CR, et al.: The Charlottesville blood pressure survey: value of repeat blood pressure measurements to determine the prevalence of labile and sus-

tained hypertension. JAMA 236: 847, 1976.
11. Levy RL, Hillman CC, Stroud W, et al.: Transient hypertension: its significance in terms of later development of sustained hypertension and cardiovascular-renal diseases. JAMA 125: 829, 1944.
12. Hines EA Jr: Range of normal blood pressure and subsequent development of hypertension: a followup study of 1,522 patients. JAMA 115: 291, 1940.
13. Vancura A: On transient hypertension in young subjects. Cardiologia (Basel) 16: 124, 1950.
14. Madsen PER, Buch J: Long-term prognosis of transient hypertension in young male adults. Aerospace Medicine 42: 752, 1971.
15. Carey RM: Unpublished observations.
16. Heyden S, Bartel AG, Hames CG, et al.: Elevated blood pressure levels in adolescents, Evans County, Georgia: a seven year followup of 30 patients and 30 controls. JAMA 209: 1683, 1969.
17. Kannel WB, Schwartz MJ, McNamara PM: Blood pressure and the risk of coronary heart disease: the Framingham study. Dis Chest 56: 43, 1969.
18. Lew EA: Blood pressure and mortality—life insurance experience. The Epidemiology of Hypertension: Proceedings of an International Symposium (Stamler J, Stamler R, Pullman TN, eds) New York, Grune & Stratton, 1967, p 392.
19. Rosenblum R, Dolman AJ: Propranolol in the treatment of hyperkinetic heart syndrome, idiopathic hypertrophic subaortic stenosis and systemic hypertension. Am Heart J 79: 134, 1970.
20. Frolich ED, Dustan HP, Page IH: Hyperdynamic beta-adrenergic circulatory state. Arch Intern Med 117: 614, 1966.
21. Frolich ED, Tarazi RC, Dustan HP: Hyperdynamic beta-adrenergic circulatory state: increased beta-receptor responsiveness. Arch Intern Med 123: 1, 1969.
22. Forsyth RP, Harris RE: Circulatory changes during stressful stimuli in Rhesus monkeys. Circ Res 26 (suppl I): 13, 1970.
23. Hilton SM: Inhibition of baroreceptor reflexes on hypothalamic stimulation. J Physiol 165: 56, 1962.
24. Gorlin R: The hyperkinetic heart syndrome. JAMA 182: 823, 1962.

Body Fat: Its Relationship to Coronary Heart Disease, Blood Pressure, Lipids and Other Risk Factors Measured in a Large Male Population

ROLAND L. WEINSIER, M.D., Dr.P.H. in Nutr.*
ROBERT J. FUCHS, M.S.
THOMAS D. KAY, R.T. (N.M.T.)
JOHN H. TRIEBWASSER, M.D.
MALCOLM C. LANCASTER, M.D.
Brooks Air Force Base, Texas

Obesity is variably considered to be a major contributor to hypertension and hyperlipidemia, and its treatment is recommended in the management of coronary heart disease. Total body fat was measured by tritium dilution in a large male population and its relationship to age, blood pressure, serum lipids, uric acid and the diagnoses of coronary heart disease, hypertension and glucose intolerance was examined. In addition, three commonly used weight: height indices of obesity were correlated with each of these parameters.

The correlation of body fat with blood pressure, serum cholesterol and triglycerides, although statistically significant, was of only small magnitude. Mean levels of body fat were not significantly different between patients with coronary disease and control subjects, whereas serum cholesterol and, to a lesser extent, systolic blood pressure were potent risk factors for the disease. It is concluded that obesity is only a minor determinant of blood pressure and lipid level, and that its contribution to coronary heart disease is small or nonexistent.

Excessive body fat has been so conspicuously associated with disorders such as coronary heart disease, hypertension and hyperlipidemia that obesity per se, by its association, is often incriminated as a major cause. However, the widely accepted beliefs that obesity is a causative factor in the diseases it is associated with and that its correction is tantamount to their control are far from being as well founded as is often believed.

Much of the dilemma stems from insurance experience data showing an increased mortality rate among policyholders whose body weight is excessive for their height [1]. The created impression that virtually all degrees of overweight constitute risks to health and longevity may be an extrapolation from the actuarial data. In fact, overweight generally had to exceed 25 per cent above average weight before appreciable increases in mortality rate were demonstrated [2]. At the same time, proof of the efficacy of weight losing maneuvers is lacking. Serious misunderstanding may also arise from the fact that overweight and obesity are not identical. However, a reliable estimate of body fat is difficult to determine in a large population, and, therefore, various indices of obesity are employed. Most commonly, these are based on various combinations of weight:height ratios, measurements of relative weight (referenced to a standard weight for a select population) and determinations of subcutaneous fat by skinfold calipers.

From the Internal Medicine Branch, Clinical Sciences Division, USAF School of Aerospace Medicine, Brooks Air Force Base, Texas. The research reported in this paper was conducted by personnel of the Clinical Sciences Division, USAF School of Aerospace Medicine, Aerospace Medical Division AFSC, United States Air Force, Brooks Air Force Base, Texas. Requests for reprints should be addressed to The Nutrition Program, University of Alabama, School of Medicine, University Station, Birmingham, Alabama 35294. Manuscript accepted March 29, 1976.

*Present address: The Nutrition Program, University of Alabama, School of Medicine, University Station, Birmingham, Alabama 35294.

Each of these estimates has limitations [3]. Thus, conclusions drawn from the large number of studies relating "obesity" to various parameters of health have been contradictory and confusing.

To resolve some of these problems, we undertook the measurement of per cent body fat by the tritium dilution technic in a large male population. The data were then examined in their relationship to age, blood pressure, serum lipids and uric acid, and to the diagnoses of coronary heart disease, hypertension and glucose intolerance.

MATERIALS AND METHODS

Patient Population and Measured Parameters. The population examined consisted of 1,483 consecutive referrals to the USAF School of Aerospace Medicine Aeromedical Consultation Service. Patients were ambulatory, male, air crewmembers, not acutely ill, who were referred from different parts of the country for evaluation of a variety of potentially disqualifying findings, generally electrocardiographic, neurologic, cardiac, ear, nose and throat, or ophthalmologic in nature. Approximately 90 to 95 per cent of those examined were white, with a mean age of 37 years. The population represented a broad spectrum of age (17 to 64 years), weight (53 to 120 kg) and height (147 to 206 cm).

The following attributes were measured: per cent body fat, nude height and weight, blood pressure, oral glucose tolerance, serum cholesterol, triglycerides and uric acid. In some cases, not all parameters were available. The height, weight and blood pressure used for reference were those taken by the flight surgeon or internist during the initial examination at the School. Serum cholesterol and triglycerides were analyzed after an overnight fast employing a modification of the Wease, Malvin and Espinosa method [4], and serum uric acid was analyzed by the Technicon® method N-13 [5]. On the same morning, a standard 2-hour oral glucose tolerance screening test (40 g glucose/m^2) was performed following three days of a 300 g carbohydrate intake.

Technic of Body Fat Measurement. Body fat content was derived from the total body water, measured by the tritium dilution technic. The tritiated water was a sterile solution containing benzyl alcohol (0.9 per cent) to prevent bacterial growth. The specific activity was 1 mc/g, with a concentration of 1 mc/ml. The radiochemical purity was 98 per cent and the pH was 7. The solution was diluted with distilled water to 25 μc/ml so that 10 ml gave a dose of 250 μc. The total body dose from tritium was 19 mrads per determination.

Each patient was instructed to avoid food, alcohol and water for at least 8 hours before the test. The test dose was 10 ml of tritiated water, taken orally, followed by 10 ml of water. After 3 hours, a 15 ml sample of whole blood was drawn, and two 1 ml aliquots of serum (one sample, one standard) were put into counting tubes.

Total body water (TBW) and per cent body fat were calculated by means of standard formulas [6], under the assumptions that water makes up 73 per cent of the lean body mass (LBM) and that body fat contains essentially no water [7].

$$\text{TBW (in liters)} = \frac{(\text{standard cpm} - \text{sample cpm})(47{,}000)}{(\text{standard cpm} - \text{background cpm})}$$

$$\text{LBM (in kg)} = \text{TBW}/0.73$$

$$\text{Per cent body fat} = \frac{\text{body weight} - \text{LBM}}{\text{body weight}} \times 100$$

If any condition existed which was suspect of altering a patient's state of hydration, he was either tested at a later time or excluded from the study.

Weight:Height Indices of Obesity. Three indices of obesity were derived from body weight (W) and height (H): W:H, W:H^2 (sometimes called Quetelet's index) and H:$W^{1/3}$ (often called the ponderal index). Each was examined for a relationship with the various measured parameters and disease states.

Disease Categories. The diagnosis of coronary heart disease was only made when there was evidence of probable or overt disease on the basis of (1) abnormal selective coronary angiography (cardiology staff concensus), (2) documented myocardial infarction or (3) classic symptoms of angina pectoris. Indications for cardiac catheterization included a history or electrocardiographic findings suggestive of coronary disease, the presence of an abnormal electrocardiographic response to treadmill exercise (performed routinely), acquired bundle branch block, supraventricular tachyarrhythmias and evidence to suggest significant valvular heart disease. Whereas the presence of electrocardiographic abnormalities was a frequent basis for referral, the diagnosis of coronary heart disease was not based on this criterion alone. Since normal selective coronary angiograms were found in approximately 60 per cent of the catheterized patients (regardless of other findings), the presence of normal or abnormal coronary angiograms was also regarded as a separate diagnostic category.

A diagnosis of hypertension was based on a three day average systolic pressure of $\geq$140 mm Hg or diastolic pressure of $\geq$90 mm Hg. A diagnosis of glucose intolerance was made only when an abnormal 2-hour glucose tolerance screen was supported by either a second abnormal test (generally 3-hour) or a prior record of glucose intolerance. Interpretation of an abnormal test response was based on one or more of the following plasma glucose values: fasting, $>$120 mg/100 ml; 1 hour, $>$220 mg/100 ml; 1 1/2 hour, $>$175 mg/100 ml; 2 hour, $>$135 mg/100 ml; 3 hour $>$120 mg/100 ml.

Analysis of Data. Correlation coefficients were calculated and scatter plots derived to describe the degree of association of both age and body fat with blood pressure, lipids and uric acid. Regression lines were purposefully omitted from the plots in order to emphasize the marked variability of the data and to avoid misinterpretation by relating observed differences between subjects to changes within an individual subject.

For each disease category, the means of each measured parameter (e.g., body fat, blood pressure) were compared between patients with and without a positive diagnosis. The effect of age was removed using stratified age categories.

RESULTS

Characteristics of Patient Population. The study population is described in Table I according to the mean, range and standard deviation for age, body fat, blood pressure, blood lipids and uric acid. The results of every parameter were not available in all cases.

Correlation of Age and Obesity with Measured Parameters. Per cent body fat had a significant positive correlation with age (r = 0.36), whereas lean body mass varied inversely with age (r = −0.19) (p <0.01).

Correlation coefficients for blood pressure and per cent body fat, controlling for age effect, were 0.18 (systolic) and 0.19 (diastolic) (Table II). Although statistically significant (p <0.01), the degree of correlation is not impressive when the data are visualized as scatter plots (Figures 1 and 2).

Correlation coefficients for blood lipids and per cent body fat, controlling for age effect, were 0.15 for cholesterol and 0.24 for triglycerides (p <0.01) (Table II). Again, however, scatter plots of the data revealed the marked variability and weakness of the associations (Figures 3 and 4).

Comparison of Measured Parameters in Patients With and Without Specific Diseases (Table III). Coronary heart disease: Per cent body fat was compared between a group of 80 patients with probable or overt coronary heart disease and 935 patients free of coronary disease, averaging differences over age categories <30, 30–39, 40–49 and ≥50 years to minimize the effect of age. Average body fat was only slightly greater in those with heart disease (23.0 per cent) than in those without (21.1 per cent) (p = 0.07). Of 48 patients with angiographically demonstrated coronary heart disease versus 94 with normal angiograms, body fat was not statistically different (21.9 per cent and 21.4 per cent, respectively), averaging differences over age categories <40 and ≥40 years.

Mean systolic blood pressure was notably higher among patients with the diagnosis of coronary heart disease (p <0.01); diastolic blood pressure differed less significantly (p = 0.09). On the other hand, no differences in average blood pressure were found between groups with and without coronary angiographic abnormalities.

Mean serum cholesterol levels were significantly higher among the younger patients with coronary heart disease, but the significance of the differences gradually fell in the older age groups (see footnote ‡, Table III). Similarly, for those with coronary angiographic abnormalities: serum cholesterol averaged 37 mg/100 ml higher among patients with coronary heart disease in the <40 year category (251 versus 214 mg/100 ml), compared to only 19 mg/100 ml higher in the ≥40 year category (246 versus 227 mg/100 ml).

Mean serum triglyceride and uric acid levels were comparable between the groups in all age categories.

Hypertension: Hypertensive patients tended to have a greater per cent body fat which, while statistically significant (p >0.001), was small in terms of its actual difference (23.0 versus 21.0 per cent). Serum cholesterol levels tended to be higher among hypertensive subjects, particularly among those receiving medical therapy, whereas triclyceride levels were similar between groups, irrespective of whether the subjects were receiving antihypertensive medication.

Mean serum uric acid levels did not differ statistically between hypertensive and normotensive patients in the younger age categories, regardless of therapy. By contrast, for the ≥40 age group uric acid levels were significantly higher among hypertensive subjects compared to control subjects, and also higher among hypertensive subjects receiving medication compared to those not receiving medication. Of particular interest is that the average uric acid concentration was greater even among untreated hypertensive patients when compared to normotensive patients (footnotes § and #, Table III).

TABLE I Characteristics of Patient Population

Parameter	Mean	Range	Standard Deviation	No. of Subjects
Age (yr)	37	17–64	9	1,483
Body fat (%)	20.6	5.2–39.5	5.5	1,015
Blood pressure (mm Hg)				
Systolic	129	90–210	14	1,299
Diastolic	82	42–118	11	1,299
Cholesterol (mg/100 ml)	217	108–516	40	1,265
Triglycerides (mg/100 ml)	110	22–612	63	1,264
Uric acid (mg/100 ml)	6.5	3.4–14.5	1.2	1,267

TABLE II Correlations of Age and Obesity with Measured Parameters

		% Body Fat	
Parameter	Age	Simple	Age-Adjusted
Age	. . .	0.36 (1,015)	. . .
Blood pressure			
Systolic	0.17 (1,299)	0.23 (866)	0.18
Diastolic	0.30 (1,299)	0.28 (866)	0.19
Cholesterol	0.34 (1,265)	0.25 (845)	0.15
Triglycerides	0.22 (1,264)	0.29 (844)	0.24
Uric acid	0.01 (1,267)	0.19 (847)	. . .

NOTE: Figures in parentheses indicate the number of observations. All correlations are significant at p <0.01, except uric acid, with age, which is not significant at the 0.05 level.

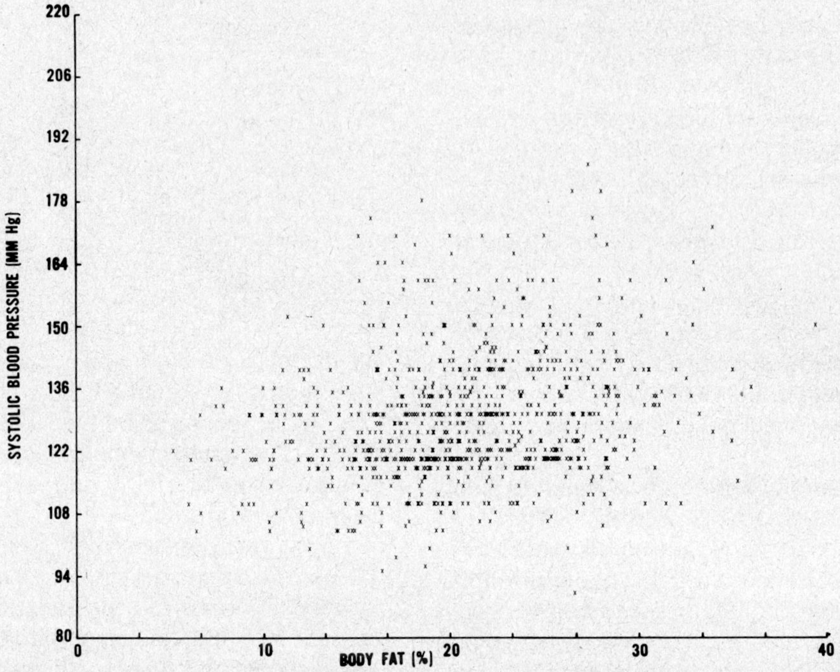

Figure 1. *Scatter plot describing the relationship between systolic blood pressure and per cent body fat. Although a statistically significant correlation exists (r = 0.18, age-adjusted), the relationship is visually unimpressive.*

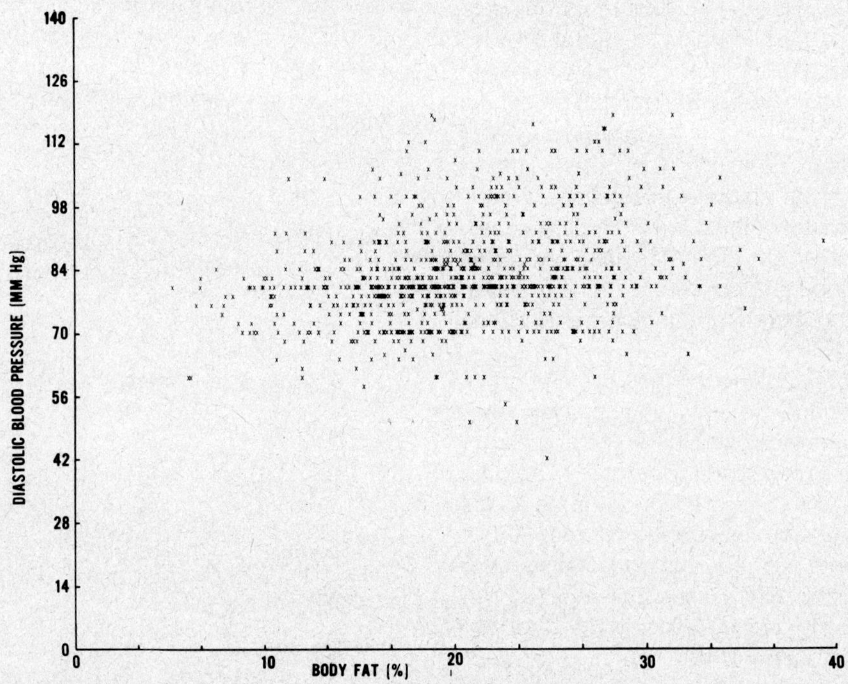

Figure 2. *Scatter plot describing the relationship between diastolic blood pressure and per cent body fat. Although a statistically significant correlation exists (r = 0.19, age-adjusted), the relationship is visually unimpressive.*

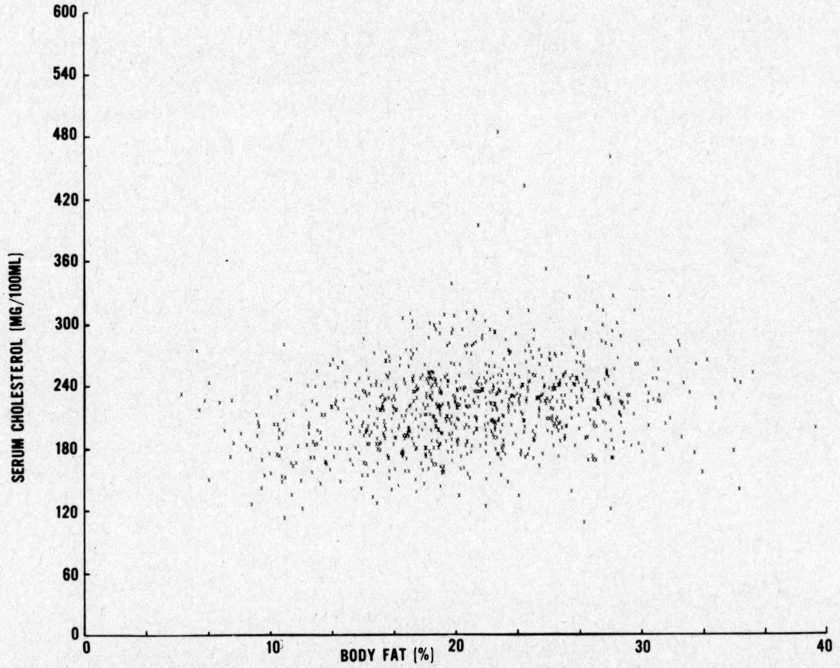

Figure 3. *Scatter plot describing the relationship between serum cholesterol and per cent body fat. Although a statistically significant correlation exists (r = 0.15, age-adjusted), the relationship is visually unimpressive.*

Figure 4. *Scatter plot describing the relationship between serum triglycerides and per cent body fat. Although a statistically significant correlation exists (r = 0.24, age-adjusted), the relationship is visually unimpressive.*

TABLE III Mean Values (Age-Adjusted) for Various Parameters in Patients With and Without Specific Diagnoses

	Coronary Heart Disease*		Coronary Angiography†		Hypertension*		Hypertensive Patients†		Glucose Intolerance†	
	Present/Absent	p	Abnormal/Normal	p	Present/Absent	p	Medical Rx/ No Medical Rx	p	Present/Absent	p
Body fat (%)	23.0/21.1 (80/935)	0.07	21.9/21.4 (48/94)	NS	23.0/21.0 (113/902)	<0.001	22.5/23.5 (38/75)	NS	23.5/20.9 (44/971)	<0.01
Systolic blood pressure (mm Hg)	137/129 (93/1,206)	<0.01	132/130 (53/123)	NS	150/127 (146/1,153)	<0.001	152/149 (36/110)	NS	137/129 (68/1,231)	<0.001
Diastolic blood pressure (mm Hg)	86/82 (93/1,206)	0.09	84/84 (53/123)	NS	96/81 (146/1,153)	<0.001	103/94 (36/110)	<0.001	89/82 (63/1,231)	<0.001
Cholesterol (mg/100 ml)	235/218 (87/1,178	‡	249/220 (50/121)	<0.001	226/219 (141/1,124)	0.06	238/222 (36/105)	0.05	231/219 (65/1,200)	0.03
Triglycerides (mg/100 ml)	122/112 (87/1,178)	NS	134/114 (50/121)	NS	121/112 (141/1,124)	NS	118/124 (36/105)	NS	144/112 (65/1,200)	<0.01
Uric acid (mg/100 ml)	6.4/6.5 (86/1,181)	NS	6.4/6.5 (49/121)	NS	7.1/6.4 (142/1,125)	§	7.5/6.9 (36/106)	#	6.6/6.5 (65/1,202)	‖

NOTE: Figures in parentheses indicate the number of observations.

* Adjusted for age categories <30, 30–39, 40–49, ≥50 years.

† Adjusted for age categories <40 and ≥40 years.

‡ Cholesterol differences significant in younger age categories only: 30–39 (260/216 mg/100 ml, $p < 0.001$); 40–49 (254/226 mg/100 ml, $p < 0.001$); ≥50 (241/232 ml/100 ml, NS). (Insufficient data for <30 category.)

§ Uric acid differences significant in older age categories only: <30 (6.7/6.6 mg/100 ml, NS); 30–39 (6.7/6.3 mg/100 ml, $p < 0.05$); 40–49 (7.4/6.3 mg/100 ml, $p < 0.001$) ≥50 (7.6/6.6 mg/100 ml, $p < 0.001$).

Uric acid differences significant in older age category only: <40 (6.8/6.7 mg/100 ml, NS); ≥40 (8.3/7.1 mg/100 ml, $p < 0.01$).

‖ Uric acid differences significant in older age category only: <40 (6.2/6.5 mg/100 ml, NS); ≥ 40 (7.0/6.5 mg/100 ml, $p < 0.01$).

Glucose intolerance: As noted in Table III, patients with glucose intolerance tended to be more obese, have higher systolic and diastolic blood pressure levels, and relatively elevated cholesterol and triglyceride levels. The mean serum uric acid level was significantly higher among older glucose intolerant patients (7.0 versus 6.5 mg/100 ml), whereas the levels did not statistically differ in the <40 year group (6.2 versus 6.5 mg/100 ml).

Weight:Height Ratios as Relative Indices of Obesity. Three indices of obesity (W:H, W:H^2, H:W$^{1/3}$) were found to be comparable in their correlation with per cent body fat (r = 0.73, 0.74 −0.70, respectively). At most, however, any one of the indices, if used as a predictor, would account for only about one-half of the variance of body fat ($r^2 = 0.74^2 = 0.55$).

The relationships of various risk parameters with body fat and weight:height indices are shown in Table IV.

TABLE IV Correlations of Body Fat and Weight: Height Indices with Measured Parameters

Parameter	% Body Fat	H:W$^{1/3}$	W:H^2	W:H
Age	0.36	−0.15	0.11	0.08
Blood pressure				
Systolic	0.23	−0.21	0.22	0.20
Diastolic	0.28	−0.27	0.26	0.22
Cholesterol	0.25	−0.20	0.17	0.13
Triglycerides	0.29	−0.28	0.27	0.23
Uric acid	0.19	−0.23	0.28	0.29

COMMENTS

A technic for direct measurement of the degree of obesity in a patient does not exist. Various anthropometric measures, and even clinical observation, permit identification of gross obesity. However, these methods are of limited value for a more accurate determination of body fat and may be grossly inaccurate for those who are above weight standards as a result of athletic conditioning. The most reliable methods available, all indirect, include measures of body density, potassium-40 and total body water. In a comparison study of the three technics, Krzywicki et al. [8] found them to be highly correlated in their estimates of body fat. To the best of our knowledge, the present study is the first large scale attempt to relate coronary heart disease and its various risk associates to obesity using one of the more reliable measures of body fat.

A general trend has been noted for body weight and subcutaneous fat to increase with age, judging at least from studies in developed countries [9,10]. Our findings showed that, in fact, there is a relatively strong positive correlation between total body fat and age (r = 0.36), whereas lean body mass tended to decrease with age (r = −0.19). These findings support the conclusions of Pierson et al. [11] that the aging process is accompanied both by an increase in body fat and a decrease in muscle mass. In studies such as ours, if account is not taken of this increase in body fat with age, it is possible to associate some attributes of ill health with obesity that are actually only related to age.

Body Fat, Blood Pressure and Lipids. The present data revealed the small degree to which obesity is associated with either the blood pressure or lipid level (Table II). The correlation coefficients are, in fact, similar to those found in previous population studies using various estimates of body fat (with blood pressure [9,10,12,13], with blood lipids [9,10,14–16]. However, upon examining the descriptive data as the scatter plots of Figures 1–4, variability is so great that no person's blood pressure or lipid level could necessarily be attributed to his degree of obesity. This clearly suggests that obesity is neither the sole nor major determinant of these variables.

By contrast, longitudinal studies have shown that weight reduction may have a significant, although quite variable, effect on lowering blood pressure [17], serum cholesterol [18–21] and triglyceride levels [20–21]. The differences seen between the present cross sectional data and those of some prospective studies can be explained in two ways: One is that a low order of correlation of obesity with blood pressure and lipid levels does not preclude the possibility that changes in body fat could have a modifying influence on these parameters. A second consideration is that the effect of weight change on blood pressure and lipidemia may only be transient with a return to base line values after weight stabilizes at a new level. In fact, weight reduction programs are generally accompanied by uncontrolled variables, besides that of body fat, which readily affect blood pressure and lipid levels. Dahl [22] has argued that the hypotensive effect of reducing regimens is only secondary to their lower salt content. The lipid changes reported to parallel weight change (not necessarily fat change) could possibly be attributed to concomitant changes in meal frequency [23,24], dietary composition of fat [21], carbohydrate [25], cholesterol [26] and calories [27], among other variables [28,29]. Reports have supported [30,31] and refuted [19–21] the transient effect of weight change on serum cholesterol. Mann [3] has contended that the effect of weight gain or loss on cholesterolemia can only be transient and that the effects of weight reduction programs on blood pressure levels remain indecisive.

The present data, relating body fat to other attributes among persons with relatively stable weight, clearly suggest that the contribution of obesity per se to blood pressure and lipid levels is necessarily small. Obesity may influence these variables, but by no means determines their level.

Coronary Heart Disease and Measured Parameters. Although life insurance statistics emphasize the relationship between overweight and death from heart disease [1], epidemiologic studies lend less credance to the association. The evidence derived from the seven-nation study conducted by Keys and his colleagues [9,32] failed to show an independent contribution of obesity (measured by skinfold thickness and the index weight:height^2) to coronary heart disease when the effect of blood pressure was removed. In the Los Angeles Study [33] and the Western Collaborative Group Study [34] the investigators came to similar conclusions, and in the Framingham Study [35] it was found that relative weight related only to angina pectoris and sudden death. The present data did not show a significant difference in the age-adjusted means of per cent body fat between patients with and without coronary heart disease, supporting Mann's contention that the contribution of obesity to coronary heart disease is either small or nonexistent [3]. The possibility that body fat bears a stronger relationship to certain specific manifestations of coronary heart disease cannot be ruled out from our data.

Interestingly, serum cholesterol alone stood out as a risk associate of coronary disease when based on the diagnostic criterion of either "probable or overt" disease or abnormal angiography. By contrast, systolic blood pressure levels and, to a lesser extent, diastolic blood pressure levels were significantly elevated only in patients in whom the diagnosis was based on the former criterion, and serum triglyceride and uric acid levels did not appear in either case as so-called risk factors for coronary heart disease. On closer examination of the cholesterol values in various age groups, it was noted that the mean levels in patients with and without coronary heart disease were highly divergent at younger ages, becoming insignificantly different in the elders. This is in agreement with the findings of the Framingham Study wherein serum cholesterol gradually lost its significance as a risk factor in the older age groups [36].

Hypertension and Measured Parameters. Studies relating estimates of obesity and blood pressure have not infrequently equated statistical significance with practical significance [10,13,17,19]. The difference we found in mean per cent body fat between hypertensive and normotensive subjects was 2 per cent (equivalent to an average difference in weight of only 1.6 kg); the correlation coefficient between body fat and blood pressure was 0.18 (Figures 1 and 2). Both values were statistically significant but of such low magnitude as to re-emphasize the weak, or negligible, contribution of body fat to blood pressure level.

The present data support the previously noted tendency to higher cholesterol levels among hypertensive patients [37]. This relative hypercholesterolemia seems to derive, however, from the higher serum values in patients receiving antihypertensive medication versus those not receiving medication (Table III). On the other hand, hyperuricemia has been found more frequently among hypertensive subjects, aside from the added effects of drug therapy [37]. Our data support this direct relationship between hypertension and hyperuricemia. This is on the basis that the average uric acid level among medically untreated hypertensive subjects tended to be higher than the level among normotensive subjects, at least in the $\geq$ 40 year age categories (footnotes § and #, Table III). That the differences in uric acid levels found within both the diagnosis and treatment categories were only significant among the older patients suggests, perhaps, that a compensatory mechanism that is operative in youth fails with aging.

Glucose Intolerance and Measured Parameters. The presence of glucose intolerance was accompanied by a greater degree of adiposity and a higher blood pressure level, both of which are recognized associates of the disorder [38]. Serum lipids, however, bear a more controversial relationship. Cholesterol levels among those with well-controlled diabetes have been reported to be normal [39,40], whereas triglyceride levels have been variably reported as being normal [40–42] or elevated [39,43], at least among older diabetic subjects [44]. In the present study, the age-adjusted mean values for serum cholesterol and triglycerides were higher among the 65 patients with decreased glucose tolerance compared to 1,200 patients with normal tolerance. The explanation for this finding, which contrasts with some previous reports, is not clear.

It was of interest to find that the mean serum uric acid level among glucose intolerant patients was significantly elevated over that in control subjects, but only in the older age group. This "protective effect" of youth is similar to the uric acid findings among hypertensive patients mentioned herein.

Weight:Height Indices of Obesity. The three most commonly used weight:height indices of obesity are W:H, W:H^2 and H:W$^{1/3}$, used because of their convenience of measurement. Which ratio best reflects body fat has been a matter of controversy, although most studies have favored Quetelet's index (W:H^2) [45–47]. In the present study, the three indices were comparable in their direct correlation with per cent body fat. However, these correlations are not high when the indices are considered as predictors of body fat. The three indices and per cent body fat all had low correlations with the risk associates we studied.

IMPLICATIONS

The present data, relating body fat to other attributes among people with relatively stable weight, clearly demonstrate the small degree to which obesity is associated with either the blood pressure or blood lipid level. This is not to say that change in body fat may not modify these variables, but that obesity per se is neither the sole nor the major determinant of their level.

The contribution of obesity to coronary heart disease appears to be small or nonexistent. By contrast, serum cholesterol continues to stand out as a potent risk factor, especially in younger persons, along with systolic blood pressure.

It is postulated that the clinically impressive effect of weight reduction on blood pressure and blood lipids may in large part be related to other attendant variables. On the other hand, maintenance of a lower body fat, without permanent changes in diet and other habits, may have relatively little effect. Although the potential benefits of weight reduction on minimizing risk factors for coronary heart disease may warrant its use in select cases, it is important to recognize the tenuous basis for its widespread recommendation.

ACKNOWLEDGMENT

We are indebted to Lt. Carl Efird, USAF, and Mr. Norman Drisco for compilation of the data for computer analysis, and to Mr. Richard McNee for his critical review and helpful suggestions.

REFERENCES

1. Society of Actuaries: Build and Blood Pressure Study, 1959, vol 1, Chicago, The Society, 1959.
2. Hutchinson JJ: Clinical implications of extensive actuarial study of build and blood pressure. Ann Intern Med 54: 90, 1961.
3. Mann GV: The influence of obesity on health. N Engl J Med 291: 178, 226, 1974.
4. Wease BS, Malvin HH, Espinosa ES: A simplified test tube method for the analysis of total cholesterol and glycerides in human serum. USAF School of Aerospace Medicine—TR-66-53, June 1966.
5. Technicon method N-13, Technicon Manual, Tarrytown, New York, Technicon Corporation, 1962.
6. Logsdon DF: Estimation of the lean body mass and per cent body fat by the tritiated water dilution technique. Radiology Tech 44: 146, 1972.
7. Prentice TC, Siri WE, Berlin NI, et al.: Studies of total body water with tritium. J Clin Invest 31: 412, 1952.
8. Krzywicki HJ, Ward GM, Rahman DP, et al.: A comparison of methods for estimating human body composition. Am J Clin Nutr 27: 1380, 1974.
9. Keys A, Aravanis C, Blackburn H, et al.: Coronary heart disease: overweight and obesity as risk factors. Ann Intern Med 77: 15, 1972.
10. Tran MH, Lellouch J, Richard JL: Fat body mass. II. Its relationship with some biological parameters, blood pressure and physical training in a population of 3660 men aged 20 to 55. Biomedicine 18: 499, 1973.
11. Pierson RN Jr, Lin D, Phillips RA: Total-body potassium in health: effects of age, sex, height and fat. Am J Physiol 226: 206, 1974.
12. Epstein FH, Francis T Jr, Hayner NS, et al.: Prevalence of chronic disease and distribution of selective physiologic variables in a total community, Tecumseh, Michigan. Am J Epidemiol 81: 307, 1965.
13. Kannel WB, Brand N, Skinner JJ Jr, et al.: The relation of adiposity of blood pressure and development of hypertension: the Framingham Study. Ann Intern Med 67: 48, 1967.
14. Motoye HJ, Epstein FH, Kjelsberg MO: Relationship between serum cholesterol and body fatness: an epidemiologic study. Am J Clin Nutr 18: 397, 1966.
15. Harlan WR Jr, Oberman A, Mitchell RE, et al.: Constitutional and environmental factors related to serum lipids and lipoprotein levels. Ann Intern Med 66: 540, 1967.
16. Albrink M, Meigs JW: The relationship between serum triglycerides and skinfold thickness in obese subjects. Ann NY Acad Sci 131: 673, 1965.
17. Chiang BN, Perlman LV, Epstein FH: Overweight and hypertension: a review. Circulation 39: 403, 1969.
18. National Diet Heart Study. Research group final report. Circulation 33 (suppl I): 1, 1968.
19. Ashley FW Jr, Kannel WB: Relation of weight change to changes in atherogenic traits: the Framingham Study. J Chronic Dis 27: 103, 1974.
20. Olefsky J, Reaven GM, Farquhar JW: Effects of weight reduction of obesity: studies of lipid and carbohydrate metabolism in normal and hyperlipoproteinemic subjects. J Clin Invest 53: 64, 1974.
21. Leelarthaepin B, Woodhill JM, Palmer AJ, et al.: Obesity, diet, and type-II hyperlipidemia. Lancet 2: 1217, 1974.
22. Dahl LK: Salt intake and salt need. N Engl J Med 258: 1152, 1205, 1958.
23. Cohn C: Feeding patterns and some aspects of cholesterol metabolism. Fed Proc 23: 76, 1964.
24. Fabry P, Hejl Z, Fodor J, et al.: The frequency of meals. Its relation to overweight, hypercholesterolaemia, and decreasing glucose-tolerance. Lancet 2: 614, 1964.
25. Roberts AM: Effects of a sucrose-free diet on the serum-lipid level of men in Antarctica. Lancet 1: 1201, 1974.
26. Keys A, Anderson JT, Grande F: Serum cholesterol response to changes in the diet. II. The effect of cholesterol in the diet. Metabolism 14: 759, 1965.
27. Nestel PJ, Carroll KF, Havenstein N: Plasma triglyceride response to carbohydrates, fats, and caloric intake. Metabolism 19: 1, 1970.
28. Trowell H: Ischemic heart disease and dietary fiber. Am J Clin Nutr 25: 926, 1972.
29. Grande F, Anderson JT, Keys A: Effect of carbohydrates of leguminous seeds, wheat and potatoes on serum cholesterol concentration in man. J Nutr 86: 313, 1965.
30. Anderson JT, Lawler A, Keys A: Weight gain from simple overeating. II. Serum lipids and blood volume. J Clin Invest 36: 81, 1957.
31. Krehl WA, Lopez SA, Good EI, et al.: Some metabolic changes induced by low carbohydrate diets. Am J Clin Nutr 20: 139, 1967.
32. Keys A: Coronary heart disease in seven countries. Circulation 12 (suppl I): 1, 1970.
33. Chapman JM, Coulson AH, Clark VA, et al.: The differential effect of serum cholesterol, blood pressure and weight on the incidence of myocardial infarction and angina pectoris. J Chronic Dis 23: 631, 1971.
34. Roseman RH, Friedman M, Straus R, et al.: Coronary heart disease in the western collaborative group study: a follow-up experience of 4 and one-half years. J Chronic Dis 23: 173, 1970.
35. Kannel WB, LeBauer EJ, Dawber TR, et al.: Relation of body weight to development of coronary heart disease: the Framingham Study. Circulation 35: 734, 1967.
36. The Framingham Study: An Epidemiological Investigation of Cardiovascular Disease, Section 27 (Kannel WB, Gordon P, eds), Superintendent of Documents, Washington, D.C.,

U.S. Government Printing Office, 1972, p 13.
37. Cannon PJ, Stason WB, Demartini FE, et al.: Hyperuricemia in primary and renal hypertension. N Engl J Med 275: 457, 1966.
38. Sharkey TP: Diabetes mellitus—present problems and new research. J Am Diet Assoc 58: 201, 336, 1971.
39. Schrade W, Boehle E, Biegler R, et al.: Fatty-acid composition of lipid fractions in diabetic serum. Lancet 1: 285, 1963.
40. Rudnick PA, Anderson PS Jr: Diabetes mellitus in Hiroshima, Japan: a detection program and clinical survey. Diabetes 11: 533, 1962.
41. Nikkila EA, Pelkonen R, Miettinen A: Relationship between glucose metabolism and serum triglyceride and cholesterol levels. Diabetologia 2: 232, 1966.
42. Albrink MJ, Lavietes PH, Man EB: Vascular disease and serum lipids in diabetes mellitus: observations over thirty years (1931–1961). Ann Intern Med 58: 305, 1963.
43. New MI, Roberts TN, Bierman EL, et al.: The significance of blood lipid alterations in diabetes mellitus. Diabetes 12: 208, 1963.
44. Bierman EL, Porte D Jr: Carbohydrate intolerance and lipemia. Ann Intern Med 68: 926, 1968.
45. Keys A, Fidanza F, Karvonen MJ, et al.: Indices of relative weight and obesity. J Chronic Dis 25: 329, 1972.
46. Billewicz WZ, Kemsley WFF, Thomson AM: Indices of obesity. Br J Prev Soc Med 16: 183, 1962.
47. Khosla T, Lowe CR: Indices of obesity derived from body weight and height. Br J Prev Soc Med 21: 122, 1967.

Plasma Arginine Vasopressin in the Syndrome of Antidiuretic Hormone Excess Associated with Bronchogenic Carcinoma

PAUL L. PADFIELD, M.R.C.P.
JAMES J. MORTON, Ph.D.
JEHOIADA J. BROWN, F.R.C.P.
ANTHONY F. LEVER, F.R.C.P.
J. IAN S. ROBERTSON, F.R.C.P.
MARTIN WOOD, M.R.C.P.
RUTH FOX, M.R.C.P.
Glasgow, Scotland

A study of plasma arginine vasopressin in 17 patients with the syndrome of inappropriate antidiuretic hormone secretion (SIADH) associated with bronchogenic carcinoma, revealed that the arginine vasopressin levels were distinctly elevated in most. In 14 patients with bronchogenic carcinoma, but without overt SIADH, plasma levels of arginine vasopressin were significantly higher than in normal subjects ($p < 0.001$). This, together with the finding of a lower than normal plasma osmolality in this group, suggests that inappropriate ADH excess might be much more common in patients with bronchogenic carcinoma than previously thought.

The normal positive correlation between plasma osmolality and plasma arginine vasopressin was found to be reversed in SIADH.

Seven of nine patients with overt SIADH, studied after fluid deprivation, showed an increase in plasma arginine vasopressin coincident with an increase in plasma osmolality ($r = +0.8$, $p < 0.01$); in one patient, plasma arginine vasopressin returned to the original level following rehydration. The possibility that this might imply a degree of physiologic control to what is generally considered an autonomous secretion is discussed. It is, however, considered more likely that other factors, including changes in plasma volume and glomerular filtration, might explain the increase in plasma levels of arginine vasopressin.

The association of hyponatremia with bronchogenic carcinoma was apparently first noted in 1938 [1], but it was not until 1957 that this was attributed to an inappropriately high level of circulating antidiuretic hormone [2] and the term "syndrome of inappropriate antidiuretic hormone secretion" (SIADH) was coined. Features of the syndrome are hyponatremia, usually with continuing urinary sodium loss, hypo-osmolar plasma and inappropriately concentrated urine [3]. The same combination occurs in normal subjects given water with ADH [4]. Since its recognition, SIADH has been described in association with a variety of conditions [3] but bronchogenic carcinoma, particularly the oat cell variety, remains by far the most commonly reported cause.

SIADH is said to occur in 1.6 per cent of patients with bronchogenic carcinoma [5] although, until the development of reliable assays for the measurement of antidiuretic activity, the diagnosis was of necessity inferential. When levels of plasma antidiuretic activity have been reported, they have generally been high, although values within the normal range have been noted (see "Comments").

From the M.R.C. Blood Pressure Unit, Western Infirmary, Glasgow, G116NT Scotland. Requests for reprints should be addressed to Dr. Paul L. Padfield. Manuscript accepted March 3, 1976.

TABLE I Patients with Overt SIADH

Case No.	Age (yr) and Sex	Serum Sodium (mmol/liter)	Plasma Osmolality (mosmol/kg)	Urine Osmolality (mosmol/kg)	Plasma Arginine Vasopressin (pg/ml)	Tumor Histology
1	45,M	123	262	788	147	Oat cell
2	68,F	118	242	684	18	Oat cell
3	53,M	106	218	638	643	Oat cell
4	60,M	121	236	...	12	Oat cell
5	49,F	118	263	537	18	Oat cell
6	60,M	120	248	641	13	Unknown
7	63,M	123	268	737	6.5	Unknown
8	45,M	117	250	489	16.5	Oat cell
9	50,F	118	248	667	32	Oat cell
10	55,M	121	258	512	51	Unknown
11	46,M	137	297	617	30	Squamous cell
12	62,F	134	304	623	87	Anaplastic
13	53,M	118	250	510	56	Oat cell
14	49,M	123	264	733	44	Oat cell
15	69,F	120	247	499	21	Oat cell
16	69,M	126	270	407	8	Unknown
17	44,M	120	252	739	170	Oat cell
Mean ± SEM	55 ± 2	121 ± 1.6	257 ± 5	614 ± 28	81 ± 37	

NOTE: Two patients (Cases 11 and 12) were studied while deprived of fluid; presenting serum sodium values were 128 and 118 mmol/liter, respectively. Plasma vasopressin in Cases 9 and 10 was measured by the method of Beardwell [37].

We report here the results obtained in patients with bronchogenic carcinoma studied under standardized conditions, using a recently developed radioimmunoassay for measuring plasma arginine vasopressin [6].

PATIENTS AND METHODS

Thirty-one patients (24 male) with a diagnosis of bronchogenic carcinoma were studied; 17 of these were referred because of distinct hyponatremia of less than 125 mmol/liter [121 ± 1.6 mmol/liter; mean ± standard error of the mean (SEM)]; each of these had plasma and urine osmolality relationships suggestive of SIADH (Table I). The remaining 14 had normal serum sodium concentrations (139 ± 0.9 mmol/liter) and were studied for comparison (Table II). Control measurements were made in a further 34 subjects (18 inpatients with psoriasis and 16 healthy volunteers).

In six patients with bronchogenic carcinoma, histologic proof of the diagnosis was not obtained.

Case 6. This patient presented with the Eaton Lambert (myasthenic) syndrome, and roentgenologic evidence of a right main stem bronchial lesion and lymphangitis carcinomatosis developed three months later.

Case 7. This patient presented in extremis with finger clubbing, a grossly enlarged uneven liver and a large opacity in the right upper zone on chest film; he died after four days.

TABLE II Patients Without Overt SIADH

Case No.	Age (yr) and Sex	Serum Sodium (mmol/liter)	Plasma Osmolality (mosmol/kg)	Urine Osmolality (mosmol/kg)	Plasma Arginine Vasopressin (pg/ml)	Tumor Histology
18	62,M	137	290	409	5.7	Unknown
19	56,M	140	279	845	8.6	Anaplastic
20	61,M	141	294	787	4.0	Anaplastic
21	69,M	137	279	596	5.0	Oat cell
22	54,F	135	277	678	7.0	Anaplastic
23	58,M	141	285	416	10.0	Oat cell
24	39,M	138	...	...	7.0	Anaplastic
25	80,M	137	278	565	7.5	Anaplastic
26	57,M	139	288	579	11.4	Squamous cell
27	61,M	141	288	721	8.5	Squamous cell
28	65,F	145	276	652	12.5	Oat cell
29	64,M	141	296	908	15.0	Unknown
30	70,M	137	284	796	10.5	Anaplastic
31	77,M	139	285	867	9.0	Squamous cell
Mean ± SEM	62 ± 3	139 ± 0.9	285 ± 2	678 ± 45	8.7 ± 0.8	

Case 10. This patient had a lesion on a chest film of the left main bronchus which, on bronchoscopy, looked malignant. Tissue damaged during fixation.

Case 16. This patient had finger clubbing, a markedly enlarged liver with roentgenologic evidence of a lesion of the right main stem bronchus and osteolytic lesions in the ribs.

Cases 18 and 29. Both of these patients had roentgenologic evidence of a bronchogenic neoplasm with bony secondaries.

All patients and normal subjects were studied between 800 and 1000 hours, in the supine position, after food and fluid deprivation from 2200 the night before. Peripheral venous blood was obtained for measurement of plasma arginine vasopressin, osmolality, urea and electrolytes. All subjects passed urine 1 hour before and immediately after venepuncture; osmolality was measured in the second specimen (Advanced Osmometer).

Nine patients (Cases 1–9, Table I) were studied again after a period of fluid restriction (12 ± two days, range four to 24 days: 450 to 750 ml/24 hours). One patient (Case 2, Table I) was reinvestigated after a further nine days during which free access to fluid was allowed. In two patients (Cases 8 and 9, Table I) plasma volume [7] was measured before and after fluid deprivation.

RESULTS

In the 34 subjects without bronchogenic carcinoma, plasma osmolality was 295 ± 0.9 mosmol/kg (range 287 to 306 mosmol/kg), urine osmolality 693 ± 38 mosmol/kg (range 348 to 1,060 mosmol/kg) and plasma arginine vasopressin 6.1 ± 0.3 pg/ml (range 3.5 to 11.9 pg/ml).

In patients with SIADH, plasma osmolality was significantly lower ($p < 0.001$) than in those with bronchogenic carcinoma without SIADH (Tables I and II), and in both groups, plasma osmolality was significantly lower than in normal subjects ($p < 0.001$). There was no significant difference in urine osmolality among the three groups (Tables I and II).

In patients with SIADH, plasma arginine vasopressin levels were generally elevated although the range was wide (Figure 1 and Table I); in four patients, levels were within the upper half of the normal range. The relationship of plasma arginine vasopressin to plasma osmolality was, however, inappropriate and these patients could be clearly separated from normal control subjects on this basis (Figure 2). In patients with bronchogenic carcinoma but without overt SIADH, mean plasma arginine vasopressin levels were also higher than in normal subjects ($p < 0.001$), although all but two values were within the upper half of the normal range (Figure 1 and Table II). Again the separation from normal subjects became more apparent with reference to plasma osmolality (Figure 2). Taking all patients with bronchogenic carcinoma together, there was a significant negative correlation between plasma arginine

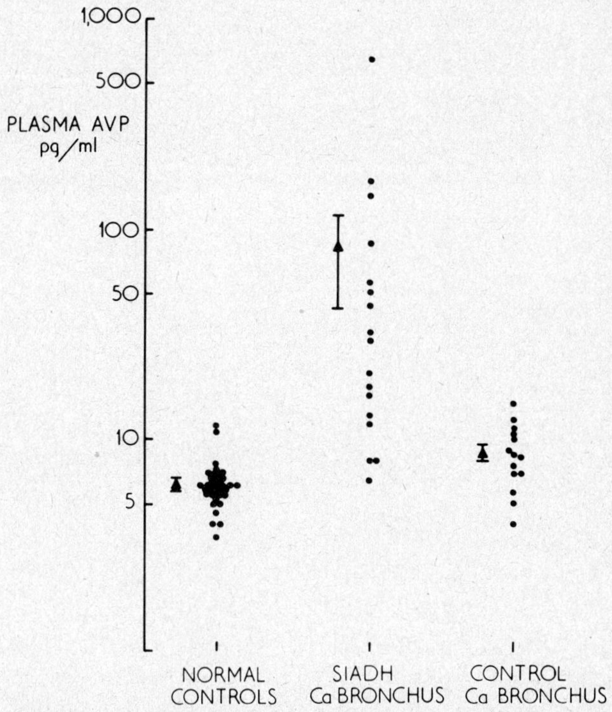

Figure 1. *Comparison of plasma arginine vasopressin (AVP) between groups. Means and standard errors indicated.*

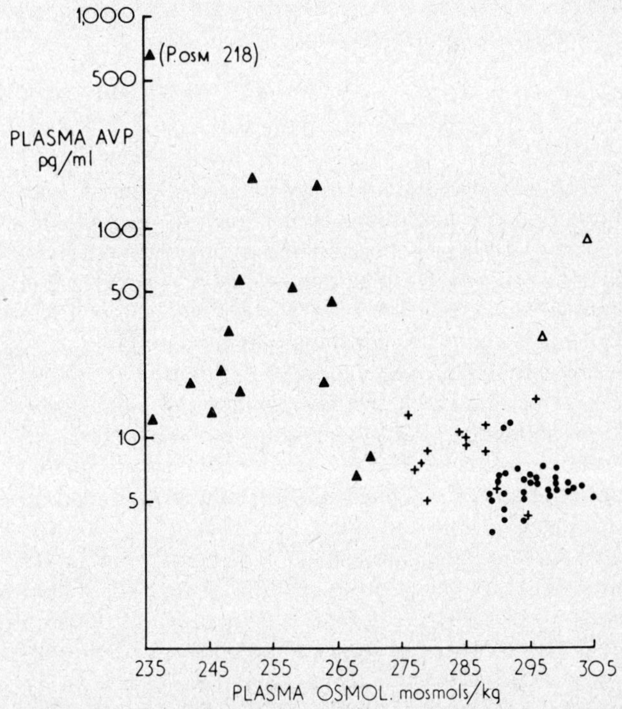

Figure 2. *Relationship between plasma arginine vasopressin (AVP) and plasma osmolality. ▲ = bronchogenic carcinoma (SIADH). △ = bronchogenic carcinoma (SIADH) — fluid deprived when studied. + = bronchogenic carcinoma (without overt SIADH). ● = normal control subjects.*

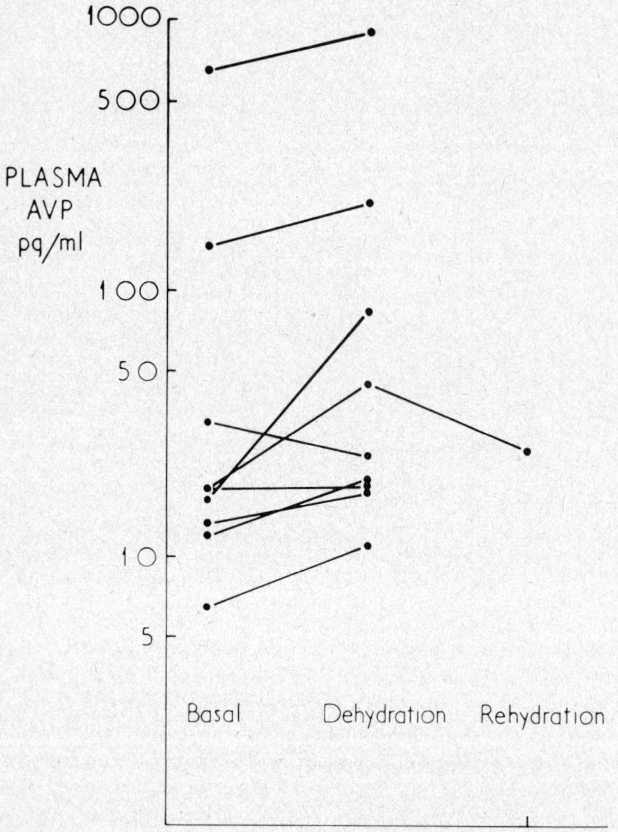

Figure 3. *Plasma arginine vasopressin (AVP) in nine patients studied before and during fluid deprivation, with one patient studied again after rehydration.*

vasopressin and plasma osmolality (r = −0.5, p <0.01).

The ADH-like material in the plasma of patients with bronchogenic carcinoma was shown to be immunologically similar to the standard arginine vasopressin in that progressive dilutions of the plasma extracts paralleled the standard curve in all but one patient (Case 8, Table I). In this patient, the plasma extract showed a cross reaction of less than 30 per cent.

Fluid Restriction. In the nine patients with SIADH who were deprived of fluid, there was a marked increase in serum sodium (118 ± 1.7 to 137 ± 1.1 mmol/liter), serum urea (23 ± 3 to 55 ± 8 mg/100 ml) and plasma osmolality (248 ± 5 to 290 ± 2 mosmol/kg) (p <0.001) with a moderate increase in urine osmolality (643 ± 38 to 847 ± 54 mosmol/kg; p <0.05) and significant weight loss (56.4 ± 7 to 52.5 ± 6 kg; p <0.05). Plasma volume decreased in the two subjects in whom measurements were made (Cases 8 and 9, Table I: 4,237 ml to 3,370 ml, and 2,405 ml to 2,286 ml, respectively).

Plasma arginine vasopressin increased in seven patients despite initially high levels in six; there was no change in one patient and a decrease in one other (Figure 3). Changes in plasma arginine vasopressin ranged from −25 per cent to +400 per cent with an average increase of 86 per cent. There was a close positive correlation between the absolute changes in plasma arginine vasopressin and plasma osmolality (r = +0.8, p <0.01). In the one patient studied again after rehydration, plasma arginine vasopressin fell to near the original level (Figure 3).

COMMENTS

Since the first demonstration of antidiuretic activity in the oat cell tumor of a patient with bronchogenic carcinoma and SIADH [8], some 50 patients have been described in whom measurements of ADH either in tumor cells, plasma or urine have been made (Table III). ADH-like activity is usually present in the tumors of patients with SIADH, although there are exceptions [9]. Plasma ADH levels are generally high (Table III).

Arginine Vasopressin Levels in SIADH. Our data provide further evidence that most patients with SIADH associated with bronchogenic carcinoma do have markedly increased circulating levels of arginine vasopressin. The finding of normal, although inappropriately high, plasma or urinary levels of arginine vasopressin in patients with distinct hyponatremia has also been described previously [10–12] and suggests that these tumors may vary in their ability to secrete ADH. As reported here, significantly high plasma levels of arginine vasopressin also occur in patients with bronchogenic carcinoma without overt SIADH. This increase in arginine vasopressin might have been explained if the patients, by virtue of their illness, were more depleted of water than normal subjects. The observation of a significantly lower than normal plasma osmolality provides strong evidence against this possibility and therefore suggests that many of these patients also have SIADH, albeit subclinical. It is thus possible that many or all bronchogenic carcinomas might be capable of secreting arginine vasopressin, and the finding of a distinctly elevated plasma level associated with SIADH in a patient with a definite squamous cell lesion (Case 11, Table I) shows that the syndrome is not confined to patients with oat cell tumors. It has been shown that, in vitro, not only tumor cells from patients with SIADH but also tumor cells from patients without the syndrome are capable of forming antidiuretic material [13]. This raises the possibility, therefore, that measurement of plasma arginine vasopressin may be helpful in the early diagnosis of bronchogenic carcinoma.

It is not known for certain that ADH measured in patients with SIADH is the same as the naturally occurring hormone (arginine vasopressin), although there is evidence that it is either this or a chemically and biologically very similar compound [13–17]. Our radioim-

TABLE III Literature Survey of Antidiuretic Activity in SIADH Associated with Bronchogenic Carcinoma

Reference	Source	Assay	No. of Cases	Amount of Antidiuretic Activity*	Comments
Amatruda et al. [8]	Tumor	BIO	1	70–350 μU/mg dry weight	Nil detected in other tissues
Bower et al. [31]	Plasma	BIO	1	3.0–8.0 μU/ml	No activity detected in plasma of normally hydrated controls
	Primary tumor			0.1–1.0 μU/mg dry weight	
	Secondary tumor			6.0–8.0 μU/mg dry weight	
Lee et al. [32]	Plasma	BIO	1	1.7 μU/ml	Nil in normally hydrated controls; normal <15 mU/24 hours; tumor weight—143 g
	Urine			100 mU/24 hours	
	Tumor			10 μU/mg dry weight	
De Sousa et al. [33]	Urine	BIO	2	1.8 U/24 hours	...
	Tumor			7.0 mU/mg dry weight	
Utiger [34]	Tumor	RIA	1	142 μU/mg wet weight	Normal pituitary 8–11 U/mg wet weight
Barraclough et al. [35]	Plasma	BIO	6	2.6–16 μU/ml	Nil in normally hydrated controls; nil detected in one necrotic tumor
	Tumor			4–75 μU/mg dry weight	
Sawyer [17]	Tumor	BIO	5	20–150 μU/mg dry weight	...
Vorherr et al. [9]	Tumor	BIO RIA	10	130–763 μU/mg dry weight	Activity detected in only 5 of 10 tumors; normal pituitary 85 ± 15 mU/mg dry weight
Lipscomb et al. [16]	Tumor	BIO	1	0.2 mU/mg dry weight	...
	Plasma			80 μU/ml	
Marks et al. [36]	Tumor	BIO	1	0.29 ± 0.03 U/mg dry weight	...
	(Pancreas)	RIA		0.38 U/mg dry weight	
Segar, Moore [23]	Tumor			525 μU/mg dry weight	Normal subjects <1.6 μU/ml
	Plasma	BIO	1	12.5 μU/ml	
Beardwell [37]	Plasma	RIA	4	24–102 pg/ml	Normal range 1–4.3 pg/ml; uncorrected for recovery (46 ± 8 per cent)
George et al. [14]	Tumor	RIA	1	23.5 μU/mg wet weight	
Baumann et al. [10]	Plasma	RIA	4	5.1–31 μU/ml	Normal range 2–12 μU/ml
Miller, Moses [11]	Urine	RIA	5	1–316 mU/24 hours	Normal range 12–108 mU/24 hours
Skowsky et al. [12]	Plasma	RIA	6	11–242 μU/ml	Normal range 4–11.5 μU/ml
Present study	Plasma	RIA	17	6.5–643 pg/ml	Normal range 3.5–12 pg/ml

NOTE: BIO = bioassay. RIA = radioimmunoassay.

*For conversion 1 μU of arginine vasopression = 2.5 pg of standard arginine vasopressin.

munologic results support this, although in the one patient whose plasma extract had a low cross reaction with the standard arginine vasopressin it is possible that there existed an antidiuretic substance chemically dissimilar from the usual human form of ADH.

Reversed Relation of Plasma Arginine Vasopressin and Osmolality. In normal subjects, studied over a wide range of water intake, there is a significant positive correlation between plasma osmolality and arginine vasopressin concentration ($r = +0.67$, $p < 0.01$) [6]. This probably reflects the ability of an increase in plasma osmolality to stimulate arginine vasopressin [18].

Taking all patients with bronchogenic carcinoma together, however, the correlation reverses and becomes significantly negative ($r = -0.5$, $p < 0.01$). This reversal might result from the autonomous nature of arginine vasopressin secretion in this syndrome. Excess arginine vasopressin would produce water retention and a hypo-osmolar plasma. Because this fails to exert its normal inhibitory influence on vasopressin release, the hypo-osmolality persists and the relationship of arginine vasopressin to osmolality reverses. However, the ability of arginine vasopressin to concentrate urine and therefore, presumably, to retain water reaches a maximum at plasma levels below 15 pg/ml (Padfield, unpublished observations). This suggests that the linearity of the negative correlation between plasma osmolality and arginine vasopressin might not persist at higher concentrations of arginine vasopressin.

An alternative explanation for the reversed relationship is that arginine vasopressin stimulates fluid intake and that this, together with increased urine concentration, produces the hypo-osmolar plasma. This seems unlikely as there is no good evidence of a direct dipsogenic effect of arginine vasopressin either in man [19] or in animals [20–22]. A patient with SIADH and bronchogenic carcinoma has been described, however, who had inappropriate thirst [23]. None of the patients we describe in this paper complained to us of thirst at any stage in their illness.

Control of Plasma Arginine Vasopressin in SIADH. There is good evidence that the bronchogenic carcinoma associated with SIADH secretes ADH [13,14], and it is generally accepted that the secretion is autonomous [24]. However, in a study including four patients with SIADH and bronchogenic carcinoma, plasma levels were found to be, at least in part, responsive to maneuvers which alter arginine vasopressin release in normal man [10]. Only one subject had a distinctly elevated basal arginine vasopressin level (31 μU/ml) which rose markedly after the administration of nicotine (>118 μU/ml). It cannot be concluded, however, that the arginine vasopressin was increased by the tumor rather than the pituitary gland. We have shown that in seven of nine patients studied, even initially very high plasma levels of arginine vasopressin can be increased still further by a period of fluid restriction involving a marked increase in plasma osmolality. This increase in arginine vasopressin is also generally accompanied by an increase in urine osmolality. The possibility that, during the period of dehydration, the underlying carcinoma enlarges and secretes more ADH is unlikely in view of the observation in one patient in whom arginine vasopressin levels fell again following free access to fluid. The decrease in plasma volume seen in two patients is not of sufficient magnitude to explain the increase in arginine vasopressin purely on the basis of hemoconcentration, although it may be partly responsible. It is, thus, possible that secretion of arginine vasopressin by tumors is not strictly autonomous but that it is, at least in part, responsive to physiologic maneuvers. However, it is known that the glomerular filtration rate is increased in patients with SIADH [25–28] and that this increase is corrected by fluid deprivation [26]. As arginine vasopressin is removed from the circulation, mainly by the kidney [29,30], it is possible that, given a fixed rate of secretion of arginine vasopressin, a lowering of the glomerular filtration rate would raise the plasma level. Although the glomerular filtration rate was not measured in our patients, the striking increase in blood urea following fluid deprivation is probably a reflection of a decrease in the glomerular filtration rate. Without data on the metabolic clearance of arginine vasopressin, therefore, we are unable to be sure that an elevated plasma level reflects increased secretion.

The appearance of overt SIADH in patients with bronchogenic carcinoma appears to herald a terminal stage in the illness, as in the 15 patients in whom details are available the mean survival time from the recognition of hyponatremia was only 16 weeks (range one to 40 weeks). In two patients the development of SIADH preceded the appearance of roentgenologic changes of the underlying bronchogenic carcinoma by three months.

In conclusion, we have shown that, under conditions least likely to pick up a difference (mild dehydration), not only do patients with SIADH have excess circulating levels of arginine vasopressin but also that patients with bronchogenic carcinoma without overt SIADH tend to have relatively high levels. The possibility that such differences from normal would be accentuated by forced hydration is currently being investigated.

REFERENCES

1. Winkler AW, Crankshaw OF: Chloride depletion in conditions other than Addison's disease. J Clin Invest 17: 1, 1938.
2. Schwartz WB, Bennet W, Curelop S, Bartter FC: A syndrome of renal sodium loss and hyponatraemia probably resulting from inappropriate secretion of antidiuretic hormone. Am J Med 23: 529, 1957.
3. Bartter FC, Schwartz WB: The syndrome of inappropriate secretion of antidiuretic hormone. Am J Med 42: 790, 1967.
4. Leaf A, Bartter FC, Santos RF, et al.: Evidence in man that urinary electrolyte loss induced by pitressin is a function of water retention. J Clin Invest 32: 868, 1953.
5. Azzopardi JG, Freeman E, Poole G: Endocrine and metabolic disorders in bronchial carcinoma. Br Med J 4: 528, 1970.
6. Morton JJ, Padfield PL, Forsling ML: A radioimmunoassay for plasma arginine vasopressin in man and dog. Application to physiological and pathological states. J Endocr 65: 411, 1975.
7. Anderson SB: Simultaneous determination of plasma volume with ^{131}I labelled gamma-globulin, ^{131}I labelled albumin and T-1824. Clin Sci 23: 221, 1962.
8. Amatruda TT, Mulrow PJ, Gallacher JC, et al.: Carcinoma of the lung with inappropriate antidiuresis. Demonstration of antidiuretic hormone-like activity in tumour extract. N Engl J Med 269: 544, 1963.
9. Vorherr H, Massry SG, Utiger RD, et al.: Antidiuretic principle in malignant tumour extracts from patients with inappropriate ADH syndrome. J Clin Endocrinol 28: 162, 1968.
10. Baumann G, Lopez-Amor E, Dingman JF: Plasma arginine vasopressin in the syndrome of inappropriate antidiuretic hormone secretion. Am J Med 52: 19, 1972.
11. Miller M, Moses AM: Urinary antidiuretic hormone in polyuric disorders and in inappropriate ADH syndrome. Ann Intern Med 77: 715, 1972.
12. Skowsky WR, Rosenbloom AA, Fisher DA: Radioimmunoassay measurement of arginine vasopressin in serum. Development and application. J Clin Endocrinol 38: 278, 1974.
13. Vorherr H, Vorherr UF, McConnell TS, et al.: Localisation and origin of antidiuretic principle in para-endocrine active malignant tumours. Oncology (Basel) 29: 201, 1974.
14. George JM, Capen CC, Phillips AS: Biosynthesis of vasopressin in vtiro and ultrastructure of a bronchogenic carcinoma. J Clin Invest 51: 141, 1972.
15. Hamilton BPM, Upton CV, Amatruda TT: Evidence for the presence of neurophysin in tumours producing the syndrome of inappropriate antidiuresis. J Clin Endocrinol 35: 764, 1972.
16. Lipscomb HS, Wilson C, Retiene K, et al.: The syndrome of inappropriate antidiuretic hormone release. A case report and characteristics of the antidiuretic hormone-like material isolated from an oat cell carcinoma of the lung. Cancer Res 28: 378, 1968.
17. Sawyer WH: Pharmacological characteristics of the antidiuretic principle in a bronchogenic carcinoma from a patient with hyponatraemia. J Clin Endocrinol 27: 1497, 1967.
18. Verney EB: The antidiuretic hormone and the factors which determine its release. Proc Roy Soc 135: 25, 1947.
19. Pasqualini RQ, Codevilla A: Thirst suppressing ("Antidipsetic")

effect of pitressin in diabetes insipidus. Acta Endocrinol 30: 37, 1959.
20. Adolph EF, Barker JP, Keller AD: Thirst tests in dogs and modifications of thirst with experimental lesions of the neurohypophyses. Am J Physiol 173: 233, 1959.
21. Fitzsimons JT: Thirst. Physiol Rev 52: 468, 1972.
22. Szczepanska SE, Kozlowski S, Sobocinska J: Blood antidiuretic hormone level and osmotic reactivity of thirst mechanism in dogs. Am J Physiol 227: 766, 1974.
23. Segar WE, Moore WW: Increased antidiuretic hormone and "inappropriate" thirst in a patient with bronchogenic carcinoma. Minerva Med 5: 625, 1968.
24. Bartter FC: The syndrome of inappropriate secretion of antidiuretic hormone (SIADH). DM p 1, Nov 1973.
25. Carter NW, Rector FC, Seldin DW: Hyponatraemia in cerebral disease resulting from the inappropriate secretion of antidiuretic hormone. N Engl J Med 264: 67, 1961.
26. Clift GV, Schletter FE, Moses AM, et al.: Syndrome of inappropriate vasopressin secretion. Arch Intern Med 118: 453, 1966.
27. De Sousa RC, Delaere J, Thaon A, Rudler JC, Mach RS: Le syndrome de Schwartz-Bartter. Carcinome du poumon avec secretion inadequate d'hormone antidiuretique. Schweiz Med Wochneschr 94: 1805, 1964.
28. Grantham JJ, Brown RW, Schloerb PR: Asymptomatic hyponatraemia and bronchogenic carcinoma. The deleterious effects of diuretics. Am J Med Sci 249: 273, 1965.
29. Ginsburg M, Heller H: The clearance of injected vasopressin from the circulation and its fate in the body. J Endocrinol 9: 283, 1953.
30. Lauson HD: Metabolism of antidiuretic hormones. Am J Med 42: 713, 1967.
31. Bower BF, Mason DM, Forsham PH: Bronchogenic carcinoma with inappropriate antidiuretic activity in plasma and tumor. N Engl J Med 271: 934, 1964.
32. Lee J, Jones JJ, Barraclough MA: Inappropriate secretion of vasopressin. Lancet 2: 792, 1964.
33. De Sousa RC, Delaere J, Berde B: Inappropriate secretion of vasopressin. Lancet 1: 436, 1965.
34. Utiger RD: Inappropriate antidiuresis and carcinoma of the lung. Detection of arginine vasopressin in tumour extract by immunoassay. J Clin Endocrinol 26: 970, 1966.
35. Barraclough MA, Jones JJ, Lee J: Production of vasopressin by anaplastic oat cell carcinoma of the bronchus. Clin Sci 31: 135, 1966.
36. Marks LJ, Berde B, Klein LA, et al.: Inappropriate vasopressin secretion and carcinoma of the pancreas. Am J Med 45: 967, 1968.
37. Beardwell CG: Radioimmunoassay of arginine vasopressin in human plasma. J Clin Endocrinol 33: 254, 1971.

Candida Peritonitis

Report of 22 Cases and Review of the English Literature

ARNOLD S. BAYER, M.D.
Torrance and Los Angeles, California

MICHAEL J. BLUMENKRANTZ, M.D.
Los Angeles, California

JOHN Z. MONTGOMERIE, F.R.A.C.P.*
Torrance, California

JEFFREY E. GALPIN, M.D.
Torrance and Los Angeles, California

JACK W. COBURN, M.D.
LUCIEN B. GUZE, M.D.
Los Angeles, California

Thirty-one patients with Candida isolated from peritoneal fluid were examined. Twenty-two were considered to have Candida peritonitis. The data on these 22 patients, plus 12 additional patients described in the literature, were reviewed. This infection was observed as a complication of peritoneal dialysis, gastrointestinal surgery or perforation of an abdominal viscus. Recent antibiotic administration seemed to be an important predisposing factor. The disease usually remained localized intra-abdominally, although disseminated candidiasis was also noted in three cases. Clinically significant infection could be differentiated from peritoneal contamination with Candida by the presence and persistence of fever, peritoneal signs, peripheral leukocytosis, positive peritoneal cultures for Candida, abnormal films of the abdomen and purulent ascitic fluid. Surgical interventions and removal of infected peritoneal fluid were the cornerstones of therapy. Short-term, low-dose systemic and/or intraperitoneally administered amphotericin B appeared promising in the treatment of unremitting infection. Mortality in treated patients was low and was comparable to that in patients with bacterial peritonitis.

The incidence of candidal infections, both focal and generalized, has been increasing rapidly in recent years [1–10]. Peritonitis due to Candida, however, has been uncommonly described, and we are aware of only 12 patients previously described in the English literature [8,11–21]. We report our experience with 22 such patients. The wide spectrum of disease as well as certain diagnostic, therapeutic and prognostic features, are emphasized.

METHODS

Records of the clinical microbiology laboratory at Harbor General Hospital (HGH) from 1970 to 1975 were examined. Twenty-five patients with Candida isolated from peritoneal fluid were identified. In addition, data on six such recent patients from the Nephrology Service of the Wadsworth Veterans Administration Hospital were analyzed. Identification and speciation of Candida were by standard fermentation reactions [22].

RESULTS

Peritoneal Contamination Versus Peritonitis. In Table I the clinical and laboratory features of 31 patients with positive peritoneal cultures

From the Department of Medicine, Harbor General Hospital, Torrance, California; the Nephrology Service, Wadsworth Veterans Administration Hospital, the Research and Medical Services, Wadsworth Veterans Administration Hospital; and the Department of Medicine, UCLA School of Medicine, Los Angeles, California. Requests for reprints should be addressed to Dr. Arnold S. Bayer, Department of Medicine, Harbor General Hospital, 1000 West Carson Street, Torrance, California 90509. Manuscript accepted March 19, 1976.

* Present address: Division of Infectious Diseases, Rancho Los Amigos Hospital, Downey, California 90242.

for Candida are summarized. The findings in nine patients were clearly distinct from those in the remaining 22 and suggested peritoneal contamination rather than frank peritonitis with Candida. All patients were afebrile, and none displayed peritoneal signs (diffuse abdominal tenderness with rebound, guarding and hypoactive or absent bowel sounds), peripheral leukocytosis, or cloudy to turbid ascitic fluid. Moreover, the cultures of peritoneal specimens were only transiently positive in all nine patients, becoming sterile within 48 hours of continued peritoneal dialysis.

In contrast, 22 patients had characteristic clinical findings of intra-abdominal sepsis and were considered to have Candida peritonitis (Table I). In 10 patients the infection was acquired during peritoneal dialysis, whereas the infection was associated with gastrointestinal surgery or perforation in the remaining 12 patients. The two groups of patients were analyzed separately.

Candida Peritonitis Associated with Peritoneal Dialysis (Cases 1–10, Table II). There were eight men and two women in this group. The average age was 40 years. Four patients had acute renal failure, whereas the other six had chronic renal insufficiency from six months to four years in duration. The time they had received peritoneal dialysis prior to the development of peritonitis varied from two days to one and a half years. All 10 patients were persistently febrile with temperatures ranging from 37.7° to 39.1°C. No episodes of hypotensive shock attributable to candidemia were observed. Routine ophthalmoscopy showed no evidence of endophthalmitis.

Laboratory Data. All the patients had leukocytosis with 12,200 to 15,800 cells/mm^3, and a neutrophilia of 75 to 92 per cent. In three of 10, abdominal roentgenograms were obtained. On each occasion an adynamic ileus was demonstrated. The dialysate was cloudy or purulent in each case. Three patients, in whom peritoneal fluid white blood cell and differential counts were performed, had more than 1,000 cells/mm^3, with greater than 90 per cent polymorphonuclear leukocytes noted. Blastospores typical of Candida were seen on microscopy of the dialysate in four of six patients so examined. Cultures of peritoneal fluid, repetitively yielded Candida for at least 96 hours after initial isolation, despite continuous peritoneal lavage.

Microbiologic Data. Cultures of the peritoneal fluid yielded Candida tropicalis on six occasions, C. albicans in three instances and C. guillieramondii once. In seven of 10 patients, the etiologic agent was also isolated from the dialysis catheter tip and/or the abdominal wound site. One patient with associated peritoneal and systemic candidiasis had positive blood cultures for Candida. The nine other patients had sterile blood cultures and no evidence of other organ involvement with Candida. In these latter patients candidiasis was considered to be localized to the abdominal cavity. No bacterial pathogens were isolated from the blood or peritoneal fluid.

TABLE I Clinical and Laboratory Features of 31 Patients with Candida Isolated from Peritoneal Fluid

	Contamination (9 cases)	Peritonitis (22 cases)
Underlying process		
Peritoneal dialysis	9	10
Gastrointestinal surgery or perforation	0	12
Fever $\geq$ 38°C*	0	20
Peritoneal signs*	0	22
Abnormal plain films of the abdomen (adynamic ileus* and/or free intraperitoneal air)	0/4	13/13
Peripheral leukocytosis* $\geq$ 12,000 white blood cells/mm^3	0	22
Turbid or purulent peritoneal fluid*	0	22

*The incidence of these features is significantly different between the two groups ($p < 0.001$) as determined by the Chi square method with Yates correction factor.

Possible Predisposing Factors. One patient who had disseminated infection was receiving a cytotoxic drug (azathioprine) plus corticosteroids at the time candidiasis was diagnosed. In six patients, systemic antibiotics had been administered for an antecedent bacterial infection within three weeks before the development of Candida peritonitis. In addition, two of these six patients had been given concomitant intraperitoneal antimicrobial therapy. There were two patients in this group with long-standing diabetes mellitus. Five patients had indwelling silastic catheters for long-term peritoneal dialysis.

Therapy and Outcome (Table II). Four patients (Cases 1, 2, 3 and 9) received no specific antifungal therapy and were treated only by continuous peritoneal lavage. One patient recovered completely; the other three died of other causes. In these latter three, the dialysate was rendered clear and culture-negative antemortem, and no evidence of Candida peritonitis was found at autopsy. The number of days of continued dialysis necessary to achieve a microbiologic cure in these four patients ranged between four and six.

Six patients (Cases 4, 5, 6, 7, 8 and 10) were treated with antifungal agents. In each case, prior to the administration of these drugs, continuous peritoneal di-

TABLE II Candida Peritonitis Complicating Peritoneal Dialysis—Clinical, Diagnostic, Therapeutic and Prognostic Features

Case	Time of Peritoneal Dialysis Prior to Peritonitis	Dialysate and Other Cultures	Antibiotics Prior to Candidiasis	Antifungal Therapy	Other	Outcome
1	7 days	C. tropicalis from dialysate and wound	10 days systemically	None	Continuous peritoneal dialysis	Dialysate clear in 4 days; recovered
2	2 days	C. albicans from dialysate and peritoneal dialysis catheter tip	4 days systemically	None	Continuous peritoneal dialysis	Dialysate clear in 4 days; died of unrelated cause
3	2 days	C. albicans from dialysate	None	None	Continuous peritoneal dialysis	Dialysate clear in 4 days; died of unrelated cause
4*	5 mo	C. tropicalis from dialysate and peritoneal dialysis catheter tip	7 days systemically	Intravenously amphotericin B— 330 mg; over 21 days	Continuous peritoneal dialysis; hemodialysis	Recovered
5*	3 mo	C. tropicalis from dialysate	None	Intraperitoneally amphotericin B—2.4 g, intravenously amphotericin B—600 mg; over 16 days	Continuous peritoneal dialysis	Recovered
6*	4 mo	C. tropicalis from dialysate	None	Intraperitoneally amphotericin B—1.5 g, intravenously amphotericin B—300 mg; over 10 days	Continuous peritoneal dialysis	Recovered
7*	1½ yr	C. tropicalis from dialysate and peritoneal dialysis catheter tip	5 days systemically	Intraperitoneally amphotericin B—1,200 mg, intravenously amphotericin B—200 mg; over 8 days	Continuous peritoneal dialysis	Died of Candida peritonitis
8*	20 days	C. tropicalis from dialysate, peritoneal dialysis tip and wound	7 days systemically and intraperitoneally	Intraperitoneally amphotericin B—1,440 mg, intravenously amphotericin B—350 mg, 5FC† orally—80 g; over 20 days	Removal of infected peritoneal dialysis catheter; continuous peritoneal dialysis	Recovered
9	2 days	C. guillieramondii in dialysate	None	None	Continuous peritoneal dialysis	Dialysate clear in 6 days; died of unrelated cause
10	2 days	C. albicans in blood, urine, dialysate, wound and peritoneal dialysis catheter tip	2½ weeks systemically and intraperitoneally	Intravenously amphotericin B—1,500 mg; over 35 days	Continuous peritoneal dialysis; hemodialysis	Recovered

* Indwelling silastic catheters used.
† 5-fluorocytosine.

TABLE III Candida Peritonitis Following Gastrointestinal Surgery or Perforation

Case	Precipitating Cause	Antibiotics Prior to Candidiasis	Peritoneal and Other Cultures	Surgery	Antifungal Therapy	Outcome
11	Perforated duodenal ulcer	None	C. albicans and Streptococcus viridans in ascitic fluid	Evacuation of peritoneal fluid; irrigation of peritoneal cavity; repair of duodenal ulcer	None	Recovered
12	Perforated small bowel and caecum 2 degrees to gunshot wound	None	Candida species in ascitic fluid	Evacuation of peritoneal fluid; irrigation of peritoneal cavity; small bowel resection and caecal repair	None	Recovered
13	Perforated colonic diverticulum	None	C. albicans in ascitic fluid	Evacuation of peritoneal fluid; irrigation of peritoneal cavity; colostomy	None	Recovered
14	Perforated dudodenal ulcer	None	C. tropicalis and Strep. viridans in ascitic fluid	None	None	Died; diagnosis confirmed at postmortem
15	Perforated duodenal ulcer	None	C. albicans in ascitic fluid	Evacuation of peritoneal fluid; irrigation of peritoneal cavity; repair of perforated duodenal ulcer	None	Recovered
16	Perforated gastric ulcer	None	C. parakreusii, Clostridium perfringens, Strep. viridans in ascitic fluid	Evacuation of peritoneal fluid; irrigation of peritoneal cavity; gastrojejunostomy	None	Recovered
17	Perforated gastric ulcer	None	C. albicans in ascitic fluid	None	None	Died; diagnosis confirmed at postmortem
18	Perforated duodenal ulcer	None	C. albicans, Veillonella species in ascitic fluid	Evacuation of peritoneal fluid; irrigation of peritoneal cavity; repair of duodenal ulcer	None	Recovered
19	Perforated duodenal ulcer	None	C. albicans in ascitic fluid	Evacuation of peritoneal fluid; irrigation of peritoneal cavity; repair of duodenal ulcer	None	Recovered
20	Perforated caecum and small bowel 2 degrees to stab wound	None	C. albicans in ascitic fluid	Evacuation of peritoneal fluid; irrigation of peritoneal cavity; repair of enteric perforations	None	Recovered
21	Carcinomatous small bowel obstruction; bowel resection	24 days systemically	C. albicans in ascitic fluid and venous catheter tip	Drainage of intra-abdominal abscess	None	Died; disseminated candidiasis at postmortem
22	Gallstone ileus	27 days systemically	C. albicans in intra-abdominal abscess, urine, wound and urinary catheter tip	Duodenal repair; cholecystectomy; drainage of subphrenic abscess	None	Died; disseminated candidiasis at postmortem

alysis, removal and replacement of an infected peritoneal catheter and/or institution of hemodialysis had been unsuccessful in eradicating the Candida peritonitis. All six patients received amphotericin B either intravenously, alone or combined with intraperitoneal therapy (see Table II). One patient additionally received 5-fluorocytosine. In five patients the infection was cured and the patient survived. Of note, in four of the five patients with long-term indwelling silastic catheters, the catheters remained patent and usable throughout the course of treatment. In Case 7, in which the patient died, peritoneal lavage could not be effectively maintained because of viscid peritoneal exudate, and Candida peritonitis was still present antemortem.

Of the five patients who responded to systemic amphotericin B therapy, four had no evidence of extraperitoneal organ involvement with Candida. The early therapeutic course (one to seven days) in these four patients was characterized by hectic fevers, severe abdominal pain and significant weight loss. However, each subsequently responded to amphotericin therapy, becoming afebrile, with disappearance of abdominal complaints and findings, and each had normal peripheral white blood cell counts and clear effluent dialysate within 21 days of initiation of treatment. In these four patients, cultures of peritoneal fluid became sterile within 14 days. The total dose of amphotericin B required for both clinical and microbiologic cure in these four cases averaged approximately 500 mg intravenously and 1,600 mg intraperitoneally.

One patient with disseminated candidiasis (Case 10) received 1,500 mg of amphotericin B intravenously over 35 days. However, this patient was clinically well within 25 days of the start of therapy, and peritoneal fluid became culture-negative after 22 days of treatment.

Candida Peritonitis Following Perforation of an Enteric Viscus or Gastrointestinal Surgery (Cases 11–22, Table III). There were eight men and four women in this group. The average age was 49 years. Candida infection followed perforation of an abdominal viscus in 10 of the 12 cases. In the remaining two cases, candidiasis complicated gastrointestinal surgery. An anastomotic or suture line leakage was demonstrated in both patients.

Eleven of 12 patients had no serious antecedant illnesses; metastatic cancer of the cervix (Case 21) was present in the remaining one.

All patients were persistently febrile, with temperatures ranging from 37.8° to 39°C. Seven patients presented with hypotensive shock; however, it could not be determined if this was due to hypovolemia or septicemia. Ophthalmoscopy disclosed no abnormalities.

Laboratory Data. All 12 patients had a peripheral leukocytosis between 12,400 and 20,000 cells/mm^3. In addition, each had a polymorphonuclear response between 82 and 95 per cent. Ascitic fluid was cloudy or purulent in every case. Ascitic fluid white blood cell and differential counts were not carried out in this group of patients. Ten of 10 patients in whom abdominal roentgenography was performed had an adynamic ileus and/or free intraperitoneal air.

Microbiologic Data. C. albicans was the etiologic agent in nine cases; C. tropicalis, C. parakrusei and Candida species were each isolated from one patient. On four occasions, Candida were present in the peritoneal fluid concurrent with a variety of aerobic and anaerobic bacteria.

Two patients (Cases 21 and 22) had disseminated candidiasis with involvement of many organ systems; blood cultures were, however, negative. Ten patients in whom the candidiasis was apparently localized to the abdomen also had sterile blood cultures.

Possible Predisposing Factors. Two of 12 patients received systemic antimicrobial agents for three weeks prior to the onset of Candida peritonitis. These agents had been initiated in each case because of evident or suspected peritoneal soiling with enteric contents. One patient (Case 21) was receiving corticosteroids at the time Candida peritonitis developed and disseminated infection occurred.

Therapy and Outcome. Eight of 10 patients with a perforated abdominal viscus were treated by operative repair with drainage of the infected peritoneal fluid and irrigation of the abdominal cavity at the time of surgery. All eight survived. The two remaining patients (Cases 14 and 17) who were not operated upon died.

In two patients (Cases 21 and 22) with postoperative suture line leakages, disseminated candidiasis developed and they died despite surgical drainage of an intra-abdominal Candida abscess. Systemic antifungal drugs were not administered in either case.

Pathology. Autopsy data were available in five cases (Cases 7, 14, 17, 21 and 22). In Cases 7, 14 and 17, purulent peritonitis with fibrous adhesions between loops of bowel was found. There was no gross evidence of Candida infection in other intra-abdominal structures or distant organ systems. Microscopic pathology of the peritoneum was available in only one of the latter three cases (Case 7) and was unremarkable.

In the remaining two patients, obvious disseminated candidiasis was confirmed at autopsy. In one of these (Case 21), liver, kidneys, spleen and heart were involved in addition to the peritoneum. In the other patient (Case 22), Candida infection was found in the peritoneum, kidneys, brain and lung. Microscopically, there were multiple, well-circumscribed acute abscesses which contained many polymorphonuclear leukocytes. The

Candida organisms were round, 5 to 7μ, with budding yeast forms producing pseudomycelia.

COMMENTS

In recent years, Candida has emerged as one of the most common pathogens in patients with serious underlying disorders. This has been most notable in patients with narcotic addiction, in patients receiving immunosuppressive therapy or prolonged antibiotic treatment and in patients with indwelling bladder catheters [1,2,5,8,9,23–31]. However, in large series of patients with candidemia, disseminated candidiasis and Candida endocarditis, peritoneal involvement has rarely been described [1,7,8,23,24,32–35,37].

In previous reports, infectious peritonitis has frequently been described as a complication of peritoneal dialysis [38–42]. Staphylococci and enteric gram-negative rods are the most common pathogens in such cases, whereas Candida have rarely been recovered [38–47].

The isolation of Candida from the abdominal fluid in patients undergoing peritoneal dialysis may create a diagnostic dilemma. A variety of clinical symptoms, signs and laboratory abnormalities mimicking peritonitis have been described in such patients in the absence of infection [38,48]. However, these findings are usually transient and respond readily to relocation of the dialysis catheter, continued dialysis or temporary discontinuation of the dialysis. In contrast, such maneuvers are often not successful in patients with Candida peritonitis. The presence and persistence of fever, peripheral leukocytosis with neutrophilia, purulent peritoneal fluid, adynamic ileus and positive cultures of peritoneal fluid for Candida were helpful factors differentiating Candida peritonitis from peritoneal contamination with this organism.

Twelve previously reported cases of Candida peritonitis were reviewed. These 12 cases were quite comparable to our 22 cases in terms of the patients' general clinical characteristics, systemic response to infection, laboratory abnormalities and antecedent antibiotic therapy. Similar to our experience, these cases followed gastrointestinal surgery or perforation, or were associated with peritoneal dialysis.

A notable difference was the finding of non-albicans strains as etiologic agents in one half of the present 22 cases, whereas C. albicans was the responsible pathogen in 11 of 12 previously reported cases. Earlier investigators had suggested that C. albicans may be the only strain of Candida pathogenic for man [49,50]. However, the isolation of Candida other than C. albicans in many of our cases is consistent with other reports that such strains may cause visceral candidiasis [1,3,8,36,37,51–53].

TABLE IV Candida Peritonitis Results of Treatment—Present Series plus Literature Cases*

Therapy	No. Patients	Infection Cured
Group I—Associated with Peritoneal Dialysis		
None	1	0
Continuous peritoneal dialysis alone	4	4
Peritoneal dialysis + amphotericin B intravenously	2	2
Peritoneal dialysis + amphotericin B intravenously and intraperitoneally†	4	3
Peritoneal dialysis + gentian violet intraperitoneally	1	1
	12	10
Group II—Associated with Gastrointestinal Surgery or Enteric Perforation		
None	3	0
Peritoneal dialysis alone	1	0
Peritoneal dialysis + gentian violet intraperitoneally	1	0
Surgical repair and drainage alone	11	9
Surgical intervention plus postoperative amphotericin B systemically	4	4
Amphotericin B intravenously alone	1	1
	21	14

*In one literature patient, insufficient data prevented assessment of therapy.
†Two patients also received 5-fluorocytosine orally.

Consideration of the present cases together with those in the literature allowed some generalizations concerning therapy, mortality (Table IV) and possible pathogeneses of this disorder. Nine of 34 patients (27 per cent) died as a result of Candida peritonitis. However, four of the nine were untreated. In addition, one patient with a perforated viscus could not be operated upon and died despite the intraperitoneal administration of gentian violet. Moreover, in three other patients (including two with disseminated disease), procedures designed to evacuate the abdominal cavity of infected ascitic fluid were unsuccessful in eradicating the candidiasis, and appropriate antifungal drugs were not provided. In the remaining patient who died, effective peritoneal lavage could not be maintained, and death ensued despite the intraperitoneal and intravenous administration of amphotericin B. Of note in this latter patient, a severely debilitated diabetic, amphotericin B levels in the peritoneal fluid (2 μg/ml) were twice the organism's minimal fungistatic concentration for this drug; yet, cultures of peritoneal fluid for Candida remained persistently positive antemortem.

In 24 of 25 patients with remitting infection, therapeutic modalities could be properly assessed. In 13 of 24 patients, surgical intervention and drainage, or continuous peritoneal dialysis were effective in controlling the infection. In 10 other patients, such procedures were not sufficient to eradicate the candidiasis and antifungal agents were thus required. In one instance, the parenteral administration of amphotericin B, alone, cured the infection.

Thus, if untreated, mortality is high in Candida peritonitis. In contrast, when abdominal drainage, surgical repair and/or antifungal therapy were provided in the appropriate clinical settings, mortality was low and not dissimilar to figures recently cited for bacterial peritonitis and intra-abdominal bacterial abscess [54,55].

Several aspects of the therapy of this infection with amphotericin B are notable. Four patients in the present series, in whom Candida peritonitis was uncontrolled by continuous peritoneal dialysis, were treated with intraperitoneally administered amphotericin B, at a final dialysate concentration of 2 to 4 μg/ml [56–58]. The intraperitoneal administration of amphotericin B in two of these four patients was associated with recovery and minimal constitutional reactions to this agent [59]. In one patient, however, abdominal pain and fever occurred coincident with the intraperitoneal instillation of amphotericin B. It should also be emphasized that the duration and total dosage of intravenously administered amphotericin B required to achieve a clinical and mycologic cure in the patients in our series so treated appear to be far less than has been recommended for effective chemotherapy of other visceral mycoses [60]. All five previously described patients treated with amphotericin B recovered. This includes four patients with Candida peritonitis following intestinal perforation and one patient in whom it was complicating peritoneal dialysis. However, insufficient data prevented determination of total dosage and duration of therapy necessary for optimum therapeutic effect in those patients.

Although the clinical settings in which this infection was seen tended to separate patients into two distinct populations, the route of infection in each group was not exactly delineated. In dialysis-associated infection, it could not be determined if the Candida peritonitis was exogenous in origin (after colonization of the abdominal wound area or via contaminated dialysate) or if the infection was endogenous, originating from the enteric flora. Local and systemic Candida infections have frequently been noted both in patients with renal failure and in those with indwelling catheters in various body sites [1,23,34,61–65]. Among the 12 patients with Candida peritonitis following dialysis, Candida were present in the abdominal wound in four.

The incidence of bacterial peritonitis during peritoneal dialysis has been declining steadily with the use of closed dialysate delivery systems and permanent indwelling silastic catheters [66]. In these patients, there is no wound site open to the environment. These observations suggest that the cases reported here of Candida peritonitis complicating chronic peritoneal dialysis probably occurred via exogenous contamination of the dialysate or during connect-disconnect procedures.

Seven of these 12 patients had received recent antibiotic therapy. Candida are found in the feces of up to 31 per cent of healthy subjects [67] and in a much higher per cent of patients receiving antibiotics [17,68–70]. Moreover, the transmural migration of intestinal microorganisms during peritoneal dialysis in uremic animals has been documented [71].

Other factors, possibly important in the development of peritoneal candidiasis in patients undergoing peritoneal dialysis, include loss of immunoglobulins into the peritoneal cavity [72], uremic enterocolitis [73,74], the existence of defective leukocyte chemotaxis and depressed lymphocyte reactivity in renal failure [75,76], and increased virulence of Candida in the presence of antimicrobial agents [77,78].

In patients in whom peritoneal candidiasis followed rupture of an abdominal viscus or intra-abdominal surgery, leakage of enteric contents through defects in the gastrointestinal tract appeared to be of paramount importance. In addition to Candida being normally found in feces, these organisms can be isolated from the oropharynx in up to 40 per cent of the normal population [67]. The rate of colonization in this site rises, as in fecal colonization, when antibiotics are utilized [8,79,80]. Eleven of 22 patients in this group received antecedent antimicrobial therapy.

An interesting phenomenon in both our series as well as in the previously reported cases was the apparent ability of the peritoneum to restrict the candidiasis intra-abdominally. Just two of 29 patients, so tested, had candidemia. In only five of the 34 patients did generalized candidiasis develop; in all five, systemic medications thought to favor dissemination of fungal infections (i.e., corticosteroids, broad-spectrum antibiotics and cytotoxic drugs [8,81]) were being administered at the time candidiasis occurred. Clinical studies have indicated that bacteremia during bacterial peritonitis is also uncommon, occurring in only 2 to 4 per cent of such cases [82,83]. The peritoneum appears to have functional stomata posessing both lymphatic and hematogenous connections [42]. The mechanisms by which these become relatively impermeable to both bacteria and fungi in cases of intra-abdominal sepsis have not been clearly defined.

ADDENDUM

Since completion of this manuscript, an abstract has appeared describing eight patients with Candida peritonitis complicating peritoneal dialysis [84]. Of interest, as in our patients, C. tropicalis was the offending organism in the majority of cases. Also, as in our report, the presence of a viscid peritoneal exudate occasionally prevented continuous dialysis. The clinical response to the administration of systemic antifungal drugs (5-fluorocytosine and/or amphotericin B) in unremitting peritonitis was favorable. However, in contrast to the experience in this study, we were generally able to successfully treat patients without the necessity of removing indwelling silastic catheters.

ACKNOWLEDGMENT

We thank Dr. Anthony W. Chow for his review of the manuscript.

REFERENCES

1. Bernhardt HE, Orlando JC, Benfield J, et al.: Disseminated candidiasis in surgical patients. Surg Gynecol Obstet 134: 819, 1972.
2. Bodey GP: Fungal infections complicating acute leukemia. J Chronic Dis 19: 667, 1966.
3. Edwards JE, Foos RY, Montgomerie JZ, et al.: Ocular manifestations of Candida septicemia. Review of 76 cases of hematogenous Candida endophthalmitis. Medicine (Baltimore) 53: 47, 1974.
4. Eras P, Goldstein MJ, Sherlock P: Candida infection of the gastrointestinal tract. Medicine (Baltimore) 51: 367, 1972.
5. Hart PD, Russell E, Remington JS: The compromised host and infection. II. Deep fungal infection. J Infect Dis 120: 169, 1969.
6. Hughes JM, Remington JS: Systemic candidiasis. A diagnostic challenge. Calif Med 116: 8, 1972.
7. Andriole VT, Kravetz HM, Roberts WC, et al.: Candida endocarditis. Clinical and pathologic studies. Am J Med 32: 251, 1962.
8. Louria DB, Stiff DP, Bennett B: Disseminated moniliasis in the adult. Medicine (Baltimore) 41: 307, 1962.
9. Taschdjian CL, Kozinn PJ, Toni EF: Opportunistic yeast infections with special reference to candidiasis. Ann NY Acad Sci 174: 606, 1970.
10. Pedraza MA: Mycotic infections at autopsy. Am J Clin Pathol 51: 470, 1969.
11. Montemartini C, Specchia G, Dander B: Peritonitis caused by Candida albicans. Digestion 3: 368, 1970.
12. Phillips I, Eykyn S, MacGregor GA, et al.: Candida peritonitis treated with 5-fluorocytosine in a patient receiving hemodialysis. Clin Nephrol 1: 271, 1973.
13. Shapiro BS: Candida peritonitis. Conn Med 30: 727, 1966.
14. Reeves KO, Ripepi AC, Carter RE, et al.: Candida peritonitis in a quadriplegic. South Med J 65: 325, 1972.
15. Reynell PC, Martin EA, Beard AW: Monilia peritonitis. Br Med J 1: 919, 1953.
16. Hurwich BJ: Monilial peritonitis. Arch Intern Med 117: 405, 1966.
17. Andreassen M, Ericksen KR, Stenderup A: Monilial peritonitis as a complication of preoperative intestinal sterilization. Lancet 2: 618, 1958.
18. Ohlwiler DA, Bricker EM: Candida albicans peritonitis successfully treated with amphotericin B. N Engl J Med 260: 488, 1959.
19. Roberts FJ: Peritonitis caused by Candida albicans. Can Med Assoc J 91: 366, 1964.
20. Palmer RA, Newell JE, Gray EJ, et al.: Treatment of chronic renal failure by prolonged peritoneal dialysis. N Engl J Med 274: 248, 1966.
21. Maryanov L: Bronchopulmonary moniliasis complicated by peritonitis. South Med J 52: 975, 1959.
22. Emmons CW, Binford CH, Utz JP: Candidiasis, chap 14. Medical Mycology, Philadelphia, Lea and Febiger, 1970.
23. Young RC, Bennett JE, Geelhoed GW, et al.: Fungemia with compromised host resistance. Ann Intern Med 80: 605, 1974.
24. Folb PI, Trounce JR: Immunological aspects of Candida infection complicating steroid and immunosuppressive drug therapy. Lancet 2: 1112, 1970.
25. Fulginiti VA, Schribner R, Groth CG, et al.: Infections in recipients of liver homografts. N Engl J Med 279: 619, 1968.
26. Hill RB, Rowlands DT, Rifkind D: Infectious pulmonary disease in patients receiving immunosuppressive therapy for organ transplantation. N Engl J Med 271: 1021, 1964.
27. Levy ES, Cohen DB: Systemic moniliasis complicating corticotropin therapy. Arch Intern Med 95: 118, 1955.
28. Levine AS, Graw RG, Young RC: Management of infections in patients with leukemia and lymphoma. Semin Hematol 9: 141, 1972.
29. Brode FR, Paré AP, Fraser RG: Pulmonary diseases in the compromised host. Medicine (Baltimore) 53: 255, 1974.
30. Cherubin CE, Baden M, Kavaler F, et al.: Infective endocarditis in narcotic addicts. Ann Intern Med 69: 1091, 1968.
31. Ramsey RG, Gunnar RM, Tobin JR: Endocarditis in the drug addict. Am J Cardiol 25: 608, 1970.
32. Medoff G, Dismukes WE, Meade RH: A new therapeutic approach to Candida infections. Arch Intern Med 130: 241, 1972.
33. Dennis D, Miller M, Peterson CG: Candida septicemia. Surg Gynecol Obstet 119: 520, 1964.
34. Richards KE, Pierson CL, Bucclarelli L, et al.: Monilial sepsis in the surgical patient. Surg Clin North Am 52: 1399, 1972.
35. Hartford CG: Postoperative fungal endocarditis. Arch Intern Med 134: 116, 1974.
36. Turnier E, Kay JH, Bernstein S, et al.: Surgical treatment of Candida endocarditis. Chest 67: 262, 1975.
37. Seelig MS, Speth PC, Kozinn PJ, et al.: Candida endocarditis after cardiac surgery. J Thorac Cardiovasc Surg 65: 583, 1973.
38. Ribot S, Jacobs MG, Frankel HJ, et al.: Complications of peritoneal dialysis. Am J Med Sci 252: 505, 1966.
39. Nienhuis LI: Clinical peritoneal dialysis. Arch Surg 93: 643, 1966.
40. Mattocks AM, el-Bassiouni EA: Peritoneal dialysis. A review. J Pharmacol Sci 60: 1767, 1971.
41. Maher JF, Schreiner GE: Hazards and complications of dialysis. N Engl J Med 273: 370, 1965.
42. Montgomerie JZ, Kalmanson GM, Guze LB: Renal failure and infection. Medicine (Baltimore) 47: 1, 1968.
43. Lankisch PG, Tonnis HJ, Fernandez-Redo E, et al.: Use of Tenckhoff catheter for peritoneal dialysis in terminal renal failure. Br Med J 4: 712, 1973.
44. Brewer TE, Caldwell FT, Patterson RM, et al.: Indwelling

peritoneal (Tenckhoff) dialysis catheter. Experience with 24 patients. JAMA 219: 1011, 1972.
45. Lasker N, Shalhoub R, Habibe O, et al.: The management of end stage kidney disease with intermittent peritoneal dialysis. Ann Intern Med 62: 1147, 1965.
46. Leigh DA: Peritoneal infections in patients on long-term peritoneal dialysis before and after cadaveric renal transplantation. J Clin Pathol 22: 539, 1969.
47. Stewart JH, Tuckwell LA, Sinnett PF, et al.: Peritoneal and hemodialysis. A comparison of the morbidity and mortality suffered by dialyzed patients. Q J Med 35: 407, 1966.
48. Oreopoulous DG, Izatt S: Infection of the peritoneum during dialysis. Br Med J 3: 592, 1972.
49. Dubos RJ: Bacterial and Mycotic Infections of Man, Philadelphia, J. B. Lippincott, 1972, p 886.
50. Conant NF, Smith DT, Baker RD: Manual of Clinical Mycology, Philadelphia, W. B. Saunders, 1954, p 456.
51. Conn NK, Crean GP, MacCabe AP, et al.: Systemic candidiasis and endocarditis due to C. tropicalis. Br Med J 1: 944, 1959.
52. Weingart JS, Wirtz DC, Irving NW: Monilia osteomyelitis. Report of a case resulting from thrush. Am J Clin Pathol 12: 597, 1942.
53. Richart R, Dammin GJ: Candida tropicalis as a pathogen for man. N Engl J Med 263: 474, 1960.
54. Storer EH: Peritonitis and intraabdominal abscesses, chap 34. Principles in Surgery (Schwartz SI, Lillehei RC, Shires GT, Spencer FC, Storer EH, eds), New York, McGraw-Hill Book Co., 1974.
55. Altemeir WA, Culbertson WR, Fullen WD, et al.: Intraabdominal abscesses. Am J Surg 125: 70, 1973.
56. Gold W, Stout HA, Pagano JF, et al.: Amphotericin A and B, antifungal antibiotics produced by streptomycete. I. In vitro studies. Antibiotics Annual 1955–1956, p 579, 1956.
57. Littman ML, Pisano MA, Lancaster RM: Induced resistance Candida species to nystatin and amphotericin B. Antibiotics Annual 1955–1958, p 981, 1958.
58. Athar MA, Winner HI: The development of resistance by Candida species to polyene antibiotics in vitro. Med Microbiol 4: 505, 1971.
59. Butler WT: Pharmacology, toxicity and therapeutc usefulness of amphotericin B. JAMA 195: 127, 1966.
60. Braude AI: Diseases caused by fungi, section II, chap 164–170. Principles of Internal Medicine (Wintrobe MM, Thorn GW, Adams RD, Braunwald E, Isselbacher KJ, Petersdorf RG, eds), New York, McGraw-Hill Book Co., 1974.
61. Franklin SS, Merrill JP: Acute renal failure. N Engl J Med 262: 761, 1960.
62. Curry CR, Quie PG: Fungal septicemia in patients receiving parenteral hyperalimentation. N Engl J Med 285: 1221, 1971.
63. Ashcraft KW, Leape LL: Candida sepsis complicating parenteral feeding. JAMA 212: 454, 1970.
64. Smith JA, Selick A, Edelist G: A clinical and microbiologic study of venous catheterization. Can Med Assoc J 109: 115, 1973.
65. Maki DG, Goldman DA, Rhame FS: Infection control in intravenous therapy. Ann Intern Med 79: 867, 1973.
66. Tenckhoff H: Peritoneal dialysis today. Nephron 12: 420, 1974.
67. Rosebury T: Microorganisms indigenous to man, chap 7. Indigenous Fungi, New York, McGraw-Hill Book Co., 1962.
68. Loh W, Baker EE: Fecal flora of man after oral administration of chlortetracycline or oxytetracycline. Arch Intern Med 95: 74, 1955.
69. Schaberg A, Hildes JA, Wilt JC: Disseminated candidiasis. Arch Intern Med 95: 112, 1955.
70. Brown RL: The gastrointestinal tract and stool following aureomycin therapy. Antibiot Chemother 2: 5, 1952.
71. Schweinberg FB, Frank HA, Frank ED, et al.: Transmural migration of intestinal bacteria during peritoneal irrigation in uremic dogs. Proc Soc Exp Biol Med 71: 150, 1949.
72. McKelvey EM, Yeoh HH, Schuster GA, et al.: Immunoglobulin and dextran losses during peritoneal dialysis. Arch Intern Med 134: 266, 1974.
73. Mason EE: Gastrointestinal lesions occurring in uremia. Ann Intern Med 37: 96, 1952.
74. Thoroughman JC, Peace RJ: Abdominal surgical emergencies caused by uremic enterocolitis. Report of 12 cases. Am J Surg 25: 533, 1959.
75. Clark RA, Hamory BH, Ford GH, et al.: Chemotaxis in acute renal failure. J Infect Dis 126: 460, 1972.
76. Newberry WM, Sanford JP: Defective cellular immunity in renal failure—depression of reactivity of lymphocytes to phytohemagglutinin by renal failure serum. J Clin Invest 50: 1262, 1962.
77. Huppert M, MacPherson D, Cazin J: Pathogenesis of Candida albicans infection following antibiotic therapy. I. The effect of antibiotics on the growth of C. albicans. J Bacteriol 65: 171, 1953.
78. Huppert M, Cazin J: Pathogenesis of Candida albicans infection following antibiotic therapy. II. Further studies on the effect of antibiotics on the in vitro growth of C. albicans. J Bacteriol 70: 435, 1955.
79. Meads M, Rowe WP, Haslam NM: Alterations in the bacterial flora of the throat during oral therapy with aureomycin. Arch Intern Med 87: 533, 1951.
80. Miller CP, Bohnhoff M: Effect of streptomycin therapy on the bacterial flora of the throat. Am J Med 6: 417, 1949.
81. Bach MC, Adler JL, Breman J, et al.: Influence of rejection therapy on fungal and nocardial infections in renal-transplant recipients. Lancet 1: 180, 1973.
82. Odel HM, Ferris DO, Power MH: Peritoneal lavage as an effective means of extrarenal excretion—a clinical appraisal. Am J Med 9: 63, 1950.
83. Stevens RE, Baskin S, Greene JA, et al.: Peritoneal dialysis in the management of chronic renal failure. JAMA 190: 1128, 1964.
84. Barnes R, Brown D, Silva J, et al.: Candida peritonitis complicating peritoneal dialysis. Abstracts of the American Society of Nephrology, 1975, p 27.

Clinical Manifestations of Mannosidosis—A Longitudinal Study

JORGE J. YUNIS, M.D.
RAYMOND C. LEWANDOWSKI, Jr., M.D.
SYLVESTER J. SANFILIPPO, M.D.
MICHAEL Y. TSAI, Ph.D.
Minneapolis, Minnesota

IANCU FONI, M.D.
HEINZ H. BRUHL, M.D.
Faribault, Minnesota

Mannosidosis is a partially defined disorder of glycoprotein metabolism; less than 20 cases have been reported in the literature. In this work, a longitudinal study of five new patients is presented in an attempt to delineate the phenotype and clinical course of this unusual storage disease. The data on our patients and those in the literature indicate that people with mannosidosis appear normal at birth and that their typical phenotype develops by two years of age. This is characterized by a distinctive coarse facies and dysostosis multiplex. Although recurrent infections, hearing loss and mental retardation occur, the course in this storage disorder generally is stable and is compatible with adult life.

The diagnosis is confirmed by the presence of a deficiency in α-D-mannosidase activity in leukocytes or fibroblasts, by the presence of vacuolated lymphocytes in peripheral blood and foam cells in bone marrow, and an increased excretion of mannose-rich oligosaccharides in urine.

Mannosidosis is an autosomal recessive storage disease [1,2], characterized by tissue accumulation of oligosaccharides rich in mannose [3]. The initial case of mannosidosis was reported by Öckerman [1] in 1967; 12 additional cases were recently described [4–8]. Four more cases previously reported as an unusual storage disease resembling the Hurler syndrome [9–11] were classified as examples of mucolipidosis I [12] and have subsequently been found to represent examples of mannosidosis (Spranger, personal communication).

In the past, mannosidosis has been described as a storage disorder of early life in which patients display coarse facies, mental retardation, impaired speech, recurrent infections of the respiratory tract and ear, mild hepatosplenomegaly, dysostosis multiplex, vacuolated lymphocytes [4,13], excessive excretion of mannose-rich oligosaccharides in urine [5,14,16] and deficiency of acid α-D-mannosidase in various tissues and blood [2,3,17,18].

The present longitudinal study of five patients together with an extensive review of those described in the literature delineate the characteristic phenotype and clinical course of this unusual disease.

CASE REPORTS

Case 1. This 20 year old white man of Scandinavian ancestry was first seen at the age of five years and eight months for evaluation of mental retardation (IQ of 39). The patient did not sit without support until he was one year of age, and he walked and spoke single words at two and a half years of age. There was no history of consanguinity, and the patient has two normal living brothers, 15 and 18 years old.

From the Medical Genetics Division, Department of Laboratory Medicine and Pathology, University of Minnesota Medical School, Box 198 Mayo Memorial Building, Minneapolis, Minnesota 55455, and the Faribault State Hospital, Faribault, Minnesota. This study was supported in part by Grants HD-01962 and GM-00025 from the National Institutes of Health. Requests for reprints should be addressed to Dr. Jorge J. Yunis. Manuscript accepted March 5, 1976.

At age 5 years and 8 months, the patient was 101 cm tall (third percentile) and weighed 17.5 kg (25th percentile). The head was dolichocephalic and disproportionately large with a head circumference of 54.5 cm (>97th percentile). There was a spacious and prominent forehead, hypertelorism, small nose, large and posteriorly rotated ears, prominent supraorbital ridges and prognathism. These findings were also observed at ages two and 20 years (Figure 1). Slit lamp examination of the eyes revealed no corneal or lens opacities. The tympanic membranes were scarred and retracted. The liver was palpable 3 to 4 cm below the right costal margin and the spleen 3 to 4 cm below the left costal margin. There was a mild thoracolumbar gibbus of the spine and an umbilical hernia. The patient had an apraxic gait characterized by awkward, wide-based, hesitant and yet purposeful steps. The neurologic examination including calorics, cerebellar testing and peripheral fine touch, vibratory sense, two point discrimination and position sense were all normal (electromyogram refused).

Complete audiologic testing at five years and eight months, repeated at ages 15 and 17 years, disclosed a moderate to severe bilateral neurosensory hearing loss with a mild conductive component. The electroencephalogram showed occasional spikes in the left frontal and mid-temporal regions. A hematologic study revealed multiple cytoplasmic vacuoles in 32 per cent of the peripheral blood lymphocytes (Figure

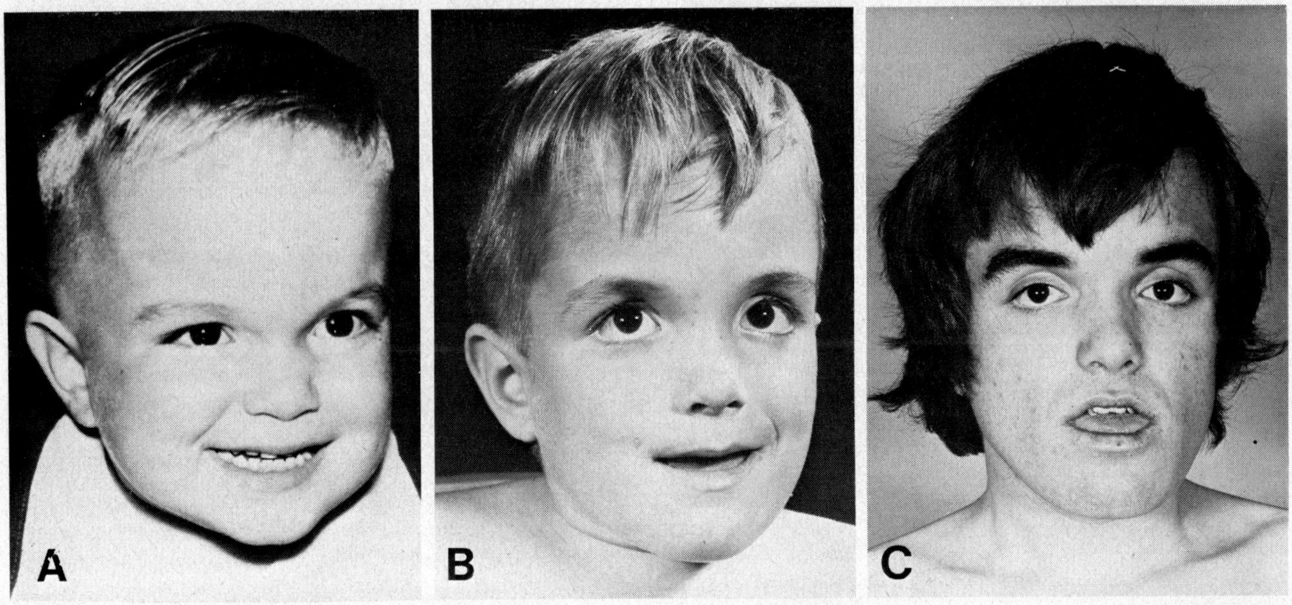

Figure 1. *Front view of face of patient (Case 1) at ages two **(A)**, five years and eight months **(B)** and 20 years **(C)**.*

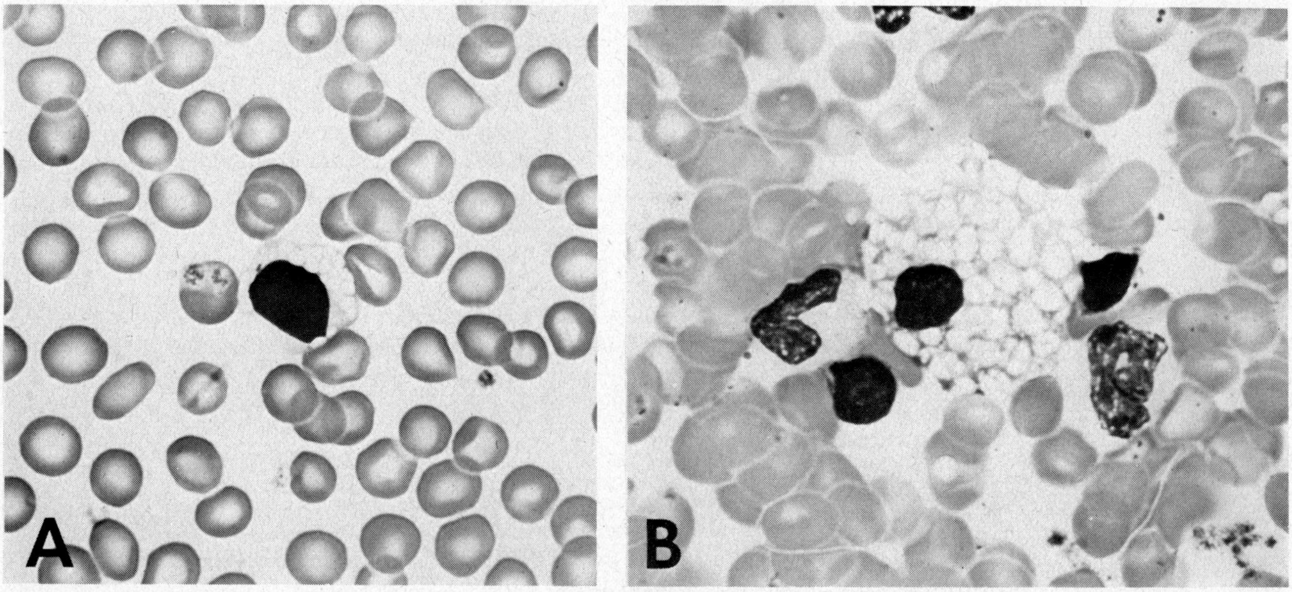

Figure 2. ***A,*** *peripheral lymphocyte of patient (Case 1) showing numerous vacuoles with generalized cytoplasmic distribution. Wright stain.* ***B,*** *large foam cell from bone marrow of same patient with eccentric nucleus. Wright stain.*

2A) and numerous large foam cells in bone marrow smears stained with Wright stain. These foam cells were about 20 to 30 μ in diameter, commonly with eccentric nuclei, and had cytoplasm packed with uniform vacuoles of 2 to 4 μ in diameter. These cells were probably reticular in origin (Figure 2B). The foam cells stained positive with periodic acid-Schiff reagent when water was avoided during fixation and staining.

Lymph node sections stained with hematoxylin and eosin revealed many foam cells in the sinusoidal areas and medulla. These cells stained moderately to strongly positive with periodic acid-Schiff. A liver biopsy specimen showed a generally well-preserved architecture with occasional small groups of foam cells in the portal areas. Kupffer cells and the foam cells stained moderately positive with periodic acid-Schiff.

At age five years and eight months, roentgenograms of the skull indicated an increased anteroposterior diameter and thickening of the calvarium (Figure 3A). The spine showed inferior-anterior beaking of the first lumbar vertebra (Figure 3B), and the ribs were broad, dense and spatulous. The hands showed slight tapering of the proximal ends of the second through fifth metacarpals and a slight increase in the width of some metacarpal and proximal phalangeal shafts accompanied by coarse trabeculation (Figure 3C). At ages 15 and 20 years, follow-up films were obtained which revealed some increased thickening of the calvarium (Figure 3D), several Schmorl's nodules and an unchanged beaking (Figure

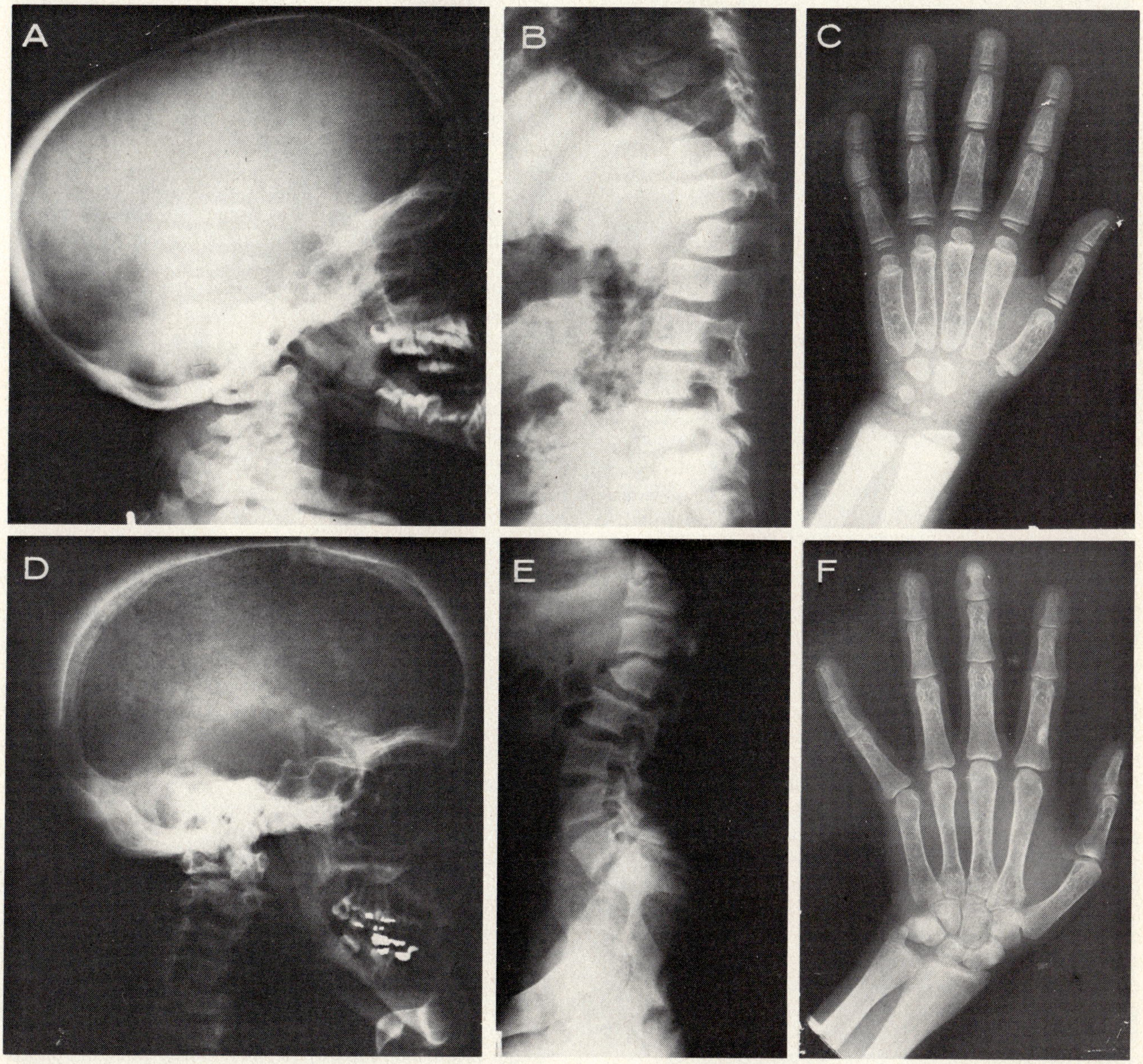

Figure 3. *Roentgenograms of patient (Case 1):* ***A*** *and* ***D,*** *skull;* ***B*** *and* ***E,*** *spine;* ***C*** *and* ***F,*** *hand; at ages five years and eight months and 20 years, respectively.*

TABLE I Ranges of α-D-Mannosidase and Hexosaminidase Activities in Serum and Leukocytes*

	Serum		Leukocytes	
	Mannosidase, pH 4.4 Activity (nmol/ml/min)	Hexosaminidase, pH 4.4 / Mannosidase, pH 4.4	Mannosidase, pH 4.4 Activity (nmol/mg protein/min)	Hexosaminidase, pH 4.4 / Mannosidase, pH 4.4
Normal controls (19)	1.7–2.4	7.2–10.8	11.0–24.2	4.0–11.4
Father, Case 1	1.1	32.0	9.0	15.4
Mother, Case 1	1.3	20.0	11.0	12.6
Case 1	0.5	88.0	0.3	294.0
Father, Cases 2–5	1.1	30.0	11.0	24.7
Mother, Cases 2–5	1.3	20.0	12.0	11.8
Case 2	0.8	60.0	0.5	220.0
Case 3	0.8	68.0	0.5	242.0
Case 4	0.8	65.0	0.5	250.0
Case 5	0.8	70.0	0.5	260.0

*By the fluorimetric method of Masson et al. [17] using 4 methylumbelliferyl α-D-mannopyranoside as substrate in 0.1 M phosphate citrate buffer.

3E). Films of the hands revealed a striking disappearance of coarse trabeculation and normalization of modeling of the metacarpal bones (Figure 3F). There was absence of frontal sinuses and there were only few air spaces in the mastoid, sphenoid and maxillary sinuses.

The statural growth paralleled the third percentile from ages seven through 14 years and then ceased, attaining an adult height of 150 cm (<third percentile). Hepatosplenomegaly, previously noted at age five years and eight months, has not been observed since age 10 years. No clinical gibbus has been noted since age 17 years. A mental age of 2.2 years at age five years and eight months rose to the four-year level at age 20 years. The patient hears only loud speech with the help of a hearing aid, is essentially mute and has learned lip reading. A marked decrease of α-D-mannosidase activity at pH 4.4 was found in leukocytes (Table I), serum immunoglobulins were normal and there was an abnormally high urinary excretion of oligosaccharides rich in mannose (Figure 4).

Cases 2, 3, 4 and 5. These four patients, two sisters 15 and a half and 17 years old (Cases 2 and 3) and two brothers 20 and 24 years old (Cases 4 and 5), were the products of a consanguineous marriage between first cousins of Germanic and Norwegian ancestry. There are four other normal sibs. These patients (Cases 2–5) appeared normal at birth and normal developmental landmarks were achieved during the first year of life. During the second year, all but one of the patients (Case 5) began to have frequent episodes of infection, especially otitis media, and all began to show evidence of hearing loss, developmental retardation and an unusual facies characterized by coarseness, protruding supraorbital ridges, hypertelorism, broad-based and saddled nose and prominent jaw. At ages one year and four months (Case 2) and three to five years (Cases 3–5), the patients had vacuolated lymphocytes in the peripheral blood, foam cells in the bone marrow and unusual findings on roentgenograms characterized by marked thickening of the calvarium, sclerosis of the base of the skull, broad, dense and spatulous ribs, beaking of the eleventh and twelfth thoracic vertebrae (Case 2), thickening of the cortex of the upper humerus, and mild coarseness and poor modeling of the metacarpals. Follow-up x-ray examinations in these patients (Cases 2–5) at ages 15 and a half, 17, 20 and 24 years, respectively, disclosed similar nonprogressive findings of the skull, ribs and spine, and normalization in modeling of the metacarpals. Other abnormalities included Schmorl's nodules and platyspondylia (Case 4), coxa valga (Cases 2 and 3), and the skulls showed obtuse angulation of the mandible, absent frontal mastoid sinuses and hypoplasia of sphenoid and maxillary sinuses.

Mental retardation is moderate in Cases 2 and 5 (mental age of eight years) and severe in Case 4 (mental age of four years). Between eight and 15 years of age, one patient (Case 3) showed slight improvement in mental age (four → six). All four patients have had a nonprogressive hearing loss with a predominant neurosensoral and a mild conductive component since ages three to five years. The hearing loss is moderate in Cases 2 and 5, and is accompanied by speech and reading abilities compatible with their functional level. It is severe in Cases 3 and 4; these patients are essentially mute. Normal statural growth patterns were observed for the first 14 years of life in all cases and then ceased at 15 to 17 years of age, resulting in adult heights within 2 standard deviations (SD) below the mean for females and less than 2 SD below the mean for the males (157, 152, 160 and 169 cm in Cases 2–5, respectively).

The most recent examination of these patients (Cases 2–5) (ages 15 and a half, 17, 20 and 24 years, respectively; Figure 5) revealed the following clinical features in common: midfrontal bossing, moderate to marked prominence of supraorbital ridges, broad nose with depressed nasal bridge, absence of corneal and lens opacities by slit lamp examination, hypertelorism and large ears (by measurement), prominent jaw, hyperconvex fingernails, minimal limitation of extension of interphalangeal joints, valgus deformity of great toes, umbilical hernia, absence of hepatosplenomegaly and gibbus deformity. The electroencephalogram and urinary mucopolysaccharides were normal. In addition, the two females (Cases 2 and 3) showed clinical evidence of coxa valga. One male (Case 4) demonstrated a gait disturbance similar to that in Case 2 with the same normal neurologic findings. The peripheral blood of all patients showed 22 to

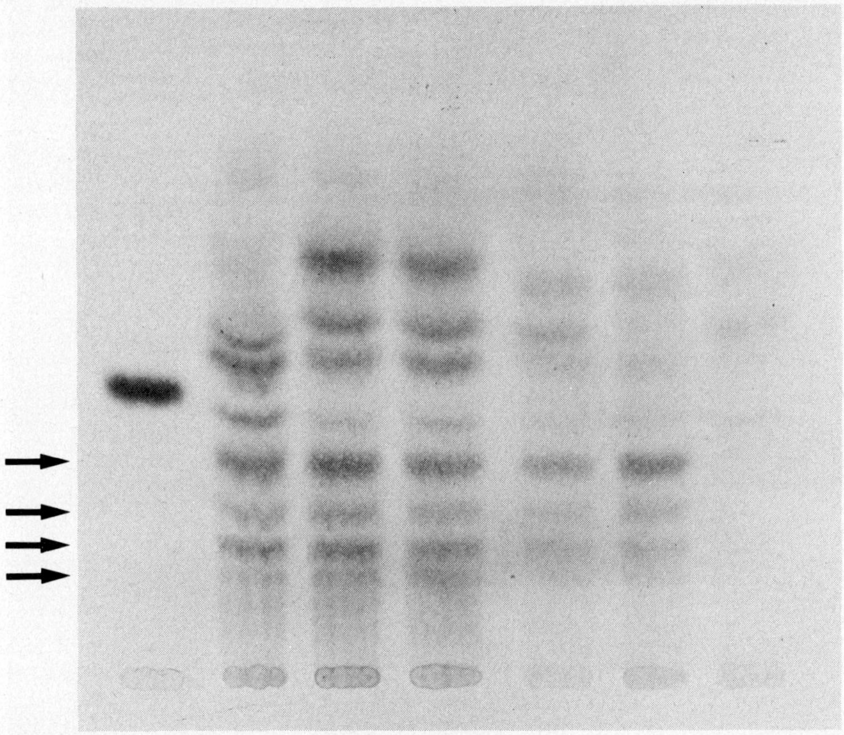

Figure 4. *Thin layer chromatography of urinary carbohydrate-containing compounds. Twenty microliters of each of the 24-hour urine samples from control (7), and the five patients with mannosidosis (2–6) were applied on a silica gel G plate. Twenty microliters of a lactose solution (mg/ml) (1) were applied as a reference. Fractionation was carried out in a solvent system of n-butanol/acetic/acid/water (2:1:1, v/v) and the plates were stained with orcinol. Note the presence of at least four abnormal bands in the five patients with mannosidosis* ***(arrows).***

33 per cent lymphocytes with multiple vacuoles and the bone marrow showed numerous foam cells similar to those found in Case 1. White blood cells gave low levels of α-D-mannosidase activity at pH 4.4 whereas serum retained a substantial amount of activity (Table I), and urinary oligosaccharides rich in mannose were increased (Figure 4).

COMMENTS

Mannosidosis results from a deficiency of acid α-D-mannosidase [2] and is biochemically characterized by a generalized accumulation in tissue [3] and an abnormally high urinary excretion of mannose-rich oligosaccharides [16,19].

Patients with mannosidosis appear normal during the first nine months to two years of life [6,10,11] (also Cases 1 and 3 of Autio et al. [4]; our Cases 1–5). They then begin to experience recurrent respiratory tract infections, otitis media, hearing loss, mild to moderate developmental retardation and slight coarsening of the facies accompanied by a broad and prominent forehead, prominent supraorbital ridges, hypertelorism, a broad-based and saddled nose, and a square and prominent jaw (our Cases 1–5). Although roentgenograms are within normal limits during the first year of life [20,21], by two years of age they show abnormalities [4] (our Case 2). The most unusual roentgenographic findings are a marked thickening of the skull, hypoplastic or absent sinuses and prognathism with obtuse angulation of the mandible. Other changes include mild to moderate dysostosis multiplex similar to that observed in the mucopolysaccharidoses (Figure 3).

By five years of age, the patients not only manifest the phenotypic and roentgenographic changes described, but they also have a clearly abnormal coarsening of their facies; they are obviously retarded; their hearing loss reaches its peak; and an apraxic gait or coxa valga may be present. From this point on, progression of the disease appears to be minimal. The prominence of supraorbital ridges and jaw, however, may become more conspicuous with age. Although prognathism has not been specifically discussed in previous papers, it appears to be a common and rela-

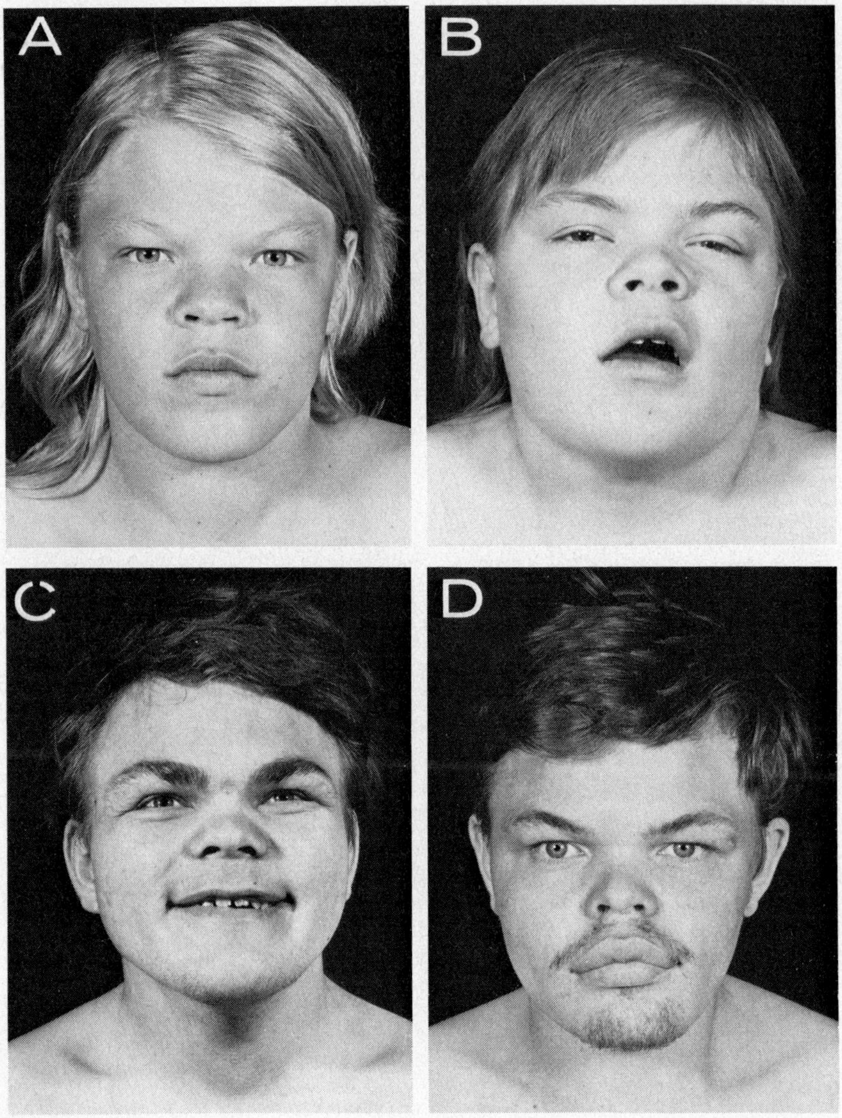

Figure 5. *Front view of face of patients: **A,** at age 15 years (Case 2); **B,** at age 17 years (Case 3); **C,** at age 19 years (Case 4); and **D,** at age 24 years (Case 5).*

tively discriminating feature, at least in patients over six years of age [4,8,11] (our Cases 1–5). The hepatosplenomegaly noted in two patients and the clinical gibbus noted in one patient disappear prior to late childhood [20] (our Case 1). Statural growth, which generally progresses at a normal rate through the early teen-age years, ceases early, resulting in an adult height of less than 2 SD below the mean for our male patients (Cases 1, 4 and 5). Interestingly, most of the roentgenologic features remain static or show little change after four years of age, the main exception being some normalization as evidenced by loss of coarse trabeculation and improved modeling of the metacarpals [20,21] (our Case 1). In their teens, platyspondylia (our Case 4) and Schmorl's nodules (our Cases 1–5) may develop.

In patients with mannosidosis, mental retardation is generally static, but occasionally mental development improves with age (our Cases 1 and 3). Patients in their teens usually have a mental age in the range of four to eight years.

Low levels of gamma globulins, reported by Kjellman et al. [20] and mentioned by Nordén et al. [5], could not be substantiated in the case studied by Farriaux et al. [8] or in our five older patients. It is not clear whether hypogammaglobulinemia is present only in severe cases of mannosidosis [20], or if hypogammaglobulinemia is present early in the disease and disappears later in life.

The clinical expression of mannosidosis may vary widely from patient to patient. This is exemplified by the differences observed among affected sibs. For example, one of our patients (Case 2) shows moderate mental retardation (mental age of eight years), moderate hearing loss, adequate speech, sporadic ear infections, gibbus, coxa valga and normal neuromotor function, whereas her brother (Case 4) shows severe mental retardation (mental age of four years), severe hearing loss and mutism, frequent ear infections and an apraxic gait. The patient (Case 3) of Nordén et al. [5] experienced repeated severe infections and stunted growth whereas his brother (Case 2) had sporadic infections and normal growth. It is possible that the frequency and severity of infections may affect growth and hearing and even the degree of apparent mental retardation.

In early childhood, the coarse facial features and roentgenographic findings may initially suggest the better-known mucopolysaccharidoses. However, the finding of normal urinary mucopolysaccharide levels and the presence of vacuolated lymphocytes in the peripheral blood smears essentially rule out these disorders. Although vacuolated lymphocytes are almost always found in mannosidosis, the age at which they appear in peripheral blood is variable. For example, they have been observed as early as six and nine months in Cases 5 and 6 of Autio et al. [4], were not seen at six months but were discovered at one year and four months in our Case 1, were not observed in the 10 and a half month old patient of Tsay et al. [6], and appeared at three years and 11 months but not at one year and eight months in the case of Perelman et al. [7]. Another crucial laboratory finding is the presence of numerous large foam cells that stain positive with periodic acid-Schiff when water is carefully avoided during fixation and staining. Similar periodic acid-Schiff–positive material has also been found in neuronal storage cells, in Kupffer and reticuloendothelial cells in the portal spaces of liver and in the sinusoidal areas and medulla of lymph nodes [3,4,22] (our Case 1). The periodic acid-Schiff–positive material apparently represents mannose-rich oligosaccharides stored in lysosomes as a result of a deficiency in glycoprotein degradation [13].

The enzyme α-D-mannosidase is known to occur in multiple molecular forms in human tissues [2,17,18,23]. In liver, there are three components, two with an optimum pH of 4.4 and one with a more neutral optimum pH of 6.0. The enzyme activity of the two acid components is markedly decreased in patients with mannosidosis [2]. A somewhat similar situation is found in leukocytes [17]. A decrease of activity of the acid α-D-mannosidase component(s) has been confirmed in serum [17], fibroblasts [8,18] and tears [8] of affected patients. The molecular basis and role of the various forms of acid mannosidase is not known [24], but it is evident that they are all equally decreased in mannosidosis.

The enzyme defect can be best detected at pH 4.4 in leukocytes or cultured fibroblasts of affected patients, whereas serum may give equivocal results due to a considerable overlap with neutral α-mannosidase at this pH [17] (Table I). Although prenatal diagnosis is considered feasible [25], detection of carriers may pose a problem since values of α-D-mannosidase activity in some of the obligate heterozygotes overlap with those of normal persons. The problem is minimized when the activity of α-D-mannosidase at pH 4.4 is compared with that of another lysosomal enzyme, such as hexosaminidase. In this manner, the ratio in heterozygotes may be intermediate between normal and deficient [17] (Table I).

Patients with mannosidosis have a high urinary excretion of mannose-containing oligosaccharides which is 15 to 65 times that observed in normal persons [5,15]. The preponderant oligosaccharides (185 to 430 mg/liter of urine) is a trisaccharide with two mannose residues, α-D-Man$p$-(1 $\rightarrow$ 3)-β-D-Man$p$-(1 $\rightarrow$ 4)-D-GlcNAc [15]. Two other types of oligosaccharides excreted in large amounts represent tetra- and penta-oligosaccharides with three and four mannose residues, respectively [19]. Recently, Humbel and Collart [16] described a simple and rapid thin-layer chromatographic technic for screening urinary oligosaccharides in patients with glycoprotein storage disease. With this technic we have observed four band components present in relatively high concentrations in the urine of our five patients (Figure 4). Analysis by column and paper chromatography of the fastest migrating band showed that it corresponds to the mannose-rich trisaccharide reported by Nordén et al. [15].

Mannosidosis appears to be an autosomal recessive disease since three of eleven sets of parents with affected children were consanguineous [7,11] (also our Cases 2–5), there is no sex predilection, and obligate carriers generally show a 50 per cent enzyme level [17]. The disease may have a universal distribution since it has already been found among people of Western, Central and Eastern European origin.

Patients with mannosidosis may live to adult life. Except for recurrent infections of the ear or respiratory tract, affected people are generally healthy retardates. They are trainable and function well in a sheltered environment. Although they continue to exhibit very low levels of α-D-mannosidase activity, evidence of continued storage material in bone marrow and peripheral blood, and an abnormally high urinary excretion of oligosaccharides, there is little, if any, evidence of clinical or roentgenologic progression of the disease beyond school age.

ACKNOWLEDGMENT

We wish to express our thanks to Oliver Cass for determining the urinary oligosaccharides and to Marylyn Hoglund for editorial assistance.

REFERENCES

1. Öckerman PA: A generalized storage disorder resembling Hurler's syndrome. Lancet 2: 239, 1967.
2. Carroll M, Dance N, Masson PK, et al.: Human mannosidosis. The enzymatic defect. Biochem Biophys Res Commun 49: 579, 1972.
3. Öckerman PA: Mannosidosis. Isolation of oligosaccharide storage material from brain. J Pediatr 75: 360, 1969.
4. Autio S, Nordén NE, Öckerman PA, et al.: Mannosidosis: clinical, fine-structural and biochemical findings in three cases. Acta Paediatr Scand 62: 555, 1973.
5. Nordén NE, Öckerman PA, Szabo L: Urinary mannose in mannosidosis. J Pediatr 82: 686, 1973.
6. Tsay GC, Dawson G, Matalon R: Excretion of mannose-rich complex carbohydrates by a patient with α-mannosidase deficiency (mannosidosis). J Pediatr 84: 865, 1974.
7. Perelman R, Nathanson M, Lepastier G, et al.: Mannosidosis associée a l'absence d'alpha-1-antitrypsine. Présentation d'une obervation. Revue de la litterature. Ann Pédiatr 22: 385, 1975
8. Farriaux JP, Legouis I, Humbel R, et al.: La mannosidase. A propos de 5 observations. Nouv Presse Med 4: 1867, 1975.
9. Sanfilippo SJ, Yunis JJ, Worthen HE: An unusual storage disease resembling the Hunter-Hurler syndrome. Am J Dis Child 104: 553, 1962.
10. Spranger JW, Wiedemann HR, Tolksdorf M, et al.: Lipomucopolysaccharidose. Eine neue Speicherkrankheit. Z Kinderheilkd 103: 285, 1968 (Patient 2).
11. Loeb H, Teppel M, Cremer H: Clinical, biochemical and ultrastructural studies of an atypical form of mucopolysaccharidosis. Acta Paediatr 58: 220, 1969.
12. Spranger JW, Wiedemann HR: The genetic mucolipidoses. Diagnosis and differential diagnosis. Humangenetik 9: 113, 1970.
13. Öckerman PA, Autio S, Nordén NE: Diagnosis of mannosidosis. Lancet 1: 207, 1973.
14. Nordén NE, Erickson O, Hultberg B, et al.: Gel chromatographic distribution of urinary carbohydrate compounds. Clin Chim Acta 44: 95, 1973.
15. Nordén NE, Lundblad A, Svensson S, et al.: A mannose-containing trisaccharide isolated from urines of three patients with mannosidosis. J Biol Chem 248: 6210, 1973.
16. Humbel R, Collart M: Oligosaccharides in urine of patients with glycoprotein storage diseases. I. Rapid detection by thin-layer chromatography. Clin Chim Acta 60: 143, 1975.
17. Masson PK, Lundblad A, Autio S: Mannosidosis: Detection of the disease and of heterozygotes using serum and leukocytes. Biochem Biophys Res Commun 56: 296, 1974.
18. Taylor HA, Thomas GH, Aylsworth A, et al.: Mannosidosis. Deficiency of a specific α-mannosidase component in cultured fibroblasts. Clin Chim Acta 59: 93, 1975.
19. Nordén NE, Lundblad A, Svensson S, et al.: Characterization of two mannose-containing oligosaccharides isolated from the urine of patients with mannosidosis. Biochemistry 13: 871, 1974.
20. Kjellman B, Gamstorp I, Brun A, et al.: Mannosidosis. A clinical and histopathologic study. J Pediatr 75: 366, 1969.
21. Spranger JW, Langer LO, Wiedemann HR: Bone dysplasia. An Atlas of Constitutional Disorders of Skeletal Development, Philadelphia, W. B. Saunders Co., 1974, p 175.
22. Freitag F, Blumcke S, Spranger J: Hepatic ultrastructure in mucolipidosis I (Lipomucopolysaccharidosis). Virchows Arch (Zellpathol) 7: 189, 1971.
23. Poenaru L, Dreyfus JC: Electrophoretic heterogeneity of human α-mannosidase. Biochim Biophys Acta 303: 171, 1973.
24. Phillips NC, Robinson D, Winchester BG: Human liver α-D-mannosidase activity. Clin Chim Acta 55: 11, 1974.
25. Butterworth J, Sutherland GR, Bradhead DM, et al.: Lysosomal enzyme levels in human amniotic fluid cells in tissue culture. III. α-glucuronidase, N-acetyl-β-D-glucosaminidase, α-mannosidase and acid phosphatase. Clin Genet 5: 356, 1974.

Chronic Neutropenia in Childhood

Analysis of 16 Cases and a Review of the Literature

STEPHANIE H. PINCUS, M.D.*
LAURENCE A. BOXER, M.D.†
THOMAS P. STOSSEL, M.D.‡
Boston, Massachusetts

We analyzed the clinical histories and hematologic information concerning 16 persons in whom chronic neutropenia was discovered early in life. Only two of them, those with the lowest mean neutrophil counts, had frequent and severe pyogenic infections. Almost all the infections were caused by Staphylococcus aureus or by enteric microorganisms and involved the skin, respiratory tract or gastrointestinal system. The prognosis in our subjects or in patients described in the literature could not be predicted from the bone marrow morphology, presence or absence of blood monocytosis, pattern of genetic transmission or results of special tests of neutrophil function.

We propose that the complex nomenclature associated with chronic neutropenic states be discarded until a better basis for classification becomes available.

The neutrophilic polymorphonuclear leukocyte is an actively phagocytic cell that is believed to play an important role in the defense against pyogenic infection. A long process of maturation from precursors in the bone marrow, a very short sojourn in the peripheral blood and irreversible entry into body tissues characterize the normal life cycle of this cell [1]. The blood level of neutrophils is maintained by a high turnover rate, controlled by poorly understood and complex factors. Although in some persons the setting of their neutrophil counts is genetically determined below the accepted "normal" range without ill effects [2–5], neutrophil counts well below the statistical limits of normal for prolonged periods is thought to predispose to pyogenic infection. This susceptibility ought to be particularly evident in childhood, when other modalities of host defense are not mature. Whereas neutropenias associated with generalized bone marrow failure, hypersplenism or the entity called cyclic neutropenia are easily diagnosed and their pathogenesis relatively well understood, other forms of neutropenia in childhood have been reported under a bewildering variety of names and speculated etiologies [6–39] (Table I).

When a child is found to have chronic neutropenia without other hematologic abnormalities or splenomegaly, two questions arise: (1) What are the etiology and pathogenesis of the condition? (2) What is the prognosis with respect to the hematologic status and the patient's susceptibility to pyogenic infection? We have analyzed the clinical and some laboratory features of children followed at the Children's Hospital Medical Center because of chronic neutropenia and have reviewed published reports of neutropenia in childhood to determine what information exists to bear on these questions.

From the Division of Hematology-Oncology, Children's Hospital Medical Center, and the Department of Pediatrics, Harvard Medical School, Boston, Massachusetts 02115. This work was supported by U.S. Public Health Service Grant HL-17742. Requests for reprints should be addressed to Dr. Thomas P. Stossel. Manuscript accepted March 19, 1976.

* Recipient of a Dermatology Foundation Fellowship. Present address: Veterans Administration Hospital, Seattle, Washington 98108.

† Present address: Department of Pediatrics, University of Indiana School of Medicine, Indianapolis, Indiana 46101.

‡ Established Investigator of the American Heart Association. Present address: Medical Oncology Unit, Massachusetts General Hospital, Boston, Massachusetts 02114.

TABLE I Summary of Reports Concerning Childhood Neutropenia

Reference	Year of Report	Name Given	No. of Patients	Range of Neutrophil Counts (per mm^3)	Monocytosis	Bone Marrow Morphology	Inheritance	Clinical Course and Special Studies
Tobler, Büser-Plüss [6]	1942	Chronic neutropenia	1	360	Yes	Maturation arrest at metamyelocyte stage*	Unknown	Boils; pneumonia
Salmonssen [7]	1948	Chronic granulocytopenia in childhood	1	0–510	Occasional	Normal	Unknown	Stomatitis; boils
Ström [8]	1949	Chronic benign granulocytopenia	1	50–4,000	No	Normal or maturation arrest at myelocyte stage	Unknown	No illness
Gasser [9]	1952	Essential chronic granulocytopenia	1	138–4,700	No	Decrease in segmented neutrophils; phagocytosis of neutrophils by monocytes	Unknown	"Susceptible to infections"
Vahlquist, Anjou [10]	1952	Chronic benign granulocytopenia	1	0–900	No	Maturation arrest at band stage	Unknown	Remission after 10 mo
			2	40–836	No	Normal	Unknown	Otitis media; pharyngitis
			3	0–336	No	Maturation arrest at myelocyte stage	Unknown	No illness
			4	96–1,029	No	Normal	Unknown	Stomatitis; pharyngitis
Vrtilek [11]	1952	Chronic granulocytopenia	1	0–2,000	Yes	Normal	Unknown	No illness
			2	0	Yes	Normal	Unknown	Remission after 4 yr
			3	0–2,200	No	"Shift to left"	Unknown	"Sickly"
			4	100–500	No	Normal	Unknown	No illness
Kostman [12]	1956	Infantile genetic agranulocytosis	1	0–150	Yes	Maturation arrest at myelocyte stage	Autosomal recessive	Died at 6 mo
			2	504 (myelocytes and metamyelocytes—lymphopenia also present)	No	Unknown	Autosomal recessive	Died at 3 mo
			3	400	Yes	Unknown	Autosomal recessive	Died at 1½ mo
			4	0–200	Yes	Maturation arrest at myelocyte stage	Autosomal recessive	Died at 3 yr
			5	900–3,300	Unknown	Maturation arrest at band stage	Autosomal recessive	"Sickly"
			6	600–3,500	Occasional	...	...	Boils
Stahlie [13]	1956	Congenital benign neutropenia	1	0–800	No	Maturation arrest at myelocyte band stage	Unknown	No illness

McLean [14]	1957	Chronic neutropenia	1	0–4,000	Yes	Normal	Unknown	Boils; pneumonia
Hedenberg [15]	1959	Infantile agranulocytosis—probably genetic	1	0–1,500	Yes	Maturation arrest at myelocyte stage	Unknown	Died at 1 yr
Hitzig [16]	1959	Familial neutropenia	1	0	Yes	Maturation arrest at myelocyte stage	Dominant	Boils; stomatitis
			2	900	Yes	Maturation arrest at myelocyte stage	Dominant	Boils; stomatitis
			3 (father of previous two)	84	Yes	Maturation arrest at myelocyte stage	Dominant	Boils; stomatitis
Levine [17]	1959	Chronic familial neutropenia	1	164	Yes	Unknown	?dominant with variable penetrance "Strong family history of neutropenia"	Gingivitis
Andrews et al. [18]	1960	Lethal congenital neutropenia	1	0–500	Yes	Maturation arrest at promyelocyte stage	Autosomal recessive	Died at 5 mo
			2	0–1,300	Yes	Maturation arrest at promyelocyte stage	Autosomal recessive	Died at 4 mo
Aarskog [19]	1961	Infantile genetic agranulocytosis	1	0–178	Yes	. . .	Unknown	Died at 4 mo
Bjure et al. [20]	1962	Familial neutropenia	1 } siblings	350–1,200	No	Decrease in mature neutrophils	Autosomal recessive	No neutrophils seen; illness said to increase after plasma infusion
			2 } siblings	160–700	No	Decrease in mature neutrophils	Autosomal recessive	
Ambs et al. [21]	1964	Chronic constitutional neutropenia	1	20–60	No	Decrease in mature neutrophils with megaloblastic changes	Unknown	No serious illness
			2	20–50	No	Decrease in mature neutrophils with megaloblastic changes	Unknown	No serious illness
McGillivray et al. [22]	1964	Congenital neutropenia	1	0–420	Yes	Decreased M:E ratio, normal neutrophil maturation	Unknown	Died at 2 yr
			2	0–100	Yes	Rare neutrophil precursors	Unknown	Died at 1 yr
			3	0–2,100	Occasional	Rare neutrophil precursors (postmortem)	Unknown	Died at 1 yr multiple abscesses
			4	64–1,564	Occasional	Decreased M:E ratio	Unknown	Pneumonia
			5	0–384	No	Decreased M:E ratio, normal neutrophil maturation	Unknown	Boils; gingivitis

TABLE I (Cont'd) Summary of Reports Concerning Childhood Neutropenia

Reference	Year of Report	Name Given	No. of Patients	Range of Neutrophil Counts (per mm³)	Monocytosis	Bone Marrow Morphology	Inheritance	Clinical Course and Special Studies
Cutting, Lang [23]	1964	Familial benign chronic neutropenia (3 generations of one family)	1	600–2,500	Yes	Maturation arrest at myelocyte stage	Dominant	Gingivitis
			2	300–2,000	Yes	Maturation arrest at myelocyte stage	Dominant	Gingivitis
			3	360	Yes	Maturation arrest at myelocyte stage	Dominant	No illness
Zuelzer [24]	1964	Myelokathexis	1	125–1,402	No	Normal with "degenerative changes" in mature neutrophils	Unknown	. . .
Krill et al. [25]	1964	Congenital idiopathic neutropenia	1	. . .	. . .	. . .	Unknown	Adenitis; pneumonia
Zuelzer, Bajoghli [26]	1964	Chronic granulocytopenia	1	100–2,000	No	Maturation arrest at meta/myelocyte stage	Unknown	Skin infections
			2	0–400	Yes	Maturation arrest at meta/myelocyte stage	Unknown	Abscesses; septicemia; ear infections
			3	0–500	No	Maturation arrest at meta/myelocyte stage	Unknown	No serious illness
			4	100–200	Yes	Maturation arrest at meta/myelocyte stage	Unknown	Stomatitis; boils
			5	40–600	No	Maturation arrest at meta/myelocyte stage	Unknown	Gingivitis; boils
Lang, Cutting [27]	1964	Infantile genetic agranulocytosis	1	240	Yes	Maturation arrest at metamyelocyte stage	Unknown	Sinusitis; boils
Miller et al. [30]	1964	Congenital neutropenia	1	0–60	Yes	Maturation arrest at myelocyte stage	Unknown	Died at 4 mo
Krill, Mauer [28]	1966	Congenital agranulocytosis	1	0	Yes	Only promyelocytes	Unknown	Died at 6 wk
Vahlquist, Verneholt [29]	1966	Agranulocytosis	1	100–400	Yes	Maturation arrest at promyelocyte stage	Unknown	No illness
Gilman et al. [31]	1970	Congenital agranulocytosis	1	250–5,000	Yes	Reduction in mature neutrophils	Unknown	Died at 14 yr of "leukemia"
			2	0–10,200	Unknown	Unknown	Unknown	Died at 13 yr of a perforated appendix
			3	0–2,210	Unknown	Unknown	Unknown	Bronchiectasis, gingivitis
Kyle, Linman [32]	1970	Chronic idiopathic neutropenia	1	85–644	Yes	Maturation arrest at metamyelocyte stage	Unknown	Gingivitis

			2	84–346	Yes	Maturation arrest at myelocyte stage	Unknown	Gingivitis
Wriedt et al. [33]	1970	Congenital neutropenia	1	0–219	Yes	Maturation arrest at myelocyte stage	Unknown	Stomatitis; died of pneumonia at 20 yr
			2	0–280	Yes	Maturation arrest at myelocyte stage	Unknown	Pneumonia; mastoiditis; boils
Miller et al. [34]	1971	Lazy leukocyte syndrome	1 } siblings	170	Unknown	Normal	Recessive	Stomatitis
			2 } siblings	135	Unknown	Normal	Recessive	Stomatitis
Barak et al. [35]	1971	Infantile genetic agranulocytosis	1	0–820	Yes	Maturation arrest at myelocyte stage	Unknown	Skin, ear, lung infections
Rodin et al. [36]	1973	Infantile genetic agranulocytosis	1 } siblings	630	No	Maturation arrest at myelocyte stage	Recessive	Died at 1 yr
			2 } siblings	24–90	Occasional	Unknown	Recessive	Died at 14 mo
			3 (distant relative)	0–3,600	Occasional	Maturation arrest at myelocyte stage	Recessive	Died at 1 yr
Deinhard, Page [37]	1974	Congenital benign neutropenia	1	<1,000	No	Normal	Unknown	No illness
Parmley et al. [38]	1975	Congenital neutropenia	1	0–130	Yes	Decreased myelocytes, markedly decreased mature neutrophils	Unknown	Chronic pneumonia, mastoiditis otitis; stomatitis
Kostman [39]	1975	Infantile genetic agranulocytosis	1	0–900	Yes	Maturation arrest at promyelocyte/myelocyte stage in all	All presumed autosomal recessive	Died at 7 mo
			2	0–400	Yes			Died at 3 mo
			3	0–250	Yes			Died at 11 mo
			4	0–300	Yes			Died at 10 mo
			5	0–250	Yes			Died at 5 mo
			6	0–650	Yes			Died at 1 yr
			7	0–1,000	Yes			Died at 6½ yr
			8	0–900	Yes			Died at 3½ yr
			9	0–150	Yes			Died at 7 mo
			10	0–400	Yes			Alive at 11 mo

MATERIALS AND METHODS

The charts of all patients seen at Children's Hospital Medical Center from 1965 to 1974 in whom the diagnosis of neutropenia was made were reviewed. Cases of bone marrow failure, of transient neutropenia associated with drug administration, viral or severe bacterial infections, of neutropenia secondary to chemotherapy for malignancy, and of neutropenia as part of a disease complex, such as neutropenia associated with pancreatic insufficiency [40], dysgammaglobulinemia [41] or systemic illnesses like systemic lupus erythematosus were excluded. No method was available for detecting patients seen at the hospital prior to 1965. However, some patients were located by means of the records of the Hematology Division.

Information collected from the charts included the age at which the diagnosis was made, the family history and a history of prior infections. The mean polymorphonuclear leukocyte, monocyte and eosinophil counts were determined by averaging all values obtained more than one week apart. During

TABLE II Information Concerning 16 Patients with Chronic Neutropenia Seen at Children's Hospital Medical Center

Case No.	Age (yr) and Sex	Age at Diagnosis (yr)	Age at First Infection (yr)	Probable Inheritance	Neutrophils Mean ± SEM	Neutrophils Range
1	26, F	1	2 wk	Dominant (mother, Case 2)	580 ± 163	0–2,500
2	5, M	3 mo	3 mo	Dominant (son, Case 1)	340 ± 140	0–2,100
3	18, M	10	Unknown	Recessive (brother, Case 4)	685 ± 293	0–3,953
4	11, F	2	Unknown	Recessive (sister, Case 3)	1,024 ± 335	0–4,582
5	11, F	1	3 mo	Unknown	312 ± 111	0–950
6	10, F	6	5 yr	Unknown	212 ± 39	0–500
7	F	2 mo	4 wk	Unknown	120 ± 15	0–425
8	3, F	1½	None†	Unknown	891 ± 311	0–2,600
9	2, F	6 mo	6 mo	Unknown	1,486 ± 96	100–3,800
10	2, M	1	1 yr	Unknown	477 ± 199	25–2,500
11	1, F	1	10 mo†	Unknown	703 ± 188	0–2,050
12	1, M	6 mo	3 wk	Unknown	147 ± 45	0–450
13	6, M	5	10 mo	Dominant (brother, Case 14; son, Case 15)	953 ± 408	350–3,186
14	5, M	4	3 yr	Dominant (brother, Case 13; son, Case 15)	870 ± 228	0–1,650
15	27, M	11	Unknown	Dominant (father, Cases 13 and 14)	1,766 ± 244	86–2,465
16	2, M	1½	7 mo	Unknown	407 ± 116	112–862

* The term maturation arrest connotes normal representation of neutrophil precursors up to and including the stage cited with few or none of later stages identifiable.
† Neutropenia was an incidental finding.

the patients' hospitalization, biweekly counts were analyzed. Mean cell counts in one patient (Case 1), who has been followed for over 20 years, were computed on the basis of bimonthly counts. If, at the time of the review, more than one year had elapsed since the last blood count, the patient was contacted and counts obtained. If available, bone marrow slides were reviewed. Otherwise, the reading listed is that made at the time of the aspiration.

Special procedures were undertaken with some patients. These included (1) infusion of plasma, 10 ml/kg, reported to increase neutrophil counts in cases of chronic neutropenia [20]; (2) administration of tetanus toxoid, 0.5 ml intramuscularly or prednisone, 40 mg/M^2 orally [42,43], agents believed to mobilize bone marrow reserves; (3) dermal abrasions, tests of inflammatory responses [44]; and (4) epinephrine administration, 0.3 ml of a 1:1000 dilution, subcutaneously thought to shift marginal neutrophils into the circulation. Tests were performed to detect antibody in some patients' serum against normal neutrophils [45]. Statistical evaluation of covariance analysis with regression and t tests

Blood Leukocyte Counts (no.)					
Eosinophils		Monocytes			
Mean ± SEM	Range	Mean ± SEM	Range	Bone Marrow Morphology	Clinical Course
244 ± 50	0–1,060	2,093 ± 259	350–4,300	Maturation arrest* at promyelocyte stage	Frequent pyoderma as a child; splenectomy age 4, occasional pyoderma
329 ± 84	50–1,400	3,084 ± 517	0–10,600	Maturation arrest at promyelocyte or myelocyte stage	Frequent pyoderma during first 2 yr of life
950 ± 145	201–1,915	572 ± 171	0–1,766	Maturation arrest at myelocyte stage	Chronic pulmonary infiltrates; 2 lung abscesses
933 ± 346	0–4,200	1,315 ± 355	70–3,924	Maturation arrest at metamyelocyte stage	Frequent pyoderma and sinusitis; Otitis media
356 ± 74	0–560	1,154 ± 207	350–1,980	Maturation arrest at myelocyte stage	Stomatitis
105 ± 37	0–380	588 ± 83	180–1,410	Maturation arrest at band stage	No serious illnesses
617 ± 60	0–2,261	1,794 ± 1,751	100–7,375	Maturation arrest at promyelocyte stage	Died age 4½ yr of liver failure; had pyoderma, pneumonia, liver abscesses, urinary tract infection; also had large ventricular septal defect
68 ± 16	0–150	551 ± 82	100–1,100	Normal	No serious illnesses
185 ± 65	0–750	480 ± 130	0–1,000	Normal	No serious illnesses
77 ± 37	0–300	458 ± 184	0–1,540	Normal twice; maturation arrest at band stage once	Occasional pyoderma
25 ± 18	0–160	660 ± 157	430–800	Normal	No serious illnesses
217 ± 71	0–725	2,972 ± 268	2,000–4,800	Maturation arrest at promyelocyte or myelocyte stage	Pyoderma, recurrent pneumonias and lung abscesses; right upper lobectomy at 6 mo
109 ± 25	25–225	358 ± 71	180–600	Maturation arrest at band stage	Haemophilus influenzae pneumonia at age 5; no other serious illnesses
153 ± 36	40–357	862 ± 454	240–4,272	Normal	No serious illnesses
281 ± 98	86–850	593 ± 317	43–2,365	Not obtained	"Frequent infections" as child
118 ± 38	0–285	768 ± 151	400–1,452	Maturation arrest at band stage	No serious illnesses

for differences between means were performed according to standard methods [46] employing a digital computer system.

RESULTS

Search of the records revealed 12 patients with persistent, noncyclic neutropenia, who were seen between 1965 and 1975. During the first four months of 1975, four additional patients with neutropenia were seen as outpatients. The information concerning the patients is summarized in Table II.

Of these 16 patients, seven were female and nine male. Their current age ranges from 27 to one year. Although neutropenia was discovered in eight patients at age 1 year or less, in one patient the diagnosis was not made until age 10 and in another not until age 11. The two patients (Cases 7 and 12) who had the most serious infections were found to have neutropenia at ages two months and six months, respectively. However, two other patients (Cases 9 and 2) without severe difficulties were found to be neutropenic at the same ages.

In three families, more than one member was affected. Two families had two neutropenic members and one family had three. One patient (Case 2) is the son of another patient (Case 1) indicating inheritance of the neutropenia as an autosomal dominant trait. Two patients (Cases 13 and 14) are the sons of another patient (Case 15) who was only mildly neutropenic at the time of the study, but was documented to have had persistent neutropenia and recurrent infections as a teenager. The low normal neutrophil count of this patient (Case 15) reflects the fact that the mean is based predominantly on values obtained during the spring of 1975.

In families with no known previous history of neutropenia, both parents and all siblings were tested to exclude occult neutropenia. Two patients (Cases 3 and 4) are two affected siblings from a family of six children. The most likely explanation is a recessive pattern of inheritance, but their father (who did not have a history of recurrent infections) died of accidental injuries at age 32 and was, therefore, not available for testing. The father of one patient (Case 7) was unknown. All the other patients were sole affected family members, suggesting a recessive inheritance, if any.

The clinical status of most patients was remarkably good. One of the 16 patients (Case 7) has died. Death was directly related to liver failure with portal hypertension and esophageal varices. The liver disease was, in part, attributable to abscesses caused by enteric bacteria which developed after thoracic surgery for consolidated staphylococcal pneumonias. However, in addition to chronic neutropenia, this patient had a large ventricular septal defect associated with severe congestive heart failure. Two other patients are chronically ill. One (Case 2) has chronic pulmonary disease manifested largely as cystic lesions visible on chest films and the other (Case 12) has had several severe episodes of Esch. coli pneumonia with abscess formation and has required a lobectomy. However, the other 13 patients lead normal lives, although several of them have had occasional episodes of pyoderma, gingivitis and stomatitis.

Hematologic Findings. Table II shows that the mean neutrophil counts in two patients were less than 200/mm^3. There is a statistically significant ($p < 0.001$) difference between these patients' counts and those of the other patients as a group. These were the two patients (Cases 7 and 12) with the most severe infections. Most patients demonstrated a wide variation in the neutrophil count. For example, one patient (Case 1), who has been followed for over 20 years, had neutrophil counts ranging from 0 to 2,500/mm^3. The highest counts were, in general, those associated with an acute infection. The two patients with the lowest mean counts and the severest clinical histories also had the least variation in individual counts. One patient (Case 6), however, also had a low variation in counts and a relatively low mean count but has not had difficulties with infections.

All but three of the patients had increased mean monocyte counts, and all but two had counts above the normal range at some time. The two patients with the most severe neutropenia (Cases 7 and 12) had increased, but not the highest, mean monocyte counts. However, there was no statistically significant inverse correlation between monocyte counts and neutrophil counts, either when comparing mean counts of all the patients or when analyzing the individual counts for individual patients.

The eosinophil counts could not be correlated with either the neutrophil counts or the monocyte counts. Of the two patients with the most severe neutropenia, only one had an increased total eosinophil count. However, two patients (Cases 3 and 4) (siblings) had markedly increased total eosinophil counts.

There were no abnormalities of the hematocrit except for one patient (Case 7) who was intermittently anemic. The anemia was ascribed to her bleeding esophageal varices. All patients had normal platelet counts, except one (Case 1) who had an increased count, possibly related to splenectomy.

Special studies to evaluate marrow reserves (response to the administration of endotoxin, prednisone or tetanus vaccine), marginal pool size (response to the administration of epinephrine) and cellular migration (skin window) were performed in a few patients (Table III). The response to the administration of epinephrine

TABLE III Results of Special Tests of Neutrophil Responses in Patients with Chronic Neutropenia Seen at Children's Hospital Medical Center

Case No.	Epinephrine	Tetanus Toxoid	Prednisone	Other
1	490 → 783*	...	...	...
3	0 → 68	...	...	...
4	0 → 336	36 → 68*	...	...
5	192 → 400	...	...	...
7	276 → 330	"No response"	No response to a therapeutic trial	Eosinophils, monocytes, but no neutrophils in a Rebuck window; few neutrophils seen in excised infected lung tissue
9	260 → 760	112 → 3,026	...	...
10	"No response"	...	440 → 626†	Monocytes but no neutrophils in Rebuck window
12	...	...	0 → 31	Monocytes, few neutrophils in Rebuck window; few neutrophils in excised infected lung tissue

*Peak change in absolute neutrophil (segmented + band) count at any time during the test if known.
†Change in absolute neutrophil count 1 hour after administration of drug.

was examined in seven patients; most responded with an increase in neutrophils at 5 to 15 minutes. Rebuck skin windows were evaluated in three patients (Cases 7, 10 and 12). Mononuclear cell reactions were noted in these patients when evaluated at 5 or 12 hours. Few or no neutrophils were identified when the slides were examined at 5 hours. All three patients were severely neutropenic ($<300/mm^3$) at the time of evaluation. Five patients had tests to evaluate the response to the administration of typhoid vaccine or prednisone. Four had poor responses, and one (Case 9) had a relatively good response in terms of the absolute number of neutrophils released into the peripheral circulation. One patient (Case 7) had no response to a single infusion of normal plasma.

Bone marrow morphology varied both between patients and between marrow aspirates obtained from the same patient at different times. For example, three different marrow specimens in one patient (Case 12) differed. The initial marrow examination revealed "poor myelocyte development." A marrow sample one month later was reported to show "arrest at the promyelocyte stage." A third marrow aspirate obtained at the age of 14 months revealed myeloid hyperplasia and showed "arrest" at the myelocyte stage, with some vacuolated lymphocytes and myeloid precursors. Two patients (Cases 1 and 7) had an "arrest" both at the promyelocyte stage and at the myelocyte stage depending on the particular marrow specimen. Three patients (Cases 1, 5 and 12) were reported to have vacuolated cells within the marrow. Four other patients (Cases 8, 9, 10 and 11) had normal marrow morphology. The severity of the clinical disease could not be correlated with the marrow morphology. One patient (Case 12) who had frequent infections had a marrow picture which was similar to that of two other patients (Cases 1 and 2), who had less difficulty with infections.

Infections (Table IV). Pyoderma and otitis media were the most frequent infections and were present at some time in 12 patients. There were 47 infections of the skin, including localized abscesses, furunculosis and cellulitis. Staph. aureus was isolated on 18 occasions. Esch. coli and Pseudomonas species were each isolated four times, and β-hemolytic streptococci was isolated once. In the remaining 20 reported episodes of cutaneous infection, no organisms were obtained.

There were 42 episodes of otitis media in 12 patients. In only seven instances were pathogens recovered. Pneumococci and Ps. aeruginosa were each isolated on two occasions, Esch. coli, Staph. aureus. and S. albus once each.

Pulmonary infections were next in frequency, occurring in 10 patients. There were 13 instances of pneumonia as evidenced by fever and findings on chest films. Pathogens included Staph. aureus and Esch. coli each on two occasions. Four lung abscesses arose in two patients (Cases 3 and 12). There were 11 episodes of "bronchitis" in 10 patients. A number of nonspecific infections of the upper respiratory tract were not included because of lack of adequate documentation.

Gingivitis and stomatitis occurred in five patients. These same patients had difficulty with dental caries, as did two additional patients. Sinusitis was also documented in two of the 14 patients.

Infections of the urinary tract and gastrointestinal system were very uncommon. Only one episode of

TABLE IV Documented Infections

Site	No. of Patients	No. of Episodes	Bacteriologic Isolates	
Skin			Staph. aureus	18
Cellulitis, pyoderma furunculosis	11	47	Pseudomonas	4
			Esch. coli	4
			Streptococcus	1
Wound	1	6 (persistent)	Esch. coli	
Ear			Pneumococcus	2
Otitis media	12	42	Pseudomonas	2
			Esch. coli	1
			Staph. aureus	1
			S. albus	1
Pulmonary	10		Staph. aureus	2
Pneumonia	8	13	Esch. coli	2
Abscess	2	4	Esch. coli	1
Bronchitis	4	11		
Dental				
Gingivitis and/or stomatitis	5	11		
Caries, severe	7			
Nasopharynx	2	4		
Sinusitis	2	4	β-streptococcus	1
Pharyngitis				
Miscellaneous				
Liver abscess	1	4 (persistent)	Strep. fecalis and Esch. coli	1
Urinary tract	1	2		

urinary tract infection was reported (Case 7). In one patient (Case 7) multiple hepatic abscesses developed. Organisms cultured from the liver abscesses were Esch. coli and Strep. fecalis. There was no case of osteomyelitis, meningitis or bacterial endocarditis.

Episodes of "infection" occurring outside the hospital were often included in patients' presenting histories and could not be assessed as to severity or microbial etiology.

Miscellaneous Laboratory Data. No consistent abnormalities of hepatic or renal failure were noted except in one patient (Case 7) who had liver failure. Of 10 patients tested all had normal stool trypsin activity. Iron deficiency, noted in one patient, responded to appropriate treatment.

Immunoglobulin determinations were performed in 10 of the patients. Three patients (Cases 2, 5 and 12) had elevated serum IgG levels (1,650 to 2,650 mg/100 ml), and one patient was reported to have an "elevated" IgA level. The serum of 15 patients (Cases 6 through 14 and Case 16) was tested for the presence of antineutrophil antibody. Antibody was not detected in any of the serums.

Treatment. In all episodes of infection the patients responded to treatment with appropriate antibiotics, except two patients (Cases 7 and 12). One patient (Case 7) required several operations for treatment of pulmonary and liver abscesses in addition to receiving large doses of intravenous antibiotics. The infections could not be completely eradicated. Another patient (Case 12) underwent a lobectomy at age 14 months for treatment of a lung abscess which failed to respond to appropriate therapy. Further infection was controlled in this patient by antibiotic treatment.

Glucocorticoids had no effect on the clinical course or neutrophil counts of four patients (Cases 1, 3, 7 and 12). One patient (Case 1) underwent splenectomy at age three years without any subsequent change in her neutrophil levels.

COMMENTS

Cases of chronic neutropenia in childhood described in this report and recorded in the literature suggest that most of the ancillary factors currently analyzed are so variable that they are of limited help in evaluating prognosis and classifying these disorders.

Neutrophil Counts. Susceptibility to pyogenic infection in syndromes of bone marrow failure has been reported to be inversely proportional to the blood neutrophil count [47]. However, both the literature and our cases demonstrate that patients with very low mean neutrophil counts may have strikingly variable clinical histories, although we note that the two patients in our series who had the greatest difficulties with infection had the lowest mean neutrophil counts. Since hemorrhage, tissue invasion, drug effects, monocytopenia and lymphopenia are associated with generalized bone marrow failure, it is not surprising that infection is a more frequent complication of this disease complex than in syndromes in which only neutropenia exists. The range or the mean values of neutrophil counts may not reflect the patients' most frequent counts or the patients' abilities to respond to infection. For this reason, tests to assess marrow reserves have been employed.

Unfortunately, almost all patients with chronic neutropenia have subnormal responses to agents which increase blood neutrophil counts in normal persons [48]. Furthermore, the results of these tests do not correlate well with more sophisticated assays for granulocyte turnover rates; and these can only be undertaken in patients with mild neutropenia. Since all neutropenic patients have diminished inflammatory responses as determined by Rebuck skin window tests [49], this procedure will not be helpful for establishing the pathogenesis of neutropenia.

Monocytosis. Since the monocyte can perform many of the antibacterial functions of neutrophils, it is possible that an increase in blood monocytes might compensate for the effects of neutropenia. Both in our series and in the literature, the presence or absence of blood monocytosis did not correlate with prognosis. It is not clear, in fact, whether the high monocyte counts in some of the sicker patients are concomitants of the neutropenic state or the consequence of the fact that the patient happened to be infected.

Bone Marrow Morphology. Both the literature and our patients attest to the variety of bone marrow morphology profiles encountered in chronic neutropenia of childhood. In patients with similar clinical histories and similar peripheral neutrophil counts, bone marrow granulocyte distributions differed. Moreover, bone marrow morphology varied even in the same patient at different times. All patients had some recognizable granulocyte precursors.

The variability encountered suggests that marrow morphology is not very useful for predicting prognosis or for determining pathogenesis, although it is vital for ruling out generalized bone marrow failure or invasion in the diagnostic work-up of the neutropenic patient. The bone marrow morphology of a group of patients with autoimmune neutropenia was indistinguishable from the morphology encountered in these children with chronic neutropenia not associated with antineutrophil antibodies [45].

Genetics. The inheritance of chronic neutropenia in childhood, if discernible, can follow either autosomal dominant or recessive patterns. Neither the peripheral blood or bone marrow picture nor the clinical course of our patients or of the patients described in the literature could be predicted by the mode of genetic transmission. A special case appears to be chronic neutropenia occurring as a recessive trait among inbred families in northern Sweden. Affected children have suffered from an unusually severe and frequently lethal clinical course [12,39].

Clinical Findings. The histories of our patients indicate that most cases of chronic neutropenia in childhood follow a benign course. This benignity contrasts sharply to that in a minority of our cases and in many cases in the literature. It is likely that the risk in the neutropenic patient has changed in recent years because of general improvement in social conditions, medical care and the availability of effective antibiotics against the pathogens which cause most of the infections in these patients, penicillinase-resistant staphylococci and gram-negative enteric organisms. The infections suffered by our patients follow the general pattern reported in the past in which infections of the skin, mucous membranes and lungs predominate. Bone and central nervous system infections have not been recorded. These facts are of some interest from the standpoint of determining the role of the neutrophil in host defense against pyogenic infection. The neutrophil appears to be responsible for preventing invasion by microorganisms in tissues interfacing with the environment. The results suggest that the neutrophil has less relevance for protection against high grade encapsulated pathogens which invade the blood and cause septicemia and meningitis. However, many factors complicate this analysis. Susceptibility to infection and the course of infection are determined by the frequency of exposure to pathogens, by the virulence of the pathogens, and by the vigor and efficacy of treatment as well as by the adequacy of host defenses.

From the foregoing we suggest that there is currently little data on which to justify the many names given to these disorders. We suggest that eponyms, terms such as "benign chronic neutropenia" and "infantile genetic agranulocytosis" and acronyms be discarded. We recommend that chrnoic neutropenia is an adequate term for cases in which no genetic transmission is documentable and that hereditary chronic neutropenia be used when inheritance is established. The term "congenital" is rarely justified by formal documentation and adds little to the understanding of the disease.

In asking for this simplification of terminology we recognize that chronic neutropenia in childhood is probably a heterogenous set of disorders. Perhaps future studies will permit a rational subdivision of the nosology of chronic neutropenias in childhood. Cultivation of bone marrow neutrophil precursors holds promise, but quite different results have been obtained in different patients, often with similar histories and hematologic pictures. For example, cultures of marrow from children with chronic neutropenia and frequent severe infections have yielded no mature granulocytes [50] or else diminished to normal numbers of mature neutrophil colonies [51–54]. Whether the discrepancies result from sampling difficulties, variation in technics or truly reflect the heterogeneity of these disorders awaits resolution. Some fraction of children with chronic neutropenia may have autoimmune neutropenia, and tests are now available for establishing this diagnosis [45].

Reports in the literature [10,11,54] indicate that some neutropenic children experience normalization of neutrophil counts when they grow older. Although neutropenia may be a manifestation of preleukemic states in adults, none of our patients has shown any signs of leukemia. Only one case reported in the literature [31] suggested that chronic neutropenia in childhood may evolve into leukemia, and the documentation of a leukemic state in that patient was incomplete. In one kindred described, pancytopenia developed [36]. In none of our patients has generalized bone marrow failure developed.

ACKNOWLEDGMENT

We thank David G. Nathan, M.D., for encouragement and support.

REFERENCES

1. Athens JW, Haab OP, Raab SO, et al.: Leukokinetic studies. IV. The total blood, circulating and marginal granulocyte pools and the granulocyte turnover rate in normal subjects. J Clin Invest 40: 989, 1961.
2. Djaldetti M, Joshua H, Kalderon M: Familial leukopenia-neutropenia in Yemenite Jews. Bull Res Counc Israel 9E: 24, 1960.
3. Broun GO Jr, Herbig FK, Hamilton JR: Leukopenia in Negroes. N Engl J Med 275: 1410, 1966.
4. Shaper AG, Lewis P: Genetic neutropenia in people of African origin. Lancet 2: 1021, 1971.
5. Caramihai E, Karayalcin G, Aballi AJ, et al.: Leukocyte count differences in healthy white and black children 1 to 5 years of age. J Pediatr 86: 252, 1975.
6. Tobler W, Buser-Plüss E: Beobachtungen in einem falle von chronischer, myelogener, hochgradiger neutropenie mit monocytärer reaktion. Ann Paediatr 159: 258, 1942.
7. Salmonssen L: Granulocytopenia in children. Acta Paediatr 35: 189, 1948.
8. Ström J: Chronic benign granulocytopenia in a child during the second year of life. Acta Paediatr 38: 590, 1949.
9. Gasser C: Die pathogenese der essentiellen chronischen granulocytopenie im kindesalter auf grund der knochenmarksbefunde. Helv Paediatr Acta 7: 426, 1952.
10. Vahlquist B, Anjou N: Granulocytopénie chronique bénigne. Acta Haematol 8: 199, 1952.
11. Vrtilek MR: Das bild der chronischen granulocytopenie im kindesalter. Helv Paediatr Acta 7: 207, 1952.
12. Kostmann R: Infantile genetic agranulocytosis. Acta Paediatr 45 (suppl 105): 1, 1956.
13. Stahlie TD: Chronic benign neutropenia in infancy and early childhood. J Pediatr 48: 710, 1956.
14. McLean M: Chronic neutropenia. Arch Dis Child 32: 431, 1957.
15. Hedenberg F: Infantile agranulocytosis of probably congenital origin. Acta Paediatr 48: 77, 1959.
16. Hitzig WH: Familiäre neutropenie mit dominantem erbgang und hypergammaglobulinämie. Helv Med Acta 5: 779, 1959.
17. Levine S: Chronic familial neutropenia with marked periodontal lesions. Oral Surg 12: 310, 1959.
18. Andrews JP, McClellan JT, Scott CH: Lethal congenital neutropenia with eosinophilia occurring in two siblings. Am J Med 29: 358, 1960.
19. Aarskog D: Infantile congenital aneutrocytosis. Arch Dis Child 36: 511, 1961.
20. Bjure J, Nilsson LR, Plum CM: Familial neutropenia possibly caused by deficiency of a plasma factor. Acta Paediatr 51: 497, 1962.
21. Ambs E, Biren P, Lange FC: Die chronische, konstitutionelle neutropenie mit lymphocytose im säuglings und kleinkindesalter. Z Kinderheilkd 91: 5, 1964.
22. MacGillivray JB, Dacie JV, Henry JRK, et al.: Congenital neutropenia: a report of five cases. Acta Paediatr 53: 188, 1964.
23. Cutting HO, Lang JE: Familial benign chronic neutropenia. Ann Intern Med 61: 876, 1964.
24. Zuelzer WW: "Myelokathexis"—a new form of chronic granulocytopenia. N Engl J Med 270: 699, 1964.
25. Krill CE, Dunlap-Smith H, Mauer AM: Chronic idiopathic neutropenia. N Engl J Med 270: 973, 1964.
26. Zuelzer WW, Bajoghli M: Chronic granulocytopenia in childhood. Blood 23: 359, 1964.
27. Lang JE, Cutting HO: Infantile genetic agranulocytosis. Pediatrics 35: 596, 1965.
28. Krill CE, Mauer AM: Congenital agranulocytosis. J Pediatr 68: 361, 1966.
29. Vahlquist B, Verneholt J: Agranulocytose im kindesalter. Z Kinderheilkd 96: 106, 1966.
30. Miller DR, Freed BA, Lapey JD: Congenital neutropenia. Am J Dis Child 115: 337, 1968.
31. Gilman PA, Jackson DP, Guild HG: Congenital agranulocytosis: prolonged survival and terminal acute leukemia. Blood 36: 576, 1970.
32. Kyle RA, Linman JW: Gingivitis and chronic idiopathic neutropenia: report of two cases. Mayo Clin Proc 45: 494, 1970.
33. Wriedt K, Kauder E, Mauer AM: Defective myelopoiesis in congenital neutropenia. N Engl J Med 283: 1072, 1970.
34. Miller ME, Oski FA, Harris MB: Lazy leukocyte syndrome. Lancet 1: 665, 1971.
35. Barak Y. Paran M, Levin S, et al.: In vitro induction of myeloid proliferation and maturation in infantile genetic agranulocytosis. Blood 38: 74, 1971.
36. Rodin AE, Haggard ME, Nichold MM, et al.: Infantile genetic agranulocytosis. Am J Dis Child 126: 818, 1973
37. Deinhard AS, Page AR: A study of steroid-induced granulocytosis in a patient with chronic benign neutropenia of childhood. Br J Haematol 28: 333, 1974.
38. Parmley RT, Ogawa M, Darby CP Jr, et al.: Congenital neutropenia: neutrophil proliferation with abnormal maturation. Blood 46: 723, 1975.
39. Kostman R: Infantile genetic agranulocytosis. Acta Paediatr Scand 64: 362, 1975.
40. Schwachman H, Diamond LK, Oski FA, et al.: The syndrome of pancreatic insufficiency and bone marrow dysfunction. J Pediatr 65: 645, 1964.
41. Ackerman BD: Dysgammaglobulinemia: report of a case with

a family history of a congenital gamma globulin disorder. Pediatr 34: 211, 1964.
42. Kauder E, Mauer AM: Neutropenias of childhood. J Pediatr 69: 147, 1966.
43. Dale DC, Fauci AS, Guerry D IV, et al.: Comparison of agents producing a neutrophilic leukocytosis in man. J Clin Invest 56: 808, 1975.
44. Rebuck JW, Crowly JH: A method of studying leukocytic functions in vivo. Ann NY Acad Sci 59: 757, 1955.
45. Boxer LA, Greenberg MS, Boxer GJ, et al.: Autoimmune neutropenia. N Engl J Med 293: 748, 1975.
46. Snedecor GW, Cochrane WG: Statistical Methods, Ames, Iowa, Iowa State University Press, 1967.
47. Bodey GP, Buckley M, Sathe YS, et al.: Quantitative relationships between circulating leukocytes and infection in patients with acute leukemia. Ann Intern Med 64: 328, 1966.
48. Bishop GR, Rothstein G, Ashenbrucker HE, et al.: Leukokinetic studies XIV. Blood neutrophil kinetics in chronic steady-state neutropenia. J Clin Invest 50: 1678, 1971.
49. Dale DC, Wolff SM: Skin-window studies of the acute inflammatory response of neutropenic patients. Blood 38: 138, 1971.
50. L'Esperance P, Brunning R, Good RA: Congenital neutropenia: in vitro growth of colonies mimicking the disease. Proc Natl Acad Sci USA 70: 669, 1973.
51. Greenberg PL, Schrier SL: Granulopoiesis in neutropenic disorders. Blood 41: 753, 1973.
52. Senn JS, Messner HA, Stanley ER: Analysis of interacting cell populations in cultures of marrow from patients with neutropenia. Blood 44: 33, 1974.
53. Mintz U, Sachs L: Normal granulocyte colony-forming cells in the bone marrow of Yemenite Jews with genetic neutropenia. Blood 41: 745, 1973.
54. Joyce RA, Boggs DR, Chervenick PA: Neutrophil kinetics in hereditary neutropenia (abstract). Blood 46: 1017, 1975.

Skin Capillary Abnormalities As Indicators of Organ Involvement in Scleroderma (Systemic Sclerosis), Raynaud's Syndrome and Dermatomyositis

HILDEGARD R. MARICQ, M.D.
Charleston, South Carolina

GEORGE SPENCER-GREEN, M.D.
New York, New York

E. CARWILE LeROY, M.D.
Charleston, South Carolina

Forty-four study patients with scleroderma (systemic sclerosis) (28 patients), Raynaud's syndrome (13 patients) or dermatomyositis (three patients) were observed for skin capillary abnormalities by widefield microscopy and compared with three control groups of 20 subjects each: (1) patients with other rheumatic disease, (2) hospitalized patients with nonrheumatic conditions, and (3) healthy volunteers. The distinctive microvascular pattern (dilated and distorted capillary loops alternating with avascular areas) previously reported in scleroderma and dermatomyositis was observed almost exclusively in the study patients. The severity of capillary abnormalities varied among the diagnostic subgroups, and a positive correlation was found between the degree and extent of abnormal microvascular patterns and multisystem involvement.

On this basis, widefield nailfold capillary observations are proposed as a simple, inexpensive, reproducible technic for making an improved early diagnosis and predicting multisystem involvement in scleroderma, Raynaud's syndrome and dermatomyositis, presently a group of loosely associated and overlapping connective tissue disorders which often defy early and precise diagnosis.

The diagnosis of rheumatic disorders has been improved by the introduction of the criteria for acute rheumatic fever, rheumatoid arthritis, systemic lupus erythematosus, gout and pseudogout. Such criteria are lacking for several loosely associated and often overlapping syndromes: scleroderma (systemic sclerosis), Raynaud's syndrome without a definable connective tissue disorder and dermatomyositis.

Raynaud's phenomenon occurs in approximately 80 to 90 per cent of the patients with scleroderma [1] and often precedes other symptoms and signs. At an early stage it is, therefore, difficult to distinguish between patients with so-called "Raynaud's disease" (pathology limited to extremities) and those in whom scleroderma later develops (a multisystem disorder whose more serious prognosis depends on visceral involvement) [2–5]. A common denominator of all target organ involvement in scleroderma appears at the microcirculatory level and consists of distinctive lesions of small arteries and arterioles [1,6,7].

As a potential diagnostic aid, the morphology of skin and other surface capillaries has been known to be abnormal in rheumatic diseases for a half century [8–10]. The favorite site of observation has been the nailfold capillary bed. Similar abnormalities of nailfold capillaries in scleroderma, Raynaud's syndrome and dermatomyositis have

From the Department of Medicine, College of Physicians & Surgeons of Columbia University, New York, New York; and the Division of Rheumatology and Immunology, Department of Medicine, Medical University of South Carolina, Charleston, South Carolina. This work was supported in part by the Sidney and Charlotte Lifschultz Foundation Gift for the Study of Scleroderma, the South Carolina State Appropriation for Research, the National Institutes of Health (Grant AM 18904), the R.G.K. Foundation Gift for the Study of Scleroderma, a grant from the Arthritis Foundation, Inc., New York Chapter, and the Grace J. Pezrow Grant for the Study of Raynaud's Syndrome. Requests for reprints should be addressed to Dr. H. R. Maricq, Division of Rheumatology and Immunology, Department of Medicine, Medical University of South Carolina, 80 Barre Street, Charleston, South Carolina 29401. Manuscript accepted March 26, 1976.

been reported by a number of investigators [8–18]; principal findings have consisted of marked dilatation of certain capillary loops. Attempts to distinguish between Raynaud's "disease" and scleroderma on the basis of capillary findings have not been conclusive, and the capillary abnormalities have not before been correlated with organ involvement.

By using widefield examination and evaluating patterns of microvascular abnormalities in several areas of finger skin rather than elementary capillary lesions in a limited area of nailfold, a characteristic and similar pattern of capillary abnormalities has been observed in scleroderma, dermatomyositis and Raynaud's syndrome which is distinct from patterns seen in systemic lupus erythematosus and rheumatoid arthritis [19–21]. The connection between small artery and arteriolar lesions observed histopathologically in internal organs, and the capillary abnormalities seen with in vivo capillaroscopic methods in the skin is not known. A correlation between visceral involvement in scleroderma-Raynaud's syndrome-dermatomyositis and the extent of finger capillary abnormalities would establish a link between the arterial and capillary abnormalities and suggest a common or related pathogenesis.

For these reasons the widefield nailfold capillary patterns of all patients with scleroderma-Raynaud's syndrome-dermatomyositis referred to a rheumatic disease clinic were studied and compared with three selected control groups to determine (1) the specificity of the abnormal capillary pattern for scleroderma-Raynaud's syndrome-dermatomyositis and (2) the relationship of the severity of capillary abnormalities to the severity of the clinical syndrome. The distinctive capillary pattern was found to be specific for scleroderma-Raynaud's syndrome-dermatomyositis and a positive correlation was found between the severity of the capillary changes and the clinical syndrome, as determined by the number of discrete organ systems involved.

TABLE I Study Group: Clinical Criteria

System	Criteria of Involvement*
Peripheral vascular	1. Presence of Raynaud's phenomenon documented by a physician other than capillary observer
Cutaneous	1. Typical symmetrical skin changes (hidebound dermis, atrophic epidermis with loss of appendages)
	2. Sclerodactyly on physical examination by physician observer
	3. Skin biopsy specimen consistent with scleroderma
Gastrointestinal	1. Decreased esophageal motility on x-ray series of upper gastrointestinal tract
	2. Widened duodenum on x-ray series of upper gastrointestinal tract
	3. Sacculations of colon on roentgenogram of lower gastrointestinal tract
Pulmonary	1. Bibasilar pulmonary markings on the roentgenogram of chest with no other underlying cause
	2. Abnormal diffusion capacity on pulmonary function tests
	3. Vital capacity <70 per cent predicted
Cardiac	1. Conduction defect on electrocardiogram
	2. Low voltage throughout on electrocardiogram
	3. Pericarditis
	4. Cardiomegaly
Muscular	1. Proximal muscle weakness by physician observer
	2. Creatine phosphokinase activity >50 IU/liter
	3. Electromyogram consistent with myositis
	4. Myositis on muscle biopsy
Renal	1. Recent onset (<6 mo) of increased blood pressure (diastolic >90 mm Hg)
	2. Elevated blood urea nitrogen and creatinine levels on >1 determination
	3. Abnormal urinalysis (>1+ proteinuria, >2 red blood cells, casts in sediment)

*A single criterion was considered positive in all systems except renal, in which two criteria were required.

PATIENTS AND METHODS

Study Patients. The study group consisted of all patients seen in the Edward Daniels Faulkner Arthritis Clinic during the 10 month period between July 1, 1973, and May 1, 1974, in whom the diagnosis of scleroderma, Raynaud's syndrome or dermatomyositis was either definite or tentative. A total of 50 patients was seen; of these, six were excluded (three with scleroderma, two with dermatomyositis, one with Raynaud's syndrome) because it was not possible to complete all examinations required. In the 44 study patients in whom complete and often repeated skin capillary observations were made, the eventual diagnosis was scleroderma in 28, Raynaud's syndrome in 13 and dermatomyositis in three. Subjects ranged in age from 20 to 71 years and consisted of 40 women (mean age 44.9 years) and four men (mean age 39.8 years).

The major criterion for the diagnosis of scleroderma was taut skin involving diffusely the fingers, hands, arms and, in some patients, the face and trunk as well.

Twenty-five of the 28 patients with scleroderma had diffuse scleroderma of the extremities and trunk. Three of the 28 had taut skin distal to the metacarpophalangeal joints only (sclerodactyly) and, on this basis, could qualify for the designation CREST syndrome (calcinosis, Raynaud's phenomenon, esophageal hypomotility, sclerodactyly and telangiectasia [22,23]). In all three of these patients, two organ systems other than skin were involved.

The diagnosis of Raynaud's syndrome was based on the observation by a physician of the characteristic biphasic vasomotor response (pallor or cyanosis during vasoconstriction and suffusion, erythema or edema during reactive vasodilatation) in a patient in whom clinical and laboratory evaluation did not support the diagnosis of rheumatoid arthritis, systemic lupus erythematosus, scleroderma or dermatomyositis, and in whom intravascular (cryoglobulin, cold agglutinin), mechanical (machine operators) and toxic (vinyl chloride) causes were not present.

The diagnosis of dermatomyositis was based on the presence of characteristic skin (dermatitis of face, trunk or hands and/or subcutaneous calcification) and muscle (criteria for myositis as specified in Table I) involvement. Although dermatitis was essential for the diagnosis of dermatomyositis, it was not included as an independent organ involvement in the data presented.

Patients in the study group were receiving a variety of symptomatic therapies. The wide variety prevented a systematic analysis of therapy. Previous observations have not suggested any specific therapy that might be correlated with capillary abnormalities of the type seen in scleroderma-Raynaud's syndrome-dermatomyositis.

Control Groups. Three separate groups of controls, each consisting of 20 subjects, were observed.

Group 1: Rheumatic controls consisted of five men (mean age 51.5 years) and 15 women (mean age 42.9 years) from the clinic, with the diagnosis of rheumatoid arthritis in nine patients, psoriatic arthritis in two patients, systemic lupus erythematosus in seven patients, Sjögren's syndrome in one patient and periarteritis nodosa in one patient. Three of the patients with systemic lupus erythematosus had skin involvement. No patient in this group had Raynaud's syndrome or sclerodactyly.

Group 2: Hospitalized control subjects consisted of 20 women from 17 to 77 years of age (mean age 46.7 years) who were hospitalized at the Columbia-Presbyterian Medical Center for other than rheumatic disease and who gave no history of inflammatory arthritis. Six were recovering from uneventful obstetrical deliveries; the remaining 14 were hospitalized for one of the following diseases: fever of unknown origin, cystitis, reticulum cell sarcoma, Hodgkin's disease, bullous pemphigoid, cancer of the breast, osteoarthritis of the spine, pyelonephritis, giardiasis, cancer of the stomach, peripheral neuropathy, macroglobulinemia, cerebellar ataxia and cerebral vascular accident.

Group 3: Healthy control subjects consisted of three men (mean age 36.3 years) and 17 women (mean age 43.5 years) who were nonhospitalized volunteers with no history of rheumatic complaints, dysphagia or Raynaud's phenomenon. Black patients were not studied because of the inability to visualize capillaries through deeply pigmented skin.

Technics. Each patient was examined by inspection for visible abnormalities of the hands and by widefield microscopy (12X) at six standard sites on each hand including the nailfold and the remainder of the dorsum of the distal phalanx, and the finger pad of the fourth finger; the nailfold-distal

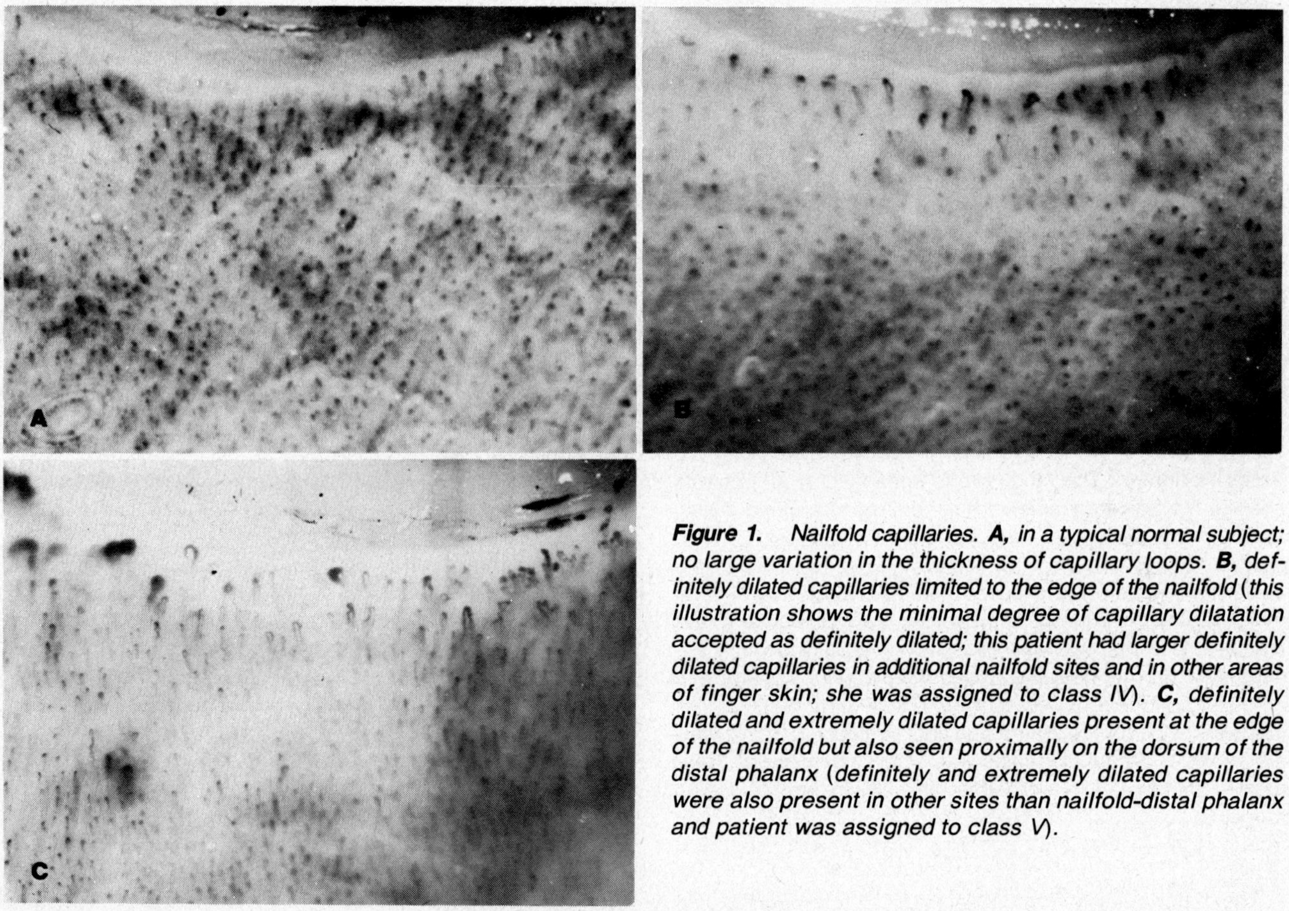

*Figure 1. Nailfold capillaries. **A**, in a typical normal subject; no large variation in the thickness of capillary loops. **B**, definitely dilated capillaries limited to the edge of the nailfold (this illustration shows the minimal degree of capillary dilatation accepted as definitely dilated; this patient had larger definitely dilated capillaries in additional nailfold sites and in other areas of finger skin; she was assigned to class IV). **C**, definitely dilated and extremely dilated capillaries present at the edge of the nailfold but also seen proximally on the dorsum of the distal phalanx (definitely and extremely dilated capillaries were also present in other sites than nailfold-distal phalanx and patient was assigned to class V).*

phalanx, the dorsum of the middle phalanx and the dorsal aspect of the middle joint of the third finger; and an area of dorsal skin 1.5 cm proximal to the fourth metacarpalphalangeal joint. Immersion oil was applied to each site prior to microscopic examination to aid in visualization of the vessels. A photographic record was made of each site examined on the left hand, using high speed Ektachrome film, a single lens reflex camera with macro lens and bellows, and a low voltage, low heat light source (to reduce local heat-induced vasodilatation) so that the results could be evaluated by a trained observer unaware of the patients' clinical status. Final magnification was between 3X and 4X on the negative. Technics were similar to those previously reported [19,20,24]. Four patients could not be fully photographed due to hand deformities secondary to scleroderma.

Observations made at each site examined included the presence or absence of dilated capillary loops, visible subpapillary plexus, relative loss of capillaries and dilated venules. These changes have previously been described in connective tissue disease [19,20]. Capillary loop size was designated normal, slightly dilated, definitely dilated (loop increased in size but loop form preserved), and extremely dilated (capillaries increased several times in size and capillary loops distorted). In addition, any areas that appeared visibly abnormal were observed microscopically; if abnormalities were seen, photographs were taken.

At the time of capillary examination, the following data were obtained from each patient: history and duration of Raynaud's phenomenon, stiffness and/or swelling of finger and wrist joints, muscle aches and weakness, dysphagia and dyspnea on exertion.

Clinical and Laboratory Evaluation. The following laboratory data, obtained from patients in the study group during the two months prior to study, were compiled: roentgenogram of the chest, pulmonary function studies, electrocardiogram, barium contrast roentgenographic study of upper and lower gastrointestinal tract, urinalysis, blood pressure, serum creatinine and blood urea nitrogen. Results of creatine phosphokinase activity, electromyogram and skin biopsy specimens obtained within the year before the examination were evaluated. Bibasilar pulmonary markings, decreased esophageal motility or widened duodenum, or colonic sacculations on roentgenographic examination at any previous time were considered positive.

Seven systems were evaluated in study patients from the clinical data. These included peripheral vascular, cutaneous, gastrointestinal, pulmonary, cardiac, muscular and renal, which were determined to be involved by the criteria listed in Table I. These criteria are similar in all respects to those proposed by Medsger et al. [4]. Data were adequate to determine system noninvolvement in 88 per cent; the remaining 12 per cent with missing data were randomly distributed with

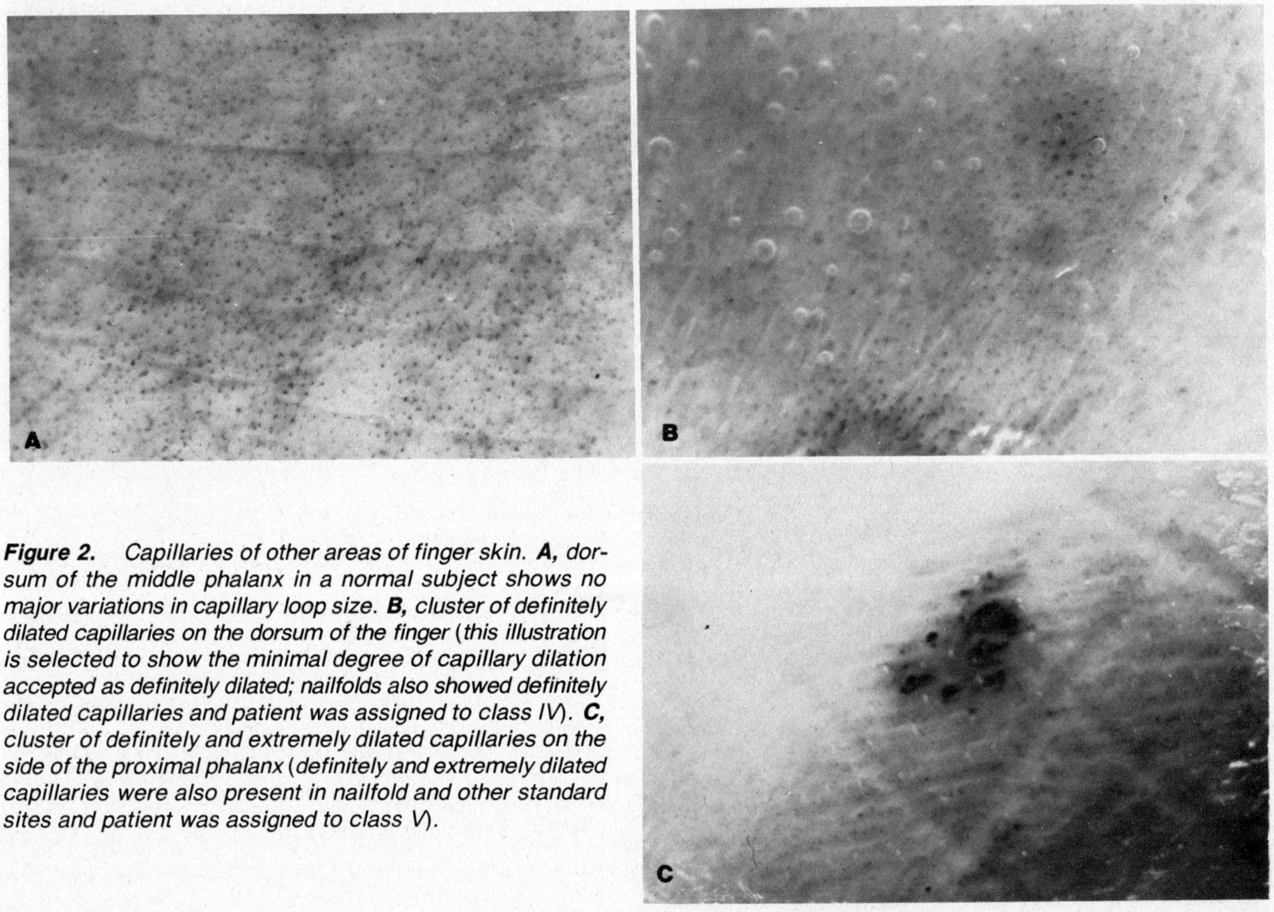

__Figure 2.__ Capillaries of other areas of finger skin. __A,__ dorsum of the middle phalanx in a normal subject shows no major variations in capillary loop size. __B,__ cluster of definitely dilated capillaries on the dorsum of the finger (this illustration is selected to show the minimal degree of capillary dilation accepted as definitely dilated; nailfolds also showed definitely dilated capillaries and patient was assigned to class IV). __C,__ cluster of definitely and extremely dilated capillaries on the side of the proximal phalanx (definitely and extremely dilated capillaries were also present in nailfold and other standard sites and patient was assigned to class V).

TABLE II Clinical Features and Capillary Class in the Study Group

Diagnosis	Total No. of Patients	Capillary Class	No. of Patients	Organs Involved Mean	Organs Involved Range	V*	Duration (yr) Mean	Duration (yr) Range
Raynaud's syndrome	13	I	6	1	1	0	7	<1 – 10
		II	6	2	1 – 3	3	8	<1 – 25
		IV	1	. . .	3	1	<1	. . .
Scleroderma	28	I	2†	. . .	2 and 5	1	<1	. . .
		II	1	. . .	2	0	>20	. . .
		III	3	4	3 – 4	3	. . .	<1 – 25
		IV	7	4	2 – 5	6	5	2 – 13
		V	15‡	4	3 – 7	15	9	<1 – 20
Dermatomyositis	3	III	1	. . .	2	1	<1	. . .
		IV	1 §	. . .	3	1	<1	. . .
		V	1	. . .	2	1	<1	. . .

* V = patients with visceral involvement (other than skin and vascular).
† Includes one patient who had five systems involved but had experienced no Raynaud's phenomenon.
‡ Includes three patients with CREST syndrome, duration three, eight and 20 years, organ involvlement three systems each; three patients without Raynaud's phenomenon.
§ Patient with Raynand's phenomenon.

respect to capillary class. No patient in the study group had inflammatory joint disease, and articular system involvement was not evaluated.

RESULTS

Study Group. The main finding in the study group was the presence of clusters of dilated capillary loops as described earlier [19,20]. These capillary findings were divided into the following five classes (Figures 1 and 2). Class I: Normal or slightly dilated capillary loops only. Class II: Definitely dilated loops confined to nailfold-distal phalanx. Class III: Extremely dilated loops confined to nailfold-distal phalanx. Class IV: Definitely dilated loops on nailfold-distal phalanx and definitely dilated loops found on at least one site other than nailfold-distal phalanx. Class V: Extremely dilated loops on nailfold-distal phalanx and extremely dilated or definitely dilated loops found at one site other than nailfold-distal phalanx.

The clinical features and the capillary class distri-

TABLE III System Involvement in Study Group

Class	No. of Patients	Peripheral Vascular	Cutaneous	Gastro-intestinal	Pulmo-nary	Cardiac	Muscular	Renal
I	8	8	2	1	1	1	. . .	. . .
II*	7	7	2	2	1	. . .	. . .	. . .
III†	4	3	3	2	2	1	2	. . .
IV‡	9	9	9	6	4	4	1	. . .
V §	16	13	14	11	11	7	2	2
Total	44	40	30	22	19	13	5	2
Per cent	100	91	68	50	43	30	11	7

(Columns Peripheral Vascular through Renal are under the heading "Involvement".)

*Three had only vascular involvement, one had vascular and cutaneous involvement, one had vascular plus gastrointestinal involvement, one had vascular and pulmonary, and a seventh had vascular, cutaneous and gastrointestinal involvement.
†One had dermatomyositis with pulmonary involvement, and the remaining three had scleroderma. Of these three, one had vascular, cutaneous and gastrointestinal involvement; one had vascular, cutaneous, gastrointestinal and muscular involvement; and one had vascular, cutaneous, cardiac and pulmonary involvement.
‡All patients had vascular and cutaneous involvement. In eight, more than these two systems were involved; three had gastrointestinal, pulmonary and cardiac involvement; one had gastrointestinal and pulmonary involvement; two had gastrointestinal involvement; and one each had cardiac or muscle involvement.
§Of these 16 patients, three denied any history of Raynaud's phenomenon. One patient had dermatomyositis with muscular and cardiac involvement. In seven patients three systems were involved: three had cutaneous, vascular and gastrointestinal involvement; two had cutaneous, vascular and pulmonary involvement; one had cutaneous, gastrointestinal and pulmonary involvement; and one had vascular, gastrointestinal and cardiac involvement. Five patients had four systems involved: three had cutaneous, vascular, gastrointestinal and pulmonary involvement; one had cutaneous, vascular, pulmonary and cardiac involvement; and one had cutaneous, gastrointestinal, pulmonary and cardiac involvement. Two patients had five systems involved: cutaneous, vascular, pulmonary, cardiac and either gastrointestinal or renal. One patient had all seven systems involved and died with malignant hypertension a week after examination. A second patient in this class with four systems involved died at another hospital with congestive heart failure, thought to be secondary to a viral infection of the respiratory tract, four months after examination.

bution among diagnostic subgroups of the 44 study patients are shown in Table II.

In the study group (Table III) 36 of 44 patients had abnormal capillary patterns (scleroderma = 26 of 28, Raynaud's syndrome = seven of 13, dermatomyositis = three of three). Furthermore, capillary class was correlated with organ involvement in the study patients (Figure 3 and Table IV). The details of patients with abnormal capillary patterns (classes II through V) are given in footnotes to Table III.

Eight study patients had class I capillary patterns (Table III). Of these eight, six had only vascular involvement, a seventh had vascular and cutaneous involvement, and the eighth had vascular, cutaneous, gastrointestinal, pulmonary and cardiac involvement, and died of malignant hypertension several months after examination, an exception to the study.

It was possible to reexamine 18 of the 44 study patients, eight with Raynaud's syndrome, nine with scleroderma and one with dermatomyositis. Follow-up observations performed nine to 22 months after the initial observations were not used in the data analyzed. Of the eight patients with Raynaud's syndrome, four showed no change in capillary class or in clinical condition. Two showed a decrease in capillary class (toward normal) with no obvious clinical change. One showed a change from class II to IV and, unfortunately, was lost to clinical evaluation. The eighth patient with Raynaud's syndrome had the most abnormal capillary findings (class IV) in the entire group with Raynaud's syndrome *and* these changed from class IV to V. In this patient pericarditis with effusion developed during the period of follow-up observation.

Of the nine patients with scleroderma, capillary class and clinical condition remained unchanged in seven. The eighth patient showed a change from class II to IV with no change in clinical condition over 21 months. The ninth patient showed a change from class V to class IV with no clinical change.

The single patient with dermatomyositis in whom repeated observations were made showed a change from class IV during active myositis to class II during a remission associated with therapy to class V during an exacerbation of her disease. Of the five patients of the study group who died during the study, class V capillary changes were observed in four (one dermatomyositis, three scleroderma) and class I capillary changes (scleroderma) in one, a previously mentioned exception to the study conclusion.

Control Groups. Group 1: Capillary findings in the rheumatic control group were in agreement with the pattern abnormalities reported previously [19,20]. Of the nine patients with rheumatoid arthritis, three showed prominent subpapillary plexus with normal vessel size in the nailfold. Four more of these revealed a plexus in

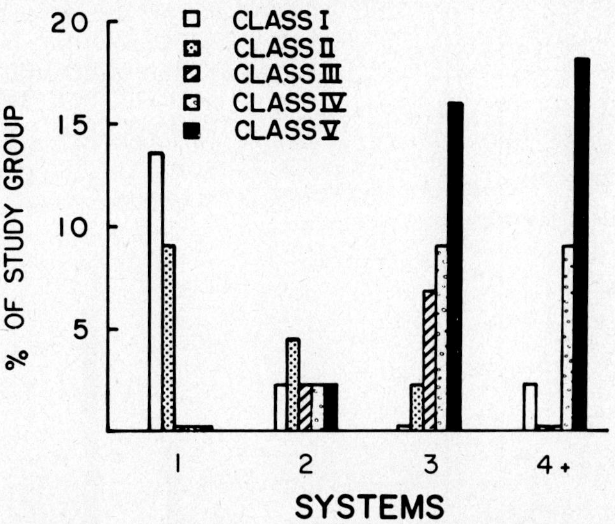

Figure 3. Correlation of capillary class and system involvement in scleroderma, Raynaud's syndrome and dermatomyositis.

the area of the dorsal skin proximal to the fourth metacarpal-phalangeal joint, a variation also seen in normal subjects. Two had no significant findings. One of the two patients with psoriatic arthritis had prominent subpapillary plexus, the second was normal. Three of seven patients with systemic lupus erythematosus showed characteristic punched-out, window lesions with loss of capillaries and prominence of subpapillary vessels in affected skin. The others showed no significant abnormalities. In one patient with Sjögren's syndrome only long, somewhat dilated loops were revealed but no visible plexus. In only one patient of this control group, a patient with periarteritis nodosa, were several unusual, large clusters of widely dilated capillary loops seen in numerous grossly visible telangiectatic spots on her hands, face and legs.

Group 2: In the hospitalized control group no markedly dilated loops were seen. Ten patients in this group had some visible subpapillary plexus in the nailfold, a nonspecific finding.

Group 3: Of the 20 healthy volunteers, one woman aged 59 had several definitely dilated loops and some loss of capillaries surrounding these in nailfold-distal phalanx

TABLE IV Correlation Between Capillary Class and System Involvement in the Study Group

No. of Systems Involved	Capillary Class			
	I–II	III–V	X^2*	P
1 or 2	13	3	21.72	<0.001
3 or more	2	26		

*With Yates correction.

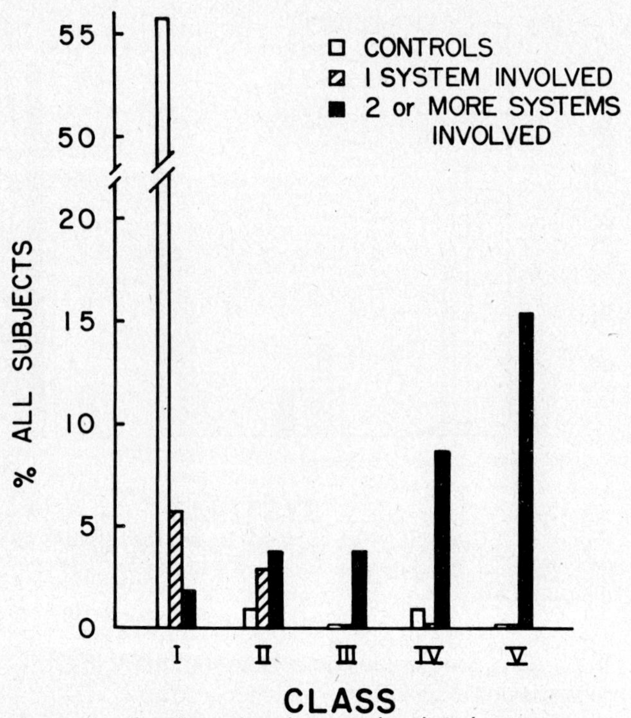

Figure 4. Capillary class in control and study groups.

TABLE V Comparison of Study Group and Control Subjects

Subjects	Capillary Class I	Capillary Class II–V	X²*	P
Study group	8	36	64.07	<0.001
Control groups	58	2		

*With Yates correction.

(class II). This patient was asymptomatic and no further evaluation was made. All other control subjects were normal, with three patients revealing subpapillary plexus in the nailfold.

Group Comparisons. Figure 3 illustrates the significant correlation between capillary class (defined herein) and number of systems involved (p <0.001, Table IV). The comparison of capillary findings between study group and control groups, shown in Figure 4 and Table V, disclosed a significant difference (p <0.001) in the prevalence of abnormal capillary patterns in these groups of subjects.

Since Raynaud's phenomenon and gastrointestinal involvement are the most frequently observed features in addition to the skin lesions in scleroderma, and since these three systems are so frequently involved together in these patients [25], the relationship between capillary abnormalities and system involvement was examined after excluding these three most commonly affected systems. Table VI demonstrates that the degree of capillary abnormality is closely associated with visceral involvement after skin, vascular and gastrointestinal involvement are excluded (p <0.001).

No relationship was found between capillary class and duration of illness (calculated from the onset of Raynaud's phenomenon and/or from the onset of skin involvement).

To remove possible observational bias, the relationship between capillary class and system involvement was also analyzed using data obtained from coded photographs. The results remained similar to the directly observed data, with p values <0.001. The correlation was high between capillary class assignments of subjects based on direct observations and those based on coded photographic data of the same subjects rated "blindly" by a different investigator (Spearman's rank correlation 0.91; p <0.0005).

TABLE VI Correlation Between Capillary Class and the Type of System Involvement

Capillary Class	Vascular, Cutaneous and/or Gastrointestinal Involvement Only (no. of patients)	Additional System Involvement* (no. of patients) 1	2	3	4	X²†	P
I	7	...	1	...	...		
II	6	1	...	...	...		
III	1	1	2	...	...	13.16	<0.001
IV	3	3	3	...	...		
V	3	7	4	1	1		

* In a total of 24 patients.

† X² between capillary classes I and II versus III, IV, V and the three common systems versus additional system involvement; with Yates correction.

COMMENTS

In the present study, patients with scleroderma, Raynaud's syndrome and dermatomyositis were considered as a single study group for the following reasons: (1) distinctive and similar skin capillary patterns had been previously observed in these disorders [19–21]; (2) the small artery lesion found in these three disorders is often indistinguishable; and (3) clinically there is an overlap, generally in the early stages, among these three disorders [1].

Concerning the second point, the small artery lesion in scleroderma has been well characterized in several viscera, especially the kidney [7], the lung [26] and, more recently, the heart [26,27]. Many classic studies of Raynaud's disease (i.e., Raynaud's phenomenon without connective tissue disease or other systemic diagnosis) have shown small artery changes similar to those seen in scleroderma [2]. More recently, patients with dermatomyositis have been shown to have small artery lesions similar to those in scleroderma [28]. Therefore, in the present investigation designed to study the association between the small artery (on the basis of organ involvement) and capillary lesions, these three overlapping disorders with similar small artery abnormalities were combined.

The results of this study confirm and extend our previous findings of characteristic microvascular abnormalities present in the finger skin of patients with scleroderma and dermatomyositis [19,20].

In addition, the results suggest that the abnormal microvascular patterns are not exclusively associated with local skin disease but reflect systemic involvement and can be seen in some patients in the absence of clinically observable skin disease. The data also suggest that capillary microscopy may be helpful for early recognition of scleroderma among subjects with Raynaud's syndrome. First, in the Raynaud's syndrome group, all subjects with involvement other than skin and vascular system had abnormal capillaries of class II or higher. Furthermore, in the patient with the highest capillary class, pericarditis and other features suggestive of scleroderma developed at follow-up, and her capillary class increased from IV to V. Secondly, in contrast, all six patients with Raynaud's phenomenon alone had class I capillaries. Follow-up examinations which were carried out in two of the six showed no change in capillary class or clinical condition. These individual observations warrant a systematic study of a larger group of patients to determine the diagnostic and prognostic role of widefield capillary observations.

Earlier workers have already suggested examination of nailfold capillaries as a useful tool [29,30], but technical problems with quantitation and photography have discouraged the use of clinical capillaroscopy. It has also been difficult to make serial observations of exactly the same area.

Current clinical practice in detecting organ involvement in Raynaud's syndrome and scleroderma consists of either the study of symptoms with standard physical and laboratory examinations or the elaborate, invasive and occasionally harmful exploration of subtle organ involvement by investigative technics. Repeated use of these investigative technics is not feasible for ethical, economic and personal reasons, unless of course new clinical features justify such procedures. Widefield capillary microscopy, on the other hand, is an inexpensive and noninvasive test which can be repeated at any desired interval. The present use of widefield microscopy and photomicrography permits ready site relocation and capillary pattern detection.

The close association between the degree of nailfold capillary abnormality and organ involvement in scleroderma is strong support for a generalized vascular pathogenesis for this disorder, as well as confirmation that the capillary abnormalities are a direct mirror of this generalized vascular derangement. Independent lines of investigation have delineated a capacity of scleroderma tissue cells to synthesize connective tissue elements, especially collagen, in increased amounts [31]. The connection between the microvascular and the biosynthetic abnormalities is uncertain. Two hypotheses could be considered: one would assume that a local primary lesion occurs at the endothelial level (which may itself be secondary to a blood-borne agent) which, in turn (together with other factors), leads to an activated state of fibroblast function. The second would ascribe a primary role to the activated fibroblast state and would attempt to understand the microvascular alterations as secondary to a generalized mesenchymal cell defect.

ACKNOWLEDGMENT

We gratefully acknowledge the technical assistance of Mrs. Karen Menth.

REFERENCES

1. Campbell PM, LeRoy EC: Pathogenesis of systemic sclerosis: a vascular hypothesis. Sem Arthritis Rheum 4: 351, 1975.
2. Rodnan G: Progressive systemic sclerosis (scleroderma), and calcinosis, chap 54. Arthritis and Allied Conditions (Hollander JL, McCarty DJ, eds), Philadelphia, Lea & Febiger, 1972.
3. Bennett R, Bluestone R, Holt PJL, et al.: Survival in scleroderma. Ann Rheum Dis 30: 581, 1971.
4. Medsger TA, Masi AT, Rodnan GP, et al.: Survival with systemic sclerosis (scleroderma). Ann Intern Med 75: 369, 1971.

5. Medsger TA, Masi AT: Survival with scleroderma. II. A lifetable analysis of clincal and demographic factors in 358 male U.S. veteran patients. J Chronic Dis 26: 647, 1973.
6. Norton WL, Nardo JM: Vascular disease in progressive systemic sclerosis. Ann Intern Med 73: 317, 1970.
7. Cannon PJ, Hassar M, Case DB, et al.: The relationship of hypertension and renal failure in scleroderma (progressive systemic sclerosis) to structural and functional abnormalities of the renal cortical circulation. Medicine (Baltimore) 53: 1, 1974.
8. Müller O: Die Kapillaren der menschlichen Körperoberfläche in gesunden und kranken Tagen. Stuttgart, Ferdinand Enke, 1922.
9. Illig L: Die terminale Strombahn. Capillarbett und Mikrozirkulation, Berlin-Göttingen, Springer-Verlag, 1961, p. 362.
10. Davis E, Landau J: Clinical Capillary Microscopy. Springfield, Charles C Thomas, 1966.
11. Brown GE: The skin capillaries in Raynaud's disease. Arch Intern Med 35: 56, 1925.
12. Brown GE, O'Leary PA: Skin capillaries in scleroderma. Arch Intern Med 36: 73, 1926.
13. Gilje O, Kierland R, Baldes EJ: Capillary microscopy in the diagnosis of dermatologic diseases. J Invest Dermatol 22: 199, 1954.
14. Kawashima Y: Capillary microscopic examination in collagen disease. Jap J Dermatol (B) 76: 24, 1966.
15. Buchanan IS, Humpston DJ: Nail-fold capillaries in connective tissue disorders. Lancet 1: 845, 1968.
16. Redisch W, Messina EJ, Hughes G, et al.: Capillaroscopic observations in rheumatic diseases. Ann Rheum Dis 29: 244, 1970.
17. Rouen LR, Terry EN, Doft BH, et al.: Classification and measurement of surface microvessels in man. Microvasc Res 4: 285, 1972.
18. Jablonska S, Bubnow B, Szczepanski A: Diffuse scleroderma and Raynaud's disease. Br J Dermatol 74: 174, 1962.
19. Maricq HR, Blume RS, LeRoy EC: Wide-field study of nailfold capillary bed in disorders of connective tissue. 6th European Conference on Microcirculation, Basel, S. Karger, 1971, p 116.
20. Maricq HR, LeRoy EC: Patterns of finger capillary abnormalities in connective tissue disease by "wide-field" microscopy. Arthritis Rheum 16: 619, 1973.
21. Maricq HR: Unpublished observations.
22. Winterbauer RH: Multiple telangiectasia, Raynaud's phenomenon, sclerodactyly and subcutaneous calcinosis: a syndrome mimicking hereditary hemorrhagic telangiectasia. Bull Johns Hopkins Hosp 114: 361, 1964.
23. Rodnan GP, Medsger TA, Buckingham RB: Progressive systemic sclerosis—CREST syndrome: observations on natural history and late complications in 90 patients. Arthritis Rheum 18: 423, 1975.
24. Maricq HR: "Wide-field" photography of nailfold capillary bed and a scale of plexus visualization scores (PVS). Microvasc Res 2: 335, 1970.
25. Stevens MB, Hookman P, Siegel CI, et al.: Aperistalsis of the esophagus in patients with connective-tissue disorders and Raynaud's phenomenon. N Engl J Med 270: 1218, 1964.
26. Sackner MA, Akgun N, Kimbel P, et al.: The pathophysiology of scleroderma involving the heart and respiratory system. Ann Intern Med 60: 611, 1964.
27. James TN: Coronary arteries and conduction system in scleroderma heart disease. Circulation 50: 844, 1974.
28. Banker BQ, Victor M: Dermatomyositis (systemic angiopathy) of childhood. Medicine (Baltimore) 45: 261, 1966.
29. Ross JB: Nail fold capillaroscopy—a useful aid in the diagnosis of collagen vascular diseases. J Invest Dermatol 47: 282, 1966.
30. Gilje O: Capillary microscopy in the differential diagnosis of skin diseases. Acta Derm Venereol 33: 303, 1953.
31. LeRoy EC: Increased collagen synthesis by scleroderma skin fibroblasts in vitro. A possible defect in the regulation or activation of the scleroderma fibroblast. J Clin Invest 54: 880, 1974.

Benign Hepatic Tumors and Oral Contraceptive Pills

TEJINDER M. S. KALRA, M.D.*
JAGDISH C. MANGLA, M.D.
ELISE W. DePAPP, M.D.
Rochester, New York

In order to consider possible environmental factors related to the development of benign hepatic tumors, all reports of this disorder in the case records of five different hospitals in Rochester, New York, during the past 10 years were reviewed. Seven patients with benign hepatic tumors of the liver and two with peliosis hepatis were identified. Among the seven with a benign hepatic tumor, four were women currently receiving oral contraceptives; one had been receiving this medication in the past, and two had no history of exposure to any steroid whatsoever. The two patients with peliosis hepatis were receiving long-term androgenic anabolic steroids. Dilated, thin-walled vessels and vascular spaces were a more prominent feature of the tumor seen in four patients receiving oral contraceptive pills. It is emphasized in this report that benign hepatic tumors do occur in men and in patients with cirrhotic liver without the use of any kind of steroids.

Hepatic adenomas, hamartomas or benign liver cell tumors were considered rare disorders. Warvi [1] reviewed 67 cases of benign hepatomas reported up until 1944 and found that in most of these cases the patients actually had multiple regenerative nodules in cirrhotic livers. Henson et al. [2] encountered only four cases of benign hepatomas at the Mayo Clinic between 1907 and 1954. Baum et al. [3] discovered only three cases of hepatic adenoma among the records kept since 1913 at St. Joseph Mercy Hospital in Ann Arbor, Michigan. Other reports [4,5] further confirm the rarity of this tumor. Since October 1973, however, 26 cases of benign liver cell tumors or hamartomas, including both adenomas and focal nodular hyperplasias, had been reported in women, 24 of whom were receiving oral contraceptive pills [3,4,6–14]. These reports call attention to a possible association, but in no way establish a definite cause and effect relationship between these hepatic tumors and oral contraceptives.

We have reviewed all cases of benign liver cell tumors seen during the past 10 years (1964 to 1974) at five hospitals in Rochester, New York, in order to determine whether we could detect any relationship between these tumors and the ingestion of oral contraceptive pills or other related steroids. We encountered and describe in this report seven patients with benign hepatic tumors of the liver and two patients with peliosis hepatis.

From the Department of Gastroenterology, Monroe Community Hospital, Rochester, New York 14603; and the University of Rochester Medical Center, Department of Pathology, Rochester, New York 14642. Requests for reprints should be addressed to Dr. Tejinder M. S. Kalra. Manuscript accepted March 30, 1976.

*Present address: St. Mary's Hospital, 89 Genesee Street, Rochester, New York 14611.

TABLE I Case Summaries

Case No.	Age (yr) and Sex	Steroid History	Clinical Presentation	Findings	Pathology	Treatment and Results
				Group A		
1	33,F	Enovid 2 yr, Ovulen 6 yr	Sudden pain, shock and signs of intraperitoneal bleeding	At laparotomy 8 cm tumor in left lobe, ruptured and bleeding into peritoneum	Benign hepatic adenoma	Left hepatectomy, well after 18 mo
2	29,F	Orthonovum 10 yr	Sudden pain in right upper quadrant, radiating to right shoulder, palpable mass in relation to right side of enlarged liver	At laparotomy 15 cm tumor in right lobe with a large subcapsular hematoma	Similar to that in Case 1	Evacuation of hematoma, right hepatectomy, well 30 mo
3	38,F	Enovid 5 yr	Elective abdominal hysterectomy	At laparotomy 3 cm tumor near triangular ligament on interior surface	Focal nodular hyperplasia	Excisional biopsy of tumor, well 24 mo
4	40,F	Birth control pills for 3 yr, name not known	Cerebrovascular accident, subarachnoid hemorrhage	At autopsy, in addition to ruptured berry aneurysm, a 2 cm tumor in right lobe of liver	Focal nodular hyperplasia	Died of cerebrovascular accident
				Group B		
5	40,F	Birth control pills for 1 yr, 9 yr ago	Recurrent episodes of cholecystitis	On laparotomy incidentally a 3 cm size nodule on liver	Focal nodular hyperplasia	Doing well
				Group C		
6	77,F	None	Portal hypertension, diabetes; liver scan: a big filling defect in middle of liver	Hepatic arteriogram quite suggestive of adenoma; at autopsy a 8 cm well encapsulated adenoma in left lobe of liver	Hepatic adenoma	Died of hepatic failure
7	42,M	None	Fever of unknown origin for 1 yr, extensive work-up and investigations—no obvious cause	On laparotomy a 5 cm size nodule on surface of liver	Focal nodular hyperplasia	No recurrence of fever since resection of tumor 8 mo before
				Group D		
8	64,M	Fluoxymesterone 2 mo (40 mg/day), oxymethalone 8 mo (140 mg/day), prednisone 1 mo (40 mg/day)	Aplastic anemia, recurrent infections, preterminal androgen refractory anemia	At autopsy, in addition to generalized plasmacytosis, pneumonia and pulmonary aspergillosis, there were 1 to 2 mm multiple blood-filled cysts in liver, also in spleen and kidney	Peliosis hepatis	Died of primary disease and its complications
9	8,M	Fluoxymesterone 20 to 40 mg/day, 4 yr; oxymethalone 100 mg/day, 1 mo; fluoxymesterone 30 mg/day, 1 yr; testosterone 15 mg/day, 2 mo; prednisone 10 to 20 mg/day for 4 yr	Aplastic anemia at age 3½	At autopsy liver studded with 4 to 7 mm blood-filled sinuses	Peliosis hepatis	Died of primary disease and its complications

MATERIALS AND METHODS

The benign tumors and tumor-like hepatic lesions considered here are of three different histopathologic types. Two of the lesions present as discrete, circumscribed liver nodules or masses; these include hepatic adenoma and focal nodular hyperplasia. The latter is a well circumscribed, sometimes encapsulated, multinodular, cirrhotic-like mass, with a distinctive histology in an otherwise normal liver: small, proliferating bile ducts and lymphocytic infiltration are common within the fibrous septums [15]. These lesions have also been referred to as abnormal liver cell hyperplasia with peliosis, benign hepatoma or hepatic cell adenoma with peliosis. The third type of lesion, peliosis hepatis, involves the liver more diffusely as multiple blood-filled spaces, sinuses or cysts. Utilizing the International coding system [16] and standard nomenclature [17] for search of benign tumors of hepatocytic origin, case records of 122 patients from five different hospitals in Rochester, New York, were scrutinized. Three cases of hepatic adenoma, four of focal nodular hyperplasia and three of peliosis hepatis were found. In two of three cases of peliosis hepatis the patients were receiving long-term androgenic anabolic steroids; these cases are reported in this study for the purposes of comparison with the other two types of lesions.

CASE REPORTS

The description of these cases (summarized in Table I) is divided into four groups: Group A: Cases in which there was a history of oral contraceptive intake (Cases 1–4). Group B: Indeterminate group—one case (Case 5) in which there was history of use of oral contraceptive pills many years ago. Group C: Cases of benign hepatic tumor in which there was no history of intake of any kind of steroid (Cases 6 and 7). Group D: Cases of peliosis hepatis related to androgenic anabolic steroids (Cases 8 and 9).

Group A

Case 1. A 33 year old white woman, mother of two, had been taking birth control pills for eight years (Enovid® for two years, Ovulen® for six years). She had been in good health until the day of admission. She had a sudden onset of severe abdominal pain about half an hour after eating a meal. She was brought to the Emergency Department of Strong Memorial Hospital where she was found to be in shock. On examination, she was found to be acutely ill, pale, cold and clammy. Her heart rate was 110/min, temperature 99°F. A chest examination did not reveal any abnormality. Her abdomen revealed diffuse tenderness and guarding. A plain film of the abdomen was within normal limits. There was no evidence of free air. The hematocrit value was 33 per cent. A complete blood count, chest film, SMA 12, electrolytes and serum amylase values were within normal limits. She was given multiple blood transfusions and an emergency exploratory laparotomy was performed. There was a large tumor, about 8 cm in diameter, in the left lobe of the liver, which had ruptured and was bleeding into the peritoneal cavity. The left lobe of the liver was resected. The patient is doing well after one and a half years of follow up. Microscopically, the tumor consisted of a benign hepatic adenoma with striking dilatation and prominence of the vascular spaces (Figure 1).

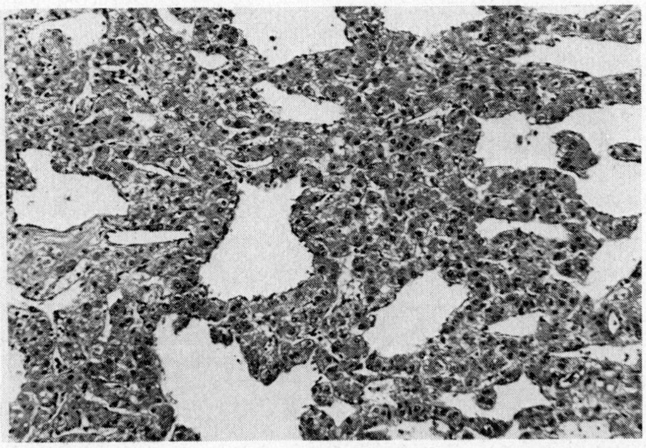

Figure 1. *Case 1. Hepatic adenoma with markedly ectatic sinusoidal vascular spaces. Hematoxylin and eosin stain; original magnification × 40, reduced by 50 per cent.*

Case 2. This 29 year old separated, white woman was admitted to Rochester General Hospital with a sudden onset of acute pain in the upper right abdominal quadrant and epigastrium. The pain was persistent with occasional radiation to the right shoulder. She had been taking birth control pills (Ortho-Novum®) for the last 10 years. She was pale and diaphoretic, with a blood pressure of 140/80 mm Hg. There was tenderness in the epigastric region and a mass in relation to the liver (occupying the entire right side of the abdomen) was felt. Peristaltic sounds were hypoactive. A plain film of the abdomen was within normal limits, along with a complete blood count, blood urea nitrogen and electrolytes. On exploratory laparotomy, the liver was enlarged down to the iliac crest. There was a soft rounded tumor about 15 cm in diameter in relation to the right lobe of the liver. The surface of the liver was covered with large vessels. There was a large

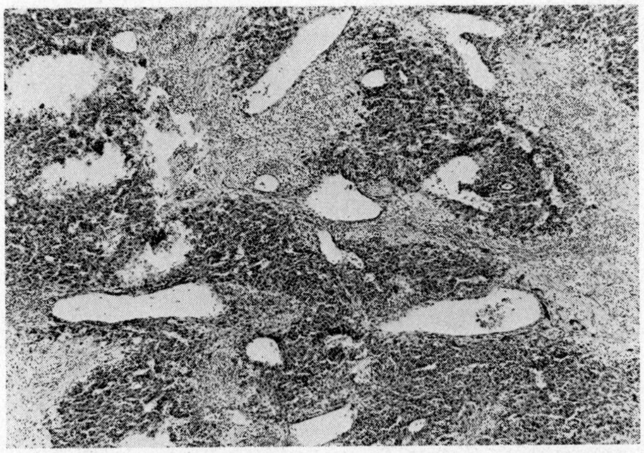

Figure 2. *Case 2. Dilated vascular spaces in hepatic adenoma suggestive of "peliosis," and fibromyxoid proliferation adjacent to many vessels. Hematoxylin and eosin stain; original magnification × 10, reduced by 50 per cent.*

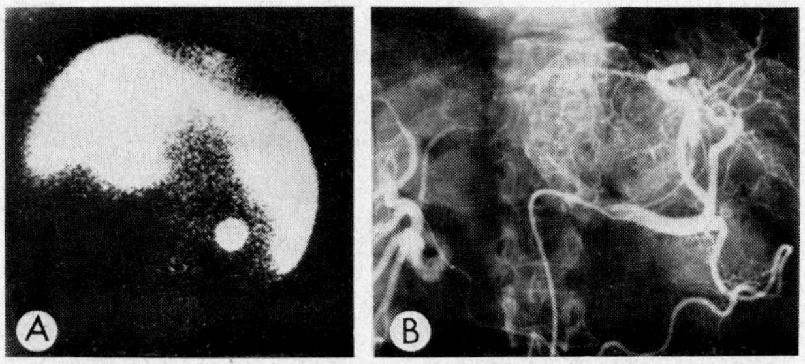

Figure 3. *Case 6.* ***A,*** *liver scan with technetium 99 shows filling defect in the left lobe of the liver.* ***B,*** *hepatic arteriogram (arterial phase)—hepatic adenoma.*

area of subcapsular hematoma. The tumor was confined and fairly well circumscribed. This was resected with a blunt dissection. The subcapsular hematoma was evacuated. She is well after two and a half years of follow up. Microscopic examination of the tumor revealed liver cell adenoma with features generally similar to those described in the first case (Figure 2).

Case 3. A 38 year old white woman, mother of three, was 18 weeks pregnant. She was admitted for elective hysterectomy and permanent sterilization for induced abortion and unwanted, accidental pregnancy. She had been taking oral contraceptive pills (Enovid) for the last five years and stopped taking them a few months before pregnancy. On laparotomy, a firm nodule measuring 3 cm in diameter was resected from the inferior lateral border near the triangular ligament of the liver. On microscopic examination, it had the features of focal nodular hyperplasia. Postoperatively the patient did quite well.

Case 4. A 40 year old white woman was brought to the Emergency Department with severe headache. She went into a coma, decerebrate rigidity developed, and she died within a few hours. A diagnosis of subarachnoid hemorrhage was made. On postmortem examination she was found to have a ruptured berry aneurysm of the right middle cerebral artery with massive subarachnoid hemorrhage and subdural extension on the right side. In addition, examination of the liver showed the presence of a subcapsular, well circumscribed nodule 2 cm in diameter on the anterior aspect of the right lobe. The histologic features of the lesion were those of focal nodular hyperplasia. Retrospectively, enquiring from the husband of the deceased, it was found that she had been taking birth control pills for about three years regularly prior to her death.

Group B

Case 5. A 40 year old white woman had recurrent episodes of symptoms suggestive of acute cholecystitis in the past year. The gallbladder did not visualize on oral cholecystography. She was operated on and had a cholecystectomy. A 2 to 3 cm in diameter well circumscribed nodule on the anterior surface of the liver was found during surgery. This tumor was excised, and microscopic examination revealed the features of focal nodular hyperplasia. This patient had taken oral contraceptive pills for one year, nine years ago.

Group C

Case 6. A 77 year old white woman was admitted to Monroe Community Hospital with multiple medical problems including atherosclerotic heart disease, congestive cardiac failure, diabetes mellitus, portal hypertension with ascites and recurrent hepatic encephalopathy. There was a questionable history of infective hepatitis three years prior to this admission. Her protein intake was restricted, and she was given neomycin therapy to avoid hepatic encephalopathic features. There was no history of alcohol ingestion. On physical examination, there was edema over the feet. The liver was slightly enlarged and felt hard in the epigastric region. The spleen was palpable about 6 cm below the left costal margin. There was a moderate amount of ascites. A grade 2/6 systolic murmur was diffusely heard over the precordial region. Results of liver function tests were abnormal. Prothrombin time was 16.3 seconds (control 13 seconds), serum bilirubin 4.0 mg/100 ml, serum glutamic oxaloacetic transaminase (SGOT) 78 IU, serum glutamic pyruvic transaminase (SGPT) 84 IU, lactic dehydrogenase (LDH) 280 IU, albumin 2.5 g/100 ml, total proteins 6.26 g/100 ml. Liver biopsy on two previous occasions was nondiagnostic because of the inadequate sample. Esophageal varices were seen on the barium swallow. A technetium 99 liver scan revealed a big filling defect (Figure 3A) in the left lobe of the liver. A hepatic arteriogram to delineate the nature of the filling defect seen on the liver scan was performed. The findings were consistent with hepatic adenoma (Figure 3B). The patient's condition deteriorated and she finally died of hepatic encephalopathy. At autopsy, the liver was enlarged and cirrhotic. There was an 8 to 9 cm in diameter discrete, encapsulated mass in the left lobe of the liver (Figure 4). The microscopic examination of the tumor revealed features of encapsulated hepatic adenoma (Figure 5).

Case 7. A 41 year old man was being investigated for chronic febrile illness of one to two years' duration; with temperature elevations as high as 102°F, mostly in the afternoon hours. There were periods of diarrhea, with five to eight loose bowel motions a day. Physical examination disclosed no abnormalities. A wide range of blood tests, roentgenograms, scans, cultures of blood, urine and sputum including bone marrow for acid-fast bacilli and other microbes, biopsy of the liver, rectal biopsy and various skin tests for possible bacterial and fungal infections were normal. On exploratory laparotomy, a 5 cm in diameter nodule was seen on the surface of the liver. Excisional biopsy of the tumor revealed focal nodular hyperplasia (Figure 6). The cause of fever, however, could not be ascertained. The patient had remission of fever and it has not recurred since then.

Group D

Case 8. A 64 year old white man was diagnosed as having aplastic anemia in April 1968. He presented with a low grade fever, generalized malaise, widespread cutaneous petechiae and pneumonic consolidation of the right lung. Therapy with Halotestin® (fluoxymesterone), 40 mg daily, was started. He remained reasonably well with a hematocrit value in the low 30's. The administration of oxymetholone, 140 mg per day, was started in May 1970. In December 1970 he was read-

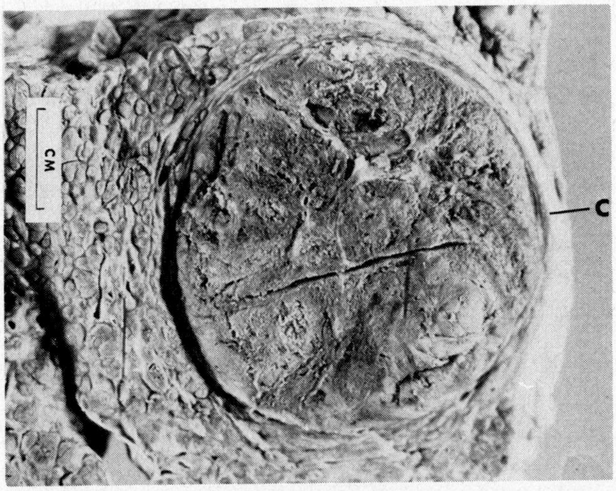

Figure 4. *Case 6. Well defined, encapsulated (C) hepatic adenoma in a cirrhotic liver.*

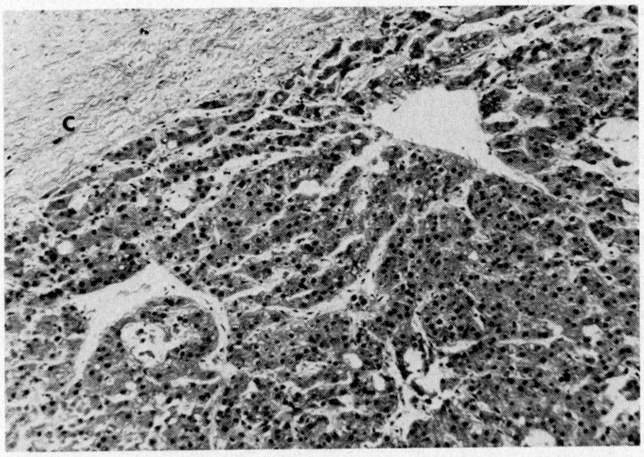

Figure 5. *Case 6. Encapsulated (C) hepatic adenoma (in cirrhotic liver) with some dilation of the vascular spaces. Hematoxylin and eosin stain; original magnification × 40, reduced by 50 per cent.*

mitted for re-evaluation of his androgen refractory aplastic anemia. He had a progressively downhill course and died. On postmortem examination there was evidence of generalized plasmacytosis, bilateral hemorrhagic pneumonia and right pulmonary aspergillosis. Examination of the liver revealed peliosis hepatis with multiple small, blood-filled cysts measuring 1 to 2 mm in their greatest diameter. Peliotic cavities were also seen in the spleen, bone marrow and kidney.

Case 9. This patient was an eight year old white boy in whom aplastic anemia was noted at age three and a half years, following complaints of easy bruising. In 1962 the pertinent data included a hemoglobin level of 3.7 g/100 ml, white blood cell count of 260/mm^3 with 86 per cent lymphocytes and 1,000 platelets. Bone marrow aspiration was markedly hypocellular. The administration of prednisone and fluoxymesterone was started and the patient was maintained with these drugs in varying doses until his death. He became and remained markedly masculinized. He also had frequent blood transfusions and numerous recurrent infections. He was admitted again as a result of fever and back pain following a fall. The patient experienced increasing abdominal pain and respiratory distress, and he died. At autopsy the liver was studded with rounded blood-filled cavities averaging 4 to 7 mm in diameter with characteristic features of peliosis hepatis on microscopic examination (Figure 7).

HISTOPATHOLOGY

In three cases (Cases 1, 2 and 6) the hepatic adenoma ranged in size from 8 to 15 cm in diameter. Each presented as a sharply circumscribed, encapsulated tumor mass. In Case 6, the adenoma was a light tan-grey in contrast to the surrounding reddish brown parenchyma (Figure 4); in this case the adenoma arose in a cirrhotic liver. In Cases 1 and 2, the remainder of the liver was

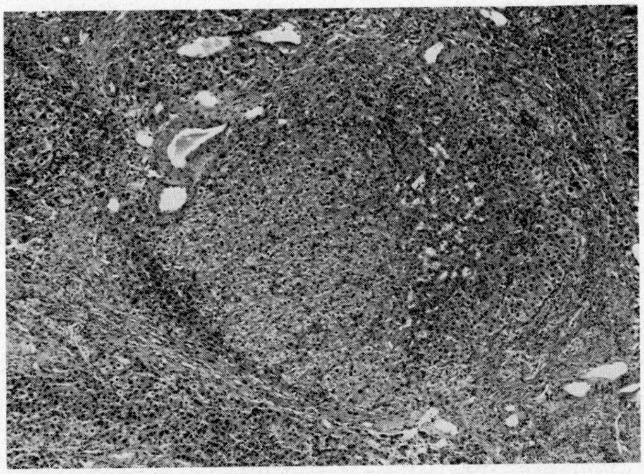

Figure 6. *Case 7. Focal nodular hyperplasia with lymphocytic infiltration of fibrous septums and parenchyma. Hematoxylin and eosin stain; original magnification × 10, reduced by 50 per cent.*

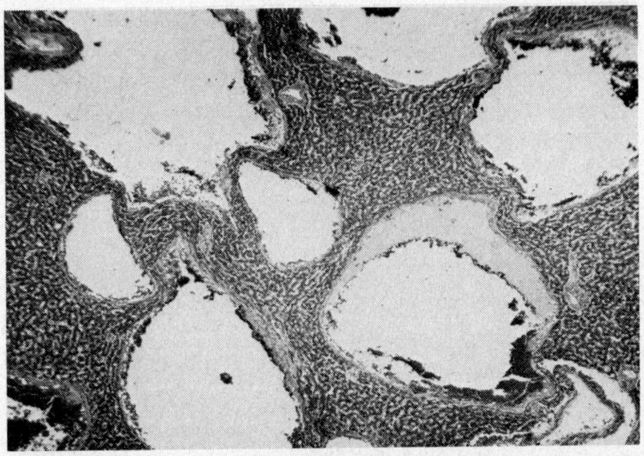

Figure 7. *Case 9. Peliosis hepatis. Hematoxylin and eosin stain; original magnification × 10, reduced by 50 per cent.*

normal. Microscopically, each adenoma was composed of sheets of normal appearing monomorphic hepatic parenchymal cells, with haphazardly arranged sinusoidal spaces. No portal triads or identifiable central veins were present in these tumors. Multiple sections revealed an intact capsule. Marked dilatation of varying sized endothelial-lined vascular spaces was prominent. In Case 2, in particular, there were many areas of loose fibromyxoid tissue in association with the large vascular spaces (Figure 2).

The four cases of focal nodular hyperplasia (Cases 3, 4, 5 and 7) were characterized grossly by sharply delineated, but not truly encapsulated, nodules varying in size from 3 to 5 cm in diameter. Microscopically, each lesion was composed of normal parenchyma cells divided into lobules by fibrous septums with varying degrees of lymphocytic infiltration. Bile duct proliferation was also present within the connective tissue component. Again, dilated, thin-walled vascular spaces were present throughout the lesion, both in the parenchyma and in the fibrous septums (Figure 6).

In general, vascularity and phlebectasia were more marked in tumors belonging to cases in group A.

In two cases (Cases 8 and 9) of peliosis hepatis, diffuse hepatomegaly was seen (Case 8, 2,500 g; Case 9, 2,440 g). On cross section, these livers had the typical spongy appearance of peliosis with numerous blood-filled cysts. Microscopically, many of the cysts had endothelial lining whereas others did not (Figure 7).

COMMENTS

In the last two years a number of cases of benign hepatic tumors have been reported [3,4,6–14]. With one exception [11], all the reports have stressed the role of oral contraceptives. This may give an undue importance to a possible increase in incidence of hepatic adenoma and an etiologic relationship to oral contraceptive pills. On the basis of present reports we cannot categorically accept or deny the previous claims, but we will make an attempt to give a balanced view.

The clinical presentation of the patients in the four cases of hepatic adenoma in group A (in which there is a definite history of oral contraceptive pill intake) is quite similar to those previously described [3,4,6–14] in the literature. One patient (Case 5) has been described in this report under a separate indeterminate group (group B) since she gave a history of the use of oral contraceptive pills for only one year and that had been nine years earlier. It would be conjectural to relate hepatic adenoma in that patient to the use of the pill. It may be postulated that the tumor was related to the use of the pill nine years ago and had persisted since then or gradually decreased in size if it had been larger to begin with.

Cases of peliosis hepatis in which the patient has a history of androgenic anabolic steroids are included in this report because of the close relationship between oral contraceptive pills and androgenic steroids chemically. It was also important to present a full spectrum of the pathologic findings in patients taking oral contraceptive pills with both peliosis hepatis and hepatic adenoma; patients taking androgenic steroids had only peliosis hepatis without hepatic adenoma.

There were two patients in group C in this report who were not receiving any kind of oral contraceptive pill or any other structurally similar steroids. In fact, one of the patients was a man (Case 7). The other was a woman with cirrhosis of the liver.

It is quite possible that some cases occurring in men or in women not receiving steroids may not be reported or published unless they manifest some "unusual, unexpected or exciting" clinical or pathologic features. Since the observation of oral contraceptive pills and benign hepatic tumors is relatively recent, it is also quite possible that in some patients with such lesions a history of oral contraceptive pills intake may not even be enquired from the patient. Recently a case of hepatic adenoma associated with diarrhea was reported in a young woman [11]; however, there is a complete omission of any history of oral contraceptive pills intake in that report.

Histologically the hepatic tumors described in this study are benign, well demarcated from the surrounding liver tissue. These are composed of cords or nodules of liver cells at places incompletely separated by fibrous trabeculae. Bile duct reduplication was prominent in cases described by O'Sullivan and Wilding [4], it was seen in all four cases of focal nodular hyperplasia in this study. All the tumors in the three groups (groups A, B and C) were vascular. The vascularity in group A, however, was quite striking. The dilated, thin-walled vessels and vascular spaces with or without endothelial lining constitute an important feature of the lesions in group A patients. This feature could be referred to as peliosis hepatis. Characteristic lesions of peliosis hepatis have been described in certain chronic debilitating conditions and in patients with aplastic anemia receiving long-term androgenic anabolic steroids [18]. In group D (Cases 8 and 9) in this report, two patients with that lesion are described. In group A patients, there were no gross cystic spaces on the external or cut surface of the liver, the suggestion of "peliosis" was only on microscopic examination of the tumor. One wonders if this common feature of "peliosis" could be linked to the basic structural resemblance of the oral contraceptive pills and the androgenic steroids. The only difference being in the spectrum of lesions from microscopic (as in group A) to grossly visible cystic spaces in liver (as in group D). There is one published report on regression of benign hepatic tumors after the stoppage of the pill [19]. Similar observations could serve as stronger evidence to incriminate the pill in the pathogenesis of hepatic neoplasia. Most of the direct evidence regarding the tumorogenic potential of oral contraceptive pills comes from animal studies in rats as it was shown [5,20] that large doses of mestranol produce liver damage and even hepatomas. Perez et al. [21] showed with electron microscopy that the liver cells of women taking the pill show hypertrophy of endoplasmic reticulum which may increase the carcinogenic potential [22–25] of many compounds.

The main aim of our report is to show that, despite such a large body of evidence to incriminate the pill, hepatic hamartomas, although rare, do occur in men (as in Case 7) and in cirrhotic liver (as in Case 6) even without a history of any steroid intake. The oral contraceptive pills, if at all associated with these lesions, is not the only cause.

ADDENDUM

Since the initial writing of this paper and submission for publication, more case reports have appeared in the literature [19,26].

REFERENCES

1. Warvi N: Primary neoplasms of the liver. Arch Pathol 37: 367, 1944.
2. Henson SW Jr, Gray HK, Dockerty MD: Benign tumors of the liver. Surg Gynecol Obstet 103: 23, 1956.
3. Baum JK, Bookstein JJ, Holtz F, et al.: Possible association between benign hepatomas and oral contraceptives. Lancet 2: 926, 1973.
4. O'Sullivan JP, Wilding RP: Liver hamartomas in patients on oral contraceptives. Br Med J 3: 7, 1974.
5. Cahal DA: Assessment of safety of drugs. Br Med J 1: 854, 1966.
6. Contostavlos DL: Benign hepatomas and oral contraceptives (Letter). Lancet 2: 1200, 1973.
7. Knapp WA, Ruebner BH: Hepatomas and oral contraceptives. Lancet 1: 270, 1974.
8. Kelso DR: Benign hepatomas and oral contraceptives (Letter). Lancet 1: 315, 1974.
9. Horvath E, Kovacs K, Ross RC: Benign hepatoma in young women on contraceptive steroids (Letter). Lancet 1: 357, 1974.
10. Antoniades K, Brooks CE: Hemoperitoneum from liver cell adenoma in a patient on oral contraceptives. Surgery 77: 137, 1975.
11. Minow RA, Tompkins RK, Gritnick GL: Diarrhea syndrome in hepatic adenoma. Am J Digest Dis 20: 182, 1975.
12. Mays ET, Christopherson WM, Barrows GH: Focal nodular hyperplasia of the liver. Possible relationship to oral contraceptives. Am J Clin Pathol 61: 735, 1974.
13. Stauffer JQ, Lapinski MW, Hanold DJ, et al.: Focal nodular hyperplasia of the liver and intrahepatic hemorrhage in young women on oral contraceptives. Ann Intern Med 83: 301, 1975.
14. Berg JW, Ketelaar RJ, Rose EF, et al.: Hepatomas and oral contraceptives (Letter). Lancet 2: 349, 1974.
15. Edmondson HA: Tumors of the liver and intrahepatic bile ducts. Atlas of Tumor Pathology, fasc 25, Washington, D.C., Armed Forces Institute of Pathology, 1958, p 193.
16. International classification of diseases, adapted. Public Health Service publication no. 1963, Dec. 1968, 8th Rev.
17. Standard Nomenclature of Diseases and Operations, issued by AMA, New York, McGraw-Hill, 5th ed, 1961.
18. Bagheri SA, Boyer JL: Peliosis hepatis associated with androgenic anabolic steroid therapy. A severe form of hepatic injury, Ann Intern Med 81: 610, 1974.
19. Ross D, Jorga P, Medo M, et al.: Regression of focal nodular hyperplasia after discontinuation of oral contraceptives. Ann Intern Med 85: 203, 1976.
20. Committee on Safety of Medicines: carcinogenicity tests of oral contraceptives. London, Her Majesty's Stationery Office, 1972.
21. Perez V, Gorosdisch S, De Martive J, et al.: Oral contraceptives: long term use produces fine structural changes in liver mitochondria. Science 165: 805, 1969.
22. Udenfriend S: Arene oxide intermediates in enzymatic hydroxylation and their significance with respect to drug toxicity. Ann NY Acad Sci 179: 295, 1971.
23. Lingeman CH: Liver-cell neoplasms and oral contraceptives. Lancet 1: 64, 1974.
24. Black NM, Leish P Jr: Mammary carcinogenesis. NY State J Med 72: 1601, 1972.
25. Herbst AI, Kurman RJ, Scully RE: Vaginal and surgical abnormalities after exposure to stilbestrol in utero. Obstet Gynecol 40: 287, 1972.
26. Edmondson HA, Henderson B, Benton B: Liver-cell adenomas associated with use of oral contraceptives. N Engl J Med 296: 470, 1976.

The Myeloproliferative Disorders

Correlation Between Clinical Evolution and Alterations of Granulopoiesis

PETER GREENBERG, M.D.*
BETH MARA, B.S.
INE BAX,
REMY BROSSEL, M.D.
Palo Alto, California

STANLEY SCHRIER, M.D.
Stanford, California

Patients with myeloproliferative disorders were prospectively studied by in vitro agar-gel marrow culture technics to evaluate factors involved in the evolution of abnormal granulopoiesis. Marrow granulocytic colony-forming capacity was determined in 78 patients with chronic myeloid leukemia, subacute myeloid leukemia, preleukemia, Di Guglielmo's syndrome, polycythemia vera or essential thrombocythemia. A wide range of marrow colony-forming capacity values was noted early in disease courses; however, in 26 of 33 patients decreased colony-forming capacity was associated with disease transformation into acute myeloid leukemia or other clinically aggressive stages. An increased proportion of abnormally light buoyant density ($<$1.062 g/cm^3) colony-forming cells was present in the marrow and peripheral blood of 15 of 16 patients with chronic myeloid leukemia, subacute myeloid leukemia, preleukemia or essential thrombocythemia; in seven of eight patients with $>$35 per cent abnormally light colony-forming cells their disease subsequently underwent transformation. Elevated levels of urinary colony-stimulating factor output were noted in 17 of 31 patients, and in 10 of 12 patients whose disease subsequently underwent acute transformation within 10 months of study. In six of seven patients who simultaneously had an increased urinary output of colony-stimulating factor and low colony-forming capacity in marrow, transformation occurred within 10 months. These findings indicate that progressive abnormalities of both marrow clonal growth patterns and levels of possible humoral regulatory substances develop during evolution of these diseases. In contrast, patients with idiopathic sideroblastic ineffective erythropoiesis had normal values for marrow colony-forming capacity, proportion of light density colony-forming cells and urinary colony-stimulating factor output, and in none has their disease transformed into acute myeloid leukemia. These in vitro studies appear useful for clinical staging, evaluating prognosis and categorizing patients with myeloproliferative disorders.

The myeloproliferative disorders provide a clinical setting for evaluating the evolution of abnormal granulopoiesis. Based on clinical and karyotypic data, several investigators have suggested that the myeloproliferative disorders result from either a growth disturbance of the multipotential hemopoietic stem cell [1–3] or of abnormalities of "myelostimulatory substances" [1,4]. The growth disturbance is manifested by excessive proliferation of mature cells of more than one committed hemopoietic cell line in the more chronic dis-

From the Department of Medicine, Veterans Administration Hospital, Palo Alto, California and Stanford University School of Medicine, Stanford, California. This study was supported by U.S. Public Health Service Research Grants CA13141 from the National Cancer Institute, RR70 General Clinical Research Centers, Division of Research Resources; American Cancer Society (California Division 577C-1); and Veterans Administration Research Funds. Requests for reprints should be addressed to Dr. Peter L. Greenberg, Veterans Administration Hospital, 3801 Miranda Avenue, Palo Alto, California 94304. Manuscript accepted May 25, 1976.

* Scholar of the Leukemia Society of America.

orders, with superimposed impairment in cellular maturation in the more acute forms [2]. The chronic myeloproliferative disorders have a propensity to undergo transformation into more acute and aggressive stages including a clinical state resembling acute myeloid leukemia.

In addition to kinetic and morphologic methods, human granulopoiesis can be further characterized by several newly introduced measurements of in vitro marrow cell growth. These measurements include evaluation of in vitro proliferation of marrow granulocytic progenitor cells to form granulocytic colonies in semi-solid agar, termed colony-forming capacity, the proportion of abnormally light buoyant density colony-forming cells, and humoral levels of the stimulus for in vitro granulopoiesis, colony-stimulating factor. Physiologic and clinical relevance of these indices have been suggested by prior studies [5–8]. Abnormalities of marrow colony-forming capacity have been reported in patients with acute myeloid leukemia and preleukemia [9–13]. Density gradient separation of marrow cells has indicated a distinctive abnormal light-density distribution pattern of colony-forming cells in patients with leukemia and certain myeloproliferative disorders [14]. Abnormal colony-stimulating factor levels have been found in serum and urine of patients with leukemia [15,16].

The purpose of this study was to evaluate these measurements of in vitro granulopoiesis in prospectively studied patients with myeloproliferative disorders, in order to determine whether these indices would provide a means for defining factors involved in the evolution of these diseases.

METHODS

Colony-Forming Capacity. Our technic for evaluating colony-forming capacity in human marrow has already been described [10,17]. Our normal values for marrow colony-forming capacity, obtained by evaluating 46 control subjects, are 14 to 44 colonies/10^5 marrow cells plated (26 $\pm$ 7.5, mean $\pm$ SD). Colonies are counted at 7 to 10 days of culture and are comprised of more than 50 cells at various stages of granulocytic differentiation (generally 150 to 1,500 cells). Clusters, or abortive colonies, consisting of aggregations of 3 to 50 cells, persisted in some of our patients.

Proportion of Abnormally Light Buoyant Density Colony-Forming Cells. The neutral density cell separation procedure used has previously been described [14]. Between 10^7 and 10^9 nucleated marrow cells were suspended in 5 ml of bovine serum albumin (pH 5.1, density 1.062 g/cm^3, 269 mosmol), layered over 2 ml of cell-free albumin of the same density, and 2 ml of unbuffered salt solution (269 mosmol) was layered over the albumin. After centrifugation at 4,000 $\times$ g for 10 minutes at 4°C the light-density ($<$1.062 g/cm^3) cell fraction and the cell pellet were recovered, washed with modified McCoy's tissue culture medium and cultured for colony-forming capacity. In marrow samples from nine normal subjects, 2.8 $\pm$ 2.6 per cent (mean $\pm$ SD) of the granulocytic colony-forming cells were of buoyant density $<$1.062 g/cm^3 (range 0.1 to 7.4 per cent).

Urinary Colony-Stimulating Factor Output. Our method of processing urine for quantitating colony-stimulating factor output essentially free of inhibitory substances has previously been described [18]. Our values for daily urinary colony-stimulating factor output in 12 normal persons 22 to 63 years old are 68,000 $\pm$ 21,000 units (mean $\pm$ SD) (range 36,000 to 97,000 units), and for eight persons 66 to 87 years old, 135,000 $\pm$ 83,000 units (31,000 to 255,000 units). This age-related increase in colony-stimulating factor excretion has been reported by other workers [19]. A unit of colony-stimulating factor has been defined as that amount necessary for stimulating the formation of one colony in vitro.

Statistical analyses have been performed utilizing the Wilcoxon two sample rank test and, when indicated, the chi-square test with Yates correction. Abnormal values of individual colony-forming capacity and colony-stimulating factor levels are considered to be those beyond $\pm$ 2 SD of the mean values for control subjects.

PATIENT SELECTION

Between April 1970 and August 1975 we evaluated 82 patients with myeloproliferative disorders (marrow colony-forming capacity values were determined in 78). All patients, or their records, were available for follow-up evaluation. In this period the disease in 33 patients transformed into aggressive stages, generally demonstrating a clinical picture consistent with acute myeloid leukemia (Table I). Twenty-four of these patients died quickly, often despite chemotherapeutic measures that are effective in inducing clinical remissions in from 61 to 78 per cent of our patients with classic acute myeloid leukemia [20]. The patients were classified on the basis of their clinical courses and marrow morphology. Multiple marrow aspirate smears and sections were examined. Evaluation of cellularity was determined on histologic sections from marrow aspirates or biopsy specimens. Sections of biopsy specimens were considered to be normocellular when 30 to 70 per cent of the section was comprised of hemopoietic cells ("Appendix"). The term "decreased late granulocytes" indicates that the specimen contained comparatively few band forms and segmented neutrophils, whereas the other granulocytic elements were distributed in a quantitatively normal manner. The term "left-shifted granulopoiesis" indicates that the marrow specimen contained a relative increase in the proportion of myeloblasts and promyelocytes. The morphologic distinctions used to define our patient groups, as based on the patient material noted in the "Appendix," is similar to clinical characterization used in prior studies [2,21]. In these disorders, abnormal proliferation and/or maturation of more than one hemopoietic cell line, and generally all lines, were noted. Frequently, proliferation of one cell line predominated and provided the basis for clinical categorization.

Chronic Myeloid Leukemia. In the patients with chronic myeloid leukemia, marrow granulocytic hyperplasia and low leukocyte alkaline phosphatase values were consistently found, and high serum muramidase levels and splenomegaly were frequently present ("Appendix"). When karyotypic studies were performed, the Philadelphia chromosome was present in marrow cells from five subjects and absent in five subjects.

Regarding the terminal phases of chronic myeloid leukemia, our experience is similar to that of others [22,23]. As

TABLE I Marrow Colony-Forming Capacity (CFC) in Relation to Disease Status of Patients with Myeloproliferative Disorders

			Time (mo) Relative to Initial in Vitro Studies				
Patient	Age (yr) and Sex	Initial CFC/10^5 Marrow Cells*	After Diagnosis	Before Acute Transformation or	To Clinical Stability	Before Death	Duration of Illness
			Chronic Myeloid Leukemia				
1	53, M	TNTC	0	51	...	53	53
2	52, M	TNTC	108	8	...	10	118
3	58, F	TNTC	12	...	+	2	14
4	35, M	120 ± 4	0	40		44	44
5	68, F	95 ± 5	0	...	18+	...	18+
6	33, F	40 ± 2	5	...	1+	...	6+
7	60, M	30 ± 5	1	...	8+	...	9+
8	67, M	16 ± 2	1	...	+	24	25
9	38, F	14 ± 1	0	3	...	5	5
10	69, M	8 ± 1	108	2	...	3	111
11	83, F	5 ± 1	7	5	...	6	13
12	36, M	5 ± 1	0	...	36+	...	36+
13	30, F	5 ± 1	24	...	12+	...	36+
14	66, M	1 ± 1.5	6	1	...	3	9
15	49, M	0	1	...	54+	...	55+
16	80, M	0	20	3	...	5	25
			Blast Crisis				
24	66, F	4 ± 2	1	NA	...	1	2
25	69, M	1 ± 0.2	1	NA	...	1	2
26	69, M	0	1	NA	...	1	2
			Subacute Myeloid Leukemia				
29	83, M	93 ± 16	24	...	+	2	26
30	49, M	27 ± 8	11	13	...	23	34
31	69, M	20 ± 2	2	...	+	4	6
32	70, F	20 ± 1	1+	...	24+	...	25+
33	50, F	14 ± 5	1	17	...	17	18
34	65, M	11 ± 2	0	...	+	1	1
35	56, M	1 ± 0.5	0	10	...	10	10
36	62, M	1 ± 0.4	1	1	...	1	2
37	57, M	1 ± 0.5	1	3	...	3	4
38	67, M	1 ± 0.5	0	...	+	8	8
39	70, M	1 ± 0.6	0	...	+	16	16
40	40, F	0	3	12	...	12	15
41	74, M	0	0	...	+	2	2
42	59, M	0†	1	6	...	6	7
43	60, F	0	6	14	...	20	20
44	68, M	0	1	6	...	11	12
			Di Guglielmo's Syndrome				
63	48, F	69† ± 5	2	2	...	6	8
64	62, M	1 ± 0.5	1	...	5	5	6
65	86, M	0	24	...	16+	...	40+
66	58, F	0†	5	13	...	15	20
67	53, F	0†	0	5	...	5	5
68	71, M	0†	0	9	...	9	9
69	57, F	0	7	...	37	37	44
70	42, M	0	0	1	...	1	1
71	70, M	0	1	...	1	1	2
			Idiopathic Ineffective Erythropoiesis				
72	57, F	80 ± 5	168	...	20	20	188
73	65, M	65 ± 10	8	...	17+	...	25+
74	63, M	28 ± 8	0	...	54+	...	54+
75	73, F	27 ± 4	60	...	51+	...	111+
76	62, F	21 ± 3	5	...	6+	...	11+
77	62, F	20 ± 4	6	...	22+	...	28+
78	65, M	13 ± 3	19	...	21+	...	40+
79	60, F	12 ± 5	13	...	56+	...	69+
80	58, F	3 ± 1	0	...	44+	...	44+
81	94, M	3 ± 1	0	...	12+	...	12+

Continued

TABLE I (Cont'd) Marrow Colony-Forming Capacity (CFC) in Relation to Disease Status of Patients with Myeloproliferative Disorders

Patient	Age (yr) and Sex	Initial CFC/10^5 Marrow Cells*	Time (mo) Relative to Initial in Vitro Studies: After Diagnosis	Before Acute Transformation or	To Clinical Stability	Before Death	Duration of Illness
		Polycythemia Vera					
82	52, M	66 ± 2	1	. . .	36+	. . .	37+
83	68, M	57 ± 5	60	. . .	2+	. . .	62+
84	62, M	53 ± 6	48	. . .	2+	. . .	50+
85	61, M	30 ± 3	1	. . .	36+	. . .	37+
86	58, M	23 ± 2	48	. . .	44+	. . .	92+
87	59, M	23 ± 3	1	. . .	16+	. . .	17+
88	42, M	17 ± 1	72	. . .	2+	. . .	74+
89	63, M	14 ± 3	0	. . .	26+	. . .	26+
90	74, F	6 ± 1	1	. . .	14+	. . .	15+
91	63, F	3 ± 1	0	. . .	10+	. . .	10+
92	61, F	1 ± 0.5	108	1	. . .	2	110
		Essential Thrombocythemia					
93	46, F	61 ± 1	96	. . .	5+	. . .	101+
94	52, M	17 ± 2	1	. . .	4+	. . .	5+

NOTE: TNTC = colonies too numerous to count. NA = not applicable.
*Mean ± standard deviation.
†Excessive clusters.

the disease in these patients transformed into the more aggressive clinical stages, two general presentations were detected. In some patients there was a gradual acceleration of the disease with progressive anemia and/or thrombocytopenia, splenomegaly, leukocytosis with only a moderate increase in the peripheral blast count, and they became refractory to previously effective therapy. Marrow morphology was not helpful in distinguishing this group from patients in the more chronic phases of their diseases. Other patients had an acute transition of abrupt onset befitting the term blast crisis, with a rapid increase in peripheral myeloblasts, associated with anemia, thrombocytopenia and frequently splenomegaly. The latter form of transformation was generally associated with gross myeloblastic infiltration in marrow, and diminution of erythroid and platelet precursors.

Of the 23 persons with chronic myeloid leukemia who were studied, the disease in 11 patients underwent acute transformation into blast crisis or their myeloid leukemia was accelerated within one to 51 months (median four months) from the time of marrow culture. The duration of the patients' illnesses ranged from five to 118 months from the time of diagnosis, with a median survival of 42 months (Table I).

Polycythemia Vera. These patients had increased red cell mass (determined by Cr^{51}-labeled red cell technics), splenomegaly, panymyelosis and no evidence for secondary polycythemia. In 10 of 11 patients the disease has remained stable for 10 to 92 months from the time of diagnosis; in one patient it has transformed into myelofibrosis (Table I).

Essential Thrombocythemia. These patients had markedly increased platelet counts, a normal red cell mass, marrow findings of megakaryocytic hyperplasia without granulocytic hyperplasia or myelofibrosis, and splenomegaly. The condition of the two patients studied has remained clinically stable (Table I).

Subacute Myeloid Leukemia. The patients with subacute myeloid leukemia comprise a group of leukemic patients with a course more indolent than acute myeloid leukemia, yet more rapid than chronic myeloid leukemia [24–26]. The patients frequently had single or multiple refractory cytopenias (anemia, thrombocytopenia and/or neutropenia) for months to years before a definitive diagnosis was made. Marrows showed granulocytic hyperplasia and a persistent increase of early myeloid precursors with between 10 and 40 per cent myeloblasts, and poor granulocytic maturation beyond the myelocyte stage, although the marrow cellularity of these patients was generally less than that of patients with chronic myeloid leukemia or acute myeloid leukemia. Qualitative abnormalities of the erythroid, granulocytic and/or megakaryocytic lines were often present. These patients generally did not receive cytotoxic therapy until an accelerated stage of their disease eventuated. The median survival in this patient group was 11 months from the time of diagnosis (Table I). In nine of 17 patients in this group the disease underwent acute transformation within one to 17 months; seven of these nine patients died shortly thereafter, being refractory to antileukemic therapy. Six of the eight patients in whom the disease did not undergo acute transformation died of infection or hemorrhage associated with their dominant cytopenia (Table I).

Preleukemia. Criteria for the diagnosis of preleukemia, which were similar to those of previous workers [27,28], consisted of relatively prolonged courses of refractory anemia, neutropenia, thrombocytopenia or monocytosis, singly or in combination, associated with characteristically abnormal marrow morphology ("Appendix"). Preleukemia is an inexact

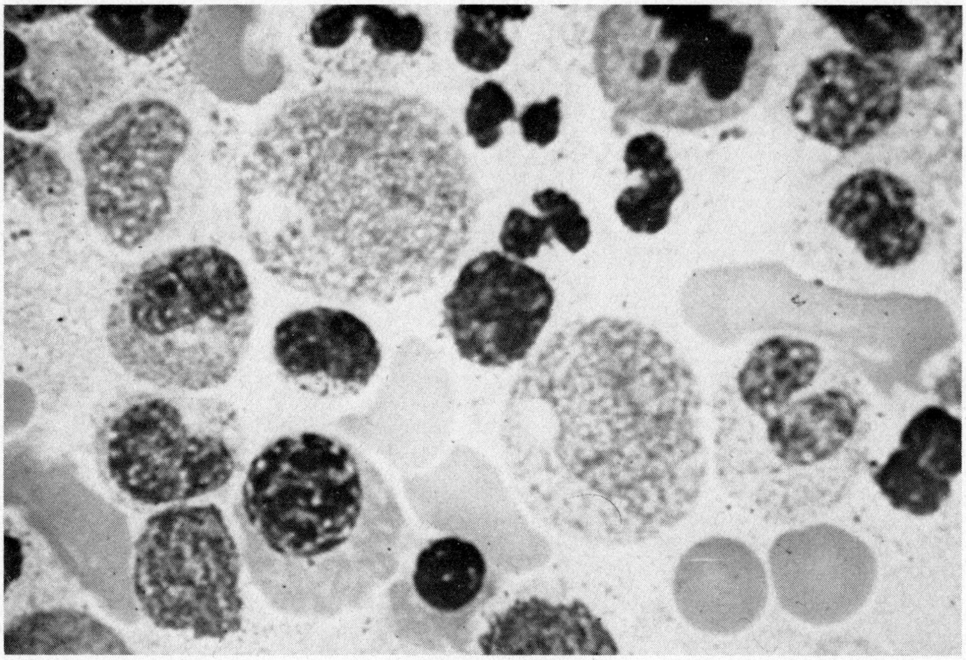

Figure 1. *Abnormal marrow mononuclear cells in patients with preleukemia. Note nucleocytoplasmic asynchrony (see text). Megaloblastoid erythroid cells are also shown.*

term since it cannot be diagnosed with certainty until leukemia develops. We have maintained the designation with the understanding that we are referring to the group of patients having myelodysplastic disorders with the clinical characteristics described in whom the disease has a propensity to terminate in acute myeloid leukemia. Marrow examination indicated dysplastic maturation of the granulocytic, erythroid and megakaryocytic cell lines, including qualitative changes such as myeloid nucleocytoplasmic asynchrony, megaloblastoid erythropoiesis, occasionally with ringed sideroblasts, and often bilobed megakaryocytes [28,29] ("Appendix"). In addition, the presence of an abnormal mononuclear cell was noted in the marrows of 15 of the 17 patients in the present study. This cell comprised approximately 5 to 10 per cent of the myeloid cells, had granular bluish grey cytoplasm with a prominent nuclear hof, and a reticulated nuclear chromatin pattern with one or two pale-staining nucleoli (Figure 1). This cell type appears similar to that previously described in other patients with preleukemia [30], and although the precise nature of this cell is unknown, it has been identified as an abnormal promyelocyte. The cellularity of the marrow sections were either normal, decreased or increased; when increased, this was due to erythroid but not granulocytic hyperplasia.

The 24 patients described with preleukemia included 17 patients in the present study and seven patients whose in vitro growth studies were reported previously [10]. These latter seven patients are included since the longer follow-up period has permitted better definition of their clinical courses. The following clinical abnormalities were found: splenomegaly in seven of 24 patients (29 per cent), low leukocyte alkaline phosphatase levels in 11 of 17 patients (65 per cent), cytopenia of more than one line in 16 of 24 patients (67 per cent) and monocytosis in five of 24 patients (20 per cent). The patients' ages ranged from 26 to 88 years (65 year median). Acute transformation into acute myeloid leukemia occurred in 10 of 24 patients (42 per cent) within two to 57 months (10 month median), and the duration of the patients' diseases ranged from two months to 15 years (1.5 year median) (Table II). In one patient, the condition evolved into preleukemia one year after idiopathic ineffective erythropoiesis was documented, and acute transformation occurred three years later. There were no obvious clinical or morphologic findings that separated the 10 patients in whom acute transformation occurred from the remaining 14 patients in this group in whom it has not as yet occurred.

Di Guglielmo's Syndrome and Idiopathic Ineffective Erythropoiesis. The patients in these two diagnostic categories were characterized by previously described criteria [31–37]. These patients had anemia, reticulocytopenia, abnormal red cell morphology, intense bone marrow erythroid hyperplasia, increased iron stores and numerous ringed sideroblasts. Ferrokinetic studies revealed increased plasma iron turnover, decreased incorporation of iron into red blood cells and progressive hepatic uptake of iron. Ineffective erythropoiesis secondary to folic acid or vitamin B_{12} deficiency, thalassemia and drug toxicity was excluded.

The nine patients with Di Guglielmo's syndrome had abnormal erythroid precursors which were megaloblastic or megaloblastoid; of major importance was the finding of dysplastic myeloid precursors with an increase of early myeloid cells and poor maturation of these cells beyond the promyelocyte or myelocyte stage. Rarely, Auer rods were present in the myeloblasts. Dysplastic megakaryocytes were present, occasionally with nucleoli or bilobed nuclei. Seven of nine patients were initially pancytopenic ("Appendix"). Eight of nine patients have died, five after acute transformation into acute myeloid leukemia within one to 18 months (nine months median) (Table I).

In the 10 patients with idiopathic ineffective erythropoiesis,

TABLE II Preleukemic Patients. Relationship Between Marrow Colony-Forming Capacity and Clinical Status

			Time (mo) Relative to Initial in Vitro Study				
Patient	Age (yr) and Sex	Colonies per 10^5 Marrow Cells*	From Diagnosis	Before Acute Transformation	or To Clinical Stability	To Death	Duration of Illness
			Present Group				
46	68,F	92 ± 8	10	37	...	39	49
47	61,F	39 ± 1	72	...	36+	...	108+
48	26,M	35 ± 5	0	50	55+	...	55+
49	88,F	14 ± 3	36	20	...	26	62
50	26,F	11 ± 2	1	...	6+	...	7+
51	63,F	10 ± 1†	72	...	12+	...	84+
52	64,F	9 ± 0.2	14	...	3+	...	17+
53	54,F	7 ± 1	180	...	8+	...	188+
54	68,M	6 ± 1	1	...	10+	...	11+
55	81,M	3 ± 0.2	0	...	12+	...	12+
56	70,M	3 ± 1	21	...	17+	...	38+
57	68,M	2 ± 1	1	...	1	1	2
58	84,M	1 ± 0.4	0	9	...	9	9
59	40,M	1 ± 0.4	1	...	2	2	3
60	75,M	1 ± 0.2	0	...	1+	...	1+
61	73,M	0	0	...	16	16	16
62	67,F	0†	1	34	...	37	38
			Previously Reported Group [10]				
95	59,M	30 ± 7	0	8	...	11	11
96	39,F	10 ± 2	9	10	38+	...	57+
97	36,M	2 ± 1	0	...	9	9	9
98	77,F	0	8	2	...	3	11
99	89,M	0	2	18	...	18	20
100	61,M	0	48	9	...	11	59
101	36,F	0	6	...	13	13	19

*Mean ± standard deviation.
†Excessive clusters.

marrow morphologic abnormalities were limited to the erythroid cells; in particular, they had normal myeloid and megakaryocytic maturation. The leukocyte counts were normal, and platelet counts in nine of 10 patients were within normal limits or increased ("Appendix"). Therefore, this latter group does not fit into the myeloproliferative disorders as defined herein, in that only one hemopoietic cell line appears to be involved. In none of these patients has acute myeloid leukemia evolved after a median of 4.5 years follow-up (range one to 15+ years). These patients have been included in this study in order to contrast their in vitro growth patterns and clinical courses with those of patients with Di Guglielmo's syndrome and other refractory anemias.

RESULTS

Marrow Granulopoiesis Colony-Forming Capacity and Proportion of Light Density Colony-Forming Cells. In 33 of the 78 patients with chronic myeloid leukemia, subacute myeloid leukemia, preleukemia, Di Guglielmo's syndrome, polycythemia vera or essential thrombocythemia in whom the colony-forming capacity was evaluated (43 determinations, including serial studies), their diseases underwent acute transformation (Tables I and II, Figure 2). Twenty-six of these 33 patients had abnormally low marrow colony-forming capacity prior to transformation ($p < 0.01$). Twenty-two patients had decreased colony-forming capacity values at initial study; the four others showed sequential diminution of colony-forming capacity as their diseases evolved (Figure 3). Of the patients in whom transformation subsequently occurred, it occurred in the 22 patients with initially low colony-forming capacity within a significantly shorter period (six months median) than in those 11 patients with initially normal or increased colony-forming capacity (17 months median) ($p < 0.05$) (Table I). Conversely, however, decreased marrow colony-forming capacity per se, as found in 47 of 78 patients, was not associated with a significantly increased incidence of acute transformation. Prior chemotherapy does not explain the in vitro abnormalities, since the majority of these patients were not treated prior to study. The in vitro growth abnormalities often were not paralleled by obvious changes of marrow morphology, particularly near the time of incipient disease transformation.

An increased proportion of abnormally light-density colony-forming cells characterized marrow and peripheral blood from 15 of 16 patients studied with chronic myeloid leukemia, subacute myeloid leukemia,

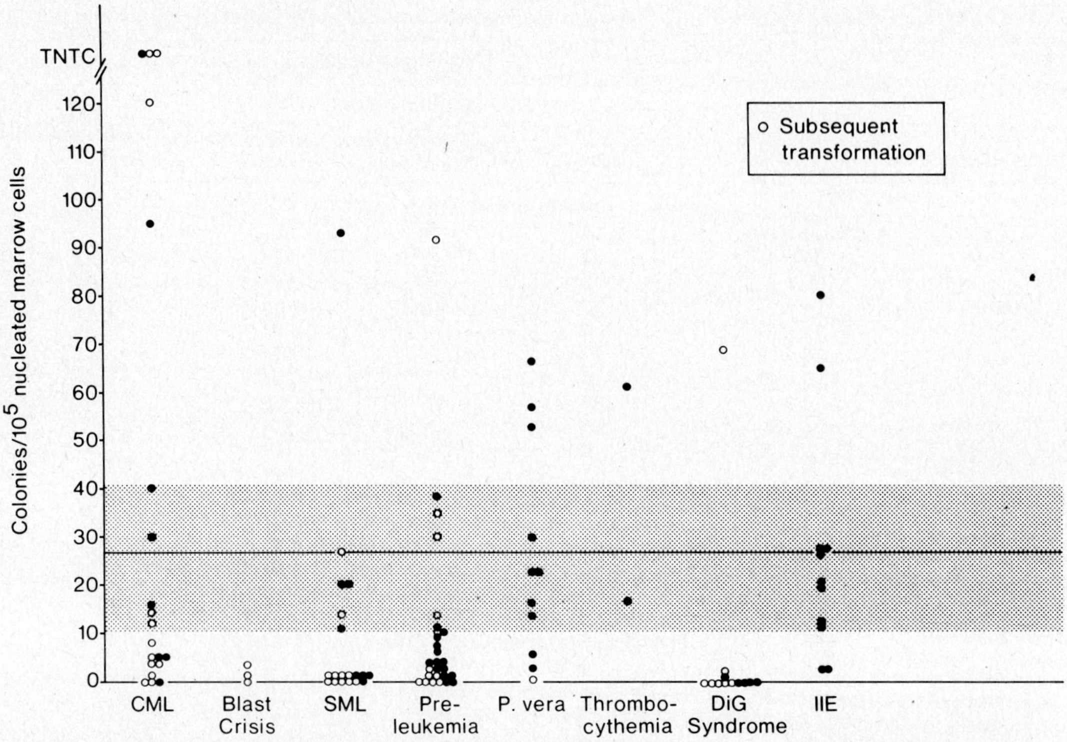

Figure 2. Marrow colony-forming capacity (CFC) in patients with myeloproliferative disorders and idiopathic ineffective erythropoiesis. TNTC denotes normal sized colonies which were too numerous to count on dishes plated with 2 × 10^5 nucleated cells. Open circles denote determinations from patients in whom the disease has subsequently undergone acute transformation. The stippled area indicates the mean ± 2 SD of control marrow CFC values. CML = chronic myeloid leukemia, SML = subacute myeloid leukemia, DiG = Di Guglielmo's syndrome, IIE = idiopathic ineffective erythropoiesis.

preleukemia and essential thrombocythemia ($p < 0.01$) (Figure 4, "Appendix"). This proportion tended to be directly related to the duration of the disease but was unrelated to the leukocyte count or prior therapy. In seven of eight patients with >35 per cent abnormally light-density colony-forming cells, their disease underwent acute transformation within one to 20 months (seven months median) (Figure 4) ($p < 0.01$). The patients with a lower proportion of light colony-forming cells have remained clinically stable ($p < 0.01$).

Chronic Myeloid Leukemia. Table I indicates the relationship between the colony-forming capacity values in the patients' marrow and their clinical status. Particular emphasis was given to determine when disease transformation occurred relative to marrow colony-forming capacity. In 22 patients with chronic myeloid leukemia, colony-forming capacity was evaluated in the marrow (16 patients, 20 determinations) (Figure 2) or peripheral blood (six patients, seven determinations). Nine patients were studied within one month of the diagnosis. Six of the eight patients in whom acute transformation occurred showed abnormally low in vitro marrow growth prior to clinical evolution (Table I, Figures 2 and 3), although as a group the colony-forming capacity values in patients with chronic myeloid leukemia did not differ significantly from those in control subjects. In two patients in whom sequential studies were performed, marrow colony-forming capacity decreased as the condition of these patients evolved toward acute transformation (Figure 3). Marrow colony-forming capacity values did not correlate with duration of prior disease, prior chemotherapy or peripheral leukocyte counts (Table I). The three patients in blast crisis at the time of their initial in vitro studies had significantly low marrow colony-forming capacity values ($p < 0.01$).

Evaluation of colony-forming cell density distribution patterns revealed that specimens from seven of eight patients with chronic myeloid leukemia (nine of 10 determinations) had an increased proportion of abnormally light-density (< 1.062 g/cm^3) granulocytic colony-forming cells ($p < 0.01$) (Figure 4).

Subacute Myeloid Leukemia. In 16 patients with subacute myeloid leukemia (20 determinations) marrow colony-forming capacity was evaluated. As shown in Figure 2, a wide range of colony-forming capacity values was found, but the predominant value was very low (median, 1 colony/10^5 marrow cells plated), and as a group these values were significantly lower than normal ($p < 0.01$). Seven of nine patients in whom acute transformation occurred showed subnormal colony-forming capacity values one to 14 months (six months median) prior to clinical evolution (Table I). An abnormally increased proportion of light-density granulocytic precursors was present in the two patients studied ($p < 0.05$) (Figure 4). Both of these patients died quickly, and in the one with 43 per cent light colony-forming cells this occurred after acute transformation occurred.

Preleukemia. The 24 patients (26 marrow colony-forming capacity determinations) in this group included 17 newly studied patients and seven patients previously described [10], (Table II, Figure 2). The median marrow colony-forming capacity value was 6 colonies/10^5 marrow cells in the present group and 0/10^5 marrow cells in the group previously reported on. These values are significantly less than normal ($p < 0.01$), but they are not significantly different from each other. Twenty-two of 24 patients had abnormally low in vitro marrow growth patterns during their course ($p < 0.01$). In two cases, marrow colony-forming capacity values were initially normal, but they decreased during evolution of the disease (Figure 3). Abnormal in vitro marrow growth patterns were present in nine of 10 subjects two to 50 months before acute transformation occurred (10 months median). There was no significant difference in marrow colony-forming capacity values in the group of 10 patients in whom acute transformation occurred when compared to the group of 14 patients who have remained clinically stable. All five patients whose marrow cells were studied by density gradient centrifugation had an increased proportion of abnormally light colony-forming cells ($p < 0.01$) (Figure 4).

Di Guglielmo's Syndrome. Nine patients in this group had 12 determinations of marrow colony-forming capacity (Figure 2). In five of these patients transformation occurred and colony-forming capacity was very low or absent. As a group, the colony-forming capacity values in the patients were lower than normal ($p < 0.01$). In four patients (five determinations) an excessive number (too numerous to count) of granulocytic clusters were found, in addition to an absence of normal-sized colonies. In all four patients with cluster formation, transformation to acute myeloid leukemia occurred within two to 13 months. In contrast, of the five patients without cluster formation, transformation to acute myeloid leukemia occurred in only one (Table I) ($p < 0.04$, Chi square test). However, three of these five patients died shortly of infection.

Idiopathic Ineffective Erythropoiesis. Marrow colony-forming capacity was evaluated in 10 patients in this group (11 determinations). Marrow colony-forming capacity in these patients varied over a wide range and as a group the colony-forming capacity values were not

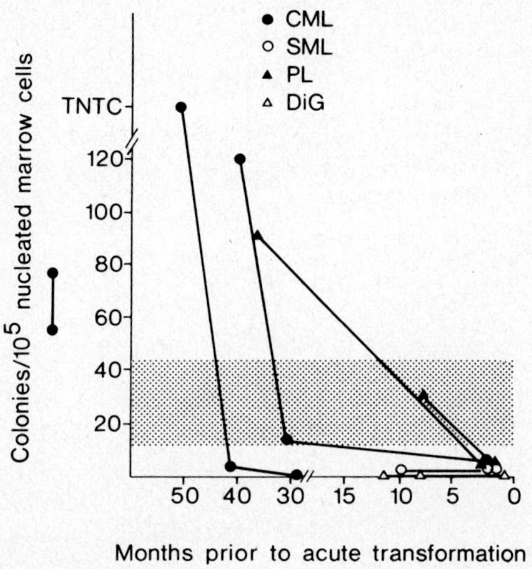

Figure 3. *Sequential values of marrow colony-forming capacity (CFC) in patients whose myeloproliferative disease underwent acute transformation. CML = chronic myeloid leukemia, SML = subacute myeloid leukemia, PL = preleukemia, DiG = Di Guglielmo's syndrome. Stippled area denotes the mean ± 2 SD of control CFC values.*

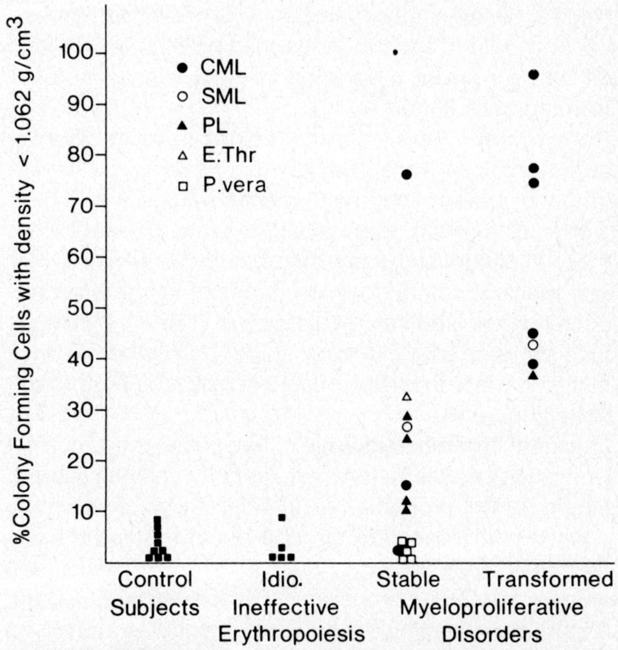

Figure 4. *Proportion of abnormally light-density colony-forming cells (density < 1.062 g/cm³) in control subjects, patients with idiopathic ineffective erythropoiesis and myeloproliferative disorders. In the latter category the patients have been divided into those whose diseases have remained clinically stable as contrasted to those in whom the disease has undergone acute transformation. CML = chronic myeloid leukemia, SML = subacute myeloid leukemia, PL = preleukemia, E.Thr = essential thrombocythemia, P. vera = polycythemia vera.*

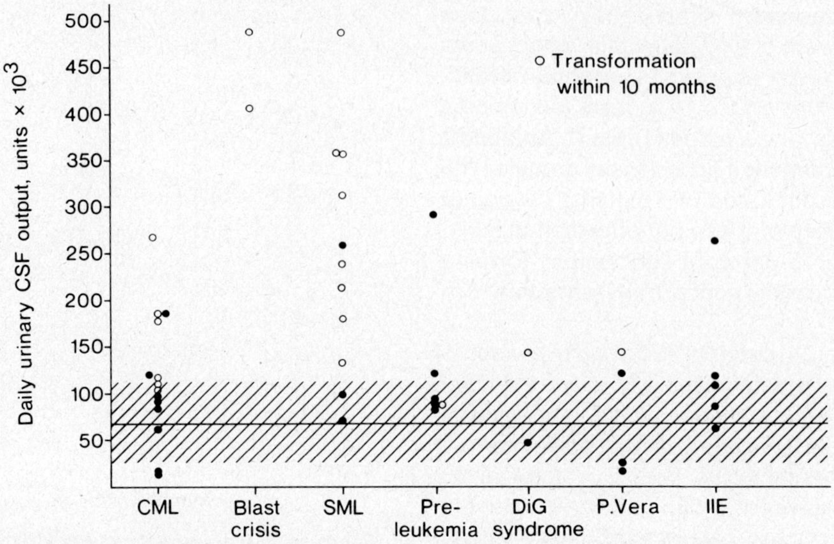

***Figure 5.** Daily urinary output of colony-stimulating factor (CSF) in patients with myeloproliferative disorders and idiopathic ineffective erythropoiesis. 0 denotes patients in whom the disease underwent acute transformation within 10 months of study. Lined area indicates the mean ± 2 SD values of normal adult subjects. CML = chronic myeloid leukemia, SML = subacute myeloid leukemia, IIE = idiopathic ineffective erythropoiesis.*

significantly different from those in control subjects. Neutral density cell separation was performed on five patients with idiopathic ineffective erythropoiesis, and all had a normal proportion of light-density colony-forming cells (Figure 4).

Polycythemia Vera. Marrow colony-forming capacity determinations were performed in 11 patients. A wide range of colony-forming capacity values was noted which, as a group, was not significantly different from those in control subjects. One of the patients had a very low marrow colony-forming capacity at the time her condition evolved into myelofibrosis (Table I, Figure 2). Five patients with clinically stable polycythemia vera had a normal proportion of light density colony-forming cells (Figure 4).

Essential Thrombocythemia. Two patients had normal or increased colony-forming capacity values (Table I, Figure 2). The proportion of light-density colony-forming cells was increased in the one person tested (Figure 4).

Urinary Colony-Stimulating Factor Output. Daily urinary colony-stimulating factor output was increased in 17 of 31 patients with myeloproliferative disorders when compared to age-related control subjects ($p < 0.05$) (Figure 5, "Appendix"). These patients had no evidence of infection or renal disease at the time of urine collection. No correlation was noted between urinary colony-stimulating factor output and total leukocyte or monocyte counts. Increased colony-stimulating factor values were present in 10 of 12 patients in whom urinary colony-stimulating factor output was determined within 10 months prior to acute transformation ($p < 0.01$) (Figure 5). Urinary colony-stimulating factor output was significantly increased ($p < 0.01$) in patients in blast crisis, in patients with chronic myeloid leukemia in whom acute transformation subsequently occurred, and in patients with subacute myeloid leukemia. In contrast, colony-stimulating factor levels in preleukemia, stable chronic myeloid leukemia, polycythemia vera, Di Guglielmo's syndrome and idiopathic ineffective erythropoiesis were not significantly elevated. Sequential studies showed rising or persistently elevated levels of colony-stimulating factor output associated with acute transformation in four patients, whereas colony-stimulating factor output has remained normal in two patients who are clinically stable (Figure 6).

Simultaneous evaluation of urinary colony-stimulating factor output and marrow colony-forming capacity were performed in 20 patients with myeloproliferative disorders. In six of seven patients with both low marrow colony-forming capacity and high urinary colony-stimulating factor output, acute transformation occurred within 10 months, the exception being a patient with polycythemia vera. Similarly six of 10 patients in whom transformation occurred within 10 months of observation had this abnormal pattern of in vitro indices ($p < 0.03$, Chi square test).

COMMENTS

Our data indicate that values for marrow colony-forming capacity and levels of urinary colony-stimulating factor

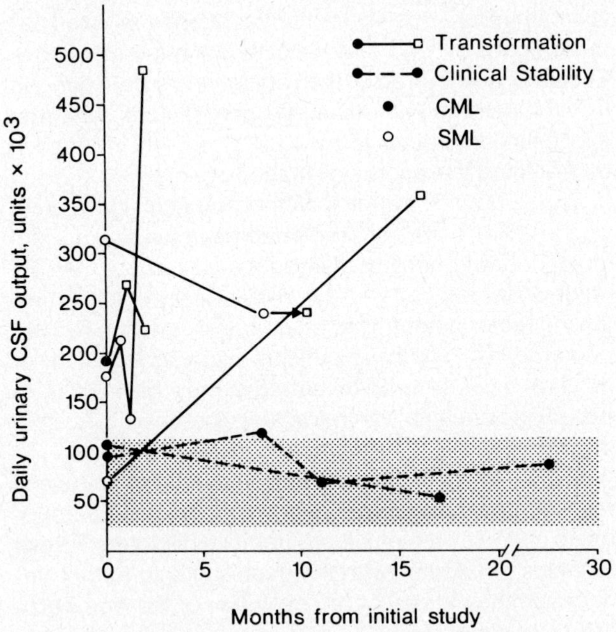

Figure 6. *Sequential changes of urinary colony-stimulating factor (CSF) output in patients whose condition has remained clinically stable (● - - - - ●), or whose disease has undergone acute transformation (○ —— □). □ denotes time of transformation. CML = chronic myeloid leukemia, SML = subacute myeloid leukemia. The stippled area indicates the mean ± 2 SD of values for normal subjects.*

output vary with disease category and clinical stage in patients with myeloproliferative disorders. Patients with chronic myeloid leukemia had a wide range of marrow colony-forming capacity, with generally high values early in the course of the disease, which decreased to subnormal levels prior to acute transformation (Figures 2 and 3). Previous workers have also shown increased colony-forming capacity values early in chronic myeloid leukemia and normal values in the chronic treated phase of the disease [38]. An increased proportion of abnormally light buoyant density colony-forming cells was present in marrow and peripheral blood cells from seven of the eight patients with chronic myeloid leukemia in whom the assay was performed.

In patients with subacute myeloid leukemia and preleukemia, marrow colony-forming capacity values were significantly lower than normal. An increased proportion of light-density colony-forming cells was also present in the patients in these groups. Acute transformation subsequently occurred in seven of eight patients with subacute myeloid leukemia, preleukemia or chronic myeloid leukemia with more than 35 per cent light colony-forming cells. These findings suggest that abnormally light colony-forming cells characterize leukemic or potentially leukemic granulopoietic precursors. These data confirm and extend prior reports in patients with certain myeloproliferative disorders [14,39].

Our prospective clinical categorization of patients as having preleukemia was borne out by the high incidence of acute myeloid leukemia. The abnormal in vitro myeloid growth patterns in these patients have provided a useful adjunct for defining this diagnostic category. Since similar clinical and in vitro marrow growth abnormalities were found in those patients whose condition has remained stable as well as in those in whom transformation has occurred, one can propose that other factors may be involved in the progression of this disorder to acute myeloid leukemia.

In eight of nine patients with Di Guglielmo's syndrome absent or nearly absent colony formation was noted. In those patients whose marrow cells showed excessive cluster formation in vitro, the incidence of acute transformation was significantly increased. Since transformation also occurred in patients with subacute myeloid leukemia and preleukemia who had cluster formation, it appears that this in vitro growth pattern is a particularly ominous finding. The prognosis in patients with acute myeloid leukemia who had small cluster formation was also previously reported to be poorer, and the clusters in those patients were shown to be generated by leukemic myeloblasts [13].

Patients with clinically stable polycythemia vera had normal marrow colony-forming capacity values and a normal proportion of light-density marrow colony-forming cells (Figures 2 and 4). Normal values were found in these patients early in their disease and up to eight years after the diagnosis was made, with or without prior alkylator or radioactive phosphorous therapy. The chronic uncomplicated stage of polycythemia vera, therefore, lacks abnormalities of granulocytic clonal growth which characterize leukemia and preleukemia. Abnormal density distribution patterns of colony-forming cells have been previously reported in polycythemia vera concomitant with acute transformation [39].

Patients with myeloproliferative disorders in whom acute transformation occurred had significantly subnormal marrow colony-forming capacity values. The lower the initial colony-forming capacity values were, the closer the disease in these patients was to transformation (Tables I and II). Sequential diminution of colony-forming capacity occurred concomitant with disease progression (Figure 3). These findings suggest that the evolution of these disorders is associated with marrow replacement by progressively more abnormal granulopoietic populations. However, low colony-forming capacity values alone were not correlated with an enhanced incidence of transformation, indicating that additional factors are involved in the evolution of these diseases.

Elevated levels of urinary colony-stimulating factor output were present in the majority of patients studied, and in 10 of 12 patients in whom acute transformation subsequently occurred within 10 months. In six of seven patients with both increased colony-stimulating factor output and low marrow colony-forming capacity transformation occurred within 10 months. These findings indicate that progressive abnormalities of levels of possible granulopoietic regulatory substances combined with alterations of marrow clonal growth occur during evolution of these diseases, and appear to be accurate predictors of impending transformation. Leukemic cells have been shown to require colony-stimulating factor for their proliferation in vitro [40]. Elevated serum and urinary colony-stimulating factor levels have been reported in patients with leukemia and certain myeloproliferative disorders [15,16]. These data are compatible with the hypothesis that the development and progression of leukemia may be significantly influenced by altered levels of humoral granulopoietic regulatory factors [41]. The pathophysiologic relevance of the altered serum and urinary levels of colony-stimulating factor remains to be clarified, particularly since these materials have relatively low stimulatory activity for human marrow in vitro [42] in comparison with their activity for mouse marrow. Exceptions occurred in the relationships between the in vitro parameters measured and clinical outcome, suggesting that other factors are also likely involved in determining the course of these patients.

The group of patients with idiopathic ineffective erythropoiesis was characterized by having a normal incidence and density distribution pattern of marrow colony-forming cells, and normal urinary colony-stimulating factor output. That acute transformation has not occurred in any of these patients suggests that study of in vitro myeloid growth patterns may be helpful in classifying patients with refractory sideroblastic anemia in whom the risk of evolution to leukemia is low.

Our data suggest that these in vitro studies are useful for clinical staging, evaluating prognosis and categorizing patients with myeloproliferative disorders. These technics provide us with the opportunity to further understand the biology of the evolution of the myeloproliferative disorders.

APPENDIX Clinical Parameters of Patients with Myeloproliferative Disorders*

Patient	Age (yr) and Sex	White Blood Cells (× 10³/mm³)	Hematocrit (%)	Platelets (× 10³/mm³)	LAP	Serum Muramidase	Splenomegaly	Prior Chemotherapy	Cellularity	Bone Marrow: Myelopoiesis Qt	Myelopoiesis Ql	Erythropoiesis Qt	Erythropoiesis Ql	Megakaryopoiesis Qt	Megakaryopoiesis Ql
						Chronic Myeloid Leukemia									
1	53,M	280	17	236	↓	↑	+	0	↑↑	↑	N	↓	N	N	N
2	52,M	6.9	35	60	...	↓	0	+	↑↑	↑	LS	↓	N	↑	N
3	58,F	26.6	31	420	↓	↑	+	0	↑↑	↑	LS	↓	N	N	N
4 † §	35,M	597	29	886	↓	↑	+	0	↑↑	↑	N	↓	N	N	N
5 §	68,F	40	49	725	...	...	+	0	↑↑	↑	N	N	N	↑	N
6 †	33,F	16	40	650	↓	N	0	0	↑↑	↑	LS	↓	N	↑	N
7 §	60,M	122	33	54	...	↑	+	0	↑↑	↑	N	↓	N	↓	N
8	67,M	8.7	49	2,720	↓	↑	0	0	↑↑	↑	N	N	N	↑	N
9 §	38,F	24	27	52	↓	↑	+	0	↑↑	↑	N	↓	N	↓	N
10 †	69,M	7.7	30	138	...	...	0	+	↑↑	↑	LS	N	N	N	N
11 §	83,F	117	27	59	...	...	+	+	↑↑	↑	N	↓	N	↓	N
12	36,M	43	36	432	↓	↑	0	0	↑↑	↑	N	N	N	N	N
13 † §	30,F	53	40	590	↓	...	0	0	↑↑	↑	N	↓	N	↑	N
14 §	66,M	12	24	100	↓	...	+	0	↑↑	↑	LS	↓	D	↑	D
15	49,M	213	37	497	↓	...	+	0	↑↑	↑	N	N	N	↑	N
16 §	80,M	38	24	290	↓	↑	+	+	↑↑	↑	LS	↓	N	N	N
17 §	48,F	252	30	260	↓	↑	+	0	↑↑	↑	N	↓	N	N	N
18	18,F	27	36	844	...	...	+	+	↑↑	↑	N	N	N	↑	N
19 †	46,F	16	16	9	...	...	+	+	↑↑	↑	LS	↓	N	↓	N
20 †	41,M	27	48	275	↓	...	+	+	↑↑	↑	N	N	N	N	N
21 † §	26,M	6	33	63	↓	...	+	+	↑↑	↑	LS	↓	N	↓	N
22 †	50,M	55	33	1,100	...	...	+	+	↑↑	↑	LS	↓	N	↑	N
23 §	30,F	85	40	560	...	...	0	+	↑↑	↑	N	↓	N	N	N
						Blast Crisis									
24	66,F	150	21	34	N	N	+	+	↑↑	↑	PM	↓	D	↓	D
25	69,M	1.8	22	8	...	...	0	+	↑↑	↑	PM	↓	D	↓	D
26	69,M	1.0	23	11	N	↓	0	+	↑↑	↑	PM	↓	D	↓	D
27 §	62,M	65	29	90	...	...	0	+	↑↑	↑	PM	↓	D	↓	D
28 §	61,M	152	34	29	...	↑	+	+	↑↑	↑	PM	↓	D	↓	D

Continued

APPENDIX (Cont'd) Clinical Parameters of Patients with Myeloproliferative Disorders

Patient	Age (yr) and Sex	White Blood Cells (× 10³/mm³)	Hematocrit (%)	Platelets (× 10³/mm³)	LAP	Serum Muramidase	Splenomegaly	Prior Chemotherapy	Cellularity	Bone Marrow: Myelopoiesis Qt	Myelopoiesis Ql	Erythropoiesis Qt	Erythropoiesis Ql	Megakaryopoiesis Qt	Megakaryopoiesis Ql
Subacute Myeloid Leukemia															
29	83,M	10	39	233	. . .	↑	0	0	↑	↑	LS	↓	N	N	N
30	49,M	6	30	350	↓	N	+	+	↑	↑	LS PM	↓	D	N	D
31	69,M	2.5	30	80	. . .	↑	0	0	↑	↑	LS	↓	N	↓	D
32	50,F	1.2	26	65	. . .	N	+	0	↑	↑	LS PM	↓	N	↑	D
33 †	65,M	2.5	24	4	↑	N	0	0	↑	↑	LS PM	↑	D	↓	D
34 §	70,F	30	35	65	↓	. . .	+	0	↑	↑	LS PM	↓	N	↓	D
35 §	56,M	4.4	19	280	↑	↓	+	0	↑	↑	LS PM	↓	D	N	D
36	62,M	1.4	22	60	↑	N	+	0	↑	↑	LS PM	↓	D	↓	D
37 †	57,M	2.1	27	99	↑	N	+	0	↑	↑	LS PM	N↑	D	N	N
38 §	67,M	1.9	32	100	. . .	↑	0	0	↑	↑	LS PM	N	D	↓	N
39	70,M	2	38	278	↑	N	0	0	↑	↑	LS PM	↓	N	N	N
40	40,F	2.2	34	35	↓	N	0	0	↑	↑	LS PM	↓	D	↓	D
41	74,M	1.2	29	42	. . .	N	0	0	↑	↑	LS PM	↓	D	↓	D
42 §	59,M	1.2	31	48	. . .	N	0	0	↑	↑	LS PM	↓	D	↓	N
43 §	60,F	2.7	35	290	. . .	. . .	0	0	↑	↑	LS PM	↓	. . .	↓	N
44	68,M	4.1	44	59	↓	↑	+	0	↑	↑	LS PM	↓	N	↓	D
45 §	63,M	3.8	27	104	. . .	↑	0	0	↑	↑	LS PM	↓	N	↓	N
Preleukemia															
46	68,F	6	33	70	↑	. . .	+	0	N	↑	D*	N	D	↑	D
47 §	61,F	1	35	50	N	↑	+	0	↑	N	LS D*	↑	D	N	D
48	26,M	6	38	84	↓	N	0	0	↑	N	LS D*	↑	D	↓	D
49 †	88,F	3	36	74	↓	↓	0	0	N	↑	LS D	N	D	N	D
50	26,F	2.6	34	227	↓	↓	0	0	N	N	D* LS	↑	D	N	D
51	63,F	3.3	26	534	↓	N	+	0	↓	N	D*	N	D	N	D
52 †	64,F	7.4	27	44	. . .	. . .	0	+	N	N	D*	↓	D LS	↓↓	D
53	54,F	3.7	35	275	N	N	0	0	↑	N	D*	N	D	N	D
54 † §‡	68,M	4.9	33	93	. . .	. . .	0	0	↓	N	D* LS, DL	↑	D	↓	D
55	81,M	2.3	31	137	. . .	. . .	0	0	N	N	DL D*	N	D LS	↓	D
56 † §	70,M	4.7	31	273	. . .	N	0	0	↑	N	D*	↑	D	N	D
57 §	68,M	2.2	22	35	↓	↑	+	0	↑	↑	LS D*	↓	D	↓	D
58 §‡	84,M	3.4	20	100	↓	↑	0	0	N	↑	DL D*	N	D LS	↓	D
59 §	40,M	3.1	36	76	. . .	N	0	0	↑	N	DL D	↑	D LS	↑	D
60 †	75,M	6.2	28	242	N	. . .	0	0	N	N	LS D*	↓	D	↑	D

Continued

APPENDIX (Cont'd) Clinical Parameters of Patients with Myeloproliferative Disorders

Patient	Age (yr) and Sex	White Blood Cells (× 10³/mm³)	Hematocrit (%)	Platelets (× 10³/mm³)	LAP	Serum Muramidase	Splenomegaly	Prior Chemotherapy	Cellularity	Bone Marrow: Myelopoiesis Qt	Myelopoiesis Ql	Erythropoiesis Qt	Erythropoiesis Ql	Megakaryopoiesis Qt	Megakaryopoiesis Ql
61	73,M	5.9	31	130	↓	↑	0	0	N	↑	LS D* DL	↓	D	↓	D
62	67,F	4.7	28	396	. . .	. . .	0	0	N	N	D* LS, DL	↓	D	↓	D
Di Guglielmo's Syndrome‡															
63 §	48,F	42	22	370	. . .	N	0	0	↑	↓	D	↑	D	N	D
64	62,M	1.7	23	112	↑	N	+	0	N	N	PL, LS PM	↑	D	↓	D
65 §	86,M	3.1	25	145	. . .	. . .	0	0	↑	↑	LS PM	↑	D	↓	D
66	58,F	1.4	28	9	↓	. . .	0	0	↑	N	LS PM	↑	D	↓	D
67	53,F	2.4	35	44	. . .	. . .	0	0	N	↓	PL PM	↑	D	↓	D
68	71,M	1.8	28	63	↓	↑	0	0	N	↓	LS, DL PM	↑	D	↓	D
69	57,F	2.2	31	140	. . .	↓	0	0	N	N	LS PM	↑	D	N	D
70	42,M	3.3	23	44	. . .	. . .	0	0	↑	N	LS PM	↑	D	↓	D
71	70,M	0.6	31	10	↓	. . .	0	0	↑	↑	LS PM	↑	D	↓	D
Idiopathic Ineffective Erythropoiesis‡															
72	57,F	10	30	730	↓	N	+	0	N	N	N	↑	D	N	N
73†	65,M	8.2	33	250	. . .	. . .	0	0	↑	N	N	↑	D	N	N
74† §	63,M	4	30	169	. . .	N	0	0	N	N	N	↑	D	N	N
75	73,F	3.5	25	180	. . .	. . .	+	0	N	N	LS	↑	D	↓	N
76 †	62,F	5.3	27	460	. . .	N	0	0	N	N	N	↑	D	↑	N
77 † §	62,F	4	32	385	N	N	+	0	↑	N	N	↑	D	N	N
78 §	65,M	5.8	26	300	N	N	0	0	↑	N	LS	↑	D	N	N
79 §	60,F	5.0	26	450	↓	N	0	0	N	N	N	↑	D	N	N
80	58,F	8.1	29	636	. . .	. . .	0	0	↑	N	N	↑	D	N	N
81 † §	94,M	7	28	132	↓	↑	0	0	↑	N	N	↑	D	N	N
Polycythemia Vera															
82	52,M	12	53	541	↑	. . .	0	0	↑	↑	N	↑	N	↑	N
83 †	68,M	19	45	314	. . .	. . .	+	+	↑	↑	N	↑	N	↑	N
84 †	62,M	22	59	1,120	↑	. . .	+	+	↑	↑	N	↑	N	↑	N
85	61,M	9.5	50	508	N	. . .	+	+	N	N	N	N	N	N	N
86	58,M	15.6	49	663	. . .	. . .	+	0	↑	↑	N	↑	N	↑	N
87 †	59,M	14	60	607	N	N	+	0	↑	↑	N	↑	N	↑	N
88 †	42,M	7.8	46	245	. . .	. . .	+	+	N	↑	N	↑	N	↑	N
89 † §	63,M	7.2	62	355	↑	. . .	0	0	↑	N	N	↑	N	↑	N
90 §	74,F	20	51	410	N	N	+	0	↑	↑	N	↑	N	↑	N
91 §	63,F	8.9	56	383	↑	N	0	0	↑	↑	LS	↑	N	↑	N
92 §	61,F	9.5	33	24	↑	↑	+	+	N	↑	LS	N	N	↓	N
Essential Thrombocythemia															
93 †	46,F	7.5	36	1,600	↓	N	+	0	↑	↑	N	↑	N	↑	N
94	52,M	10.3	36	1,198	. . .	N	+	0	↑	↑	N	↑	N	↑	N

NOTE: Qt = quantitative. Ql = qualitative. LAP = leukocyte alkaline phosphatase. ↑ = increased. ↓ = decreased. PM = poor maturation. N = normal. LS = left-shifted granulopoiesis. DL = decreased late granulopoiesis. D = dysplastic maturation. D* = abnormal mononuclear cells (see text).

*Data obtained at time of initial in vitro study.

† Per cent light-density colony-forming cells determined (see Figure 4).

‡ Ringed sideroblasts present in patients in these groups.

§ Urinary colony-stimulating factor output determined (see Figures 5 and 6).

REFERENCES

1. Dameshek W: Some speculations on the myeloproliferative syndromes. Blood 6: 372, 1951.
2. Gilbert HS, Dameshek W: The myeloproliferative disorders. DM p 43, 1970.
3. Gilbert HS: A reappraisal of the "myeloproliferative disease" concept. J Mt Sinai Hosp 37: 426, 1970.
4. Ward H, Block M: The natural history of agnogenic myeloid metaplasia and a critical evaluation of its relationship with the myeloproliferative syndrome. Medicine (Baltimore) 50: 357, 1971.
5. Rickard KA, Morley A, Howard D, et al.: The in vitro colony forming cell and the response to neutropenia. Blood 37: 6, 1971.
6. Morley A, Rickard KA, Howard D, et al.: Studies on the regulation of granulopoiesis. IV. Possible humoral regulation. Blood 37: 14, 1971.
7. Metcalf D, Stanley ER: Haematological effects on mice of partially purified colony stimulating factor (CSF) prepared from human urine. Br J Haematol 21: 481, 1971.
8. Greenberg P, Schrier S: Clinical utility of in vitro evaluation of granulopoiesis. Ann Rev Med 25: 269, 1974.
9. Pike B, Robinson W: Human bone marrow colony growth in agar-gel. J Cell Physiol 76: 77, 1970.
10. Greenberg PL, Nichols WC, Schrier SL: Granulopoiesis in acute myeloid leukemia and preleukemia. N Engl J Med 284: 1225, 1971.
11. Bull J, Duttera M, Stashick E, et al.: Serial in vitro marrow culture in acute myelocytic leukemia. Blood 42: 679, 1973.
12. Senn J, Pinkerton P: Defective in vitro colony formation by human bone marrow preceding overt leukemia. Br J Haematol 23: 277, 1972.
13. Moore M, Spitzer G, Williams N, et al.: Agar culture studies in 127 cases of untreated acute leukemia. Blood 44: 1, 1974.
14. Moore M, Williams N, Metcalf D: In vitro colony formation by normal and leukemic human hemopoietic cells. Characterization of the colony forming cells. J Natl Cancer Inst 50: 603, 1973.
15. Foster R, Metcalf D, Robinson WA, et al.: Bone marrow colony-stimulating activity in human sera. Results of two independent surveys in Buffalo and Melbourne. Br J Haematol 15: 147, 1968.
16. Metcalf D, Chan SH, Gunz FW, et al.: Colony stimulating factor and inhibitor levels in acute granulocytic leukemia. Blood 38: 143, 1971.
17. Greenberg PL, Schrier SL: Granulopoiesis in neutropenic disorders. Blood 41: 753, 1973.
18. Greenberg PL, Bax I, Mara B, et al.: Alterations of granulopoiesis following chemotherapy. Blood 44: 375, 1974.
19. Stanley ER, Metcalf D, Maritz J, et al.: Standardized bioassay for bone marrow colony stimulating factor in human urine. J Lab Clin Med 79: 657, 1972.
20. Embury S, Hood C, Greenberg PL, et al.: Maintenance chemotherapy. Effect on length of complete remission in acute myelogenous leukemia. Proceedings of the American Society of Hematology meeting, Atlanta, December 1974, p 102.
21. Gunz FW, Baikie AC: Leukemia, 3rd ed, New York, Grune & Stratton, 1974, pp 327, 377.
22. Gunz FW, Baikie AC: Ibid, p 330.
23. Schwartz J, Canellos G: Hydroxyurea in the management of the hematologic complications of chronic granulocytic leukemia. Blood 46: 11, 1975.
24. Rheingold J, Kaufman R, Adelson E, et al.: Smoldering acute leukemia. N Engl J Med 268: 812, 1963.
25. Sexauer J, Kass L, Schnitzer B: Subacute myelomonocytic leukemia. Am J Med 57: 853, 1974.
26. Knospe WH, Gregory SA: Smoldering acute leukemia. Clinical and cytogenetic studies in six patients. Arch Intern Med 127: 910, 1971.
27. Block CA, Jacobson LO, Bethard WF: Preleukemic acute leukemia. JAMA 152: 1018, 1953.
28. Saarni M, Linman J: Preleukemia. The hematologic syndrome preceding acute leukemia. Am J Med 55: 38, 1973.
29. Smith W, Ablin A, Goodman J, et al.: Atypical megakaryocytes in the preleukemic phase of AML. Blood 42: 535, 1973.
30. Fisher W, Armentrout S, Weisman R, et al.: "Preleukemia." A myelodysplastic syndrome often terminating in acute leukemia. Arch Intern Med 132: 226, 1973.
31. Schwartz S, Critchlow J: Erythremic myelosis (Di Guglielmo's disease). Blood 7: 765, 1952.
32. Scott R, Ellison R, Ley A: A clinical study of twenty cases of erythroleukemia (Di Guglielmo's syndrome). Am J Med 37: 162, 1964.
33. Gilbert H, Dameshek W: op cit, p 23.
34. Gunz F, Baikie AC: op cit, p 404.
35. Eastman P, Schwartz R, Schrier S: Distinctions between idiopathic ineffective erythropoiesis and Di Guglielmo's disease. Clinical and biochemical differences. Blood 40: 487, 1972.
36. Dacie JV, Smith M, White J, Mollin D: Refractory normoblastic anemia. A clinical and haematological study of seven cases. Br J Haematol 5: 56, 1959.
37. Kushner J, Lee G, Wintrobe M, et al.: Idiopathic refractory sideroblastic anemia. Medicine (Baltimore) 50: 139, 1971.
38. Goldman J, Th'ng K, Lowenthal R: In vitro colony forming cells and colony stimulating factor in chronic granulocytic leukemia. Br J Cancer 30: 1, 1974.
39. Moore M, Spitzer G: In vitro studies in the myeloproliferative disorders. 8th Leukocyte Culture Conference (Lindahl Kiessling K, ed), New York, Academic Press, 1974, p 431.
40. Metcalf D, Moore M, Sheridan J, et al.: Responsiveness of human granulocytic leukemic cells to colony-stimulating factor. Blood 43: 847, 1974.
41. Metcalf D: Human leukemia: recent tissue culture studies on the nature of myeloid leukemia. Br J Cancer 27: 191, 1973.
42. Metcalf D, Moore M: Growth and responsiveness of human granulocytic leukemic cells in vitro. Bibl Haematol 40: 235, 1975.

Mediastinal Irradiation for Chronic Lymphocytic Leukemia

ARTHUR SAWITSKY, M.D.
KANTI R. RAI, M.D.
ISAMETTIN ARAL, M.D.
RICHARD T. SILVER, M.D.
ARVIN S. GLICKSMAN, M.D.
ROBERT W. CAREY, M.D.
SALVATORE SCIALLA, M.D.
C. J. CORNELL, Jr., M.D.
BARBARA SELIGMAN, M.D.
LORNE SHAPIRO, M.D.
For Cancer and Leukemia Group B
New Hyde Park, New York

Thirty-one patients with chronic lymphocytic leukemia were treated with mediastinal radiation. In none of the patients was complete remission achieved; either partial remission or clinical improvement was achieved in 52 per cent, but the duration of response was short. The response rate was 77 per cent for the patients receiving a total radiation dose greater than 3,000 rads and 45 per cent for those receiving less than 3,000 rads. Severe life-threatening toxicity was noted in 11 patients and seven of these patients died; two patients died with progressive disease. Severe toxicity was manifested by one or more of the following: bone marrow aplasia, pancytopenia, gram-negative sepsis, generalized herpes zoster and severe esophagitis. Neither the total dose of radiation nor the dose per week correlated with the severity of reaction or death.

Richards et al. [1] have reported that "thymic" irradiation administered to patients with active chronic lymphocytic leukemia resulted in a partial or full response in 21 of a total of 22 patients. Richards et al. noted that in general the treatment was well tolerated; a few patients exhibited a mild, transient dysphagia, nausea, vomiting and cough. Eight institutional members (Appendix I) of the Cancer and Leukemia Group B (CALGB) collaborated in a study to test the effectiveness of "thymic" (we prefer the term "mediastinal") irradiation. Preliminary results, suggesting a high incidence of life-threatening toxicity and treatment-associated deaths, prompt a word of caution at this time.

METHODS AND MATERIALS

Patients with chronic lymphocytic leukemia manifesting active and/or progressive disease were chosen at the discretion of the senior investigators at each participating institution for treatment with mediastinal irradiation. All patients were treated with mega voltage irradiation to the mediastinum as described by Richards et al. [1]. No patient had previously received radiation to this area.

APPENDIX I Collaborating Institutions (CALGB)

Institution	No. of Patients
Long Island Jewish-Hillside Medical Center	8
New York Hospital-Cornell Medical Center	5
Rhode Island Hospital	5
Massachusetts General Hospital	4
Walter Reed Army Medical Center	4
Dartmouth Medical School	2
Jewish Hospital of Brooklyn	2
Royal Victoria Hospital-Montreal	2

This investigation was supported by the following grants from the National Cancer Institute: CA 11028, CA 07968, CA 08025, CA 12449, CA 04326, CA 12886, and by grants from the Helena Rubinstein Foundation, the National Leukemia Association, Inc. and the United Leukemia Fund, Inc. Requests for reprints should be addressed to Dr. Arthur Sawitsky, Long Island Jewish-Hillside Medical Center, New Hyde Park, New York 11040. Manuscript accepted August 18, 1976.

TABLE I Mediastinal Radiation

		Clinical Response			Degree of Toxicity		Deaths	
	No.	Partial Remission	Clinical Improvement	No Response	1+ to 2+	3+ to 4+	Toxic	Progressive Disease
All patients	31	9	8	14	6	11	7	2
No previous Rx	5	2	1	2	3	2	1	0
Previous Rx	26	7	7	12	3	9	6	2
Male	23	8	5	10	5	9	6	2
Female	8	1	3	4	1	2	1	0
Under age 60 yr	17	6	4	7	4	7	4	1
Over age 60 yr	14	3	4	7	2	4	3	1
Clinical stage 1 + 2	15	6	5	4	3	3	1	0
Clinical stage 3 + 4	16	3	3	10	3	8	6	2
Radiation therapy								
Rads/wk								
<800	18	6	6	6	3	6	3	0
>800	13	3	2	8	3	5	4	2
Total dose (rads)								
<3,000	18	4	4	10	2	10	7	1
>3,000	13	5	4	4	4	1	0	1

NOTE: Rx = therapy.

The characteristics of the 32 patients entered into the study are given in Table I. One patient was dropped from analysis because of insufficient data. The criteria for staging of chronic lymphocytic leukemia in these patients were those described by Rai et al. [2].

The criteria of response were as follows: Complete remission is defined as complete disappearance of all objective and subjective evidence of the disease (as in CALGB criteria, December 1969). Partial remission status was achieved with fulfillment of all the following criteria: (1) hemoglobin level maintained above 12 g/100 ml (males) and 11 g/100 ml (females), (2) platelets above 100,000/mm^3, (3) blood lymphocyte count less than 15,000/mm^3, (4) neutrophils above 2,000/mm^3, (5) reduction in the size of the spleen and nodes (if originally enlarged) to at least 50 per cent of the status before treatment and (6) significant diminution of all symptoms. Clinical improvement is defined as a reduction in the blood lymphocyte count to less than 15,000/mm^3, with a reduction in node and spleen size if initially enlarged, and diminution in the symptoms. Those patients in whom clinical improvement was not achieved were considered nonresponders.

RESULTS AND COMMENTS

In no patient was complete remission achieved, and 52 per cent of the patients showed partial remission or clinical improvement. All the responses were reported to be short, but the range in weeks could not be computed. Patients who had stages 1 and 2 disease had a response rate of 73 per cent as compared to those whose disease was in stages 3 and 4 who had a response rate of 37 per cent. The response rate was 77 per cent for the patients receiving a total radiation dose greater than 3,000 rads and 45 per cent for those receiving less than 3,000 rads (Table I).

Of great concern, however, was the finding of severe life-threatening toxicity in 11 of the 31 patients. More severe toxicity was found in patients with stage 4 disease (thrombocytopenia) than in those whose disease was in other clinical stages. Although 90 per cent of the severe toxicity occurred in previously treated patients, life-threatening toxicity was also noted in two of five patients not previously treated. Treatment-associated deaths occurred in seven patients (22.5 per cent). All the deaths were in males; all but one had received previous chemotherapy, but none had received previous radiation therapy. In two patients radiation pneumonitis developed; one of these patients died. The clinical data and course of the 11 patients who experienced severe toxicity are given in Table II. Two patients died in complete bone marrow aplasia, one patient died after the development of leukopenia with overwhelming gram-negative sepsis, and one patient died with generalized herpes zoster, first detected one week after completion of mediastinal radiation. Other types of severe toxicity included severe and prolonged esophagitis in one patient, thrombocytopenia in six patients, anemia in four patients, leukopenia in four patients and life-threatening infection in five patients. Neither the total dose of radiation nor the dose per week correlated with the severity of reaction or death.

TABLE II Clinical Data and Course in Patients with Severe Toxicity

							Hematologic Data		
							Pretreatment Values		
Case No.	Age (yr) and Sex	Date Dx	Previous Therapy and Date of Last Treatment	Clinical Stage at Time of This Treatment	Date Mediastinal Radiation Begun	Port Size (cm), Total Dose (rads)	Hemoglobin (g/100 ml)	White Blood Cells (per mm³)	Platelets (per mm³)
1	68,F	July 1974	CLB Pred 12/7/74	4	12/26/74	18 × 10 450/3 wk	11.0	177,000	50,000
2	70,M	1972	Splenectomy 2/75 CLB Pred 5/20/75	3	6/30/75	18 × 8 1,200/7 days	9.0	300,000	240,000
3	57,M	1970	CLB	4	3/27/75	14 × 10 2,700/4 wk	8.5	43,000	70,000
4	62,F	1968	CLB	2	2/14/75	15 × 9 2,600/4 wk	13.0	36,000	125,000
5	62,M	1970	Pred CLB Cytoxan® 8/21/75	4	8/27/75	17 × 10 2,400/3+ wk	4.5	200,000	60,000
6	59,M	1974	None	4	7/31/75	15 × 10 1,980/2+ wk	10.0	30,000	100,000
7	54,M	1971	CLB Pred 3/21/75	2	3/27/75	16 × 10 2,625/3 wk	11.0	140,000	200,000
8	57,M	Oct 1970	CLB Pred 7/21/75	4	8/19/75	17 × 10 2,000/3 wk	9.0	103,000	100,000
9	55,M	March 1974	CLB Pred 2/27/75	2	3/27/75	17 × 10 2,800/3 wk	10.0	110,000	130,000
10	50,M	1971	CLB 7/19/75	4	8/6/75	16 × 10 1,000/2 wk	9.0	54,400	30,000
11	45,M	1970	CLB 4/8/75	4	4/14/75	16 × 10 3,100/6 wk	10.5	80,000	60,000

NOTE: CLB = chlorambucil; Pred = prednisone; AIHA = autoimmune hemolytic anemia, direct and indirect antiglobulin test positive.

Hematologic Data					
Nadir of Values					
Hemoglobin (g/100 ml)	White Blood Cells (per mm^3)	Platelets (per mm^3)	Toxicity	Remarks	Results
8.3	100,000	10,000	Severe sepsis	No decrease in liver or spleen size	No response, death 1/15/75
9.0	3,420	200,000	Sepsis, agranulocytosis	Role of splenectomy?	No response, death 7/18/75
11.0	14,400	45,000	Radiation pneumonitis	Decrease in nodes, spleen	No response, death
10.0	10,700	120,000	Radiation pneumonitis	Steroid, recovered	No response
Transfusion	7,700	20,000	Sepsis	Positive blood culture Esch. coli, Klebsiella, pseudomonas	No response, death 10/8/75
6.5	0,700	30,000	Esophagitis, sepsis, aplasia	Nodes and spleen to normal	No response, death 10/8/75
11.0	5,000	100,000	Severe and prolonged esophagitis	AIHA, excellent hematologic recovery	Poor response
9.0	50,000	30,000	Systemic herpes zoster	Onset 1 wk after completion of radiotherapy	No response, death 10/7/75
6.0	10,000	10,000	Mild esophagitis	Postmortem mycelial esophagitis	No response, death
6.0	14,700	12,000	Persistent anemia and thrombopenia 5+ months	Spleen size decreased, nodes not palpable	Improved
Transfusion X 6	18,000	20,000	Severe marrow hypoplasia	Persistent thrombopenia	No response

The high incidence of severe toxicity and treatment-associated deaths in patients with chronic lymphocytic leukemia undergoing mediastinal radiation suggests that caution must be exercised in the selection of such patients for this type of treatment. This is particularly true for patients who are anemic and/or thrombocytopenic, and for patients who have had previous chemotherapy.

REFERENCES

1. Richards FT, Spurr CL, Pajak TF, et al.: Thymic Irradiation: an approach to chronic lymphocytic leukemia. Am J Med 57: 862, 1974.
2. Rai KR, Sawitsky A, Cronkite EP, et al.: Clinical staging of chronic lymphocytic leukemia. Blood 46: 218, 1975.

Are Agents Affecting Platelet Functions Clinically Useful?

M. VERSTRAETE, M.D.
Leuven, Belgium

Many studies have been performed recently on the usefulness of drugs affecting platelet functions in the prevention of arterial and venous thrombosis. This work is reviewed here and some clinical recommendations are made.

Unbalanced activation of coagulation factors (sometimes referred to as hypercoagulability) and stasis are the key factors leading to most instances of a venous thrombosis, not changes or injury of the venous wall. A typical venous thrombus contains an alternating area of platelet aggregates and fibrin; platelet mass adhering to the vessel wall, mainly in the valve pocket, is limited [1]. The platelets are aggregated by the local generation of thrombin; drugs which impede the formation or concentration of this enzyme, such as heparin and coumarins, respectively, are effective clinical agents for preventing venous thrombosis and pulmonary embolism.

In contrast, thrombi in arteries tend to occur at sites of endothelial damage or on prosthetic surfaces; the interaction of platelets with the arterial wall and their adherence to each other are the first of a series of events leading to the formation of an arterial thrombus. This initial platelet nidus plays a major and possibly trigger role, and is not adequately prevented by the oral administration of anticoagulants. The question at issue is whether drugs that affect platelet function can prevent the interaction of platelets with the arterial wall, and subsequent macrothrombosis and microembolization from these sites.

Numerous substances impede the aggregation of human platelets. It is surprising that dipyridamole and other pyrimido-pyrimidine compounds have no effect on the bleeding time or on tests of platelet aggregation after in vivo ingestion of the drug, but they do reduce platelet adhesiveness to glass-bead columns in certain patients [2–5]. Aspirin has no effect on decreased platelet survival [6–9], but it clearly prolongs the bleeding time; it suppresses platelet aggregation with collagen and adrenaline (second wave), and aggregation by ADP becomes reversible [10,11]; its effect on platelet-adhesiveness is not clear cut [12]. Sulfinpyrazone also normalizes decreased platelet survival and reduces platelet glass adhesiveness, but it affects neither the bleeding time in man nor the collagen-induced platelet aggregation and the release reaction after in vivo ingestion of the drug [13,14]. This suggests that sulfinpyrazone acts on the vessel wall rather than on the platelets themselves. The administration of clofibrate can prolong a shortened platelet survival [15] and decrease "ex vivo" the adhesiveness of platelets to glass [16]. Also, the glucose polymers, dextrans, seem to have little effect on platelet function in vitro, and their in vivo activity may result from reduced platelet adhesiveness

From the Medical Research Department, Laboratory Blood Coagulation, University of Leuven, Belgium. Requests for reprints should be addressed to Dr. M. Verstraete, Laboratorium Bloedstolling, Capucijnenvoer 35, B-3000 Leuven, Belgium. Manuscript accepted January 30, 1976.

and impaired release reaction and aggregation due to retarded platelet-surface interaction [17]. After the infusion of low-molecular weight dextran, decreased levels of factor VIII, fibrinogen and factor V and IX have been described [18]. The lysability of thrombi formed after the infusion of dextran is increased, but there is no effect after the addition of dextran in vivo [19,20].

DRUGS INHIBITING PLATELET FUNCTION AND PERIPHERAL ARTERIAL DISEASE

Platelet survival studies were performed in patients with recurrent arterial thrombosis or prosthetic aortofemoral grafts; they were repeated during treatment with one of four drug combinations: dipyridamole (0.4 g), aspirin (4 g), and the combination of dipyridamole (0.1 or 0.4 g) and aspirin (1.2 g) daily. Except for aspirin, all these drug regimens were able to normalize platelet survival in this group of patients [7]. Surprisingly, in other syndromes associated with arterial occlusions (thrombotic thrombocytopenic purpura, hemolytic uremic syndrome), steroids also (1 to 2 mg prednisone/kg/day) corrected platelet survival toward normal [7]. These results do not demonstrate the clinical usefulness of these drugs.

The antithrombotic protective value of aspirin was tested in patients after brachial arteriotomy for coronary arteriography [21]. Two doses of aspirin were used (0.325 g and 0.650 g) and given once the night before catheterization. The aspirin had no effect on the incidence of either thrombus formation or pulse rate reduction (admitted by a less specific end-point) after catheterization, but the administration of oral anticoagulants was capable of reducing both. The number of cases was too small to show a more potent antithrombotic effect with anticoagulants plus aspirin than with either drug on its own. Another randomized trial also failed to show a beneficial effect of aspirin (15 mg/kg/day) after catheterization in children [22].

A larger dose of aspirin (1.5 g/day) was used in a controlled trial in patients with diabetic angiopathy. Over a two year period a significant reduction of the vascular occlusion rate from 40 per cent in 50 control patients to 16 per cent in 50 patients treated with aspirin was noted; the patients of the two groups were also treated with oral anticoagulants [23].

The evaluation of any treatment in patients with chronic obliterative disease of limb arteries is difficult indeed. The ultimate criterion for judging the efficacy of a new drug in modifying the natural course of the ailment is the clinical outcome among patients in a randomized clinical trial adequately performed and pursued over some years, and carefully interpreted. It is firmly hoped that the double-blind trials in patients with severe peripheral arterial insufficiency and the trials in patients subjected to surgical vascular repair, which are presently being conducted with aspirin alone or in combination with dipyridamole, will comply with the stringent rules of clinical pharmacology.

ESTABLISHED CEREBRAL VASCULAR DISEASE

Vascular disease of the brain is the third leading cause of death after coronary artery disease and hypertensive cardiovascular disease. No major advance in the treatment of permanent stroke has been made in the last decades. It is now well established that the prodromal symptoms of transient cerebral ischemia are often caused by emboli from atheromatous ulcers located in the carotid arteries [24–27]. Because these ulcers are often shallow or filled with platelets and other elements, they may not be visible on angiograms. The causal relationship between platelet emboli and transient ischemic attacks suggested that an attempt to decrease their incidence with drugs suppressing platelet function might be successful.

The results of the first controlled prospective double-blind trials were disappointing: the incidence of transient neurologic episodes, stroke or death during treatment with dipyridamole (0.4 or 0.8 g daily for an average period of 11 months) or placebo was similar [28]. The administration of clofibrate (1.5 g daily for 60 months) did not affect the incidence of further episodes of cerebral ischemia or the mortality rate in 47 patients with focal cerebral vascular disease [29]. One study was suggestive of a favorable effect of an agent affecting platelet function: in a double-blind cross-over study on 20 patients with transient ischemic attacks, the administration of sulfinpyrazone (0.8 g daily for six weeks) was shown to decrease the number of amaurosis attacks significantly (50 per cent reduction) compared with the placebo period [30]. Using the same drug, Blakely et al. [31] carried out a double-blind trial in 291 elderly men who had survived a stroke (0.6 g sulfinpyrazone daily for four years). A statistically significant reduction in terms of mortality due to cardiovascular causes was found only in that subgroup of patients who already had clinical evidence of arterial disease at entry to the study. In another prospective trial carried out on 450 geriatric patients, the effect of aspirin (1 g daily for one year) was compared to that of placebo; there was no evidence of any prophylactic effect on the thromboembolic-arteriosclerotic diseases of either the coronary or the cerebral arteries [32]. Less weight can be given to a retrospective study [33] and to isolated case studies, also performed with aspirin with similar conclusions, suggesting that aspirin decreased the incidence of transient ischemic attacks [34,35].

In conclusion, it can be said that these trials have so far generated more questions than answers, leaving the issues unsettled at present. In the Canadian Cooperative

Study of Recurrent Cerebral Emboli (RRPCE), sulfinpyrazone, aspirin, the two drugs together, or placebo are used [36]. The objectives of this trial are to determine whether the drugs used significantly reduce the frequency of cerebral ischemic attacks, prevent strokes or increase survival. The effect of aspirin alone is being tested in two separate double-blind clinical trials. One is being performed in America in surgical and nonsurgical patients with transient cerebral ischemia who are receiving 1.3 g aspirin or placebo/day (AITIA study). In France, a large scale trial is underway to determine whether aspirin or aspirin and dipyridamole are more effective in preventing transient ischemic attacks when used in combination with hydrogenated ergot alkaloids (Hydergine®) than when the latter is used alone [37].

CORONARY ARTERY DISEASE

Among other drugs, anticoagulants and clofibrate have been tried to prevent the clinical counterparts of coronary artery disease. It is probably fair to say that long-term treatment with oral anticoagulants, when administered at the usual dosage, did not dramatically decrease progression of the disease. There was a significant reduction in mortality, especially in sudden deaths, and in nonfatal recurrence of myocardial infarction when clofibrate was given to patients with angina in two prospective secondary prevention trials with clofibrate [38,39]. Most surprising was that this beneficial effect did not correlate with the initial cholesterol level or its reduction; as clofibrate also affects platelet function it was suggested that the latter effect may be related to the clinical gain [40]. It must, however, be realized that the role of platelets in the pathogenesis of a myocardial infarction is still unclear; the chain of causality not being established. Moreover, the results mentioned with clofibrate in patients who survived a myocardial infarction could not be confirmed by the Coronary Drug Project Research Group [41].

A clinical trial with dipyridamole was performed in 1968 in 103 patients with a recent myocardial infarction. This drug, administered in a daily dose of 0.4 g over one month, did not decrease the mortality rate or the incidence of thromboembolic complications [42]. Four other double-blind trials in patients with ischemic heart disease also failed to reveal a beneficial effect of dipyridamole therapy in coronary artery disease [43–46]. It should be emphasized that a small daily dose of 0.1 g dipyridamole was used in the latter trials.

Pathologists reported that patients with rheumatoid arthritis who might be expected to be aspirin takers had an exceedingly low incidence of myocardial infarction or cerebrovascular accidents [47]. A retrospective epidemiologic study also revealed a strong negative association between regular aspirin users and apparent signs of myocardial infarction [48], but this could not be confirmed in a similar study on 1,000,000 men and women followed for up to six years [49].

There is one report on aspirin given to a large number of patients over several years in which the incidence of coronary or cerebral thrombosis was surprisingly low; unfortunately, this retrospective study does not have a control group [50].

The outcome of patients who were discharged from the hospital after their first myocardial infarction was investigated by Elwood et al. [51] in a prospective study. The patients were instructed to take a rather small dose of aspirin (0.3 g) daily; after 30 months 1,239 patients had been admitted to the trial; fewer patients in the aspirin group died in the first 12 months, but the difference is not significant. It, therefore, seems reasonable to undertake prospective controlled trials with a larger dose of aspirin for the prophylaxis of ischemic heart disease. Similar double-blind, randomized studies are underway in middle-aged men who are either considered at high or moderate risk of ischemic heart disease or who suffer from unstable angina, and in patients who have survived a recent myocardial infarction.

It was shown in man that increased platelet turnover can be corrected by the administration of dipyridamole (0.4 g daily) alone and that this effect is potentiated by the administration of aspirin (1 g daily), which on its own has no effect on platelet utilization, even when used in larger doses (4 g daily) [6–8,11]. Groups are now studying the effect of dipyridamole and aspirin therapy in patients with angina who were shown to have a short platelet survival, in patients subjected to coronary artery surgery and in patients who survived a myocardial infarction (Persantin-Aspirin-Reinfarction Study or PARIS.).

It can be concluded that the published prospective trials with clofibrate, dipyridamole or aspirin in the primary or secondary prevention of myocardial infarction did not reveal a significant reduction of the morbidity or mortality in the experimental group. There was a positive trend in some trials in which a larger dose of either drug was used alone or the latter two used in combination, and this seems to be confirmed in some still unpublished trials. There is some evidence that patients with angina only may benefit from treatment with clofibrate. Apart from these results, no practical recommendations can at present be made and hard data are needed to prove the hypothesis that platelet affecting drugs protect against fatal or nonfatal infarction.

THROMBOEMBOLISM IN PATIENTS WITH PROSTHETIC HEART VALVES

In patients with valvular disease of the heart, the prevalence of thromboembolism is high, especially when the mitral valve is stenosed. Valvular repair improves the function of the heart, but patients who have been operated on are still susceptible to the complications of thrombosis and embolism despite long-term anticoagulation and often for a long time after surgery. Although it is true that the newer prosthetic materials used in the more recent valves are less frequently associated with systemic emboli than those previously used, it is now known that the surface area and shape of the poppet, the disc in the valve [6], but not the presence of hemolysis [14,52] are contributing factors to thrombosis. It is also likely that a more intensive treatment with oral anticoagulants would result in a more efficient antithrombotic protection, but at the cost of frequent and accurate checking of the anticoagulation obtained and probably with a higher incidence of bleeding. Another drawback is that oral anticoagulants are known to be potentially teratogenic in the first weeks of pregnancy; this constitutes a problem in young women with cardiac valve replacement who wish to become pregnant [53].

In fact, before platelet survival studies were routinely performed, Sullivan et al. [54] had already shown in a controlled study that dipyridamole (0.4 g/day) given in addition to warfarin resulted in a greater protection against thromboembolism than anticoagulation alone. The same investigators later confirmed their initial findings: 14.3 per cent of 84 patients with prosthetic valves who were treated with anticoagulants had, one year after surgery, clinical evidence of arterial emboli compared to 1.3 per cent of 79 patients who, in addition to receiving oral anticoagulants, received 0.4 g of dipyridamole daily; there was no difference in mortality between the two groups [55]. The superiority of oral anticoagulants and dipyridamole over anticoagulants alone was also reported in two other controlled trials [56,57].

It was surprising to find that although results of glass-bead retention tests and aggregation of platelets to ADP and collagen are normal, platelet turnover is increased in patients with old style prosthetic heart valves, but not with homograft valves [58], and the newer Starr-Edwards prosthesis model 6,000 [59,62]. Shortened platelet survival in these patients can be brought to normal either by the administration of sulfinpyrazone (provided 0.8 g daily is given) [14,60,61], dipyridamole (0.4 g daily) [6] or aspirin plus dipyridamole [65,66] but not by aspirin alone (even 4 g daily) [6,7,63]. These results still leave open the issue of whether a reduced platelet survival is caused by the thrombotic consumption of platelets or whether it indicates a predisposition to thrombosis.

It was important to investigate whether platelet survival time can predict the likelihood of systemic emboli in patients with substituted valves. Weily et al. [60] found that patients with short platelet survival have a 45 per cent incidence of thromboembolism compared to a 7 per cent incidence in those with normal platelet survival. Further studies of the same group demonstrated that in patients with mitral valve disease the incidence of preoperative thromboembolism correlates well with postoperative platelet survival time [64]. The mean postoperative platelet survival in 14 patients without previous thromboembolism was 6.8 days and in those with preoperative thromboembolism 5.0 days; this difference is significant. Also, after the insertion of a substitute valve there was a close correlation between the reduction of platelet survival and the incidence of thromboembolism [60]. Patients with severe rheumatic heart disease have an increased number of megathrombocytes (i.e., evidence for shortened platelet survival) which returns to normal after valve substitution [65]. If these findings are further confirmed, patients with shortened platelet survival would constitute a subgroup in which prophylactic therapy may be particularly indicated prior to as well as after cardiac surgery.

Prospective trials in a large group of patients with prosthetic heart valves observed for a long period are presently investigating the effectiveness of sulfinpyrazone, aspirin or aspirin combined with oral anticoagulants in preventing thromboembolism.

DRUGS INHIBITING PLATELET FUNCTION IN RENAL DISEASES

Fibrin thrombi, platelet aggregates and subendothelial deposits have been demonstrated in glomerulonephritis, more particularly of the proliferative mesangioproliferative type, but also in active lipid nephrosis and in the nephrotic syndromes due to other causes [66–68]. These findings have prompted the use of anticoagulants in patients with acute and chronic glomerulonephritis. Heparin was often the agent of choice because, in addition to its antithrombotic property, it also has antibody eluting action and can also block, at a certain dose, C'3 activity; an interesting feature as the complement-fixing antigen-antibody reaction is held responsible for part of the tissue destruction [69,70].

Most of the reports on anticoagulants and drugs inhibiting platelet function, used alone or combined with immunosuppressive agents in patients with renal diseases, concern isolated cases or are retrospective and largely uncontrolled trials [71–75].

Aspirin has been used in a prospective double-blind cross-over trial in 12 patients with idiopathic nephrosis (who were maintained on steroid treatment) and 27 patients with proliferative glomerulonephritis [76]. Placebo or aspirin (15 mg/kg/day) was administered at random during 16 weeks and then the alternate drug was used. Despite unequivocal evidence of suppression of platelet aggregation during aspirin treatment, there were no statistically significant changes in the clinical course or laboratory parameters suggesting a favorable change in glomerular function.

A randomized blind trial in patients with membranous or mesangiocapillary glomerulonephritis is presently being performed. The objective of this trial is to compare the effectiveness of combined cyclophosphamide, dipyridamole (0.4 g/day) and warfarin therapy with no treatment, on renal function, microscopic appearance of the kidney and mortality rate; the preliminary results appear to be very encouraging [77].

THE ROLE OF ANTIPLATELET DRUGS ON REJECTION OF ORGAN TRANSPLANTS

The initial description of thrombosis of small cortical vessels and cortical necrosis in immediate renal allograft rejection was first reported by Porter et al. [78], and this form of platelet deposition and intravascular coagulation have been amply confirmed since [79–85]. Why platelets aggregate in immediate rejection is uncertain. It is known that platelets aggregate on antigen-antibody complexes, and the release of vasoactive agents and lysozymes from the platelets may cause vascular disruption resulting in rejection; fibrin deposition is probably a secondary and later process.

In dogs, presensitized by several skin grafts, heparin treatment improved the function of cadaveric renal transplants [86,87]. This anticoagulant had to be administered immediately at the reestablishment of the arterial blood supply to the allograft kidney to avoid thrombotic lesions in the graft and hyperimmune rejection; a more delayed heparin administration offered, in this experimental model, no protection.

Although aspirin used in large doses (2.4 g) in presensitized dogs could delay the onset of hyperimmune rejection [87] and reduce the incidence of fibrinoid necrosis of medium-sized vessels, there was no significant difference in survival times between the group given aspirin and the control group of presensitized dogs [88]. Using sulfinpyrazone in the same experimental model, immediate rejection was prevented in the treated dogs, but the renal transplants were later rejected by primary cellular rejection [89]. In pigs, the administration of dextran 60 delayed rejection of dog xenografts [90]; also Claes [91], using dextran 70 in dogs, demonstrated promising results similar to those obtained by him previously with cyproheptadine, a deaggregating agent having few side effects. Also, the administration of a combination of aspirin and dextran produced a significantly longer survival of xenogeneic kidney graft in dogs than the use of either aspirin or dextran alone [92].

The present prevention of rejection in transplant recipients with the use of steroids and immunosuppressive drugs is full of complications (e.g., peptic ulcer, tuberculosis and neoplasia); therefore, newer approaches are being sought. Moreover, it is gradually becoming recognized that arterial thrombosis is a more frequent and often fatal event in renal allograft patients than in the population at large [93–96]. Coronary and cerebral arterial thrombosis occur more often in the early post-transplantation period, suggesting that stress, immunosuppressive drugs and corticosteroid treatment are among the factors contributing to arterial thrombosis in a population already at high risk due to preexisting hypertension, hypertriglyceridemia and hyperparathyroidism. The prevention of thrombus formation with the use of antiaggregating agents may, therefore, not only improve the function of an allograft kidney, and for a longer period of time, but also be of benefit because of its retarding effect on the over-all thrombotic process in vital arteries [90,97,98]. Mathew et al. [99] have, over four years, allocated at random 45 transplant patients either to treatment or no treatment with a combination of dipyridamole and anticoagulants. In addition, all patients were receiving standard treatment with azathioprine and prednisone. Only two of 26 patients died of renal failure in the treated group followed for a mean of 33.5 months, versus five of 28 in the untreated group which was followed for a mean of 29.6 months; with larger numbers this difference in mortality could become significant. This study is still in progress; the blind gradings of glomerular and vessel lesion in regular renal biopsy specimens from these patients show a significant difference between the two groups, but there is no difference in interstitial changes. A prospective double-blind study is in progress to evaluate the effects of cyproheptadine on platelet function and renal rejection in man.

A preliminary report has been presented by Griepp et al. [100] who have followed 42 patients for three years after they received a heart transplant. Sixteen patients received only the usual immunosuppressive drugs, 26 patients received a combined treatment of immunosuppressive drugs, oral anticoagulants and dipyridamole. The patients who survived more than three months were considered at risk for atheromatosis and underwent either coronary angiography or postmortem examination. It appeared that the patients who received the combined drug regimen had a delay of coronary arteriosclerosis in the transplanted human heart.

DRUGS AFFECTING PLATELET FUNCTION IN THROMBOTIC THROMBOCYTOPENIC PURPURA AND HEMOLYTIC UREMIC SYNDROME

Thrombotic microangiopathy (Moschcowitz syndrome) and the hemolytic uremic syndrome (Gasser syndrome) differ in their long-term prognosis but have several characteristics in common; they also show glomerular and vascular lesions resembling those of graft rejection.

The pathogenesis of these and closely related disorders is still unknown; whether a vascular disease or a disorder of coagulation is the primary event has been debated for years. Among the numerous forms of therapy, anticoagulation at various levels of intensity, but in a limited number of patients, has also been instituted. The clinical responses to anticoagulation in each syndrome were variable as was supportive treatment and even the final diagnosis of the patients thus far treated.

So far, there is only suggestive evidence that inhibitors of platelet function used in association with other drugs may be of benefit in these patients [101–106].

TRIALS WITH DRUGS INHIBITING PLATELET FUNCTION IN POSTOPERATIVE DEEP VENOUS THROMBOEMBOLISM

Oral anticoagulants offer a certain protection against venous thrombosis and have been the mainstay in prophylaxis until low-dosage heparin therapy was recommended. Notwithstanding the high incidence of deep venous thrombosis in the postoperative state (circa 35 per cent as can be seen in the control groups, Tables I, II and III), and the risk of massive pulmonary embolism, most surgeons and obstetricians are unwilling to risk the possible bleeding complications of oral anticoagulants for the uncertain protection from venous thromboembolism. It is, therefore, not surprising that in the search for a safer agent, many clinical trials with antiaggregating drugs were performed in patients who were operated on [107,108]. It seems self-evident that a reduction of thrombosis in ileofemoral veins will be accompanied by a reduction of pulmonary embolism.

Tables I to III summarize the evidence so far available; only the published results of prospective, controlled trials are listed. Several of these trials were conducted in patients admitted for hip surgery, an operation known to carry a high risk of venous thromboembolism. The homogeneity of the group of patients subjected to hip surgery is only apparent; in some trials, mainly mold arthroplasty and femoral head replacement were performed; in others, total hip replacement. Moreover, there are important differences in the design and execution of all these trials, and it would therefore be unfair to give them all the same weight. In Table IA trials are shown in which the diagnosis of deep venous thrombosis was only ascertained by clinical signs and symptoms; Tables IB to III give the results of trials in which the effect of treatment was judged by radioactive fibrinogen scanning of the legs and/or phlebography.

These results must be viewed within the limitations of the technical problems of diagnosing deep venous thrombosis. It is not surprising that the isotopic diagnosis of deep vein thrombosis is about 10 times greater than

TABLE I Clinical Trials with Oral Drugs Inhibiting Platelet Function in Operated Patients

Source	Type of Surgery	Biometry	No. of Patients	Daily Dose/Administration Time	Deep Vein Thrombosis (%)	Pulmonary Embolism (%)	Mortality Due to Pulmonary Embolism (%)
A. Clinical Diagnosis of Deep Vein Thrombosis							
Browse et al. 1969 [109]	Major surgery	Double-blind	334	Placebo	2.1	0.6	. . .
		At random	315	Dipyridamole 0.4 g/11 days	3.8	0.3	. . .
Weber et al. 1971 [110]	Mainly operated patients (88%)	Open	448	Placebo	2.9	1.3	4
		Alternating	454	ASA 1.5 g/10 days	0.66*	0.6	. . .
Salzman et al. 1971 [111]	Vitalium, mold arthroplasty of the hip	Open	67	Previous control group	34.3	10.4	. . .
		At random	43	ASA 1.2 g/3 weeks	9.3	9.3	0
			34	Dipyridamole 0.4 g/3 weeks	17.6	8.8	0
			43	Warfarin	9.3*	4.6	0
			49	Dextran 40, 500 ml/4 days	10.2*	4.0	0
Harris et al. 1972 [112]	Total hip replacement	Open	114	Warfarin	2.6	5.3	0
		At random	113	Dextran 40, 500 ml/4 days	6.1	6.1	0
Zekert et al. 1974 [113]	Hip fracture	Double-blind	120	Placebo	14.1	11.6	6.6
		At random	120	ASA 1.5 g/14 days	5.8*	2.5	0.8
Loew et al. 1974 [114]	Any operation	Double-blind	527	Placebo	2.5	3.4	. . .
		At random	510	ASA 1.5 g/10 days	1.0*	1.2*	. . .
B. Detection of Deep Venous Thrombosis by Radioactive Fibrinogen Scanning or Phlebography							
Carter et al. 1971 [115]	Major surgery (phlebography)	At random	26	Placebo	23.0	5.6 of 281 patients	. . .

			28	Hydroxychloroquine 200 mg intravenously before operation and 8 hourly thereafter	0*	0.7 of 284 patients	. . .
O'Brien et al. 1971 [116]	Thoracotomy (fibrinogen scan)	Open	20	Placebo	65.0	. . .	. . .
		Not at random	19	ASA 0.6 g/5 days	74.6	. . .	. . .
			19	ASA 2.4 g/5 days	74.6	. . .	. . .
B.M.R.C. 1972 [117]	General surgery (fibrinogen scan)	Double-blind	150	Placebo	22.0	. . .	. . .
			153	ASA 0.6 g/5 days	27.5	. . .	. . .
O'Sullivan et al. 1972 [118]	Any operation (fibrinogen scan)	Open	75	Placebo	47.0	. . .	. . .
		At random	75	ASA 1 g + dipyridamole 0.1 g/7 days	17.5*	. . .	. . .
Parodi et al. 1973 [119]	Any operation (fibrinogen scan)	At random	22	Placebo	40.9	. . .	. . .
			19	Dipyridamole 0.45 g operative day and 0.15 g intravenously thereafter	21.1	. . .	. . .
			21	As in previous group but in addition ASA 1 g	9.5*	. . .	. . .
Wood et al. 1973 [120]	Femur fracture (fibrinogen scan)	Double-blind	9	Placebo	55.5	. . .	. . .
		At random	9	RA 233 0.75 g + ASA 0.6 g/14 days	77.7	. . .	. . .
			12	RA 233 0.75 g + placebo/14 days	83.3	. . .	. . .
Harris et al. 1974 [121]	Total hip replacement (phlebography)	At random	55	Warfarin	18.1*	0	. . .
			51	ASA 1.2 g day before operation/ambulation	36.0*	0	. . .
			61	Dextran 10%, 500 ml first 3 postoperative days; 3 days, subsequently alternate days	22.9*	3.2	. . .
			20	Heparin 10,000 U/day or 15,000 U/day subcutaneously	55.0	5	. . .
Carter et al. 1974 [122]	General surgery (fibrinogen scan) (phlebography)	At random	97	Controls	17.5	. . .	. . .
			107	Hydroxychloroquine 1.2 g before operation and 0.8 g daily until discharge	4.6	. . .	. . .
Clagett et al. 1975 [108]	General surgery (fibrinogen scan) (phlebography)	Double-blind	49	Placebo	20.4	. . .	. . .
		At random	56	ASA after operation 1.3 g/8 days	6.1*	. . .	. . .
Weiss et al. 1975 [123]	Mainly hysterectomy (fibrinogen scan)	Open	19	Controls	. . .	30.5	. . .
			36	Dipyridamole 0.225 g and ASA 1 g daily from 4th postoperative day	. . .	5.2*	. . .

NOTE: ASA = acetylsalycyclic acid; RA 233 = 2,6-bio(diethanolamino)-4-piperidinopyrimido-(5,4,-d) pyrimidine.

* $p < 0.05$.

TABLE II Clinical Trials with Dextran Detection of Deep Venous Thrombosis by Radioactive Scanning or Phlebography

Source	Type of Surgery	Biometry	No. of Patients	Daily Dose/Administration Time	Deep Vein Thrombosis (%)	Pulmonary Embolism (%)	Mortality Due to Pulmonary Embolism (%)
			A. General Surgery				
Jansen 1972 [126]	Major surgery (phlebography)	Double-blind	301	Glucose	9.9	...	1.3
		At random	304	Dextran 70, 500 ml during operation	5.9*	...	0.3
			296	Dextran 40, 500 ml during operation	4.4*	...	...
Carter et al. 1973 [127]	Major surgery (scanning)	At random	101	Dextrose-saline	9.9	...	...
			106	Dextran 70, 500 ml during and on alternate days after operation	0.9*	...	...
Stephenson et al. 1973 [128]	Major abdominal operation (scanning)	At random	46	Controls	35	10.8	...
			34	Dextran 70, 500 ml on 1st and 2nd day after operation	29	8.8	...
Becker et al. 1972 [129]	Cholecystectomy or transvesical prostatectomy (scanning and phlebography)	At random	35	Early ambulation	31.4	...	...
			39	Electrical stimulation of calf muscles during anesthesia	5.1	...	...
			42	Dextran 70, 500 ml immediately before operation and the day after	30.9	...	...
Edinburgh trial Ruckley 1974 [130]	Major operation (scanning)	At random	128	Controls	37	3.1	1.5
			128	Dextran 70, 500 ml before operation and the 1st and 2nd day after operation	25	2.3	0
			125	Heparin, 2,500 U before operation and 5,000 U twice daily (7 days)	12*	0.8	0
Kline et al. 1975 [124]	Elective surgery of stomach, colon, biliary system (scanning and phlebography)	Blind	435	Saline solution	26.4	3.0	1.6
		At random	396	Dextran 70, 1,000 ml at operation	21.3	0.8*	0.2*
Gruber 1975 [131]	General surgery (leg scanning)	Open	95	Controls	35.8	10.5	5.3
		At random	83	Heparin, 5,000 U 2 hours before operation and 12 hourly for 7 days	13.2*	7.2	7.2
			83	Dextran 40, 500 ml before and after operation and first 2 postoperative days	20.5*	7.2	1.2
			B. Gynecologic or Urologic Surgery				
Lambie et al. 1970 [132]	Gynecologic surgery (scanning)	At random	40	Warfarin	30.0	...	...
			40	Dextran 70, 10 ml/kg during operation and 3.5 ml/kg/day the first 3 postoperative days	10.0*	...	...
Davidson et al. 1972 [133]	Gynecologic surgery (scanning)	At random	30	Warfarin 36 hours before operation	13.3	...	...
			30	Dextran 70, 500 ml during operation and 250 ml daily the first two 24 hours after operation	10.0	...	...

Bonnar et al. 1972 [134]	Hysterectomy for benign conditions (scanning and phlebography)	Blind	140	Placebo	10.7	. . .	. . .
		At random	120	Dextran 70, 1,000 ml during operation	0.8*	. . .	. . .
Bonnar et al. 1973 [135]	Radical resection for malignant disease (scanning)	Blind	42	Placebo	33.0	. . .	. . .
		At random	20	Dextran 70, 1,000 ml during operation	5.0*	. . .	. . .
McCarthy et al. 1974 [136]	Gynecologic surgery (scanning)	At random	64	Heparin, 5,000 U subcutaneously before operation and 12 hourly for 7 days	10.9	1.5	. . .
			68	Dextran 70, 500 ml during and the day after operation	16.2	1.4	. . .
Hedlund 1975 [137]	Urologic operation (scanning)	Double-blind	40	Placebo injections (intravenously or subcutaneously), 12 hourly	45.0	. . .	. . .
		At random	38	Heparin, 10,000 U subcutaneously from 1st until 5th postoperative day	34.2	. . .	. . .
			37	Dextran 70, 10 ml/kg before operation and 250 ml on 1st, 3rd and 5th postoperative day	27.0	. . .	. . .

* p <0.05.

TABLE III Clinical Trials with Dextran in Orthopedic Patients. Detection of Deep Venous Thrombosis by Phlebography or/and Radioactive Scanning

Source	Type of Surgery	Biometry	No. of Patients	Daily Dose/Administration Time	Deep Vein Thrombosis (%)	Pulmonary Embolism (%)	Mortality Due to Pulmonary Embolism (%)
Johnsson 1968 [138]	Femoral neck fracture (phlebography)	Random binominal sequence	25	Saline solution	52.0	. . .	. . .
			27	Dextran 70, 500 ml during operation, first 2 days thereafter and every 3rd day	4.0*	. . .	. . .
Ahlberg 1968 [139]	Hip fracture (phlebography)	At random (?)	45	Saline solution	35.5	4.4	4.4
			39	Dextran 70, 500 ml during operation, and 2nd and 5th postoperative day	12.8*	0	0
Ahlberg 1969 [140]	Hip fracture (phlebography)	At random (?)	95	Saline solution	42.1	. . .	3.5
			70	Dextran 70, 500 ml before and 1st, 3rd, 5th and 7th postoperative day	18.5*	. . .	1.1
Myhre at al. 1969 [141]	Hip fracture (phlebography)	At random	55	Dextrose 10%	40	. . .	3.6
			50	Warfarin	18*	. . .	0
			55	Dextran 70, 500 ml at admission and approximately every 2nd day	20	. . .	0
Evarts et al. 1971 [142]	Elective hip surgery	Blind	36	Dextrose 5%	55.6	13.85	. . .
		Alternate	19	Dextran 40, 500 ml postoperatively	26.3*	10.5	. . .

(Continued)

TABLE III (Cont'd) Clinical Trials with Dextran in Orthopedic Patients. Detection of Deep Venous Thrombosis by Phlebography and/or Radioactive Scanning

Source	Type of Surgery	Biometry	No. of Patients	Daily Dose/Administration Time	Deep Vein Thrombosis (%)	Pulmonary Embolism (%)	Mortality Due to Pulmonary Embolism (%)
	(phlebography)			and daily for 10–12 days			
			31	Dextran 40, 1,000 ml pre- and post-operative and daily for 10 days	6.4*	0	...
Bronge et al. 1971 [143]	Femoral neck fracture (phlebography)	Year of birth	61	Oral anticoagulants	34.4	...	1.6
			74	Dextran 70, 500 ml during operation and 2nd, 4th and 6th postoperative day	36.5	...	2.7
Daniel et al. 1972 [144]	Femoral neck fracture (scanning)	At random	31	Dextrose 5%	61.3	...	...
			55	Dextran 70, 500 ml during and 3 subsequent days after operation	60.0	...	...
Bergquist et al. 1972 [145]	Femoral neck fracture (phlebography)	Year of birth	75	Oral anticoagulants	30.2	4.0	1.3
			63	Dextran 70, 500 ml before and every 2nd day after operation (3 times)	33.3	1.5	0
Myrvold et al. 1973 [146]	Femoral neck fracture (scanning and phlebography)	Year of birth	39	Heparin, 5,000 U subcutaneously, 12 hourly from admission until operative day; 10,000 U subcutaneously, 12 hourly the first 4 postoperative days and 5,000 U subcutaneously, 12 hourly the 5th to 7th postoperative day	41.0	...	...
			55	Dextran 70, 1 g/kg on admission and 500 ml every second day before and after operation until 6th postoperative day	36.3	...	...
Korvald et al. 1973 [147]	Hip fracture (phlebography)	At random	43	Dextran 70, 500 ml on admission, day of operation and 1st, 3rd and 5th day after	34.9	...	1
			39	Dextran 70, as above and warfarin-sodium	10.2*	...	0
Bergquist et al. 1973 [148]	Femoral neck fracture (scanning)	Year of birth	32	Oral anticoagulants	50.0	...	3.1
			43	Dextran 70, 500 ml before and every 2nd day after operation	44.2	...	0
Harris et al. 1974 [121]	Total hip replacement (phlebography)	At random	55	Oral anticoagulants	31.3*	0	...
			51	ASA 1.2 g/day before operation until ambulation	36.0*	0	...
			61	Dextran 40, 500 ml during operation and first 2 postoperative days, subsequently alternate days	25.0*	3.2	...
			20	Heparin, 10,000 U/day or 15,000 U/day subcutaneously until ambulation	55.0	5	...
Harper et al. 1973 [149]	Patients with leg amputation (phlebography)	Not stated	15	Saline solution	66.6	26.6	6.6
			12	Dextran 70, 500 ml after amputation and the 1st, 3rd and 5th postoperative day	0*	0	0

*p <0.05.

the clinical diagnosis. The reason is that the radiofibrinogen method detects even minor degrees of calf vein thrombosis. This was clearly demonstrated by Kline et al. [124] who found that 77 per cent of the patients without clinical signs of deep venous thrombosis had a positive scan, but also were shown to have phlebographic evidence of venous thrombosis. From necropsy studies and venography it is known that pulmonary embolism is related to thrombosis in the ileofemoral segments and that calf vein thrombosis has little clinical significance except in its relation to major vein thrombosis [125].

It is remarkable that in the six trials [109–114] in which the diagnosis of deep venous thrombosis in *general surgery* was made on clinical grounds only (Table IA), all four trials conducted with aspirin reveal a significant difference [110,111,113,114] but not the two trials performed with dipyridamole [109,111]. It is indeed known that aspirin prevents the synthesis and release of prostaglandins from platelets, and prostaglandins are known to be mediators of the inflammatory response. When the diagnosis was based on leg scanning (Table IB) the three trials using the combination aspirin plus dipyridamole appear to give significantly better results than placebo [118,119,123]; aspirin used alone in small or large doses (0.6 to 1.2 g/day) [116,117] or dipyridamole alone [119,120] appeared not to protect the patients adequately except in one trial with aspirin [100]. Hydroxychloroquine was tested in two trials and the incidence of deep vein thrombosis was significantly lower than in the placebo group [115,122]. In *orthopedic surgery,* when deep vein thrombosis was detected phlebographically, large doses of aspirin seem to be less effective than oral anticoagulants or dextran but superior to small doses of heparin [121].

Numerous trials have been carried out with the two commercial forms available of dextran; one with a mean molecular weight distribution of 40,000 (Rheomacrodex) and the other of 70,000 (Macrodex). Results in *general surgery* were evaluated on leg scanning or (and) phlebography and are not clearly in favor of dextran, as in four clinical trials dextran did not protect the patient significantly better than placebo [124,128–130]. In three trials dextran was significantly superior to placebo [126,127,131] (Table IIA).

In two trials comparing dextran and a placebo in *gynecologic surgery* there was a significant reduction of deep venous thrombosis as judged by leg scanning [134,135] and the protection offered by dextran or anticoagulants appeared to be better or similar in three other trials [132,133,136] (Table IIB). Only one trial has so far been conducted in urologic surgery, and it failed to show a significant reduction of deep vein thrombosis in the dextran group [137].

Table III lists the controlled clinical trials with dextran evaluating the incidence of postoperative deep vein thrombosis with phlebography in orthopedic patients. There appears to be a significant reduction of deep venous thrombosis in the eight trials in which the results in patients given dextran infusions were compared to those in an untreated control group [121,138–141,147,149]. In three other trials, the incidence of deep vein thrombosis in those treated with dextran was compared to that in an anticoagulated group and found to be similar [143,145,146]. No significant difference in positive radioscans of the legs of orthopedic patients was observed when dextran was compared to dextrose [144] or to oral anticoagulants [148].

At the moment it seems that the incidence of deep venous thrombosis is highest during operation and on the first day after. It is most fortunate that dextran can be given safely before operation because surgeons are reluctant to do this with oral anticoagulants which, to be fully effective, should be given at least 30 hours before surgery.

The phlebographic evaluation of deep venous thrombosis is not easy, and the various studies based on this criterion differ in several respects, including the technic, interpretation and timing after operation of the phlebography. Becker et al. [129] have shown that one third of the thrombi found by radioscanning of the legs could not be demonstrated by phlebography in patients treated with dextran. One of the explanations given is that dextran changes the structure of the thrombus and makes it more susceptible to endogenous fibrinolysis. This difference between the two methods used to judge the incidence of deep venous thrombosis offers a possible explanation why clinical trials with dextran result in a higher protection against venous thrombosis when the latter is assessed by phlebography (mainly Table III) rather than by radioscanning of the legs (mainly Table II). One of the requirements for success seems to be that 500 to 1,000 ml of a 6 per cent dextran 70 solution should be administered immediately before or after anesthesia and 500 ml should be given on the following and next three alternate days. Using this scheme, the prophylaxis of postoperative deep vein thrombosis appears to be as effective with dextran as with oral anticoagulants in all trials.

Whether dextran protects postoperative patients from pulmonary embolism could not be established with certainty in the trials so far published, as the clinical diagnosis of pulmonary embolism is difficult and fatal embolism is relatively uncommon. To pool the data from different trials is a debatable exercise. A well designed and controlled recent trial on 831 surgical patients at high risk revealed, in patients given dextran 70, a nonsignificant reduction in deep venous thrombosis judged by fibrinogen scanning, but the incidence and fatality rate of pulmonary embolism decreased significantly [124]. These findings support the concept that calf vein thrombosis has limited clinical morbidity [150] in contradistinction to thrombosis in the ileofemoral segments (which is not detected by radioactive scanning) and tend to confirm the findings of Sevitt and Gallagher [151] that oral anticoagulant therapy reduces the incidence of and mortality from pulmonary embolism without a corresponding diminution of small calf vein thrombosis at autopsy.

Compared to dextran, the protection offered by the administration of small doses of subcutaneous heparin against postoperative deep calf vein thrombosis is better documented in all types of surgery except suprapubic urologic surgery and possibly hip surgery; moreover, the administration of a small dose of heparin significantly reduces fatal pulmonary embolism [152,153].

Considering the uncertainties about orally administered drugs inhibiting platelet function, it is hoped that the on-going trials will help to decide to what extent these drugs, when used alone or in combination, can offer the same protection in the postoperative state as the use of small doses of heparin without inducing complications of their own.

IDIOPATHIC RECURRENT VENOUS THROMBOSIS

Patients with idiopathic recurrent venous thrombosis belong to an ill-defined group which will eventually be split up into subgroups once the pathogenesis is better known. Steele et al. [154] have already made the first step in this direction; they followed, over a three year period, 28 patients with recurrent venous thrombosis who had all had at least one pulmonary embolism. Platelet survival studies, which confirmed similar experiments of Abrahamsen [155] allowed them to distinguish two subgroups: those with a short platelet survival who were also refractory to oral anticoagulant therapy (seven of 28) and a second group with normal platelet survival who had had no arterial thrombosis in the past and responded clinically to anticoagulant therapy (21 of 28). The administration of sulfinpyrazone, in a dose of 800 mg/day, was accompanied by a dramatic reduction in episodes of venous and arterial thrombosis in all seven patients, and platelet survival (but not fibrinogen turnover) became significantly prolonged in several, and even normal in a few, patients. These clinical results were confirmed in a randomized controlled study [30]. In these two studies the diagnosis of recurrent venous thrombosis was made on clinical grounds but the objection that the treatment could mask the symptoms is unlikely since sulfinpyrazone has little anti-inflammatory action. Sulfinpyrazone also lengthens the reduced platelet survival found in patients with gout [156]. All these findings should encourage investigators to test, in prospective and controlled trials, the long-term effect of drugs affecting platelet function in patients with recurrent thrombosis with normal or reduced platelet survival, and to correlate the clinical results with the effect on platelet and fibrinogen survival.

Harker and Slichter [7] have given dipyridamole to a few patients with recurrent venous thrombosis who also had shortened platelet and fibrinogen survival; administration of this drug was even unable to significantly prolong these survivals which nevertheless were normalized during heparin therapy. These results are at variance with the conclusions of Steele et al. [154]; the discrepancy might be explained if the first group of investigators studied the patients when the thrombosis occurred but the second group followed patients in whom the venous thrombosis was quiescent, with apparent clinical success. Other studies are not controlled clinical trials and tend to confuse, rather than clarify, a difficult issue [157–161]. A large scale trial in which aspirin was used to prevent thrombophlebitis after phlebography unfortunately did not include a simultaneously assessed control group [162].

PREVENTION OF OCCLUSION IN ARTERIOVENOUS SHUNTS, ARTIFICIAL VESSELS OR OF RENAL DIALYSIS MEMBRANE

Thrombosis of arteriovenous shunts in patients with renal failure is a major problem as it increases the burden to nephrologists and patients in terms of thrombus removal, shunt reconstruction and delay in hemodialysis. Oral anticoagulant therapy can to some extent prevent the occlusion of Cimino-shunts or Scribner-shunts; it is difficult to maintain these severely affected patients at the desired low prothrombin level for years without risk of bleeding.

Drugs inhibiting platelet function were shown to prevent clotting in plastic shunts implanted in swine [163], Teflon®-shunts in rats [164] or silicone rubber shunts in dogs [165]. Furthermore an increased turnover of autologous platelets in patients with arteriovenous silastic cannulas [7] or with Scribner-shunts was described; in the latter cases dipyridamole was given alone or combined with aspirin (4.6 g/day) [166]. Several investigators had already mentioned that the administration of aspirin can prevent closure of arteriovenous fistulas in man [167] or clot formation on dialyzer membrane [168].

These findings prompted several clinicians to start prospective clinical trials with drugs inhibiting platelet function in patients with shunts connected to the vascular system. A prospective double-blind trial with sulfinpyrazone (0.6 g daily) versus a placebo was performed over a six month period in 52 patients undergoing renal hemodialysis [169]. Half of the patients receiving sulfinpyrazone had thrombotic episodes in their arteriovenous shunt as compared to 86 per cent of the group receiving placebo ($p < 0.01$). A further extension of this trial confirmed the initial conclusions and showed that sulfinpyrazone therapy is effective within a week of its start and that it loses its effectiveness after the same time interval when treatment is withdrawn [170].

Aspirin therapy (1 g every second day) was tried during the first 28 postoperative days in a group of renal patients with an arteriovenous fistula (Brescia-Cimino fistulas) [171]. Shunt closure was observed in 11 of the 47 patients given a placebo and in two of the 45 patients of the experimental group ($p < 0.05$). It, therefore, seems that treating uremic patients a small dose of aspirin is effective in preventing shunt occlusion in the postoperative period. There was, however, even at this dose, more severe wound hemorrhage and more frequent epistaxis in the group treated with aspirin.

There is limited experience with antiaggregating agents in patients with a silastic shunt between the lateral ventricle and jugular vein for the relief of hydrocephalus [172]. The survival of platelets was found to be reduced in some of these patients and could be normalized with the administration of dipyridamole (1.5 mg/kg/day). It was shown by Friedman et al. [173] that 57 per cent of a large number of patients with ventriculojugular shunts had pulmonary changes secondary to embolization of clots. The use of drugs inhibiting platelet function may, therefore, be advantageous in patients with a ventriculojugular shunt.

The use of the Gambro-Alwall dialyzer in patients with chronic renal insufficiency is associated with considerable blood loss due to thrombus formation in the dialysis membrane. Nine patients received dipyridamole (0.6 g daily) and/or a pyrimido-pyrimidine derivative (1 g RA-233 daily), these two drugs combined or a placebo, during the week preceding dialysis. There was a significant reduction of blood loss in the first three groups due to platelet and red cell accretion on the renal dialysis membrane [168].

SUMMARY

Notwithstanding the large number of clinical trials, most of them designed and performed according to the requirements of modern clinical pharmacology, only a few firm clinical recommendations on drugs affecting platelet function in the prevention of arterial or venous thrombosis can be made at present.

There is no good evidence for the clinical effectiveness of aspirin or any other drug affecting platelet function in patients with peripheral arterial occlusion or after vascular grafting. In cerebrovascular disease there is reasonable evidence that the administration of sulfinpyrazone can significantly reduce cerebral ischemia or mortality, but similar trials performed with aspirin, dipyridamole or clofibrate failed to reveal a significant difference in favor of the experimental treatment.

Patients with angina only were shown to benefit from treatment with clofibrate, but prospective trials with dipyridamole or aspirin in the primary or secondary prevention of myocardial infarction did not reveal a significant reduction in morbidity or mortality in the experimental group. Use of a combination of the latter two drugs did, however, reveal a reduction in morbidity and mortality.

In patients with prosthetic heart valves, there is firm evidence that dipyridamole and sulfinpyrazone therapy can normalize decreased platelet survival, an effect which has been shown to correlate well with the incidence of thromboembolism. Provided further trials lead to confirmatory conclusions, drugs inhibiting platelet function associated or not with oral anticoagulants may constitute an ideal prophylaxis in patients with a substitute valve.

There is still much uncertainty as to whether dipyridamole, given in addition to conventional treatment, benefits patients with membranous or mesangiocapillary glomerulonephritis. The same holds for drugs inhibiting platelet function after kidney or heart transplantation in man.

Only scanty reports are available on the usefulness of drugs affecting platelet function in thrombotic thrombocytopenic purpura and the hemolytic uremic syndrome.

Three different types of antiplatelet drugs are available for the prevention of postoperative deep vein thrombosis: dextran, oral drugs also affecting platelet function and heparin administered subcutaneously in small doses. In *orthopedic surgery,* dextran 70 administered before and every second day after surgery was the drug showing the most convincing reduction in the incidence of phlebographically proved deep vein thrombosis. Major orthopedic surgery is precisely the type of surgery in which the effectiveness of small dose heparin is much in doubt and in which the effectiveness of aspirin and dipyridamole is still to be confirmed. In *general surgery,* use of a combination of 1 g aspirin and 0.225 g dipyridamole daily was shown to offer approximately the same level of protection as small doses of heparin, and these two forms of prevention seem to offer a greater degree of protection than dextran. However, so far only the administration of a small dose of heparin was shown to prevent fatal pulmonary infarction in patients subjected to general surgery.

There is only circumstantial evidence that therapy with sulfinpyrazone, dipyridamole and aspirin may be useful in preventing recurrent venous thrombosis.

The prophylactic value of drugs affecting platelet

function has also been studied in artificial vessels. There is definite proof that the administration of aspirin or sulfinpyrazone can reduce the occlusion of Brescia-Cimino fistulas and that the administration of aspirin or pyrimido-pyrimidine derivatives prevent platelet accretion on a dialyzing membrane.

The relationship between changes in platelet survival, platelet glass adhesiveness and platelet aggregation, and clinical thrombotic events is unclear. Experience has shown that the presumed biologic effect is not necessarily the one which provides the clinical usefulness of a given drug.

REFERENCES

1. Havig O: Pathogenesis of peripheral venous thrombosis. An autopsy study. Proceedings of the 4th International Congress on Thrombosis and Haemostasis, Vienna, 1973, p 275.
2. Emmons PR, Harrison MJG, Honour AJ, et al.: Effect of dipyridamole on human platelet behavior. Lancet 2: 603, 1965.
3. Sullivan JM, Kagnoff MF, Gorlin R: Reduction of platelet adhesiveness in patients with coronary artery disease. Am J Med Sci 255: 292, 1968.
4. Bouvier CA, Rosner P, Berthoud S, et al.: Anomalies du comportement plaquettaire lors d'infarctus du myocarde. Cardiologia 50: 232, 1967.
5. Gray GR, Wilson PA, Douglas AS: The effect of dipyridamole on platelet aggregation and adhesiveness. Scott Med J 13: 409, 1968.
6. Harker LA, Slichter SJ: Studies of platelet and fibrinogen kinetics in patients with prosthetic heart valves. N Engl J Med 283: 1302, 1970.
7. Harker LA, Slichter SJ: Platelet and fibrinogen consumption in man. N Engl J Med 287: 999, 1972.
8. Harker LA, Slichter SJ, Scott CR, et al.: Homocystinemia. Vascular injury and arterial thrombosis. N Engl J Med 291: 537, 1974.
9. Harker LA: In vivo evaluation of antithrombotic therapy in man. Platelets, Thrombosis and Inhibitors (Didisheim P, Shimamoto T, Yamazaki H, eds), Stuttgart-New-York, F.K. Schattauer Verlag, 1974, p 481.
10. O'Brien JR: Effect of salicylates on human platelets. Lancet 1: 779, 1968.
11. Zucker MB, Peterson J: Inhibition of adenosine diphosphate-induced secondary aggregation and other platelet functions by acetylsalicylic acid ingestion. Proc Soc Exp Biol Med 127: 547, 1968.
12. Stuart RKJ: Platelet function studies in human beings receiving 300 mg of aspirin per day. J Lab Clin Med 75: 463, 1970.
13. Smythe HA, Ogryzlo MA, Murphy EA, et al.: The effect of sulfinpyrazone (Anturan) in platelet economy and blood coagulation in man. Can Med Assoc J 92: 818, 1965.
14. Weily HS, Genton E: Altered platelet function in patients with prosthetic mitral valves: effects of sulfinpyrazone therapy. Circulation 42: 967, 1970.
15. Gilbert JB, Mustard JF: Some effects of Atromid on platelet economy and blood coagulation in man. J Atheroscler Res 3: 623, 1963.
16. Carson P, MacDonald L, Pickard S, et al.: Effect of Atromid on platelet stickiness. J Atheroscl Res 3: 619, 1963.
17. Cronberg S, Robertson B, Nilsson IM, et al.: Suppressive effect of dextran on platelet adhesiveness. Thromb Diath Haemorrh 16: 384, 1966.
18. Perkins HA, Rolfs MR, McBride A: Low molecular weight dextran in open heart surgery: effect on coagulation factors and on red cell antibody activity. Transfusion 4: 10, 1964.
19. Muzaffar TZ, Stalker AL, Bryce WAJ, et al.: Dextran and fibrin morphology. Nature (Lond) 238: 288, 1972.
20. Metcalf MJ, Arfors KE, McKenzie FN, et al.: Effect of dextran on the lysis of artificial thrombi. Europ Surg Res 6 (suppl 1): 28, 1974.
21. Hynes KM, Gau GT, Rutherford BD, et al.: Effect of aspirin on brachial artery occlusion following brachial arteriotomy for coronary arteriography. Circulation 47: 554, 1973.
22. Freed MD, Rosenthal A, Fyler D: Attempts to reduce arterial thrombosis after cardiac catheterization in children: use of percutaneous technique and aspirin. Am Heart J 87: 283, 1974.
23. Linke H: Langzeitprophylaxe mit ASS (Colfarit) bei arteriellen Angiopathien. Therapeutische Berichte 47: 33, 1975.
24. Kurtzke JP, Kurland LT: Epidemiology of cerebrovascular disease. Cerebrovascular Survey Report, Subcommittee on Cerebrovascular Disease NINDS, Washington DC, 1970, p 163.
25. Barnett HJM: Platelets, drugs and cerebral ischemia. Platelets, Drugs and Thrombosis (Hirsch J, Cade JF, Gallus AS, Schönbaum E, eds), Basel, S. Karger, 1975, p 233.
26. Baker RN, Broward JA, Fant HC, et al: Anticoagulant therapy in cerebral infarction. Neurology (Minneap) 12: 823, 1962.
27. Friedman GD, Wilson S, Mosier JM, et al.: Transient ischemia attacks in a community. JAMA 210: 1428, 1969.
28. Acheson J, Danta G, Hutchinson EC: Controlled trial of dipyridamole in cerebral vascular disease. Br Med J 1: 614, 1969.
29. Acheson J, Hutchinson EC: Controlled trial of clofibrate in cerebral vascular disease. Atherosclerosis 15: 177, 1972.
30. Evans G, Gent M: Effect of platelet suppressive drugs on arterial and venous thromboembolism. Platelets, Drugs and Thrombosis (Hirsch J, Cade JF, Gallus AS, Schönbaum E, eds), Basel, S. Karger, 1975, p 258.
31. Blakely JA, Gent M: Platelets, drugs and longevity in a geriatric population. Platelets, Drugs and Thrombosis (Hirsh J, Cade JF, Gallus AS, Schönbaum, E, eds), Basel, S. Karger, 1975, p 284.
32. Heikinheimo R, Jarvinen K: Acetylsalicylic acid and arteriosclerotic-thromboembolic diseases in the aged. J Am Geriat Soc 19: 403, 1971.
33. Dyken ML, Kolar OJ, Jones FH: Differences in the occurrence of carotid transient ischemic attacks associated with antiplatelet aggregation therapy. Stroke 4: 732, 1973.
34. Harrison MJG, Marshall J, Meadows JC, et al.: Effect of aspirin in amaurosis fugax. Lancet 2: 743, 1971.
35. Mundall J, Quintero P, Von Kaulla KN, et al.: Transient monocular blindness and increased platelet aggregability treated with aspirin—a case report. Neurology (Minneap) 21: 402, 1971.
36. Gent M, Barnett HJM: The Canadian Cooperative study of recent recurrent presumed cerebral emboli (RRPCE). A progress report (Abstract), IVth Congress of the International Society of Thrombosis and Haemostasis, Vienna, 1973, p 165.
37. Boneu B, Guiraud B, Fernet P: Traitement anti-agrégant plaquettaire par l'aspirine. Bases biologiques. Application,

aux accidents vasculaire cérébraux. Nouv Presse Méd 1: 863, 1972.
38. Newcastle upon Tyne Physicians: Trial of clofibrate in the treatment of ischemic heart disease. Br Med J 4: 1767, 1971.
39. Scottish Society of Physicians: Ischemic heart disease: a secondary prevention trial using clofibrate. Br Med J 2: 775, 1971.
40. Gilbert JB, Mustard JF: Some effects of Atromid on platelet economy and blood coagulation in man. J Atheroscler Res 3: 623, 1963.
41. Coronary drug project research group: clofibrate and niacin in coronary heart disease. JAMA 27: 360, 1975.
42. Gent AE, Brook CGD, Foley TH, et al.: Dipyridamole: a controlled trial of its effect in acute myocardial infarction. Br Med J 4: 366, 1968.
43. Foulds T, Mackinnon J: Controlled double-blind trial of "Persantin" in treatment of angina pectoris. Br Med J 2: 835, 1960.
44. Zion MM, Bradlow BA: A controlled clinical trial of "Persantin" (RA8) in angina pectoris. S Afr Med J 35: 11, 1961.
45. Soloff LA, Gimenez JL, Winters WL Jr: Experimental and clinical observations on 2,6-bis(diethanolamino)-4,8-dipiperidino-pyrimido-(5,5-d) pyrimidine (Persantin). Am J Med Sci 243: 783, 1962.
46. Sbar S, Schlant RC: Dipyridamole in the treatment of angina pectoris: a double-blind evaluation. JAMA 201: 865, 1967.
47. Cobb S, Anderson F, Bauer W: Length of life and causes of death in rheumatoid arthritis. N Engl J Med 249: 553, 1953.
48. Boston Collaborative Drug Surveillance Group: Regular aspirin intake and acute myocardial infarction. Br Med J 1: 440, 1974.
49. Hammond EC, Sarfinkel L: Aspirin and coronary heart disease: findings of a prospective study. Br Med J 1: 269, 1975.
50. Craven LL: Experiences with aspirin (acetylsalicylic acid) in nonspecific prophylaxis of coronary thrombosis. Mississipi Valley Med J 75: 38, 1953.
51. Elwood PC, Cochrane AL, Burr ML, et al.: A randomized controlled trial of acetylsalicylic acid in the secondary prevention of mortality from myocardial infarction. Br Med J 1: 436, 1974.
52. Weily HS, Steele PP, Genton E: Platelet survival in patients with a Beall valve. Relation to low incidence of thromboembolism. Am J Cardiol 30: 229, 1972.
53. Warkany J: Warfarin embryopathy. Am J Dis Childr 129: 287, 1975.
54. Sullivan JM, Harken DE, Gorlin R: Pharmacologic control of thromboembolic complications of cardiac-valve replacement. N Engl J Med 279: 576, 1968.
55. Sullivan JM, Harken DE, Gorlin R: Pharmacologic control of thromboembolic complications of cardiac-valve replacement. N Engl J Med 284: 1391, 1971.
56. Arrants JE, Hairston P, Lee WH Jr: Use of dipyridamole (persantine) in preventing thromboembolism following valve replacement. Chest 58: 275, 1970.
57. Rabello C, Rivas JA, Rocha F, et al.: Estudo da ação de Dipiridamol na evolução de pacientes submetiødos à substituiçao de próteses valvares. Rev Bras clin ter 2: 95, 1973.
58. Lander H, Kinlough RL, Robson HN: reduced platelet survival in patients with Starr-Edwards prostheses. Br Med J 1: 688, 1965.
59. Manohitharajah SM, Rahman AN, Donnely RJ, et al.: Platelet survival in patients with homograft and prosthetic heart valves. Correlation with incidence of thromboembolism. Thorax 29: 639, 1974.
60. Weily HS, Steele PP, Davies H, et al.: Platelet studies in patients with substitute heart valves. N Engl J Med 290: 534, 1974.
61. Steele PP, Davies H, Genton E: Platelet function studies in coronary artery disease. Circulation 48: 1194, 1973.
62. Kummer H, Hunziker HR, Althaus U: Medicamentöse Beeinflüssung des Thrombocytenumsatzes bei Patienten mit künstlichen Herzklappen. Schweiz Med Wochenschr 104: 142, 1974.
63. Stuart RK, McDonald JWD, Ahujy SP, et al.: Platelet survival in prosthetic heart valve patients (abstract), IIIrd Congress of the International Society of Thrombosis and Haemostasis, Washington DC, 1972, p 384.
64. Genton E, Steele P: Platelets, drugs and heart disease. Platelets, Drugs and Thrombosis (Hirsh J, Cade JF, Gallus AS, Schönbaum E, eds), Basel, S. Karger, 1975, p 263.
65. Garg SK, Lackner H, Karpatkin S: The increased percentage of megacaryocytes in various clinical disorders. Ann Intern Med 77: 361, 1972.
66. Farquhar MG, Vernier RL, Good RA: Electron microscopy of the glomerulus in nephrosis, glomerulonephritis and lupus erythematosus. J Exp Med 106: 649, 1957.
67. Koffler D, Paronetto F: Immunofluorescent localization of immunoglobulins, complement and fibrinogen in human disease. II. Acute, subacute, and chronic glomerulonephritis. J Clin Invest 44: 1665, 1965.
68. Duffy JL, Cinque T, Grisham E, et al.: Intraglomerular fibrin, platelet aggregation and subendothelial deposits in lipoid nephritis. J Clin Invest 49: 251, 1970.
69. Fischel EE: Immune reactions in human glomerulonephritis. J Chronic Dis 5: 34, 1957.
70. Friedman P, Markowitz AA: Gamma globulin and complement in diseased kidney. J Clin Invest 41: 328, 1962.
71. Kincaid-Smith P, Saker BM, Fairly KF: Anticoagulants in "irreversible" acute renal failure. Lancet 2: 1360, 1968.
72. Herdman RC, Edson JR, Pickering RJ, et al.: Anticoagulation in renal diseases in children. Am J Dis Child 119: 27, 1970.
73. Cade JR, De Quesada AM, Shires DL, et al.: The effect of long term high dose heparin treatment on the course of chronic proliferative glomerulonephritis. Nephron 8: 67, 1971.
74. Kincaid-Smith P: Coagulation and renal disease. Kidney Int 2: 183, 1972.
75. Bello E, Reuss L, Lazcano F, et al.: Tratamiento de glomerulopatias proliferativas y mesengioproliferativas con heparina-deipiridamol. Rev Méd Chile 101: 279, 1973.
76. Trygstad CW, Bang NU, Heidenreich RO, et al.: A controlled trial of aspirin in childhood glomerular disorders. Thromb Diath Haemorrh 30: 12, 1973.
77. Kincaid-Smith P: Platelets, drugs and the kidney. Platelets, Drugs and Thrombosis (Hirsh J, Cade JF, Gallus AS, Schönbaum E, eds), Basel, S. Karger, 1975, p 301.
78. Porter KA, Calne RY, Zukoski CF: Vascular and other changes in 200 canine renal homotransplants treated with immunosuppressive drugs. Lab Invest 13: 810, 1964.
79. Kissmeyer-Neilsen F, Olsen S, Petersen VP, et al.: Hyperacute rejection of kidney allografts associated with preexisting humoral antibodies against donor cells. Lancet 2: 662, 1966.
80. Mowbray JF: Methods of suppression of immune response. Proceedings of the 9th International Congress on Internal Medicine, vol 137, Amsterdam, Excerpta Medica, 1966, p 106.
81. Lowenhaupt RW, Nathan P: Platelet accumulation observed by electron microscopy in the early phase of renal allotransplant rejection. Nature (Lond) 220: 822, 1968.
82. Busch GJ, Braun WE, Carpenter CB, et al.: Intravascular

coagulation (IVC) in human renal allograft rejection. Transplantation 1: 267, 1969.
83. Kincaid-Smith P, McKenzie IFC, Morris PJ, et al.: Biopsy features of early acute rejection in cadaveric renal grafts. Transplantation 1: 287, 1969.
84. Simpson KM, Bunc DL, Amemiya H, et al.: Humerol antibodies and coagulation mechanisms in the accelerated or hyperacute rejection of renal homografts in sensitized canine recipients. Surgery 68: 77, 1970.
85. Kincaid-Smith P: The pathogenesis of the vascular and glomerular lesions of rejection in renal allografts and their modification by antithrombotic and anticoagulant drugs. Aust Ann Med 3: 201, 1970.
86. McMillan R: Heparin in delayed transplant function. Lancet 1: 1178, 1968.
87. Macdonald A, Busch GJ, Alexander JL, et al.: Heparin and aspirin in the treatment of hyperacute rejection of renal allografts in presensitized dogs. Transplantation 9: 1, 1970.
88. Mathew TH, Hogan GP, Lewers DT, et al.: Controlled, double-blind trial of antiplatelet aggregating agents in vascular renal allograft rejection. Transplant Proc 3: 901, 1971.
89. Sharma HM, Moore S, Merrick HW, et al.: Platelets in early hyperacute allograft rejection in kidneys and their modification by sulfinpyrazone (Anturan) therapy. Am J Pathol 66: 445, 1972.
90. Messmer K, Hammer C, Land W, et al.: Modification of hyperacute xenogeneic kidney rejection. Transplant Proc 3: 542, 1971.
91. Claes G: Studies on platelets and fibrin during rejection of canine allografts. Scand J Urol Nephrol (suppl) 10: 1, 1972.
92. Shons AR, Navajarian JS: Modification of xenograft rejection by aspirin, dextran, and cinanserin: the importance of platelets in hyperacute rejection. Transplant Proc 6: 435, 1974.
93. Australian National Renal Transplantation Survey: Second report by a subcommittee. Med J Aust 2: 605, 1971.
94. Advisory Committee to the Renal Transplant Registry: The ninth report of the human renal transplantation registry. JAMA 220: 253, 1972.
95. Lowrie EG, Lazarus JH, Mocellin AJ, et al.: Survival of patients undergoing chronic hemodialysis and renal transplantation. N Engl J Med 288: 863, 1973.
96. Ibels LS, Stewart JH, Mahony JF, et al.: Deaths from occlusive arterial disease in renal allograft recipients. Br Med J 2: 552, 1974.
97. Kincaid-Smith P: Modification of the vascular lesions of rejection in cadaveric renal allografts by dipyridamole and anticoagulants. Lancet 2: 920, 1969.
98. Aledort LM, Taub R, Burrows L, et al.: Use of inhibitors of platelet function in renal rejection phenomena. Platelets and Thrombosis (Sherry S, Scriabine A, eds), München, Urban and Schwarzenberg, 1974, p 263.
99. Mathew TH, Clyne DH, Nanra RS, et al.: A controlled trial of oral anticoagulants and dipyridamole in cadaveric renal allografts. Lancet 1: 1307, 1974.
100. Griepp RB, Stinson EB, Dong E, et al.: The influence of warfarin and dipyridamol on coronary arteriosclerosis in the transplanted human heart. Circulation 7-8 (suppl 4): 98, 1973.
101. Giromini M, Bouvier CA, Dami R, et al.: Effect of dipyridamole and aspirin in thrombotic microangiopathy. Br Med J 1: 545, 1972.
102. Utting JA, Shreeve DR: Haemolytic-uraemic syndrome in an adult with pericarditis and pleurisy. Br Med J 2: 591, 1973.
103. Amir J, Krauss S: Treatment of thrombotic thrombocytopenic purpura with antiplatelet drugs. Blood 42: 27, 1973.
104. Rossi EC, Redondo D, Borges WH: Thrombotic thrombocytopenic purpura survival following treatment with aspirin, dipyridamole and prednisone. JAMA 228: 1141, 1974.
105. Powell HR, Ekert H: Streptokinase and anti-thrombotic therapy in the hemolytic-uremic syndrome. J Pediatr 84: 345, 1974.
106. Howard DJ, Roberts AB, Page FT: Late recurrence of thrombotic thrombocytopenic purpura after splenectomy. Br Med J 1: 317, 1975.
107. O'Brien JR: Effects of salicylates in human platelets. Lancet 1: 779, 1968.
108. Clagett GP, Schneider P, Rosoff CB, et al.: The influence of aspirin on postoperative platelet kinetics and venous thrombosis. Surgery 77: 61, 1975.
109. Browse NL, Hall JH: Effect of dipyridamole on the incidence of clinically detectable deep-vein thrombosis. Lancet 2: 718, 1969.
110. Weber W, Wolff U, Bromig G: Postoperative Thromboembolieprophylaxe mit Colfarit. Ther Berichte (Bayer, Leverkusen) 43: 229, 1971.
111. Salzman EW, Harris WH, DeSanctis RW: Reduction in venous thromboembolism by agents affecting platelet function. N Engl J Med 284: 1287, 1971.
112. Harris WH, Salzman EW, DeSanctis RW, et al.: Prevention of venous thromboembolism following total hip replacement. JAMA 220: 1319, 1972.
113. Zekert F, Kohn P, Vormittag E, et al.: Thromboembolieprophylaxe mit Acetylsalicylsäure bei Operationen wegen hüftgelenksnaher Frakturen. Mschr Unfallheilk 77: 97, 1974.
114. Loew D, Wellmer HK, Baer U, et al.: Postoperative Thromboembolie-Prophylaxe mit Acetylsalicylsäure. Dtsch Med Wochenschr 99: 565, 1974.
115. Carter AE, Eban R, Perrett RD: Prevention of postoperative deep vein thrombosis and pulmonary embolism. Br Med J 1: 312, 1971.
116. O'Brien JR, Tulevski VG, Etherington M: Two in-vivo studies comparing high and low aspirin dosage. Lancet 2: 388, 1971.
117. British Medical Research Council: Effect of aspirin on postoperative venous thrombosis. Lancet 2: 441, 1972.
118. O'Sullivan EF, Vellar IDA: Assessment of the efficacy of antiplatelet drugs in the prevention of postoperative deep vein thrombosis. IIIrd Congress International Society of Thrombosis and Haemostasis, Washington DC, 1972, p 438.
119. Parodi JC, Grandi A, Font E, et al.: El dipyridamol y el acido acetilsalicilico en la profilaxis de las thrombosis venosas postoperatorias de los membros inferiores. Dia méd. 44: 92, 1973.
120. Wood EH, Prentice CRM, McGrouther DA, et al.: Trial of aspirin and RA-233 in prevention of post-operative deep vein thrombosis. Thromb Diath Haemorrh 30: 18, 1973.
121. Harris WH, Salzman EW, Athanasoulis C, et al.: Comparison of warfarin, low-molecular-weight dextran, aspirin, and subcutaneous heparin in prevention of venous thromboembolism following total hip replacement. J Bone Joint Surg 56: 1552, 1974.
122. Carter AE, Eban R: Prevention of postoperative deep venous thrombosis in legs by orally administered hydroxychloroquine sulphate. Br Med J 2: 94, 1974.
123. Weiss V, Jekiel M, Bouvier CA: Preventive effects of dipyridamole and ASA on postoperative thrombo-embolic disease in gynaecological surgery. J Int Fed Obst Gynecol, to be published.
124. Kline A, Hughes LE, Campbell H, et al.: Dextran 70 in prophylaxis of thromboembolic disease after surgery: a clinically oriented randomized double-blind trial. Br Med

J 2: 109, 1975.
125. Kakkar VV: Review of present status of prophylaxis of venous thromboembolism. Proc Roy Soc Med 67: 706, 1974.
126. Jansen H: Postoperative thromboembolism and its prevention with 500 ml dextran given during operation. Acta Chir Scand suppl 427, p 86, 1972.
127. Carter AE, Eban R: The prevention of postoperative deep venous thrombosis with dextran 70. Br J Surg 60: 681, 1973.
128. Stephenson CBS, Wallace JC, Vaughan JV: Dextran 70 in the prevention of post-operative deep vein thrombosis with observations on pulmonary embolism: report on a pilot study. NZ Med J 77: 302, 1973.
129. Becker J, Schampi B: The incidence of postoperative venous thrombosis of the legs. Acta Chir Scand 139: 357, 1972.
130. Ruckley CV: Heparin versus dextran in the prevention of deep-vein thrombosis. Lancet 2: 118, 1974.
131. Gruber UF, Sturm V, Rem J, et al.: The present state of prevention of postoperative thromboembolic complications. Intentional Hemodilution (Messmer K, Schmid-Schönhein H, eds). Bibl Haematol 41: 98, 1975.
132. Lambie JM, Barber DC, Dhall DP, et al.: Dextran 70 in prophylaxis of postoperative venous thrombosis. A controlled trial. Br Med J 2: 144, 1970.
133. Davidson AI, Brunt MEA, Matheson NA: A further trial comparing Dextran 70 with Warfarin in the prophylaxis of postoperative venous thrombosis. Br J Surg 59: 314, 1972.
134. Bonnar J, Walsh J: Prevention of thrombosis after pelvic surgery by British Dextran 70. Lancet 1: 614, 1972.
135. Bonnar J, Walsh JJ, Haddon M, et al.: Coagulation system changes induced by pelvic surgery and the effect of Dextran 70. Bibl Anat 12: 351, 1973.
136. McCarthy TG, McQueen J, Johnstone FD, et al.: A comparison of low-dose subcutaneous heparin and intravenous dextran 70 in the prophylaxis of deep venous thrombosis after gynecological surgery. J Obstet Gynaecol Br 81: 486, 1974.
137. Hedlund PO: Postoperative venous thrombosis in benign prostatic disease. A study of 316 patients with the ^{125}I-fibrogen uptake test. Scand J Urol Nephrol suppl 27, p 1, 1975.
138. Johnsson SR, Bygdeman S, Eliasson R: Effect of dextran on postoperative thrombosis. Acta Chir Scand suppl 387: 80, 1968.
139. Ahlberg A, Göran N, Robertson B, et al.: Dextran in prophylaxis of thrombosis in fractures in the hip. Acta Chir Scand suppl 387, p 83, 1968.
140. Ahlberg A: Thromboprofylaxe med Macrodex i ett collumfrakturmaterial. Symposium (Haeger K, Robertson B, eds), Studentlitteratur, Lund, 1969, p 89.
141. Myhre HO, Holen A: Thromboseprofylakse. Dextran eller Warfarin-natrium? Et kontrolleert klinisk forsok. Nord Med 82: 1534, 1969.
142. Evarts CM, Feil EI: Prevention of thromboembolic disease after elective surgery of the hip. J Bone Joint Surg 53 1271, 1971.
143. Bronge A, Dahlgren S, Lindquist B: Prophylaxis against thrombosis in femoral neck fracture—a comparison between dextran 70 and dicumarol. Acta Chir Scand 137, 29, 1971.
144. Daniel WJ, Moore AR, Flanc C: Prophylaxis of deep vein thrombosis (DM) with dextran 70 in patients with a fractured neck of femur. Austr NZ J Surg 41: 289, 1972.
145. Bergquist E, Bergquist D, Bronge A, et al.: An evaluation of early thrombosis prophylaxis following fracture of the femoral neck. Acta Chir Scand 138: 689, 1972.
146. Myrvold HE, Persson JE, Svensson B, et al.: Prevention of thromboembolism with dextran 70 and heparin in patients with femoral neck fractures. Acta Chir Scand 139: 609, 1973.
147. Korvald E, Støren EJ, Ongre A: Simultaneous use of warfarin—sodium and dextran 70 to prevent postoperative venous thrombosis in patients with hip fractures. J Oslo City Hosp 23: 25, 1973.
148. Bergqvist D, Dahlgren S: Leg vein thrombosis diagnosed by ^{125}I-fibrinogen test in patients with fracture of the hip: a study of the effect of early prophylaxis with dicoumarol or dextran 70. VASA 2: 121, 1973.
149. Harper DR, Dhall DP, Woodruff PWTT: Prophylaxis in iliofemoral venous thrombosis. The major amputee as a clinical research model. Br J Surg 60: 831, 1973.
150. Mavor GE, Golloway JMD: Iliofemoral venous thrombosis. Pathological considerations and surgical management. Br J Surg 56: 45, 1969.
151. Sevitt S, Gallagher N: Prevention of venous thrombosis and pulmonary embolism in injured patients. A trial of anticoagulant prophylaxis with phenindione in middle-aged and elderly patients with fractured necks of femur. Lancet 2: 981, 1959.
152. Kakkar VV, Field ES, Nicolaides AN, et al.: Low dose of heparin in the prevention of deep vein thrombosis. Lancet 2: 699, 1971.
153. An International Multicentre Trial: Prevention of fatal postoperative pulmonary embolism by low doses of heparin. Lancet 2: 45, 1975.
154. Steele PP, Weily HS, Genton E: Platelet survival and adhesiveness in recurrent venous thrombosis. N Engl J Med 288: 1148, 1973.
155. Abrahamsen AF: Platelet survival studies in man: with special reference to thrombosis and atherosclerosis. Scand J Haematol suppl 3, p 1, 1968.
156. Smythe HA, Ogryzlo MA, Murphy EA, et al.: The effect of sulphinpyrazone (Anturan) in platelet economy and blood coagulation in man. Can Med Assoc J 92: 818, 1965.
157. Tautz I: Die Behandlung der oberflachigen Thrombophlebitis mi colfarit. Therapiewoche 22: 1407, 1972.
158. Sellier W: Erfahrungen mit dem Thrombozytenaggregationshemmer Colfarit bei thromboembolischen Erkrankungen in der Praxis. Med Welt 22: 2013, 1971.
159. Knappmann J: Erfahrungen mit dem Acetylsalicyl-Säurepräparat "Colfarit." Beobachtungen an 112 Patienten. Med Welt 48: 1929, 1971.
160. Joist JH: Medikamentöse Hemmung der Blutplättchenfunktion. Med Welt 27: 1247, 1970.
161. Scharrer I, Schepping M, Breddin K: Thromboseprophylaxe mit Aspirin der Einfluss von Acetylsalicylsaüre auf die Thrombocytenaggregaten in vitro and in vivo. Klin Wochenschr 24: 1318, 1969.
162. Hach W: Thromboseprophylaxe nach Phlebographie. Proceedings of the Colfarit symposium II, Bayer Pharma, 1973, p 53, September 28, 1973; Pharma-Forschungszentrum, Wuppertal; Bayer.
163. Mustard JF, Rowsell HC, Smythe HA, et al.: The effect of sulfinpyrazone on platelet economy and thrombus formation in rabbits. Blood 29: 859, 1967.
164. Didisheim P: Inhibition by dipyridamole of arterial thrombosis in rats. Thromb Diath Haemorrh 20: 257, 1968.
165. Benis AM, Nossel HL, Aledorf LM, et al.: Thrombus formation in flow chambers studied with dogs having long-term extracorporeal shunts. Abstracts, IIIrd Congress International Society of Thrombosis and Haemostasis, Washington DC, 1972, p 352.
166. Scribner BH, Thomas GI, Slichter SJ, et al.: Studies of platelet destruction due to prosthetic arterio-venous cannulas. Fourth Annual Contractors Conference of the Artificial

Kidney Program of the National Institute of Arthritis and Metabolic Diseases, Washington DC, 1971.
167. Koestering H, Mietzsch G, Wigger W, et al.: Thrombolyse zur Beseitigung thrombotischer Verschlüsse beim cimino-shunt bei Hämodialysepatienten. Med Klin 67: 945, 1972.
168. Lindsay RM, Ferguson D, Prentice CR, et al.: Reduction of thrombus formation on dialyser membranes by aspirin and RA-233. Lancet 2: 1287, 1972.
169. Kaegi A, Pineo GF, Shimizu A, et al.: Arterio-venous shunt thrombosis. Prevention by sulfinpyrazone. N Engl J Med 290: 304, 1974.
170. Hirsh J, Gent M, Genton E: The current status of platelet suppressive drugs in the treatment of thrombosis. Thromb Diath Haemorrh 33: 406, 1973.
171. Andrassy K, Ritz E, Schoeffner W, et al.: The influence of acetylsalicylic acid on platelet adhesiveness and thrombotic fistula complications in hemodialysed patients. Klin Wochenschr 3: 166, 1971.
172. Stuart M, Stockman J, Murphy S, et al.: Shortened platelet lifespan in patients with hydrocephalus and ventriculojugular shunts: results of preliminary attempts at correction. J Pediatr 80: 21, 1972.
173. Friedman S, Zita-Gozum C, Chatten J: Pulmonary vascular changes complicating ventriculovascular shunting for hydrocephalus. J Pediatr 64: 305, 1964.

Decisions Regarding the Provision or Withholding of Therapy

Stenographic reports, edited by Philip E. Cryer, M.D. and John M. Kissane, M.D., of weekly clinicopathologic or clinicosociologic conferences held in Barnes and Wohl Hospitals, are published in each issue of the Journal. These conferences are participated in jointly by members of the Departments of Internal Medicine and Pathology of Washington University School of Medicine.

Dr. Gerald Perkoff: In the Clinicosociologic Conferences presented previously we have directed our discussions to the social issues which related to the medical conditions of individual patients. Although each patient was an example of problems and approaches which might have general application, in only one of the earlier conferences—that on long-term hemodialysis [1]—did we deal with complex ethical issues.

In the present conference we discussed extremely controversial but day to day decisions in patient care. The topic is a broad one, i.e., the choice between two alternatives: to treat a patient aggressively at all costs or to judge the over-all value of therapy on some larger social scale and treat the patient less aggressively or not at all. We purposely avoided the topics of abortion or of maintenance of body functions through technology since both subjects have been widely discussed and since neither is encountered frequently in the average physician's practice. Instead, we chose two patients in whom the therapeutic decisions that were made in the course of ambulatory and hospital care are similar to those encountered by every physician. It should be evident that these were controversial topics and that both those involved in the care of these patients and those who later discussed them had widely divergent opinions. It should also be clear that the conference provides no definite answers which would satisfy everyone and that the actions taken and the positions presented represent the views of individual physicians; they should not be interpreted as the policies of the Washington University School of Medicine or of *The American Journal of Medicine.* Indeed, the purpose of the conference was to provide a forum for discussing the uncertainties and insecurities in therapeutics which reflect real clinical situations. There are no certain answers to many serious ethical issues shared by all physicians and their patients.

PATIENT PRESENTATIONS

Patient 1. An 86 year old retired secretary was first seen in the Medical Care Group (MCG) of Washington University in the spring of 1975 complaining of lack of memory. She had been in a hospital only once for some unknown cause as a young woman. She gave a history of labile blood pressure, nervousness and memory loss. The latter had been severe enough to lead her to assign power of attorney to a third party who made her financial and other decisions. Despite this, she was able to communicate directly with the examining physician and to give an adequate history. She had no living relatives and lived by herself in a home for the aged. She went to the theater occasionally and sometimes received visiting friends. Positive physical findings included a blood pressure of 170/82 mm Hg, bilateral carotid bruits, a grade 2/6 systolic murmur along the left sternal border and a very firm, 7 to 8 cm pulsatile mass in the upper mid-abdomen with an overlying harsh, systolic bruit. Laboratory data were unremarkable except that a roentgenogram of the abdomen confirmed the presence of a large, mid-abdominal aortic aneurysm.

A surgeon was contacted and the patient's problems were discussed by telephone. The surgeon believed that an 86 year old woman with labile hypertension was not a candidate for aortic aneurysm replacement. The patient's guardian was informed of this view and accepted it; the patient was not included in this decision.

Nothing more was heard from the patient until the evening of October 24, 1975, when a call was received from the nursing home stating that the patient had experienced sudden, severe back pain, that she had become cold, sweaty and weak, and that she had collapsed to the floor. The patient was brought to the emergenc room by ambulance. The blood pressure was 70/40 mm Hg and increased to 140/80 mm Hg following the intravenous infusion of saline solution. The patient was alert and able to converse. The abdomen was firm and tender with a very large palpable mass in the upper abdominal quadrant; the stool was guaiac positive. The hematocrit value had fallen to 25 per cent. The diagnosis of rupturing abdominal aortic aneurysm was made. In the emergency room, the situation was discussed with the patient who elected to have surgery even though it was made clear that the chances for success were small. The guardian was not available.

The patient was taken to the operating room and a 7 cm graft was placed in the abdominal aorta after the removal of a large, ruptured aneurysm. The patient was in the surgical intensive care unit for approximately 30 hours during which time progressive obtundation and, despite apparent graft function, mottling of the lower extremities and progressive acidosis developed. She died the morning of October 27, 1975.

Patient 2. A 90 year old man presented for his first and only visit to MCG on August 14, 1975, complaining of weight loss and anorexia for two months. The patient lived alone and had taken care of himself for many years, although he had only minimal vision and very poor hearing. In June 1975 he noticed a decrease in appetite and subsequently lost approximately 20 pounds. He had not had nausea, vomiting or a change in bowel habits. He had been hospitalized elsewhere in 1954 and was told that he had a "lump" in the large intestine which should be removed, but he chose not to have surgery.

Physical examination showed an elderly man with an irregular pulse of 76/min, normal temperature and respirations, a weight of 109 pounds and a blood pressure of 180/90 mm Hg. There were bilateral dense cataracts, and both ears showed severe chronic otitis media. The heart was slightly enlarged with a grade 4/6 crescendo-decrescendo systolic murmur at the aortic area and along the left sternal border. All pulses were palpable. Examination of the abdomen revealed a hard, 10 by 15 cm mass in the midline below the umbilicus. Rectal examination disclosed a markedly enlarged prostate and a negative stool guaiac. The neurologic examination was within normal limits, and the patient was oriented and mentally clear.

Upon admission to the hospital, a catheter inserted into the bladder yielded 1,600 ml of bloody urine which was removed in several stages; the midline abdominal mass disappeared. The hematocrit value was 34.5 per cent. Urinalysis showed numerous red blood cells. The serum creatinine was 1.9 mg/100 ml and the albumin 3.4 g/100 ml, but the results of all other routine serum chemistry studies were normal. Cystoscopy showed grade 4 trabeculation of the bladder; an intravenous urogram and retrograde studies did not reveal any abnormalities. The patient was scheduled for a transurethral prostatectomy.

The night after cystoscopy the patient's temperature rose to 38.5°C and he felt chilly, but the findings on physical examination and urinalysis were unchanged. The next morning, left pleuritic chest pain developed, the arterial oxygen tension (pO_2) was 55 mm Hg and, upon repeat, 53 mm Hg. A ventilation-perfusion lung scan showed defects in the lower field of both lungs compatible with pulmonary emboli, and the patient was given heparin. Over the next two days he continued to complain of pleuritic chest pain, but he was not dyspneic and his heparin therapy proceeded without difficulty. Because of the past history of a colonic mass, a barium enema was performed on August 21; it revealed only diverticulosis. By August 24, however, the patient had not had a bowel movement, and abdominal distention and cramping abdominal pain had developed. Increased infiltrates in the lower lobe of the left lung and upper lobe of the right lung were evident on a chest film, and hyponatremia was present. Repeat x-ray examination of the abdomen showed a large impaction of retained barium in the colon extending to the cecum. Repeated enemas and laxatives relieved only part of the obstruction. Following preoperative anesthesiology evaluation the patient was classified as a grade 4 risk, unacceptable for transurethral prostatectomy, and surgery was cancelled.

The fever continued, the chest infiltrates increased and the abdominal pain became so severe that the patient required meperidine. He began to state repeatedly that he wanted no additional therapy and that he wished to die; he refused all further diagnostic procedures. By August 29 he was coughing steadily and had bilateral, diffuse pulmonary rales. New infiltrates had appeared in the middle and upper lobes of the right lung. It was believed that he had pneumonia. After considerable discussion, it was decided to treat the patient with penicillin. On August 30 the abdominal pain increased, the hematocrit value decreased suddenly from 30 per cent to 22 per cent, and the stools became guaiac positive. It was believed that retroperitoneal and gastrointestinal hemorrhage had developed secondary to anticoagulation, and heparin therapy was discontinued. After further discussion, it was decided not to give the patient any blood transfusions but to continue the administration of fluids and penicillin. By September 3 the patient was semicomatose. He had bilateral diffuse rales and persistent anemia with a hematocrit value of 18 per cent. The abdomen had become less distended; the patient occasionally was roused from his stupor, but he refused to accept any fluids or other personal ministrations. He died on September 7, 1975.

CLINICAL DISCUSSION

Dr. Gerald Perkoff: Both of these patients presented difficult problems during their care. The first patient, an 86 year old woman, had been essentially well except for poor memory; she had assigned legal responsibility for her affairs to a guardian. However, she was able to communicate well with her physician and to give an accurate history. She was found to have an asymptomatic abdominal aortic aneurysm. After initial evaluation and consultation, it was decided that the patient's age and her history of hypertension made the surgical risks of elective aneurysm replacement too high, and it was decided not to perform surgery. Although this decision was discussed with the guardian, it was not discussed with the patient.

Approximately six months later the aneurysm ruptured. Hypotension responded initially to the intravenous administration of saline solution, and the patient was alert and mentally clear when a different surgeon discussed the problem with her, pointing out the low probability of surgical success. Despite the risks, the patient desired surgery. The guardian was not available. The patient died 30 hours after surgery.

The second patient was a 90 year old man who had poor vision due to cataracts and who was nearly deaf due to chronic otitis. He had anorexia with a 20 pound weight loss and was found to have a bladder neck obstruction due to prostatic hypertrophy. A transurethral prostatectomy was planned but was never performed. Following cystoscopy, the patient had fever, chest pain, hypoxemia, pulmonary infiltrates and abnormal ventilation-perfusion lung scans, and he was treated with heparin for pulmonary emboli. Because of the history of a bowel mass, a barium enema was performed; it revealed only diverticulosis. The barium was not expelled and produced obstipation with increasingly severe abdominal pain for which he required narcotics. The patient refused further diagnostic procedures and stated repeatedly that he wanted no additional therapy, that he wished to die. When pneumonia developed, a minimal course of therapy with penicillin was chosen. When he had a retroperitoneal hemorrhage, he continued to refuse therapy. It was decided not to give him blood transfusions. He became obtunded, then comatose and, after several days, died

I would like to begin our discussion with the first patient. Dr. Jaffe, what is the prognosis in patients with a recognized abdominal aortic aneurysm who are not operated upon?

Dr. Bernard Jaffe: It is quite difficult to get good current data because the great majority of patients are now treated. In the mid-1950's a series of 68 cases was published in which it was shown that patients with untreated abdominal aortic aneurysms had a five year life expectancy of only 5 per cent and that 60 per cent of patients died within one year of diagnosis [2]. Since the first patient had a 7 to 8 cm aneurysm, her five year life expectancy, based on nothing else but the aneurysm, was about 5 per cent without an operation.

Dr. Perkoff: The life expectancy of anyone at 86 or 87 years probably averages about six years, so this risk is greater than the risk of death from other causes. In general, then, do you believe 86 year old people with aortic aneurysms should be operated upon? Our patient was asymptomatic; she had a murmur, mild hypertension and memory loss at the time the decision was made not to operate.

Dr. Jaffe: I think that any patient with a large abdominal aortic aneurysm whose general medical condition or coronary artery disease is not so severe as to preclude long-term survival should be operated upon. In this hospital, the operative mortality rate in patients undergoing elective aneurysm resection is 3 per cent, and there are a number of 80 plus year old survivors.

Dr. Perkoff: What is the expected mortality rate when

such a patient is operated upon after aneurysm rupture with shock?

Dr. Jaffe: In otherwise healthy people, the mortality in patients with a ruptured abdominal aneurysm is 50 per cent. In an 86 year old patient, the mortality rate would be significantly greater.

Dr. Perkoff: Dr. Vavra, what should we make of the fact that this woman had given a third party the authority to make major decisions? How does the guardian figure into this?

Dr. John Vavra: It sounds to me that this woman did not want to make any foolish mistakes with her estate and, because of memory loss, sought power of attorney to protect her from some bad decisions. It does not sound as though she was unable to make certain kinds of decisions for herself, or that she was incapable of understanding medical problems.

The decision not to perform the elective operation was made with the knowledge and approval of the guardian, but without the patient's knowledge. On the other hand, the emergency operation was performed with the patient's consent, but without the guardian's consent. This brings up a problem now being debated—what is a physician's responsibility to his patient? There are three views. The physician's primary responsibility to the patient is (1) to keep "the contract," or to keep promises, which means to involve the patient in all important information obtained during the medical work-up and to permit the patient to be involved in decisions about what ought to be done; (2) the duty not to harm the patient; and (3) the duty to protect other people who are involved. If we are not to harm a patient, then when medical decisions are made complicated information must be interpreted to the patient. He cannot just be given all the data as raw facts. The obligation to protect implies that other people may be involved who need to be protected in the course of the medical work-up. Other personal relationships and factors, such as the family finances, need to be considered. If you ask a patient what the primary responsibility of the physician is, he will state that the primary responsibility of the physician is to keep promises, to keep the contract and to provide information. If you ask a physician what his primary responsibility is, he is likely to emphasize to be sure not to harm the patient and to protect all people involved. In the case of the first patient, the decision not to operate was made on the physician's premise not to harm. The guardian and the physician discussed the medical problem, and the decision was made without involving the patient. There is no reason to believe that the patient was unable to understand or that she could not have been involved in the decision about surgery; she probably should have been consulted. Very interestingly, when the patient returned with her aneurysm bleeding, the opposite decision was made. The patient was supplied with information, and gave her consent to surgery. The guardian was not involved; there obviously was a disparity in the way the physician's obligation was formulated during the course of the patient's illness.

Dr. Perkoff: Dr. LeFrak, would you comment on this patient? In this instance there was a certain diagnosis, sound knowledge about the prognosis, and a specific form of therapy with a known outcome was available.

Dr. Stephen LeFrak: I believe that the elderly make up the group that is most discriminated against in hospitals. Many health professionals are willing to say, "this patient is very old and has lived a full life; let him die in peace." I think we owe the elderly a great deal more than that. We must not invoke age alone as a rationale for not providing intensive care, surgery or other treatment modalities for them. Because of their age, the elderly deserve the best of modern medicine, humanistically and technically.

I think every physician ought to take a look at the Metropolitan Life actuarial tables. An 86 year old women is expected to live a little over five years, a fairly long time. Medical decisions should be based on that life expectancy. If an aneurysm ruptures, we have heard that mortality exceeds 50 per cent. Since age is not a contraindication to aneurysmectomy, medical judgement would seem to dictate that this woman should have undergone an elective surgical procedure before her aneurysm ruptured.

Dr. Perkoff: Basically, the question I asked myself when the issue was presented to us and subsequently, is "Can a physician do other than treat a patient if the patient is completely informed and desires treatment?" The answer I gave was that there is no other choice but to treat such a patient. I think the qualifications I stated before I asked Dr. LeFrak to comment are of some importance here. This woman presented a much simpler problem than the second patient. We knew exactly what was wrong with her, we knew the diagnosis early and a standard form of therapy was available with a known outcome. Whether the patient was 50 or 90 years of age mattered less than that the outcome could be predicted in a reasonable way and that a logical decision could be made about therapy. That being the case, it was appropriate to operate even when the risks were the highest. By the same token, it was a mistake not to have operated earlier when she was well. Further, a telephone consultation is not the appropriate way to confront anyone with a patient. Had this patient interacted personally with the surgeon at the time of her first visit, it clearly would have been preferable. All of us wish to make decisions under the best possible circumstances; these were not provided to this patient at the time. Either the internist or the surgeon, or both, should have insisted upon a consultation visit.

The second patient is much more complex. He was too ill to receive definitive surgical treatment for his primary problem, prostatic hypertrophy. He literally had complications of every diagnostic and therapeutic procedure which was carried out. Until he became comatose, he was actively involved in discussions about his problems and clearly stated that he did not wish to receive treatment; he wished to die. At best, successful aggressive therapy would have left him chronically bedridden and unacceptable for surgery. These facts were clearly involved in the course followed by his physicians, of whom I was one. Dr. Vavra, two major views have been developed in this situation; would you outline them and expand upon them for us?

Dr. Vavra: Let me start by saying that one of the important aspects of this protocol was that the patient was given information, and he made fairly definite statements that he did not want to be treated and that he wanted to die. Is that correct?

Dr. Perkoff: Yes.

Dr. Vavra: He was also informed, as complications arose, that if he did survive he would likely end up in a nursing home, with a catheter, and of the problems likely to ensue?

Dr. Perkoff: No, I do not believe I ever told him that. You did not either, did you Dr. Rudnick?

Dr. Seth Rudnick: No, he did not know that, or if he knew it, he knew it on his own and not from us.

Dr. Paula Clayton: Did he come in wanting to die or was it only as complications arose that he expressed this idea?

Dr. Perkoff: It was only as the complications occurred that he said he wanted to die. However, he was brought to MCG much in the same manner as many patients are brought to the emergency room of a hospital and left there. He had no family; an elderly friend, who believed he could no longer care for himself in his apartment, had helped him get to MCG and then had left. He did not seek medical attention of his own free will.

Dr. Vavra: Before commenting on how to deal with dying patients, I would like to indicate that at times it is very difficult to understand why a patient asks a physician to discontinue treatment and to do nothing more. It is not usually clear, particularly when the physician has not seen the man before, whether the patient is really speaking out of some sense of violation of his dignity, whether it is the "disease" speaking, or whether he is depressed and has had enough of procedures and manipulation.

The two different points of view in the medical and ethical debate as to the physician's responsibility to the dying patient have been best articulated by Robert Morison and Leon Kass [3]. Leon Kass states that the physician's responsibility is to the patient and to the patient alone. Robert Morison states that patients cannot be abstracted from the community to which they belong and the environment in which they live, so that it is not possible to talk about them either alive or dead without seeing them in relation to other people and to the environment. Robert Morison has a broader focus than Leon Kass.

From Kass' point of view it is the physician's responsibility to use his medical skills to the utmost to save the life of the patient, to keep his pain and suffering to a minimum, and to continue to treating him until it is quite clear that his pain and suffering cannot be alleviated and that there is almost nothing else to offer in terms of useful therapy. Patients may make statements that life is not worth living and that they should be permitted to die, but after treatment is instituted they are usually glad that things were done and that they are still alive. There is always the anticipation that disorders not treatable now may be controllable in the very near future, as we all know from the very rapid recent advances in medical science. From Kass' point of view everything possible should be done for sick people, and the physician has no right to withhold therapy unless he is certain it would not be successful.

Morison states the obligation differently. Morison says that physicians obviously have to be sensitive to the dying patient but when the patient is on the downward projectory of his life, he and his family may indicate clearly that important relationships are being compromised and that the patient's dignity is being violated much as Jonathan Swift's was; Swift was kept alive by his doctors for several years despite his wishes to be permitted to die. Morison states that the cost of maintaining life with dignity for the person or for the family includes an appreciation not only of medical factors but also of social and economic factors within the larger contextual framework. Kass rejects outright the view that economic and social factors are important and that physicians have a right to face their decisions to stop therapy upon them. In the second patient it was decided not to give him antibiotics other than penicillin and not to give him blood transfusions. Morison says that if physicians are allowed to make decisions of this type, they need to find a way to talk about these decisions rather than following their "conscience." The two points of view revolve on whom the physician is responsible to: the patient alone, or the patient in the larger context of his environment. With regard to the second patient, it is very difficult to tell what the proper decision should have been. The patient's statements were made when he was seriously ill and there were valid reasons for treating him vigorously. We believe that he was a person with a fairly strong sense of his integrity who earlier had refused surgery out of a sense of his own dignity.

Once patients are in the hospital, it is very hard for

physicians not to do something. It is much easier to make these decisions outside the hospital environment. Once a patient is admitted to the hospital, a lot of people are involved in their care and physicians very frequently will do more then than they might have if they knew the patient better or if he were still at home.

Dr. Perkoff: This man was treated with penicillin but he was not given any transfusions. This difference in decision making is an example of both the emotional and factual confusion with which we approached this particular patient.

Dr. LeFrak, I know that the Kass view is the one you hold over the Morison view. Would you comment?

Dr. LeFrak: I think that it is fallacious to contrast the physician's responsibility to his patient with his responsibility to society. This is a false distinction. The only way we fulfill our responsibility to society is by fulfilling our responsibility to the individual patient. Once society becomes "more important than the individual" and once "cost-benefit analysis" becomes more important than the individual, our whole society as we have known it changes. So, to contrast the interests of the individual with that of "society as a whole" is not only wrong but also has far reaching consequences. Although I do not think that Kass and Morison are opposed in quite this way, this is not a simple distinction to make, nor one that should be made.

It is very difficult to define dying in the dying patient. It appears that the second patient was not dying when he came to the hospital. He started to die while he was in the hospital. Very few people bring themselves to the hospital to die or wanting to die. If they want to die, they do not come to the hospital. So, by the very act of presenting themselves at the hospital, they have already made a decision, "I want to live, I want to get better, do the most you can for me." I think we have the obligation to do all we can. There is always time to allow the patient to die with dignity tomorrow. To allow someone to die one day too soon is a mistake that cannot be rectified.

Dr. Vavra: Being sensitive to the relativistic ethic of Morison, I think it is very important to keep the patient's needs in primary view, but it is also important to be cognizant of the consequences to other people. To overemphasize unlikely consequences is the camel's nose or slippery slope argument, i.e., if you let a camel get his nose into a tent then the rest of the camel will go in, or if you do not plant your feet firmly on the ice you will slide to the bottom. I think it unlikely that patients will be denied good medical care if the physician considers the social and economic consequences as well as the important medical and psychologic problems of dying patients.

Dr. Clayton: I think that when you talk about this patient you have to consider that he certainly was a very independent man. He was 90 years old, had no family, lived by himself and had a great deal of pride in his independence. He made a decision years earlier not to undergo surgery that had been recommended. When you talk about responsibility to the patient, you should consider that if he then sees himself as losing his independence in the hospital and this leads him to want to die, a part of your responsibility may be to let him die.

Dr. Perkoff: As Dr. Vavra mentioned earlier, a physician who is faced with a situation in which there is no reasonable likelihood of success has a difficult time. One of the things that impressed us was that everything that had been done to this man made his condition worse rather than better. In fact, other than choosing a more potent group of antibiotics or giving him a transfusion, we really had no therapy to offer him. That may not be adequate justification for the course that was followed, but recognition of those feelings surely influenced the decisions which were made. Dr. Rudnick, you were directly involved with this man. I know there was a great difference of opinion and much concern on the part of the house staff about the care of this patient. Would you comment, please?

Dr. Rudnick: I think that, in a sense, it is a bit easier for a house officer to approach the problem of the patient who is critically and probably terminally ill. The house officer's prime concern is to the patient. The societal concern that intrudes upon him is limited to the family. I think I am less concerned than the patient's primary physician with cost effectiveness or a general consideration of what the patient will do when he returns to society.

However, we are faced with life and death decisions daily. Our entire training is to prolong life, to do everything we can to improve the patient's care. I do not think any of us ever consciously consider doing anything that would allow the patient's life to be shortened. Yet there is a conflict for all of us, and it usually occurs in a case like that of the second patient. The patient or the family make certain demands on us. Those demands can be quite divergent, either to do everything for the patient or to do nothing for the patient. We are never quite sure what "nothing" or "everything" is. We are confronted with critical questions and decisions. Am I doing this for the patient's benefit? Am I killing him by not performing some procedure or by performing it? Active or passive euthanasia is almost a useless distinction for us. We are quite aware of the potentially fatal consequence of withholding an antibiotic. Conversely if we put the patient through innumerable procedures and therapies, and all the complications of heparinization or of a barium enema develop we also know we have contributed to his death. Recently, another complication has been presented, "Am I going to be sued if I do not do exactly what the patient and/or his family desires?"

A final element of our quandry, one that crosses our

minds all the time, is if we know that the patient is going to die, do we back off a little bit? Do we say "I am not going to do quite everything I can, I am not going to remain awake until 5 o'clock in the morning with this one patient, because I know no matter what I do he will die?" No where in this decision making process are there formal guidelines. We perform in this situation on the basis of our knowledge, intuition and, occasionally, prayer.

Dr. Perkoff: I think that is a very accurate description of the way most of us feel. But, even feeling the way we do, we end up with very different views.

Dr. Clayton, one of the questions that Dr. Vavra raised, and which certainly must be considered whenever a patient says he or she wants to die, is the difficulty of distinguishing the person from the illness. There are some who believe that if a person wants to die, this is in fact one form of suicide. Since suicide is an unacceptable thing in society, it a priori becomes a manifestation of mental illness. If the patient is mentally ill, his statements must be discounted. How does mental illness fit in here?

Dr. Clayton: I guess I was shocked when it was said that no patient wants to die. In psychiatry we see a lot of patients who are depressed; their chief complaint is that they want to die. What I was getting at when I asked if the patient expressed the idea that he wanted to die on admission is that, with anorexia and weight loss that were never explained, it is important to determine whether or not this man was suffering from a depression when he came to you in the first place. The problems are different when someone with an affective disorder wants to die, when someone who is gravely medically ill wants to die, or when someone who is dying wants to die.

Patients who do not have what you consider adequate medical justification for wanting to die, that is, you cannot understand why they may say they want to die as their medical condition does not include imminent death, are probably suffering from psychiatric illness, and the illness most likely is an affective disorder which should be treated. Patients who are going downhill rapidly and who then express a wish not to be treated are probably not mentally ill. But, I do not know of any good studies which would indicate what really is the case in terminally ill patients. People who study terminally ill patients discuss the fear of dying and the thoughts about dying, but they do not actually ask the patients if they want to die or if they have thoughts of suicide. Suicide is extremely rare in dying patients. Only 4 per cent of suicides are committed because the patient is terminally ill [4].

Dr. Perkoff: Are interviewing technics and diagnostic criteria good enough to permit adequate recognition of an affective disorder in a person with a complicated illness?

Dr. Clayton: I think that if this patient had been seen at the beginning of his illness this decision could have been made. Depression is a mood change and a cluster of psychologic and somatic symptoms, usually of relatively recent onset. Past history and family history are important. After all the procedures, and when his condition was worsening day by day and he had further symptoms which may have indicated to him that he was dying, it would have been very difficult to decide whether the depression was primary or secondary to his worsening condition.

Dr. Perkoff: Dr. LeFrak, do you want to add something?

Dr. LeFrak: I think Dr. Clayton has confirmed what I said, that the so-called dying patient rarely wants to die and rarely attempts suicide. When we have a patient who is inappropriately suicidal, we take steps to insure his life. So, medical patients really do not come to the hospital because they want to die.

Dr. Rudnick's comment concerning holding back, even unconsciously, in the terribly ill patient needs to be stressed. This can become a self-fulfilling prophecy, i.e., this patient is so sick that no matter what we do he will die, so we do less, and the patient dies. At the time it is easier to let a patient die. It is easier emotionally, because we all can breathe a sigh of relief. It is physically less taxing and less time-consuming, and we can rationalize this type of inaction with our philosophical arguments and commend ourselves on our sensitivity and humanity. Frankly, we have to be very aware of what goes on inside of ourselves before we make these kinds of decisions.

Lastly, I would like to suggest that it may almost be impossible to truly communicate with the critically ill patient or his family in the midst of a life-threatening illness. We talk to patients and their families, and I really wonder how, in the midst of terrible emotional upset, either the family or the patient can really communicate in a meaningful way as to whether therapy, especially extraordinary therapy, should be instituted or maintained. I think it is unfair to place this burden on the family or at times even on the patient. I think that one of the jobs of physicians is to bear the guilt for making certain decisions and not to place this burden on the family. We get paid for that while the family has to live with that decision forever, and the patient may not live at all. This is not to say that we should not inform the patient and the family as best we can, but it is a plea to shoulder the burden for these decisions which are our responsibility.

Dr. Perkoff: Now I would like to get the opinions of those in the audience. Dr. Binder, do you want to start?

Dr. Morton Binder: I think that it is often easier to let a patient live than to let him die. It takes less thinking and less decision making to keep a patient alive than to decide that the best thing is to let him die. I think that people do come to the hospital to die. We bring patients to the hospital all the time to die; they come for help including relief of pain.

In a sense, the patients discussed here were poor examples because no one knew them. I think that when patients have signed a so-called living-will and have very strong feelings about how they want to be treated in their last illness, you can respect that decision even in the emergency room. Did somebody tell the first patient what the morbidity of the operation was like, how she would feel, what she would be like after the surgery? Or, was she quoted a 50 per cent chance to live?

Dr. Perkoff: Dr. Jaffe, can you answer that question?

Dr. Jaffe: The patient was told in detail what she would feel postoperatively and exactly what the possibilities were should she survive.

Age is something we, as all physicians, must deal with routinely. Occasionally, we mistakenly deny patients the advantages of operation merely because of advanced age.

Dr. Perkoff: Are there other comments from the audience?

Dr. Philip Majerus: I wonder if Dr. Binder has not hit upon the point that these patients are examples of a different social problem from that of the dying patient per se, namely, that of institutional medical care. If the second patient had had a physician who knew him well, he might have been better off not being admitted to the hospital in the first place or having been discharged immediately after being catheterized. That kind of medical decision is very hard to make in this hospital. Yet, it might have been better for him.

Dr. Edward Reinhard: I think this brings up Dr. Binder's point again. It really is much more difficult to let a patient die than it is to keep him alive. I think it is much more difficult to recognize the fact that the patient's life is a great burden to him and to base therapeutic decisions on that recognition. This is something you learn progressively with experience. It is our obligation at times to recognize the fact that the patient wants to die, that the patient's life is terrible to him and that it is destroying the family not only by its psychologic effects but also by its financial effects. Even if you can keep him alive a few more months by heroic efforts it is a mistake to do it if the quality of life is unbearable; you have to overcome your feelings and allow the patient to die.

Dr. LeFrak: I would like to ask Dr. Reinhard two questions. First, if patients really want to die, why do they come back to see you and accept treatment? We all know, or they should know, that if they do not come back they can die. Secondly, there is a growing image in our society, propagated by the media, that our patients are dying in great pain, great agony and great suffering, and that the hospitals are filled with these people, all in pain and being artifically supported. I do not think that is true. Do your patients die in great pain?

Dr. Reinhard: That is a very good point. The idea that patients should be relieved of their suffering by allowing them to die is not correct. I will agree with you that relief of pain is not an adequate reason to withhold therapy, because you can relieve pain. But, the quality of life that progressively deteriorates, should also be considered.

Dr. Ernest Rouse, III: A lot of us do not want to get overly aggressive with patients and yet we have a real problem. When Dr. Reinhard, with his clinical experience, says a patient is going to die, everybody believes him. Yet, in my limited clinical experience, I have seen patients whom I never thought would survive get well. I think that is the time when we have to turn to the attending physicians and, as Dr. Reinhard indicated, learn from experience.

Dr. Gail Clark: We have been talking a lot about what the patient said and how the patient said it and what a lot of other people have to say about the patient. I just wondered, Dr. Rudnick, when the patient was saying "I want to die," did anybody actually go in and say to the patient, "You know, if you were not bleeding, if you were not impacted and if you were not infected, and if you felt like you did when you came in the door, would you still want to die?" I was impressed with Victor Frankel's approach to suicidal patients. When a patient came into his office and said "I want to commit suicide" he would not ask, "why do you want to," but rather, "Why didn't you?"

Dr. Perkoff: I do not think any of us asked him the specific question in the way in which you outlined it, Dr. Clark.

Dr. Kenneth Ludmerer: Like everyone here, I believe that a decision to let a patient go is probably a more difficult decision than one to go all out for him. But a related question, once that decision is made, is how to let a patient go. In other words, recognizing a terminally ill patient, preferably before he is in the final stages, when his resources are together, and recognizing that medical science will not permit the patient to survive, how can we as physicians and human beings help this patient, and his family and his friends accept his death?

Dr. LeFrak: I just want to respond to two things that are implied in your question, Dr. Ludmerer. One is what is "terminally ill?" This is a term that is used frequently and it upsets me. We all have a terminal illness; we are all going to die. And I do not understand what people mean by "terminal illness." Secondly, I do not think the decision to let a patient die needs to be made today. I always think it is worthwhile to give him at least another

24 hours; we can always make that decision tomorrow. That may mean I have difficulty facing those kinds of decisions, but I am always uncomfortable making a decision which is unalterable. Once the patient is dead, it is unalterable.

Dr. Perkoff: I do not know of anyway to summarize this discussion. Many issues have been raised today and we find ourselves unable to resolve them, This inability reflects the true state of affairs in this area. It is important to know that house officers and senior physicians alike share insecurity and uncertainty with these problems. We must become able to verbalize the feeling all of us have when we deal with patients, especially with patients like these. Science for its own sake is terribly important, but the application of science to our patients involves our feelings as well as our factual knowledge. The decisions we make are in good measure emotional as well as scientific. If that much has become clear through this discussion, then we have accomplished much of what we set out to do today.

REFERENCES

1. Clinicosociologic Conference: Long-term dialysis. Am J Med 59: 702, 1975.
2. Wright IS, Urdaneta E, Wright B: Re-opening the case of the abdominal aortic aneurysm. Circulation 13: 754, 1956.
3. Morison RS, Kass LR: Death: process and event. Science 173: 694, 1971.
4. Robins E, Murphy GE, Wilkinson RH Jr, et al.: Some clinical considerations in the prevention of suicide based on a study of 134 successful suicides. Am J Pub Health 49: 888, 1959.

INFORMATION FOR AUTHORS

PREPARATION OF MANUSCRIPTS

Manuscripts should be typed on one side of the sheet, doublespaced, on white bond paper, 8½ by 11 inches, with margins of 1 inch. Two copies of the manuscript and illustrations should be sent to the Editor at 666 Fifth Avenue, New York, New York 10019. Title page should include full name, degrees and affiliation of all authors, the source from which the article emanates, and the name and address of the person to whom requests for reprints should be addressed.

All manuscript pages including tables and legends should be numbered consecutively in the upper right hand corner.

The number of manuscript pages, the number of illustrations and the number of tables should be indicated at the bottom of the covering letter.

Every article must be preceded by an abstract (not to exceed 350 words). This obviates the need for a summary. In addition, for the convenience of our readers, we require a brief abstract (not exceeding 100 to 125 words) and key words for indexing purposes. These brief abstracts appear in the back of the *Journal* in the same issue in which the paper appears.

Since all manuscripts submitted for publication in the *Journal* are sent out for review before a final decision is made, there is generally a lapse of three to six weeks before contributors are notified. If you have received an acknowledgment of receipt, there is no need to call the *Journal* office; your manuscript has not gone astray. The decision will be forthcoming shortly.

PREPARATION OF ILLUSTRATIONS AND TABLES

Illustrations must be black and white glossy prints or professional drawings in india ink; they should be unmounted. The name of the lead author and the title of the article should be typed on a label and affixed to the back of each illustration; the top should be indicated.

Reference to all illustrations should be inserted in the text in consecutive order. Legends for the illustrations should be typed, double spaced, on a separate sheet with numbers corresponding to those on the photographs or drawings. They should not be attached to the pictures.

Tables should be typed on separate sheets and should be set up in accordance with the style of the Journal. Units of measure should be confined to column headings. Abbreviations should be kept to a minimum and should conform with those used by the *Journal* or listed as acceptable in the Council of Biology Editors Style Manual. Any variations should be explained. All vertical rules should be omitted.

The publisher allows a fixed amount towards the reproduction of illustrations and tables. Charges in excess of this amount must be assumed by the authors. The Editor reserves the right to limit the number of illustrations and/or tables.

PREPARATION OF BIBLIOGRAPHY

Bibliographic references should be listed chronologically on a separate sheet (not in footnotes) as referred to in the text and should be typed (double-spaced) in accordance with the style and abbreviations (open punctuation) used by Index Medicus; only the first page of the journal citation is necessary. Examples follow:

For periodical references:

22. Theologides A, Kennedy BJ: Toxoplasmic myocarditis and pericarditis. Am J Med 47: 169, 1969.

For book references (with chapter):

18. Schiebler GL, Van Mieron LHS, Krovetz LJ: Diseases of the tricuspid valve, chap 2. Heart Disease in Infants, Children and Adolescents (Moss AJ, Adams F, eds), Baltimore, Williams & Wilkins, 1968.

For book references (without chapter):

13. Berne E: Principles of Group Treatment, New York, Oxford University Press, 1966, p 26.

Authors are responsible for the accuracy of all references.

REPRINTS

Price schedules and order cards for reprints are mailed to the person so listed in the footnote on the title page.

The American Journal of Medicine, **666 Fifth Avenue, New York, New York 10019**

Factors Involved in Immunization Program for Swine Influenza

GORONWY O. BROUN, Sr., M.D.
DENNIS O'CONNOR, M.D.
ROSE RITA SCHMIDT, M.A.
BARBARA PUDER, B.S.
St. Louis, Missouri

The decision to undertake a nationwide program of vaccination against swine influenza requires assessment of the status of immunity of those in various age groups in our population against this agent. Pools of serum were collected from persons born in the years from 1889 to 1943; they were tested for hemagglutinin inhibiting (HI) antibody against the HSW1N1 influenza virus strains isolated in 1931 and 1976. The titers secured serve as an indication of the average level of immunity of those of different ages. Persons less than 43 years of age are found to be without antibody protection. The need for vaccination of people in different age groups based on mortality statistics of previous epidemics is evaluated. It is realized that no epidemic may occur and that a reduced virulence of the viral agent and use of antibiotics may reduce the death rate if the infection recurs. The extraordinary high mortality in 1918 in people between 15 and 44 years of age deserves recognition together with the fact that those in the same age group are now without protection. The fact that women of childbearing age fall into this group deserves special consideration in view of increased mortality in puerperal women observed in the pandemics of 1918 and 1957. The degree of protection afforded the newborn by transplacental transmission of maternal antibodies is discussed. The need of increasing the level of immunity in those who have varying titers of HI antibodies is considered in relation to the prevalence of cardiopulmonary complications and other chronic diseases in older subjects.

The appearance of a strain of influenza virus at Fort Dix, New Jersey, antigenically identical to the HSW1N1 strain generally accepted as the cause of the pandemic of 1918–1920, and evidence of its spread by human contact, have led to the establishment of a national program of vaccination against this agent. Francis and Magill [1] reported as early as 1944 that those born before and during the period of the pandemic had antibodies against this virus, which, by the time of his observations, remained prevalent only in swine. He also showed that those born subsequent to the disappearance of this agent from the human population had no immunologic protection. In more recent years, there have been reports of evidence of spread of HSW1N1 from swine to human beings based on serologic studies [2] and at least one isolation of HSW1N1 from lung tissue at autopsy [3].

The strain of HSW1N1 influenza virus isolated at Fort Dix in 1976 so far has caused only a single death, and spread of the infection was

From the Departments of Internal Medicine and Pediatrics of St. Louis University School of Medicine, St. Louis, Missouri. Requests for reprints should be addressed to Dr. Goronwy O. Broun, Sr., St. Louis University, 1325 South Grand Boulevard, St. Louis, Missouri 63104. Manuscript accepted September 29, 1976.

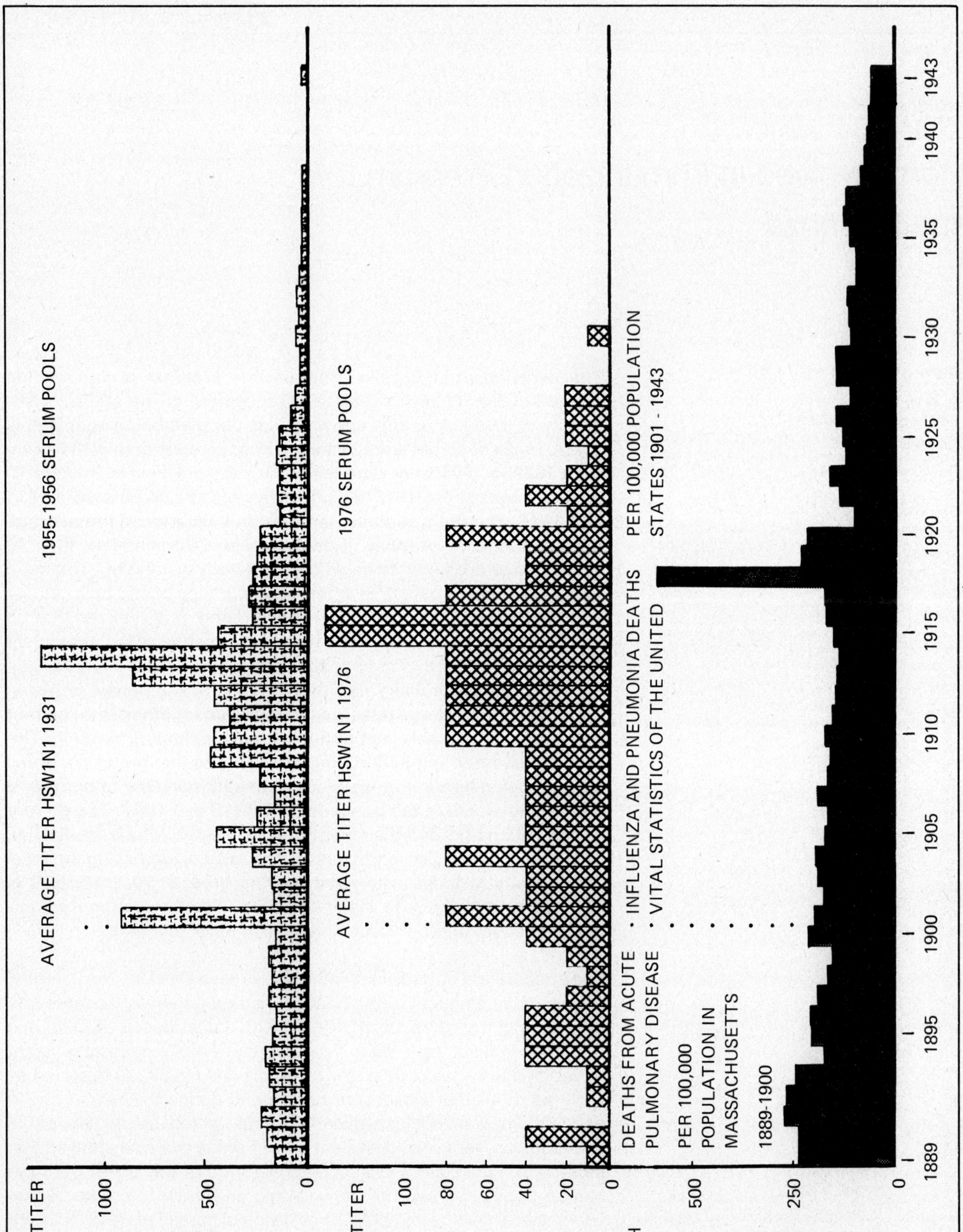

Figure 1. *Antihemagglutinin titer against 1931 and 1976 HSW1N1 influenza virus strains in serum pools, collected from patients by year of birth, compared to annual death rates from influenza and pneumonia.*

TABLE I Antihemagglutinin Titer of Serum Pools of Specimens from People Born in Certain Age Periods. Specimens for Pools Collected Between 1951 and 1956, and Between 1956 and 1959 Tested Against 1931 HSW1N1 Influenza Virus Strain and in 1976 Against the 1976 HSW1N1 Strain

St. Louis University Hospital Population Collected 1951–1956			Black Population Collected 1956–1959			St. Louis University Hospital Population Collected in 1976			
Years of Birth Covered by Pool*	Number of Serums in Pool	Average HI Titer for HSW1N1 1931	Years of Birth Covered by Pool*	Number of Serums in Pool	Average HI Titer for HSW1N1 1931	Years of Birth Covered by Pool*	Number of Serums in Pool	Average HI Titer for HSW1N1 1976	Prevalent Influenza Virus
			1869–1878	4	0				Strain causing 1875 epidemic
1875–1889	241	117	1879–1888	68	11	1880–1889	13	10	Strain causing 1875 epidemic
1890–1898	292	195	1888–1898	169	25	1890–1898	47	24	Strain causing pandemic of 1890–1893
1899–1910	456	297	1898–1908	243	26	1899–1910	140	51	Strain causing epidemic of 1899–1901
1911–1917	320	512	1906–1918	488	48	1911–1917	134	74	Strain causing epidemic of 1899–1901
1918–1920	161	315	1916–1928	730	23	1918–1920	57	55	HSW1N1
1921–1928	549	91				1921–1928	192	18	HSW1N1
1929–1932	628	129	1926–1938	813	0	1929–1932	77	2	HON1
1933–1938	787	5	1938–1944	206	0	1933–1938	54	0	HON1
1939–1943	366	0				1939	11	0	HON1
1946–1956	511	0				1940–1965	312	0	H1N1
1890–1928	1,778	258	1888–1928	1,630	31	1890–1928	570	44	...

*Year of birth of people whose serum is included in pools.

sharply limited to the military post. An additional fatal infection probably acquired directly from swine occurred in Minnesota in a person who also suffered from Hodgkin's disease [3]. Only the occurrence of a widespread epidemic with high mortality due to the swine virus will establish it as a serious danger to the country as a whole. Protective measures are justified only because this possibility cannot be excluded.

We have studied influenza infection in the St. Louis area continuously for the past 33 years. Previous publications have included observations on the antigenic variations in influenza virus strains isolated in this vicinity [4] and the use of serum pools to demonstrate the exposure of the population to the various virus strains and the level of immunity of the local population [5,6]. The pathology caused by H2N2 influenza in 1957 in pregnant women has been studied [7], and maternal transmission of influenza antibodies during pregnancy has been observed [8].

In the St. Louis population we will demonstrate the distribution of antibodies against the HSW1N1 virus isolated from swine in the 1930's and the recent New Jersey isolate. Not only the presence or absence of antibodies but also the variations in titer which may affect the need of immunization of people in different age groups will be considered.

Data will be presented indicating the danger posed to pregnant women by influenza infections. Possible protection of the newborn by transplacental transmission of maternal antibodies will be discussed.

METHODS OF PROCEDURE

The antibody levels were measured by the hemagglutinin inhibition (HI) test of Hirst [9] as modified by Salk [10]. Serums used in the study were treated with receptor destroying enzymes of vibreo cholera, RDE, to eliminate nonspecific inhibitors in tests for HSW1N1, H1N1 and H3N2 virus, and with periodate and trypsin in the case of the H2N2 strains.

In the period since 1950, we have assembled into pools, according to the date of birth of each individual, serum specimens submitted to the St. Louis University Hospital laboratory for various serologic examinations. These pools were then examined utilizing the antihemagglutinin test for influenza antibodies using a number of antigens including the HSW1N1 strain. The level of HI antibodies in serum pools collected from persons born each year from 1889 to 1943 is shown in Figure 1. The upper graph illustrates the HI titers of serums collected in 1955 and 1956 against the HSW1N1 isolated in 1931. The central graph shows the titers of serum specimens collected in 1976 against the New Jersey 1976 HSW1N1 isolate. The number of serums in the pools illustrated in the upper graph varied from 10 to 161 with an average of 54 serums. The number of serums in the pools

TABLE II Present Status of Immunity Against HSW1N1 Influenza Virus in the General Population

Subjects	Results
Women of childbearing age	No immunologic protection
Newborn and children, ages 1–4 years	No immunologic protection
Children	
Age 5–14 years	No immunologic protection
Age 15–43 years	No immunologic protection
Age 44–55 years	HI titer 1/13
Age 56–65 years	HI titer 1/68
Over 65 years	HI titer 1/40

shown in the center graph varied from 3 to 34, with an average of 14 serums.

In order that the variations in titer in the serum pools can be correlated with the incidence of influenza infection, the bottom graph illustrates the deaths per 100,000 population due to acute respiratory tract infections in Massachusetts as recorded in the *Boston Medical and Surgical Journal* from 1889 to 1900 and the deaths attributed to "influenza and pneumonia" in the Vital Statistics of the United States from 1901 to 1943. The latter figure, gathered each year from a number of cities, is still used by the U.S. Public Health Service as an index of the occurrence of influenza infection. The marked increase in mortality during the 1918 pandemic is clearly seen.

In Table I are shown the results secured with three groups of serum pools collected so as to include serums obtained from people born in periods varying between three and 10 years as indicated in the first or left-hand column of each of the three subdivisions. The serums in subdivisions 1 and 3 were collected from people in the St. Louis University Hospital in which the majority of patients were white; those in subdivision 2 were collected from St. Mary's Infirmary where the majority of patients were black. The titer of antihemagglutinins found in the serum pools are shown in the third column of each subdivision of the table. The titers recorded in subdivisions 1 and 2 were secured by use of the antigen of the HSW1N1 strain of influenza virus isolated from hogs in 1931, and those in subdivision 3 were obtained by use of the antigen prepared from the influenza virus strain of human origin isolated at Fort Dix, New Jersey, in 1976.

TITERS OF SWINE ANTIBODIES IN THE POPULATION BY AGE GROUPS AND YEAR OF COLLECTION OF SPECIMEN

The data in Figure 1 and Table I show the following facts in regard to the distribution of antihemagglutinins against swine virus in our population:

(1) The highest HI titers against HSW1N1 influenza virus are found in people born between 1901 and 1920; particularly in those born between 1909 and 1917.

(2) The titer of antihemagglutinins of people born in 1918 and 1919 is lower than that of those born in the 1909–1917 period.

(3) The antibody levels in people born prior to 1901 decrease in a number of years below the level of the 1901–1917 pools.

(4) In the decade following the pandemic, the antibody levels are lower than those in serum collections before the pandemic.

(5) Between 1929 and 1933 swine antibody titers decreased rapidly, and after 1943 they disappeared almost completely.

COMMENTS

Many questions can be raised regarding the background of the distribution of swine influenza antibodies as shown in our data, but the titers found to be present at this time give information of practical value in planning an immunization program. In Table II, the antibody levels found in recent months in people in various age groups are summarized. It is realized that in utilizing the titers found in pooled serums two factors are operative. One is that a certain percentage of people may have no antibodies and the other is the height of the titer of each person contributing to the serum pool. However, the result does indicate the average levels of immunity supplied by antibodies for the entire group.

The immunologic picture as presented in this table has a strong resemblance to that which must have existed prior to the pandemic of 1918. Normally, the very young and the old, the two extremes of age, have higher death rates from influenza as well as from other causes. In 1918, the peak of the mortality curve was in those between 14 and 34 years f age. This group of people, as well as those of still younger age, is now without immunologic protection against the HSW1N1 virus strain. Certain factors affecting the need of vaccination in various population groups will be considered.

Effect of Influenza Infections on Mortality of Puerperal Women. Of great importance in planning an immunization program against influenza is whether this infection poses a particular hazard for pregnant women. In the relatively mild outbreaks of influenza that occur every two or three years, we have observed no evidence that this is the case. Pandemic outbreaks, however, require special consideration. In personal conversation with obstetricians during the 1918–1920 pandemic, a high mortality in puerperal women was well recognized and was a cause of deep concern. The statistical proof that this danger existed is well documented by Dublin and Lotka [11] in their analysis of the countrywide statistics of the Metropolitan Life Insurance Co.

They record that white women of childbearing age showed a 49 per cent increase in total puerperal death rate over the mean before the pandemic. Black women experienced a much less striking increase, namely, 20 per cent. This is the only period between 1911 and 1935 that the mortality of puerperal white women exceeded that of black women. It was the so-called accidents of pregnancy, "abortion," "miscarriage" and "premature births" which showed the greatest increase although deaths at term, due to "childbirth," "labor" and "parturition" also were at record high levels. Deaths in these two general categories tripled the average before the pandemic in white women and doubled that in black women. Despite the lowering of resistance to bacterial infection caused by influenza, the deaths from puerperal septicemia were actually decreased during the 1918 pandemic.

Dublin [12], in a later report based on the Metropolitan Life Insurance Co. records for the years 1936 through 1945, covers mortality statistics during the period of the last large epidemic of influenza due to the H0N1 strain of that virus. This occurred in the winter of 1943–1944.

Comparing the mortality in the year 1942 with the two following years, this report shows that deaths attributed to influenza in white women increased 53 per cent in 1943 and 96 per cent in 1944. The corresponding figures for black women was a 16 per cent increase in 1943 and a 33 per cent increase in 1944.

The general mortality for people with puerperal diseases shows no increase in mortality in white women during this influenza epidemic. Black women showed a very small 4 per cent increase in 1943 but a 19 per cent increase in 1944.

Deaths in puerperal women are further subdivided in this report into three categories, those due to "puerperal septicemia," "puerperal albuminuria and convulsions" and "other diseases of the puerperal state." It would seem most likely that deaths in puerperal women associated with a respiratory tract infection would be included in the third category. The mortality in black women due to "other diseases of the puerperal state" showed a 17 per cent increase in 1943 and a 40 per cent increase in 1944 over the level recorded in 1942. These data suggest that in black women, but not in white women, the H0N1 epidemic of 1943–1944 resulted in an increased mortality in pregnant women. This is a reversal of the ethnic incidence compared to the 1918 pandemic in which, as previously mentioned, white women showed a much higher mortality. We have no evidence that outbreaks of influenza which occurred between 1946 and 1956, when the H1N1 strain was prevalent, caused any increase in mortality of puerperal women.

At the time of the H2N2 pandemic of 1957and 1958, virologic and pathologic studies in nine fatal cases of influenza were carried out in our laboratories [7]. Of these nine cases, four were associated with pregnancy. In one patient, death occurred at the 26th week of pregnancy and in another during the seventh month. Two patients died shortly after delivery, one on the second and the other on the seventh day postpartum. In both, the influenza infection began prior to delivery. H2N2 virus was isolated from the lungs in each instance.

One patient was hospitalized in the St. Louis University Hospital and another in St. Mary's Hospital. Both of these institutions were served by our laboratories. The statistics of these two hospitals show that in a five year period, 1955–1959, there were six deaths in puerperal women in 27,748 admissions for pregnancy. Only two of these deaths were associated with acute respiratory tract infections. Both occurred in 1957 during the pandemic and were shown to be due to influenza by isolation of virus from the lungs.

In 1956, in these same two hospitals, there were 313 admissions for acute respiratory tract infections. In 1957, there were 613 admissions under this category. Six deaths attributed to influenza occurred during November and December of 1957. One third of all deaths in puerperal women in these two hospitals, in the five year period centering on 1957, were due to influenza. One third of all deaths due to influenza during the pandemic of 1957 were associated with pregnancy.

In the other two fatal cases of influenza associated with pregnancy the patients were referred from other hospitals from which we do not have accurate statistics. Influenza virus was isolated from the lungs at postmortem examination in both cases. This indicates that the fatal results of influenza in pregnancy were not limited to the two previously named hospitals.

In two of the fatal cases of influenza associated with the puerperal state the patients also had valvular heart disease in the form of mitral stenosis. This complication obviously adds to the danger of death in pregnant women.

Mulder and Hers [13] reported on 25 fatalities due to influenza studied virologically during the pandemic of 1957–1958. Eight of these were in pregnant women. In 11 of these cases the patients had valvular heart disease. These experiences suggest that in the H2N2 pandemic of 1957–1958, a considerable percentage of fatal cases were in pregnant women and that valvular heart disease was a common complication.

In the 1957–1958 pandemic, in cases that were not studied virologically, Greenberg et al. [14] found a significant increase in mortality in puerperal women during October and November of 1957 compared to the previous five year period.

In our study of the pathology of the 1957 H2N2 influenzal pneumonias [7], we suggested that anoxemia caused by mechanical block of gaseous exchange due to the hyaline membrane found covering the surfaces of the pulmonary alveoli was an important cause of death due to the viral infection. Cardiac and long-term pulmonary disease would still further impair respiratory function. Superimposed bacterial infection is involved in the fatal termination in many cases. In later outbreaks of influenza due to the H2N2 strain and the more recent infection due to the H3N2 virus, there has been no evidence of increased mortality in puerperal women.

Fetal Mortality and Possible Protection of Newborn by Transplacental Transmission of Antibodies During Pregnancy. The anoxemia caused by the influenza infection also may cause distress and even death of the fetus. Bass [15] states that influenza, although rarely if ever teratogenic, may cause fetal deaths. MacKenzie and Houghton [16] reviewed nine studies of the occurrence of congenital deformities in infants born to mothers who suffered an attack of influenza during pregnancy in 1957. Five studies reported a positive association and four found no evidence that this occurred. We have no evidence of teratogenesis or increased fetal mortality in our hospital statistics.

In studies we have made of maternal transmission of influenza antibodies to the fetus [8], we found that when antibodies were present in maternal blood during pregnancy over 50 per cent of the offspring would show such antibodies in the cord blood at the time of delivery. Presence of HSW1N1 antibodies was, of course, limited to women born prior to 1940. Even in the early 1960's, the titer of maternal antibodies was in most instances low, and titers above 1/10 in the fetal blood were rare. In our experience, the persistence of these antibodies after birth is brief, in many instances, no more than one month. It would appear, therefore, that the degree of immunity afforded by maternal antibodies is limited. Nevertheless, some protection may be conferred by maternal vaccination.

Infants. Ages six months to four years: In ordinary years, young infants have relatively few lower respiratory tract infections in a nonvirulent influenza outbreak [17]. However, in the statistics from the 1918–1920 pandemic reported by Dublin and Lotka [11] white infants between the ages of one and four years showed a threefold increase in deaths, and black infants showed a twofold increase. In planning protection against the possible return of this infection, complacency in regard to this age group is scarcely justified. Since recently prevalent strains of influenza have not produced a high mortality in infants, the vaccine considered for use should be of the HSW1N1 type. Serologic studies of infants between six months and four years of age show that they readily produce antibodies when exposed to prevalent influenza virus strains. To justify immunization in this group, a vaccine free of serious toxic reactions must be available.

Children. Ages five to 14 years: Although it is true that for unknown reasons the minimal mortality in the great pandemic was in children between five and 14 years of age, there still was a sufficiently high death rate to justify protection [11]. Moreover, we have no logical basis for assuming that children in this group will show a natural immunity to a similar infection. If the severity of reactions to the vaccine can be kept low, this group of children should be immunized against the HSW1N1 strain.

Ages 15 to 44 years: In the 1918 pandemic, the highest mortality occurred in this age group [11]. Once the safety and proper dosage of the swine vaccine are established, this segment of the population should be given a high priority in receipt of this immunization. The group includes women of childbearing age. The phenomenon known as "original antigenic sin" results in a greater anamnestic increase in antibody titer against the influenza virus strain to which an individual subject is first exposed when contact is made later with a different but related strain. This suggests that there may be some advantage in using for the first vaccination an agent of the potential virulence of the HSW1N1 strain.

Adults. 45 to 55 years of age: Antibodies against swine influenza are found in serum pools collected from people in this age group. The titer, however, is quite low. It is likely that this indicates that a considerable percentage of these people escaped exposure, rather than presence of a low titer in those who were exposed. Since it is not practical to determine the presence or absence of antibodies individually, the entire group should be offered immunization. Since present practice does not recommend vaccination against the currently prevalent influenza virus strains except in those at high risk, monovalent swine vaccine would be the agent employed.

Ages 56 to 65 years: The serum pools in this age bracket show the highest titers of all those tested. This probably indicates a high percentage of exposure to the 1918 strain. Some of these people, however, may have escaped exposure and others may now have only a low titer. Although people in this age group should have a lower infection and mortality rate than any others, they should be offered the protection of a vaccine injection as a booster for their present immunity. People at high risk should be vaccinated not only against the swine virus but also the recently prevalent strains.

The H2N2 and H3N2 strains may act as a less potent stimulus of anamnestic increases in swine antibodies than the H1N1 strains. Webster [18] has reported this difference in regard to H2N2 viruses. In a study of 30 persons showing swine antibodies in their serum, we found that less than one-third showed an anamnestic increase after vaccination with H3N2 vaccine. This indicates that little reliance can be placed on vaccines prepared from current strains to increase immunity against swine virus.

Over 65 years of age: We found a titer against HSW1N1 virus of 1/40 in the pooled serum from people in this age group. All were living during the time that this strain was prevalent. Since age and the frequency of various health complications places these individuals in a high risk category, they should receive immunization against recently prevalent strains as well as the swine vaccine.

Use of Influenza Vaccines in Pregnant Females. We have indicated that we have no definite evidence that endemic or locally epidemic influenza infections increase the mortality of pregnant women. There is substantial evidence that the pandemic of influenza due to the HSW1N1 virus in 1918 did cause a marked increase in puerperal deaths. A limited study, which we carried out during the pandemic of H2N2 influenza in 1957, leads us to believe that an increased risk for pregnant women also was caused by that virus strain. As stated previously, there is no certainty that a large outbreak of swine influenza will occur in the immediate future or, if it does occur, that the virulence of the infectious agents will equal that of the 1918 pandemic. The justification for use of HSW1N1 vaccine rests on our inability to exclude the occurrence of such an outbreak. To guard against this possibility, the protection that can be afforded by vaccination against swine influenza appears to be indicated.

The usual reactions of a young adult to the vaccine may be expected. There is no evidence that the vaccine would produce harmful effects on the fetus. Since the strains of influenza virus present in recent years have not increased mortality of puerperal women, use of vaccine against these strains would only be required in people with complications such as cardiopulmonary disease.

Medical Personnel. One of the serious problems encountered in the great pandemic was the high percentage of physicians, nurses and other auxilliary medical personnel disabled by influenza when their services were desperately needed. A special effort should be made to protect those participating in the care of the sick to avoid a repetition of this situation.

SUMMARY

We have outlined the need for immunization against influenza in various population groups. The projected vaccination program in our opinion is justified as a precaution against a repetition of the disastrous pandemic of 1918, although no one can predict that this will occur. Moreover, this nationwide program should not be considered a waste of our resources since it may be an initial step in our efforts to control this still dangerous plague. There should be considerable value in building a widespread immunity in our population against the potentially lethal HSW1N1 strain. As a follow-up, similar programs employing the more recently prevalent strains, given systematically, so that all of the known hemagglutinin and neuraminidase components are covered every few years, might well be a notable contribution to the conquest of influenza.

REFERENCES

1. Francis R Jr, Magill R: The incidence of neutralizing antibody in the serum of human individuals of different ages. J Exp Med 79: 301, 1944.
2. Schnurronberger PR, Woods GT, Marin RI: Serologic evidence of human infection with swine influenza virus. Am Rev Respir Dis 102: 356, 1970.
3. Smith TF, Burgert EO Jr, Dowdle WR, et al.: Isolation of swine influenza virus from autopsy lung tissue of man. N Engl J Med 294: 708, 1976.
4. Broun GO, Muether RO, Shrader EL, et al.: Characteristics of influenza virus infections observed in St. Louis from 1943 to 1957. Arch Intern Med 101: 203, 1958.
5. Broun GO, Schmidt RR: A study of the epidemiology of influenza by use of serum pools. AMA Scientific Exhibits, New York, Grune & Stratton, 1956, p 150.
6. Broun GO, Oligschlager D, LeGier M, et al.: Studies of the epidemiology of influenza as demonstrated by serum pools. Arch Intern Med 106: 496, 1960.
7. Soto PJ Jr, Broun GO, Wyatt JP: Asian influenzal pneumonitis. Am J Med 27: 18, 1959.
8. Broun GO, Mier T, Schmidt RR, et al.: Relationships of influenza antibody pattern of cord serum to that of maternal and paternal serum. J Lab Clin Med 62: 5, 862, 1963.
9. Hirst GK: The quantitative determination of influenza virus and antibodies by means of red cell agglutination. J Exp Med 75: 49, 1942.
10. Salk JE: A simplified procedure of titrating the hemagglutinating capacity of influenza virus and the corresponding antibody. J Immunol 49: 87, 1944.
11. Dublin LI and Lotka AJ: Twenty-five years of health progress. New York, Metropolitan Life Insurance Co., 1937, p 129.
12. Dublin LI: Health progress 1936–1945. New York, Metropolitan Life Insurance Co., 1948.
13. Mulder J, Hers JF: Influenza. Groningen, Wolters-Noordhoff Publishing, 1972.
14. Greenberg MG, Jacobziner H, Pakter J, et al.: Influenza mortality in the epidemic of asian influenza. New York City, 1957. Am J Obstet Gynecol 76: 897, 1958.
15. Bass MA: Diseases of pregnant women affecting the offspring. Adv Intern Med 5: 15, 1952.
16. MacKenzie JS, Houghton M: Influenza infections during pregnancy. Bacteriol Rev 38: 356, 1974.
17. Kilbourne ED: Epidemiology of influenza. The Influenza Viruses and Influenza, New York, Academic Press, 1975, p 525.
18. Webster RG: Original antigenic sin in ferrets. J Immunol 97: 177, 1966.

Recommendations for Screening Programs for Congenital Hypothyroidism

Report of a Committee of the American Thyroid Association

D. A. FISHER, M.D.
Torrance, California

G. N. BURROW, M.D.
New Haven, Connecticut

J. H. DUSSAULT, M.D.
Quebec, Canada

D. R. HOLLINGSWORTH, M.D.
Lexington, Kentucky

P. R. LARSEN, M.D.
Boston, Massachusetts

E. B. MAN, Ph.D.
North Stonington, Connecticut

P. G. WALFISH, M.D.
Ontario, Canada

Requests for reprints should be addressed to Dr. D. A. Fisher, Harbor General Hospital, 1000 West Carson Street, Torrance, California 90509.

The importance of early treatment of congenital hypothyroidism has been emphasized by many investigators. Currently, however, we usually rely on physician acumen for early diagnosis. Since the majority of cases are sporadic with subtle and nonspecific manifestations appearing early in the course, the diagnosis often is not suspected before six to eight weeks of age and may be delayed until three to six months of age. In the past, the placenta has been considered to be permeable to thyroid hormones so that the hypothyroid fetus was expected to have normal circulating levels of thyroxine (T4). This assumption, coupled with inherent limitations in the protein-bound iodine and butanol extractable iodine procedures, largely precluded attempts at screening newborns for hypothyroidism. Recent evidence that the placental transfer of thyrotropin (TSH) and thyroid hormones is markedly limited, as well as the recent availability of highly sensitive and specific radioimmunoassay systems for measuring thyroid hormones and TSH in biologic fluids, have made screening of newborns for congenital hypothyroidism feasible.

During the past three years, pilot screening programs have been established in Quebec, Pittsburgh and Toronto; and The American Thyroid Association appointed a Committee on Newborn Screening for Hypothyroidism to monitor these programs and to make recommendations regarding screening based on the accumulated results of these pilot programs. The committee and the Association believe that enough evidence has accumulated to make preliminary recommendations which are included in this report. This report was approved for publication by the members of The American Thyroid Association at the business meeting on June 12, 1975.

Dr. Dussault and colleagues [1,2] in Quebec adapted the T4 radioimmunoassay system to eluates of filter paper blood spots already in use for phenylketonuria screening. Dr. Larsen [3] has further simplified the filter paper spot T4 method. Dr. Foley and colleagues [1–4] in Pittsburgh have screened cord blood using a conventional TSH radioimmunoassay system. Dr. Walfish and collaborators [1,5] in Toronto have screened newborns using the filter paper spot T4 method at three to five days of age and utilizing T4 and TSH radioimmunoassay of cord blood samples. In the Quebec program approximately 100,000 infants had been screened by June 1975, and 15 hypothyroid newborns and six infants with low thyroxine-binding globulin (TBG) levels were detected. In Pittsburgh, 15,000 infants had been screened; four hypothyroid newborns and one infant with a low TBG level were detected. In the Toronto program 6,000 infants had been screened and two hypothyroid newborns and six infants with low TBG levels were detected. The total number of newborn infants screened approximated 121,000, and 21 infants with congenital hypothyroidism had been detected (Table I), an incidence of one in 5,760 newborns.

Analysis of the test results from the 21 infants with proved congenital hypothyroidism (Table II) detected by the screening programs revealed the following:

(1) Measured or estimated cord serum T4 values in all were <7 μg/100 ml. Estimates were based on the measured filter paper spot result at two to four days. This method may overestimate somewhat.

(2) In five of six infants with cord blood TSH measurements TSH levels were >100 μU/ml. In seven of the 10 infants in the Quebec study with serum TSH measurements conducted on recall between two and four weeks, levels were in excess of 50 μU/ml. One other had a modestly elevated level (32 μU/ml). One of the remaining two infants was hypopituitary with a low serum TSH, and one was euthyroid with a normal serum TSH concentration and a high serum triiodothyronine (T3) level.

(3) Five of six infants had low serum T3 values (<50 ng/100 ml). One other infant with dyshormonogenesis had a high serum T3 level at three weeks.

Logistical difficulties in recall for retesting can be significant. From 0.7 to 1.0 per cent of samples require retesting in the filter paper T4 screening programs, and from 2.0 to 2.5 per cent of samples require retesting in cord blood T4 screening programs. Very preliminary evidence suggests that cord blood TSH screening may miss a few infants with hypothyroidism secondary to TSH deficiency. Filter paper spot T4 screening may miss a few infants with compensated or partial thyroid insufficiency, although the proportion of such cases is not yet clear. Finally, the effects of early thyroid hormone treatment (begun before one month) have yet to be defined. It is anticipated, however, that results will be at least as good as those obtained with therapy begun before three months of age; 85 per cent of such infants have IQ values >85 [6].

The cost of T4 screening using filter paper spots or cord blood samples approximates 60 cents a test whereas the cost of cord blood or filter paper TSH screening is approximately $1.50 a test. The cost of detecting each congenitally hypothyroid newborn by T4 screening approximates $4,000 and by TSH screening $12,000. Assuming, conservatively, that 30 per cent of the infants in whom the diagnosis is delayed will require institutional care at $10,000 yearly for 30 years and that only 10 per cent of the infants in whom the diagnosis is made at birth will require such care, a

TABLE I Results of Preliminary Screening Programs for Congenital Hypothyroidism

	No. of Infants Screened	No. of Abnormal Infants Detected: Hypothyroid	No. of Abnormal Infants Detected: Low TBG	Type of Screening
Dussault et al. Quebec	100,000	15	6	Filter paper spot, 2 to 4 days
Foley et al. Pittsburgh	15,000	4	1	Cord blood TSH
Walfish et al. Toronto	6,000	2	6	Cord blood T4 and TSH; filter paper blood spot at 3 to 5 days
Totals	121,000	21	13	

NOTE: TBG = thyroxine-binding globulin.

TABLE II T4, T3 and TSH Measurement Results in Infants with Hypothyroidism Detected by Several Preliminary Screening Programs

	Cord Serum Concentration*: T4 (μg/dl)		Cord Serum Concentration*: T3 (ng/dl)			Cord TSH (μU/ml)		Later TSH (μU/ml)†			
	<5.0	5.0–7.0	<50	50–100	>100	50–100	>100	<20	20–50	>50	>100
Dussault et al. Quebec	11/15‡	4/15	2/3	...	1/3†	...	...	2/10	1/10	2/10	5/10
Foley et al. Pittsburgh	2/4	2/4	3/3	...	...	...	4/4	...	...	...	...
Walfish et al. Toronto	...	2/2	...	...	...	1/2	1/2	...	...	1/2	1/2

* Measured directly or estimated from 2 to 4 day filter paper spot sample.
† Measurements conducted between two and four weeks.
‡ Eleven of 15 samples tested.

screening program can save $600,000 for each 10 infants detected.

Thus, there now is good evidence for an incidence of congenital hypothyroidism of at least one in 6,000 births in North America, and evidence that screening newborns for this disorder can be effective and cost accounted. The American Thyroid Association recommends:

(1) The establishment and expansion of preliminary screening programs for congenital hypothyroidism.

(2) Combining testing for hypothyroidism with existing newborn screening programs to improve cost effectiveness and to help guarantee quality control and efficient follow-up. The advantages of a regional approach to screening have been demonstrated in Quebec, and this experience can serve as a model for other areas.

(3) Screening for congenital hypothyroidism using a filter paper T4 method with filter paper TSH testing of suspicious samples. This approach is particularly applicable when samples must be mailed to a central laboratory, or

(4) Screening for congenital hypothyroidism using cord blood T4 testing when samples can be processed locally. Suspicious samples should be retested using a TSH radioimmunoassay.

(5) Further development of TSH measurement methods for screening newborns for hypothyroidism, particularly for filter paper samples. Recent studies have shown that such measurements are feasible [7,8].

(6) Study of screening for hypothyroidism using reverse T3 measurements [9]. This method may be applicable to in utero screening of high risk mothers as well as screening of newborns.

(7) Development of adequate pools of T4 and TSH antiserums to support widespread public screening programs for congenital hypothyroidism.

REFERENCES

1. (a) Newborn screening for hypothyroidism. Perinatal Thyroid Physiology and Disease (Fisher DA, Burrow GN, eds), New York, Raven Press, 1975.
   (b) Fisher DA, Sack J: Idem, p 197.
   (c) Larsen PR, Abuid J: Idem, p 211.
   (d) Dussault JH, Coulombe P, Laberge C: Idem, p 221.
   (e) Foley TP Jr, Klein AH, Agustin AV, Hopwood N: Idem, p 255.
   (f) Walfish PG: Idem, pp 239, 249, 263.
2. Dussault JH, Coulombe P, Laberge C, et al.: Preliminary report on a mass screening for neonatal hypothyroidism. J. Pediatr 86: 670, 1975.
3. Larsen PR, Broskin K: Thyroxine immunoassay using filter paper blood samples for screening of neonates for hypothyroidism. Pediatr Res 9: 604, 1975.
4. Klein AH, Agustin AV, Foley TP Jr: Successful laboratory screening for congenital hypothyroidism. Lancet 1: 77, 1974.
5. Walfish PG, O'Donnell J, Ulbright T, et al.: Screening for neonatal hypothyroidism. Comparison of neonatal dried capillary blood thyroxine (T4) to cord serum T4 and thyrotropin (TSH). Proceedings of the VII International Congress, Boston, June 1975. Thyroid Research (Robbins J, Braverman LE, eds), Amsterdam, Excerpta Medica, International Congress Series, 1976, p 601.
6. Klein A, Meltzer S, Kenny MD: Improved prognosis in congenital hypothyroidism treated before age three months. J Pediatr 81: 912, 1972.
7. Irie M, Enomoto K, Naruse H: Measurement of thyroid-stimulating hormone in dried blood spot. Lancet 2: 1233, 1975.
8. Grajwer LA, Lam RW, Bruce VA, et al.: A sensitive TSH radioimmunoassay for newborn thyroid screening. Clin Res 24: 192A, 1976.
9. Chopra IJ, Crandall BF: Thyroid hormones and thyrotropin in amniotic fluid. N Engl J Med 293: 740, 1975.

Propionibacterium acnes: Pathogen in Central Nervous System Shunt Infection

Report of Three Cases Including Immune Complex Glomerulonephritis

B. A. BEELER, M.D.
J. G. CROWDER, M.D.
J. W. SMITH, M.D.
A. WHITE, M.D.
Indianapolis, Indiana

Propionibacterium acnes is a pleomorphic gram-positive anaerobic rod usually isolated as a contaminant from skin. We report three cases of P. acnes infection of central nervous system shunts for hydrocephalus. The organism was seen repeatedly on gram stain in a specimen of shunt fluid in all three cases; initially, it was regarded as a contaminant. In addition, two of the patients had precipitins to extracts of their organism. Serum from normal control subjects had no such precipitins. One of the patients had an immune-complex glomerulonephritis—an entity not previously associated with anaerobic organisms. All three patients recovered after removal of the shunt and treatment with antibiotics. P. acnes is a significant pathogen in patients with central nervous system shunts.

P. acnes is a pleomorphic gram-positive anaerobic rod which is a frequent contaminant in cultures of skin obtained percutaneously [1]. This organism has been recognized as a pathogen in the past [2–4]. Until recently, there has been disagreement as to whether this organism is distinct from the aerobic diphtheroids, the Corynebacterium sp. Recent evidence suggests that anaerobic diphtheroids are indeed distinct and as such are designated Propionibacterium [5].

We have recently seen three cases in which the central nervous system shunts for hydrocephalus were infected with P. acnes. In all three cases diagnosis was delayed by failure to recognize the clinical significance of gram-positive, nonspore-forming rods on smear.

MATERIALS AND METHODS

P. acnes was obtained from the clinical laboratory as a subculture from each culture of cerebrospinal fluid from each patient. It was identified as a gram-positive pleomorphic rod which on gas liquid chromatography gave a major propionic acid and lesser acetic acid peak. The organism was then grown for 12 to 14 days in 1,000 ml of Brewer's modified thioglycolate medium. The organisms were removed from the medium by centrifugation at 10,000 g, washed by mixing with 0.9 per cent sodium chloride and centrifuged. The excess fluid was decanted. This was repeated three times. The packed cell volume was determined in a graduated cylinder, and sufficient saline solution (0.9 per cent) was added to make a 20 per cent solution v/v. This mixture of cells was then disrupted by 10 minutes of sonication (Biosonik). The mixture

From the Departments of Medicine and Clinical Pathology, Indiana University School of Medicine, Indianapolis, Indiana 46202. Requests for reprints should be addressed to Dr. Arthur White, Indiana University School of Medicine, 1100 West Michigan Street, Indianapolis, Indiana 46202. Manuscript accepted January 28, 1976.

was centrifuged at 10,000 g, and the supernatant was used as the antigen source. The antigens thus prepared will be referred to as antigens I, II and III to correspond to the patients in the respective case reports.

Serum was examined for precipitins to P. acnes in Ouchterlony plates to 0.9 per cent Noble's agar. P. acnes antigen was placed into the center well and the antibody sources were placed into the peripheral wells. The plates were incubated at 37°C for 24 hours and examined for precipitin lines.

CASE REPORTS

Case I. This patient was noted to have hydrocephalus shortly after his birth in 1954. A right nephrectomy was performed and a shunt placed between the lumbosacral subarachnoid space and the right ureter. This was replaced, at age 13, with a ventriculoatrial shunt with a Spitz-Holter valve because of signs of increased intracranial pressure. At age 17, fever, chills, gross hematuria and ankle edema developed. The patient's blood urea nitrogen was 45 mg/100 ml, creatine 2.2 mg/100 ml and 24 hour urine protein 9 g. A retrograde pyelogram showed the left kidney to be enlarged. The patient was treated for 10 days with ampicillin and referred to the Indiana University Medical Center (IUMC). On admission at IUMC, he was afebrile, his blood pressure was 150/100 mm Hg, and pedal edema was still present. The rest of the physical examination was within normal limits. Laboratory data included a hemoglobin level of 8.9 g/100 ml, a white blood count of 10,500/mm^3 with a normal differential, and a reticulocyte count of 3.1 per cent. Hemolytic studies were normal.

Serum complement (C'3) was 30 per cent of normal. A positive lupus erythematosus preparation was noted, and 2+ speckling was seen on the antinuclear antibody determination. Cold agglutinins were positive at 1:16 dilution and later increased to a titer of 1:128. The antistreptolysin O titer was not elevated. The lowest creatinine clearance was 36 ml/min. Urinalysis showed a specific gravity of 1.005, 4 to 6 coursely granular casts, 10 to 11 finely granular casts, 5 white blood cells, 35 to 40 red cells, 1 to 3 white cell casts and 4 to 5 red cell casts/hpf. Gram-positive rods were seen on stain of fluid from the Spitz-Holter valve and these were subsequently identified on culture as P. acnes. Culture of the lumbar spinal fluid yielded no growth. During the patient's hospitalization, 13 blood cultures were obtained, 11 of which grew P. acnes. After he failed to respond to the administration of 8 million units of penicillin G daily, he was treated with erythromycin 2 g daily. With erythromycin, his serum inhibited the organism at a dilution of 1:256, but he continued to have positive blood cultures and his renal disease did not diminish until the shunt was removed.

The patient completely recovered from his renal disease; 18 months after admission, his blood pressure, serum creatinine, creatinine clearance, urine protein and urinary sediment were within normal limits.

Case II. This patient had a cerebral astrocytoma removed at age five and a ventriculoatrial shunt for hydrocephalus placed at age 31. At age 36, she was admitted for evaluation of severe headache. Although she was afebrile, the shunt was found to be infected with Staphylococcus epidermidis (coagulase-negative). This shunt was replaced and her symptoms were temporarily resolved. She returned two months later, again with headaches. At this time, the shunt fluid contained pleomorphic gram-positive rods, culturally identified as P. acnes, on three separate examinations. Blood cultures were negative on three occasions. She was treated with replacement of the shunt and 12 g of ampicillin daily and has done well for one year.

Case III. This patient is a 61 year old white man who had a venticuloperitoneal shunt inserted for low pressure hydrocephalus in December 1973. Two weeks after discharge, he returned complaining of severe generalized abdominal pain. The pain eventually localized in the area of the right paramedian mid-abdominal incision over the peritoneal end of his shunt. No abnormality of the wound was noted. There was no rebound tenderness, and bowel sounds were present. The shunt fluid contained gram-positive rods on direct smear which were culturally identified as P. acnes on three occasions. Six days after admission, the Spitz-Holter valve was removed under general anesthesia without difficulty. While in the recovery room, the patient had a shaking chill with a temperature of 103.6°F; confusion, disorientation and nuchal rigidity developed. Lumbar spinal fluid revealed 37,062 white blood count/mm^3, 100 per cent being polymorphonuclear leukocytes. The cerebrospinal fluid protein was 410 mg/100 ml and glucose 59 mg/100 ml. The gram stain and culture were both negative as were three blood cultures. He was treated with chloramphenicol 4 g daily, gentamicin 5 mg/kg/day in three doses, and gentamicin 5 mg in 5 cc saline solution intrathecally. Over the next seven days, he became afebrile. The patient's hospital course was one of steady improvement and he was discharged after two weeks of therapy.

RESULTS

Serums from the patients were tested to determine if detectable antibody to P. acnes was present (Table I). Serum from one patient (Case I) developed precipitin lines with antigen I in 1:4 dilution of serum. Undiluted serum from this patient collected 18 months after his discharge developed precipitins with antigens from the organisms isolated from the other two patients (Cases II and III). Serum from one of these (Case II) was not tested against antigen I but developed precipitin lines with the patient's own organism's antigens in 1:16 dilution of serum and against antigen III in a 1:8 dilution of serum (Figure 1). Serum from the third patient (Case III) was not tested against antigen from the first patient (Case I), and no precipitins were detectable in this patient's serum using either antigen II or antigen III. Therefore, precipitins to P. acnes were detectable in the serums of the first patient (Case I), both during the acute phase of illness and 18 months after he was cured, and the serum from the second patient (Case II). No precipitins were detectable in the serum of the third patient (Case III).

TABLE I Titers of P. acnes Precipitins in Patients with Infections

Antigen	Case I	Case II	Case III
I	1:4	ND*	ND
II	U+	1:16	0
III	U	1:8	0

* ND = not done.
+ Undiluted.

TABLE II Titers of Precipitins to P. acnes in Control Subjects

Antigen	Serum Source	No.	Titer
I	Normal	5	0
II	Normal	12	0
II	Patients*	5	0
II	Acne	2	U* 1:8

*Patients infected with organism other than P. acnes.

Serums from a group of control subjects were studied to see if they contained precipitating antibodies to this organism (Table II). Five normal serums were tested against antigen I; no precipitins were detectable. Serums from 12 normal subjects and five patients infected with other bacteria had no detectable precipitins against antigen II. Two patients with moderately severe acne had detectable precipitins.

COMMENTS

In the past, Propionibacterium acnes has been referred to as Corynebacterium acnes. This organism was described by Unna [6] as being present in acne comodoes in 1896. Current evidence based on biochemical differences and DNA base homology studies suggest that the aerobic Corynebacterium species is distinct from the anaerobic Propionibacterium species [5]. The literature has been confusing in the past in differentiating these species.

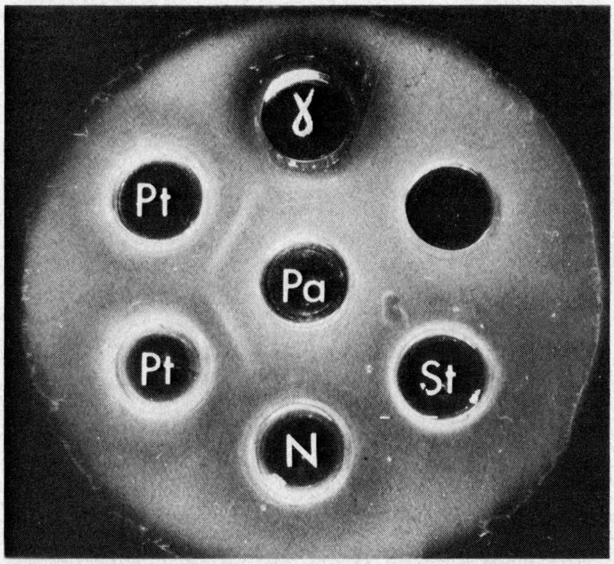

Figure 1. Precipitins in Ouchterlony plates in serum from two patients (Cases I and II) against antigen II. γ = pooled concentrated human gamma globulin, Pa = antigen extract, Pt = serum from patients (either in Case I or Case II), N = serums from uninfected subjects, St = serums from patient with staphylococcal infection with high titers of staphylococcal teichoic acid antibodies.

P. acnes was the most common organism isolated from anaerobic blood cultures. In one series [1], 360 positive anaerobic blood cultures grew P. acnes. However, only one of these isolates was considered to be clinically significant, and in most instances P. acnes isolated from blood cultures are contaminants from the skin.

There are sufficient data in the literature to confirm that both aerobic and anaerobic diphtheroids are potential pathogens [2–4]. Anaerobic diphtheroids have been reported as a cause of bacterial meningitis, endocarditis, wound infection and hepatitis. Recently, they were among the organisms isolated from prepackaged plastic catheters [7].

There is also a report of P. acnes as a cause of chronic meningitis in a series of three patients [4], all of whose serums contained elevated titers of P. acnes agglutinins. Therefore, a positive culture for P. acnes cannot be disregarded as a contaminant without first considering the circumstances. The consistent finding of gram-positive rods on stain of cerebrospinal fluids, as in these three patients, should certainly suggest more than contamination as did repeated isolation of this organism. The findings of specific antibody to their own organism in our two patients (Cases I and II), and the clinical course in the three patients confirm the role of P. acnes in their disease.

Only with good anaerobic cultures can P. acnes be identified as the etiology of shunt infections. Most hospital laboratories do not do anaerobic cultures routinely on cerebrospinal fluid; therefore, the clinician must specifically request them in patients suspected of being infected with P. acnes. The present study suggests that gram-positive rods on gram stain and perhaps negative aerobic cultures of suspected infected fluids without organisms on gram stain should be cultured anaerobically.

Infection of the shunt placed to control hydrocephalus occurs with an incidence ranging in various recent series from 15.7 per cent [8] to 27 per cent [9]. Infection is also a significant cause of mortality in these patients. Coagulase-negative staphylococci are the most common infecting organisms, infections with Staph. aureus are the second most frequent [9,10]. Other organisms, including rare pathogens such as Bacillus cereus, have also been reported [11]. These patients may present with sepsis, signs of increased intracranial pressure [12] or the nephrotic syndrome [13]. There has also been a description of an asymptomatic state in which cultures of shunt fluid are positive and associated with leukocytosis and hypoglycorachia in patients whose shunts were tapped as part of a prospective study [14].

Central nervous system shunt infection has been associated with the nephrotic syndrome in the past [13,15–25]. It has been suggested that this process is secondary to immune-complex disease. In one of our patients, the findings were suggestive of an immune-complex glomerulonephritis which has not been previously associated with an anaerobic shunt infection. The findings of circulating antigen (positive blood cultures), antibody (precipitins) and low serum complement, all tend to support this diagnosis. Cold agglutinins were also noted to be present. The presence of cryoglobulins has been reported previously, but their significance is not known [23,24].

This patient's (Case I) renal disease was completely resolved after removal of the P. acnes infected shunt. A renal biopsy specimen showing immune-complexes would have been more definitive evidence; however, the patient had only one remaining kidney which, in our opinion, contraindicated a percutaneous biopsy.

In summary, P. acnes is an anaerobic diphtheroid which is a normal inhabitant of human skin and is most frequently cultured as a contaminant. As in the three cases of central nervous system shunt infection reported here, it is also a significant pathogen capable of causing sepsis and immune-complex glomerulonephritis. Infection with this organism should be considered whenever gram-positive rods are seen on stain of central nervous system shunt fluid. Shunt fluid should be cultured anaerobically if infection is suspected. In patients with diseases due to P. acnes, precipitating antibody may develop.

REFERENCES

1. Wilson WR, Martin WJ, Wilkowske CJ, et al.: Anaerobic bacteremia. Mayo Clin Proc 47: 639, 1972.
2. Johnson WD, Kaye D: Serious infections caused by diphtheroids. Ann NY Acad Sci 174: 568, 1970.
3. Kaplan K, Weinstein L: Diphtheroid infections in man. Ann Intern Med 70: 919, 1969.
4. French RS, Ziter FA, Spruance SL, et al.: Chronic meningitis caused by P. acnes. A potentially important clinical entity. Neurology 24: 624, 1974.
5. Johnson JL, Cummins CS: Cell wall composition and deoxyribonucleic acid similarities among the anaerobic coryneforms, classical propionibacteria and strains of Arachnia propionica. J Bacteriol i09: 1047, 1972.
6. Unna G: Histopathology of Diseases of the Skin (translated from German with the assistance of the author by Norman Walker, Edinburgh and William F. Clay and J. Cohen, New York), New York, MacMilliam Publishers, 1896.
7. Recall of contaminated intravenous cannulae. Morbidity and Mortality Weekly Reports 23: 57, 1974, Center for Disease Control, U.S. Department of Health, Education and Welfare.
8. Shurtleff DB, Christie D, Foltz EL: Ventriculoauriculostomy associated infection (a 12 year study). J Neurosurg 35: 686, 1971.
9. Schoenbaum SC, Gardner P, Shillito J; infections of cerebrospinal fluid shunts. Epidemiology, clinical manifestations and therapy. J Infect Dis 131: 543, 1975.
10. McLaurin RL, Dodson D: Infected ventriculo-atrial shunts. Some principles of treatment. Dev Med Child Neurol 13 (suppl 25): 71, 1971.
11. Leffert HL, Baptist JN, Gidez LY: Meningitis and bacteremia after ventriculoatrial shunt revision. Isolation of a lecithinase producing Bacillus cereus. J Infect Dis 122: 547, 1970.
12. Nulsen FE, Becker DP: Control of hydrocephalus by valve regulated shunt. Infections and their prevention. Clin Neurosurg 14: 256, 1966.
13. Black JA, Challcombe DN, Ockenden BG: Nephrotic syndrome associated with bacteremia after shunt operations for hydrocephalus. Lancet 2: 921, 1965.
14. Folkes EC: Occult infections of ventriculoatrial shunts. J Neurosurg 33: 517, 1970.
15. Stidkler GB, Shin MH, Burke EC, et al.: Diffuse glomerulonephritis associated with infected ventriculoatrial shunt. N Engl J Med 279: 1077, 1968.
16. McKenzie SA, Hayden K: Two cases of "shunt nephritis." Pediatrics 54: 806, 1974.
17. Luthardt T: Bacterial infections in ventriculo-auricular shunt systems. Dev Med Child Neurol 12 (suppl 22): 110, 1960.
18. Holland N: Hypocomplementemic glomerulonephritis associated with micrococcus infection of ventriculo-atrial shunt. 37th Annual Meeting of the Society for Pediatric Research, Atlantic City, New Jersey, April 1967.
19. Northway JD, McAdams AJ, West CD: Sepsis, nephritis and hypocomplementemia. Paper read at the 37th Annual Meeting of the Society for Pediatric Research, Atlantic City, New Jersey, April 1967.
20. Hansen MF: Nephritis complicating ventriculo-vascular shunts. 35th Annual Meeting of the Society for Pediatric Research, Philadelphia, Pennsylvania, May 1965.
21. Stauffer UG: Shunt nephritis. Diffuse glomerulonephritis complicating ventriculoatrial shunts. Dev Med Child Neurol 12 (suppl 22): 161, 1970.
22. Kaufman DB, McIntosh R: The pathogenesis of the renal lesion in a patient with streptococcal disease, infected ventriculoatrial shunt, cryoglobulinemia and nephritis. Am J Med 50: 262, 1971.
23. McLaurin RL: Infected cerebrospinal fluid shunts. Surg Neurol 1:191, 1973.
24. Dobrin RS, Day NK, Quie PG, et al.: The role of complement, immunoglobulin and bacterial antigen in coagulase-negative staphylococcal shunt nephritis. Am J Med 59: 660, 1975.
25. Yu HC: Prophylactic antimicrobial agents after ventriculoatriostomy for hydrocephalus. J Pediatr Surg 8: 881, 1973.

Extrinsic Allergic Alveolitis After Aspergillus fumigatus Inhalation

Evidence of a Type IV Immunologic Pathogenesis

MICHAEL W. YOCUM, M.D.*
ALAN R. SALTZMAN, M.D.
DOUGLAS M. STRONG, Ph.D.
JOHN C. DONALDSON, M.D.
Bethesda, Maryland

GEORGE W. WARD, Jr., M.D.
Washington, D.C.

FRANCIS M. WALSH, M.D.
ORR M. COBB, Jr., M.D.
ROBERT C. ELLIOTT, M.D.
Bethesda, Maryland

Three weeks after a massive inhalation of mold present on infected oats, a farmer's wife had extrinsic allergic alveolitis. Aspergillus fumigatus was cultured from the moldy oats and from deep bronchial washings obtained at fiberoptic bronchoscopy. Spores and hyphae characteristic of Aspergillus species were demonstrated within granulomas in the pulmonary tissue obtained by transbronchial biopsy. Serum precipitins, delayed (48 hour) cutaneous hypersensitivity and in vitro lymphocyte transformation to A. fumigatus were demonstrated. The findings in this case suggest that a type IV immunologic response and subsequent (lymphocyte-mediated) tissue inflammation may underlie the pathogenesis of this and other forms of hypersensitivity pneumonitis.

Three distinct forms of pulmonary hypersensitivity reaction occur upon inhalation of Aspergillus mold spores. The first form, occurring in patients with atopic asthma, is manifested by immediate bronchoconstriction and is characterized by a type I, wheal and flare, immunoglobulin E (IgE)-mediated skin test [1]. A second form, allergic bronchopulmonary aspergillosis [2,3], also occurs in patients with atopic asthma and is characterized by wheezing, fever, expectoration of fungus-laden mucous plugs, subsegmental pulmonary infiltrates, eosinophilia of sputum and blood and serum precipitins to Aspergillus fumigatus [4]. Intradermal tests elicit a type I and a 4 to 6 hour type III or Arthus [1] reaction; inhalation challenge elicits immediate as well as 4 to 6 hour episodes of bronchoconstriction with functional abnormalities of large airway obstruction. A third form of pulmonary hypersensitivity reaction to Aspergillus spore inhalation, extrinsic allergic alveolitis [4–7], occurs predominantly in nonatopic patients and is characterized by dyspnea, dry cough, malaise, myalgia, rales, diffuse micronodular pulmonary infiltrates and serum precipitins to Aspergillus. Intradermal tests elicit an Arthus reaction which may or may not be preceded by a wheal and flare reaction, and inhalation challenge elicits only a 4 to 8 hour reaction of fever, leukocytosis, dyspnea, and rales with functional abnormalities of restrictive and diffusion defects. Other examples of extrinsic allergic alveolitis include farmer's lung [8,9], maple bark disease [10], pigeon breeder's disease [11–13] and bagassosis [14,15].

From the Department of Medicine, National Naval Medical Center, Bethesda, Maryland; the Clinical and Experimental Immunology Department, Naval Medical Research Institute, Bethesda, Maryland; and the Allergy Immunology Service, Walter Reed Army Medical Center, Washington, D.C. This work was supported by the U.S. Navy Bureau of Medicine and Surgery, Clinical Investigation Program CICC No. 4-06-305 and CICC No. 4-06-381. The opinions or assertions contained herein are the private views of the authors and are not to be construed as official or as reflecting the views of the Department of the Navy or the Department of Defense. Requests for reprints should be addressed to Dr. John C. Donaldson, LCDR, MC, USN, Box 298, National Naval Medical Center, Bethesda, Maryland 20014. Manuscript accepted January 23, 1976.

* Present address: Allergy-Immunology Division, Henry Ford Hospital, 2799 West Grand Boulevard, Detroit, Michigan 48202.

Because serum precipitins are usually demonstrable in allergic bronchopulmonary aspergillosis and extrinsic allergic alveolitis, type III immunologic tissue injury has been postulated as the pathogenesis of these pulmonary hypersensitivity diseases [4]. However, recent reports concerning delayed (48 hour) cutaneous hypersensitivity [16,17], histopathology of pulmonary tissue [18–20], in vitro lymphocyte studies [21–23] and animal models [24,25] suggests that type IV [1] with or without type III immunologic injury may best explain the pathogenesis of these diseases.

We describe a patient in whom extrinsic allergic alveolitis developed secondary to massive inhalation of A. fumigatus spores from moldy oats. We present evidence from delayed cutaneous hypersensitivity, in vitro lymphocyte transformation and histopathologic studies to implicate a type IV immunologic response and subsequent tissue inflammation as the pathogenesis of this patient's disease.

CASE REPORT

A 37 year old farmer's wife was admitted to the National Naval Medical Center (NNMC) on July 5, 1974, because of fever and malaise of three week's duration. Six weeks before admission, she was bagging oats covered with a black mold which filled the air, and she was forced to leave the barn several times "to get air." Three weeks later, she had a temperature of 103°F, dyspnea, malaise, headaches, lightheadedness, nausea, anorexia and dry cough. She had had a similar but milder illness of two weeks' duration after bagging oats in June 1973.

The patient's history included tuberculous peritonitis in 1950 and pulmonary tuberculosis in 1954; for each illness she had been treated with isoniazid, para-aminosalicylic acid and streptomycin for 18 months. There was no history of rhinitis, asthma, eczema or parasitic disease.

On examination the patient had a temperature of 100°F, and scattered pulmonary rales without rhonchi or wheezes. The hematocrit value was 40 per cent, white blood cell count 13,700/mm^3 with 79 per cent neutrophils, 14 per cent lymphocytes, 5 per cent monocytes and 2 per cent eosinophils. The erythrocyte sedimentation rate was 72 mm/hour. A chest film revealed bilateral miliary interstitial fibronodular infiltrates (Figure 1A). Cultures of urine, cerebrospinal fluid, blood, sputum and bone marrow were negative for bacterial or fungal pathogens; the reaction to an intradermal test to tuberculoprotein, intermediate strength, was negative.

On July 10, the patient's temperature rose to 103°F, and striking dyspnea and cyanosis developed. Arterial blood gases revealed a pH of 7.47, oxygen tension of 60 torr, carbon dioxide tension of 25 torr and bicarbonate ion of 25 meq/liter. Treatment for miliary tuberculosis was initiated with rifampin, ethambutol and isoniazid. On July 11, a fiberoptic bronchoscopy with transbronchial biopsy of the lower lobe of the right lung was performed. Histopathologic examination of the pulmonary biopsy material revealed consolidation of the parenchyma with an infiltration of plasma cells, lymphocytes and a moderate number of eosinophils. Throughout the lobule were numerous granulomas with focal areas of central necrosis (Figure 2). These necrotic zones contained leukocytes, eosinophils and necrotic debris. Epithelial cells and occasional foreign body giant cells surrounded the granulomas which appeared to be confined to respiratory bronchioles and alveolar ducts. Gomori methenamine silver stain revealed branching septate hyphae characteristic of A. fumigatus within the necrotic centers of granulomas (Figure 3). Vessels revealed mild edema and infiltration of plasma cells and lymphocytes into media and adventitia. Acid-fast and immunofluorescent tissue stains for Mycobacteria tuberculosis gave negative results but A. fumigatus was cultured from the deep bronchial washings obtained during bronchoscopy.

The patient's temperature diminished, and on July 16, antituberculosis therapy was discontinued. On July 18, a prick skin test reaction to an Aspergillus mixture (1/10 weight by

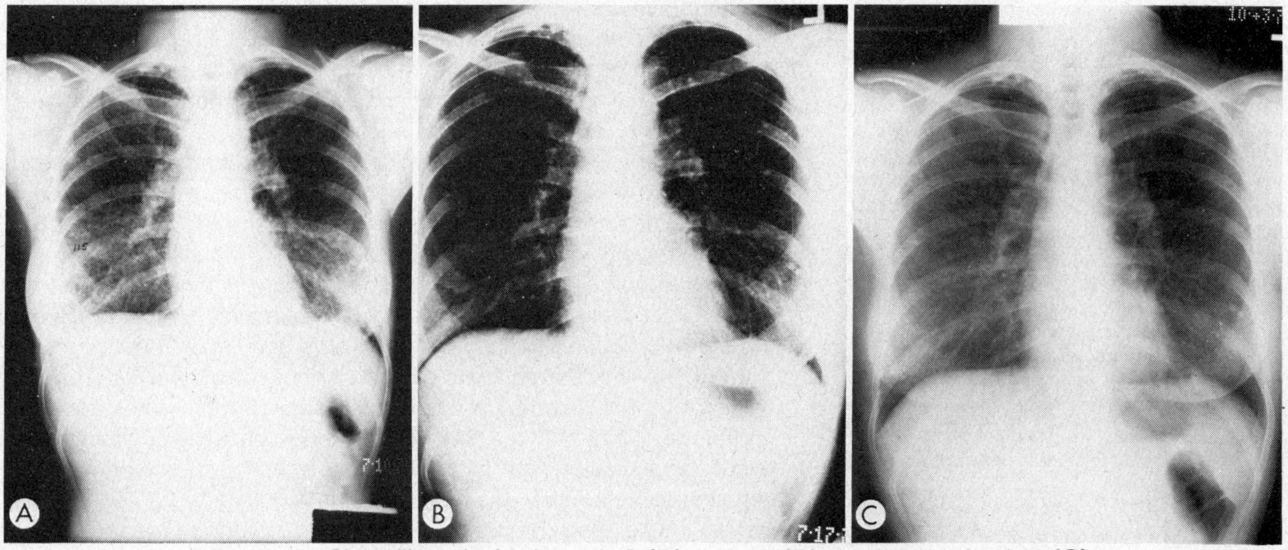

Figure 1. *Chest films obtained on July 5* ***(A)****, July 23* ***(B)*** *and October 3, 1974* ***(C)****.*

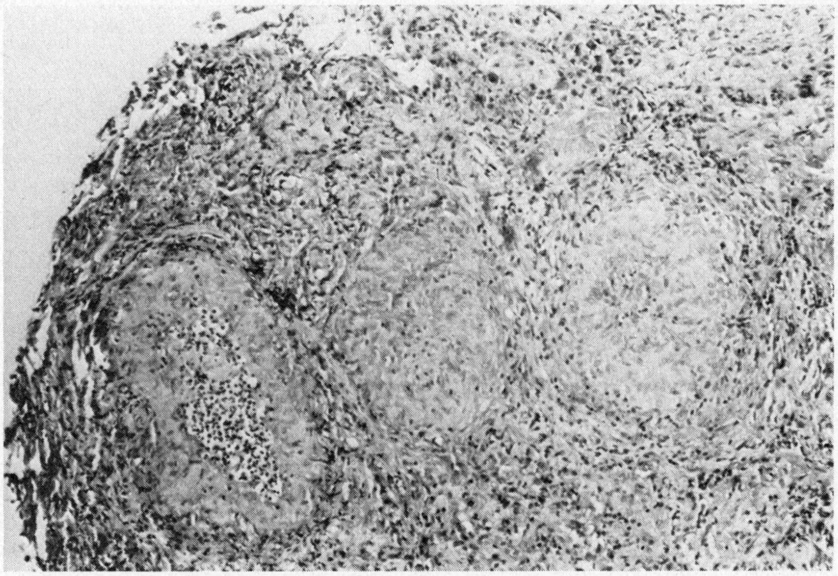

Figure 2. *Transbronchial biopsy specimen of pulmonary tissue demonstrated multiple granulomas. Note central necrosis of granuloma on the left. Hematoxylin and eosin stain; original magnification × 32, reduced by 38 per cent.*

volume, w/v) and the reaction to an intradermal test of 0.02 ml (1,000 protein nitrogen units/ml, PNU/ml) were negative at 20 minutes and at 8 hours; however, at 36 hours a 9 by 10 mm indurated skin reaction was observed. A repeat intradermal test with intermediate strength tuberculoprotein elicited 14 by 14 mm of induration. On July 23, the patient was afebrile and asymptomatic. On pulmonary testing, lung volumes and flow rates were normal, but oxygen tension was 73 torr, and single breath diffusion capacity was 64 per cent of predicted. A chest film revealed marked clearing of the previous infiltrates (Figure 1B). Culture of the moldy oats grew A. fumigatus, and serum precipitins were strongly positive to Aspergillus but negative to thermophilic actinomycetes. All Myco. tuberculosis cultures were negative at six weeks.

Our patient was readmitted to the NNMC on October 3, 1974, because of a seven day history of fever, malaise, myalgia, arthralgia, dyspnea and cough. One week before these symptoms, she had cut and stored field oats, some of which were moldy, in the barn. On examination she had a temperature of 100°F and rales over the bases of the lungs without wheezes or rhonchi. A chest film revealed new miliary interstitial fibronodular infiltrates (Figure 1C). The white blood cell count was 10,400/mm^3 with 2 per cent band forms,

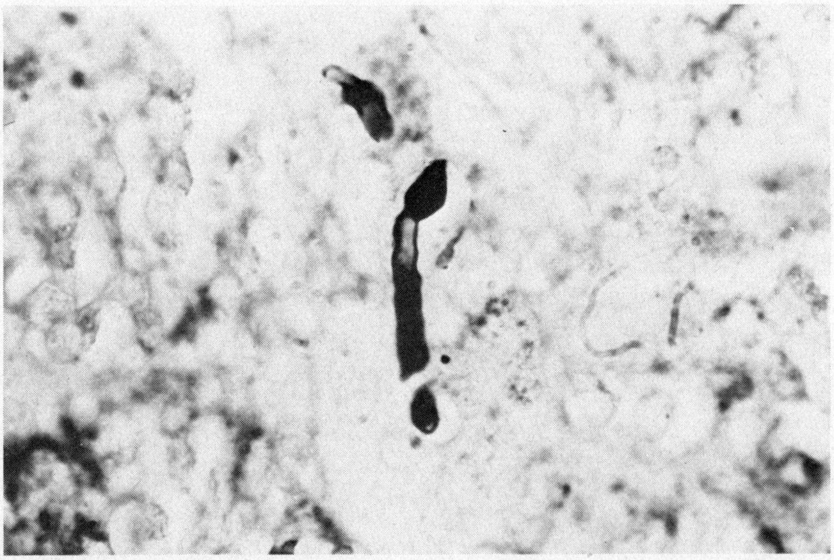

Figure 3. *Branching septate hyphae present in granulomas. Gomori methenamine silver stain; original magnification × 1,000, reduced by 38 per cent.*

TABLE I Results of Intradermal Skin Test to Fungal Antigens

Antigen	20 Minutes*	8 Hours	48 Hours†
A. fumigatus	9 x 10	0	15 x 15
Alternaria	5 x 5	0	0
Hormodendrum	6 x 7	0	0
Penicillium	8 x 8	0	0
Pullularia	6 x 6	0	0
Helminthosporium	6 x 6	0	0
Rhizopus	5 x 5	0	0
Fusarium	0	0	0
Epicoccum	0	0	0
Botrytis	0	0	0

*Size of wheal in millimeters.
†Millimeters of induration.

72 per cent neutrophils, 20 per cent lymphocytes, 3 per cent monocytes and 3 per cent eosinophils; the erythrocyte sedimentation rate was 60 mm/hour. Fiberoptic bronchoscopy and transbronchial biopsy were performed; subsequently, sputum and tissue cultures were negative for fungi and Myco. tuberculosis. Histopathologic examination of the pulmonary biopsy material did not reveal any granulomas, fungi, acid-fast organisms or angiitis, but there was moderate edema of bronchial submucosa with vascular congestion and infiltration of lymphocytes and plasma cells. Peribronchial smooth muscle and elastic tissue were moderately fragmented and focally hypertrophied; surrounding alveolar septa had moderate fibrous thickening; and alveolar lining cells showed a type II reactivity with foamy macrophages in alveolar sacs. On October 10, the patient became afebrile without any antibiotic therapy, chest examination revealed clearing of rales, and a chest film disclosed clearing of the pulmonary infiltrates.

When seen as an outpatient on November 4, 1974, the patient was asymptomatic, free of pulmonary rales and showed complete resolution of the previous pulmonary infiltrates on chest film. By avoiding barn work and grain handling she has remained well for 16 months.

IMMUNOLOGIC STUDIES AND RESULTS

Skin Tests. Results of prick tests performed with several tree, grass and weed pollens, molds, housedust and animal epidermal inhalants of 1/10 w/v concentration (Hollister-Steir Laboratories, Yeadon, Pa.) were all negative at 20 minutes. Intradermal tests employed 0.02 ml volumes of fungal antigens (1,000 PNU/ml concentration), and the results at 20 minutes, 8, 24 and 48 hours are shown in Table I. A. fumigatus was the only fungus to elicit a positive reaction to a 48-hour skin test.

Serum Studies. Immunoglobulins G (IgG), A (IgA), M (IgM) and D (IgD) were quantitated by single radial immunodiffusion (Kallestad Laboratories, Minneapolis, Minn.), and IgE was quantitated by the method of Gleich et al. [26]. There was diffuse elevation of all serum immunoglobulin levels as shown in Table II. Serum precipitins to fungal antigens were performed by the Ouchterlony double diffusion in agarose and by the counterelectrophoresis methods of Gordon et al. [27] and Ward and associate [28]. Cultures of A. fumigatus, A. flavus and A. niger were kindly provided by the Communicable Disease Center, Atlanta, Ga. at a 1,500 μg/ml carbohydrate concentration [29]. Other fungal and thermophilic actinomycetes antigens were provided by Hollister-Steir Laboratories. Results, shown in Table III, revealed that the precipitins were negative to thermophilic actinomycetes both by double diffusion in agarose gel and by counterelectrophoresis.

TABLE II Serum Immunoglobulin Concentrations

	IgG (mg/dl)	IgA (mg/dl)	IgM (mg/dl)	IgD (mg/dl)	IgE (IU/ml)
Patient	1,850	420	300	9	1,300
Normal range	600–1,600	200–400	60–200	0–6	0–90

In Vitro Lymphocyte Studies. Blood collection, preparation of mononuclear cell suspensions, mitogen and antigen stimulations are described in detail elsewhere [30]. Fungal antigens were dialyzed exhaustively to remove phenol. For antigen stimulation, 2×10^5 cells were cultured for 120 hours with media or media plus serial dilutions of fungal antigens (initial concentration 20,000 PNU/ml or 1/10 w/v). Lymphocyte transformation was measured by the incorporation of radiolabelled thymidine. Results of lymphocyte transformation to A. fumigatus and Penicillium antigens after 120-hour incubation in heterologous plasma and to phytohemagglutinin (PHA) concanavallin-A (CON-A) and pokeweed mitogen (PWM) after 72-hour incubation are shown in Table IV. The patient had definite lymphocyte transformation to A. fumigatus antigen over a 3 log dilution range; however, maximum transformation occurred at a 200 PNU/ml (1/100 w/v) concentration. Other fungal antigens tested in this patient (Rhizopus,

TABLE III Serum Fungal Precipitins

	DD*	CEP†
A. fumigatus	+	+
A. clavatus	+	–
A. nidulens	+	–
A. niger	–	ND
A. flavus	–	ND
A. glaucus	–	ND
Micropolyspora faeni	–	–
Thermoactinomyces vulgaris	–	–
Penicillium	–	ND
Hormodendrum	–	ND
Rhizopus	–	ND
Alternaria	–	ND

NOTE: ND = not done.
*Double diffusion in agar gel.
†Counterelectrophoresis.

TABLE IV Lymphocyte Transformation

	Media	Aspergillus*	Penicillium	PHA	CON-A	PWM
Patient	1,165 ± 245†	30,383 ± 1,193	4,002 ± 654	104,366 ± 11,708	144,776 ± 10,484	65,244 ± 3,096
Normal control	1,721 ± 169	5,680 ± 510	3,779 ± 293	97,845 ± 15,469	84,170 ± 2,875	38,628 ± 2,825

*Antigen concentration was 200 PNU/ml or 1/100 weight by volume.
†^{3}H-thymidine uptake in counts per minute ± standard error of the mean for triplicate cultures.

Alternaria, Helminthosporium and Hormodendrum) failed to elicit significant lymphocyte transformation.

COMMENTS

A. fumigatus spore inhalation may result in aspergilloma formation in pulmonary cavities or cysts, invasive aspergillosis in immunodeficient patients, extrinsic bronchial asthma or allergic bronchopulmonary aspergillosis in atopic patients and extrinsic allergic alveolitis in nonatopic patients [4]. We describe a patient in whom there was no evidence of cavitary lung disease, aspergilloma on chest films or invasive aspergillosis. Our patient did, however, have a pulmonary hypersensitivity reaction to the inhalation of A. fumigatus corroborated by three episodes of self-limited illness and a sustained remission with avoidance of mold exposure. She did not have extrinsic asthma by history, clinical findings or pulmonary function tests nor did she have any evidence of allergic bronchopulmonary aspergillosis, as she did not expectorate fungal-laden mucous plugs, have eosinophilia in her peripheral blood or sputum, an Arthus skin test or segmental pulmonary infiltrates. Despite an elevation of the total serum IgE level, our patient was nonatopic as evidenced by a negative history and skin tests to multiple aeroallergens. Serum IgE levels are frequently elevated in allergic bronchopulmonary aspergillosis [31], but the levels of serum IgE, IgG and IgA may also be elevated in patients with extrinsic allergic alveolitis [32], as was demonstrated in our patient.

Our patient appeared to have an extrinsic allergic alveolitis due to massive inhalation of A. fumigatus spores which measure from 2.5 to 5.0 μ in diameter and may be deposited in peripheral pulmonary tissue as was seen in the pulmonary biopsy material. Cultures of the moldy oats and deep bronchial washings were positive for A. fumigatus, and the demonstration of aspergillus spores in pulmonary tissue clearly implicated this fungus in the etiology of our patient's illness. The clinical findings of fever, myalgia, headache, malaise, dyspnea, pulmonary rales, leukocytosis, miliary fibronodular interstitial infiltrates and hypoxia concurrent with a diffusion defect support the diagnosis of extrinsic allergic alveolitis. Similar findings have been described in maltworker's lung due to inhalation of A. clavatus [6,7] and in a patient who inhaled A. flavus from moldy corn [5]. Cryptostroma corticale [10] and A. fumigatus [33] have previously been demonstrated within pulmonary granulomas, and our case constitutes an additional report of this unusual histopathologic finding.

The pathogenesis of our patient's illness, however, did not appear to result from type III immunologic tissue injury. Despite the fact that serum precipitins to A. fumigatus were present, their pathogenic significance is diminished because they are often found in similarly exposed but asymptomatic subjects [4]. Furthermore, the absence of an Arthus skin test reaction and vasculitis with polymorphonuclear leukocytic infiltration in pulmonary tissue make it extremely unlikely that a type III immune response and precipitin-mediated tissue inflammation contributed to our patient's illness. The histopathology of pulmonary tissue was more compatible with a type IV (lymphocyte-mediated) immunologic inflammatory response and resembled the histopathology seen in several forms of extrinsic allergic alveolitis [10,18,20,34–36]. Additional support for a type IV immune pathogenesis was the demonstration on two occasions of a 36 to 48 hour skin test reaction and in vitro lymphocyte transformation to A. fumigatus antigen. The absence of delayed cutaneous hypersensitivity, serum precipitins and lymphocyte transformation to other cereal molds, and the absence of precipitins to thermophilic actinomycetes weigh against other ubiquitous fungi as etiologic agents of the illness in our patient.

There are suggestions in the literature that a type IV rather than a type III immune response may underlie the pathogenesis of extrinsic allergic alveolitis and perhaps allergic bronchopulmonary aspergillosis. Positive 48-hour intradermal tests have been reported in maple bark disease [10], pigeon breeder's disease [16] and allergic bronchopulmonary aspergillosis [17]. Turner-Warwick [17] described a unique subset of otherwise typical patients with allergic bronchopulmonary aspergillosis who responded to A. fumigatus inhalation challenge with 6-hour reactions of fever, myalgia, malaise, leukocytosis, pulmonary restrictive and diffusion defects, and diffuse pulmonary micronodular infiltrates. Some patients had negative reactions to prick skin tests and negative serum precipitins to A. fumigatus antigen, but they did have positive reactions to 48-hour intradermal tests and produced migration inhibitory factor to this antigen. The reported pulmonary histopathologic findings of epithelioid tubercles, foreign body and Langhans' giant cells, alveolar fibrosis and interstitial pneumonitis with histiocytes, lymphocytes and foamy macrophages, as was seen in our patient and in patients with farmer's lung [18,20], allergic bronchopulmonary aspergillosis [19], maple bark disease [10], pigeon breeder's disease [34] and humidifier lung [35,36], are more compatible with type IV, rather than type III immunologic inflammation. Finally, in vitro lymphocyte transformation reported previously in pigeon breeder's disease [21–23] and in this report is additional evidence of a type IV immunologic pathogenesis in extrinsic allergic alveolitis. The serum precipitins in our patient signified that exposure to A. fumigatus had occurred and that this exposure had been immunogenic; however, these precipitins could not be definitely implicated in the pathogenesis of her disease. An alternative and more probable pathogenesis of this patient's extrinsic allergic alveolitis appeared to be a type IV immune response and subsequent lymphocyte-mediated inflammation secondary to massive inhalation of A. fumigatus as evidenced by delayed cutaneous hypersensitivity, pulmonary histopathology and in vitro lymphocyte transformation. Additional reports in the literature provide evidence of a type IV immunologic pathogenesis of extrinsic allergic alveolitis and, perhaps, allergic bronchopulmonary aspergillosis.

Further investigation of cell-mediated immunity by in vivo and particularly in vitro methods is urged in all forms of extrinsic allergic alveolitis and allergic bronchopulmonary aspergillosis to elucidate more fully the pathogenesis of these diseases.

REFERENCES

1. Gell PGH, Coombs RPA: Clinical Aspects of Immunology, Philadelphia, F.A. Davis Co., 1968, p 575.
2. Hinson KFW, Moon AJ, Plummer NS: Bronchopulmonary aspergillosis: a review and a report of eight new cases. Thorax 7: 317, 1952.
3. Salvin RG, Stanczyk DJ, Lonigro AJ, et al.: Allergic bronchopulmonary aspergillosis—a North American rarity: clinical and immunologic characteristics. Am J Med 47: 306, 1969.
4. Pepys J: Hypersensitivity diseases of the lungs due to fungi and organic dusts. Monographs in Allergy, vol 4, Basel, S. Karger, 1969.
5. Patterson R, Sommers H, Fink JN: Farmer's lung following inhalation of Aspergillus flavus growing in mouldy corn. Clin Allergy 4: 79, 1974.
6. Riddle HFV, Channell S, Blyth W, et al.: Allergic alveolitis in a maltworker. Thorax 23: 271, 1968.
7. Riddle HFV: Prevalence of respiratory symptoms and sensitization by mould antigens among a group of maltworkers. Br J Industr Med 31: 31, 1974.
8. Dickie HA, Rankin J: Farmer's lung: an acute granulomatous interstitial pneumonitis occurring in agricultural workers. JAMA 167: 1069, 1958.
9. Emanuel DA, Wenzel FJ, Bowerman CI, et al.: Farmer's lung: clinical, pathologic and immunologic study of twenty-four patients. Am J Med 37: 392, 1964.
10. Emanuel DA, Wenzel FJ, Lawton BR: Pneumonitis due to Cryptostroma corticale (maple bark disease). N Engl J Med 274: 1413, 1966.
11. Reed CE, Sosman A, Barbee RA: Pigeon-breeders' lung: a newly observed interstitial pulmonary disease. JAMA 193: 261, 1965.
12. Hargreave FE, Pepys J, Longbottom JL, et al.: Bird breeder's (fancier's) lung. Lancet 1: 445, 1966.
13. Fink JN, Sosman AJ, Barboriak JJ, et al.: Pigeon breeders' disease: a clinical study of a hypersensitivity pneumonitis. Ann Intern Med 68: 1205, 1968.
14. Buechner HA, Prevatt AL, Thompson J, et al.: Bagassosis: a review with further historical data, studies of pulmonary function and results adrenal steroid therapy. Am J Med 25: 234, 1958.
15. Salvaggio JE, Buechner HA, Seabury JH, et al.: Bagassosis. I. Precipitins against extracts of crude bagasse in the serum of patients. Ann Intern Med 64: 748, 1966.
16. Warren WP, Woolf CR: Avian-induced hypersensitivity pneumonitis. Can Med Assoc J 107: 1196, 1972.
17. Turner-Warwick M: Immunology of the lower respiratory tract. Clin Allergy 3 (suppl): 653, 1973.
18. Seal RME, Hapke EJ, Thomas GO, et al.: The pathology of acute and chronic stages of farmer's lung. Thorax 23: 469, 1968.
19. Chan-Yeung M, Chase WH, Trapp W, et al.: Allergic bronchopulmonary aspergillosis: clinical and pathological study of three cases. Chest 59: 33, 1971.
20. Wenzel FJ, Emanuel DA, Gray RL: Immunofluorescent studies in patients with farmer's lung. J Allergy Clin Immunol 48: 224, 1971.
21. Caldwell JR, Pearce DE, Spencer C, et al.: Immunologic mechanisms in hypersensitivity pneumonitis. I. Evidence for cell-mediated immunity and complement fixation in pigeon breeder's disease. J Allergy Clin Immunol 52: 225, 1973.
22. Hansen PJ, Penny R: Pigeon breeder's disease: study of the cell-mediated immune response to pigeon antigens by the lymphocyte culture technique. Int Arch Allergy Appl Immunol 47: 498, 1974.
23. Moore VL, Fink JN, Barboriak JJ, et al.: Immunologic events in pigeon breeder's disease. J Allergy Clin Immunol 53: 319, 1974.
24. Kawai T, Salvaggio J, Lake W, et al.: Experimental production of hypersensitivity pneumonitis with bagasse and thermophilic actinomycete antigen. J Allergy Clin Immunol 50: 276, 1972.
25. Richerson HB, Cheng FHF, Bauserman SC: Acute experimental hypersensitivity pneumonitis in rabbits. Am Rev Respir Dis 104: 568, 1971.
26. Gleich GJ, Averbeck AK, Swedlund HA: Measurement of IgE in normal and allergic serum by radioimmunoassay. J Lab Clin Med 77: 690, 1971.
27. Gordon MA, Almy RE, Greene CH: Diagnostic mycoserology by immunoelectro-osmophoresis. Am J Clin Pathol 57: 471, 1971.
28. Ward GW Jr, Kohler PF: Counterelectrophoresis as a rapid method for the detection of aspergillus precipitins in pulmonary disease. Chest 63 (suppl): 49, 1973.
29. Coleman RM, Kaufman L: Use of the immunodiffusion test in

the serodiagnosis of aspergillosis. Appl Microbiol 23: 301, 1972.

30. Strong DM, Woody JN, Facktor MA, et al.: Immunological responsiveness of frozen-thawed human lymphocytes. Clin Exp Immunol 21: 442, 1975.
31. Patterson R, Fink JN, Pruzansky JJ, et al.: Serum immunoglobulin levels in pulmonary allergic aspergillosis and certain other lung diseases, with special reference to immunoglobulin E. Am J Med 54: 16, 1973.
32. Roberts RC, Wenzel FJ, Emanuel DA: Serum immunoglobulin levels in farmer's lung disease. J Allergy Clin Immunol 52: 297, 1973.
33. Riley DJ, Mackenzie JW, Uhlman WE, et al.: Allergic bronchopulmonary aspergillosis: evidence of limited tissue invasion. Rev Respir Dis 111: 232, 1975.
34. Hensley GT, Garancis JC, Cherayil GD, et al.: Lung biopsies of pigeon breeders' disease. Arch Pathol 87: 572, 1969.
35. Fink JN, Banaszak EF, Thiede WH, et al.: Interstitial pneumonitis due to hypersensitivity to an organism contaminating a heating system. Ann Intern Med 74: 80, 1971.
36. Sweet LC, Anderson JA, Callies QC, et al.: Hypersensitivity pneumonitis related to a home furnace humidifier. J Allergy Clin Immunol 48: 171, 1971.

Tuberculous Pseudotumors of the Liver

ROBERT D. ZIPSER, M.D.
JAMES E. RAU, M.D.*
RICHARD R. RICKETTS, M.D.
LYNN C. BEVANS, M.D.
Los Angeles, California

A 35 year old man presented with fever, weight loss and adenopathy. The clinical presentation, laboratory studies, liver scan and laparotomy all suggested metastatic carcinoma. Bacteriologic and pathologic studies established a diagnosis of macronodular tuberculosis isolated to the liver. Response to antituberculous drug therapy was rapid. Review of the literature revealed this case to be a rare example of tuberculous pseudotumors of the liver.

Tuberculosis of the liver usually occurs in a miliary form. Uncommonly, large nodules, greater than 2 or 3 cm in diameter, are present. In 1952 Leader [1] made an extensive review of the world literature and documented 80 cases of hepatic tuberculosis with large abscesses or nodules. In most of these cases tuberculosis was present elsewhere in the body. Rarely does tuberculosis present as isolated liver involvement with multiple large nodules. This form resembles metastatic cancer in that the clinical presentation, liver function tests, liver scan and gross appearance of the liver are similar and has been described as pseudotumoral by Debray et al. [2]. The American literature contains no reports of this form of tuberculosis, but there are a few recent reports in the foreign literature [2–8].

We describe a patient with isolated tuberculous pseudotumors of the liver (diagnosis is made by laparotomy) who subsequently responded rapidly to antituberculous therapy.

CASE REPORT

A 35 year old Mexican-American man was admitted to Los Angeles County-University of Southern California Medical Center on June 28, 1975, with a six week history of daily fever, night sweats, malaise and a 20 pound weight loss. Five months earlier he had noticed painless adenopathy in the left side of his neck, which had persisted unchanged until his admission. He denied cough, dyspnea or a history of exposure to tuberculosis. He also denied any change in bowel habits or abdominal discomfort. He came to the United States from Mexico in 1968, but he returned to Mexico in 1971 where he remained until six months prior to admission.

Physical examination revealed a mildly cachectic, chronically ill appearing man. Temperature was 100.4°F, pulse rate 112 beats/min, respirations 18/min and blood pressure 120/75 mm Hg. Four firm, 2 cm in diameter, nontender lymph nodes were palpable in the left supraclavicular and posterior cervical areas. Chest examination revealed no abnormalities. The liver was palpable 4 cm below the right costal margin during quiet respiration. The edge was firm, nontender and slightly nodular. The remainder of the abdominal examination was within normal limits.

Laboratory data included a hematocrit value of 35 per cent, a hemoglobin level of 12.1 g/100 ml and a white cell count of 9,900/mm^3 with 55 per cent neutrophils, 30 per cent lymphocytes and 9 per cent monocytes. The urinalysis was within normal limits. Blood urea nitrogen, serum glucose, elec-

From the Departments of Medicine, Surgery, and Pathology, Los Angeles County-University of Southern California Medical Center, Los Angeles, California. Requests for reprints should be addressed to Dr. Robert D. Zipser, Department of Medicine, Los Angeles County-University of Southern California Medical Center, 1200 North State Street, Los Angeles, California 90033.
Manuscript accepted January 23, 1976.
* Present address: Southern California Permanente Medical Group, Inglewood, California 90305.

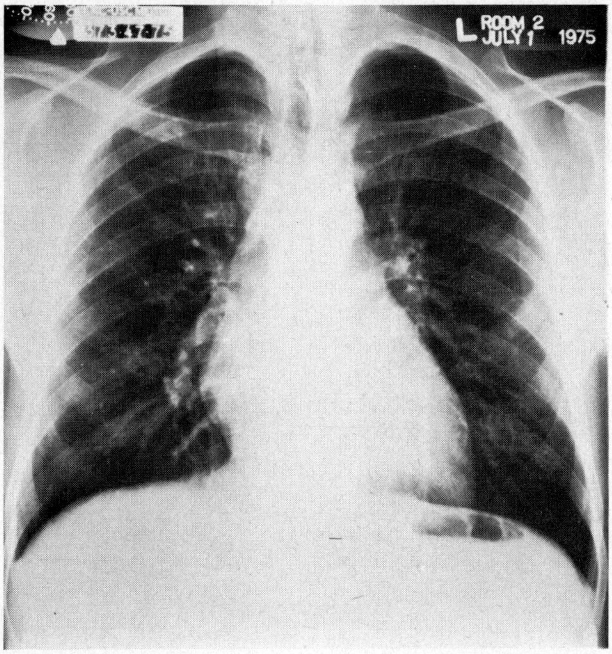

Figure 1. *Chest roentgenogram shows no evidence of active tuberculosis.*

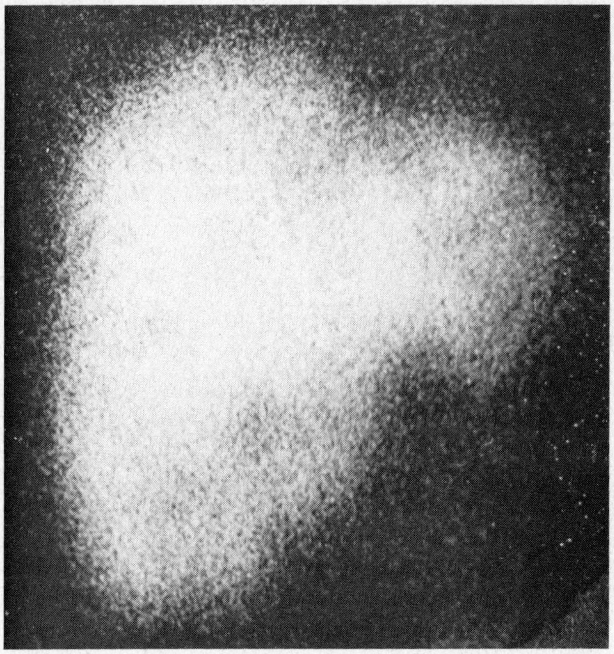

Figure 2. *^{99m}Tc sulfur-colloid liver scan shows multiple large filling defects.*

trolytes, serum glutamic oxaloacetic transaminase (SGOT), serum glutamic pyruvate transaminase (SGPT), lactic dehydrogenase (LDH) and bilirubin were within normal limits. The alkaline phosphatase was 5.9 Bessey-Lowry-Brock units (normal 1 to 3 units). The prothrombin time was 62 per cent of control. The albumin was 2.7 g/100 ml and the globulins 6.3 g/100 ml. An immunoglobulin assay showed the immunoglobulin A level to be 1,425 mg/100 ml, immunoglobulin G level 1,650 mg/100 ml and immunoglobulin M level 310 mg/100 ml. Routine blood cultures were negative. Concentrated smears of urine were negative for acid-fast bacilli.

Multiple roentgenographic views of the chest disclosed no abnormalities (Figure 1). An intermediate strength purified protein derivative skin test gave 10 mm induration at 48 hours. The amebic indirect hemagglutination test was negative. A technetium sulfur-colloid liver scan disclosed numerous filling defects in the liver with mild increased bone marrow uptake (Figure 2). On July 8, a lymph node biopsy specimen revealed a cystic, purulent node which, on microscopic examination, showed stellate-shaped necrosis surrounded by histiocytes and lymphocytes (Figure 3). Acid-fast and gram stains were negative. On July 11, a Menghini needle biopsy specimen of the liver was obtained that revealed nonspecific changes of hepatocyte necrosis with round cell infiltration of sinusoids, but no true epithelioid granulomas, fatty change, fibrosis or cholestasis (Figure 4). Acid-fast and gram stains were again negative.

The patient continued to have night sweats and daily temperatures to 102°F. On July 11, in consideration of the patient's poor condition, positive purified protein derivative skin test and necrotizing lymphadenitis, it was decided to begin therapy with isoniazid and ethambutol. After seven days there was only a minimal reduction in the frequency of the patient's spikes in temperature. He then underwent laparotomy; the liver surface contained multiple nodules, varying in diameter from 2 mm to 5 cm (Figure 5). The larger nodules were fluctuant to palpation. Further exploration revealed numerous firm para-aortic nodes measuring approximately 2 cm in diameter and a firm mass in the region of the head of the pancreas. The remainder of the intra-abdominal examination disclosed no abnormalities. The initial impression at that time was metastatic carcinoma, possibly originating in the pancreas. A wedge biopsy specimen of the liver was obtained and revealed fibrocaseous granuloma by rapid frozen section. A second wedge biopsy specimen was obtained for culture and special stains.

On the fourth postoperative day, acid-fast stains confirmed the presence of tuberculous bacilli in the liver tissue, and rifampin was added to the antibiotic regimen. Two days later the patient became afebrile and showed a markedly improved appetite and sense of well being. He was discharged on the tenth postoperative day. Two weeks later culture of liver tissue became positive and Mycobacterium tuberculosis was identified. Cultures from the needle liver biopsy specimen, the lymph node biopsy specimen and multiple urine specimens remained negative. Two months after discharge the patient continued to feel well. He had regained the lost weight. The liver was no longer enlarged, but the elevated alkaline phosphatase and globulin levels persisted.

PATHOLOGIC FINDINGS

Microscopic examination of liver tissue obtained at laparotomy revealed numerous small granulomas composed of epithelioid cells without giant cells or

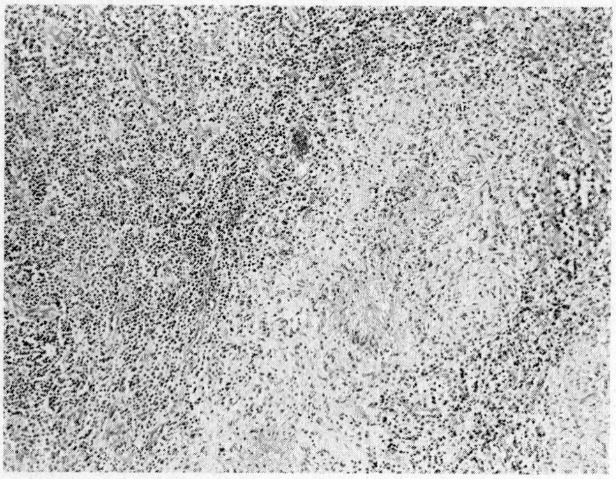

Figure 3. *Cervical lymph node biopsy tissue shows stellate-shaped necrosis. Hematoxylin and eosin stain; original magnification × 100, reduced by 30 per cent.*

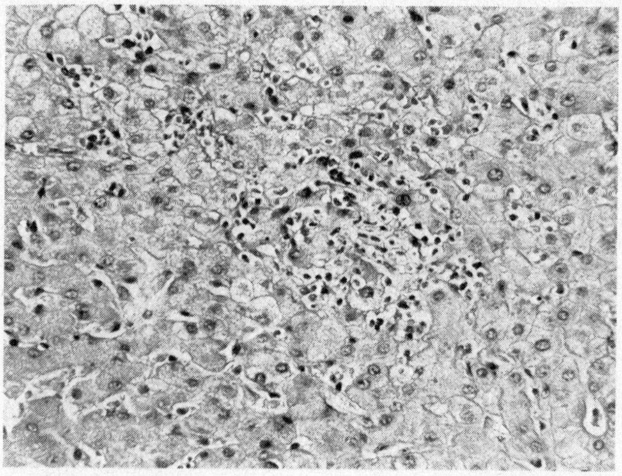

Figure 4. *Needle biopsy specimen of the liver shows mild hydropic change with focal hepatocyte necrosis and round cell infiltration. Hematoxylin and eosin stain; original magnification × 300, reduced by 30 per cent.*

caseation. They were similar to those described by Haex and VonBeek [9] as epithelioid cell subtubercles and by Korn et al. [10] as microgranulomas. The granulomas grouped, coalesced and formed large conglomerate tubercles; the larger of which had central caseation (Figure 6). Acid-fast bacilli were identified in the caseous portions of several conglomerate tubercles. Rare Langhans' giant cells were present in single and conglomerate tubercles (Figure 7). The over-all appearance suggested a progressive phenomenon beginning with the small tubercles, forming in groups with a single peripheral border of lymphocytes and histiocytes, then developing central caseation (Figures 6 and 8). The larger the tuberculoma, the more extensive was the central caseation. It was the larger conglomerate tuberculomas that appeared as yellow-white tumors and resembled metastatic carcinoma.

That portion of the wedge biopsy specimen without epithelioid granulomas was characterized by bile duct proliferation, sinusoidal lymphocytosis, Kupffer cell hyperplasia and irregular hepatocellular damage.

COMMENTS

Hepatic tuberculosis occurs in several forms. The most common form, miliary hepatic tuberculosis with nodules from 0.5 to 2 mm in diameter, is found in 80 to 100 per cent of autopsied patients with disseminated miliary tuberculosis and in 50 to 80 per cent of autopsied patients with nonmiliary pulmonary tuberculosis [11–15]. Miliary hepatic tuberculosis with minimal or no apparent

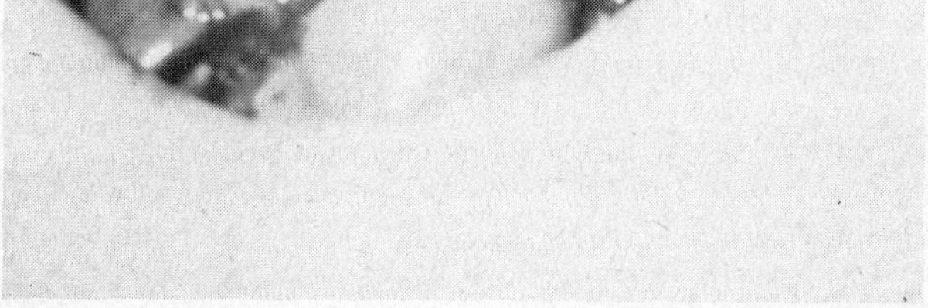

Figure 5. *Intra-operative photograph of the liver shows large conglomerate tuberculomas. Intestines are in foreground.*

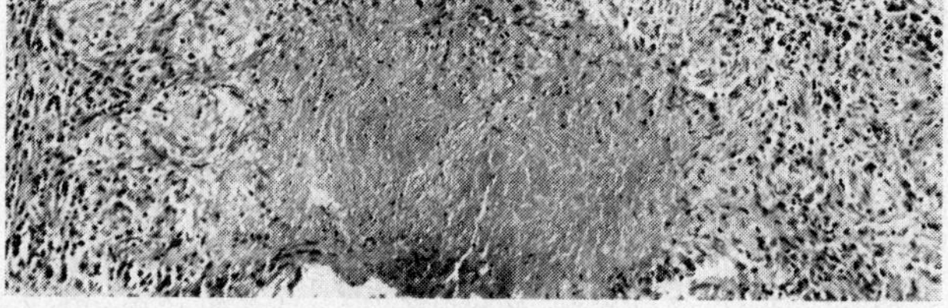

Figure 6. *Wedge biopsy specimen of the liver shows multiple granulomas coalesced into a conglomerate tubercle with central caseation. Hematoxylin and eosin stain; original magnification × 120, reduced by 30 per cent.*

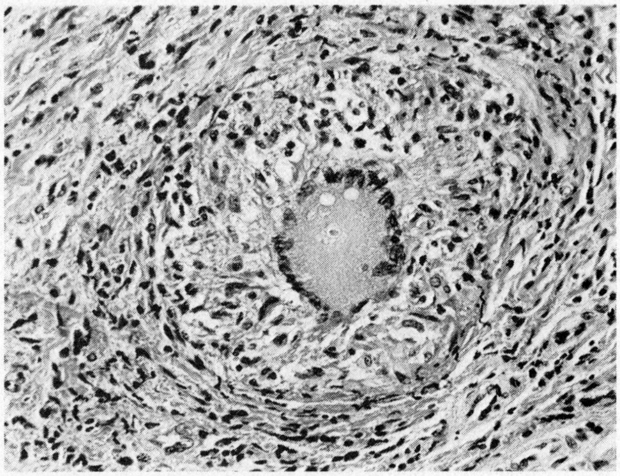

Figure 7. Wedge biopsy specimen of the liver shows epithelioid granuloma and Langhan's giant cell. Hematoxylin and eosin stain; original magnification × 300, reduced by 30 per cent.

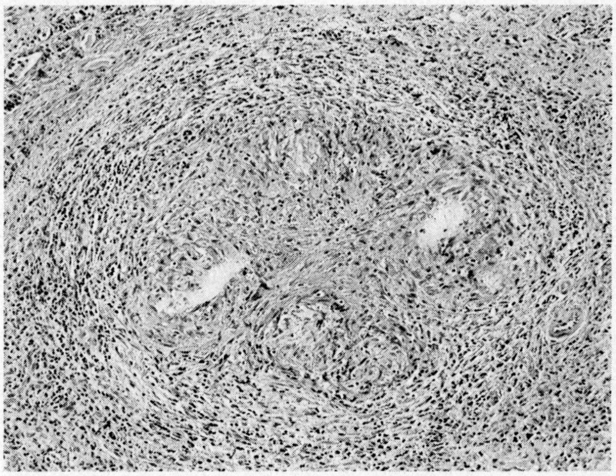

Figure 8. Wedge biopsy specimen of the liver shows multiple epithelioid granulomas forming an early conglomerate tubercle. Note the peripheral lymphocyte and histiocyte response encircling the entire tubercle. Hematoxylin and eosin stain; original magnification × 120, reduced by 30 per cent.

pulmonary or gastrointestinal involvement has rarely been reported [16–20].

Macronodular hepatic involvement with tuberculous nodules of several centimeters in diameter is much less common. It was first described by Bristowe [21] in 1858 who found cavitary hepatic tuberculosis in 12 of 167 autopsied patients with tuberculous ulcerations of the intestines. Rolleston [12] in 1905 called this form local tuberculosis and subdivided cases into those that involved the bile ducts and those in which tuberculomas formed. Tuberculomas were either solitary or multiple. Solitary tuberculomas up to 12 cm in diameter have been reported frequently [22–28]. Multiple tuberculomas appear as large nodules that often have central caseation. Macronodular hepatic tuberculosis has been diagnosed in patients who had no apparent pulmonary involvement as well as in patients with disseminated pulmonary tuberculosis.

Our case represents the macronodular type with multiple tuberculomas appearing as tumors on the liver surface. Because of its close resemblance to cancer on liver scan and at surgery, the term pseudotumoral seems most appropriate. The hepatic involvement was undoubtedly part of widespread tuberculosis as suggested by supraclavicular, cervical and para-aortic adenopathy, and diffuse lymphohematogenous spread seems the most likely origin of hepatic disease. However, the absence of detectable pulmonary or gastrointestinal disease and the nonspecific lymph node histology justifies comparison to other cases of apparent isolated hepatic tuberculosis.

The hepatic nodules ranged in diameter from less than 1 cm to 5 cm; this is similar to that reported in the foreign literature [2–8,29,30]. The only similar reports in the American literature were by Leader [1] in 1952 and by Morris [31] in 1930, however, in both of these cases the patients had cavitary pulmonary disease as well.

Our patient had the characteristic presentation of chills and fever, weight loss, malaise and hepatomegaly. Unusual presentations have included diarrhea, palpable abdominal mass, abdominal pain, portal hypertension and jaundice [5,8,29,32]. Jaundice may be intermittent and is usually attributed to tuberculomas of the porta hepatis obstructing bile flow. Patients with isolated solitary tuberculomas tended to have more localizing signs with enlarging abdominal masses and pain.

The results of the liver function studies in our patient were similar to those of other patients with macronodular tuberculosis. The results were nonspecific and common to most space occupying lesions. Transaminase levels are usually normal or minimally elevated. Alkaline phosphatase is moderately increased, albumin decreased, globulin increased and prothrombin time slightly prolonged. Bilirubin levels are variable, but are rarely highly elevated.

The diagnosis of isolated macronodular hepatic tuberculosis has usually been made only at laparotomy or at autopsy. Recently, Debray et al. [2] and Traissac et al. [33] used laparoscopy to diagnose and to follow this disease. The preoperative or premorbid diagnoses were consistently either metastatic carcinoma, amebic abscess or empyema of the gallbladder. Two patients underwent surgery only after a course of therapy for suspected amebic abscess was unsuccessful [6,34]. The close resemblance of the findings at surgery to metastatic carcinoma is striking. In our case, the multiple nodules on the liver surface were also initially thought to be metastatic carcinoma. Only after rapid frozen section revealed granulomas were further specimens obtained for culture. In a similar case reported by Neill [35], an intraoperative diagnosis of neoplasm was made. A biopsy specimen revealed necrosis and fibrous replacement of liver. Ten months later the diagnosis of tuberculosls was made at autopsy.

Needle biopsy of the liver is an excellent means of diagnosing miliary tuberculosis [10,16,36]. However, in several of the reported cases of macronodular tuberculosis the liver biopsy specimen was nondiagnostic [8,34]. It is, of course, possible that tuberculosis is diagnosed by liver biopsy in some cases without awareness of its macronodular characteristics. The needle biopsy specimen from our patient was not diagnostic nor did Mycobacterium tuberculosis grow on culture.

Even with liver specimens obtained at laparotomy, the diagnosis is sometimes difficult. The most common microscopic findings are nonspecific with Kupffer cell hyperplasia, focal hepatocyte necrosis with round cell infiltration and portal inflammation. Popper [37] has suggested that these nonspecific changes may be one mechanism of granuloma formation in the liver; histiocytic accumulation without the preexisting hepatocyte necrosis may be another mechanism. Epithelioid granulomas are seen in many other granulomatous diseases as well. Conglomerate tubercles with caseation, although suggestive, have not been proved pathognomonic of tuberculosis. Acid-fast stains and culture are required to positively confirm the diagnosis.

Hersch [7] has noted that the tubercles in the miliary form tend to predominate inside the hepatic lobules, whereas the tubercles in the local forms occur mainly in the portal regions. Thus, we can speculate that such local factors as greater oxygen tension in the portal area as compared to the central area favor bacillus growth and may promote conglomerate tubercle formation and subsequent caseation. Indeed, acid-fast bacilli are more prevalent in specimens with caseation than in those with epithelioid granulomas [7]. In our case, the acid-fast bacilli were also demonstrated in the caseous portions of the conglomerate tubercles.

We were fortunate to culture Mycobacterium tuberculosis from the liver tissue obtained at surgery despite seven days of antituberculous therapy. Few others have been able to bacteriologically confirm the diagnosis. In most cases, the diagnosis was made by acid-fast stains of tissue or, more commonly, suggested by the microscopic appearance of caseating granulomas. In some cases, antituberculous therapy prevented bacteriologic confirmation. Because of the resemblance to carcinoma, cultures were not obtained in other cases.

In the era before effective antituberculous drugs, hepatic tuberculosis was usually fatal. Death was often a result of miliary spread. Surgical cures were attempted in some cases of solitary tuberculomas; a few were successful [27,28]. With effective therapy the prognosis is good. Patients become afebrile in a few weeks, and resolution of nodules is complete in six to nine months [2,33].

Our case demonstrates a rare presentation of tuberculosis, pseudotumors of the liver. The initial diagnosis was pancreatic carcinoma. This is unusual in a 35 year old man. We suggest that such unusual presentations of "metastatic carcinoma" to the liver be thoroughly investigated with pathologic and bacteriologic studies.

ACKNOWLEDGMENT

We gratefully acknowledge Dr. Telfer B. Reynolds for his assistance in the care of the patient and preparation of the manuscript.

REFERENCES

1. Leader SA: Tuberculosis of the liver and gall-bladder with abscess formation. A review and case report. Ann Intern Med 37: 594, 1952.
2. Debray J, Krulik M, Bernard J-F: La tuberculose pseudotumorale du foie. A propos d'une observation personnelle. Sem Hop Paris 48: 3165, 1972.
3. Joseph R, Nezelof C, Job J-C, et al.: La tuberculose macronodulaire du foie. Une observation avec revue de la litterature. Ann Pediatr (Paris) 6: 342, 1959.
4. De Rosa F, Guglielmi A: Tubercolosi nodosa del fegato clinicamente primitiva. Omnia Med Ther 47: 707, 1969.
5. Pineda FM, Dalmacio-Cruz A: Tuberculosis of the liver and the porta hepatis. Report of 9 cases. Acta Med Philipp 2: 128, 1966.
6. Gulati PD, Vyas PB: Tuberculosis of the liver. J Indian Med Assoc 45: 144, 1965.
7. Hersch C: Tuberculosis of the liver. A study of 200 cases. S Afr Med J 38: 906, 1964.
8. Bhargava SP, Sharma ML: Multiple tuberculoma of liver. A case report. J Indian Med Assoc 38: 552, 1962.
9. Haex AJC, Van Beek C: Tuberculosis and the Aspiration Liver Biopsy. Haarlem, The Netherlands, Bohn Publishing Co., 1955, p 77.
10. Korn RJ, Kellow WF, Heller P, et al.: Hepatic involvement in extrapulmonary tuberculosis. Histologic and functional characteristics. Am J Med 27: 60, 1959.
11. Saphir O: Changes in the liver and in the pancreas in chronic pulmonary tuberculosis. Arch Pathol 7: 1026, 1929.
12. Rolleston HD: Tuberculosis of the liver and bile-ducts. Diseases of the Liver, Gallbladder and Bile Ducts, Philadelphia, W. B. Saunders & Co., 1905.
13. Curry FJ, Alcott D: Tuberculous hepatitis with jaundice. Gastroenterology 28: 1037, 1955.
14. Torrey RG: The occurrence of miliary tuberculosis of the liver in the course of pulmonary tuberculosis. Am J Med Sci 151: 549, 1916.

15. Ullom JT: The liver in tuberculosis. Am J Med Sci 136: 694, 1909.
16. Frank BB, Raffensperger EC: Hepatic granulomata. Report of a case with jaundice improving on antituberculous therapy and review of the literature. Arch Intern Med 115: 223, 1965.
17. Cinque TJ, Gary NE, Palladino VS: Primary miliary tuberculosis of the liver. Am J Gastroenterol 42: 611, 1964.
18. Gold J, Wigderson A, Lehman E, Schwartz IR: Tuberculous hepatitis. Report of a case with review of the literature. Gastroenterology 33: 113, 1957.
19. Terry RB, Gunnar RM: Primary miliary tuberculosis of the liver. JAMA 164: 150, 1957.
20. Cleve EA, Gibson JR, Webb WM: Atypical tuberculosis of the liver with jaundice. Ann Intern Med 41: 251, 1954.
21. Bristowe JS: On the connection between abscess of the liver and gastrointestinal ulceration. Trans Path Soc 9: 241, 1858.
22. Chimene DR, Roberts TW, Rohman M: Solitary tuberculoma of the liver. NY State J Med 65: 2479, 1965.
23. Grave GF: Mpilo hospital case report. Tuberculoma of the liver. Cent Afr J Med 18: 148, 1972.
24. Armstrong JR: Tuberculoma of the liver successfully treated with streptomycin. Tubercle 34: 191, 1953.
25. Gracey L: Tuberculous abscess of the liver. Br J Surg 52: 442, 1965.
26. Herrell WE, Simpson WC: Recurrent hyperpyrexia due to solitary tuberculoma of the liver with review of the literature. JAMA 111: 517, 1938.
27. Ransohoff J: Hepatectomy for tuberculoma of the liver. Medical News 84: 727, 1904.
28. Robson M: Three cases of abdominal section for unusual conditions. Tubercular disease of the liver. Trans Clin Soc 28: 83, 1895.
29. Sheldon WPH: A case of massive tuberculosis of the liver. Lancet 2: 1343, 1927.
30. Ashton N: A case of multiple tuberculomata of the liver. J Pathol 58: 95, 1946.
31. Morris E: Tuberculosis of the liver. Am Rev Tuberc 22: 585, 1930.
32. DeCrespigny CT, Cleland JB: A case of primary multiple tuberculomata of the liver with a degenerated hydatid cyst. Med J Aust 1: 151, 1923.
33. Traissac FJ, Doutre LP, Paccalin J, Perissat J, Gratadour P, Terme: Tuberculose hepatique autonome. Forme miliaire et forme tumorale abcedee. Arch Fr Mal App Dig 60: 487, 1971.
34. Duckworth WC: Tuberculosis of the liver. S Afr Med J 38: 945, 1964.
35. Neill DG: Tuberculosis of the liver. Including a report of five cases. Med J Aust 1: 893, 1951.
36. Alexander JF, Galambos JT: Granulomatous hepatitis. The usefulness of liver biopsy in the diagnosis of tuberculosis and sarcoidosis. Am J Gastroenterol 59: 23, 1973.
37. Popper H, Schaffner F: Liver: Structure and Function, New York, McGraw-Hill, 1957, p 555.

Multiple Endocrine Adenomas in a Patient with the Maffucci Syndrome

ADRIAN M. SCHNALL, M.D.
SAUL M. GENUTH, M.D.
Cleveland, Ohio

A patient with multiple cutaneous hemangiomas and skeletal dyschondroplasia (the Maffucci syndrome) was found to have a pituitary chromophobe adenoma, a parathyroid adenoma and two other neoplasms. The presence of two endocrine tumors suggested the syndrome of multiple endocrine adenomatosis, and raised the issue of an etiologic relationship between this disease and the Maffucci syndrome. Dyschondroplasia, however, has no known influence on the secretion of parathyroid hormone or any of the pituitary hormones. The Maffucci syndrome is associated with a high incidence of malignancy, but it involves primarily mesodermal derivatives, whereas multiple endocrine adenomatosis affects tissues of ectodermal origin. The association of the two in our patient is probably fortuitous.

The occurrence of multiple hemangiomas and dyschondroplasia in the same patient was first described by Maffucci [1] in 1881. By 1973, 105 documented cases had been described [2]; since then at least five further reports of the Maffucci syndrome have appeared [3–7]. Many investigators have emphasized the high incidence of tumors in patients with the Maffucci syndrome; in some instances, they are the malignant counterparts of the tumors of cartilage and vessel wall essential to the syndrome, but in many cases the neoplasms involve completely different organs and are of different cell types [2,8,9]. The patient we describe is unique in that he had a documented parathyroid adenoma associated with the Maffucci syndrome. Since he has also had a pituitary chromophobe adenoma, he may have a sporadic case of multiple endocrine adenomatosis (MEA type I). A sigmoid polyp and a neurilemmoma involving nerve roots have also been found in this person.

CASE REPORT

A 37 year old man was admitted to the Saltzman Institute of Mt. Sinai Hospital of Cleveland for evaluation of hypercalcemia. For the three weeks prior to his admission, he had noted weakness and nausea. One year before this admission, a renal stone was demonstrated on an intravenous pyelogram after an episode of flank pain. The patient had previously been apprised of hypercalcemia at age 12, age 25 (calcium 12.5 mg/100 ml) and age 31 (calcium 12.6 mg/100 ml), but he had refused evaluation. There was no family history of endocrine tumors, hypercalcemia, peptic ulcer disease, soft tissue tumors or bony abnormalities. He was an only child. He had been normal at birth, but his parents noticed that he had some difficulty in walking in the

From the Saltzman Institute for Clinical Investigation, the Mt. Sinai Hospital of Cleveland, and the Case Western Reserve University, Cleveland, Ohio. Requests for reprints should be addressed to Dr. Saul M. Genuth, The Mt. Sinai Hospital of Cleveland, 1800 East 105 Street, Cleveland, Ohio 44106. Manuscript accepted January 30, 1976.

second or third year of his life. By age three, his left leg was shorter than the right. Subsequently, the right leg became progressively more angulated in a valgus deformity of about 30 degrees, and the patient fell frequently. At age 12, surgery was performed on the right femur, resulting in a significant reduction in the angulation of the leg and an increase of 2 inches in height. Since that time, there had been no bone pain or further deformity of bone, but the patient required a 3 inch lift on the left shoe. He did not grow significantly in height after age 13 or 14; pubic and axillary hair development and penile enlargement had occurred at age 12 or 13. He first noted purple, raised, skin discolorations at age 14, initially on the lateral aspect of the left foot, over the line of maximal weight-bearing. New similar lesions appeared regularly as time passed, involving both hands and feet, the left hip, chest and buttocks. All such lesions were painless, but they bled profusely on minor trauma.

At age 22, the patient noticed decreased peripheral vision. Ophthalmologic evaluation revealed a bitemporal hemianopsia, and craniotomy was recommended but declined. At age 25, because of progression of the visual loss, he underwent transfrontal hypophysectomy with removal of a chromophobe adenoma. His vision improved postoperatively but worsened again during the subsequent two years, despite a course of cobalt treatment (5,500 rads) to the pituitary area. At age 27, a second transfrontal hypophysectomy was performed; histologic examination again demonstrated a chromophobe adenoma. Subsequently, there was no functional vision in the right eye or the left temporal field. During the next year, the patient noticed thinning of his pubic and axillary hair and a definite decrease in the volume of his ejaculate.

At age 31, he underwent a laminectomy because of pain and weakness in the right leg and lower trunk. An extramedullary neurilemmoma was found, involving nerve roots at the level of the sixth thoracic vertebra. At age 36, after recurrent rectal bleeding, a 3 cm pedunculated polyp was excised from the sigmoid colon; pathologically, it was an adenomatous polyp with cystic changes.

Examination revealed a white man with torso and arms of normal appearance but with disproportionately short legs. The head was slightly squared and elongated. Height was 60 inches, weight 141 pounds. Mental status examination was within normal limits; he was of above-average intelligence. Vision was normal in the nasal half of the left visual field; otherwise, he had light-dark perception only. Bilateral optic atrophy was present. No conjunctival or corneal calcifications were seen. There were no signs of acromegaly, hyperthyroidism or hypothyroidism. The thyroid was not palpable and no masses were felt in the neck. The middle phalanx of the right fourth finger was bowed, the radial aspect concave. The third and fourth digits of the left hand extended incompletely at the distal and proximal interphalangeal joints. The left leg was 3 inches shorter than the right. The left foot was enlarged and club-shaped, partly because of a bony enlargement 9 to 10 cm in diameter in the area of the lateral malleolus, and partly because of 20 to 25 soft superficial lesions over the dorsal surfaces of the toes and the lateral border of the foot (Figure 1). These ranged in diameter from 0.5 to 2 cm, were purple in color, had a mottled surface and irregular margins; they were pedunculated in some cases. All such lesions were nontender; some blanched on pressure. Similar lesions were scattered over the trunk, the right foot, the left hip area and the skin overlying the right medial malleolus. No axillary or chest hair was present; pubic hair was sparse.

Films (Figure 2) showed cystic enlargement of the left second, fifth and sixth ribs anteriorly, and the right 10th and 11th ribs, all near the costochondral junctions, with multiple punctate calcifications within the cystic areas. Multiple lucent cystic areas were seen throughout the phalanges of most of the fingers of both hands (Figure 3). There was no evidence of subperiosteal bone resorption (Figure 3). Irregular calcification, cystic areas and focal areas of enlargement were seen in the pelvis, femurs, and left tibia and fibula. Skull films showed a normal sella turcica except for a small calcification posterior and superior to the dorsum sellae.

Numerous serum calcium values ranged from 10.9 to 12.4 mg/100 ml, phosphorus from 2.1 to 2.7 mg/100 ml and alkaline phosphatase from 47 to 70 IU/liter (normal $<$50 IU/liter). Tubular reabsorption of phosphate was 93 per cent (four days after the discontinuation of a long-term dose of triamcinolone, 4 mg every three days) and 87 per cent (on the 11th day after withdrawal). Serum parathyroid hormone ranged from 2.4 to 3.4 ng/ml (normal $<$0.4 ng/ml) and serum calcium from 11.2 to 12.4 mg/100 ml. No localizing increase in parathyroid hormone was demonstrated on neck vein catheterization studies. Twenty-four hour urinary hydroxyproline levels were 66, 59 and 35 mg (normal $<$40 mg), and 24-hour urinary calcium levels, with the patient adhering to a 150 mg calcium diet, ranged from 173 to 361 mg, with a mean value of 257 mg.

Results of pituitary function studies were as follows: basal human growth hormone, 1 ng/ml, with no increase during insulin-induced hypoglycemia (minimum glucose 39 mg/100 ml) or L-DOPA stimulation; serum luteinizing hormone, 2.5 and 1.6 mIU/ml (normal 6 to 18 mIU/ml); serum follicle-stimulating hormone $<$1.5 mIU/ml (normal 5 to 40 mIU/ml); serum thyroxine 5.9 μg/100 ml (normal 6 to 13 μg/100 ml); resin triiodothyronine uptake 72 per cent (normal 80 to 120 per cent); radioactive iodine uptake 14 per cent; serum thyroid-stimulating hormone 3 μU/ml (normal $<$10 μU/ml); plasma testosterone 56 ng/100 ml (normal 300 to 1,000 ng/100 ml); morning cortisol level 17 μg/100 ml with no rise during insulin hypoglycemia; 24-hour urinary 17-hydroxysteroids (17-OHCS) 0.5 mg basal, 3.3 mg on the day of metyrapone administration and 1.6 mg on the day after. Serum gastrin levels were 100 and 110 pg/ml (normal $<$150 pg/ml) when the serum calcium level was 11.4 to 12.4 mg/100 ml.

On neck exploration a 5 g right superior parathyroid adenoma (chief cell) was removed, and two normal parathyroid glands were identified. The serum calcium level fell rapidly and stabilized at 8.7 to 9.0 mg/100 ml. A 24-hour urinary calcium determination two days postoperatively was 36 mg. A tubular reabsorption of phosphate determined three days after surgery was 85 per cent (during treatment with 150 mg/day of cortisone acetate). The patient was discharged with instructions to take replacement doses of cortisone acetate; he was asymptomatic and normocalcemic three months later. Six months postoperatively, his serum calcium was 10.1 mg/100 ml, phosphate 2.8 mg/100 ml, alkaline phosphatase 41 IU/liter and 24-hour urine hydroxyproline 31 mg.

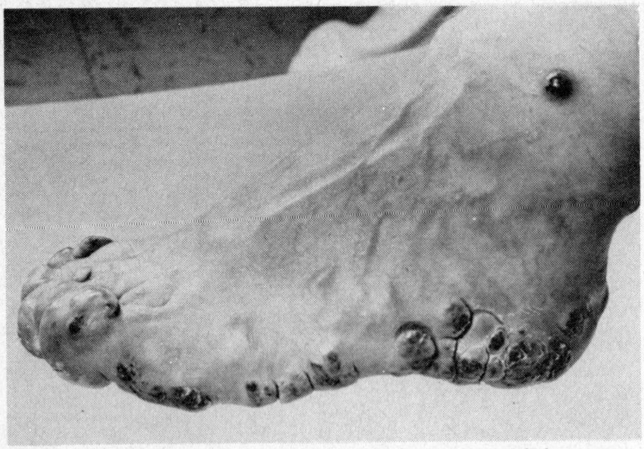

Figure 1. *Lateral aspect of left foot. Note multiple superficial hemangiomas.*

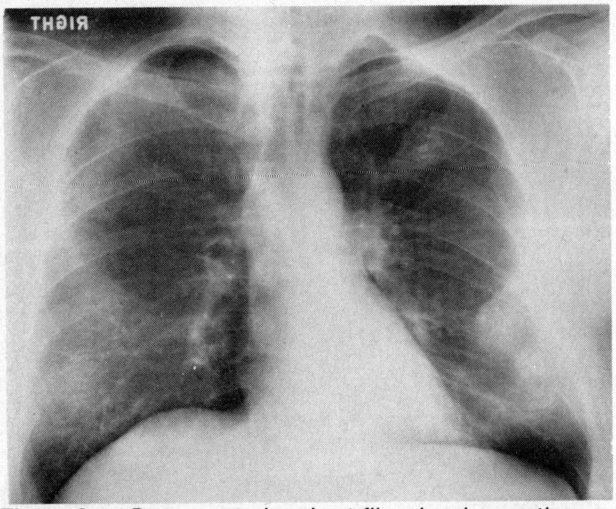

Figure 2. *Posteroanterior chest film showing cystic enlargement of the anterior second, fifth and sixth ribs, with multiple punctate calcifications within the cystic areas.*

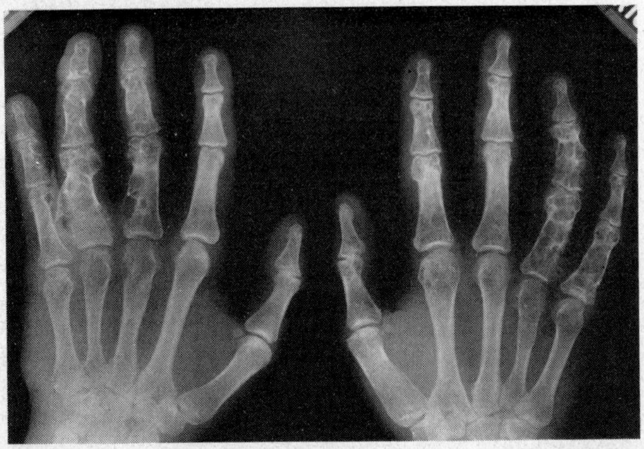

Figure 3. *Anteroposterior film of both hands. Irregular cystic lucencies have replaced the normal bone structure in most of the phalanges. The metacarpals and the phalanges of the left second digit are relatively spared. There is no evidence of subperiosteal bone resorption.*

COMMENTS

The skeletal component of the Maffucci syndrome (or the pure skeletal form, Ollier's disease) is characterized by masses of uncalcified cartilage isolated within the shafts of long bones. These islands of cartilage are composed of immature cells which otherwise appear normal but for unknown reasons have failed to ossify [10,11]. Because such areas are frequently multiple and widespread, and because bony deformities usually are noted early in life, many investigators have considered the underlying abnormality one of development; hence, the term "dyschondroplasia." Although the skeletal disease frequently begins at an early age, the condition is not inherited. In the Maffucci syndrome, multiple hemangiomas accompany the abnormality of cartilage cells, and since both blood vessel wall and chondrocyte are of mesodermal origin, many have postulated a generalized mesodermal dysplasia as the pathogenesis of the disease. The isolated masses of cartilage also proliferate, however, frequently deforming the long bones, and are classified pathologically as enchondromas. Their histologic structure is indeed similar to that of solitary enchondromas, and their frequently asymmetric distribution and great propensity for malignant change suggest that they be viewed as neoplastic rather than as a developmental anomaly. The high incidence of associated tumors also suggests that these patients have at least an unusual susceptibility to neoplastic disease.

The roentgenographic appearance in skeletal dyschondroplasia is characteristic; the areas in which ossification has failed appear as multiple irregular cystic lucencies, especially in the phalanges, and cause gross derangement of bony architecture in the long bones and pelvis. In addition to these typical features of dyschondroplasia, our patient's films also showed prominent mottled calcifications within areas of involved bone, as reported in a number of other cases of the Maffucci syndrome.

The patient we describe is of special interest for several reasons. First, might there be a causal relationship between his congenital skeletal disease and the parathyroid adenoma? Historically, no consistent abnormality of serum calcium or of calcium metabolism has been reported in the Maffucci syndrome. Published calcium values [12–19] have been normal in all but one case, in a 19 year old woman with a serum calcium of 12.1 mg/100 ml. In this woman a 2 kg ovarian teratocarcinoma was removed, following which new lytic bone lesions appeared as well as intra-abdominal metastases within the next year. Andren et al. [20] found a normal calcium accretion rate, normal rapidly and slowly exchangeable calcium spaces, and normal urinary and fecal calcium clearances in one patient. In one report, the patient had renal colic and an elevated alkaline phosphatase level, but widespread metastatic chondrosarcoma and marked abnormalities of liver function attributable to metastases in the liver were found postmortem; permission for postmortem examination of the head and neck was specifically denied in this case [21]. No other patient with the Maffucci syndrome has been said to have any symptoms or signs of hyperparathyroidism.

The known actions of parathyroid hormone on bone produce a diffuse resorptive process rather than a spotty failure of calcification as seen in dyschondroplasia, and the absence of dyschondroplasia in previous reports of primary hyperparathyroidism further argues against a causative role for parathyroid hormone in this disease. The initial increase in alkaline phosphatase and urinary hydroxyproline in our patient, and the decrease postoperatively in both measurements, suggests a parathyroid hormone effect upon bone. This patient's films, however, did not show even early signs of osteitis fibrosa cystica (Figure 3). It is very doubtful that dyschondroplasia is simply an advanced stage of the bone disease of parathyroid hormone excess.

Although hypercalcemia was present at least 12 and possibly 25 years before the patient underwent parathyroid surgery, the dyschondroplasia had been known to be present for 35 of his 37 years and very likely preceded the hypercalcemia. This raises the possibility that the primary skeletal abnormality somehow induced hypersecretion of parathyroid hormone. A simple failure of ossification of cartilage, however, would not be expected to act as a stimulus to parathyroid hormone secretion, since such a failure of ossification should not in itself produce hypocalcemia. Further, there is no current reason to believe that proliferation of cartilage cells would lead to parathyroid stimulation. It is conceivable that the accumulation of calcium in the soft tissue lesions and areas of involved bone might cause a transient hypocalcemia, but neither hypocalcemia nor hyperparathyroidism has been reported in other patients with the Maffucci syndrome in whom tissue calcifications were comparable to those of our patient. Finally, the lack of generalized parathyroid hyperplasia in all four glands, the fact that a single huge adenoma was found and the rapid decrease in serum calcium postoperatively all argue against any general metabolic stimulus to parathyroid hormone secretion in the patient we describe.

A second point of interest involves the apparent lack of progression of our patient's cartilaginous lesions since age 12, shortly before puberty. Several investigators have commented that the bone lesions in many instances of the Maffucci syndrome seem to stabilize at puberty [2]; a review of individual case reports, however, reveals that when growth of the cartilage masses ceases the patient is often over age 18, and in at least two such cases chondromatous enlargement recurred at the age of 30 [12]. In one case, the cartilaginous lesions seemed to enlarge *more rapidly* at puberty and did not stabilize until several years later [12]. In these last three cases, the patients were all male, as is our patient. He had clear-cut evidence of androgen stimulation in the development of secondary sex characteristics at puberty, and these changes did roughly correlate with the cessation of growth of his skeletal lesions. One possible unifying hypothesis is that the chondrocytes which form the skeletal "lesion" in the Maffucci syndrome proliferate rapidly during rapid linear bone growth but much more slowly after the closure of epiphyses under continuing androgen stimulation. The cells apparently retain their potential for rapid growth, however, as recrudescences may occur. Since postpubertal loss of androgen effect would have no effect on linear bone growth or epiphyseal closure, it is not surprising that in our patient the androgen deficiency that occurred after hypophysectomy (at age 27) was without apparent effect upon his dyschondroplasia.

The effects of growth hormone on cartilaginous and skeletal growth are well known. The somatomedins, under the influence of growth hormone, have been shown to stimulate cartilage synthesis as measured by several specific parameters: the incorporation of sulfate into chondroitin sulfate, thymidine into DNA, uridine into RNA and proline into cartilaginous hydroxyproline [23–25]. Growth hormone deficiency was documented in our patient at age 37, was very likely present after hypophysectomy at ages 25 to 27, and may have been present at or before the onset of visual symptoms from his chromophobe adenoma at age 22. The cartilaginous lesions had not apparently progressed since the age of 12, but it is conceivable that lack of growth hormone prevented recrudescent growth of these lesions in the third and fourth decades. As noted herein, such reactivation has been reported in the Maffucci syndrome. Growth hormone levels have not been previously reported in this disease, but the few patients with coexisting pituitary lesions have demonstrated neither acceleration nor regression of their bone disease [5,16,17,22]. To our knowledge, growth hormone deficiency has not been associated with the regression of any preexisting tumor primary to cartilage or bone, and any relationship between growth hormone secretion and the progression of dyschondroplasia must remain speculative.

The final point of interest raised by our patient is that, in addition to the Maffucci syndrome, he has had two of the tumors integral to the syndrome of multiple endocrine adenomatosis (type I), a pituitary adenoma and a parathyroid adenoma [26]. In addition, he was found to have a third tumor sometimes associated with this syndrome—a Schwannoma [27]. He had no abnormal findings on roentgenograms of the gastrointestinal tract, normal serum gastrin levels and no symptoms of peptic ulcer disease. He had no evidence, therefore, of a gastrin-secreting neoplasm, the third common component of the MEA type I syndrome. Although this syndrome is often familial, there have been reports of sporadic occurrences, as appears to be the case here. Two other pituitary chromophobe adenomas have been reported in patients with the Maffucci syndrome. In von Baradnay's case [22], a chromophobe adenoma (and an adrenal cortical adenoma) was found incidentally postmortem. Jingu et al. [5], however, described a man with the Maffucci syndrome since the age of one in whom bitemporal hemianopsia developed when he was 39, and he was found to have the pituitary tumor at craniotomy. Our case brings the incidence of chromophobe adenomas in the Maffucci syndrome to three of 114 reported cases, certainly much greater than the incidence among the general population. It is difficult to accept any causal relationship between the dyschondroplasia and such tumors, since the pituitary lesions have not been associated with excessive trophic hormone production in any case. Although there has been no previous report of multiple endocrine tumors in the Maffucci syndrome, the incidence of neoplasia in general is greatly increased. The majority of associated tumors have consisted of malignant transformation of the initially benign enchondromas (16 cases) or blood vessel tumors (3 cases), but there have also been associated tumors of both endodermal and ectodermal origin [8]. In our patient a sigmoid polyp (endodermal) was removed as well as the other neoplasms noted. Since anterior pituitary, parathyroid and Schwann cells are all derived from ectoderm, one cannot postulate a common primitive pathway for endocrine tumors and the anomalies of cartilage cells and vessel walls in our patient. It seems clear, however, that the basic abnormality in the Maffucci syndrome not only leads to dysplasia of mesodermal tissue but also predisposes to neoplastic change in other tissues. The present case notwithstanding, there is no convincing evidence that dyschondroplasia leads to any consistent abnormality of endocrine function.

REFERENCES

1. Maffucci A: Di un caso di enchondroma ed angioma multiplo. Mov Med Chir Nap 3: 399, 565, 1881.
2. Lewis RJ, Ketcham AS: Maffucci's syndrome: functional and neoplastic significance. J Bone Joint Surg (Am) 55: 1465, 1973.
3. Kennedy JG: Dyschondroplasia and hemangiomata (Maffucci's syndrome). Br Dent J 135: 18, 1973.
4. Raff M: Unilateral enchondromatosis with multiple lymphangiokermatomas. Nosology of Maffucci's syndrome. Hautarzt 24: 309, 1973.
5. Jingu K, Katayama J, Takahashi M, Chin C: A case of Maffucci's syndrome. Jap J Clin Radiol 18: 281, 1973.
6. Grimmer H: Vascular diseases of the vulva. 3. Maffucci syndrome (Maffucci-Kast syndrome). Z Haut Geschlechtskr 46 (suppl): 45, 1971.
7. Wickenhauser J, Canigiani G, Czech W: Beitrag zum Maffucci-Syndrom. Radiol Clin Biol 43: 155, 1974.
8. Anderson IF: Maffucci's syndrome. S African Med J 39: 1066, 1965.
9. (a) Bean WB: Dyschondroplasia and hemangiomata. Arch Intern Med 95: 767, 1955.
   (b) Ibid. Arch Intern Med 102: 544, 1958.
10. Speiser F: Ein Fall von systematischer Enchondromatose des Skelette. Virchows Arch Path Anat 258: 126, 1925.
11. Jaffe H: Tumors and Tumorous Conditions of the Bones and Joints, Philadelphia, Lea & Febiger, 1958, p 184.
12. Carleton A, Elkington JSt.C, Greenfield JG, Robb-Smith AHT: Maffucci's syndrome (dyschondroplasia and hemangiomata). Q J Med 11: 203, 1942.
13. Nardell SG: Ollier's disease: dyschondroplasia. Br Med J 2: 555, 1950.
14. Cecchi E, Baccarini V: Syndrome de Maffucci. Rev Rhum 29: 190, 1962.
15. Ikram-ul-Haq, Tait GB, Stuart CE: Maffucci's syndrome. J Int Coll Surg 43: 133, 1965.
16. Kuzma JF, King JM: Dyschondroplasia with hemangiomatoses (Maffucci's syndrome) and teratoid tumor of the ovary. Arch Pathol 46: 74, 1948.
17. Strang C, Rannie I: Dyschondroplasia with hemangiomata (Maffucci's syndrome). J Bone Joint Surg 32-B: 376, 1950.
18. Mullins JF, Livingood CS: Maffucci's syndrome (dyschondroplasia with hemangiomas). A case with early osseous changes. Arch Dermatol Syph 63: 478, 1951.
19. Piquet B, Medioni L: Remarques a propos d'un syndrome de Maffucci-Kast. Rev Rhum 28: 27, 1960.
20. Andren L, Dymling JF, Elner A, Hogeman KE: Maffucci's syndrome. Acta Chir Scand 126: 397, 1963.
21. Johnson JL, Webster JR, Sippy HI: Maffucci's syndrome. Am J Med 28: 864, 1960.
22. Baradnay G, Hoffmann J, Oekroes J: Dyschondroplasia und Hemangiomata (Maffucci Syndrom). Zentralbl Allg Pathol 101: 296, 1960.
23. Daughaday WH, Hall K, Raben MS, et al.: Somatomedin: proposed designation for sulphation factor. Nature (Lond) 235: 107, 1972.
24. Hall K: Human somatomedin. Acta Endocrinol Scand 163 (suppl): 1, 1972.
25. Uthne K: Human somatomedins: purification and some studies on their biological action. Acta Endocrinol Scand 175 (suppl): 1, 1973.
26. Ballard H, Frame B, Hartsock RJ: Familial multiple endocrine adenoma-peptic ulcer complex. Medicine (Baltimore) 43: 481, 1964.
27. Kipnis D, Black W: Clinicopathologic conference: multiple endocrine adenomatosis. Am J Med 47: 608, 1969.

Monoclonal IgE with Renal Failure

ADRIAN O. VLADUTIU, M.D.
ROMESH K. KOHLI, M.D.
ANTHONY P. PREZYNA, M.D.
Buffalo, New York

Only four cases of immunoglobulin E (IgE) monoclonal "gammapathies"* have been reported previously. Discussed here is a 57 year old man who presented with hypertension and the nephrotic syndrome. A monoclonal IgE-kappa component (0.6 mg/ml), which did not appear as an M spike on protein electrophoresis, was demonstrated by immunoelectrophoresis in the serum and urine. The patient's condition deteriorated rapidly due to renal failure, and he died five weeks after the diagnosis was made. Pathologic examination disclosed extensive glomerular lesions, but amyloid was not detected by light or electron microscopy. The possible relationship between the monoclonal gammapathy and kidney impairment is discussed.

The frequency with which M components occur among immunoglobulin classes corresponds to the concentration of the various classes in normal serum. Immunoglobulin E (IgE) is present in the lowest concentration in normal serum, which probably accounts for the rarity of IgE myeloma [1–5].

In the first reported cases of IgE myeloma the patients had features in common, such as a high number of plasma cells in the peripheral blood and lambda Bence Jones proteinuria [1,2], but subsequent cases [3–5] showed that these similarities were merely coincidental.

Our case differs from the other reported cases of IgE myeloma in that the serum concentration of monoclonal IgE was much lower and hypertension, the nephrotic syndrome and renal failure were also present.

CASE REPORT

A 57 year old man (Case 1) was admitted to The Buffalo General Hospital on July 9, 1975, because of renal failure and hypertension. Approximately six months previously, he had complained of increasing weakness, and a month before admission he had headaches, weight gain, swelling of the legs and paroxysmal nocturnal dyspnea. Two weeks before this hospitalization he was admitted to another hospital because of shortness of breath and blurred vision where the diagnosis of congestive heart failure and renal failure was made; he was subsequently transferred to our hospital.

His past medical history and family history were noncontributory. There was no history of allergy or parasitic infestation. The patient's weight was 84 kg, the temperature 37.6°C, the pulse rate 88/min and the respiratory rate 18/min. The blood pressure was 210/110 mm Hg. Funduscopic examination showed grade 4 hypertensive retinopathy. No lymphadenopathy was

From the Departments of Immunopathology, Medicine and Pathology, The Buffalo General Hospital, Buffalo, New York. Requests for reprints should be addressed to Dr. A. O. Vladutiu, Department of Immunopathology, The Buffalo General Hospital, 100 High Street, Buffalo, New York 14203. Manuscript accepted January 30, 1976.

* The term "gammapathy" is used throughout since Waldenström, who first introduced the term gammopathy, subsequently changed it to gammapathy.

found. The heart was slightly enlarged; an atrial gallop and a grade 2/6 systolic murmur were heard maximal at the left sternal border. A soft liver edge was palpated 3 cm below the right costal margin. There was 2+ edema of the ankles and legs.

On the first admission the hemoglobin level was 10.1 g/100 ml, the hematocrit value 30.8 per cent, the white blood cell count 5,400/mm^3 and the platelet count 140,000/mm^3. On blood smear there were 78 per cent neutrophils, 17 per cent lymphocytes, 13 per cent monocytes, 5 per cent eosinophils and 2 per cent basophils. The erythrocyte sedimentation rate was 75 mm/hour (Wintrobe) and the Sia test was positive. Cryoglobulins were not detected. The serum viscosity was 1.4 U (normal 1.4 U to 1.8 U). Coagulation studies revealed no abnormalities. The blood group was O, the Rh genotype R_1R_1. No irregular isoantibodies were found.

Urinalysis disclosed a specific gravity of 1.021, pH of 5.0 and 4+ proteinuria. The urine osmolality was 235 mOsm/kg. The Addis count revealed 3,000,000 red cells, 5,000,000 white cells, 4,000,000 hyaline casts and many double refractile fat bodies. The protein content in a 24-hour specimen was 15.12 g in 970 ml.

The blood urea nitrogen was 71 mg/100 ml; serum bicarbonate was 14 meq/liter, chloride 108 meq/liter, sodium 141 meq/liter, potassium 5 meq/liter, the blood glucose 102 mg/100 ml, uric acid 7.1 mg/100 ml, calcium 8.1 mg/100 ml, phosphate 15 mg/100 ml, cholesterol 232 mg/100 ml and bilirubins 0.4 mg/100 ml. The alkaline phosphatase level was 64 μmol/min/liter at 37°C (normal 30 to 105 μmol/liter), aspartate aminotransferase 6 μmol/min/liter at 37°C (normal 5 to 50 μmol/min), lactic dehydrogenase (LDH) 550 μmol/min/liter at 37°C (normal 200 to 700 μmol/min/liter) and acid phosphatase 6.2 μmol/min/liter 37°C (normal 0.5 to 10 μmol/min/liter). The serum total protein was 5.1 g/100 ml (albumin 1.84 g/100 ml and gamma globulin 0.31 g/100 ml). The latex fixation and antistreptolysin O tests were negative and the antihyaluronidase titer was 64. Hb_sAg was negative by radioimmunoassay. The glomerular filtration rate [6] was 1 ml/min and the renal plasma flow [7] 4 ml/min. A bone marrow aspirate showed slightly increased cellularity, increased iron and 39 per cent of both mature and immature plasma cells. An electrocardiogram disclosed left ventricular hypertrophy. The chest films revealed an enlarged heart, increased pulmonary vasculature and a small amount of pleural effusion bilaterally. Skeletal roentgenograms were within normal limits. Cystoscopic examination and retrograde pyelogram revealed enlarged kidneys. A percutaneous kidney biopsy was performed (see "Results").

Our patient was treated daily for four days with melphalan (16 mg) and prednisone (120 mg). He was also given aluminum hydroxide, alpha methyl dopa, digoxin and furosemide, and his salt intake was restricted. During hospitalization his blood pressure decreased to 160/80 mm Hg; however, no improvement in renal function was noted. One of many peripheral blood smears showed 3 per cent plasma cells. Due to a progressive rise in urea nitrogen levels reaching 125 mg/100 ml and a decrease in urinary volume (300 ml/day), peritoneal dialysis was instituted twice during the initial 16 days of hospitalization. After discharge, the patient was not dyspneic and his blood pressure was 160/80 mm Hg. He was readmitted three times for peritoneal dialysis. On the last admission his condition suddenly deteriorated, he became comatose and died on August 16, 1975. The immediate cause of death was hypertensive encephalopathy.

MATERIALS AND METHODS

Electrophoresis. Microzone electrophoresis of serum, concentrated urine and peritoneal washings was performed in a thin layer of 1 per cent agarose gel in barbital buffer, pH 8.6, at 7 V/cm and stained with Amido black. High voltage electrophoresis was carried out at 19 V/cm for 17 minutes at 4°C in 0.2 per cent agarose gel ("Seakem"; Marine Colloids Inc., Rockland, Mass.) in sodium phosphate buffer, pH 8.5 and scanned at 205 nm without previous staining (Spectrophor I, Bausch & Lomb, Rochester, N.Y.).

Immunochemical Analysis. Several antiserums to each immunoglobulin and to kappa and lambda light chains were obtained from Behring Diagnostics (Sommerville, N.J.), Hyland (Costa Mesa, Calif.), Cappel (Downingtown, Pa.), and Melloy Laboratories (Springfield, Va.). Antiserums to free kappa and lambda light chains (Bence Jones proteins) were obtained from Behring Diagnostics and did not show any reaction in double diffusion with normal human serum or with purified IgG kappa or lambda. All antiserums were tested for specificity by immunoelectrophoresis and double diffusion in agarose gel and were monospecific. Immunoelectrophoreses of serum, concentrated urine and peritoneal washings were performed by a modified micromethod [8] in 1.2 per cent agar gel ("Agar Noble," Difco, Detroit, Mich.) in sodium barbital buffer, pH 8.6 at 7 V/cm for 60 minutes at room temperature. Immunoelectrophoresis was also carried out in a thin layer of 1 per cent agarose gel in the same buffer at 7 V/cm and in sodium dodecyl sulfate agarose gel [9]. Immunodiffusion studies were performed in agarose gel [10] using rabbit anti-IgE (Case 2) (Behring Diagnostics), goat anti-IgE (Case 2) (Hyland), goat anti-F_c ϵ (Case 2) (kindly supplied by Dr. J. Wipich) and rabbit anti-kappa and anti-lambda serums (Behring Diagnostics). Serum samples of IgE lambda (Case 2) [2] and IgE kappa (Case 3) [3] were kindly donated by Drs. K. Ishizaka and H. Spiegelberg. Serum levels of IgG, IgM, IgD, third and fourth components of complement (C3 and C4) were determined by radial immunodiffusion [11] with commercial reagents (Behring Diagnostics and Hyland). The IgE level was determined by radioimmunoassay (Phadebas IgE, Pharmacia Laboratories Inc., Piscataway, N.J.) and by radial immunodiffusion [11] using known amounts of IgE from Cases 3 and 4 as standards.

Immunohistology and Electron Microscopy. Smears of bone marrow from our patient (Case 1) and from patients without multiple myeloma were dried, fixed in acetone for 10 minutes, rinsed with phosphate-buffered saline solution, pH 7.2, and incubated with appropriate dilutions (1:3 to 1:10) of fluorescein-isothiocyanate-labelled anti-IgG, IgA, IgM, IgE, kappa and lambda (Cappel and Melloy Laboratories) for direct fluorescence, and with goat anti-F_c ϵ (Case 2), followed by fluorescent rabbit antigoat serum for indirect fluorescence. The kidney biopsy specimen was examined for the presence of IgG, IgA, IgM, IgE and C3 using the same fluorescent technic.

Specimens of kidney tissue were fixed in 10 per cent buffered formalin and embedded in paraffin for light microscopy. Specimens stained with thioflavin and crystal violet, and Congo red were examined under polarized light for amyloid. Other specimens of the kidney tissue were fixed in 2 per cent buffered glutaraldehyde and embedded in Epon® 812 for electron microscopy. The thin sections were examined with a Siemens 101 electron microscope.

RESULTS

Microzone serum electrophoresis showed decreased albumin and gamma globulins (Figure 1). A very small peak representing IgE protein was observed between the beta and gamma regions on high voltage electrophoresis. Urine electrophoresis showed all serum protein fractions of which albumin represented 50 per cent (about 7 g/day), and an extra spike in the fast gamma region, due to Bence Jones protein, accounting for 2 per cent of proteins in the urine (about 0.3 g/day). Immunoelectrophoresis in agarose gel revealed a precipitin arc in the beta region, developed with anti-IgE serum. This protein had a slightly faster (alpha$_2$) mobility in agar gel immunoelectrophoresis. An abnormal arc in the same region, having a configuration similar to that of the IgE arc, also developed with anti-kappa serum (Figure 2). A faint, elongated arc developed with anti-lambda serum which did not have a configurational change in the region of the IgE arc, thus showing that the IgE was only of kappa type, i.e., monoclonal. The monoclonality of our patient's IgE was confirmed by immunoelectrophoresis in sodium dodecyl sulfate agarose gel. An arc in the fast gamma region was revealed by anti-free kappa light chain serum in agar gel electrophoresis both in the patient's serum and urine. This kappa Bence Jones protein moved faster in agarose gel, very close to the IgE protein. The mobility of the IgE in our case (Case 1) was much faster than that in Case 2 and slightly faster than that in Case 3. Immunoelectrophoresis of the peritoneal washings showed IgE, kappa Bence Jones protein and other serum proteins with the exception of IgM.

Immunologic identity of our patient's serum (Case 1) with serum from the other two patients (Cases 2 and 3) was demonstrated by double diffusion (Figure 3). Further data on the IgE isolated from our patient's serum will be reported elsewhere.

Quantitation of immunoglobulins yielded the following results: IgG 1.35 mg/ml, IgA 0.24 mg/ml and IgM 0.35 mg/ml. The IgD was below the level of detection by our immunodiffusion method. At the time of admission IgE was 0.6 mg/ml and decreased to about 0.3 mg/ml two weeks after treatment. Serum C3 concentration was 1.32 mg/ml and C4 concentration was 0.84 mg/ml.

Virtually no cells in bone marrow smears stained with fluorescent anti-IgM, IgG or IgA, 3 to 4 cells/hpf stained

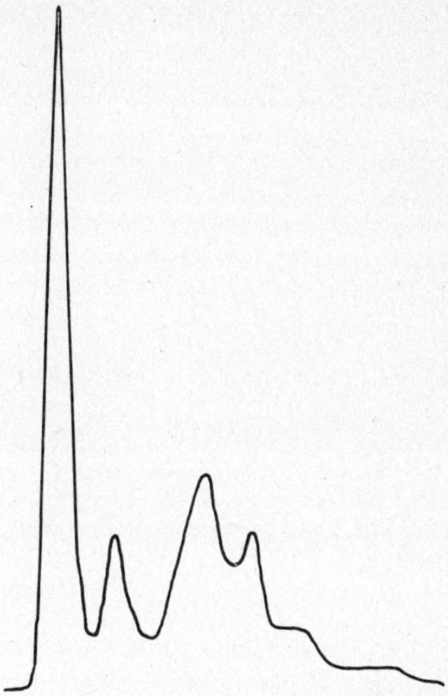

Figure 1. Densitometric scan of the serum electrophoresis.

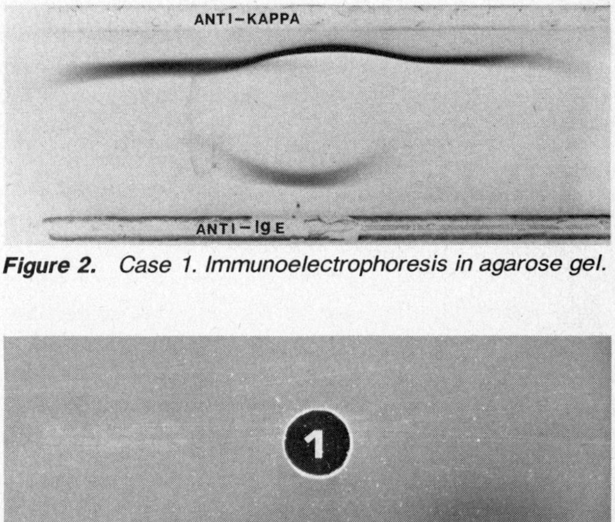

Figure 2. Case 1. Immunoelectrophoresis in agarose gel.

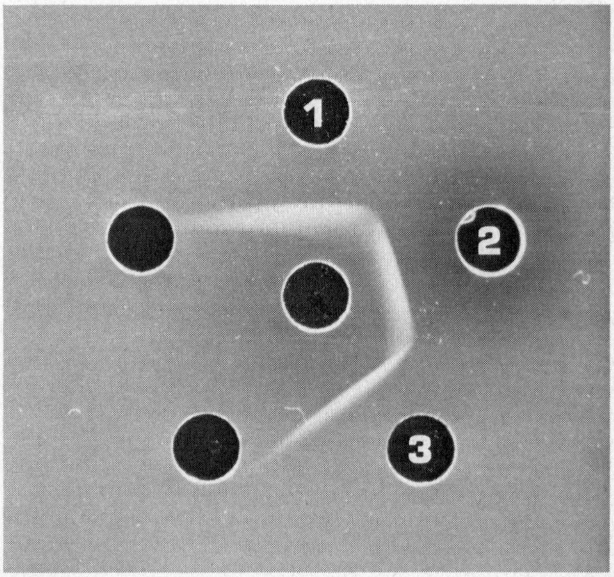

Figure 3. Double diffusion in agarose gel. Center well: goat anti-$F_{c}\epsilon$. Wells: 1 = Case 1, 2 = Case 2 and 3 = Case 3.

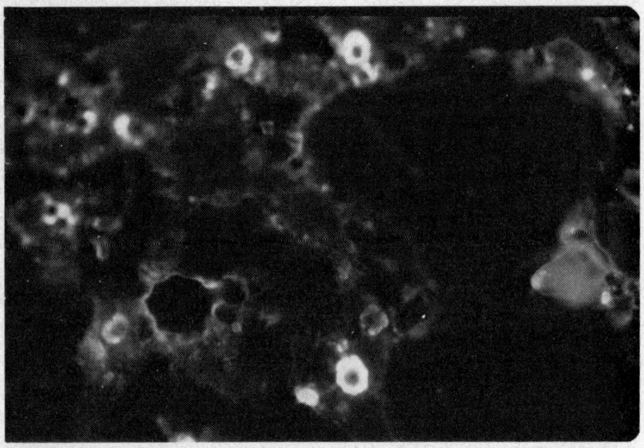

Figure 4. *Indirect immunofluorescence of bone marrow smear incubated with goat anti-$F_c\epsilon$ and fluorescent rabbit antigoat serums. Original magnification × 400, reduced by 27 per cent.*

with anti-IgE (Figure 4) and 10 to 12 cells/hpf stained with anti-kappa serum. Control smears, from patients without multiple myeloma, were negative with anti-IgE or anti-kappa serums. The kidney biopsy tissue showed mesangial sclerosis in the majority of the glomeruli, thickening of the glomerular basement membrane, and wrinkling and splitting of the glomerular and tubular basement membranes. No IgG, IgA, IgM, IgE or C3 deposits were demonstrable by immunofluorescence. The kidney biopsy specimen did not show amyloid by light or electron microscopy.

At autopsy, hemorrhagic infarction was noted in the left and right temporal and occipital lobes of the brain secondary to cerebral edema, as well as brainstem compression secondary to herniation of the cerebrum, and cerebellar tonsillar herniation. The spleen was markedly congested and lymphoid tissue had relatively decreased. Lymph nodes in the retroperitoneal area were slightly enlarged. Their architecture was generally preserved, and only occasional plasma cells were noted in the lymphoid parafollicular population. The small venules in the lymph nodes had hyaline infiltrates. The bone marrow had about 50 per cent plasma cells, many being atypical, "in sheets" and some in mitosis. Occasional small focal infiltrates of lymphocytes and petechial hemorrhages were seen in visceral organs. Small vessels in spleen, lymph nodes and kidneys showed hyaline infiltrates which were negative for amyloid. The kidneys weighed 300 g each; they had extensive lobular glomerulosclerosis, and thickening of the tubular basement membrane and Bowman's capsule (Figure 5). The proximal tubules showed variable degrees of epithelial cell degeneration. Hyaline and occasional granular and large, laminated casts were seen in some tubules. No giant cell reaction was observed in the tubules.

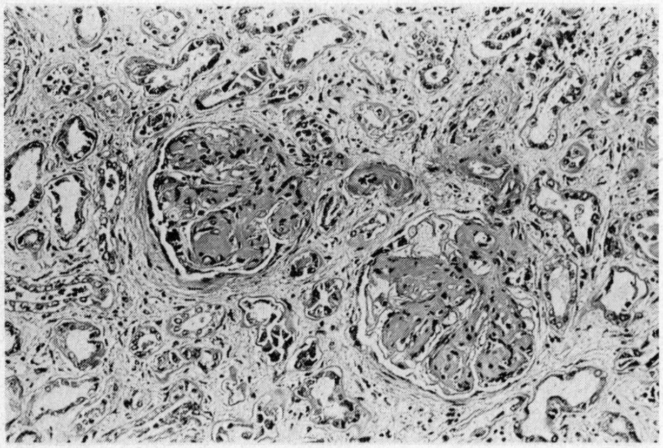

Figure 5. *Pattern of extensive lobular sclerosis in glomeruli. Hematoxylin and eosin stain; original magnification × 120, reduced by 30 per cent.*

COMMENTS

The serum microzone electrophoresis pattern in our patient did not show an M component. In a study of 858 cases of myelomatosis, the electrophoretic pattern was normal in 15 per cent [12]. The absence of an M component in the serum electrophoresis is not uncommon in IgD myeloma [13] but has not been reported in IgE myeloma.

Increased serum IgE concentrations have been found in patients with parasitism [14], bronchopulmonary allergic aspergillosis [15], acral dermatitis [16] and a new syndrome in children characterized by recurrent pyogenic infections [17]. However, in our patient the concentration of IgE was higher than the values found in patients with these diseases. A patient described by Patterson et al. [18] had an extremely high level of IgE (0.48 mg/ml), increased peripheral lymphocytes which stained for surface IgE and marked eosinophilia. The patient was in relatively good health, his bone marrow showed only an increase in mature eosinophils, and the IgE had both kappa and lambda light chains, i.e., polyclonal. High levels of IgE were reported in four patients with multiple myeloma without M components [19]. Since the IgE found in these patients was not typed for light chains, its monoclonal character cannot be ruled out. The highest IgE level in these patients was about 90 times lower than the IgE level in our patient.

Cases of myeloma with hypogammaglobulinemia, Bence Jones proteinuria and lack of M component were grouped as "light chain disease" [20]. It seems unlikely that our patient had light chain disease with a coincidental monoclonal increase of IgE since hypercalcemia and bone lesions, not found in our patient, are common in light chain disease whereas the concentrations of IgE are undetectable in this disease [21]. IgE levels have been decreased in patients with various monoclonal gammapathies, regardless of the presence or absence of Bence Jones proteinuria [22].

TABLE I **Clinical Features of IgE Monoclonal Gammapathies**

References	Case No.	Age (yr) and Sex	Hemoglobin (g/100 ml)	M Component (mg/ml)	Bone Lesions	Bence Jones Proteinuria	Renal Failure
[1]	4	50,M	10.2	45 (lambda)	–	+	–
[2]	2	60,M	4.0	75 (lambda)	+	+	–
[3]	3	65,F	5.0	27 (kappa)	+	+	–
[4]	5	51,M	7.0	1.8 (kappa)*	+	?	–
Present study	1	57,M	10.1	0.8 (kappa)	–	+	+

*Calculated from [5].

Serum immunoelectrophoresis in our patient revealed a homogeneous protein which reacted specifically with anti-IgE and anti-kappa serums, and which showed antigenic identity with the IgE of two patients known to have IgE myeloma (Cases 2 and 3). Five cases in which glomerular lesions were associated with benign monoclonal gammapathies have been reported [23,24]. However, in our patient, serum protein abnormalities (presence of a monoclonal IgE and kappa light chains and marked depression of the other immunoglobulins), Bence Jones proteinuria, anemia and bone marrow findings strongly suggest the diagnosis of plasma cell myeloma, not benign gammapathy.

In the reported cases of IgE myeloma the concentration of serum IgE was much higher than in our case. The stage of the disease in our patient could not be assessed on the basis of the amount of abnormal protein since the serum IgE was not the true representative of the plasma cell mass because of renal loss.

Our patient had hypertension and the nephrotic syndrome which are rarely found in patients with multiple myeloma [25]. In the majority of cases of myeloma with the nephrotic syndrome the patients had renal amyloidosis [26]; in cases of myeloma without amyloidosis the relationship between myeloma and the nephrotic syndrome was not clearly understood [27]. Hobbs [28] mentioned three patients with IgG myeloma and the nephrotic syndrome, whose kidneys appeared normal by light and electron microscope. Similarly, kidney lesions were also absent in cases of lymphoma associated with the nephrotic syndrome [29]. A secondary development of the nephrotic syndrome was recently described in a patient with monoclonal IgG-cryoglobulins and deposition of IgG and C3 on the glomerular basement membrane [30]. Serum hyperviscosity and immune complexes between monoclonal and polyclonal immunoglobulins [31] could also damage the glomeruli. Rosen et al. [32] reported a case of IgA myeloma in which complexes of IgA and low density lipoproteins presumably led to glomerular changes.

In our patient glomerular damage was found in the absence of serum hyperviscosity, cryoglobulins, or demonstrable immune complexes, immunoglobulins deposits and amyloid. It is unlikely that the amyloid disappeared from the patient's kidney since in experimental animals amyloid deposits regressed in the spleen but persisted in the kidney [33]. Couchie et al. [34] discussed three patients with multiple myeloma who did not have amyloid but who did have nodules of eosinophilic material in the mesangial areas, resembling the findings in our patient. Conceivably, the renal impairment in our patient was related to the monoclonal gammapathy, but a direct relationship between the two could not be demonstrated. Therefore it remains possible that the gammapathy appeared coincidentally in a hypertensive patient with already advanced renal disease.

Attempts have been made to correlate clinical aspects, frequency and severity of complications in cases of multiple myeloma with the immunoglobulin class and/or subclass of the M component [35,36]. The data in Table I show that only anemia, relatively earlier age of onset and perhaps Bence Jones proteinuria are features in common in all patients with IgE myeloma. In fact, it is premature to look for features in common in such myeloma when only a few cases are known. It is likely that other cases of IgE myeloma have been misdiagnosed as light chain disease. Hopefully, more cases of IgE myeloma will be detected, thus permitting a better characterization of this very rare disease.

ACKNOWLEDGMENT

We are greatly indebted to Dr. Guiseppe Andres for his invaluable help and to Drs. K. Ishizaka, H. Spiegelberg and J. Wipich for providing some of the antiserums used in this study. Mr. Paul Bronson performed the immunoelectrophoresis in sodium dodecyl sulfate agarose gel. The technical assistance of Mrs. Marion Sepulveda and Mrs. Barbara Winiarski is also acknowledged.

ADDENDUM

Since this paper was submitted for publication, two new cases of IgE myelomas with bone lesions [37,38] and a case of light chain deposition in the kidney with a nodular glomerulosclerosis pattern [39] have been reported.

REFERENCES

1. Johansson SGO, Bennich H: Immunological studies of an atypical (myeloma) immunoglobulin. Immunology 99: 1187, 1968.
2. Ogawa M, Kochwa S, Smith C, et al.: Clinical aspects of IgE myeloma. N Engl J Med 281: 1217, 1969.
3. Fishkin BG, Orloff N, Scaduto LE, et al.: IgE multiple myeloma: a report of the third case. Blood 39: 361, 1972.
4. Stefani DV, Makeeva RA: Two rare cases of myeloma disease (type D and E). Probl Haematol Blood Transf USSR 6: 44, 1972.
5. Stefani DV, Gusev AJ, Makeeva RA: Isolation of immunochemically pure IgE from serum of E myeloma patient Yu. Immunochemistry 10: 559, 1973.
6. Sigman DM, Elwood CM, Knox F: The measurement of glomerular filtration rate in man with sodium iodothalamate 1^{131} (Conray). J Nucl Med 7: 60, 1965.
7. Elwood C, Armenia J, Orman D, et al.: Measurement of renal plasma flow by iodopyracet 1^{131}. JAMA 193: 771, 1965.
8. Scheidegger JJ: Une micromèthode d'immunoelectrophorèse. Int Arch Allergy Appl Immunol 7: 103, 1955.
9. Shapiro AL, Vinnelo E, Maizel JV: Molecular weight estimation of polypeptide chains by electrophoresis in SDS polyacrylamide gel. Biochem Biophys Res Commun 28: 815, 1967.
10. Ouchterlony O: Diffusion-in-gel methods for immunological analysis. Prog Allergy 7: 103, 1955.
11. Mancini G, Carbonara AO, Heremans JF: Immunochemical quantitation of antigens by single radial immunodiffusion. Immunochemistry 2: 235, 1965.
12. Kyle RA: Multiple myeloma. Review of 869 cases. Mayo Clin Proc 50: 29, 1965.
13. Fine JM, Rivat C, Lambin P, et al.: Monoclonal IgD. A comparative study of 60 sera with IgD "M" component. Biomedicine (Express) 21: 119, 1974.
14. Johansson SGO, Melbin J, Vahlquist B: Immunoglobulin levels in Ethiopian preschool children, with special reference to high concentration of immunoglobulin E (IgND). Lancet 1: 1118, 1968.
15. Patterson R, Fink JN, Pruzanski JJ, et al.: Serum immunoglobulin levels in pulmonary allergic aspergillosis and certain other lung disease, with special reference to immunoglobulin E. Am J Med 54: 16, 1973.
16. Winkelman RK, Gleich GJ: Chronic acral dermatitis. Association with extreme elevation of IgE. JAMA 225: 378, 1973.
17. Buckley RH, Wray BB, Belmaker EZ: Extreme hyperimmunoglobulinemia E and undue susceptibility to infection. Pediatrics 49: 59, 1972.
18. Patterson R, Oh SH, Roberts M, et al.: Massive polyclonal hyperimmunoglobulinemia E, eosinophilia and increased IgE-bearing lymphocytes. Am J Med 58: 553, 1975.
19. Heiner DC, Rose B: Elevated levels of γ E (IgE) in conditions other than classical allergy. J Allergy Clin Immunol 45: 30, 1970.
20. Williams RC Jr, Brunning RD, Wolheim IA: Light chain disease—an abortive variant of multiple myeloma. Ann Intern Med 65: 471, 1966.
21. Stone MJ, Frenkel EP: The clinical spectrum of light chain myeloma. A study of 35 patients with special reference to the occurrence of amyloidosis. Am J Med 58: 601, 1975.
22. Grove DI, Burston TO, Forbes IJ: Serum IgE levels in paraproteinemia. Int Arch Allergy Appl Immunol 49: 564, 1975.
23. Kaplan NJ, Kaplan KC: Monoclonal gammopathy, glomerulonephritis and the nephrotic syndrome. Arch Intern Med 125: 696, 1970.
24. Jensen H, Wiik A: Monoclonal immunoglobulinaemia associated with glomerulopathy. Acta Med Scand 197: 265, 1975.
25. Waldenström J: Diagnosis and Treatment of Multiple Myeloma, New York, Grune & Stratton, 1970, p 53.
26. Martinez-Maldonado M, Yium J, Suki WN, et al.: Renal complications in multiple myeloma: pathophysiology and some aspects of clinical management. J Chronic Dis 24: 221, 1971.
27. Healy JK: Acute oliguric renal failure associated with multiple myeloma. Br Med J 2: 1126, 1963.
28. Hobbs JR: Immunoglobulins in clinical chemistry. Adv Clin Chem 14: 219, 1971.
29. Ghosh L, Muehrcke RC: The nephrotic syndrome: a prodrome to lymphoma. Ann Intern Med 72: 379, 1970.
30. Bengtsson U, Larsson O, Lindstedt G, et al.: Monoclonal IgG cryoglobulinemia with secondary development of glomerulonephritis and nephrotic syndrome. Q J Med 44: 991,1975.
31. Gray HM, Kohler PF, Terry WD, et al.: Human monoclonal γ G-cryoglobulins with anti- γ globulin activity. J Clin Invest 47: 1875, 1968.
32. Rosen S, Cortell S, Adner MM, et al.: Multiple myeloma and the nephrotic syndrome. A biochemical and morphologic study. Am J Clin Pathol 47: 567, 1967.
33. Richter GW: The resorption of amyloid under experimental conditions. Am J Pathol 30: 239, 1954.
34. Couchie C, Kenis Y, Potoliège P, et al.: Les manifestations rénales des dysglobulinémies. Les manifestations renales du myèlome. J Urol Nephrol (Paris) 68: 89, 1962.
35. Hobbs JR: Immunochemical classes of myelomatosis. Br J Haematol 16: 599, 1969.
36. Schur PH, Kyle RA, Bloch KJ, et al.: IgG-subclasses: relationship to clinical aspects of multiple myeloma and frequency distribution among M-components. Scand J Haematol 12: 60, 1974.
37. Mills RJ, Fahie-Wilson MN, Carter PM, et al.: IgE myelomatosis. Clin Exp Immunol 23: 228, 1976.
38. Knedel M, Fateh-Moghadam, Edel H, et al.: Multiples Myelom mit monoklonaler IgE-Gammopathie. Dtsch Med Wochenschr 101: 496, 1976.
39. Randal ER, Williamson WC, Mullinax F, et al.: Manifestations of systemic light chain deposition. Am J Med 60: 293, 1976.

AUTHOR INDEX—VOLUME 61

A

Abbott, J. A., 641
Abdallah, P. S., 326
Adler, R. A., 52
Agodoa, L. C. Y., 407
Aisner, J., 23
Alderman, M., 731
Alexander, J. W., 703
Aloia, J. F., 59
Alvarez-de la Cadena, O., 504
Alvira, M. M., 703
Ames, R. P., 748
Andersen, J. C., 553
Anderson, E. T., 493
Anthonisen, N., 85
Anthony, B. F., 498
Antic, R., 85
Appel, G. B., 129
Aral, I., 892
Arevalo-Toledo, N., 504
Armstrong, P. W., 215
Arnold, T., 333
Aronson, M. D., 295
Askari, A., 485
Aungst, C. W., 14
Austen, G., Jr., 351
Avramides, A., 136
Ayers, C. R., 811

B

Bale, G. F., 424
Banka, V. S., 650
Bankhurst, A. D., 303
Bartlett, R. C., 340
Bartter, F. C., 43
Barzel, U. S., 134
Basta, L. L., 420
Bax, I., 878
Bayer, A. S., 346, 498, 832
Beeler, B. A., 935
Bentley, D. W., 298
Beretta-Piccoli, C., 739
Berl, T., 119
Bernheim, J., 145
Betts, R. F., 298
Bevans, L. C., 946
Bhathena, D., 401
Blajchman, M. A., 572
Blinderman, A., 103
Blumenkrantz, M. J., 832
Bode, F., 85
Bodenheimer, M. M., 650
Bone, R. C., 585
Bowden, R. E., 43
Boxer, L. A., 849
Boylan, J. W., 308
Braylan, R. C., 553
Breslau, N., 184
Brine, J. A. S., 439
Brossel, R., 878
Broun, G. O., Sr., 925
Browman, G. P., 572
Brown, J. J., 825
Bruhl, H. H., 841
Bryon, P. A., 145
Buckman, M. T.,124
Bulkley, B. H., 361
Burkholder, P. M., 471
Burrow, G. N., 932
Burton, J. R., 215
Buselmeier, T. J., 190

C

Cagin, N. A., 449
Calderon, J., 273
Calle, G., 33
Cannom, D. S., 452
Carey, R. M., 811
Carey, R. W., 892
Carlow, T. J., 124
Carter, A. C., 136
Carvalho, A., 179
Casali, R. E., 190
Case, D. B., 790
Cassidy, E., 615
Catto, G. R. D., 64
Choi, E. Y. C., 560
Chow, A. W., 346, 498
Christian, C. L., 385
Chulay, J. D., 513
Chung, E. K., 537
Cobb, O. M., Jr., 939
Coburn, J. W., 832
Cohen, A. S., 277
Cohen, L. S., 452
Cohn, P. D., 119
Cohn, S. H., 59
Colon, S., 145
Corey, L., 615
Cornell, C. J., Jr., 892
Côté, J., 459
Coulson, R., 184
Crede, R. H., 156
Crowder, J. G., 935
Curtis, J. J., 401
Cutillo, A., 74

D

Davidson, C., 709
de Chatel, R., 739
Dechavanne, M., 145
Delorme, A., 725
DePapp, E. W., 871
de Torrente, A., 119
Devynck, M-A., 758
Diaz-Buxo, J. A., 221
Dickson, E. R., 414
Donaldson, J. C., 939
Douglas, R. G., Jr., 298
Drayer, J. I. M., 790
Dussault, J. H., 932

E

Eide, I., 608
Elliott, R. C., 939
Ellis, K., 59
Ellman, L., 179
Enger, E., 608
Ettinger, B., 200

F

Faas, F. H., 533
Falls, W. F., Jr., 111
Fanning, W. L., 295
First, M. R., 703
Fisher, D. A., 932
Fisher, R. I., 553
Fleming, C. R., 414
Foni, I., 841
Foster, D. W., 9
Fox, R., 825
Francis, P. B., 585
Frantz, A. G., 590
Freedman, M. H., 572
Friedman, H. S., 273
Frölich, J. C., 43
Fuchs, R. J., 815

G

Galgiani, J. N., 632
Galla, J. H., 401
Galpin, J. E., 346, 832
Gardner, B., 136
Genecin, A., 140
Genuth, S. M., 952
Gentry, L. O., 283
George, C. R. P., 407

German, H. J., 547
Gewurz, H., 560
Ghaed, N., 52
Gill, J. R., Jr., 43
Giraldo, R., 33
Glassock, R., 407
Glicksman, A. S., 892
Goldstein, N. P., 170
Gomes, J. A. C., 273
Gomez, G. A., 14
Gotloib, L., 465
Grajower, M., 134
Greenberg, P., 878
Gupta, R. C., 29
Gutiérrez, F., 33
Guyene, P. T., 725
Guze, L. B., 346, 498, 832

H

Hanson, R. F., 393
Harrison, E. G., Jr., 414
Hatch, F. E., 697
Hattwick, M. A. W., 615
Heinemann, H. O., 681
Helfant, R. H., 650
Henle, G., 333
Henle, W., 333
Hermann, G. A., 650
Hermans, P. E., 221
Hernández, H., 33
Hertel, B. F., 716
Hertz, P., 119
Hewitt, W. L., 493
Hill, P., 748
Hirschfeld, D. S., 641
Hofeldt, F. D., 52
Hollingsworth, D. R., 932
Holub, D. A., 129
Holzbach, R. T., 367
Horwitz, C. A., 333
Huet, P.-M., 459
Huffer, W. E., 478
Hultgren, H. N., 665
Husain, M., 124
Hutchins, G. M., 361

I

Ibarra-Perez, C., 504
Imperato-McGinley, J., 251
Irwin, E. S., 295
Isenberg, J. N., 393

J

Jackson, J. M., 439
Jaffe, E. S., 553
Johnson, R. H., 632
Joly, J.-G., 459

K

Kalra, T. M. S., 871
Kao, J. J., 665
Kawamoto, E., 119
Kay, T. D., 815
Kean, B. H., 159
Keane, W. F., 207
Kelm, H. J., 790
Keiser, H. R., 43
Khan, M. A., 151
Kioschos, J. M., 420
Kjellstrand, C. M., 190
Kleid, J. J., 449
Kleve, L., 437
Klimek, J. J., 340
Kohli, R. K., 957
Kryger, M., 85
Kunkel, F. W., 641
Kurnick, J. E., 29

L

Lafortune, M., 459
Lagarde, M., 145
Lajam, F., 273
Lancaster, M. C., 815
Lankerani, M. R., 513
Laragh, J. H., 721, 731, 790, 797
Larsen, P. R., 932
Lavoie, P., 459
Leach, R. P., 401
Leary, M. C., 316
Lee, J. B., 681
Légaré, A., 459
Leonard, A., 207
LeRoy, E. C., 862
Lever, A. F., 825
Levitt, B., 449
Levy, J. V., 779
Levy, W., 452
Lewandowski, R. C., Jr., 841
Lewis, F. B., 333
Lindenbaum, J., 547
Linnemann, C. C., Jr., 703
Londoño, F., 33
López, R., 33
Lowy, K., 298
Lucas, B. A., 401
Luke, R. G., 401
Lutwick, L. I., 632

M

MacGregor, R. R., 597
Macklem, P. T., 165
MacLeod, M., 64
Man, E. B., 932
Mangla, J. C., 871
Mann, J. J., 140
Mara, B., 878
Marder, R. J., 560
Maricq, H. R., 862
Mark, J. B. D., 326
Marleau, D., 459
Marsik, F. J., 340
Masi, A. T., 424
Matas, A. J., 716
Mathew, M. T., 215
McBride, J. A., 572
McCann, S. R., 316, 321
McCowen, K. D., 52
McGarry, J. D., 9
McKusick, V. A., 140
McNitt, T. R., 283
Menard, J., 725
Mendelow, H., 433
Merigan, T. C., 326
Meyer, P., 758
Mittelman, A., 14
Moake, J. L., 437
Modin, G., 641
Montgomerie, J. Z., 832
Monti, S., 74
Moon, C., 731
Moore, M., 316
Moore, W. L., Jr., 283
Moorthy, A. V., 471
Morgan, D. B., 709
Morton, J. J., 825
Moses, A. M., 184
Moskowitz, R. W., 485
Moylan, R. A., 351
Murray, H. W., 140

N

Najarian, J. S., 190, 716
Noble, G. R., 615
Noreiga-Guerra, L., 504

O

Oates, J. A., 43
O'Connor, D., 925
O'Duffy, J. D., 170
Oken, M. M., 316, 321
Olsson, C. A., 351
Omvik, P., 608
O'Neil, J. P., 537

P

Padfield, P. L., 825
Page, A. R., 393
Pasdar, H., 650
Peake, G. T., 124
Peress, L., 165

Perondi, R., 74
Peters, R. W., 641
Peterson, R. E., 251
Petrak, Z., 59
Pierce, A. K., 585
Pincus, S. H., 849
Podleski, W. K., 1
Popovtzer, M. M., 478
Pozet, N., 145
Prezyna, A. P., 957
Pruitt, A. W., 579
Puder, B., 925

Q

Quadracci, L. J., 407
Quintiliani, R., 340

R

Rai, K. R., 892
Raij, L., 207
Rau, J. E., 946
Rau, J. M., 566
Redman, J. F., 533
Reilly, P. C., Jr., 159
Rent, R., 560
Restrepo, A., 33
Reubi, F., 739
Reynolds, P. M., 439
Reynolds, R. C., 657
Ricketts, R. R., 946
Ridolfi, R. L., 361
Robertson, C. H., Jr., 657
Robertson, J. I. S., 825
Robinson, W. A., 29
Robledo, M., 33
Rockwell, D., 433
Rosai, J., 716
Rose, H. D., 626
Rose, H. J., 579
Ruben, F. L., 433
Rubin, R. J., 615

S

Sakurai, H., 273
Saltzman, A. R., 939
Sanfilippo, S. J., 841
Sawitsky, A., 892
Scheinman, M. M., 641
Schiff, G. M., 703
Schimpff, S. C., 23
Schmidt, R. R., 925
Schnall, A. M., 952
Schoenfeld, P. L., 641
Schrier, R. W., 119
Schrier, S., 878
Schroeder, J. S., 665
Scialia, S., 892
Sealey, J. E., 731, 790
Seehafer, J. R., 541
Segal, M., 333
Seligman, B., 892
Sergent, J. S., 385
Servadio, C., 465
Seyberth, H. W., 43
Shaeffer, J. R., 437
Shapiro, F. L., 207
Shapiro, L., 892
Sharp, H. L., 393
Shea, P., 340
Shenouda, A., 697
Shideman, J. R., 190
Sieger, B. E., 283
Sierra, F., 33
Silver, R. T., 892
Simmons, R. L., 190, 716
Sinha, A. A., 321
Siroky, M. B., 351
Smith, D., 709
Smith, J. A., 547
Smith, J. W., 935
Snider, G. L., 151
Soderstrom, C. W., 541
Sokal, J. E., 14
Somberg, J. C., 449
Spector, A. A., 420
Spencer-Green, G., 862
Spicer, T. E., 566
Steele, R. W., 283
Stevens, D. A., 632
Stjernholm, M., 478
Stobo, J. D., 221
Stossel, T. P., 849
Striker, G. E., 407
Strong, D. M., 939
Stubbert, J., 295
Sutherland, J. C., 23
Swaim, W. R., 316
Sybrecht, G., 165

T

Tan, H. K., 553
Tatz, J. S., 273
Taylor, A. A., 43
Thurau, K., 308
Thurston, H., 768
Tilkian, A. G., 665
Tomko, D. J., 111
Traeger, J., 145
Trentham, D. E., 424
Triebwasser, J. H., 815
Trout, R. G., 650
Tsai, M. Y., 841
Turiel, M., 74

U

Utsinger, P. D., 287

V

Varkey, B., 626
Verdon, T., 52
Verstraete, M., 897
Viallet, A., 459
Vichayanrat, A., 136
Vignos, P. J., Jr., 485
Villeneuve, J. P., 459
Vivian, A. B., 439
Vladutiu, A. O., 957

W

Walfish, P. G., 932
Wallace, J. M., 790
Wallace, R., 277
Wallach, S., 136
Walsh, F. M., 939
Ward, G. W., 939
Ward, P. C. J., 333
Weber, M. A., 790
Weidmann, P., 739
Weinsier, R. L., 815
Weir, B., 340
Weisberg, L. A., 590
Whitcomb, M. E., 151
White, A., 935
White, R. P., 790
Wiernik, P. H., 23
Williams, C., 420
Williams, G. C., 393
Williams, R. C., Jr., 303
Wilson, J. E., III, 657
Winkelstein, A., 433
Wood, M., 825

Y

Yeh, B. P. Y., 111
Yocum, M. W., 939
Young, L. S., 493
Young, V. M., 23
Yount, W. J., 287
Yunis, J. J., 841

Z

Zaky, D. A., 298
Zanick, D., 333
Zavoral, J., 393
Zimmerman, E. A., 590
Zimmerman, S. W., 471
Zinneman, H. H., 316, 321
Zipser, R. D., 946

SUBJECT INDEX—VOLUME 61

E = Editorial; CPC = Clinicopathologic Conference; CSC = Clinicosociologic Conference; CCBSS = Combined Clinical and Basic Science Seminar; LE = Letters to the Editor.

A

Abdomen, acute pain in, associated with intestinal anthrax, 968
Abscess, splenic, 513
Acromegaly, body composition and skeletal metabolism after pituitary irradiation in, 59
ACTH administration followed by acute unilateral adrenal hemorrhage in Cushing's syndrome, 533
Adenomas
  hepatic, and oral contraceptive pills, 871
  multiple endocrine, in Maffucci syndrome, 952
Adrenal hemorrhage following ACTH administration in Cushing's syndrome, 533
Adrenergic beta receptor blockade, effect of sodium depletion on plasma renin before and after, 608
Airways, upper and central, diagnosis of obstruction of, 85
Allescheria boydii, visceral fungal infections due to, 632
Allopurinol hypersensitivity, granular deposition of IgM at dermal-epidermal junction, 287
Alprenolol, effect on blood pressure, 779
Alveolitis, extrinsic allergic, after Aspergillus fumigatus inhalation, 939
American Burkitt's lymphoma (CPC), 377
American Thyroid Association, report of committee on screening programs for congenital hypothyroidism, 932
Amphotericin B in treatment of Candida peritonitis, 832
Anemia, refractory, complement independent erythropoietic inhibitor acting on progenitor cell in, 572
Aneurysm, dissecting, of the aorta with fever, 140
Angiotensin
  blockade in renovascular hypertension with high plasma renin activity, 790
  receptors
    vascular, role in blood pressure control, 768
    in vascular tissue, 758, 768
Angiotensin II
  vascular response to, 758, 768
Antidiuretic hormone excess, syndrome of, and bronchogenic carcinoma, 825
Anti-inflammatory agents, effect on granulocyte adherence, 597
Antithrombin III deficiency, hereditary, effect on platelet function, 179
Aorta, dissecting aneurysm of, with fever, 140
Arteritis, temporal, bilateral scalp necrosis in, 541
Arthritis
  tuberculous, 277
  with inflammatory dermatosis, 424
Ascites in patients undergoing maintenance hemodialysis, 465
Aspergillus fumigatus inhalation followed by extrinsic allergic alveolitis, 939
Aspergilloma, pulmonary, rational approach to treatment, 626
Asthma, acute, mechanism of increase in total lung capacity during, 163
Atherosclerotic lesions, regression through control of hyperlipidemia, 420
Atrial pacing in sinus node dysfunction, 641
Autoantibody, cellular origins of (E), 303
Autoimmunity, cellular role in (E), 303
Autotransplantation of splenic tissue, 414

B

B thalassemia variant with high hemoglobin F and mild clinical course, 437
Bacteremia, "breakthrough" gram-negative rod, subinhibitory antibiotic levels in, 493
Bartter's syndrome
  defect in proximal tubular sodium readsorption in, 111
  high urinary prostaglandins in, 43
Behçet's disease, neurologic involvement in, 170
Beta-adrenergic receptor blocking drugs in spontaneous hypertension, 779
Bifascicular block due to hyperkalemia, 537
Biopsy findings in tuberculous arthritis, 277
Blood pressure
  control
    and prostaglandins (CCBSS), 681
    vascular angiotensin receptors and their role in, 768
  effect of dextra-propranolol on, 779
  relationship of body fat to, 815
Body composition following pituitary irradiation in acromegaly, 59
Body fat; relation to coronary heart disease, blood pressure and lipids, 815
Body weight and water and electrolyte excretion in idiopathic orthostatic hypotension, 709
Bone disease, renal, investigation and treatment of, 64
Breast cancer and primary hyperparathyroidsim, 136
Bronchodilator, inhaled, effect in chronic obstructive pulmonary disease, 74
Bronchogenic carcinoma, syndrome of antidiuretic hormone excess associated with, 825
Bronchoscopy, flexible fiberoptic (E), 151
Burkitt's lymphoma, American (CPC), 377

C

C1q deficiency associated with urticarial-like lesions and cutaneous vasculitis, 560

Calcium and phosphorus infusions, alternating, effects on osteoporosis, 478
Cancer
bronchogenic, associated with syndrome of antidiuretic hormone excess, 825
of breast and primary hyperparathyroidism, 136
thyroid, low dose radioiodide thyroid ablation in, 52
Torulopsis glabrata infections in patients with, 14, 23
Candida peritonitis, 832
Carcinoma, bronchogenic, plasma arginine vasopressin levels in, 825
Cardiac
see also Heart
Cardiac catheterization in documentation of pulmonary hypertension and granulomas in intravenous drug abusers, 657
Cardiac conduction system in progressive systemic sclerosis, 361
Cardiac death, sudden, and ventricular rhythm disorders (E), 449
Cardiovascular effects of lithium in man, 665
Catecholamine-secreting paraganglioma, metastatic (CPC), 523
Cellular origins of autoantibody (E), 303
Central nervous system shunt infection with Propionibacterium acnes, 935
Childhood neutropenia, 859
Chlorambucil in IgM pyroglobulinemia, 316, 321
Cholestasis of pregnancy, recurrent, 367
Clinicopathologic Conferences
American Burkitt's lymphoma, 377
Decisions regarding the provision or withholding of therapy, 915
Hodgkin's disease with nervous system manifestations, 239
Metastatic catecholamine-secreting paraganglioma (extra-adrenal pheochromocytoma), 523
Mixed cryoimmunoglobulinemia, 95
Systemic mastocytosis, 671
Combined clinical and basic science seminars
Prostaglandins and blood pressure control, 681
Vasculitis syndromes; clinical and experimental models, 385
Coagulation disorder in chronic myelocytic leukemia, heparin therapy for, 547
Coccidioidomycosis, disseminated, treated with transfer factor from related donor, 283
Complement components in patient with urticarial-like lesions and cutaneous vasculitis, 560
Complement-independent erythropoietic inhibitor acting on progenitor cell in refractory anemia, 572
Conduction block in progressive systemic sclerosis, 361
Congenital hypothyroidism, screening programs for, 932
Connective tissue disease, steroid myopathy in, 485
Contraceptive pills, oral, and benign hepatic tumors, 871
Converting enzyme inhibitor, superiority of, over saralasin in evaluating renin dependency in hypertension, 790
Cryoimmunoglobulinemia (CPC), 95
Cushing's syndrome, adrenal hemorrhage following ACTH administration in, 533
Cyst, solitary renal, hypertension and hyperreninemia in an adolescent, 579
Cytomegalovirus pneumonia, diagnosis of, in compromised hosts, 326

D

Deafness, nephritis, macrothrombocytopathia and thrombocytopenia, 145
Decubitus ulcers and sepsis, 346
Dermatoses, inflammatory, and arthritis, 424
Dermatomyositis, skin capillary abnormalities as indicators of organ involvement in, 862
Dextro-propranolol, effect on blood pressure, 779
Diabetes, malignant external otitis in, 298
Disseminated coccidioidomycosis treated with transfer factor from related donor, 283
Diuretic therapy of hypertension, elevation of serum lipid levels during, 748
Dying, coronor describes manner of, in New York City 1784–1816, 103

E

Echocardiographic detection of fungal vegetations in Candida parasilopsis endocarditis, 273
Echymosis, cutaneous, intravascular coagulation and purpura fulminans, 566
Editorials
Acute renal success; the unexpected logic of oliguria in acute renal failure, 308
Cellular origins of autoantibody—a perplexing question, 303
Cytodestructive mechanisms provoked by lymphocytes, 1
Flexible fiberoptic bronchoscopy, 151
Intravascular coagulation associated with the adult respiratory distress syndrome, 585
Ketogenesis and its regulation, 9
Labile hypertension; precursor of sustained essential hypertension, 811
Ventricular rhythm disorders and sudden cardiac death, 449
Elderly patients, heterophil-antibody positive infectious mononucleosis in, 333
Electrolyte and water excretion, diurnal pattern of, in idiopathic orthostatic hypotension, 709
Empty sella syndrome, primary, with visual field defects, 124
Endocarditis, Candida parasilopsis, echocardiographic detection of fungal vegetations in, 273
Endocrine gland insufficiency, syndrome of, 129
Endocrine tumors, multiple, in Maffucci syndrome, 952
Endophthalmitis, bilateral Escherichia coli endogenous, 295
Epstein-Barr virus infections in heterophil-antibody positive infectious mononucleosis, 333
Erythropoietic inhibitor in refractory anemia, 572
Escherichia coli endogenous endophthalmitis, bilateral, 295
Esophageal malignancy, ectopic hyperparathyroidism in, 134

F

Felty's syndrome, effect of lithium on granulopoiesis, 29
Fetal hemoglobin concentrations in sickle cell-β^0 thalassemia variant, 437
Fever with dissecting aneurysm of the aorta, 140
Fiberoptic bronchoscopy, flexible (E), 151
Fungal infections, visceral, due to Petriellidium boydii, 632
Fungal vegetations in Candida parasilopsis endocarditis, 273

G

Gas distribution, effects of inhaled bronchodilator on, in chronic obstructive pulmonary disease, 74
Genitourinary tract sepsis, metastatic infection secondary to, 351
Glomerulonephritis
  immune complex, and central nervous system shunt infection, 935
  with pulmonary hemorrhage and antiglomerular basement membrane antibodies, 407
Glycoprotein metabolism and mannisidosis, 841
Goodpasture's syndrome
  and nail-patella syndrome, 401
  nonlinear deposits of immunoglobulins in, 407
  pulmonary hemorrhage in, 407
Granulocyte adherence, effect of anti-inflammatory agents and inflammation on, 597
Granulomas, foreign body, and pulmonary hypertension in intravenous drug abusers, 657
Granulopoiesis
  correlation between clinical evolution and alterations of, 878
  effect of lithium on, in Felty's syndrome, 29

H

Heart
  see also Cardiac
  disease, coronary, relationship of body fat to, 815
  valves, artificial, course of pregnancy in patients with, 504
Hemodialysis, maintenance, ascites in patients undergoing, 465
Hemodynamics, comparative effects of lidocaine and procainamide on, 215
Hemoglobin F in sickle cell-β^0 thalassemia variant, 437
Hemorrhage
  acute unilateral adrenal, following ACTH administration in Cushing's syndrome, 533
  pulmonary, in Goodpasture's syndrome, 407
Heparin
  therapy for coagulation disorder in chronic myelocytic leukemia, 547
Heparin
  use in purpura fulminans, 566
  use in connection with surgical procedure in patients with intravascular coagulation, 547
Hepatic
  see also Liver
Hepatic adenomas and oral contraceptive pills, 871
Hepatic function, physiologic alterations in, during pregnancy, 367
Hepatic tuberculosis, 946
Hepatic tumors, benign, and oral contraceptive pills, 871
Hepatitis, viral, in pregnancy, 367
Herpesvirus homonis type 2 meningoencephalitis following renal transplantation, 703
Heterophil-antibody positive infectious mononucleosis in elderly patients, 333
Hodgkin's disease
  nephrotic syndrome in, 471
  with nervous system manifestations (CPC), 239
Hormone-related (pseudo) hypoparathyroidism, renal response to PTH in, 184
Horton's disease, bilateral scalp necrosis in, 541
Hypercalcemia of acute renal failure, 119
Hyperkalemia, bifascicular block due to, 537
Hyperlipidemia
  chronic obstructive liver disease and immunodeficiency, 393
  regression of atherosclerotic lesions and spontaneous cure of systemic hypertension through control of, 420
Hyperparathyroidism
  ectopic, in esophageal malignancy, 134
  primary, and breast cancer, 136
Hyperreninemia, hypertension and a solitary cyst in an adolescent, 579
Hypersensitivity, allopurinol, granular deposition of IgM at dermal-epidermal junction in, 287
Hypertension
  and early stage kidney disease, 739
  elevation of serum lipid levels during diuretic therapy of, 748
  hyperreninemia and a solitary renal cyst in an adolescent, 579
  idiopathic portal, 459
  labile, precursor of sustained essential hypertension (E), 811
  pulmonary, and foreign body granulomas in intravenous drug abusers, 657
  spontaneous, beta-adrenergic receptor blocking drugs in, 779
  sustained essential, labile hypertension as precursor of (E), 811
  symposium, 721–810
    introduction to part II, 721
  systemic, spontaneous cure through control of hyperlipidemia, 420
Hyperthyroidism (CPC), 523
Hyperviscosity and pyroglobulin, 316
Hyperviscosity syndrome, IgM pyroglobulinemia with erythrocytosis presenting as, 316, 321
Hyponatremia and bronchogenic carcinoma, arginine vasopressin levels in, 825

Hypoparathyroidism, hormone-related (pseudo), renal response to PTH in, 184
Hypotension, idiopathic orthostatic, diurnal pattern of water and electrolyte excretion and body weight in, 709
Hypothyroidism, congenital, screening programs for, 932

I

Immune complex deposition, 471
Immune deficiencies, absence in progressive multifocal leukoencephalopathy, 433
Immunoglobulin deficiency, idiopathic late-onset, 221
Immunoglobulin E, monoclonal, with renal failure, 957
Immunoglobulin M
  granular deposition of, at dermal-epidermal junction in allopurinol hypersensitivity, 387
  pyroglobulinemia with erythrocytosis presenting as hyperviscosity syndrome, 316, 321
  with kappa light chain macroglobulinemia and hyperviscosity syndrome, 316
Immunoglobulins, nonlinear deposits of, in Goodpasture's syndrome, 407
Immunization program for swine influenza, factors involved in, 925
Immunodeficiency, xanthomas and obstructive liver disease, 393
Infectious mononucleosis, heterophil-antibody positive, in elderly patients, 333
Inflammation, effect on granulocyte adherence, 597
Influenza A viral infection associated with acute renal failure, 697
Influenza B, epidemiologic relationship to Reye's syndrome, 615
Influenza, swine, factors involved in immunization program for, 925
Internal medicine, general, primary medical care and training programs in (E), 156
Intravascular coagulation
  and adult respiratory distress syndrome (E), 585
  chronic, associated with chronic myelocytic leukemia, 547
  disseminated, characteristic of purpura fulminans, 566

J

Jaundice in pregnancy, 367

K

Ketogenesis and its regulation (E), 9
Ketosis, hormonal control of, 9
Kidney
  see also Renal
  disease, and hypertension, 739
  solitary cysts of, 579
KO 1366 and KO1313, effect on blood pressure, 779

L

Lead nephropathy (LE), 683
Left ventricle, normal and asynergic, local characteristics of, 650
Letters to the editor, 583
  Lead nephropathy, 583
  Lung biopsy in immunocompromised hosts, 584
Leukemia
  chronic lymphocytic, mediastinal irradiation for, 892
  chronic myelocytic
    associated with chronic intravascular coagulation, 547
    splenectomy for palliation, 14
Leukoencephalopathy, progressive multifocal, absence of immune deficiencies in, 433
Lidocaine and procainamide, comparative effects on acutely impaired hemodynamics, 215
Lipids, relationship of body fat to, 815
Lithium
  cardiovascular effects of, 665
  effects on granulopoiesis in Felty's syndrome, 29
Liver
  see also Hepatic
  acute fatty, of pregnancy, 367
  disease and secondary hyperlipidemia, immunodeficiency and xanthomas in, 393
  tuberculous pseudotumors of, 946
Lung
  biopsy
    in immunocompromised hosts (LE), 584
    in documentation of pulmonary hypertension and granulomas in intravenous drug abusers, 657
  capacity, total, mechanism of increase in acute asthma, 165
  tissue, antemortem findings in, in cytomegalovirus pneumonia, 326
Lymphadenopathy, immunoblastic, evolution into malignant lymphoma with plasmacytoid features, 553
Lymphocytes
  cytodestructive mechanisms provoked by (E), 1
  transformation in extrinsic allergic alveolitis, 939
Lymphoma
  American Burkitt's, in childhood (CPC), 377
  malignant, with plasmacytoid features, 553
  post-transplant malignant, 716

M

Macroglobulinemia, IgMK and hyperviscosity syndrome, 316
Macrothrombocytopathia, thrombocytopenia, nephritis and deafness, 145
Maffucci syndrome, multiple endocrine adenomas in, 952
Malaria—the mime, 159
Male phenotypic development, complexities of, 251
Malignant external otitis in diabetic patients, 298
Mannose-rich oligosaccharides, increased excretion of, in mannosidosis, 841
Mannosidosis, a longitudinal study, 841

Mastocytosis, systemic (CPC), 671
Mediastinal irradiation for chronic lymphocytic leukemia, 892
Medical care, primary, and training programs in general internal medicine (E), 156
Meningoencephalitis, herpesvirus hominis type 2, following renal transplantation, 703
Metastatic infection from genitourinary sources, 351
Methicillin-resistant Staphylococcus aureus outbreak at large community hospital, 340
Metoprolol, effect on blood pressure, 779
Myeloproliferative disorders, correlation between clinical evolution and alterations of granulopoiesis, 878
Myocardial fibrosis, focal, and progressive systemic sclerosis, 361
Myocardial infarction, transmural and nontransmural, short and long-term prognosis of patients with, 452
Myopathy, steroid, in connective tissue disease, 485

N

Nail-patella syndrome, end-stage renal failure in, 401
Necrosis, bilateral scalp, in temporal arteritis, 541
Nephritis, deafness, thrombocytopenia and macrothrombocytopathia, 145
Nephrolithiasis, recurrent, effect of phosphate therapy in, 200
Nephrotic syndrome
idiopathic, irreversible acute renal failure in, 207
in Hodgkin's disease, 471
Nervous system manifestations in Hodgkin's disease (CPC), 239
Neurologic involvement in Behçet's disease, 170
Neutropenia, chronic, in childhood, 859

O

Obesity, relationship to coronary heart disease, blood pressure and lipids, 815
Obstruction of upper and central airways, diagnosis of, 85
Oliguria in acute renal failure, 308
Organ involvement, skin capillary abnormalities as indicators of, 862
Organ manifestations of mastocytosis (CPC), 671
Osteoporosis, effects of alternating phosphorus and calcium infusions on, 478
Otitis, external malignant, in diabetes, 298
Otitis media in chronic neutropenia of childhood, 849

P

Paracoccidioidomycosis, gamut of, 33
Paraganglioma, metastatic catecholamine-secreting (CPC), 523
Parathyroid hormone, renal response to, in pseudohypoparathyroidism, 184
Peritoneum, infection of, with Candida, 832
Petriellidium boydii, visceral fungal infections due to, 632
Pheochromocytoma, extra-adrenal (CPC), 523
Phosphorus and calcium infusions, effects of alternating, on osteoporosis, 478
Phosphate therapy, effect in nephrolithiasis, 200
Pindolol, effect on blood pressure, 779
Pituitary irradiation in acromegaly, body composition and skeletal metabolism following, 59
Plasma arginine vasopressin in syndrome of antidiuretic hormone excess associated with bronochogenic carcinoma, 825
Plasma prorenin; cryoactivation and relationship to renin substrate, 731
Plasma renin activity measurements, methodological problems in, 725
Plasma renin concentration, effect of sodium depletion on, 608
Platelet functions
are agents affecting, clinically useful, 897
effect of antithrombin III deficiency on, 179
Pneumonia, cytomegalovirus, diagnosis of, in compromised hosts, 326
Pneumocystis carinii in pulmonary infections, 326
Pneumonitis, hypersensitivity, type IV immunologic response in pathogenesis, 939
Practolol, effect on blood pressure, 779
Pregnancy
cholestasis of, recurrent, 367
course in patients with artificial heart valves, 504
in Hodgkin's disease (CPC), 239
jaundice in, 367
physiologic alterations in hepatic function during, 367
Primary medical care and training programs in general internal medicine (E), 156
Procainamide and lidocaine, comparative effects on acutely impaired hemodynamics, 215
Propionibacterium acnes, pathogen in central nervous system shunt infection, 935
Propranolol
effect on blood pressure, 779
effect of sodium depletion on plasma renin before and after adrenergic beta receptor blockade with, 608
Prorenin, plasma, and renin substrate in normal subjects, 731
Prostaglandins
and blood pressure control (CCBSS), 681
high urniary, disorder in Bartter's syndrome, 43
Pseudohermaphroditism, male, 251
Pseudohyperparathyroidism in esophageal malignancy, 134
Pseudotumors, tuberculous, of the liver, 946
PTH, renal response to, in hormone-related (pseudo) hypoparathyroidism, 184
Pulmonary aspergilloma, rational approach to treatment, 626
Pulmonary disease, chronic obstructive, effects of bronchodilator on gas distribution and ventilatory efficiency in, 74
Pulmonary hemorrhage in Goodpasture's syndrome, 407
Pulmonary hypersensitivity reactions following Aspergillus fumigatus inhalation, 939

Pulmonary hypertension and foreign body granulomas in intravenous drug abusers, 657
Pulmonary infection with cytomegalovirus, 326
Purpura fulminans in an adult, 566
Purpura, thrombotic thrombocytopenic, remission following splenectomy, 439
Pyogenic infections in childhood neutropenia, 849
Pyrogel formation in IgM pyroglobulinemia, 321
Pyroglobulin and hyperviscosity, 316
Pyroglobulin and pyrogel formation, 321
Pyroglobulinemia, IgM, with erythrocytosis presenting as hyperviscosity syndrome, 316, 321

R

Radioiodide, low dose, thyroid ablation in thyroid cancer, 52
Raynaud's syndrome, skin capillary abnormalities as indicators of organ involvement in, 862
Renal
  see also Kidney
Renal arteries, atherosclerotic stenosing lesions of, regression through control of hyperlipidemia, 420
Renal bone disease, investigation and treatment of, 64
Renal disease and Proprionibacterium acnes infected central nervous system shunt, 935
Renal failure
  acute
    associated with influenza A viral infection, 697
    hypercalcemia of, 119
    irreversible, in idiopathic nephrotic syndrome, 207
    post-transplant, etiology and prognosis in, 190
    unexpected logic of oliguria in (E), 308
  end-stage, in nail-patella syndrome, 401
  monoclonal IgE with, 957
Renal response to PTH in hormone-resistant (pseudo) hypoparathyroidism, 184
Renal success, acute (E), 308
Renal transplantation followed by herpesvirus hominis type 2 meningoencephalitis, 703
Renin
  angiotension system, receptor modulation of, 768
  dependency in hypertension, superiority of converting enzyme inhibitor over saralasin in evaluating, 790
  levels, relationship to blood pressure responses, 790
  plasma, effect of sodium depletion on, 608
  substrate and plasma prorenin in normal subjects, 731
Respiratory distress syndrome, adult, and intravascular coagulation (E), 585
Reye's syndrome, nationwide outbreak of, 615

S

Saralasin, superiority of converting enzyme inhibitor over, in evaluating renin dependency in hypertension, 790
Sarcoma, immunoblastic, evolution into malignant lymphoma, 553
Scalp necrosis, bilateral, in temporal arteritis, 541
Scleroderma, skin capillary abnormalities as indicators of organ involvement in, 862
Screening programs for congenital hypothyroidism, 932
Sella turcica, enlarged, diagnosis and evaluation of, 590
Sepsis
  associated with decubitus ulcers, 346
  of genitourinary tract, metastatic infection secondary to, 351
Serum lipid levels during diuretic therapy of hypertension, 748
Shunt infection, central nervous system, with Propionibacterium acnes, 935
Sickle cell-β^0 thalassemia variant with high hemoglobin F and mild clinical course, 437
Sinus node dysfunction, atrial pacing in, 641
Skeletal metabolism following pituitary irradiation in acromegaly, 59
Skeletal metastases and genitourinary tract sepsis, 351
Skin
  capillary abnormalities, indicators of organ involvement, 862
  infections in chronic neutropenia, 849
  manifestations in mastocytosis (CPC), 671
  tests in extrinsic allaergic alveolitis, 939
Sodium
  depletion, effect on plasma renin concentration, 608
  readsorption, proximal tubular, evidence for defect in, in Bartter's syndrome, 111
Sotalol, effect on blood pressure, 779
Splenectomy
  remission of thrombotic thrombocytopenic purpura following, 439
  survival after, in chronic myelocytic leukemia, 14
Splenic abscess, 513
Splenosis: autotransplantation of splenic tissue, 414
Staphylococcus aureus, methicillin-resistant, outbreak at large community hospital, clinical, epidemiologic and bacteriologic observations of, 340
Steroid myopathy in connective tissue disease, 485
Survival after splenectomy in chronic myelocytic leukemia, 14
Sweet's syndrome, arthritis with inflammatory dermatosis resembling, 424
Swine influenza, factors involved in immunization program for, 925
Symposium on hypertension
  Angiotensin receptors in vascular tissue, 758
  Beta-adrenergic receptor blocking drugs in spontaneous hypertension, 779
  Elevation of serum lipid levels during diuretic therapy of hypertension, 748
  Hypertension associated with early stage kidney disease; complementary roles of circulating renin, the body sodium/volume state and duration of hypertension, 739
  Introduction to part II of the hypertension symposium: prorenin, renal hypertension, diuretics and hyperlipidemia, angiotensin receptors and blocking drugs, a new treatment system, 721
  Methodological problems in plasma renin activity measurements, 725

Modern system for treating high blood pressure based on renin profiling and vasoconstriction-volume analysis; a primary role for beta blocking drugs such as propranolol, 797
Plasma prorenin: cryoactivation and relationship to renin substrate in normal subjects, 731
Estimating renin participation in hypertension: superiority of converting enzyme inhibitor over saralasin, 790
Vascular angiotensin receptors and their role in blood pressure control, 768
Synovial fluid findings in tuberculous arthritis, 277
Systemic mastocytosis (CPC), 671
Systemic sclerosis
progressive, cardiac conduction system in, 361
skin capillary abnormalities as indicators of organ involvement, 862

T

Therapy, decisions regarding the provision or withholding of (CSC), 915
Thrombocytopenia, macrothrombocytopathia, nephritis and deafness, 145
Thrombotic thrombocytopenic purpura, remission following splenectomy, 439
Thyroid ablation, low dose radioiodide, in thyroid cancer, 52
Thyrotoxicosis (CPC), 523
Torulopsis glabrata as etiologic factor in infections in patients with cancer, 23
Total lung capacity, mechanism of increase in acute asthma, 165
Training programs and primary medical care in general internal medicine (E), 156
Tuberculosis of the liver, pseudotumors in, 946
Tuberculous arthritis, 277
Tuberculous pseudotumors of the liver, 946
Tumor tissue in liver, gallbladder and duodenum (CPC), 377
Tumors, benign hepatic, and oral contraceptive pills, 871

U

Ulcers, decubitus, and sepsis, 346
Urticaria pigmentosa in systemic mastocytosis (CPC), 671
Urticarial-like lesions associated with C1q deficiency, 560

V

Vascular angiotensin receptors and their role in blood pressure control, 758, 768
Vascular response to angiotensin II, 758
Vascular tissue, angiotensin receptors in, 758, 768
Vasculitis
clinical classification of, and presenting manifestations (CCBSS), 385
cutaneous, associated with C1q deficiency, 560
Vasopressin, plasma arginine, in syndrome of antidiuretic hormone excess associated with bronchogenic carcinoma, 825
Ventilatory efficiency, effects of inhaled bronchodilator on, in chronic obstructive pulmonary disease, 74
Ventricle, left, normal and asynergic, local characteristics of, 650
Ventricular rhythm disorders and sudden cardiac death (E), 449
Viral hepatitis in pregnancy, 367
Viral infection, influenza A, associated with acute renal failure, 697
Visceral fungal infections due to Petriellidium boydii, 632
Viscometric studies in IgM pryoglobulinemia, 316
Visual field defects in primary empty sella syndrome, 124

W

Water and electrolyte excretion, diurnal pattern of, in idiopathic orthostatic hypotension, 709

X

Xanthomas, immunodeficiency and obstructive liver disease, 393